Cardiology
An Illustrated Textbook

System requirement:
- Operating System—Windows XP or above
- Web Browser—Internet Explorer 8 or above, Google Chrome, Mozilla Firefox and Safari
- Essential plugins—Java and Flash Player
  - Facing problems in viewing content—may be your system does not have java enabled.
  - If videos do not show up—may be your system requires Flash player or needs to manage flash setting. To learn more about flash setting click on the link in the troubleshoot section.
  - You can test java and flash by using the links from the troubleshoot section of the CD/DVD.

Accompanying CD/DVD-ROM is playable only in Computer and not in DVD player.

CD/DVD has autorun function—may take few seconds to load on your computer. If it does not work, then follow the steps below to access the contents manually:
- Click on my computer
- Select the **CD/DVD drive** and click open/explore—this will show list of files in the **CD/DVD**
- Find and double click the file—launch.html

DVD Contents

Cardiology
An Illustrated Textbook

VOLUME 1

Editors

Kanu Chatterjee
Clinical Professor of Medicine
The Carver College of Medicine
University of Iowa
United States of America
Emeritus Professor of Medicine
University of California, San Francisco
United States of America

Mark Anderson
Professor
Departments of Internal medicine and
Molecular Physiology and Biophysics
Head
Department of Internal Medicine
Francois M Abboud Chair in Internal Medicine
The Carver College of Medicine
University of Iowa
United States of America

Donald Heistad
Professor of Medicine
The Carver College of Medicine
University of Iowa
United States of America

Richard E Kerber
Professor of Medicine
The Carver College of Medicine
University of Iowa
United States of America

JAYPEE BROTHERS MEDICAL PUBLISHERS (P) LTD

New Delhi • Panama City • London • Dhaka • Kathmandu

Jaypee Brothers Medical Publishers (P) Ltd.

Headquarter

Jaypee Brothers Medical Publishers (P) Ltd
4838/24, Ansari Road, Daryaganj
New Delhi 110 002, India
Phone: +91-11-43574357
Fax: +91-11-43574314
Email: jaypee@jaypeebrothers.com

Overseas Offices

J.P. Medical Ltd.,
83 Victoria Street London
SW1H 0HW (UK)
Phone: +44-2031708910
Fax: +02-03-0086180
Email: info@jpmedpub.com

Jaypee-Highlights Medical Publishers Inc.
City of Knowledge, Bld. 237, Clayton
Panama City, Panama
Phone: 507-301-0496
Fax: +507-301-0499
Email: cservice@jphmedical.com

Jaypee Brothers Medical Publishers (P) Ltd
17/1-B Babar Road, Block-B, Shaymali
Mohammadpur, Dhaka-1207
Bangladesh
Mobile: +08801912003485
Email: jaypeedhaka@gmail.com

Jaypee Brothers Medical Publishers (P) Ltd
Shorakhute, Kathmandu
Nepal
Phone: +00977-9841528578
Email: jaypee.nepal@gmail.com

Website: www.jaypeebrothers.com
Website: www.jaypeedigital.com

Cardiology: An Illustrated Textbook (Volume 1)

First Edition : **2013**

ISBN 978-93-5025-275-8

Printed at: Ajanta Offset & Packagings Ltd., New Delhi

Contributors

Harold P Adams MD
Professor of Medicine
The Carver College of Medicine
University of Iowa, USA

Bilal Aijaz MD
Associate Professor of Medicine
University of Alabama, USA

Masood Akhtar MD
Clinical Professor of Medicine
University of Wisconsin Medical School and Public Health
Department of Medicine
Cardiovascular Disease Section Electrophysiology
Sinai/St Luke's Medical Centers
Milwaukee, Wisconsin, USA

Suhail Allaqaband MD
University of Wisconsin Medical School and Public Health
Milwaukee Clinical Campus, Wisconsin, USA

Mark Anderson MD PhD
Professor, Departments of Internal Medicine and
Molecular Physiology and Biophysics
Head, Department of Internal Medicine
Francois M Abboud Chair in Internal Medicine
The Carver College of Medicine
University of Iowa, USA

Franca S Angeli MD
University of California
San Francisco, USA

Aarthi Arasu MD
University of California
San Francisco, USA

Reza Ardehali MD
Stanford University School of Medicine, USA

Ehrin J Armstrong MD
University of California, San Francisco, USA

Alejandro C Arroliga MD
Professor of Medicine
Dr A Ford Wolf and Brooksie Nell Boyd Wolf Centennial
Chair of Medicine
Scott and White Health Care and Texas A&M Health
Science Center College of Medicine

Nitish Badhwar MD
Associate Professor of Medicine
University of California, San Francisco, USA

Aaron L Baggish MD
Cardiovascular Division
Massachusetts General Hospital
Harvard Medical School
Boston, MA, USA

Tanvir Bajwa MD
Professor of Medicine
University of Wisconsin Medical School and Public Health
Department of Medicine
Sinai/St Luke's Medical Centers
Milwaukee Clinical Campus

Dipanjan Banerjee MD
Assistant Professor of Medicine
Stanford University School of Medicine, USA

Mohamad Barakat MD
University of Southern California Keck School of Medicine
Los Angeles, California, USA

Joaquin Barnoya MD MPH
Research Director
Cardiovascular Unit of Guatemala
Guatemala City
Guatemala
Research Assistant Professor
Department of Surgery, Prevention and Control
Washington University School of Medicine
St Louis, MO, USA

Kevin Barrows MD
Associate Professor of Medicine
University of California, San Francisco, USA

Lisa Bauer RN PhD ANP-BC
Assistant Professor of Medicine
University of California, San Francisco, USA

Edwin JR van Beek MD
Professor of Medicine
Chair of Clinical Radiology
Clinical Research Imaging Centre
Queen's Medical Research Institute
University of Edinburgh, United Kingdom

Christopher Benson MD
Associate Professor of Medicine
The Carver College of Medicine
University of Iowa, USA

Philip F Binkley MD
Wilson Professor of Medicine and Public Health
Davis Heart Lung Research Institute
The Ohio State University of Medicine and Public Health
Columbus, Ohio, USA

Vera Bittner MD
Professor of Medicine
University of Alabama, USA

Ann Bolger MD
Professor of Medicine
University of California, San Francisco, USA

Elias H Botvinick MD
Professor of Medicine and Radiology
University of California
San Francisco, USA

Andrew Boyle MD
Assistant Professor of Medicine
University of California
San Francisco, USA

Mohan Brar MD
Assistant Clinical Professor of Medicine
The Carver College of Medicine
University of Iowa, USA

Theresa M Brennan MD
Associate Professor of Medicine
The Carver College of Medicine
University of Iowa, USA

Donald Brown MD
Professor of Medicine
The Carver College of Medicine
University of Iowa, USA

Manjula V Burri MD
Department of Cardiology
The Carver College of Medicine
University of Iowa, USA

Dwayne N Campbell MD
The Carver College of Medicine
University of Iowa, USA

Blasé A Carabello MD
Professor of Medicine
Baylor College of Medicine
Houston, Texas, USA

Enrique V Carbajal MD
University of California
San Francisco
Fresno Campus, USA

Naima Carter-Monroe MD
CV Path Institute
Gaitersburg, MD, USA

Clay A Cauthen MD
Cleveland Clinic Foundation
Cleveland, Ohio, USA

Henry F Chambers MD
Professor of Medicine
University of California
San Francisco, USA

Kanu Chatterjee MBBS
Professor of Medicine
The Carver College of Medicine
University of Iowa
Emeritus Professor of Medicine
University of California
San Francisco, USA

Ahsan Chaudhary MD
Kaiser Permanente Hospitals
San Francisco, USA

Melvin D Cheitlin MD
Emeritus Professor of Medicine
University of California
San Francisco, USA

Indrajit Choudhuri MD
University of Wisconsin Medical School and Public Health
Department of Medicine
Cardiovascular Disease Section
Sinai/St Lukes Medical Centers
Milwaukee, Wisconsin, USA

Timothy AM Chuter MD
Professor of Surgery
Division of Vascular Surgery
University of California
San Francisco, USA

Moniek GJP Cox
University of Arizona College of Medicine
Tucson Arizona, USA

Michael H Crawford MD
Professor of Medicine
University of California
San Francisco, USA

Bharat V Dalvi MD
Professor of Medicine
The University of Mumbai, Mumbai, Maharashtra, India

Samir B Damani MD
Scripps Medical Center
San Diego, California, USA

Prakash C Deedwania MD
Professor of Medicine
University of California
San Francisco
Fresno Campus, USA

Teresa De Marco MD
Professor of Medicine
University of California
San Francisco, USA

Elaine M Demetroulis MD
Associate Professor of Medicine
The Carver College of Medicine
University of Iowa, USA

John A Dodson
The Columbia University of Medicine
New York, USA

Victor J Dzau MD
Professor of Medicine
Duke School of Medicine
Durham North Carolina, USA

Uri Elkayam MD
Professor of Medicine
University of Southern California
Keck School of Medicine
Los Angeles, California, USA

Michael E Ernst PharmD
Professor of Medicine
Department of Pharmacy Practice and Science
College of Pharmacy
Department of Family Medicine
The Carver College of Medicine
University of Iowa, USA

Gordon A Ewy MD
Professor of Medicine
University of Arizona College of Medicine
Director, University of Arizona Sarver Heart Center
Tucson, Arizona, USA

Robert Saeid Farivar MD PhD
Professor of Surgery
Department of Cardiothoracic Surgery
University of Iowa Hospitals and Clinics
The Carver College of Medicine
University of Iowa, USA

Joss Fernandez MD
Department of Cardiothoracic Surgery
University of Iowa Hospitals and Clinics
The Carver College of Medicine
University of Iowa, USA

Peter J Fitzgerald MD
Professor of Medicine
The Stanford University School of Medicine
Pala Alto, California, USA

Kirsten E Fleischmann MD MPH FACC
Professor of Medicine
University of California
San Francisco, USA

Elyse Foster MD
Professor of Medicine
University of California
San Francisco, USA

Michael B Fowler MD
Professor of Medicine
The Stanford University School of Medicine
Palo Alto, California, USA

Mony Fraer MD
Professor of Medicine
The Carver College of Medicine
University of Iowa, USA

Gary S Francis MD
Professor of Medicine
University of Minnesota
Minnesota, USA

Victor F Froelicher MD
Professor of Medicine
The Stanford University School of Medicine
Pala Alto, California, USA

Edward D Frohlich MD
Professor of Medicine
Ochshner Medical Center
Ochshner Clinic
New Orleans, LA

Milena A Gebska MD PhD
Cardiology Division
The Carver College of Medicine
University of Iowa, USA

Jalal K Ghali MD
Professor of Medicine
DMC Cardiovascular Institute
Wayne State University, USA

Mihai Gheorghiade MD
Professor of Medicine
North Western University
Chicago, USA

Geoffrey S Ginsburg MD PhD
Duke University School of Medicine
Durham, North Carolina, USA

Saket Girotra MBBS
Cardiology Division
The Carver College of Medicine
University of Iowa, USA

Stanton A Glantz PhD
Professor of Medicine
University of California
San Francisco, USA

Nora A Goldschlager MD
Professor of Medicine
University of California
San Francisco, USA

James A Goldstein MD
Professor of Medicine
William Buomont Hospital
University of Michigan, USA

Rakesh Gopinathannair MD MA
University of Kentucky
Kentucky, USA

Ellen El Gordon MD
Associate Professor of Medicine
The Carver College of Medicine
University of Iowa, USA

Mary Gray MD
Professor of Medicine
University of California
San Francisco, USA

Gabriel Gregoratos MD
Emeritus Professor of Medicine
University of California
San Francisco, USA

Hjalti Gudmundsson MD
Department of Cardiology
The Carver College of Medicine
University of Iowa, USA

Ashrith Guha MBBS MPH
Cardiology Division
The Carver College of Medicine
University of Iowa, USA

Dipti Gupta MD MPH
Cardiology Division
The Carver College of Medicine
University of Iowa, USA

Rajeev Gupta MD
Professor of Medicine
University of Jaipur, Jaipur, Rajasthan, India

Garrie J Haas MD
Professor of Medicine
Division of Cardiovascular Medicine
Davis Heart Lung Research Institute
The Ohio State University of Medicine and Public Health
Columbus, Ohio, USA

Babak Haddadian MD
University of Wisconsin Medical School and Public Health
Department of Medicine
Sinai/St Luke's Medical Centers
Milwaukee Clinical Campus, Wisconsin, USA

Jonathan L Halperin MD
Robert and Harriet Heilbrunn Professor of Medicine
(Cardiology)
Mount Sinai School of Medicine
The Zena and Michael A Wiener Cardiovascular Institute
The Marie-Josee and Henry R Kravis Center for
Cardiovascular Health
Mount Sinai Medical Center, Yew York, USA

Seyed M Hashemi MD
Division of Cardiology
The Carver College of Medicine
University of Iowa, USA

Samad Hashimi MD
Department of Cardiothoracic Surgery
University of Iowa Hospitals and Clinics
The Carver College of Medicine
University of Iowa, USA

Richard NW Hauer MD
University of Arizona School of Medicine
Tucson, Arizona, USA

Paul A Heidenreich MD MS
Professor of Medicine
Stanford School of Medicine, Palo Alto, California, USA

Donald Heistad MD
Professor, Dept of Internal Medicine
Division of Cardiovascular Medicine
University of Iowa, Iowa City

J Thomas Heywood MD
Professor of Medicine
Scripps Medical Center
University of California
San Diego, USA

Arthur Hill MD
Professor of Surgery
University of California
San Francisco, USA

Jennifer E Ho MD
Cardiology Division
Brigham and Women's Hospital
Harvard Medical School
Boston, MA

Jullien Hoffman MD
Professor of Pediatrics and Medicine
University of California
San Francisco, USA

Yasuhiro Honda MD
Stanford School of Medicine
Palo Alto, California, USA

Philip A Horwitz MD
Professor of Medicine
The Carver College of Medicine
University of Iowa, USA

Priscilla Y Hsue MD
Professor of Medicine
University of California
San Francisco, USA

Nkechinyere Ijioma MD
Department of Medicine
The Carver College of Medicine
University of Iowa, USA

Eugen Ivan MD
The Utah School of Medicine
University of Utah, USA

Farouc A Jaffer MD PhD
Cardiovascular Research Center
Cardiology Division and Center for
Molecular Imaging Research
Massachusetts General Hospital
Harvard Medical School
Boston, MA, USA

M Fuad Jan MD
University of Wisconsin Medical School and Public Health
Department of Medicine, Cardiovascular Disease Section
Sinai/St Lukes Medical Centers
Milwaukee, Wisconsin, USA

Cardiology: An Illustrated Textbook

Jooby John MD
Interventional Cardiology
Lenox Hill Hospital
New York, USA

Frances Johnson MD
Associate Professor of Medicine
The Carver College of Medicine
University of Iowa, USA

V Jacob Jose MD
Professor of Medicine
Vellore Medical College
Vellore, Tamil Nadu, India

Stefanie Kaiser MD
San Francisco Kaiser Permanente

John Kane MD
Professor of Medicine
University of California
San Francisco, USA

Karam Karam MD
Department of Cardiothoracic Surgery
University of Iowa Hospitals and Clinics
The Carver College of Medicine
University of Iowa, USA

Joel S Karliner MD
Professor of Medicine
University of California
San Francisco, USA

Wassef Karrowni MD
Division of Cardiology
The Carver College of Medicine
University of Iowa, USA

Arthur C Kendig MD
Associate Professor of Medicine
The Carver College of Medicine
University of Iowa, USA

Richard E Kerber MD
Professor of Medicine
The Carver College of Medicine
University of Iowa, USA

Masud H Khandaker MD
Mayo Clinic College of Medicine
Rochester, Minnesota

Nudrat Khatri MD
University of Southern California
Keck School of Medicine
Los Angeles, California, USA

Louis P Kohl MD
University of California
San Francisco, USA

Michel Komajda MD
Northwestern University
School of Medicine
Chicago, USA

Tomas Konecny MD
Mayo School of Medicine
Rochester, Minnesota, USA

Suma Konety MD MS
University of Minnesota
School of Medicine
Minnesota, USA

Diane C Kraft MD
Cardiology Division
The Carver College of Medicine
University of Iowa, USA

Ameya Kulkarni MD
University of California
San Francisco, USA

Teruyoshi Kume MD
Stanford School of Medicine
Palo Alto, California, USA

Fred Kusumoto MD
Professor of Medicine
Mayo Clinic
Jacksonville, Florida, USA

Elena Ladich MD
CV Path Institute
Gaithersburg, MD, USA

Carl V Leier MD
The James W Overstreet Professor of Medicine and
Pharmacology
Division of Cardiovascular Medicine
Davis Heart Lung Research Institute
The Ohio State University of Medicine and Public Health
Columbus, Ohio, USA

Wei Wei Li MD PhD
Fellow in Cardiology
Electrophysiology Section
The Carver College of Medicine
University of Iowa, USA

KellyAnn Light-McGroary MD
The Carver College of Medicine
University of Iowa, USA

Paul Lindower MD
Professor of Medicine
The Carver College of Medicine
University of Iowa, USA

Patricia Lounsbury RN BC BSN
The Carver College of Medicine
University of Iowa, USA

David Majure MD
Clinical Instructor of Medicine
University of California
San Francisco, USA

Mary Malloy MD
Professor of Medicine
University of California
San Francisco, USA

Cardiology: An Illustrated Textbook

x **Anne Mani** MD
Jefferson Medical College
Philadelphia, USA

Nestor Mercado MD
Scripps Medical Center
University of California, San Diego, USA

Frank I Marcus MD
Professor of Medicine
University of Arizona School of Medicine
Tucson, Arizona, USA

James B Martins MD
Professor of Medicine
The Carver College of Medicine
University of Iowa, USA

Umesh Masharani MD
Professor of Medicine
University of California
San Francisco, USA

Barry M Massie MD
Professor of Medicine
University of California
San Francisco, USA

Mathew S Maurer MD
Professor of Medicine
Columbia University School of Medicine
New York, USA

Alexander Mazur MD
Associate Professor of Medicine
The Carver College of Medicine
University of Iowa, USA

Patrick McBride MD MPH
University of California
San Francisco, USA

Dana McGlothlin MD
Associate Professor of Medicine
University of California
San Francisco, USA

Kunal Mehtani MD
Kaiser Permanente Medical Center
San Francisco, California, USA

Bernardo Menajovsky MD MS
Department of Medicine and the Division of Pulmonary
Critical Care
Scott and White Health Care and Texas A&M Health
Science Center
College of Medicine

Andrew D Michaels MD
Chief Cardiology
Director, Cardiac Catheterization Laboratory
St Joseph Hospital
Eureka, CA, USA

Rakesh K Mishra MD
University of California
San Francisco, USA

Christine Miyake MD
The Carver College of Medicine
University of Iowa, USA

Peter J Mohler PhD
Professor of Medicine
The Ohio State University of Medicine and Public Health
Columbus, Ohio, USA

Jagat Narula MD PhD
Cardiology Division
University of California
Irvine School of Medicine
Irvin, CA

Tamara Nelson MD
Associate Professor of Medicine
Department of Internal Medicine
The Carver College of Medicine
University of Iowa, USA

Ariane Neyou MD
Department of Cardiology
University of Texas Health Science
Houston, TX, USA

Hoang Nguyen MD
Kaiser Permanente Medical Center
San Francisco, California, USA

Rick A Nishimura MD
Professor of Medicine
Mayo Clinic College of Medicine
Rochester, Minnesota, USA

Eveline Oestreicher Stock MD
Department of Cardiology
University of California
San Francisco, USA

Isidore C Okere MBBS
The Carver College of Medicine
University of Iowa, USA

Jeffrey E Olgin MD
Ernest Gallo-Kanu Chatterjee Distinguished
Professor of Medicine
Director, Chatterjee Center for Cardiac Research
Professor of Medicine
University of California
San Francisco, USA

Brian Olshansky MD
Professor of Medicine
The Carver College of Medicine
University of Iowa, USA

Eric A Osborn MD PhD
Cardiology Division
Beth Israel Deaconess Medical Center
Harvard Medical School, Boston, MA
Cardiovascular Research Center
Cardiology Division, and Center for Molecular Imaging
Research, Massachusetts General Hospital
Harvard Medical School, Boston, MA, USA

Raveen Pal MD FRCP(C)
Assistant Professor of Medicine
Division of Cardiology
Queen's University
FAPC3-Kingston General Hospital

Peter S Pang MD
North Western University
Chicago, USA

William Parmley MD
Emeritus Professor of Medicine
University of California, San Francisco, USA

Ileana L Piña MD
Professor of Medicine and Epidemiology/Biostatistics
Case Western Reserve University
Cleveland, Ohio, USA

James Prempeh MD
St Mary's Good Samaritan Regional Health Center
Mount Vernon, Illinois, USA

Vijay Ramu MD
Mayo Clinic Medical Center
Jacksonville, Florida

Vijay U Rao MD PhD
Department of Cardiology
University of California
San Francisco, USA

Rita Redberg MD MSc
Professor of Medicine
University of California
San Francisco, USA

Jennifer G Robinson MD MPH
Professor of Medicine
Departments of Epidemiology and Medicine
The Carver College of Medicine
University of Iowa, USA

Melvin Scheinman MD
Professor of Medicine
University of California
San Francisco, USA

Nelson B Schiller MD
Professor of Medicine
University of California
San Francisco, USA

John Speer Schroeder MD
Professor of Medicine
Stanford School of Medicine
Palo Alto, California, USA

PK Shah MD
Professor of Medicine
Cedars Sinai Medical Center
Los Angeles, California, USA

Pravin M Shah MD
Professor of Medicine
Hoag Medical Center
Newport Beach, CA, USA

Sanjay K Shah MD
Department of Cardiology
University of Utah, USA

Satyavan Sharma MD
Professor of Medicine
University of Mumbai, Mumbai, Maharashtra, India

Gardar Sigurdsson MD
Associate Professor of Medicine
The Carver College of Medicine
University of California
San Francisco, USA

Amardeep K Singh MD
Department of Cardiology
University of California
San Francisco, USA

David Singh MD
Department of Cardiology
University of California
San Francisco, USA

S Sivasankaran MD
Professor of Medicine
Sree Chitra Tirunal Institute of Medical Sciences
and Technology
Trivandrum, Kerala, India

Virend Somers MD
Professor of Medicine
Mayo Clinic School of Medicine
Rochester, Minnesota, USA

Christopher Spradley MD
Department of Medicine and the Division of Pulmonary
and Critical Care
Scott and White Health Care and Texas A&M Health
Science Center, College of Medicine
Texas, USA

Matthew L Springer PhD
Associate Professor of Medicine
University of California
San Francisco, USA

Renee M Sullivan MD
Department of Cardiology
The Carver College of Medicine
University of Iowa, USA

A Jamil Tajik MD
Professor of Medicine
University of Wisconsin Medical School and Public Health
Department of Medicine
Cardiovascular Section
Sinai/St Lukes Medical Centers
Milwaukee, Wisconsin, USA

WH Wilson Tang MD
Professor of Medicine
Cleveland Clinic
Cleveland, Ohio, USA

Brad H Thompson MD
Professor of Medicine
The Carver College of Medicine
University of Iowa, USA

Paul D Thompson MD
Professor of Medicine
Director of Cardiology, Henry Low Heart Center
Hartford Hospital
Hartford, CT, USA

Eric J Topol MD
Professor of Medicine
Division of Cardiovascular Diseases, Scripps Clinic
Scripps Translational Science Institute and
the Scripps Research Institute
La Jolla, California, USA

Jose Torres MD
Department of Cardiothoracic Surgery
University of Iowa Hospitals and Clinics
The Carver College of Medicine
University of Iowa, USA

Abhimanyu (Manu) Uberoi MD
Department of Cardiology
The Stanford School of Medicine
Palo Alto, California, USA

Deepa Upadhyaya MD
Department of Cardiology
University of California
San Francisco, USA

Philip C Ursell MD
Professor of Pathology
University of California
San Francisco, USA

Byron F Vandenberg MD
Associate Professor of Medicine
The Carver College of Medicine
University of Iowa, USA

Vasanth Vedantham MD PhD
Division of Cardiology
Electrophysiology Section
University of California, San Francisco, USA

Jorge Velazco MD
Department of Medicine and
the Division of Pulmonary and Critical Care
Scott and White Health Care and Texas A&M Health
Science Center
College of Medicine, Texas, USA

G Vijayaraghavan MD
Professor of Medicine
Vice Chairman and Director
Kerala Institute of Medical Sciences
Kerala, India

Renu Virmani MD
Professor of Medicine
CV Path Institute
Gaithersburg, MD, USA

Ernesto Viteri MD
Cardiovascular Unit of Guatemala
Guatemala City, Guatemala

Scott A Vogelgesang MD
Professor of Medicine
M Paul Strottmann Family Chair of Medical Student Education
Department of Internal Medicine
The Carver College of Medicine
University of Iowa, USA

Deepak Voora MD
Duke University School of Medicine
Durham, North Carolina

Robert M Wachter MD
Professor of Medicine
University of California, San Francisco, USA

Ethan Weiss MD
Associate Professor of Medicine
University of California, San Francisco, USA

Robert M Weiss MD
Professor of Medicine
The Carver College of Medicine
University of Iowa, USA

Hugh H West MD
Professor of Medicine
University of California, San Francisco, USA

David J Whellan MD
Associate Professor of Medicine
Director of Coordinating Center for Clinical Research
Jefferson Medical College
Philadelphia, USA

Ronald Witteles MD
Stanford School of Medicine
Palo Alto, California, USA

Yanfei Yang MD
Department of Cardiology
Electrophysiology Section
University of California
San Francisco, USA

Yerem Yeghiazarians MD
Associate Professor of Medicine
University of California, San Francisco, USA

Jonathan Zaroff MD
Kaiser Permanente Medical Center
San Francisco, California, USA

Susan Zhao MD
Department of Cardiology
University of California, San Francisco, USA

Jeffrey Zimmet MD
VA Medical Center
University of California
San Francisco, USA

Cardiology: An Illustrated Textbook

Foreword

It is a privilege to write this foreword for this comprehensive *Cardiology—An Illustrated Textbook*. Because of the excessive morbidity and mortality from cardiovascular disease, the subject is extensively discussed in the world's literature and existing textbooks. A fair question from the reader is: why do we need another textbook of cardiology? That question can be answered in different ways.

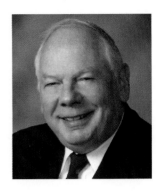

First of all, our knowledge and ability to treat all kinds of cardiovascular diseases have expanded exponentially in the past few decades. I recall when I was a cardiology fellow at the Peter Bent Brigham Hospital, Boston (USA), and watched my first Vineberg procedure as an attempt to revascularize the heart. It was a brutal punishing treatment for the myocardium, and was a great disincentive to the cardiologist to refer such patients to the cardiac surgeon. Now, when we approach coronary artery disease, we have so many options available to us; including angioplasty, stents, "keyhole" surgery and potent pharmacologic ways to alter the lipid profile. Rapid advances in noninvasive imaging and electrophysiology remind us how quickly our knowledge base is changing.

Second, it is always useful to know and compare the different approaches to cardiovascular disease at world-class institutions. The Contributors and Editors of this textbook are primarily based at the University of Iowa and the University of California, San Francisco, USA, two well-known centers for research and treatment of cardiovascular disease. Many other institutions are also represented. This unique blending of knowledge and expertise also reflects the fact that the principal editor, Dr Kanu Chatterjee, has spent most of his career at University of California, San Francisco (UCSF) and the University of Iowa, USA. It was my privilege to be associated with him as a colleague at UCSF, and to appreciate his broad knowledge of cardiology. His receipt of "best teacher" awards from the Department of Medicine attest to his ability to transmit that knowledge to students, housestaff, fellows and faculties.

Third, we are part of the fast-food generation. We are bombarded by so much information that we frequently are more attentive to our electronic devices than we are to the real people around us. We love photographs and graphs which can tell a whole story at a glance. I think that the reader will be pleased with the quality of the illustrations in the textbook, and find it easy-to-learn from them. I suppose that a few people (perhaps cardiology fellows and those studying for the cardiovascular boards) will sit down and read the textbook from cover to cover. More likely, however, it will serve as a reference text, wherein the reader can go to a specific chapter, and benefit from a concise and informative discussion of the particular problem at hand.

Fourth, every textbook of Cardiology has its strengths and weaknesses, and its distinctive sections. I believe that the reader will be pleased to review the Section on Evolving Concepts. Subjects such as the genomics of cardiovascular disease, gene therapy and angiogenesis, and stem cell therapy, to mention but a few chapters, will be of interest to all those concerned with cardiovascular disease.

Overall, the comprehensive textbook will continue the tradition of excellent textbooks of cardiology. It will be of great interest not only to the cardiologist but also to all those interested in cardiovascular disease including internists and other specialists. I am pleased to recommend the book most highly.

William W Parmley MD MACC
Emeritus Professor of Medicine
University of California, San Francisco, USA
Ex-President
American College of Cardiology
Ex-Editor-in-Chief
Journal of American College of Cardiology

Preface

Cardiology—An Illustrated Textbook is a revived but really a new textbook in cardiology. "Cardiology" was initially published as a loose-leaf referenced textbook. In 1993, it was published as a hard copy illustrated and referenced textbook. Since its publication, almost two decades ago, there have been enormous advances in every aspect of cardiology. Substantial progress has occurred in the understanding of coronary circulation, the molecular mechanisms of myocyte function and in the assessment of regional and global ventricular functions in physiologic and pathologic conditions. In this textbook, these advances have been emphasized.

The advances in cardiovascular pharmacology have also been considerable. The advantages and disadvantages of diuretic therapy, vasodilators, neurohormone modulators, positive inotropic agents, antilipid, antithrombotic and antiplatelet agents have been discussed. The clinical pharmacology of these agents in the management of various cardiovascular disorders has been emphasized. In the textbook, these advances are the subject of entirely new chapters.

We have witnessed the development of newer diagnostic techniques and the refinement of older diagnostic methods for detection of cardiovascular pathology. Molecular imaging and three-dimensional echocardiography and intravascular ultrasound imaging have been introduced. Advances have occurred in nuclear, cardiovascular computerized tomographic and magnetic resonance imaging. In the textbook, the advances in these diagnostic techniques and their clinical applications in the practice of cardiology have been extensively discussed. The role of rest and stress and electrocardiography and echocardiography has been emphasized.

During last two decades, we have witnessed enormous advances in the understanding of the genesis of atrial and ventricular arrhythmias, in the techniques of electrophysiologic and the pharmacologic and nonpharmacologic treatment of arrhythmias. The function and dysfunction of ion channels and the diagnosis and management of supraventricular and ventricular arrhythmias have been presented in details.

There have been revolutionary changes in the understanding of the pathophysiologic mechanisms and management of acute coronary syndromes. The new therapeutic modalities for the management of chronic coronary artery diseases have been discovered and devoted to discuss.

The diagnosis and management of valvular heart disease and heart failure are discussed in detail as well as chemotherapy and radiation-induced cardiovascular disorders. The progress in vascular biology, in genetics and pharmacogenomics in cardiology has also been considerable. In recent years, awareness of the cost of health care, errors in the practice of cardiology and gender and geographic differences in the incidence, diagnosis and management of cardiovascular disorders has risen. In the textbook, we have addressed these important and controversial topics.

We have also added modified guidelines for the management of angina, arrhythmias, heart failure, valvular heart diseases and perioperative cardiac evaluations.

All the chapters in the textbook have been written by the nationally and internationally recognized experts in their respective fields. The editors are very appreciative of and grateful to the contributors.

We sincerely thank Mr Joseph Gallo for his generous support enabling publication of the textbook of cardiology. We also acknowledge the help of all our administrative assistants and colleagues.

We also sincerely thank Shri Jitendar P Vij (Chairman and Managing Director), Mr Tarun Duneja (Director-Publishing), Mrs Samina Khan (PA to Director-Publishing), Dr Richa Saxena and the expert team of M/s Jaypee Brothers Medical Publishers (P) Ltd, New Delhi, India. Without their hard work, the textbook could not have been published.

Kanu Chatterjee
Mark Anderson
Donald Heistad
Richard E Kerber

Volume 1

Cardiology: An Illustrated Textbook

**Section 4
ELECTROPHYSIOLOGY**

Cardiology: An Illustrated Textbook

Volume 2

Contents

Section 9
MYOCARDIAL AND PERICARDIAL DISEASES

Cardiology: An Illustrated Textbook

BASIC CARDIOLOGY

Chapter 1

Cardiac Anatomy

Melvin D Cheitlin, Philip C Ursell

Chapter Outline

INTRODUCTION

Knowledge of the intimate anatomy of the heart was mostly of academic interest, known mainly to anatomists and pathologists, until nearly the middle of the 20th century. From the late 19th century, the heart could be imaged by the chest X-ray as a shadow projection on a 2-dimensional plane from several angles. Only the outline of the heart projected against the more radiolucent lungs is discernable by this method, and estimates of chamber enlargement can be made if the increased dimensions are prominent enough. For surgeons operating inside the heart, however, this 2-dimensional representation was not good enough.

With the advent of cardiac catheterization and angiocardiography in clinical practice in the mid-20th century, knowledge of internal cardiac anatomy became essential both to the cardiac surgeons and to the cardiologists. From the 1970s the utility of echocardiography as a diagnostic tool necessitated a detailed understanding of the 3-dimensional anatomy of the heart by all cardiologists and even physicians in many other fields. Shortly thereafter development of computed tomography and magnetic resonance imaging enabled 3-dimensional reconstruction of the heart, one layer at a time, so that the detailed internal anatomic structures could be visualized with a precision approaching that seen by anatomic dissection.

Knowledge of the intimate relationships of the internal structure of the heart permits the clinician to explain pathologic complications that occur during cardiac disease. For instance, the proximity of the aortic annulus to the conduction system (atrioventricular or His bundle passing through the right fibrous trigone) explains the common complication of various degrees of heart block in the patient with infective endocarditis and ring abscess. Similarly, calcification of the valvular annuli commonly associated with advanced age can lead to conduction system disorders, and aortic valve surgery for calcific aortic stenosis can be complicated by heart block and bundle branch block. Further, the proximity of structures to the sinuses of Valsalva can explain the development of fistulous communications following rupture of a sinus of Valsalva aneurysm or outflow tract fistulas after penetrating injury to the heart.

Instead of describing every aspect of cardiac anatomy in exhaustive detail as is done in many anatomy textbooks, this chapter describes the features of cardiac anatomy that are of particular importance to the clinician. It focuses on details that aid in understanding the cardiac anatomy visualized in the various diagnostic imaging techniques, in devising cardiac interventional procedures and in explaining the complications seen in patients with cardiac disease. Unless otherwise noted, the dimensions listed apply to normal adult human hearts of average size.

PERICARDIUM AND HEART IN THE MEDIASTINUM

The most anterior structure in the anterior mediastinum is the thymus gland remnant, anterior to the ascending aorta. Deep to the thymus is the pericardial sac containing the heart. Even when enclosed by the sac, the position and shape of the heart is discernible in the opened thorax. The heart essentially is a conical structure composed of layers of myocardium enclosing the atrial and ventricular chambers. The atrial and ventricular walls are anchored to the fibrous atrioventricular valve annuli. The aorta and main pulmonary artery arise from their respective fibrous valve rings, and these four fibrous rings together are termed the fibrous skeleton of the heart.

Located in the central chest, the heart within the pericardial sac resides in the middle mediastinum, with two-thirds of its volume to the left and one-third to the right of center (Fig. 1). The parietal pleura lie completely adjacent to the right and left lateral pericardium, so that only a small retrosternal portion of heart anteriorly on the left is uncovered by pleura. The two phrenic nerves pass through the middle mediastinum on the right and left surfaces of the pericardial sac, slightly posteriorly. The position of the phrenic nerves limits the extent of pericardiectomy done for constrictive pericarditis. Injury to the phrenic nerves can also occur during open-heart surgery, causing diaphragmatic paralysis and great difficulty in ventilating the patient postoperatively. The esophagus passes posterior to the heart, close to the left atrium. Superior and posterior to the left atrium is the bifurcation of the trachea. In the early days of catheterization, the left mainstem bronchus lying on the left atrium provided bronchoscopic access to the left atrium via needle puncture through the bronchus.

The myocardial wall consists of three layers: (1) the epicardium; (2) the myocardium and (3) the endocardium. The epicardium is comprised of a fatty connective tissue layer subjacent to the visceral pericardium. The myocardium comprises the bulk of the heart wall consisting of interdigitating layers of myocardial cells with accompanying vasculature and lymphatics. The endocardium consists of a thin layer of fibrocellular connective tissue with a single layer of endothelial cells lining the chambers of the heart. Developmentally, the growing heart in the embryo invaginates the pericardial sac, so that the mature heart becomes suspended only by the reflections of pericardium around the great vessels. These attachments of pericardial reflections form the dorsal mesocardium, one site at the sinoatrial surface around the venous inlets into the atria and the other at the great arteries as they exit the ventricles to form an arterial or conotruncal mesocardium. The autonomic nerves to the heart enter through these mesocardial attachments.

Although the parietal pericardium is fixed in position by attachments to the sternum anteriorly and diaphragm inferiorly, the heart suspended at the pericardial reflections is somewhat moveable within the pericardial space; the pericardial surfaces are lubricated by a small amount of serous fluid to reduce friction during systole and diastole. Other functions of the pericardium are: (1) to isolate the heart from mediastinal and pulmonary infection and (2) to stabilize the heart in the mediastinum with changes in body position or more violent trauma. The reflections of the pericardium on the great vessels are such that two-thirds of the ascending aorta and the main pulmonary artery are intrapericardial (Fig. 1). The pericardial reflections at the great veins place half of the superior vena cava and only a short segment of inferior vena cava within the pericardial sac.

Many pericardial recesses are formed as a result of the pericardial reflections around the great vessels (Figs 2A and B). One such recess is formed on the inferoposterior surface of the heart by the continuous reflection from the inferior vena cava to each of the right pulmonary veins and leftward to the left pulmonary veins. This semicircle of pericardial reflection encloses a small recess within the posteroinferior pericardial sac known as the oblique sinus. A larger recess within the pericardial sac is that potential space between the great arteries superiorly and the atria inferiorly, the transverse sinus (Fig. 3).

The clinical importance of these pericardial reflections is apparent in the high mortality rate seen in rupture of the ascending aorta (type A aortic dissection). Since the ascending aorta is mostly intrapericardial (Fig. 1), aortic rupture results in hemorrhage into the pericardial space. The normal pericardium is fibrous and relatively noncompliant, and sudden increases in intrapericardial volume may rapidly produce cardiac tamponade. Type B aortic dissection involves the descending aorta distal to the take-off of the left subclavian artery, so rupture and hemorrhage are contained by the posterior mediastinal structures and the pleura which almost completely surrounds the aorta. This type of dissection is less likely to be rapidly fatal.

The pericardial blood supply derives from the internal mammary arteries, which pass posterior to the rib cage 0.5 cm lateral to the right and left sternal borders. On reaching the diaphragm, the internal mammary arteries divide into the musculophrenic and the superior epigastric branches. Other blood supply to the pericardium is supplied by the intercostals, subclavian and posterior mediastinal arteries. In the pericardial reflections at the root of the great arteries are small connections between the epicardial coronary arteries and the internal mammary arteries; before the development of coronary bypass surgery, these connections were the basis for a fanciful idea of ligating the internal mammary arteries in patients with coronary artery disease to divert blood to the coronary arteries, a procedure that was proved ineffective.

The thoracic cage is supplied by blood from the intercostal arteries arising from the descending aorta and from the internal mammary arteries anteriorly. The veins of the thoracic cage follow the arterial distribution. The ten lower intercostal veins on the right enter the azygous vein that passes superiorly and anteriorly to connect with the superior vena cava (Fig. 4A).

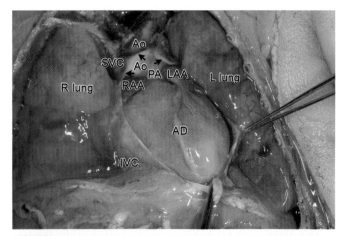

FIGURE 1: Pericardial sac and the cardiac silhouette. In the open thorax of a newborn infant, the parietal pericardium is reflected to expose the epicardial surface, showing the majority of the heart located to the left of the midline. The pericardial reflection over the great arteries (arrows) shows that portions of these vessels lie within the pericardial sac. Although the atrial appendages are the only portion of atriums visible, the anterior aspect of the ventricular surfaces are shown with the anterior descending branch of the left coronary artery as the landmark delimiting the interventricular septum. The connections of the superior vena cava (SVC) and inferior vena cava (IVC) with the right atrium are aligned vertically. (Abbreviations: AD: Anterior descending coronary artery; Ao: Ascending aorta; L: Left; LAA: Left atrial appendage; PA: Main pulmonary artery; R: Right; RAA: Right atrial appendage)

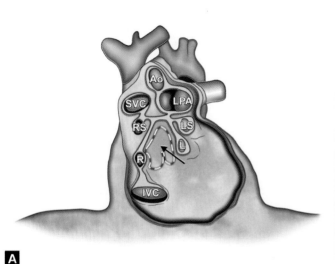

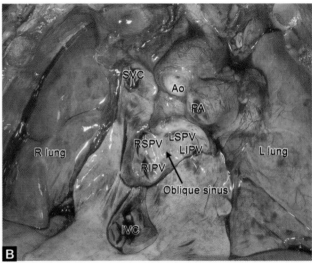

FIGURES 2A AND B: Pericardial reflections and the oblique sinus. The neonatal heart has been removed from the thorax to show the pericardial reflections around the great veins and the pulmonary veins posteriorly. A reflection of pericardium extends between the vertically aligned superior vena cava (SVC) and the inferior vena cava (IVC). The oblique sinus (arrow) is a potential space resembling a cul-de-sac formed by the continuous reflection of the pericardium from the IVC around each of the pulmonary veins. (Abbreviations: Ao: Ascending aorta; L: Left; LIPV: Left inferior pulmonary vein; LSPV: Left superior pulmonary vein; PA: Main pulmonary artery; R: Right; RIPV: Right inferior pulmonary vein; RSPV: Right superior pulmonary vein)

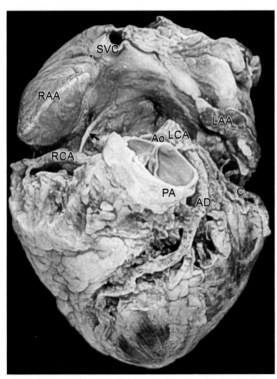

FIGURE 3: Epicardial anatomy: extramural coronary arteries and the transverse sinus. In this view of the isolated heart, the atria have been reflected posteriorly to exaggerate the transverse sinus between the atria and the great arteries. After epicardial fat has been dissected from the interventricular and atrioventricular sulci, the extramural coronary arteries can be identified as they course over the surface of the heart. Barely visible behind the pulmonary artery (PA), the aortic aorta (Ao) gives rise to the right coronary artery (RCA) and the left coronary artery (LCA). The relatively short left coronary artery divides into the circumflex (C) branch within the left atrioventricular sulcus and the anterior descending (AD) branch within the anterior interventricular sulcus. The sulcus terminalis marks the position of the sinoatrial node (*). In the transverse sinus an early atrial branch (arrow) of the right coronary artery provides a branch to the sinoatrial node. (Abbreviations: AD: Anterior descending coronary artery; LAA: Left atrial appendage; SVC: Superior vena cava; RAA: Right atrial appendage)

The two upper intercostal veins on the right enter the azygos or the right innominate vein. On the left side, the lower intercostal veins lead into the hemiazygos vein or the accessory hemiazygos vein (Fig. 4B). The hemiazygos vein crosses the midline behind the descending aorta at about the level of the eighth thoracic vertebral body and enters the right-sided azygos vein. With congestive heart failure and associated venous dilatation, the azygos vein can be seen as a round structure on the postero-anterior chest X-ray as it joins the superior vena cava.

The relationship of the great veins in the superior media-stinum is clinically important. The innominate (brachiocephalic) veins are formed by the confluence of the subclavian veins (passing over the first rib and posterior and inferior to the clavicles) and the internal jugular veins just behind the sternoclavicular joints. The left innominate vein passes anterior to the aortic arch, crossing the midline and joining the right innominate vein to form the superior vena cava. Deep to the venous structures are the great arteries arising from the aortic arch. The first branch from the aorta is the innominate or brachiocephalic artery, dividing behind the right sternoclavicular joint into the right subclavian artery (deep to the subclavian vein) and the right common carotid artery. The second great artery from the aortic arch is the left common carotid artery, and the third major branch is the left subclavian artery.

From the description of the thoracic great veins and arteries, it is apparent that the venous structures are superficial to the arteries and that both the left innominate vein and the aortic arch cross the midline. The position of the left innominate vein deep to the sternum explains the potential for injury to this vessel during a thoracotomy through a midline incision, especially during a repeat thoracotomy where adhesions are likely. Also, the relationship between the left innominate vein and the aortic arch explains the possibility of an aortoinnominate vein fistula after penetrating trauma. The relationship of the great veins to the clavicle and sternoclavi-cular joints makes these easily palpable bony structures

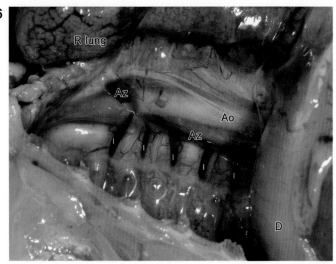

FIGURE 4A: Thoracic veins. With the right lung reflected out of the thorax (patient's head out of field at left), a lateral view of the posterior mediastinum shows intercostal veins (I) connecting with the azygos vein (Az) abutting the spine. More superiorly, the azygos vein will connect with the superior vena cava. (Abbreviations: Ao: Descending thoracic aorta; D: Right diaphragm; R: Right)

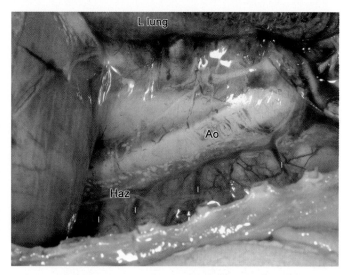

FIGURE 4B: With the left lung reflected out of the thorax (patient's head at right), a lateral view of the posterior mediastinum shows the highest intercostal veins (I) that will connect with the left innominate (brachiocephalic) vein superiorly. The lower intercostal veins connect with the hemiazygos vein (Haz) that will drain into the azygos vein

valuable landmarks for the percutaneous placement of central venous catheters into the internal jugular and subclavian veins.

CARDIAC SURFACE ANATOMY

With the pericardium opened and the heart exposed anteriorly, the right atrium forms the right lateral border with the superior vena cava superiorly and the thoracic segment of the inferior vena cava as it enters the right atrium inferiorly (Fig. 2). Further superiorly the ascending aorta forms the right border and on the left, the knob of the aortic arch; below the aortic arch and to the left, the main pulmonary artery is seen as it courses leftward and posteriorly. Just below the bulge of the main pulmonary artery on the cardiac silhouette is the left atrial appendage, and below that the muscular left ventricle forms the left cardiac border including the apex near the diaphragm. The right atrial appendage is not a border-forming structure, because it protrudes medially as a superior triangular structure anterior to and hiding the root of the ascending aorta. In fact from an anterior view, the great arteries are embraced on either side by the right and left atrial appendages, the right abutting the aorta as mentioned and the left next to the main pulmonary artery (Figs 1 and 5). On a posterior-anterior chest X-ray, the cardiac silhouette is formed by the same structures, and distortion of the image can indicate individual chamber or vessel enlargement.

Similarly, the epicardial surface provides clues as to the internal anatomy of the heart. A straight line between the two vena cavae indicates the inlet portion of the right atrium (sinus venarum) (Figs 1 and 2). The inferolateral border of the right atrium is marked on the cardiac surface by the right atrioventricular sulcus. Although not a border-forming structure the right atrial appendage overhangs the right atrioventricular groove in which the right coronary artery runs, the vessel usually being buried in epicardial fat. The position of the heart

in the chest is such that the right atrioventricular groove is almost vertical, and this groove marks the position of the tricuspid annulus. The right ventricle is an anterior structure that in the frontal plane roughly projects as a triangle with the inlet as one side and the outlet as another side; its most superior angle marks the right ventricular outflow tract leading to the main pulmonary artery anteriorly. About 1 cm medial of the left cardiac border lies the interventricular sulcus marking the interventricular septum and thus the anterior portions of the right and left ventricles. In this groove lies the anterior descending coronary artery, again covered by fat (Fig. 5).

Observing the heart in the frontal plane, the superior parallel vascular structures from right to left are the superior vena cava, the ascending aorta and the main pulmonary artery (Fig. 5). The main pulmonary artery is 4–5 cm in length and bifurcates into the right pulmonary artery that passes transversely posterior to the ascending aorta (Fig. 6) and the left pulmonary artery which passes posteriorly and inferiorly. Posterior to the right atrial-superior vena caval junction, the right pulmonary artery divides into a superior and an inferior branch at the hilum of the right lung. At the right lung hilum, the superior branch of the right pulmonary artery courses under or side by side with the bronchus to the right upper lobe; this airway-vessel relationship is termed eparterial. In line with the main pulmonary artery, the left pulmonary artery arches leftward and posteriorly toward the hilum of the left lung. Just distal to the bifurcation of the main pulmonary artery, the ligamentum arteriosum connects the superior surface of the left pulmonary artery to the proximal descending aorta (Fig. 5). At the left lung hilum, the left pulmonary artery courses *over* the bronchus (hyparterial relationship).

The ascending aorta arises from the aortic fibrous annulus and passes superiorly. The root of the aorta refers to the aortic origin where the three semilunar leaflets of the closed aortic valve define three cup-like spaces bounded by the aortic walls

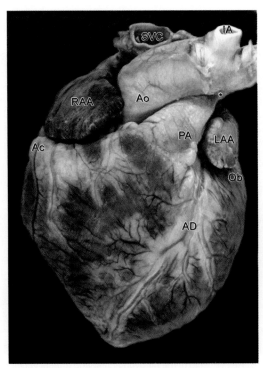

FIGURE 5: Epicardial anatomy: anterosuperior surface of the heart. The anterosuperior surface of the heart shows the great arteries crossed at their roots. The right atrial appendage abuts the ascending aorta, and the left atrial appendage is adjacent to the pulmonary artery. (Abbreviations: *: Ligamentum arteriosum; Ac: Acute margin of heart; AD: Anterior descending coronary artery; Ao: Ascending aorta; IA: Innominate (or brachiocephalic) artery; LAA: Left atrial appendage; PA: Main pulmonary artery; Ob: Obtuse margin of heart; RAA: Right atrial appendage; SVC: Superior vena cava)

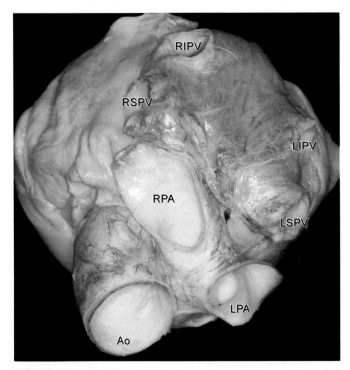

FIGURE 6: Relationship between the right pulmonary artery and the left atrium. The superior aspect of the heart shows the right pulmonary artery (RPA) between the ascending aorta (Ao) and the left atrium with the pulmonary vein connections. (Abbreviations: LIPV: Left inferior pulmonary vein; LSPV: Left superior pulmonary vein; RIPV: Right inferior pulmonary vein; RSPV: Right superior pulmonary vein; LPA: Left pulmonary artery)

(sinuses of Valsalva). The first arteries arising from the aorta are the right and left coronary arteries, their ostia usually being located in the sinuses. As the aorta passes superiorly, leftward and posteriorly forming the aortic arch it gives rise to the innominate (or brachiocephalic) (Fig. 5), left common carotid and left subclavian arteries. The aortic arch passes over the left mainstem bronchus, thus marking this arch as "left-sided". In a small percentage of patients the aortic arch passes over the right mainstem bronchus ("right-sided" aortic arch). After the left subclavian artery arises, the descending aorta assumes a left paravertebral position and courses caudally in the posterior mediastinum to the left of the spine (Fig. 4 lower panel). Twelve paired intercostal arteries arise from the descending aorta, and a variably placed anterior spinal artery and several bronchial arteries arise from the anterior descending aorta.

In the frontal view of the heart, the acute angle defined by the atrioventricular groove anteriorly and the right edge of the right ventricle is the basis for references to the "acute margin" of the heart (Fig. 5). On the left side of the heart the corresponding heart border is the "obtuse margin" of the heart.

Viewed from the right lateral aspect as in a chest X-ray, the anterior heart border is formed by the right ventricle and the posterior border by the right atrium inferiorly and the left atrium superiorly (Fig. 5). The right ventricular outflow tract and the initial part of the main pulmonary artery form the superior portion of the anterior aspect of the right ventricle. Above the pulmonary artery is the ascending aorta. From the left lateral aspect, the right ventricle is anterior and the posterior border is formed by the left atrium superiorly and the left ventricle inferiorly. Thus, orienting the heart in space, the right ventricle is rightward and anterior and the left ventricle is leftward and posterior. The atria are posterior and superior to the ventricles, with the right atrium anterior and rightward and the left atrium posterior and leftward.

From the posterior aspect, the aortic arch rises superior to the root of the left lung. The main pulmonary artery bifurcates into the right and left pulmonary artery branches above the left atrium. The left atrium receives four pulmonary veins, the right and left superior and inferior pulmonary veins (Figs 6 and 7). The right pulmonary veins pass posteriorly into the left atrium between the superior vena cava above and the inferior vena cava below. This close relationship explains the developmental error of the right superior pulmonary vein draining into the superior vena cava or the right atrium instead of the left atrium (anomalous pulmonary venous connection).

From the posterior aspect to the right of the connection of the pulmonary veins with the left atrium is a long-axis depression known as Sondergaard's groove, a shallow epicardial indentation marking the position of the interatrial septum internally (Fig. 7). In accessing the mitral valve, surgeons use Sondergaard's groove as a landmark to enter the left atrium from the posterior or right thoracotomy approach by making an incision just to the left of the groove. To the right of Sondergaard's groove there is another indentation, the sulcus terminalis denoting the site of the specialized muscle of the sinoatrial node. Marking the outlet portions of the atria is the posterior atrioventricular groove. In the right side of this groove the right coronary artery passes posteroinferiorly to the crux of the heart and then turns to course within the posterior

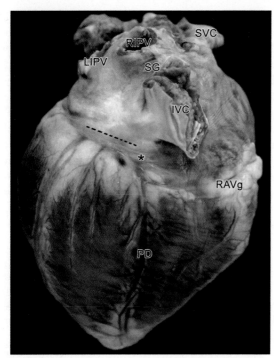

FIGURE 7: Epicardial anatomy: inferior (diaphragmatic) surface of the heart. The inferior (diaphragmatic) surface of the heart shows the posterior descending coronary artery (PD) as the landmark for the interventricular septum. The right pulmonary veins are just leftward of an imaginary line drawn from the caval veins. Between the right pulmonary veins and this line is Sondergaard's groove (SG) marking the interatrial septum. (Abbreviations: *: Crux of heart;- - - - -: Position of coronary sinus within left atrial wall; IVC: Inferior vena cava; LIPV: Left inferior pulmonary vein; RAVg: Fat-filled right atrioventricular groove; RIPV: Right inferior pulmonary vein; SVC: Superior vena cava)

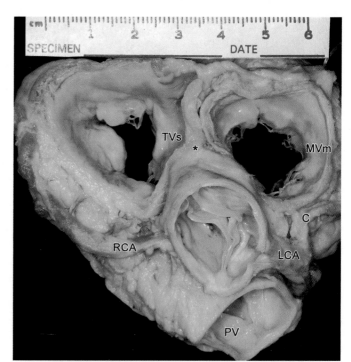

FIGURE 8: Relationship of the atrioventricular and arterial valves. Viewed from the superior aspect, the base of the heart with most of the atria cut away shows the aortic valve wedged between the two atrioventricular valves. Deep to the dissection plane illustrated, the three valves come together at the right fibrous trigone or central fibrous body (*), while the pulmonary valve (PV) is separate from the fibrous skeleton of the heart. (Abbreviations: C: Circumflex coronary artery within left atrioventricular groove; LCA: Left coronary artery; MVm: Mural leaflet of mitral valve; RCA: Right coronary artery within right atrioventricular groove; TVs: Septal leaflet of tricuspid valve)

interventricular groove toward the apex as the posterior descending coronary artery. The crux of the heart is the point at which Sondergaard's groove, the right and left atrioventricular grooves and the posterior interventricular groove all intersect (Fig. 7). In other words, the crux (represented by a shallow dimple) is the point on the inferior surface at which all four chambers of the heart meet. The coronary sinus runs in the left side of the atrioventricular groove along the diaphragmatic surface. This conduit passes rightward and empties into the right atrium through the coronary sinus orifice.

INTERNAL STRUCTURE OF THE HEART

The heart can be said to have a fibrous "skeleton" on which the muscles of the atria and the ventricles are anchored. The "skeleton" consists of fibrous connective tissue that forms the valvular annuli and electrically isolates the atrial and ventricular muscles except in one small area. The only normal muscular connection between atrial and ventricular myocardium is via the atrioventricular (His) bundle, a tiny cord-like isthmus of specialized myocardial cells with conduction properties that propagates the electrical impulse from the atrioventricular node to the right and left bundle branches. The fibrous "skeleton" consists of the mitral, tricuspid and aortic annuli in a close triangular arrangement (Fig. 8); the separate pulmonic annulus is anterior and leftward of the aortic annulus. The small fibrous junction between the mitral, tricuspid and aortic annuli is called

the right fibrous trigone (central fibrous body), and the small fibrous junction between the mitral and aortic annuli on the left behind the left atrial appendage is called the left fibrous trigone. Thus, the atrioventricular bundle penetrates the right fibrous trigone in coursing toward the left side of the interventricular septum.

RIGHT ATRIUM

The right atrium is anterior and rightward of the left atrium, the two chambers being separated by the interatrial septum. Embryologically the atria become partitioned by the sequential ingrowth of two muscular septa. During development the septum primum grows from the roof of the atrium toward the atrioventricular region. Closure of the septum primum is completed by tissue contributions from the endocardial cushions. Prior to closure, a second opening in the midportion of the septum primum appears, the foramen ovale, allowing blood to continue to flow from the right atrium to the left atrium. To the right of the septum primum, a second partition, the septum secundum, grows down as a superior and posterior crescent. The septum secundum finally grows to overlap the foramen ovale in such a way that greater left atrial pressure can close the opening. The fossa ovalis, a crater-like depression in the atrial septum as seen from the right atrial aspect, is the site at which the two septa overlap. Thus, normally, with the first breaths by the newborn infant, the left atrial pressure comes to exceed the right atrial pressure during all phases of the cardiac cycle, and the flap against the foramen ovale is closed, allowing no shunting between the atria. In most individuals the foramen ovale becomes permanently sealed during infancy. In approximately 20% of individuals, however, the two septae never completely fuse, allowing a slit-like potential communication at the foramen ovale throughout life, usually at the anterior margin of the fossa ovalis. Under some circumstances, for instance after release of a Valsalva maneuver, the right atrial pressure transiently exceeds that of the left and a right-to-left shunt occurs. This is the basis for a potential paradoxical embolism in patients with a patent foramen ovale but an otherwise normal heart. Other circumstances in which a patent foramen ovale can result in a right-to-left shunt include tricuspid regurgitation or right ventricular diastolic dysfunction with right ventricular hypertrophy or failure where right atrial pressure is abnormally elevated.

When formed abnormally the atrial septal partition can be the site of at least three distinctive malformations. The commonest defect, the secundum atrial septal defect, results from a failure of the septum primum to cover the foramen ovale. Less common is the ostium primum defect, a result of failure of the endocardial cushions to fuse with the inferior edge of the septum primum. A rare third defect, the sinus venosus atrial septal defect, results from a failure of the embryonic sinus venosus to be incorporated into the embryonic right atrium; the defect is usually located at the posterosuperior or, less commonly, at the posteroinferior aspect of the atrial septum. This defect often is associated with anomalous pulmonary venous connection to the superior vena cava or the right atrium.

In the adult heart, the fossa ovalis is about the size of a dime (Fig. 9). Surrounding the membranous tissue in the base of the crater, there is a ridge of atrial muscle superiorly and posteriorly called the limbus of the fossa ovalis, an important

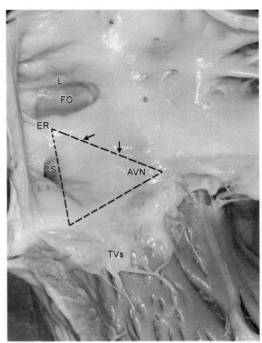

FIGURE 10: Right atrium and landmarks for the atrioventricular node. A close-up view of the right atrial septum and vestibule of the tricuspid valve discloses the Eustachian ridge (ER, or sinus septum) separating the fossa ovalis (FO) and coronary sinus. The tendon of Todaro courses along the crest of the ridge subendocardially (arrows). The triangle of Koch (dashed lines) is the landmark for the atrioventricular node (AVN) and bundle: at the angle formed by the tendon of Todaro and the annulus of the septal leaflet of the tricuspid valve, the atrioventricular bundle penetrates the central fibrous body on its way to the left side of the septum. (Abbreviations: CS: Coronary sinus os; L: Limbus of fossa ovalis; TVs: Septal leaflet of tricuspid valve)

landmark in performing a trans-septal left-sided cardiac catheterization (Figs 10 and 11). In this procedure, a Brockenbrough needle with a curve at its end sheathed within a catheter is placed into the superior vena cava and rotated so that the needle is pointed posteromedially; it then is slowly pulled back until it

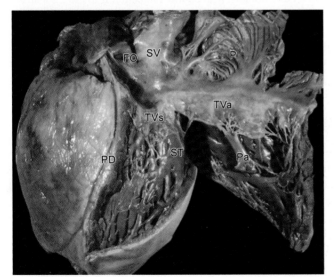

FIGURE 9: Right atrium and right ventricular inlet. The opened right atrium (including right atrial appendage) and right ventricular inlet demonstrates the pectinate muscles (P) of the "rough" part of the right atrium and the smooth endocardial surface of the sinus venarum portion (SV). Within the ventricle, the free wall thickness is less than 0.4 cm. (Abbreviations: FO: Fossa ovalis; Pa: Anterior papillary muscle; PD: Posterior descending coronary artery; ST: Septomarginal trabeculum; TVa: Anterior leaflet of tricuspid valve; TVs: Septal leaflet of tricuspid valve)

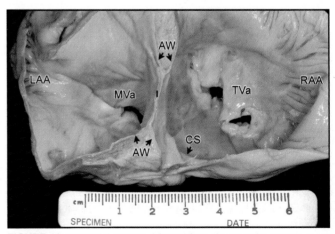

FIGURE 11: Interatrial septum. Viewed from the superior aspect, a cut through the fossa ovalis demonstrates the primary atrial septum (I) essentially as a membrane, while the adjacent tissue is comprised of the infolded atrial walls (AW). Thus, the blade septostomy should be performed in the fossa ovalis without deviation into the limbus. (Abbreviations: CS: Coronary sinus os; LAA: Opened left atrial appendage; MVa: Anterior leaflet of mitral valve; RAA: Opened right atrial appendage; TVa: Anterior leaflet of tricuspid valve)

passes across the limbus and springs into the fossa ovalis, causing a sharp movement of the needle which can be both seen under fluoroscopy and felt. At that point the needle is in the fossa ovalis and can be safely advanced through the septum into the left atrium. Deviation outside of this dime-sized oval may result in complications; because the limbus marks the boundary of the true atrial septum and the infolded atrial walls (Fig. 11), puncturing the limbus results in the blade coursing outside of the atrial wall into epicardial tissue (where there are vessels and nerves) before entering the left atrium.

The inner surface of the right atrium has a smooth part and a "rough" part (Fig. 9). The smooth part of the right atrium is that part of the wall between the vena cavae. In contrast, the free wall of the right atrium including the atrial appendage has numerous muscle ridges known as pectinate muscles. The relatively large number of pectinate muscles and the fact that they extend beyond the appendage is one feature that distinguishes the right atrium from the left atrium. This "rough" part of the chamber represents the contribution of the embryonic atrium. Very thin walls, much less than a millimeter thick, separate the fine muscle ridges. If a catheter is pressed against the lateral wall of the right atrium and under fluoroscopy does not appear to be almost pressing against the lung, then the wall is abnormally thick; usually this means a thickened pericardium as seen in constrictive pericarditis, or a pericardial effusion. Another consequence of the thin atrial wall is the danger of cardiac perforation when maneuvering within the right atrium with a stiff catheter.

After passing through the diaphragm the inferior vena cava connects with the right atrium. In some hearts the right atrium has a thin, crescentic membrane coursing anteromedially from the inferior vena cava within the cavity; this structure is known as the valve of the inferior vena cava or the Eustachian valve, a vestige of an embryologic venous valve that guarded the inferior vena cava orifice. On occasion a more substantial, cobweb-like remnant of the Eustachian valve called a Chiari network can extend into the lumen of the right atrium, and in some cases this structure can be discerned echocardiographically as moving erratically in the cavity of the right atrium. The orifice of the inferior vena cava is rightward and inferior to the fossa ovalis (Fig. 12). In the fetus, oxygenated umbilical vein blood from the inferior vena cava is directed at the foramen ovale, creating a shunt of oxygenated blood to the left heart and head and neck, bypassing the developing lung. The proximity and orientation of the inferior vena caval orifice to the fossa ovalis facilitates a catheter from the inferior vena cava passing through an atrial secundum defect.

The superior vena cava connection with the right atrium superiorly is aligned with the atrial connection of the inferior vena cava, but is slightly anterior in position. On the inner surface of the right atrium at the junction between the superior vena cava and the right atrium laterally, the crista terminalis is a robust ridge of muscle that corresponds to the sulcus terminalis seen on the epicardial surface (Fig. 12). As the crista terminalis courses inferiorly, it flattens and becomes indistinct near the inferior vena cava. Between the crista terminalis and the interatrial septum posteriorly, the right atrial wall is smooth (without pectinate muscles) and is called the sinus venarum cavarum (Fig. 12). This smooth part of the right atrium is derived

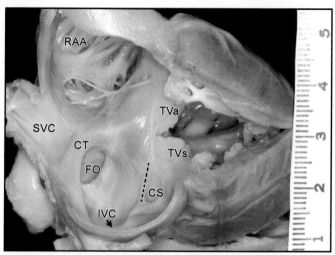

FIGURE 12: Sinus venarum ("smooth" part of the right atrium). En face the opened right atrium of a newborn's heart demonstrates the adjacent relationship between the inferior vena cava (IVC) and fossa ovalis (FO) where the fetal interatrial shunt occurs. (Abbreviations: - - - - - -: Subendocardial position of tendon of Todaro on the Eustachian ridge; CS: Coronary sinus os; CT: Crista terminalis; RAA: Right atrial appendage; SVC: Superior vena cava; TVa: Anterior leaflet of tricuspid valve; TVs: Septal leaflet of tricuspid valve)

from the right horn of the embryonic sinus venosus. Immediately anterior to the inferior vena caval orifice and between the fossa ovalis and the tricuspid annulus is the orifice of the coronary sinus. It is "guarded" by another vestigial valvular structure, the valve of the coronary sinus or thebesian valve. Coursing from the inferior vena cava in an anteromedial direction, a subendocardial fibrous ligament termed the tendon of Todaro passes to the right fibrous trigone (Figs 10 and 12). Opening into the right atrial cavity are a variable number of small orifices from the thebesian veins, especially on the anterior and lateral walls. Occasionally with contrast injection into the right atrium, contrast can be seen entering these vessels retrograde.

The floor of the right atrium (vestibule of the tricuspid valve) is comprised of a circumferential wall of atrial muscle that funnels blood toward the outlet. Situated on the floor of the right atrium, the right atrioventricular orifice is directed anteriorly and leftward and is guarded by the tricuspid valve.

TRICUSPID VALVE

From the right atrioventricular annulus the tricuspid valve leaflets hang into the cavity of the right ventricle (Fig. 9). The leaflet attachment is continuous around the right atrioventricular ring; however, the hinge line varies from segment to segment. Medially, the hinge of the tricuspid valve crosses the middle of the membranous portion of the interventricular septum (Fig. 13). The fibromembranous tissue comprising the leaflets can be divided roughly into three leaflets, the largest being the anterior leaflet and the smallest the posterior, with the septal leaflet being intermediate in size (Fig. 9). The notched or undulating leaflet edges or free margins are attached to the papillary muscles by fibrous cords called chordae tendineae that branch once or twice before their leaflet attachments at variable distances from the edge. The chordae are thinnest at the leaflet edge and thicker in attaching on the

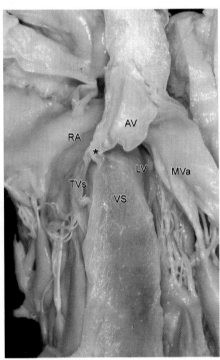

FIGURE 13: In this simulated four-chamber view, the attachment of the septal leaflet of the tricuspid valve (TVs) to the membranous portion of the interventricular septum (*) can be the basis for a left ventricular (LV)-to-right atrial (RA) shunt in patients with a malformation in this region. (Abbreviations: AV: Aortic valve; MVa: Anterior leaflet of mitral valve; VS: Ventricular septum)

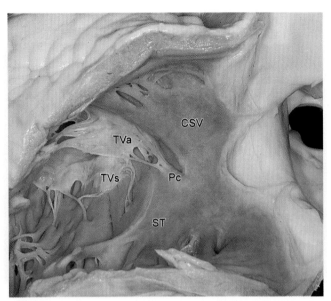

FIGURE 14: Right ventricular outlet (infundibulum). The transition between the inlet and outlet portions of the right ventricle is marked by the papillary muscle of the conus (muscle of Lancisi) (Pc). In the right ventricular outflow tract, the crista supraventricularis (CSV) separates the pulmonary valve from the other three valves. (Abbreviations: ST: Septomarginal trabeculum; TVa: Anterior leaflet of tricuspid valve; TVs: Septal leaflet of tricuspid valve)

ventricular aspect of the leaflets. Each leaflet receives chordae from more than one papillary muscle.

The smooth atrial surface of each leaflet is the surface that coapts (or fits together) during systole. The anterior leaflet is situated subjacent to the sternocostal area where it is tethered by chordae primarily from the anterior papillary muscle, with a limited contribution of chordae from a small papillary muscle near the outlet septum (papillary muscle of the conus or muscle of Lancisi) (Fig. 14). The septal leaflet has chordae that insert directly into the interventricular septum. The posterior leaflet is positioned inferiorly and is tethered by chordae from a variable number of very small papillary muscles along the right ventricular inlet inferiorly. There can be supernumerary leaflets at the intervalvular spaces. Of clinical significance is the attachment of the tricuspid valve at the commissure between the anterior and septal leaflets, across the membranous septum (Fig. 13). Due to this attachment, it is possible to have a perimembranous septal defect with a left ventricle-to-right atrial shunt.

RIGHT VENTRICLE

The right atrioventricular orifice is inferior and faces anteriorly and slightly leftward into the inflow portion of the right ventricle. The free wall of the normal right ventricle is thin (up to 0.4 mm) and lined by muscle columns called trabeculae carneae that make up two-thirds of the wall's thickness with a narrow layer of compact muscle subjacent to the epicardium (Fig. 9). The right ventricle may be thought of as roughly triangular, with one side the right atrioventricular orifice, the second side the diaphragmatic aspect and the third side the

one adjacent to the interventricular septum (Fig. 15). The superior extent of the triangle leads to the right ventricular outflow tract. Seen echocardiographically, the robust interventricular septum bulges into the cavity of the right ventricle, because the pressure during ventricular systole is so much higher in the left as compared with the right ventricle. The short-axis cross section of the right ventricle is therefore crescentic, and the right ventricle can be considered as "wrapping around" the more round left ventricle (Fig. 16). Separating the inflow and the outflow tracts of the right ventricle is a muscle ridge called the crista supraventricularis (Figs 14 and 15); this structure forms an arch with one arm

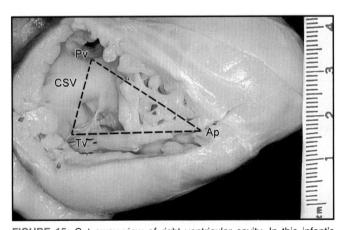

FIGURE 15: Cut away view of right ventricular cavity. In this infant's heart, a frontal view of the right ventricle with the free wall removed discloses a triangular cavity with the inlet inferiorly and the outlet superiorly. The inlet and outlet dimensions intersect at the apex (Ap). The third side of the triangle is an imaginary line through the crista supraventricularis (CSV). (Abbreviations: Pv: Pulmonary valve; Tv: Tricuspid valve)

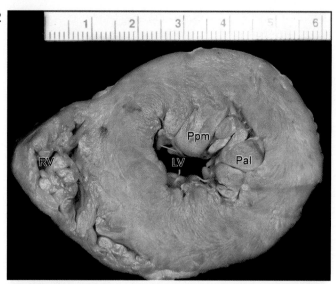

FIGURE 16: Venticles in short axis. A slice of heart in the short axis demonstrates the crescentic shape of the right ventricle adjacent to the more spherical left ventricle. At this level the prominence of the trabeculae carneae in the right ventricle can be appreciated. The increased wall thickness of the left ventricle and septum reflects myocardial hypertrophy. (Abbreviations: LV: Left ventricle; Pal: Anterolateral papillary muscle; Ppm: Posteromedial papillary muscle; RV: Right ventricle)

Many of these features can be visualized by echocardiography, computed tomography and magnetic resonance imaging. In patients with congenital heart disease, recognizing features that characterize a ventricle as being an anatomic right or left ventricle often is key to understanding the congenital anomaly.

PULMONIC VALVE

Situated superior-most in the right ventricular triangle and separating the right ventricle from the main pulmonary artery is the pulmonic valve that faces posteriorly and superiorly. This semilunar valve has three leaflets, right and left anterior leaflets and a single posterior leaflet, named according to their orientation to the main axis of the body when the heart is *in situ* (Figs 17 and 18). The valve leaflets are thin and translucent, with a fibrous thickening at the midpoint of the free margin, the nodulus Arantius. Radiating from the nodule over each leaflet are fibrous thickenings. Along the leaflet edge, these crescentic thickenings are called lunulae. Of similar configuration as the aortic leaflets, the pulmonic valve leaflets are thinner due to the lower forces sustained by the pulmonic

on the interventricular septum (the septal band) and the other on the free wall of the right ventricle (the parietal band). Anatomically distinctive of the right ventricle, the crista supraventricularis is derived from the inferior margin of the embryologic conus arteriosus. Also characteristic of the right ventricle is the trabeculated septal surface (Fig. 9), unlike the left ventricular septal surface that is smooth. One of the more prominent trabeculums, the septomarginal trabeculum, courses in the long axis along the anterior septum (Figs 9 and 14). At its apical end, a short muscular trabecular bridge called the moderator band courses between the distal septum and the free right ventricular wall. Visible by echocardiography the moderator band carries right bundle branches of the conduction system. The papillary muscles of the right ventricle are somewhat variable in configuration. An anterior papillary muscle arises on the free wall of the right ventricle (Fig. 9). Also distinctive the papillary muscle of the conus (muscle of Lancisi) arises from the superior end of the septomarginal trabeculum and can be considered the start of the right ventricular outflow tract (Fig. 14).

In summary the right ventricle is distinctive anatomically because of a number of features:

- Its roughly triangular shape enabling it to "wrap around" the left ventricle.
- The coarse trabeculation of the ventricular septal surface.
- The septal leaflet of the tricuspid valve with chordae tendinae tethering it to the septal surface.
- The configuration of the septomarginal trabeculum and moderator band.
- The papillary muscle of the conus (muscle of Lancisi).
- The separation of inflow and outflow tracts by the crista supraventricularis that separates the pulmonary valve from the other three valves.

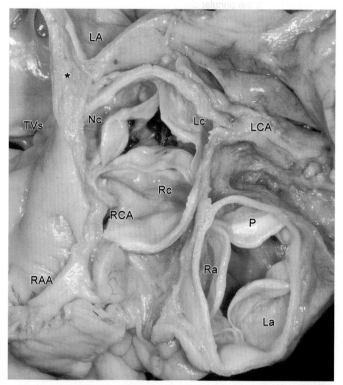

FIGURE 17: Relationship between aortic and pulmonary valves. Because of the crista supraventricularis and right ventricular conus, the pulmonary valve is a little more superior to the aortic valve. A close-up view of the two semilunar valves shows the right coronary (Rc), left coronary (Lc) and noncoronary (Nc) leaflets of the aortic valve. The noncoronary leaflet of the aortic valve is closest to the atrial septum. The adjacent leaflets of the pulmonary valve are designated differently. (Abbreviations: *: Fused medial walls of the left and right atria near interatrial septum; La: Left anterior leaflet of pulmonary valve; LA: Left atrium; LCA: Left coronary artery; P: Posterior leaflet of pulmonary valve; Ra: Right anterior leaflet of pulmonary valve; RAA: Right atrial appendage; RCA: Right coronary artery os; TVs: Septal leaflet of tricuspid valve)

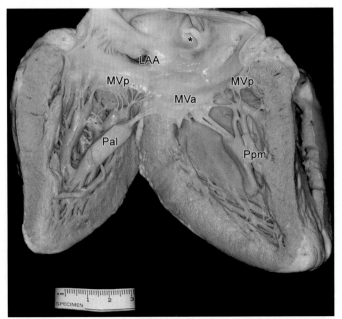

FIGURE 18: Left atrium and left ventricular inlet. The opened left atrium is notable for the pulmonary vein connections, left aspect of the interatrial septum (*) and the relatively narrow orifice that communicates with the left atrial appendage. Pectinate muscles are limited to the left atrial appendage, with only few visible around the orifice. The mitral orifice is guarded by a two-leaflet valve. The septal or aortic leaflet subtends roughly one-third of the annular circumference and has a greater height than the shallower posterior or mural leaflet that subtends two-thirds of the circumference. (Abbreviations: LAA: Orifice of left atrial appendage; MVa: Anterior leaflet of mitral valve; MVp: Posterior (or mural) leaflet of mitral valve; Pal: Anterolateral papillary muscle; Ppm: Posteromedial papillary muscle)

valve as compared with the aortic valve during diastole. In systole the leaflets flex at their wall attachments to form a rounded triangular orifice, about 3 cm² in diameter. In diastole the leaflets close by coapting along their ventricular surface.

PULMONARY ARTERIES

The main pulmonary artery arises above the pulmonic valve annulus and passes leftward first superiorly and then posteriorly around the medial (left-facing) aspect of the ascending aorta. Normally the artery is approximately 3 cm in diameter and 4–5 cm long (Fig. 5). When the valve is closed, the pulmonic valve leaflets define three cup-like sinuses at which the pulmonary artery wall bulges slightly outward. Beyond the level of the left atrium the pulmonary artery divides into the right and left pulmonary arterial branches. The right pulmonary arterial branch passes rightward behind the ascending aorta just above the left atrium, and the left pulmonary arterial branch, essentially a continuation of the main pulmonary artery, passes over the left mainstem bronchus. This leftward superior orientation of the left pulmonary artery is fixed by the attachment of the ligamentum arteriosum (Fig. 5). Distal to the ligament, the left pulmonary artery courses sharply inferiorly. From the superior and anterior surface of the left pulmonary artery, there are four branches to the upper lobe of the left lung. The remainder of the left pulmonary artery passes inferiorly into the left lower pulmonary lobe. Coursing rightward and slightly posterior behind the ascending aorta, the right pulmonary artery

lies anterior to the right mainstem bronchus and posterior to the superior vena cava and the right superior pulmonary vein. At the hilum of the right lung the pulmonary artery divides into two major branches, the superior or ascending branch supplying the upper lobe of the right lung, and the descending or interlobular branch supplying the middle and lower lobes of the right lung.

The branches of the pulmonary artery generally follow the branches of the bronchial system and supply similar pulmonary segments. The relationship of the various pulmonary artery branches to the bronchi at the lung hilums is important, since their positions can be visualized on chest X-ray and can identify the "anatomical" left and right lungs, critical in some cardiovascular malformations. As noted above, the right pulmonary artery passes anteriorly and inferiorly to the right mainstem bronchus, therefore the right bronchus is "eparterial" at the right hilum. On the left, the left upper lobe bronchus is inferior to the left pulmonary artery, making this the "hyparterial" bronchus.

LEFT ATRIUM

The left atrium is posterior and leftward of the right atrium and posterior to the aortic root. The right pulmonary artery is directly superior to the left atrium. The left atrial appendage lies to the left and anterior to the main pulmonary artery (Figs 1 and 5). The left atrial inner wall is smooth with the exception of the tubular left atrial appendage that has some pectinate muscles; however, the narrow orifice of the atrial appendage hides these ridges (Fig. 18). Viewed en face, the endocardium of the left atrium is thicker and more opaque than that of the right atrium. The four pulmonary veins, two right and two left, superior and inferior veins, connect with the left atrium posteriorly. The two right pulmonary vein ostia are near the left side of the atrial septum, and the left pulmonary vein ostia are posterior on the lateral wall of the left atrium. The left side of the atrial septum is smooth, but there is a flap of membranous tissue that corresponds to the fossa ovalis where the septum primum fused to the septum secundum (Fig. 18). At the atrial outlet, the vestibule of the mitral valve consists of a circumferential wall of muscle that funnels blood toward the valve orifice.

MITRAL VALVE

The mitral valve, so-called because of its fancied resemblance to a Bishop's miter, guards the entrance to the left ventricle. Hanging from the annulus, the leaflet tissue includes the anterior (or aortic) leaflet and the posterior (or mural) leaflet. The leaflets are anchored to the left ventricular wall by chordae tendineae that originate from papillary muscles. In addition, the mural leaflet has some chordae that come directly from the left ventricular wall. Due to the junction between the aortic and mitral annuli (left fibrous trigone), the anterior leaflet of the mitral valve contacts the noncoronary and left coronary portions of the aortic annulus (Figs 19 and 20). Thus, there is fibrous continuity between the mitral and aortic valves, unlike the right ventricular outlet where the tricuspid and pulmonary valves are separated by the crista supraventricularis. The part of the anterior leaflet from its aortic ring attachment to its point of flexion is known as the intervalvular membrane. In a superior view onto

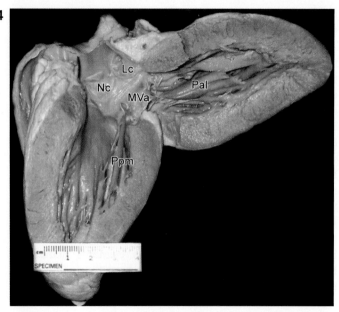

FIGURE 19: Left ventricular outlet. In this view of the left ventricular outlet, the free wall of the left ventricle has been retracted to show the smooth septal surface near the base of the heart. The noncoronary (Nc) and left coronary (Lc) leaflets of the aortic valve are visible. In contrast to the outlet of the right ventricle, there is no muscle between the mitral valve and the aortic valve; thus, there is fibrous continuity between the mitral and aortic valves. (Abbreviations: MVa: Anterior leaflet of mitral valve; Pal: Anterolateral papillary muscle; Ppm: Posteromedial papillary muscle)

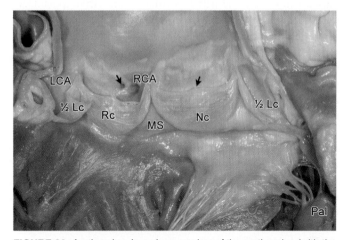

FIGURE 20: Aortic valve. In a close-up view of the aortic valve (with the left coronary leaflet (Lc) cut in half), the membranous portion of the interventricular septum (MS) is present between the noncoronary (Nc) and right coronary (RC) leaflets. In addition to the ostia leading to the main coronary arteries, a separate tiny ostium (short arrow) leading to the conal branch of the right coronary artery is identified as a normal variant. Facilitating valve closure, a tiny midline fibrous nodule on the free margin of each semilunar leaflet is known as the nodule of Arantius. Fibrous thickenings termed lunulae are barely visible in the noncoronary and right coronary leaflets, and two small fenestrations may be identified near the free margin of the right coronary leaflet. (Abbreviations: LCA: Left coronary artery os; Pal: Posterolateral papillary muscle; RCA: Right coronary artery os)

the isolated left ventricle, the "orifice" of the left ventricle, known as the left ventricular OS, contains the nonmuscular fibrous mitral valve to the left and posterior and the aortic valve to the right and anterior. With the anterior leaflet of the mitral

valve hanging into the left ventricle, the chamber of the left ventricle is divided into the inflow tract posteriorly and the outflow tract anteriorly.

The mitral leaflets are somewhat scalloped (Fig. 18). At the commissures fan-like arrangements of chordae can be identified on the ventricular aspect. The two major commissures separating the anterior and posterior leaflets are the anterolateral and posteromedial commissures. The posterior leaflet is seen to have two other minor commissures subdividing the leaflet into anterolateral, medial and posteromedial scallops. The clinical significance of this minor anatomical point is that each of these scallops can prolapse back into the left atrium during systole, forming a distinct angiographic and echocardiographic picture. In the majority of cases mitral regurgitation caused by mitral valve prolapse is amenable to mitral valve repair rather than replacement.

The chordae originating from the papillary muscles attach to the free margins of the leaflets and also onto the ventricular surface of the leaflet beyond the free edge. This architecture subdivides the septal leaflet into a rough crescentic area adjacent to the free edge (1 cm wide at the center of the leaflet, narrowing as it approaches the commissures) and a smooth portion that extends medially and superiorly; in the anterior leaflet, the smooth portion becomes the intervalvular membrane that attaches to the noncoronary and left coronary portion of the aortic annulus. The posterior leaflet hangs from that portion of the mitral annulus that is adjacent to the position of the coronary sinus.

Closure of the mitral valve during systole is accomplished by coapting the atrial surfaces of the two leaflets. The overlap of the closed leaflets is important to the proper seal of the valve. The chordae tendineae keep the mitral leaflets from prolapsing into the left atrium. The chordae originate from the anterolateral and posteromedial papillary muscles and distribute to both leaflets. In contrast to the tricuspid valve, there are no mitral valve chordae that attach to the ventricular septum in the normal heart. The mitral valve apparatus includes three groups of chordae:

1. First-order chordae arise as fibroelastic cords from the tips of the papillary muscles and insert into the free margin of the valve. These chordae can divide two or three times before their leaflet attachment.
2. Second-order chordae at or near the tips of the papillary muscles arise as strong tendinous cords and attach to the ventricular surface or rough area of the anterior leaflet.
3. Third-order chordae originate from the left ventricular wall near the atrioventricular ring and attach to the ventricular surface of the posterior leaflet only.

LEFT VENTRICLE

The left ventricle has an oblong, truncated shape with an open end (prolate ellipsoid), the left ventricular OS, which contains the mitral valve posteriorly and the aortic valve anteriorly. The ventricle tapers from the OS to the apex (Figs 5, 7 and 19). Viewing the heart from its anterior aspect, the left ventricular wall forms the gently curving obtuse margin of the heart (Fig. 5). The ventricular wall extends anteriorly to the interventricular sulcus, and the right anterior wall of the left ventricle is formed by the interventricular septum. As evident in the short axis, the wall of the left ventricle is thicker than that of the right ventricle (Fig. 16), normally about 1 cm thick, and is divided into an outer two-thirds zone of compact muscle and an inner one-third trabeculated zone. The trabeculae carneae of the left ventricular inner surface are thinner and more delicate than those of the right ventricle; at the apex they can have the configuration of a rope hammock. Remodeled overtime by high left ventricular systolic pressures, these muscle ridges may become flattened, but in hypertrophied hearts they can be quite robust. Without many trabeculae carneae superiorly, the left ventricular aspect of the septum in the outflow tract appears smooth as compared with the septum of the right ventricle (Fig. 19).

In diastole, the half-football-shaped left ventricle approximates an ellipsoid of revolution. The two papillary muscles project into the left ventricular cavity from their anterolateral and posteromedial positions (Figs 18 and 19). Although the number and positions of the papillary muscles are constant, there are a variable number of papillary muscle heads, usually two or three, with the posteromedial one more variable than the anterolateral.

The ventricles viewed in short axis show the left ventricle to be circular (Fig. 16). Recall that the anterior wall being the interventricular septum bulges toward the right, making the cross section of the right ventricular cavity crescentic. The outflow tract of the left ventricle shows the smooth surface of the muscular septum superiorly. Just proximal to the aortic valve the interventricular septum includes the membranous portion that abuts the aortic annulus (Fig. 20). The opposing margin of the left ventricular outflow tract is the anterior leaflet of the mitral valve, especially at its junction with the annulus. From the left ventricular outflow tract, the membranous septum appears as a small rhomboid membrane present between the lines of attachment of the right and noncoronary leaflets at the aortic annulus. Viewing the opaque membrane en face, it is difficult to appreciate the proximity of the septal leaflet of the tricuspid valve on the right ventricular aspect (Fig. 13). In fact, on the right side the septal leaflet and anterior leaflet of the tricuspid valve attach to the middle of the membranous septum. Therefore, part of the membranous septum on the right is above the attachment of the tricuspid valve and is called the atrioventricular portion of the membranous septum. Congenital defects in this area of the septum can result in a left ventricle-to-right atrial shunt. Defects in other areas of the membranous septum produce a purely interventricular shunt.

As in the right ventricle, the anatomic left ventricle is characterized by a number of distinctive anatomic features:
- The shape is oblong, shaped like a prolate ellipsoid.
- The interventricular septal surface is smooth.
- There is fibrous continuity between the mitral and the aortic valves. Thus, the inflow and outflow tracts of the left ventricle are separated only by the anterior leaflet of the mitral valve.
- The apical trabeculae are thin and cobweb like.
- The left atrioventricular valve, the mitral valve, is bicuspid and its chordae insert only into papillary muscles, not the ventricular septum.

The clinical importance of these differences is that many can be recognized by echocardiography and other imaging

techniques. These anatomic details are keys to discerning congenital malformations.

The orientation of the muscle bundles of the left ventricle is critical to understanding the mechanics of left ventricular contraction. Fiber orientation is a complex topic, however, beyond the scope of this anatomy chapter. In simple terms, the compact outer two-thirds of the left ventricular free wall are comprised of syncytial layers of myocardial cells supported loosely by a continuous matrix of fibrous tissue. The great majority of the muscular septum is compact, with myofiber contributions from both ventricles. In general the muscle layers of the left ventricle are oriented orthogonally, each layer spiraling toward the cardiac apex. This arrangement is responsible for the pump function of the ventricles—the longitudinal shortening that pulls the base of the left ventricle toward the apex and the circumferential shortening that rapidly reduces the left ventricular volume and ejects the stroke volume during systole. At the same time the orthogonal spiral arrangement of myofibers generates a twisting motion of the left ventricle during systole. Thus, the muscle bundles are arranged such that they form superficial and deep layers as well as circumferential bands that with ventricular contraction shorten both the minor as well as the major (longitudinal) axis of the left ventricle. These motions allow for the estimation of stress in different layers of the left ventricle by speckle-tracking Doppler echocardiography and magnetic resonance imaging.

AORTIC VALVE

The aortic valve guards the outlet from the left ventricle. The valve is semilunar with three leaflets suspended from the aortic annulus (Figs 8, 17 and 20). The leaflets are named for their positions in situ relative to the body axis—right (or anterior) coronary leaflet and left (or left posterior) coronary leaflet and noncoronary (or right posterior) leaflet. During diastole the aortic walls in the root of the aorta expand well-beyond the limits of the aortic annulus, increasing the volumes of the three sinuses of Valsalva and visible angiographically. The coronary arteries usually arise from the aortic wall that surrounds these sinuses. Like the pulmonary valve leaflets, the aortic leaflets have noduli Arantius at the midportion of the free margin and crescentic lunulae (Fig. 20).

The anatomic relationships of the sinuses of Valsalva are of clinical importance. The right coronary's sinus bulges into the posterior aspect of the right ventricular outflow tract (Fig. 8). The left coronary's sinus abuts the outlet septum anteriorly and faces the transverse sinus posteriorly, as well as the right pulmonary artery as it passes posterior to the ascending aorta. The noncoronary sinus is adjacent to the medial wall of the right atrium and the interatrial septum. Injury or aneurysmal formation and rupture in each of these sinuses can result in fistulous communication into these respective cardiac chambers or even into the pericardial space.

In diastole, the three aortic leaflets close by apposition of their ventricular surfaces. Along the edges near the commissures, the leaflets commonly contain holes or fenestrations (Fig. 20). Normally these do not cause valvular regurgitation, because they are above the line of closure. Nonetheless, these fenestrations as well as incomplete aortic leaflet coaptation are considered the cause for the small aortic regurgitation jets seen in about 5% of normal hearts by Doppler echocardiography. In systole, the opening of the aortic valve forms a rounded triangular orifice with flexion at the wall attachments of the leaflets. If this flexion area becomes calcified (as is often seen in advanced age), various degrees of aortic valve stenosis occur.

The fibrous aortic annulus or ring forms the junction between the outflow tract (or subaortic sinus) of the left ventricle and the aorta. The transition from cardiac muscle to the smooth muscle of the aortic media occurs at this junction. The actual attachments of the aortic leaflets at the aortic annulus form crescents, the highest points being the attachments at the commissures. Thus, the composition of the heart muscle-smooth muscle interface in the wall varies according to the level.

CONDUCTION SYSTEM

Although the work of the heart is dependent on myocardial contractility, the mechanism that initiates and provides order to the phasic contraction and relaxation of the cardiac muscle is dependent on the other two fundamental properties of cardiac muscle, automaticity and conductivity. The conduction system—including nodes, bundle branches and Purkinje fibers—consists of modified myocardial cells that are positioned to either facilitate or slow impulse conduction. Both the sinoatrial node and the atrioventricular node are comprised of specialized myocardial cells with highly developed automaticity, and the myocardial cells of the His bundle, bundle branches and Purkinje fibers have the specialized property of rapid conductivity.

None of the collections of specialized muscle in the heart is discernible grossly. All were discovered through tedious dissection and microscopy. The major portion of the adult sinoatrial node, a 3 by 10 mm body of pacemaker nodal cells, normally initiates the depolarization that causes the atrial muscle to contract. The node is situated in subepicardial tissue superolaterally near the junction between the superior vena cava and the right atrial appendage; in other words, the specialized muscle lies within the sulcus terminalis (Figs 3 and 5). The sinoatrial node, also called the SA node, is derived from the right horn of the embryonic sinus venosus.[1] The SA node receives its blood supply from the sinoatrial nodal artery (Fig. 3). This small artery is located in a relatively constant position centrally within the specialized muscle (Figs 21A and B—histology of SAN). Although the SA node is often considered as a discrete sausage-shaped mass, an attenuated extension of specialized muscle trails inferiorly along the sulcus terminalis.[2] The electrical impulse initiated in the specialized muscle spreads over the working atrial muscle in organized fashion along preferential pathways; however, there are no histologically recognizable anatomic tracts between the SA node and the atrioventricular or AV node.[3] Thus, the preferential conduction likely occurs along bundles of working muscle in particular orientation. For example, along the anterior aspect of the transverse sinus, a fascicle of atrial muscle serving as a pathway carrying the impulse from the right atrium to the left atrium is called Bachmann's bundle.

After the impulse spreads through the atrium, it reaches the atrioventricular node (AV node) (Figs 10 and 22). From the

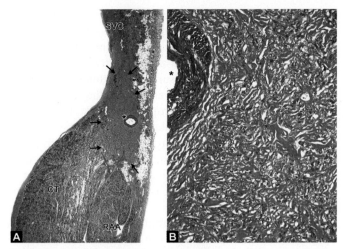

FIGURES 21A AND B: Histology of sinoatrial node. At low magnification (A), the sinoatrial node (outlined by arrows) is seen on the epicardial aspect between the superior vena cava (SVC) and the right atrial appendage (RAA). Relatively constant in position, the artery to the SA node indicated by the stars courses within the specialized muscle. At high magnification (B), the specialized muscle fibers (red in this trichrome stain) are coursing in haphazard array, separated by collagen (blue). (Abbreviations: CT: Crista terminalis; RAA: Right atrial appendage)

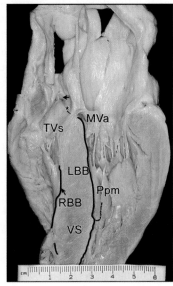

FIGURE 22: Position of atrioventricular node and course of atrioventricular bundle. In a simulated four-chamber view with the inferior side of Koch's triangle represented by the coronary sinus os (arrow), the more anterior atrioventricular node (*) abuts the central fibrous body and connects with the atrioventricular bundle (- - - - -). The bundle courses anteriorly along the inferoposterior margin of the membranous portion of the interventricular septum (not shown) and projects left and right bundle branches (LBB and RBB) subendocardially on either side of the muscular septum. (Abbreviations: MVa: Anterior leaflet of mitral valve; Ppm: Posteromedial papillay muscle; TVs: Septal leaflet of tricuspid valve; VS: Ventricular septum)

endocardial aspect within the right atrium, the landmarks for the AV node form Koch's triangle bounded by the tendon of Todaro superiorly, the annulus of the septal leaflet of the tricuspid valve apically and an imaginary line in the long axis through the coronary sinus ostium inferiorly (Fig. 10). The AV node is comprised of a small bean-shaped mass of specialized myocardial cells that abuts the right fibrous trigone between the right and left atria (Figs 23A and B). In 90% of hearts, the

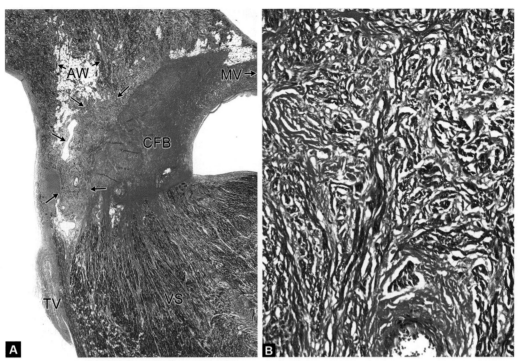

FIGURES 23A AND B: At low magnification (A), the atrioventricular node is seen abutting the central fibrous body (CFB). Somewhat variable in its course, the artery to the AV node is present within the specialized muscle. At high magnification (B), the narrow-caliber specialized muscle fibers (red in this trichrome stain), similar to the SA node, appear haphazard in orientation and are separated by collagen (blue). (Abbreviations: AW: Atrial wall; MV: Mitral valve; TV: Tricuspid valve; VS: Ventriculum septum)

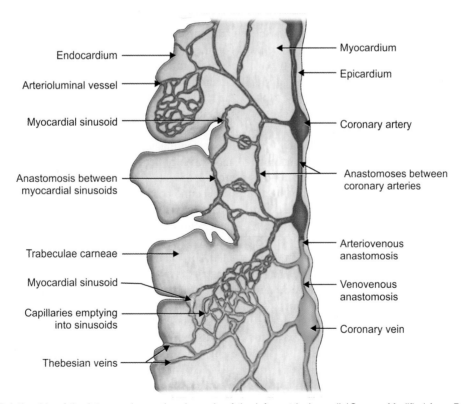

FIGURE 24: Relationship of the intramural vascular channels of the left ventricular wall (*Source:* Modified from Barry A, Patten BM. Structure of the human heart. In: Gould SE (Ed). Pathology of the Heart. Springfield, IL: Charles C. Thomas; 1968)

AV nodal artery originates from the right coronary artery near the crux of the heart. In the other 10% of hearts, the artery arises from the left circumflex coronary artery.

Slowing conduction, the AV node conveys the impulse to the His (or atrioventricular) bundle that is approximately

10–20 mm in length and 1–3 mm in diameter (Fig. 24). From the apex of Koch's triangle (angle formed by the junction between the tendon of Todaro and the annulus of the septal leaflet of the tricuspid valve, Fig. 10), the His bundle courses anteriorly within the right fibrous trigone and passes down to the crest of the muscular interventricular septum, posterior and inferior to the membranous septum. Within the His bundle is an artery arising from either branches of the left anterior descending coronary artery or posterior ventricular branches of the right or left circumflex coronary artery. At the crest of the muscular interventricular septum, the His bundle divides into the right and left bundle branches.

The left bundle branches spread out in a subendocardial fan-like distribution posteroinferior to the membranous portion of the interventricular septum. Although the subendocardial left bundle fibers are not so discrete anatomically, they function as anterior and posterior fascicles (or divisions), with possibly an intermediate fascicle. The anterior fascicles fan out toward the apex, forming a subendocardial plexus that branches at the anterolateral papillary muscle. The posterior fascicles reach the area of the posteromedial papillary muscle and spread out as Purkinje fibers to the rest of the left ventricular muscle. The Purkinje fibers spread from the subendocardium intramurally to the subepicardium.

From the His bundle the right bundle branch continues 10–20 mm as a discrete 1–3 mm diameter structure deeply buried in the muscle of the interventricular septum; it resurfaces near the papillary muscle of the conus (muscle of Lancisi) superiorly on the septomarginal trabeculum. The subendocardial right bundle branch becomes more compact in passing down this robust trabeculum toward the apex. The right bundle can pass over the moderator band to the right ventricular free wall or, more frequently, passes over one of the trabeculae carneae to reach the ventricular wall near the anterior papillary muscle of the right ventricle. When it reaches the free wall, it branches into a finely distributed, subendocardial anastomosing plexus. A small branch bends sharply back along the upper interventricular septum to the conus. The blood supply to the right bundle branch is principally from the septal branches of the left anterior descending coronary artery.

In some hearts there are accessory muscle bundles that span the fibrous atrioventricular rings, connecting atrial to ventricular muscle directly and thus bypassing the AV node. Called bundles of Kent,[4] these muscle bridges offer low-resistance pathways for the impulse to travel from atrium to ventricle, and they form the anatomic basis for the Wolff-Parkinson-White syndrome or accelerated atrioventricular conduction. Kent bundles can be situated anywhere along the atrioventricular annuli. In 1931, Mahaim[5] described "paraspecific" septal fibers leaving the left side of the His bundle at the membranous septum and reaching the upper left septal muscle, and James[6] described fibers that bypass the AV node and join the His bundle. These muscle fiber bridges that bypass the AV node form the anatomic basis for the described elecrocardiographic abnormalities.

CORONARY ARTERIES

The main coronary arteries arise from funnel-like openings in the aortic wall at the right coronary leaflet and the left coronary leaflet, most often in the midline of the sinuses (Figs 17 and 20). There is usually a single ostium for each main coronary artery, left and right; however, occasionally there will be a separate small ostium near the right coronary ostium for the conus branch of the right coronary artery. Another common variant is a separate ostium for the left anterior descending and the left circumflex coronary artery. Thus, at coronary arteriography, the perceived absence of a left anterior descending or a left circumflex coronary may be due to the selective catheterization of one of the two ostia.

Arising from the left posterior aortic sinus of Valsalva, the left main coronary artery is a muscular artery that passes anterior and somewhat leftward, posterior to the right ventricular outflow tract and anterior to the left atrium (Fig. 8). The left main coronary artery is short (usually less than 1 cm) and bifurcates into the left anterior descending and left circumflex coronary arteries. The coronary arteries are enveloped by loose connective tissue and epicardial fat. The left anterior descending coronary lies in the anterior interventricular sulcus, extending down the anterior surface of the heart inferiorly to the apex and frequently around the apex to the distal part of the inferior cardiac surface (Figs 3 and 5). The anterior descending coronary artery gives off a number of branches including a first and often a second diagonal branch that supply the anterior left ventricular free wall, one or more large septal perforator branches and a number of septal branches that supply the anterior two-thirds of the muscular interventricular septum. On the cardiac surface there are small ventricular branches that supply the medial aspect of the right ventricular free wall.

Frequently there is a prominent coronary artery (the intermedius coronary artery) arising from the bifurcation of the left main coronary. This artery supplies the anterolateral portion of the left ventricle.

Coursing in the left atrioventricular sulcus, the circumflex coronary artery gives off superiorly 1–3 anterior branches, one lateral and one posterior branch to the left atrial wall. The circumflex artery continues in the atrioventricular groove around the left lateral aspect of the heart. Several branches called obtuse marginal arteries supply the anterolateral wall of the left ventricle. Deep to the coronary sinus, the circumflex coronary artery continues posteroinferiorly to the crux of the heart. In about 15% of hearts, the circumflex coronary artery crosses the crux on the diaphragmatic surface and turns toward the apex to become the posterior descending coronary artery supplying the inferior wall of the left ventricle and also portions of the inferior right ventricle adjacent to the posterior interventricular sulcus. With this coronary artery arrangement the heart is said to have a left-dominant circulation. In about 25% of hearts, the superior vena caval ostial artery that gives rise to the sinoatrial nodal artery is a branch of the circumflex coronary artery, but in 70% of hearts the sinoatrial artery arises from the proximal portion of the right coronary artery. In the remaining 5% of hearts, the blood supply to the sinoatrial node has a dual source from both right and left circumflex coronary arteries.

The right coronary artery originates from the anterior or right coronary sinus of Valsalva and passes rightward under the right atrial appendage in the right atrioventricular sulcus (Figs 3, 8 and 17). The first branch is the right ventricular conal artery that passes anteriorly to the right ventricular outflow tract. In about 20% of hearts, the conal artery arises from a separate orifice in the right coronary sinus (Fig. 20). This clinically important vessel becomes the major source of collateral circulation to the left anterior descending coronary system when that vessel is occluded. At catheterization of patients with obstructed left anterior descending arteries, the conal branch should be visualized to see if the distal anterior descending is patent beyond the obstruction. Another early branch from the right coronary artery is the artery to the superior vena caval orifice that gives rise to the sinoatrial nodal artery (Fig. 3). The right coronary artery gives branches superiorly to the right atrial wall and one to three branches inferiorly to the free wall of the right ventricle. At the acute margin of the heart, the acute marginal artery is a large vessel supplying the anterior wall of the right ventricle. The right coronary artery continues inferiorly in the right atrioventricular sulcus, passing under the inferior vena cava at its connection with the right atrium. The right coronary artery continues posteriorly to the crux of the heart and makes an anterior loop into the posterior atrial septum. In 90% of hearts, a branch—the AV nodal artery—passes in the inferior interatrial septum superiorly to supply the AV node. After giving off the AV nodal artery, the right coronary artery turns toward the apex to course in the posterior interventricular sulcus as the posterior descending coronary artery that supplies the posteroinferior surface of the left ventricle, parts of the posterior right ventricle adjacent to the posterior interventricular sulcus and, by small septal perforators, the posterior one-third of the interventricular septum (Figs 7 and 9). When the posterior descending coronary artery is a continuation of the right coronary artery as occurs in 75% of hearts, the heart is said to have a right-dominant circulation. In some hearts, the posterior descending coronary artery wraps around the apex and supplies the distal portion of the anterior left ventricular wall. The terminal distribution of the left circumflex and the right coronary arteries posteriorly are reciprocally related, and the blood supply to the posterior wall of the left ventricle depends on whether there is a right dominant or a left dominant circulation. In 5% of hearts, the right coronary artery is a congenitally small vessel, supplying only branches to the right ventricle, with the entire left ventricle supplied by the left coronary artery.

INTRAMURAL VESSELS

The extramural coronary arteries that lie on the epicardial surface give off branches that penetrate the walls of all four cardiac chambers. These intramural resistance vessels do not develop atherosclerosis. A complex meshwork of anastomosing vessels arises from these perforating arteries, eventually supplying capillary vessels that form a network around the myocardial muscle fibers. The pattern of this branching varies, some extending down to the subendocardial areas where they spread out, others arising at right angles from the perforating arteries in a comb-like pattern at all levels of the ventricular wall (Fig. 24). There is controversy as to whether there are anastomosing connections between the perforating arteries in the subendocardial region or whether they are end-arteries. Most likely, there are both patterns present. The endocardium, especially in the papillary muscles, are supplied either through the distal portion of the epicardial coronary arteries or from the left ventricular cavity through luminal channels. In fact arterioluminal channels between the arteriolar arteries and the left ventricular cavity via intertrabecular spaces have been described.[7]

There have been many reports of direct connections of arteriolar vessels emptying into ventricular and atrial cavities,

the names of these vessels depending on the connections and the histology of the small vessels involved. Other vessels or channels called sinusoids are thin walled and capillary like, but with lumens of variable size and shape; some of these vessels connect directly to the ventricular chambers and some to venous structures that then empty into the ventricles. These have been called venoluminal channels. The ostia of these various vessels can be seen on careful inspection of the endocardium of the right and left ventricles, and collectively they are called thebesian veins or, more appropriately, thebesian vessels. They are more numerous or at least visible in the atria than in the ventricles.

Postmortem radiographic and dissection studies have documented subarteriolar collateral connections from about 100 μm to over 200 μm between the coronary arterial systems. These collateral vessels are most numerous near the apex and through the muscular interventricular septum, but they may also be identified in the interatrial septum, at the crux of the heart, between the sinoatrial nodal artery and other atrial arteries, as well as over the anterior surface of the right ventricle. In the human with nonobstructed coronary arteries, there are only rarely epicardial collateral vessels. When atherosclerosis results in progressive obstruction to the epicardial coronary arteries, the intramural potential collateral vessels enlarge and become clinically important. There are also extracoronary anastomotic connections between the coronary arteries and the systemic arteries, primarily at the base of the great vessels and around the ostia of the pulmonary veins and vena cavae. The systemic arteries involved are primarily the pericardial vessels derived from the internal mammary and intercostal arteries, usually at the pericardial reflections. In general, these systemic-to-coronary artery collaterals are clinically unimportant, even in obstructive coronary artery disease.

CORONARY VEINS

The cardiac veins generally follow the epicardial distribution of the coronary arteries. They lie embedded in epicardial fat and are superficial to the coronary arteries. They receive blood from the myocardial capillaries and carry it back to the right atrium. Most of the venous return to the right atrium is via the coronary sinus (Figs 25 and 26).

The great cardiac vein accompanies the anterior descending coronary artery in the anterior interventricular sulcus. It drains toward the base of the heart and then follows the left circumflex coronary artery posteriorly in the left atrioventricular sulcus, joining the coronary sinus just beneath the left inferior pulmonary vein. The great cardiac vein has valves at its connection with the coronary sinus. Throughout its course it receives veins from the anterior muscular interventricular septum, the anterior and lateral walls of the right and left ventricles, and the left atrium. Coursing on the diaphragmatic surface of the left ventricle, the posterior cardiac vein of the left ventricle accompanies the circumflex coronary artery to connect with the coronary sinus at its distal end.

The middle cardiac vein lies in the posterior interventricular sulcus overlying the posterior descending coronary artery; it receives tributaries from the posterior muscular interventricular septum and posterior ventricular walls and empties into the

Basic Cardiology

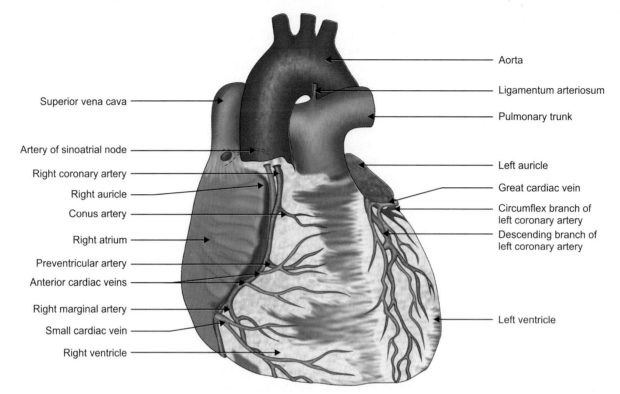

FIGURE 25: Ventral surface of the heart showing coronary arteries and veins (*Source:* Modified from Barry A, Patten BM. Structure of the human heart. In: Gould SE (Ed). Pathology of the Heart. Springfield, IL: Charles C. Thomas; 1968)

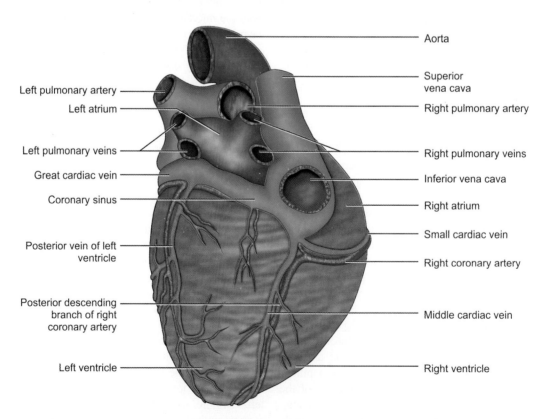

FIGURE 26: Dorsocaudal surface of the heart showing coronary arteries and veins (*Source:* Modified from Barry A, Patten BM. Structure of the human heart. In: Gould SE (Ed). Pathology of the Heart. Springfield, IL: Charles C. Thomas; 1968)

coronary sinus close to the coronary sinus ostium. The small cardiac vein on the surface of the right ventricle accompanies the acute marginal artery and drains the anterolateral wall of the right ventricle. It follows the course of the right coronary artery in the right atrioventricular sulcus, receives tributaries from the right atrium and empties into the coronary sinus near its ostium at the right atrium. On the anterior aspect of the right ventricle there are 3–12 anterior cardiac veins that empty through the ventricular wall in the conal region, into the small cardiac vein, or directly into the right atrium through separate orifices.

The coronary sinus is the continuation of the great cardiac vein; it is 3–5 mm in diameter and 2–5 cm in length. It courses in the left atrioventricular sulcus inferiorly, receiving veins from the left atrial and ventricular walls. A small vein draining from the roof of the posterior left atrium between the left and right pulmonary veins, called the oblique vein of the left atrium or vein of Marshall, is the remnant of the embryologic left common cardinal vein. When this cardinal vein remains patent, it is called a persistent left superior vena cava and connects the left innominate vein with the coronary sinus. This is clinically important in that catheters passed through the left median basilic vein enter the right atrium through the coronary sinus and are difficult to maneuver into the right ventricle and out the pulmonary artery.

CARDIAC LYMPHATICS

In the subendocardial connective tissue of all four cardiac chambers there is a plexus of valved lymphatic vessels. These channels drain through a web of anastomosing lymphatic vessels that envelop the myocardial fibers. The lymphatics course through the interstitial connective tissue, draining toward the epicardium where they form an epicardial lymphatic plexus. These vessels join on the epicardium to form several large lymphatic vessels that follow the course of the epicardial coronary arteries and veins. The major lymphatic trunks drain into the atrioventricular sulcus and form a single large trunk that passes over the top of the left main coronary artery and under the arch of the main pulmonary artery. This trunk courses to the left of the aortic root where it exits the pericardial sac to join the left mediastinal lymphatic plexus, draining into the mediastinal lymph nodes and finally into the thoracic duct.

CARDIAC INNERVATION

Both sympathetic and parasympathetic afferent and efferent nerves innervate the heart. The preganglionic neurons of the sympathetic chain are located in the upper five or six thoracic levels of the spinal cord and synapse with second-order neurons in the cervical sympathetic ganglia. The postganglionic sympathetic axons terminate in the heart and on the adventitia of the great vessels. The parasympathetic preganglionic neurons are located in the dorsal efferent nucleus of the medulla; these axons project as branches of the vagus nerve to the heart and great vessels where they synapse with second-order neurons in epicardial ganglia and adventitia of the great vessels (Fig. 27).

Both sympathetic and parasympathetic fibers enter the heart for the most part by common autonomic nerve trunks from the mediastinum by way of the dorsal mesocardia. The autonomic nerves are interdigitated within two neuroplexuses, divided for convenience into a superficial cardiac plexus on the anterior

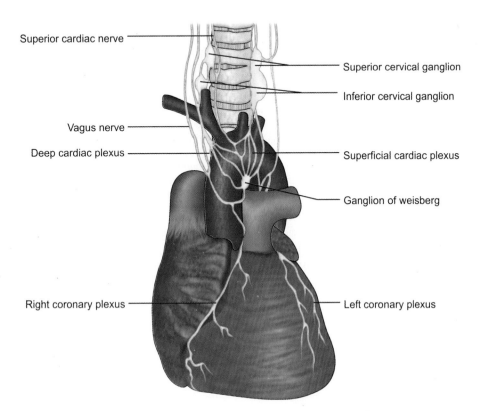

FIGURE 27: Autonomic nerve supply to the heart (*Source:* Modified from Tandler J. In: Anson BJ (Ed). Lehrbuch der Systematischen Anatomie. Berlin: Springer-Verlag; 1926)

ascending aorta, the aortic arch and the pulmonary trunk, as well as a deep cardiac plexus located above the bifurcation of the trachea on the right between the trachea and the right side of the aortic arch.

Since the left fourth and sixth embryonic aortic arches develop into the left aortic arch and the ductus arteriosus, cardiac branches of the left vagus nerve and left-sided sympathetic nerves distribute primarily to the aortic arch and pulmonary trunk, forming the arterial and conotruncal plexi. Embryologically the venous side favors the right-sided structures, since the right superior vena cava is retained, and the sinus venosus shifts to the right from midline and is incorporated into the right atrium. Therefore, the venous part of the heart is associated with cardiac nerves from the right cardiac sinoatrial plexus.

The sympathetic nerves arise from the superior and middle cervical ganglia, giving off the superior and middle cardiac nerves respectively. The inferior cardiac nerve originates from the fusion of the inferior cervical ganglion and the first thoracic ganglion, called the stellate ganglion. Each vagus nerve contributes to the cardiac plexuses by way of the superior and inferior cervical nerves, as well as a thoracic cardiac branch arising from the recurrent laryngeal nerve. The superficial cardiac plexus receives its contributions from the inferior cervical cardiac branch of the left vagus and the left superior cardiac nerves of the sympathetic nervous system. The ganglion of Wrisberg is associated with this plexus and lies between the aortic arch and the pulmonary trunk to the right of the ligamentum arteriosum.

The deep cervical plexus receives contributions from three right-sided sympathetic cardiac nerves, three cardiac branches of the right vagus nerve, three superior cervical and thoracic cardiac branches of the left vagus nerve, the middle and upper cardiac nerves from the sympathetic trunk, and direct branches from the five or six thoracic sympathetic ganglia.

From these autonomic nervous system plexi, the sympathetic and vagal nerves distribute to the walls of the great vessels, including the SA and AV nodes and the bundle of His. Sympathetic nerves and some parasympathetic nerves accompany the coronary arteries and innervate the ventricles. In the same nerves and through the same pathways, both afferent sympathetic and parasympathetic fibers pass back to the central nervous system.

CONCLUSION

Cardiac anatomy is complex and a thorough understanding requires detailed knowledge on a number of levels from gross relationships to histology and ultrastructure. The field has evolved over centuries, and information continues to accrue, stimulated in large part by clinical advances. This chapter provides an overview of cardiac anatomy that is relevant to general cardiology practice. This anatomical information forms the basis for an understanding of not only radiographic studies but also cardiac pathophysiology and the approach to therapeutic interventions. For various subspecialty works, more detailed information is available in the published literature.

REFERENCES

1. Mommersteeg MT, Hoogaars WM, Prall OW, et al. Molecular pathway for the localized formation of the sinoatrial node. Circ Res. 2007;100:354-62.
2. Sánchez-Quintana D, Cabrera JA, Farre J, et al. Sinus node revisited in the era of electroanatomical mapping and catheter ablation. Heart. 2005;91:189-94.
3. Ho SY, Anderson RH, Sánchez-Quintana D. Atrial structure and fibres: morphologic bases of atrial conduction. Cardiovasc Res. 2002;54:325-36.
4. Kent AFS. Observations on the auriculoventricular junction of the mammalian heart. Q J Exp Physiol. 1913;7:193-5.
5. Mahaim I. Les Maladies Organiques du Faisceau de HisTawara. Paris: Masson; 1931.
6. James TN. The connecting pathways between the sinus node and AV node and between the right and left atrium in the human heart. Am Heart J. 1963;66:498-508.
7. Wearn JT, Mettier SR, Klump TG, et al. The nature of the vascular communications between the coronary arteries and the chambers of the heart. Am Heart J. 1933;9:143-64.

GENERAL REFERENCES

1. Barry A, Patten BM. The structure of the adult heart. In: Goul SE (Ed). Pathology of the Heart, 3rd edition. Springfield, IL: Charles C Thomas; 1968.
2. Licata RH. Anatomy of the heart. In: Liusada AA (Ed). Development and Structure of the Cardiovascular System. New York: McGraw-Hili; 1961.
3. McAlpine WA. Heart and Coronary Arteries: An Anatomical Atlas for Clinical Diagnosis, Radiological Investigation, and Surgical Treatment. Berlin: Springer; 1975.
4. Netter FH. The Ciba Collection of Medical Illustrations, Vol 5 Heart. Summit, NJ: Ciba; 1969.
5. Patten BM. The heart. In: Anson BJ (Ed). Human Anatomy: A Complete Systematic Treatise, 12th edition. Philadelphia: Blakiston; 1966.
6. Virmani R, Ursell PC, Fenoglio JJ. Examination of the heart. Hum Pathol. 1987;18:432-40.
7. Mommersteeg MT, Hoogaars WM, Prall OW, et al. Molecular pathway for the localized formation of the sinoatrial node. Circ Res. 2007;100:354-62.
8. Ho SY, Anderson RH, Sánchez-Quintana D. Atrial structure and fibres: morphologic bases of atrial conduction. Cardiovasc Res. 2002;54:325-36.
9. Sánchez-Quintana D, Cabrera JA, Farre J, et al. Sinus node revisited in the era of electroanatomical mapping and catheter ablation. Heart. 2005;91:189-94.

Chapter 2

Cardiac Function in Physiology and Pathology

Joel S Karliner, Jeffrey Zimmet

Chapter Outline

INTRODUCTION

Synchronous cardiac contraction and relaxation require the coordination of numerous complex systems both within and without the cardiac myocyte. The human heart has evolved to integrate these pathways to provide efficient energy production and utilization in order to maintain blood supply to other vital organs as well as to the heart itself. Disruption of these pathways can be both cause and effect of cardiac injury and failure. Among the two most prominent pathways that require moment to moment coordination and integration are the beta-adrenergic signaling pathway and calcium handling. Both are central to cardiac contraction and relaxation, are abnormal in pathophysiologic states, and are targets for therapeutic intervention.

BETA-ADRENERGIC RECEPTOR-MEDIATED SIGNALING

Located on the cell surface, β-adrenoceptors are prototypical G-protein coupled receptors. They are liganded by the naturally occurring catecholamines, norepinephrine and epinephrine. Norepinephrine is released from synaptic vesicles of sympathetic nerves that innervate the heart and is principally responsible for cardiac chronotropy and contractility. Signaling results from the downstream activation of cyclic adenosine monophosphate (cAMP), initiated by liganding of the receptor by the catecholamine. Through a series of complex interactions, cAMP activates the contractile apparatus and also influences the conductance of ion channels that govern heart rate.

Numerous studies have established that the β-adrenergic receptor is highly regulated. After the receptor binds to a stimulatory guanine nucleotide regulatory protein (Gs), adenylyl cyclase is activated to hydrolyze ATP and produce cAMP. The G-protein-receptor complex can be uncoupled from its downstream signaling effectors by a molecule called G-protein receptor kinase-2 (GRK-2, aka β-arrestin) in a process termed desensitization. The receptor then can recycle to the cell surface. These uncoupling proteins also target receptors to clathrin-coated pits resulting in receptor downregulation and eventual proteolysis. It has recently been shown that GRKs by themselves can activate parallel signaling pathways such as stretch-associated angiotensin-II activation.[1]

In the mid-20th century it was observed that catecholamines were elevated in patients with chronic congestive heart failure (CHF) and that this abnormality could be a cause of cardiac dysfunction in such individuals. This hypothesis led to the idea that blocking β-adrenoceptors might be a useful strategy in heart failure. Although it took many years to prove this hypothesis, β-blocker therapy is now routine in heart failure patients. Along the way, much was learned about β-receptors.

There are two principal types of β-receptors: β_1 and β_2. Early studies by Bristow and his colleagues in tissue obtained from advanced heart failure patients revealed that β_1 receptor density was reduced, while β_2 receptor density actually increased and switched its coupling to a guanine nucleotide inhibitory protein (Gi).[2] In heart failure the increase in β_2 receptor density is thought to be a compensatory response which is aimed at retaining adrenergic drive but which instead may result in further cardiotoxicity.

What adverse mechanisms are mediated by β-receptors in heart failure? Polymorphisms in the β_1- and α_{2C}-adrenergic receptors may play a role in some patients.[3,4] Another recently described mechanism in a rodent model may provide at least a partial answer.[5] β_1 and β_2 receptors are normally distributed differently in cardiomyocyte T-tubules, such that β_2-mediated signaling is spatially restricted compared to β_1 signaling. In heart failure, where β_1 signaling induces cell remodeling and programmed cell death, this spatial restriction is lost, such that β_1 and β_2 signaling resemble each other.

Another area of basic pathophysiology that has drawn much attention is the relation between β-adrenergic receptor signaling and calcium regulation. Calcium was first found to exert an influence on the heart in the second decade of the 20th century. Subsequently it has become clear that calcium is a universal second messenger and in the heart exerts effects on contractility, mitochondrial function, transcriptional regulation and action potential generation. Calcium control is tightly linked to β-adrenoceptor signaling via intracellular mechanisms that take up and release ionic calcium.

The sarcoplasmic reticulum (SR), equivalent to the endoplasmic reticulum in other cells, lies just beneath the sarcolemma, which consists of the cell surface and invaginated T tubules. Each junction between the sarcolemma and the SR, where L-type calcium channels and ryanodine receptors are clustered, constitutes a local calcium signaling complex or couplon.[6] Type 2 ryanodine receptors, named after their affinity to the plant alkaloid ryanodine, are located in close proximity in the SR, and govern calcium storage and release from the SR via chemical coupling. When calcium enters the cell via sarcolemmal L-type calcium channels, adjacent ryanodine receptors are activated. This leads to SR calcium release and a marked increase in intracellular calcium concentration. This process has been termed calcium-induced calcium release and results in enhanced cardiac muscle contraction. Calcium is then removed via an SR calcium ATPase (SERCA-2), which in turn is under the control of an adjacent protein called phospholamban, which tonically inhibits SERCA. This inhibition decreases the rate of muscle relaxation and contractility. In humans, SERCA accounts for 70% of cytoplasmic calcium removal. Most of the remaining cytoplasmic calcium is removed via the sodium-potassium exchanger. Inhibition of this exchanger resulting in increased cytosolic calcium is the basis of the action of digitalis glycosides, which for almost two centuries was the only effective heart failure treatment available.

When phospholamban is phosphorylated by protein kinase A (PKA) or by calcium/calmodulin kinase II (CamKII), both of which are activated by sympathetic stimulation, its ability to inhibit SERCA is lost. Thus, activators of PKA and CamKII, such as β-adrenergic agonists, enhance the rate of cardiac myocyte relaxation. In addition, since SERCA is more active, the next action potential will cause increased calcium release, resulting in augmented contraction. It has been found that SERCA protein and activity are diminished in heart failure, and replenishing this protein using gene therapy is a current therapeutic goal. Animal experiments have been successful, and a human clinical trial is under way.

LINKS BETWEEN β-ADRENERGIC SIGNALING AND CALCIUM REGULATION

As noted above, β-adrenergic blockade has emerged as successful conventional therapy for heart failure. Why this should be so has elicited considerable interest. In a canine model of myocardial infarction, upregulation of previously down-regulated β-receptors in response to β-blockade has been reported.[7] One concept has elicited considerable interest as well

as controversy. This involves the consequences of altered ryanodine receptor function and SR calcium loss. Studies have described increased ryanodine receptor open probability in isolated preparations and increased calcium loss from SR vesicles isolated from failing hearts. These findings point to a possible common mechanism underlying alterations of systolic and diastolic function seen in heart failure. The underlying hypothesis is that hyperphosphorylation of the L-type calcium channel, the ryanodine receptor and the SERCA/phospholamban complex by PKA and CamKII may lead to chronic calcium loss. Calcium channel hyperphosphorylation can also result in increased calcium current that predisposes to arrhythmias. Excess phosphorylation in the SR complex can result in depletion of SR calcium stores, causing impaired cytosolic calcium transients resulting in systolic and diastolic dysfunction. Thus, inhibition of excess β-adrenergic drive would be expected to reduce these responses and improve cardiac function, which indeed appears to be the case as documented by randomized, controlled clinical trials. As CamKII is upregulated both in hypertrophy and in heart failure, small molecule inhibitors of CamKII are being developed but to date remain at the preclinical stage.

Calcium is also involved in myofilament function via a calcium-dependent ATPase. It is required for ATP generation by mitochondria, which is the source of the ATP hydrolyzed by SERCA, sodium/potassium ATPase, as well as by myofilament ATPase. Thus, augmented or reduced mitochondrial generation of ATP under normal and pathological circumstances is dependent on calcium availability, and the relation between calcium flux and ATP generation is critical for fundamental processes such as contraction, relaxation and electrical activity.

The localization of mitochondria near calcium release sites on the SR places these organelles in position to accumulate calcium, thereby regulating the level of calcium in the cytosol. Conversely, mitochondria can prevent SR calcium depletion by recycling this ion to the SR. Mitochondrial calcium uptake is also necessary for dehydrogenase activation in the mitochondrial matrix which regulates the NADH/NAD⁺ ratio. The role of calcium in oxidative phosphorylation and the production of ATP in the mitochondria are exquisitely balanced with the energy required for myocyte crossbridge cycling that is fueled by the hydrolysis of MgATP and regulated by calcium.[8,9] Thus, dysregulation of mitochondrial calcium can contribute to cell demise under pathophysiological conditions.

MITOCHONDRIA

Cardiac myocytes are richly endowed with mitochondria which, as noted, supply ATP which in turn provides energy to drive contraction of the heart. Mitochondria have two membranes: an outer membrane permeable to molecules of 10 kilodaltons or less and an inner membrane permeable only to oxygen, carbon dioxide and water. The inner membrane, which is layered and invaginated, forms cristae, thereby markedly increases its surface area. This membrane is home to the complexes of the electron transport chain (ETC), the ATP synthase complex, and transport proteins (Fig. 1). The space between the two membranes (intermembrane space) has an important role in the mitochondrion's

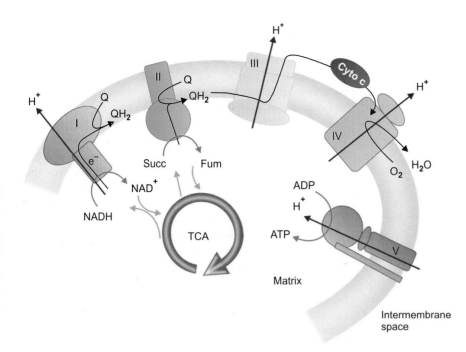

FIGURE 1: Electron transport chain and generation of ATP within the mitochondria. The Krebs (TCA) cycle takes place within the mitochondrial matrix. The cycle results in complete oxidation of the carbon atoms of the acetyl groups from acetyl-CoA. The net result of one turn of the cycle is the production of three molecules of NADH, 1 GTP and 1 FADH$_2$, and release of two molecules of CO$_2$. NADH generated from the cycle is oxidized by complex I (NADH:ubiquinone oxidoreductase), resulting in regeneration of NAD$^+$ needed as a cofactor for various steps of the cycle. Membrane-bound Complexes I, III and IV of the respiratory chain generate the proton gradient used by complex V (ATP synthase) to generate ATP. Complex II (succinate:ubiquinone oxidoreductase) is the only membrane-bound component of the TCA cycle. (Abbreviations: NAD$^+$: Nicotine adenine dinucleotide; NADH: Reduced nicotine adenine dinucleotide; Succ: Succinate; Fum: Fumarate; Q: Ubiquinone oxidoreductase; QH$_2$: Reduced ubiquinone oxidoreductase; e$^-$: Electrons; Cyto c: Cytochrome C; ATP: Adenosine triphosphate; ADP: Adenosine diphosphate)

raison d'etre which is the process of oxidative phosphorylation resulting in the generation of ATP. The inner membrane surrounds another compartment called the matrix which contains the enzymes responsible for citric acid (Krebs) cycle reactions. The folded cristae provide both a large surface area and intimate contact with the matrix, so that matrix components can rapidly diffuse to inner membrane complexes.

It should be noted that the only Krebs cycle reaction that occurs in the inner membrane itself is the oxidation of succinate to fumarate catalyzed by succinate dehydrogenase. This succinate dehydrogenase complex, which is composed of the enzyme, succinate and the energy carrier flavin adenine dinucleotide (FAD), is also called complex II of the ETC. This system accepts energy from carriers in the matrix and stores it in a form that can be used to phosphorylate ADP. Two carriers donate free energy to the ETC. These are nicotine adenine dinucleotide (NAD) and FAD. Reduced NAD carries energy to complex I (NADH-coenzyme Q reductase), while as noted above FAD is part of complex II.

NADH binds to a prosthetic group on complex I called flavin mononucleotide (FMN) and is reoxidized to NAD, which acts as an energy shuttle via recycling. FMN receives the resulting hydrogen from NADH and two electrons; it also garners a proton from the matrix and passes the electrons to iron-sulfur clusters that are part of the complex and forces two protons into the intermembrane space. Electrons pass to a carrier located in the membrane (Coenzyme Q) and are passed to complex III, which is associated with a further hydrogen translocation event. The next step in the pathway is cytochrome C and then further on to complex IV (cytochrome oxidase), where more protons are translocated. It is at this site that oxygen binds along with protons. Using the remaining pair of electrons and free energy, oxygen is reduced to water. This last step is diatomic, requiring two electron pairs and two cytochorme oxidase complexes. Thus, oxygen serves as an electron acceptor so that electron

transport can operate continuously. From succinate, there is a similar pathway, but protons are not translocated at complex II.

What is the purpose of this complicated schema? It is to drive the activity of ATP synthase (complex V) which is dependent on the proton (chemiosmotic) gradient created by the ETC between the matrix and the intermembrane space. ATP forms spontaneously in the presence of ATP synthase, but the chemiosmotic gradient is necessary to cause the release of bound ATP, so that the cycle can continue and ATP can be continuously generated. When there is a threat that the gradient will be dissipated by the need for more ATP, electron transport is increased so that the gradient is maintained. As oxygen is the ultimate electron acceptor, the process of ATP generation is termed oxidative phosphorylation. All of the above reactions are summarized schematically in Figure 1. Much of mitochondrial pathophysiology revolves around the inability to maintain the chemiosmotic gradient and the consequences of this failure.

For mitochondria to maintain this proton-mediated pH gradient and the resulting membrane potential ($\Delta\psi_m$) necessary to drive oxidative phosphorylation, the inner mitochondrial membrane must remain impermeable to all, but a few ions and metabolites for which specific transport mechanisms have evolved. It has been hypothesized that water and restricted metabolites can pass through the inner membrane via a "pore", also called the permeability transition pore. The physical characterization of this permeability barrier remains controversial. Nevertheless, persistent opening of this barrier under oxidative stress causes collapse of the proton gradient and $\Delta\psi_m$ across the inner mitochondrial membrane, resulting in uncoupling of oxidative phosphorylation and initiation of a series of biochemical changes which lead to cell death.

As a normal byproduct of the electron transfer activity described above, mitochondria generate reactive oxygen species (ROS). The primary sources are complexes I and III. Thus, somewhere between 0.2–2% of molecular oxygen consumed by mitochondria is converted to superoxide. Excess superoxide is toxic to the mitochondria, so its generation is kept in check by antioxidant enzymes located in the mitochondria, including manganese superoxide dismutase (MnSOD), catalase and glutathione peroxidase. MnSOD dismutes superoxide to hydrogen peroxide, which is converted to water by catalase and glutathione peroxidase. During oxidative stress these cardioprotective enzymes are overwhelmed and excess ROS are generated.

CARDIAC HYPERTROPHY

Physiologic cardiac muscle hypertrophy is a normal response to repetitive exercise. When hypertrophy occurs in disease states it is termed pathologic. Hypertrophy may be concentric, due to pressure overload (hypertension, aortic stenosis), or eccentric due to volume overload (mitral or aortic insufficiency, dilated cardiomyopathy). In some instances the cause is genetic and numerous mutations in cardiac muscle proteins, especially in the β-myosin heavy chain gene, have been found in humans. These are often familial, but how these mutations lead to hypertrophy remain largely mysterious.

Regardless of how hypertrophy is initiated, certain characteristic responses have been identified. These include reactivation of a fetal gene program, especially of β-myosin heavy chain and natriuretic peptides. The re-expression of β-myosin heavy chain is especially prominent in rodent models of hypertrophy, where the α-isoform predominates. However, in humans 90% of the myosin heavy chain pool consists of the β-isoform. Thus the isoform switch in humans is of problematic importance. Natriuretic peptide hormones are expressed in the atria and ventricles. The increase in these peptides, which in experimental settings inhibit the hypertrophic response via activation of cyclic guanosine monophosphate (cGMP), also serve as markers for heart failure. One postulated mechanism for the mechanism of cGMP is via cGMP-dependent protein kinase which inhibits L-type calcium channels, thus reducing calcium transient amplitude. This could result in inhibition of calcineurin-mediated activation of nuclear factor of activated T cells (NFAT), a nuclear transcription factor that is obligatory for hypertrophy. However, the counter-regulatory effect of natriuretic peptides is insufficient to inhibit the progression of hypertrophy in humans.

As the result of extensive experimental studies, especially employing genetically altered mice, numerous other pathways have been implicated in the pathogenesis of cardiac muscle hypertrophy.[10,11] Among these mediators of hypertrophy are pathways stimulated by norepinephrine, angiotensin II, the IL-6 family of cytokines, MAP kinases, Janus kinases (JAKs) and Cam kinases. One well-established mechanism of hypertrophy in rodent models is via the heterotrimeric G-protein Gq. Activation of Gq by norepinephrine, angiotensin II or endothelin results in PKC and inositol trisphosphate-mediated calcium release due to activation of phospholipase Cβ. As noted above, calcium release activates the protein phosphatase calcineurin and its target NFAT, which in cooperation with the cardiac-restricted zinc finger transcription factor GATA4 is a critical nuclear mediator of pathologic hypertrophy. It should be noted

that the calcineurin-NFAT pathway can be activated by CamKII and inhibited by FOXO-3, a member of the Forkhead/winged helix family of transcription factors, which contain a conserved DNA binding domain called the Forkhead box (Fox). Norepinephrine and angiotensin II also activate α$_1$-adrenergic and angiotensin receptors, respectively. These are linked to Gq and subsequently to activation of extracellular signal-regulated kinases (ERKs). The latter then activate the protein kinase mammalian target of rapamycin (mTOR) which regulates protein translation and ultimately, hypertrophy. Another pathway that negatively regulates hypertrophy is mediated by glycogen synthase kinase-3β (GSK-3β).[12]

A number of other regulators of cardiac hypertrophy have also been experimentally determined. Among these are microRNAs, such as miR199a,[13] PKCβ[14] and histone acetylation/deacetylation. It has been found that class II histone deacetylases (HDACs) associate with the MEF2 transcription factor, among others, to maintain normal cardiac size and function. Stress signals result in the phosphorylation of class II HDACs and their export from the nucleus to the cytoplasm resulting in activation of genes involved in cardiac growth.[15] Thus, HDAC knockout mice develop massive cardiac hypertrophy in response to stress stimuli.[12] Sirtuins are histone deacetylases that have been implicated in aging, resistance to oxidative stress and blockade of hypertrophy in the heart.[16-18] Another process that may contribute to hypertrophy is autophagy, which is a complex process of cellular degradation that is initiated in response to nutrient limitation, cellular stress, ROS or accumulation of protein aggregates of damaged organelles.[19]

Cardiac fibroblasts are the most numerous cell types in the heart and contribute to the regulation of cardiac hypertrophy via paracrine mechanisms. Prominent among the factors involved in this molecular crosstalk that result in cardiomyocyte hypertrophy are TGFβ1, fibroblast growth factor 2 and members of the IL-6 cytokine family.[20] Agonists that stimulate fibroblasts to release these mediators are angiotensin II and norepinephrine. All of these interactions become more prominent during stress conditions such as pressure overload and left ventricular remodeling. A recently discovered member of the IL-1 family, interleukin-33, represents a novel paracrine signaling system that is antihypertrophic and antifibrotic.[20]

α$_1$-ADRENERGIC RECEPTORS AND HYPERTROPHY

Evidence from rodent studies has indicated that stimulation of α$_1$-adrenergic receptors causes cardiac myocyte hypertrophy and augments cardiac contractility. Such stimulation is also cardioprotective. In contrast to β-adrenergic receptors, which are downregulated by chronic agonist exposure, α-adrenergic receptors do not downregulate. Recent studies in humans have confirmed that α-adrenergic receptors, predominately the α$_{1A}$ and α$_{1B}$ subtypes, are present in human myocardium. In failing hearts, these receptors were not downregulated, similar to findings in rodent models of heart failure.[21] In right ventricular trabeculae from normal mouse hearts α-adrenergic stimulation produced a negative inotropic response, but this response was reversed in trabeculae from failing hearts. These findings were attributed in part to increased myofilament calcium sensitivity caused by a more abundant smooth muscle isoform of myosin light chain kinase.[22] In contrast, α_1-mediated inotropic responses did not differ between normal and failing left ventricles. Both smooth muscle myosin light chain kinase mRNA protein levels were increased in right ventricles from failing human hearts. The risk of treating heart failure with an α-adrenergic antagonist was evident in a landmark primary prevention hypertension trial in which the α_1-adrenergic antagonist doxazosin was stopped early due to lack of any benefit for the primary outcome (fatal coronary heart disease or nonfatal myocardial infarction combined) and a signal suggesting potential harm in one of the secondary outcomes (heart failure).[23] It should be noted that the cardiovascular risk of using α-adrenergic blockers in patients with prostate enlargement has never been evaluated in a randomized, controlled clinical trial.

As noted above, myocardial hypertrophy is a well-described response to pressure-overload states. Of these conditions, the most prevalent is systemic arterial hypertension. Patients with hypertension who develop left ventricular hypertrophy have an increased risk of developing cardiovascular complications, including heart failure, atrial fibrillation and sudden cardiac death. Effective treatment of hypertension has long been known to result in regression of left ventricular hypertrophy. Early trials in humans demonstrated that antihypertensive therapy resulted in a decrease in left ventricular mass, and that patients who did show such a decrease also had improvements in measures of diastolic filling.[24] While multiple classes of medications have been studied, and for the most part all seem to be effective, there is evidence of a differential effect on left ventricular mass. Meta-analyses of randomized trials of the effects of antihypertensive agents on left ventricular mass showed that the reduction in hypertrophy was greatest with angiotensin II receptor antagonists (13% of patients showing a reduction in left ventricular mass index), followed closely by calcium channel blockers (11% of patients) and ACE inhibitors (10% of patients); beta-blockers seemed to be consistently less effective in this regard (6% of patients).[25,26]

CONGESTIVE HEART FAILURE

As noted above patients with persistent and progressive volume or pressure overload exhibit left ventricular hypertrophy and are at risk for congestive heart failure (CHF). Other patients suffer a myocardial infarction and develop compensatory left ventricular hypertrophy and dilatation which leads to CHF. Heart failure is the result of macrostructural changes collectively called remodeling. Other patients with cardiomyopathy due to various causes (e.g. hypertension, alcohol, myocarditis, diabetes, peripartum, amyloid) also develop CHF. For patients with valvular heart disease, effective treatment consists in valve replacement. For many patients with coronary heart disease revascularization is effective, but a minority of these individuals exhibit progressive CHF. Regardless of the cause, CHF which progresses to class IV and is refractory to medical therapy is one indication for cardiac transplantation. Due to the relative paucity of available hearts, many patients are placed on a waiting list. In the meantime, an increasing number are being treated with devices that augment their cardiac output, so-called left ventricular assist devices (LVADs). The use of LVADs has provided a platform to examine changes in myocardial structure

and function brought about by chronic left ventricular unloading. Biopsy material and larger portions of hearts removed at the time of transplantation have been studied. In a few instances, the LVAD evolved to "destination therapy", i.e. was removed because of persistent recovery, but such instances are rare. In most cases, LVADs have been installed as a "bridge" to transplant.

The mechanism by which left ventricular hypertrophy and/or dilatation evolves into CHF is not clear. By looking through the large end of the LVAD "telescope" it is possible to study "reverse remodeling" and compare changes associated with CHF before treatment and the structural, molecular and biochemical alterations produced by this therapy.[27] Such studies in humans have revealed that LVAD treatment reduces cardiac pressure and volume overload. This leads to diminished wall tension and lessened myocardial oxygen demand thereby reducing the ischemic burden in patients with coronary artery obstruction. Hypertrophy regresses as evidenced by reduced echocardiographic left ventricular wall thickness.

The effect of LVAD support on improving distorted ventricular geometry has been well-described, and many LVAD-supported hearts show improvement in LV chamber dilatation and LV mass. Analysis of cardiac myocytes obtained at the time of cardiac transplantation has demonstrated that long-term LVAD support results in reductions in myocyte volume, length, width and cell length-to-thickness ratio, compared with unsupported hearts.[28] These observations suggest that favorable effects of the LVAD on the failing heart result at least in part from regression of hypertrophy at the cellular level. In patients with nonischemic cardiomyopathy, LVADs have shown promise in reversing clinical heart failure, allowing for later explantation of the device as described above.[29] Cardiac myocytes taken from LVAD-supported hearts at the time of transplant have subsequently been compared with those from hearts that recovered sufficiently to allow LVAD explantation.[30] Both groups showed a decrease in myocyte size, but only the recovery group showed improvements in indices of SR calcium handling. Thus, although LVAD support seems to consistently lead to regression of cellular hypertrophy, this is not necessarily associated with clinical recovery.

However, changes in fibrosis have not been consistently reported as a result of LVAD treatment. Similarly, changes in matrix metalloproteinases (MMPs), especially MMP-9, have been variable, while reductions in tissue inhibitors of metalloproteinases (TIMP-1 and TIMP-3) have been observed. Regardless of these variable alterations, total collagen content remains unchanged. Other ventricular properties that do not regress to normal during LVAD support include increased tissue angiotensin levels, myocardial stiffening and fetal gene expression.[31,32]

As noted above, heart failure causes β_1-adrenoceptor downregulation without a change in β_2-receptor density. However, the latter are functionally uncoupled. Chronic LVAD unloading reverses these changes and restores a normal inotropic response to the nonselective β-adrenergic receptor agonist isoproterenol. LVAD treatment also increases the gene expression and protein level of SERCA-2, restores the force-frequency relation of isolated trabeculae and normalizes the magnitude and time course of the intracellular calcium transient. LVAD support returns natriuretic peptides and their signaling to normal. It also augments antiapoptotic signaling pathways and negatively regulates NF-κB which is responsible for activation of several factors contributing to the pathogenesis of CHF, such as interleukin-6, TNFα and Bcl-x$_L$.[27]

Additional understanding of the mechanism of evolution of CHF has been provided by experiments involving G-protein receptor kinase (β-arrestin) mentioned above. It is well-recognized that β$_1$-adrenergic receptors signal through a G-protein-mediated pathway that can be harmful under-conditions of chronic catecholamine stimulation as occurs in CHF.[33] Recent data indicate that β$_1$-receptors can also activate epidermal growth factor receptors in a β-arrestin dependent process called transactivation, which confers cardioprotection in response to a chronic increase in catecholamines.[34] Additionally it has been found that GRK-2 is upregulated in rats with chronic CHF due to myocardial infarction leading to enhanced catecholamine release via desensitization/down-regulation of the chromaffin cell α$_2$-adrenergic receptors that normally inhibit catecholamine secretion.[35] Experiments using gene-targeting of adrenal GRK-2 decreased circulating catecholamines and led to improved cardiac function and β-adrenergic reserve in postmyocardial infarction heart failure in a mouse model.[36] In rats with postinfarction heart failure, exercise training lowered GRK-2 and reduced sympathetic overdrive.[37] Thus, GRK-2 is a potential therapeutic target for the treatment of chronic CHF.

MICRO-RNAs

Micro-RNAs (miRs) are small, noncoding RNAs. They are short ribonucleic acid molecules, on average only 22 nucleotides in length and function as post-transcriptional regulators that bind to complementary sequences in the three prime untranslated regions of target messenger RNA transcripts, usually resulting in gene silencing. The human genome encodes over 1,000 miRNAs, which may target more than half of mammalian genes. Each miRNA may repress hundreds of mRNAs. Specific miRs have been implicated in the regulation of cardiac hypertrophy and ischemia/reperfusion injury.[38] Both antagonists of miRs, called antagomiRs, and miR mimetics, called agomiRs, have been synthesized to inhibit and enhance miR actions, respectively. The biology of miRs is an exciting new area which is likely to have important therapeutic implications.

ISCHEMIA/REPERFUSION INJURY

As coronary blood flow is abruptly decreased, cardiac myocytes are subjected to progressive oxygen deprivation. This results in disruption of the mitochondrial membrane gradient ($\Delta\psi_m$) described above, which is required to maintain oxidative phosphorylation, and eventually results in cessation of this process. Absent generation of sufficient ATP, the contractile elements are no longer able to function. Further injury occurs as a result of the decline in pH associated with increased lactate levels. As hydrogen ion concentration increases, the sodium/hydrogen antiporter is activated in an attempt to restore pH levels. This results in an increase in sodium levels and

dysfunction of the sodium/calcium exchanger that results in increased intracellular calcium, causing calcium overload. As a result degradative enzymes, such as calpain, are activated. Simultaneous with these events, ROS generation from complexes I and III of the ETC increases and the mitochondrial transition barrier opens leading to release of cytochrome C. The latter associates with other proteins including caspase-9 to form a macromolelcular complex called the apoptosome, which in turn activates the effector, caspase-3. Caspases inactivate crucial cellular targets including essential subunits in complex 1. A major defense against ROS-induced damage, glutathione, is oxidized. This coincides with cleavage of BID, a proapoptotic protein, which transduces signals from the cytosol to the mitochondria, leading to caspase activation.

During ischemia/reperfusion injury, several other proapoptotic factors that have nuclear effects are also released from mitochondria, including Smac/Diablo and apoptosis inducing factor (AIF), among others. Release of AIF into the cytosol is followed by rapid translocation to the nucleus where it facilitates chromatin condensation and DNA fragmentation. Excessive oxidative stress also results in the activation of poly (ADP-ribose) polymerase 1 (PARP-1). Protein poly (ADP-ribosylation) is crucial for genomic integrity and cell survival and is catalyzed by PARP-1, which is a nuclear enzyme that functions as a DNA damage sensor and signaling molecule. PARP-1 binds to DNA strand breaks and participates in DNA repair processes. It utilizes NAD$^+$ to form poly (ADP-ribose) (PAR) polymers on specific acceptor proteins. Under conditions of moderate oxidative stress, PARP-1 activation facilitates DNA repair. However, excessive PARP-1 activation depletes the intracellular pool of its substrate NAD$^+$, thereby impairing glycolysis, decoupling the Krebs cycle and mitochondrial electron transport (Fig. 1), and eventually causing ATP depletion and consequent cell dysfunction and death by necrosis.

MECHANISMS OF CARDIOPROTECTION

Concurrent with an understanding of the mechanisms of cell death, both necrotic and apoptotic, described above, there has been an intensive effort to determine how the heart can be protected from injury. It would be desirable to have available approaches that can protect vulnerable tissue before damage occurs due to oxidative stress, such as frequently happens during cardiac or vascular surgery. Such protection before, during or immediately after catheter interventions would also be welcome. One approach that has proved successful is periprocedural β-blockade, which reduces myocardial oxygen demand by lowering heart rate and blood pressure. Another approach, still largely experimental, but beginning to have clinical application, is the concept of myocardial conditioning. Just as the well-trained athlete has learned to "warm-up" before a foot race or other strenuous activity, the heart (and other organs) can be "preconditioned". This phenomenon was first described by Murry et al. in 1986.[39] In a canine model, it was found that several brief periods of ischemia/reperfusion preceding a much more prolonged bout of ischemia/reperfusion could substantially reduce myocardial injury. This intervention was termed ischemic preconditioning. Its effect lasts for 1–3 hours. A delayed effect of preconditioning, occurring 24–72 hours following acute ischemic preconditioning, called the second window of protection, has been recognized.[40] Subsequently, in 2003, an identical beneficial effect occurred when the conditioning stimulus was applied at the onset of reperfusion and has been called postconditioning.[41]

The mechanisms of these responses have been extensively studied and a variety of pathways have been elucidated, presumably many or all of them having evolved as redundant responses to cellular injury. A number of endogenous mediators that transduce signals via G-protein coupled receptors have been found to produce cardioprotection, including adenosine, brady-kinin, opioids[42] and sphingosine 1-phosphate.[43] One such pathway activated by these endogenous mediators is called the reperfusion injury salvage kinase (RISK) pathway[44] and involves phosphorylation and activation of prosurvival kinases such as Erk 1/2, PI-3 kinase/Akt and GSK-3β (Fig. 2). Another separate but complementary pathway has been called the survivor activating factor enhancement (SAFE) pathway[45] (Fig. 2). This mechanism is activated by liganding of cytokine receptors on the cell surface thereby conveying signals to the nucleus via the JAK-STAT pathway, a process that rapidly results in activation of various cardioprotective effectors such as manganese superoxide dismutase, iNOS and COX-2.[46] The activation of both these enzymes, the former resulting in the production of NO, has been implicated as mechanisms of the second window of protection described above.

A recently described third pathway is activation of the enzyme sphingosine kinase which phosphorylates endogenous sphingosine to produce the second messenger sphingosine 1-phosphate (S1P). S1P is exported from the cell and ligands cognate cell surface receptors in an autocrine or paracrine manner to couple with the guanine nucleotide inhibitory protein (Gi) to initiate cardioprotection via PI3-K/Akt, Erk1/2 and GSK-3β as described above.[43,47] The sphingolipid pathway is also illustrated in Figure 2.

The importance of the sphingosine kinase/S1P axis in cardioprotection is further supported by measurements of S1P and sphingosine kinase activity in preconditioned hearts[48] and by abolition of the cardioprotective effect of ischemic precondi-tioning in sphingosine kinase isoform 1 knockout hearts.[49] Of note is that sphingosine, which has previously thought to be deleterious to the heart, is cardioprotective in low concentrations and utilizes cyclic nucleotide-dependent pathways that are independent of G-protein coupled receptors[50] (Fig. 2). Recent evidence indicates that endogenous cardioprotectants such as adenosine and S1P are released from cells via pannexin-I/P_2X_7 purinergic receptor channels[51] (Fig. 2). Volatile anesthetics are also preconditioning agents that activate sphingosine kinase and result in release of cytoprotective S1P.[52]

As summarized in Figure 2, all of the molecular prosurvival pathways described above converge on mitochondria. An alternative or parallel mechanism advanced by Garlid et al.[53] is that occupied receptors for the agonists described above migrate to caveolae, where signaling enzymes are scaffolded into signalosomes that bud off the plasma membrane and then continue their migration to mitochondria. Regardless of the mechanism involved, an initial mitochondrial event in this prosurvival cascade is opening of mitochondrial inner membrane K_{ATP} channels, although not all subscribe to this hypothesis.[54]

Nevertheless, the following events occur after ischemic or pharmacologic preconditioning are: increased mitochondrial potassium uptake, matrix alkalinization, volume increase, ROS production, especially by complex I and mitochondrial permeability transition inhibition. The latter occurs via ROS-mediated activation of PKCε that resides in mitochondria and/or has been translocated to these organelles.[53] Thus, increased low-level ROS generation activated by either ischemic and/or pharmacologic preconditioning enhances myocardial cell survival. For each intervention, or their combination, there is a ROS threshold beyond which the conditioning stimulus is ineffective and excess ROS release results in cell necrosis. In this connection, it has been suggested that another response to preconditioning in ischemia/reperfusion is upregulation of autophagy.[19] Under these conditions acutely enhanced autophagy would result in removal of unstable mitochondria thereby lowering cellular ROS production and reducing the likelihood of mPTP opening. Thus, Sirt 1, which upregulates autophagy through deacetylation of several autophagy proteins, has been linked to cardioprotection.[19]

Of special note is the translocation of PKCε to the mitochondria. Previous work had proposed a number of cytoprotective mechanisms resulting from this translocation, including inhibition of mitochondrial permeability transition, opening of K_{ATP} channels, and phosphorylation of cytochrome oxidase subunit IV. Recently, a new mitochondrial substrate for PKCε, aldehyde dehydrogenase 2, has been described.[55] The function of this enzyme is to detoxify toxic aldehydes that are produced by lipid peroxidation during ischemia/reperfusion, such as the reactive 4-hydroxy-2-nonenal and its adducts. There is a strong inverse correlation between aldehyde dehydrogenase 2 and infarct size. A small molecule activator of aldehyde dehydrogenase 2 had a similar effect[55] (Fig. 3) and also conferred cardioprotection in PKCε knockout mice.[56]

Of interest, it has recently been reported in mouse cardiac myocytes that connexin 43 residing in or transported to mitochondria is a cytoprotective mediator of signal transduction by stimulating mitochondrial K_{ATP} channel opening.[57] Another recently described protector of mitochondrial integrity downstream of JAK/STAT and Akt signaling is Pim kinase-1.[58] The prosurvival Pim kinases are a family of three vertebrate protein serine/threonine kinases (Pim-1, -2 and -3) belonging to the CaMK (calmodulin-dependent protein kinase-related) group. Pim-1 translocates to mitochondria in response to ischemia/reperfusion injury and enhances expression of antiapoptoic Bcl-x_L and Bcl-2. It also preserves Δψ_m during oxidative stress, attenuates mitochondrial swelling in response to calcium overload and reduces cytochrome C release in response to a proapoptotic challenge.[58]

All of the interventions described above substantially, but not completely, prevent many of the harmful effects of oxidative stress, such as mitochondrial permeability transition, cytochrome C release, calcium overload and depression of oxidative phos-phorylation. To achieve maximal cardioprotection, a combina-tion of these approaches requires rigorous testing in animal models and ultimately in patients.

Postconditioning shares many if not all of the mechanisms attributed to preconditioning and holds promise to be an effective clinical strategy. Experimentally, using a "cocktail" approach,

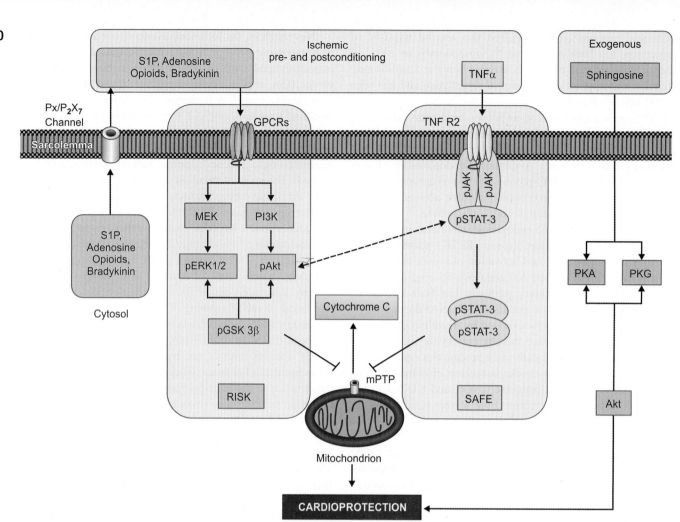

FIGURE 2: Pathways leading to cardioprotection following ischemic pre- and postconditioning. Pre- and postconditioning lead to intracellular generation of agonists such as S1P, adenosine, opioids and bradykinin which are exported across the sarcolemma via pannexin/P$_2$X$_7$ channels. Once these molecules have gained access to the outer surface of the sarcolemma they activate G-protein coupled receptors in an autocrine or paracrine fashion to generate the signals shown. Similarly, low concentrations of TNFα can be generated intracellularly and released or given exogenously to activate the pathway shown. Low dose exogenous sphingosine also has cardioprotective effects. See text for details. (Abbreviations: Px/P$_2$X$_7$: Pannexin/purinergic$_2$X$_7$ channels; S1P: Sphingosine 1-phosphate; GPCRs: G-protein coupled receptors; TNFα: Tumor necrosis factor alpha; TNF R2: Tumor necrosis factor receptor 2; MEK: Mitogen-activated protein kinase 1; pERK: Phosphorylated extracellular signal-related kinase; PI3K: Phosphoinositide 3-kinase; pAkt: Phosphorylated serine-threonine kinase also known as protein kinase B; pGSK 3β: Phosphorylated glycogen synthase kinase 3-beta; mPTP: Mitochondrial transition "pore"; pJAK: Phosphorylated Janus kinase; pSTAT: Phosphorylated signal transducer and activator of transcription; PKA: Protein kinase A; PKG: Protein kinase G; RISK: Reperfusion injury salvage kinase pathway; SAFE: Survivor activating factor enhancement pathway)

the combination of ischemic postconditioning, and infusion of both sphingosine and sphingosine 1-phosphate, salvaged rat myocardium subjected to as much as 90 min of global ischemia.[59] Postconditioning can be applied acutely in patients undergoing percutaneous coronary interventions. In over 400 patients in 8 studies, favorable results using a variety of short-term outcome measures have been reported.[42] The use of pharmacologic therapy for postconditioning has had mixed results, but the combination approach described above, which mimics the endogenous release of multiple effectors, has never been reported in humans.

AGING

Cardiac aging has been examined largely in rodent models. These studies reveal impairment of most of the mechanisms

regulating cardiac myocyte function which is described above. Beta-adrenergic responses are diminished, including chronotropic and contractile responses. Coupling of β-adrenoceptors to the guanine nucleotide regulatory protein Gs is reduced and less cAMP is generated for a given stimulus. Decreased chronotropic responses to exercise are another feature of aged myocardium. With advancing age, SERCA-2 protein is reduced in rats, but not in mice. As noted above SERCA function is impaired in CHF in humans. During aging, the calcium sequestering properties of myocyte SERCA-2 protein are reduced, perhaps in part because of defective PKA-dependent phosphorylation of phospholamban. Calcium release (ryanodine) channels are also dysfunctional, possibly because of decreased phosphorylation by PKA and CaMK. This results in increased SR calcium leak that may contribute to both systolic and diastolic dysfunction with age. It is of considerable interest that

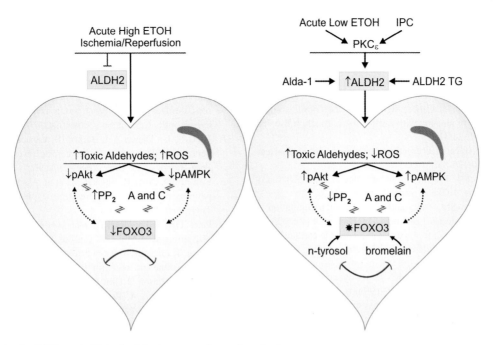

FIGURE 3: New roles for PKCε and aldehyde dehydrogenase in cardioprotection.

Depicted in the left panel is the "sad" heart, which is acutely depressed by ischemia/reperfusion injury. Toxic aldehydes and reactive oxygen species are produced that among other effects; reduce prosurvival signals such as those transduced by Akt, AMP-activated protein kinase and FOX3. In the "happy" heart on the right, these adverse responses can be prevented by overexpression of aldehyde dehydrogenase 2 or by a small molecule activator of this enzyme. During ischemic preconditioning PKCε is translocated to the mitochondria (or PKCε resident in the mitochondria is activated) and stimulates the activity of aldehyde dehydrogenase 2 in the mitochondria, which results in detoxification of toxic aldehydes. (Abbreviations: Alda-1: Small molecule activator of aldehyde dehydrogenase 2; ALDH2: Aldehyde dehydrogenase 2; FOX3: Forkhead transcription factor of the O subtype; IPC: Ischemic; pAkt: Phosphorylated prosurvival serine-threonine kinase also known as protein kinase B; pAMPK: Phosphorylated adenosine monophosphate kinase; PKCε: Protein kinase C epsilon; PP₂ A and C: Protein phosphatase A and C; ROS: Reactive oxygen species; TG: Transgenic)

in male nonfailing aged human hearts there is extensive myocyte loss and hypertrophy of the surviving myocytes.[60] In contrast, this is not the case in females. In rats, the activity of telomerase, which correlates with cell replication, was decreased in aging male myocytes, but increased in females.[61]

In mitochondria prepared from old rat hearts the majority of genes whose expression is altered are those coding for proteins involved in oxidative phosphorylation, substrate metabolism and the tricarboxylic acid cycle, and most of these are downregulated.[62] This results in reduced mitochondrial functional capacity as manifested by diminished complex I and V activities leading to diminished ATP synthesis. There is also a substantial loss of cardioprotection with aging as indicated by the inability of aged rat myocardium to undergo successful ischemic pre and postconditioning as well as pharmacologic preconditioning with a variety of agents.[63] Of note is that sphingosine protects both old and young hearts from ischemia/reperfusion injury and in hearts from 27-month-old rats sphingosine is superior to S1P and ischemic pre and post-conditioning.[64] As noted above, there has been considerable interest in sirtuins as regulators of aging, and the heart is no exception.[16]

Human studies are sparse. One of two studies in isolated right atrial appendages showed a negative response to IPC and two other studies in humans with variable outcome measurements could not document any effect of IPC in older patients (>65 years of age compared with younger patients). These results are consistent with diminished mitochondrial functional capacity. Experimentally, this loss of cardioprotection with aging can be reversed by caloric restriction and exercise in rodents, and in one retrospective analysis by exercise in humans.[65]

ACKNOWLEDGMENT

The authors thank Drs Elena Maklashina and Gary Cecchini for providing Figure 1 and Mr Norman Honbo for artwork on Figures 2 and 3.

REFERENCES

1. Rakesh K, Yoo BS, Kim I-M, et al. β-arrestin-biased agonism of the angiotensin receptor induced by mechanical stress. Science Signalling. 2010;3:ra46.
2. Port JD, Bristow MR. Altered beta-adrenergic receptor gene regulation and signaling in chronic heart failure. J Mol Cell Cardiol. 2001;33:887-905.
3. Liggett SB, Mialet-Perez J, Thaneemit-Chen S, et al. A polymorphism within a conserved β₁-adrenergic receptor motif alters cardiac function and β-blocker response in human heart failure. PNAS. 2006;103:11288-93.
4. Liggett SB, Mialet-Perez J, Thaneemit-Chen S, et al. An α₂C-adrenergic receptor polymorphism alters the norepinephrine-lowering effects and therapeutic response of the β-blocker bucindolol in chronic heart failure. Circ Heart Fail. 2010;3:21-8.
5. Nikolaev VO, Moshkov A, Lyon AR, et al. β₂-adrenergic receptor redistribution in heart failure changes cAMP compartmentation. Science. 2010;327:1653-7.

6. Bers DM. Calcium cycling and signaling in cardiac myocytes. Annu Rev Physiol. 2008;70:23-49.

7. Karliner JS, Stevens MB, Honbo N, et al. Effects of acute ischemia in the dog on myocardial blood flow, beta-receptors, and adenylate cyclase activity with and without chronic beta-blockade. J Clin Invest. 1989;83:474-81.

8. Balaban RS. The role of Ca(2+) signaling in the coordination of mitochondrial ATP production with cardiac work. Biochim Biophys Acta. 2009;1787:1334-41.

9. Maughan DW. Kinetics and energetics of the crossbridge cycle. Heart Fail Rev. 2005;10:175-85.

10. Dorn GW II, Force T. Protein kinase cascades in the regulation of cardiac hypertrophy. J Clin Invest. 2005;115: 527-37.

11. Barry SP, Davidson SM, Townsend PA. Molecular regulation of cardiac hypertophy. Internat J Biochem Cell Biol. 2008;40:2023-39.

12. Trivedi CM, Luo Y, Yin Z, et al. Hdac2 regulates the cardiac hypertrophic response by modulating Gsk3 beta activity. Nat Med. 2007;13:324-31.

13. Song X, Li Q, Lin L, et al. MicroRNAs are dynamically regulated in hypertrophic hearts, and miR-199a is essential for the maintenance of cell size in cardiomyocytes. J Cell Physiol. 2010;225:437-43.

14. Palaniyandi SS, Sun L, Ferreira JCB, et al. Protein kinase C in heart failure: a therapeutic target? Cardiovasc Res 2009;82:229-39.

15. Olsen EN, Backs J, McKinsey TA. Control of cardiac hypertrophy and heart failure by histone acetylation/deacetylation. Novartis Found Sympo. 2006;274:3-12.

16. Alcendor RR, Gao S, Zhai P, et al. Sirt1 regulates aging and resistance to oxidative stress in the heart. Circ Res. 2007;100:1512-21.

17. Sundaresan NR, Gupta M, Kim G, et al. Sirt3 blocks the cardiac hypertrophic response by augmenting Foxo3a-dependent antioxidant defense mechanisms in mice. J Clin Invest. 2009;119:2758-71.

18. Pillai VB, Sundaresan NR, Kim G, et al. Exogenous NAD blocks cardiac hypertrophic response via activation of the SIRT3-LKB1-AMP-activated kinase pathway. J Biol Chem. 2010;285:3133-44.

19. Gottlieb RA, Mentzer Jr. RM. Autophagy during cardiac stress: joys and frustrations of autophagy. Annu Rev Physiol. 2010;72:45-59.

20. Kakkar R, Lee RT. Intramyocardial fibroblast myocyte communication. Circ Res. 2010;106:47-57.

21. Jensen BC, Swigart PM, DeMarco T, et al. α_1-adrenergic receptor subtypes in nonfailing and failing human myocardium. Circ Heart Fail. 2009;2:654-63.

22. Wang GY, Yeh CC, Jensen BC, et al. Heart failure switches the RV alpha1-adrenergic inotropic response from negative to positive. Am J Physiol Heart Circ Physiol. 2010;298:H913-20.

23. ALLHAT Officers and Coordinators for the ALLHAT Collaborative Research Group. Major outcomes in high-risk hypertensive patients randomized to angiotensin-converting enzyme inhibitor or calcium channel blocker vs diuretic: the Antihypertensive and Lipid-Lowering Treatment to Prevent Heart Attack Trial (ALLHAT). JAMA. 2002;288:2981-97.

24. Schulman SP, Weiss JL, Becker LC, et al. The effects of antihypertensive therapy on left ventricular mass in elderly patients. New England Journal of Medicine. 1990;322:1350-6.

25. Schmieder RE, Martus P, Klingbeil A. Reversal of left ventricular hypertrophy in essential hypertension. A meta-analysis of randomized double-blind studie. JAMA. 1996;275:1507-13.

26. Klingbeil AU, Schneider M, Martus P, et al. A meta-analysis of the effects of treatment on left ventricular mass in essential hypertension. American Journal of Medicine. 2003;115:41-6.

27. Wohlschlaeger J, Schmitz KJ, Schmid C, et al. Reverse remodeling following insertion of left ventricular assist devices (LVAD): a review of the morphological and molecular changes. Cardiovasc Res. 2005;68:376-86.

28. Zafeiridis A, Jeevanandam V, Houser, SR, et al. Regression of cellular hypertrophy after left ventricular assist device support. Circulation. 1998;98:656-62.

29. Birks EJ, Tansley PD, Hardy J, et al. Left ventricular assist device and drug therapy for the reversal of heart failure. New England Journal of Medicine. 2006;355:1873-84.

30. Terracciano CM, Hardy J, Birks EJ, et al. Clinical recovery from end-stage heart failure using left-ventricular assist device and pharmacological therapy correlates with increased sarcoplasmic reticulum calcium content but not with regression of cellular hypertrophy. Circulation. 2004;109:2263-5.

31. Klotz S, Jan Danser AH, Burkoff D. Impact of left ventricular assist device (LVAD) support on the cardiac reverse remodeling process. Prog Biophys Mol Biol. 2008;97:479-96.

32. Lowes BD, Zolty R, Shjakar SF, et al. Assist devices fail to reverse patterns of fetal gene expression despite beta-blockers. J Heart Transplant. 2007;26:1170-6.

33. Patek OA, Tilley DG, Rockman HA. Physiologic and cardiac roles of β-arrestins. J Mol Cell Cardiol. 2009;46:300-8.

34. Noma T, Lemaire A, Naga Prasad SV, et al. Beta-arrestin-mediated beta$_1$-adrenergic receptor transactivation of the EGFR confers cardioprotection. J Clin Invest. 2007;117: 2445-58.

35. Lymperopoulos A, Rengo G, Funakoshi H, et al. Adrenal GRK2 upregulation mediates sympathetic overdrive in heart failure. Nat Med. 2007;13:315-23.

36. Lymperopoulos A, Rengo G, Gao E, et al. Reduction of sympathetic activity via adrenal-targeted GRK2 gene deletion attenuates heart failue progression and improves cardiac function after myocardial infarction. J Biol Chem. 2010;285:16378-86.

37. Rengo G, Leosco D, Zincarelli C, et al. Adrenal GRK2 lowering is an underlying mechanism for the beneficial sympathetic effects of exercise training in heart failure. Am J Physiol Heart Circ Physiol. 2010;298:H2032-8.

38. Small EM, Frost RJ, Olson EN. MicroRNAs add a new dimension to cardiovascular disease. Circulation. 2010;121: 1022-32.

39. Murry CE, Jennings RB, Reimer KA. Preconditioning with ischemia: a delay of lethal cell injury in ischemic myocardium. Circulation. 1986;74:1124-36.

40. Housenloy DJ, Yellon DM. The second window of preconditioning (SWOP). Where are we now? Cardiovasc Drugs Ther. 2010;24:235-54.

41. Zhao ZQ, Corvera JS, Halkos ME, et al. Inhibition of myocardial injury by ischemic postconditioning during reperfusion: comparison with ischemic preconditioning. Am J Physiol Heart Circ Physiol. 2003;285:H579-88.

42. Ovize M, Baxter GF, Di Lisa F, et al. Postconditioning and protection from reperfusion injury: where do we stand? Position paper from the working group of cellular biology of the heart of the European Society of Cardiology. Cardiovasc Res. 2010;87:406-23.

43. Vessey DA, Li L, Honbo N, et al. Sphingosine 1-phosphate is an important endogenous cardioprotectant released by ischemic pre- and postconditioning. Amer J Physiol Heart Circ Physiol. 2009;297:H1429-35.

44. Housenloy DJ, Yellon DM. New directions for protecting the heart against ischaemia-reperfusion injury: targeting the reperfusion injury salvage kinase (RISK)-pathway. Cadiovasc Res. 2004;61: 448-60.

45. Lacerda L, Somers S, Opie LH, et al. Ischaemic postconditioning protects against reperfusion injury via the SAFE pathway. Cardiovasc Res. 2009;84:201-8.

46. Barry SP, Townsend PA, Latchman DS, et al. Role of the JAK-STAT pathway in myocardial injury. Trends in Molecular Medicine. 2006;13:83-9.

47. Tao R, Zhang J, Vessey DA, et al. Deletion of the sphingosine kinase-1 gene influences cell fate during hypoxia and glucose deprivation in adult mouse cardiomyocytes. Cardiovasc Res. 2007;74:56-63.

48. Vessey DA, Kelley M, Li L, et al. Role of sphingosine kinase activity in protection of heart against ischemia reperfusion injury. Med Sci Monit. 2006;12:BR318-24.

49. Jin ZQ, Zhang J, Huang Y, et al. A sphingosine kinase 1 mutation sensitizes the myocardium to ischemia/reperfusion injury. Cardiovasc Res. 2007;76:41-50.

50. Vessey DA, Li L, Kelley M, et al. Sphingosine can pre and post-condition heart and utilizes a different mechanism from sphingosine 1-phosphate. J Biochem Mol Toxicol. 2008;22:113-8.

51. Vessey DA, Li L, Kelley M. Pannexin-I/P_2X_7 purinergic receptor channels mediate the release of cardioprotectants induced by ischemic pre- and postconditioning. J Cardiosvasc Pharmacol Ther. 20J0;15:190-5.

52. Kim M, Kim M, Park SW, et al. Isoflurane protects human kidney proximal tubule cells against necrosis via sphingosine kinase and sphingosine-1-phosphate generation. Am J Nephrol. 2010;31:353-62.

53. Garlid KD, Costa ADT, Qinlan CL, et al. Cardioprotective signaling to mitochondria. J Mol Cell Cardiol. 2009;46:858-66.

54. Halestrap AP, Clarke SJ, Khaliulin I. The role of mitochondria in protection of the heart by preconditioning. Biochim Biophys Acta. 2007;1767:1007-31.

55. Chen CH, Budas GR, Churchill EN, et al. Activation of aldehyde dehydrogenase-2 reduces ischemic damage to the heart. Science. 2008;321:1493-5.

56. Budas GR, Disatnik MH, Chen CH, et al. Activation of aldehyde dehydrogenase 2 (ALDH2) confers cardioprotection in protein kinase C epsilon (PKCε) knockout mice. J Mol Cell Cardiol. 2010;48:757-64.

57. Rottlaender D, Boengler K, Wolny M, et al. Connexin 43 acts as a cytoprotective mediator of signal transduction by stimulating mitochondrial K_{ATP} channels in mouse cardiomyocytes. J Clin Invest. 2010;120:1441-53.

58. Borillo GA, Mason M, Quijada P, et al. Pim-1 kinase protects mitochondrial integrity in cardiomyocytes. Circ Res. 2020;106:1265-74.

59. Vessey DA, Li L, Kelley M, et al. Combined sphingosine, S1P and ischemic postconditioning rescue the heart after protracted ischemia. Biochem Biophys Res Commun. 2008;375:425-9.

60. Janczewski AM, Lakatta EG. Modulation of sarcoplasmic reticulum Ca^{2+} cycling in systolic and diastolic heart failure associated with aging. Heart Fail Rev. 2010;15:431-45.

61. Leri A, Malhotra A, Liew CC, et al. Telomerase activity in rat cardiac myocytes is age and gender dependent. J Mol Cell Cardiol. 2000;32:385-90.

62. Preston CC, Oberlin AS, Holmuhamedov EL, et al. Aging-induced alterations in gene transcripts and functional activity of mitochondrial oxidative phosphorylation complexes in the heart. Mech Ageing Develop. 2008;129:304-12.

63. Boengler K, Schulz R, Heusch G. Loss of cardioprotection with ageing. Cardiovasc Res. 2009;83:247-61.

64. Vessey DA, Kelley M, Li l, et al. Sphingosine protects aging hearts from ischemia/reperfusion injury. Superiority to sphingosine 1-phosphate and ischemic pre- and post-conditioning. Oxidative Medicine and Cellular Longevity. 2009;2:146-51.

65. Abete P, Ferrara N, Cacciatore F, et al. High level of physical activity preserves the cardioprotective effect of preinfarction angina in elderly patients. J Am Coll Cardiol. 2001;38:1357-65.

Chapter 3

Coronary Circulation in Physiology and Pathology

Kanu Chatterjee

Chapter Outline

INTRODUCTION

Coronary circulation in physiologic and pathologic states is related to coronary vascular anatomy and factors that modulate coronary blood flow. Coronary blood flow changes in response to various coronary vascular intrinsic and extrinsic stimuli. The modulating and regulating mechanisms of coronary circulation, however, differ in different pathologic conditions.

CORONARY VASCULAR ANATOMY

The coronary vascular system consists of coronary arteries and veins. The epicardial coronary arteries are muscular arteries and serve as conduit vessels. The epicardial coronary arteries give rise to intramural branches that also contain smooth muscle cells. There are two types of branches that arise from these penetrating intramural arteries. The first type rapidly branches into an arterial network which provides blood flow to the outer two-thirds, approximately 60–70%, of the left ventricular myocardium; the second type courses to the endocardium and forms an arcade of anastomotic channels called the subendocardial plexus.[1] The endocardium and subendocardium, which constitute approximately 20–30% of the inner walls of the left ventricle, receive blood flow from the anastomotic arterial system. The intramyocardial arteries and the arterioles constitute the resistance vessels of the coronary circulation.

The arteriovenous and venovenous anastomotic channels form the cardiac venous system. The epicardial and myocardial veins usually run parallel to and accompany the coronary arteries. The larger veins form coronary sinus which drains into the right atrium. A substantial increase in right atrial pressure is associated with a similar increase in coronary sinus and intra-myocardial venous pressures which impedes myocardial venous drainage and may impair myocardial perfusion.

REGULATION OF CORONARY BLOOD FLOW

MYOCARDIAL OXYGEN DEMAND

Coronary blood flow and myocardial oxygen supply is primarily determined by myocardial oxygen demand. The major determinants of myocardial oxygen demand are summarized in Table 1. The major determinants of myocardial oxygen demand and oxygen consumption (MVO_2) are heart rate, contractility and wall stress.[2] The faster is the heart rate, the higher is the myocardial oxygen requirement. Increase in oxygen demand is not only due to increased frequency of contraction but also to increased contractility resulting from positive force-frequency relation. In the failing myocardium, however, the contractility decreases with increasing heart rate due to inverse force

TABLE 1

The major determinants of myocardial oxygen demand

The major determinants of myocardial oxygen demand:
• Heart rate
• Contractility
• Wall stress
• Ventricular pressure
• Ventricular volumes
• Ventricular wall thickness

frequency relation. The slower heart rate is associated with improved left ventricular perfusion due to longer perfusion time. Myocardial oxygen consumption is directly proportional to changes in contractility. During dobutamine infusion or exercise, MVO_2 increases due to increase in contractility.[3] The myocardial oxygen demand and MVO_2 are also directly proportional to wall stress. The wall stress is directly related to ventricular volume and systolic blood pressure, and is inversely related to wall thickness. The larger the ventricular volume, the higher the arterial pressure and thinner the ventricular wall, and higher is the wall stress which is associated with increased myocardial oxygen demand and MVO_2.

MYOCARDIAL OXYGEN SUPPLY

Myocardial oxygen supply is the product of coronary blood flow and myocardial oxygen extraction. Myocardial oxygen extraction is the difference in the coronary arterial—venous oxygen content. Even at basal metabolic demand, myocardial oxygen extraction is near maximum. Usually coronary sinus venous oxygen saturation at basal conditions is between 20% and 30%, corresponding to a partial arterial oxygen pressure (PaO_2) of about 20 mm Hg. Even at a very high and super-normal PaO_2, the dissolved arterial oxygen content increases only minimally. Thus, myocardial oxygen supply is primarily dependant on coronary blood flow. The factors that regulate coronary blood flow and myocardial oxygen supply and perfusion are summarized in Table 2. The perfusion pressure is the difference between aortic diastolic pressure and the coronary sinus venous pressure (right atrial pressure). However, it should be appreciated that left ventricular diastolic pressure and intramyocardial tissue pressure also offer resistance to forward coronary blood flow and myocardial perfusion. To maintain forward coronary blood flow, aortic diastolic pressure needs to be at least a few mm Hg higher than right atrial and left ventricular diastolic pressures. The transmyocardial pressure gradient is defined as the pressure difference between aortic diastolic pressure and left ventricular diastolic and coronary venous pressures. Myocardial perfusion is related to changes in transmyocardial perfusion pressure gradient. Transmyocardial pressure gradient may decrease either due to reduction in aortic diastolic pressure or due to an increase in left ventricular diastolic pressures. In many pathologic states, such as severe aortic stenosis, both hemodynamic abnormalities occur concurrently.

TABLE 2

The major determinants of coronary blood flow

- Perfusion pressure
- Epicardial coronary artery resistance
- Compressive resistance
- Basal viscous resistance
- Autoregulatory resistance
- Coronary arteriolar resistance
- Extravascular resistance
- Ventricular diastolic pressure
- Coronary sinus venous pressure

Coronary vascular resistance consists of epicardial coronary artery resistance, intramyocardial coronary arterial resistance, coronary arteriolar resistance and resistance related to left ventricular diastolic and coronary venous pressures.

There are several functional components that influence resistance in the coronary vascular bed.

VISCOUS RESISTANCE

The basal viscous resistance is the resistance in the coronary vascular bed when the coronary vessels are fully dilated. Since coronary arteries are distensible, the viscous resistance varies with changes in the distending pressures.[4] It also varies with changes in coronary vascular cross-sectional area and changes in the caliber of the epicardial conduit arteries and blood viscosity. Normally, the basal viscous resistance is less in the inner portion than in the outer portion of the left ventricular wall. In contrast, the compressive component of the coronary vascular resistance, which involves intramyocardial coronary arteries and arterioles, is less in the inner portion than in the outer portion of the ventricular walls. This difference in the transmyocardial resistance contributes to maintaining the normal coronary blood flow distribution. The myocardial oxygen demand is greater in the subendocardium than in the outer layers of the ventricular wall. Normally, the differences in transmyocardial resistance contribute to maintaining adequate subendocardial blood flow. In the pathologic states, the alteration in the distribution of transmyocardial coronary blood flow can induce subendocardial ischemia.

COMPRESSIVE RESISTANCE

The compressive resistance results from compression of coronary arteries by myocardium. It varies during cardiac cycle and is higher during systole than in diastole. Compressive resistance decreases total coronary blood flow only slightly. Most myocardial blood flow occurs during diastole. Normally, the compressive resistance in diastole is of small magnitude; however, it increases with increase in ventricular diastolic pressure and in pericardial pressure.

AUTOREGULATORY RESISTANCE

Autoregulatory resistance is the principal mechanism by which coronary blood flow is maintained constant at a constant level of myocardial oxygen demand despite changes in perfusion pressure. Autoregulatory resistance is primarily determined by the caliber of the arterioles. The arteriolar resistance is inversely proportional to the fourth power of arteriolar radius. Thus, a slight change in the caliber of the arterioles is associated with a substantial change in autoregulatory resistance. The autoregulatory resistance is high at basal conditions but decreases when there is an increase in metabolic demand during exercise. During exercise, coronary blood flow may increase 4- to 6-fold. With intact autoregulation, coronary blood flow remains relatively unchanged with perfusion pressure ranging 60–120 mm Hg.

The normal resting coronary blood flow in humans is about 70–100 ml/min/100 gm of tissue. The normal weight of human

CHAPTER 3

Coronary Circulation in Physiology and Pathology

heart is approximately 300 gm and total coronary blood flow is about 250 ml/min. The endocardial and epicardial flows also have been estimated and are approximately 83 and 75 ml/min/100 gm.[1] The flow ratio of endocardium to epicardium usually ranges 1.06–1.16. With maximal coronary vasodilatation, this ratio is close to 1.0.[1] The autoregulatory coronary vascular resistance is modulated by metabolic, neurohormonal and myogenic factors.

MYOGENIC RESISTANCE

The myogenic mechanism involves spontaneous contraction or relaxation of the coronary vascular smooth muscles in response to changes in intraluminal pressure. There is a positive correlation between myogenic response and changes in intraluminal pressure.[5] The myogenic vascular constriction serves to protect distal vessels in response to a sudden increase in arterial pressure.[6] The myogenic resistance is substantial and tightly regulated in the coronary microcirculation, including arterioles.[7] The human coronary microcirculation also responds by vasoconstriction, with increasing intraluminal pressure.[6,8] Several mechanisms for regulation of myogenic resistance have been proposed.[6] It has been suggested that the cell membrane depolarization due to stretch-activated *cation* channels play a role.[6,9] The activation of protein kinase C (PKC) signaling pathways are also involved.[6,8] The activation of other protein kinases, such as mitogen-activated protein kinase (MAPK), have also been implicated.[6,10,11] In the animal studies the reactive oxygen species (ROS) appear to contribute to the regulation of myogenic resistance.[12] The elevated intramural pressure is associated with ROS production and contributes to myogenic microvascular constriction.

MODULATION OF CORONARY BLOOD FLOW

FLOW MEDIATED REGULATION

The flow-mediated vasodilatation (FMD) is an important mechanism of relaxation of the coronary vascular bed. A change in shear stress is associated with release of NO and other endothelium-derived relaxing factors which cause dilatation of the vascular smooth muscles. Human coronary conduit and resistance vessels dilate in response to shear stress. In absence of atherosclerotic coronary artery disease, the dilatation of the resistance vessels is not attenuated by indomethacin, an inhibitor of cyclooxygenase but significantly reduced by L-NAME, a nitric oxide (NO) synthase inhibitor, which suggests that NO release mediates coronary arteriolar dilatation.[12] In patients with coronary artery disease, however, the FMD is not affected by inhibition of synthesis of NO or of cyclooxygenase, suggesting that neither NO nor prostaglandins are involved in dilatation of the resistance vessels.[12] The FMD is inhibited, however, by blocking Ca^{+2} activated K^+ channels, which suggests that endothelium-derived hyperpolarizing factors (EDHF) play an important role in inducing coronary arteriolar smooth muscle relaxation.[13] Endothelial-derived hydrogen peroxide, as an EDHF, contributes to dilatation of the human coronary resistance vessels in response to shear stress.[14] Hydrogen peroxide has been shown to reduce production of inhibitors of EDHF epoxyeico-

satrienoic acids (EETs) in human coronary arterioles.[14,15] Bradykinins also produce endothelium-dependent coronary vasodilatation which is partly due to release of hydrogen peroxide and inhibition of EETs.[6]

METABOLIC FACTORS

The metabolic factors contribute substantially in autoregulation of coronary circulation. A number of metabolic factors, such as adenosine, oxygen and carbon dioxide tensions, pH, lactic acid, and potassium and phosphate concentrations, influence metabolic regulation of coronary circulation. Adenosine is an important metabolic mediator and causes coronary vasodilatation in response to increase in myocardial metabolic demand during exercise. Adenosine causes vasodilatation by activating adenosine receptors, and there are at least four subtypes: (1) A1; (2) A2A; (3) A2B and (4) A3. The regulation of coronary blood flow is primarily mediated by A2A adenosine receptor.[16] Adenosine decreases coronary vascular resistance which is associated with increased coronary blood flow. Adenosine dilates primarily resistance vessels (Fig. 1). The epicardial coronary artery cross-sectional area remains unchanged during adenosine infusion, whereas the average peak velocity measured by intracoronary Doppler ultrasound technique is increased and suggesting dilatation of the coronary resistance vessels. The magnitude of coronary vasodilatation in response to adenosine is not uniform in all vascular beds. In the presence of significant epicardial coronary artery stenosis, the vascular bed in the distribution of more severely stenosed epicardial coronary artery is already dilated. The magnitude of increase in coronary blood flow during a further increase in metabolic demand is less in this area than that in the area of distribution of normal or less severely stenosed epicardial coronary arteries. Thus, the perfusion of the different myocardial segments is not uniform, and forms the basis of stress perfusion imaging. The metabolic factors affect microarteries which are of 30–100 micrometers diameters.[16]

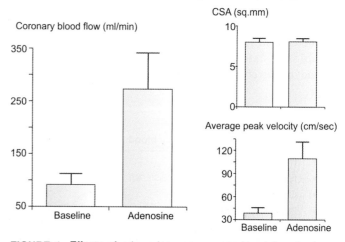

Effect of adenosine on coronary dimensions and flow

FIGURE 1: Effects of adenosine on coronary blood flow in dogs. Average peak velocity increased suggesting dilatation of the resistance vessels. There was very little change in coronary artery diameter suggesting that conduit artery resistance is relatively unaffected. Thus increased coronary blood flow is primarily due to reduction in arteriolar resistance

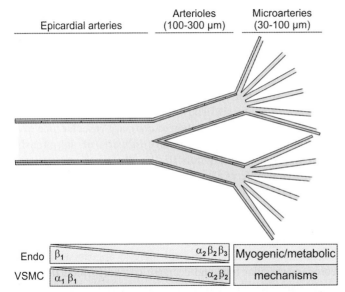

| | Epicardial arteries | Arterioles (100-300 μm) | Microarteries (30-100 μm) | |

Endo	β_1	$\alpha_2 \beta_2 \beta_3$	Myogenic/metabolic
VSMC	$\alpha_1 \beta_1$	$\alpha_2 \beta_2$	mechanisms

FIGURE 2: The schematic illustration of the coronary arterial system which consists of epicardial coronary arteries, arterioles (100–300 micrometers) and microarteries (30–100 micrometers). The adrenergic receptors are located primarily in the arterioles and the epicardial arteries. The metabolic and the myogenic factors affect the micro-arteries. (Abbreviation: VSMS: Vascular smooth muscle cells). (*Source:* Barbato E, Heart. 2009;95:603-8; Ref 16)

NEUROGENIC MODULATION

The neurogenic modulation of coronary vascular resistance is related to activation of vasoconstrictor alpha-adrenergic and vasodilator beta-adrenergic receptors. These adrenergic receptors are located primarily in the coronary arterioles which have diameters of 100–300 micrometers and also are present in the epicardial coronary arteries[17] (Fig. 2).

The adrenergic alpha-receptor subtypes—alpha-1 and alpha-2—are present in the vascular smooth muscle cells, and activation of these alpha receptors causes vasoconstriction. The distribution of the alpha-receptor subtypes is not uniform: alpha-1 receptors are present predominantly in the larger caliber arteries including epicardial coronary arteries, whereas the alpha-2 receptors density is higher in the arterioles. The alpha-2 receptors are also present in the vascular endothelium, and the activation of the endothelial alpha-2 receptors is associated with NO mediated vasodilatation.

The subtypes of beta-adrenergic receptors—beta-1, beta-2 and beta-3—are present in the vascular smooth muscle cells of the coronary vasculature and in the myocardium. The density of beta-2 receptors is highest in the arterioles and their stimulation is associated with coronary vasodilatation. The beta-1 receptors are present predominantly in the epicardial coronary arteries and their activation is associated with dilatation of the epicardial coronary arteries. The beta-3 receptors are present mostly in the endothelial cells of the arterioles, and activation of these receptors produce coronary vasodilatation via NO and hyperpolarization mechanisms. The beta-1 and beta-2 receptors are also present on endothelial cells but their functional significance remains unclear.

The coronary vasodilatation mediated by increased adrenergic activity stimulates cardiac metabolic activity. The phenomenon of coronary vasodilatation mediated by increased

sympathetic and cardiac metabolic activity is called "feed forward sympathetic vasodilation".[18] The "feed forward coronary vasodilation" is partly mediated by activation of beta-1 and beta-2 adrenergic receptors.[19] The disturbances of this phenomenon may influence myocardial perfusion. In human studies, it has been reported that alpha-adrenergic receptors activation contributes to vasoconstrictor tone in the coronary vascular bed under basal conditions.[20] The beta-adrenergic receptors exert a minor vasodilatory effect at rest.

The activation of adrenergic activity during cold pressor test, mental stress or exercise causes vasodilatation of both the epicardial and coronary microvasculature in the presence of normal coronary arteries. Intravenous administration of dobutamine, a predominantly beta-adrenergic receptor agonist, causes dilatation of the epicardial coronary arteries and coronary arterioles. Coronary vasodilatation during dobutamine infusion is also meditated by increased metabolic demand. Nebivolol, which is a selective beta-1 receptor blocking agent with beta-3 receptor stimulating property, induces coronary vasodilatation and increases coronary flow reserve.[17] Thus, alpha-receptor blockade and stimulation of beta-1, beta-2 and beta-3 receptors are associated with coronary vasodilatation. In the presence of normal endothelial function, stimulation of cholinergic receptors causes coronary vasodilatation by releasing acetylcholine. Acetylcholine-mediated coronary vasodilatation is related to release of endothelium-dependant relaxing factors including NO (Figs 3 and 4). However, following inhibition of NO synthesis by LNAME, intracoronary infusion of acetylcholine is associated with a significant increase in the cross-sectional area of the epicardial coronary arteries. But the average peak velocity flow does not increase significantly suggesting that NO predominantly affects the conductance vessels and not the resistance vessels. Atherosclerotic coronary artery disease is associated with endothelial dysfunction, and acetylcholine causes paradoxical response.[21] It causes epicardial coronary artery constriction and increases coronary arteriolar resistance and decreases coronary blood flow.

Simultaneous 2-D and Doppler ultrasound: effect of Acetylcholine

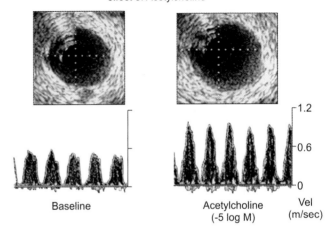

FIGURE 3: Effects of intracoronary infusion of acetylcholine in normal dogs. The intracoronary ultrasound imaging demonstrates an increase in coronary artery cross-sectional area indicating dilatation of the conduit vessels. There was also an increase in the average peak velocity (intracoronary Doppler technique) indicating dilatation of the resistance vessels in response to intracoronary infusion of acetylcholine

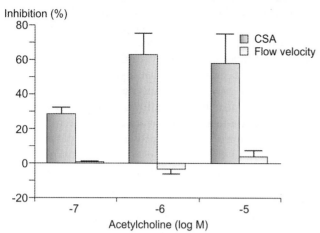

Effect of L-NAME (100 μM) on vasodilator response to Acetylcholine

FIGURE 4: Effects of nitric oxide (NO) synthase inhibitor LNAME on coronary artery cross-sectional area (CSA) and average peak velocity. The magnitude of the increase in CSA was markedly attenuated after LNAME suggesting that NO pathway dilates the conductance vessels. The AVP was not substantially involved, indicating that the coronary resistance vessel dilatation is little affected by NO

In the presence of atherosclerotic coronary artery disease, coronary vasoconstriction also occurs in response to stimulation of alpha-adrenergic receptors. Coronary vasoconstriction during percutaneous coronary intervention has been observed, and it is reversed by the administration of alpha-adrenergic receptors antagonists.[22]

HORMONAL MODULATION

Hormonal modulation of coronary circulation in physiologic and pathologic states is related to activation of various neurohormonal systems. The renin-angiotensin-aldosterone system, catecholamines, endothelins, bradykinins, NO and natriuretic peptides influence coronary vascular tone. In the basal state, angiotensin appears to exert coronary vasoconstriction as

angiotensin II receptor-1 (AT-1) blocking agent induces dilatation of the conduit and resistance vessels[23] (Fig. 5). The coronary vasodilatation induced by angiotensin receptor blockade is partly mediated by NO as LNAME, an NO synthase inhibitor which attenuates coronary vasodilatation (Fig. 6).[23] However, it is not abolished by inhibition of bradykinin or prostacyclin synthesis. Thus, it appears that the angiotensin system is involved in regulation of coronary vascular tone even at basal conditions. Intracoronary infusion of angiotensin-converting enzyme inhibitors that do not cause any systemic hemodynamic effects also cause coronary vasodilatation, which is markedly attenuated by bradykinin inhibition with administration of bradykinin-2 receptor antagonists[24] (Figs 7A to C). Thus, bradykinins also contribute in regulation of coronary vascular tone.[24]

In experimental studies, aldosterone appears to increase coronary vascular tone and decrease coronary blood flow.[25] In cardiac-specific, aldosterone synthase transgenic mice, the basal coronary blood flow decreased by more than 50% compared to that in the wild type mice. The decrease in coronary blood flow was attenuated in response to acetylcholine, bradykinin and sodium nitroprusside, suggesting that the decrease in basal coronary blood flow by aldosterone is mediated by both endothelium-dependent and endothelium-independent mechanisms.

Vasopressins are potent vasoconstrictors and vasoconstriction is caused by stimulation of vascular smooth muscles by activation of vasopressin-1 receptors. Vasopressins increase not only systemic vascular resistance but also coronary vascular resistance. In experimental animals, vasopressins cause coronary vasoconstriction and impair myocardial perfusion.[26]

Endothelins—primarily endothelin-1—are also potent coronary vasoconstrictors, increasing coronary vascular resistance and decreasing coronary blood flow.[27] Endothelins cause constriction of vascular smooth muscle cells primarily of the coronary resistance vessels. The endothelins exert their vasoconstrictive effects by activating specific receptors Endothelin-A and Endothelin-B. Endothelin-1 induces an

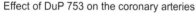

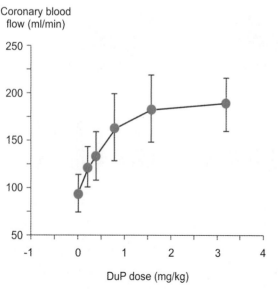

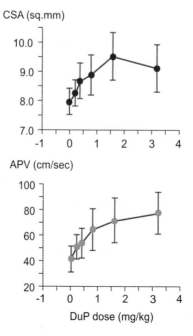

FIGURE 5: Effects of angiotensin receptor subtype-1 blocking agent DUP-753 (Losartan) on epicardial coronary artery cross-sectional area (CSA) and the average peak velocity (APV). There was dilatation of both conductance and resistance vessels and increase in coronary blood flow. (*Source:* Modified from Sudhir K, MacGregor JS, Gupta M, et al. Effect of selective angiotensin II receptor antagonism and angiotensin converting enzyme inhibition on the coronary vasculature in vivo: intravascular two-dimensional and Doppler ultrasound studies. Circulation. 1993;87(3):931-8)

SECTION 1

Basic Cardiology

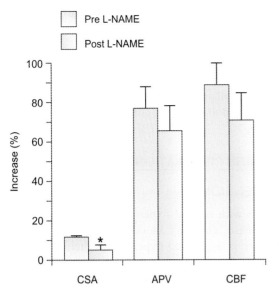

FIGURE 6: Effects of NO-synthase inhibitors on losartan induced dilatation of the conductance and resistance vessels. The magnitude of dilatation of the conductance vessels was attenuated by NO-synthase inhibition suggesting that NO pathway dilates the conductance vessels. There was no effect on resistance vessels. (Abbreviations: CSA: Cross-sectional area; APV: Average peak velocity; CBF: Coronary blood flow). (*Source:* Modified from Sudhir K, Chou T, Hutchison S, et al. Coronary vasodilation induced by angiotensin-converting enzyme inhibition in vivo: differential contribution of nitric oxide and bradykinin in conductance and resistance arteries. Circulation. 1996;93:1734-9)

exaggerated vasoconstrictor response in atherosclerotic coronary arteries.[27-31] Norepinephrine also increases coronary vascular resistance by activating alpha-adrenergic receptors of the coronary arteries.

The B-type natriuretic peptide (BNP) causes relaxation of the coronary conduit and resistance vessels and increases coronary blood flow without any concomitant increase in myocardial oxygen demand[32,33] (Fig. 8). The exogenous administration of BNP is associated with both systemic arterial and venous dilatation. The coronary vascular relaxation by BNP is partially attenuated by indomethacin and NO synthase inhibitors suggesting that both prostaglandins and NO

systems are involved. It remains unclear whether natriuretic peptides play a physiologic role in the regulation of coronary vascular tone.

The sex hormones estrogen and testosterone acutely cause coronary vasodilatation.[34-38] The mechanisms of coronary vasodilatation remain unclear. Activation of nuclear receptor mechanisms appears unlikely as vasodilatation occurs very quickly after their administration. The physiologic role of sex hormone-mediated coronary vasodilatation also remains unclear.

CORONARY COLLATERAL CIRCULATION

Coronary collateral vessels are anastomotic channels and serve as alternative sources of blood flow and myocardial perfusion in presence of obstructive coronary artery disease. Although anastomotic channels are normally present in the coronary circulation, collateral arteries that develop in obstructive coronary disease are larger muscular arteries have the anatomic composition similar to those of epicardial coronary arteries, and are present predominantly in the epicardium.[39] Like epicardial coronary arteries, collateral arteries are conductance arteries and connect the territory of one epicardial coronary artery to that of another.[40] The collateral vessels may also develop in the same epicardial coronary artery connecting the proximal to the distal segment across severely or totally occluded segments.

A number of factors have been identified which influence development of collateral vessels. The presence, severity and duration of ischemia have been documented as important stimuli.[41-43] More severe and longer duration of myocardial ischemia is more likely to cause development of significant coronary collateral vessels. The severity of the coronary artery stenosis, as assessed by the transstenotic pressure gradient, is another stimulus. A substantial pressure gradient is required to induce development of the collateral vessels. Slower induction of myocardial ischemia, as occurs when severe coronary artery occlusion develops gradually, is more likely to be associated with development of collateral vessels than when severe ischemia occurs suddenly following total occlusion of an epicardial coronary artery.[44]

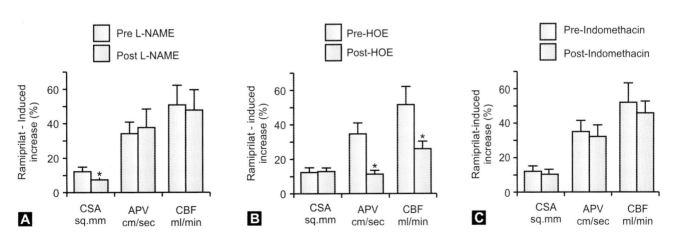

FIGURES 7A TO C: Effects of angiotensin converting enzyme inhibitor on coronary circulation. It dilates both coronary conductance and resistance vessels. The conductance vessels dilatation is attenuated by NO-synthase inhibitor. Resistance vessels dilatation is attenuated by bradykinin inhibition suggesting that bradykinin is involved in angiotensin converting enzyme inhibitors mediated coronary vasodilatation. (Abbreviations: CSA: Cross-sectional area; APV: Average peak velocity; CBF: Coronary blood flow). (*Source:* Modified from Sudhir et al., Circulation, Ref. 22)

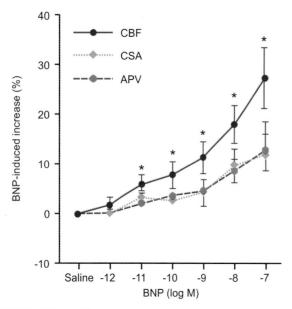

FIGURE 8: Effects of B-type natriuretic peptide on coronary circulation. There is a significant increase in coronary blood flow (CBF) due to dilatation of the conductance (CSA) and the resistance (AVP) vessels. (*Source:* Modified from Christian Zellner, Andrew A. Protter, Eitetsu Ko, et al. Coronary vasodilator effects of BNP: mechanisms of action in coronary conductance and resistance arteries. Am J Physiol- Heart and Circulatory Physiology. 1999:276)

Although the magnitude of collateral blood flow following epicardial coronary artery occlusion may be adequate in absence of increased myocardial oxygen demands, it is insufficient when oxygen demand is increased during exercise.[45] Coronary blood flow per gram of myocardium, dependent on collateral flow, is reduced compared to normally perfused myocardium.[46] One of the mechanisms of reduced flow is the reduced perfusion pressure of the collateral blood vessels. The pressure in the collateral arteries is similar to that in the arterial segment distal to the coronary artery stenosis. Coronary artery pressure distal to severe stenosis may be only 25–50% of aortic pressure.[47,48]

Neurohormonal regulation of collateral circulation may be contributing mechanisms to maintain adequate collateral blood flow. NO-mediated endothelium-dependent vasodilatation and its inhibition by NO synthase inhibitor in collateral blood vessels have been observed.[49,50] The release of vasoconstrictors thromboxane A2 and serotonin with platelet activation in the collateral vessels may decrease collateral blood flow particularly during increased oxygen demand at the time of exercise.[51]

The beta-adrenergic receptors have been identified in the collateral vessels and their activation causes dilatation of these vessels.[52] The beta blockade therapy is associated with impaired vasodilatation and reduced collateral blood flow during exercise.[53]

The precise mechanisms for the formation of collateral vessels remain unclear. The various growth factors, such as basic fibroblast growth factor (bFGF) and vascular endothelial growth factor (VEGF) known to promote vasculogenesis, have been implicated.[54,55]

The existence and regulation of coronary collateral circulation has several clinical significances. In patients with acute coronary syndromes pre-existence of collateral blood vessels have been shown to reduce infarct size after reperfusion.[56] The ventricular function is better in patients with collateral vessels than without collateral vessels.[57] The prognosis of patients with collaterals appears to be better in patients than without collaterals.[58] However, no controlled studies have been performed to assess the clinical significance of collateral vessels.

CORONARY CIRCULATION IN PATHOLOGIC STATES

HYPERTENSION

In patients with arterial hypertension but without coronary artery disease, coronary blood flow reserve is reduced.[59] When there is associated hypertrophy, there is microvasculature rarefaction which contributes to reduced coronary flow reserve. Coronary vascular resistance is elevated in hypertension due to impaired endothelium-dependent coronary vasodilatation.[59,60] There is impairment of vasodilatation of both coronary conductance and resistance vessels. Intracoronary infusion of both acetylcholine and substance P produced blunted vasodilatory response of conductance and resistance vessels in patients with hypertension compared to patients without hypertension.[61] Both acetylcholine and substance P produce endothelium-dependent vasodilatation but by different mechanisms. Acetylcholine and substance P activate different muscarinic receptors. Both acetylcholine and substance P-induced vasodilatation is blunted by NO synthase inhibitors, suggesting that the NO pathway is involved.[62] In hypertensive patients with subclinical renal damage, coronary flow reserve is impaired usually in patients with left ventricular hypertrophy.[63] Several potential anatomic and physiologic mechanisms have been proposed that include smooth muscle cell hypertrophy and impaired vasodilator reserve. In hypertension with hypertrophy, there is considerable medial hypertrophy of the coronary resistance vessels which is associated with impaired coronary blood flow reserve.[64] With long-term pharmacotherapy there may be regression of medial hypertrophy.[64] In hypertensive patients without coronary artery disease, coronary flow velocity reserve and aortic distensibility is reduced as measured by transesophageal echocardiography.[65]

Myocardial blood flow distribution is altered in hypertrophy. In absence of hypertrophy, the blood flow is higher in the endocardial layers. When there is concentric hypertrophy, for example, in response to pressure overload, the blood flow is higher in subepicardial and epicardial layers than in the endocardium.[66] The endothelium-dependent vasodilatation is impaired both in patients with concentric and eccentric left ventricular hypertrophy.[67,68] The endothelium-independent vasodilatation of the resistance vessels is impaired predominantly in patients with eccentric hypertrophy.[67]

In experimental animals with pressure-overloaded left ventricular hypertrophy, the subendocardial flow reserve is impaired at rest.[69] During induced stress, there is further reduction in subendocardial flow reserve which may cause diastolic dysfunction due to subendocardial ischemia.[69]

The changes in coronary microvascular function have been observed in patients with hypertension by positron emission tomography (PET) studies.[70] At rest coronary flow response remains normal but it is blunted in response to increased metabolic demand.[70] The potential mechanisms of myocardial ischemia in hypertension are summarized in Table 3.

VALVULAR HEART DISEASE

In aortic valve stenosis, there is microvascular dysfunction which is associated with reduced subendocardial blood flow which can induce subendocardial ischemia and necrosis even in absence of epicardial coronary artery disease.[71] In patients with hemodynamically significant aortic stenosis without epicardial coronary artery disease, coronary sinus blood flow which approximates global coronary blood flow is increased both at rest and during isometric exercise.[72] However, normalized for left ventricular mass, coronary blood flow remains within normal limits. The ratio of the diastolic pressure time index and the systolic pressure time index (DPTI/SPTI), which reflects the myocardial oxygen supply/demand relation, is reduced, indicating that myocardial oxygen supply is inadequate for the oxygen demand.[72] In patients who had angina during isometric exercise, the DPTI/SPTI ratio decreased to a greater extent compared to those who did not experience angina suggesting that the myocardial oxygen supply and demand mismatch was higher in patients with angina.[72] In patients with severe aortic stenosis, coronary flow reserve is reduced due to decreased coronary blood flow as a result of reduced perfusion pressure and a concomitant increase in myocardial oxygen demand.[73] The decreased coronary flow reserve in aortic stenosis may reflect coronary microcirculatory dysfunction.[74] Reduced coronary flow reserve may be associated with myocardial ischemia, left ventricular dysfunction, and worse prognosis.[75]

Transthoracic Doppler and myocardial contrast echocardiography and myocardial biopsy during surgical interventions revealed that in patients with aortic stenosis, there was impaired coronary flow reserve, compared to the patients without aortic stenosis and in these patients, there was increased myocyte apoptosis.[76] Decreased coronary flow reserve is also associated with a long-term worse prognosis.[77] In severe aortic stenosis, transmyocardial perfusion pressure gradient is reduced as the aortic diastolic pressure is low and left ventricular diastolic pressure is increased. The coronary blood flow reserve is impaired in patients with significant aortic stenosis due to impaired coronary vasodilation which improves after aortic valve replacement.[78] It should be appreciated that coronary flow reserve may be impaired in patients with aortic sclerosis in absence of significant aortic valve stenosis and in absence of obvious epicardial coronary artery stenosis, suggesting that microvascular-endothelial dysfunction may be present during the early stages of the calcific aortic valve disease.[79]

In severe aortic regurgitation, a potential exists for myocardial ischemia due to increased myocardial oxygen demand and impaired myocardial perfusion.[71] In chronic severe aortic regurgitation, the left ventricular volume is increased. Although there is eccentric hypertrophy, the wall stress is increased due to disproportionate increase in left ventricular volume and dimensions. Thus, myocardial oxygen demand is increased. In severe chronic aortic regurgitation, aortic diastolic pressure, which is the myocardial perfusion pressure, is also low. If there is an increase in left ventricular diastolic pressure, the transmyocardial pressure gradient is reduced and subendocardial ischemia may occur. The slower heart rate can also be detrimental due to increased time for continuing regurgitation. In experimental volume overloaded model

TABLE 3

The potential mechanisms of myocardial ischemia in hypertension, valvular heart disease and hypertrophic cardiomyopathy

Hypertension:

Changes in the determinants of myocardial oxygen demand

Left ventricular systolic pressure	increased
Wall stress	decreased
Heart rate	unchanged
Contractility	unchanged or increased

Changes in the determinants of oxygen supply

Perfusion pressure	normal or increased
Left ventricular diastolic pressure	normal or increased
Transmyocardial pressure gradient	unchanged or increased
Coronary vascular resistance	increased
Coronary vasodilatory reserve	impaired
Rarefaction of microvessels	
Redistribution of blood flow from endocardium to epicardium	

Valvular Heart Disease

Aortic Stenosis:

Changes in determinants of oxygen demand

Left ventricular systolic pressure	increased
Wall stress	decreased
Heart rate	unchanged
Contractility	unchanged

Changes in the determinants of oxygen supply

Perfusion pressure	normal or decreased
Left ventricular diastolic pressure	unchanged or increased
Transmyocardial pressure gradient	unchanged or decreased
Coronary vasodilatory reserve	impaired

Chronic aortic regurgitation

Changes in determinants of oxygen demand

Left ventricular systolic pressure	increased
Wall stress	increased
Heart rate	unchanged
Contractility	unchanged

Changes in the determinants of oxygen supply

Perfusion pressure	decreased
Left ventricular diastolic pressure	unchanged or increased
Transmyocardial pressure gradient	unchanged or decreased
Coronary vasodilatory reserve	impaired

Hypertrophic cardiomyopathy

Changes in determinants of oxygen demand

Left ventricular systolic pressure	normal or decreased
Wall stress	decreased
Heart rate	unchanged
Contractility	normal or decreased

Changes in determinants of oxygen supply

Perfusion pressure	normal or decreased
Left ventricular diastolic pressure	unchanged or increased
Transmyocardial pressure gradient	unchanged or decreased
Coronary vasodilatory reserve	impaired

CHAPTER 3

Coronary Circulation in Physiology and Pathology

following creation of complete heart block, there is a little change in left ventricular coronary flow reserve after 6–7 weeks of creating complete heart block.[80] Thus, some increase in heart rate may be beneficial as it reduces total regurgitant volume. The potential mechanisms of myocardial ischemia in aortic valve disease are summarized in Table 3.

HYPERTROPHIC CARDIOMYOPATHY

Hypertrophic cardiomyopathy is a genetic disorder characterized by primary myocardial hypertrophy. The hypertrophy is usually asymmetric and left ventricular wall thickness is not uniform. A substantial abnormality of coronary circulation has been observed in patients with hypertrophic cardiomyopathy.[81-91]

The global myocardial oxygen demand is decreased in hypertrophic cardiomyopathy. Although the left ventricle is hypercontractile, left ventricular wall stress is reduced as left ventricular volume and systolic pressure in general are normal and its wall thickness is increased. However, regional and global coronary blood flow can be impaired particularly during stress.[83-86] Cardiac magnetic resonance studies have reported that in patients with hypertrophic cardiomyopathy, resting myocardial blood flow was similar to those of healthy controls.[88] However, hyperemic myocardial blood flow was lower in patients with hypertrophic cardiomyopathy compared to controls. The endocardial and epicardial blood flow ratio decreased in patients with hypertrophic cardiomyopathy during induced hyperemia. The reduction of subendocardial blood flow was greater with increasing wall thickness. In general, the magnitude of fibrosis was also greater with impaired hyperemic blood flow.[88]

The PET, with the use of 13N-ammonia to measure myocardial blood flow at rest and after dipyridamole, reported that the minimal coronary vascular resistance was higher in patients with hypertrophic cardiomyopathy. These findings suggest that there is impaired coronary vasodilatory reserve in hypertrophic cardiomyopathy.[87] Impaired coronary vasodilatation in the presence of normal epicardial coronary arteries may induce myocardial ischemia and reflects dysfunction of the microcirculation.[86] Reversible myocardial ischemia has also been documented during exercise by thallium 201 myocardial perfusion studies.[85] Abnormal myocardial lactate extraction during pacing has been observed in patients with hypertrophic cardiomyopathy which also indicates stress induced myocardial ischemia.[85] Impaired coronary flow reserve due to microvascular dysfunction not only contributes to myocardial ischemia but also to adverse ventricular remodeling, and worse long-term prognosis of patients with hypertrophic cardiomyopathy.[89]

Coronary flow reserve determined by intracoronary Doppler technique has reported an immediate improvement after alcohol septal ablation in patients with obstructive hypertrophic cardiomyopathy.[90] These findings suggest that hemodynamic causes such as severe left ventricular outflow gradient also contribute to coronary microvascular dysfunction.[90,91] The potential mechanisms for myocardial ischemia are summarized in Table 3.

METABOLIC DISORDERS

Anemia

In chronic anemia, there are changes both in the determinants of myocardial oxygen demand and oxygen supply. Due to reduced hemoglobin and decreased oxygen carrying capacity, there is a compensatory increase in coronary blood flow and increased oxygen extraction. There is an inverse relation between the hemoglobin level and coronary blood flow.[92] The coronary vascular resistance is also markedly decreased. Decreased viscosity is the predominant mechanism for the reduction of coronary vascular resistance.

Diabetes

Irrespective of the type of diabetes, coronary microvascular dysfunction has been observed.[93-95] In both type 1 and type 2 diabetes, endothelium-dependent and endothelium-independent coronary blood flow reserve is impaired. Thus, hyperglycemia appears to produce a direct adverse effect on coronary microvascular function.

ISCHEMIC HEART DISEASE

In acute coronary syndromes, there is a primary decrease in coronary blood flow without any significant changes in the determinants of myocardial oxygen demand. There is inadequate coronary vasodilatation related to impaired endothelial function. After percutaneous coronary intervention, there may be activation of alpha-adrenergic receptors inducing constriction of coronary vessels.

In patients with chronic stable angina, there are changes in both the determinants of myocardial oxygen demand and oxygen supply. However, the predominant changes in oxygen supply or in demand are related to the clinical subsets.

In patients with classic angina (Heberden's angina), there is an increase in heart rate, blood pressure and contractility during exercise or emotional stress that is associated with increased myocardial oxygen demand. There is also a decrease in coronary blood flow reserve due to endothelial dysfunction. Inadequate vasodilatation of the coronary conductance and resistance vessels result in a reduction in coronary blood flow. Thus, ischemic threshold is significantly lowered and ischemia occurs at a lower level of myocardial oxygen demand (Fig. 9).

In patients with vasospastic angina, the principal mechanism of myocardial ischemia is primary decrease of coronary blood flow due to "spasm" of the epicardial coronary arteries, and appears to be related to decreased NO.[96] The endothelium-dependent vasodilatation in response to acetylcholine is impaired at the site of vasospasm compared to that in normal segments.[97] But the magnitude of bradykinin-induced coronary vasodilatation of the epicardial coronary arteries at the spastic site is similar to that of a non-spastic site. Nitrate-induced vasodilatation was also similar in the spastic and non-spastic sites. These findings suggest that NO-mediated endothelium-dependent vasodilatation is impaired at the site of spasm of the epicardial coronary arteries but the bradykinin-mediated

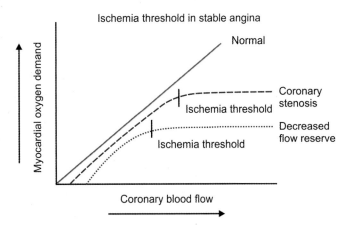

Ischemia threshold in stable angina

FIGURE 9: Effects of increased myocardial oxygen demand on coronary blood flow. With increasing myocardial oxygen demand there is demand-mediated increase in coronary blood flow. In presence of epicardial coronary artery stenosis when coronary blood flow cannot increase anymore and ischemia is precipitated (ischemia threshold). Due to associated endothelial dysfunction in presence of atherosclerosis coronary blood flow reserve is impaired and ischemia threshold occurs at a lower level of oxygen demand

TABLE 4

Changes in coronary circulation in clinical subsets of stable angina

Classic (Heberden's) angina	Demand and supply ischemia
Vasospastic (Prinzmetal's) angina	Supply ischemia
Mixed angina	Demand and supply ischemia
Linked angina	Supply ischemia
Cardiac syndrome X	Supply ischemia

endothelium-dependent vasodilatation is maintained. Intracoronary infusion of isosorbide dinitrate dilates the conductance vessels without a significant change in microvascular resistance in patients with vasospastic angina.[98]

Mixed angina is characterized by variable exercise level that precipitates angina. The changes in coronary blood flow with same degree of anatomic epicardial coronary artery stenosis may be related to endothelial dysfunction which decreases coronary blood flow due to increase in the microvascular resistance.

In linked angina, there is a disproportionate increase in coronary vascular resistance associated with a decrease in coronary blood flow. The increase in coronary microvascular resistance results from centrally mediated increase in sympathetic activity during visceral stimulation such as esophageal reflux. Increased coronary vascular resistance occurs in presence or absence of atherosclerotic coronary artery disease.

The cardiac "syndrome X" is characterized by exercise-induced angina with evidence of myocardial ischemia in absence of atherosclerotic obstructive coronary artery disease.[99] This clinical subset has been subsequently termed "microvascular angina".[100] Inappropriate increase in coronary microvascular resistance and a decrease in coronary flow reserve have been proposed as the potential mechanism. Both endothelium-dependent and endothelium-independent coronary vasodilatations are impaired.[99-103]

In response to vasoconstrictor stimuli during hyperventilation, mental stress and exposure to cold, an exaggerated response of coronary microcirculation may occur.[104-106] Abnormal cardiac adrenergic nerve function has also been observed in patients with cardiac syndrome X. A higher cardiac defect during 123-metaiodobenzylguanidine (MIBG) uptake has been observed in patients with syndrome X compared to healthy subjects.[106] The changes in coronary circulation in various subsets of angina are summarized in Table 4.

The effects of commonly used antianginal drugs on coronary circulation are summarized in Table 5. Beta-adrenergic receptors antagonists primarily decrease the determinants of myocardial oxygen demand. There is a substantial decrease in heart rate and contractility and less changes in arterial blood pressure. Coronary vascular resistance may increase due to activation of alpha-adrenergic receptors in the coronary vessels. Myocardial perfusion may increase slightly due to an increase in diastolic perfusion time if there is a substantial decrease in heart rate.[107,108]

Nitrates decrease ventricular volumes due to dilatation of the systemic veins. There is also a decrease in arterial pressure. Thus, there is reduction in wall tension and myocardial oxygen demand. An increase in heart rate and contractility may occur from reflex activation of sympathetic system if there is a significant hypotension. These reflex increase in heart rate partly offset reduction in myocardial oxygen demand resulting from decreased wall tension.[108]

The non-dihydropyridine heart rate regulating calcium channel blockers decreases coronary blood flow due to decrease in myocardial oxygen demand. Contractility and heart rate decrease reduce myocardial oxygen consumption.[109] In contrast, dihydropyridine calcium channel blockers decrease myocardial oxygen demand by decreasing contractility and arterial pressure. However, there is also dilatation of the coronary conductance and resistance vessels.[110] The mechanism of decrease in myocardial ischemia by ranolazine has not been clearly determined. There is no change in heart

TABLE 5

The effects of commonly used antianginal drugs on coronary circulation

Beta adrenoreceptor blocking agents
- Decreased coronary blood flow and myocardial oxygen consumption predominantly due to decreased heart rate and contractility
- Increased coronary vascular resistance due to activation of alpha adrenergic receptors

Nitrates:
- Decreased myocardial oxygen consumption due to decreased ventricular volumes and pressure due to decreased venous return resulting from systemic venodilatation
- Dilatation of the conductance vessels

Calcium channel blocking agents

Dihydropyridines:
- Decreased myocardial oxygen demand due to decreased arterial pressure and contractility
- Dilatation of the conductance and resistance vessels

Heart rate regulating calcium channel blocking agents:
- Decreased coronary blood flow and myocardial oxygen consumption predominantly due to decreased heart rate, and contractility

Ranolazine:
- No direct effects on myocardial oxygen demand or coronary blood flow
- Inhibition of late sodium current resulting in a decreased calcium overload, improved diastolic tension and secondary increase in myocardial blood flow and perfusion

44 rate, arterial pressure or contractility. Thus, there is no change in myocardial oxygen demand. Ranolazine also does not increase coronary blood flow directly but it improves myocardial perfusion. In presence of myocardial ischemia, there is increased activation of late sodium current which stimulates the sodium/calcium exchange mechanism. Thus, there is myocardial cellular calcium over load which increases left ventricular diastolic tension and coronary vascular compressive resistance. Coronary blood flow and myocardial perfusion are reduced in endocardial and subendocardial layers. Ranolazine inhibits late sodium current and reverses ischemia-induced cellular calcium overload and improves myocardial blood flow and myocardial perfusion.[111]

SYSTOLIC HEART FAILURE

Abnormalities of coronary circulation are common in systolic heart failure. There are changes in myocardial oxygen demand and in coronary blood flow (Table 6).[112] The heart rate/systolic blood pressure product usually remains unchanged. The global contractile function is reduced. Left ventricular volume is markedly increased and the wall thickness is decreased or

TABLE 6

Changes in coronary circulation in systolic heart failure

Determinants of myocardial oxygen demand and consumption	
Heart rate x blood pressure	unchanged
Contractility	decreased
Wall stress	decreased (primarily due to increased volume)
Determinants of coronary blood flow	
Perfusion pressure	unchanged or decreased
End diastolic pressure (subendocardial compressive resistance)	increased
Transmyocardial perfusion pressure gradient	decreased
Coronary sinus venous pressure (resistive resistance)	increased
Microvascular resistance	increased
Coronary vasodilatory reserve	decreased

remains unchanged.[112] The net effect is increased myocardial oxygen demand and consumption (Fig. 10). Increased

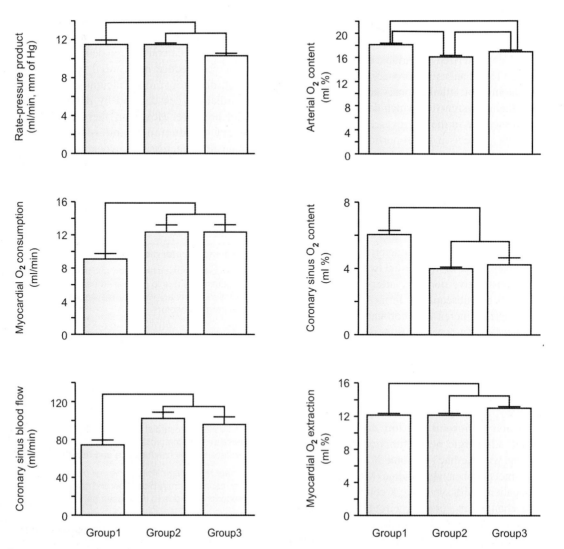

FIGURE 10: Changes in coronary circulation in patients with systolic heart failure. Rate-pressure product (rate x pressure) remains unchanged. Coronary sinus blood flow (CSBF) and myocardial oxygen consumption (MVO$_2$) were increased in both ischemic and non-ischemic dilated cardiomyopathy compared with patients without heart failure. (*Source:* Modified from Chatterjee, J Cardiac Fail, Ref. 112)

myocardial oxygen consumption is observed both in patients with ischemic and nonischemic dilated cardiomyopathy. The coronary sinus oxygen content decreases with increased myocardial oxygen consumption. The prognosis of patients with lower coronary sinus oxygen content is worse than that in patients with higher coronary sinus oxygen content (Fig. 11).

The coronary blood flow is increased parallel to the increase in myocardial oxygen demand. Coronary blood flow normalized for left ventricular mass, however, may remain normal or even decreased.[113] The perfusion pressure may remain unchanged or decrease depending on the severity of heart failure. Severe systolic heart failure is associated with a substantial increase in left ventricular diastolic pressure which increases endocardial and subendocardial compressive resistance and decrease subendocardial blood flow.[115]

Coronary blood flow reserve is impaired in patients with ischemic and nonischemic dilated cardiomyopathy. Both endothelium-dependent and endothelium-independent mechanisms of coronary vasodilatation are impaired.[112,114] Furthermore, increased release of cytokines and neurohormones enhance coronary vascular tone and decrease coronary blood flow reserve. Increased wall stress also contributes to impaired coronary blood flow reserve.[115]

There is a substantial activation of neurohormones in systolic heart failure. The enhanced adrenergic activity, renin-angiotensin-aldosterone system, vasopressin and endothelins exert adverse effects on coronary circulation (Table 7). Increased adrenergic activity is associated with increased coronary vascular resistance and decreased coronary blood flow. Angiotensins and endothelins also cause constriction of coronary resistance vessels, increase coronary vascular resistance and decrease coronary blood flow.

Vasopressin causes constriction of both conductance and resistance vessels by activating vasopressin 1A receptors which is associated with decreased coronary blood flow.

Myocardial metabolic function can be impaired in systolic heart failure. The serum levels of nonesterified free fatty acids are increased. Myocardial glucose and nonesterified fatty acid

uptake and ATP concentrations are decreased. There is a shift from nonesterified fatty acid uptake to glucose uptake for myocardial substrate utilization which is associated with increased myocardial oxygen consumption.[112] During increased stress there is a marked increase in myocardial lactate release suggesting myocardial ischemia.[116]

Some compensatory mechanisms occur to maintain myocardial oxygen delivery when coronary blood flow becomes inadequate for myocardial oxygen demand. Myocardial oxygen extraction is increased. Blood levels of 2,3-diphosphoglycerate

---

TABLE 7

The effects of neurohormonal abnormalities on coronary circulation in heart failure

Activation of alpha-1 receptors—Coronary vasoconstriction
  Increased coronary vascular resistance
  Decreased coronary blood flow

Activation of alpha-2 receptors—NO-mediated coronary vasodilatation
- Myocardial beta-1 receptor—
  Demand mediated increase in coronary blood flow
- Beta-2 receptors—
  Primary coronary vasodilatation
  Increased coronary blood flow
- Angiotensin—
  Increased coronary vascular resistance
  Decreased coronary blood flow
- Aldosterone—
  Increased coronary vascular resistance
  Decreased coronary flow reserve
- Vasopressin—
  Coronary vasoconstriction
  Decreased coronary blood flow
- Endothelins—
  Coronary vasoconstriction
  Increased coronary vascular resistance
  Decreased coronary flow

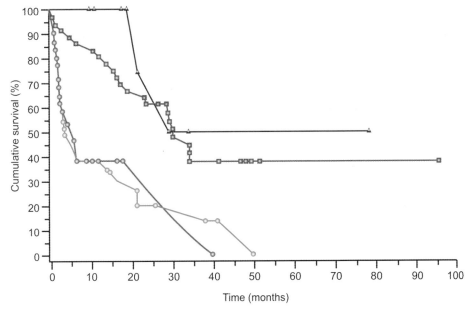

FIGURE 11: Survival curves for patients in group 1 (coronary artery disease) with high (squire) and low (triangle) coronary sinus oxygen content and in group 2 (idiopathic cardio myopathy) with high (diamond) and low (circle) coronary sinus oxygen content. In patients with low coronary sinus oxygen content (< 4.44 vol. percent) the survival was lower than in patients with high coronary sinus oxygen content (> 4.44 vol. percent) (p < 0.001). (*Source:* Modified from Chatterjee K. Coronary hemodynamics in heart failure and effects of therapeutic interventions. J Cardiac Fail. 2009;15:116-23)

46 (2,3-DPG) are increased. Oxygen tension for 50% oxygen saturation (P50) is increased, and there is a rightward shift of the oxygen dissociation curve which facilitates oxygen delivery and myocardial oxygen transport.[112]

The effects of commonly used therapies in systolic heart failure are summarized in Table 8.[112] Angiotensin inhibition with the use of converting enzyme inhibitors is associated with decrease in myocardial oxygen consumption and also a primary increase in coronary blood flow. In general, beta-adrenergic receptor antagonists decrease myocardial oxygen consumption. Some beta-adrenergic antagonists also decrease oxidative stress.

Aldosterone antagonists have the potential to decrease coronary vascular resistance by decreasing perivascular fibrosis. Hydralazine causes demand-related changes in coronary blood flow. There may also be an increase in coronary blood flow/demand ratio. Nitrates, in general, decrease myocardial oxygen demand and consumption. There is also dilatation of the conductance vessels.

Changes in coronary blood flow and myocardial oxygen consumption in response to angiotensin converting enzyme inhibitor captopril, alpha-adrenergic blocking agent prazosin and direct acting vasodilator hydrazaline are illustrated in Figures 12 and 13. Coronary blood flow and myocardial oxygen consumption decrease in response to captopril and prazosin. However, in response to prazosin, coronary blood flow may increase despite a decrease in myocardial oxygen demand suggesting a primary coronary vasodilatory effect of prazosin. In response to hydralazine, coronary blood flow and myocardial oxygen consumption changes in parallel to changes in myocardial oxygen demand. In experimental studies in dogs, intracoronary infusion of ramiprilat, an angiotensin converting

TABLE 8

Effects of commonly used therapies in systolic heart failure on coronary circulation

Angiotensin–converting enzyme inhibitors:	
Decreased myocardial oxygen demand and consumption	
Improved myocardial efficiency	
Primary coronary vasodilatation	
Beta-adrenergic antagonists	
Nebivolol	Decreased myocardial oxygen demand and consumption
	Improved coronary flow reserve
Metoprolol	Improved myocardial energetics
Carvedilol	Decreased oxidative stress
	Improved coronary hemodynamic
Aldosterone antagonists	Not adequately studied in patients
	Has potential to decrease coronary vascular resistance
Hydralazine	Demand mediated changes in coronary blood flow and consumption
	Increased myocardial flow/demand
Nitrates	Decreased myocardial oxygen demand and consumption
Exogenous B-type natriuretic peptides	Primary coronary vasodilatation
	No increase in myocardial oxygen consumption
Beta receptor agonist	Increased myocardial oxygen demand and consumption
	Demand mediated increase in coronary blood flow
Phosphodiesterase inhibitors	Primary coronary vasodilatation
	Decreased coronary vascular resistance
	Increased coronary blood flow
Levosimendan	Primary increase in coronary blood flow
	No increase in myocardial oxygen consumption
Chronic resynchronization	Increased coronary flow reserve
	Increased coronary blood flow

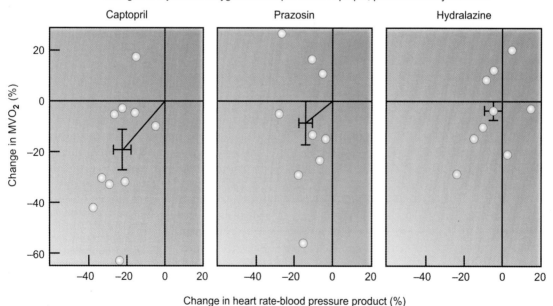

Changes in myocardial oxygen consumption with captopril, prazosin and hydralazine

FIGURE 12: Effect of captopril, an angiotensin converting enzyme inhibitor, prazosin, an alpha-adrenergic blocking agent and hydralazine, a direct acting vasodilator on coronary hemodynamics in patients with systolic heart failure. With captopril and hydralazine changes in myocardial oxygen consumption (MVO$_2$) paralleled to the changes in heart rate blood pressure product indicating demand mediated changes in MVO$_2$. With prazosin, in some patients, there was an increase in MVO$_2$ despite a decrease in heart rate blood pressure product (myocardial oxygen demand)

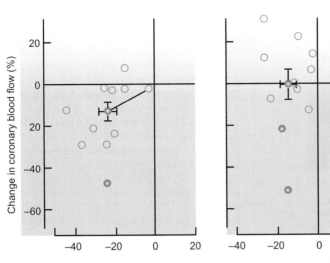
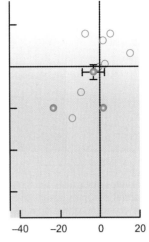

FIGURE 13: Effect of captopril, an angiotensin converting enzyme inhibitor, prazosin, an alpha-adrenergic blocking agent and hydralazine, a direct acting vasodilator on coronary blood flow in patients with systolic heart failure. In response to captopril and hydralazine changes in coronary blood flow paralleled to the changes in heart rate blood pressure product indicating changes in coronary blood flow were primarily demand mediated. In response to prazosin, there was an increase in coronary blood flow despite a decrease in heart rate blood pressure product indicating a direct coronary vasodilatory effect

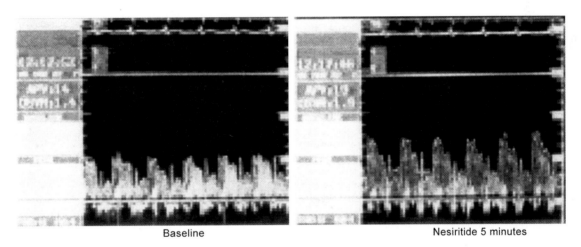

FIGURE 14: Effect of intravenous administration of nesiritide (exogenous BNP) on coronary hemodynamics. Intracoronary Doppler flow studies demonstrate an increase in coronary blood flow (*Source:* Michaeles AD et al. Circulation. 2003;107:2697-701)

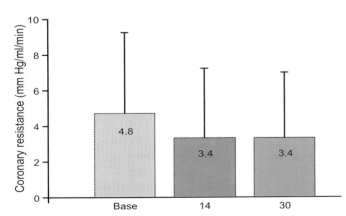

FIGURE 15: Effect of intravenous administration of nesiritide (exogenous BNP) on coronary vascular resistance which decreased indicating coronary vasodilatation (*Source:* Michaeles AD et al. Circulation. 2003;107:2697-701)

enzyme inhibitor is associated with increased coronary blood flow, average peak velocity and coronary artery cross sectional area. This coronary vasodilatory effect of ramiprilat is partially inhibited by nitric oxide synthase inhibitors and by bradykinin inhibitors but not by indomethacin. These findings suggest that coronary vasodilatation by angiotensin converting enzyme inhibitors is partly mediated by nitric oxide and bradykinins but not by prostacyclins.

Intravenous administration of exogenous BNP (B-type natriuretic peptide) is associated with a primary increase in coronary blood flow without an increase in myocardial oxygen consumption (Figs 14 to 16). Beta-receptors agonists increase myocardial oxygen demand and there is demand-related increase in coronary blood flow.

Phosphodiesterase inhibitors cause coronary vasodilatation and a primary increase in coronary blood flow without a significant increase in myocardial oxygen demand.

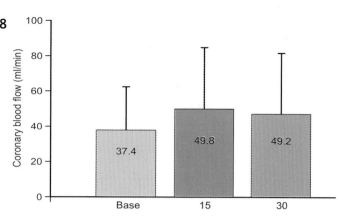

FIGURE 16: Effect of intravenous administration of nesiritide (exogenous BNP) on the epicardial coronary artery diameter which increased indicating dilatation of the coronary conductance vessels (*Source:* Michaeles AD et al. Circulation. 2003;107:2697-701)

The calcium sensitizing agent also causes a primary increase in coronary blood flow without an increase in myocardia oxygen consumption. Chronic resynchronization treatment, usually employed in patients with refractory heart failure, increases coronary flow reserve and coronary blood flow.

REFERENCES

1. Andrew G Wallace. Pathophysiology of cardiovascular disease. In: Smith LH, Their SO (Eds). Pathophysiology: The Biological Principles of Disease. Philadelphia: WB Saunders Co, Publisher; 1981. pp. 1072-86.
2. Feliciano L, Henning RJ. Coronary blood flow: physiologic and pathophysiologic regulation. Clin Cardiol. 1999;2:775-86.
3. Chatterjee K. Effects of dobutamine on coronary hemodynamics and myocardial energetics. In: Kanu Chatterjee (Ed). Dobutamine: A Ten-Year Review. New York: mNCM Publishers Inc.;1989. pp. 49-67.
4. Liu Y, Gutterman DD. Vascular control in humans: focus on the coronary microcirculation. Basic Res Cardiol. 2009;104:211-27.
5. Miller FJ, Dellsperger KC, Gutterman DD. Myogenic vasoconstriction of human coronary arterioles. Am J Physiol. 1997;273:H257-64.
6. Meininger GA, Davis MJ. Cellular mechanisms involved in the vascular myogenic response. Am J Physiol. 1992;263: H647-59.
7. Wang SY, Friedman M, Franklin A, et al. Myogenic reactivity of coronary resistance arteries after cardiopulmonary bypass and hyperkalemic cardioplegia. Circulation. 1995;92:1590-6.
8. Rouleau J, Boerboom LE, Surjadhana A, et al. The role of autoregulation and tissue diastolic pressures in the transmural distribution left ventricular blood flow in anesthetized dogs. Circ Res. 1979;45:804-15.
9. Davis MJ, Wu X, Nurkiewicz TR, et al. Integrins and mechanotransduction of vascular myogenic response. Am J Physiol Heart Circ Physiol. 2001;280:H1427-33.
10. Chilian WM, Kuo L, DeFily DV, et al. Endothelial regulation of coronary microvascular tone under physiological and pathophysiological conditions. Eur Heart J. 1993;14:55-9.
11. Marcus M, Wright C, Doty D, et al. Measurement of coronary velocity and reactive hyperemia in the coronary circulations of humans. Circ Res. 1981;49:877-91.
12. Norwicki PT, Flavahan S, Hassanain H, et al. Redox signaling of the arteriolar myogenic response. Circ Res. 2001;89:114-6.
13. Miura H, Wachtel RE, Loberiza FR, Jr, et al. Flow-induced dilation of human coronary arterioles: important role of Ca^{+2} activated K^+ channels. Circulation. 2001;103:1992-8.
14. Shimookawa H, Morilkawa K. Hydrogen peroxide is an endothelium-derived hyperpolarizing factor in animals and humans. J Mol Cell Cardiol. 2005;39:725-32.
15. Gauthier KM, Deeter C, Krishna UM, et al. 14,15-Epoxyeicosa-5(Z)-enoic acid: a selective epoxyeicsatrienoic acid antagonists that inhibit endothelium-dependent hyperpolarization and relaxation in coronary arteries. Circ Res. 2002;90:1028-36.
16. Mustafa SJ, Morrison RR, Teng B, et al. Adenosine receptors and the heart: role in regulation of coronary blood flow and cardiac electrophysiology. Adenosine Receptors in Health and Disease. Springer Berlin Heidelberg Publishers; 2009. pp. 161-88.
17. Barbato E. Role of adrenergic receptors in human coronary vasomotion. Heart. 2009;95:603-8.
18. Miyashiro JK, Feigl EO. Feedforward control of coronary blood flow via coronary beta-receptor stimulation. Circ Res. 1993;73:252-63.
19. Fen G, de Beer VJ, Hoekstra M, et al. Both beta-1-and beta-2-adrenoreceptors contribute to feed-forward coronary resistance vessel dilation during exercise. Am J Physiol Heart Circ Physiol. 2009, Dec 24 (epub ahead of print).
20. Orlick AE, Ricci DR, Alderman EL, et al. Effects of alpha adrenergic blockade upon coronary hemodynamics. J Clin Invest. 1978;62: 459-67.
21. Ludmer PL, Selwyn AP, Shook TL, et al. Paradoxical vasoconstriction induced by acetylcholine in atherosclerotic coronary arteries. N Engl J Med. 1986;315:1046-51.
22. Gregorini L, Fajadet J, Robert G, et al. Coronary vasoconstriction after percutaneous transluminal coronary angioplasty is attenuated by antiadrenergic agents. Circulation. 1994;90:895-907.
23. Sudhir K, MacGregor JS, Gupta M, et al. Effect of selective angiotensin II receptor antagonism and angiotensin converting enzyme inhibition on the coronary vasculature in vivo: intravascular two-dimensional and Doppler ultrasound studies. Circulation. 1993;87:931-8.
24. Sudhir K, Chou T, Hutchison S, et al. Coronary vasodilation induced by angiotensin-converting enzyme inhibition in vivo: differential contribution of nitric oxide and bradykinin in conductance and resistance arteries. Circulation. 1996;93:1734-9.
25. Garnier A, Bendall JK, Fuchs S, et al. Cardiac specific increase in aldosterone production induces coronary dysfunction in aldosterone synthase-transgenic mice. Circulation. 2004;110:1819-25.
26. Muller S, How OJ, Hermansen SE, et al. Vasopressin impairs brain, heart and kidney perfusion: an experimental study in pigs after transient myocardial ischemia. Critical Care. 2008;12:R20.
27. Kinlay S, Behrendt D, Wainstein M, et al. Role of endothelin-1 in the active constriction of human atherosclerotic coronary arteries. Circulation. 2001;104:1114-8.
28. Wu GF, Wykrzykowska JJ, Rana JS, et al. Effects of B-type natriuretic peptide (nesiritide) on epicardial coronary arteries, systemic vasculature, and microvessels. J Invasive Cardiol. 2008;20:76-80.
29. Larose E, Behrendt D, Kinlay S, et al. Endothelin-1 is a key mediator of coronary vasoconstriction in patients with transplant coronary arteriosclerosis. Circ Heart Fail. 2009;2:409-16.
30. Kyriakides ZS, Kremastinos DT, Bofills E, et al. Endogenous endothelin maintains coronary artery tone by endothelin type A receptor stimulation in patients undergoing coronary arteriography. Heart. 2000;84:176-82.
31. Halcox JP, Nour KR, Zalos G, et al. Coronary vasodilation and improvement in endothelial dysfunction with endothelin ET(A) receptor blockade. Circ Res. 2001;89:969-76.
32. Zellner C, Protter AA, Ko E, et al. Coronary vasodilator effects of BNP: mechanisms of action in coronary conductance and resistance vessels. Am J Physiol: Heart. 1999;276:H1049-57.
33. Michaels AD Klein A, Madden JA, et al. Effects of intravenous nesiritide on human coronary vasomotor regulation and myocardial oxygen uptake. Circulation. 2003;107:2697-701.

34. Hutchison SJ, Chou TM, Chatterjee K, et al. Tamoxifen is an acute, estrogen-like coronary vasodilator of porcine coronary arteries in vitro. J Cardiovasc Pharmacol. 2001;38:657-65.

35. Chou TM, Sudhir K, Hutchison S, et al. Testosterone induces dilation of canine coronary conductance and resistance arteries in vivo. Circulation. 1996;94:2614-9.

36. Sudhir K, Ko E, Zellner C, et al. Physiological concentrations of estradiol attenuate endothelin 1-induced coronary vasoconstriction in vivo. Circulation. 1997;96:3626-32.

37. Jiang C, Sarrel PM, Poole-Wilson PA, et al. Acute effect of 17 beta-estradiol on rabbit coronary artery contractile response to endothelin-1. Am J Physiol: Heart. 1992;263:H271-5.

38. Yue P, Chatterjee K, Beale C, et al. Testosterone relaxes rabbit coronary arteries and aorta. Circulation. 1995;91:1154-60.

39. Schaper W. Collateral vessel growth in the human heart: role of fibroblast growth factor-2. Circulation. 1996;94:600-1.

40. Levine DC. Pathways and functional significance of the coronary collateral circulation. Circulation. 1974;50:831-7.

41. Tayebjee MH, Lip GYH, MacFadyen RJ. Collateralization and the response to obstruction of epicardial coronary arteries. Q J Med. 2004;97:259-72.

42. Piek JJ, van Liebergen RA, Koch KT, et al. Clinical, angiographic and hemodynamic predictors of recruitable collateral flow assessed during balloon angioplasty coronary occlusion. J Am Coll Cardiol. 1997;29:275-82.

43. Pohl T, Seiler C, Billinger M, et al. Frequency distribution of collateral flow and factors influencing collateral channel development. Functional collateral channel measurement in 450 patients with coronary artery disease. J Am Coll Cardiol. 2001;38:1872-8.

44. Foreman BW, Dai XZ, Bache, RJ. Vasoconstriction of coronary collateral vessels with vasopressin limits blood flow to collateral-dependent myocardium during exercise. Circ Res. 1991;69:657-64.

45. Bache RJ, Schwartz JS. Myocardial blood flow during exercise after gradual coronary occlusion in the dog. Am J Physiol Heart. 1983;245:H131-8.

46. Arani DT, Greene DG, Bunnel IL, et al. Reductions in coronary flow under resting conditions in collateral-dependent myocardium of patients with complete occlusion of the left anterior descending coronary artery. J Am Coll Cardiol. 1984;3:668-74.

47. Smith Sc, Gorlin R, Herman MV, et al. Myocardial blood flow in man: effects of coronary collateral circulation and coronary artery bypass surgery. J Clin Invest. 1972;51:2556-65.

48. Goldstein RE, Stinson EB, Scherer JL, et al. Intraoperative coronary collateral function in patients with coronary occlusive disease: nitroglycerin responsiveness and angiographic correlations. Circulation. 1974;49:298-308.

49. Frank MW, Harris KR, Ahlin KA, et al. Endothelium-derived relaxing factor (nitric oxide) has atonic vasodilating action on coronary collateral vessels. J Am Coll Cardiol. 1996;27:658-63.

50. Traverse JH, Kinn JW, Klassen C, et al. Nitric oxide inhibition impairs blood flow during exercise in hearts with a collateral-dependent myocardial region. J Am Coll Cardiol. 1998;31:67-74.

51. Kinn JW, Bache RJ. Effect of platelet activation on collateral blood flow. Circulation. 1998;98:1431-7.

52. Feldman RD, Christy JP, Paul ST, et al. Beta-adrenergic receptors on canine collateral vessels: characterization and function. Am J Physiol Heart. 1989;257:H1634-9.

53. Traverse JH, Altman JD, Kinn J, et al. Effect of beta-adrenergic receptor blockade on blood flow to collateral dependent myocardium during exercise. Circulation. 1995;91:1560-7.

54. Fujita M, Ikemoto M, Kishihita M, et al. Elevated basic fibroblast growth factor in pericardial fluid of patients with unstable angina. Circulation. 1996;94:610-3.

55. Fleisch M, Billinger M, Eberli FR, et al. Physiologically assessed coronary collateral flow and intracoronary growth factor concentrations in patients with 1- to 3-vessel coronary artery disease. Circulation. 1999;100:1945-50.

56. Cheirif J, Narkiewicz-Jodko JB, Hawkins HK, et al. Myocardial contrast echocardiography: relation of collateral perfusion to extent of injury and severity of contractile dysfunction in a canine model of coronary thrombosis and reperfusion. J Am Coll Cardiol. 1995;26:537-46.

57. Nicolau JC, Pinto MA, Nogueira PR, et al. The role of antegrade and collateral flow in relation to left ventricular function post-thrombolysis. Int J Cardiol. 1997;61:47-54.

58. Elsman P, van't Hof AWJ, de Boer MJ, et al. Zwolle Myocardial Infarction Study Group. Role of collateral circulation in the acute phase of ST-segment-elevation myocardial infarction treated with primary coronary intervention. Eur Heart J. 2004;25:854-8.

59. Motz W, Vogt M, Scheler S, et al. Coronary circulation in arterial hypertension. J Cardiovasc Pharmacol. 1991; 17:S35-9.

60. Hoeing MR, Bianchi C, Rosenzweig A, et al. The cardiac microvasculature in hypertension, cardiac hypertrophy and diastolic heart failure. Curr Vasc Pharmacol. 2008;6:292-300.

61. Levy AS, Chung JC, Kroetsch JT, et al. Nitric oxide and coronary vascular endothelium adaptations in hypertension. Vasc Health Risk Manag. 2009;5:1075-87.

62. Egashira K, Suzki S, Hirooka Y, et al. Impaired endothelium-dependent vasodilation of large epicardial and resistance coronary arteries in patients with essential hypertension. Different responses to acetylcholine and substance P. Hypertension. 1995;25:201-6.

63. Quyyumi AA, Mulcahy D, Andrews NP, et al. Coronary vascular nitric oxide activity in hypertension and hypercholesterolemia. Comparison of acetylcholine and substance P. Circulation. 1997;95:104-10.

64. Bezante GP, Viazzi F, Leoncini G, et al. Coronary flow reserve is impaired in hypertensive patients with subclinical renal damage. Am J Hypertens. 2009;22:191-6.

65. Strauer BE. Significance of coronary circulation in hypertensive heart disease for development and prevention of heart failure. Am J Cardiol. 1990;65:34G-41G.

66. Nemes A, Forster T, Csanády M. Simultaneous echocardiographic evaluation of coronary flow velocity reserve and aortic distensibility indices in hypertension. Heart Vessels. 2007;22:73-8.

67. Remert JC, Kleinman LH, Fedor JM, et al. Myocardial blood flow distribution in concentric left ventricular hypertrophy. J Clin Invest. 1978;62:379-86.

68. Sekiya M, Funada J, Suzuki J, et al. The influence of left ventricular geometry on coronary vasomotion in patients with essential hypertension. Am J Hypertens. 2000;13:789-95.

69. Vatner SF, Shannon R, Hittinger L. Reduced subendocardial coronary reserve. A potential mechanism for impaired diastolic function in hypertrophied and failing heart. Circulation. 1990;81:III8-14.

70. Parodi O, Sambuceti G. The role of coronary microvascular dysfunction in the genesis of cardiovascular diseases. Q J Nucl Med. 1996;40:9-16.

71. Miyagawa S, Masai T, Fukuda H, et al. Coronary microcirculatory dysfunction in aortic stenosis: myocardial contrast echocardiography study. Ann Thorac Surg. 2009;87:715-9.

72. Bertrand ME, LaBlanche JM, Tilmant PY, et al. Coronary sinus blood flow at rest and during isometric exercise in patients with aortic valve disease. Mechanisms of angina pectoris in presence of normal coronary arteries. Am J Cardiol. 1981;47:199-205.

73. Garcia D, Camici PG, Durand LG, et al. Impairment of coronary flow reservation in aortic stenosis. J Appl Physiol. 2009;106:113-21.

74. Julius BK, Spillmann M, Vassalli G, et al. Angina pectoris in patients with aortic stenosis and normal coronary arteries. Mechanisms and pathophysiological concepts. Circulation. 1997;95:892-8.

75. Rajappan K, Rimoldi OE, Dutka DP, et al. Mechanisms of coronary microcirculatory dysfunction in patients with aortic stenosis and angiographically normal coronary arteries. Circulation. 2002;105:470-6.

76. Galiuto L, Lotrionte M, Crea F, et al. Impaired coronary and myocardial flow in severe aortic stenosis is associated with increased apoptosis: a transthoracic Doppler and myocardial contrast echocardiography study. Heart. 2006;92:208-12.

77. Nemes A, Balázs E, Csanády M, et al. Long-term prognostic role of coronary flow velocity reserve in patients with aortic valve stenosis—Insights from the SZEGED Study. Clin Physiol Funct Imaging. 2009;29:447-52.

78. Ben-Dor I, Goldstein SA, Waksman R, et al. Effects of percutaneous aortic valve replacement on coronary blood flow assessed with transesophageal Doppler echocardiography in patients with severe aortic stenosis. Am J Cardiol. 2009;104:850-5.

79. Bozbas H, Pirat B, Yidirir A, et al. Coronary flow reserve is impaired in patients with aortic valve calcification. Atherosclerosis. 2008;197:846-52.

80. Gascho JA, Mueller TM, Easthan C, et al. Effect of volume-overload hypertrophy on the coronary circulation awake dogs. Cardiovasc Res. 1982;16:288-92.

81. Cannon RO III, Rosing DR, Maron BJ, et al. Myocardial ischemia in patients with hypertrophic cardiomyopathy: contribution of inadequate vasodilator reserve and elevated left ventricular filling pressures. Circulation. 1985;71:234-43.

82. Camici PG, Chiriatti G, Lorenzoni R, et al. Coronary vasodilation is impaired in both hypertrophied and non-hypertrophied myocardium of patients of patients with hypertrophic cardiomyopathy: a study with nitrogen-13 ammonia and positron emission tomography. J Am Coll Cardiol. 1991;17:879-86.

83. Olivotto I, Cecchi F, Gistri R, et al. Relevance of coronary microvascular flow impairment to long-term remodeling and systolic dysfunction in hypertrophic cardiomyopathy. J Am Coll Cardiol. 2006;47: 1043-8.

84. Cortigiani L, Rigo F, Gherardi S, et al. Prognostic implications of coronary flow reserve on left anterior descending coronary artery in hypertrophic cardiomyopathy. Am J Cardiol. 2008;102:1718-23.

85. Cannon RO III, Dilsizian V, O'Gara PT, et al. Myocardial metabolic, hemodynamic, and electrocardiographic significance of reversible thallium-201 abnormalities in hypertrophic cardiomyopathy. Circulation. 1991;83:1660-7.

86. Olivotto I, Cecchi F, Camici PG. Coronary microvascular dysfunction and ischemia in hypertrophic cardiomyopathy. Mechanisms and clinical consequences. Ital Heart J. 2004;5:572-80.

87. Pedrinelli R, Spessot M, Chiriatti G, et al. Evidence for a systemic defect of resistance-sized arterioles in hypertrophic cardiomyopathy. Coron Artery Dis. 1993;4:67-72.

88. Petersen SE, Jerosch-Herold M, Hudsmith LE, et al. Evidence for microvascular dysfunction in hypertrophic cardiomyopathy: new insights from multiparametric magnetic resonance imaging. Circulation. 2007;115:2418-25.

89. Nemes A, Balázas E, Soliman OI, et al. Long-term prognostic value of coronary flow velocity reserve in patients with hypertrophic cardiomyopathy: 9-year follow-up results from SZEGED study. Heart Vessels. 2009;24:352-6.

90. Jaber WA, Yang EH, Nishimura RA, et al. Immediate improvement in coronary flow reserve after alcohol septal ablation in patients with hypertrophic obstructive cardiomyopathy. Heart. 2009;95:564-9.

91. Sekine T, Daimon M, Hasegawa R, et al. Cibenzoline improves coronary flow velocity reserve in patients with hypertrophic cardiomyopathy. Heart Vessels. 2006;21:350-5.

92. von Restorff W, Höfling B, Holtz J, et al. Effect of increased blood fluidity through hemodilution on coronary circulation at rest and during exercise in dogs. Pflugers Arch. 1975;357:15-24.

93. Iltis I, Kober F, Desrois M, et al. Defective myocardial blood flow and altered function of the left ventricle in type 2 diabetic rats: a noninvasive in vivo study using perfusion and cine magnetic resonance imaging. Invest Radiol. 2005;40:19-26.

94. Di Carli MF, Jainisse J, Grunberger G, et al. Role of chronic hyperglycemia in the pathogenesis of coronary microvascular dysfunction in diabetes. J Am Coll Cardiol. 2003;16:1387-93.

95. Strauer BE, Motz W, Vogt M, et al. Evidence for reduced coronary flow reserve in patients with insulin dependent diabetes. A possible cause for diabetic heart disease in man. Exp Clin Endocrinol Diabetes. 1997;105:15-20.

96. Hori T, Matsubara T, Ishibashi T, et al. Decrease of nitric oxide end-products during coronary circulation reflects elevated basal coronary artery tone in patients with vasospastic angina. Jpn Heart J. 2000;41:583-95.

97. Kuga T, Egashira K, Mohri M, et al. Bradykinin-induced vasodilation is impaired at the atherosclerotic site but preserved at the spastic site of human coronary arteries in vivo. Circulation. 1995;92:183-9.

98. Yamada T, Okamoto M, Sueda T, et al. Response of conductance and resistance vessels of the coronary artery to intracoronary isosorbide dinitrate in patients with variant angina. Intern Med. 1996;35:844-8.

99. Lanza GA. Cardiac syndrome X: a critical overview and future perspectives. Heart. 2007;93:159-66.

100. Maseri A, Crea F, Kaski JC, et al. Mechanism of angina pectoris in syndrome X. J Am Coll Cardiol. 1991;17:499-506.

101. Cannon RO III. Microvascular angina and the continuing dilemma of chest pain with normal coronary angiograms. J Am Coll Cardiol. 2009;54:877-85.

102. Bottcher M, Botker He, Sonne H, et al. Endothelium-dependent and -independent perfusion reserve and the effect of L-arginine on myocardial perfusion in patients with syndrome X. Circulation. 1999;99:1795-801.

103. Chauhan A, Mullins PA, Taylor G, et al. Both endothelium-dependent and -independent function is impaired in patients with angina pectoris and normal coronary angiograms. Eur Heart J. 1997;18:60-8.

104. Cannon RO, Epstein SE. Microvascular angina as a cause of chest pain with angiographically normal coronary arteries. Am J Cardiol. 1988;61:1338-43.

105. Chauhan A, Mullins PA, Taylor G, et al. Effect of hyperventilation and mental stress on coronary blood flow in syndrome X. Br Heart J. 1993;69:516-24.

106. Di Monaco A, Bruno I, Sestito A, et al. Cardiac adrenergic nerve function and microvascular dysfunction in patients with cardiac syndrome X. Heart. 2009;95:550-4.

107. Yabe Y, Morishita T. Systemic and coronary hemodynamic effects of beta-adrenoreceptor blocking agents in coronary artery disease. Jpn Heart J. 1987;28:675-86.

108. Katzung BG, Chatterjee K. Vasodilators and the treatment of angina pectoris. In: Katzung BG (Ed). Basic and Clinical Pharmacology, 10th edn. New York: McGraw Hill Lange Publishers; 2007. pp. 183-97.

109. Rouleau J-L, Chatterjee K, Ports TA, et al. Mechanism of relief of pacing-induced angina with oral verapamil: reduced oxygen demand. Circulation. 1983;67:94-100.

110. Kramer PH, Chatterjee K, Schwartz A, et al. Alterations in angina threshold with nifedipine during pacing induced angina. Br Heart J. 1984;52:308-13.

111. Venkataraman R, Belardinelli L, Blackburn B, et al. A study of the effects of ranolazine using automated quantitative analysis of serial myocardial perfusion images. JACC Cardiovasc Imaging. 2009;2: 1301-9.

112. Chatterjee K. Coronary hemodynamics in heart failure and effects of therapeutic interventions. J Cardiac Fail. 2009;15:116-23.

113. Parodi O, De Maria R, Oltrona L, et al. Myocardial blood flow distribution in patients with ischemic heart disease or dilated cardiomyopathy undergoing heart transplantation. Circulation. 1993;88:509-22.

114. Traverse JH, Chen YJ, Crampton M, et al. Increased extravascular forces limit endothelium-dependent and -independent coronary vasodilation in congestive heart failure. Cardiovasc Res. 2001;52: 454-61.

115. Dini FL, Ghiadoni L, Conti U, et al. Coronary flow reserve in idiopathic dilated cardiomyopathy: relation with left ventricular wall stress, natriuretic peptides and endothelial dysfunction. J Am Soc Echocardiogr. 2009;22:354-60.

116. Neglia D, De Caterina A, Marraccini P, et al. Impaired myocardial metabolic reserve and substrate selection flexibility during stress in patients with idiopathic dilated cardiomyopathy. Am J Physiol Heart. 2007;293:H3270-8.

Section 2

CARDIOVASCULAR PHARMACOLOGY

Chapter 4

Diuretics

Michael E Ernst

Chapter Outline

- Normal Renal Solute Handling
- History and Classification of the Diuretic Compounds
- Clinical Pharmacology of the Diuretic Compounds
  - General Pharmacokinetic and Pharmacodynamic Principles
- Adaptive Responses to Diuretic Administration
- Individual Diuretic Classes

- Carbonic Anhydrase Inhibitors
- Loop or High-ceiling Diuretics
- Thiazide and the Thiazide-like Diuretics
- Potassium-sparing Diuretics
- Clinical use of Diuretics in Cardiovascular Diseases
  - Diuretic Use in Hypertension
  - Diuretic Use in Edematous Disorders
- Adverse Effects of Diuretics

INTRODUCTION

The era of modern diuretic therapy in cardiovascular disease emerged in the late 1950s with the development of effective oral agents with improved tolerability. Until then, the only diuretics available had been intravenous or intramuscular mercurial derivatives, limited by difficulty in use and an unfavorable toxicity profile.

Today, the diuretic compounds are recognized as powerful tools that impair sodium reabsorption in the renal tubules. In doing so, they increase the fractional excretion of sodium, affect the rate of urine formation and alter long-term sodium balance. These are desirable therapeutic approaches for treating a variety of conditions involving abnormal fluid and electrolyte balance. After more than 50 years in clinical use, diuretics remain of considerable importance in the management of cardiovascular diseases. Diuretics have uses other than in hypertension and edematous disorders, such as in the treatment of hypercalcemia, diabetes insipidus, glaucoma and cerebral edema. This chapter will focus primarily on the pharmacology and clinical use of diuretics in the cardiovascular patient.

NORMAL RENAL SOLUTE HANDLING

Under conditions of normal physiology and sodium intake, nearly 100% of the sodium load is filtered through the glomerulus and progressively reabsorbed throughout different segments of the nephron, the basic urine-forming unit of the kidney. Each anatomic segment is highly specialized in function and the mechanism of action of each diuretic agent is best understood appreciating the relationship of both its site of action in the nephron and the normal physiology of the involved segment.

Reabsorption of sodium occurring throughout the nephron is controlled through the Na^+/K^+-ATPase pump located in the basolateral membrane of tubular epithelial cells. This pump is responsible for moving sodium from the cell into the interstitium and blood, and potassium from interstitium to cell, a process that maintains the cell interior in an electrically negative state in relation to the extracellular fluid.[1] The resulting electro-chemical gradient drives sodium intracellularly across the apical membrane, a process accomplished through specific transport pathways of the luminal membrane which are unique between various segments of the nephron. As the sodium load passes through these segments, movement of sodium down the electrochemical gradient, from lumen to tubular cells and to interstitium, is coupled by movement of water and other solutes against or in parallel to their electrochemical gradient.[1]

In the absence of a specific pharmacologic intervention, up to 90% of the filtered load of sodium is reabsorbed in upstream segments of the nephron, primarily in the proximal tubule (65–70%) via a carbonic anhydrase pathway. An additional 20–30% is reabsorbed in the next segment, the loop of Henle, regulated by a $Na^+/K^+/2Cl^-$ exchange symporter. Reabsorption of the remaining filtered sodium reaching the distal segments, approximately 5%, is mediated through the Na^+/Cl^- exchange symporter.[2] The combined effects of these segments serve to tightly regulate the overall physiologic handling of sodium, achieving a remarkable consistently low sodium excretion despite fluctuations in the amounts ingested.

HISTORY AND CLASSIFICATION OF THE DIURETIC COMPOUNDS

A chance discovery in 1937 that the antibiotic, sulfanilamide, caused a mild diuresis accompanied by a metabolic acidosis,

54 presented an important finding which suggested that oral diuretic therapy might, in fact, be conceivable.[2] Shortly thereafter, the mechanism of sulfanilamide's diuretic and acidotic effects was determined to result from inhibition of carbonic anhydrase in the proximal tubule.[3] In hopes of developing an oral agent with improved diuretic efficacy, researchers quickly synthesized and screened numerous compounds for greater potency and specificity as inhibitors of carbonic anhydrase. In the process, chlorothiazide, both sulfonamide and a carbonic anhydrase inhibitor was discovered; however, unlike other carbonic anhydrase inhibitors, it unexpectedly increased chloride rather than bicarbonate excretion.[2] This key finding prompted the realization that sites other than the proximal tubule could also be pharmacologically targeted and eventually led to the development of the thiazides and other diuretic agents still in primary therapeutic use today.

Modern diuretic compounds are now viewed as a heterogeneous class of drugs that differ remarkably in several aspects, including their chemical derivation, mechanism and therapeutic efficacy. As the amount of sodium reabsorbed varies between the different segments of the nephron, the site of action, natriuretic and therapeutic efficacy, and ultimately the specific clinical indication of each class of diuretic is determined by the specific tubular ion transport systems with which they interfere.

The most common and clinically useful classification of diuretics is to group them into one of several categories on the basis of the primary site of their interference with sodium reabsorption (Fig. 1):

- Carbonic anhydrase inhibitors (e.g. acetazolamide), acting in the proximal tubule
- High-ceiling or "loop" diuretics (e.g. furosemide, bumetanide, torsemide), acting in thick ascending limb of the loop of Henle
- Thiazide and thiazide-like diuretics (e.g. hydrochlorothiazide, chlorthalidone, metolazone, indapamide) acting in the early portion of the distal convoluted tubule
- A fourth category, which are primarily utilized for their potassium-sparing capabilities, can further be subclassified into the sodium channel blockers (e.g. amiloride, triamterene) and the mineralocorticoid antagonists (e.g. spironolactone, eplerenone). These agents act in the late distal tubule and collecting duct.
- A final category of diuretics, the osmotic agents (e.g. mannitol), interfere with sodium reabsorption throughout all segments of the nephron by creating an osmotic force throughout the length of the renal tubule.

Distinguishing the diuretic compounds according to their primary site of action is important, as their therapeutic efficacy

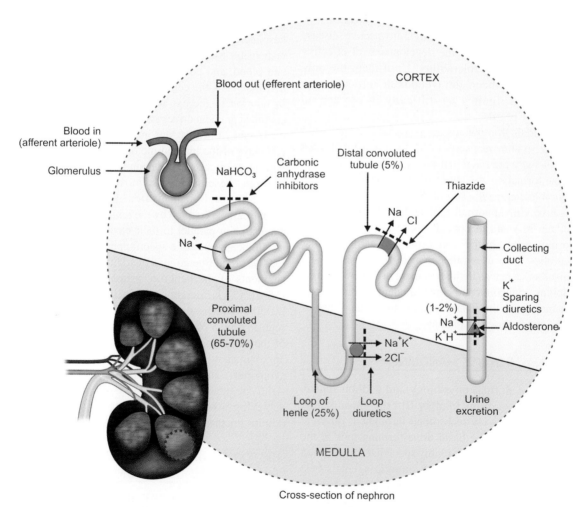

FIGURE 1: Diuretic sites of action in the nephron (Na^+: Sodium; Cl^-: Chloride; K: Potassium; $NaHCO_3$: Sodium bicarbonate; numbers in parentheses reflect the relative percentage of the sodium load reabsorbed in that segment)

TABLE 1

Characteristics of diuretics: classification, site and mechanism of action, clinical uses

Diuretic classification	Major site of action	Enzyme/Channel inhibited	Maximum effect (% of filtered sodium load)	Clinical uses
Carbonic anhydrase inhibitors	Proximal tubule	Carbonic anhydrase	3–5	Glaucoma, metabolic alkalosis, high altitude sickness
High-ceiling or Loops	Thick ascending limb of loop of Henle	$Na^+/K^+/2Cl^-$ symporter	20–25	Edematous disorders (congestive heart failure, cirrhosis, nephrotic syndrome), renal insufficiency, hypertension in kidney disease
Thiazide and Thiazide-like*	Early distal convoluted tubule	Na^+/Cl^- symporter	5–8	Hypertension, hypercalciuria, diabetes insipidus, pseudohypoaldosteronism type 2 (Gordon's syndrome)
Potassium-Sparing	Cortical collecting duct		2–3	
Pteridine derivatives		Epithelial sodium channel		Pseudoaldosteronism (Liddle syndrome), thiazide or loop diuretic-induced hypokalemia or hypomagnesemia
Aldosterone receptor antagonists		Aldosterone receptor		Primary and secondary aldosteronism, congestive heart failure, hyperandrogen states, thiazide or loop diuretic-induced hypokalemia or hypomagnesemia, resistant hypertension (independent of primary aldosteronism), Barrter syndrome
Osmotic agents	Multiple segments	Sugar acts as non-absorbable solute		Cerebral edema, intracranial hypertension

*The terms *thiazide* and *thiazide-like* are used to group thiazides based on the presence of a benzothiadiazine molecular structure. *Thiazide-like* diuretics lack the benzothiadiazine structure but share a similar mechanism of action.
(*Source:* Reference 4)

and primary clinical indications are not completely interchangeable (Table 1). Recognizing their sites of action also provides an avenue for additive effects that can be obtained when the different classes of diuretics are used in combination (i.e. "sequential nephron blockade") in certain types of patients.[4]

CLINICAL PHARMACOLOGY OF THE DIURETIC COMPOUNDS

GENERAL PHARMACOKINETIC AND PHARMACODYNAMIC PRINCIPLES

Some generalizations can be made about the pharmacology of the diuretics, despite heterogeneity by class and agent. At physiologic pH, diuretics are either organic anions (loops and thiazides) or cations (amiloride and triamterene). All diuretics, except mannitol, are highly protein bound, which limits filtration at the glomerulus and traps the diuretic in the vascular space; therefore, they must be actively secreted into the proximal tubule lumen to exert their effect. Active transport into the lumen occurs via an organic acid secretory pathway for the carbonic anhydrase inhibitors, loops and thiazides, and a parallel pathway for organic bases. Mannitol and spironolactone are exceptions; mannitol is freely filtered at the glomerulus and passes through the nephron, acting as a nonreabsorbable solute drawing water along with it, while

spironolactone (although protein-bound) enters the renal tubules from plasma by competitively inhibiting the binding of aldosterone to the mineralocorticoid receptor at the basolateral surface.[4]

For the most part, diuretics have direct actions that are site-specific, acting on one or another of the tubular segments but not all of them. A few agents maintain a degree of secondary activity at another segment (e.g. some thiazides also inhibit carbonic anhydrase), but it is generally considered an irrelevant contribution to their overall therapeutic effect. This is because diuretic action at one site induces important adaptive changes in other segments of the kidney that attempt to preserve sodium, thereby minimizing the contribution of any secondary site of action to the overall natriuretic effect.

As diuretics are a heterogeneous class, discussion of their pharmacodynamics must occur in the context of distinguishing the features that constitute a clinically relevant response. In general, the desired response is to obtain some meaningful level of natriuresis, which can either correspond to a significant diuresis and reduction in extracellular volume as in the case of loop diuretics to relieve edematous states or a more prolonged low-level diuresis which reduces systemic vascular resistance and lowers blood pressure, as in the use of thiazides for hypertension. Regardless of the indication for use and desired effect, the pharmacodynamic characteristics of diuretics are influenced by a number of factors. Most importantly, a threshold quantity of the drug must be achieved at the site of action before a clinically relevant response can be obtained.[5] When administered intravenously, bioavailability issues are not present; however, when given orally, diuretic response will be influenced by the rate and extent of absorption which can be highly variable among diuretic compounds and individual patients. The best index approximating diuretic drug delivery to the intraluminal site of action is its urinary excretion rate, as this corresponds to the observed natriuretic response.[5] This relationship exists for both loops and thiazides (although shallower for thiazides) and can be illustrated using a typical sigmoidal curve (Fig. 2) where the critical determinants are basal response, dose causing 50% response, upper asymptote (maximal response) and slope.

The plasma half-life of a diuretic governs both its expected duration of action and dosing frequency. Loop diuretics have very short half-lives and must be dosed multiple times per day, while thiazides and other distally acting diuretics have half-lives that are sufficient for them to be dosed once or twice daily. Empiric dosing of diuretics is generally based on expected population responses, but considering the pharmacodynamic relationship illustrated in Figure 2, diuretic dosing can be individualized to find the dose that delivers enough drug to the site of action to reach the steep portion of the dose-response curve as well as the lowest dose eliciting a maximal response. In normal subjects, there is a little need for such tailoring. One merely selects a typical starting dose and, if necessary, adjusts upward or downward based on the intended response. For thiazides (with a shallower dose/response curve) in the treatment of hypertension, this will be a limited range of 12.5–50 mg/day of hydrochlorothiazide or its equivalent. For loops, where more appreciable volume contraction and diuresis are desired, a starting intravenous dose of 40 mg of furosemide or its equivalent generally results in a maximal excretion of 200–250 mmol sodium in 3–4 liters of urine over 3–4 hours.[5]

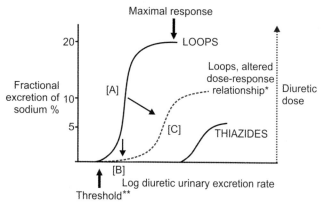

FIGURE 2: Pharmacodynamic illustration of the relationship between diuretic dose and response (adapted from reference 10)
* Nephrotic syndrome, congestive heart failure, cirrhosis
** Determinants of diuretic threshold and efficacy include: dose, bioavailability; tubular secretory capacity rate of absorption and time course of delivery. After identifying the threshold dose to achieve effect, a higher diuretic concentration [A] leads to significant natriuresis. When severe sodium retention occurs or sodium intake is reduced, the curve shifts to the right and the previous diuretic serum concentration achieved by the dose in [A] is no longer effective [B]. The dose of the diuretic must be increased to achieve clinically effective natriuresis [C]. Increasing the frequency of doses has no effect on sodium excretion as long as each dose is below the threshold

Under conditions of normal health, the maximal natriuretic response will be the same for all diuretic agents within a class, in any one patient. Once the diuretic threshold is met (as depicted in Figure 2), there is an optimal rate of delivery leading to maximal response, above which additional diuretic delivery does not result in greater diuresis. Several conditions may distort this diuretic dose-response relationship, such as congestive heart failure, cirrhosis and nephrotic syndrome, shifting the curve downward and to the right.[5] In such conditions, it becomes more important for the dose of the diuretic to be sequentially titrated in the individual to determine the dose that will deliver enough drug to the site of action to reach the steep portion of the curve and elicit the intended response. Such tailoring in these situations allows one to obtain a maximal response using the lowest effective dose, thereby minimizing unnecessary risks associated with more arbitrarily selected higher doses.

ADAPTIVE RESPONSES TO DIURETIC ADMINISTRATION

The "braking" phenomenon is a term, commonly used to refer to the short-term and long-term adaptive changes observed in the nephron as a result of diuretic administration. These changes are natural compensations intended to protect intravascular volume. Their net result is to stabilize volume losses that lead to the tolerance of the diuretic effect. Diuretic tolerance should be distinguished clinically from diuretic resistance states, the latter describing a phenomenon occurring in conjunction with pathophysiologic conditions such as renal failure, nephrotic syndrome, congestive heart failure and cirrhosis.[5] The mechanism of resistance in the setting of these comorbidities is more aptly explained by altered pharmacokinetics and pharmacodynamics rather than physiologic adaptations.

Two concepts are fundamental for understanding the adaptations to diuretic administration. First, because the various segments of the nephron are arranged in a series, a change in behavior of one segment, such as that induced by a diuretic, alters conditions for the downstream segments. For example, administration of a loop diuretic will cause more solute to be delivered to the distal segment. Chronic exposure to this higher solute load leads to structural hypertrophy of the distal segment, which enhances its overall resorptive capacity.[6] Secondly, diuretic-induced diminution of extracellular fluid stimulates hemodynamic, neural and endocrine mechanisms designed to conserve water and solutes. The sum of these conservative mechanisms results in increased reabsorption of salt and water at sites proximal and distal to the site of action of the administered diuretic, thereby limiting the overall amount of diuresis. A practical example of this can be seen in the normal subject, where administration of a diuretic results in an appreciable diuresis on the first day, less on the second day and essentially no effect on the third day.

Short-term tolerance to diuretics stems from a period of post-dose sodium retention, triggered by the initial reduction in extracellular fluid volume. Generally short plasma half-lives of most diuretics contribute to this mechanism.[7] Although the phenomenon is classically observed with the shorter-acting loop diuretics, it also applies to thiazides. Ordinarily, an initial diuretic-induced diuresis results in a net negative sodium balance.[8] However, in the absence of continuous infusion, the diuretic effect dissipates before the next dose is administered. A period of rebound sodium retention follows when the drug concentration in plasma and tubular fluid declines below the diuretic threshold. Using furosemide as an example, the brisk natriuresis resulting in a negative sodium balance for six hours after the initial dose is followed by a compensatory 18-hour post-diuresis sodium retention period in which sodium excretion is reduced to a level lower than intake.[8] The degree of sodium retention may be of sufficient magnitude to nullify prior natriuresis, such that within a matter of days in nonedematous patients, weight loss is limited to 1–2 kg.[9] Dosing intervals for diuretics should generally exceed the duration of time when effective amounts of the drug are at the site of action, in order to avoid or limit this post-dose antinatriuresis period.

Short-term adaptations to diuretics are not explained solely by limitations imposed by their pharmacokinetic parameters or dosing strategies. Important contributors to the short-term adaptations also include activation of the renin-angiotensin-aldosterone (RAAS) and sympathetic nervous systems, suppression of atrial natriuretic peptide secretion and suppression of renal prostaglandin secretion.[10] The degree of post-dose sodium retention is significantly influenced by dietary sodium intake. Restriction of dietary sodium promotes overall negative sodium balance and enhances the therapeutic response to diuretics, while persistently high-dietary sodium offsets this effect by leading to net neutral salt balance.[11] Stated another way, the more sodium ingested, the more frequent is the need for the diuretic.[4]

Long-term diuretic tolerance is marked by a gradual return of sodium chloride balance to neutral. Many of the same mediators involved in post-diuretic sodium retention are also responsible for the chronic adaptations. Persistent volume removal triggers chronic activation of the RAAS-system and increases circulating angiotensin-II and aldosterone levels, both of which promote increased sodium reabsorption in the proximal and distal tubules. Interestingly, administration of α-adrenergic antagonists and RAAS-blockers do not appear to appreciably modify these processes.[12] This finding likely suggests the involvement of volume-independent mechanisms.[13,14] Such mechanisms include structural hypertrophy of distal nephron segments which enhances distal sodium reabsorption (occurring in response to long-term loop administration) as well as upregulation of sodium transporters downstream from the primary site of diuretic action.[6] For thiazides, micropuncture studies have shown that persistent volume contraction also leads to increased proximal solute reabsorption, limiting the overall delivery of sodium and chloride to the primary thiazide site at the distal tubule.[15]

INDIVIDUAL DIURETIC CLASSES

CARBONIC ANHYDRASE INHIBITORS

Carbonic anhydrase catalyzes the hydration of bicarbonate in the proximal tubule; thereby facilitating its reabsorption.[4] Normally sodium reabsorption accompanies bicarbonate in this process. Inhibitors of carbonic anhydrase (Table 1) interfere with this enzyme activity in the brush border and inside the epithelial cells of the proximal tubule, resulting in impaired sodium,

bicarbonate and water reabsorption, as well as a brisk alkaline diuresis. As the majority of the filtered sodium load is reabsorbed in the proximal tubule, one would ordinarily expect a proximally acting agent to produce a substantial diuretic response. However, the net diuretic effect of carbonic anhydrase inhibitors is limited because sodium that is reabsorbed distal to the proximal tubule (mainly in the thick ascending limb of the loop of Henle) offsets these losses.

Additionally, the kidney compensates in several ways which serve to diminish the overall carbonic anhydrase-dependent component of sodium reabsorption. Sodium rejected proximally increases its delivery to the macula densa which activates the tubuloglomerular feedback mechanism, suppressing the glomerular filtration rate and amount of solutes filtered. Furthermore, the alkaline diuresis caused by the carbonic anhydrase inhibitor reduces bicarbonate levels in the serum, which results in overall less bicarbonate filtration.[1]

Acetazolamide (Table 2) demonstrates the most favorable diuretic features among several chemical derivatives of sulfanilamide that were synthesized while searching for more potent carbonic anhydrase inhibitors. Developed in 1945, it remains the prototype in the class, although it is now rarely used because of its nominal diuretic capabilities and the development of metabolic acidosis occurring with prolonged administration. Acetazolamide is completely absorbed orally, with a half-life of about 6–9 hours, reaching steady state after two days. It can be dosed twice daily. It is entirely renally excreted and should be used carefully, if at all, in those with compromised renal function.[4]

Acetazolamide's diuretic legacy is primarily one of historical significance in having helped elucidate the process of urinary acidification and diuresis in renal tubules rather than in any major clinical application in cardiovascular disease. Rarely, a case can be made for a minor role in heart failure patients which are refractory to loop diuretics, where proximal tubular reabsorption of sodium is increased and less sodium overall is delivered to the loop of Henle. The addition of acetazolamide can increase diuresis in some of these patients.[16]

Today, the primary uses of acetazolamide are not directly related to its diuretic action, but rather in the systemic metabolic acidosis induced as a byproduct. This can be helpful in remedying iatrogenic metabolic alkalosis occasionally caused by high doses of loop diuretics (typically in patients with cardiogenic pulmonary edema). Metabolic alkalosis can result in hypoventilation, a reflex designed to raise blood carbon dioxide concentrations to correct the systemic pH. In some patients, such as those with chronic obstructive pulmonary disease, this hypoventilation may compromise respiratory drive and lead to further hypoxemia.[4] Correcting alkalosis in these situations may improve oxygenation.[17]

Additionally, other clinical applications of acetazolamide involve carbonic anhydrase-dependent bicarbonate transport occurring outside the kidney. As carbonic anhydrase is involved in intraocular fluid formation, acetazolamide and its derivatives can be used to decrease intraocular pressure in patients with glaucoma. Acetazolamide has also proven effective in treatment and prophylaxis of acute mountain sickness. The exact mechanism is unknown, but is perhaps related to the iatrogenic metabolic acidosis induced by the drug.

TABLE 2

Approximate pharmacokinetic parameters of the commonly available diuretics

Diuretic class	Oral bio-availability (%)	Vd (L/kg)	Protein binding (%)	Fate	$T_{1/2}$ (hr) (normal)	Duration of action (hr)* (normal)	Additional notes
Carbonic Anhydrase Inhibitors							
Acetazolamide	100	0.2	70–90	R (100%)	6–9	8–12	Metabolic acidosis with prolonged use
Thiazide-type							
Chlorothiazide	15–30	1	70	R (100%)	1.5–2.5	6–12	Rarely used anymore
Hydrochlorothiazide	60–70	2.5	40	R (100%)	3–10	6–12	Increased absorption with food
Bendroflumethiazide	90	1–1.5	94	R (30%), M (70%)	2–5	18–24	Primarily used outside the US
Thiazide-like							
Chlorthalidone	65	3–13	99	R (65%)	50–60	24–72	Binds to carbonic anhydrase in erythrocytes
Metolazone	65	113 (total)	95	R (80%)	8–14	12–24	Retains efficacy in renal insufficiency
Indapamide	71–79	25 (total)	75	M (70%), R (5%)	14	24–36	Possible vasodilatory properties
High-ceiling or loops							
Furosemide	10–100	0.15	91–99	R (50%), 50% conjugated in kidneys	1.5	6	Slightly prolonged $T_{1/2}$ in renal insufficiency
Bumetanide	80–100	0.15	90–99	R (60%), M (40%)	1.5	3–6	Slightly prolonged $T_{1/2}$ in renal insufficiency
Torsemide	80–100	0.2	99	R (20%), M (80%)	3–4	8–12	Slightly prolonged $T_{1/2}$ in renal insufficiency
Ethacrynic acid	100	—	90	R (67%), M (33%)	1	4–8	Higher risk of ototoxicity; reserve for patients with documented allergy to other loops
Distal/Collecting duct							
Amiloride	15–25	350 (total)	0	R (50%), 50% fecal	17–26	24	$T_{1/2}$ = 100 hours in end stage renal disease
Triamterene	50	—	55–67	M (80%), R (10)	3	7–9	$T_{1/2}$ of active metabolite = 3 hours
Spironolactone	65	—	90	M (extent unknown)	1.5	16–24	$T_{1/2}$ of active metabolite = 15 hours
Eplerenone	69	43–90 (total)	50	M (extent unknown)	5	24	Less affinity for androgen receptors
Osmotic							
Mannitol	17–20	0.5	0	R (100%)	1	2–8	$T_{1/2}$ = 36 hours in end stage renal disease

* refers to natriuretic effect; — indicates insufficient data; R = renal excretion as intact drug; M = hepatically metabolized; V_d = volume of distribution; $T_{1/2}$ = elimination half-life
(*Source:* References 2 and 4)

LOOP OR HIGH-CEILING DIURETICS

Loop diuretics (Table 1), so named for their site of action in the thick ascending limb of the loop of Henle, were developed in the 1960s while searching for less toxic agents than the organic mercurials. Two agents, furosemide and ethacrynic acid, were developed independently around the same time.

Ethacrynic acid was synthesized following the strategy based on mercurial diuretics that assumed diuresis occurred as a result of inhibiting sulfhydryl groups in the kidney.[4] Screening of other compounds for diuretic activity identified a group of active sulfamoylanthranilic acids substituted on the amine group of the aromatic ring.[4] Among this group, furose-mide was introduced first, followed later by bumetanide and torsemide. The identification and development of these compounds were heralded as major advances in diuretic therapy, as their sizeable effect proved useful in renal insufficiency and heart failure patients unresponsive to other agents. Loop diuretics are often referred to as "high-ceiling" agents due to the substantial diuresis they can cause; maximally effective doses can lead to excretion of 20–25% of filtered sodium, blocking nearly all of the reabsorption occurring in this segment.

Located within the apical membrane of epithelial cells of the thick ascending limb is the electroneutral $Na^+/K^+/2Cl^-$ cotransporter, which passively carries sodium, potassium and chloride ions into the cell based on the electrochemical Na$^+$ gradient generated by the Na$^+$/K$^+$-ATPase pump of the basolateral membrane.[1] Some potassium is returned to the lumen via K$^+$-channels of the luminal membrane, such that the net effect of this pathway is Na$^+$Cl$^-$ reabsorption and a voltage across the tubular wall oriented with the lumen positive in relation to the interstitium.[18] Mechanistically, loop diuretics bind to Na$^+$/K$^+$/2Cl$^-$ cotransporter at the chloride site, causing a diuresis of Na$^+$Cl$^-$ and K$^+$Cl$^-$. In addition to prevent its reabsorption, potassium secretion from distal tubular sites is also promoted by loop diuretics by virtue of the increased delivery of sodium to these sites. The lumen positive charge at the thick ascending limb is also important for calcium and magnesium reabsorption; administration of a loop diuretic increases the fractional calcium excretion as well as a significant increase in magnesium excretion. The former may be useful in treating hypercalcemia.

The thick ascending limb is an important segment responsible for concentrating the urine. Since it is impermeable to water, solute removal from this area of the nephron generates the hypertonic medullary interstitium that serves as the osmotic force driving water reabsorption across the collecting duct, regulated under the influence of antidiuretic hormone. Loop diuretics prohibit solute removal at the thick ascending limb and decrease this osmotic force, thus impairing the ability of the kidney to generate concentrated urine.[1] In addition, solute removal at the thick ascending limb normally dilutes the tubular fluid, allowing free water generation during water deficits. By prohibiting solute removal, loop diuretics impair the kidney's ability to produce maximally diluted urine as well as prevent free water excretion during water loading.

Loop diuretic administration induces hemodynamic changes within the systemic and renal microcirculations. Within minutes, intravenous loop diuretics stimulate the RAAS at the macula densa, which can cause vasoconstriction, increased afterload and decreased renal blood flow.[19] This action is short lived, but can diminish the effectiveness of the diuretic briefly and may explain why certain patients fail to respond to bolus diuretic therapy, but experience effective diuresis with infusions. A second-phase response, characterized by an increase in renal release of vasodilating prostaglandins, such as prostacyclin, occurs within approximately 15 minutes of intravenous loop diuretic administration.[20] The accompanying venodilatation decreases cardiac preload and ventricular filling pressures, probably explaining the immediate symptomatic improvement often observed in patients with acute pulmonary edema even before diuresis has commenced.[4] A compensatory activation of the sympathetic nervous system can be triggered with increased afterload and decreased cardiac function as a result; however, the need to quickly induce diurese generally prevails over these concerns. The final stage of neurohormonal activation follows after prolonged volume removal and occurs with both intravenous and oral administration. This stage is characterized by chronic activation of the RAAS and increased circulating concentrations of angiotensin II and aldosterone, leading to the chronic adaptations to therapy as previously described in the earlier section.

The available loop diuretics include furosemide, bumetanide, torsemide and ethacrynic acid (Table 2). All are extensively bound to serum albumin (> 95%) and must gain access to the tubular lumen by active secretion through probenecid-sensitive organic anion transporters located in the proximal tubule. This process may be slowed by elevated levels of endogenous organic acids such as in chronic kidney disease as well as drugs that share the same transporter including salicylates and nonsteroidal anti-inflammatory drugs.

A number of important pharmacokinetic features must be considered when selecting among the available loop diuretics; among them are bioavailability, half-life and routes of metabolism. Furosemide is the most widely used of the class, but is subject to erratic within and between subject absorption, ranging from 10% to 100%.[21] In addition concomitant administration with food decreases the bioavailability. This wide degree of variability in absorption makes it difficult to reliably predict response, such that one must try different doses before the drug is judged to be ineffective.[4] The absorption of bumetanide and torsemide are more predictable, ranging from 80% to 100%.[22] For these agents, the dose is approximately the same when switching from intravenous to oral dosing. Assuming an average absorption of 50% for furosemide, the oral dose should be approximately twice the intravenous dose when switching routes.

The half-life of loop diuretics dictates their duration of action and frequency of dosing. Furosemide and bumetanide are rapidly acting, but have very short half-lives. Therapeutic response occurs within minutes after intravenous administration, while peak response is noted 30–90 minutes after oral dosing. With both routes of administration, response continues for approximately 2–3 hours, lasting up to 6 hours.[4] As their action is brief, loop diuretics are subjected to a significant post-dose rebound sodium retention. Furosemide and bumetanide must be given multiple times per day, which helps to ensure that adequate amounts of drug are maintained at the site of action, thereby minimizing the impact of the post-dose antinatriuresis period. Torsemide has somewhat a longer plasma half-life and duration of action, and can therefore be dosed less frequently.

Approximately 50% of a dose of furosemide is excreted unchanged in the urine and the remainder is conjugated to glucuronic acid in the kidney.[23] In contrast, bumetanide and torsemide are substantially metabolized (60% and 80%, respectively), primarily through hepatic routes.[24] In hepatic disease, the plasma half-life of bumetanide and torsemide are prolonged and their effects paradoxically enhanced.[25] Similarly, renal insufficiency will alter the pharmacokinetics of furosemide by prolonging both the plasma half-life and duration of action due to decreased urinary excretion and renal conjugation. Although bumetanide and torsemide are hepatically metabolized, their pharmacokinetic profiles in renal insufficiency will also change, but only as a function of decreased renal clearance of intact drug.[26] This is because renal disease impairs the delivery of all loop diuretics into the tubular lumen due to competition by endogenous organic acids that accumulate in renal disease. As a result, larger doses of all loops may be necessary in the presence of renal disease to effectively reach the site of action. Due to its greater ototoxic potential than other loops diuretics, ethacrynic acid should be reserved for use in patients with documented allergic reaction to other loops.[4]

Thiazide diuretics (Table 1) were serendipitously discovered while chemically modifying the sulfa nucleus of acetazolamide in an attempt to develop more potent inhibitors of carbonic anhydrase.[2] The finding that it produced increased chloride rather than bicarbonate accompanying sodium in the urine was an unanticipated consequence, but a major advancement that paved the way for further advances in diuretic therapy. Chlorothiazide, the prototype of the class, became available in 1957, effectively beginning the modern era of diuretic therapy and rendering obsolete the organometallic compounds previously available.

As a group, the thiazides are more properly designated as benzothiadiazines, because most of the compounds are analogs of 1,2,4-benzothiadiazine-1,1-dioxide. Although there is a significant variation in the substitutions and nature of the heterocyclic rings between the different thiazide congeners, all of them retain an unsubstituted sulfonamide group in common with the carbonic anhydrase inhibitors. As such, thiazides retain a wide range of potency with regard to carbonic anhydrase inhibition; however, their diuretic effect has clearly been dissociated from this activity.[2] This is because any solute rejected in the proximal tubule through carbonic anhydrase inhibition continues to downstream segments, where most is picked up by the large capacity thick ascending limb, thereby obviating any relevant clinical effect of action in the proximal tubule.[2]

Thiazide diuretics inhibit sodium reabsorption from the luminal side in the early segments of the distal tubule, by interfering with the electroneutral Na^+Cl^- symporter located in the apical membrane. The increased delivery of sodium to the collecting duct also increases the exchange with potassium, leading to potassium depletion. Magnesium excretion is also increased with thiazide administration. Adaptive mechanisms, as discussed earlier, result in increased proximal tubular solute reabsorption with chronic thiazide use. As the normal Na^+Cl^- reabsorption in the distal tubule contributes to tubular fluid dilution, thiazides impair the diluting capacity of the kidney, but preserve urinary concentrating mechanisms. The former characteristic can prove useful in paradoxically diminishing urinary output to half its pretreatment value in patients with diabetes insipidus.[4] In contrast to loop diuretics, thiazides actually enhance calcium reabsorption and can be used to treat nephrolithiasis due to hypercalciuria.

With few exceptions, the pharmacokinetic parameters of thiazides are not uniformly characterized (Table 2). Generally, all are orally absorbed, have volumes of distribution equal to or greater than equivalent body weight and are extensively bound to plasma proteins.[2] Thiazides must actively be secreted into the proximal tubule, as they are highly protein bound and subject to limited glomerular filtration. Thiazides compete with uric acid for secretion into the proximal tubule by the organic acid secretory system; this leads to reduced uric acid excretion and can precipitate gout in predisposed individuals.

Despite heterogeneity in their structure-activity relationships, which has given rise to designations of the analogs as either being thiazide-type or thiazide-like, the general designation of thiazide diuretic is inclusive of all diuretics sharing primary action in the distal tubule.[2] An exception is indapamide, which has less direct evidence for activity at the Na^+Cl^- symporter and has been suggested to possess vasodilatory effects.[27] All thiazides have demonstrated parallel dose-response curves and comparable maximal chloruretic effects. In general, their dose-response curve is much shallower than that of loops (Fig. 2), such that there is a little difference in efficacy between the lowest and maximally effective doses. Although the various analogs differ by potency in the dose required to produce their therapeutic effects, they do not differ in their optimal therapeutic or maximal responses and there is no direct evidence for superiority of effect of any particular thiazide when equipotent dosing is considered.

The average thiazide onset of action is approximately 2–3 hours, peaking at 3–6 hours, with progressively diminishing natriuretic effect occurring beyond 6 hours for most agents; chlorthalidone, as discussed later, is an exception.[2] There is a significant variation in the metabolism, bioavailability and plasma half-lives of the thiazides (Table 2). The latter two pharmacokinetic features are the most clinically relevant parameters as they influence the dose and frequency of administration. Chlorothiazide is relatively lipid insoluble and requires large doses to achieve concentrations, which are high enough for the drug to arrive at its site of action. Hydrochlorothiazide, the most widely used thiazide in the United States, has improved bioavailability with approximately 60–70% absorbed orally.[28] Coadministration of food slightly enhances absorption, most likely through interference with gastric emptying.

Several thiazides undergo hepatic metabolism (e.g. bendroflumethiazide, polythiazide, methyclothiazide, indapamide), while others are excreted nearly complete as intact drug in urine (e.g. chlorothiazide, hydrochlorothiazide). Chlorthalidone and metolazone are subjected to a mixed pathway of primarily renal (50–80%) with minor biliary excretion (10%).[28] Other than the 50% reduction in hydrochlorothiazide absorption, noted in patients with heart failure, almost no information exists regarding the influence of disease on the pharmacokinetics of thiazides.[28]

As the distal tubule only reabsorbs about 5% of the filtered sodium load, the overt diuretic efficacy of thiazides for volume removal in edematous disorders is limited. However, relative to the loop and other diuretics, an advantage of the thiazides is their long duration of action. This property is a major determinant allowing them to distinguish themselves primarily for their use as antihypertensive agents. Early studies assigned short elimination half-lives (1–3 hours), but most are now generally accepted to begin around 8–12 hours, approximating the threshold for effective once-daily dosing.[28] Chlorthalidone distinguishes itself from other thiazides as a true long-acting agent, possessing a significantly longer elimination half-life that averages 50–60 hours.[29] It has a larger volume of distribution than other thiazides with ≥ 99% of drug bound to erythrocyte carbonic anhydrase.[29] This strong binding affinity accounts for the lengthy half-life of chlorthalidone, with erythrocyte carbonic anhydrase functioning as a storage reservoir enabling a constant backflow of chlorthalidone into plasma to sustain a prolonged low level of diuresis and minimize the post-diuretic anti-natriuresis period.[2] This property may have important clinical relevance in distinguishing chlorthalidone as a more effective antihypertensive agent in the typical dosing range of thiazides utilized today.[30,31]

The duration of antihypertensive effect for thiazides exceeds that of their diuretic effect, mainly due to the important hemodynamic changes induced by the prolonged low-level diuresis. These hemodynamic effects can be separated into acute (1–2 weeks) and chronic (several months) periods (Fig. 3).[32] After commencing regular dosing of a thiazide, blood pressure-lowering is initially attributed to extracellular fluid contraction and reduction in plasma volume.[33] The accompanying decrease in venous return depresses cardiac preload and output, thereby reducing blood pressure. However, there is a clear dissociation between the degree of initial diuresis and antihypertensive effect, as the eventual chronic response to thiazides cannot be reliably predicted by the degree of initial fall in plasma volume.[34] Other significant changes occurring acutely include a transient rise in peripheral vascular resistance, likely the result of counter-regulatory activation of sympathetic nervous and RAAS systems. This transient rise in systemic resistance is not usually sufficient to negate the diuretic-induced blood pressure reduction and the counter-regulatory increases in sympathetic nervous and RAAS systems can be opposed by combining thiazides with RAAS-blocking agents such as angiotensin converting enzyme (ACE) inhibitors or angiotensin-II receptor blockers (ARBs).[2]

In the chronic phase of thiazide use, effects on plasma volume and cardiac output are insufficient to explain the antihypertensive response as these parameters return to near-normal levels.[35] The most likely explanation for the persistent blood pressure-lowering effects of thiazides is an overall reduction in total peripheral resistance. The exact mechanisms responsible for this change are unclear. Evidence for direct vasodilatory properties or a reverse autoregulation phenomenon is not definitive and factors such as structural membrane changes and altered ion gradients have been hypothesized, but not well studied. A more simple explanation may be that long-term thiazide administration induces a low level of prolonged diuresis,

maintaining a nominal state of volume contraction which would promote downward shift in vascular resistance.[2]

The residual effects of thiazides following their discontinuation are significant and persistent. Rapid volume expansion, weight gain and fall in renin levels occur, but blood pressure rises slowly and does not immediately return to pretreatment levels.[32] In fact, with adherence to lifestyle modifications (weight loss, reduction in sodium and alcohol), nearly 70% of patients remained free of antihypertensives for up to one year after being withdrawn from thiazide-based therapy in the "Hypertension Detection and Follow-up Program".[36]

POTASSIUM-SPARING DIURETICS

In the distal tubule and collecting ducts, sodium is reabsorbed through an aldosterone-sensitive sodium channel and by activation of an ATP-dependent sodium-potassium pump. With the help of both mechanisms, potassium and hydrogen are secreted into the lumen to preserve electroneutrality.[2] Potassium-sparing diuretics are divided into two distinct classes: (1) those acting as direct antagonists of cytoplasmic mineralocorticoid receptors and (2) those acting independent of mineralocorticoids. All potassium-sparing diuretics act primarily at the cortical part of the collecting duct and to a lesser extent in the final segment of the distal convoluted tubule and connecting tubule. As only a small amount of sodium is reabsorbed here, these agents are capable of limited natriuresis (excluding states of mineralocorticoid excess) in most patients. Their primary clinical utility resides in their potassium-sparing capabilities and to a lesser extent, their ability to correct magnesium deficiencies.

Spironolactone and eplerenone (Table 2) are competitive antagonists of aldosterone, the most potent of the naturally occurring mineralocorticoids and thereby interfere with the aldosterone mediated exchange of sodium for potassium and hydrogen. Spironolactone is well-absorbed orally and highly protein bound. The compound itself has a short half-life of only 1.5 hours, but it is extensively metabolized in the liver and its therapeutic action resides mainly in that of its several metabolites.[5] Among them, 7-α-thiomethylspirolactone and canrenone are the most well-characterized, with half-lives of about 15–20 hours, which are sufficiently long enough to permit once-daily dosing. As time must be allowed to accumulate active metabolites, spironolactone has a characteristically slow onset, up to 48 hours before becoming maximally effective.[4] Since spironolactone gains access to its site of action independent of glomerular filtration, it remains active in renal insufficiency. However, it must be used very carefully in this setting due to the propensity for hyperkalemia to occur.

Spironolactone has been available for use in hypertension for many years, while eplerenone is a newer agent demonstrating similar efficacy. Both drugs are rarely used alone, but rather in combination with other diuretics to avoid potassium deficiency. Their aldosterone-blocking capabilities also makes them a primary therapy in patients with essential hypertension due to mineralocorticoid excess such as in primary aldosteronism due to bilateral adrenal hyperplasia or in patients with aldosterone producing adrenal adenomas awaiting surgical resection, or those who are nonsurgical candidates. Additionally, patients with secondary hyperaldosteronism such as that

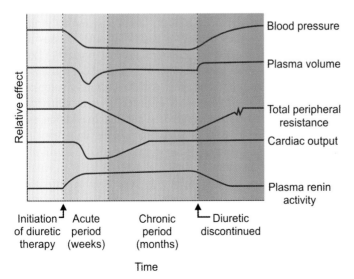

FIGURE 3: Time course of hemodynamic responses to thiazides
(*Source:* Reference 32)

observed in hepatic cirrhosis and ascites, benefit from spirono-lactone. The major adverse effects of spironolactone are antiandrogenic and stem from the fact that it is a steroid that competitively inhibits testosterone and progesterone at the cellular level. In particular, gynecomastia can become a concern, especially with high doses. In the dose range of 12.5–50 mg/day, it is rarely a problem. Eplerenone appears to have more selectivity for aldosterone receptors and less affinity for androgen and progestin receptors than spironolactone.[2] Cost differences have traditionally favored spironolactone and it remains to be determined whether eplerenone's safety and efficacy constitute significant advancements over spironolactone.

The actions of amiloride and triamterene (Table 2) are quite different than spironolactone and eplerenone. Both are pteridine derivatives and exert their action by blocking epithelial sodium channels in the luminal membrane. In this manner, the electrical potential across the tubular epithelium falls, which reduces the driving force for secretion of potassium into the lumen.[4] About 50% of an oral dose of either agent is absorbed. Triamterene is the older of the two drugs in the class; both are rarely used strictly as antihypertensives because of their weak ability to lower blood pressure. Rather, they are most often used in fixed-dose combinations with a thiazide diuretic to offset the potassium and magnesium losses induced by thiazides.

Triamterene has a short half-life (3–6 hours) and duration of effect.[4] Ideally it should be dosed multiple times per day; however, because it is most commonly used in a fixed-dose combination with hydrochlorothiazide, it is rarely dosed more frequently than once-daily. Triamterene is converted to an active phase II sulfate-conjugated metabolite by the liver and the metabolite is then secreted into the proximal tubular fluid.[5] Both renal and liver disease significantly affect the disposition of triamterene; the former by impairing tubular secretion of the active metabolite and the latter by reducing formation of metabolite. Triamterene is a potential nephrotoxin associated with formation of crystals, nephrolithiasis, interstitial nephritis and acute renal failure. It must be used carefully when other potentially nephrotoxic drugs are coadministered.

Amiloride has a much longer half-life (17–26 hours) and can be dosed once or twice daily, achieving steady state in approximately two days.[4] It is preferred in patients with liver disease as there is no required metabolic activation. However, it is extensively renally cleared and accumulates rapidly when administered in patients with chronic kidney disease. In these situations, the dose and/or dosing frequency of amiloride should be reduced to avoid the potential for hyperkalemia.

OSMOTIC DIURETICS

The osmotic diuretic, mannitol (Table 2), is freely filtered through the glomerulus and poorly absorbed. As it is not reabsorbed in the nephron, mannitol does not interfere with specific tubular electrolyte transport systems. Rather it increases osmolality, as it remains in the tubule lumen and thus impairs the tubular water reabsorption normally driven by the osmotic gradient. As the medullary solute gradient is lost, the urinary concentrating ability of the kidney is greatly reduced and tubular fluid is diluted. The osmotic diuresis that prevails is similar to the glucose-mediated osmotic polyuria and diuresis observed in patients with uncontrolled diabetes.[4] Although some excretion of bicarbonate occurs in the proximal tubule, mannitol's effect is largely in promoting sodium and chloride wasting in the loop of Henle. The increased delivery of sodium to distal sites increases the exchange for potassium, such that potassium is also lost in the process. The onset of mannitol is quick, with a half-life of approximately one hour in patients with normal renal function.[37] The offset is equally fast and for this reason, it is best administered as a continuous infusion.

Mannitol is effective in reducing cerebral edema, first by osmotic fluid removal from the brain and then by osmotic diuresis, making it useful in neurosurgical procedures, head trauma and in other conditions of increased intracranial pressure.[1] Mannitol has been used as a preventive measure against acute renal failure in patients receiving cisplatin, radiocontrast exposure or other high-risk situations; however, there is no evidence that it is any more effective than insuring adequate volume status with parenteral fluids, a more appropriate strategy. In the same manner, mannitol has been investigated for use in oliguric acute renal failure to promote diuresis; again, limited data support this strategy and insuring adequate volume status is a more appropriate approach.[38] Furthermore, the half-life of mannitol is markedly prolonged in renal insufficiency (up to 36 hours). In this situation, mannitol remains in the vascular space and the osmotic effect can expand blood volume and is a concern for precipitating heart failure. Given its significant limitations, mannitol should be only rarely used as a diuretic.

CLINICAL USE OF DIURETICS IN CARDIOVASCULAR DISEASES

Aside from their chemical and mechanistic classifications, diuretics can be categorized functionally into one of three primary uses—treatment of essential hypertension, volume removal in edematous disorders, and correction of potassium and magnesium deficiencies. Thiazide diuretics appear to be the most effective diuretics over the long term in lowering blood pressure in patients with hypertension. Not only do they result in significant lowering of blood pressure as monotherapy, thiazides enhance the efficacy of nearly all other classes and they reduce hypertension-related morbidity and mortality.[2] Loop diuretics are the most powerful diuretics to evoke a substantial diuresis; therefore, they are agents of choice for symptomatic relief in patients with edematous disorders such as congestive heart failure, cirrhosis and nephrotic syndrome. In addition, they are used in preference to thiazides in patients with impaired renal function [glomerular filtration rate (GFR) < 40 ml/min/1.73 m^2], where thiazides are unlikely to be as effective. Finally, potassium-sparing agents are largely reserved for correcting potassium and magnesium deficiencies associated with thiazide diuretic administration and in other less common situations, including hyperaldosteronism and rare genetic conditions such as Liddle or Bartter syndromes.

While only one type of diuretic is generally used at a time, there are several conditions where diuretic tolerance is encountered. In these situations, combinations of two different types of diuretics are often employed to improve response. Thus, to effectively utilize diuretics in the patient with cardiovascular disease, a clinician needs to first appreciate their unique interclass and intraclass characteristics and couple this with knowledge of the pathophysiology of the condition being treated. If both are considered in tandem, one can reliably predict the expected therapeutic response to diuretic administration.

DIURETIC USE IN HYPERTENSION

General Considerations

Thiazides have been a mainstay in the treatment of hypertension for many years and are preferred agents for chronic therapy in most hypertensive patients where a diuretic is indicated.[31] Thiazide administration typically results in a 10–15/5–10 mm Hg reduction in blood pressure compared to placebo.[2] Thiazide responders are often referred to as having low-renin or salt-sensitive hypertension, in deference to the large contribution volume and sodium play in the maintenance of their blood pressure. These patients typically include the elderly, blacks and high cardiac output states such as obesity. Although the aforementioned groups are often considered more likely to respond to thiazides, an advantage of thiazides is that they can be effectively combined with nearly any antihypertensive, producing a blood pressure-lowering effect that is additive of the two individual components in almost all cases.[2] Importantly, racial differences observed in the monotherapy response to RAAS-blocking agents, such as ACE inhibitors or ARBs (blacks often do not respond as well to monotherapy with these agents), are minimized. Combining thiazides with RAAS blocking agents also has the added practical advantage of minimizing potassium wasting and metabolic adverse effects caused by thiazides. Data from clinical trials indicate that most of the patients eventually require 2–3 antihypertensives to achieve their blood pressure goal. Given their ability to augment efficacy of nearly all other types of antihypertensives, thiazides are powerful tools which improve the capability of achieving blood pressure goals.[39] In patients considered to have resistant hypertension, lack of appropriate diuretic use has been identified as the primary drug-related cause.[40,41]

Thiazide dosing has evolved in parallel to our progressive understanding of their mechanism of action and dose-response relationships. When first introduced, thiazides were used in much higher doses than today, stemming from the belief that efficacy was directly linked to the amount of renal sodium excretion and reduction in plasma volume obtained; the larger the dose, the greater the assumed reduction in blood pressure.[31] However, the dose-response curve is much shallower than originally believed. Thiazides are now utilized in significantly lower doses and the term low-dose thiazide has become synonymous with 12.5–25 mg/day of hydrochlorothiazide or its equivalent.[2] Approximately 50% of patients will respond initially, even to these small doses. Increasing the dose of hydrochlorothiazide to 25 mg/day may add approximately 20% to the responders, while at 50 mg/day 80–90% of possible responders should experience measurable blood pressure decreases.[42]

Comparative Efficacy

The ability of thiazides to effectively lower blood pressure translates into reductions in cardiovascular events. Beginning with the completion of the landmark Veteran's Affairs Cooperative Group study in 1967 and continuing through the early 1990s, a series of randomized placebo-controlled trials involving more than 47,000 hypertensive patients convincingly demonstrated these effects. Most of these studies employed a stepped-care approach, beginning initially with a diuretic, followed by an adrenergic inhibitor (beta-blocker), then vasodilator. Combined meta-analyses and systematic review show that thiazide-based regimens reduce relative rates of heart failure by 41–49%, stroke by approximately 29–38%, coronary heart disease by 14–21% and overall mortality by 10–11% compared to placebo.[2] Effect sizes are homogeneous throughout major subgroups of patients, including by gender, age and presence of diabetes.[43-45] The results of these studies have collectively formed the basis for the recommendations contained in the first seven guideline reports of the Joint National Committee, all advocating thiazides as initial therapy for most patients.[39]

With the introduction in the 1980s and early 1990s of a host of "newer" antihypertensives (ACE inhibitors, ARBs, calcium channel blockers), comparative studies of their efficacy began with thiazide diuretic/beta-blocker regimens as the standard of comparison. Most of these studies were not sufficiently powered to identify small to moderate differences in risk reduction among the regimens, but rather to identify any large disparities. The Blood Pressure Lowering Treatment Trialists' collaboration was developed to maximize information obtained from these and future trials. Against active comparators, meta-analyses from this collaboration demonstrate lack of superiority of any antihypertensive class over thiazides, including within subgroups of age and gender.[44,45] Nevertheless, the 1980s and 1990s saw diminished use of diuretics as they were no longer patented and were subject to an active negative campaign of marketing which overemphasized their adverse metabolic and electrolyte effects, in contrast to those more neutral effects of the newer agents.[31]

In response to allegations that diuretics would be inferior to the newer agents, the largest randomized comparative study to date in hypertension was undertaken. The Antihypertensive and Lipid-lowering to prevent Heart Attack Trial (ALLHAT) has provided the most comprehensive information regarding the overall benefit of thiazides evaluated against other therapies.[46] The ALLHAT compared first-step treatment using chlorthalidone 12.5 mg daily to amlodipine, lisinopril or doxazosin in 42,418 high-risk participants aged 55 and older, including an oversampling of African Americans (35%). No differences were observed in the composite primary endpoint of fatal coronary heart disease or nonfatal myocardial infarction for all treatments; however, chlorthalidone was superior in several predefined secondary endpoints including heart failure (versus amlodipine, lisinopril, doxazosin) and stroke (versus lisinopril). Numerous analyses stratifying by race and metabolic status have consistently shown that none of the agents surpassed chlorthalidone in antihypertensive efficacy or event reduction.[47]

The efficacy of thiazides, both in lowering blood pressure and in reducing cardiovascular disease events, has typically been considered a "class effect" despite absence of any substantial direct comparison studies within the class to validate this assumption.[2] Class effects can only be substantiated after determination of equipotent dosing; and when not directly compared in a cardiovascular event trial, assume that if both achieve similar blood pressure lowering, then both can achieve similar reduction in cardiovascular events. With regard to thiazides, this rationale is flawed because fundamental differences exist in their pharmacokinetics and pharmacodynamics. On the basis that it has reduced cardiovascular events in every study where used, some hypertension experts preferentially recommend chlorthalidone, while noting that other thiazide regimens have resulted in less consistent benefit in clinical trials.[2] The few trials of hydrochlorothiazide in which it has successfully lowered cardiovascular disease events have typically used higher doses ($\geq$ 25–50 mg/day) than commonly used today.[30] This detail is widely underappreciated and the popular belief of thiazide interchangeability is reinforced by the exclusivity of fixed-dose combinations containing hydrochlorothiazide 12.5–25 mg doses. Interestingly, the only two comparative trials to actually use low-dose hydrochlorothiazide regimens found they were inferior to the comparator regimens in reducing cardiovascular disease events.[48,49]

The reason for the disparate findings is unclear, but may simply relate to differences in potency and blood pressure-lowering efficacy between the two drugs in low doses commonly employed. Despite the misperception of equipotency among hydrochlorothiazide and chlorthalidone at low doses, chlorthalidone is actually 1.5–2 times more potent than hydrochlorothiazide, based on doses required to achieve similar levels of blood pressure reduction.[50-52] Comparison using ambulatory blood pressure monitoring data suggests the antihypertensive efficacy of chlorthalidone (25 mg) may even exceed that of hydrochlorothiazide (50 mg).[51] These findings are attributed to the long-acting nature of chlorthalidone in maintaining its efficacy throughout the nighttime period, blunting "escape" in blood pressure occurring during the interval between daily dosages. It is possible that the exuberance for using low doses to minimize the adverse metabolic and electrolyte disturbances of thiazides may leave some patients without adequate volume contraction. Evidence for this can be found in a study of resistant hypertensives, where most demonstrated high systemic resistance despite already taking 3 or 4 antihypertensive medications including low-dose hydrochlorothiazide in more than 90% of patients.[53]

Whether a diuretic class effect exists with regard to cardiovascular protection is not easily resolved as there are no direct comparative outcome studies. In the absence of such data, clinicians should rely on the fact that cardiovascular events are lowered as a direct function of the degree of blood pressure lowering achieved. Since most patients require multiple agents to control blood pressure, a diuretic will likely be part of the regimen and it may be irrelevant which agent is selected as long as the desired level of blood pressure control can be achieved. As an example, a sustained-release indapamide regimen was reportedly associated with reductions of 39%, 64% and 21% in fatal stroke, heart failure and death in elderly patients over 80 years old.[54] Although tempting as it may be, relevant differences between thiazides, after accounting for equipotency, can only be viewed as speculative.

Special Considerations

An important clinical issue with thiazides is that they are generally considered less effective in renal insufficiency, particularly when GFR falls below 40 ml/min/1.73 m^2. This is a somewhat arbitrary cutoff, as research has not clearly answered the question of the exact level of GFR at which point the efficacy of each thiazide compound is abolished. Thus, in patients with chronic kidney disease, it is advisable to use a loop diuretic instead, keeping in mind that it may need to be dosed two or three times daily to maintain efficacy. Larger doses of thiazides have been shown to induce diuresis in patients with chronic kidney disease,[55,56] but the efficacy of thiazides in this setting has a specific ceiling, which is controlled by several factors including the reduced delivery of filtered solute and drug to the distal tubule site of action and the fact that the distal tubule is responsible for only a small amount of sodium reabsorption even under normal circumstances. Additionally, increasing the doses of thiazides is impractical given the risk of metabolic and electrolyte side effects. Metolazone, a thiazide-like quinazoline derivative, is an exception among thiazides as it retains efficacy in patients with renal insufficiency and other diuretic-resistance states. As it is limited by slow and erratic absorption, the more predictable bioavailability of other thiazides makes them better suited for chronic therapy of hypertension. Metolazone is generally reserved in combination with loop diuretics in volume-overloaded patients undergoing close monitoring of fluid and electrolyte balance. It is usually administered daily for a short period (3–5 days) with frequency of administration reduced to thrice weekly once euvolemia is achieved.[10]

In the absence of states of mineralocorticoid excess or certain rare genetic conditions, the primary role of potassium-sparing diuretics, such as triamterene or amiloride, in the treatment of hypertension is that of an ancillary to help offset the potassium and magnesium wasting induced by thiazides. Spironolactone is advantageous not only in that it can correct thiazide-induced potassium and magnesium wasting, but low doses of 12.5–50 mg daily show significant additive hypotensive effects in patients resistant to treatment regardless of ethnicity or baseline aldosterone level.[40,57] This finding likely reflects the importance of aldosterone's effect in supporting elevated blood pressure in hypertensive patients treated with RAAS-blocking agents. Amiloride, which is an epithelial sodium channel blocker, demonstrated greater efficacy than spironolactone in blacks resistant to treatment.[58] It is available as both a single agent and in combination with hydrochlorothiazide.

DIURETIC USE IN EDEMATOUS DISORDERS

General Considerations

Loop diuretics are the most potent diuretics available, making them agents of choice in patients with edematous disorders such as renal insufficiency, hepatic cirrhosis, congestive heart failure and nephrotic syndrome. As previously stated, when GFR falls to less than 40 ml/min/1.73 m^2, other diuretics used as single agents are less likely to be effective owing to diminished delivery of drug to the site of action. Thus, loop diuretics are preferred for hypertension or volume control in patients with chronic kidney disease.

Several principles must be considered when using diuretics in the treatment of edematous disorders. First, while a cornerstone of therapy, diuretics themselves are not definitive therapy and the primary treatment of edema should be directed at correction of the underlying disorder whenever possible. As an ancillary strategy, sodium restriction should be promoted when edema accumulates, as this may be sufficient enough to correct the problem in patients with mild edema, in addition to enhancing the natriuretic efficacy of diuretics if administered.[59] Finally, it should be recognized that all patients with edema do not require treatment with diuretics. As an example, in the absence of pulmonary congestion and comprised respiratory function, peripheral edema itself is mainly a cosmetic issue and poses no immediate threat to the patient.

In most cases, the removal of excess extracellular fluid volume with diuretics should be gradual. This is necessary both to avoid precipitous electrolyte imbalances as well as reductions in effective blood volume that would be of sufficient magnitude to impair tissue perfusion. Thus, the rate of removal is critical. Initial losses in response to diuretic administration occur from the plasma volume. The rate at which vascular space is refilled by fluid mobilized from the interstitium is variable and this ultimately directs the maximal rate of diuresis that can be tolerated.[59] For generalized edema, interstitial fluid is rapidly mobilized and a diuresis of 1–2 l/day can be safely achieved.[59] Mobilization is much slower and diuresis must therefore be approached more gradually, for edema that is sequestered as ascites or in the pleural space.

As previously discussed, the pharmacodynamics of diuretics is altered in most edematous conditions; namely, such that maximal response is lower (Fig. 2). The mechanisms underlying this decreased responsiveness are uncertain, but may relate to increased proximal or distal reabsorption of sodium or an upregulation of the Na$^+$/K$^+$/2Cl$^-$ transporter.[4] From a clinical perspective, this means that administering larger single doses will not improve the diuretic response. As in normal patients, it is best to first start with small doses and then titrates upward according to response. This can be achieved practically by sequentially doubling the dose until response is observed or a ceiling dose is reached (Table 3). Escalating doses above these ceiling doses will result in no additional benefit, but an increase in side effects. If response is suboptimal, other strategies, such as continuous infusion or using combinations of diuretics as outlined below, may be tried.

Renal Insufficiency

In the absence of heart failure, cirrhosis or nephrotic syndrome, dysregulation of volume homeostasis is usually a late manifestation of renal insufficiency, often not developing until GFR falls to less than 10 ml/min.[59] As renal function declines, the ability to maintain sodium balance diminishes and the fraction of filtered sodium that must be excreted to maintain sodium balance rises progressively. In the setting of constant sodium intake, fractional excretion of sodium must increase fivefold when GFR falls to 20% of normal and tenfold when GFR is 10% of normal.[59] Normal kidneys are able to accommodate this over a wide range of sodium intake, but patients with renal insufficiency have limited ability to raise the fractional excretion of sodium above 50%.[59] Assuming sodium intake

TABLE 3

Ceiling doses and therapeutic regimens for loop diuretics in normal patients and in conditions with reduced diuretic response

Clinical scenario	Furosemide IV	Furosemide PO	Bumetanide IV and PO	Torsemide IV and PO
Continuous Infusion Rates (mg/hr)	40 mg loading dose		1 mg loading dose	20 mg loading dose
CrCl < 25	20, then 40		1, then 2	10, then 20
CrCl 25–75	10, then 20		0.5, then 1	5, then 10
CrCl > 75	10		0.5	5
Single-dose ceilings (mg)				
Renal insufficiency*				
Moderate (CrCl 20–50)	80–160	160	2–3	20–50
Severe (CrCl < 20)	160–200	400	8–10	50–100
Congestive heart failure** (preserved renal function)	40–80	80–160	1–2	20–40
Cirrhosis** (preserved renal function)	40	80	1	10–20
Nephrotic Syndrome** (preserved renal function)	80–120	240	2-3	40–60

*Mechanism of reduced effect is impaired delivery to the site of action. The therapeutic strategy is to use sufficiently high enough doses to attain effective amounts at the site of action, and increase frequency of administration of the effective dose.
**Mechanism of reduced effect is diminished nephron response (and binding of diuretic to urinary albumin in nephrotic syndrome). The therapeutic strategy is to increase the frequency of the effective dose.
(*Source:* References 5 and 10)

exceeds this reduced maximal excretion, extracellular fluid volume expands and edema develops.

Large doses of thiazides can induce a modest diuresis in patients with renal disease, but loop diuretics are preferred because they produce a more vigorous and reliable response. Renal clearance of loops falls in parallel with GFR because of decreased renal mass and accumulation of organic acids that compete for proximal secretion. Only 10–20% as much drug may be secreted into the tubular lumen in a patient with a creatinine clearance of 15 ml/min, compared to one with normal renal function.[5] That said, response to the diuretic expressed as fractional excretion of sodium is similar for patients with renal insufficiency to that of healthy patients; thus, residual nephrons seem to respond normally,[60] but the problem is in getting enough drug to the site of action to achieve the diuretic threshold.

As less diuretic reaches the urine in renal disease, there is a need to administer larger doses to attain adequate amounts at the site of action. Patients should be given increasing doses of a loop diuretic until an effective dose is identified (or a specific ceiling dose achieved). This is a key step in the process; otherwise, administering multiple small doses of a diuretic will be ineffective because adequate urinary concentrations will not be achieved. Once the effective dose is determined, it should be given as frequently as necessary to maintain response, which will be determined according to the duration of action of the drug in the particular patient as well as the extent of their ability to comply with sodium restrictions.[5] If intermittent doses are not sufficient, a continuous infusion may be tried. Before using a continuous infusion, a loading dose should be given first to reduce the time necessary to achieve a steady state therapeutic drug concentration. The rate of the continuous infusion is then determined based on renal function (Table 3).[5]

Patients with inadequate natriuresis despite the use of maximal doses of loop diuretics may benefit from the sequential nephron blockade brought about by using combinations of diuretic agents.[10] Addition of a distally acting diuretic, such as a thiazide, to the loop agent is the most common strategy. Several mechanisms contribute to the enhanced response with combination use in refractory states. First, the longer half-life of distally acting agents may decrease the effect of the post-dose sodium retention observed with the shorter-acting loops. Secondly, chronic administration of loop diuretics can induce hypertrophy of distal tubule cells, enhancing their reabsorption of sodium and blunting the response to loops.[10] As most thiazides retain minor effects on carbonic anhydrase in addition to their main site of action in the distal tubule, the addition of a thiazide can block reabsorption at these sites and usually increase the diuretic response.[61]

Of the thiazides, metolazone is frequently selected for use in combination with a loop because of its long half-life and preserved activity in renal insufficiency. Other thiazides can be used as well, but will require larger doses (e.g. hydrochlorothiazide 25–100 mg daily or equivalent) since they must reach the lumen of the nephron to be effective.[5] Rarely acetazolamide and collecting duct agents, such as spironolactone and amiloride, are used, but their response is less dramatic than that of a thiazide. Regardless of which agent is selected, combination diuretic therapy must be cautiously employed owing to the increased possibility of hyperkalemia or hypokalemia (depending on underlying renal function and which type of agent is added) as well as circulatory collapse resulting from too vigorous of a reduction in extracellular fluid volume.

Cirrhosis

Secondary hyperaldosteronism plays an important role in the pathogenesis of sodium retention in patients with cirrhotic edema. Spironolactone, a competitive inhibitor of aldosterone, is a mainstay of therapy in such patients. Not only it increases patient comfort, but it can also eliminate the need or reduce the interval between paracenteses, an advantage is that protein normally removed during paracenteses can also be spared. The usual dosing range of spironolactone is 50–400 mg/day, but doses above 200 mg/day are often not well tolerated due to painful gynecomastia.[5] An advantage of spironolactone is the once-daily dosing made possible by the sufficiently long half-lives of its active metabolites. As the onset of natriuresis may take 2–4 days, as a result dose adjustments should therefore not be more frequent than every 4–5 days.[59] Spironolactone itself is capable of only moderate diuresis; thus, edematous cirrhotic patients often require the addition of other diuretics, along with occasional paracentesis. Although either a thiazide or loop diuretic can be added, the presence of renal insufficiency usually necessitates the use of a loop diuretic.

The pharmacokinetics and pharmacodynamics of loop diuretics in cirrhotic patients are well characterized.[5] In the absence of concomitant renal insufficiency, the diuretic concentration in tubular fluid is normal.[62] However, for unknown reasons, cirrhosis shifts the dose-response curve downward and to the right (Fig. 2), such that tubular responsiveness remains diminished even in the presence of normal renal function. Since the decreased response does not result from inadequate delivery of drug to the site of action, larger doses will not increase the diuretic response; rather, more frequent doses alone or with a thiazide, may be effective.[5]

Cirrhotic patients with edema receiving diuretics are prone to complications such as intravascular volume depletion and pre-renal azotemia, in up to 20% of patients.[59] Once euvolemia is achieved, maximal diuresis should be limited to 500 ml/day. As in other conditions in which combinations of diuretics are used, close monitoring of electrolytes is necessary. Diuretic therapy should be reduced or discontinued if azotemia develops.[59]

Congestive Heart Failure

Patients with mild heart failure may not have appreciable edema and diuretic therapy is not an absolute necessity, particularly if patients can restrict sodium intake. If hypertension coexists, it is sensible to employ a thiazide diuretic, which may be sufficient to control mild edema, if present. However, most patients with congestive heart failure will eventually develop edema to the extent that requires the use of a loop diuretic.

Responsiveness to oral loop diuretics in patients with heart failure is dependent on several factors including gastrointestinal absorption and tubular secretion. The absolute bioavailability of the diuretic is unchanged, but the rate of absorption is slowed such that the peak response may not be observed for several hours after the dose is administered.[5] The unpredictability of diuresis with furosemide in this situation may portend a worse outcome. Torsemide has a higher bioavailability than furosemide and evidence exists for less fatigue and readmittance for decompensated heart failure in patients receiving torsemide compared to furosemide, a finding potentially attributable to better bioavailability and more predictable response.[63]

As long as renal function remains preserved, delivery of diuretic into the tubular fluid remains normal in heart failure. However, renal responsiveness to loops as measured by the natriuretic response to maximally effective doses can be one-third to one-fourth than that of healthy individuals.[64] Larger doses will therefore not overcome this diminished response, unless renal insufficiency is present. Rather, the natriuretic response may be increased by giving moderate doses more frequently.[5] In this manner, intravenous therapy is often appropriate in patients with severe heart failure or acute pulmonary edema. In addition to avoiding troughs in drug concentration that can lead to intermittent periods of positive sodium balance, it also has the added advantage of bypassing the delayed gut absorption of the diuretic. A loading dose followed by a continuous infusion (Table 3) is preferred, as they seem to provide greater natriuresis with a lower incidence of toxicity than intermittent bolus injections.[65]

A thiazide diuretic can be added in combination to a loop diuretic in situations where the loop diuretic and sodium restriction are not adequate to control the edema.[10] The synergy provided by such combinations can result in profound diuresis and patients must be followed closely to prevent severe hypokalemia and volume depletion to the extent that could induce circulatory collapse.[5]

Distally acting, potassium-sparing agents may increase sodium excretion slightly in some patients. Potential responders can be identified by measuring urinary electrolytes. Low urinary sodium output in the presence of high urinary potassium concentrations indicate that sodium is being exchanged for potassium distally; the addition of a distally acting diuretic in this situation may enhance the natriuretic response.[5] More importantly, the empiric addition of spironolactone 25 mg/day to the standard regimen of an ACE-inhibitor and loop diuretic in patients with severe heart failure (ejection fraction < 35%) reduced death by 30% and hospitalizations by 35% in a pivotal trial.[66] These findings occurred independently of changes in body weight or urinary sodium excretion, suggesting that the blockade of aldosterone's effect on cardiac and vascular tissues is an important strategy in the management of these patients.

Nephrotic Syndrome

Diuretic resistance is often encountered in the nephrotic syndrome; a constellation of findings characterized by proteinuria, hypoalbuminemia and generalized edema. As serum albumin concentrations are low, there is an increase in the permeability of the glomerular basement membrane to plasma proteins.[59] The resulting decrease in plasma oncotic pressure alters Starling forces in the peripheral capillary beds, favoring fluid transudation into the interstitial compartment.[59] Since diuretics are primarily bound to albumin, hypoalbuminemia also causes more diffusion of diuretic into the extracellular fluid, leading

to reduction in delivery to the secretory sites and ultimately, the diuretic site of action.[5] In severely hypoalbuminemic patients (< 2 g/dL), coadministration of albumin with the loop diuretic (30 mg furosemide mixed with 25 g albumin) may increase the diuretic response.[5] However, since tubular secretion of the diuretic is normal in the majority of patients with nephrotic syndrome (unless there is accompanying renal insufficiency), combined infusions are not necessary. Additionally, albumin administration can exacerbate hypertension and pulmonary congestion.

Despite adequate tubular secretion, diuretic response in the nephrotic syndrome is diminished. This is the result of increased binding of the diuretic to albumin in the tubular fluid, which reduces the amount of unbound, active drug available to exert its effect.[5] Nearly one-half to two-third of the diuretics reaching tubular fluid is bound to albumin when urinary albumin concentrations exceed 4 g/l.[5] As a result, the dose of diuretic must be increased twofold or threefold that is given to normal patients in order to deliver adequate amounts of unbound, active drug to the site of action. Additionally, the natriuretic response in nephrotic patients is further impaired by decreased cellular responsiveness in the loop of Henle and increased sodium retention in the distal tubule.[5] Doses of the loop diuretic must therefore be sufficient not only to overcome urinary binding, but they must also be administered more frequently. Metozalone or another thiazide diuretic may be combined with the loop diuretic as an additional strategy in nephrotic patients.[59]

ADVERSE EFFECTS OF DIURETICS

A number of important and predictable adverse effects can occur with diuretics. Flow chart 1 illustrates some of the more commonly noted effects and the pathways by which they can occur. For the most part, adverse effects of diuretics are minimized by using lower doses as well as ensuring appropriate monitoring vigilance on the part of the clinician.

Both thiazide and loop diuretics increase potassium and magnesium excretion. On an average, potassium will fall by 0.3–0.4 mEq/l with typical dosing.[2] Among thiazides, chlorthalidone is commonly believed to cause more hypokalemia, but there is no compelling evidence of this finding when low doses are used.[52] The incidence of clinically relevant hypokalemia with thiazides is further reduced when they are combined with ACE-inhibitors or ARBs. Diuretic-induced hypokalemia can be managed by coadministering a potassium-sparing diuretic or oral potassium supplements. Potassium-sparing diuretics are generally more effective since they correct the underlying etiology and have the additional effect of reducing magnesium excretion.[2] The latter point is often unrecognized in its importance; magnesium deficiencies must be corrected first, otherwise potassium supplementation will be ineffective in normalizing potassium levels. Additionally, dietary sodium restriction can also help in minimizing the loss of potassium occurring with diuretics.[11]

Maintenance of potassium homeostasis is important, since epidemiologic evidence implicates hypokalemia in the pathogenesis of diuretic dysglycemia and new-onset diabetes.[67] It is important to recognize that new-onset diabetes will occur over time in many hypertensive patients regardless of type of

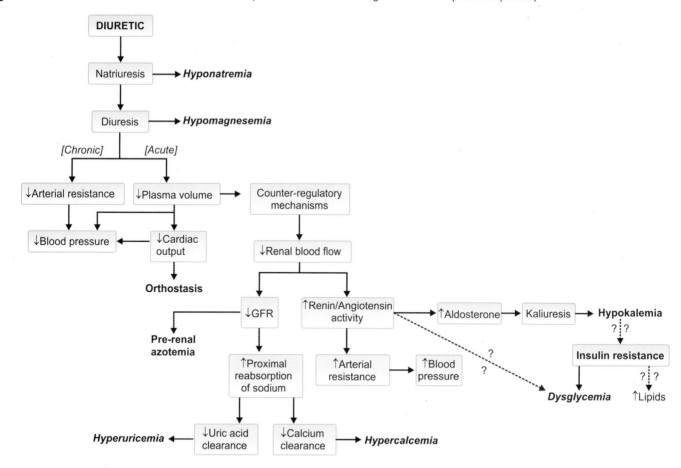

antihypertensive used. Data suggest long-term diuretic therapy over several years that may lead to an excess of 3–4% in diabetes cases as compared to other antihypertensives, but there is no evidence that it obviates their proven benefit in reducing CVD events.[2]

Hyponatremia is often caused by diuretics. Thiazides seem to have a greater propensity than loops, but its all diuretics are implicated.[68] Thiazide-induced hyponatremia usually manifests within the first two weeks of therapy, while loops can occur after a longer interval. Several risk factors predispose patients to diuretic-induced hyponatremia; these include older age, female gender, psychogenic polydipsia and concurrent antidepressant use (in particular, selective serotonin reuptake inhibitors).[68] In the presence of these conditions, hyponatremia can occur at any time. Most patients are asymptomatic, but careful monitoring of serum sodium should occur as well as counseling patients to avoid excessive free-water intake in order to minimize risks of its occurrence.

Diuretics can increase serum lipid levels, primarily total cholesterol and low-density lipoproteins, approximately 5–7% in the first year of therapy.[69] However, these increases are short lived and the high prevalence of statin background therapy in hypertensive patients generally makes this an inconsequential finding.

Few clinically relevant drug interactions occur with diuretics. As they compete with uric acid for secretion by the organic acid pathway, diuretics can increase serum uric acid and precipitate gout in some patients.[2] Nonsteroidal anti-inflammatory drugs can antagonize their therapeutic effects by causing sodium retention. Additionally, they can also increase the risk of hyperkalemia when combined with potassium-sparing agents, by decreasing secretion of renin and aldosterone. Likewise, the use of potassium-sparing diuretics with ACE-inhibitors or ARBs also entails an increased risk for hyperkalemia.

Other adverse effects of diuretics can include interstitial nephritis, ototoxicity (particularly with high-dose loop therapy), sun sensitivity, skin reactions and uropathy. Contrary to popular belief, diuretics do not need to be avoided in patients with a history of allergy to sulfonamide-based antibiotics.[70]

SUMMARY

For over 50 years, diuretic therapy has remained an important component of the management plan for a variety of cardiovascular-related disorders including hypertension and volume overload states such as congestive heart failure, cirrhosis, chronic kidney disease and the nephrotic syndrome. Few drugs in any class can boast of maintaining such prominence in therapy as when they were originally introduced.

Mutual attention paid to the diuretic site of action as well as an underlying knowledge of renal physiology and the pathophysiology of the disease provide a context in which to apply diuretic pharmacology in a manner that enables reliable prediction of their therapeutic and adverse effects. Tailoring therapy to the disease and the individual patient in this manner insures that an effective diuresis can be achieved under a variety of circumstances.

REFERENCES

1. Sarafidis PA, Georgianos PI, Lasaridis AN. Diuretics in clinical practice. Part I: mechanisms of action, pharmacological effects and clinical indications of diuretic compounds. Expert Opin Drug Saf. 2010;9:243-57.
2. Ernst ME, Moser M. Use of diuretics in patients with hypertension. N Engl J Med. 2009;361:2153-64.
3. Strauss MB, Southworth H. Urinary changes due to sulfonamide administration. Bull Johns Hopkins Hosp. 1938;63:41-5.
4. Brater DC. Pharmacology of diuretics. Am J Med Sci. 2000;319:38-50.
5. Brater DC. Diuretic therapy. N Engl J Med. 1998;339:387-95.
6. Kim GH. Long-term adaptation of renal ion transporters to chronic diuretic treatment. Am J Nephrol. 2004;24:595-605.
7. Ferguson JA, Sundblad KJ, Becker PK, et al. Role of duration of diuretic effect in preventing sodium retention. Clin Pharmacol Ther. 1997;62:203-8.
8. Loon NR, Wilcox CS, Unwin RJ. Mechanism of impaired natriuretic response to furosemide during prolonged therapy. Kidney Int. 1989;36:682-9.
9. Wilcox CS, Mitch WE, Kelly RA, et al. Response of the kidney to furosemide. I. Effects of salt intake and renal compensation. J Lab Clin Med. 1983;102:450-8.
10. Ellison DH. Diuretic resistance: physiology and therapeutics. Sem Nephrol. 1999;19:581-97.
11. Ram CV, Garrett BN, Kaplan NM. Moderate sodium restriction and various diuretics in the treatment of hypertension. Arch Intern Med. 1981;141:1015-9.
12. Wilcox CS, Guzman NJ, Mitch WE, et al. Na^+, K^+, and BP homeostasis in man during furosemide: effects of prazosin and captopril. Kidney Int. 1987;31:135-41.
13. Ellison DH, Velazquez H, Wright FS. Adaptation of the distal convoluted tubule of the rat: structural and functional effects of dietary sodium intake and chronic diuretic infusion. J Clin Invest. 1989;83:113-26.
14. Almeshari K, Ahlstom NG, Capraro FE, et al. A volume-independent component to post-diuretic sodium retention in man. J Am Soc Nephrol. 1993;3:1878-83.
15. Walter SJ, Shirley DG. The effect of chronic hydrochlorothiazide administration on renal function in the rat. Clin Sci. 1986;70:379-87.
16. Brater DC, Kaojarern S, Chennavasin P. Pharmacodynamics of the diuretic effects of aminophylline and acetazolamide alone and combined with furosemide in normal subjects. J Pharmacol Exp Ther. 1983;227:92-8.
17. Mazur JE, Devlin JW, Peters MJ, et al. Single versus multiple doses of acetazolamide for metabolic alkalosis in critically ill medical patients: a randomized, double-blind trial. Crit Care Med. 1999;27:1257-61.
18. Shankar SS, Brater DC. Loop diuretics: from the Na-K-2Cl transporter to clinical use. Am J Physiol Renal Physiol. 2003;284:F11-21.
19. Francis GS, Siegel RM, Goldsmith SR, et al. Acute vasoconstrictor response to intravenous furosemide in patients with chronic congestive heart failure. Activation of the neurohumoral axis. Ann Intern Med. 1985;103:1-6.
20. Dikshit K, Vyden JK, Forrester JS, et al. Renal and extrarenal hemodynamic effects of furosemide in congestive heart failure after acute myocardial infarction. N Engl J Med. 1973;288:1087-90.
21. Murray MD, Haag KM, Black PK, et al. Variable furosemide absorption and poor predictability of response in elderly patients. Pharmacotherapy. 1997;17:98-106.
22. Vargo DL, Kramer WG, Black PK, et al. Bioavailability, pharmacokinetics, and pharmacodynamics of torsemide and furosemide in patients with congestive heart failure. Clin Pharmacol Ther. 1995;57:601-9.
23. Pichette V, Du SP. Role of the kidneys in the metabolism of furosemide: its inhibition by probenecid. J Am Soc Nephrol. 1996;7:345-9.
24. Brater DC, Leinfelder J, Anderson A. Clinical pharmacology of torasemide, a new loop diuretic. Clin Pharmcol Ther. 1987;42:187-92.
25. Schwartz S, Brater DC, Pound D, et al. Bioavailability, pharmacokinetics, and pharmacodynamics of torsemide in patients with cirrhosis. Clin Pharmacol Ther. 1993;54:90-7.
26. Voelker JR, Cartwright-Brown D, Anderson S, et al. Comparison of loop diuretics in patients with chronic renal insufficiency. Kidney Int. 1987;32:572-8.
27. Zempel G, Ditlevsen J, Hoch M, et al. Effects of indapamide on Ca^{2+} entry into vascular smooth muscle cells. Nephron. 1997;76:460-5.
28. Welling PG. Pharmacokinetics of the thiazide diuretics. Biopharm Drug Dispos. 1986;7:501-35.
29. Riess W, Dubach UC, Burckhardt D, et al. Pharmacokinetic studies with chlorthalidone (Hygroton) in man. Eur J Clin Pharmacol. 1977;12:375-82.
30. Ernst ME, Carter BL, Basile JN. All thiazide-like diuretics are not chlorthalidone: putting the accomplish study into perspective. J Clin Hypertens (Greenwich). 2009;11:5-10.
31. Ernst ME, Grimm RH. Thiazide diuretics: 50 years and beyond. Curr Hypertens Rev. 2008;4:256-65.
32. Tarzi RC, Dustan HP, Frohlich ED. Long-term thiazide therapy in essential hypertension. Evidence for persistent alterations in plasma volume and renin activity. Circulation. 1970;41:709-17.
33. Wilson IM, Freis ED. Relationship between plasma and extracellular fluid volume depletion and the antihypertensive effect of chlorothiazide. Circulation. 1959;20:1028-36.
34. Gifford RW, Mattox VR, Orvis AL, et al. Effect of thiazide diuretics on plasma volume, body electrolytes, and excretion of aldosterone in hypertension. Circulation. 1961;24:1197-205.
35. Roos JC, Boer P, Koomans HA, et al. Haemodynamic and hormonal changes during acute and chronic diuretic treatment in essential hypertension. Eur J Clin Pharmacol. 1981;19:107-12.
36. Stamler R, Stamler J, Grimm R, et al. Nutritional therapy for high blood pressure. Final report of a four-year randomized controlled trial—The Hypertension Control Program. JAMA. 1987;257:1484-91.
37. Cloyd JC, Snyder BD, Cleeremans B, et al. Mannitol pharmacokinetics and serum osmolality in dogs and humans. J Pharmacol Exp Ther. 1986;236:301-6.
38. Thadhani R, Pascual M, Bonventre JV. Acute renal failure. N Engl J Med. 1996;334:1448-60.
39. Carter BL, Ernst ME. Should diuretic therapy be first step therapy in all hypertensive patients? In: Toth PP, Sica DA (Eds). Clinical Challenges in Hypertension II, 1st edition. Oxford: Atlas Medical Publishing; 2010.
40. Calhoun DA, Jones D, Textor S, et al. Resistant hypertension: diagnosis, evaluation, and treatment. A scientific statement from the American Heart Association Professional Education Committee of the Council for High Blood Pressure Research. Hypertension. 2008;51:1403-19.
41. Trewet CB, Ernst ME. Resistant hypertension: identifying causes and optimizing treatment regimens. South Med J. 2008;101:166-73.
42. Materson BJ, Reda DJ, Cushman WC, et al. Single-drug therapy for hypertension in men. A comparison of six antihypertensive agents with placebo. N Engl J Med. 1993;328:914-21.
43. Effects of different blood-pressure-lowering regimens on major cardiovascular events: results of prospectively-designed overviews of randomised trials. Lancet. 2003;362:1527-35.
44. Blood Pressure Lowering Treatment Trialists' Collaboration. Do men and women respond differently to blood pressure-lowering treatment?

Results of prospectively designed overviews of randomized trials. Eur Heart J. 2008;2:2669-80.

45. Blood Pressure Lowering Treatment Trialists' Collaboration. Effects of different regimens to lower blood pressure on major cardiovascular events in older and younger adults: meta-analysis of randomised trials. BMJ. 2008;336:1121-3.

46. ALLHAT Officers and Coordinators for the ALLHAT Collaborative Research Group. Major outcomes in high-risk hypertensive patients randomized to angiotensin-converting enzyme inhibitor or calcium channel blocker vs diuretic: the Antihypertensive and Lipid-Lowering Treatment to Prevent Heart Attack Trial (ALLHAT). JAMA. 2002;288: 2981-97.

47. Wright JT, Probstfield JL, Cushman WC, et al. ALLHAT findings revisited in the context of subsequent analyses, other trials, and meta-analyses. Arch Intern Med. 2009;169: 832-42.

48. Wing LM, Reid CM, Ryan P, et al. A comparison of outcomes with angiotensin-converting enzyme inhibitors and diuretics for hypertension in the elderly. N Engl J Med. 2003;348:583-92.

49. Jamerson K, Weber MA, Bakris GL, et al. Benazepril plus amlodipine or hydrochlorothiazide for hypertension in high-risk patients. N Engl J Med. 2008;359:2417-28.

50. Carter BL, Ernst ME, Cohen JD. Hydrochlorothiazide versus chlorthalidone: evidence supporting their interchangeability. Hypertension. 2004;43:4-9.

51. Ernst ME, Carter BL, Goerdt CJ, et al. Comparative antihypertensive effects of hydrochlorothiazide and chlorthalidone on ambulatory and office blood pressure. Hypertension. 2006;47:352-8.

52. Ernst ME, Carter BL, Zheng S, et al. Meta-analysis of dose-response characteristics of hydrochlorothiazide and chlorthalidone: effects on systolic blood pressure and potassium. Am J Hypertens. 2010;23:440-6.

53. Taler SJ, Textor SC, Augustine JE. Resistant hypertension. Comparing hemodynamic management to specialist care. Hypertension. 2002;39:982-8.

54. Beckett NS, Peters R, Fletcher AE, et al. Treatment of hypertension in patients 80 years of age and older. N Engl J Med. 2008;358:1887-98.

55. Knauf H, Mutschler E. Diuretic effectiveness of hydrochlorothiazide and furosemide alone and in combination in chronic renal failure. J Cardivasc Pharmacol. 1995;26:394-400.

56. Dussol B, Moussi-Frances J, Morange S, et al. A randomized trial of furosemide vs hydrochlorothiazide in patients with chronic renal failure and hypertension. Nephrol Dial Transplant. 2005;20:349-53.

57. Nishizaka MK, Zaman MA, Calhoun DA. Efficacy of low-dose spironolactone in subjects with resistant hypertension. Am J Hypertens. 2003;16:925-30.

58. Saha C, Eckert GJ, Ambrosius WT, et al. Improvement in blood pressure with inhibition of the epithelial sodium channel in blacks with hypertension. Hypertension. 2005;46:481-7.

59. Rasool A, Palevsky PM. Treatment of edematous disorders with diuretics. Am J Med Sci. 2000;319:25-37.

60. Van Olden RW, Van Meyel JJM, Gerlag PGG. Sensitivity of residual nephrons to high dose furosemide described by diuretic efficiency. Eur J Clin Pharmacol. 1995;47:483-8.

61. Oster JR, Epstein M, Smoller S. Combined therapy with thiazide-type and loop diuretic agents for resistant sodium retention. Ann Intern med. 1983;99:405-6.

62. Villeneuve JP, Verbeeck RK, Wilkinson GR, et al. Furosemide kinetics and dynamics in patients with cirrhosis. Clin Pharmacol Ther. 1986;40:14-20.

63. Murray MD, Deer MM, Ferguson JA, et al. Open-label randomized trial of torsemide compared with furosemide therapy for patients with heart failure. Am J Med. 2001;111:513-20.

64. Brater DC, Chennavasin P, Seiwell R. Furosemide in patients with heart failure: shift in dose-response curves. Clin Pharmacol Ther. 1980;28:182-6.

65. Dormans TP, Van Meyel JJ, Gerlag PG, et al. Diuretic efficacy of high dose furosemide in severe heart failure: bolus injection versus continuous infusion. J Am Coll Cardiol. 1996;28:376-82.

66. Pitt B, Zannad F, Reme WJ, et al. The effect of spironolactone on morbidity and mortality in patients with severe congestive heart failure. N Engl J Med. 1999;341:709-17.

67. Carter BL, Einhorn PT, Brands M, et al. Thiazide-induced dysglycemia: review of the literature and call for research. A report from a working group from the National Heart, Lung, and Blood Institute. Hypertension. 2008;52:30-6.

68. Sarafidis PA, Georgianos PI, Lasaridis AN. Diuretics in clinical practice. Part II: electrolyte and acid-base disorders complicating diuretic therapy. Expert Opin Drug Saf. 2010;9:259-73.

69. Savage PJ, Pressel SL, Curb JD, et al. Influence of long-term, low-dose, diuretic-based, antihypertensive therapy on glucose, lipid, uric acid, and potassium levels in older men and women with isolated systolic hypertension: the systolic hypertension in the elderly program. Arch Intern Med. 1998;158:741-51.

70. Strom BL, Schinnar R, Apter AJ, et al. Absence of cross-reactivity between sulfonamide antibiotics and sulfonamide nonantibiotics. N Engl J Med. 2003;349:1628-35.

Chapter 5

Vasodilators and Neurohormone Modulators

Gary S Francis, Suma Konety

Chapter Outline

INTRODUCTION

It has long been recognized that impedance to left ventricular (LV) outflow is a critical determinant of cardiac performance.[1–4] This is especially true of patients with impaired LV systolic performance such as in systolic heart failure (Fig. 1).[5] Ultimately, the failing heart loses its natural ability

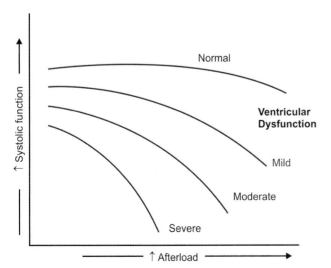

FIGURE 1: The relationship between various degrees of left ventricular dysfunction and afterload stress. (*Source:* Modified from Cohn JN, Franciosa JA. Vasodilator therapy of cardiac failure. N Engl J Med. 1977;297:27-31, 254-8, with permission)

to respond to increased impedance to ejection (i.e. loss of homeometric autoregulation), although lowering systemic resistance by drugs can rescue myocardial systolic function to some extent.

Heightened resistance or impedance to LV ejection is often referred to as "afterload", but the term afterload originates from isolated muscle studies done in the mid-1970s and is not, strictly speaking, appropriately applied to the clinical setting. Afterload is defined as ventricular wall stress during shortening and cannot easily be measured in the intact circulation. Afterload is a product of LV cavity size (La Place relationship) and is inversely related to wall thickness or hypertrophy. In clinical practice, systemic vascular resistance (SVR) is frequently calculated [SVR = (mean arterial pressure – CVP) x 80/cardiac output] from right heart catheterization data, but this calculation is largely an estimate of small peripheral vessel caliber resistance. SVR is therefore only a part of the total impedance (Table 1) that the LV sees during ejection. Aortic impedance is also not typically measured as part of clinical care. Most bedside estimates of afterload are still derived by measuring SVR. The failing ventricles (both left and right) are exquisitely sensitive to afterloading conditions, and it is a logical extension of this concept that drugs that reduce aortic impedance will improve cardiac systolic performance, independent of any effect on myocardial contractility. Since aortic impedance is not routinely measured, SVR is used as a surrogate for impedance and tends to be equated with "afterload" by clinicians, but strictly

TABLE 1

Components of aortic impedance

- Large vessel distensibility
- Small vessel caliber (systemic vascular resistance)
- Small vessel compliance
- Blood viscosity
- Inertia

(*Source:* Tang WH, Young JB. Chronic heart failure management. In: EJ Topol (Ed). Textbook of Cardiovascular Medicine, 3rd edition. Philadelphia: Lippincott Williams and Wilkins; 2007. pp. 1373-405)

speaking, aortic impedance is a much more comprehensive concept than SVR.

VASODILATOR DRUGS AND LOW BLOOD PRESSURE

Patients with moderate-to-severe heart failure often have low blood pressure (BP) that is asymptomatic. Low brachial systolic pressure is sometimes perceived by physicians as a contraindication to the use of arteriolar dilator drugs such as nitrates, angiotensin converting enzyme (ACE) inhibitors, angiotensin receptor blockers (ARBs) or carvedilol. However, vasodilator drugs can maintain or even increase systolic BP by increasing stroke volume in patients with systolic heart failure. Observations from large clinical trials have challenged the belief that vasodilators are deleterious in patients with low systolic BP.[6–8] Generally speaking, vasodilator drugs should be continued in patients with systolic heart failure and asymptomatic low systolic BP in the range of 90–110 mm Hg. Severe, symptomatic hypotension can sometimes occur in a volume deplete patient in response to an ACE inhibitor, e.g. following a robust diuresis. Such brisk falls in BP are now less common, as clinicians recognize that symptomatic hypotension is a well-described adverse event that can occur when ACE inhibitors or ARBs are used in the context of hypovolemia and an activated renin-angiotensin-aldosterone system (RAAS). Symptomatic reduction in systolic BP in response to vasodilators in a euvolemic or volume-overloaded patient with severe LV dysfunction is another matter. Such patients are said to be truly intolerant of vasodilators, and symptomatic hypotension in response to drug therapy is a very powerful sign of poor prognosis. Low BP without symptoms is far more common and can usually be ignored when using vasodilator drugs.

ARTERIAL VERSUS VENOUS EFFECTS OF VASODILATOR DRUGS IN PATIENTS WITH SYSTOLIC HEART FAILURE

Arteriolar dilating drugs, such as hydralazine or amlodipine, reduce aortic impedance and thereby increase the velocity of shortening during LV ejection. LV end-systolic volume is thus reduced and LV ejection fraction increases. With hydralazine, LV end-diastolic volume (i.e. preload) may not acutely be altered, so the stroke volume response can be markedly increased.[9] When vasodilator drugs, such as nitrates, are employed in patients with systolic heart failure, blood volume

may acutely redistribute into the large capacitance veins and LV end-diastolic volume or preload may be reduced. The reduced LV end-diastolic volume may limit the increase in stroke volume to some extent.[10] With balanced arteriolar-venous vasodilator drugs, such as sodium nitroprusside, typically venous pressure falls (decongestion) and stroke volume still improves as a consequence of marked reduction in aortic impedance. Essentially, the hemodynamic effects of vasodilator drugs are dependent on the relative effects of the drug on resistance and capacitance vessels. In patients with severe regurgitant lesions, such as mitral or aortic regurgitation, vasodilator drugs reduce the regurgitant fraction and increase forward cardiac output, thus adding to their beneficial effects.

The reflex tachycardia observed in normal subjects in response to arteriolar dilating drugs is not seen in patients with advanced systolic heart failure.[11] This is likely due to the reduced cardiac norepinephrine spillover rate that occurs with unloading of the baroreceptors and low-pressure mechanoreceptors in response to systemic vasodilation in heart failure.[12] In fact, the magnitude of the blunted neurohumoral response to nitroprusside infusion in patients with systolic heart failure (i.e. lack of reflex tachycardia) may be a marker of the severity and prognosis of heart failure.[11]

In general, the beneficial response to vasodilator drug therapy is most obvious in patients with systolic heart failure and a dilated LV. Patients with normal LV cavity size may be more sensitive to changes in preload reduction, and hypotension can occur in response to reduced SVR if the heart is small or there is a relatively reduced preload.

ARTERIOLAR VASODILATORS

HYDRALAZINE

Hydralazine is an old drug, one of the first to be used to treat hypertension in the 1950s. Its mechanism of action is still not completely elucidated, but it appears to be a direct acting, potent arteriolar dilator that relaxes the smooth muscles of small resistance vessels. It has essentially no venodilating effects. Hydralazine primarily dilates the renal- and peripheral-resistant arterioles and has little effect on coronary or liver blood flow. It may also have antioxidant effects and can prevent tolerance to nitrates (Fig. 2).

It has been known for years that when hydralazine is used in non-systolic heart failure patients, e.g. in patients with systemic hypertension, large doses can produce reflex tachycardia, edema and even worsen angina. Reflex tachycardia in response to hydralazine is not typically observed in patients with more advanced systolic heart failure because of a blunted baroreceptor response.

Hydralazine can be given orally where it is rapidly absorbed from the gastrointestinal tract. However, the bioavailability is highly variable and depends on the rapidity that is acetylated by the liver, a genetically determined trait. In the United States, about half of the people are fast acetylators and half are slow acetylators. Acetylation activity is not routinely measured in patients. A lupus-like syndrome is more likely to occur in slow acetylators and this typically wanes when hydralazine is stopped. Fast acetylators may

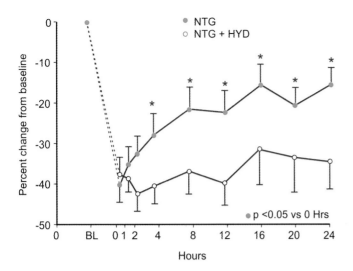

FIGURE 2: Nitroglycerin (NTG) alone is associated with the development of early tolerance, whereas the combination of NTG and hydralazine (HYD) 75 mg four times per day is associated with less NTG tolerance. (*: Statistically significant changes). (*Source:* Modified from Elkayam U. Nitrates in the treatment of congestive heart failure. Am J Cardiol. 1996;77:41C-51C, with permission).

require higher doses of hydralazine. Chronic hydralazine use can cause vitamin B6 deficiency.

The hemodynamic response to chronic oral hydralazine therapy in patients with systolic heart failure is usually characterized by no change in heart rate, a fall in SVR and about a 50% increase in cardiac output.[13] Usually, BP does not change much. Patients with chronic mitral or aortic regurgitation demonstrate a reduction in the regurgitant jet by echo and auscultation, and forward stroke volume is markedly increased. There is no long-term improvement in exercise capacity despite a modest, persistent improvement in EF. The combination of hydralazine and isosorbide dinitrate ushered in the vasodilator era for the treatment of heart failure (Fig. 3).

Even today we do not know entirely how to dose hydralazine for individual patients with advanced heart failure. Because of the high success rate of other vasodilator drugs, such as ACE inhibitors and ARBs, hydralazine has been relegated to second-tier therapy. The one important exception is featured by the results of the African-American Heart Failure Trial (A-HeFT) (Fig. 4).[14] In this trial, the combination of hydralazine and isosorbide dinitrate in a combination of fixed-dose drug (BiDil®) added to standard therapy improved survival and other outcomes among black patients with systolic heart failure. One rationale for the trial was that isosorbide dinitrate might augment nitric oxide production, and therefore improve endothelial function. Hydralazine may also work as an antioxidant and can reduce nitrate tolerance.[15] The combination of hydralazine and isosorbide dinitrate today should be considered as an add-on therapy, superimposed on more conventional therapy, when patients are demonstrating signs and symptoms of worsening heart failure.

Typically, hydralazine is prescribed along with isosorbide dinitrate to improve cardiac output and reduce pulmonary capillary wedge pressure (PCWP). The initial hydralazine dose used in A-HeFT was 37.5 mg three times per day and gradually increased to 75 mg three times per day. Isosorbide dinitrate was titrated to a dose of 80 mg three times per day. Hydralazine and

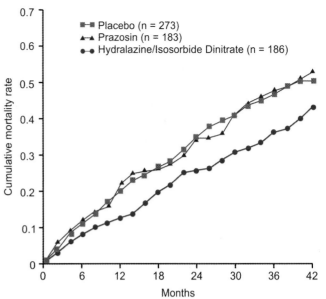

FIGURE 3: Mortality curves of patients with heart failure randomized to placebo, prazosin or isosorbide dinitrate/hydralazine in the first Vasodilator Heart Failure Trial (V-HeFT 1); p= 0.046 on the generalized Wilcoxan test, which gives more weight to the treatment differences in the early part of the mortality curves. (*Source:* Modified from Cohn JN, Archibald DG, Ziesche S, et al. Effect of vasodilator therapy on mortality in chronic congestive heart failure. Results of a Veterans Administration Cooperative Study. N Engl J Med. 1986;314:1547-52, with permission)

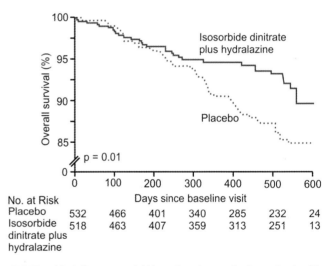

No. at Risk						
Placebo	532	466	401	340	285	232	24
Isosorbide dinitrate plus hydralazine	518	463	407	359	313	251	13

FIGURE 4: Mortality curves of African-American patients randomized to placebo or isosorbide dinitrate/hydralazine in addition to standard therapy for heart failure in the African-American Heart Failure Trial (A-HeFT). (*Source:* Modified from Taylor AL, Zliesche S, Yancy C, et al. Combination of isosorbide dinitrate and hydralazine in blacks with heart failure. N Engl J Med. 2004; 351:2049-57, with permission)

isosorbide dinitrate were combined in the drug BiDil®. Doses of hydralazine, as high as 1,200 mg/day, have been used to treat systolic heart failure, but onset of lupus syndrome is seen in 15–20% of patients receiving more than 400 mg/day. Fluid retention is also common when higher doses of hydralazine are used. There is likely a survival advantage associated with long-term hydralazine therapy when taken with isosorbide dinitrate to treat systolic heart failure.

Amlodipine is a dihydropyridine L-type calcium channel blocking agent that is widely used to treat hypertension and angina. It is a long-acting, potent, arteriolar dilating drug that is well tolerated. The typical starting dose is 2.5 or 5 mg/day and the target dose for many patients is 10 mg/day. Calcium channel drugs are vasodilators and have anti-ischemic effects, so it is logical that they would be investigated in patients with systolic heart failure. The most promising calcium channel blocker to emerge from these studies as potential heart failure therapy was amlodipine. The only drawback to amlodipine is the frequent development of pedal edema with the higher dose, but this is assumed to be due to benign vasodilation in the small arterioles and venules in the ankles, and not due to heart failure *per se*. Other non-dihydropyridine calcium channel blockers, such as verapamil and diltiazem, may either have negative inotropic properties, cause cardiac electrical conduction problems, or are simply not very powerful vasodilators. They do not play any role in the treatment of heart failure.

The effect of amlodipine on outcomes in patients with chronic systolic heart failure was evaluated in the two prospective randomized amlodipine survival evaluation (PRAISE) studies.[16,17] The earlier of the two studies demonstrated that all-cause mortality might be lower in a subset of patients with nonischemic dilated cardiomyopathy treated with amlodipine, although overall, the trial was neutral. A second PRAISE trial was then done solely in patients with nonischemic dilated cardiomyopathy. In PRAISE II, an overall neutral effect of amlodipine was once again observed. It seems clear that amlodipine is safe to use in patients with systolic heart failure when needed to control hypertension or angina. However, amlodipine is not effective as primary therapy for the treatment of systolic heart failure, despite its powerful vasodilating properties. Several other potent vasodilators have failed to improve mortality in patients with heart failure, including prazosin, flosequinan, nesiritide, and synthetic prostacyclin (epoprostenol) or Flolan. These observations suggest that vasodilation alone is not enough to provide a mortality benefit. Presumably it is not simple "vasodilation" that provides for the survival benefit, but there should be some neurohumoral modulation property or some other mechanisms beyond simple reduction in SVR.

ORAL NITRATES

Nitrates have been widely used to treat angina by physicians for well over 100 years. It is only in the past 25 years that they have been used to treat systolic heart failure. Their favorable effects on angina, systolic heart failure, mitral regurgitation and coronary spasm are now well known. The mechanism of action of nitrates is complex, but these molecules appear to undergo a metabolic biotransformation in vascular smooth muscle which leads to the formation of nitric oxide (NO) or a related S-nitrosothiol. These breakdown products of nitrates stimulate the enzyme guanylate cyclase, leading to the formulation of cyclic-guanosine monophosphate (c-GMP). c-GMP in turn reduces calcium influx, which leads to venous and arterial vasodilation.[18] It is also likely that the vascular endothelium responds to nitrates with the synthesis and release of prosta-

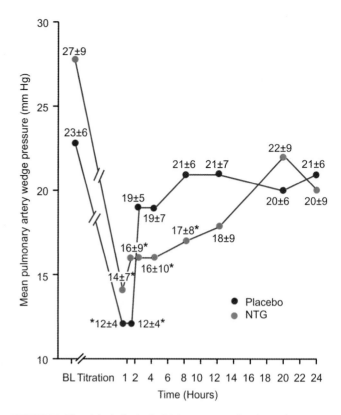

FIGURE 5: The data indicate that tolerance can develop to intravenous nitroglycerin (NTG) over 24 hours. There is a brisk initial response to IV NTG manifested by a fall in pulmonary capillary wedge pressure (PCWP) during titration; but during 24 hours of infusion, PCWP increases back toward control in both the NTG and the placebo arms of the study. (*Source:* Modified from Elkayam U, Kulick D, McIntosh N, et al. Incidence of early tolerance to hemodynamic effects of continuous infusion of NTG in patients with coronary artery disease and heart failure. Circulation. 1987;76:577-84, with permission)

cyclin,[19] thus improving endothelial function. Nitrates primarily cause venodilation, which typically increases capacitance and reduces preload, thus lowering end-diastolic volume, reducing cardiac wall tension and diminishing PCWP. Dyspnea is relieved. Larger doses lead to arteriolar dilation, further reducing afterload and improving forward flow. LV cavity size diminishes, reducing mitral regurgitation.[20] It is not surprising that oral nitrate therapy has emerged as an important treatment for systolic heart failure. Nitrates are among the few vasodilators that are able to increase exercise tolerance in patients with systolic heart failure.[21,22] However, nitrate tolerance occurs in many patients (Fig. 5), thus casting suspicion on long-term efficiency. This can be offset to some extent by hydralazine.[15]

RENIN-ANGIOTENSIN-ALDOSTERONE SYSTEM (RAAS) BLOCKERS

ANGIOTENSIN CONVERTING ENZYME INHIBITORS (ACE INHIBITORS)

ACE inhibitors were introduced into clinical practice in the 1980s for the treatment of hypertension and heart failure. This class of drug therapy has revolutionized therapy for these two conditions, and has been demonstrated to improve survival in patients with systolic heart failure (Figs 6A and B). The development of this class of drugs for the treatment of heart

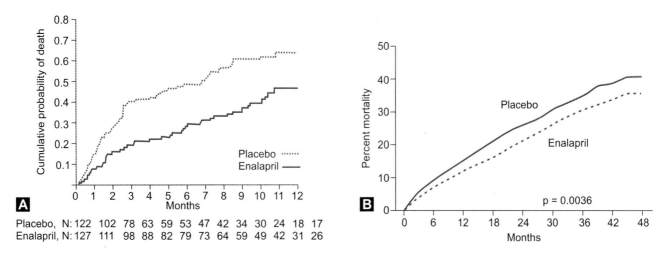

FIGURES 6A AND B: In the CONSENSUS Trial, the difference between treatments is even more striking, as the patients likely had more advanced heart failure. Kaplan-Meier survival curves (A) from The CONSENSUS Trial Study Group. Effects of enalapril on mortality in severe congestive heart failure. Results of the Cooperative North Scandinavian Enalapril Survival Study (CONSENSUS). (*Source:* Modified from N Engl J Med. 1987;316:1429-35, with permission). (B) From the SOLVD Investigators. Effect of enalapril on survival in patients with reduced left ventricular ejection fractions and congestive heart failure. (*Source:* Modified from N Engl J Med. 1991;325:293-302, with permission)

failure was predicated on the observation that the RAAS is activated in chronic heart failure,[23] and contributes importantly to heightened afterload and to the LV remodeling process.

Angiotensinogen is produced in the liver and is converted in the blood by renin to form a small peptide, angiotensin I (Flow chart 1). Angiotensin I is then further cleaved to form angiotensin II, a very small peptide, but potent arteriole constrictor. Angiotensin II subserves a host of other biological activities primarily through the angiotensin II receptor, including promotion of volume retention, activation of and sensitization

FLOW CHART 1: The renin-angiotensin-aldosterone system

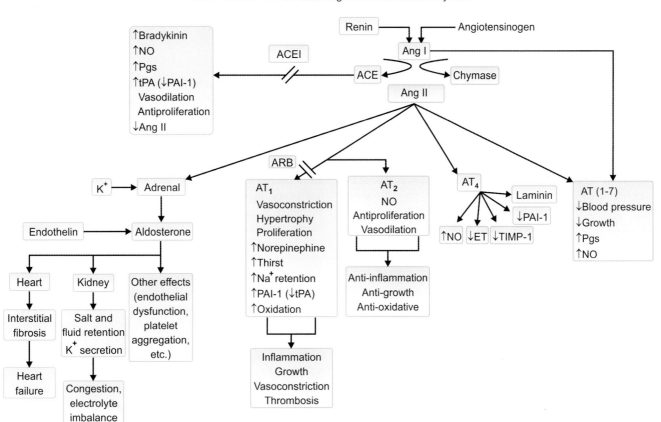

(Abbreviations: ACE: Angiotensin-converting-enzyme; ACEI: Angiotensin-converting-enzyme-inhibitor; ang I: Angiotensin I; ang II: Angiotensin II; AT: Angiotensin receptor; ET: Endothelin; NO: Nitric oxide; PAI: Plasminogen activator inhibitor; PGs: Prostaglandins; TIMP: Tissue inhibitor of metalloproteinase; tPA: Tissue plasminogen activator). (*Source:* Modified from Kalidindi SR, Tang WH, Francis GS. Drug insight: Aldosterone-receptor antagonists in heart failure—The journey continues. Nat Clin Pract Cardiovasc Med. 2007;4(7):368-78, with permission)

CHAPTER 5

Vasodilators and Neurohormone Modulators

to the sympathetic nervous system (SNS), thirst, regulation of salt and water balance, modulation of potassium balance, cardiac myocyte and vascular smooth muscle growth, to name a few. Its actions are central to the development of acute and chronic systolic heart failure.

Early, overly simplistic thinking was that systolic heart failure was essentially a vasoconstricted state caused by excessive SNS activity and heightened levels of other vasoconstrictor neurohormones, including angiotensin II, arginine vasopressin (AVP) and endothelin. When it became apparent that ACE inhibitors could block the production of angiotensin II, ACE inhibitors became an attractive candidate for the treatment of patients with systolic heart failure. ACE inhibitors would be expected to reduce SVR, and in turn would increase cardiac output and forward flow. Although the initial clinical studies indeed supported this hypothesis,[24] it soon became clear that ACE inhibitors were doing much more than reducing SVR. Long-term clinical improvement was accompanied by reduced LV remodeling and improved patient survival when applied to post-myocardial infarction patients,[25] very similar to the seminal animal work of Pfeffer and his colleagues.[26] ACE inhibitors were no longer thought of as simple arteriolar dilators, but were neurohormone modulators that could very favorably alter the natural history of systolic heart failure and improve survival by inhibiting the progression of LV remodeling (Figs 6A and B).

We now recognize that neurohormonal activation plays a key role in the initiation and progression of heart failure. The RAAS is central to this neurohormonal cascade, as patients with systolic heart failure and high renin levels seemingly derive the most acute benefit from blocking the RAAS.[27] It is now well established that ACE inhibitors slow the progression of heart failure and improve survival in patients with a reduced ejection fraction and congestive heart failure.[28] Much of this improvement is believed to be due to "reverse remodeling". Even patients with a reduced ejection fraction, but few or no heart failure symptoms, derive clinical benefit from ACE inhibitor therapy.[29] The development of symptomatic heart failure is delayed in these patients. The activation of neurohormones (renin, norepinephrine and AVP) appears to occur early in the natural history of the syndrome, before symptoms occur.[30] This observation suggested that early introduction of neurohormonal blocking drugs before symptoms ensue may slow the progression of systolic heart failure or even delay its onset of signs and symptoms.[29] Indeed, today neurohumoral modulating drugs are recommended in patients who demonstrate impaired LV systolic function in the absence of symptoms. Many investigators observed that the RAAS was markedly activated during decompensated heart failure, but returns to normal once the patient clinically stabilizes, even though severe LV dysfunction may persist.[31] The concept that blocking the RAAS improved patients with systolic heart failure became widely recognized in the 1990s.

In the 1980s a number of hypotheses and concepts emerged that challenged the long-standing notion that systolic heart failure was fundamentally a mechanical problem. Katz introduced the idea that heart failure may be a disorder of abnormal gene expressional growth response to injury,[32] and many others believed that the myocardial remodeling was at least in part due to activation of neurohormonal systems,[33] which

FLOW CHART 2: Heart failure is a complex clinical syndrome characterized by extensive neuroendocrine activation. The release of neurohormones appears to be in response to reduced cardiac function and a perceived reduction in effective circulatory volume. It is as if neuroendocrine activity is attempting to protect the blood pressure and maintain circulatory homeostasis. Although this may be adaptive early on, chronic neuroendocrine activation leads to peripheral vasoconstriction, left ventricular remodeling and worsening left ventricular performance, and thus becomes an attractive therapeutic target. Drugs designed to block the exuberant neuroendocrine response, such as ACE inhibitors, have now becomes the cornerstone of treatment for heart failure

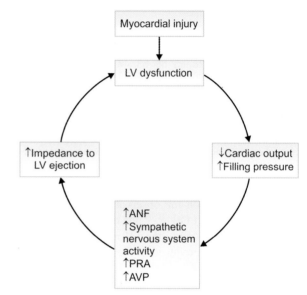

(Abbreviations: LV: Left ventricle; AVP: Arginine vasopressin; ANF: Atrial natriuretic factor; PRA: Plasma renin activity). (*Source:* Francis GS, Tang WH. In: JD Hosenpud, BH Greenberg (Eds). Congestive Heart Failure, 3rd edition. Philadelphia: Lippincott Williams and Wilkins; 2007. pp. 602-19)

were also well known to be the cardiac growth factors when studied *in vitro*.[34] Alteration of loading conditions due to increased LV chamber size and increased wall stress also undoubtedly led to progressive LV remodeling.[34] Both mechanical and neurohormonal signals regulated the remodeling process, as did altered gene expression. It became clear that the all-important LV remodeling process was largely structural and not functional.[35] Additional data emerged indicating that excessive angiotensin II caused cardiac myocyte necrosis under experimental conditions.[36] Eventually a coherent story emerged suggesting that systolic heart failure was at least in part driven by excessive neurohormonal activation,[37,38] setting up a vicious cycle of worsening heart failure and death (Flow chart 2). Even though these neurohormonal systems are likely adaptive in an evolutionary sense,[39] and are not simple biomarkers or epiphenomena, they are known to directly contribute to LV remodeling[40–42] and even patient mortality.[43] The strong notion emerged that pharmacological inhibition of the RAAS (and the SNS) might reduce the progression of LV remodeling,[44–47] and therefore such drugs should improve patient survival.[28]

The ACE inhibitors were the first class of drugs to really test the neurohumoral hypothesis (Figs 6A and B). Needless to say, they have now become a standard of care for patients with hypertension, systolic heart failure, acute myocardial infarction and advanced cardiovascular disease. Their role in the treatment of patients with systolic heart failure is now undoubted. The ACE inhibitor class of drugs reduces SVR, presumably by inhibiting angiotensin II arteriolar constriction reducing sympathetic tone. There is also marked venodilation with a fall in PCWP, presumably due to reduction in sympathetic activity to veins and desensitization of venous capacitance vessels to norepinephrine. Angiotensin II does not directly dilate veins, so there is no direct effect of ACE inhibitors on venous capacitance vessels. Venous capacitance vessels dilate in response to ACE inhibitors due to reduced sympathetic activity at the neuroeffector level. There is modest improvement in cardiac index with ACE inhibitors and the heart rate may be slightly slow. As previously mentioned, if the patient is acutely hyperreninemic from recent vigorous diuresis, there can be a substantial and prolonged fall in BP with even small doses of ACE inhibition. This is why many physicians prefer to use short-acting ACE inhibitors, such as captopril, in hospitalized patients with acute systolic heart failure, as patients are less likely to develop prolonged symptomatic hypotension. If symptomatic hypotension ensues, the patient should lie down and the feet should be elevated until these symptoms resolve and the BP improves. Usually a sense of well-being is established with the use of ACE inhibitors despite chronically low arterial pressures. Rarely, dysgeusia or loss of taste occurs, sometimes requiring withdrawal of the drug. Rash is uncommon with the smaller doses of ACE inhibitors used today. A dry, nonproductive cough occurs in some patients receiving ACE inhibitors, and the drug is discontinued in 5–10% of patients for this reason. The mechanism of cough is not entirely clear, but is believed to be due to the effects of bradykinin on sensory neurons in the proximal airways.

There is now a long list of ACE inhibitors to choose from (Table 2). They have somewhat dissimilar pharmacodynamics, pharmacokinetics and rates of elimination. In general, it is best to start with small doses of ACE inhibitors that have been tested in a large clinical trial and slowly titrate up over days to weeks to a target dose established as safe and effective by use in large clinical trials. It is expected that many patients with advanced systolic heart failure will have about a 20% increase in serum creatinine with ACE inhibitor use. This is usually not a reason to discontinue or lower the dose of the ACE inhibitor. However, this class of drug is contraindicated in patients with cardiogenic shock or acute renal failure, and can cause renal insufficiency when used in patients with renal artery stenosis. Occasionally, hyperkalemia can occur requiring alteration of the dose or temporary/permanent discontinuation of the ACE inhibitor. Careful, regular follow-up with a check on electrolytes, blood urea nitrogen (BUN) and serum creatinine is important in the care of these patients when making decisions about altering the dose of ACE inhibitors.

ANGIOTENSIN RECEPTOR BLOCKERS (ARBs)

Angiotensin receptors of the AT_1 subtype bind angiotensin II with a high structural specificity but limited binding capacity.[48] The remarkable success of ACE inhibitors in the treatment of hypertension, arterial disease, myocardial hypertrophy, heart failure and diabetic renal disease encouraged the development of alternative drugs to block the RAAS. It was eventually recognized that ACE inhibitor drugs blocked only one of several pathways that reduces angiotensin II activity, and that angiotensin II could "escape" from chronic ACE inhibition. ARBs do not demonstrate this "escape" phenomenon. ARBs do not cause cough. They can be used safely in patients who develop angioedema during treatment with an ACE inhibitor. Increased levels of angiotensin II peptides seen with the use of ARBs does not appear to have unexpected off-target effects despite activating AT_2 receptors. First-dose hypotension is not typically seen when ARBs are given to diuretic-treated patients, as often occurs with ACE inhibitors. This is probably because ARBs have a much slower onset of action. Orthostatic hypotension is rare. Rebound hypertension upon withdrawal of ARBs does not appear to be a problem. As with ACE inhibitors, acute renal failure may occur with ARBs if they are administered to patients with renal artery stenosis or cardiogenic shock. The incidence of renal dysfunction and hyperkalemia is comparable with ARBs and ACE inhibitors.[49] It is now reasonably clear that ACE inhibitors and ARBs should not be used together, as the likelihood of hyperkalemia, hypotension and worsening renal function is greater.[50]

Many randomized controlled trials of ARBs have been performed in patients with chronic systolic heart failure,[51,52] in patients with acute myocardial infarction complicated by heart failure or LV dysfunction[53] and in patients at high risk for vascular events.[54] Several important points have emerged from these large trials: (1) ARBs and ACE inhibitors appear to have very similar efficiency in these patient groups; (2) if the patient does not tolerate an ACE inhibitor, an ARB is a suitable substitution; (3) although generally more expensive, ARBs are better tolerated than ACE inhibitors and (4) the combination of an ACE inhibitor and an ARB (dual RAAS blocking effect) does not lead to more efficiency and is associated with more hypotension, worsening renal function and hyperkalemia.[55] Despite earlier favorable reports, ARBs do not appear to prevent recurrent atrial fibrillation.[56]

The dose of ARBs has generally been determined by pharmaceutical-generated data and subsequent verification of these doses in large clinical trials (Table 2). Extensive experience with RAAS blockers over the years has led to changes in dose recommendations. For example, a recent clinical trial demonstrated that losartan 150 mg daily reduced the rate of death or admission for heart failure to a greater extent than a dose of 50 mg per day.[57]

ACE inhibitors have been shown to attenuate LV enlargement and reduce mortality following myocardial infarction. We now have data to suggest that inhibition the RAAS with ARBs also results in favorable structural and functional changes. Treatment with the ACE inhibitor captopril, the ARB valsartan, or the combination of captopril plus valsartan resulted in similar changes in cardiac volume, ejection fraction and infarct segment length in a patient 20 months following acute myocardial infarction.[58] These observations suggest that ARBs have similar anti-remodeling properties as ACE inhibitors, and thus have added to their popularity for the treatment of hypertension and systolic heart failure. Unfortunately, their efficiency for the treatment of heart failure with preserved ejection fraction, as with ACE inhibitors, has not met with similar success.[59]

TABLE 2

Common drugs used in managing chronic heart failure in the United States

Drug	Trade name	Heart failure indication	Post-myocardial infarction indication	Dosing
Angiotensin-converting enzyme (ACE inhibitors)				
Benazepril	*Lotensin*	No	No	5-40 mg QD
Captopril	Capoten	Yes	No	6.25-150 mg TID
Enalapril	Vasotec	Yes	No	2.5-20 mg BID
Fosinopril	Monopril	Yes	No	10-80 mg QD
Lisinopril	Prinivil, Zestril	Yes	No	5-20 mg QD
Moexipril	*Univasc*	No	No	7.5-60 mg QD
Perindopril	*Aceon*	No	No	2-16 mg QD
Quinapril	Accupril	Yes	No	5-20 mg BID
Ramipril	Altace	Yes	Yes	2.5-20 mg QD
Trandolapril	*Mavik*	No	Yes	1-4 mg QD
Zofenopril	*Bifril*	NA	NA	7.5-60 mg QD
Angiotensin II receptor blockers (ARBs)				
Candesartan	Atacand	Yes	No	8-32 mg QD/BID
Eprosartan	*Teveten*	No	No	400-800 mg QD
Irbesartan	*Avapro*	No	No	150-300 QD
Losartan	*Cozaar*	No	No	50-100 mg QD/BID
Telmisartan	*Micardis*	No	No	40-80 QD
Olmesartan	*Benicar*	No	No	20-40 mg QD
Valsartan	Diovan	Yes	No	80-320 mg QD
β-Adrenergic receptor antagonists				
Carvedilol	Coreg	Yes	Yes	3.125-25 mg BID
Metoprolol succinate	Toprol XL	Yes	No	25-200 mg QD
Bisoprolol	*Zebeta*	No	No	1.25-10 mg QD
Nebivolol	*Nabilet*	No	No	1.25-10 mg QD
Aldosterone receptor antagonists				
Spironolactone	Aldactone	Yes	No	25-50 mg QD
Eplerenone	Inspra	No	Yes	25-50 mg QD
Others				
Amlodipine	*Norvasc*	No	No	2.5-10 mg QD
Hydralazone-isosorbid dinitrate	BiDil (37.5/20)	Yes	No	1-2 tablets TID
Digoxin	Digitek	Yes	No	0.125-0.25 mg QD

(Abbreviations: BID: Twice daily; QD: Once daily; TID: Three times daily. Italics indicate a drug that is currently not indicated by the US Food and Drug Administration for treating patients with heart failure). *Source:* Tang WH, Young JB. Chronic heart failure management. In: EJ Topol (Ed). Textbook of Cardiovascular Medicine, 3rd edition. Philadelphia: Lippincott Williams and Wilkins; 2007. pp. 1373-405)

MINERALOCORTICOID (ALDOSTERONE) RECEPTOR BLOCKERS

ALDOSTERONE AND SYSTOLIC HEART FAILURE

Aldosterone was structurally identified more than 50 years ago, and was soon after designated as mineralocorticoid due to its salt retaining properties. It also releases potassium from the kidney, gastrointestinal tract, sweat and salivary glands. It has long been known to play a pathophysiologic role in cardiovascular disease, including congestive heart failure (Flow chart 3).[60,61] In addition to its mineralocorticoid properties, which can cause hypokalemia and hypomagnesemia, aldosterone contributes in many ways to the development of heart failure.

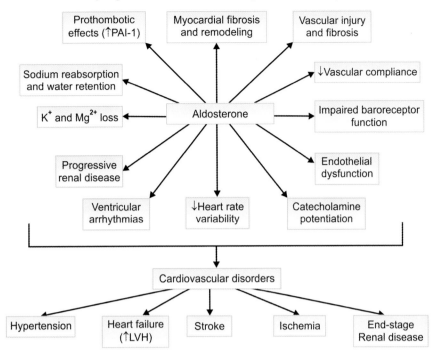

(Abbreviations: LVH: Left ventricular hypertrophy; PAI-1: Plasminogen activator inhibitor-1). (*Source:* Modified from Struthers AD, MacDonald TM. Review of aldosterone and angiotensin-II-induced target organ damage and prevention. Cardiovasc Res. 2004;61:663-70, with permission)

It likely causes vascular and cardiac remodeling, endothelial dysfunction, inhibits norepinephrine reuptake and causes baroreceptor dysfunction (Flow chart 3). It expands intravascular and extravascular volume. Inhibition of aldosterone is believed to be favorable due to: (1) reduced collagen deposition and possibly anti-remodeling effects; (2) BP reduction; (3) prevention of hypokalemia and associated arrhythmias and (4) modulation of nitric oxide synthesis (Flow chart 3). The major mineralocorticoid in heart failure is cortisol and not aldosterone. Serum aldosterone levels are not consistently elevated in patients with heart failure in the absence of diuretics. Accordingly, it is not aldosterone blockade *per se*, but mineralocorticoid receptor blockade that is important. Spironolactone and eplerenone are thus mineralocorticoid receptor blockers more than simply aldosterone receptor blockers.

ACE inhibitors were originally believed to persistently suppress angiotensin II in patients with heart failure, a major determinant of aldosterone production by the adrenal glands. This notion probably led to some initial loss of interest in aldosterone receptor inhibitors for the treatment of systolic heart failure. We now know that ACE inhibitors do not persistently suppress angiotensin II, and that there is aldosterone escape. There is now much greater interest in studying aldosterone receptor blockers. Two landmark studies, the randomized aldosterone evaluation study (RALES) (Fig. 7)[62] and the myocardial infarction heart failure efficacy and survival study (EPHESUS) (Fig. 8)[63] have remarkably increased the role of aldosterone mineralocorticoid antagonists for the everyday treatment of systolic heart failure. The drugs spironolactone[62] and eplerenone[63] are now widely used to treat chronic systolic heart failure and post-myocardial infarction heart failure. Despite their greater use today, in the United States it is estimated that less

than one-third of eligible patients hospitalized for heart failure receive appropriate, guideline-recommended aldosterone antagonist therapy.[64] Some of the reluctance to use aldosterone blockers in patients with systolic heart failure may be justified because of the advanced age of patients, the frequency of chronic renal insufficiency, other common comorbidities such as diabetes mellitus and the serious threat of hyperkalemia.[65] However, when used according to the protocol, hyperkalemia is seemingly not such a major problem. Careful follow-up of patients and frequent measurement of renal function and serum potassium are necessary to ensure safety when using aldosterone receptor blocking drugs.

The RAAS is likely an ancient (~400–600 million years) system that evolved in mammals in such a way as to allow them to adapt salt and volume depletion, as might have occurred during transition from the sea to land eons ago. The notion is that regulation of salt and water retention is adaptive, perhaps by protecting intravascular volume, BP and perfusion to vital organs. We now know that chronic stimulation of the RAAS in patients with heart failure can be maladaptive, and that pharmacologically blocking the RAAS can improve patient survival. Blockade of aldosterone membrane receptors is a widely accepted form of therapy for systolic heart failure. The RALES and EPHESUS studies provide strong evidence that aldosterone mineralocorticoid receptor blockade is an effective therapy for patients with advanced heart failure and early post-myocardial infarction heart failure, respectively. The role of nuclear aldosterone receptors is less clear, but given the complex array of regulatory properties that angiotensin II and aldosterone demonstrate, including inflammation, collagen synthesis, cytokine production, regulation of nitric oxide and cell adhesion molecules, one has to suspect that the activation

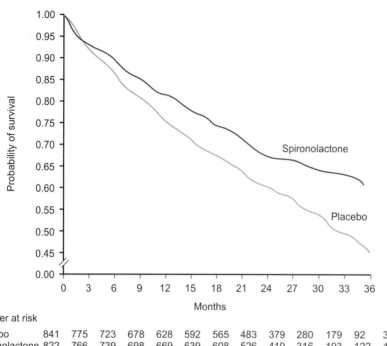

FIGURE 7: Survival curves of patients with advanced heart failure randomly allocated to spironolactone or placebo. Most patients were not receiving β-adrenergic blockers. There was a 30% reduction in mortality in patients randomized to spironolactone compared to patients in the placebo group. From the Randomized Aldactone Evaluation Study (RALES). (*Source:* Modified from Pitt B et al. The effect of spironolactone on morbidity and mortality in patients with severe heart failure. N Engl J Med. 1999;341:709-17, with permission)

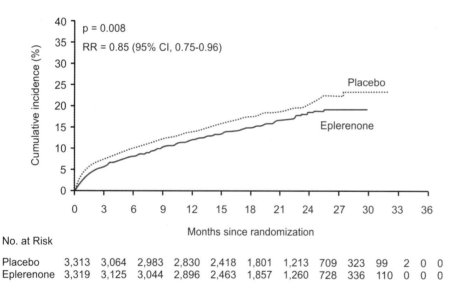

FIGURE 8: Kaplan-Meier estimates of the rate of death from any cause in the EPHESUS trial (Abbreviations: RR: Relative risk; CI: Confidence interval) (*Source:* Modified from Pitt B, Remme W, Zannad F, et al. Eplerenone, a selective aldosterone blocker, in patients with left ventricular dysfunction after myocardial infarction. N Engl J Med. 2003;348:1309-21, with permission)

of nuclear aldosterone receptors with resultant regulation of selective gene expression is also responsible for many of the biological activities of aldosterone, some of which are seen in systolic heart failure.

SPIRONOLACTONE AND EPLERENONE IN CHRONIC HEART FAILURE

The mechanism of action of spironolactone is complex, as aldosterone mineralocorticoid modulates many features of the heart failure syndrome. Although spironolactone is still used as an antihypertensive agent, it is not considered to be a "vasodilator" in the usual sense. Patients taking spironolactone need to be frequently and carefully monitored (patients in RALES were seen monthly for the first 12 weeks), as hyperkalemia and azotemia can occur with spironolactone,[65]

particularly if nonsteroidal anti-inflammatory drugs are used concomitantly. Diabetes mellitus, chronic kidney disease, volume depletion, advanced age and use of other potassium sparing agents, and nonsteroidal anti-inflammatory drugs are all risk factors for the development of hyperkalemia when using RAAS blocking drugs.[61] With careful monitoring, however, serious hyperkalemia is uncommon.[62]

Because of the central importance of aldosterone in the pathophysiology of heart failure, it is not surprising that the aldosterone receptor blocker spironolactone has emerged as an important therapy. Spironolactone is an old drug that was primarily used in large doses to treat ascites, edema and refractory hypertension. Excessive mineralocorticoid, common in patients with heart failure, promotes sodium retention, loss of magnesium and potassium, SNS activation, parasympathetic nervous system inhibition, myocardial and vascular fibrosis, baroreceptor dysfunction and impaired arterial compliance.[66] With the widespread emergence of ACE inhibitors, however, there was a common belief that ACE inhibitor therapy would also block aldosterone synthesis, so that there would be no need to add a drug-like spironolactone to an ACE inhibitor. However, it was eventually recognized that ACE inhibitors only transiently suppress the formation of aldosterone.[67] A small pilot study of 12.5–25 mg per day of spironolactone in conjunction with an ACE inhibitor, loop diuretic and digoxin-proved spironolactone was effective, well tolerated and did not cause serious hyperkalemia.[68] A much larger study was then launched.

The definitive RALES was published in 1999[62] and clearly demonstrated that spironolactone (25–50 mg per day) added to standard therapy (β-blockers were not yet in widespread use) was safe and reduced mortality by 30% (Fig. 7). Death from progressive heart failure and sudden death were both reduced by spironolactone. The patients who participated in RALES were primarily NYHA class III (70%) and IV (30%).

Eplerenone, a newer, more selective aldosterone mineralocorticoid receptor blocker, causes less gynecomastia and breast tenderness than spironolactone. It is more mineralocorticoid specific than spironolactone. EPHESUS[63] was conducted in patients who experienced a recent acute myocardial infarction with an EF of 40% or less who had heart failure, or had a history of diabetes mellitus. The patients in EPHESUS were randomly allocated to eplerenone or placebo in addition to standard therapy for acute myocardial infarction.

In EPHESUS, eplerenone (average dose 42.6 mg per day) reduced all-cause mortality by 15%, cardiovascular mortality by 17% and significantly lowered the need for subsequent hospitalization (Fig. 8). Sudden cardiac death was also reduced. As with RALES, serious hyperkalemia was unusual. The EMPHASIS-HF trial (Effect of Eplerenone versus Placebo on Cardiovascular Mortality and Heart Failure Hospitalization in Subjects with NYHA Class II Chronic Systolic Heart Failure) which employed eplerenone in a large double-blinded trial of patients with more mild (NYHA class II) heart failure was recently stopped prematurely when a favorable response was noted. This would suggest that eplerenone may be effective in patients with systolic heart failure and more mild symptoms.

Today, aldosterone mineralocorticoid antagonists are widely used to treat advanced heart failure and for selected patients with acute myocardial infarction. However, less than one-third of eligible patients hospitalized for heart failure are receiving guideline-recommended aldosterone receptor blocking drugs.[64] This is perhaps due in part to the need for more frequent and careful follow-up and the fear of hyperkalemia. There is a perception by some physicians that this class of drugs poses more risk than other RAAS blockers. Nevertheless, aldosterone receptor blockers are effective and safe when properly prescribed and monitored and their indications are seemingly expanding. There appears to be considerably less reverse remodeling in patients with mild-to-moderate heart failure and LV systolic dysfunction randomly assigned to eplerenone, even though there is a reduction in collagen turnover and a reduction in brain natriuretic factor (BNP).[69] Despite these surprising neutral effects on reverse remodeling, the results of the EMPHASIS-HF trial suggest that patients with mild-to-moderate

systolic heart failure still derive a favorable effect on morbidity and mortality from eplerenone.

PHOSPHODIESTERASE TYPE 5 INHIBITORS

SILDENAFIL AND TADALAFIL

Phosphodiesterases are enzymes that hydrolyze the cyclic nucleotides—c-GMP and cyclic adenosine monophosphate (cAMP). At least 11 families of phosphodiesterase isoenzymes have been identified. Phosphodiesterase 5 (PDE 5) degrades c-GMP via hydrolysis, thus influencing c-GMP's ability to modulate smooth muscle tone,[70] particularly in the venous system of the penile corpus cavernosum and in the pulmonary vasculature. The discovery of sildenafil, a highly selective inhibitor of PDE 5, was initially aimed to be a novel treatment for coronary artery disease. The initial clinical studies in the early 1990s were not promising for this target, but the off-target effect of the enhancement of penile erections did not escape the notice of investigators. The use of PDE 5 inhibitors was then redirected toward erectile dysfunction and more recently pulmonary hypertension.

Nitric oxide (NO) activates soluble guanylate cyclase, stimulating the production of c-GMP. PDE 5 normally hydrolyzes c-GMP. Sildenafil inhibits PDE 5, leading to increased c-GMP and vasodilation in response to NO. For years it was known that PDE 5 was not present in normal cardiac myocytes, and the heart itself was not considered an appropriate target. This was recently challenged by Kass and his colleagues[71] who demonstrated that inhibiting PDE 5 in hypertrophied RVs induces a positive inotropic response.[71,72] In fact, PDE 5 is markedly upregulated in hypertrophied ventricles, and PDE 5 inhibition may lead to regression of RV hypertrophy.[72] PDE 5 has long been known to be highly expressed in the lung vasculature, and so it is not surprising that sildenafil may be beneficial for the treatment of patients with pulmonary hypertension. As of this writing, it is still not clear if normal cardiac myocytes express PDE 5, but hypertrophied and/or failing myocytes do express it, and PDE 5 inhibition can be clinically helpful in patients with pulmonary hypertension and some element of right ventricular hypertrophy or failing right ventricle.

Sildenafil and tadalafil are both PDE 5 inhibitors that are useful in patients with pulmonary arterial hypertension who have mild to moderately severe symptoms.[73] Preliminary data on sildenafil suggest that its use may also be safe and even beneficial in patients with disproportionate pulmonary hypertension and LV dysfunction.[74,75] Sildenafil citrate (Revatio®) is prescribed in doses of 20 mg TID and tadalafil (Adcirca®) is much longer acting and is prescribed in doses of 5 mg per day as needed to control pulmonary hypertension. Hypotension can occur with PDE 5 inhibitors, especially when they are used with nitrates. There is no specific antidote for PDE 5 induced hypotension. Sildenafil and tadalafil are not approved for use in patients with heart failure, but they are being investigated. A small case series (three patients) has recently implied that a combination of sildenafil and nitrates can be used in patients with heart failure and pulmonary hypertension,[76] although clearly more robust clinical trials are needed. Experimental data indicate that PDE 5 levels are increased in severely failing hearts[77] and that sildenafil reduces myocardial remodeling.[78] Recent data also suggest that PDE 5 is regulated in the LV by oxidative stress.[79] Clearly this story is still unfolding and we have much to learn. Nevertheless, drugs such as sildenafil and tadalafil that selectively restore right ventricular contractility, limit right ventricular hypertrophy and reduce pulmonary artery remodeling are intriguing as potential therapy for right heart failure due to disproportionately increased pulmonary artery pressure. Perhaps PDE 5 inhibitors will also favorably affect left-sided systolic heart failure, particularly if there is associated pulmonary hypertension. More studies are needed, and use of these drugs for the treatment of heart failure remains investigational for now.

INTRAVENOUS VASODILATORS

NITROPRUSSIDE

Sodium nitroprusside can be dramatic in reversing the deleterious hemodynamics of acute systolic heart failure. Those who have had experience using the drug in this setting are often astonished how quickly the drug lowers PCWP and improves cardiac output, leading to prompt and often striking clinic improvement. The drug is usually started as doses of 10 mcg/min, and gradually titrated up to not more than 400 mcg/min, as needed to control hemodynamic abnormalities and symptoms. Some clinicians give nitroprusside according to body weight, with the typical dose starting at 10–20 mcg/kg/min. Our extensive experience with nitroprusside suggests that with low-dose infusion rates (less than 3 mcg/kg/min) used for less than 72 hours, toxicity is almost never observed.[80] The systolic BP should not be allowed to be less than 90 mm Hg or to a level that includes hypotensive symptoms. Invasive monitoring with a pulmonary artery catheter and an arterial catheter can be useful if the patient has marginal BP. When nitroprusside induces hypotension prior to the desired hemodynamic improvement, the additional administration of dopamine in doses greater than 3 mcg/kg/min will usually correct the problem.[81] Persistent or severe hypotension will nearly always dissipate as soon as nitroprusside is stopped.

METABOLISM AND TOXICITY OF NITROPRUSSIDE

Nitroprusside has been used to treat severe heart failure for many years,[82] although the Food and Drug Administration (FDA) has approved it only for severe hypertension and hypotensive surgery. It must be used carefully by experienced nurses and clinicians. Thiocyanate toxicity can occur, and thiocyanate levels should be checked as needed. Measurement of thiocyanate is a simple, inexpensive colorimetric test, normal levels being less than 10 mg/ml. Metabolic acidosis, anuria and a prolonged high dose of nitroprusside (> 400 mcg/min) can predispose to thiocyanate toxicity, prompting the measurement of thiocyanate levels. The thiocyanate ion is also readily removed by hemodialysis. When thiocyanate toxicity does occur, the patient may present with confusion, hyperreflexia and convulsions. Occasionally, mild hypoxemia occurs from nitroprusside due to ventilation-perfusion mismatch, but it is of little clinical consequence, as cardiac output rises and the delivery of oxygen to tissues increases. Coronary "steal" can occur when nitroprusside is used in the setting of acute myocardial infarction, and it should not be used routinely in this setting.[83] If intravenous vasodilator therapy is used for patients with acute myocardial infarction and severe heart failure, intravenous nitroglycerin may be preferred. Nevertheless, nitroprusside has been used successfully in this setting when given late.[82] If nitroprusside is used to treat severe heart failure related to acute myocardial infarction, it should be given later, perhaps 12 hours after admission to the hospital.[83]

NITROPRUSSIDE AND SEVERE HEART FAILURE

Nitroprusside quickly improves hemodynamics and symptoms in patients with severe heart failure.[84] Even patients with hypotension and shock may improve with nitroprusside,[85] as BP may stabilize or even improve with a large increase in cardiac output. Patients with severe mitral regurgitations or aortic regurgitation may also demonstrate dramatic reversal of serious hemodynamic perturbations with nitroprusside. Patients with severe aortic stenosis and worsening heart failure can be improved with nitroprusside used prior to aortic value replacement,[86] provided they are not hypotensive. It can also be used to stabilize acute heart failure in patients who demonstrate a ruptured interventricular septum following acute myocardial infarction. Recent data indicate that in patients hospitalized with advanced, low-output heart failure, those stabilized in the hospital with nitroprusside may have a more favorable long-term clinical outcome.[87]

INTRAVENOUS NITROGLYCERIN

Similar to nitroprusside, intravenous nitroglycerin has an immediate onset and offset of action. The infusion rate is usually initiated at 10–20 mcg/min and titrated slowly to 200–500 mcg/min as needed to control symptoms and improve hemodynamic parameters. It is not approved by the FDA for the treatment of heart failure, but has been widely used for this indication over the past 20 years. Intravenous nitroglycerin is endothelium dependent, and unlike nitroprusside, it has more effect on the venous circulation than on the arterial circulation. However, higher doses of intravenous nitroglycerin decrease SVR, as well as increase venous capacity. Therefore, cardiac output increases and BP can be maintained. PCWP is reduced. Mitral regurgitation improves. There are few data available on the effects of intravenous nitroglycerin on coronary circulation in patients with heart failure. Coronary blood flow appears to improve. This suggests that both the epicardial conductance vessels and the coronary arteriolar resistance vessels are favorably influenced by intravenous nitroglycerin.

LIMITATIONS OF INTRAVENOUS NITROGLYCERIN IN THE TREATMENT OF PATIENTS WITH HEART FAILURE

Intravenous nitroglycerin causes headache in about 20% of patients and, when severe, may require cessation of the infusion. Hypotension (10%), nausea and bradycardia occasionally occur. Some patients are relatively resistant to intravenous nitroglycerin and seemingly require very large doses to afford a hemodynamic effect. The reason for this is not particularly clear, but very large doses in excess of 500 mcg/min are best avoided. Nitrate tolerance is said to occur when there is a robust initial hemodynamic response, but by 1–2 hours the dose of intravenous nitroglycerin must be increased to establish a continued hemodynamic response. About one-half of patients develop nitrate tolerance, and it cannot be predicted by baseline hemodynamic values (Fig. 5). The mechanism of resistance to intravenous nitroglycerin is not clear, but it is possibly prevented by the concomitant use of oral hydralazine (Fig. 2).

NESIRITIDE

Nesiritide is a pure, human Brain Natriuretic Peptide (BNP) synthesized using recombinant DNA techniques. It has the same 32-amino acid sequence as endogenous BNP released from the heart. When infused intravenously into the circulation of patients with heart failure, the mean terminal elimination half-life of nesiritide is about 18 minutes. Plasma BNP levels increase about three-fold to six-fold with a nesiritide infusion. Human BNP is eliminated from the circulation through complex, multiple mechanisms. Most of the BNP is cleared by c-receptors on cell surfaces, but some is cleared by neutral endopeptidases in renal tubular and vascular cells, and a smaller amount is cleared by renal filtration that is proportional to body weight.

The largest clinical trial of nesiritide, Vasodilation in the Management of Acute CHF (VMAC), was a comparison study with intravenous nitroglycerin.[88] It demonstrated that nesiritide-improved hemodynamic function and self-reported symptoms are more effective than intravenous nitroglycerin or placebo (Figs 9A and B). On this basis, nesiritide was approved by the FDA for heart failure and became widely used for the treatment

of acute heart failure. Nesiritide has venous, arterial and coronary vasodilator properties. Cardiac output improves and PCWP is reduced. Hypotension occurs in about 4% of patients, and unlike intravenous nitroglycerin, it can be prolonged (~20 min) because of nesiritide's relatively longer half-life. The effects of nesiritide on renal function are variable, but generally only a modest or neutral renal effect is observed, though worsening renal function has been reported.[89,90]

In 2005, Sackner-Bernstein and his colleagues reported that nesiritide may be associated with an increased risk of death after treatment for acute decompensated heart failure.[91] At about this time, infusions of nesiritide were also being widely performed in outpatient clinics, and the drug came under severe criticism.[92] Ultimately, a randomized controlled trial of nesiritide versus placebo was performed, which demonstrated that serial outpatient nesiritide infusions did not provide a demonstrable clinical benefit over standard therapy.[93] Rapid de-adoption of nesiritide was observed.[94] A large randomized mortality trial of nesiritide for acute heart failure has shown that the role of nesiritide for the treatment of acute decompensated heart failure will likely diminish.

ORAL β-ADRENERGIC BLOCKING DRUGS

There is a fundamental belief that the biologically powerful adrenergic nervous system compensates the failing heart by increasing myocyte size (hypertrophy), heart rate and force of contraction (inotropy). The SNS also activates the RAAS, thus conserving intravascular volume and redirecting blood flow to vital organs. However, an overly active SNS has repeatedly been shown to be essentially toxic to myocardial cells in both animals and humans.[95] There have been numerous large randomized

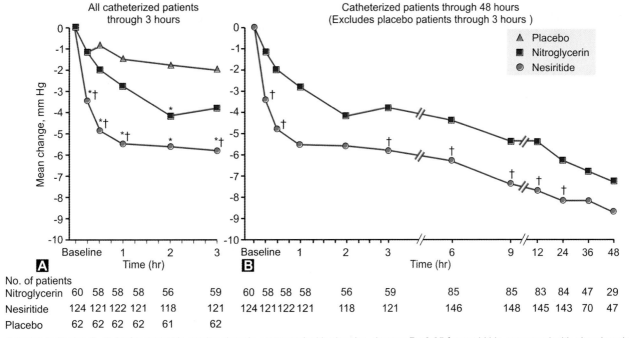

No. of patients													
Nitroglycerin	60	58	58	58	56	59							
Nesiritide		124	121	122	121	118	121						
Placebo		62	62	62	62	61	62						

Asterisk indicates P <0.05 for nesiritide or nitroglycerin compared with placebo, dagger, P <0.05 for nesiritide compared with nitroglycerin

FIGURES 9A AND B: Changes in pulmonary capillary wedge pressure from baseline in response to intravenous nitroglycerin, nesiritide and placebo in patients with heart failure [*Source:* Modified from Publication Committee for the VMAC Investigators (Vasodilatation in the management of Acute CHF). Intravenous nesiritide vs nitroglycerin for treatment of decompensated congestive heart failure: A randomized controlled trial. JAMA. 2002;287:1531-40, with permission)

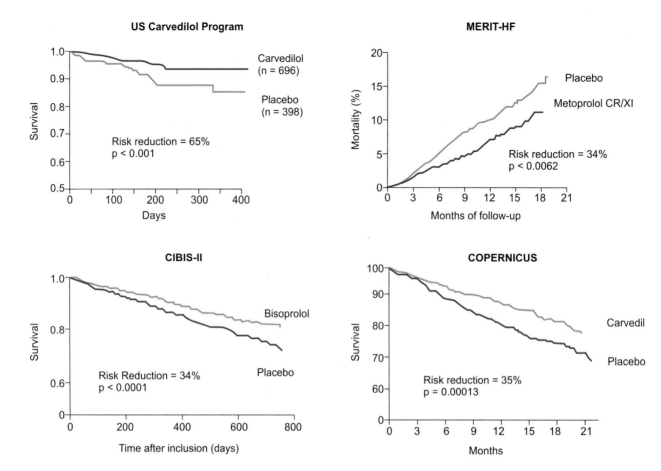

FIGURE 10: Placebo-controlled studies of beta blocker therapy (*Source:* Harry Krum. In: JD Hosenpud, BH Greenberg (Eds). Congestive Heart Failure, 3rd edition. Philadelphia: Lippincott Williams and Wilkins; 2007. pp. 510-20)

trials supporting the concept that blocking the SNS with β-adrenergic blocking drugs in patients with systolic heart failure slows the progression of systolic heart failure and improves patient survival (Fig. 10).

The importance of dysfunctional adrenergic activation in heart failure was first elucidated by the work of Braunwald and his colleagues at the National Institutes of Health in the 1960s.[96] Since then, there has been an enormous basic and clinical research effort testing the rather counterintuitive concept that blocking the β_1- and β_2-adrenergic receptors will benefit patients with systolic heart failure.[97] It is well known that β-adrenergic receptors downregulate in response to excessive sympathetic drive,[98] presumably in an attempt to protect the cardiac myocyte from overstimulation. Such biological behavior suggests that blocking the receptors pharmacologically may also protect the heart.[99] Moreover, pheochromocytoma (a classic example on long-term hyperadrenergic activity) is well known to express itself as dilated or hypertrophic cardiomyopathy.[100] This provides proof of concept that the overly active SNS and its dysfunctional status are central to the pathophysiology of heart failure,[101–104] similar to the overly active RAAS.

The first use of β-adrenergic blockers to treat patients with heart failure was the product of a series of carefully written case reports from Göteborg, Sweden.[105–107] This experience was a source of both great excitement and profound skepticism. Eventually, a small clinical trial [Metoprolol in Dilated Cardiomyopathy (MDC)] was launched, and showed only

marginal benefit of metoprolol in patients with heart failure.[108] Other clinical trials were performed using bisoprolol [The Cardiac Insufficiency Bisoprolol Study (CIBIS) and CIBIS II][109,110] and metoprolol succinate [the Metoprolol CR/XL Randomized Intervention Trial in Congestive Heart Failure (MERIT-HF)].[111] Carvedilol, an α_1 and nonselective β-adrenergic blocker, was also demonstrated to improve survival in patients with moderate and even very severe heart failure [The Carvedilol Prospective Randomized Cumulative Survival (COPERNICUS) Trial].[112] Some would argue that the α_1-adrenergic receptor blockade induced by carvedilol provides an additional advantage to the standard β-adrenergic blockade,[113,114] but this has remained controversial. Today β-adrenergic blockers are widely used throughout the world to treat patients with systolic heart failure.[115] They are considered "evidence-based" therapy. The suggested initial dose and evidence-based maximal dose are shown in Table 2.

Although it is unusual nowadays to see patients with heart failure who are naive to either RAAS blockers or β-blockers, occasionally the issue of which class of drug to start first arises. Experience indicates that either RAAS blockers (i.e. ACE inhibitor or ARB) or a β-blocker may be initiated first,[116] but eventually full doses of both classes of drugs should be attempted. The titration schedule of β-adrenergic drugs should be slow, that is over several weeks. The magnitude of heart rate reduction is significantly associated with the survival benefit of β-blockers in patients with systolic heart failure, whereas the dose of β-blocker is not.[116,117] There is also a strong correlation between change in heart rate and improvement in LV ejection fraction.[118] It appears as though decreased heart rate, improved chamber contractility and afterload reduction each contribute to the improved LV ejection fraction with use of carvedilol.[119]

β-adrenergic blocking drugs are now widely used to treat all stages of heart failure. Some patients admitted to the hospital with NYHA class III or IV systolic heart failure may not tolerate β-blockers because of symptomatic hypotension or low cardiac output, but most hospitalized patients with acute heart failure do tolerate these drugs. The continuation of β-blocker therapy in patients hospitalized with acute decompensated systolic heart failure is associated with lower postdischarge mortality risk and improved treatment rates.[120] Withdrawal of β-blocker therapy in the hospital is associated with a higher risk. β-blocker therapy before and during hospitalization for acute systolic heart failure is associated with improved outcomes.[121] In our experience, the most common documented cause of discontinuance of β-blockers in patients with heart failure is failure to restart β-blockers after they have been stopped during hospitalization.[122]

Not all patients with systolic heart failure improve with β-blocking therapy. One possibility is that functional improvement from β-blockers may be related to changes in myocardial contractile protein gene expression,[123] which could vary from patient to patient. Another possibility is that β-blocking drugs are quite different from each other. Metoprolol and bisoprolol are both β-receptor subtype selective (i.e. β_1). Bucindolol, labetalol and carvedilol are each nonselective, and labetalol and carvedilol have α_1-blocking properties that produce ancillary vasodilation. Bucindolol, although not available, has been intensely studied and has mild vasodilator properties, probably mediated by c-GMP. Additionally, bucindolol has meager "inverse agonism", so there is less negative chronotropism and inotropic effects. Bucindolol can also lower systemic norepinephrine levels substantially in some patients, and therefore has the potential to be a powerful sympatholytic agent. The norepinephrine lowering effects of bucindolol, as well as the clinical response to the drug, are strongly influenced by the presynaptic α_2c-adrenergic receptors, which modulate exocytosis and exhibit substantial genetic variation in humans. It is believed that a α_2c-adrenergic receptor polymorphism affects the sympatholytic effects of bucindolol in patients with systolic heart failure.[124] Patients with the α_2c-Del 322-325 polymorphism appear to have a marked increased in the sympatholytic response to bucindolol, and these carriers exhibit no evidence of clinical efficacy when treated with bucindolol. This concept is consistent with observations from other studies that indicate a marked decrease in plasma norepinephrine levels as a consequence of certain drug therapy, such as moxonidine, is associated with increased mortality and more heart failure hospitalizations. This also seems true with regard to the response to bucindolol where carriers of the α_2c-Del 322-325 variant exhibit very low plasma norepinephrine levels during bucindolol use and a poor response to treatment. The frequency of this genetic variant is ~0.04 in whites and ~0.40 in blacks.

In addition to their favorable effects on LV performance and patient survival, β-adrenergic blockers, like RAAS blockers, slow the progression of LV remodeling. This occurs in patients with heart failure secondary to acute myocardial infarction and in patients with chronic heart failure from dilated cardiomyopathy. LV end-diastolic volume tends to improve the LV becomes less spherical and assumes a more natural ellipsoid shape. Mitral regurgitation is ameliorated or improved, and on an average the LV ejection fraction goes up by about 5–7 ejection fraction units. In some cases there is spectacular reverse remodeling, and in other cases this is less apparent or may not be seen at all. Reverse remodeling of the LV is associated with improved survival. We now have three major heart failure therapeutic strategies aimed at producing reverse remodeling: (1) RAAS blocking drugs; (2) Cardiac Resynchronization Therapy (CRT) and (3) β-adrenergic blocking drugs. Of course, coronary revascularization can also improve LV size and performance in selected patients. These therapies have proven to be the powerful drivers of improved patient survival.

CONCLUSION

Neurohumoral modulating drugs now have a central role in the treatment of patients with systolic heart failure. This was not the case 35 years ago when only digitalis and diuretics were used. Annualized mortality has fallen from ~20% to less than 10% per year commensurate with the use of RAAS and SNS blocking drugs. Of course, ICDs and CRT have also importantly contributed to this mortality reduction. The total cardiovascular death rate burden has fallen substantially in accordance with the widespread use of these therapies. Although, the incidence of ST segment elevation myocardial infarction (STEMI) has also fallen dramatically, incident heart failure continues to increase. There is now much better treatment for hypertension and hyperlipidemia. Paradoxically, as people live longer, we are now seeing a wave of heart failure in the elderly, the fastest growing segment of our population. The scourge of heart failure has not gone away, but has rather been shifted to people in their 70s, 80s and 90s. In the end, prevention of heart failure by lifelong control of known risk factors and mechanistic enlightenment although additional genomic studies may reduce the burden of heart failures even more, as systolic heart failure is likely a largely preventable disorder.

ACKNOWLEDGMENT

We acknowledge the outstanding help of Lindsay Hoke in the preparation of this manuscript.

REFERENCES

1. Imperial ES, Levy MN, Zieske H. Outflow resistance as an independent determinant of cardiac performance. Circ Res. 1961;9:1148-55.
2. Sonnenblick EH, Downing SE. Afterload as a primary determinant of ventricular performance. Am J Physiol. 1963;204:604-10.
3. Wilcken DE, Charlier AA, Hoffman JI. Effects of alterations in aortic impedance on the performance of the ventricles. Circ Res. 1964;14:283-93.
4. Ross J, Braunwald E. The study of left ventricular function in man by increasing resistance to ventricular ejection with angiotensin. Circulation. 1964;29:739-49.
5. Cohn JN. Blood pressure and cardiac performance. Am J Med. 1973;55:351-61.

6. Meredith PA, Ostergren J, Anand I, et al. Clinical outcomes according to baseline blood pressure in patients with a low ejection fraction in the CHARM (Candesartan in Heart Failure: Assessment of Reduction in Mortality and Morbidity) program. J Am Coll Cardiol. 2008;52:2000-7.

7. Anand IS, Tam SW, Rector TS, et al. Influence of blood pressure on the effectiveness of a fixed-dose combination of isosorbide dinitrate and hydralazine in the African-American Heart Failure Trial. J Am Coll Cardiol. 2007;49:32-9.

8. Rouleau JL, Roecker EB, Tendra M, et al. Influence of pretreatment systolic blood pressure on the effect of carvedilol in patients with severe chronic heart failure: the Carvedilol Prospective Randomized Cumulative Survival (COPERNICUS) study. J Am Coll Cardiol. 2004;43:1423-9.

9. Franciosa JA, Pierpont G, Cohn JN. Hemodynamic improvement after oral hydralazine in left ventricular failure: a comparison with nitroprusside infusion in 16 patients. Ann Intern Med. 1977;86:388-93.

10. Franciosa JA, Blank RC, Cohn JN. Nitrate effects on cardiac output and left ventricular outflow resistance in chronic congestive heart failure. Am J Med. 1978;64:207-13.

11. Olivari MT, Levine TB, Cohn JN. Abnormal neurohumoral response to nitroprusside infusion in congestive heart failure. J Am Coll Cardiol. 1983;2:411-7.

12. Kaye DM, Jennings GL, Dart AM, et al. Differential effect of acute baroreceptor unloading on cardiac and systemic sympathetic tone in congestive heart failure. J Am Coll Cardiol. 1998;31:583-7.

13. Chatterjee K, Parmley WW, Massie B, et al. Oral hydralazine therapy for chronic refractory heart failure. Circulation. 1976;54:879-83.

14. Taylor AL, Ziesche S, Yancy C, et al. Combination of isosorbide dinitrate and hydralazine in blacks with heart failure. N Engl J Med. 2004;351:2049-57.

15. Elkayam U. Nitrates in the treatment of congestive heart failure. Am J Cardiol. 1996;77:41C-51C.

16. Packer M. Prospective Randomized Amlodipine Survival Evaluation 2. Presented at the 49th American College of Cardiology meeting, Anaheim CA. March 2000.

17. Packer M, O'Conner CM, Ghali JK, et al. Effect of amlodipine on morbidity and mortality in severe chronic heart failure. N Engl J Med. 1996;335:1107-14.

18. Ignarro LJ, Lippton H, Edwards JC, et al. Mechanism of vascular smooth muscle relaxation by organic nitrates, nitrites, nitroprusside and nitric oxide: evidence for the involvement of S-nitrosothiols as active intermediates. J Pharmacol Exp Ther. 1981;218:739-49.

19. De Caterina R, Dorso CR, Tack-Goldman K, et al. Nitrates and endothelial prostacyclin production: studies in vitro. Circulation. 1985;71:176-82.

20. Franciosa JA, Nordstrom LA, Cohn JN. Nitrate therapy for congestive heart failure. JAMA. 1978;240:443-6.

21. Leier CV, Huss P, Magorien RD, et al. Improved exercise capacity and differing arterial and venous tolerance during chronic isosorbide dinitrate therapy for congestive heart failure. Circulation. 1983;67:817-22.

22. Franciosa JA, Goldsmith SR, Cohn JN. Contrasting immediate and long-term effects of isosorbide dinitrate on exercise capacity in congestive heart failure. Am J Med. 1980;69:559-66.

23. Chatterjee K, Parmley WW. Vasodilator therapy for acute myocardial infarction and chronic congestive heart failure. J Am Coll Cardiol. 1983;1:133-53.

24. Captopril Multicenter Research Group. A placebo-controlled trial of captopril in refractory chronic congestive heart failure. J Am Coll Cardiol. 1983;2:755-63.

25. Pfeffer MA, Braunwald E, Moyé LA, et al. Effect of captopril on mortality and morbidity in patients with left ventricular dysfunction after myocardial infarction. Results of the survival and ventricular enlargement trial. The SAVE Investigators. N Eng J Med. 1992;327:669-77.

26. Pfeffer JM, Pfeffer MA, Braunwald E. Influence of chronic captopril therapy on the infarcted left ventricle of the rat. Circ Res. 1985;57:84-95.

27. Curtiss C, Cohn JN, Vrobel T, et al. Role of the renin-angiotensin system in the systemic vasoconstriction of chronic congestive heart failure. Circulation. 1978;58:763-70.

28. The SOLVD Investigators. Effect of enalapril on survival in patients with reduced left ventricular ejection fraction and congestive heart failure. N Engl J Med. 1991;325:293-302.

29. The SOLVD Investigators. Effect of enalapril on mortality and the development of heart failure in asymptomatic patients with reduced left ventricular ejection fractions. N Engl J Med. 1992;327:685-91.

30. Francis GS, Benedict C, Johnstone DE, et al. Comparison of neuroendocrine activation in patients with left ventricular dysfunction with and without congestive heart failure. Circulation. 1990;82:1724-9.

31. Dzau VJ, Colucci WS, Hollenberg NK, et al. Relation of the renin-angiotensin-aldosterone system to clinical state in congestive heart failure. Circulation. 1981;63:645-51.

32. Katz AM. Molecular biology in cardiology, a paradigmatic shift. J Mol Cell Cardiol. 1988;20:355-66.

33. Packer M. The neurohormonal hypothesis: a theory to explain the mechanism of disease progression in heart failure. J Am Coll Cardiol. 1992;20:248-54.

34. Hill JA, Olson EN. Cardiac plasticity. N Engl J Med. 2008;358:1370-80.

35. McDonald KM, Garr M, Carlyle PF, et al. Relative effects of α_1-adrenoceptor blockade, converting enzyme inhibitor therapy, and angiotensin II sub-type 1 receptor blockade on ventricular remodeling in the dog. Circulation. 1994;90:3034-46.

36. Tan L, Jalil JE, Pick R, et al. Cardiac myocyte necrosis induced by angiotensin II. Circ Res. 1991;69:1185-95.

37. Levine TB, Francis GS, Goldsmith SR, et al. Activity of the sympathetic nervous system and renin-angiotensin system assessed by plasma hormone levels and their relation to hemodynamic abnormalities in congestive heart failure. Am J Cardiol. 1982;49:1659-66.

38. Packer M. Neurohormonal interactions and adaptations in congestive heart failure. Circulation. 1988;77:721-30.

39. Harris P. Evolution and the cardiac patient. Cardiovasc Res. 1983;17:313-445.

40. Pfeffer MA, Braunwald E. Ventricular remodeling after myocardial infarction. Experimental observations and clinical implications. Circulation. 1990;81:1161-72.

41. Cohn JN. Structural basis for heart failure. Ventricular remodeling and its pharmacological inhibition. Circulation. 1995;91:2504-7.

42. Cohn JN, Ferrari R, Sharpe N. Cardiac remodeling-concepts and clinical implications: a consensus paper from an international forum on cardiac remodeling. J Am Coll Cardiol. 2000;35:569-81.

43. Packer M, Lee WH, Kessler PD, et al. Role of neurohormonal mechanisms in determining survival in patients with severe chronic heart failure. Circulation. 1987;75:IV80-92.

44. Pfeffer MA, Lamas GA, Vaughan DE, et al. Effect of captopril on progressive ventricular dilation after anterior myocardial infarction. N Engl J Med. 1988;319:80-6.

45. Konstam MA, Kronenberg MW, Rousseau MF, et al. Effects of the angiotensin converting enzyme inhibitor enalapril on the long-term progression of left ventricular dilation in patients with asymptomatic systolic dysfunction. Circulation. 1993;88:2277-83.

46. Greenberg B, Quinones MA, Koilpillai C, et al. Effects of long-term enalapril therapy on cardiac structure and function in patients with left ventricular dysfunction. Results of the SOLVD echocardiography substudy. Circulation. 1995;91:2573-81.

47. St John Sutton M, Pfeffer MA, Plappert T, et al. Quantitative two-dimensional echocardiographic measurements are major predictors of adverse cardiovascular events after acute myocardial infarction. The protective effects of captopril. Circulation. 1994;89:68-75.

48. Goodfriend TL, Elliott ME, Catt KJ. Angiotensin receptors and their antagonists. N Engl J Med. 1996;334:1649-54.

49. Burnier M, Brunner HR. Angiotensin II receptor antagonists. Lancet. 2000;355:637-45.

50. Phillips CO, Kashani A, Ko DK, et al. Adverse effects of combination angiotensin II receptor blockers plus angiotensin-converting enzyme inhibitors for left ventricular dysfunction: a quantitative review of

data from randomized clinical trials. Arch Intern Med. 2007;167: 1930-6.

51. Cohn JN, Tognoni G. A randomized trial of the angiotensin-receptor blocker valsartan in chronic heart failure. N Engl J Med. 2001;345:1667-75.

52. Young JB, Dunlap ME, Pfeffer MA, et al. Mortality and morbidity reduction with Candesartan in patients with chronic heart failure and left ventricular systolic dysfunction: results of the CHARM low-left ventricular ejection trials. Circulation. 2004;110:2618-26.

53. Pfeffer MA, McMurray JJ, Velazquez EJ, et al. Valsartan, captopril, or both in myocardial infarction complicated by heart failure, left ventricular dysfunction, or both. N Engl J Med. 2003;349:1893-906.

54. ONTARGET Investigators. Telmisartan, ramipril, or both in patients at high risk for vascular events. N Engl J Med. 2008;358:1547-59.

55. Messerli FH. The sudden demise of dual renin-angiotensin system blockade or the soft science of the surrogate end point. J Am Coll Cardiol. 2009;53:468-70.

56. GISSI-AF Investigators. Valsartan for prevention of recurrent atrial fibrillation. N Engl J Med. 2009;360:1606-17.

57. Konstam MA, Neaton JD, Dickstein K, et al. Effects of high-dose versus lose-dose losartan on clinical outcomes in patients with heart failure (HEAAL study): a randomized, double-blind trial. Lancet. 2009;374:1840-8.

58. Solomon SD, Skali H, Anavekar NS, et al. Changes in ventricular size and function in patients treated with valsartan, captopril, or both after myocardial infarction. Circulation. 2005;111:3411-9.

59. Massie BM, Carson PE, McMurray JJ, et al. Irbesartan in patients with heart failure and preserved ejection fraction. N Engl J Med. 2008;359:2456-67.

60. Weber KT. Aldosterone in congestive heart failure. N Engl J Med. 2001;345:1689-97.

61. Tang WH, Parameswaran AC, Maroo AP, et al. Aldosterone receptor antagonists in the medical management of chronic heart failure. Mayo Clin Proc. 2005;80:1623-30.

62. Pitt B, Zannand F, Remme WJ, et al. The effect of spironolactone on morbidity and mortality in patients with severe heart failure. N Engl J Med. 1999;341:709-17.

63. Pitt B, Remme W, Zannand F, et al. Eplerenone, a selective aldosterone blocker in patients with left ventricular dysfunction after myocardial infarction. N Engl J Med. 2003;348:1309-21.

64. Albert NM, Yancy CW, Liang L, et al. Use of aldosterone antagonists in heart failure. JAMA. 2009;302:1658-65.

65. Juurlink DN, Mamdani MM, Lee DS, et al. Rates of hyperkalemia after publication of the Randomized Aldactone Evaluation Study. N Engl J Med. 2004;351:543-51.

66. Weber KT, Villarreal D. Aldosterone and anti-aldosterone therapy in congestive heart failure. Am J Cardiol. 1993;71:3A-11A.

67. Staessen J, Lijnen P, Fagard R, et al. Rise in plasma concentration of aldosterone during long-term angiotensin II suppression. J Endocrinol. 1981;91:457-65.

68. The RALES Investigators. Effectiveness of spironolactone added to an angiotensin converting enzyme inhibitor and a loop diuretic for severe chronic congestive heart failure [the Randomized Aldactone Evaluation Study (RALES)]. Am J Cardiol. 1996;78:902-7.

69. Udelson JE, Feldman AM, Greenberg B, et al. Randomized, double blind, multicenter, placebo-controlled study evaluating the effect of aldosterone antagonism with eplerenone on ventricular remodeling in patients with mild-to-moderate heart failure and left ventricular systolic dysfunction. Circ Heart Fail. 2010;3:347-53.

70. Kumar P, Francis GS, Tang WH. Phosphodiesterase 5 inhibition in heart failure: mechanisms and clinical implications. Nat Rev Cardiol. 2009;6:349-55.

71. Takimoto E, Champion HC, Li M, et al. Chronic inhibition of cyclic GMP phosphodiesterase 5A prevents and reverses cardiac hypertrophy. Nat Med. 2005;11:214-22.

72. Kass DA. Hypertrophied right hearts get two for the price of one: can inhibiting phosphodiesterase type 5 also inhibit phosphodiesterase type 3? Circulation. 2007;116:233-5.

73. Archer SL, Michelakis ED. Phosphodiesterase type 5 inhibitors for pulmonary arterial hypertension. N Engl J Med. 2009;361:1864-71.

74. Semigran MJ. Type 5 phosphodiesterase inhibition: the focus shifts to the heart. Circulation. 2005;112:2589-91.

75. Guazzi M, Samaja M, Arena R, et al. Long-term use of sildenafil in the therapeutic management of heart failure. J Am Coll Cardiol. 2007;50:2136-44.

76. Stehlik J, Movsesian MA. Combined use of PDE5 inhibitors and nitrates in the treatment of pulmonary arterial hypertension in patients with heart failure. J Card Fail. 2009;15:31-4.

77. Pokreisz P, Vandenwijngaert S, Bito V, et al. Ventricular phosphodiesterase-5 expression is increased in patients with advanced heart failure and contributes to adverse ventricular remodeling after myocardial infarction in mice. Circulation. 2009;119:408-16.

78. Nagayama T, Hsu S, Zhang M, et al. Sildenafil stops progressive chamber, cellular and molecular remodeling and improves calcium handling and function in hearts with pre-existing advanced hypertrophy caused by pressure overload. J Am Coll Cardiol. 2009;53:207-15.

79. Lu Z, Xu X, Hu X, et al. Oxidative stress regulates left ventricular PDE5 expression in the failing heart. Circulation. 2010;121:1474-83.

80. Cohn JN, Burke L. Nitroprusside. Ann Intern Med. 1979;91:752-7.

81. Mikulic E, Cohn J, Franciosa JA. Comparative hemodynamic effects of inotropic and vasodilator drugs in severe heart failure. Circulation. 1977;56:528-33.

82. Franciosa JA, Guiha NH, Limas CJ, et al. Improved left ventricular function during nitroprusside infusion in acute myocardial infarction. Lancet. 1972;1:650-4.

83. Cohn JN, Franciosa JA, Francis GS, et al. Effect of short-term infusion of sodium nitroprusside on mortality rate in acute myocardial infarction complicated by left ventricular failure: results of a Veterans Administration cooperative study. N Engl J Med. 1982;306:1129-35.

84. Guiha NH, Cohn JN, Mikulic E, et al. Treatment of refractory heart failure with infusion of nitroprusside. N Engl J Med. 1974; 291:587-92.

85. Cohn JN, Mathew KJ, Franciosa JA, et al. Chronic vasodilator therapy in the management of cardiogenic shock and intractable left ventricular failure. Ann Intern Med. 1974;81:777-80.

86. Khot UN, Novaro GM, Popovic ZB, et al. Nitroprusside in critically ill patients with left ventricular dysfunction and aortic stenosis. N Engl J Med. 2003;348:1756-63.

87. Mullens W, Abrahams Z, Francis GS, et al. Sodium nitroprusside for advanced low-output heart failure. J Am Coll Cardiol. 2008;52:200-7.

88. VMAC. Intravenous nesiritide vs nitroglycerin for treatment of decompensated congestive heart failure: a randomized controlled trial. JAMA. 2002;287:1531-40.

89. Sackner-Bernstein JD, Skopicki HA, Aaronson KD. Risk of worsening renal function with nesiritide in patients with acutely decompensated heart failure. Circulation. 2005;111:1487-91.

90. Teerlink JR, Massie BM. Nesiritide and worsening renal function: the emperor's new clothes? Circulation. 2005;111:1459-61.

91. Sackner-Bernstein JD, Kowalski M, Fox M, et al. Short-term risk of death after treatment with nesiritide for decompensated heart failure: a pooled analysis of randomized controlled trials. JAMA. 2005;293:1900-5.

92. Topol EJ. Nesiritide—Not verified. N Engl J Med. 2005;353:113-6.

93. Yancy CW, Krum H, Massie BM, et al. Safety and efficacy of outpatient nesiritide in patients with advanced heart failure: results of the Second Follow-Up Serial Infusions of Nesiritide (FUSION II) trial. Circ Heart Fail. 2008;1:9-16.

94. Hauptman PJ, Schnitzler MA, Swindle J, et al. Use of nesiritide before and after publications suggesting drug-related risks in patients with acute decompensated heart failure. JAMA. 2006;296:1877-84.

95. Mann DL, Kent RL, Parsons B, et al. Adrenergic effects on the biology of the adult mammalian cardiocyte. Circulation. 1992;85:790-804.

96. Braunwald E, Chidsey CA, Pool PE, et al. Congestive heart failure—Biochemical and physiological considerations: combined clinical staff conference at the National Institutes of Health. Ann Intern Med. 1966;64:904-41.

97. Braunwald E, Bristow MR. Congestive heart failure: fifty years of progress. Circulation. 2000;102:IV14-23.

98. Bristow MR, Ginsburg R, Umans V, et al. β_1- and β_2-adrenergic-receptor subpopulations in nonfailing and failing human ventricular myocardium: coupling of both receptor subtypes to muscle contraction and selective β_1-receptor down-regulation in heart failure. Circ Res. 1986;59:297-309.

99. Eichhorn EJ, Bristow MR. Medical therapy can improve the biological properties of the chronically failing heart. A new era in the treatment of heart failure. Circulation. 1996;94:2285-96.

100. Dalby MC, Burke M, Radley-Smith R, et al. Pheochromocytoma presenting after cardiac transplantation for dilated cardiomyopathy. J Heart Lung Transplant. 2001;20:773-5.

101. Cohn JN. Sympathetic nervous system in heart failure. Circulation. 2002;106:2417-8.

102. Bristow M. Antiadrenergic therapy of chronic heart failure: surprises and new opportunities. Circulation. 2003;107:1100-2.

103. Triposkiadis F, Karayannis G, Giamouzis G, et al. The sympathetic nervous system in heart failure physiology, pathophysiology and clinical implications. J Am Coll Cardiol. 2009;54:1747-62.

104. Floras JS. Sympathetic nervous system activation in human heart failure: clinical implications of an updated model. J Am Coll Cardiol. 2009;54:375-85.

105. Waagstein F, Hjalmarson A, Varnauskas E, et al. Effect of chronic beta-adrenergic receptor blockade in congestive cardiomyopathy. Br Heart J. 1975;37:1022-36.

106. Swedberg K, Hjalmarson A, Waagstein F, et al. Beneficial effects of long-term beta-blockade in congestive cardiomyopathy. Br Heart J. 1980;44:117-33.

107. Swedberg K, Hjalmarson A, Waagstein F, et al. Adverse effects of beta-blockade withdrawal in patients with congestive cardiomyopathy. Br Heart J. 1980;44:134-42.

108. Waagstein F, Bristow MR, Swedberg K, et al. Beneficial effects of metoprolol in idiopathic dilated cardiomyopathy. Lancet. 1993;342:1441-6.

109. CIBIS Investigators and Committees. A randomized trial of β-blockade in heart failure. The Cardiac Insufficiency Bisoprolol Study (CIBIS). Circulation. 1994;90:1765-73.

110. CIBIS-II Investigators and Committees. The Cardiac Insufficiency Bisoprolol Study II (CIBIS-II): a randomized trial. Lancet. 1999;353:9-13.

111. Hjalmarson A, Goldstein S, Fagerberg B, et al. Effects of controlled-release metoprolol on total mortality, hospitalizations, and well-being in patients with heart failure: the Metoprolol CR/XL Randomized Intervention Trial in congestive heart failure (MERIT-HF). JAMA. 2000;283:1295-302.

112. Packer M, Fowler MB, Roecker EB, et al. Effect of carvedilol on the morbidity of patients with severe chronic heart failure: results of the carvedilol prospective randomized cumulative survival (COPERNICUS) study. Circulation. 2002;106:2194-9.

113. Poole-Wilson PA, Swedberg K, Cleland JG, et al. Comparison of carvedilol and metoprolol on clinical outcomes in patients with chronic heart failure in the Carvedilol Or Metoprolol European Trial (COMET): randomized controlled trial. Lancet. 2003;362:7-13.

114. Packer M. Do β-blockers prolong survival in heart failure only by inhibiting the β_1-receptor? A perspective on the results of the COMET trial. J Card Fail. 2003;9:429-43.

115. Klapholz M. β-blocker use for the stages of heart failure. Mayo Clin Proc. 2009;84:718-29.

116. Willenheimer R, van Veldhuisen DJ, Silke B, et al. Effect on survival and hospitalization of initiating treatment for chronic heart failure with bisoprolol followed by enalapril, as compared with the opposite sequence: results of the randomize Cardiac Insufficiency Bisoprolol Study (CIBIS) III. Circulation. 2005;112:2426-35.

117. McAlister FA, Wiebe N, Ezekowitz JA, et al. Meta-analysis: β-blocker dose, heart rate reduction, and death in patients with heart failure. Ann Intern Med. 2009;150:784-94.

118. Flannery G, Gehrig-Mills R, Billah B, et al. Analysis of randomized controlled trials on the effect of magnitude of heart rate reduction on clinical outcomes in patients with systolic chronic heart failure receiving beta-blockers. Am J Cardiol. 2008;101:865-9.

119. Maurer MS, Sackner-Bernstein JD, El-Khoury Rumbarger L, et al. Mechanisms underlying improvements in ejection fraction with carvedilol in heart failure. Circ Heart Fail. 2009;2:189-96.

120. Fonarow GC, Abraham WT, Albert NM, et al. Influence of beta-blocker continuation or withdrawal on outcomes in patients hospitalized with heart failure: findings from the OPTIMIZE-HF program. J Am Coll Cardiol. 2008;52:190-9.

121. Butler J, Young JB, Abraham WT, et al. Beta-blocker use and outcomes among hospitalized heart failure patients. J Am Coll Cardiol. 2006;47:2462-9.

122. Parameswaran AC, Tang WH, Francis GS, et al. Why do patients fail to receive β-blockers for chronic heart failure over time? A "real-world" single-center, 2-year follow-up experience of β-blocker therapy in patients with chronic heart failure. Am Heart J. 2005;149:921-6.

123. Lowes BD, Gilbert EM, Abraham WT, et al. Myocardial gene expression in dilated cardiomyopathy treated with beta-blocking agents. N Engl J Med. 2002;346:1357-65.

124. Bristow MR, Murphy GA, Krause-Steinrauf H, et al. An α_2c-Adrenergic receptor polymorphism alters the norepinephrine-lowering effects and therapeutic response of the β-blocker bucindolol in chronic heart failure. Circ Heart Fail. 2010;3:21-8.

Cardiovascular Pharmacology

Positive Inotropic Drugs

Carl V Leier, Garrie J Haas, Philip F Binkley

Chapter Outline

INTRODUCTION

Positive inotropic drugs (aka, positive inotropes) are agents that increase the velocity and strength of contraction of the cardiac myocyte and as a consequence, the myocardium and the heart as an organ unit; a few of the measurements of contractility or inotropy include Δ LV systolic upstroke pressure/Δ time, peak slope of LV developed pressure and end-systolic elastance. This chapter will focus on pharmacologic agents used primarily to augment inotropy. While the positive inotropic drugs also increase the amount or magnitude of contraction, this effect can also be attained to a certain extent by various non-inotropic agents (e.g. unloading vasodilating drugs) and thus, is not a unique property of positive inotropes.

Positive inotropic drugs are, therefore, generally directed at patients whose overall cardiovascular function is compromised by loss of cardiac contractility resulting in symptoms and signs of depressed stroke volume, cardiac output, hypoperfusion of vital organs and systems and often, hypotension.

In general, positive inotropes enhance cardiac contractility via modulation of calcium handling by the cardiomyocyte. The cellular mechanisms of action of the major inotropic drugs are illustrated in Figure 1.

Enhancement of cardiac contractility by positive inotropes with consequent improvement of compromised hemodynamics is not achieved without a cost. Unless the agent also possesses substantial cardiac unloading properties (preload and afterload reduction) or substantially evokes other favorable effects (e.g. improvement of autonomic balance), positive inotropes increase the oxygen and metabolic demands of the heart. This unfavorable property is exacerbated by other pharmacologic effects not uncommonly associated with inotropic agents such as positive chronotropy (increase in heart rate), cardiac dysrhythmias and a rise in vascular resistance afterload. These undesirable effects can be particularly troublesome in the setting of occlusive coronary artery disease, where the oxygen metabolic supply can be limited. For these reasons, intravenously administered inotropic therapy should generally be reserved for acute, short-term intervention. Chronic oral inotropic therapy is, thus far, relegated to an agent (currently digoxin) with a mild positive inotropic effect, accompanied by other favorable properties (refer to the digoxin section below). The development of newer inotropic agents to expand these application profiles has, to date, been mired in adverse effects and outcomes.

INTRAVENOUSLY ADMINISTERED, SHORT-TERM POSITIVE INOTROPIC THERAPY

The agents placed under this heading represent a spectrum of pharmacologic properties in addition to their positive inotropic effects. The predominant distinguishing feature among these agents is their effect on vasculature, which can range from vasodilatation to balanced vascular tone to vasoconstriction (Fig. 2 and Table 1). The pharmacologic mechanisms for their positive inotropy center on increasing intracellular cyclic adenosine monophosphate (cAMP) by either adrenergic receptor stimulation or inhibition of cAMP degradation (Fig. 1).

ADRENERGIC RECEPTOR AGONISTS

Although the adrenergic agonists can evoke tachycardia and dysrhythmias, they do have short elimination half-lives, an ideal pharmacologic property in the monitored critical care setting where a quick "turn on" and "turn off" of cardiovascular effects allow immediate and tightly controlled hemodynamic support.

The catechols (3,4-hydroxyphenyl ring) are the major drug group in the adrenergic family used for positive inotropic therapy. The molecular structures of those most commonly employed clinically are shown in Figure 3.

The adrenergic agonists evoke most of their pharmacologic effects through stimulation of beta- and alpha-adrenergic receptors. The myocardium is heavily populated with beta-receptors and to a lesser extent, alpha-receptors; all capable of augmenting cardiac contractility in varying degrees. Stimulation of β_1- and β_2-adrenergic receptors increases the inotropic (and chronotropic) state of the cardiomyocyte via mechanisms shown in Figure 1. Beta-adrenergic receptors are also located in other organs and regions of the body with the β_2-receptor being the

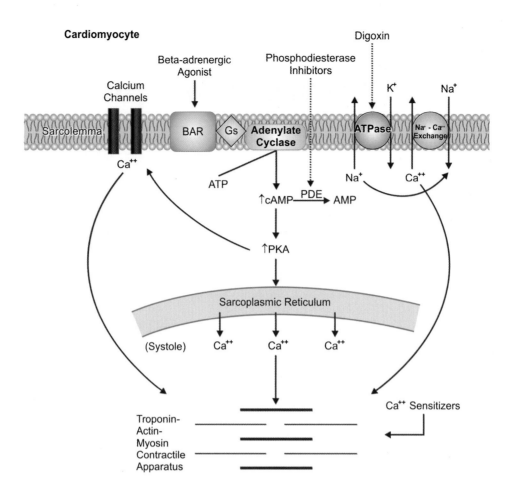

FIGURE 1: The major positive inotropic groups generally act through mechanisms that increase the concentration and availability of intracellular calcium for the actin-myosin contractile apparatus. Beta-adrenergic agonists attach to the beta-adrenergic receptor, activating the Gs protein-adenylate cyclase complex to convert ATP to cAMP. cAMP activates protein kinase A, which phosphorylates several intracellular sites resulting in an influx and release of Ca++ for systole. Phosphodiesterase inhibitors retard the breakdown of cAMP. Calcium sensitizers act by making the troponin-actin-myosin complex more responsive to available Ca++. By blocking the Na/K ATPase pump, digoxin increases intracellular Na+ loading of the Na+-Ca++ exchanger, resulting in less extrusion of Ca++ from the myocyte. Dashed arrow indicates inhibition. While this illustration depicts the major pharmacologic actions of these positive inotropic groups, their comprehensive mechanisms are considerably more numerous and complex. (Abbreviations: ATP: Adenosine triphosphate; cAMP: Cyclic adenosine monophosphate; AMP: Adenosine monophosphate; PDE: Phosphodiesterase; BAR: Beta-adrenergic receptor; PKA: Protein kinase A)

TABLE 1

The hemodynamic profiles of the agents currently employed to deliver short-term inotropic and vasoactive support

| | Phosphodiesterase Inhibitor | Adrenergic agonists | | | | |
| | | | Dopamine | | | |
	Milrinone	Dobutamine	Low dose	Higher dose	Norepinephrine	Phenylephrine
Contractility (inotropy)	↑	↑↑↑	↑	↑↑	→↑	╱
Cardiac output	↑↑	↑↑↑	↑	↑	→↑	╱
Heart rate (chronotropy)	→↑	→↑	→↑	↑↑	→↑	→╱
LV filling pressure	↓↓↓	↓↓	↓	→↑	→↑	→↑
Systemic blood pressure	→↓	→↑	→	↑↑	↑↑↑	↑↑↑
Systemic vascular resistance	↓↓↓	↓↓	→	↑↑	↑↑↑	↑↑↑
Pulmonary vascular resistance	↓↓↓	↓↓	→	→↑	↑	↑
↓ decrease; → minimal to no change; ╱ mild increase; ↑ increase						

most ubiquitous, accounting for concomitant vasodilatation and bronchodilatation during β₂-receptor agonism. Alpha-adrenergic receptors are predominantly located in the vasculature, such that their stimulation evokes vasoconstriction in excess of any positive inotropic effect. The cardiovascular effects of adrenergic agents used clinically for inotropic and hemodynamic support are individually presented under the heading of each and summarized in Table 1.

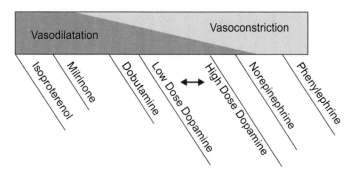

FIGURE 2: The spectrum of net vascular properties of the agents currently available for short-term positive inotropy and cardiovascular support. The vascular effects and responses are a major determinant for selection in individual patients

Dobutamine

Dobutamine is presented first because at this time, it is the agent most commonly used for short-term intravenous inotropic support and its net cardiovascular effects in the setting of left ventricular systolic failure result predominantly from positive inotropic enhancement of depressed cardiac contractility.

Dobutamine was developed from methodical manipulation and substitutions on the basic catechol-phenylethylamine molecule.[1] Out of over 15 molecules formulated and then tested in the animal model, dobutamine achieved the greatest augmentation of cardiac contractility and performance with the least net vasoactivity and chronotropy.

Dobutamine, a racemic compound (+ and – enantiomers), activates myocardial β_1- and β_2-adrenergic receptors and, via cAMP and the downstream mechanisms depicted in Figure 1, increases the velocity and extent of myocardial contraction. In chronic heart failure, the number and inotropic responsiveness of β_1-receptors are reduced[2] such that dobutamine's cardiac effects in this clinical setting are, in large part, rendered by agonism of β_2-receptors. Beta-receptor stimulation also accounts for the chronotropic properties of dobutamine.

In the setting of systolic heart failure, dobutamine generally evokes a mild net vasodilatory effect, reducing vascular resistance, through arteriolar β_2-receptor stimulation exceeding the modest vasoconstricting effects of its alpha-receptor agonism. Studies by Binkley and his colleagues[3–5] indicate that the cardiovascular pharmacology of dobutamine in human heart failure is considerably more complex. Dobutamine's favorable effects on aortic impedance and vascular-ventricular coupling allow further enhancement of ventricular contractility and performance.[4,5] In the total artificial heart model (calf), dobutamine increases cardiac output in the absence of myocardium and positive inotropic mechanisms.[5] This response is likely rendered by the vascular properties of dobutamine; its dextro-isomer (+enantiomer) reduces systemic vascular resistance and afterload via β_2-receptor stimulation and its levo-isomer (–enantiomer) reduces venous capacitance with enhanced venous return via alpha-receptor agonism.[5,6]

The major clinical indication for dobutamine administration is short-term inotropic support in patients compromised by ventricular systolic dysfunction, which has resulted in a problematic reduction in blood pressure and systemic perfusion (Table 2). "Short-term" until the patient recovers adequately or

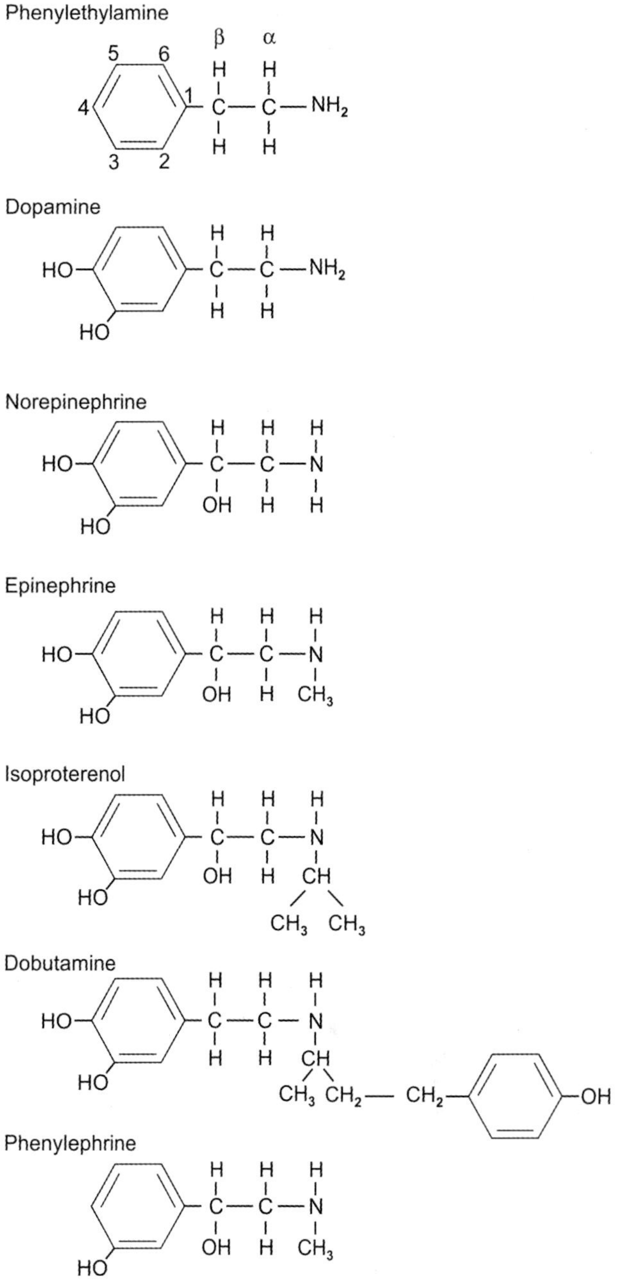

FIGURE 3: The phenylethylamine molecule is the basic structure for the adrenergic compounds under discussion. Variations in the hydroxyl attachment at the β site and the groups at the amino end determine the pharmacologic properties and consequent clinical applications of the catechols. Very little modification of the molecular structure is needed to change a strong vasodilator (isoproterenol) to a strong vasopressor (norepinephrine). Deletion of the 4-hydroxyl group from the epinephrine molecule results in phenylephrine, a powerful vasoconstrictor

is moved into more advanced interventions (e.g. mechanical support, remedial cardiac surgery). The typical patient presents with decompensated chronic or acute systolic heart failure, reduced stroke volume and cardiac output, elevated ventricular filling pressures, mild-to-moderate reduction in systemic blood pressure (systolic blood pressure 70–100 mm Hg) and impaired systemic perfusion (e.g. prerenal azotemia, elevated liver enzymes, impaired mentation); the clinical setting of "cold and wet".[7] The non-inotropic spectrum of intervention in this general clinical setting can include diuretics for volume overload and

TABLE 2

The clinical applications of dobutamine administration

Major indication:

Short-term (hours to days) inotropic and hemodynamic support for patients with ventricular systolic dysfunction resulting in a depressed stroke volume and cardiac output, systemic hypoperfusion, mild-to-moderate systemic hypotension (systolic blood pressures of 70–100 mm Hg) and an elevated left ventricular diastolic filling pressure (> 18 mm Hg). This support is maintained until the patient recovers or is directed into more advanced cardiovascular support (e.g. intra-aortic balloon counterpulsation, ventricular assist device) and/or remedial intervention (e.g. coronary artery intervention, valvular repair or replacement, cardiac transplantation).

Additional considerations:

A. Pharmacologic support as needed for patients with severe heart failure undergoing major diagnostic or surgical procedures
B. Cardiovascular hemodynamic support for the heart failure patient through the course of a major illness
C. Pharmacologic bridge in severe heart failure to standard therapies (e.g. angiotensin-converting enzyme inhibitor, beta-adrenergic blocker)
D. As a continuous infusion via indwelling central venous catheter to provide the only means of stabilizing an unstable or decompensated heart failure patient to allow discharge from the hospital (to extended care, home or hospice)
E. For hemodynamic support during weaning from cardiopulmonary bypass and during recovery from cardiac surgery
F. To facilitate recovery of myocardial stunning in the setting of low output cardiac failure
G. As a means of improving renal function and urine output in patients hospitalized for low output, systemic hypoperfusion and volume-overloaded congestive heart failure when renal responsiveness to standard therapy and diuretics is impaired
H. For hemodynamic support during management of cardiac transplant rejection complicated by hemodynamic decompensation
I. To augment systolic function of problematic systolic failure of the right ventricle
J. To assess ventricular (right or left) contractile reserve
K. To evaluate the severity of low-flow, low-gradient aortic valvular stenosis
L. As pharmacologic stress for myocardial perfusion imaging

Section 2 — Cardiovascular Pharmacology

elevated ventricular filling pressures (> 18 mm Hg), vasopressor infusion (e.g. moderate- to high-dose dopamine, norepinephrine, phenylephrine) for marked hypotension and shock, and inodilator or vasodilator therapy (e.g. milrinone, nitroprusside, nitroglycerin,) for patients with systemic systolic blood pressure more than 90–100 mm Hg. It is not unusual to administer two of these agents simultaneously to achieve and maintain optimal clinical and hemodynamic stability on the way to more definitive intervention.

In the appropriate patient, namely the patient with ventricular systolic dysfunction resulting in a fall in stroke volume and cardiac output, an elevation in left ventricular end-diastolic filling pressure, systemic hypoperfusion and mild-to-moderate reduction in systemic blood pressure, dobutamine increases stroke volume, cardiac output, systemic systolic blood pressure and pulse pressure, and systemic perfusion, while decreasing pulmonary and systemic vascular resistance and left ventricular filling pressure[8–10] (Fig. 4). In patients with concomitant mitral regurgitation, the decrease in systemic vascular resistance, ventricular volume and mitral orifice area likely accounts for the reduction in mitral regurgitation with additional augmentation of stroke volume and cardiac output during

dobutamine administration.[10] While there appears to be a dose-related separation of positive inotropy and beneficial hemodynamic effects from positive chronotropy, higher dosing will evoke a faster heart rate and can provoke ectopic beats and tachydysrhythmias[8] (Fig. 4).

Regional blood flow studies in patients with decompensated chronic heart failure revealed that dobutamine increases limb blood flow proportional to any increase in cardiac output with a less predictable augmentation in renal blood flow and no statistical change in hepatic-splanchnic flow.[11] Dobutamine favorably affects renal function, glomerular filtration rate and urine output.[8]

In patients with ventricular systolic dysfunction and patent coronary arteries, dobutamine increases coronary blood flow proportional to or greater than the increase in cardiac output and myocardial oxygen consumption.[12,13] This favorable effect on myocardial energetics is likely related to several mechanisms, including dobutamine-induced increase of coronary perfusion pressure (drop in left ventricular diastolic pressure more than the reduction in systemic diastolic pressure) and coronary diastolic perfusion time and a reduction in coronary vascular resistance.[8,12–14] The decrease in systemic and pulmonary vascular resistance, ventricular systolic (+diastolic) volume and ventricular afterload with dobutamine reduces myocardial oxygen consumption. Positive inotropy by itself generally causes an increase in myocardial oxygen consumption. At doses short of provoking a clinically significant rise in heart rate (> 10% above baseline), the coronary blood flow and myocardial oxygen delivery are equal to or exceeds the increase in myocardial oxygen consumption evoked by the positive inotropic effects of dobutamine.[12,13] However, these favorable coronary-myocardial energetic properties of dobutamine can be disrupted in the setting of occlusive coronary artery disease, whereby fixed obstructive lesions can prevent augmentation of coronary blood flow to match the rise in contractility and oxygen consumption. Any substantial elevation in the heart rate imposes a particular threat to coronary perfusion and the balance of oxygen demand and delivery by increasing myocardial oxygen consumption without an increase (or even a decrease) in coronary flow through shortening of the coronary diastolic perfusion time.[14] The positive chronotropic (in addition to inotropic) effect of high-dose dobutamine is now regularly employed during dobutamine stress myocardial imaging to elicit evidence of ischemia in patients with suspected occlusive coronary artery disease.

The chronotropic properties are of extreme importance in all patients, but particularly in patients with occlusive coronary disease where tachycardia will overtake the aforementioned favorable coronary-myocardial effects to provoke myocardial ischemia. For these reasons, proper patient and dose selection is of marked importance in patients with ventricular systolic dysfunction and occlusive coronary artery disease. Using these pharmacotherapeutic considerations as a guide, dobutamine can be safely administered to heart failure patients with occlusive coronary disease to attain and maintain a stable clinical and hemodynamic short-term course until the patient is directed to more advanced management (e.g. intra-aortic balloon counterpulsation, coronary angiography and intervention, coronary bypass surgery).[15–22] During this short-term "pharmacologic bridge", dobutamine, for safe effective therapy, has to

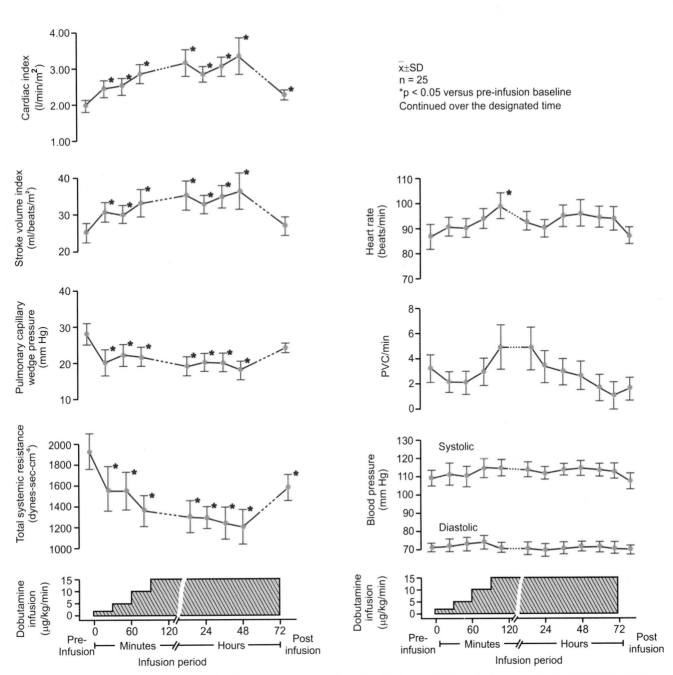

x̄±SD
n = 25
*p < 0.05 versus pre-infusion baseline
Continued over the designated time

CHAPTER 6 · Positive Inotropic Drugs

FIGURE 4: Pharmacodynamic curves for the dose-response and sustained infusions (72 hours) of dobutamine in chronic low output congestive heart failure. The infused dose is presented in the bottom panel (*Source:* Modified from reference 8, with permission)

be able to favorably affect the determinants of oxygen metabolic consumption and delivery (reduce elevated ventricular diastolic pressures, vascular resistance, ventricular volume and wall stress and increase coronary perfusion pressure and time) equal to and greater than the rise in myocardial oxygen consumption of positive inotropy. Nevertheless, even with proper patient and dose selection, some patients with occlusive coronary artery disease can develop myocardial ischemia + infarction during dobutamine administration.[16–18]

Dobutamine may have a favorable effect on myocardial stunning beyond the simple increase in coronary blood flow and myocardial perfusion of the affected region or whole heart.[23–25]

Clinical indications and applications: The most common clinical scenarios for appropriate dobutamine administration (to improve

and stabilize hemodynamic and clinical status) include patients managed for decompensated, hypoperfused, often hypotensive chronic systolic heart failure, acute systolic heart failure (e.g. acute myocardial infarction, acute myocarditis), or immediately following cardiac surgery + cardiopulmonary bypass. The various considerations for the administration of dobutamine are presented in Table 2.

Administration and dosing: Although the usual dose range for dobutamine is 2.0–15.0 mcg/kg/min, many patients can experience clinical and hemodynamic benefit at a lower starting dose of 0.5–1.0 mcg/kg/min and do so with minimal to no increase in heart rate or dysrhythmias. Dosing can be advanced by 1.0–2.0 mcg/kg/min increments every 12–15 or more minutes until the desired clinical and hemodynamic effects are attained, but short of increasing heart rate more than 10% above baseline, provoking dysrhythmias or eliciting side effects. In the absence of beta-adrenergic blockade, the inability to improve hemodynamics, stroke volume, cardiac output and clinical parameters in symptomatic systolic heart failure during incremented dobutamine infusion rates up to 15 mcg/kg/min portends a poor prognosis.[8]

Once the decision is made to discontinue the dobutamine infusion, maintenance doses of less than or equal to 2.0 mcg/kg/min can usually be stopped without difficulty. Higher infusion rates over an extended period generally require weaning over 12–72 hours to avert clinical and hemodynamic deterioration with more abrupt discontinuation.[8,26] Prolonged, higher dose infusions in patients treated for decompensated chronic systolic heart failure often require a longer weaning period or incremental oral dosing of hydralazine to achieve withdrawal of dobutamine without difficulty.[26] Although tolerance can occur to a mild-moderate degree during a prolonged continuous infusion, it is generally not enough to facilitate weaning.[27]

The pharmacokinetic and pharmacodynamic properties of dobutamine endorse its application as a short-term positive inotropic agent. In heart failure patients, its half-life averages 2.37 + 0.07 minutes[28] indicating that steady state for any dose is achieved in about 12–13 minutes, an invaluable characteristic if positive inotropy is urgently needed. And most of the drug is eliminated within 12–13 minutes upon discontinuation of the infusion, allowing a rapid dissipation of adverse effects if encountered during the infusion. In human heart failure, there is a direct near-linear relationship between the infusion dose of dobutamine, its plasma levels and hemodynamic responses[29] (Fig. 5).

Concomitant administration of a phosphodiesterase inhibitor (e.g. milrinone) enhances the inotropic effect of dobutamine by retarding the breakdown of intracellular cAMP generated by dobutamine.[30] The inotropic and hemodynamic effects of dobutamine are predictably blunted in patients receiving beta-adrenergic blocking agents, particularly the nonselective adrenergic blockers (e.g. carvedilol);[31,32] this interaction can be readily overcome with incremental dosing of dobutamine,[33] which competitively replaces the adrenergic blocker at the receptor site. It is usually not necessary to replace dobutamine with a non-adrenergic agent (e.g. milrinone) in most of these patients.

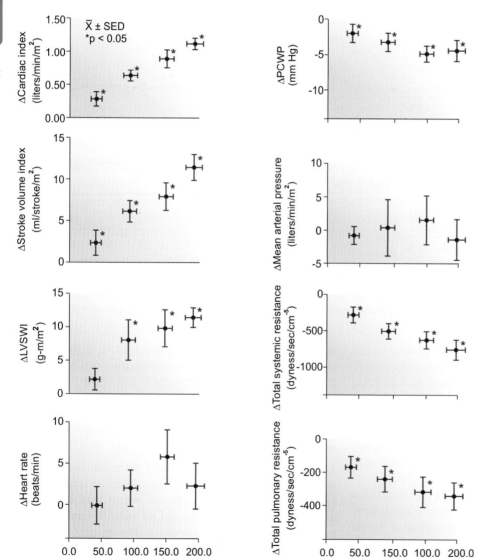

FIGURE 5: Graphs depicting the relationship of dobutamine infusion dose, plasma concentration and hemodynamic effects in patients with moderate-to-severe heart failure. The infusion rates for the 4 data points of each graph are 2.5, 5.0, 7.5 and 10.0 mcg/kg/min incremented every 20–30 minutes. Key: Δ: Change in; LVSWI: Left ventricular stroke work index; *: Indicates a significant change from baseline. (*Source:* Modified from ref 29)

Adverse and undesirable effects: The most common adverse effects of dobutamine are tachycardia and dysrhythmias. From comparative studies and registries, it is clear that improper patient and/or dose selection will evoke sinus tachycardia, atrial and ventricular dysrhythmias, other undesirable effects and adverse clinical outcomes.[34–37] In retrospective studies, the apparent dobutamine-induced adverse effect on outcomes is largely attributable to its administration in a more ill and compromised patient population than that served by the comparator.[37–39] Nevertheless, these reports[34–39] serve to emphasize the importance of proper patient, drug and dose selection.

Other side effects, also generally dose related, include headache, tremor, anxiety, palpitations and nausea. A hypertensive response (elevated systemic systolic blood pressure) can be observed when dobutamine is administered to patients with a history of systemic hypertension or peripheral vascular disease. Patients with high-grade occlusive coronary artery disease can experience angina, myocardial ischemia and infarction, particularly in patients who don't meet the primary indication for use (Table 2) and/or receive excessive initial dosing or excessively rapid advancement of dose. Dobutamine infusions can lower plasma potassium concentrations.[40] Less common side effects include generalized erythema/flushing, eosinophilia and hypersensitivity myocarditis;[41,42] reactions likely related to a bisulfite adjuvant. Dobutamine has been reported to induce stress cardiomyopathy (aka, Takotsubo cardiomyopathy) in patients undergoing pharmacologic stress testing with this agent.[43]

Dopamine

While dopamine, an endogenous precursor of epinephrine and norepinephrine, is the simplest molecule of the adrenergic agents, it has the most complex pharmacology (Figs 2 and 3 and Table 1). In general, dopamine elicits its pharmacodynamic effects through stimulation of dopaminergic receptors (D_1 and D_2) and adrenergic receptors (β_1, β_2 and α) and through the neuronal release and reduced neuronal uptake of endogenous norepinephrine.[44–46] At lower infusion rates (< 4.0 mcg/kg/min) in human heart failure, dopamine behaves as a mild vasodilator (dopaminergic), particularly of visceral and renal arterial-arteriolar vascular beds. With increased dosing, this effect is overtaken by dopamine's agonism of adrenergic receptors directly and through its release of norepinephrine from nerve endings; vasodilatation gives way to a net-balanced vascular effect and some positive inotropy at moderate dosing (4.0–8.0 mcg/kg/min) and to considerable vasoconstriction and some retained inotropy at higher doses (> 8.0 mcg/kg/min).

In states of low cardiac output, systemic hypoperfusion, and adequate or elevated left ventricular filling pressures, dopamine at less than 4.0 mcg/kg/min can augment ventricular contractility, stroke volume and cardiac output, and reduce systemic and pulmonary vascular resistance; all to a modest degree without a substantial change in systemic blood pressure.[11,47–50] As infusion rates move to more than 4.0 mcg/kg/min, vascular resistance, stroke volume and cardiac output plateau and there occurs a substantial dose-related rise in systemic blood pressure. Positive chronotropy and provocation of dysrhythmias are also dose related and can become an undesirable effect at more than

or equal to 6.0 mcg/kg/min. Ventricular filling pressure can drop in some patients, but generally does not change or can increase with higher dosing. Indices of ventricular contractility (positive inotropy) are blunted at higher dosing and during continuous infusion,[11] presumably secondary to the rise in blood pressure, vascular resistance and ventricular afterload and depletion of myocardial norepinephrine stores from dopamine-induced release (and reduced uptake) at nerve endings during high-dose or prolonged infusions.

The vasoconstricting properties of moderate to high doses of dopamine are employed clinically to increase and stabilize systemic blood pressure in cardiogenic or vasodilatory (e.g. septic) hypotension and shock.[51–55] This clinical application predominates over its use as a primary inotropic agent and represents its principal indication (vasopressor). Interestingly, the results of a recently performed multicenter trial on shock showed that dopamine offers little advantage over norepinephrine and may even be less effective in the cardiogenic subgroup.[55] (see Norepinephrine on the next page).

Much of the appeal for dopamine administration in problematic hypotension and shock emanates from what are believed to be favorable dopaminergic renal effects. It has been shown that dopamine, particularly at lower doses (< 5.0 mcg/kg/min), can augment renal blood flow equal to or greater than the percentage increase in cardiac output.[11,56–58] Whether this augmentation in renal blood flow evokes an increase in glomerular filtration rate, natriuresis and diuresis in heart failure, hypotension or shock remains controversial and burdened by conflicting published results.[11,47,56–61]

The most common adverse effects of dopamine administration are similar to those of dobutamine, namely positive chronotropy and dysrhythmias, both dose related.[11] Dopamine crosses the blood-brain barrier to provoke nausea and vomiting in some patients. Intense vasoconstriction by dopamine can lead to ischemia of digits and various organ systems. Subcutaneous infiltration at the infusion site can provoke pain and ischemic changes, potentially reversible with local instillation of phentolamine. Dopamine has been reported to depress minute ventilation in heart failure.[62]

Other Adrenergic Agents

These agents are used in various clinical settings for various indications. Due to over-riding vascular effects, they are not employed as primary positive inotropic drugs.

Isoproterenol: This drug is perhaps the purest beta-adrenergic receptor agonist (β_1 and β_2) available for clinical use. However, its positive inotropic properties are largely overshadowed by strong vasodilatory and positive chronotropic effects (Table 1). Its principal clinical application is rather narrow, namely to increase heart rate in the short term (until recovery or definitive intervention) in patients with problematic bradycardia or inadequate heart rate response; particularly in clinical situations where intravenous atropine is contraindicated, inadequate or ineffective. In view of other available, generally safer vasodilating agents (e.g. milrinone, nesiritide, nitrates), isoproterenol is rarely used as a primary vasodilating agent. Adverse effects

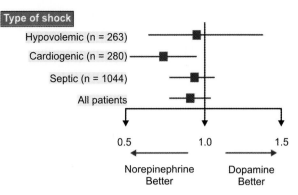

FIGURE 6: A forest plot showing the hazard ratio (± 95% confidence intervals) of norepinephrine versus dopamine support during shock management of the three major shock subgroups studied. While there were no differences between the two treatments for all shock patients combined or for septic and hypovolemic subgroups, the hazard ratio of the cardiogenic shock subgroup favored norepinephrine over dopamine based on dysrhythmic events during treatment and mortality at 28 days following the shock episode (*Source:* Modified from reference 55)

include flushing, tremor, anxiety, tachycardia, dysrhythmias and hypotension.

Epinephrine: This endogenous catecholamine stimulates β_1, β_2 and α_1 adrenergic receptors. Epinephrine differs from dobutamine in that its administration is modulated by neuronal uptake and its β_2 and α_1 effects are more intense than those of dobutamine. In cardiovascular medicine, epinephrine is most often employed during cardiopulmonary resuscitation or as a global hemodynamic support drug during withdrawal for cardiopulmonary bypass and recovery from cardiac surgery. Adverse effects include those described above for dobutamine, dopamine and isoproterenol.

Norepinephrine and phenylephrine: These agents are predominant α_1-adrenergic agonists with mild beta-receptor agonism and thus, they are viewed as vasopressors (Fig. 2 and Table 1). As such, these compounds are used for vasoconstriction to increase and stabilize systemic blood pressure in states of marked hypotension and shock (vasodilatory and cardiogenic).[55,63] The results of a large multicenter trial (1,679 patients) conducted in Europe on the treatment of shock states showed no difference in overall mortality at 28 days (primary endpoint) between dopamine and norepinephrine when used to stabilize blood pressure and clinical status.[55] However, for comparable blood pressure responses, dopamine appeared to be more chronotropic and arrhythmogenic. In the cardiogenic subgroup of 280 patients, the 28-day survival outcome favored norepinephrine as the preferred stabilizing vasopressor[55] (Fig. 6).

Norepinephrine dosing in hypotension and shock generally ranges 0.02–0.40 mcg/kg/min. In addition to the adverse effects described for dopamine, norepinephrine can evoke dose-related systemic hypertension and bradycardia.

More intense vasoconstriction with minimal positive inotropy is rendered by phenylephrine.

PHOSPHODIESTERASE INHIBITORS

Drugs under this grouping are often referred to as "inodilators" because vasodilation is a major component of their pharma-

cology. In fact, amrinone, studied early in this category, is principally a vasodilator with little to no ability to augment ventricular contraction beyond its unloading effects on the ventricle.[64–66] Thrombocytopenia during prolonged administration tempered its clinical application. As a therapeutic modality, amrinone has largely been replaced by milrinone.

Milrinone

While milrinone can elicit some positive inotropy through other cellular mechanisms (e.g. activation of the calcium release channel), its cardiovascular effects are principally rendered through inhibition of Phosphodiesterase III (PDE III) with consequent impairment of the breakdown metabolism of cAMP[67] (Fig. 1).

In contrast to dobutamine, a positive inotrope with mild vasodilating properties, milrinone is a vasodilator with mild positive inotropic properties. Therefore, for any matched degree of enhanced contractility, milrinone evokes a greater reduction in pulmonary and systemic vascular resistance, systemic blood pressure and ventricular filling pressures[68–73] (Figs 7A and B). As a vasodilator, proper dosing of milrinone can improve hemodynamics with little to no increase in myocardial oxygen consumption.[73,74] Its ability to lower pulmonary vascular resistance and pressure makes it a favorable agent for augmentation of central hemodynamics in patients with elevated pulmonary artery pressures.[71,72] Bolus milrinone has become one of the vasodilating agents used to determine reversibility of pulmonary hypertension in patients with advanced heart failure under evaluation for cardiac transplantation.[75,76]

In patients with severe low output congestive heart failure, milrinone augments the hemodynamic effects of dobutamine and vice versa. It is not unusual to employ this combination in patients with markedly compromised hemodynamics, generally in the setting of advanced, end-stage heart failure, as a pharmacologic bridge to placement of a ventricular assist device and/or cardiac transplantation. Parenthetically, without these advanced interventions, the requirement for this drug combination to clinically stabilize the patient portends a poor outcome.

Since, milrinone does not act through adrenergic receptors, it can augment hemodynamics in patients on beta-adrenergic antagonists; this is particularly important for the nonselective beta-blockers (e.g. carvedilol), which competitively interfere with low-dose dobutamine.[77]

While vasodilatation is a favorable property of milrinone when administered properly to the appropriate patient, vasodilation also renders its limitations. This agent is generally not employed in patients with systemic systolic blood pressure less than 90 mm Hg and thus, milrinone is not a first-line agent for the management of low output hypotension or shock. Extensive vasodilatation, hypotension and its cellular PDE III inhibition can elevate heart rate and provoke dysrhythmias.[78] Some patients experience a generalized warmth and flushing at moderate-to-high infusion rates or during bolus administration. Fluid retention is not uncommon during continuous infusions.[78]

Milrinone is generally started at 0.20–0.30 mcg/kg/min and gradually advanced as needed to achieve the intended hemodynamic and clinical endpoints and short of evoking tachycardia, dysrhythmias or hypotension. Milrinone has a half-life of

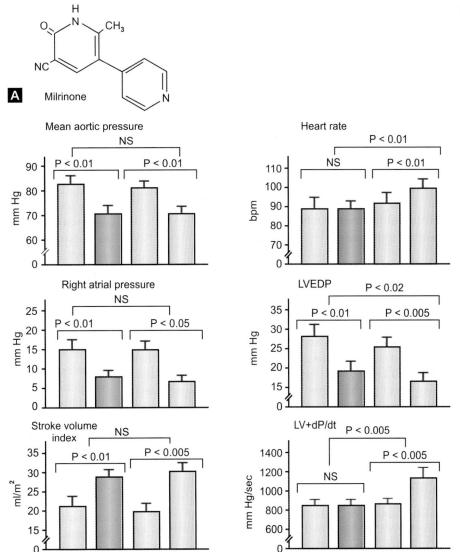

FIGURES 7A AND B: (A) The molecular structure of milrinone. (B) Comparison of the hemodynamic effects of milrinone (ML) at the maximal dose administered and nitroprusside (NP) at the dose selected to match the reduction in mean aortic pressure by milrinone. For comparable ventricular unloading, milrinone evoked positive inotropy (increased + dP/dt—change in LV developed systolic pressure over change in time) and positive chronotropy. (Abbreviations: LVEDP: Left ventricular end-diastolic pressure; NS: Not statistically significant). (*Source:* Modified from reference 69)

CHAPTER 6

Positive Inotropic Drugs

1–3 hours[79,80] and thus, the onset of action and equilibration is not as prompt as that seen with the catechol inotropes. Although infrequently required, an initial bolus dose of 20–80 mcg/kg infused over 10–15 minutes accelerates the onset of action in situations where a more rapid effect is needed.[81] The lengthy elimination half-life (1–3 hours) results in a more prolonged recovery from adverse effects once milrinone is discontinued. Some pharmacodynamic tolerance can occur with prolonged administration.

OTHER INTRAVENOUSLY ADMINISTERED POSITIVE INOTROPIC INTERVENTIONS

A number of additional pharmacologic interventions are known to enhance myocardial contractility.

Calcium Sensitizers

Calcium sensitizers (e.g. levosimendan) augment cardiac contractility by modulating intracellular mechanisms of contraction at the same concentrations of intracellular calcium (Fig. 1).

Levosimendan: Although some of its positive inotropic effect is probably rendered through phosphodiesterase inhibition, levosimendan is reported to enhance myocardial contractility through sensitization of the contractile apparatus to available calcium by increasing or stabilizing calcium binding to troponin C.[82,83]

Levosimendan behaves as an inodilator in human heart failure; it reduces vascular resistance and ventricular filling pressures, and by unloading the ventricle and some positive inotropy, it augments stroke volume and cardiac output.[84–87] Compared to dobutamine, levosimendan predictably causes a greater reduction in systemic blood pressure and B-type natriuretic peptide during infusions, but with identical all-cause mortality and comparable secondary clinical outcomes at 180 days postinfusion.[86] As a predominant vasodilator, levosimendan should theoretically have a favorable effect on myocardial energetics and oxygen balance; although this consideration has not been adequately studied in human systolic heart failure. For patients on nonselective adrenergic blockers (e.g. carvedilol), levosimendan can render its hemodynamic effects without having to compete for adrenergic receptors.[88] Because of its prominent vasodilating properties, levosimendan should not be considered a first-line drug for low output hypotension or shock.

Levosimendan itself has an elimination half-life of 1–2 hours, but a primary active metabolite (OR-1896) has a half-life of more than 75 hours. A sustained hemodynamic effect long after the infusion, which stopped may be favorable in some instances, but when accompanied by tachycardia, dysrhythmias, hypotension or other undesirable effects, the lengthy and somewhat unpredictable elimination is a shortcoming, particularly in critical care.

Levosimendan is available for clinical use in some countries of Europe, Asia and South America.

Additional Intravenously Administered Positive Inotropes

Preliminary studies of istaroxime, an inhibitor of sarcolemmal Na/K ATPase and activator of calcium ATPase of the sarcoplasmic reticulum, show promise as an agent to enhance cardiac systolic and diastolic performance.[89]

Intravenously administered thyroxine or triiodothyronine can improve hemodynamics and blood pressure with a reasonable safety margin, even in patients with advanced, end-stage heart failure and cardiogenic shock.[90,91] Historically, intravenously administered glucagon has been used to augment myocardial contractility in patients with low output hypotension or shock refractory to adrenergic stimulation or treated with moderate to high doses of beta-adrenergic blocking agents.

ORALLY ADMINISTERED POSITIVE INOTROPIC AGENTS

Oral inotropes have not fared well over the past two decades as intervention to improve myocardial contractility and performance. While digitalis (currently digoxin) has been used for over 200 years to treat cardiac failure and "dropsy", this coveted role has been reined in by the Digitalis Investigation Group (DIG) trial published in 1997.[92] Many orally administered, non-digitalis agents have been formulated over the past four decades to replace digoxin in the therapeutics of human heart failure; examples include amrinone, milrinone, vesnarinone, pimobendan and butopamine. But all were found to be ineffective, to provoke undesirable effects or to adversely affect outcomes.

Digitalis-Digoxin

Most of the enhancement of myocardial contractility by digoxin appears to be generated by inhibiting the Na/K ATPase pump of the cardiomyocyte sarcolemma (Fig. 1). This inhibition results in elevation of intracellular sodium, which increases (via blunting of the sodium-calcium exchanger) the intracellular calcium available for contraction.[93] Digitalis may also direct calcium into the myocyte via modulation of the voltage-sensitive sodium channels.[93]

Some of the clinical benefits of digitalis therapy in heart failure likely occur through alteration of sympathetic tone. Heart failure increases sympathetic nervous system tone and reduces parasympathetic tone, resulting in a number of undesirable effects including increased vascular resistance, tachycardia,

renin release and diminished baroreceptor sensitivity; many of these undesirable responses are favorably suppressed or reversed by chronic digitalis administration.[94–101] It is likely that any clinical or hemodynamic benefit noted during chronic digoxin administration is attributable to a varying combination of a direct effect on the cardiomyocyte and improvement of autonomic tone and balance.

Intravenously administered digoxin in heart failure evokes a modest increase in mean stroke volume, cardiac output and systemic blood pressure, a modest decrease in heart rate and ventricular filling pressures, and little change in vascular resistance; although individual responses can vary widely with better hemodynamic effects noted in the more hemodynamically compromised patients.[101–103] The nonpredictable variability of hemodynamic responses and potential undesirable effects (e.g. dysrhythmias) for a drug with a relatively low therapeutic index and long elimination half-life have limited the use of intravenous digoxin and its congeners. Intravenous digoxin is reserved as an option to slow an elevated ventricular rate in patients with decompensated heart failure and rapidly conducting atrial fibrillation or flutter.

The results of noncontrolled or relatively small (low number of enrolled patients) studies over the years have suggested that long-term, orally administered digoxin in heart failure can favorably affect clinical status, augment ventricular ejection fraction, increase exercise performance, and improve hemodynamics at rest and during exercise.[104–111] Again, the clinical and hemodynamic responses are individually quite variable with improvement more noteworthy in patients with severe decompensation.[105–107,110]

Two digoxin withdrawal studies, both double blind, randomized and placebo controlled, published in 1993 provide evidence supporting the merits of chronic digoxin administration in patients with mild-moderate heart failure (FC II-III) and sinus rhythm.[111,112] The Prospective Randomized Study of Ventricular Failure and the Efficacy of Digoxin (PROVED) study[111] was performed in patients chronically treated with diuretics and digoxin and the Randomized Assessment of the effect of Digoxin in Inhibitors of the Angiotensin-Converting Enzyme (RADIANCE) study[112] in patients chronically treated with diuretics, digoxin and angiotensin-converting enzyme inhibitors. In both studies, compared to continued digoxin therapy, the patients randomized to withdrawal of digoxin to placebo experienced, over a three-month period, a reduction in left ventricular ejection fraction, clinical status, functional capacity and exercise performance and an increase in heart rate and body weight. This deterioration was most notable in patients with more severe heart failure, but also occurred in patients with a milder course.[113,114] Both trials were performed prior to standard background beta-blocker therapy.

Studies examining the use of digoxin in patients with ventricular dysfunction following acute myocardial infarction showed minimal benefit and a high potential for adverse outcomes.[115–121]

The DIG trial[92] has overshadowed all prior studies regarding the use of digitalis chronically in patients with heart failure and sinus rhythm, and has now provided the framework for current digoxin use. Six thousand eight hundred patients with symptoms and signs of heart failure, LV ejection fraction less than or equal to 0.45 and in sinus rhythm were randomized 1:1 to digoxin (median dose 0.25 mg/day) or placebo. Patients with heart failure and ejection fraction, more than 0.45 were enrolled in a parallel ancillary study. About 95% of the study population was chronically taking an angiotensin-converting enzyme inhibitor, 82% a diuretic and 78% both agents. Chronic digoxin therapy in the DIG Trial had no effect on total mortality, but tended to reduce mortality attributable to heart failure and statistically reduced the combined endpoints of heart failure mortality or hospitalization for heart failure[92] (Fig. 8). While this benefit was greatest in patients with lower ejection fractions and worse clinical status, modest improvement was also noted for patients with an LV ejection fraction more than 0.45.[92,122,123]

The DIG Trial has since undergone considerable scrutiny, re-analysis and post-hoc analysis. Major limitations of the trial include absence of concomitant beta-blocker therapy and in retrospect, excessively high digoxin dosing and serum levels. Two percent of digoxin-treated patients in the trial were hospitalized for suspected digoxin toxicity compared to 0.9% for placebo (p < 0.001). Higher serum concentrations of digoxin (> 1.2 ng/ml) were associated with increased mortality over a mean follow-up of 37 months.[124] Importantly, improved heart failure mortality and hospitalization outcomes were maintained at lower digoxin levels (< 1.0 ng/ml).[124–126] The initial concern for a higher digoxin-related mortality for women[127] was later shown to be related to higher serum digoxin concentrations; outcomes improved at less than 1.0 ng/ml with a progressive rise in mortality and morbidity at levels more than or equal to 1.2 ng/ml.[128]

The DIG Trial was performed prior to routine beta-adrenergic blocker therapy in heart failure.[92] The results of two retrospective studies on populations far smaller than that of the DIG Trial suggest that chronic digoxin therapy may be of little benefit in heart failure patients in sinus rhythm on current, optimal therapeutic management including angiotensin-converting enzyme inhibition or angiotensin receptor blockade, beta-adrenergic blockade, diuretic, spironolactone and biventricular pacing for ventricular resynchronization.[129,130]

Indications and application: For the overall heart failure population, long-term digoxin administration has a Class IIa indication (level of evidence: B) from the 2009 ACC/AHA Task Force, which stated "Digitalis can be beneficial in patients with current or prior symptoms of heart failure and reduced left ventricular ejection fraction to decrease hospitalizations in heart failure.[131] Chronic digoxin therapy remains an option to control ventricular rate in the heart failure patient with atrial fibrillation, although this consideration has been challenged.[132]

With the exception of blocking AV nodal conduction in rapidly conducting atrial fibrillation or flutter in heart failure patients for whom other AV blocking agents (e.g. beta-adrenergic blockers, calcium channel blockers) may be problematic, there is hardly ever a need for accelerated or high-dose digoxin administration (historically termed "digitalization"). The initial and maintenance oral dose is 0.0625–0.25 mg/day. The 0.125 mg/day dose has largely replaced 0.25 mg/day as the standard maintenance dose because at the lower dose, serum digoxin levels (drawn > 8 hours after dosing) typically remain less than or equal to

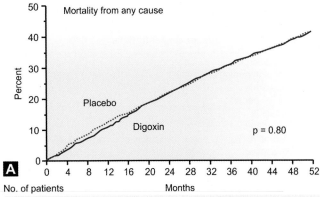

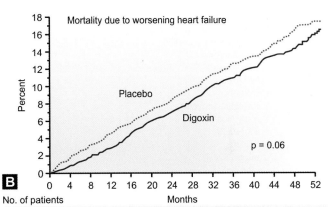

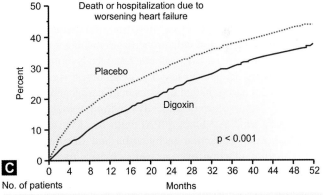

FIGURES 8A TO C: Graphs showing selected results of the Digitalis Investigation Group (DIG) Trial. (A) Long-term digoxin therapy did not impact total mortality. (B) Digoxin tended to favorably affect heart failure mortality at borderline statistical significance. (C) Chronic digoxin administration favorably affected (p < 0.001) the combined outcomes of mortality or hospitalization when attributable to worsening heart failure (*Source*: Modified from reference 92)

1.0 ng/ml in patients with normal renal function and clearance. Fifty to eighty percent of orally administered digoxin is absorbed with an elimination half-life of 36–48 hours, largely via renal excretion. Dose reduction or discontinuation becomes important in patients with renal dysfunction and/or during

TABLE 3

A partial list of agents known to affect, through a number of different mechanisms, serum digoxin concentrations

A. Decrease levels
  Cholestyramine
  Sucralfate
  Kaolin-pectin
  Antacids
  Salbutamol
  Rifampin
  Thyroxine

B. Increase levels
  Antiarrhythmic agents
    Amiodarone
    Propafenone
    Quinidine
  Calcium channel blocking agents
    Verapamil
    Diltiazem
    Dihydropyridines (e.g. nifedipine)
  Potassium-sparing diuretics
    Spironolactone
    Triamterene
    Amiloride
  Antimicrobials
    Macrolides (-mycin)
    Tetracycline
    Itraconazole
  Other
    Captopril
    Carvedilol
    Cyclosporine
    Indomethacin
    Omeprazole
    St. John's wort

concomitant administration of medications known to elevate digoxin concentrations (Table 3).

Digoxin's direct effect on sinoatrial and atrioventricular nodal cells and its autonomic properties (reducing sympathetic tone and enhancing parasympathetic tone) leads to many of the manifestations of digoxin toxicity, generally at serum levels more than 2.0 ng/ml, including sinus bradycardia and AV nodal blockade. Other digoxin-toxic dysrhythmias include atrial tachycardia with AV block ("PAT with block"), ventricular ectopic beats, ventricular tachycardia and fibrillation, and accelerated conduction over accessory bypass tracts. Nausea, vomiting, mental disturbances and visual aberrations are some of the systemic manifestations of toxicity. Digitalis, a sterol molecule, is a common cause of gynecomastia and breast discomfort in men taking this agent long term. To suppress some of the problematic toxic dysrhythmias, the intravenous administration of atropine, potassium and/or magnesium when appropriate, can be employed until serum digoxin concentrations fall to acceptable levels and the adverse effects dissipate. Severe, life-threatening toxicity often necessitates the administration of anti-digoxin Fab-fragment immunotherapy.[133,134]

Other Orally Administered Positive Inotropic Agents

Hydralazine has positive inotropic properties in human heart failure in addition to its well-established vasodilating, ventricular unloading effects.[12,26,135] These inotropic and hemodynamic effects can be employed to wean dobutamine (and perhaps,

milrinone and low-dose dopamine) from heart failure patients who appear hemodynamically dependent on the intravenous inotrope.[26]

Absolute and relative hypothyroidism can play a major role in the clinical course and outcomes in heart failure.[136–141] Thyroid hormone replacement enhances myocardial contractility through a number of mechanisms and is of particular clinical importance in these specific patient groups. Whether thyroid hormone intervention merits consideration as a means of augmenting cardiac performance and clinical outcomes in patients with heart failure beyond these groups remains unanswered.

REFERENCES

1. Tuttle RR, Mills J. Dobutamine: development of a new catecholamine to selectively increase cardiac contractility. Circ Res. 1975;36:185-96.

2. Bristow MR, Ginsburg R, Umans V, et al. B$_1$- and B$_2$-adrenergic-receptor subpopulations in nonfailing and failing human ventricular myocardium: coupling of both receptor subtypes to muscle contraction and selective B$_1$-receptor downregulation in heart failure. Circ Res. 1986;59:297-309.

3. Binkley PF, VanFossen DB, Nunziata E, et al. Influence of positive inotropic therapy on pulsatile hydraulic load and ventricular-vascular coupling in congestive heart failure. J Am Coll Cardiol. 1990;15:1127-35.

4. Binkley PF, VanFossen DB, Haas GJ, et al. Increased ventricular contractility is not sufficient for effective positive inotropic intervention. Am J Physiol. 1996;271:H1635-42.

5. Binkley PF, Murray KD, Watson KM, et al. Dobutamine increases cardiac output of the total artificial heart. Circulation. 1991;84:1210-5.

6. Ruffalo RR, Spradlin TA, Pollock D, et al. Alpha and beta adrenergic effects of the stereoisomers of dobutamine. J Pharmacol Exp Ther. 1981;219:447-52.

7. Nohria A, Tsang S, Fang J, et al. Clinical assessment identifies hemodynamic profiles that predict outcomes in patients admitted with heart failure. J Am Coll Cardiol. 2003;41:1797-804.

8. Leier CV, Webel J, Bush CA. The cardiovascular effects of the continuous infusion of dobutamine in patients with severe heart failure. Circulation. 1977;56:468-72.

9. Beregovich J, Bianchi C, D'Angelo R, et al. Hemodynamic effects of a new inotropic agent (dobutamine) in chronic heart failure. Brit Heart J. 1975;37:629-34.

10. Keren G, Lanaido S, Sonnenblick E, et al. Dynamics of functional mitral regurgitation during dobutamine therapy in patients with severe congestive heart failure. Am Heart J. 1989;118:748-54.

11. Leier CV, Heban PF, Huss P, et al. Comparative systemic and regional hemodynamic effects of dopamine and dobutamine in patients with cardiomyopathic heart failure. Circulation. 1978;58:466-75.

12. Magorien RD, Unverferth DV, Brown GP, et al. Dobutamine and hydralazine: comparative influences of positive inotropy and vasodilation on coronary blood flow and myocardial energetics in nonischemic congestive heart failure. J Am Coll Cardiol. 1983;1:499-505.

13. Leier CV, Binkley PF. Parenteral inotropic support for advanced congestive heart failure. Prog Cardiovasc Dis. 1998;41:207-24.

14. Boudoulas H, Rittgers SE, Lewis RP, et al. Changes in diastolic time with various pharmacologic agents: implication for myocardial perfusion. Circulation. 1979;60:164-9.

15. Krivokapich J, Czernin J, Schelbert HR. Dobutamine positive emission tomography: absolute quantitation at rest and dobutamine myocardial blood flow and correlation with cardiac work and percent diameter stenosis in patients with and without coronary artery disease. J Am Coll Cardiol. 1996;28:565-72.

16. Pacold I, Kleinman B, Gunnar R, et al. Effects of low-dose dobutamine on coronary hemodynamics, myocardial metabolism, and anginal threshold in patients with coronary artery disease. Circulation. 1983;68:1044-50.

17. Pozen RG, DiBianco R, Katz RJ, et al. Myocardial and hemodynamic effects of dobutamine in heart failure complicating coronary artery disease. Circulation. 1981;63:1279-85.

18. Bendersky R, Chatterjee K, Parmley WW, et al. Dobutamine in chronic ischemic heart failure: alterations in left ventricular function and coronary hemodynamics. Am J Cardiol. 1981;48:554-8.

19. Beanlands RS, Bach DS, Raylman R, et al. Acute effects of dobutamine on myocardial oxygen consumption and cardiac efficiency measured using Carbon-11 acetate kinetics in patients with dilated cardiomyopathy. J Am Coll Cardiol. 1993;22:1389-98.

20. Fowler MB, Alderman EL, Osterle SN, et al. Dobutamine and dopamine after cardiac surgery: greater augmentation of myocardial blood flow with dobutamine. Circulation. 1984;70:I-103-11.

21. Gillespie TA, Ambos HD, Sobel BE, et al. Effects of dobutamine in patients with acute myocardial infarction. Am J Cardiol. 1977;39:588-94.

22. Keung EC, Siskind SJ, Sonnenblick EH, et al. Dobutamine therapy in acute myocardial infarction. JAMA. 1981;245:144-6.

23. Sun KT, Czernin J, Krivokapich J, et al. Effects of dobutamine on myocardial blood flow, glucose metabolism, and wall motion in normal and dysfunctional myocardium. Circulation. 1996;94:3146-54.

24. Rahimtoola SH. Hibernating myocardium has reduced blood flow at rest that increases with low-dose dobutamine. Circulation. 1996;94:3055-61.

25. Barilla F, DeVincentis G, Mangieri E, et al. Recovery of viable myocardium during inotropic stimulation is not dependent on an increase in myocardial blood flow in the absence of collateral filling. J Am Coll Cardiol. 1999;33:697-704.

26. Binkley PF, Starling RC, Hammer DF, et al. Usefulness of hydralazine to withdraw from dobutamine in severe congestive heart failure. Am J Cardiol. 1991;68:1103-6.

27. Unverferth DV, Blanford M, Kates RE, et al. Tolerance to dobutamine after a 72 hour continuous infusion. Am J Med. 1980;69:262-6.

28. Kates RE, Leier CV. Dobutamine pharmacokinetics in severe heart failure. Clin Pharmacol Therap. 1978;24:537-41.

29. Leier CV, Unverferth DV, Kates RE. The relationship between plasma dobutamine concentrations and cardiovascular responses in cardiac failure. Am J Med. 1979;66:238-42.

30. Colucci WS, Denniss AR, Leatherman GF, et al. Intracoronary infusion of dobutamine in patients with and without severe congestive heart failure. J Clin Invest. 1988;81:1103-10.

31. Metra M, Nodari S, D'Aloia A, et al. Beta-blocker therapy influences the hemodynamic response to inotropic agents in patients with heart failure: a randomized comparison of dobutamine and enoximone before and after chronic treatment with metoprolol or carvedilol. J Am Coll Cardiol. 2002;40:1248-58.

32. Bollano E, Tang MS, Hjalmarson A, et al. Different responses to dobutamine in the presence of carvedilol or metoprolol in patients with chronic heart failure. Heart. 2003;89:621-4.

33. Waagstein F, Malek I, Hjalmarson AC. The use of dobutamine in myocardial infarction for reversal of the cardiodepressive effect of metoprolol. Br J Clin Pharmac. 1978;5:515-21.

34. Silver MA, Horton DP, Ghali JK, et al. Effect of nesiritide versus dobutamine on short-term outcomes in the treatment of acutely decompensated heart failure. J Am Coll Cardiol. 2002;39:798-803.

35. Gheorghiade M, Stough WG, Adams K, et al. The pilot randomized study of nesiritide versus dobutamine in heart failure (PRESERVD-HF). Am J Cardiol. 2005;96(6A):18G-25G.

36. Burger AJ, Horton DP, LeJemtel TH, et al. Effect of nesiritide (B-type natriuretic peptide) and dobutamine on ventricular arrhythmias in the treatment of patients with acutely decompensated congestive heart failure: the PRECEDENT study. Am Heart J. 2002;144:1102-8.

37. Abraham WT, Adams KF, Fonarow GC, et al. In hospital mortality in patients with acute decompensated heart failure requiring intravenous vasoactive medications: an analysis from the acute decompensated heart failure national registry (ADHERE). J Am Coll Cardiol. 2005;46:57-64.

38. O'Connor CM, Gattis WA, Uretsky B, et al. Continuous dobutamine is associated with increased risk of death in patients with advance heart failure: insights from the Flolan International Randomized Trial (FIRST). Am Heart J. 1999;138:78-86.

39. Elkayam U, Tasissa G, Binanay C, et al. Use and impact of inotropes and vasodilator therapy in hospitalized patients with severe heart failure. Am Heart J. 2007;153:98-104.

40. Goldenberg IF, Olivari MT, Levine TB, et al. Effect of dobutamine on plasma potassium in congestive heart failure secondary to idiopathic or ischemic cardiomyopathy. Am J Cardiol. 1989;63:843-6.

41. El-Sayed OM, Abdelfattah RR, Barcelona R, et al. Dobutamine-induced eosinophilia. Am J Cardiol. 2004;93:1078-9.

42. Hawkins ET, Levine TB, Goss SG, et al. Hypersensitivity myocardium in the explanted hearts of transplant recipients. Pathol Annu. 1995;30:287-304.

43. Abraham J, Mudd JO, Kapur NK, et al. Stress cardiomyopathy after intravenous administration of catecholamines and beta-agonists. J Am Coll Cardiol. 2009;53:1320-5.

44. Goldberg LI, Rajfer SI. Dopamine receptors: application in clinical cardiology. Circulation. 1985;72:245-8.

45. Brown L, Lorenz B, Erdmann E. The inotropic effects of dopamine and its precursor levodopa in isolated human ventricular myocardium. Klin Wochenschr. 1985;63:1117-23.

46. Anderson FL, Port JD, Reid BB, et al. Myocardial catecholamine and neuropeptide Y depletion in failing ventricles of patients with idiopathic dilated cardiomyopathy. Correlation with beta-adrenergic receptor downregulation. Circulation. 1992;85:46-53.

47. Beregovich J, Bianchi C, Rubler S, et al. Dose-related hemodynamic and renal effects of dopamine in congestive heart failure. Am Heart J. 1974;87:550-7.

48. Durairaj SK, Haywood LJ. Hemodynamic effects of dopamine in patients with resistant congestive heart failure. Clin Pharmacol Ther. 1978;24:175-85.

49. Maskin CS, Kugler J, Sonnenblick EH, et al. Acute inotropic stimulation with dopamine in severe congestive heart failure: beneficial hemodynamic effect at rest and during maximal exercise. Am J Cardiol. 1983;52:1028-32.

50. Rajfer SI, Borow KM, Lang RM, et al. Effects of dopamine on left ventricular afterload and contractile state in heart failure. J Am Coll Cardiol. 1988;12:498-506.

51. MacCannell KL, McNay JL, Meyer MD, et al. Dopamine in the treatment of hypotension and shock. N Engl J Med. 1966;275:1389-98.

52. Loeb HS, Winslow EBJ, Rahimtoola SH, et al. Acute hemodynamic effects of dopamine in patients with shock. Circulation. 1971;44:163-73.

53. Holzer J, Karliner JS, O'Rourke RA, et al. Effectiveness of dopamine in patients with cardiogenic shock. Am J Cardiol. 1973;32:79-84.

54. Winslow EJ, Loeb HS, Rahimtoola SH, et al. Hemodynamic studies and results of therapy in 50 patients with bacteremic shock. Am J Med. 1973;54:421-32.

55. De Backer D, Biston P, Devriendt J, et al. Comparison of dopamine and norepinephrine in the treatment of shock. N Engl J Med. 2010;362:779-89.

56. McDonald RH, Goldberg LI, McNay JL, et al. Dopamine in man: augmentation of sodium excretion, glomerular filtration rate and renal plasma flow. J Clin Invest. 1964;43:1116-24.

57. Ulkayam U, Ng TMH, Hatamizadeh P, et al. Renal vasodilating action of dopamine in patients with heart failure. Circulation. 2008;117:200-5.

58. Ungar A, Fumagalli S, Marini M, et al. Renal, but not systemic hemodynamic effects of dopamine are influenced by the severity of congestive heart failure. Crit Care Med. 2004;32:1125-9.

59. Goldberg LI, McDonald RH, Zimmerman AM. Sodium diuresis produced by dopamine in patients with congestive heart failure. N Engl J Med. 1963;269:1060-4.

60. Vargo DL, Brater DC, Rudy DW, et al. Dopamine does not enhance furosemide-induced natriuresis in patients with congestive heart failure. J Am Soc Nephrol. 1996;7:1032-7.

61. Varriale P, Mossavi A. The benefit of low-dose dopamine during vigorous diuresis for congestive heart failure associated with renal insufficiency: does it protect renal function? Clin Cardiol. 1997;20:627-30.

62. van de Borne P, Oren R, Sowers VK. Dopamine depresses minute ventilation in patients with heart failure. Circulation. 1998;98:126-31.

63. Dellinger RP, Levy MM, Carlet JM, et al. Surviving Sepsis Campaign: international guidelines for management of severe sepsis and septic shock. Intensive Care Med. 2008;34:17-60.

64. Benotti JR, Grossman W, Braunwald E, et al. Hemodynamic assessment of amrinone, a new inotropic agent. N Engl J Med. 1978;299:1373-7.

65. Hermiller JB, Leithe ME, Magorien RD, et al. Amrinone in severe congestive heart failure: another look at an intriguing new cardioactive drug. J Pharmacol Exp Ther. 1984;228:319-26.

66. Wilmshurst PT, Thompson DS, Juul SM, et al. Effects of intracoronary and intravenous amrinone in patients with cardiac failure and patients with near normal cardiac function. Br Heart J. 1985;53:493-506.

67. Holmberg SR, Williams AJ. Phosphodiesterase inhibitors and cardiac sarcoplasma reticulum calcium release channel: differential effects of milrinone and enoximone. Cardiovasc Res. 1991;25:537-45.

68. Baim DS, Edelson J, Braunwald E, et al. Evaluation of a new bipyridine inotropic agent-milrinone in patients with severe congestive heart failure. N Engl J Med. 1983;309:748-56.

69. Jaski BE, Fifer MA, Wright RF, et al. Positive inotropic and vasodilator actions of milrinone in patients with severe congestive heart failure. J Clin Invest. 1985;75:643-9.

70. Monrad ES, McKay RG, Baim DS, et al. Improvement in indices of diastolic performance in patients with severe congestive heart failure treated with milrinone. Circulation. 1984;70:1030-7.

71. Eichhorn EJ, Konstam MA, Weiland DS, et al. Differential effects of milrinone and dobutamine in right ventricular preload, afterload, and systolic performance in congestive heart failure secondary to ischemic or idiopathic dilated cardiomyopathy. Am J Cardiol. 1987;60:1329-33.

72. Monrad ES, Baim DS, Smith HS, et al. Milrinone, dobutamine, and nitroprusside: comparative effects on hemodynamics and myocardial energetics in patients with severe congestive heart failure. Circulation. 1986;73:III168-74.

73. Pfugfelder PW, O'Neill BJ, Ogilive RI, et al. Canadian multicenter study of a 48 hour infusion of milrinone in patients with severe heart failure. Can J Cardiol. 1991;7:5-10.

74. Monrad ES, Baim DS, Smith HS, et al. Effects of milrinone on coronary hemodynamics and myocardial energetics in patients with congestive heart failure. Circulation. 1985;71:972-9.

75. Givertz MM, Hare JM, Loh E, et al. Effect of bolus milrinone on hemodynamic variables and pulmonary vascular resistance in patients with severe left ventricular dysfunction: a rapid test for reversibility of pulmonary hypertension. J Am Coll Cardiol. 1996;28:1775-80.

76. Pamboukian SV, Carere RG, Cook RC, et al. The use of milrinone in pre-transplant assessment of patients with congestive heart failure and pulmonary hypertension. J Heart Lung Transplant. 1999;18:367-71.

77. Lowes BD, Tsvetkova T, Eichhorn EJ, et al. Milrinone versus dobutamine in heart failure subjects treated chronically with carvedilol. Int J Cardiol. 2001;81:141-9.

78. Simonton CA, Chatterjee K, Cody RJ, et al. Milrinone in congestive heart failure: acute and chronic hemodynamic and clinical evaluation. J Am Coll Cardiol. 1985;6:453-9.

79. Benotti JR, Lesko LJ, McCue JE, et al. Pharmacokinetics and pharmacodynamics of milrinone in chronic congestive heart failure. Am J Cardiol. 1985;56:685-9.

80. Edelson J, Stroshane R, Benziger DP, et al. Pharmacokinetics of the bipyridines amrinone and milrinone. Circulation. 1986;73:III145-52.

81. Baruch L, Patacsil P, Hameed A, et al. Pharmacodynamic effects of milrinone with and without a bolus loading infusion. Am Heart J. 2001;141:266-73.

82. Endoh M. Cardiac Ca^{2+} signaling and Ca^{2+} sensitizers. Circ J. 2008;72:1915-25.

83. Hasenfuss G, Pieske B, Castell M, et al. Influence of the novel inotropic agent levosimendan on isometric tension and calcium cycling in failing human myocardium. Circulation. 1998;98:2141-7.

84. Slawsky MT, Colucci WS, Gottlieb SS, et al. Acute hemodynamic and clinical effects of levosimendan in patients with severe heart failure. Circulation. 2000;102:2222-7.

85. Givertz MM, Andreon C, Conrad CH, et al. Direct myocardial effects of levosimendan in humans with left ventricular dysfunction. Circulation. 2007;115:1218-24.

86. Mebazaa A, Nieminen MS, Packer M, et al. Levosimendan vs dobutamine for patients with acute decompensated heart failure. JAMA. 2007;297:1883-91.

87. Nieminen MS, Akkila J, Hasenfuss G, et al. Hemodynamic and neurohumoral effects of continuous infusion of levosimendan in patients with congestive heart failure. J Am Coll Cardiol. 2000;36:1903-12.

88. Mebazza A, Nieminen MS, Filippatos GS, et al. Levosimendan vs dobutamine: outcomes for acute heart failure patients on β-blockers in SURVIVE. J Heart Fail. 2009;11:304-11.

89. Gheorghiade M, Blair JEA, Filippatos GS, et al. Hemodynamic, echocardiographic, and neurohormonal effects of istaroxime, a novel intravenous inotropic and lusitropic agent. J Am Coll Cardiol. 2008;51:2276-85.

90. Malik FS, Mehra MR, Uber PA, et al. Intravenous thyroid hormone supplementation in heart failure with cardiogenic shock. J Card Fail. 1999;5:31-7.

91. Hamilton MA, Stevenson LW, Fonarow GC, et al. Safety and hemodynamic effects of intravenous triiodothyronine in advanced heart failure. Am J Cardiol. 1998;81:443-7.

92. The Digitalis Investigation Group. The effect of digoxin on mortality and morbidity in patients with heart failure. N Engl J Med. 1997;336:525-33.

93. Hauptman PJ, Kelly RA. Digitalis. Circulation. 1999;99:1265-70.

94. Ferrari A, Gregorini L, Ferrari MC, et al. Digitalis and baroreceptor reflexes in man. Circulation. 1981;63:279-85.

95. Ferguson DW, Berg WJ, Sanders JS, et al. Sympathoinhibitory responses to digitalis glycosides in heart failure patients: direct evidence from sympathetic neural recordings. Circulation. 1989;80:65-77.

96. Schobel HP, Oren RM, Roach PJ, et al. Contrasting effects of digitalis and dobutamine in baroreflex sympathetic control in normal humans. Circulation. 1991;84:1118-29.

97. Brouwer J, van Veldhuisen DJ, Man in't Veld AJ, et al. Heart rate variability in patients with mild to moderate heart failure: effects of neurohormonal modulation by digoxin and ibopamine. J Am Coll Cardiol. 1995;26:983-90.

98. Newton GE, Tong JH, Schofield AM, et al. Digoxin reduces cardiac sympathetic activity in severe congestive heart failure. J Am Coll Cardiol. 1996;28:155-61.

99. Krum H, Bigger JT, Goldsmith RL, et al. Effect of long-term digoxin therapy on autonomic function in patients with chronic heart failure. J Am Coll Cardiol. 1995;25:289-94.

100. Covit AB, Schaer GL, Sealey JE, et al. Suppression of the renin-angiotensin system by intravenous digoxin in chronic congestive heart failure. Am J Med. 1983;75:445-7.

101. Ribner HS, Plucinski DA, Hsieh AM, et al. Acute effects of digoxin on total systemic vascular resistance in congestive heart failure due

to dilated cardiomyopathy: a hemodynamic-hormonal study. Am J Cardiol. 1985;56:896-904.

102. Gheorghiade M, St Clair J, St Clair C, et al. Hemodynamic effects of intravenous digoxin in patients with severe heart failure treated with diuretics and vasodilators. J Am Coll Cardiol. 1987;9:849-57.

103. Cohn K, Selzer A, Kersh ES, et al. Variability of hemodynamic responses to acute digitalization in chronic heart failure patients due to cardiomyopathy and coronary artery disease. Am J Cardiol. 1975;35:461-8.

104. Arnold SB, Byrd RC, Meister W, et al. Long-term digitalis therapy improves left ventricular function in heart failure. N Engl J Med. 1980;303:1443-8.

105. Lee DCS, Johnson RA, Bingham JB, et al. Heart failure in outpatients: a randomized trial of digoxin versus placebo. N Engl J Med. 1982;306:699-705.

106. The Captopril-Digoxin Multicenter Research Group. Comparative effects of therapy with captopril and digoxin in patients with mild to moderate heart failure. JAMA. 1988;259:539-44.

107. Guyatt GH, Sullivan MJJ, Fallen EL, et al. A controlled trial of digoxin in heart failure. Am J Med. 1988;61:371-5.

108. DiBianco R, Shabetai R, Kostuk W, et al. A comparison of oral milrinone, digoxin, and their combination in the treatment of patients with chronic heart failure. N Engl J Med. 1989;320:677-83.

109. Sullivan M, Atwood JE, Myers J, et al. Increased exercise capacity after digoxin administration in patients with heart failure. J Am Coll Cardiol. 1989;13:1138-43.

110. Davies RF, Beanlands DS, Nadeau C, et al. Enalapril versus digoxin in patients with congestive heart failure: a multicenter study. J Am Coll Cardiol. 1991;18:1602-9.

111. Uretsky BF, Young JB, Shahidi FE, et al. Randomized study assessing the effect of digoxin withdrawal in patients with mild to moderate chronic congestive heart failure: rtesults of the PROVED trial. J Am Coll Cardiol. 1993;22:955-62.

112. Packer M, Gheorghiade M, Young JB, et al. Withdrawal of digoxin from patients with chronic heart failure treated with angiotensin-converting-enzyme inhibitors. RADIANCE study. N Engl J Med. 1993;329:1-7.

113. Adams KF, Gheorghiade M, Uretsky BF, et al. Clinical predictors of worsening heart failure during withdrawal from digoxin therapy. Am Heart J. 1998;135:389-97.

114. Adams KF, Gheorghiade M, Uretsky BF, et al. Patients with mild heart failure worsen during withdrawal from digoxin therapy. J Am Coll Cardiol. 1997;30:42-8.

115. Goldstein RA, Passamani ER, Roberts R. A comparison of digoxin and dobutamine in patients with acute infarction and cardiac failure. N Engl J Med. 1980;303:846-50.

116. Hodges M, Friesinger GC, Riggins RCK, et al. Effects of intravenously administered digoxin on mild left ventricular failure in acute myocardial infarction in man. Am J Cardiol. 1972;29:749-56.

117. Moss AJ, Davies HT, Conard DL, et al. Digitalis-associated cardiac mortality after myocardial infarction. Circulation. 1981;64:1150-6.

118. Madsen EB, Gilpin E, Henning H, et al. Prognostic importance of digitalis after acute myocardial infarction. J Am Coll Cardiol. 1984;3:681-9.

119. Bigger JT, Fleiss JL, Rolnitzky LM, et al. Effect of digitalis treatment on survival after acute myocardial infarction. Am J Cardiol. 1985;55:623-30.

120. Muller JE, Turi ZG, Stone PH, et al. Digoxin therapy and mortality after myocardial infarction. N Engl J Med. 1986;314:265-71.

121. Ryan TJ, Bailey KR, McCabe CH, et al. The effects of digitalis on survival in high-risk patients with coronary artery disease: the Coronary Artery Surgery Study (CASS). N Engl J Med. 1983;67:735-42.

122. Meyer P, White M, Mujib M, et al. Digoxin and reduction of heart failure hospitalization in chronic systolic and diastolic heart failure. Am J Cardiol. 2008;102:1681-6.

123. Ahmed A, Rich MW, Fleg JL, et al. Effects of digoxin on morbidity and mortality in diastolic heart failure: the ancillary Digitalis Investigation Group Trial. Circulation. 2006;114:397-403.

124. Rathore SS, Curtis JP, Wang Y, et al. Association of serum digoxin concentration and outcomes in patients with heart failure. JAMA. 2003;289:871-8.

125. Ahmed A, Pitt B, Rahimtoola SH, et al. Effects of low serum concentrations on mortality and hospitalization in heart failure: a propensity matched study of the DIG Trial. Int J Cardiol. 2008;123:138-46.

126. Ahmed A, Waagstein F, Pitt B, et al. Effectiveness of digoxin in reducing one-year mortality in chronic heart failure in the Digitalis Investigation Group Trial. Am J Cardiol. 2009;103:82-7.

127. Rathore SS, Wang Y, Krumholz HM. Sex-based differences in the effect of digoxin for treatment of heart failure. N Engl J Med. 2002;347:1403-11.

128. Adams KF, Patterson JH, Gattis WA, et al. Relationship of serum digoxin concentration to mortality and morbidity in women in the Digitalis Investigation Group Trial. J Am Coll Cardiol. 2005;46:497-504.

129. Dhaliwal AS, Bredikis A, Habib G, et al. Digoxin and clinical outcomes in systolic heart failure patients on contemporary background heart failure therapy. Am J Cardiol. 2008;102: 1356-60.

130. Georgiopoulou VV, Kalogeropoulos AP, Giamouzis G, et al. Digoxin therapy does not improve outcomes in patients with advanced heart failure on contemporary medical therapy. Circ Heart Failure. 2009;2:90-7.

131. Jessup M, Abraham WT, Casey DE, et al. 2009 Focused Update: ACCF/AHA Guidelines for the diagnosis and management of heart failure in adults. Circulation. 2009;119:1977-2016.

132. Fauchier L, Grimard C, Pierre B, et al. Comparison of beta blocker and digoxin alone and in combination for management of patients with atrial fibrillation and heart failure. Am J Cardiol. 2009;103:248-54.

133. Smith TW, Haber E, Yeatman L, et al. Reversal of advanced digoxin intoxication with Fab fragments on digoxin-specific antibodies. N Engl J Med. 1976;294:797-800.

134. Antman EM, Wenger TL, Butter VP, et al. Treatment of 150 cases of life-threatening digitalis intoxication with digoxin-specific Fab antibody fragments. Circulation. 1990;81:1744-52.

135. Leier CV, Desch CE, Magorien RD, et al. Positive inotropic effects of hydralazine in human subjects. Am J Cardiol. 1980;46:1039-44.

136. Ievasi G, Pingitore A, Landi P, et al. Low-T_3 syndrome: a strong prognostic predictor of death in patients with heart disease. Circulation. 2003;107:708-13.

137. Ascheim DD, Hryniewicz K. Thyroid hormone metabolism in patients with congestive heart failure: the low triiodothyronine state. Thyroid. 2002;12:511-5.

138. Mariotti R, Ievasi G. Acute effects of triiodothyronine (T_3) replacement therapy in patients with chronic heart failure and low-T_3 syndrome: a randomized, placebo-controlled study. J Clin Endocrinol Metab. 2008;93:1351-8.

139. Iacoviello M, Guida P, Guastamacchia E, et al. Prognostic role of sub-clinical hypothyroidism in chronic heart failure outpatients. Curr Pharm Des. 2008;14:2686-92.

140. Kahaly GJ, Dillmann WH. Thyroid hormone action in the heart. Endocr Rev. 2005;26:704-28.

141. Klein I, Danzi S. Thyroid hormone treatment to mend a broken heart. J Clin Endocrinol Metab. 2008;93:1172-4.

Antilipid Agents

Jennifer G Robinson

Chapter Outline

Over 150 years ago, Virchow and his colleagues described the accumulation of lipid as the hallmark of the atherosclerotic plaque. Since then, an extensive body of evidence has shown a direct relationship between blood cholesterol levels and atherosclerotic cardiovascular diseases. Causality has been proven in numerous clinical trials showing that lowering total and low density lipoprotein cholesterol (LDL-C) slows the development of atherosclerotic disease and prevents clinical events. The large majority of clinical data comes from statin trials. Other lipid modifying drugs have demonstrated more modest cardiovascular benefits. This chapter will review appropriate uses, mechanisms of action, lipid-modifying efficacy, cardiovascular benefits and safety for each class of lipid-modifying drugs.

APPROPRIATE USES

The National Cholesterol Education Program Adult Treatment Panel (NCEP ATP III) has identified two lipid targets for the prevention of cardiovascular diseases, LDL-C and non-high-density lipoprotein cholesterol (non-HDL-C) (Table 1).[1] The first target of therapy is *LDL-C,* with treatment goals based on the risk of a coronary heart disease event in the next 10 years. The second target of therapy is non-*HDL-C*. Non-HDL-C is calculated by subtracting HDL-C from total cholesterol and reflects circulating levels of atherogenic apolipoprotein-B containing lipoproteins. The non-HDL-C goal is 30 mg/dL

higher than the LDL-C goal. Although the NCEP ATP III guidelines recommended using non-HDL-C when triglycerides are 150–500 mg/dL, recent evidence suggests that this recommendation can be simplified to using the non-HDL-C goal when triglycerides are less than 500 mg/dL.[2]

In those with triglyceride levels more than 500 mg/dL, prevention of pancreatitis is the initial objective. Once triglycerides are less than 500 mg/dL, attention can then turn to addressing LDL-C and non-HDL-C levels for cardiovascular prevention. Although low levels of HDL-C and high levels of triglycerides are markers of increased cardiovascular risk, specific treatment targets have not been identified due to the lack of evidence that pharmacologically altering the levels of these two factors *per se* reduces cardiovascular risk.[3] Cardiovascular prevention efforts in patients with low HDL-C should focus on lifestyle and drug therapy to achieve LDL-C and non-HDL-C goals. In the NCEP ATP III 2004 update, statins were recommended as first line therapy for cardiovascular prevention.[4]

Similar treatment strategies are used to lower LDL-C and non-HDL-C. All patients should be advised to undertake therapeutic lifestyle changes. *Statins* are the drugs of choice based on an extensive record of safely reducing cardiovascular events and overall mortality. Bile acid sequestrants and niacin also reduce cardiovascular risk, although they are less effective and have more adverse effects than statins. Ezetimibe is a well tolerated

TABLE 1

Overview of lipid treatment goals and strategies

	1st target LDL-C	Triglycerides (mg/dL)	
		< 500 2nd target Non-HDL-C	> 500
Objective	Prevent CVD	Prevent CVD	Prevent pancreatitis
Treatment goals	LDL-C goal High risk: CHD/CHD risk equivalents* < 100 (optional < 70) mg/dL Moderately high risk: > 2 risk factors** with 10-20% 10-year CHD risk† < 130 mg/dL (optional < 100 mg/dL) Moderate risk: > 2 risk factors** with < 10% 10-year CHD risk < 130 mg/dL Lower risk: 0–1 risk factor < 160 mg/dL (consider drug therapy LDL > 190 mg/dL/optional LDL > 160 mg/dL)	Non-HDL-C goal 30 mg/dL higher than LDL goal	Triglycerides < 500 mg/dL
Lifestyle	Therapeutic lifestyle changes	Therapeutic lifestyle changes	Therapeutic lifestyle changes Very low-fat (< 15%) diet
Drug 1st choice	Statins	Statins	Fibrates
Drug add-on or 2nd choice	Niacin bile-acid sequestrant Ezetimibe	Niacin Ezetimibe Fibrate	Omega-3 fish oil Niacin Statins (high dose)

* Coronary heart disease (CHD) includes a history of myocardial infarction, stable or unstable angina, coronary artery revascularization, or clinically significant myocardial ischemia; CHD risk equivalents include other cardiovascular disease, including peripheral arterial disease, abdominal aortic aneurysm, carotid artery disease (stroke of carotid or intracerebral origin, transient ischemic attack, or > 50% carotid artery stenosis), diabetes, and > 2 risk factors with > 20% 10-year CHD risk

** Risk factors include age (men > 45 years, women > 55 years), cigarette smoking, hypertension (blood pressure > 140/90 mm Hg or antihypertensive therapy), low HDL-C (< 40 mg/dL) and family history of premature CHD (onset in male first degree relative < 55 years; first degree female relative < 65 years)

† 10-year risk of nonfatal myocardial infarction and CHD death estimated by Framingham Scoring

CHAPTER 7

Antilipid Agents

drug that lowers LDL-C and non-HDL-C but has yet to be established whether ezetimibe reduces cardiovascular risk.

Fibrates are generally the first choice for triglyceride-lowering to prevent pancreatitis. However, fibrates reduce cardiovascular risk less than statins and have safety concerns when used in combination with statins. High doses of omega-3 fish oil, niacin or statins also effectively lower elevated triglycerides. The mechanisms of action, efficacy and safety for each class of drug will now be reviewed.

STATINS

Statins are the foundation of cardiovascular risk reduction. Consistent evidence from more than 100,000 clinical trial participants has shown statins reduce the risk of coronary heart disease and stroke in direct proportion to the magnitude of LDL-C lowering. Statins inhibit 3-hydroxy-3-methylglutarul coenzyme A (HMG CoA) reductase, the rate-limiting step in cholesterol synthesis (Fig. 1). A lower concentration of intracellular cholesterol upregulates LDL receptors on the cell surface and enhances removal of circulating LDL-C. Downstream products of HMG CoA also influence inflammatory, thrombotic and vasodilatory factors, although the impact of these "pleiotropic" effects on clinical cardiovascular events remains to be determined.[5]

EFFICACY

A dose of statin should be used that will lower LDL-C by at least 30–40%. Starting doses of statins generally achieve this degree of LDL-C lowering (pitavastatin 2 mg, atorvastatin 10 mg, lovastatin or pravastatin 40 mg, rosuvastatin 10 mg, simvastatin 40 mg and fluvastatin 80 mg) (Table 2). Reducing LDL-C by more than or equal to 50% or more may be desirable, but usually requires the highest doses of atorvastatin (40–80 mg), rosuvastatin (20–40 mg), or a statin used in combination with another LDL-C lowering agent. Each doubling the statin dose will result in an additional 6% reduction in LDL-C and non-HDL-C ("rule of sixes"). Moderate doses of statins lower triglycerides by about 15–20%, while the highest doses of atorvastatin, rosuvastatin, and simvastatin can lower triglycerides by up to 30%. Statins modestly raise HDL-C by 2–10%. Although HDL-C and triglyceride levels predict cardiovascular risk, it does not appear that the increases in HDL-C or decreases in triglyceride decreases from statin, or any other drug, therapy contribute further cardiovascular reduction beyond that obtained from LDL-C lowering.[3]

MUSCLE SAFETY

The majority of patients tolerate statins without difficulty.[6] Although commonly reported, muscle complaints are usually not related to statin use. Rhabdomyolysis occurs very rarely

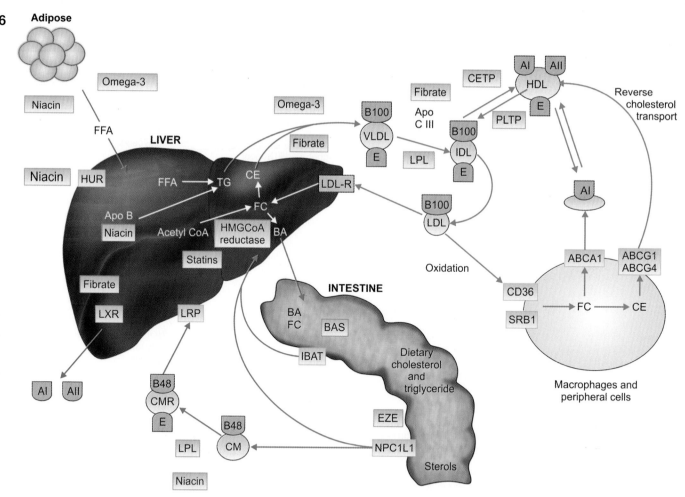

FIGURE 1: Overview lipid-modifying drug mechanisms

Statins inhibit the rate-limiting step in cholesterol synthesis, 3-hydroxy-3-methylglutaryl coenzyme A reductase (HMGCoA reductase) which binds acetyl CoA to free cholesterol to create cholesterol esters. Reduction in intrahepatic free cholesterol (FC) increases the number of LDL-receptors (LDL-R) on the cell membrane, faciliating removal of LDL-C from plasma. *Bile-acid sequestering agents (BAS)* and *ezetimibe (EZE)* lower plasma LDL-C by lowering intracellular free cholesterol levels. BAS bind bile acids via the intestinal bile acid transporter (IBAT), interrupting the enterohepatic circulation of bile acid FC. EZE acts on the Niemann-Pick C1-Like 1 (NPC1L1) transporter in at the intestinal wall to prevent absorption of dietary and biliary cholesterol. EZE also blocks uptake of plant sterols. *Dietary sterol/stanols* competitively inhibit the uptake of cholesterol in the intestine. The efficacy of all three intestinally active agents is limited since there is a compensatory increase in hepatic cholesterol synthesis. *Niacin* acts through a unknown and known mechanisms, including partially inhibiting the release of free fatty acids (FFA) from adipose; increasing lipoprotein lipase (LPL) activity thereby enhancing removal of chylomicron (CM) triglyceride from plasma; decreasing apolipoprotein B (apo B) synthesis which lowers very low density lipoprotein cholesterol (VLDL-C) and intermediate density lipoprotein cholesterol (IDL-C), and thus plasma triglcyerides; and increasing high density lipoprotein cholesterol (HDL-C) levels through decreased hepatic uptake, likely through the holouptake receptor (HUR) and catabolism. Increased levels of HDL-C may increase reverse cholesterol transport from peripheral cells to the liver. *Fibrates* lower triglyceride levels by decreasing VLDL secretion and increasing catabolism of triglyceride-rich particles via several mechanisms, including reduced apolipoprotein C (apo C) production which upregulates lipoprotein-lipase-mediated lipolysis and increased cellular FFA uptake as well as increasing FFA catabolism. Fibrates increase HDL-C induce apolipoprotein A-I and A-II (AI & AII) synthesis via the liver X receptor/retinoid X receptor heterodimer (LXR), *Omega-3 fatty acids (O-3)* reduce the rate of VLDL synthesis through a number of putative mechanisms inhibiting release of FFA from adipose, inhibiting FFA synthesis, and increasing apo B degradation (Abbreviations: ABC: ATP-binding cassette; B48 or B100: Apolipoprotein B48 or B100; CETP: Cholesterol ester transfer protein; CMR: CM remnant; E: Apolipoprotein E; LRP: LDL receptor-related protein 1; PLTP: Phospholipid transport protein; SRB-1: Steroid receptor binding protein)

and generally in patients with multiple factors predisposing to decreased clearance such as advanced age, diminished renal function, and medications interfering with statin metabolism. Notably, currently marketed statins are much safer than low-dose aspirin, which has more than 200-fold higher rate of major bleeding than statins have of inducing rhabdomyolysis. In properly selected patients participating in long-term clinical trials of statin therapy, myopathy (muscle symptoms with creatine kinase elevations more than 10 times the upper limit of normal) and rhabdomyolysis occurred in less than 0.2% of

subjects, with the exception of a higher rate of approximately 0.9% observed with simvastatin 80 mg.[7,8] The higher rate of muscle injury with simvastatin 80 mg has resulted in a communication from the US Food and Drug Administration regarding the safety of this dose.[7,8]

STATIN DRUG INTERACTIONS

Risk of myopathy and rhabdomyolysis is related to circulating drug levels. Three statins are metabolized by hepatic cytochrome P450 enzyme (CYP) 3A4 and have the most potential for drug

TABLE 2

Percent change in lipids and lipoproteins from baseline for various doses of statins, and statins coadministered with ezetimibe, niacin or fenofibric acid. Doses achieving a 30% to less than 50% reduction in LDL-C are highlighted in light gray and doses achieving more than or equal to 50% reductions are highlighted in dark gray.[14,27-33]

Statin dose	Fluvastatin	Pitavastatin	Pravastatin	Simvastatin	Atorvastatin	Rosuvastatin	Simvastatin + Ezetimibe 10 mg	Rosuvastatin + Fenofibric acid 135 mg	Lovastatin + ER Niacin 2 gm
LDL-C									
2 mg		-36							
4 mg		-43							
10 mg	NR		-20	-28	-37	-46	-46	-37	NR
20 mg	-22		-24	-35	-43	52	-50	-39	NR
40 mg	-25		-30	-39	-48	-55	-56	NR	-42
80 mg	-35		-37	-46	-51	NA	-59	NA	NA
Non-HDL-C									
2 mg		-33							
4 mg		-36							
10 mg	NR		-19	-26	-34	-42	-42	-45	NR
20 mg	NR		-22	-33	-40	-48	-47	-45	NR
40 mg	NR		-27	-36	-45	-51	-51	NR	NR
80 mg	NR		NR	-42	-48	NA	-55	NA	NR
Triglycerides									
2 mg		-19							
4 mg		-18							
10 mg	NR		-8	-12	-20	-20	-24	-47	NR
20 mg	-12		-8	-18	-23	-24	-26	-43	NR
40 mg	-14		-13	-15	-27	-26	-29	NR	-44
80 mg	-19		-19	-18	-28	—	-26	NA	NR
HDL-C									
2 mg		+7							
4 mg		+5							
10 mg	NR		+3	+5	+6	+8	+8	+20	NR
20 mg	+3		+4	+6	+5	+10	+9	+19	NR
40 mg	+4		+6	+5	+4	+10	+9	NR	+30
80 mg	+11		+3	+7	+2		+7	NA	NR

(Abbreviations: ER: Extended release; NA: Dose not approved; NR: Not reported).

CHAPTER 7

Antilipid Agents

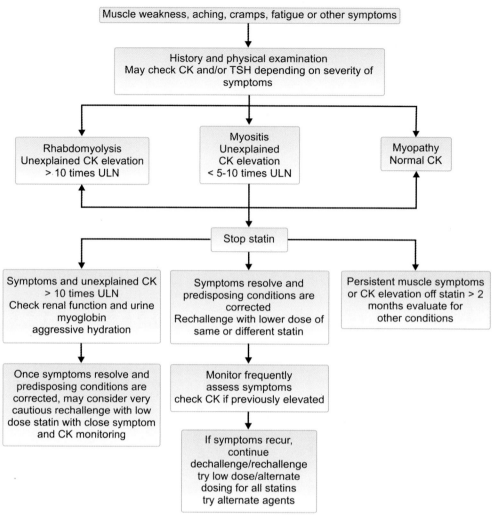

(Abbreviations: CK: Creatine kinase; TSH: Thyroid stimulating hormone; ULN: Upper limit of normal range).

interactions—atorvastatin, lovastatin and simvastatin (remember as "A, L, S") (Table 3). Avoid concomitant use of these three statins with potent inhibitors of CYP3A4, including use with azole antifungals (ketoconazole and itraconazole; alternative— fluconazole), macrolide antibiotics (erythromycin and clarithromycin; alternative—azithromycin), rifampicin and protease inhibitors (alternative—indinavir) (Table 4). Lower doses of simvastatin and lovastatin are recommended for patients receiving weaker CYP3A4 inhibitors amiodarone, calcium channel blockers diltiazem and verapamil (alternatives— amlodipine and nifedipine). Interactions with some antidepressants (alternatives—paroxetine and venlafaxine) have also been reported. Alternatives to CYP3A4 metabolized statins include rosuvastatin, which is minimally metabolized, pravastatin which has no cytochrome P450 metabolism, fluvastatin, which is metabolized by the 2C9 pathway and pitavastatin which has no significant CYP3A4, 2C9 or 2C8 metabolism. All statins are glucuronidated, increasing the potential for interaction with gemfibrozil. Cyclosporine raises blood levels of virtually all statins by both cytochrome P450 and other pathways, and low doses of statins should be titrated carefully, if needed.

RENAL EXCRETION

Although statins are primarily metabolized by the liver, some statins have relatively greater renal excretion—lovastatin, pitavastatin, pravastatin, rosuvastatin and simvastatin. Dose adjustment may be considered in those with markedly impaired renal excretion. All statins should be used with caution in patients with a glomerular filtration rate less than 30 since substantially impaired renal excretion is also a marker for other patient characteristics that may increase the potential for adverse muscle effects, including advanced age, frailty and polypharmacy.

MANAGING MUSCLE SYMPTOMS

An approach to the management of muscle and other symptoms in statin-treated patients is provided in Flow chart 1. Persistent muscle pain or weakness affecting the proximal muscles is the most common manifestation of statin intolerance. Intermittent or nocturnal muscle cramps and localized joint pain are not uncommon. Generalized fatigue may be the presenting complaint for elderly patients. The general approach is to discontinue the statin until symptoms resolve, and then rechallenge

TABLE 3

Summary of comparative pharmacokinetics of statins in healthy volunteers

	Atorvastatin	Fluvastatin	Lovastatin	Pitavastatin	Pravastatin	Rosuvastatin	Simvastatin
Major metabolic enzyme	CYP3A4	CYP2C9	CYP3A4 Glucuronidation	Minimal CYP450 Glucuronidation	No CYP450 Glucuronidation	Some CYP 2C8 Glucuronidation	CYP3A4 Glucuronidation
Renal excretion (%)	≤ 2	< 6	≥ 10	15	20	10	13
Absorption (%)	30	98	30–31	51	34	40–60	60–80
Prodrug	No	No	Yes	No	No	No	Yes
t_{max} (h)	1.0–2.0	0.5–1.0	2.0–4.0	1.0	1.0–1.5	3.0–5.0	1.3–3.0
$T_{1/2}$ (hours)	14–15	3.0	2.0	12	2.0	20	1.4–3.0
Lipophilicity (logP)	4.06	3.24	4.30	—	−0.23	—/33	4.68
Protein binding (%)	> 98	> 98	> 95	99	43–54	88	95
Affinity for Pgp transporter	Yes	No	Yes	—	Yes	No	Yes
Hepatic first-pass metabolism (%)	20–30	40–70	40–70	—	50–70	50–70	50–80
Systemic active metabolites (no.)	Yes (2)	No	Yes (3)	No	No	Minimal	Yes (3)
Bioavailability (%)	12–14	29	<5	51	18	20	<5

TABLE 4

Selected clinically relevant statin drug interactions

Drug interactions	Atorvastatin	Fluvastatin	Lovastatin	Pitavastatin	Pravastatin	Rosuvastatin	Simvastatin
Gemfibrozil Alternative: Fenofibrate	+	+	++	+	++	+	++
Cyclosporine	++		++	++	++	++	++
HIV protease inhibitors Alternative: Indinavir	+		+	+		+	+
Ketoconazole, itraconazole Alternative: Fluconazole	+		+				+
Erythromycin, clarithromycin, telithromycin Alternative: Azithromycin	+		++				+
Rifampicin	+		+			+	+
Diltiazem, verapamil Alternatives: Amlodipine, nifedipine			+				+, ++
Amiodarone			+				+
Digoxin	+						+
Fluoxetine, fluvoxamine, sertraline, nefazodone Alternative: paroxetine, venlafaxine	+	+	+			+	

CHAPTER 7

Antilipid Agents

with a low dose of the same or another statin. Creatine kinase levels are usually normal in statin-intolerant patients but may be helpful if symptoms are severe. Patients with recurrent muscle symptoms on statin rechallenge may tolerate alternate dosing strategies including alternate day or weekly dosing intervals, with up-titration as tolerated. For example, rosuvastatin 5–10 mg once a week, or 2.5 mg every other day, can lower LDL-C by 25%. Patients reliably developing muscle symptoms after a discrete time period, for example, 3 months, may tolerate a statin, if taken for 2½ months with a 2 week statin-free holiday. Regular or extended-release fluvastatin 80 mg is also an option. Even a low dose of a statin will be more effective than alternative LDL-C lowering therapies. Additional strategies include improving diet and lifestyle habits plant stanol/sterol supplementation, ezetimibe and bile acid sequestering agents.

Coenzyme Q10 has been shown in a few, but not most, randomized studies to improve statin tolerance when given in higher doses of 100–200 mg/day. Vitamin D supplementation has also been proposed for Vitamin D deficient patients suffering muscle symptoms, but randomized trials have not yet been performed. Red yeast rice, which contains a low dose of naturally occurring lovastatin, may be tolerated by some patients otherwise intolerant of statins, although the usual cautions regarding efficacy and safety apply as they do to other over-the-counter remedies.

Creatine kinase levels should not be monitored on a routine basis in statin-treated patients, although creatine kinase levels should be evaluated in patients developing severe or recurrent muscle symptoms. Muscle symptoms that fail to resolve within 2 months of statin discontinuation are likely due to another etiology. Rheumatologic disorders (including polymyalgia rhuematica), hypothyroidism, chronic sleep deprivation, sleep apnea, underlying muscle disorders, among others, are not uncommon. These conditions may also lower the threshold for statin-related muscle symptoms and once treated, statin therapy can then be resumed.

LIVER SAFETY

Abnormal liver function tests are also common among patients receiving statins but are not usually related to statin use.

Persistent elevations in hepatic alanine transaminase (ALT; which is the most specific test for drug-related hepatotoxicity) in long-term clinical trials are uncommon and related to increasing statin dose. Over a period of 2–5 years, persistent ALT elevations greater than 3 times the upper limit of normal occurred in approximately 1% of study participants receiving 80 mg of atorvastatin or simvastatin. Persistent ALT elevations less than 3 times the upper limit of normal are usually due to non-alcoholic steatohepatitis, or fatty liver, related to insulin resistance. As long as a stable pattern of ALT elevation has been established, statins can still be used in these patients for cardiovascular prevention with regular ALT monitoring. Often ALT levels improve with long-term statin therapy. In patients with unexplained ALT elevations greater than 3 times the upper limit of normal, the statin should be discontinued along with other potential hepatotoxic prescription and over-the-counter agents. The patient monitored until levels return to baseline or an etiology is established. Except for bile acid sequestrants, statins and other lipid-lowering therapies are generally contraindicated in patients with severe liver disease and the value of preventive therapy should be carefully evaluated in such patients.

ADD-ON TO STATIN THERAPY

Consideration may be given to adding a second agent to a statin in patients who have not achieved their LDL-C and non-HDL-C goals and for whom more aggressive therapy is deemed appropriate. It should be noted, however, at this time there is insufficient clinical trial evidence that adding a second agent to statin therapy will result in additional cardiovascular event reduction. Until evidence from ongoing trials is available, selection of one agent over another can only be guided by considerations of LDL-C and non-HDL-C lowering efficacy, safety and cost.

Ezetimibe, bile acid sequestrants and niacin 2 gm will lower LDL-C, an additional 15% when added to statin therapy (Table 5). Niacin is more effective than other agents for lowering non-HDL-C due to greater increases in HDL-C. Bile acid-sequestrants are less effective for lowering non-HDL-C due to

TABLE 5

Lipid lowering options for patients who have not achieved LDL-C and non-HDL-C goals on statin therapy[11,34-36]

Drug	Percent changes from baseline			
	LDL-C	Non-HDL-C	Triglyceride	HDL-C
Double statin dose	−6%	−6%	−2 to −12%	−2 to +2%
Ezetimibe 10 mg	−15 to −20%	−12%	−9%	NS
Niacin 2 gr	−1 to −8%	−15 to −31%*	−24%	+18 to +21%
Bile acid binding agent Colestipol 2 scoops (6 gr) Cholestyramine 2 scoops (8 gr) Coleselvalam 6 tabs or suspension (3.75 gr)	−6 to −16%	−5 to −8%	0 to +23%	+1 to +7%
Fenofibrate 145 mg Fenofibric acid 135 mg	−6 to +4%	−3 to −23%*	−15 to −27%	+10 to +13%
Gemfibrozil 600 mg BID	+7%	+2%	−18%	0%
Marine omega-3 fatty acids	−6 to +10%	−7 to −9%	0 to −27%	+2 to +4%
*Calculated by subtracting mean HDL-C from mean total cholesterol				

their very low density lipoprotein cholesterol (VLDL-C) raising effects. Fibrates have variable effects on LDL-C, and may raise it in patients with elevated triglyceride levels. Fenofibrate will lower LDL-C and non-HDL-C somewhat more than gemfibrozil, and appears to be safer than gemfibrozil when used with a statin. Omega-3 fatty acids may increase LDL-C and have modest effects on non-HDL-C, despite significant triglyceride lowering.

The term "residual risk" has been used to describe patients who have achieved their LDL-C and non-HDL-C goals on statin therapy yet still experience a cardiovascular event. Typically, these patients have low HDL-C and elevated levels of triglycerides, LDL-C particles and apolipoprotein B. An evidence-based strategy has yet to be determined for these patients since drug-related changes in HDL-C and triglyceride have not been associated with cardiovascular risk reduction.[3] Fenofibrate added to moderate dose simvastatin therapy did not result in additional cardiovascular risk reduction in the action to control cardiovascular risk in diabetes (ACCORD) trial, although a subgroup analysis did suggest those with elevated triglycerides and low HDL-C levels experienced greater risk reduction.[9] It should be noted, however, that high-dose statin therapy reduces cardiovascular risk compared to moderate dose statin therapy regardless of the type of lipid disorder present.[10] Two ongoing clinical trials are evaluating the additive benefit of extended-release niacin to background statin therapy. Until clinical trial data are available, it is just as likely that the residual lipid abnormalities present in the inflammatory state of insulin resistance and obesity are just as likely to be markers, rather than causes, of increased cardiovascular risk.

BILE ACID SEQUESTRANTS

Bile acid sequestrants interrupt the enterohepatic recirculation of cholesterol-rich bile acids by irreversibly binding them in the intestinal lumen (Fig. 1). Bile acid sequestrants are not systemically absorbed. Cholestyramine and colestipol modestly decrease CHD risk in long-term clinical trials, as would be expected from their modest effect on LDL-C. No long-term clinical outcomes data are available for colesevelam.

EFFICACY

As monotherapy, bile acid sequestrants at the recommended dosage [colestipol 2 scoops (6 gr), cholestyramine 2 scoops (8 gr) or colesevelam 6 tabs or suspension (3.75 gr)] will lower LDL-C by about 15% and non-HDL-C by about 10%.[11] Bile acid sequestrants increase triglycerides on average by 15–30% and the largest triglyceride increases occur in patients with more severe hypertriglyceridemia. Bile acid sequestrants are contraindicated in those with triglyceride levels more than 400 mg/dL and should be used with caution when triglycerides are 200–400 mg/dL. Colesevelam has been shown to reduce hemoglobin A_{1C} levels by about 0.5% in diabetics with inadequate glycemic control, with greater benefit in those with hemoglobin A_{1C} levels more than 8.0%.[12] Notably, average triglyceride levels were less than 200 mg/dL in these studies.

SAFETY

Adverse intestinal effects, such as bloating, constipation and bowel obstruction, limit their use, although these effects are less common with colesevelam.[13] Colestipol and cholestyramine decrease the absorption of anionic drugs and vitamins (vitamins A, D and K, and folic acid) and should be administered 1 hour after or 4 hours before estrogen, progestin, warfarin, digoxin, thyroxine, phenobarbitol, propranolol, thiazide diuretics, tetracycline, vancomycin, penicillin G, niacin or ezetimibe. Colesevelam has much higher specificity for bile acids than the other sequestrants and does not interfere with the absorption of warfarin, digoxin or several other anionic drugs.

EZETIMIBE

Ezetimibe also acts in the intestine. Ezetimibe selectively inhibits uptake of cholesterol by blocking Niemann-Pick C1-Like 1 receptor, a critical mediator of cholesterol absorption, at the brush border of the small intestine (Fig. 1). By reducing cholesterol absorption from bile acids and diet, ezetimibe reduces intracellular cholesterol levels which in turn up-regulates LDL receptors to lower plasma cholesterol levels. Statins and bile acid sequestrants act similarly through this final cholesterol-lowering pathway. Ezetimibe and its active metabolites undergo extensive enterohepatic recirculation limiting systemic exposure. Ezetimibe has no effect on the metabolism of statins, fibrates, warfarin or a number of other drugs studied. Combination of ezetimibe with cyclosporine increases the blood concentrations of both drugs.

EFFICACY

As monotherapy, ezetimibe lowers LDL-C and non-HDL-C by about 20%. When used with a statin, ezetimibe lowers LDL-C by 15–20% with a lesser effect on non-HDL-C (Table 4).[14] A combination of tablet of ezetimibe 10 mg and simvastatin 80 mg lowers LDL-C by about 60%, similar to the highest doses of atorvastatin and rosuvastatin.

SAFETY

Ezetimibe has minimal adverse effects and does not appear to increase the risk of myopathy when used in conjunction with a statin.[13] No dose adjustments are needed in patients with renal or hepatic insufficiency. Statin-ezetimibe combinations cause persistent hepatic ALT elevations greater than 3 times the upper limit of normal at a rate similar to atorvastatin 80 mg. The value of ezetimibe when added to statin therapy for cardiovascular prevention is unclear. Two of three surrogate endpoint trials showed ezetimibe had no additional effect on carotid intimal medial thickness over statin therapy alone, and one long-term endpoint trial demonstrated a less than expected cardiovascular risk reduction benefit from the combination of ezetimibe and simvastatin compared to placebo.[15] Methodologic problems limit conclusions from the surrogate endpoint trials and the aortic stenosis population studies in the clinical endpoint trial may have unique characteristics. Two large outcomes trials better designed to evaluate ezetimibe added to statin therapy are ongoing. Until data are available from these trials, ezetimibe can still be considered an option if LDL-C and non-HDL-C goals have not been met on maximal statin therapy, or in the statin intolerant patient.

NIACIN

Niacin can improve all lipid parameters, although effects are highly variable between patients. Therefore, niacin should only be continued in those experiencing a significant therapeutic response in the targeted lipid parameter(s) until clinical trial data are available regarding its cardiovascular risk reduction benefits added to a statin. Not all of niacin's mechanisms of action have been elucidated. Niacin lowers LDL-C and VLDL-C by decreasing apolipoprotein B synthesis. Triglyceride reductions result from partial inhibition of fatty acid release from adipose tissue, leading to decreased hepatic triglyceride synthesis, as well as through increased lipoprotein lipase activity which increases the rate of chylomicron triglyceride removal from plasma (Fig. 1). Niacin-induced increases in HDL-C levels are likely related to decreased triglyceride levels, and may result from decreased hepatic uptake and catabolism of HDL-C. Niacin undergoes extensive first pass metabolism in the liver, through enzymatic pathways separate from those metabolizing statins, and is rapidly excreted in urine. Niacin has few important drug interactions although it is extensively bound to cholestyramine.

In the Coronary Drug Project trial, niacin reduced the risk of coronary heart disease by 17% over a period of approximately 6 years. This is about the risk reduction expected from a 15% reduction in LDL-C and non-HDL-C from the average 2 gm of niacin used in this trial.[5,16] Six trials of niacin used in combination with a colestipol or a statin have demonstrated a benefit on coronary or carotid atherosclerotic plaque.[17,18] Two of these very small trials reported a significant reduction in cardiovascular events. A trial is underway to evaluate whether niacin-induced HDL-C increases and triglyceride reductions further reduce cardiovascular events over LDL-C lowering. Another trial is evaluating the incremental cardiovascular benefit of adding niacin combined with laropriprant, described below, to background statin therapy.

EFFICACY

One gram of niacin will raise HDL-C by 15% and lower triglycerides by 25%, but has little effect on LDL-C or non-HDL-C levels. At the 2 gm dose, niacin will lower LDL-C by about 15%, and further increase HDL-C (+ 25%) and lower triglycerides (- 30%). Niacin 2 gm will also lower lipoprotein by about 20%, although it is not known whether this will further reduce cardiovascular risk. When added to a statin, niacin retains the HDL-C raising and non-HDL-C and triglyceride lowering properties for niacin monotherapy, although some attenuation of LDL-C lowering may occur.

Extended-release niacin in doses greater than 2 gm/day are not recommended due to serious concerns about hepatoxicity. Immediate-release, or crystalline, niacin more than 3 gm/day may further lower LDL-C (> 20%), raise HDL-C (> 35%), and lower triglycerides (> 40%). Nicotinamide and inositol hexanicotinate, marketed as "no-flush" niacin, have no lipid effects.

FLUSHING

Immediate-release, or crystalline, niacin may have substantial cutaneous effects, such as flushing and itching, that are reduced with extended-release niacin formulations. Nicotinic acid receptors in the skin release prostaglandin D_2 which results in vasodilatation and histamine release. Tachyphylaxis to these effects develops with consistent dosing over a period of weeks to months. A higher dose of aspirin (325 mg), ibuprofen 200 mg, or another nonsteroidal anti-inflammatory drug (NSAID) taken 30–60 minutes prior to niacin administration can alleviate flushing, redness, itching, rash and dryness.[19] These drugs should be limited to short-term use due to concerns about gastrointestinal and cardiovascular toxicity with long-term NSAID use. Laropriprant, which reduces niacin flushing by blocking prostaglandin D_2 release, is under development.

Niacin adherence may be improved titrating the dose gradually over a period of weeks to months. The starting dose of extended release niacin is 500–1000 mg at bedtime, and for immediate-release niacin is 125–250 mg twice daily. Niacin should be retitrated when switching between brands or forms of niacin or after missing more than three doses. Patients find it helpful to hear a description of niacin flushing symptoms prior to the first use: flushing usually starts 30–120 minutes after ingestion of extended-release niacin, and 15–30 minutes after the ingestion of immediate-release niacin; episodes typically last 5–60 minutes. During a flushing episode, chewing as aspirin or taking diphenhydramine may decrease severity. Flushing rates usually substantially diminish after 4 weeks of extended-release niacin use, and rarely occur after 1 year of use. Ingestion with a snack or meal slows absorption. Spicy foods, alcohol, hot beverages and hot baths or showers can exacerbate flushing.

SAFETY

Doses of extended-release niacin greater than 2 gm/day are contraindicated due to a very high rate of serious hepatotoxicity, including liver failure, reported with the sustained-release formulation of niacin at 1.5-3 gm/day. Sustained-release niacin, which is available over the counter, should be avoided, especially in doses of more than 1.5 gm daily. In contrast, immediate-release niacin appears to have no significant hepatotoxcity in doses up to 3 gm/day. Rates of persistent hepatic transaminase elevations with extended-release niacin-statin combinations appear to be similar to that of moderate-dose statins (< 1%).

No evidence of serious hepatoxicity has been reported to date for extended-release niacin used with moderate dose statins. Few data are available for extended release niacin used with the highest doses of statin, or the long-term safety of higher doses of immediate-release niacin used concomitantly with a statin.

Serum ALT should be monitored every 6–12 weeks during the first 6–12 months of niacin treatment, and every 6 months thereafter. Niacin should be discontinued if hepatic transaminase levels are persistently more than 3 times the upper limit of normal, bilirubin is more than 3 mg/dL, prothrombin time is elevated, or symptoms of nausea, vomiting or malaise are present. Niacin rechallenge should be undertaken only with careful monitoring, if at all.

Rhabdomyolysis has not been reported for niacin mono-therapy and has been rarely reported with niacin used in combination with a statin. Although few patients have been studied in long-term clinical trials, the myopathy rate of niacin combined with a statin appears to be similar to that of a statin alone. The exception is for patients of Chinese descent who are significantly increased risk of myopathy when niacin more than or equal to 1 gm is used concomitantly with simvastatin more than or equal to 40 mg.[8] In patients of Chinese descent, simvastatin 80 mg should not be used with niacin.

Niacin may worsen insulin resistance and cause diabetes, especially in those with impaired fasting glucose or abnormal glucose tolerance. Fasting glucose levels should be monitored after each dose titration and annually thereafter. Although niacin reduces cardiovascular events in patients with diabetes, diabetic therapy may need intensification to maintain patients at their hemoglobin A_{1c} goals.

Uncommon adverse effects of niacin include intermittent atrial fibrillation, exacerbation of gout (consider allopurinol if a history of gout and serum uric acid levels exceed 10 mg/dL), hyperpigmentation of skin-fold areas (acanthosis nigricans), upper gastrointestinal bleeding (niacin is contraindicated in patients with active peptic ulcer disease), mildly decreased platelet counts, and rarely blurred vision (cystoid macular degeneration reported with niacin > 3 grams).

TRIGLYCERIDE-LOWERING THERAPY

Triglycerides are not a target of therapy for cardiovascular risk reduction. Although those with triglyceride levels more than 150 mg/dL are at increased cardiovascular risk, adjustment for low HDL-C levels and insulin resistance eliminates the majority of the risk associated with elevated triglycerides. Nor are triglyceride changes from drug therapy associated with reduced cardiovascular risk.[3] In those with severe hypertriglyceridemia (> 500 mg/dL), triglycerides are the target of therapy to prevent pancreatitis.

Patients should fast for at least 8 hours prior to obtaining the blood sample for triglyceride measurement. Secondary causes of hypertriglyceridemia should be evaluated in all patients. Particular attention should be paid to detecting undiagnosed or poorly controlled diabetes or hypothyroidism. Once these conditions are adequately treated, triglyceride levels usually fall to less than 500 mg/dL.

All patients should see a dietitian for counseling on a diet very low in fat (< 15%) and refined carbohydrates, and obese patients should be counseled to lose weight. When triglycerides are more than 1000 mg/dL, a triglyceride-lowering drug is usually started simultaneously with diet and lifestyle changes. Fibrates are considered first-line therapy and lower triglycerides by 20–50%. Higher doses of niacin, omega-3 fish oil and statins also lower triglycerides. Bile acid sequestrants are absolutely contraindicated in severely hypertriglyceridemic patients since they can markedly exacerbate hyper-triglyceridemia. Ezetimibe has only modest triglyceride-lowering effects. Once triglyceride less than 500 mg/dL are achieved, attention should then turn to treating LDL-C and non-HDL-C to reduce cardiovascular risk.

Fibrates are nuclear peroxisome proliferator-activated (PPAR) receptor-α agonists that upregulate the gene for lipoprotein lipase and downregulate the gene for apolipoprotein C-III, an inhibitor of lipoprotein lipase. Lipoprotein lipase increases triglyceride hydrolysis (which decreases VLDL-C secretion) and increases catabolism of triglyceride-rich particles (Fig. 1). Fibrates modestly raise HDL-C by lowering triglycerides and by increasing synthesis of apolipoproteins A-I and A-II. Fibrates variably influence LDL-C levels depending on the type of dyslipidemia and which fibrate is used.

Gemfibrozil undergoes glucuronidation in the liver and is 70% renally excreted. Gemfibrozil potently inhibits glucuroni-dation of other drugs, including all statins. Fenofibrate is also metabolized via glucuronidation and is primarily renally excreted. However, fenofibrate and fenofibric acid, its active metabolite, are much less potent inhibitors of glucuronidation than gemfibrozil, and have little effect on statin levels. Fibrates may substantially increase prothrombin time and international normalized ratios in patients receiving warfarin. Warfarin dose may need to be decreased by 25–35%.

Fenofibrate very modestly reduces cardiovascular risk to the degree expected from the magnitude of its modest LDL-C and non-HDL-C changes.[9,16] Conversely, gemfibrozil reduces cardiovascular risk more than expected from the minimal changes observed in LDL-C and non-HDL-C. The risk reduction with gemfibrozil is independent of triglyceride changes and has been largely attributable to the use of gemfibrozil itself.[20]

EFFICACY

Lipid effects may vary substantially depending on the type and severity of the dyslipidemia present. As monotherapy, fenofibrate is slightly more effective than gemfibrozil for lowering LDL-C (11% vs 1%, respectively) and non-HDL-C (18% vs 13%), although both may increase LDL-C levels in hypertriglyceridemic patients.[21] Both drugs lower triglycerides by about 45% and raise HDL-C by about 10%.

SAFETY

Fibrates increase the risk of myopathy, abnormal transaminase levels, and creatinine elevations.[22] Fibrate monotherapy increases the risk of myopathy five-fold (number needed to harm 3500) over statins alone. The risk for gemfibrozil is two-fold higher than for fenofibrate. When used with a statin, gemfibrozil has a 33-fold higher risk of myopathy than fenofibrate, in part due to greater inhibition of glucuronidation. Gemfibrozil increases blood levels of all statins, with a lesser impact on fluvastatin. Fenofibrate appears to have little impact on statin blood levels, and so is the drug of choice for combination with low-to-moderate dose statins. Fenofibrate has not been evaluated with the highest doses of statins. Although fenofibrate-statin combinations have acceptable muscle safety, it should be noted their value has not yet been demonstrated in clinical outcomes trials.

In patients at increased risk for myopathy, the potential benefits of fibrates should be carefully weighed against their risks, especially in combination with a statin. Myopathy risk characteristics include advancing age, female sex, renal or hepatic dysfunction, hypothyroidism, debilitation, surgery, trauma, excessive alcohol intake or heavy exercise. Extensive patient education and regular creatine kinase monitoring should be considered in such cases. For severely hypertriglyceridemic patients for whom the safety of fibrates is a concern, high doses of marine omega-3 fatty acids (> 3 gm) should be strongly considered.

Rises in creatinine levels can occur in patients taking fenofibrate, although the clinical significance of this is unclear. Fenofibrate often improves proteinuria with long-term use, and no cases of renal failure have been reported. However, the dose of fenofibrate should be reduced if creatinine rises above the normal range, and the patient carefully monitoring for adverse effects. Fenofibrate dose should be reduced in patients with glomerular filtration rates less than 60 ml/min/1.73 m^2, and fenofibrate completely avoided when it is less than 15 ml/min/1.73 m^2. Fenofibrate is nondialyzable and must be avoided in dialysis and renal transplant patients. A reduced dose of gemfibrozil can be used in these patients. Gemfibrozil also has significant renal excretion and concomitant use with statins with renal clearance should be avoided. The maximum dose for elderly patients is one-third of the full dose of fenofibrate.

Although gemfibrozil more frequently increases hepatic transaminase levels than fenofibrate, the rates of hepatic and total adverse events are lower for gemfibrozil than fenofibrate. Both fibrates are contraindicated in the setting of severe liver disease. Fibrates predispose to gallstones but are only contraindicated in untreated gallbladder disease. Increased risk of deep vein thrombosis and pulmonary embolism has been observed in some fibrate trials, but no increase was observed when fenofibrate was added to simvastatin in the ACCORD trial.[9] Unlike the earlier fenofibrate intervention and event lowering in diabetes (FIELD) trial of fenofibrate monotherapy,[23] no increase in coronary mortality was noted in ACCORD.

OMEGA-3 FATTY ACIDS

The omega-3 fatty acids eicosopentanoic acid (EPA) and docohexanoic acid (DHA) in doses more than 3 gm daily can lower triglyceride levels about as much as a fibrate.[24] EPA and DHA come from marine sources (fish and seaweed) and are the only omega-3 fatty acids that lower triglycerides. α-linolenic acid is an omega-3 fatty acid derived from land-based plant sources is minimally converted to EPA and DHA and has minimal lipid effects.

EPA and DHA, including intake from fatty fish once or twice a week, have been shown to reduce the risk of coronary death, although the mechanisms through which this occur is unclear.[25] Triglyceride-lowering *per se* does not appear to reduce cardiovascular risk in studies to date.[3] The mechanisms through which omega-3 fatty acids lower triglycerides have not been fully elucidated, but the ultimate result is a reduced rate of VLDL-triglyceride secretion (Fig. 1). EPA and DHA are rapidly absorbed with a long half-life due to extensive incorporation into cell membranes. Omega-3 fatty acids have no effects on cytochrome P450 metabolism and no apparent drug interactions.

EFFICACY

A 3–4 gm dose of EPA/DHA is needed to lower triglycerides by 30–45%. Very concentrated fish oil is available over-the-counter or by prescription (four 1 gm capsules = 3.4 gm EPA + DHA). Care must be taken with over-the-counter preparations to ensure they are highly purified and free of significant contamination.

SAFETY

The most common adverse effects of omega-3 fish oil are fishy eructation, nausea and intestinal complaints. Pharmaceutical grade fish oil is highly refined and has fewer adverse gastrointestinal effects. Environmental toxins such as mercury, dioxins, polychlorinated biphenyls, may be present in fish oil and oily fish, and premenopausal women and children should limit consumption. Doses of omega-3 fatty acids less than 6 gm daily do not increase glucose levels or the risk of bleeding with aspirin or anticoagulants.

DRUGS IN DEVELOPMENT

Several drugs with novel mechanisms influencing the metabolism of LDL-C, VLDL-C and HDL-C are in development.[26] Several at-risk populations may benefit from LDL-C and non-HDL-C lowering agents, including those who are intolerant of statins, those with familial hypercholesterolemia or other forms of severe hyperlipidemia, and those needing additional lipid modification to reach their treatment targets. Although low HDL-C levels are a marker for increase risk, it remains to be determined whether raising HDL-C pharmacologically will reduce cardiovascular events. The long-term safety of these new agents will need to be established, and clinical trials evaluating their additive benefit over current evidence-based therapies will likely be required before they are approved for clinical use.

ACKNOWLEDGMENT

Jennifer G Robinson, MD, MPH has received research grants in the past year from Abbott, Bristol-Myers Squibb, Daiichi-Sankyo, Glaxo-Smith Kline, Hoffman la Roche, Merck, Merck Schering Plough, and the National Institutes of Health.

REFERENCES

1. National Cholesterol Education Panel. Third Report of the National Cholesterol Education Program (NCEP) Expert Panel on Detection, Evaluation, and Treatment of High Blood Cholesterol in Adults (Adult Treatment Panel III) Final Report. Circulation. 2002;106:3143-421.
2. Robinson JG. Are you targeting non-high-density lipoprotein cholesterol? J Am Coll Cardiol. 2009;55:42-4.
3. Briel M, Ferreira-Gonzalez I, You JJ, et al. Association between change in high density lipoprotein cholesterol and cardiovascular disease morbidity and mortality: systematic review and meta-regression analysis. BMJ. 2009;338 (Feb 16_1):b92.
4. Grundy SM, Cleeman JI, Merz CNB, et al. Implications of recent clinical trials for the National Cholesterol Education Program Adult Treatment Panel III guidelines. Circulation. 2004;110:227-39.

5. Robinson JG, Smith B, Maheshwari N, et al. Pleiotropic effects of statins: benefit beyond cholesterol reduction? A meta-regression analysis J Am Coll Cardiol. 2005;46:1855-62.

6. Vandenberg B, Robinson J. Management of the patient with statin intolerance. Curr Atheroscler Rep. 2010;12:48-57.

7. Davidson M, Robinson JG. Safety of aggressive lipid management. J Am Coll Cardiol. 2007;49:1753-62.

8. US Food and Drug Administration. FDA Drug Safety Communication: ongoing safety review of high-dose Zocor (simvastatin) and increased risk of muscle injury. March 19, 2010; http://www.fda.gov/Drugs/DrugSafety/PostmarketDrugSafety InformationforPatientsand Providers/ucm204882.htm Accessed June 2010.

9. The Accord Study Group. Effects of Combination Lipid Therapy in Type 2 Diabetes Mellitus. N Engl J Med. 2010: NEJMoa1001282.

10. Cannon CP, Steinberg BA, Murphy SA, et al. Meta-analysis of cardiovascular outcomes trials comparing intensive versus moderate statin therapy. J Am Coll Cardiol. 2006;48:438-45.

11. Ijioma N, Robinson J. Current and emerging therapies in hypercholesterolemia: focus on colesevelam. Clin Med Rev Vasc Health. 2010;2:21-40.

12. Manghat P, Wierzbicki AS. Colesevelam hydrochloride: a specifically engineered bile acid sequestrant. Fut Lipidol. 2008;3:237-55.

13. Jacobson TA, Armani A, McKenney JM, et al. Safety considerations with gastrointestinally active lipid-lowering drugs. Am J Cardiol. 2007;99:S47-S55.

14. Robinson J, Davidson M. Combination therapy with ezetimibe and simvastatin to acheive aggressive LDL reduction. Expert Rev Cardiovasc Ther. 2006;4:461-76.

15. Howard W. The role of ezetimibe in the prevention of cardiovascular disease: where do we stand after ARBITER-6 HALTS. Nutr Metab Cardivoasc Dis. 2010;20:295-300.

16. Robinson JG, Wang S, Smith BJ, et al. Meta-analysis of the relationship between non-high-density lipoprotein cholesterol reduction and coronary heart disease risk. J Am Coll Cardiol. 2009;53:316-22.

17. Bruckert E, Labreuche J, Amarenco P. Meta-analysis of the effect of nicotinic acid alone or in combination on cardiovascular events and atherosclerosis. Atherosclerosis. 2010;210:353-61.

18. Taylor AJ, Villines TC, Stanek EJ, et al. Extended-release niacin or ezetimibe and carotid intima-media thickness. N Engl J Med. 2009;361:2113-22.

19. Guyton JR, Bays HE. Safety considerations with niacin therapy. Am J Cardiol. 2007;99:S22-S31.

20. Robinson JG. Should we use PPAR agonists to reduce cardiovascular risk? PPAR Res. 2008: doi:10.1155/2008/891425.

21. Birjmohun RS, Hutten BA, Kastelein JJP, et al. Efficacy and safety of high-density lipoprotein cholesterol-increasing compounds: a meta-analysis of randomized controlled trials. J Am Coll Cardiol. 2005;45:185-97.

22. Davidson MH, Armani A, McKenney JM, et al. Safety considerations with fibrate therapy. Am J Cardiol. 2007;99:S3-S18.

23. The FIELD study investigators. Effects of long-term fenofibrate therapy on cardiovascular events in 9795 people with type 2 diabetes mellitus (the FIELD study): randomised controlled trial. Lancet. 2005;366:1849-61.

24. Robinson JG, Stone NJ. Antiatherosclerotic and antithrombotic effects of omega-3 fatty acids. Am J Cardiol. 2006;98(4, Suppl. 1):39-49.

25. Leon H, Shibata MC, Sivakumaran S, et al. Effect of fish oil on arrhythmias and mortality: systematic review. BMJ. 2008;337 (Dec23_2):a2931.

26. Stein EA. Other therapies for reducing low-density lipoprotein cholesterol: medications in development. Endocrinol Metab Clin N Amer. 2009;38:99-119.

27. Jones PH, Davidson MH, Stein EA, et al. Comparison of the efficacy and safety of rosuvastatin versus atorvastatin, simvastatin, and pravastatin across doses (STELLAR Trial). Am J Cardiol. 2003;92:152-60.

28. Robinson J. Management of complex lipid abnormalities with a fixed dose combination of simvastatin and extended release niacin. Vasc Health Risk Man. 2009;5:31-43.

29. Bristol Myers Squibb Co. Pravachol (pravastatin sodium) [prescribing information]. March 2007; http://packageinserts. bms.com/pi/pi_pravachol.pdf Accessed May 2009.

30. Novartis Pharmaceuticals. Lescol (fluvastatin sodium) [prescribing information]. October 2006; http://www.pharma.us. novartis.com/product/pi/pdf/Lescol.pdf Accessed May 2009.

31. Jones PH, Davidson MH, Kashyap ML, et al. Efficacy and safety of ABT-335 (fenofibric acid) in combination with rosuvastatin in patients with mixed dyslipidemia: a phase 3 study. Atherosclerosis. 2009;204:208-15.

32. Abbott Laboratories. Advicor (extended-release niacin) [prescribing information]. February 2010; http://www.rxabbott.com/pdf/advicor.pdf Accessed June 2010.

33. Kowa Pharmaceuticals. Livalo (pitivastatin) prescribing information. 7/30/09; http://cardiobrief.files.wordpress. com/2009/08/pitavastatinapfinal080309.pdf

34. Robinson JG. Pharmacologic treatment of dyslipidemia and cardiovascular disease. In: Kwiterovich P (Ed). The Johns Hopkins Textbook of Dyslipidemia. Phildelphia: Wolters Kluwer;2010. pp. 266-76.

35. Chan DC, Nguyen MN, Watts GF, et al. Effects of atorvastatin and n-3 fatty acid supplementation on VLDL apolipoprotein C-III kinetics in men with abdominal obesity. Am J Clin Nutr. 2010;91:900-6.

36. Bays H, McKenney J, Maki K, et al. Effects of prescription omega-3-Acid ethyl esters on non-high-density lipoprotein cholesterol when coadministered with escalating doses of atorvastatin. Mayo Clin Proc. 2010;85:122-8.

Chapter 8

Antithrombotic and Antiplatelet Agents

Louis P Kohl, Ethan Weiss

Chapter Outline

INTRODUCTION

Arterial and venous thromboses are a major cause of death and disability worldwide. A majority of myocardial infarctions (MI) and cerebrovascular accidents (CVA) are caused by unregulated arterial thrombosis after rupture of an atherosclerotic plaque. Venous thromboembolism (VTE)—deep vein thrombosis (DVT) and pulmonary embolism (PE)—and embolic stroke secondary to atrial fibrillation (AF) are the result of pathologic venous clot. As prevention and treatment of these entities are fundamental to the discipline, anticoagulants are an elemental component of the cardiologist's armamentarium. Warfarin, heparin and aspirin have been the standards of antithrombotic and antiplatelet therapeutics, but in the past 15 years low molecular weight heparins (LMWH) and the platelet ADP receptor antagonist clopidogrel have markedly altered the standards of treatment. A new wave of antithrombotic and antiplatelet drugs have been developed that, if approved, may similarly alter the standards of care. In this chapter, we have focused on the mechanisms and potential applications of these new agents, contrasting with the current standards.

CLOTTING, A PRIMER

Prior to discussing individual agents, a brief update on thrombosis: the classic, waterfall cascade, as described by Davie and Ratnoff in 1964,[1] served as a useful basis for understanding the mechanisms underlying clotting (Fig. 1). The addition of an "extrinsic" pathway, triggered by tissue factor (TF) activation of factor VII after endothelial injury, and recognition of factors V and VIII as cofactors transformed the linear cascade into a Y. This new schema placed factor Xa (fXa) in a central position as the first, integrative step of a common pathway. Conveniently, the activated partial thromboplastin time (aPTT) and prothrombin time (PT) are well suited to interrogate for gross abnormalities in the enzymes constituting the intrinsic and extrinsic portions of the cascade. This new formulation has provided an intuitive framework that allows medical students and non-specialist physicians to understand clotting disorders and apply antithrombotic and antiplatelet drugs rationally.

Subsequent research has revealed additional components of the clotting system and highlighted the importance of feedback and inhibition (Fig. 2). Two developments deserve specific mention: First, thrombin has been recognized as an integrating

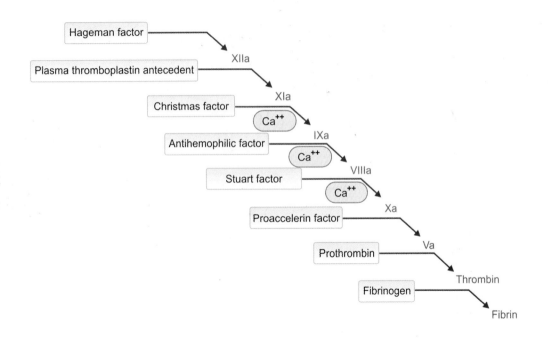

FIGURE 1: Classic waterfall cascade: initially conceived as a linear series of reactions in which each enzyme activated the next to produce fibrin. Original enzyme names are denoted in black with conversion to active enzyme in red using current nomenclature. Although TF and factor VII were not recognized as part of the original clotting cascade, it depicted the sequence of reactions of the intrinsic pathway quite accurately

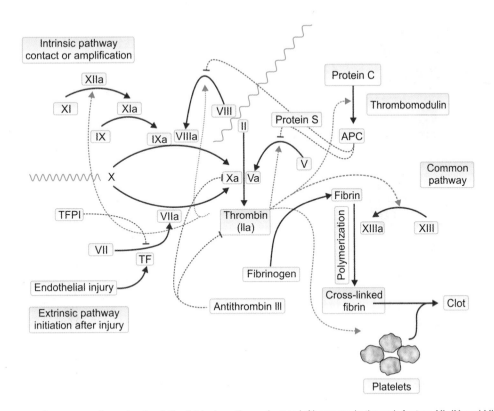

FIGURE 2: Clotting cascade as currently understood: the intrinsic pathway (upper left) proceeds through factors XI, IX and VIII to activation of fX. Activation of fXI can occur through fXIIa, as occurs after addition of a negatively charged trigger in the aPTT, or through thrombin feedback. After endothelial injury, exposed tissue factor complexes with and activates fVII via the extrinsic pathway, which activates fX in turn. The common pathway integrates procoagulant signal and leads to conversion of fibrinogen to fibrin by thrombin. Thrombin and fXa, the two principal anticoagulant targets, are components of the common pathway. *Legend*: Inactive pro-enzymes are gray. Active enzymes are black and denoted with an a. Black arrows signify activation reactions. Molecules astride the arrows are activating protases. Enzymes depicted in smaller type act as cofactors for coagulation proteases. Green, dotted arrows signify action by thrombin as an activating enzyme. Antithrombotic molecules are written in red and their sites of action are denoted by red dotted lines

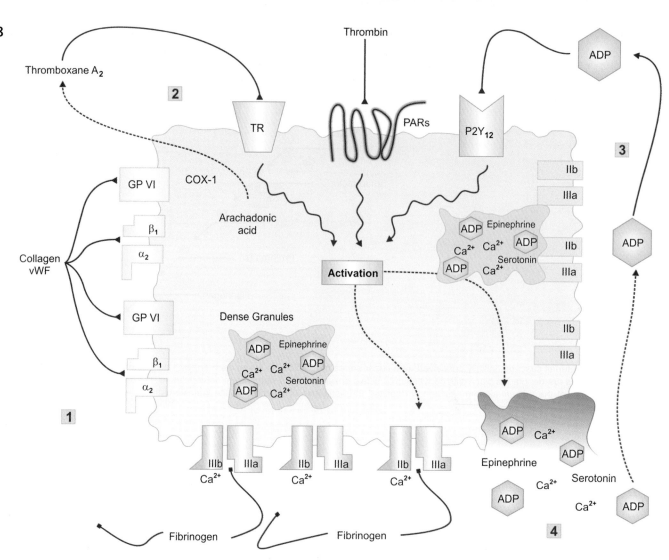

FIGURE 3: Mechanisms of platelet activation: proceeding clockwise, the first step in activation is adhesion (1). After injury, exposed components of the extracellular matrix and subendothelium, such as collagen and vWF, bind to GPVI and integrin $\alpha_2\beta_1$ on the platelet surface. Binding arrests platelet movement at sites of injury and begins the sequence of platelet activation through intracellular signal transduction. Platelet activation and recruitment occur through several signaling pathways. The three major pathways are depicted here (2). Thromboxane A_2, generated from arachidonic acid by COX-1, signals through the thromboxane receptor (TR). The ADP, released from platelets, signals through the $P2Y_{12}$ receptor. Thrombin cleaves the PAR-1 and PAR-4 receptors, leading to intracellular signaling. Of the three, thrombin is the most powerful activating agent. *Activation* (3) occurs through a number of intracellular pathways in response to thrombin, TxA_2 or ADP signaling. As a result, dense granules are released and conformational changes of GP IIb/IIIa occur, making them highly avid for fibrinogen. Other cellular changes, including platelet flattening and exposure of negatively charged phospholipids, also result. The final step is *aggregation* (4). Divalent fibrinogen molecules bind to the GP IIb/IIIa receptors of adjacent platelets. Given the high density of this receptor on the platelet surface, adjacent platelets become multiply interconnected, forming a platelet plug[3]

enzyme in the coagulation pathway. In addition to its principal role converting fibrinogen to fibrin, it forms positive feedback loops to the intrinsic arm of the clotting cascade, activating factors V, VIII and XI (as well as XIII). Rather than an orphan arm of the clotting cascade, the intrinsic pathway is now viewed as the site of feedback amplification in thrombosis—after initiation via the quickly inhibited extrinsic pathway—and a promising target for future anticoagulants.[2] Understanding of the central role played by thrombin has lead to the development of new direct thrombin inhibitors (DTI) that show promise in treating venous and arterial thrombi. The second development is discovery of multiple platelet signaling pathways. The recognition of additional activating pathways—unaffected by aspirin—has lead to the development of new antiplatelet agents that are essential for treatment of arterial thrombi.

Arterial and venous thrombi are composed of identical components; platelet aggregates, fibrin and jailed red cells, but the relative proportions in each are distinct.

Arterial thrombi are composed primarily of platelet aggregates and fibrin, in contrast to platelet-poor venous thrombi. Under the high-shear conditions of the arterial circulation, platelets serve as the stable foundation for clot propagation (Fig. 3). Platelet movement is arrested at sites of injury by adherence of constitutively expressed platelet receptors GPVI, GPIb and $\alpha_2\beta_1$ to newly exposed, subendothelial von Willebrand Factor (vWF) and collagen. Receptor binding initiates platelet activation. Adherent platelets release dense granules that contain ADP and ionized Ca, synthesize and release thromboxane A_2 (TXA_2). The adherent platelet also alters its conformation, flattening against the damaged vessel wall to provide a phospholipid and Ca^{2+} rich surface on which the clotting cascade can function efficiently. Via their respective receptors, ADP, TXA_2 and thrombin activate and recruit additional platelets at the site of injury. In activated platelets, conformational change of the abundant cell-surface receptor GPIIb/IIIa markedly increases its affinity for fibrinogen.[4] The plug is reinforced as fibrinogen molecules, produced via the clotting cascade, cross-link platelets.

ANTITHROMBOTIC AGENTS

THE HEPARINS AND INDIRECT Xa INHIBITORS

Unfractionated heparin (UFH) is the prototype intravenous anticoagulant. Derived from porcine intestinal mucosa, UFH is a polysaccharide with average molecular weight of 15 kDa. A specific pentasaccharide sequence within this polymer binds to antithrombin III (AT), inducing a conformational change that allows direct and potent fXa inhibition. The AT-heparin complex also inhibits thrombin. The UFH does not enhance AT inhibition of thrombin, but rather serves as a physical bridge, approximating the two molecules. A heparin must have 18 or more saccharide units (MW ~ 5.4 kDa) to facilitate AT-thrombin interaction. Given the average size of a UFH molecule, the vast majority can inhibit thrombin and fXa (an inhibition ratio of 1:1). Prothrombinase bound Xa or fibrin bound thrombin are relatively inaccessible to the AT-heparin complex due to its large size.[5]

Indications

Unfractionated heparin can be used in any situation in which parenteral anticoagulation is required. UFH is well suited to short-term or high-risk anticoagulation due to its short half-life (1–2 hrs) and potential for reversal with protamine. This salmon sperm derived protein binds avidly to long-chain heparins, forming complexes that are cleared via the kidney, extinguishing its anticoagulant effect. UFH is appropriate for a wide range of situations, including anticoagulation during acute coronary syndrome (ACS), maintenance of anticoagulation for high-risk patients in the perioperative setting and DVT prophylaxis. In many of these situations, heparin has been replaced by LMWH due to ease of administration. There are a small number of indications in which heparin is the current standard of care (bivalirudin, discussed below, may replace UFH for indication 4):

1. Patients with a high bleeding risk with indication for short-term anticoagulation.
2. Patients with renal impairment; as LMWH is cleared by the kidneys, it is contraindicated in patients with CrCl < 30 ml/min. UFH is not dependent on renal excretion.
3. Massive PE or extensive DVT; LMWH was not studied in these populations.
4. PCI; short half-life, ease of point-of-care monitoring with aPTT or activated clotting time (ACT).

5. Cardiopulmonary bypass (CPB) and other extracorporeal circuits due to experience and full reversibility.

Limitations, Monitoring and Adherence

The UFH is extensively bound to plasma proteins (including platelet factor 4 (PF4) and high molecular weight vWF multimers) whose concentrations vary from patient to patient. The effect on individual patients is variable and UFH must be monitored to achieve appropriate anticoagulation. As a strictly parenteral and subcutaneously (SQ) administered anticoagulant, out of hospital uses are rare and monitoring occurs as a part of inpatient care. The aPTT should be tested 4–6 hours after the initiation of therapy. Once the therapeutic aPTT is reached, usually 1.5–2 times reference, UFH can be safely monitored on a daily basis so long as dosing remains constant. The UFH also requires regular monitoring of platelet count due to the risk of heparin-induced thrombocytopenia (HIT, also known as HTTS).

The HIT is a principal adverse effect of UFH given its potential severity. Antibodies against the heparin-PF4 complex cause HIT by activating the cascade of platelet activation described above. The indiscriminate activation of platelets causes an initial drop in platelet count, usually occurring by week two of therapy, and is followed by widespread arterial thrombosis if the condition is not recognized and UFH withdrawn.[6] Other limitations of UFH include a greater risk of subtherapeutic anticoagulation, resulting less efficacious anticoagulation. When compared to LMWH in the treatment of acute VTE, meta-analyses have found increased total morality and risk of patient bleeding.[7] Although a lesser concern, long-term treatment with UFH has been associated with osteoporosis, through a direct inhibitory effect on osteoblasts.

LOW MOLECULAR WEIGHT HEPARINS

Low molecular weight heparins (LMWH) including enoxaparin, dalteparin and nadroparin are commercial preparations produced by controlled depolymerization (shortening) of UFH to an average MW of 5 kDa. Due to its shorter average molecular length, few molecules are able to bridge AT to thrombin. Therefore, LMWH exerts majority of its effect through indirect inhibition of fXa with an anti-Xa/anti-IIa ratio of ~3.8. In contrast to heparin, exclusively renal excretion occurs in a dose-dependent fashion.

Advantages and Indications

The LMWH has high (90%) bioavailability, which translates to predictable plasma levels after SQ administration. The half-life of most LMWH is approximately 4 hours, which allows daily or BID administration. These properties allow weight-based administration without a daily monitoring requirement, a significant convenience and cost advantage. The LMWH is also better suited for long-term therapy, as patients can self-administer SQ injections. Furthermore, when compared to UFH, incidences of HIT and osteoporosis are significantly lower.[8]

Most studies comparing LMWH to UFH have measured asymptomatic venous thrombosis as a primary endpoint, rather than fatal thromboembolism, due to low incidence of the latter.

The LMWH has been found non-inferior to UFH with respect to prevention of DVT in a wide range of clinical settings, with equivalent safety profiles. The LMWH, specifically enoxaparin, has shown equivalency with UFH in ACS. The appropriate use of LMWH in the catheterization lab remains unsettled, due to potential increased bleeding risk, and falls outside the scope of this chapter. A full discussion can be found in other sections of this text. On the strength of these studies, LMWH have the following FDA indications:[9,10]

- Prophylaxis of DVT in patients undergoing abdominal surgery (40 mg SQ daily), total knee replacement or total hip replacement (30 mg SQ BID) and medically ill patients (40 mg SQ daily) with limited mobility.
- Inpatient treatment of acute DVT with or without PE.
- Outpatient treatment of acute DVT without PE.
- Prophylaxis of recurrent ischemia in patients with unstable angina and NSTEMI in conjunction with aspirin.[11]
- Treatment of acute STEMI with thrombolysis in conjunction with aspirin; whether managed medically or subsequent PCI.[12]
- Extended treatment of VTE in patients with cancer (dalteparin).

Despite the lack of US clinical indication, LMWH are used (off-label) for treatment of VTE in pregnancy and for "bridging" during temporary discontinuation of warfarin in patients with prosthetic heart valves who are preparing to undergo a surgical procedure.

Limitations, Monitoring and Adherence

Two important situations exist in which weight-based dosing does not produce levels of anticoagulation; in patients with renal failure (CrCl < 30 ml/min) and individuals more than 100 kg of weight. The LMWH is contraindicated in these situations given the difficulty of monitoring. Unlike UFH, the aPTT does not reflect the level of anticoagulation after administration of LMWH. When monitoring is required, an anti-fXa level is the most accurate measure of anticoagulation, but this test is infrequently available. The LMWH is only partially reversible with protamine (~ 60%); therefore it is relatively contraindicated in settings that may require rapid reversal, such as PCI. Finally, LMWH carries a black box warning due to increased risk of epidural hematoma in patients who are under treatment or will be treated with LMWH. Repeated attempts at spinal puncture, concurrent treatment with other medications affecting hemostasis, including NSAIDs, and indwelling spinal catheters further increase the risk for this complication.

FONDAPARINUX

Fondaparinux is a synthetic analogue of the ATIII binding pentasaccharide sequence found in heparins, producing equivalent fXa inhibition to LMWH. Administered in IV form only, it is 100% bioavailable.

Advantages and Indications

Although theoretic advantages of fondaparinux exist, including more predictable dosing, evidence is lacking that fondaparinux is superior to LMWH. Nevertheless, the drug is broadly approved for treatment of acute DVT, PE[13] and DVT prophylaxis in a manner similar to LMWH. The OASIS-5 study compared outcomes of ACS patients treated with 6 days of either fondaparinux to LMWH. The investigators found fondaparinux non-inferior at 9 days with respect to patient outcomes with fewer bleeding episodes and improved 30 days mortality.[14] Based on these findings, fondaparinux receives a class 1 indication as alternative therapy to either UFH or LMWH in the recent ACCF/AHA Focused Update of the Guidelines for the Management of Patients with Unstable Angina/Non-ST Elevation Myocardial Infarction.[14a] However, guiding catheter thrombosis and other intra-procedural thrombotic effects were increased in patients treated solely with fondaparinux who underwent subsequent PCI.[15] This finding greatly tempered enthusiasm for the drug as a potential UFH replacement in ACS. Recently, the CALISTO trial demonstrated a beneficial effect of fondaparinux 2.5 mg daily (over 45 days) for the treatment of symptomatic superficial thrombophlebitis, when compared to placebo.[16] Fondaparinux has been used for the treatment of HIT, as thrombocytopenia and thrombosis are less likely than with LMWH. In theory, the small molecule is less likely to activate preformed PF4 antibodies, but case reports of HIT after fondaparinux use do exist.[17] Finally, as a synthetic molecule, there is no risk for bacterial contamination, as has occurred with UFH.

Limitations, Monitoring and Adherence

Overall, similar to LMWH, fondaparinux is principally cleared by the kidneys, and is contraindicated in patients with CrCl less than 30. Unlike LMWH, it is contraindicated in patients less than 50 kg, which may exclude a large number of elderly patients and women.

IDRABIOTAPARINUX

Idrabiotaparinux is a hypermethylated fondaparinux derivative with half-life of 130 hours, designed as a once weekly drug. Like fondaparinux, it is primarily excreted via the kidney.[18] Originally developed as idraparinux, the drug was tested as extended therapy for prevention of VTE in patients with acute DVT or PE.[19] In this study, idraparinux 2.5 mg SQ weekly was equivalent to standard therapy (LMWH and warfarin) with less observed bleeding in patients with DVT, but inferior to standard therapy after PE. A study of extended prophylaxis versus placebo (12 months) found reduced thromboembolism but with increased risk of major bleeds, including intracranial hemorrhage (ICH).[20] Subsequently, an open label trial of idraparinux in AF was stopped early given increased major bleeding events, also including ICH.[21] The development of idraparinux was halted due to the increased risk of bleeding, long half-life and irreversibility.

Renamed idrabiotaparinux after addition of a biotin moiety, the compound was now reversible by IV administration of avidin, a protein derived from eggs. Like protamine, avidin binds tightly to idrabiotaparinux, leading to rapid clearance. An initial bioequivalence study found the two molecules equivalent, with respect to clinical outcome, in treatment of acute DVT. Fewer major bleeding episodes were reported in the idrabiotaparinux group.[22] Avidin produced marked (~ 80%) and sustained reduction in anti-Xa levels, a surrogate for effect as a reversal agent. Based on this finding, new studies of idrabiotaparinux are underway in the treatment of PE (CASSIOPEA study; NCT00345618) and AF (BOREALIS-AF; NCT00580216).

AVE5206

AVE5206 is a "hemisyntheic" molecule produced by depolymerization of heparin with an enzyme that selectively spares bonds included in the AT-binding sequence. This ultra low molecular weight heparin has a molecular weight of 2.4 kDa and anti-Xa/IIa ratio of ~ 80.[23] Like fondaparinux, the lower molecular weight and more specific AT binding are thought to produce higher bioavailability by lowering non-specific binding. Initial in vitro comparison to enoxaparin showed greater anti-Xa activity. Equivalent in vivo activity was observed in a rat model of venous thrombosis and canine model of arterial thrombosis. An initial dose finding study in post-total knee replacement patients showed that AVE5026 prevented DVT in a dose-dependent manner. Once daily 20 mg and 40 mg SQ doses were significantly more efficacious than enoxaparin 40 mg SQ daily, which is lower than the FDA-approved dose.[24] The rates of bleeding in these groups were comparable. The performance of this drug in other clinical settings remains untested.

VITAMIN K ANTAGONISTS (VKA)

WARFARIN

Warfarin is the oral anticoagulant against which all newer anticoagulants are measured. Despite its many drawbacks (see below), it has been successfully used to treat a wide range of thrombotic conditions. A significant infrastructure for monitoring now exists and clinicians are comfortable with use of the drug.

Mechanism and Indications

Warfarin sodium is a dicurmarol[25] derivative that blocks addition of g-carboxyglutamic acid (Gla) to factors II, VII, IX, X, protein C and protein S by the vitamin K epoxide reductase (VKOR) enzyme complex. Inhibition of this reaction impairs the final, activating step in hepatic synthesis of these vitamin K-dependent clotting factors (Fig. 4).

The VKA are currently indicated for the treatment of the following conditions:

- Antiphospholipid antibody syndrome (APLAS)
- Primary prevention of stroke or systemic embolism in patients with atrial fibrillation
- Secondary prevention of recurrent CVA
- Secondary CAD prophylaxis after ACS or MI
- Heparin-induced thrombocytopenia (HIT)
- Impaired LV function[26]
- Peripheral arterial occlusive disease
- Prosthetic cardiac valve[27]
- Endocarditis without intra-cerebral abscess[28]
- Protein C deficiency
- Protein S deficiency
- Pulmonary embolism—acute treatment and secondary prophylaxis
- Venous thromboembolism (VTE, including DVT)—acute treatment and secondary prophylaxis

Given the extensive number of indications, a dosing discussion for each is beyond the scope of this chapter and best obtained from disease specific resources, such as AHA/ACC guidelines (e.g. AF, heart failure, valvular heart disease, etc.), ACCP evidence-based clinical practice guidelines (e.g. PE, VTE, etc.)[29] and Micromedex.

Limitations, Monitoring and Adherence

The significant cost and burden of monitoring, numerous drug interactions and a narrow therapeutic window make warfarin therapy challenging for patients and providers. Recent studies have shown that, on average, the typical patient on long-term anticoagulation for AF is within the therapeutic range just over 50% of the time. In specialized anticoagulation clinics, this percentage increases to 63%.[30] This difference has clinical significance, as a 10% improvement of time in therapeutic range (TTR) correlates with a 29% reduction in all-cause mortality.[31,32]

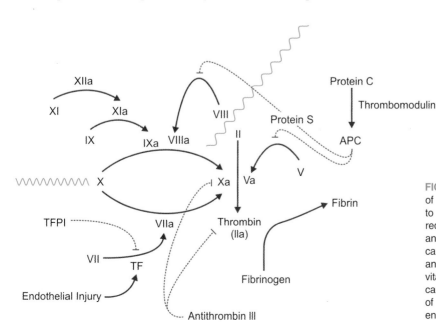

FIGURE 4: Sites of warfarin effect: vitamin K is a cofactor of γ-glutamyl carboxylase, which adds a carboxyl moiety to several proteases of the clotting cascade. Proteases requiring carboxylation are II (prothrombin), VII, IX, X and anticoagulant proteins C and S. Without addition of the carboxyl group, these enzymes are inactive. Warfarin is an inhibitor of vitamin K epoxide reductase (VKOR). If vitamin K remains oxidized through inhibition of VKOR, it cannot function as a cofactor and hepatic carboxylation of these enzymes is decreased. The names of affected enzymes are blurred in the figure

Conversely, elevated INR (especially > 4.0) places patients at risk for bleeding complications.[33] Patient adherence is an additional barrier to successful therapy with VKAs. A significant number of patients (22–33%) newly started on warfarin therapy for AF discontinue treatment by the end of year one. Several factors are associated with poor adherence to warfarin; younger age, males, poverty and homelessness, but also higher educational achievement and employment.[34] The difficulty of maintaining patient adherence and concerns about bleeding complications dissuade many clinicians from initiating warfarin therapy when treatment is indicated.

These reasons have spurred the search for new, oral anticoagulants that will maintain treatment efficacy, improve patient adherence, minimize monitoring and maximize safety. The following sections discuss new therapies that have shown promise as potential replacements for warfarin.

ATI-5923

ATI-5923 also known as tecarfarin, this new VKA also acts as a VKOR and is a structural analogue of warfarin. As such, it can be monitored via the INR. Unlike warfarin, it is a single enantiomer that is highly protein bound and metabolized by carboxyesterases in the liver to a single, inactive metabolite. This single enantiomer is not metabolized by the CYP450, potentially avoiding the many drug-drug interactions that complicate warfarin therapy. A phase IIA study of tecarfarin found that, over a 6–12 period, patients had a TTR exceeding 71%. More impressive, patients were found to be in the extremes on INR (< 1.5 or > 4.0) at a 1.2% rate.[35] The authors of this study argue that this medication may offer the same proven efficacy of warfarin with more predictable patient response and fewer complex drug interactions. Recently, investigators administered tecarfarin and warfarin to healthy volunteers in before and after fluconazole, a potent CYP2C9 and CYP3A4 inhibitor. They found that the serum levels of tecarfarin were unaffected while levels of warfarin increased 213% when given in conjunction with fluconazole.[36] Despite these promising preliminary results, the results of a phase II/III trial in 600 patients with prosthetic heart valves (EmbraceAC) did not demonstrate improved TTR in tecarfarin when compared to warfarin.[37]

DIRECT FACTOR Xa INHIBITORS

The direct fXa inhibitors are a new class of (primarily) orally formulated anticoagulants that have pharmacologic profiles similar to that of LMWH. The promise of this class lies in its potential to replace warfarin for long-term indications without need for routine monitoring or "bridging" during the perioperative period. Early studies indicate that the direct fXa inhibitors may also replace LMWH in some settings such as postoperative DVT prophylaxis.[38] It remains to be seen whether the therapeutic index of these drugs is wide enough to permit use of in a broad range of clinical settings.

RIVAROXABAN

Rivaroxaban, an oral agent, is the prototype drug in this class and was approved by the FDA in late 2011 for prevention of stroke and systemic embolism in persons with atrial fibrillation.

Mechanism

In contrast to the heparins, this new class of inhibitors directly inhibits fXa without involvement of AT III. Direct inhibitors can bind to the prothrombinase complex, not accessible AT III-mediated indirect inhibitors, with resultant reduction in thrombin generation. Rivaroxaban binds to the S1 side pocket of fXa rather than the active site.[39] The small molecule binds rapidly and reversibly, inhibiting fXa in a dose-dependent manner. Rivaroxaban prolongs PT to a greater extent than aPTT, but due to variable interaction with assay reagents these values cannot be used reliably for monitoring. The compound has high oral bioavailability (> 80%), reaches maximum concentration in 2–4 hours with a 7–11 hour terminal half-life. These properties permit daily, weight-based dosing, obviating the need for monitoring in many patients.

Efficacy

The first phase III studies compared oral rivaroxaban to SQ enoxaparin in orthopedic postoperative DVT prophylaxis. The RECORD1 study demonstrated that rivaroxaban treatment for 1 month after THA reduced asymptomatic and major VTE with rates of bleeding equivalent to once daily LMWH, an EU-approved dosing regimen.[40] In the RECORD 4 study, rivaroxaban provided superior protection from VTE when compared to enoxaparin 30 mg SQ BID (FDA approved dose) after TKA.[41] There were trends toward increased bleeding in the rivaroxaban groups, but they did not reach significance. Based on these studies, rivaroxaban is approved in the EU and Canada for VTE prophylaxis after orthopedic surgery at the 10 mg daily dose.[42] Methodological concerns regarding two additional RECORD studies[43,44] and evidence of increased bleeding in rivaroxaban-treated groups, when adjusted for covariates, has led the FDA to delay drug approval.[45]

Phase three studies of rivaroxaban have now been completed. ROCKET AF is the most significant of these trials.[46] In this non-inferiority study, fixed dose oral rivaroxaban (20 mg daily) was compared to adjusted dose warfarin for the prevention of stroke and systemic embolism in patients with non-valvular atrial fibrillation. Over 14,000 patients were enrolled and median follow up was 590 days. The patients included in this study were at high risk of stroke, as evidenced by mean $CHADS_2$ score of 3.5. Rivaroxaban was found to be noninferior to warfarin in the intention-to-treat analysis with significant reductions in intracranial hemorrhage and fatal bleeding. The absolute number of strokes and systemic emboli observed in the rivaroxaban arm was lower than in the warfarin arm, but debate persists regarding the statistical significance of this finding.[47] The EINSTEIN study of rivaroxaban for the treatment of acute symptomatic DVT was reported in late 2010.[48] In the open-label, randomized portion of the non-inferiority study, rivaroxaban (15 mg orally BID for 3 weeks, followed by 20 mg daily) was found to be non-inferior to standard therapy with subcutaneous enoxaparin followed by VKA. In the rivaroxaban treatment arm, there was no increase in the incidence of major bleeding and fewer recurrent DVT were observed. Superiority was reported with respect to recurrent VTE in a randomized, double-blind extension study (versus placebo), but at the expense of increased major and clinically relevant bleeding episodes. The most recently reported phase III trial is ATLAS ACS 2-TIMI 51, a double-blind, placebo controlled evaluation of rivaroxaban for secondary prevention of death from cardiovascular causes, MI or stroke after acute coronary syndrome (ACS).[49] The authors reported a reduction in the primary, composite endpoint in both the 2.5 mg PO BID and 5 mg PO BID treatment arms. When compared to placebo, significantly lower rates of death secondary to cardiovascular causes and significantly lower rates of all-cause death were observed in the 2.5 mg PO BID treatment arm. Significantly higher rates of TIMI major bleeding and ICH were reported in rivaroxaban-treated patients. Finally, the MAGELLAN study of VTE prevention in medically ill patients has been presented in abstract, but has not been published in a peer-reviewed journal at the time of writing.[50]

Limitations, Monitoring and Adherence

Rivaroxaban undergoes hepatic metabolism (via CYP3A4/A5 and CYP2J2) and renal excretion of active and inactive metabolites. Initial studies of rivaroxaban have found minimal interaction with clinically important medications; atorvastatin, ASA and NSAIDs, clopidogrel, ranitidine and digoxin. However, strong inhibitors of CYP3A4 and P-glycoprotein, such as azole antimycotics and protease inhibitors (PI), significantly raise plasma concentrations of rivaroxaban.[34] Due to significant renal excretion, rivaroxaban is contraindicated in patients with creatinine clearance < 30 ml/min, similar to LMWH. Drug levels were unaltered in patients with Child-Pugh A hepatic impairment, but patients with more severe liver disease have not been studied. A weight-based daily dose can be administered to all patients without significant liver or kidney impairment.

APIXABAN

Apixaban is a second direct fXa inhibitor in advanced stages of testing. Like rivaroxaban, the molecule is a selective, reversible fXa inhibitor that reaches maximum plasma concentrations quickly (~ 3 hrs) after administration, and has a prolonged half-life (8–14 hrs). About 50% of absorption occurs after oral administration. The drug is metabolized, predominantly, through non-hepatic pathways with renal excretion a major (~ 30%) route of elimination.[51,52] CYP3A4 mediates hepatic metabolism. Uses of potent inhibitors (azole antifungals, macrolide antibiotics and PI) are contraindicated in conjunction with apixaban.[53] The advantages (oral dosing without routine monitoring) and disadvantages (possible increased bleeding, limitation of use in renal impairment and drug interactions) of apixaban appear similar to those of rivaroxaban.

Efficacy

Its development has followed a trajectory similar to that of rivaroxaban. Dose ranging studies for DVT prophylaxis after orthopedic surgery,[54] DVT treatment[55] and ACS[56] demonstrated prevention of thrombosis efficacy and acceptable safety profile. An initial comparison of apixaban (2.5 mg PO BID) to enoxaparin (30 mg SQ BID) after TKA did not demonstrate non-inferiority due to an unexpectedly low event rate.[57]

Nevertheless, less bleeding was observed in the apixaban group and the drugs' safety profiles were comparable. A follow-up, post-TKA study in comparison to enoxaparin 40 mg SQ daily over 10–14 days, demonstrated a significant decrease in rate of VTE without an increase in bleeding.[58] Ongoing trials will compare apixaban to enoxaparin in post-THA (ADVANCE-3; NCT00423319), prevention of VTE in patients with metastatic cancer (NCT00320255) and medically ill patients (ADOPT; NCT00457002).

Two phase III stroke prevention studies with apixaban have recently been reported. The first, AVERROES, compared apixaban 5 mg twice daily with aspirin for stroke prevention in patients with atrial fibrillation in whom warfarin therapy was "unsuitable".[59] The rate of stroke or systemic embolism in patients treated with apixaban was significantly reduced when compared to patients treated with ASA (relative risk 0.45). The rates of major bleeding and intracranial hemorrhage were not increased in the apixaban treatment arm. A decreased rate of all-cause death (non-significant) was observed in the apixaban treatment arm. This result was not surprising in light of the well established superiority of therapeutic anticoagulation, in comparison to aspirin, in patients with atrial fibrillation and elevated risk of stroke. The subsequent ARISTOTLE study compared apixaban 5 mg twice daily to warfarin in patients with atrial fibrillation.[60] The mean stroke risk of the large study population (CHADS2 2.1) was lower than that of ROCKET AF. Apixaban was superior to warfarin in the prevention of stroke and systemic embolism with rates of major bleeding that were significantly decreased. Additionally, the rates of death from any cause were significantly decreased in the apixaban treatment arm. A placebo-controlled trial of apixaban for secondary prevention of recurrent ischemic events after ACS did not show a reduction of events and was associated with an increase in of major bleeding.[61]

Finally, studies of acute DVT treatment (AMPLIFY and AMPLIFY-EXT; NCT00633893 and NCT00643201, respectively) are underway.

Several other direct fXa inhibitors are in various stages of development. Below are brief summaries of three:

- Edoxaban (DU-176b) has reached late-stage testing in a number of clinical settings. Phase II studies showed efficacy in TKA, THA (v. dalteparin) and AF.[62] In the ENGAGE-AF TIMI 48 trial (NCT00781391), two doses of edoxaban will be compared to standard warfarin therapy for stroke prevention in AF. Phase III trials of DVT prophylaxis after THA, TKA, hip fracture and acute treatment of symptomatic DVT/PE are underway.

- Betrixaban is at an earlier stage of development, but has shown efficacy in prevention of DVT after TKA.[63] Extrarenal clearance sets betrixaban apart from other drugs in the class. A preliminary study in patients with mild, moderate and severe renal impairment is underway (NCT00999336).

- Otamixaban is parenteral in formulation. It was developed as a potential replacement for heparin in ACS. The phase II SEPIA-ACS TIMI 42 trial compared five doses of otamixaban doses to heparin plus eptifabitide. Intermediate doses showed efficacy and bleeding rates comparable to standard therapy. Lower doses of otamixaban were associated with increased thrombotic complications while the highest dose was associated with excess bleeding.[64]

DIRECT THROMBIN INHIBITORS

Thrombin is a key point of propagation in thrombosis and hemostasis (as discussed above). Not only does active thrombin convert fibrinogen to fibrin but also creates a positive feedback loop by activating factors V, VIII and XI. It also acts as a potent activator of platelets.[65] Given this central location in the clotting cascade, it is an attractive anticoagulant target. UFH indirectly inhibits thrombin, mediated by AT III, but this complex has limited activity against fibrin-bound thrombin. The inability to inhibit fibrin-bound thrombin, the site of clot propagation, is a potentially significant limitation. The direct thrombin inhibitors (DTI) are designed to overcome this limitation.

Thrombin's activity can be inhibited at three separate locations on the molecule: (1) the active, catalytic site; (2) exosite 1, the dock for substrates such as fibrin and (3) exosite 2, the heparin binding domain. Two classes of DTI are distinguished by their mechanism of inhibition. The bivalent DTI are derived from hirudin, a naturally occurring compound that was isolated from the leech in 1905—the first anticoagulant. The bivalent DTI, as the name suggests, exert their inhibitory effect through binding to exosite 1 and the catalytic site. Univalent DTI, in contrast, are small synthetic molecules that bind only to the active site.[66] None of the DTI bind at exosite site 2, the heparin-binding site. The bivalent DTI are parenteral in formulation and have limited clinical application outside the catheterization lab. The first oral DTI, dabigatran, has been approved by the FDA and, along with the direct fXa inhibitors, may significantly change standards of anticoagulation.

HIURDIN

Hiurdin, isolated from *Hirudo medicinalis*—the medicinal leech, is not used as a commercial anticoagulant. Two recombinant hirudins (r-hirudin or lepirudin and desulfato-hirudin or desirudin) differ at a single amino acid and are used in clinical practice. Referred to generically as hirudin, the three molecules are pharmacologically interchangeable.

Mechanism and Monitoring

Hirudin forms an irreversible 1:1 complex with thrombin and interacts minimally with plasma proteins. Hirudin has a short half-life in patients with normal renal function. Therapeutic levels are reached in 30–60 minutes after beginning IV infusion. Excretion is predominantly renal. Functional half-life is extended in patients with renal dysfunction and can reach 5 days in patients with absent kidney function. The aPTT is the test for choice of monitoring hirudin anticoagulation, but the response is linear only to 60–70 seconds. Beyond that point, the aPTT will underestimate the level of coagulation. If higher levels of anticoagulation are desired, such as during CPB, the ecarin clotting time (ECT), a thrombin-based measure of clotting, is the appropriate test. Both tests have the potential to underestimate degree of anticoagulation in patients with reduced levels of prothrombin (e.g. severe liver disease, diffuse intravascular coagulation (DIC) or concurrent VKA treatment),

and in patients with fibrinogen depletion (e.g. post-thrombolysis or hemodilution during CPB).[67]

Indications

Hirudins have two specific indications. Based on the HAT trials, lepirudin is approved for treatment of HIT complicated by thrombosis. In these studies, the incidence of new thrombosis was significantly lowered, by 93%, in the hirudin groups as compared to historical controls.[68,69] The risks for limb amputation or death were equivalent in the two groups. Current standards advocate immediate heparin withdrawal, regardless of thrombosis at the time of diagnosis; followed by immediate parenteral anticoagulation until a therapeutic INR has been reached with a VKA.[70] In this setting, the use of hirudin is appropriate in patients with preserved renal function. Given its ability to inhibit clot-bound thrombin, lepirudin was also studied as an alterative to heparin during PCI.[71] In these studies, hirudin was more effective in prevention of ischemic endpoints but not significantly better than heparin in prevention of cardiovascular death or MI at 1 week. Higher rates of bleeding and increased transfusion requirements observed in the studies negated the potential beneficial effects. Hirudin is an appropriate alternative during PCI in patients with HIT and has demonstrated efficacy in this population.[72] The second, but little used, indication for desirudin is prophylaxis and treatment of DVT.[73] This is appropriate only in patients with confirmed or suspected HIT/HTTS given the often-used alternatives. Hirudin has been employed in CPB complicated by HIT, where it provided effective anticoagulation but increased postoperative blood loss.[74,75]

Limitations

The two primary limitations of hirudins are mutually reinforcing. The extreme dependence on normal renal function to maintain predictable anticoagulation can make avoiding over anticoagulation difficult. Given the increased rate of bleeding, for which the greatest risk factor is impaired renal function, treatment of elderly or critically ill patients is challenging and requires close monitoring. There is no antidote to hirudin. When bleeding is life-threatening and occurs after hirudin use, only specific HD filters are effective for removal.[76] Greater than 44% of patients exposed to lepirudin develop antibodies, which have little clinical effect and may enhance the antithrombotic effect.[77] Despite the frequent development of antibodies, the risk of true anaphylactic reaction is extremely low (estimated at 0.015% after first exposure) and manifests within minutes of IV administration.[78]

BIVALIRUDIN

Bivalirudin (Angiomax, formerly Hirulog) is a synthetic, bivalent DTI and hirudin analogue. Unlike hirudin, the molecule is cleaved after binding, producing transient inhibition of thrombin.[79] Bivalirudin has a lower affinity for thrombin than hirudin by 1000-fold and does not spur antibody formation. The drug is degraded by proteolytic and hepatic mechanisms. Because it is cleared by glomerular filtration alone, dose adjustment is required in patients with renal impairment.

Indications and Efficacy

Due to short half-life and IV formulation, bivalirudin is administered as a continuous infusion after an initial bolus. The principal indication is as an alternative anticoagulant during PCI. Bivalirudin can also be used for treatment of HIT/HTTS, but its mode of administration makes use impractical in non-critical care settings. Current FDA indications are:[80]

- Use as an anticoagulant in patients with unstable angina undergoing percutaneous transluminal coronary angioplasty (PTCA).
- Use as an anticoagulant in patients undergoing percutaneous coronary intervention (PCI) with provisional use of glycoprotein IIb/IIIa inhibitor (GPI) is indicated.
- Bivalirudin is indicated for patients with or at risk of HIT/HITTS undergoing PCI.

Bivalirudin has been studied in conjunction with optimal antiplatelet therapy, including aspirin (and clopidogrel, if indicated). The drug has not been studied in patients with ACS who are not undergoing intervention.

Discussion regarding the choice of heparin versus bivalirudin in PCI can be found in other chapters, but the studies supporting these indications are discussed briefly below. The REPLACE-2 study was the first to evaluate bivalirudin as compared to standard therapy; heparin and scheduled glycoprotein IIb/IIIa inhibitor (GPI), during scheduled PCI.[81] The study found that bivalirudin, with optional use of GPI for intra-procedural complication, was non-inferior to the standard of care with respect to the primary endpoint through 6 months. Significantly lower rates of bleeding were noted in the bivalirudin-treated group. Patients with unstable angina or NSTEMI were randomized to one of three groups in the ACUITY trial; bivalirudin alone, bivalirudin plus GPI or heparin plus GPI.[82] Bivalirudin alone was equivalent to either GPI-containing regimen with respect to MI, revascularization and death at 30 days and 1 year. As in the REPLACE-2 study, rates of bleeding were significantly lower in the unaccompanied bivalirudin group. This result underlines the import of thrombin in pathologic platelet activation. Most recently, the HORIZONS-AMI trial evaluated bivalirudin alone in comparison to heparin and GPI in STEMI.[83] Significantly lower rates of bleeding during hospitalization, cardiac and all cause death at 30 days were observed in the bivalirudin group. Increased acute stent thrombosis was observed at 24 hours in bivalirudin treated patients, but a significant difference was not observed at 30 days. Bivalirudin has shown efficacy comparable to heparin when used during on-pump and off-pump CABG, with lower rates of bleeding and decreased transfusion requirements.[84–87]

Limitations and Monitoring

The two main limitations of bivalirudin are its exclusively parenteral formulation and its route of excretion, requiring dose adjustment patients with renal dysfunction. Assuming normal renal function, the half-life of bivalirudin is approximately 25 minutes. Coagulation parameters return to normal 1 hour after cessation of IV infusion. In patients with moderate, severe or dialysis-dependent renal impairment, clearance is prolonged by 20%, 60% and 80%, respectively.[88] The drug is 25% cleared by hemodialysis. As with all anticoagulants, it confers an

increased risk of bleeding, but the lower rates of bleeding in the aforementioned trials make it an appropriate alternative during PCI, PTCA or CABG. The aPTT can be used for monitoring at lower levels of anticoagulation; up to 3 times the upper limit of normal. Above this limit, the test is no longer sensitive.[89] In practice, the ACT is used for monitoring during catheterization and coronary bypass due to the high levels of anticoagulation required. In this setting, target ACT range is over 200 seconds.[90]

ARGATROBAN

Argatroban is a synthetic, small molecule derived from L-arginine. This univalent DTI, as a prototype of the class, reversibly inhibits only the active site of thrombin. Argatroban otherwise behaves similarly to bivalirudin, inhibiting both free and clot-bound thrombin. The molecule is metabolized in the liver and excreted, principally, in the feces without significant renal involvement.[91] Argatroban is administered intravenously. The plasma half-life is 45 minutes and steady-state anticoagulation is reached in 1–3 hours.

Indications and Efficacy

Argatroban has two FDA indications and is used principally in patients with HIT and significant renal dysfunction:

- Prophylaxis or treatment of thrombosis in patients with HIT
- Use during PCI in patients with documented or at risk for HIT.

The principal data for efficacy of argatroban in HIT are derived from two, historically controlled prospective studies.[92,93] In these studies, prompt treatment with intravenous argatroban (to an INR of 1.5–3 for 5–7 days) resulted in a significant decrease in new thrombosis (28% vs 38.8%) when compared to historical HIT controls treated with placebo. Authors reported a decrease in thrombosis-related death in the argatroban-treated HITTS group, but treatment with argatroban produced no difference in all-cause mortality in either group. A subsequent subgroup analysis of this data, with respect to demographic variables and platelet count, found no differences in treatment effect or rates of bleeding.[94] A subsequent comparison of argatroban to desirudin in the treatment of HIT was recently abandoned due to low enrollment.[95] An initial, retrospective study of argatroban demonstrated acceptable rates of adverse events; death, MI, urgent revascularization or major bleeding, when argatroban was used for PCI in patients with HIT.[96] As was observed with bivalirudin, the addition of GPI did not improve clinic outcomes. A subsequent, single-center study of argatroban use in patients with ACS, STEMI or NSTEMI and history of HIT reported fewer adverse outcomes and a low rate of bleeding when used for PCI in a cohort of patients with HIT.[97] Argatroban has shown promise in a number of additional clinical situations where HIT is a consideration; mechanical heart valves,[98] left ventricular-assist devices and pre-heart transplant,[99,100] thrombolysis after stroke[101] and renal replacement therapy.[102,103]

Limitations and Monitoring

The principal advantage of argatroban is ease of use in patients with impaired renal function. In treatment of HIT[104] and during

PCI,[105] no dose-adjustment of argatroban for renal dysfunction is required. Argatroban treatment of HIT in patients with mild hepatic dysfunction is possible with dose adjustment,[106] but other treatment options likely obviate use in this clinical scenario. In patients with HIT, the level of anticoagulation can be safely monitored using the aPTT so long as the desired therapeutic range in less than 3 times the upper limit of normal. A target ACT of 300–450 seconds is recommended in PCI but is derived from a small evidence base. A retrospective analysis of ACT in PCI showed that times greater than 450 seconds were associated with greater risks of bleeding, without improvement in thrombotic outcome.[107] Argatroban also prolongs the INR, a fact that can complicate transition to long-term warfarin therapy. When an infusion rate of 2 mcg/kg/min or less is used, the INR directly attributable to warfarin can be calculated from the following equation: 0.19 + 0.57 (Measured INR). In patients transitioning from argatroban to warfarin, a measured INR of 5 or less is not associated with increased bleeding.[108]

Allergic reactions after argatroban administration have manifested in a variety of clinical settings. Greater than 95% of these reactions occurred in patients who were concomitantly treated with thrombolytic therapy (e.g. streptokinase) or iodine-based contrast media. Coadministration with other antithrombotic or antiplatelet agents is associated with an increased risk of bleeding. Although partially metabolized by CYP450 enzymes, no clinically significant drug interactions have been identified.

XIMELAGATRAN

Ximelagatran was the first oral, univalent direct thrombin inhibitor to reach advanced stages of pre-clinical testing.[109] By 2005, phase III trials of ximelagatran had demonstrated efficacy in several clinical settings: postoperative DVT prophylaxis,[110–114] acute DVT treatment,[115] secondary prevention of ACS[116] and stroke prevention in patients with AF.[117] Ximelagatran had received approval in several European and South American countries for postoperative VTE prophylaxis. A British meta-analysis comparing ximelagatran to standard dose enoxaparin showed improved VTE prophylaxis, but increased serious bleeding.[118] Despite these promising results, development was halted in 2006 (and the drug was withdrawn from foreign markets) when significant hepatotoxicity and fulminant liver failure were noted in extended (> 35 days) phase III trials.

This episode merits discussion due to the increased scrutiny that future anticoagulants will face during the approval process. No elevations in liver enzymes were observed during the first trials of ximelagatran, in which the drug was tested for 2 weeks or less. The Thrive III study, in which ximelagatran was tested for an extended period (18 months) versus placebo, was the first to report significant ALT elevations.[119] The first case of fatal hepatotoxicity was reported in the SPORTIF V trial, which also confirmed that ximelagatran was as effective as warfarin for stroke prevention in AF with less bleeding.[120] The same year, an analysis of hepatotoxicity in extended clinical trials found ALT elevation in approximately 8% of treated patients. It was suggested that monitoring of ALT during the first 6 months of therapy would be sufficient to identify at-risk patients.[121] Further follow-up indicated that liver dysfunction could develop

after withdrawal of ximelagatran and that elevation of ALT was not a consistent predictor of severe hepatic dysfunction.[122] The mechanism of hepatocyte injury remains unknown but genomic studies indicate a possible association with major histocompatability complexes (MHC). Taken together, these findings indicate an idiosyncratic toxicity rather than a class effect.

DABIGATRAN

Dabigatran is a univalent, oral DTI that potently inhibits thrombin, similar to ximelagatran. Like rivaroxaban, dabigatran is approved in the EU (Pradaxa) and Canada (Pradax) for perioperative DVT prophylaxis in orthopedic patients. The structure of dabigatran etexilate, the orally formulated pro-drug, is distinct from ximelagatran. Metabolism proceeds through plasma esterases, rather than hepatic enzymes.[123] Preclinical testing and surveillance during clinical trials have revealed no hepatotoxicity. It is theorized that rapid plasma metabolism quickly lowers inactive precursor concentrations, preventing a ximelagatran-like toxicity.[124] The drug reaches peak plasma concentrations in 1.5 hours and exhibits a 14–17 hour half-life. Twice-daily dosing is standard. Dabigatran is contraindicated in severe renal impairment as 80% of active drug is cleared via the kidneys. To date, clinical trials have excluded patients with renal dysfunction and no reliable dose-reduction regimes have been examined. Greater than 60% of the drug is removed during hemodialysis,[125] but safety in this population cannot be recommended without further investigation.

Efficacy

Initial studies found dabigatran effective for postoperative VTE prevention in orthopedic patients and comparable to daily enoxaparin over a wide dose range.[126] In the RE-MODEL trial, dabigatran 150 mg or 220 mg orally BID were non-inferior to enoxaparin SQ 40 mg daily for VTE prevention after TKR.[127] Similarly, dabigatran was non-inferior to enoxaparin for VTE prevention after THR in the RE-NOVATE trial.[128] The three preceding trials reported safety profiles of dabigatran that were comparable to daily enoxaparin and formed the basis for approval in the EU and Canada. It is questionable whether US approval is imminent for this indication, as RE-MOBILIZE found dabigatran inferior to US standard, BID enoxaparin dosing after TKR.[129] A second trial of dabigatran 220 mg orally BID is ongoing (RE-NOVATE II; NCT00657150).

Following recent positive trials, dabigatran became the first, FDA-approved oral and anticoagulant since warfarin in fall of 2010. The most important of these trials is the RE-LY trial, in which dabigatran was compared to dose adjusted warfarin for stroke prevention in patients with AF and elevated $CHADS_2$ risk score.[130] Two doses of dabigatran were used in the trial. The first, 110 mg orally BID, was non-inferior to warfarin with respect to embolic stroke and all-cause mortality while the yearly rate of major bleeding significantly decreased. The second dose, dabigatran 150 mg orally BID, was superior to warfarin and reduced rates of stroke and systolic embolism. The mortality rate in patients treated with dabigatran approached statistical superiority ($p = 0.051$) when compared to warfarin while rates of major bleeding were equivalent. In both doses, lower rates of ICH were observed. Based on these findings, the FDA advisory panel has unanimously recommended approval the 150 mg PO BID dose of dabigatran for stroke prevention in AF.[131] Additional recommendations include: manufacture of a 75 mg tablet for daily use in renal impairment, use of 110 mg PO BID dose for patients with elevated bleeding risk and phase IV testing of higher dose dabigatran in this clinical setting. Finally, dabigatran 150 mg orally BID has demonstrated equivalence to standard therapy (SQ enoxaparin followed by dose adjusted warfarin) in 6 month treatment of acute VTE, both DVT and PE in the RE-COVER study.[132] A duplicate trial (RE-COVER II; NCT00680186) and two extension studies (RE-MEDEY, comparison to warfarin for 18 months; NCT00329238) and (RE-SONATE; NCT00558 259) may determine whether dabigatran replaces warfarin as the drug of choice for treatment and long-term prevention of VTE.

A site-by-site, post-hoc analysis of the RE-LY data with respect to time in therapeutic range (TTR) —in warfarin-treated patients—demonstrated that outcome discrepancies were greatest at the treatment centers with the poorest TTR.[133] This analysis suggests that the advantages of dabigatran were accentuated at sites where warfarin monitoring was most problematic. Dabigatran should immediately fill a need for patients with inadequate access to an anticoagulation clinic or for whom increased bleeding risk makes warfarin therapy unacceptable.

Limitations and Monitoring

As noted above, no excess ALT elevations, or hepatic toxicity, were noted in these studies. The main adverse effect in dabigatran treated groups was dyspepsia. The authors of the RE-LY study postulate that the acidity of dabigatran which facilitates absorption may be the cause of dyspepsia and increased rates of gastrointestinal (GI) bleeding. It was specifically formulated with tiny, acidic pellets inside a capsule to mitigate the effects of proton pump inhibitors (PPIs).[134] Two excess MI were observed per 1,000 patients in the RE-LY trial, but the significance of this finding is unclear given reductions in MI observed in trials of ximelagatran. An ongoing trial of dabigatran for secondary prevention of ACS (RE-DEEM; NCT00621855) should provide a definitive answer. Dabigatran etexilate is a P-glycoprotein efflux substrate. Plasma concentrations increase when administered in conjunction with P-glycoprotein inhibitors amiodarone and verapamil. Use of the strong P-glycoprotein inhibitor quinidine is contraindicated with dabigatran. At present, no other medications are known to interact with dabigatran. Monitoring of dabigatran is not needed in patients with normal renal function. Interestingly, subgroup analysis indicated that mild renal impairment correlated with improved outcomes in the RE-LY trial. Recommendations regarding dosing in renal impairment have yet to be finalized. Although monitoring of anticoagulation should not be required for the vast majority of patients, the ECT and thrombin time (TT) were found to be the most sensitive and precise in the therapeutic range.[135] Concern has been raised regarding the lack of an established reversal agent for dabigatran in cases of uncontrolled bleeding, especially amongst elderly patients.[135a]

ANTIPLATELET AGENTS

Platelets instigate and catalyze arterial thrombosis in a stepwise process (Fig. 5). Each step presents a potential therapeutic target for inhibition of thrombosis. At injury outset, platelets adhere to subendothelial matrix components, minimizing the breach in the endothelial wall. Although few therapeutics that interrupt adherence have been studied, development potential will be discussed briefly. Also exposed by endothelial injury, TF binds factor VII, initiates the clotting cascade and generates thrombin, which is a potent activator of platelets. ADP and TxA_2 are also crucial signals that lead to platelet activation and recruitment. The most established antiplatelet therapies, aspirin (an inhibitor of TXA_2 synthesis) and clopidogrel (an ADP/$P2Y_{12}$ antagonist), aim to disrupt this second step. New therapeutics aim to improve ADP inhibition and inhibit thrombin signaling. Once activated, intracellular signaling produces a conformational change in the GP IIb/IIIa ($\alpha_{IIb}\beta_3$) receptor that favors fibrinogen binding (as well as vWF and fibronectin). *Aggregation* is the result of avid platelet binding, via the abundant $\alpha_{IIb}\beta_3$, to many fibrinogen molecules. The two $\alpha_{IIb}\beta_3$ binding regions of fibrinogen produce extensive platelet cross-linking. This final step is inhibited by the parenteral glycoprotein IIb/IIIa inhibitors (GPI), which will be discussed only briefly in this section, due to their limited use outside the catheterization lab.

INHIBITORS OF PLATELET ADHESION

At present, there are no clinically available inhibitors of platelet adhesion. In vitro and animal models have demonstrated that inhibition of multiple receptors can reduce platelet adhesion to the subendothelial matrix.[136] Animal models have demonstrated protection from arterial thrombosis when adhesion is inhibited. For example, murine GPVI knockout mice demonstrate only a moderate bleeding phenotype but significant protection from experimentally induced, arterial thrombosis.[137] A monoclonal antibody directed against the murine GPVI receptor led to a long-term prevention from thrombosis.[138] Together, these findings make inhibitors of adhesion an attractive target for drug development. Molecules currently under investigation include naturally derived compounds, including those from the leech and the mosquito, as well as synthetic molecules.

Aegyptin, a mosquito derived molecule, displays high in vitro affinity for vWF and binds, with lower affinity, to the GPVI and $\alpha_2\beta_1$-binding sites of collagen. In vivo, the molecule prevents platelet aggregation and thrombosis after laser-induced carotid injury in rats without excess bleeding.[139] Saratin, a leech derived compound, prevents platelet and vWF binding to collagen under high-shear conditions.[140] A small molecule inhibitor of integrin $\alpha_2\beta_1$ has also shown efficacy in an animal model of arterial thrombosis.[141] Finally, ARC1779 is an intravenous, oligonucleotide-based aptamer that inhibits the A1 domain of vWF and prevents binding to platelet GP1b. Of current adhesion inhibitor candidates, it has reached most advanced stage of development. Administration of ARC1779 prevented occlusive thrombi in a simian model of carotid injury.[142] A human dose-ranging study demonstrated a dose-dependent inhibition of platelet function without increased bleeding in a cohort of healthy subjects.[143] An ex vivo study of

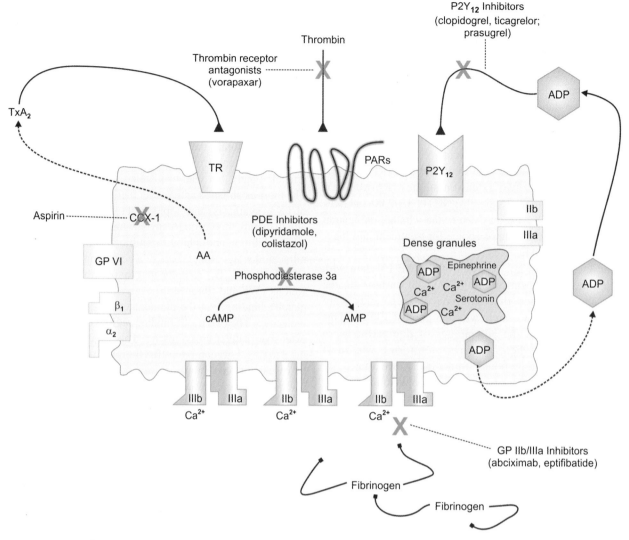

FIGURE 5: Antiplatelet agents: Depicted at right are the major sites of action of the five extant classes of antiplatelet drugs. Aspirin is the major inhibitor of the TxA$_2$ pathway. Clopidogrel and ticagrelor inhibit P2Y$_{12}$ activation by ADP. GP IIb/IIIa inhibitors inhibit fibrinogen binding and platelet aggregation

blood drawn from acute MI subjects demonstrated that ARC1779 reduced platelet activation to the level of controls despite a twofold increase in vWF activity.[144] The drug has also been administered experimentally, with apparent success, to a patient with refractory thrombotic thrombocytopenia purpura.[145]

INHIBITORS OF PLATELET ACTIVATION

TXA$_2$ Pathway Inhibitors

Aspirin or acetylsalicylic acid (ASA) is the prototype TXA$_2$ pathway inhibitor. NSAIDs ibuprofen and naproxen, which reversibly inhibit cyclooxygenase (COX), and selective COX-2 inhibitors, such as celecoxib, are members of the class, as are ridogrel and terbogrel, which combine a TxA$_2$ synthase inhibitor and TxA$_2$/prostaglandin endoperoxide receptor antagonist. While these combination drugs have theoretic advantages over aspirin, they have not proven clinically more efficacious[146] and have produced untoward side effects.[147]

Mechanism: ASA, a modification salicylic acid, was first synthesized in 1897 by Felix Hoffman of Bayer and subse-

quently marketed as Aspirin.[148] Widely used as a pain reliever, its effect on platelets and bleeding were not described until 1967.[149,150] Vane and others reported impaired prostaglandin synthesis as the biochemical mechanism of ASA shortly thereafter.[151] Aspirin acts by irreversibly acetylating cyclooxygenase-1 (COX-1), inhibiting the synthesis of prostaglandin H$_2$, a TxA$_2$ precursor. ASA is rapidly absorbed and reaches peak plasma levels in less than 1 hour. Enteric-coated ASA is absorbed at a slower rate and peak plasma levels are reached in 3–4 hours, hence the instruction to chew ASA when administered for ACS. The half-life of ASA is short, 15–20 minutes, but given irreversible platelet inactivation the functional duration of action is 5–10 days, the life span of a platelet.[152]

Indications and efficacy: The first published reports of ASA use for prevention of heart disease predate the mechanistic discoveries by nearly two decades.[153] Lawrence Craven, a general practitioner in Glendale, CA, had reasoned that ASA may prevent MI when administered daily at moderate dose, given its propensity cause bleeding. It became his practice to advise daily aspirin to overweight and sedentary men between the ages of 45 and 65.[154] Indeed, ASA has proven a highly effective therapy in prevention of thrombotic outcomes.[155,156] A recent meta-analysis estimated that daily ASA use in high-risk patients reduced serious vascular events, including MI and CVA, by one quarter.[157] The current indications for ASA use include:

- 325 mg daily for 1 month followed by 81 mg daily for life—ACS, including STEMI, NSTEMI and UA[158–160]
- 325 mg daily for 1 month followed by 81 mg daily for life—following PCI
- 81 mg daily for life—for secondary prevention of MI in patients with CAD, PAOD or documented pulmonary artery disease
- 81 mg daily for life—after CABG, carotid endarterectomy or peripheral vascular bypass[161]
- 1300 mg daily—for symptomatic intracranial arterial stenosis[162]
- 81–325 mg daily—prevention of embolic stroke in patients with AF and CHADS$_2$ score of 1 or contraindications to warfarin use[163]
- 50–325 mg daily, preferably in combination with dipyridamole 200 mg twice daily—secondary prevention of CVA after stoke or TIA[164]
- 325 mg once—administered 24–48 hours after acute stroke (of note, ASA is not recommended within 24 hours of thrombolytic therapy)[165]
- 81–162 mg daily—for patients with heart failure and reduced ejection fraction[166]
- 100 mg daily—for patients with polycythema vera and no contraindication to ASA use.[167]

The recently published CURRENT-OASIS 7 study stratified patients with ACS, scheduled to undergo early-invasive PCI, to either low or full dose ASA from the outset of therapy. The investigators found that use of low dose ASA did not alter the rates of death, MI or CVA at 30 days.[168] This result is provocative, but will likely not alter recommendations until long-term follow-up data is available. The concept of aspirin resistance; that certain individuals are resistant to the platelet inhibitory effects of ASA, has generated much discussion in the past decade. The topic is plagued by non-standard testing, conflicting results of observational or retrospective trials and possible confounding by suboptimal patient adherence. No recommendations will be included here due to lack of consensus regarding testing and treatment.[169]

Of note, ASA is not formally indicated for primary prevention. In 2009, the US Preventative Services Task Force recommended encouragement of daily, low-dose ASA use for primary prevention of cardiovascular disease (CVD) in men aged between 45 and 79 years and women between 55 and 79 years without mention of risk factors or diabetes (DM).[170] Recently published meta-analyses and RCT have questioned the benefit of ASA for primary prevention due to a poor risk-benefit ratio.[171–177] Given these contradictory recommendations, a 2010 position statement of the American Diabetes Association (ADA) and American Heart Association was released.[178] The final statement included the provision that recommendation of low dose (75–162 mg) ASA in patients with DM and an elevated ten-year risk for CVD is "reasonable". It continued that ASA should *not* be recommended for primary prevention in men with

age less than 50 years and women less than 60 years with DM without additional CVD risk factors.

Limitations and adverse effects: The main adverse effect of ASA is bleeding, most commonly GI, although rates are low. The yearly risk of major GI bleed is 0.05–0.1% among patients treated with low-dose ASA, twice the baseline rate.[179] Factors that increase the risk of bleeding are increasing age, previous GI bleeding (GIB) or peptic ulcer disease and concomitant use of warfarin, NSAIDs or steroids. The most recent AHA/American College of Gastroenterology guidelines advocate GI prophylaxis for any patient prescribed long-term antiplatelet therapy.[180] For patients on dual antiplatelet therapy, such as ASA and clopidogrel after drug-eluting stent (DES) placement, a PPI is the recommended agent to prevent GI bleeding. For patients on single antiplatelet therapy, PPI is recommended when gastroesophageal reflux disease or the above risk factors are present. After the publication of this guideline, the FAMOUS trial, an RCT of famotidine for prevention of GI sequelae in patients on chronic low-dose ASA, reported protection from ulcer, esophagitis and GIB versus placebo.[181]

Increased postoperative bleeding, but not death, has also been reported after CABG in patients with preoperative ASA use. A systematic review found that this effect was observed only in conjunction with doses greater than or equal to 325 mg daily.[182] This finding would indicate that continuation of low-dose ASA, rather than cessation 5 days prior, would be appropriate therapy for patients undergoing CABG. Cessation of antiplatelet therapy after MI or stent placement, especially within the recommended treatment windows, is associated with elevated risk of thrombosis.[183] Prior to any procedure that requires cessation of antiplatelet therapy, consultation with the primary (or consulting) cardiologist should be obtained to minimize this risk. "Rebound hypercoagulability" leading to increased rates of ischemic stroke has also been reported.[184]

A final precaution is aspirin sensitivity; a non-IgE mediated hypersensitivity-like reaction to ASA that is noted in concert with nasal polyps, asthma and chronic hyperplastic eosinophilic sinusitis.[185] Patients with this condition have respiratory exacerbations resembling asthma attacks within 3 hours of ASA (or other COX-1 selective NSAID) ingestion. The incidence is low, ~ 2.5% in the general population, but above 10% in patients who carry an asthma diagnosis. Aspirin desensitization, followed by daily use, effectively abolishes symptoms for patients who require daily use.

Inhibitors of ADP/P2Y$_{12}$ Signaling

Clopidogrel: Clopidogrel (Plavix) is the prototype P2Y$_{12}$ inhibitor, a second-generation thienopyridine. The first generation drug of this class, ticlopidine, is discussed subsequently.

Mechanism: Thienopyridines selectively and irreversibly inhibit the P2Y$_{12}$ receptor, reducing ADP-dependent platelet aggregation.[186] After ingestion, 15% of clopidogrel is converted to an active metabolite by the hepatic CYP system. Within 2 hours of a 300 mg oral dose, the active metabolite produces 40% inhibition of ADP-induced platelet aggregation.[187] Due to irreversible P2Y$_{12}$ inhibition, platelet inhibition is maintained for 48 hours, despite the 8-hour half-life of the active metabolite. After loading, daily administration of 75 mg increases platelet inhibition to approximately 60%, the maximum achievable. A larger loading dose; 600 mg, achieves maximum platelet inhibition in 2 hours.[188,189] Loading doses above 600 mg do not appear to produce provide additive benefit.[190] Clinically, loading with 600 mg prior to PCI improves 30-day clinical outcome without increasing rates of bleeding.[191,192]

Indications and efficacy: Clopidogrel was approved on the basis of a single large trial, in which it (75 mg daily) was compared directly with ASA 325 mg daily for secondary prevention of CVD in patients with symptomatic peripheral arterial disease (PAD), recent MI or recent ischemic stroke (both < 35 days).[193] The CAPRIE study reported a significant decrease in recurrent MI, stroke or vascular death favoring clopidogrel at nearly 2 years. Also reported was a trend toward fewer episodes of major bleeding in the clopidogrel group. Subgroup analysis, however, demonstrated that differential outcomes in PAD accounted for a majority of the observed effect.[194] Differences in outcome were minimal when analysis was limited to patients with recent MI. Clopidogrel was approved in 1997 for secondary prevention of CVD as an alternative to, but not replacement for, ASA. Clopidogrel has proven broadly efficacious in prevention of recurrent CVD.[195] Based on subsequent trials, notably PCI-CURE and CREDO, dual antiplatelet therapy (ASA plus clopidogrel) has become the standard of care after PCI.[196,197] Current indications for clopidogrel include:

1. ACS:
- For patients with NSTEMI or unstable angina, a 300 mg loading dose followed by 75 mg daily in combination with daily ASA
- For patients with STEMI; 75 mg daily in combination with ASA, with or without thrombolytics. Loading dose is optional in this setting, but 600 mg appears appropriate for patients proceeding to PCI

2. Secondary prevention of CVD with documented MI, stroke or PAD.

CHARISMA, a trial of clopidogrel plus ASA for primary and secondary prevention, found that medical management with long-term dual antiplatelet therapy did not benefit a high-risk population when compared to low-dose ASA.[198] Dual antiplatelet therapy may improve secondary prevention in the highest risk patients, but increased bleeding has limited wide use. Current indications do not specify duration of dual antiplatelet therapy, but the recommended minimum length of therapy for patients implanted with bare metal stents is 1 month.[199] Optimal duration of dual antiplatelet therapy after DES remains uncertain due to reports of stent thrombosis beyond 1 year.[200] However, a recent study suggests that no clinical benefit was derived from dual antiplatelet therapy beyond 12 months in conjunction with DES.[201] The importance of 12 months of uninterrupted dual antiplatelet therapy after DES is undisputed and has become a point of emphasis.

Limitations and adverse effects: Incidence of bleeding increases when clopidogrel is added to ASA as part of dual antiplatelet therapy.[202–204] In the CHARISMA trial, risk of bleeding was highest during the first year of therapy.[205] This was predominantly moderate bleeding, but maintained a strong association with increased mortality. As discussed above, PPI is currently indicated for all patients receiving dual antiplatelet therapy. Concern has arisen that concomitant use of PPI and clopidogrel attenuates the effect of the latter.[206] Inhibition of CYP450 2C19 by omeprazole, reducing the conversion of clopidogrel to its active metabolite, is the most frequently postulated mechanism for this effect. No adverse affect was observed, retrospectively, when clopidogrel was prescribed in conjunction with pantoprazole, which does not inhibit 2C19.[207] At present, the ACC/AHA does not find the data sufficient to recommend a change in clinical practice. Low rates of several life-threatening adverse events have been reported in association with clopidogrel.[208] The most important of these events is TTP, which can occur after as little as 2 weeks of treatment.

A black box warning was recently added to clopidogrel, warning of adverse events among patients with genetic polymorphisms of 2C19 that impair metabolism. In a sample of 162 healthy subjects, at least one reduced-function 2C19 allele was associated with impaired in vitro platelet aggregation and reduced blood levels of the active clopidogrel metabolite.[209] Investigators then analyzed data from the previously completed TRITON-TIMI 38 trial with respect to the presence or absence of a reduced function 2C19 allele in patients treated with clopidogrel. The reduced function allele was associated with a 4.1% absolute increase in rate of stroke, MI or death from cardiovascular causes when compared to 'noncarriers'. The incidence of this allele in the general population is 2% and 30% for homozygotes and heterozygotes respectively. An ACCF/AHA response did not advise routine CYP testing or alteration of clinical practice, citing a paucity of prospective outcome data or predictive value of routine genetic testing. [210] They emphasized the importance of clinical judgment and advised that the use of prasugrel or double-dose of clopidogrel would be reasonable for selected patients.

Ticlopidine was the first available P2Y$_{12}$ inhibitor. In patients with recent embolic stroke or cerebral ischemia, ticlopidine (250 mg twice daily) was superior to ASA in secondary prevention of stroke, MI or CV death.[211,212] Excess rates of bleeding were not observed in these studies. Due to higher rates of potentially fatal adverse effects, including neutropenia, thrombocytopenia, aplastic anemia and TTP, ticlopidine has largely been replaced by clopidogrel. It remains clinically available for dual antiplatelet therapy after PCI in patients with documented clopidogrel allergy. Ticlopidine is also approved for secondary prevention of ischemic stroke in patients with aspirin intolerance, but clopidogrel offers comparable efficacy with improved safety.[59]

Prasugrel

Prasugrel (Effient) is a third generation thienopyridine. Like clopidogrel, an active metabolite irreversibly inhibits the P2Y$_{12}$ receptor. In contrast to clopidogrel, the liver converts prasugrel more efficiently to its active metabolite. Whereas clopidogrel reaches peak effect in 4–6 hours, producing 60% inhibition of platelet aggregation, prasugrel produces complete inhibition of platelet aggregation by 1 hour.[213] Despite structural similarities, prasugrel is unaffected by common polymorphisms of 2C19 and 2C9, another CYP450 enzyme implicated in reduced clopidogrel metabolism.[214,215] These pharmacologic distinctions have correlated with increased in vivo platelet inhibition when compared to clopidogrel.[216]

Indications and efficacy: Prasugrel was approved for clinical use in 2009 on the basis of TRITON-TIMI 38 trial data. Prasugrel is currently indicated for:

- Patients with unstable angina or NSTEMI
- Patients with STEMI when managed with immediate or delayed PCI.

The original study compared prasugrel (60 mg loading dose followed by 10 mg daily) to clopidogrel (with 300 mg bolus followed by 75 mg daily) when used in patients presenting with ACS and planed PCI.[217] Prasugrel was associated with a significant decrease in the primary end-point at 15 months: death from cardiovascular causes, nonfatal MI and nonfatal stoke. Rates of urgent vessel revascularization and stent thrombosis were also reduced through 15 months. Increased rates of major bleeding were observed in the treatment group. An editorial accompanying the article observed a one-to-one correlation between cardiovascular deaths prevented and episodes of fatal bleeding.[218] Subgroup analyses of the TIMI 38 data describe superior efficacy in a number of specific populations; STEMI, DM and in conjunction with GPI, with or without stent use.[219] No differences in clinical outcome were observed in prasugrel patients treated with PPI.[220]

Limitations and adverse effects: A class III recommendation (indicating harm) regarding prasugrel has been included in the most recent STEMI and UA/SNTEMI guidelines.[160,281] It should not be used in patients with *"history of stroke and transient ischemic attack for whom primary PCI is planned, prasugrel is not recommended as part of a dual-antiplatelet therapy regimen."* Prasugrel received an extensive black box warning based on the increased risks for bleeding. Treatment with prasugrel is contraindicated in patients with age more than 75 years, except for those at highest risk, due to increased risk of fatal and ICH. The drug is contraindicated if urgent CABG is 'likely' and should be discontinued 7 days prior to any surgery. Dose adjustment of maintenance therapy is suggested for patients weighing under 60 kg or with a 'propensity to bleed'.[221] Limited experience with this drug limits estimation of TTP rates in comparison to clopidogrel.

Two additional $P2Y_{12}$ inhibitors have reached phase III testing. These new agents are non-thienopyridine agents that potently and reversibly inhibit ADP signaling.

Ticagrelor: (Brillanta, formerly AZD 6140) is an oral, reversible ATP analogue that acts as a $P2Y_{12}$ inhibitor. Unlike the thienopyridines, this drug inhibits the $P2Y_{12}$ receptor as a non-competitive inhibitor to ADP.[222,223] Ticagrelor is a direct acting compound that does not require metabolism for activation. Excretion of ticagrelor and a single active metabolite occur via the fecal route with negligible renal involvement.[224]

Efficacy: The PLATO study compared ticagrelor to clopidogrel in patients admitted to the hospital with ACS irrespective of ST elevation.[225] At 12 months patients in the ticagrelor group had significantly lower rates of a composite end point (death from vascular causes, MI and stroke). All-cause death and MI, but not stroke, were reduced in the ticagrelor group as well. Authors theorized that intensive $P2Y_{12}$ inhibition by ticagrelor produced

the observed benefit. The RESPOND study supports this assertion. In the study, clopidogrel non-responders, as described by Gurbel et al.,[226] were switched to ticagrelor. Platelet reactivity decreased by greater than 10% in all patients and over 30% in three quarters of patients treated with ticagrelor.[227] Although mechanistically plausible, platelet reactivity after administration of clopidogrel and ticagrelor has not been directly correlated to clinical outcome.

Limitations and adverse effects: The overall rates of bleeding observed in PLATO were comparable, but higher rates of intracranial bleeding were noted in association with ticagrelor. Three additional major adverse effects were noted in the ticagrelor group; dyspnea, which drove increased rates of drug discontinuation, asymptomatic cardiac pauses and increased levels of creatinine and uric acid. Concern that dyspnea was indicative of pulmonary disease prompted ONSET/OFFSET. In this small study, stable CAD patients treated with ASA were randomized to ticagrelor, clopidogrel or placebo for 6 weeks, including a loading dose for patients not in the placebo arm. A 40% incidence of dyspnea was noted among ticagrelor-treated patients, including three who discontinued therapy. However, no changes in pulmonary function tests, transthoracic echocardiography, EKG or BNP were noted in patients with dyspnea, as compared to controls.[228]

Currently available clinical data appears to favor ticagrelor over prasugrel for use in high-risk or clopidogrel-resistant patients.[229] In July 2010, the FDA advisory panel overseeing approval of ticagrelor recommended approval of the drug.[230] Contingent on approval, two post-approval studies will be required: (1) of patients with moderate and severe hepatic impairment and (2) of the US patients with ACS, as subgroup analysis of PLATO failed to demonstrate benefit for American subjects.

Cangrelor is an intravenous inhibitor of the $P2Y_{12}$ receptor with a 3–6 minute half-life and 60-minute duration of action after cessation of infusion. Two randomized, placebo-controlled trials of cangrelor were recently reported.[231,232] Parenteral cangrelor was administered at or before PCI in comparison to a 600 mg loading dose of oral clopidogrel. Treatment with cangrelor did not lead to a significant decrease in the primary end point; death from any cause, MI or ischemia-driven revascularization at 48 hours, in either study. Secondary endpoints were met but at the cost of increased major bleeding. The continued development of cangrelor as an intra-procedural $P2Y_{12}$ inhibitor is uncertain. A phase II trial of cangrelor use in the pre- and post-surgical settings is underway (BRIDGE; NCT00767507). A second direct parenteral $P2Y_{12}$ inhibitor, elinogrel, has reached phase II testing of use in patients with non-urgent PCI (INNOVATE-PCI; NCT00751231).

Phosphodiesterase (PDE) Inhibitors

Dipyridamole: The prototype drug in the class, acts by increasing intracellular levels of cyclic adenosine monophosphate (cAMP). Increased cAMP levels, in turn, reduce platelet activation by inhibiting calcium mobilization. Several in vitro mechanisms of action have been demonstrated; inhibition of platelet PDE, reduction of adenosine uptake by platelets and stimulation of prostacyclin (PGI_2) release by endothelial cells.[233] The dug also acts as a direct vasodilator (used as Persantine in stress echocardiography and thallium imaging) through inhibition of endothelial cyclic guanosine monophosphate phosphodiesterase (cGMP-PDE). Inhibition of cGMP-PDE potentiates the vascular effects of nitric oxide.[234] The mechanism of dipyridamole at clinical dosages remains indeterminate.

Indications and efficacy: Dipyridamole was introduced in 1959 for treatment of angina. The antiplatelet properties of the drug were discovered later, leading to its repurposing as an antithrombotic agent. It has proven ineffective as a lone anticoagulant.[235] Discussion of use in stress testing can be found elsewhere. The current indications for dipyridamole are:

- 100 mg four times daily in conjunction with warfarin to reduce thrombotic complications after implantation of a mechanical heart valve.[236]
- Extended-release dipyridamole (ERDP) 200 mg in conjunction with ASA 25 mg used twice daily for secondary prevention of stroke after TIA or completed ischemic stroke due to thrombosis.

Combination ERDP-ASA, marketed as Aggrenox, is the preferred agent for stroke prophylaxis and accounts for nearly all use.[237] This recommendation is based on two foundational trials. The ESPS 2 study reported a roughly 20% reduction in recurrent ischemic stroke in patients treated with the ERDP-ASA combination, compared to low-dose ASA.[238] The combination did not effect rates of bleeding, MI or death. The ESPRIT study reported a 1% absolute risk reduction in yearly stroke rate among patients treated with ERDP-ASA when compared to ASA alone.[239] A subsequent comparison of ERDP-ASA and clopidogrel for prevention of recurrent ischemic stroke demonstrated equivalent efficacy.[240]

Limitations and adverse effects: Headache is principal adverse effect of dipyridamole treatment, affecting one-third of treated patients and a leading cause of drug discontinuation. A pilot study has reported decreased rates of headache in patients in whom the dose of dipyridamole, as a component of ERDP-ASA, was titrated over 2 weeks.[241] Increased rates of diarrhea and other GI complaints have been reported in association with Aggrenox. The risks of ERDP-ASA beyond headache are similar to those of ASA alone. The ECDP-ASA administration is contraindicated in patients with severe hepatic impairment or severe renal impairment (GFR < 10 ml/min).

Cilostazol: Cilostazol is an inhibitor of platelet PDE3A that, like dipyridamole, also acts as a vasodilator. Thrombin activates PDE3A (via PAR-1, below), reducing the intracellular cAMP concentration and promoting platelet activation.[242] Given the antagonism of thrombin signaling in platelets, it is not surprising that cilostazol exerts antiplatelet effects. The principal route of drug metabolism is hepatic (CYP3A4 and 3A5) and fecal excretion predominates.[243]

Indications and efficacy: Cilostazol was granted FDA approval in 1999 for a single clinical indication: 50–100 mg twice daily for treatment of symptomatic claudication. In randomized, placebo controlled trials, cilostazol treatment produced significant increases in pain-free walking distance for patients with disabling disease (but without limb ischemia or pain at rest).[244,245] Current ACCP guidelines advocate for cilostazol use

only in patients with moderately disabling disease who are ineligible for surgical or catheter-based treatment.[246] They specifically recommend against use in patients with mild disease as exercise therapy and lifestyle modifications may be similarly efficacious. While cilostazol use is associated with symptomatic improvement, it has no proven benefit in secondary prevention of cardiovascular events.[247]

More recently, cilostazol has been tested as an adjunctive antiplatelet therapy after PCI. The addition of cilostazol to dual antiplatelet therapy after bare metal stent placement was associated with decreased angiographic stenosis at 6 months.[248] No reduction in MI or mortality was reported in the association with the reduction in stenosis. The effect was most pronounced in diabetic subjects, long lesions and small-diameter vessels, situations in which DES would be preferentially used. Addition of cilostazol to clopidogrel and ASA, dubbed triple therapy, was subsequently shown to reduce stenosis in patients with long (> 25 mm) lesions and DES placement.[249] No MI or mortality benefit was demonstrated, but triple therapy was associated with reduced target vessel revascularization. A similar effect was observed in diabetic patients treated with cilostazol in addition to standard therapy.[250] A more recent retrospective analysis of patients treated for ACS with primary PCI and DES in Korea reported improved clinical outcomes, including cardiac and total death, among patients treated with triple therapy for at least 1 month.[251] In vitro measures of platelet reactivity are decreased after 30 days of cilostazol when compared to dual antiplatelet therapy.[252] Prospective trials of triple therapy in a heterogeneous population showing clinical benefit are needed before cilostazol use after PCI becomes standard practice.

Limitations and adverse effects: The principal adverse effects of cilostazol are headache and diarrhea, as with dipyridamole. Palpitations are the unique side effect associated with cilostazol. As a PDE3A inhibitor, like milrinone, cilostazol acts as a dromotropic agent, increasing conduction velocity of the AV node. Cilostazol has been used for treatment of bradyarrhythmia, including slow AF.[253,254] Caution should be exercised when cilostazol is used in concert with inhibitors of CYP3A4/5 such as macrolide antibiotics, selective serotonin reuptake inhibitors, azole antifungals and warfarin. Additionally, grapefruit juice was associated with purpura in a patient using cilostazol.[255]

Thrombin Receptor Antagonists

Thrombin signaling via PARs appears to be the most potent of the three parallel platelet activation pathways. The PARs do not employ ligand-receptor binding. Rather, thrombin cleaves an exposed, N-terminal portion of the PAR, which leads to conformational change and exposure of a previously buried protein moiety. The newly exposed moiety is mobile and acts as a tethered ligand, activating the PAR.[256] After tethered ligand binding, the intracellular portion of the receptor effects platelet activation; shape change, TxA_2 synthesis and release, activation of $\alpha_{IIb}\beta_3$, through G-protein signaling. An excellent review of thrombin signaling through PARs can be found.[121]

Vorapaxar: Vorapaxar (SCH 530348) is an oral inhibitor of PAR_1 and prototype thrombin receptor antagonists (TRA). Vorapaxar was derived from himbacine, a compound isolated from the bark of the Australian magnolia.[257] Vorapaxar dose-dependently inhibited platelet aggregation in vitro and does not affect traditional measures of coagulation. The drug is rapidly absorbed but slowly eliminated with a half-life of 165–311 hours. Return of platelet function occurs, on average, 1 month after drug cessation.[258] The drug is excreted in the feces and dose adjustment for renal function in not required.

Efficacy: A large phase II has demonstrated that coadministration of vorapaxar with standard dual antiplatelet therapy does not increase bleeding risk.[259] In this placebo-controlled trial, a loading dose of vorapaxar was administered prior to planned PCI and a lower, maintenance dose for 2 months thereafter. A second, smaller phase II trial confirmed the safety of vorapaxar after PCI in patients with NSTEMI.[260] In this trial, standard therapy was defined as ASA, ticlopidine and heparin during catheterization. A significant reduction in periprocedural MI was reported in the treatment group. Phase III studies are underway to determine whether promising preclinical and animal studies translate to reduced MI and death in a clinical setting. The first, TRA 2°P-TIMI 50, will compare a 2.5 mg daily dose to placebo in secondary prevention of CVD over a period of 2.5 years (NCT00526474).[261] The second, TRA*CER, will randomize patients presenting with high-risk NSTEMI to placebo or 40 mg oral vorapaxar followed by 2.5 mg daily for at least 1 year (NCT00527943).[262]

A second TRA, atopaxar (E5555), is also in development. Recently released phase II data indicate that, when used in patients with ACS, atopaxar does not increased major bleeding.[263] Higher doses fully inhibited platelet function but were also associated with dose-dependent increased in liver function tests and QTc.

INHIBITORS OF PLATELET AGGREGATION

Three glycoprotein IIb/IIIa inhibitors (GPI) have received FDA approval for use in ACS or adjunctive therapy during PCI. In aggregate, these agents significantly reduce death and MI through 6 months.[264] Oral GPI have shown no clinical benefit and are associated with increased mortality.[265,266] Despite initial widespread use, the clinical indications for GPI use have become more limited. In 2004, GPI were found to provide no benefit compared to placebo when given in combination with ASA and clopidogrel prior to PCI, as had become standard.[267,268] The utility of GPI was called into further question in 2007 when bivalirudin was shown to obviate the need for either heparin or GPI during PCI, as discussed above. A complete discussion of GPI indications and use is located in sections discussing catheterization and PCI. Each agent is briefly introduced below in conjunction with significant adverse effects or limitations. All GPI are contraindicated in patients with an active bleed or elevated risk for severe bleeding.

The first approved agent, *abciximab (ReoPro)*, is a chimeric protein composed of Fab (fragment, antigen binding) regions from the murine 7E3 antibody and the Fc of human immunoglobulin. The first trial of abciximab in conjunction with coronary stenting found a marked improvement in clinical outcome at both 30 days and 6 months.[269] Abciximab has demonstrated benefit over placebo in patients with elevated troponin at the time of PCI.[270] Abciximab is not cleared by the kidneys and is safe in patients with CKD or ESRD. In EPIC, the first GPI trial, abciximab use was associated with a 50% increase in major bleeding, an absolute 11% incidence. Improvements in catheterization technique have decreased bleeding risk, but it remains the major adverse event associated with GPI. The high affinity binding of abciximab may play a role. The dissociation half-life from platelets is 4 hours, but it persists in blocking 13% of $\alpha_{IIb}\beta_3$ at 15 days.[271] Finally, abciximab doubles the risk of severe thrombocytopenia (defined as plt < 20,000).

Eptifibatide: Eptifibatide (Integrilin) is small molecule GPI modeled after a component of pigmy rattlesnake (Sistrurus miliarius barbouri) venom. A peptide-based compound, eptifibatide binds tightly to $\alpha_{IIb}\beta_3$, producing dose-dependent reversible inhibition. Significantly lower rates of MI and death occurred in patients with ACS who were treated with eptifibatide, in addition to heparin and ASA, with or without subsequent PCI.[272,273] The ESPRIT trial demonstrated reduced rates of MI and death at 1 year when used in conjunction with standard therapy during PCI.[274,275] Subsequently no benefit was reported with scheduled eptifibatide prior to PCI as compared to provisional use after procedural thrombotic complication.[276] As with abciximab, eptifibatide use is associated with increased risk of bleeding. In particular, the incidence pulmonary hemorrhage after eptifibatide (0.33%) is higher than after abciximab (0.14%). Renal clearance accounts for greater than 50% of eptifibatide elimination. Therefore, the dose must be adjusted in patients with CrCl less than 50 ml/min. It is contraindicated in patients with creatinine above 4 mg/dL or in ESRD.

Tirofiban: Tirofiban (Aggrastat) is a second small molecule, non-peptide GPI.[277,278] Although never compared directly with eptifibatide, it is used interchangeably due to similar mechanisms of action and clearance. When compared directly to abciximab, tirofiban use was associated with increased rates of MI.[279]

REFERENCES

1. Davie, EW, Ratnoff OD. Waterfall sequence for intrinsic blood clotting. Science. 1965;145:1310-2.
2. Gailani D, Renne´ T. The intrinsic pathway of coagulation: a target for treating thromboembolic disease? J Thromb Haemost. 2007; 5:1106-12.
3. Freiman, DG. The structure of thrombi. In: Colman RW, Hirsh J, Marder VJ, Salzman E (Eds). Hemostasis and Thrombosis: Basic Principles and Clinical Practice. Philadelphia: JB Lippincott; 1987. pp. 766-80.
4. Gross PL, Weitz JL. New antithrombotic drugs. Clinical Pharmacology & Therapeutics. 2009;86:139-46.
5. Weitz DS, Weitz JI. Update on heparin: what do we need to know? J Thromb Thrombolysis. 2010;29:199-207.
6. Greinacher A. Heparin-induced thrombocytopenia. J Thromb Haemost. 2009;7:9-12.
7. Dolovich LR, Ginsberg JS, Douketis JD, et al. A meta-analysis comparing low-molecular-weight heparins with unfractionated heparin in the treatment of venous thromboembolism: examining some unanswered questions regarding location of treatment, product type, and dosing frequency. Arch Intern Med. 2000;160:181-8.
8. Eikelboom JW, Hankey GJ. Low molecular weight heparins and heparinoids. MJA. 2002;177:379-83.
9. Sanofi-aventis. Lovenox Prescribing Information, 2009.

10. Pfizer. Fragmin Prescribing Information, 2007.

11. Cohen M, Demers C, Gurfinkel EP, et al. Efficacy and safety of subcutaneous enoxaparin in non–Q-wave coronary events study group. A comparison of low-molecular-weight heparin with unfractionated heparin for unstable coronary artery disease. N Engl J Med. 1997;337:447-52.

12. Antman EM, Morrow DA, McCabe CH, et al. ExTRACT-TIMI 25 investigators. Enoxaparin versus unfractionated heparin with fibrinolysis for ST-elevation myocardial infarction. N Engl J Med. 2006;354:1477-88.

13. The Matisse Investigators. Subcutaneous fondaparinux versus intravenous unfractionated heparin in the initial treatment of pulmonary embolism. N Engl J Med. 2003;349:1695-702.

14. The Fifth Organization to Assess Strategies in Acute Ischemic Syndromes Investigators. Comparison of fondaparinux and enoxaparin in acute coronary syndromes. N Engl J Med. 2006;354: 1464-76.

14a. Wright RS, Anderson JL, Adams CD, et al. 2011 ACCF/AHA focused update of the guidelines for the management of patients with unstable angina/non–ST-elevation myocardial infarction (updating the 2007 guideline): a report of the American College of Cardiology Foundation/ American Heart Association Task Force on Practice Guidelines. Circulation. 2011;123:2022-60.

15. Yusuf S, Mehta SR, Chrolavicius S, et al. Effects of fondaparinux on mortality and reinfarction in patients with acute ST-segment elevation myocardial infarction: the OASIS-6 randomized trial. JAMA. 2006;295:1519-30.

16. Decousus H, Prandoni P, Mismetti P, et al. Fondaparinux for the treatment of superficial-vein thrombosis in the legs. N Engl J Med. 2010;363:1222-32.

17. Warkentin TE, Maurer BT, Aster RH. Heparin-induced thrombocytopenia associated with fondaparinux. N Engl J Med. 2007;356:2653–5.

18. Hernberg J. Development of idraparinux and idrabiotaparinux for anticoagulant therapy. Thromb Haemost. 2009;102:811–5.

19. The van Gogh Investigators. Idraparinux versus standard therapy for venous thromboembolic disease. N Engl J Med. 2007;357:1094-104.

20. The van Gogh Investigators. Extended prophylaxis of venous thromboembolism with idraparinux. N Engl J Med. 2007;357:1105-12.

21. The Amadeus Investigators. Comparison of idraparinux with vitamin K antagonists for prevention of thromboembolism in patients with atrial fibrillation: a randomized, open-label, non-inferiority trial. The Lancet. 2008;371(9609): 315-21.

22. Buller HR, Destors JM, Gallus AS, et al. Idrabiotaparinux, a biotinylated long-acting anticoagulant, in the treatment of deep venous thrombosis (EQUINOX study): safety, efficacy, and reversibility by Avidin. Blood. 2008;112:18(abstract 32).

23. Viskov C, Just M, Laux V, et al. Description of the chemical and pharmacological characteristics of a new hemisynthetic ultra-low-molecular-weight heparin, AVE5026. Journal of Thrombosis and Haemostasis. 2009;7:1143-51.

24. Lassen MR, Dahl OE, Mismetti P, et al. AVE5026, a new hemisynthetic ultra-low-molecular-weight heparin for the prevention of venous thromboembolism in patients after total knee replacement surgery—TREK: a dose-ranging study. Journal of Thrombosis and Haemostasis. 2009;7:566-72.

25. Link KP. The discovery of dicumarol and its sequels. Circulation. 1959;19:97-107.

26. Jessup M, Abraham WT, Casey DE, et al. Focused update: ACCF/ AHA guidelines for the diagnosis and management of heart failure in adults: a report of the American College of Cardiology Foundation/ American Heart Association Task Force on Practice Guidelines. Circulation. 2009;119: 1977-2016.

27. Bonow RO, Carabello BA, Chatterjee K, et al. ACC/AHA 2006 guidelines for the management of patients with valvular heart disease: executive summary: a report of the American College of Cardiology/ American Heart Association Task Force on Practice Guidelines

(Writing Committee to Develop Guidelines for the Management of Patients with Valvular Heart Disease). Circulation. 2006;114:450-527.

28. Nishimura RA, Carabello BA, Faxon DP, et al. ACC/AHA 2008 guideline update on valvular heart disease: focused update on infective endocarditis: a report of the American College of Cardiology/American Heart Association Task Force on Practice Guidelines. Circulation. 2008;118:888-96.

29. Ansell J, Hirsh J, Hylek E, et al. Pharmacology and management of the vitamin K antagonists: American College of Chest Physicians evidence-based clinical practice guidelines (8th edition). Chest. 2008;133:160S-98S.

30. Baker WL, Cios DA, Sander SD, et al. Meta-analysis to assess the quality of warfarin control in atrial fibrillation patients in the United States. J Manag Care Pharm. 2009;15:244-52.

31. Hylek EM, Go AS, Chang Y, et al. Effect of intensity of oral anti-coagulation on stroke severity and mortality in atrial fibrillation. N Engl J Med. 2003;349:1019-26.

32. White HD, Gruber M, Feyzi J, et al. Comparison of outcomes among patients randomized to warfarin therapy according to anticoagulant control: results from SPORTIF III and V. Arch Intern Med. 2007;167:239-45.

33. Connoly SJ, Laupacis A, Gent M, et al. Canadian Atrial Fibrillation Anticoagulation (CAFA) Study. J Am Coll Cardiol. 1991;18:349-55.

34. Kneeland PP, Fang MA. Current Issues in patient adherence and persistence: focus on anticoagulants for the treatment and prevention of thromboembolism. Patient Prefer Adherence. 2010;4:51-60.

35. Ellis DJ, Usman MH, Milner PG, et al. The first evaluation of a novel vitamin K antagonist, tecarfarin (ATI-5923), in patients with atrial fibrillation. Circulation. 2009;120:1029-35, 2 p following 1035. Epub 2009.

36. Bavisotto LM, Ellis DJ, Milner PG, et al. Tecarfarin, a novel vitamin K reductase antagonist, is not affected by CYP2C9 and CYP3A4 inhibition following concomitant administration of fluconazole in healthy participants. J Clin Pharmacol. 2010 [Epub ahead of print].

37. Kakashi A. http://saveheart.wordpress.com. [Accessed 8/13/2010].

38. Garcia D, Libby E. Crowther MA. The new oral anticoagulants. Blood. 2010;115:15-20.

39. Perzborn et al. Rivaroxaban: a new oral factor Xa inhibitor. Arterioscler Thromb Vasc Biol. 2010;30:376-81.

40. Eriksson BI, Borris LC, Friedman RJ, et al. Rivaroxaban versus enoxaparin for thromboprophylaxis after hip arthroplasty. N Engl J Med. 2008;358:2765-75.

41. Turpie AGG, Lassen MR, Davidson BL, et al. Rivaroxaban versus enoxaparin for thromboprophylaxis after total knee arthroplasty (RECORD-4). Lancet. 2009;373;1673-80.

42. Summary of Product Caracterictics—EU. Bayer Schering Pharma, May 2009.

43. Lassen MR, Ageno W, Borris LC, et al. Rivaroxaban versus enoxaparin for thromboprophylaxis after total knee arthroplasty. N Engl J Med. 2008;358:2776-86.

44. Kakkar AK, Brenner B, Dahl OE, et al. Extended duration rivaroxaban versus short-term enoxaparin for the prevention of venous thromboembolism after total hip arthroplasty: a double-blind, randomised controlled trial. Lancet. 2008;72:31-9.

45. Xu Q. Xarelto (Rivaroxaban) Cardiovascular and Renal Drugs Advisory Meeting, 2009. http://www.fda.gov/downloads/ AdvisoryCommittees/CommitteesMeeting Materials/Drugs/Cardio-vascularandRenalDrugsAdvisory Committee/UCM143660.pdf. [Acessed 8/30/10].

46. Patel MR, Mahaffey KW, Garg J, et al. Rivaroxaban versus warfarin in nonvalvular atrial fibrillation. N Engl J Med. 2011;365:883-91.

47. Niessner A, Rose A. Correspondence: Rivaroxaban versus warfarin in nonvalvular atrial fibrillation. N Engl J Med. 2011;365:2333-4; author reply 2335.

48. The EINSTEIN Investigators. Oral rivaroxaban for symptomatic venous thromboembolism. N Engl J Med. 2010;363:2499-2510.

49. Mega JL, Braunwald E, Wiviott SD, et al. Rivaroxaban in patients with a recent acute coronary syndrome. N Engl J Med. 2012;366: 9-19.

50. Cohen, Alexander. The Magellan Study Methodology: Rivaroxaban compared with enoxaparin for the prevention of venous thromboembolism in hospitalized medically ill patients. Abstract presented at European Hematology Association meeting (10–13 Jun, Barcelona, Spain. 2010).

51. Raghavan N, Frost CE, Yu Z, et al. Apixaban metabolism and pharmacokinetics following oral administration to humans. Drug Metab Dispos. 2009;37:74-81.

52. Ufer M. Comparative efficacy and safety of the novel oral anticoagulants dabigatran, rivaroxaban and apixaban in preclinical and clinical development. Thromb Haemost. 2010;103:572-85.

53. Eikwlboon JW, WEitz JI. Update on antithrombotic therapy. Circulation. 2010;121:1523-32.

54. Lassen MR, Davidson BL, Gallus A, et al. The efficacy and safety of apixaban, an oral, direct factor Xa inhibitor, as thromboprophylaxis in patients following total knee replacement. J Thromb Haemost. 2007;5:2368-75.

55. Buller H, Deitchman D, Prins M, et al. Efficacy and safety of the oral direct factor Xa inhibitor apixaban for symptomatic deep vein thrombosis: the Botticelli DVT dose-ranging study. J Thromb Haemost. 2008;6:1313-8.

56. APPRAISE Steering Committee and Investigators. Apixaban, an oral, direct, selective factor Xa inhibitor, in combination with antiplatelet therapy after acute coronary syndrome: results of the apixaban for prevention of acute ischemic and safety events (APPRAISE) trial. Circulation. 2009;119:2877-85.

57. Lassen MR, Raskob GE, Gallus A, et al. Apixaban or enoxaparin for thromboprophylaxis after knee replacement. N Engl J Med. 2009;361:594-604.

58. Lassen M, Raskob G, Gallus A, et al. Apixaban versus enoxaparin for thromboprophylaxis after knee replacement (ADVANCE-2): a randomised double-blind trial. *The Lancet.* 2010;375:807-15.

59. Connolly SJ, Eikelboom J, Joyner C, et al. Apixaban in patients with atrial fibrillation. N Engl J Med. 2011;364:806-17.

60. Granger CB, Alexander JH, McMurray JJV, et al. Apixaban versus warfarin in patients with atrial fibrillation. N Engl J Med. 2011;365: 981-92.

61. Alexander JH, Lopes RD, James S, et al. Apixaban with antiplatelet therapy after acute coronary syndrome. N Engl J Med. 2011;365: 699-708.

62. Perzborn E. Faktor-Xa-inhibitoren—neue antikoagulanzien der sekundären hämostase hämostaseologie. 2009;29:260-7.

63. Turpie AG, Bauer KA, Davidson BL, et al. A randomized evaluation of betrixaban, an oral factor Xa inhibitor, for prevention of thromboembolic events after total knee replacement (EXPERT). Thromb Haemost. 2009;101:68-76.

64. Marc S Sabatine, Elliott M Antman, Petr Widimsky, et al. Otamixaban for the treatment of patients with non-ST-elevation acute coronary syndromes (SEPIA-ACS1 TIMI 42): a randomised, double-blind, active-controlled, phase 2 trial. Lancet. 2009;374:787-95.

65. Coughlin SR. Thrombin signalling and protease-activated receptors. Nature. 2000;407:258-64.

66. Di Nisio M, Middeldorp S, Büller HR. Direct thrombin inhibitors. N Engl J Med. 2005;353:1028-40.

67. Greinacher A, Warkentin TE. The direct thrombin inhibitor hirudin. Thromb Haemost. 2008;99:819-29.

68. Lubenow N, Eichler P, Lietz T, et al. Lepirudin inpatients with heparin-induced thrombocytopenia—results of the third prospective study (HAT-3) and a combined analysis of HAT-1, HAT-2, and HAT-3. J Thromb Haemost. 2005;3:2428-36.

69. Lubenow N, Eichler P, Lietz T, et al. Lepirudin for prophylaxis of thrombosis in patients with acute isolated heparin-induced thrombocytopenia: an analysis of 3 prospective studies. Blood. 2003;104:3072-7.

70. Shantsila E, Lip GYH, Chong BH. Heparin-induced thrombocytopenia; a contemporary clinical approach to diagnosis and management. Chest. 2009;135:1651-64.

71. Organisation to Assess Strategies for Ischemic Syndromes (OASIS-2) Investigators. Effects of recombinant hirudin (lepirudin) compared with heparin on death, myocardial infarction, refractory angina, and revascularisation procedures in patients with acute myocardial ischaemia without ST elevation: a randomised trial. Lancet. 1999;353:429-38.

72. Cochran K, DeMartini TJ, Lewis BE, et al. Use of lepirudin during percutaneous vascular interventions in patients with heparin-induced thrombocytopenia. J Invasive Cardiol. 2003;15:617-21.

73. Schiele F, Lindgaerde F, Eriksson H, et al. Subcutaneous recombinant hirudin (HBW 023) versus intravenous sodium heparin in treatment of established acute deep vein thrombosis of the legs: a multicentre prospective dose-ranging randomized trial. International Multicentre Hirudin Study Group. Thromb Haemost. 1997;77:834-8.

74. Warkentin TE, Greinacher A. Heparin-induced thrombocytopenia and cardiac surgery. Ann Thorac Surg. 2003;76:2121-31.

75. Riess FC, Poetzsch B, Madlener K, et al. Recombinant hirudin for cardiopulmonary bypass anticoagulation: a randomized, prospective, and heparin-controlled pilot study. Thorac Cardiovasc Surg. 2007;55:233-8.

76. Frank RD, Farber H, Stefanidis I, et al. Hirudin elimination by haemofiltration: a comparative in vitro study of different membranes. Kidney Int Suppl. 1999;56:S41-S45.

77. Eichler P, Friesen HJ, Lubenow N, et al. Antihirudin antibodies in patients with heparin-induced thrombocytopenia treated with lepirudin: incidence, effects on aPTT, and clinical relevance. Blood. 2000;96:2373-8.

78. Greinacher A, Lubenow N, Eichler P. Anaphylactic and anaphylactoid reactions associated with lepirudin in patients with heparin-induced thrombocytopenia. Circulation. 2003;108:2062-5.

79. Parry MA, Maraganore JM, Stone SR. Kinetic mechanism for the interaction of hirulog with thrombin. Biochemistry. 1994;33:14807-14.

80. Angiomax (bivalirudin) Prescribing Information. Parsippany, NJ: the Medicines Company. 2005.

81. Lincoff AM, Bittl JA, Harrington RA, et al. Bivalirudin and provisional glycoprotein IIb/IIIa blockade compared with heparin and planned glycoprotein IIb/IIIa blockade during percutaneous coronary intervention: REPLACE-2 randomized trial. JAMA. 2003;289:853-63.

82. Stone GW, McLaurin BT, Cox DA, et al. Bivalirudin for patients with acute coronary syndromes. N Engl J Med. 2006;355:2203-16.

83. Stone GW, Witzenbichler B, Guagliumi G, et al. Bivalirudin during primary PCI in acute myocardial infarction. N Engl J Med. 2008;358:2218-30.

84. Dyke CM, Smedira NG, Koster A, et al. A comparison of bivalirudin to heparin with protamine reversal in patients undergoing cardiac surgery with cardiopulmonary bypass: the EVOLUTION-ON study. J Thorac Cardiovasc Surg. 2006;131:533-9.

85. Smedira NG, Dyke CM, Koster A, et al. Anticoagulation with bivalirudin for off-pump coronary artery bypass grafting: the results of the EVOLUTION-OFF study. J Thorac Cardiovasc Surg. 2006;131:686-92.

86. Koster A, Dyke CM, Aldea G, et al. Bivalirudin during cardiopulmonary bypass in patient with previous or acute heparin-induced thrombocytopenia and heparin antibodies: results of the CHOOSE-ON trial. Ann Thorac Surg. 2007;83:572-7.

87. Merry AF, Raudkivi PJ, Middleton NG, et al. Bivalirudin versus heparin and protamine in off-pump coronary bypass surgery. Ann Thorac Surg. 2004;77:925-31.

88. Shammas NW. Bivalirudi pharmacology and clinical applications. Cardiovascular Drug Reviews. 2005;23:345-60.

89. Hirsh J, Bauer KA, Donati MB, et al. Parenteral anticoagulants. American College of Chest Physicians Evidence-Based Clinical Practice Guidelines. Chest. 2008;133:141S-59S.

CHAPTER 8

Antithrombotic and Antiplatelet Agents

90. Gibson CM, Morrow DA, Murphy SA, et al. A randomized trial to evaluate the relative protection against post-percutaneous coronary intervention microvascular dysfunction, ischemia and inflammation among antiplatelet and antithrombotic agents: the PROTECT–TIMI-30 trial. J Am Coll Cardiol. 2006;47:2364-73.

91. Argatroban Prescribing Information. GlaxoSmithKline, 2009.

92. Lewis BE, Wallis DE, Berkowitz SD, et al. Argatroban anticoagulant therapy in patients with heparin-induced thrombocytopenia. Circulation. 2001;103:1838-43.

93. Lewis BE, Wallis DE, Leya F, et al. Argatroban anticoagulation in patients with heparin-induced thrombocytopenia. Arch Intern Med. 2003;163:1849-56.

94. Lewis BE, Wallis DE, Hursting MJ, et al. Effects of argatroban therapy, demographic variables, and platelet count on thrombotic risks in heparin-induced thrombocytopenia. Chest. 2006;129:1407-16.

95. Frame JW, Rice L, Bartholomew JR, et al. Rationale and design of the PREVENT-HIT study: a randomized, open-label pilot study to compare desirudin and argatroban in patients with suspected heparin-induced thrombocytopenia with or without thrombosis. Clinical Therapeutics. 2010;32:626-36.

96. Cruz-Gonzalez I, Sanchez-Ledesma M, Baron SJ, et al. Efficacy and safety of argatroban with or without glycoprotein IIb/IIIa inhibitor in patients with heparin-induced thrombocytopenia undergoing percutaneous coronary intervention for acute coronary syndrome. J Thromb Thrombolysis. 2008;25:214-8.

97. Yeh R W, Baron SJ, Healy JL, et al. Anticoagulation with the direct thrombin inhibitor argatroban in patients presenting with acute coronary syndromes. Catheterization and Cardiovascular Interventions. 2009;74:359-64.

98. Maegdefessel L, Linde T, Michel T, et al. Argatroban and bivalirudin compared to unfractionated heparin in preventing thrombus formation on mechanical heart valves. Results of an in-vitro study. Thromb Haemost. 2009;101:1163-9.

99. Samuels LE, Kohut J, Cassanova-Ghosh E, et al. Aargatroban as a primary or secondary postoperative anticoagulant in patients implanted with ventricular assist devices. The Annals of Thoracic Surgery. 2008;85:1651-5.

100. Costanzo MR et al. The international society of heart and lung transplantation guidelines for the care of heart transplant recipients. The Journal of Heart and Lung Transplantation. 2010;29:914-56.

101. Sugg RM, Pary JK, Uchino K, et al. Argatroban tPA stroke study: study design and results in the first treated cohort. Arch Neurol. 2006;63:1057-62.

102. Murray PM, Reddy BV, Grossman EJ, et al. A prospective comparison of three argatroban treatment regimens during hemodialysis in end-stage renal disease. Kidney Int. 2004;66:2446-53.

103. Link A, Girndt M, Selejan S, et al. Argatroban for anticoagulation in continuous renal replacement therapy. Crit Care Med. 2009;37:105-10.

104. Guzzi LM, McCollum DA, Hursting MJ. Effect of renal function on argatroban therapy in heparin-induced thrombocytopenia. J Thromb Thrombolysis. 2006;22:169-76.

105. Hursting MJ, Jang IK. Impact of renal function on argatroban therapy during percutaneous coronary intervention. J Thromb Thrombolysis. 2009;22:169-76.

106. Levine R, Hursting MJ, McCollum D. Argatroban therapy in heparin-induced thrombocytopenia with hepatic dysfunction. Chest. 2006;129:1167-75.

107. Cruz-Gonzalez I, Sanchez-Ledesma M, Osakabe M, et al. What is the optimal anticoagulation level with argatroban during percutaneous coronary intervention? Blood Coag Fibrinolysis. 2008;19:401-4.

108. Hursting MJ, Lewis BE, Macfarlane DE. Transitioning from argatroban to warfarin therapy in patients with heparin-induced thrombocytopenia. Clin Appl Thromb Hemost. 2005;11:279-87.

109. Gustafsson D, Elg M. The pharmacodynamics and pharmacokinetics of the oral direct thrombin inhibitor ximelagatran and its active metabolite melagatran: a mini-review. Thromb Res. 2003;109:S9-S15.

110. Francis CW, Davidson BL, Berkowitz SD, et al. Ximelagatran versus warfarin for the prevention of venous thromboembolism after total knee arthroplasty: a randomized, double-blind trial. Ann Intern Med. 2002;137:648-55.

111. Francis CW, Berkowitz SD, Comp PC, et al. Comparison of ximelagatran with warfarin for the prevention of venous thromboembolism after total knee replacement. N Engl J Med. 2003;349:1703-12.

112. Eriksson BI, Agnelli G, Cohen AT, et al. Direct thrombin inhibitor melagatran followed by oral ximelagatran in comparison with enoxaparin for prevention of venous thromboembolism after total hip or knee replacement. Thromb Haemost. 2003;89:288-96.

113. Eriksson BI, Dahl OE, Buller HR, et al. A new oral direct thrombin inhibitor, dabigatran etexilate, compared with enoxaparin for prevention of thromboembolic events following total hip or knee replacement: the BISTRO II randomized trial. J Thromb Haemost. 2005;3:103-11.

114. Eriksson BI, Agnelli G, Cohen AT, et al. The direct thrombin inhibitor melagatran followed by oral ximelagatran compared with enoxaparin for the prevention of venous thromboembolism after total hip or knee replacement: the EXPRESS study. J Thromb Haemost. 2003;1:2490-6.

115. Fiessinger J-N, Huisman MV, Davidson BL, et al. Ximelagatran vs low-molecular-weight heparin and warfarin for the treatment of deep vein thrombosis: a randomized trial. JAMA. 2005;293:681-9.

116. Wallentin L, Wilcox RG, Weaver WD, et al. Oral ximelagatran for secondary prophylaxis after myocardial infarction: the ESTEEM randomised controlled trial. Lancet. 2003;362:789-97.

117. Olsson SB. Stroke prevention with the oral direct thrombin inhibitor ximelagatran compared with warfarin in patients with non-valvular atrial fibrillation (SPORTIF III): randomised controlled trial. Lancet. 2003;362:1691-8.

118. Cohen AT, Hirst C, Sherrill B, et al. Meta-analysis of trials comparing ximelagatran with low molecular weight heparin for prevention of venous thromboembolism after major orthopaedic surgery. British Journal of Surgery. 2005;92:1335-44.

119. Schulman S, Wahlander K, Lundstrom T, et al. Secondary prevention of venous thromboembolism with the oral direct thrombin inhibitor ximelagatran. N Engl J Med. 2003;349:1713-21.

120. Albers GW, Diener HC, Frison L, et al. Ximelagatran vs warfarin for stroke prevention in patients with nonvalvular atrial fibrillation: a randomized trial. JAMA. 2005;293:690-8.

121. Lee WM, Larrey D, Olsson R, et al. Hepatic findings in long-term clinical trials of ximelagatran. Drug Safety. 2005;28:351-70.

122. Keisu M, Andersson TB. Drug-induced liver injury in humans: the case of ximelagatran. Handb Exp Pharmacol. 2010;196:407-18.

123. Eisert WG, Hauel N, Stangier J, et al. Dabigatran: an oral novel potent reversible nonpeptide inhibitor of thrombin arterioscler. Thromb Vasc Bio. 2010;30:1885-9.

124. Sergent O, Ekroos K, Lefeuvre-Orfila L, et al. Ximelagatran increases membrane fluidity and changes membrane lipid composition in primary human hepatocytes. Toxicol in Vitro. 2009;23:1305-10.

125. Stangier J, Rathgen K, Stähle H, et al. Influence of renal impairment on the pharmacokinetics and pharmacodynamics of oral dabigatran etexilate: an open-label, parallel-group, single-centre study. Clin Pharmacokinet. 2010;49:259-68.

126. Eriksson BI, Dahl OE, Buller HR, et al. A new oral direct thrombin inhibitor, dabigatran etexilate, compared with enoxaparin for prevention of thromboembolic events following total hip or knee replacement: the BISTRO II randomized trial. Journal of Thrombosis and Haemostasis. 2005;3:103-11.

127. Eriksson BI, Dahl OE, Rosencher N, et al. Oral dabigatran etexilate vs subcutaneous enoxaparin for the prevention of venous thromboembolism after total knee replacement: the RE-MODEL randomized trial. Journal of Thrombosis and Haemostasis. 2007;5:2178-85.

128. Eriksson BI, Dahl OE, Rosencher N, et al. Dabigatran etexilate versus enoxaparin for prevention of venous thromboembolism after total

hip replacement: a randomised, double-blind, non-inferiority trial. Lancet. 2007;370:949-56.

129. RE-MOBILIZE Writing Committee, Ginsberg JS, Davidson BL, et al. Oral thrombin inhibitor dabigatran etexilate vs North American enoxaparin regimen for prevention of venous thromboembolism after knee arthroplasty surgery. J Arthroplasty. 2009;24:1-9.

130. Connolly SJ, Ezekowitz MD, Yusuf S, et al. Dabigatran versus warfarin in patients with atrial fibrillation. N Engl J Med. 2009;361:1139-51.

131. Briefing Information for the September 20, 2010 Meeting of the Cardiovascular and Renal Drugs Advisory Committee. http://www.fda.gov/AdvisoryCommittees/Committees MeetingMaterials/Drugs/CardiovascularandRenal DrugsAdvisoryCommittee/ucm226008.htm. [Accessed 9/23/2010].

132. Schulman S, Kearon C, Kakkar AK, et al. Dabigatran versus warfarin in the treatment of acute venous thromboembolism. N Engl J Med. 2009;361:2342-52.

133. Wallentin L, Yusuf S, Ezekowitz MD, et al. Efficacy and safety of dabigatran compared with warfarin at different levels of international normalised ratio control for stroke prevention in atrial fibrillation: an analysis of the RE-LY trial. Lancet. 2010;376:975-83.

134. Stangier J, Stähle H, Rathgen K, et al. Pharmacokinetics and pharmacodynamics of the direct oral thrombin inhibitor dabigatran in healthy elderly subjects. Clin Pharmacokinet. 2008;47:47-59.

135. Stangier J, Rathgen K, Stähle H, et al. The pharmacokinetics, pharmacodynamics and tolerability of dabigatran etexilate, a new oral direct thrombin inhibitor, in healthy male subjects. British Journal of Clinical Pharmacology. 2007;64:292-303.

135a. Legrand M, Mateo J, Aribaud A, et al. The use of dabigatran in elderly patients. Arch Intern Med. 2011;171:1285-6.

136. Nieswandt B, Aktas B, Moers A, et al. Platelets in atherothrombosis: lessons from mouse models. Journal of Thrombosis and Haemostasis. 2005;3:1725-36.

137. Nieswandt B, Watson SP. Platelet-collagen interaction: is GPVI the central receptor? Blood. 2003;102:449-61.

138. Nieswandt B, Schulte V, Bergmeier W, et al. Long-term antithrombotic protection by in vivo depletion of platelet glycoprotein VI in mice. J Exp Med. 2001;193:459-70.

139. Calvo E, Tokumasu F, Mizurini DM, et al. Aegyptin displays high-affinity for the von Willebrand factor binding site (RGQOGVMGF) in collagen and inhibits carotid thrombus formation in vivo. FEBS Journal. 2010;277:413-27.

140. White TC, Berny MA, Robinson DK, et al. The leech product saratin is a potent inhibitor of platelet integrin $\alpha_2\beta_1$ and von Willebrand factor binding to collagen. FEBS Journal. 2007;274:1481-91.

141. Miller MW et al. Small-molecule inhibitors of integrin $\alpha_2\beta_1$ that prevent pathological thrombus formation via an allosteric mechanism. Proc Natl Acad Sci. 2009;106:719-24.

142. Diener JL, Daniel Lagasse H, Duerschmied D, et al. Inhibition of von Willebrand factor-mediated platelet activation and thrombosis by the anti-von Willebrand factor A1-domain aptamer ARC1779. Journal of Thrombosis and Haemostasis. 2009;7:1155-62.

143. Gilbert JC et al. First-in-human evaluation of anti-von Willebrand factor therapeutic aptamer ARC1779 in healthy volunteers. Circulation. 2007;116:2678-86.

144. Spiel AO, Mayr FB, Ladani N, et al. The aptamer ARC1779 is a potent and specific inhibitor of von Willebrand factor mediated ex vivo platelet function in acute myocardial infarction. Platelets. 2009;5:334-40.

145. Mayr FB, Knöbl P, Jilma B, et al. The aptamer ARC1779 blocks von Willebrand factor-dependent platelet function in patients with thrombotic thrombocytopenic purpura ex vivo. Transfusion. 2010;50:1079-87.

146. RAPT Investigators. Randomized trial of ridogrel, a combined thromboxane A2 synthase inhibitor and thromboxane A2/prostaglandin endoperoxide receptor antagonist, versus aspirin as adjunct to thrombolysis in patients with acute myocardial infarction. The Ridogrel versus Aspirin Patency Trial (RAPT) Circulation. 1994;89:588-95.

147. Langleben D, Christman BW, Barst RJ, et al. Effects of the thromboxane synthetase inhibitor and receptor antagonist terbogrel in patients with primary pulmonary hypertension. Am Heart J. 2002;143:E4.

148. Raju NC, Eikelboom JW. Cyclooxygenase inhibitors. In: Wiviot S (Ed). Antiplatelet Therapy in Ischemic Heart Disease. American Heart Association; 2009.

149. Weiss HJ, Aledort LM. Impaired platelet-connective tissue reaction in man after aspirin ingestion. Lancet. 1967;2:495-7.

150. Weiss HJ. The discovery of the antiplatelet effect of aspirin: a personal reminiscence. J Thromb Haemost. 2003;1:1869-75.

151. Vane JR. Inhibition of prostaglandin synthesis as a mechanism of action for aspirin-like drugs. Nature New Biol. 1971;231:232-5.

152. Patrono C, Garcia Rodriguez LA, Landolfi R, et al. Low dose ASA for the prevention of atherothrombosis. New Eng J Med. 2005;353:2373-83.

153. Miner J, Hoffhines A. The discovery of aspirin's antithrombotic effects. Tex Heart Inst J. 2007;34:179-86.

154. Craven LL. Experiences with aspirin (acetylsalicylic acid) in the nonspecific prophylaxis of coronary thrombosis. Mississippi Valley Med J. 1953;75:38-44.

155. Lewis HD, Davis JW, Archibald DG, et al. Protective effects of aspirin against acute myocardial-infarction and death in men with unstable angina—results of a 'Veterans-Administration-Cooperative Study'. N Engl J Med. 1983;309:396-403.

156. ISIS-2 Collaborative Group. Randomized trial of intravenous streptokinase, oral aspirin, both or neither among 17,187 cases of suspected acute myocardial infarction: ISIS-2. Lancet. 1988;2:349-60.

157. Antithrombotic Trialists' Collaboration. Collaborative meta-analysis of randomised trials of antiplatelet therapy for prevention of death, myocardial infarction, and stroke in high risk patients. BMJ. 2002;324:71-86.

158. Anderson JL, Adams CD, Antman EM, et al. ACC/AHA 2007 guidelines for the management of patients with unstable angina/non-ST-elevation myocardial infarction: executive summary: a report of the American College of Cardiology/American Heart Association Task Force on Practice Guidelines (Writing Committee to Revise the 2002 Guidelines for the Management of Patients with Unstable Angina/Non-ST-Elevation Myocardial Infarction). Circulation. 2007;116:803-77.

159. Antman EM, Anbe DT, Armstrong PW, et al. ACC/AHA guidelines for the management of patients with ST-elevation myocardial infarction: executive summary: a report of the ACC/AHA Task Force on Practice Guidelines (Committee to Revise the 1999 Guidelines on the Management of Patients with Acute Myocardial Infarction). Circulation. 2004;110:588-636.

160. Kushner FG, Hand M, Smith SC Jr, et al. 2009 Focused updates: ACC/AHA guidelines for the management of patients with ST-elevation myocardial infarction (updating the 2004 guideline and 2007 focused update) and ACC/AHA/SCAI guidelines on percutaneous coronary intervention (updating the 2005 guideline and 2007 focused update): a report of the American College of Cardiology Foundation/American Heart Association Task Force on Practice Guidelines. Circulation. 2009;120:2271-306.

161. Hirsh J, Guyatt G, Albers GW, et al. Antithrombotic and thrombolytic therapy: American College of Chest Physicians Evidence-Based Clinical Practice Guidelines. Chest. 2008;133:110S-2S.

162. The Warfarin-Aspirin Symptomatic Intracranial Disease Trial Investigators. Comparison of warfarin and aspirin for symptomatic intracranial arterial stenosis. N Engl J Med. 2005;352:1305-16.

163. Fuster V, Rydén LE, Cannom DS, et al. ACC/AHA/ESC 2006 guidelines for the management of patients with atrial fibrillation—executive summary: a report of the American College of Cardiology/American Heart Association Task Force on Practice Guidelines and the European Society of Cardiology Committee for Practice Guidelines (Writing Committee to Revise the 2001 Guidelines for the Management of Patients with Atrial Fibrillation). Circulation. 2006;114:700-52.

164. Adams RJ et al. Update to the AHA/ASA recommendations for the prevention of stroke in patients with stroke and transient ischemic attack. Stroke. 2008;39:1647-52.

165. Adams Jr, HP et al. Guidelines for the early management of adults with ischemic stroke. Stroke. 2007;38:1655-711.

166. The Watch Trial Investigators. Randomized trial of warfarin, aspirin, and clopidogrel in patients with chronic heart failure. Circulation. 2009;119:1616-24.

167. European Collaboration on Low-Dose Aspirin in Polycythemia Vera Investigators. Efficacy and safety of low-dose aspirin in polycythemia vera. N Engl J Med. 2004;350:114-24.

168. The CURRENT-OASIS 7 Investigators. Dose comparisons of clopidogrel and aspirin in acute coronary syndromes. N Engl J Med. 2010;363:930-42.

169. Chen W-H, Simon DI. Aspirin response variability and resistance. Wiviot S (Ed). Antiplatelet Therapy in Ischemic Heart Disease. American Heart Association; 2009.

170. US Preventive Services Task Force. Aspirin for the prevention of cardiovascular disease: U.S. Preventive Services Task Force recommendation statement. Ann Intern Med. 2009;150:396-404.

171. Antithrombotic Trialists' Collaboration. Aspirin in the primary and secondary prevention of vascular disease: collaborative meta-analysis of individual participant data from randomised trials. Lancet. 2009;373:1849-60.

172. Berger JS, Roncaglioni MC, Avanzini F, et al. Aspirin for the primary prevention of cardiovascular events in women and men: a sex-specific meta-analysis of randomized controlled trials. JAMA. 2006;295:306-13.

173. De Beradis G, Sacco M, Strippoli GFM, et al. Aspirin for primary prevention of cardiovascular events in people with diabetes: meta-analysis of randomised controlled trials. BMJ. 2009;339:b4531.

174. Aspirin for Asymptomatic Atherosclerosis Trialists. Aspirin for prevention of cardiovascular events in a general population screened for a low ankle brachial index: a randomized controlled trial. JAMA. 2010;303:841-8.

175. Barnett H, Burrill P, Iheanacho I. Don't use aspirin for primary prevention of cardiovascular disease. BMJ. 2010;340:c1805.

176. Ridker PM, Cook NR, Lee I-M, et al. A randomized trial of low-dose aspirin in the primary prevention of cardiovascular disease in women. N Engl J Med. 2005;352:1293-304.

177. Ogawa H, Nakayama M, Morimoto T, et al. Japanese Primary Prevention of Atherosclerosis with Aspirin for Diabetes (JPAD) Trial Investigators. Low-dose aspirin for primary prevention of athero-sclerotic events in patients with type 2 diabetes: a randomized controlled trial. JAMA. 2008;300:2134-41.

178. Pignone M, Alberts MJ, Colwell JA, et al. Aspirin for primary prevention of cardiovascular events in people with diabetes: a position statement of the American Diabetes Association, a scientific statement of the American Heart Association, and an expert consensus document of the American College of Cardiology Foundation. Circulation. 2010;121:2694-701.

179. Laine L. Review article: gastrointestinal bleeding with low-dose ASA-what's the risk? Aliment Pharm Therap. 2006;24: 896-908.

180. Bhatt DL, Scheiman J, Abraham NS, et al. ACCF/ACG/AHA 2008 expert consensus document on reducing the gastrointestinal risks of antiplatelet therapy and NSAID use: a report of the American College of Cardiology Foundation Task Force on Clinical Expert Consensus Documents. J Am Coll Cardiol. 2008;52:1502-17.

181. Taha AS, McCloskey C, Prasad R, et al. Famotidine for the prevention of peptic ulcers and oesophagitis in patients taking low-dose aspirin (FAMOUS): a phase III, randomised, double-blind, placebo-controlled trial. The Lancet. 2010;374:119-25.

182. Sun JCJ, Whitlock R, Cheng J, et al. The effect of preoperative aspirin on bleeding, transfusion, myocardial infarction, and mortality in coronary artery bypass surgery: a systematic review of randomized and observational studies. Eur Heart J. 2008;29:1057-71.

183. Grines CL, Bonow RO, Casey Jr. DE, et al. Prevention of premature discontinuation of dual antiplatelet therapy in patients with coronary artery stents: a science advisory from the American Heart Association, American College of Cardiology, Society for Cardiovascular Angiography and Interventions, American College of Surgeons, and American Dental Association, with Representation from the American College of Physicians. Circulation. 2007;115:813-8.

184. Maulaz AB, Bezerra DC, Michel P, et al. Effect of discontinuing aspirin therapy on the risk of brain ischemic stroke. Arch Neurol. 2005;62:1217-20.

185. Stevenson DD, Szczeklik A. Clinical and pathologic perspectives on aspirin sensitivity and asthma. The Journal of Allergy and Clinical Immunology. 2006;118:773-86.

186. Collet J-P, Aiiel B, Gachet C, et al. P2Y12 inhibitors: Thienopyridines and direct oral inhibitors. Wiviot S (Ed). Antiplatelet Therapy in Ischemic Heart Disease. American Heart Association; 2009.

187. Herbert J, Frehel D, Vallee E, et al. Clopidogrel, a novel antiplatelet and antithrombotic agent. Cardiovasc Drug Rev. 1993;11:180-98.

188. Hochholzer W, Trenk D, Frundi D, et al. Time dependence of platelet inhibition after a 600-mg loading dose of clopidogrel in a large, unselected cohort of candidates for percutaneous coronary intervention. Circulation. 2005;111: 2560-4.

189. von Beckerath N, Taubert D, Pogatsa-Murray G, et al. Absorption, metabolization, and antiplatelet effects of 300-, 600-, and 900-mg loading doses of clopidogrel: results of the ISAR-CHOICE (Intracoronary Stenting and Antithrombotic Regimen; Choose between 3 High Oral Doses for Immediate Clopidogrel Effect) Trial. Circulation. 2005;112:2946-50.

190. Montalescot G, Sideris G, Meuleman C, et al. A randomized comparison of high clopidogrel loading doses in patients with non-ST-segment elevation acute coronary syndromes: the ALBION (Assessment of the Best Loading Dose of Clopidogrel to Blunt Platelet Activation, Inflammation and Ongoing Necrosis) Trial. J Am Coll Cardiol. 2006;48:931-8.

191. Cuisset T, Frere C, Quilici J, et al. Benefit of a 600-mg loading dose of clopidogrel on platelet reactivity and clinical outcomes in patients with non-ST-segment elevation acute coronary syndrome undergoing coronary stenting. J Am Coll Cardiol. 2006;48:1339-45.

192. JM Siller-Matula JM, Huber K, Christ G, et al. Impact of clopidogrel loading dose on clinical outcome in patients undergoing percutaneous coronary intervention: a systematic review and meta-analysis. Heart. 2010; Epub ahead of print: 195438v1.

193. CAPRIE Steering Committee. A randomised, blinded, trial of clopidogrel versus aspirin in patients at risk of ischaemic events (CAPRIE). Lancet. 1996;348:1329-39.

194. Patrono C, Biagent C, Hirsh J, et al. Antiplatelet drugs. American College of Chest Physicians Evidence-Based Clinical Practice Guidelines (8th Edition). Chest. 2008;133:199S-233S.

195. Meadows TA, Bhatt DL. Clinical aspects of platelet inhibitors and thrombus formation. Circ Res. 2007;100:1261-75.

196. Mehta SR, Yusuf S, Peters RJ, et al. Effects of pretreatment with clopidogrel and aspirin followed by long-term therapy in patients undergoing percutaneous coronary intervention: the PCI-CURE study. Lancet. 2001;358:527-33.

197. Steinhubl SR, Berger PB, Mann JT 3rd, et al. Early and sustained dual oral antiplatelet therapy following percutaneous coronary inter-vention: a randomized controlled trial. JAMA. 2002;288:2411-20.

198. Bhatt DL, Fox KA, Hacke W, et al. Clopidogrel and aspirin versus aspirin alone for the prevention of atherothrombotic events. N Engl J Med. 2006;354:1706-17.

199. Grines CL, Bonow RO, Casey DE, et al. Prevention of premature discontinuation of dual antiplatelet therapy in patients with coronary artery stents a science advisory from the American Heart Association, American College of Cardiology, Society for Cardiovascular Angiography and Interventions, American College of Surgeons, and American Dental Association, with Representation from the American College of Physicians. Circulation. 2007;115:813-8.

200. Eisenstein EL, Anstrom KJ, Kong DF, et al. Clopidogrel use and long-term clinical outcomes after drug-eluting stent implantation. JAMA. 2007;297:159-68.

201. Park SJ, Park DW, Kim YH, et al. Duration of dual antiplatelet therapy after implantation of drug-eluting stents. N Engl J Med. 2010;362:1374-82.

202. MATCH investigators. Aspirin and clopidogrel compared with clopidogrel alone after recent ischaemic stroke or transient ischaemic attack in high-risk patients (MATCH): randomised, double-blind, placebo-controlled trial. Lancet. 2004;364:331-7.

203. The ACTIVE Investigators. Effect of clopidogrel added to aspirin in patients with atrial fibrillation. N Engl J Med. 2009;360:2066-78.

204. Oral Anticoagulant and Antiplatelet Therapy and Peripheral Arterial Disease. July 19, 2007 The Warfarin Antiplatelet Vascular Evaluation Trial Investigators. N Engl J Med 2007; 357:217-227

205. Bergen PB, Bhatt DL, Fuster V, et al. Bleeding Complications with Dual Antiplatelet Therapy among Patients with Stable Vascular Disease or Risk Factors for Vascular Disease Results from the Clopidogrel for High Atherothrombotic Risk and Ischemic Stabilization, Management, and Avoidance (CHARISMA) Trial. Circulation. 2010;121:2575-83.

206. Ho PM, Maddox TM, Wang L, et al. Risk of adverse outcomes associated with concomitant use of clopidogrel and proton pump inhibitors following acute coronary syndrome. JAMA. 2009;301:937-44.

207. Juurlink DN, Gomes T, Ko DT, et al. A population-based study of the drug interaction between proton pump inhibitors and clopidogrel. CMAJ. 2009;180:713-8.

208. Plavix Prescribing Information. Bristol-Myers Squibb/Sanofi Pharmaceuticals Partnership; 2010.

209. Mega JL, Close SL, Wiviott SD, et al. Cytochrome P-450 polymorphisms and response to clopidogrel. N Engl J Med. 2009;360:354-62.

210. Holmes DR Jr, Dehmer GJ, Kaul S, et al. ACCF/AHA clopidogrel clinical alert: approaches to the FDA "Boxed Warning": a report of the American College of Cardiology Foundation Task Force on Clinical Expert Consensus Documents and the American Heart Association. Circulation. 2010;122:537-57.

211. Gent M, Blakely JA, Easton JD, et al. The Canadian American Ticlopidine Study (CATS) in thromboembolic stroke. Lancet. 1989;1:1215-20.

212. Hass WK, Easton JD, Adams HP, et al. A randomized trial comparing ticlopidine hydrochloride with aspirin for the prevention of stroke in high-risk patients. Ticlopidine aspirin stroke study group. New Engl J Med. 1990;322:404-5.

213. Angiolillo DJ, Bates ER, Bass TA. Clinical profile of prasugrel, a novel thienopyridine. Am Heart J. 2008;156:S16-S22.

214. Brandt JT, Close SL, Iturria SJ, et al. Common polymorphisms of CYP2C19 and CYP2C9 affect the pharmacokinetic and pharmacodynamic response to clopidogrel but not prasugrel. J Thromb Haemost. 2007;5:2428-36.

215. Price MJ. Bedside evaluation of thienopyridine antiplatelet therapy. Circulation. 2009;119:2625-32.

216. Wiviott SD, Trenk D, Frelinger AL, et al. Prasugrel compared with high loading- and maintenance-dose clopidogrel in patients with planned percutaneous coronary intervention. The prasugrel in comparison to clopidogrel for inhibition of platelet activation and aggregation-thrombolysis in myocardial infarction 44 trial. Circulation. 2007;116:2923-32.

217. Wiviott SD, Braunwald E, McCabe CH, et al. Prasugrel versus clopidogrel in patients with acute coronary syndromes. N Engl J Med. 2007;357:2001-15.

218. Bhatt DL. Intensifying platelet inhibition—navigating between scylla and charybdis. N Engl J Med. 2007;357:2078-81.

219. Wiviott SD, Antman EM, Braunwald E. Prasugrel. Circulation. 2010;122:394-403.

220. O'Donoghue ML, Braunwald E, Antman EM, et al. Pharmaco-dynamic effect and clinical efficacy of clopidogrel and prasugrel with or without a proton-pump inhibitor: an analysis of two randomised trials. Lancet. 2009;374:989-97.

221. Effient Prescribing Information. Daiichi Sankyo, Inc. and Eli Lilly and Company; 2009.

222. Husted S, Emanuelsson H, Heptinstall S, et al. Pharmacodynamics, pharmacokinetics, and safety of the oral reversible P2Y12 antagonist AZD6140 with aspirin in patients with atherosclerosis: a double-blind comparison to clopidogrel with aspirin. Eur Heart J. 2006;27:1038-47.

223. Van Giezen JJJ, Nilsson L, Berntsson P, et al. Ticagrelor binds to human P2Y12 independently from ADP but antagonizes ADP-induced receptor signaling and platelet aggregation. Journal of Thrombosis and Haemostasis. 2009;7:1556-65.

224. Teng R, Oliver S, Hayes MA, et al. Absorption, distribution, metabolism and excretion of ticagrelor in healthy subjects. Drug Metab Dispos. 2010;38:1514-21.

225. Wallentin L, Becker RC, Budaj A, et al. Ticagrelor versus clopidogrel in patients with acute coronary syndromes. N Engl J Med. 2009;361:1045-57.

226. Gurbel PA, Bliden KP, Hiatt BL, et al. Clopidogrel for coronary stenting. Circulation. 2003;107:2908-13.

227. Gurbel PA, Bliden KP, Butler K, et al. Response to ticagrelor in clopidogrel nonresponders and responders and effect of switching therapies: the RESPOND study. Circulation. 2010;121:1188-99.

228. Storey RF, Bliden KD, Patil SB, et al. Incidence of dyspnea and assessment of cardiac and pulmonary function in patients with stable coronary artery disease receiving ticagrelor, clopidogrel or placebo in the ONSET/OFFSET study. J Am Coll Cardiol. 2010;56:185-93.

229. Serabruany VL. The TRITON versus PLATO trials: differences beyond platelet inhibition. Thromb Haemost. 2010;103:259-61.

230. Briefing Information for the July 28, 2010 Meeting of the Cardiovascular and Renal Drugs Advisory Committee. http://www.fda.gov/AdvisoryCommittees/Committees MeetingMaterials/Drugs/CardiovascularandRenal DrugsAdvisoryCommittee/ucm220190.htm. [Accessed Sept. 25, 2010].

231. Harrington RA, Stone GW, McNulty S, et al. Platelet inhibition with cangrelor in patients undergoing PCI. N Engl J Med. 2009;361:2318-29.

232. Bhatt DL, Lincoff AM, Gibson CM, et al. Intravenous platelet blockade with cangrelor during PCI. N Engl J Med. 2009;361:2330-41.

233. Sudlow C. What is the role of dipyridamole in long term secondary prevention after an ischaemic stroke or transient ischaemic attack? CMA J. 2005;173:1024-6.

234. Aggrenox Prescribing Information. Boehringer Ingelheim International GmbH; 2009.

235. Gibbs CR, Lip GYH. Do we still need dipyridamole? British Journal of Clinical Pharmacology. 1998;45:323-8.

236. Sullivan JM, Harken DE, Gorlin A. Pharmacologic control of thromboembolic complications of cardiac-valve replacement. N Engl J Med. 1971;284:1391-4.

237. De Schryver ELLM, Algra A, van Gijn J. Dipyridamole for preventing stroke and other vascular events in patients with vascular disease. Cochrane Database of Systematic Reviews; 2007, Issue 3. Art. No. CD001820.

238. Diener HC, Cunha L, Forbes C, et al. European secondary prevention study 2: dipyridamole and acetylsalicylic acid in the secondary prevention of stroke. J Neurol Sci. 1996;143:1-13.

239. ESPRIT Study Group. Aspirin plus dipyridamole versus aspirin alone after cerebral ischaemia of arterial origin (ESPRIT): randomised controlled trial. Lancet. 2006;367:1665-73.

240. Sacco RL, Diener HC, Yusuf S, et al. Aspirin and extended-release dipyridamole versus clopidogrel for recurrent stroke. N Engl J Med. 2008;359:1238-51.

241. Lindgren A, Husted S, Staaf G, et al. Dipyridamole and headache: a pilot study of initial dose titration. J Neurol Sci. 2004;223:179-84.

242. Zhang W, Colman RW. Thrombin regulates intracellular cAMP concentration in human platelets through phosphorylation/activation of PDE3A. Blood. 2007;110:1475-82.

243. Hiratsuka M, Hinai Y, Sasaki T, et al. Characterization of human cytochrome p450 enzymes involved in the metabolism of cilostazol. Drug Metab Dispos. 2007;35:1730-2.

244. Dawson DL, Cutler BS, Meissner MH, et al. Cilostazol has beneficial effects in treatment of intermittent claudication: results from a multicenter, randomized, prospective, double-blind trial. Circulation. 1998;98:678-86.

245. Beebe HG, Dawson DL, Cutler BS, et al. A new pharmacologic treatment for intermittent claudication: results of a randomized, multicenter trial. Arch Intern Med. 1999;159:2041-50.

246. Clagett GP, Sobel M, Jackson MR, et al. Antithrombotic therapy in peripheral arterial occlusive disease: the Seventh ACCP Conference on Antithrombotic and Thrombolytic Therapy. Chest, 2004;126:609S-26S.

247. Robless P, Mikhailidis DP, Stansby GP. Cilostazol for peripheral arterial disease. Cochrane Database of Systematic Reviews; 2008, Issue 1, Art. No.: CD003748.

248. Douglas JS Jr, Holmes DR Jr, Kereiakes DJ, et al. Coronary stent restenosis in patients treated with cilostazol. Circulation. 2005;112:2826-32.

249. Lee SW, Park SW, Kim YH, et al. Comparison of triple versus dual antiplatelet therapy after drug-eluting stent implantation (from the DECLARE-Long trial). Am J Cardiol. 2007;100:1103-8.

250. Lee SW, Park SW, Kim YH, et al. Drug-eluting stenting followed by cilostazol treatment reduces late restenosis in patients with diabetes mellitus the DECLARE-DIABETES Trial (A Randomized Comparison of Triple Antiplatelet Therapy with Dual Antiplatelet Therapy after Drug-Eluting Stent Implantation in Diabetic Patients). J Am Coll Cardiol. 2008;51:1181-7.

251. Chen KY, Rha SW, Li YJ, et al. Triple versus dual antiplatelet therapy in patients with acute ST-segment elevation myocardial infarction undergoing primary percutaneous coronary intervention. Circulation. 2009;119:3207-14.

252. Jeong Y-H, Hwang J-Y, Kim I-S, et al. Adding cilostazol to dual antiplatelet therapy achieves greater platelet inhibition than high maintenance dose clopidogrel in patients with acute myocardial infarction: results of the adjunctive cilostazol versus high maintenance dose clopidogrel in patients with AMI (ACCEL-AMI). Study Circ Cardiovasc Interv. 2010;3:17-26.

253. Atarashi H, Endoh Y, Saitoh H, et al. Chronotropic effects of cilostazol, a new antithrombotic agent, in patients with bradyarrhythmias. J Cardiovasc Pharmacol. 1998;31:534-9.

254. Madias JE. Cilostazol: an "Intermittent Claudication" Remedy for the Management of Third-Degree AV Block. Chest. 2003;123:979-82.

255. Taniguchi K, Ohtani H, Ikemoto T, et al. Possible case of potentiation of the antiplatelet effect of cilostazol by grapefruit juice. Journal of Clinical Pharmacy and Therapeutics. 2007;32:457-9.

256. Coughlin SR. Protease-activated receptors in hemostasis, thrombosis and vascular biology. J Thromb Haemost. 2005;3:1800-14.

257. Chackalamannil S, Wang Y, Greenlee WJ, et al. Discovery of a novel, orally active himbacine-based thrombin receptor antagonist (SCH 530348) with potent antiplatelet activity. J Med Chem. 2008;51:3061-4.

258. Angiolillo DJ, Capodanno D, Goto S. Platelet thrombin receptor antagonism and atherothrombosis. Eur Heart J. 2010;31:17-28.

259. Becker RC, Moliterno DJ, Jennings LK, et al. Safety and tolerability of SCH 530348 in patients undergoing non-urgent percutaneous coronary intervention: a randomised, double-blind, placebo-controlled phase II study. Lancet. 2009;373:919-28.

260. Goto S, Yamaguchi T, Ikeda Y, et al. Safety and exploratory efficacy of the novel thrombin receptor (PAR-1) antagonist SCH 530348 for non-ST-segment elevation acute coronary syndrome. J Atheroscler Thromb. 2010;17:156-64.

261. Morrow DA, Scirica BM, Fox KA, et al. Evaluation of a novel antiplatelet agent for secondary prevention in patients with a history of atherosclerotic disease: design and rationale for the thrombin-receptor antagonist in secondary prevention of atherothrombotic ischemic events (TRA 2°P)-TIMI 50 trial. Am Heart J. 2009;158:335-41.

262. TRA*CER Executive and Steering Committees. The thrombin receptor antagonist for clinical event reduction in acute coronary syndrome (TRA*CER) trial: study design and rationale. Am Heart J. 2009;158:327-34.

263. Goto S, Ogawa H, Takeuchi M, et al. Double-blind, placebo-controlled phase II studies of the protease-activated receptor 1 antagonist E5555 (atopaxar) in Japanese patients with acute coronary syndrome or high-risk coronary artery disease. Eur Heart J. 2010 [Epub ahead of print].

264. Kong DF, Califf RM, Miller DP, et al. Clinical outcomes of therapeutic agents that block the platelet glycoprotein IIb/IIIa integrin in ischemic heart disease. Circulation. 1998;98:2829-35.

265. Chew DP, Bhatt DL, Sapp S, et al. Increased mortality with oral platelet glycoprotein IIb/IIIa antagonists: a meta-analysis of phase III multicenter randomized trials. Circulation. 2001;103:201-6.

266. Gross PL, Weitz JI. New antithrombotic drugs. Clinical Pharmacology & Therapeutics. 2009;86:139-46.

267. Kastrati A, Mehilli J, Schuhlen H, et al. A clinical trial of abciximab in elective percutaneous coronary intervention after pretreatment with clopidogrel. N Engl J Med. 2004;350:232-8.

268. Mehilli J, Kastrati A, Schuhlen H, et al. Randomized clinical trial of abciximab in diabetic patients undergoing elective percutaneous coronary interventions after treatment with a high loading dose of clopidogrel. Circulation. 2004;110:3627-35.

269. Montalescot G, Barragan P, Wittenberg O, et al. Platelet glycoprotein IIb/IIIa inhibition with coronary stenting for acute myocardial infarction. N Engl J Med. 2001;344:1895-903.

270. Kastrati A, Mehilli J, Neumann FJ, et al. Abciximab in patients with acute coronary syndromes undergoing percutaneous coronary intervention after clopidogrel pretreatment: the ISAR-REACT 2 randomized trial. JAMA. 2006;b295:1531-8.

271. Blankenship JC, Berger PB. Pharmacology of intravenous glycoprotein IIb/IIIa antagonists. Wiviot S (Ed). Antiplatelet Therapy in Ischemic Heart Disease. American Heart Association; 2009.

272. The PURSUIT Investigators. Inhibition of platelet glycoprotein IIb/IIIa with eptifibatide in patients with acute coronary syndromes. N Engl J Med. 1998;339:436-43.

273. Roe MT, Harrington RA, Prosper DM, et al. Clinical and therapeutic profile of patients presenting with acute coronary syndromes who do not have significant coronary artery disease. The platelet glycoprotein IIb/IIIa in unstable angina: receptor suppression using integrilin therapy (PURSUIT) trial investigators. Circulation. 2000;102:1101-6.

274. ESPRIT Investigators. Enhanced suppression of the platelet IIb/IIIa receptor with integrilin therapy. Novel dosing regimen of eptifibatide in planned coronary stent implantation (ESPRIT): a randomised, placebo-controlled trial. Lancet. 2000;356:2037-44.

275. O'Shea JC, Buller CE, Cantor WJ, et al. Long-term efficacy of platelet glycoprotein IIb/IIIa integrin blockade with eptifibatide in coronary stent intervention. JAMA. 2002;287:618-21.

276. Giugliano RP, White JA, Bode C, et al. Early versus delayed, provisional eptifibatide in acute coronary syndromes. N Engl J Med. 2009;360:2176-90.

277. The Platelet Receptor Inhibition in Ischemic Syndrome Management in Patients Limited by Unstable Signs and Symptoms (PRISM-PLUS) Study Investigators. Inhibition of the platelet glycoprotein IIb/IIIa receptor with tirofiban in unstable angina and non-Q-wave myocardial infarction. N Engl J Med. 1998;338:1488-97.

278. The Platelet Receptor Inhibition in Ischemic Syndrome Management (PRISM) Study Investigators. A comparison of aspirin plus tirofiban with aspirin plus heparin for unstable angina. N Engl J Med. 1998;338:1498-505.

279. Topol EJ, Moliterno DJ, Herrmann HC, et al. Do tirofiban and ReoPro give similar efficacy trial. Comparison of two platelet glycoprotein IIb/IIIa inhibitors, tirofiban and abciximab, for the prevention of ischemic events with percutaneous coronary revascularization. N Engl J Med. 2001;344:1888-94.

Section 3

DIAGNOSIS

Chapter 9

History

Kanu Chatterjee

Chapter Outline

■ The History

— General Approach
— Analysis of Symptoms

The history and physical examination are essential, not only for the diagnosis of cardiovascular disorders but also to assess its severity, to establish a plan of its management and to assess the prognosis. Appropriate history and physical examination are also essential to decide what tests are necessary for a patient as presently a plethora of tests is available for the diagnosis and management of the same cardiac disorder. For example, for the diagnosis of the etiology of chest pain due to coronary artery disease, one can perform many noninvasive, semi-invasive and invasive tests to establish or exclude the presence of obstructive coronary artery disease. It should also be appreciated that "history and physical examination" are cost-effective. Many tests that are frequently performed today are unnecessary and are much more expensive. During examination of the patient, the physician can gain the confidence of the patient and of the family and can establish a good rapport that is necessary for the appropriate management of the problem of the patient. During examination, the physician has the opportunity to demonstrate sincerity which facilitates to gain trust of the patient and the family.

In today's electronic age the patients and their relatives are often more familiar than the physicians about the recent developments in the diagnostic techniques and therapies. It is thus preferable (but some times impossible) to have this knowledge before examining the patient. In today's health care environment there are severe constraints on time available for taking appropriate history and to do adequate physical examination.[1] Frequently, the physicians have to order the "tests" because of time constraints even before examining the patient. Furthermore, there is a growing concern about malpractice suits and the medical and paramedical personnels are frequently forced to perform the investigations, which are otherwise would not have been necessary.

THE HISTORY

GENERAL APPROACH

During taking history, it is desirable to allow the patient to present the symptoms without interruption. Frequent interruptions give the impression that the physician is in hurry and impatient and disinterested. While taking history, the physician can observe the manner in which the patient describes the symptoms and the patient's emotional state and mood.

After the patient describes the symptoms, it is appropriate to discuss with the patient and the family to ascertain the chronology of symptoms and their severity. The patient may present with many symptoms. It is pertinent to enquire about each symptom. The major symptoms associated with cardiovascular disorders are chest pain or discomfort, dyspnea, palpitations, dizziness and syncope.

ANALYSIS OF SYMPTOMS

Chest Pain or Discomfort

Chest pain is one of the very common presenting symptoms that patients present to the cardiologists for their expert views for the diagnosis of its etiology and management. The chest pain or discomfort can be caused by various cardiac and noncardiac causes, which are summarized in Tables 1 to 4.

"Cardiac pain" may be due to myocardial ischemia or it can be nonischemic in origin. The cardiac pain resulting from myocardial ischemia is called "Angina pectoris". The precise mechanism of cardiac pain due to myocardial ischemia has not been elucidated. It has been postulated that small nonmedullated sympathetic nerve fibers, which are present in the epicardium along the coronary arteries, serve as the afferent pathways for angina pectoris. The afferent impulses enter the spinal cord in C8 to T4 segments, and are transmitted to the sympathetic

TABLE 1

Cardiac chest pain

- Coronary artery disease
- Acute coronary syndromes
- Stable angina
- Ischemic cardiomyopathy
- Noncoronary artery disease
- Aortic dissection
- Acute pulmonary embolism

TABLE 2

Noncardiac chest pain

Pulmonary
- Pleuritis
- Pneumonia
- Tracheobronchitis
- Pneumothorax
- Mediastinitis
- Tumor

TABLE 3

Cardiac causes of chest discomfort

- Aortic Stenosis
- Aortic regurgitations
- Hypertrophic cardiomyopathy
- Restrictive cardiomyopathy
- Pulmonary hypertension

TABLE 4

Noncardiac chest pain

Musculoskeletal
- Costochondritis
- Intercostal muscle cramps
- Cervical disc disease

Other causes
- Herpes zoster
- Emotional
- Chest wall tumor
- Disorders of breast

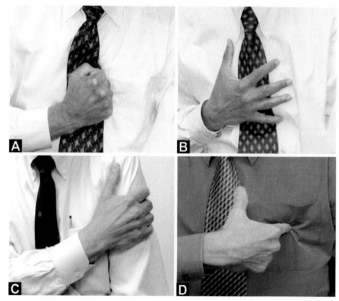

FIGURES 1A TO D: Illustrations of (A) the Levine Sign, (B) the Palm Sign, (C) the Arm Sign, (D) the Pointing Sign [*Source:* Marcus GM, et al. Am J Med. 2007;120:83-9 (Ref 3)]

ganglia of the same segments. The impulses then travel by spinothalamic tract to the thalamus. The pain perception requires activation of the specific cortical centers.

Angina pectoris is a symptom of both of chronic coronary artery disease and of acute coronary syndromes. For the diagnosis of angina pectoris, it is imperative to inquire about the character, location, site of radiation, duration, and precipitating and relieving factors of the chest discomfort.

The character of the discomfort is usually not severe pain. More frequently, it is described as "heaviness", "pressure", "tightness", "squeezing" or "band across the chest". Sometimes the patients have difficulty describing precisely the character of the chest discomfort. The character of angina pectoris is usually "dull and deep" and not "sharp and superficial". The "elephant sitting on the chest" is a typical textbook description, and frequently a knowledgeable patient uses this phrase to describe the character of the chest discomfort. However, such description is rather infrequently associated with coronary artery disease.

The location of the chest discomfort can be retrosternal, epigastric or left pectoral. It is infrequently located in the left axilla. Occasionally the initial location of angina can be left arm and hands, interscapular or left infrascapular area. When the character of pain is stabbing and pleuritic and it is positional or reproducible with palpation, it is unlikely to be angina and

the likelihood ratio is 0.2:0.3.[2] When chest pain is much localized and can be indicated by one or two finger tips, it is unlikely to be angina pectoris.

The radiation of angina pain may be to one or both shoulders, one or both arms and hands, one or both sides of the neck, lower jaw and interscapular area. The radiation can also occur to armpits, epigastrium and subcostal areas. The radiation is usually from the center to the periphery (centripetal) and rarely from the periphery to center (centrifugal). The radiation to one or both shoulders is associated with the likelihood ratios of 2.3:4.7.[2]

Patient's gestures during describing the chest discomfort have been thought to be useful in the diagnosis of its etiology. The prevalences, specificities and positive predictive values of the Levine Sign, the Palm Sign, the Arm Sign and the Pointing Sign (Figs 1A to D) have been assessed in a prospective observational study.[3] The prevalence of the Levine, Palm, Arm and Pointing Signs was 11%, 35%, 16% and 4%, respectively. The specificities of Levine Sign and Arm Sign were 78% and 86%, respectively, but the positive predictive values were only 50% and 55%, respectively. The Pointing Sign had a specificity of 98% for nonischemic chest discomfort.

The intensity of angina increases slowly and reaches its peak in minutes, not instantaneously. Similarly it is relieved gradually, not abruptly. Analysis of the duration of chest discomfort is also helpful to decide whether it is ischemic or nonischemic pain. When the duration is extremely short, only 1–2 seconds, it cannot be angina pectoris. Similarly, if the chest pain lasts continuously without remission for several hours and without evidence for myocardial necrosis, it is unlikely to be angina.

The precipitating and relieving factors of the chest discomfort should be analyzed to determine its etiology. The classic angina (Heberden's angina) is precipitated by exercise or by emotional stress and is relieved when the exercise is discontinued. It tends to occur often after meals. The original description of classic angina pectoris by William Heberden is shown in Figure 2.[4]

Chronic stable angina

Angina Pectoris: "Strangulation "in the chest Willian Heberden-1768-Those who are afflicted with it, are seized, while they are walking, and more particularly when they walk soon after eating, with painful and most disagreeable sensation in the breast, which seems as if it would take their life away, if it were to increase or to continue: the moment they stand still all this uneasiness vanishes.

FIGURE 2: Description of effort angina by Sir William Heberden in 1768 (Ref 4)

The effort angina is also relieved with sublingual nitroglycerin. The time for relief after using nitroglycerin sublingually is not instantaneous. It takes a few seconds (usually 30 seconds or longer). It should be appreciated that chest pain due to esophageal spasm is also relieved by nitroglycerin.

Exposure to cold weather precipitates angina more easily in patients with classic angina. Similarly, carrying heavy objects and heavy meals are also frequent precipitating factors. The character location and radiation of chest discomfort are similar in the different clinical subsets of angina. However, some distinctive features can be recognized in various subsets.

In patients with vasospastic angina, angina occurs at rest and usually not during exercise. The duration is variable. It tends to have cyclic phenomenon and, in the individual patient, it tends to occur more or less at the same time.

In patients with acute coronary syndromes, the duration is usually longer. In patients with ST Segment Elevation Myocardial Infarction (STEMI), the relief of chest pain may not occur until reperfusion therapy is established.

The atypical presentations frequently called "anginal equivalents" are dyspnea, indigestion and belching, and dizziness and syncope without chest pain. The atypical presentations are more common in diabetics, women and the elderly. The few clinical features of angina are summarized in Tables 5 and 6. The chest pain due to acute pericarditis, acute pulmonary embolism or acute aortic dissection may be similar to that of acute coronary syndromes.

The pericardial pain is usually superficial and sharp and may have a pleuritic quality. It can radiate to both shoulders and infraspinatus areas. Generally, pericardial pain is worse in supine position and less severe in sitting and leaning forward position. Occasionally pericardial pain waxes and wanes with cardiac systole and diastole.

The location of pain of acute pulmonary embolism can be retrosternal and may not have a pleuritic quality. It is frequently associated with tachypnea.

The chest pain resulting from acute aortic dissection is usually severe. The location can be anterior chest. Radiation to the back is common. The downward radiation along the spine is very suggestive of aortic dissection. The onset of pain is frequently instantaneous and the maximal severity may occur at the onset. The character of the pain is "shearing or tearing". A few clinical features of pain of acute pericarditis, pulmonary embolism and acute aortic dissection are summarized in Table 7.

TABLE 5

The clinical features of stable angina

Location
- Usually retrosternal, can be epigastric, interscapular

Localization
- Usually diffuse, difficult to localize
- When is very localized (point sign)—unlikely to be angina

Quality
- Pressure, heaviness, squeezing, indigestion

Radiation
- One or both arms, upper back, neck, epigastrium, shoulder
- Lower jaw (upper jaw, head, lower back, lower abdomen or lower extremities radiation is not feature of angina)

Duration
- Usually 1–10 minutes (not a few seconds or hours)

Precipitating factors
- Physical activity, emotional stress, sexual intercourse

Aggravating factors
- Cold weather, heavy meals

Relieving factors
- Cessation of activity, nitroglycerin (if relief is instantaneous it is unlikely to be angina)

Associated symptoms
- Usually none, occasionally dyspnea

TABLE 6

Few clinical features of chest pain in acute coronary syndromes

Location
- Same as stable angina

Quality
- Same as stable angina

Duration
- Usually longer than stable angina

Relieving factors
- Usually unrelieved by rest or nitroglycerin

Associated symptoms
- Dyspnea, sweating, weakness, nausea, vomiting presyncope or syncope

The severity of angina is assessed by the Canadian Cardiovascular Society (CCS) Functional Classification[5] (Table 8) or Specific Activity Scale[6] (Table 9). The use of CCS is most frequently used to assess the severity of angina, and has been proven to be useful to assess its prognosis.[7] The Specific Activity Scale, which is a more quantitative assessment of the severity of angina, is not used in the clinical trials.

In patients with suspected or documented coronary artery disease, inquiries should be made about the risk factors. The modifiable and nonmodifiable risk factors for atherosclerotic coronary artery diseases are summarized in Table 10.

TABLE 7

Few clinical features chest pain due to acute pericarditis, acute pulmonary embolism and acute aortic dissection

Acute pericarditis

Location
- Anterior chest, superficial

Character
- Sharp, can be pleuritic

Radiation
- Supraspinatus areas, shoulders, back

Relieving factors
- Worse in supine position, less severe in sitting and leaning forward position, relieved by analgesics, non steroidals and steroids

Acute pulmonary embolism

Location
- Usually retrosternal

Quality
- Deep, may be similar to acute coronary syndromes

Associated symptoms
- Tachypnea and dyspnea

Acute aortic dissection

Location
- Chest, back

Quality
- Shearing, tearing

Onset
- Instantaneous

Radiation
- Downwards along the spine

TABLE 8

Canadian cardiovascular society (CCS) functional classification

Class I
- Ordinary physical activity, such as walking and climbing stairs, does not cause angina
- Angina with strenuous or rapid or prolonged exertion at work or recreation

Class II
- Slight limitation of ordinary activity. Walking or climbing stairs rapidly, walking uphill, walking or stair climbing after meals, in cold, in wind or when under emotional stress, or only during the few hours after awakening
- Walking more than two blocks on the level, and climbing more than one flight of ordinary stairs at a normal pace and in normal conditions

Class III
- Marked limitation of ordinary physical activity
- Walking 1–2 blocks on the level and climbing more than one flight in normal conditions

Class IV
- Inability to carry on any physical activity without discomfort—anginal syndrome may be present at rest

TABLE 9

Specific activity scale

Class I
- Patients can perform to completion any activity requiring ≤ 7 metabolic equivalents [e.g. can carry 24 lbs up eight steps; carry objects that weigh 80 lbs, do outdoor work (shovel snow, spade soil); do recreational activities (skiing, basketball, squash, handball, jog/walk 5 mph)]

Class II
- Patients can perform to completion any activity requiring ≤ 5 metabolic equivalents (e.g. have sexual intercourse without stopping, garden, rake, weed, roller skate, dance fox trot, walk 4 mph on level ground), but cannot and do not perform to completion activities requiring ≥ 7 metabolic equivalents

Class III
- Patients can perform to completion any activity requiring ≥ 2 metabolic equivalents (e.g. shower without stopping, strip and make bed, clean windows, walk 2.5 mph, bowl, play golf, dress without stopping), but cannot and do not perform to completion any activities requiring ≥ 5 metabolic equivalents.

Class IV
- Patients cannot or do not perform to completion activities requiring ≥ 2 metabolic equivalents. Cannot carry out activities listed above (Specific Activity Scale Class III)

TABLE 10

Cardiac and pulmonary causes of dyspnea

Differential diagnosis of dyspnea	
Cardiac	Pulmonary
CHF	COPD
CAD	Asthma
Cardiomyopathy	Restrictive lung diseases
Valvular dysfunction	Hereditary lung diseases
LVH	Pneumothorax
Pericardial diseases	
Arrhythmias	
Congenital HD	

(Abbreviations: CHF: Congestive heart disease; HD: Heart disease; CAD: Coronary heart disease; LVH: Left ventricular hypertrophy

higher risk of coronary artery disease. These risk factors are modifiable.

Older age, male gender and family history of atherosclerotic cardiovascular disease are also risk factors for coronary artery disease, but these risk factors are not modifiable.

Dyspnea

Dyspnea is an uncomfortable sensation of breathing. It is also defined as "labored" breathing. The precise mechanism of dyspnea has not been established. It has been suggested that activation of the mechanoreceptors in the lungs, pulmonary artery and heart and activation of the chemoreceptors are involved in inducing dyspnea. Dyspnea can occur during exertion (exertional), during recumbency (orthopnea) or even with standing (platypnea).

There are both cardiac and noncardiac (Table 10) causes of dyspnea. Pulmonary disease, such as chronic obstructive lung disease, is one of the common noncardiac causes of dyspnea. Many patients have both cardiac and pulmonary disease. It is not uncommon in clinical practice to encounter patients who have coronary artery disease and chronic obstructive

Smoking, hypertension, diabetes, obesity, metabolic syndrome, hyperlipidemia and physical inactivity are risk factors for coronary artery disease. History of peripheral vascular and cerebrovascular disease and stroke is also associated with a pulmonary disease. In such patients, to determine the cause of dyspnea appropriate history and physical examination are essential. To distinguish between cardiac and noncardiac dyspnea, the measurements of serum B-type Natriuretic Peptide (BNP) or N-Terminal ProBNP (NTBNP) is helpful. In noncardiac dyspnea, the natriuretic peptide levels are normal, and in patients with heart failure, they are substantially elevated.

Exertional dyspnea can be caused by both cardiac and noncardiac causes. Exertional dyspnea is an important symptom of chronic heart failure. However, it is also a symptom of chronic pulmonary diseases and of metabolic disorders such as obesity and hyperthyroidism. Dyspnea is also a common symptom of anxiety disorders. Cardiac dyspnea gets worse with physical activity. Dyspnea of functional origin frequently improves after exercise.

Orthopnea is defined when patients develop dyspnea lying flat and feel better when the upper part of the torso is elevated. Although orthopnea is a symptom of heart failure, it also occurs in patients with pulmonary disease such as emphysema and chronic obstructive pulmonary disease.

Paroxysmal nocturnal dyspnea is virtually diagnostic of cardiac cause. After being in the recumbent position for about 15 minutes to 2 hours, the patient develops shortness of breath and has to sit or stand up to get relief. The hemodynamic mechanism is that after assuming the recumbent position, there is an increase in the intravascular and intracardiac volumes, which is associated with an increase in pulmonary venous pressure and transient hemodynamic pulmonary edema. The sitting and/or upright position is associated with a reduction of intravascular and intracardiac volumes due to decreased venous return and reduction of pulmonary venous pressure and relief of dyspnea. Left ventricular systolic and diastolic heart failure and aortic and mitral valve diseases are the common causes of paroxysmal nocturnal dyspnea.

Sleep-disordered breathing, which may be associated with dyspnea, can occur in cardiac patients. Cheyne-Stokes respiration is a specific type of periodic breathing that is characterized by alternating periods of apnea and hyperpnea. During hyperpneic phases there is a progressive decrease in PCO_2 with increased pH, which inhibits the respiratory drive; during apneic phase CO_2 accumulates with an increase in respiratory acidosis and the respiratory center is stimulated and breathing is initiated. It appears that chemoreceptors-mediated stimulation of the respiratory centers is blunted in patients with Cheyne-Stokes respiration. Patients feel shortness of breath during the hyperpneic phase. Central, obstructive and mixed types of sleep apnea are observed in patients with heart failure. The hemodynamic causes of sleep-disordered breathing in heart failure have not been clearly elucidated. Initially, the Cheyne-Stokes respiration was thought to be due to low cardiac output;[8] however, there does not appear to be a good correlation between any hemodynamic changes of systolic heart failure and Cheyne-Stokes respiration. History of sleep-disordered breathing should be enquired as it is associated with worsening heart failure, pulmonary hypertension, and increased risks of arrhythmias and sudden cardiac death.

Wheezing due to constriction of the bronchial smooth muscles associated with dyspnea does not always imply pulmonary diseases. It may be caused by hemodynamic pulmonary edema in patients with systolic and diastolic heart failure and valvular heart diseases (cardiac asthma).

There are many cardiac conditions which can be associated with episodic severe dyspnea. In between the episodes of dyspnea, these patients are relatively asymptomatic and may have good exercise tolerance. In patients with episodic dyspnea, intermittent severe mitral regurgitation due to papillary muscle dysfunction should be considered in the differential diagnosis. Intermittent mitral valve obstruction due to left atrial myxoma or ball valve thrombus is a rare cause of this syndrome. In patients with left atrial myxoma, dyspnea may be positional and may be associated with syncope. Another cause of episodic severe dyspnea is "stiff heart syndrome".[9] These patients usually have normal left ventricular ejection fraction and have history of hypertension and coronary artery disease (diastolic heart failure). Fluid retention, either from the increased salt intake or from the lack of use of the diuretics, precedes the onset of dyspnea.

Atrial or ventricular tachyarrhythmias usually do not produce episodic severe dyspnea in absence of valvular or myocardial disease. However, it can occur in patients with left ventricular dysfunction and in patients with mild-to-moderate mitral stenosis.

In patients with massive or submassive pulmonary embolism, tachypnea and dyspnea are common presenting symptoms. There may be associated chest pain and wheezing. Patients with pulmonary embolism prefer the supine position as opposed to patients with hemodynamic pulmonary edema who prefer the upright position. Arterial desaturation may be present in both conditions. A plain chest X-ray may be useful to establish the diagnosis. In patients with pulmonary embolism, the chest X-ray is clear and does not demonstrate radiologic evidences of pulmonary venous hypertension. In patients with hemodynamic pulmonary edema, prominent upper lobe vessels, perihilar haziness, and Kerley lines and frank pulmonary edema may be present (Fig. 3).

A careful cardiovascular examination may also reveal the etiology of dyspnea. For example, evidence of valvular and

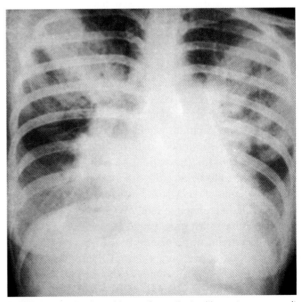

FIGURE 3: A plain chest X-ray of a patient with acute severe mitral regurgitation showing florid hemodynamic pulmonary edema

TABLE 11

Cardiac cause of dyspnea

Dyspnea
Cardiac or noncardiac dyspnea
Physical examination: Signs of heart failure—diagnostic of cardiac cause, e.g. S3, elevated JVP, positive HJR
Presence of cardiac pathology: Very suggestive of cardiac cause
Chest X-ray: Very helpful when findings of pulmonary venous congestion or pulmonary hypertension are present
ECG: Normal electrocardiogram A negative predictive value has over 90%
(Abbreviations: JVP: Jugular venous pressure; HJR: Hepatojugular refulx

myocardial heart diseases suggests cardiac cause of dyspnea (Table 11). The presence of S3 gallop usually indicates increased left ventricular diastolic pressures except in young people and patients with chronic primary mitral regurgitation. In patients with heart failure, presence of S3 is also associated with the increased levels of B-type natriuretic peptides. The presence of characteristic physical findings of significant valvular heart disease also suggests cardiac dyspnea. The absence of these signs, however, does not exclude cardiac dyspnea.

Palpitation

Palpitation is perceived as an uncomfortable sensation in the chest associated with heartbeats. The most frequent cause of palpitation is premature atrial or ventricular contractions. The premature beat itself is not felt; the normal beat following the compensatory pause is felt as a strong beat. The patients usually describe this uncomfortable sensation as "a thump", "skipped beat", "the heart is coming out of chest", "heart stops" and "heart stops beating".

The frequent premature beats may also be associated with other symptoms such as dizziness, sinking feeling, shortness of breath and chest pain. The chest pain can be troublesome and anxiety provoking. The mechanism of chest pain remains unclear; it is possible that the beat following the compensatory pause is associated with activation of myocardial afferent stretch receptors causing chest pain. The same mechanism can be hypothesized for dyspnea associated with premature beats.

During taking history about palpitation, it is desirable to enquire about the duration, whether it is regular or irregular, fast or slow, and the mode of onset and termination. It is sometimes easier for the patient to recognize the type of arrhythmia if the physician taps with the fingers to describe the type of arrhythmia. If it is fast and irregular, the likely diagnosis is atrial fibrillation; although rarely it can be due to multifocal atrial tachycardia. A fast irregular palpitation can be due to atrial flutter or very frequent premature beats.

An abrupt onset and abrupt termination of fast regular or irregular tachycardia is a common feature of supraventricular tachycardia, although it may also occur in ventricular tachycardia. The associated symptoms of supraventricular tachycardia, besides palpitation, are dyspnea, chest pain,

presyncope or even syncope. Some patients also experience polyuria during prolonged episodes of supraventricular tachycardia. The mechanism of polyuria is probably due to stimulation of release of atrial natriuretic peptide and suppression of vasopressins. The vasodilatory effects of atrial natriuretic peptides may also contribute to hypotension and presyncope.

Syncope

Syncope is defined as transient loss of consciousness. Patients with presyncope complain of dizziness and near fainting, although they do not loose consciousness completely. The mechanism of cardiac syncope is reduced cerebral perfusion resulting from decreased cardiac output and hypotension.

A large number of cardiac and noncardiac conditions can cause syncope (Chapter "Syncope"). Dysrhythmias, abnormalities of function of the autonomic nervous system, anatomic conditions such as left or right ventricular outflow obstruction, vascular disorders such as severe pulmonary arterial hypertension, acute coronary syndromes, aortic dissection and acute massive or submassive pulmonary embolism can be associated with syncope.

Acute coronary syndromes, aortic dissection or pulmonary embolism do not cause recurrent syncope. However, when syncope is the presenting symptom in these patients, the prognosis is poor.

A careful history is helpful for the diagnosis of the cause of syncope. Inquiry should be made about the circumstances in which syncope occurred, whether it was accompanied or preceded by palpitation, whether it occurs during exertion or it can also occur at rest, and whether it occurs only during upright position or it is unrelated to body position.

Stokes-Adams-Morgagni syndrome occurs due to ventricular asystole (cardiac standstill) in patients with advanced atrioventricular block. The syncope is unrelated to body position or exertion. The onset is sudden and recovery is also abrupt. During asystole the skin is pale and white and with the return of circulation, the skin appears red and flushed. There are no premonitory symptoms and after recovery of consciousness, the patients are not confused and are immediately aware of the surroundings. Stokes-Adams-Morgagni syndrome may be familial, suggesting a genetic abnormality may be present.

Vasovagal or neurocardiogenic syncope occurs during upright position and frequently after remaining in a standing position for a few minutes. The onset is not abrupt and premonitory symptoms, such as nausea, abdominal discomfort and urge for bowel movement, may precede syncope. The recovery of consciousness is gradual and patients may appear confused after recovery of consciousness.

Syncope resulting from supraventricular tachyarrhythmias is usually not of abrupt onset. Supraventricular tachycardia more frequently causes presyncope rather than frank syncope. It is associated with fast palpitations and usually occurs during upright position. Some patients with brady-tachy syndrome give history of syncope after the fast palpitations stop and the mechanism appears to be due to prolonged sinus node recovery time. Paroxysmal Orthostatic Tachycardia Syndrome (POTS) syncope usually occurs in patients during exercise and is caused by inappropriate sinus tachycardia.

There are other types of syncope which are due to stimulation of the parasympathetic nervous system that is associated with cardioinhibitory and vasodepressor response. The history of syncope precipitated by sudden movement of the head, rubbing or shaving the neck, or wearing a tight collar suggests carotid sinus syncope. The history of syncope while swallowing or drinking cold water (glossopharyngeal syncope) is due to stimulation of the ninth cranial nerves, and it may also be associated with neuralgic pain.[10]

Micturition syncope occurs during or immediately after voiding and is caused by reflex stimulation of the parasympathetic nervous system.[11] The posttussive syncope, also known as cough syncope, occurs during or immediately after paroxysms of violent cough.[12] The mechanisms of cough syncope remain unclear. A decrease in cardiac output due to decreased venous return resulting from increased intrathoracic pressure during paroxysms of prolonged cough is a potential mechanism.

In patients with orthostatic hypotension, syncope occurs in the upright position and the onset is gradual. Enquiries should be made about the use of antihypertensive drugs and sublingual nitroglycerin preceding syncope. Orthostatic hypotension may also occur in patients with diabetes, amyloidosis and other disorders of autonomic function and there may be history of impotence, sphincter disturbances and anhidrosis.

A history of presyncope, blurring of vision with or without arm claudication during exercise of the upper extremities is very suggestive of "subclavian steal" syndrome.[13]

Syncope due to anatomic causes (aortic stenosis, hypertrophic obstructive cardiomyopathy, pulmonary hypertension) usually occurs during exercise. The mechanism appears to be the inability to increase cardiac output during exercise and disproportionate decrease in metabolically mediated peripheral vascular resistance.

The convulsive disorders, such as epilepsy, can also cause syncope. It can occur in any position. There is usually a history of prodromal aura preceding the seizure. Urinary and bowel incontinence and biting of tongue and other involuntary injuries support the diagnosis of epilepsy.

Edema

Patients with edema present with the symptom of "swelling", usually of the lower extremities. Both cardiac and noncardiac conditions may be associated with edema. Enquiries should be made regarding the initial location and progression of edema. Right heart failure with systemic venous hypertension causes dependant edema such as in the ankles, feet and legs. In patients with worsening right heart failure, edema can extend to the thighs, genitalia and abdomen. In patients who are bedridden, edema can be predominantly in the back.

Chronic venous insufficiency may also be associated with lower extremity edema and a bluish discoloration of the skin may be present. In patients with idiopathic lower extremity edema, symptoms and signs of systemic venous hypertension are absent.

Generalized edema is uncommon in heart failure and usually suggests permeability edema such as in patients with hypoalbuminemia.

The history of edema localized in the upper extremity should raise the suspicion of upper extremity venous obstruction such

as subclavian, innominate and superior vena cava thrombosis. These patients may also complain of facial edema with bluish discoloration.

Non-pitting lymphedema of the upper extremity is occasionally observed in patients who had a mastectomy and axillary lymph node removal for breast malignancy.

Cough

The paroxysms of cough may be the presenting symptoms of cardiac and noncardiac patients. Patients with left heart failure may complain of nocturnal cough with or without dyspnea. Paroxysms of nonproductive cough are bothersome complications of angiotensin-converting enzyme inhibitor therapy.

Cough with or without expectoration is also a frequent presenting symptom of pulmonary diseases.

Hoarseness with or without cough is a rare complication of mitral stenosis (Ortner's syndrome). A markedly enlarged left atrium and pulmonary artery compress the left recurrent laryngeal nerve causing hoarseness.[14] Hoarseness also occurs in patients with aortic aneurysm if it compresses the left recurrent laryngeal nerve.

Hemoptysis

Hemoptysis is an uncommon presenting symptom of cardiac patients. Patients with hemodynamic pulmonary edema may present with history of frothy pink, blood-tinged sputum. These patients also have dyspnea.

Rarely, in patients with mitral stenosis and severe pulmonary hypertension, profuse hemoptysis (pulmonary apoplexy) can occur due to rupture of the bronchopulmonary venous anastomotic vessels. If profuse hemoptysis occurs in a patient instrumented with a balloon flotation catheter, pulmonary artery rupture should be suspected.

Recurrent hemoptysis may be a presenting symptom in patients with precapillary pulmonary arterial hypertension and Eisenmenger's syndrome. The thrombosis in situ of pulmonary vessels appears to be the mechanism.

Hemoptysis associated with pleuritic chest pain should raise the suspicion of pulmonary embolism.

Patients on anticoagulation therapy may present with hemoptysis. It should be appreciated, however, that frank hemoptysis is an uncommon presenting symptom of cardiac patients and primary bronchopulmonary disease, such as malignancy, should always be suspected.

REFERENCES

1. Laukkanen A, Ikaheimo M, Luukinen H. Practices of clinical examination of heart failure patients in primary health care. Cent Eur J Public Health. 2006;14:86-9.
2. Swap CJ, Nagurney JT. Value and limitations of chest pain history in the evaluation of patients with suspected acute coronary syndromes. J Am Med Assoc. 2005;294:2623-9.
3. Marcus GM, Cohen J, Varosy P, et al. The utility of gestures in patients with chest discomfort. Am J Med. 2007;120:83-9.
4. Heberden W. Some accounts of a disorder of the breast. Med Trans. 1772;2:59.
5. Campeau L. Grading of angina pectoris. Circulation. 1975;54:522-3.

6. Goldman L, Hashimoto B, Cook EF, et al. Comparative reproducibility and validity of systems for assessing cardiovascular functional class: advantages of a new specific activity scale. Circulation. 1981;64:1227-34.

7. The Criteria Committee of the New York Association. Nomenclature and Criteria for Diagnosis, 9th edition. Boston: Little Brown;1994. pp. 253-6.

8. Gottlieb SS, Kessler P, Lee WH, et al. Cheyne-Stokes respiration in severe chronic heart failure. Hemodynamic and clinical correlates in 167 patients. J Am Coll Cardiol. 1986;7:43A.

9. Dode KA, Kasselbaum DG, Bristow JD. Pulmonary edema in coronary disease without cardiomegaly. Paradox of the stiff heart. N Engl J Med. 286:1347-50.

10. Kong Y, Heyman A, Entman MI, et al. Glossopharyngeal neuralgia associated with bradycardia, syncope and seizures. Circulation. 1964;30:109-13.

11. Lyle CB, Monroe JT, Flinn DE, et al. Micturition syncope: report of 24 cases. N Engl J Med. 1961;265:982-6.

12. MacIntosh HD, Estes EH, Warren JV. The mechanisms of cough syncope. Am Heart J. 1956;52:70-82.

13. Mannick JA, Suter CG, Hume DG. The "subclavian steal" syndrome: a further documentation. J Am Med Assoc. 1962;182:254-8.

14. Fetterolf G, Norris GW. The anatomical explanation of the paralysis the left recurrent laryngeal nerve found in certain cases of mitral stenosis. Am J Med Sci. 1911;141:625-38.

Physical Examination

Kanu Chatterjee

Chapter Outline

The physical examination, like taking history, is an integral part of evaluation of a patient with suspected or established cardiovascular disorders. It also allows the physician to decide about what investigations are appropriate for establishing the diagnosis and for assessing the management strategies and prognosis.

GENERAL APPEARANCE

The physical examination starts with the inspection of the general appearance of the patient. During inspection, the physician has the opportunity to observe the patient's expression, skin color, posture and general health status. If the patient is restless and anxious, it may indicate that the underlying disorder is severe or it might be due to anxiety. In a patient presenting with chest pain, pale skin, diaphoresis, restlessness may suggest acute coronary syndrome. Pale skin may indicate anemia or peripheral vasoconstriction. Spontaneous diaphoresis is due to excessive activation of the sympathetic adrenergic system.

The presence and type of dyspnea can be determined during inspection. Tachypnea with labored breathing and inability to lie down is usually due to cardiac dyspnea associated with pulmonary venous congestion. In contrast, "puffing"—breathing with prolonged expiration—indicates chronic obstructive pulmonary disease. During inspection, the type of disordered breathing can also be diagnosed. For example, Cheyne-Stokes respiration, which is common in patients with advanced heart failure, can be apparent.

During inspection, the nutritional status of the patient can be determined. Obesity or cachexia can easily be recognized. Obesity is a risk factor for metabolic syndrome, coronary artery disease and heart failure. Cachexia is indicative of severe end-stage heart failure or other systemic disorders such as malignancy. The fragility may also be obvious during inspection

of the general appearance of the patient. It is associated with increased morbidity following cardiac and noncardiac surgery.

Mental status evaluation can be performed during inspection of the patient. Mental confusion may indicate reduced cerebral perfusion due to reduced cardiac output such as in patients with cardiogenic shock. It may also be due to primary cerebrovascular diseases such as subdural hematoma. In patients with sleep-disordered breathing, somnolence and mental confusion during the day is common.

Abnormal gait, dysphasia, dysarthria, motor weakness and other manifestations of neurologic deficits can be detected during inspection of the general appearance. These neurologic abnormalities may indicate prior cardioembolic stroke.

The Parkinsonian gait and other manifestations of Parkinsonism may indicate Shy-Drager syndrome in patients with orthostatic hypotension and syncope.[1] The patients with pseudohypertrophic muscular dystrophy, which can be associated with dilated cardiomyopathy, have characteristic abnormality of the gait. The patients with Friedreich's ataxia with ataxic gaits are occasionally associated with hypertrophic cardiomyopathy.

EXAMINATION OF THE SKIN

Examination of the color of the skin can reveal presence of cyanosis, jaundice and slaty, and bronze discoloration.

Cyanosis is characterized by bluish discoloration of the skin and mucous membrane. Most frequently cyanosis is due to presence of abnormal amount of reduced hemoglobin. If the amount of reduced hemoglobin is less than 4 g/dL, cyanosis does not develop. Cyanosis can be central or peripheral or mixed. The central cyanosis is due to intracardiac or intrapulmonary right-to-left shunt. The amount of desaturated hemoglobin is increased in central cyanosis and best recognized inspecting the buccal mucous membrane, tongue and oropharyngeal mucous membrane. The desaturation does not improve with supplemental oxygen treatment in patients with intracardiac right-to-left shunt. In Eisenmenger's syndrome due to atrial or ventricular septal defects, central cyanosis and clubbing are present in fingers and toes. However, in Eisenmenger's syndrome, due to patent ductus arteriosus, cyanosis and clubbing are present only in the toes (differential cyanosis) because desaturated blood is shunted to descending thoracic aorta via patent ductus arteriosum. The peripheral cyanosis usually reflects reduced cardiac output. A sluggish peripheral circulation, irrespective of the mechanism, can be associated with peripheral cyanosis as there is increased time available for oxygen extraction.

The bluish discoloration of the skin is also a manifestation of methemoglobinemia and argyria. Methemoglobinemia may be hereditary or acquired resulting from overdose of nitrates, nitrites or nitroprusside.

Argyria is characterized by slate-blue discoloration of the skin and results from the deposition of melanin stimulated by silver iodide.[2]

Jaundice due to hyperbilirubinemia is occasionally seen in patients with severe right heart failure associated with congestive hepatopathy. Patients with portopulmonary hypertension may also have jaundice. Malfunctions of the prosthetic valves can be associated with hemolysis and jaundice. The cardiologists are frequently consulted for preoperative clearance of the patients before liver transplantation and these patients usually have jaundice.

Bronze discoloration of the skin in unexposed areas suggests primary or secondary hemochromatosis. However similar discoloration of the skin is also observed in patients on long-term amiodarone treatment after exposure to sun.

A butterfly rash of the face is seen in patients with lupus erythematosus, which can be associated with valvular heart disease (Libman-Sachs endocarditis) and precapillary pulmonary arterial hypertension. A malar flush with cyanotic lips is seen in some patients with severe mitral stenosis.

However, it can also be seen in patients with chronic severe precapillary pulmonary arterial hypertension.

Palmer and planter keratoses and woolly hair are characteristic features of Naxos Disease, a genetically inherited form of arrhythmogenic right ventricular dysplasia/cardiomyopathy.[3]

Telangiectasia of tongue, buccal mucosa and lips may indicate Osler-Weber-Rendu syndrome, which is associated with pulmonary arteriovenous malformations.[4]

Tendon xanthoma, xanthoma within palmer creases and subcutaneous lipid nodules indicate familial hyperlipidemia, which is associated with premature coronary artery disease.

Multiple cutaneous lentigines may indicate LEOPARD syndrome, which is associated with conduction defects and congenital pulmonary stenosis.[5]

Petechiae and purpuric rash with or without Osler and Janeway nodes are features of bacterial endocarditis. Funduscopic examination may reveal "Roth spots" (retinal hemorrhagic areas with clear centers).

Carcinoid heart disease may be associated with blotchy cyanotic discoloration and also episodes of diarrhea.

Livido reticularis is a common skin manifestation of many conditions such as lupus erythematosus and the blue toes syndrome. The blue toes syndrome is due to cholesterol emboli and is characterized by cyanosis of the toes and preserved peripheral pulses and is a complication of left heart catheterization and descending aortic surgery.[6]

Diabetes can be associated with atrophic skin lesions in the legs, called necrobiosis diabeticorum and it is rather an uncommon complication of diabetes.

Lyme disease, which can be associated with pericarditis, heart block and myocarditis, is characterized by an annular skin rash with a clear central area.

Tightening of the skin, flexion contractures of the fingers causing claw-like deformity of hands are features of advanced scleroderma. The CREST syndrome (calcinosis, Raynaud phenomenon, esophageal motility disorder, sclerodactyly and telangiectasia) is a variant of scleroderma. Both scleroderma and CREST syndrome are causes of precapillary pulmonary hypertension. A few conditions of abnormalities of skin that can be associated with cardiovascular disorders are summarized in Table 1.

EXAMINATION OF THE MUSCULOSKELETAL SYSTEM

The majority of congenital heart disease with musculoskeletal abnormalities is encountered in the pediatric population. In adult cardiology practices a few conditions, although distinctly uncommon, may be seen (Chapter "Congenital Heart Disease in the Adult Patient") (Table 2).

Patients with Marfan's syndrome are tall and usually have kyphoscoliosis and pectus deformities. The arm span exceeds the height, and the upper head to pubis segment is longer than lower pubis to feet segment. The lax joints, arachnodactyly and high-arched palate are also features of Marfan's syndrome.

Marfan's syndrome is associated with aortic regurgitation and mitral regurgitation. It can also be associated with aortic root disease. The patients with Ehler-Danlos syndrome, which can be associated with mitral regurgitation due to mitral valve prolapse, arterial dilatation and aortic root disease, have hyperextensible joints and friable hyperelastic skin.

The Turner's syndrome, which is associated with coarctation of aorta, has a webbed neck, small jaw, high-arched palate, hypertelorism and low-set ears.

The Holt-Oram syndrome is characterized by the secundum atrial septal defect and absent thumbs with or without hypoplastic radial bones.

The patients with Down syndrome (trisomy 21) may have various congenital heart defects, including ventricular septal defect and endocardial cushion defects. The musculoskeletal abnormalities include a small head, slanting eyes with epicanthal folds, hypertelorism and low-set ears.

The cardiac involvement can occur in various types of acquired musculoskeletal arthritic disorders.

In patients with rheumatoid arthritis, aortic regurgitation and heart block can be observed. The coronary artery small vessel disease can cause myocardial microinfarcts.

Ankylosing spondylitis can be associated with aortic regurgitation, mitral regurgitation and atrioventricular block.[7] Valvular involvements due to verrucous endocarditis (Libman-Sacks endocarditis) and pulmonary arterial hypertension are cardiac complications of systemic lupus erythematosus.

TABLE 1

Skin abnormalities and cardiovascular disorders

- Cyanosis
  Central—intracardiac and intrapulmonary right-to-left shunt
  Peripheral—low cardiac output, increased peripheral oxygen extraction
- Methemoglobinemia—bluish discoloration of the skin
  Hereditary (rare) and acquired (nitrate and nitrite toxicity)
- Jaundice—yellow discoloration
  Prosthetic valve malfunction-hemolysis
  Portopulmonary hypertension
  Severe congestive hepatopathy
- Bronze discoloration—slaty color of the skin
  Primary or secondary hemochromatosis
  Atrial or ventricular arrhythmias
  Restrictive cardiomyopathy, dilated cardiomyopathy
- Amiodarone skin toxicity—benign
- Butterfly rash of the face—lupus erythematosus
  Valvular disease (Libman-Sack endocarditis)
  Pulmonary arterial hypertension
- Malar flush of the face—
  Severe mitral stenosis
  Severe precapillary pulmonary hypertension
- Planter and palmer keratosis and wooly hair—naxos disease
  Arrhythmogenic right ventricular dysplasia
- Telangiectasia of lips, tongue and buccal mucous membrane—
  Osler-Weber-Rendu syndrome
  Arteriovenous malformations
- Xanthomatosis—tendon xanthoma, xanthoma in the palmer crease, with or without xanthelasma—familial hyperlipidemia
  Premature coronary artery disease
- Cutaneous lentiginosis—LEOPARD syndrome
  Conduction defects, congenital pulmonary stenosis
- Petechiae and purpuric skin rash—bacterial endocarditis
  Valvular heart disease
- Blotchy cyanosis—carcinoid heart disease
  Right-sided valvular heart disease
- Livid reticularis—reticular purplish skin rash
  Lupus erythematosus
  Valvular heart disease, pulmonary hypertension
  Blue toes syndrome
  Cholesterol emboli
- Atrophic skin lesions—necrobiosis-diabeticorum
  Increased risks of cardiovascular disease
- Annular skin rash with clear center—lyme disease
  Heart block, myocarditis
- Tightening of the skin, flexion contractures of the fingers, telangiectasia-Scleroderma, CREST syndrome
  Pulmonary arterial hypertension

TABLE 2

A few musculoskeletal abnormalities associated with cardiovascular disorders

- Marfan's syndrome
  Aortic regurgitation, mitral regurgitation, aortic disease
- Ehler-Danlos syndrome
  Mitral regurgitation, aortic disease
- Turner's syndrome
  Coarctation of aorta
- Holt-Oram syndrome
  Atrial septal defect
- Down's syndrome
  Ventricular septal defect, atrioventricular cushion defects
- Rheumatoid arthritis
  Aortic regurgitation, heart block
- Ankylosing spondylosis
  Aortic and mitral valve disease, heart block
- Clubbing of the fingers and toes
  Congenital cyanotic heart disease, bacterial endocarditis
- Straight back syndrome
  Mitral valve prolapse
- Clubbing of fingers and toes
  Congenital cyanotic heart disease, bacterial endocarditis

MEASUREMENT OF ARTERIAL PRESSURE

At present, in most institutions, automated techniques are used for the measurement of blood pressure. The various techniques of measuring blood pressure, their advantages and disadvantages and pitfalls are discussed in the section of clinical hypertension.

The cuff technique is preferable to digital technique. The cuff wrist systolic pressure is higher than the arm systolic pressure and the wrist diastolic pressure is lower than the arm diastolic pressure.

The blood pressure measured by the physician is usually higher than when it is measured by the nurses.

Higher blood pressure recorded by physicians is sometimes referred as "White coat hypertension". Controversy exists about the prognostic significance of white coat hypertension.

When blood pressure is determined by auscultatory methods, the Korotkoff Phase I indicates systolic blood pressure. The disappearance of the sound (Korotkoff V) indicates diastolic blood pressure. Occasionally Korotkoff sounds disappear soon after the first sound and reappear after the release of cuff pressure. The difference of pressure at the first appearance and the reappearance of the Korotkoff sounds is called auscultatory gap. The mechanism and significance remain unclear.

The blood pressure should be recorded initially 2–3 times at 1–5 minutes intervals. The first recorded blood pressure is frequently higher than the second or the third time recording. The lowest recorded blood pressure should be used to determine the blood pressure. The mechanism of this phenomenon is not clear but it may be due to conditioning of the muscular and vascular receptors.

During the initial visit, it is desirable to determine blood pressure in both arms. The difference between the two arms pressure should be less than 10 mm Hg. In a considerable number of subjects, the pressure difference exceeds 10 mm Hg

There is higher association of straight back, pectus excavatum and scoliosis with mitral valve prolapse syndrome.

Finger and toes should be examined for clubbing. The drumstick type of clubbing is seen in cardiovascular diseases such as congenital cyanotic heart disease and bacterial endocarditis.

The bacterial endocarditis can be also associated with splinter hemorrhage, Janeway and Osler nodes and valvular regurgitations.

The Heberden's nodes, which are usually seen in the fingers, result from osteoarthritis and are not associated with cardiovascular disorder.

CHAPTER 10

Physical Examination

in absence of any cardiovascular abnormalities.[8] A significant difference in the pressure in the two arms may occur in subclavian artery obstruction, supravalvular aortic stenosis, presubclavian coarctation, pseudocoarctation and aortic dissection.

Simultaneous palpation of radial and femoral arteries may reveal a delayed onset and decreased amplitude of femoral pulse, which may indicate coarctation or pseudocoarctation of aorta and abdominal aortic and femoral atherothrombotic obstruction.

In patients with stiff calcified upper extremity arteries, cuff pressure may be much higher than the intraarterial pressure (pseudohypertension). After obliterating the pulse during pressure measurement, if the radial pulse is still palpable, it indicates stiff arteries (Osler maneuver).[9]

EXAMINATION OF THE JUGULAR VENOUS PULSE

Careful examination of the jugular venous pulse and pressure provides information regarding the hemodynamic changes in the right side of the heart. There is controversy regarding whether external or the internal jugular veins should be examined. It has been suggested that for estimation of jugular venous pressure it is easier and preferable to examine the external jugular vein.[10] However, it has also been suggested that if pulsation is present and visible, the examination of the internal jugular veins is preferable to that of the external jugular veins as the internal jugular veins are in a direct line with the superior vena cava.[11] The external jugular veins are not in a direct line with the superior vena cava and it drains into superior vena cava after negotiating two 90 degree angles.[11] Thrombus formation in the external jugular venous bulb is not uncommon, particularly in older people which may cause its partial obstruction. The lateral movement of the head may also cause partial obstruction of the external jugular veins due to contraction of the platysma muscles and cause a spurious increase in venous pressures. Occasionally the left internal jugular venous pressure is higher than the right internal jugular venous pressure because of the compression of the left innominate vein by the unfolded aorta. During inspiration, with the descent of the aorta and decompression of the left innominate vein, the pressures of both internal jugular veins are equal. However, in some elderly patients, the partial compression of the left innominate vein by the aorta may persist, impairing transmission of right atrial pressure to the left innominate vein and causing unequal pressures between right and left internal jugular veins. The right internal jugular vein is in direct line with the right innominate vein and superior vena cava. Thus it is preferable to examine the right internal jugular vein.

ESTIMATION OF JUGULAR VENOUS PRESSURE

The jugular venous pressure can be estimated by examining either external or internal jugular veins (Fig. 1). Conventionally the upper torso is elevated to 30–40 degrees and the top of the venous pulsation is determined and 5 cm is added to the height assuming that right atrium is located 5 cm below the sternal angle (angle of Louis).[12] However, a computerized tomographic study to determine the distance between the sternal angle and level of the right atrium demonstrated that the distance varies according to the body position.[13] In the supine position, the

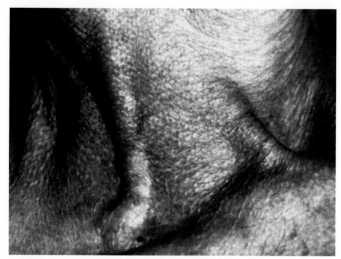

FIGURE 1: The courses of the external and internal jugular veins. The external jugular vein runs from lateral to the medial side of the neck across the sternocleidomastoid muscle. The internal jugular vein starts at the root of the neck in between the two heads of the sterno-cleidomastoid muscle runs superiorly toward the angle of the jaw

average vertical distance was 5.4 cm. However, with upper torso elevated to 30, 45 and 60 degrees the average vertical distance was 8, 9.7 and 9.8 cm respectively.[13] Thus, it has been suggested that 10 cm should be added rather than 5 cm, if the torso is elevated to 45 degree or greater.[14]

The methods of qualitative measurement of jugular venous pressure have been proposed.[11] With upper torso elevated to 30–40 degrees, if the venous pulse, the central venous pressure is usually between 7–10 cm water which is in the normal range. If the top of the venous column is more than 3 cm, the venous pressure is likely to be increased.[15]

The other qualitative techniques have been proposed. In the supine position or torso slightly elevated such as with one pillow, and the head turned very slightly to the opposite side of the neck that to be examined, the external jugular vein can be more easily recognized when a beam of light is shined across the neck. When light pressure is applied at the root of the neck, the external jugular vein is distended as the venous return is obstructed and it can be easily seen as it runs across the midportion of the sternocleidomastoid muscle, which is approximately at the same level as the sternal angle. When the inflow to the vein is obstructed by exerting pressure at the angle of the jaw, the top of the venous pulse represents the transmitted right atrial pressure and thus a rough estimation of right atrial pressure is feasible by this technique.[11] If the external jugular venous pulse is not visible in supine position above the clavicle, particularly during abdominal compression, it is very likely that the central venous and right atrial pressures are low. When the external jugular venous pulse is visible and collapses during inspiration, it is likely that that the right atrial pressure is normal. When the venous pulse does not collapse during inspiration, it is assumed that the central venous and right atrial pressures are elevated.[11]

It should be appreciated that the external jugular venous pulse may not be recognized in patients with a fat and short neck. Kinking and thrombotic obstruction of the external jugular veins may also cause a spuriously higher central venous pressure.

Sometimes central venous pressure can be estimated by examining the veins on the dorsum of the hands. These veins are distended when the hands are below the level of right atrium. The hands and arms are gently raised from the dependant position. If the right atrial pressure is normal, the veins of the dorsum of the hands collapse when the hands are at the level of sternal angle of Louis. When the right atrial pressure is high, the veins do not collapse even when the hands are raised above the sternal angle. Like external jugular veins, the veins of the upper extremity can be partially obstructed by thrombi and they are also tortuous which can impede the outflow that may be associated with spurious measurements of central venous pressures.

Thus, whenever possible, internal jugular veins should be examined not only for analysis of the character of the venous pulse but also for estimation of the central venous pressure.

Elevated central venous pressure suggests that the right atrial pressure is elevated. The upper limit of normal right atrial pressure in the supine position is about 7 mm Hg. The central venous pressure estimated in centimeter water which is converted to mm Hg by multiplying it by 0.74. In a number of clinical conditions right atrial pressures are elevated. It might be caused by obstruction of the tricuspid valve. In absence of tricuspid valve obstruction it reflects elevated right ventricular diastolic pressure, which results from right ventricular systolic or diastolic failure. In adult patients, the most common cause of right ventricular failure is left ventricular failure. Elevated jugular venous pressure is associated with a worse prognosis of patients with systolic heart failure.[16] Some of the causes of increased central venous pressure are summarized in Table 3.

In some patients the jugular venous pulsations are not visible because of the variety of reasons. In these patients venous pressures can be approximately estimated by determining the changes of the size of the inferior vena cava during inspiration. A decrease in the diameter of the inferior vena cava by 50% or greater during inspiration suggests normal right atrial pressure.[17] Lack of respiratory variation of the size of the inferior vena cava suggests increased right atrial pressure.

JUGULAR VENOUS PULSATIONS

The jugular venous pulse characters are best analyzed by examining the internal jugular veins. When the right atrial pressure waveforms are recorded during cardiac catheterization, three positive waves (a, c and v) and two negative waves (X and Y descents) are recognized. The "a" wave occurs during atrial systole with increased right atrial pressure due to atrial contraction (Fig. 2). The "c" wave is related to bulging of the closed tricuspid valve into the right atrium at the beginning of the right ventricular systole. The "x" descent is primarily due to atrial relaxation with a fall in right atrial pressure. The downward descent of the tricuspid valve apparatus also contributes to the genesis of the "x" descent.

After complete relaxation of the right atrium and the nadir of "x" descent, the right atrial pressure rises as the systemic venous return to the right atrium continues. With the onset of right ventricular systole when the tricuspid valve closes, the right atrial pressure rises and the "v" wave begins. The right atrial pressure continues to rise as the systemic venous return to the right atrium continues.

TABLE 3

A few causes of increased central venous and right atrial pressures

- Tricuspid valve obstruction—
  Rheumatic tricuspid valve stenosis (usually associated with mitral and/or aortic valve disease)
  Right atrial myxoma
  Carcinoid heart disease
  Neoplastic disease
- Right ventricular failure—
  Systolic—
      Primary-RV infarction
      Secondary-pulmonary hypertension
  Diastolic—
      Right ventricular hypertrophy
  Pericardial disease
  Pericardial effusion
  Constrictive pericarditis
- Primary tricuspid regurgitation—
  Traumatic
  Ruptured chordae
  Ebstein's anomaly
  Carcinoid heart disease
  Rheumatic heart disease
  Neoplastic disease
- Generalized volume overload—
  Glomerulonephritis
  Anemia
  Large atriovenous communications
  Isolated right ventricular volume overload
  Atrial septal defects

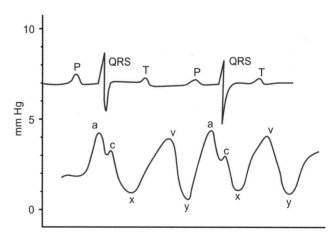

FIGURE 2: The schematic illustrations of right atrial pressure waveforms, which reveal three positive "a", "c" and "v" waves and two negative waves "x" and "y" descent. The "a" wave occurs during atrial systole following P wave of the electrocardiogram. The "c" wave occurs at the onset of right ventricular systole when the closed tricuspid valve bulges into the right atrium. It occurs just after the QRS complex of the electrocardiogram. The "x" descent is related to atrial relaxation. The peak of the "v" wave coincides with the end of right ventricular systole. It coincides with the end of the T-wave of the electrocardiogram. The "y" descent is caused by the opening of the tricuspid valve and during the rapid filling phase (P = P wave; QRS = QRS complex; T-wave. Normally the magnitude of "a" wave is greater than "v" wave and is less than 7 mm Hg)

The peak of the "v" wave coincides with the end of the right ventricular systole and can be recognized by timing with the down slope of the carotid pulse. The "y" descent begins with the opening of the tricuspid valve and continues during the rapid filling phase of the right ventricle with a concurrent pressure decline in the right atrium.

The jugular venous pulsations closely reflect transmitted right atrial pressure changes. It should be recognized that there are delays in the transmission of the right atrial pulse waves to the jugular veins (60–110 m/sec).[18]

It should be appreciated that in the jugular venous pulse the right atrial "c" wave is not transmitted. Occasionally during the jugular venous "x" descent transmitted carotid pulse induces an artifact. In absence of sinus rhythm, there is no "a" wave or "x" descents.

At the bedside, it is necessary to distinguish between jugular venous pulsation and carotid arterial pulsation. During inspection, the venous pulsation is characterized by the dominant inward movement, whereas the arterial pulse is characterized by the dominant outward movement. In the jugular venous pulse, an undulating character with two peaks and two troughs is recognized. In the carotid artery pulse there is one positive wave. Furthermore, a gentle pressure at the root of the neck obliterates the venous pulsation and the arterial pulsation becomes more obvious. The jugular venous pulsations and pressures can be varied with changes in the body position such as during sitting and standing. The changes in arterial pulsation do not occur with changes in the body position. There are respiratory variations in the jugular venous pulse. In the arterial pulse, there are respiratory changes.

A number of clinical conditions are associated with a prominent "a" wave (increased amplitude) in the jugular venous pulse. The increased amplitude of the "a" wave is primarily due to increased resistance of the right atrial emptying during right atrial systole. However, shortening of the right ventricular filling time may also be contributory.[19,20]

A prominent "a" wave is observed in patients with tricuspid valve obstruction. In absence of tricuspid valve obstruction, a prominent "a" wave results from increased resistance to right ventricular filling during atrial systole, which is almost always due to right ventricular hypertrophy. In patients with pulmonary arterial hypertension and in patients with systolic heart failure due to dilated cardiomyopathy, shortening of the right ventricular filling time is also a contributing mechanism.[19,20]

In a few arrhythmias, abnormalities of "a" wave can be appreciated. In patients with a very short PR interval, a prominent presystolic "a" wave is recognized. In atrioventricular nodal reentrant tachycardia and ventricular tachycardia with retrograde conduction, atria contract during ventricular systole due to almost simultaneous activation of atria and ventricles. In atrioventricular dissociation or complete heart block, right atrial systole can occur during ventricular systole and as right atrium contracts when the tricuspid valve is closed, a prominent "a" wave, often called cannon wave, is observed. In these patients the cannon waves occur irregularly but the arterial pulse is regular. In patients with a markedly prolonged PR interval, if atrial systole occurs during preceding ventricular systole, a prominent "a" waves occur due to a similar mechanism. The most common causes of prominent "a" waves, however, are atrial and ventricular premature beats. A few clinical conditions which can be associated with a prominent "a" wave are summarized in Table 4.

TABLE 4

A few conditions that can be associated with a prominent "a" wave

- Tricuspid valve obstruction—
  Rheumatic tricuspid stenosis
  Right atrial myxoma
  Right atrial mass
- Increased resistance distal to the tricuspid valve—
  Right ventricular hypertrophy—
      Pulmonary valve stenosis
      Pulmonary arterial hypertension
  Left ventricular hypertrophic cardiomyopathy
- Dysrhythmias—
  Atrial or ventricular premature beats
  Atrioventricular dissociation and complete heart block
  Markedly prolonged PR interval
  Very short PR interval (accessory pathway)
  Atrioventricular reentrant tachycardia
  Ventricular tachycardia with retrograde atrial activation

In a few rare conditions, the "a" wave may be absent. In patients with giant silent right atrium and severe Ebstein's anomaly, the "a" waves may not be recognized.

A prominent tall "v" wave (Lancisi sign) followed by a sharp "y" descent are characteristic features of moderate-to-severe tricuspid valve regurgitation and can be easily recognized by examining the internal jugular venous pulse. The onset of the regurgitant "v" wave is earlier and occurs with the beginning of right ventricular ejection, which coincides with the carotid pulse upstroke. The amplitude of the "v" wave is related to regurgitant volume and right atrial compliance. It should be recognized that in presence of a markedly enlarged right atrium, even severe tricuspid regurgitation may not cause a prominent "v" wave. The sharp "y" descent following the large "v" wave results from the increased transtricuspid pressure gradient at the onset of right ventricular filling, which causes a rapid decline in right atrial pressure.

In some patients with atrial septal defect, without pulmonary hypertension and tricuspid regurgitation, a prominent "v" wave may occur. The mechanism remains unclear. It has been postulated that the concomitant systemic venous return and left-to-right shunting across the defect may cause an increase in the right atrial pressure during systole causing a prominent "v" wave.

In occasional patients with a large arteriovenous fistula for hemodialysis, a prominent "v" wave is seen due to shunting of a large volume of arterial blood to the systemic venous system.[14]

A prominent "x" descent is observed in some patients with atrial septal defect. In the very early stage of cardiac tamponade, a prominent "x" descent may be seen. In severe cardiac tamponade, the "x" descent is attenuated. An attenuated "x" descent also occurs in severe tricuspid regurgitation.

A sharp "y" descent preceded by a large "v" wave is a characteristic of severe tricuspid regurgitation. A sharp "y" descent without a prominent "v" wave occurs in constrictive pericarditis, restricted cardiomyopathy and severe right heart failure with markedly increased jugular venous pressure. In both constrictive pericarditis and restrictive cardiomyopathy, the

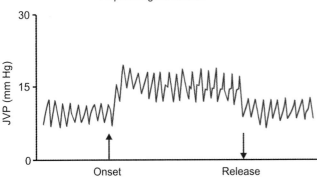

Hepato Jugular Reflux

FIGURE 3: Schematic illustration of positive hepatojugular reflux. With the onset of abdominal compression the jugular venous pressure rises and remains elevated during the period of compression. (Abbreviation: JVP: Jugular venous pressure)

mean jugular venous pressures are elevated and the amplitude of the "a" and "v" waves are similar. The most striking feature is the sharp "y" descent in the jugular venous pulse.

Bedside distinction between constrictive pericarditis and restrictive cardiomyopathy is difficult. In constrictive pericarditis, the precordium is quiet. In restrictive cardiomyopathy, a left parasternal (right ventricular) lift may be present if there is pulmonary hypertension and secondary tricuspid regurgitation. In these patients the intensity of the pulmonic component of the second heart sound is increased. In constrictive pericarditis, a pericardial knock can be heard along the lower left sternal border. In restrictive cardiomyopathy with pulmonary hypertension and severe tricuspid regurgitation, hepatic pulsation may be present. It should be appreciated that pulsatile hepatomegaly may be present in constrictive pericarditis.[21] Although the mechanism remains unclear, pulsatile hepatomegaly is no longer appreciated after successful pericardiectomy.[21]

The hepatojugular reflux, also called abdominojugular reflux, is assessed during sustained abdominal compression by applying firm pressure over the abdomen for 10–15 seconds. Normally during abdominal compression, the jugular venous pressure increases transiently by 1–3 cm. In patients with right ventricular failure, the jugular venous pressure increases by more than 3 cm and remains elevated (Fig. 3). The mechanism of the positive hepatojugular reflux remains unclear. It is likely that the failing right ventricle is unable to respond normally during volume load (increased preload) and abdominal compression. Furthermore, abdominal compression increases the level of the diaphragm which increases right ventricular afterload.[22] In adults, in absence of isolated right heart failure, a positive hepatojugular reflux is associated with pulmonary capillary wedge pressure of 15 mm Hg or higher.[23] It is likely due to decreased right ventricular compliance in patients with left heart failure due to dilated cardiomyopathy.

Kussmaul's sign is defined as when there is a lack of fall or an increase in the jugular venous pressure during inspiration. It occurs in a number of clinical conditions (Table 5). The mechanism of Kussmaul's sign in constrictive pericarditis remains unclear. It is possible that during inspiration, with the descent of the diaphragm, there is partial obstruction of the venae cavae. The physical findings of constrictive pericarditis are summarized in Table 6. In addition to elevated jugular venous

TABLE 5

A few conditions in which Kussmaul's sign can be present

- Constrictive pericarditis
- Restrictive cardiomyopathy
- Right ventricular myocardial infarction
- Massive pulmonary embolism
- Partial obstruction of the venae cavae
- Right atrial and right ventricular tumors

TABLE 6

Constrictive pericarditis—physical findings

- Elevated jugular venous pressure
- Sharp "Y" descent
- Kussamul's sign
- Accemtuated reduction of arterial
- Pulse amplitude during inspiration
- Quiet precordium
- Distant heart sounds
- Pericardial knock
- Absence of pulmonary hypertension
- Pulsus paradoxus is uncommon

TABLE 7

Restrictive cardiomyopathy—physical findings

- Kussamul's sign
- Active precordium-sustained RV and LV impulse
- Apical impulses
- Signs of pulmonary arterial hypertension
- Right and left sided S3 gallops

(Abbreviations: RV: Right ventricle; LV: Left ventricle)

pressure and Kussmaul's sign, the precordium is quiet, and the features of significant pulmonary hypertension are absent. In restrictive cardiomyopathy, in conditions associated with partial obstruction of the venae cavae, and the space occupying lesions of the right atrium and right ventricle the jugular pressure increases during the venous return to the right atrium. In patients with acute pulmonary embolism, right ventricular myocardial infarction and chronic severe tricuspid regurgitation Kussmaul's sign may be present. However, in clinical practice, the two common causes are constrictive pericarditis and restrictive cardiomyopathy. The clinical features of restrictive cardiomyopathy are summarized in Table 7. In addition to Kussmaul's sign, the evidences of pulmonary hypertension, a prominent left parasternal lift, secondary tricuspid regurgitation and occasionally systolic pulsation of the liver are present.

ARTERIAL PULSE

The contour, character and amplitude of the arterial pulses are related to left ventricular stroke volume, left ventricular velocity of ejection, aortic dP/dT, systemic vascular resistance, and the capacity and compliance of the arterial vascular system. The antegrade pulse wave (percussion wave) velocity is about

CHAPTER 10 Physical Examination

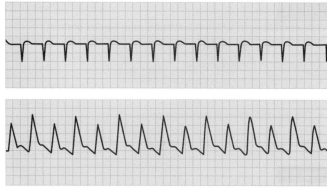

FIGURE 4: The characteristic "strong and weak alternating sequences of arterial pulses" in a patient with systolic heart failure are illustrated. The upper panel is an electrocardiogram showing normal sinus rhythm. The lower panel is directly recorded arterial pressure, showing alternating higher and lower arterial pressure

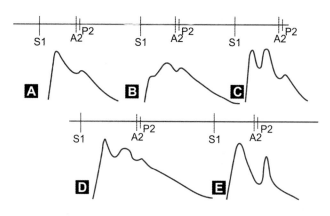

FIGURES 5A TO E: The characters of the normal (A), anacrotic (B), bisferiens (C and D) and dicrotic (E) pulse are illustrated. (Abbreviations: S1: First heart sound; A2: Aortic valve closure sound; P2: Pulmonary valve closure sound)

4 m/sec and the reflected pulse wave (tidal wave) propagates centrally from the periphery with similar velocity. As the antegrade pulse wave propagates to the periphery, it fuses with the reflected wave causing its peripheral amplification. The onset of the reflected wave occurs at the site where the antegrade pulse wave meets the resistance usually at the bifurcation of aorta. If the resistance occurs more proximally as in coarctation of aorta, the fusion of the percussion and tidal waves occur earlier and it may occur during systole. The central propagation of the reflected wave is faster with increased stiffness of the aorta as with aging and the fusion of the percussion and tidal waves occur during systole—a major determinant of systolic hypertension.

Examination of the volume and contours of arterial pulses provides important diagnostic clues regarding the underlying etiology of the pathophysiologic condition. Decreased amplitude may reflect reduced stroke volume irrespective of its etiology. Pulsus alternans in presence of regular rhythm indicates reduced left ventricular ejection fraction (Fig. 4). It should be recognized that pulsus alternans should be diagnosed only in presence of a regular rhythm. The strong beat results from the decreased afterload resulting from lower arterial pressure in the preceding cardiac cycle. The strong beat is associated with a higher arterial pressure which increases the afterload for the next beat and the stroke volume decreases and the phenomenon continues. Frequently pulsus alternans is initiated by a premature beat. Following a premature beat, left ventricular preload is increased due to the longer duration of diastole and stroke volume and the arterial pressure increase. As the increase in arterial pressure is associated with increased left ventricular afterload, the stroke volume and arterial pressure decrease and the sequence of the strong and weak beats of pulsus alternans continue despite no further appreciable changes in preload.

It should be appreciated that the absence of pulsus alternans does not exclude systolic heart failure. However, the presence of pulsus alternans is almost diagnostic of reduced left ventricular ejection fraction although it is present in only about 10% of patients with chronic systolic heart failure. In patients with acute coronary syndrome, in approximately 25% of patients pulsus alternans can be appreciated.[24]

The different pulse contours and characters are illustrated in Figures 5A to E.

The carotid pulse contour is similar to that of central aortic pressure waveform. The delay in the upstroke of the carotid pulse compared to the onset of the central aortic pulse wave is only about 20 m/sec. Thus, the examination of the carotid pulse provides an accurate assessment of the central aortic pulse.

The normal carotid pulse upstroke occurs immediately after the first heart sound. At the bedside, it is felt almost at the same time with the first heart sound. The anacrotic wave, which can be almost always recorded in the central aortic pressure tracing in its ascending limb, is not appreciated in the normal carotid pulse. The peak of the normal carotid pulse occurs in early systole and long before the second heart sound. Normally the dicrotic notch or the dicrotic wave is not appreciated (Fig. 5A).

The anacrotic pulse is characterized by the presence of a prominent positive wave during the ascending limb of the arterial pulse (Fig. 5B). It is appreciated best by examining the central arterial pulse such as the carotid pulse. The anacrotic pulse is an important physical finding of fixed left ventricular outflow tract obstruction such as aortic valve stenosis. The more severe the aortic stenosis the earlier is the anacrotic wave in the ascending limb of the carotid pulse. In very severe aortic stenosis the anacrotic wave is absent. A clinically appreciable anacrotic pulse in radial artery almost always suggests hemodynamically significant aortic valve stenosis.

The pulsus bisferiens is characterized by two peaks: (i) prominent percussion and (ii) tidal waves during systole (Fig. 5C). It is appreciated in patients with hemodynamically isolated, aortic regurgitation and in patients with mixed aortic valve disease when aortic regurgitation is the predominant lesion. It should be recognized that an absence of pulsus bisferiens does not exclude significant aortic regurgitation. The Corrigan or "water-hammer" pulse is appreciated in patients with significant aortic regurgitation. The maneuver that demonstrates the presence of water-hammer pulse is when the arm raised abruptly and filling for the changes of the radial pulse in its rise and fall. The characteristic features of the water-hammer pulse are an abrupt, very rapid upstroke of the radial pulse and a very rapid collapse of the pulse. The bounding pulse is also a feature of severe aortic regurgitation. However, it is also present in patients with severe chronic anemia, in patients with a large left-to-right shunt due to a patent ductus arteriosus and in patients with large arteriovenous fistulae.

In patients with acute severe aortic regurgitation, these changes in the arterial pulse are not observed. The pulse amplitude may be decreased.

In patients with hypertrophic obstructive cardiomyopathy, pulsus bisferiens is rarely appreciated although it can be recorded in the central aortic pressure tracing. The first peak is due to percussion wave (spike) and the second peak is due to delayed slow ejection (dome) resulting from left ventricular outflow tract obstruction (Fig. 5D).

The dicrotic pulse is characterized by an accentuated dicrotic wave which occurs in diastole (Fig. 5E). It may be observed in patients with high cardiac output as in sepsis and also when the systemic vascular resistance is high as in low output states. It is also occasionally appreciated in the immediate postoperative period after aortic valve replacement. The precise mechanisms of dicrotic pulse in these patients remain unclear.

The pulsus paradoxus is characterized by a fall in arterial pressure during inspiration more than 10 mm Hg. Normally systolic arterial pressure falls during inspiration by an average of 8–12 mm Hg. In cardiac tamponade there is a substantially greater decrease in the arterial pressure during inspiration (Fig. 6). The magnitude of the pulsus paradoxus can be better appreciated if the blood pressure is recorded by the sphygmomanometer. The cuff pressure should be decreased slowly. The systolic pressure at expiration is noted. With a further reduction of cuff pressure, the systolic pressure during inspiration is noted and the difference between these two systolic blood pressures provides an estimate of pulsus paradoxus. More severe the tamponade, a greater fall in arterial pressure occurs during inspiration.

EXAMINATION OF THE PRECORDIAL PULSATION

Precordial cardiovascular pulsations are best appreciated with the patient in supine position with the upper torso elevated not more than 45 degree. During inspection, the left ventricular apical impulse is usually visible over the left fifth intercostal space medial to the anterior axillary line. In patients with severe volume overload of the left ventricle, such as due to severe mitral or aortic regurgitation, an accentuated left ventricular apical impulse along with pulsation of the entire precordium may be visible.

The leftward displacement of the cardiac impulse can be caused by right-side tension pneumothorax, left-side pulmonary fibrosis, massive right pleural infusion and absent left precordium.

A visible subxiphoid impulse is usually due to right ventricular failure with or without hypertrophy.

An ascending aortic aneurysm may be associated with a visible pulsation over the right second intercostal space. The pulsation in the suprasternal notch may be caused by the aneurysm of the arch of the aorta. However the most common cause of supraclavicular pulsation is the kinked carotid artery.

A visible pulsation over the left second or third intercostal space is usually due to dilated pulmonary artery, which may result from pulmonary artery hypertension, poststenotic dilatation and increased flow. The retraction of the ribs in the left axilla (Broadbent's sign) is usually due to adhesive pericarditis, which is not associated with any clinical relevance.

The left parasternal impulse is best appreciated over the third and fourth interspace along the sternal border with patient in the supine position and the upper torso slightly elevated. A sustained palpable impulse during systole, also called right ventricular lift, usually indicates right ventricular systolic or diastolic failure with or without hypertrophy. Right ventricular lift is usually secondary to pulmonary hypertension. Thus other physical findings of pulmonary hypertension, such as increased intensity of the pulmonic component of the second heart sound (P2) and tricuspid regurgitation, may be present. Occasionally a palpable right ventricular gallop is also appreciated along with sustained right-left parasternal lift.

An easily palpable systolic but not sustained, right ventricular impulse is appreciated in some patients with severe

CHAPTER 10

Physical Examination

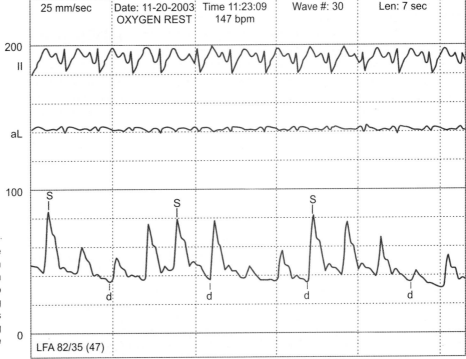

| 25 mm/sec | Date: 11-20-2003 OXYGEN REST | Time 11:23:09 147 bpm | Wave #: 30 | Len: 7 sec |

LFA 82/35 (47)

FIGURE 6: The marked decrease in the systolic blood pressure during inspiration (pulsus paradoxus) in a patient with tamponade is illustrated. The upper two panels are electrocardiogram showing normal sinus rhythm. The lower panel is directly recorded arterial pressure showing a marked decrease in arterial pressure during inspiration

tricuspid regurgitation.[25] A sustained left parasternal systolic lift is occasionally palpable in patients with severe mitral regurgitation. This impulse is due to atrial expansion during ventricular systole.[26]

Very rarely an outward diastolic and systolic right ventricular impulse, associated with constrictive pericarditis, is felt over the lower left parasternal area.[27] The diastolic impulse coincides with the pericardial knock. The mechanism for this unusual precordial impulse in constrictive pericarditis is unknown.

The left ventricular apical impulse, also called apex beat, is examined with the patient in a partial left lateral decubitus position. It is normally located in the fourth or fifth intercostal space just medial to the left mid-clavicular line. Normally it is localized and not more than 2–3 cm in diameter. The left ventricular apical impulse is usually the Point of Maximal Impulse (PMI). However, the amplitude of the epigastric or lower left sternal impulse, which is usually of right ventricular in origin, may be greater than the left ventricular apical impulse. In a number of clinical conditions when the right ventricle is markedly dilated, such as in patients with a large atrial septal defect or severe mitral stenosis, the left ventricular apical impulse may not be palpable as the left ventricle is displaced posteriorly.

The location of the left ventricular apical impulse can be displaced laterally due to left or right ventricular enlargement, right tension pneumothorax or a large pleural effusion. In patients with complete congenital absence of the left pericardium, the left ventricular apical impulse is displaced laterally in the supine position but it is moved medially in the left lateral decubitus.[28]

The genesis of the left ventricular apical impulse remains unclear. It appears to be related to the phenomenon of cardiac torsion. The normal character of the left ventricular apical impulse results from the counterclockwise movement of the basal segments as viewed from the base and clockwise movement of the apical segments.[29] The torsion characteristics are altered in various pathologic conditions.

An apex cardiogram (rarely performed in the present era) provides insights into the pathophysiological correlates of left ventricular function and hemodynamics. The initial upstroke of the left ventricular apex cardiogram coincides with the onset of the isovolumic phase of the left ventricular systole. The left ventricular ejection starts at the E point of the apex cardiogram. The normal left ventricular apical impulse during palpation coincides with the beginning of ejection, and it occurs almost

TABLE 8

Cardiovascular physical examination

Palpable precordial impulses
- Prominent systolic left parasternal impulse
  - RV failure
- Sustained LV apical impulse
  - Reduced LVEF
  - Increased LV mass
- Palpable PA impulse
  - Left to right shunt
  - Pulmonary hypertension
  - Pulmonary stenosis

(Abbreviations: LV: Left ventricle; RV: Right ventricle; LVEF: Left ventricle ejection fraction; PA: Pulmonary artery)

simultaneously with the carotid pulse upstroke or the first heart sound. The normal character of the apical impulse is usually associated with a normal left ventricular ejection fraction. The hyperdynamic apical impulse has increased amplitude (more easily palpable) but maintains the normal characters.

A sustained apical impulse is diagnosed when the impulse is felt during the entire ejection phase. The most common cause of a sustained left ventricular apical impulse is reduced left ventricular ejection fraction. A significant left ventricular hypertrophy as in patients with hypertrophic cardiomyopathy or severe aortic regurgitation can be associated with a sustained left ventricular apical impulse. Rarely in patients with severe obstructive hypertrophic cardiomyopathy will have the apical impulse bifid outward movement.[30] A few clinical conditions and mechanisms of precordial impulses are summarized in Table 8.

A palpable presystolic "a" wave or an early diastolic palpable S3 gallop is almost always associated with an abnormally elevated left ventricular diastolic pressure. The features of the left ventricular apical impulse as recorded by the apex cardiogram are illustrated in Figure 7.

AUSCULTATION

The heart sounds are schematically illustrated in Figure 8. The analysis of the heart sounds should precede analysis of the heart murmurs. The high-frequency heart sounds such as first (S1) and second (S2) and murmurs such as due to aortic and

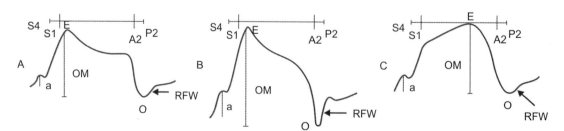

FIGURE 7: The schematic illustration of the apex cardiogram. The "E" point reflects the beginning of the ejection. The "O" point coincides with the end of the rapid filling phase and S3. The hyperdynamic impulse is characterized by normal duration of the apical impulse but the amplitude is increased. A sustained apical impulse is characterized by the continued ejection phase after the "E" point. (Abbreviations: A: Normal apical impulse; B: Hyperdynamic apical impulse; C: Sustained apical impulse; OM: Outward movement; "a": Presystolic "a" wave; S4: Fourth heart sound; A2: Aortic component of the second heart sound; P2: Pulmonic component of the second heart sound; RFW: Rapid filling wave)

SECTION 3

Diagnosis

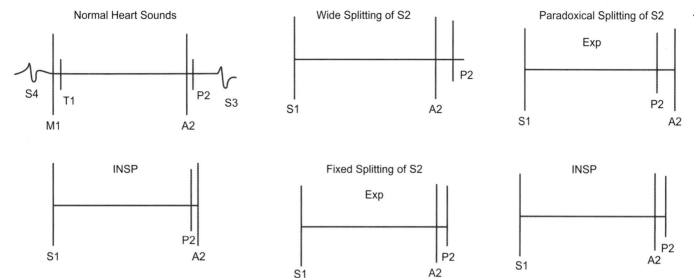

FIGURE 8: The schematic illustration of the heart sounds. S4 is the presystolic low pitch atrial sound. The S1 consists of higher pitch mitral (M1) and tricuspid valve (T1) closure sounds. The S2 consists of higher pitch closure sounds of aortic (A2) and pulmonary (P2) valves. The S3 is a lower pitch early diastolic filling sound. The wide splitting of S2 is defined when the interval between A2 and P2 is longer than normal. The A2 precedes P2 and during inspiration the interval between A2 and P2 widens. The paradoxical splitting is defined when P2 precedes A2 during the expiratory phase of the respiratory cycle and during inspiration the P2-A2 interval shortens. The "fixed splitting" is defined when the A2-P2 interval remains relatively unchanged during expiration and inspiration. (Abbreviations: S4: Fourth heart sound; M1: Mitral valve closure sound; T1: The tricuspid valve closure sound; A2: The aortic valve closure sound; P2: The pulmonary valve closure sound; S3: The third heart sound)

mitral regurgitation are better appreciated with the use of the diaphragm of the stethoscope.

The lower frequency heart sounds such as third (S3) and fourth (S4) and mid-diastolic rumbles are better heard with the bell of the stethoscope.[24]

The precise mechanisms of the genesis of the heart sounds remain unknown. The classic hypothesis for the origin of S1 is that its high-frequency components are related to the mitral and tricuspid valve closures.[31] Another hypothesis is that the high-frequency components of S1 are due to movement and acceleration of blood flow in the left ventricle and ejection of blood into the aorta.[32] In support of the classic hypothesis, in right bundle branch block, the first and the second components of S1 coincide with mitral and tricuspid valve closures.[33]

The S1 occurs just before the upstroke of the carotid pulse at the beginning of the isovolumic systole. At the bedside S1 and S2 are best recognized by timing with carotid pulse upstroke and down stroke, respectively.

The maximal intensity of S1 is appreciated over the cardiac apex. The rate of mitral valve closure is the major determinant of the intensity of S1. Left ventricular contractile function influences the rate of mitral valve closure. The position of the mitral valve before its complete closure also contributes to the intensity of S1. The longer the distance from the open to the close position, louder is S1. The shorter distance is associated with reduced intensity of S1. The mobility of the mitral valve leaflets also determines the intensity of S1. The calcified immobile mitral valve is associated with reduced intensity of S1. The PR interval influences the intensity of S1. A very short PR interval as in patients with accessory pathway, the S1 is louder than normal. The first-degree atrioventricular block is associated with decreased intensity of S1. The changing intensity of S1 can occur in AV dissociation and atrial fibrillation.

The most common cause of widely split S1 is right bundle branch block but it may also occur in atrial septal defect. In patients with severe mitral stenosis, rarely reversed splitting of S1 is appreciated. A relatively loud S4 and S1 may appear as splitting of S1 (pseudo splitting of S1). However, when the bell of the stethoscope is used, S4 and S1 can be easily appreciated. When the diaphragm is used, S1 appears as single. A systolic ejection sound following S1 may also appear as splitting of S1. However, in splitting of S1, the interval between the first and the second component is narrower than the interval between S1 and ejection sound. Furthermore, the splitting of S1 is best heard along the lower left sternal border. In contrast, the aortic ejection sound is heard over the right second interspace, along the left sternal border and over the cardiac apex. A Midsystolic Click (MSC) following S1 may appear as widely split S1. However, S1-MSC interval is much longer than splitting of S1. The S1-MSC interval varies with maneuvers (supine and standing); the interval between the two components of S1 usually remains unchanged.

In Ebstein's anomaly the closure of the tricuspid valve is characterized by a scratchy sound which is termed as "sail sound". The sail sound is widely separated from M1 partly due to the abnormality of the tricuspid valve and partly due to the presence of right bundle branch block.[34]

The auscultatory alternans is a sign of large pericardial effusion, although it may also occur in association with electrical alternans. The clinical conditions that can be associated with altered intensity and splitting of S1 are summarized in Table 9.

There are two components of the second heart sound (S2): (i) one related to closure of the aortic valve designated as A2 and (ii) the other to closure of the pulmonary valve designated as P2. At the bedside, S2 occurs with the downslope of the carotid pulse. The A2 coincides with the dicrotic notch of aortic

TABLE 9

A few clinical conditions that can be associated with altered intensity and splitting of the first heart sound

- Increased intensity—
  - Mitral valve obstruction
  - Short PR interval
  - Enhanced left ventricular contractile function
  - Holosystolic mitral valve prolapse
- Decreased intensity—
  - Long PR interval
  - Decreased left ventricular contractile function
  - Increased left ventricular diastolic pressure
  - Premature closure of the mitral valve (severe acute aortic regurgitation)
  - Immobile mitral valve
  - Large pericardial effusion
- Changing intensity—
  - AV dissociation
  - Atrial fibrillation
- Wide splitting—
  - Right bundle branch block
  - Premature ventricular contractions
  - Ventricular tachycardia
  - Atrial septal defect
- Reversed splitting—
  - Severe mitral stenosis
  - Auscultatory alternans
  - Tamponade
  - Electrical alternans

pressure tracing and P2 with the dicrotic notch of pulmonary artery pressure tracing. The ventricular ejection ends before the closure of the aortic and pulmonary valves. The intervals between the end of ejection and the closure of the aortic and pulmonary valves are called "the hang out times". The hang out times are influenced by stroke volume and aortic and pulmonary artery compliance. Normally aorta is stiffer than the pulmonary artery. The aortic hang out time is thus shorter than the pulmonary artery hang out time. The differences between the aortic and pulmonary hang out times account for most of the normal A2-P2 intervals. In pulmonary artery hypertension, the pulmonary artery stiffness increases and the pulmonary artery hang out time shortens and the splitting of S2 becomes narrower despite increased resistance to right ventricular ejection.

The isolated changes in left or right ventricular stroke volume influence aortic and pulmonary hang out times, respectively. In patients with significant aortic regurgitation or a patent ductus arteriosus with a large left-to-right shunt, there is a selective increase in left ventricular stroke volume that prolongs the aortic hang out time. In patients with atrial septal defects with large left-to-right shunts, right ventricular stroke volume increases without a significant change in left ventricular stroke volume. Thus the pulmonary artery hang out time is prolonged.

The intensity of the components of S2 is primarily determined by the pressures beyond the semilunar valves against which they close. Normally the aortic pressure is higher than the pulmonary artery pressure, and thus A2 is louder than P2.

In pulmonary arterial hypertension, the intensity of P2 is increased as the pulmonary arterial pressure increases.

There are a number of clinical conditions in which the intensity of A2 is altered. The intensity of A2 is increased in systemic hypertension, adult type of coarctation of aorta and ascending aortic aneurysm. The intensity of P2 is increased in pulmonary arterial hypertension, irrespective of its cause. The decreased intensity of A2 may be caused by a lack of appropriate coaptation of the aortic valve. In calcific aortic stenosis, the mobility of the aortic valve is markedly restricted which is associated with decreased intensity of A2. In patients with severe aortic stenosis or regurgitation, aortic diastolic pressure may decrease and the intensity of A2 is reduced.

The decreased intensity of P2 is recognized in patients with pulmonary valve stenosis and congenital absence of the pulmonary valves. Significant pulmonary regurgitation following corrective surgery is also associated with reduced intensity of P2.

The physiologic splitting of the second heart sound is defined when the A2-P2 interval increases during inspiration. During inspiration with increased systemic venous return, right ventricular stroke volume is increased. The inspiratory increase in the A2-P2 interval results primarily due to the increased pulmonary hang out time, although slight prolongation of right ventricular ejection time may also be contributory. The paradoxical or reversed splitting of S2 is defined when A2 follows P2 during expiration and the P2-A2 interval decreases during inspiration. The most common cause of paradoxical splitting of S2 is left bundle branch block.

It is also appreciated in patients with right ventricular pacing and accessory pathway with right ventricular connection. Paradoxical splitting also occurs when there is a selective increase in left ventricular stroke volume as in patients with severe aortic regurgitation or with a large patent ductus arteriosus. The increase in left ventricular stroke volume is associated with prolongation of left ventricular ejection time as well as increased aortic hang out time. A substantial increase in left ventricular outflow resistance, such as severe aortic stenosis, hypertrophic obstructive cardiomyopathy and hypertension, may also be associated with paradoxical splitting of S2.

The fixed splitting of S2 is defined when the variation in the A2-P2 interval is 20 m/sec or less during the inspiratory and expiratory cycles of respiration. The secundum type of atrial septal defect is the most common cause of fixed splitting of S2. During inspiration the magnitude of left-to-right shunt decreases and during expiratory phase the left-to-right shunt increases. A large atrial septal defect is associated with shortening of left ventricular ejection time without any change in right ventricular ejection time.[35] However, the increase in pulmonary artery hang out time due to decreased pulmonary vascular impedance appears to be the principal mechanism of the "fixed splitting" of S2.

Severe right ventricular failure may also be associated with fixed splitting of S2. Right ventricle is unable to handle the inspiratory increase in the systemic venous return. Thus, there is very little variation in right ventricular ejection time during the respiratory cycle.

The wide splitting of S2 is most common in patients with conduction abnormalities such as right bundle branch block.

TABLE 10

A few clinical conditions that may be associated with changes in intensity and splitting of the second heart sound

Increased intensity of A2:	Systemic hypertension
	Coarctation of the aorta
	Ascending aortic aneurysm
Decreased intensity of A2:	Calcific aortic stenosis
	Severe aortic regurgitation
Increased intensity of P2:	Pulmonary arterial hypertension
	Peripheral pulmonary artery branch stenosis
	Idiopathic dilatation of the pulmonary artery
Decreased intensity of P2:	Pulmonary valve stenosis
	Congenital absence of pulmonary valve
Wide splitting of S2:	Right bundle branch block
	Left ventricular pacing
	Accessory pathway with left ventricular preexcitation
	Premature beats of left ventricular origin
	Fascicular tachycardia
	Right ventricular outflow obstruction
	Pulmonary arterial hypertension
Wide and "fixed" splitting of S2:	Atrial septal defects
	Common atrium
	Right ventricular failure
Reversed (paradoxic) splitting of S2:	Left bundle branch block
	Right ventricular pacing
	Accessory pathway with right ventricular preexcitation
	Premature beats of right ventricular origin
	Right ventricular tachycardia
	Severe aortic regurgitation
	Large patent ductus arteriosus
	Left ventricular outflow obstruction
	Systemic hypertension
	Severe tricuspid regurgitation (rare)
Single S2:	Eisenmenger syndrome with ventricular septal defect
	Single ventricle

(Abbreviations: A2: Aortic component of the second heart sound; P2: Pulmonic component of the second heart sound; S2: Second heart sound)

It is also appreciated in some patients with accessory pathways with initial activation of the left ventricle.

A single S2 can occur when A2 and P2 are fused due to almost equal right and left ventricular ejection time as in patients with Eisenmenger's syndrome with ventricular septal defect or a single ventricle. In some conditions A2 may be absent such as severe aortic regurgitation resulting from bacterial endocarditis. In congenital absence of the pulmonary valve, P2 is absent. In patients with severe right ventricular outflow obstruction, the intensity of P2 is markedly reduced and S2 may appear single. A few clinical conditions which may be associated with changes in the intensity and splitting of S2 are summarized in Table 10.

THIRD (S3) AND FOURTH (S4) HEART SOUNDS

The S3 and S4 are low pitch sounds and originate in the ventricles. They are often termed ventricular filling sounds and are associated with ventricular filling and an increase in ventricular dimensions. The S3 occurs with the beginning of passive ventricular filling after the relaxation is completed. It coincides with end of the rapid filling phase of the apex-cardiogram. The S4 occurs during atrial systole. Both S3 and S4 are better appreciated with the bell of the stethoscope. The S3 is close to the second heart sound and occurs after the down stroke of the carotid pulse. The S4 is close to the first heart sound and occurs just before the upstroke of the carotid pulse.

The left ventricular S3 and S4 are best heard over cardiac apex in the left lateral decubitus position. The right ventricular S3 and S4 are best heard along the lower left sternal border. Occasionally right ventricular filling sounds are also heard over the lower right sternal border. The intensity of right ventricular S3 and S4 increases during inspiration. The S3 can be appreciated in healthy adults younger than 40 years old. It is considered abnormal if it is heard in subjects older than 40 years. The S4 is usually abnormal in children and young adults. With decreased left ventricular compliance as occurs with aging, S4 can be appreciated in many older individuals without any cardiac abnormality.

It may be sometimes difficult to distinguish between splitting of S2 from S2-S3 when S3 is present. Similarly, splitting of S1 may be difficult to distinguish from S4-S1. The bell-diaphragm technique of auscultation may be useful. As both S3 and S4 are low pitch sounds, when the bell of the stethoscope is used, these sounds become more obvious. When the diaphragm of the stethoscope is used, S3 and S4 low pitch sounds are either no longer heard or become very muffled. As the M1 and T1 components of S1 and A2 and P2 components of S2 are high-pitch sounds, they become sharper and more easily heard.

When S3 or S4 are louder and have relatively higher pitch, they sound like gallops (like horse's gallop) and are called gallop sounds. The S3 and S4 are ventricular and atrial gallops, respectively. The gallop sounds usually reflect elevated ventricular end-diastolic pressures. Left ventricular S3 gallop is also associated with elevated plasma levels of B-type natriuretic peptide.[36,37] Both presence of S3 and elevated jugular venous pressure are also associated with worse prognosis in patients with systolic heart failure.[38]

Pericardial Knock

It is a common auscultatory finding in constrictive pericarditis. It occurs in diastole and its timing is earlier than that of S3.

Ejection Sounds

The ejection sounds are related to the opening of the semilunar valves at the beginning of the ventricular ejection. The aortic ejection sound is related to the opening of the aortic valve and the pulmonary ejection sound is that of opening of the pulmonary valve. The intensity of the aortic ejection sound does not vary during the respiratory phase. The intensity of the pulmonary ejection sound however decreases during inspiration. During inspiration there is a slow upward movement of the pulmonary valve before it starts opening. This slow ascent of the pulmonary valve is associated with decreased intensity of the pulmonary ejection sound as the sudden "halting" is the mechanism of the ejection sound.

The conditions that may be associated with aortic ejection sound are aortic valve stenosis, aortic regurgitation and bicuspid aortic valve. The conditions that may be associated with pulmonary ejection sound are pulmonary valve stenosis, pulmonary hypertension, pulmonary regurgitation and idiopathic dilatation of the pulmonary artery.

In some patients with hypertrophic obstructive cardio-myopathy, a nonejection sound is heard which is called pseudoejection sound. It coincides with anterior systolic motion of the mitral valve.[39] This sound occurs later than aortic ejection sound. It has been suggested that it may result from the contact of the mitral valve with the interventricular septum during systole or from the deceleration of blood flow in the left ventricular outflow tract.

Midsystolic Click

The prolapse of the mitral valve is the most common cause of midsystolic clicks. The S1-MSC interval is longer than the S4-S1 or M1-T1 intervals. In mitral valve prolapse, in a given patient the click diameter of the left ventricle is fixed. The S1-

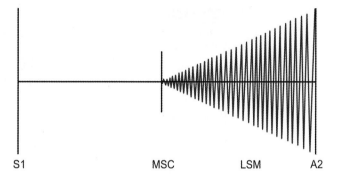

FIGURE 9: The schematic illustration of the auscultatory findings of midsystolic click—late systolic murmur syndrome due to mitral valve prolapse. (Abbreviations: S1: The first heart sound; MSC: Midsystolic click; LSM: Late systolic murmur)

TABLE 11

The maneuvers that influence the S1 and midsystolic click interval and the duration of the late systolic murmur in mitral valve prolapse are summarized

MSC-LSM	
Supine S1	MSC increased, LSM shorter
Standing S1	MSC shorter, LSM longer
Squatting S1	MSC increased, LSM shorter
Post-PMB S1	MSC shorter, LSM longer
S1-MSC = the first heart sound midsystolic click interval;	
LSM = late systolic murmur;	
PMB = post-premature beat	

(Abbreviations: MSC: Midsystolic click; S1: First heart sound)

MSC intervals vary with changes in left ventricular volumes. During the supine position the S1-MSC interval is longer because the left ventricular end-diastolic volume is larger and the click diameter is reached later. The duration of the late systolic murmur is shorter. In the upright position the left ventricular end-diastolic volume is smaller and the click diameter is reached earlier and the S1-MSC interval is shorter. The duration of the late systolic murmur is longer. Following a post-ectopic beat, the click diameter is reached earlier because of more rapid ejection due to post-ectopic potentiation and the S1-MSC interval is shorter and the duration of the late systolic murmur is longer. In Figure 9, the auscultatory findings of mitral valve prolapse are schematically illustrated. In Table 11, the maneuvers that change the S1-MSC interval and the duration of the late systolic murmur are summarized.

In some patients with mitral valve prolapse, brief musical systolic murmurs often preceded by clicks are heard in mid-systole or late systole. These murmurs are called systolic "whoop" or "precordial honk".[40]

Early Diastolic High-Frequency Sounds

The high-pitch sounds associated with the opening of the mitral or tricuspid valves are called opening snaps and occur in early diastole. These sounds coincide with their rapid opening to the maximal open position and are appreciated in patients with mitral or tricuspid valve stenosis. The opening snaps are best heard with the diaphragm of the stethoscope.

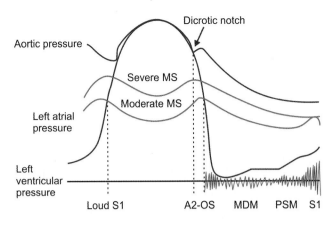

FIGURE 10: The schematic illustrations of aortic, left atrial and left ventricular pressure tracings in patients with mitral stenosis. The A2-OS interval is shorter in patients with more severe mitral stenosis than in patients with milder mitral stenosis. (Abbreviations: A2: Aortic valve closure; OS: Opening snap; MDM: Mid-diastolic murmur; PSM: Pre-systolic murmur; MS: Mitral stenosis; S1: The first heart sound)

The opening snap of mitral stenosis is better appreciated over the mitral area just medial to the apex with the patient in the left lateral position. It can be widely transmitted and can be heard over the left second intercostal space. The opening snap following A2 can be mistaken as widely split S2. However, widely split S2 is uncommon in absence of right bundle branch block. Furthermore, if the intensity of P2 is increased, three high-pitch sounds, A2, P2 and opening snap, can be appreciated over the left second intercostal space particularly during inspiration.

A mobile mitral valve leaflet is necessary for the genesis of the opening snap. It is absent in patients with a heavily calcified immobile mitral valve.

However, opening snap is present in the majority of patients with mitral stenosis and its presence along with a loud S1 provides a clue to its diagnosis.

The interval between A2 and the opening snap (A2-OS) is inversely related to the severity of mitral stenosis. The shorter the A2-OS interval, more severe is the mitral stenosis. With severe mitral stenosis, the gradient across the mitral valve is increased and the interval between closing pressure of the aortic valve and opening pressure of the mitral valve is shorter (Fig. 10). When the mitral stenosis is mild the A2-OS interval is longer. It should be appreciated that A2-OS interval should be assessed when the heart rate is relatively normal. Tachycardia is associated with a shorter A2-OS interval for the same severity of mitral stenosis.

As the A2-OS interval is also related to the closing pressure of the aortic valve, the conditions that are associated lower aortic valve closing pressure such as severe aortic stenosis or regurgitation. The A2-OS interval is shorter despite mild mitral stenosis. Thus, severity of mitral stenosis cannot be assessed in patients with coexisting aortic stenosis or regurgitation.

The tricuspid valve opening snap is usually heard in significant tricuspid valve stenosis. It is localized and associated with low pitch mid-diastolic murmur and best heard over the lower left sternal border.

Occasionally, tricuspid opening snap is appreciated in patients with an atrial septal defect and a large left-to-right

shunt.[41]

In atrial myxoma, the movement of the tumors into the ventricle with the opening of the mitral or tricuspid valve may be associated with a high-pitch sound, which is termed as "tumor plop". Similarly, the movement of large mobile vegetation can be associated with a similar sound, which is called "vegetation plop".

A high-frequency sound associated with a rapid inward movement of the prolapsed mitral valve may appear as opening snap.[42]

In occasional patients with hypertrophic cardiomyopathy with a small left ventricular cavity, high-pitch sounds are heard in early diastole coinciding with the time of contact of the anterior leaflet of the mitral valve to the interventricular septum.[43] This sound is often termed "opening slap".

The friction rub associated with pericarditis is produced by the friction of the parietal and visceral layers of the pericardium, and has a scratchy quality. It can be heard during atrial systole, ventricular systole and the rapid filling phase (three-component rub). However, it can be heard only during one or two phases of the cardiac cycle. A firm pressure with the diaphragm of the stethoscope frequently increases its intensity. The intensity may also increase during held inspiration with the patient leaning forward. The pericardial rub may be localized or widespread. Occasionally it is heard only along the lower right sternal border.

Overt hyperthyroidism is occasionally associated with a superficial "scratchy" high-pitch sound, which is called Means-Lerman scratch.

Mediastinal emphysema can cause crunching sounds, which are called mediastinal crunch. It occurs not infrequently after open heart surgery and it is benign.

Superficial scratchy sounds during systole due to the movement of the transvenous pacemakers or balloon floatation catheters across the tricuspid valve can be heard in some patients along the lower left sternal border and should not be confused with tricuspid regurgitation murmur or pericardial friction rub.

The pacemaker sounds are high-frequency sounds which occur due to stimulation of the intercostal muscles and they are unrelated to the cardiac cycle.

The presence of a relatively large amount of air (not small air bubbles) in the right ventricular cavity is associated with loud sloshing noises, which can be heard over the entire precordium. These noises sound like loud peculiar murmur and are called "mill wheel murmur".[44]

Artificial Valve Sounds

The opening and closing sounds of both mechanical and bioprosthesis are high-pitch sounds. The closing and opening sounds of mechanical prosthesis have a "clicky" character and there may be multiple clicks. The intensity of the closing clicks is louder than that of opening clicks in bileaflet mechanical prosthesis. With ball and cage mechanical valves, the closing and opening clicks are loud and may be of similar intensity. The closing or opening sounds with bioprosthesis do not have a "clicky" character but the closing sound is much louder.

TABLE 12

The timing and characters of the various types of murmurs

Systolic murmurs
- Ejection systolic starts after S1 and does not extend to S2
- Pansystolic starts with S1 and extends to S2 (mitral, tricuspid regurgitation, VSD)
- Early systolic starts with S1 and does not extend to S2 (mitral, tricuspid regurgitation, VSD)
- Late systolic starts after S1 and extends to S2 (mild MR or TR)

Diastolic murmurs
- Early diastolic starts with S2 (AI, PI)
- Mid diastolic starts after S2 (MS, TS, AFM)
- Presystolic starts after S2 and extends to S1 (MS, AFM)
- Continuous murmurs—encompass both systole and diastole (arteriovenous communication—PDA, AV fistula, mammary shuffle)

Abbreviations: PDA: Patent ductus arteriosus; AV: Atrioventricuar; AFM: Austin-Flint murmur; TS: Tricuspid stenosis; MS: Mitral stenosis; AI: Aortic insufficiency; PI: Pulmonary insufficiency; MR: Mitral regurgitation; TR: Tricuspid regurgitation; VSD: Ventricular septal defect; AS: Aortic stenosis; PS: Pulmonary stenosis

The changes in the normal sounds associated with prosthetic valves may indicate their malfunction. However, malfunction of the prosthetic valve can exist without any changes in the prosthetic sounds.

AUSCULTATION OF HEART MURMURS

The various types of cardiac murmurs and some of their causes are summarized in Table 12. In clinical practice, significant valvular heart disease is first diagnosed by detecting a murmur. Detection of murmur by auscultation has a sensitivity of 70% and a specificity of 98%.[45] The guidelines recommend that all patients with suspected valvular heart disease should have echocardiography for establishing the cause of the murmur.[46]

The murmurs can be systolic, diastolic or continuous. The systolic murmurs are further classified as midsystolic (ejection) murmurs or regurgitant murmurs. The ejection systolic murmurs are related to left or right ventricular ejection to aorta or pulmonary artery, respectively. By definition, ejection systolic murmur begins after S1 and at the end of isovolumic systole. The interval between S1 and the onset of the murmur is related to the duration of the isovolumic systole. It ends at the end of ejection and before the closure of the semilunar valves, i.e. before A2 and P2. The interval between the end of the murmur and A2 or P2 is related to the duration of aortic or pulmonary hang out times. The intensity of the ejection systolic murmur increases (crescendo) during acceleration of blood flow in early systole and the intensity decreases (decrescendo) with deceleration of flow in late systole (the crescendo-decrescendo murmurs).

The regurgitant systolic murmurs are classified into: (1) holosystolic or pansystolic—the murmur starts with S1 and terminates at or after S2; (2) the early systolic murmur starts with S1 and ends before S2 and (3) the late systolic murmur starts after S1 and terminates at S2.

The diastolic murmurs are classified into: (1) early diastolic murmur which begins with S2 and terminates before S1; (2) mid-diastolic murmur which starts after S2 and ends at or before

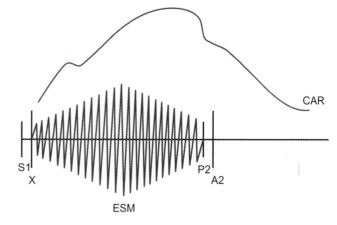

FIGURE 11: The schematic illustrations of the characters of the ejection systolic murmur and changes in carotid pulse in aortic valve stenosis. (Abbreviations: S1: First heart sound; A2: Aortic valve closure sound; P2: Pulmonary valve closure sound; ESM: Ejection systolic murmur; X: Aortic ejection sound; CAR: Carotid pulse)

S1 and (3) late diastolic or presystolic murmur which starts in late diastole after S2 and terminates at S1.

The continuous murmurs begin in systole and continue into diastole.

The intensity of a murmur is conventionally graded into six grades. Grade I is the faintest murmur that can be heard. Grade II is also a faint murmur but can be heard easily. Grade III is a moderately loud murmur. Grade IV murmur is a loud murmur associated with a palpable thrill. Grade V is a very loud murmur but cannot be heard without the stethoscope. Grade VI is the loudest murmur and can be heard without a stethoscope.

It should be appreciated that the grading of the murmurs is purely subjective and depends on many factors including the hearing of the auscultators. Furthermore, the intensity of the murmur does not always correlate with the severity of valvular heart disease.

Ejection Systolic Murmurs

The ejection systolic murmurs may result from fixed or dynamic obstruction of the left ventricular outflow tract. The murmurs are of harsh quality. The fixed obstruction may be at the level of aortic valve, or it can be supravalvular or subvalvular. The characters and duration of the murmur may be similar in valvular, supravalvular and subvalvular aortic stenosis. However, there are other distinctive features of valvular, supravalvular and subvalvular aortic stenosis. Aortic valve stenosis is frequently associated with an anacrotic carotid pulse, delayed upstroke and delayed peak (Fig. 11). The murmur radiates to both carotids. In mild to moderately severe aortic valve stenosis, an ejection sound may be heard at the onset of the ejection systolic murmur. In severe aortic stenosis, aortic ejection sound is usually absent. In older patients with calcific trileaflet aortic valve stenosis, the ejection systolic murmur may have a musical quality (Gallavardin sign), which is frequently heard over the cardiac apex or along lower left sternal border. This musical murmur is related to vibrations of the subvalvular structures. In supravalvular aortic stenosis, the right carotid pulse amplitude is frequently greater than that of the left. The intensity of the radiated murmur over the right carotid artery is often

TABLE 13

Physical findings of hemodynamically significant aortic valve stenosis

- Slow rising delayed peaking small amplitude carotid pulse
- Anacrotic carotid pulse
- Anacrotic radial pulse
- Late peaking harsh ejection systolic murmur
- Palpable systolic thrill
- Sustained left ventricular apical impulse
- Paradoxical splitting of S2 in absence of left bundle branch block or right ventricular pacing
- Evidence of pulmonary hypertension

greater than over the left. The supravalvular, valvular and subvalvular aortic stenosis may all be associated with murmurs of aortic regurgitation. The presence of an aortic ejection sound excludes the diagnosis of fixed supravalvular or subvalvular aortic stenosis. The physical findings of hemodynamically significant aortic valve stenosis are summarized in Table 13.

Aortic valve sclerosis is associated with a short ejection systolic murmur. The murmur is best heard over the right second intercostal space and generally is not loud. It may be heard along the left sternal border and over cardiac apex. In aortic sclerosis there is no significant aortic valve obstruction. The carotid pulse upstroke and S2 are normal and aortic regurgitation murmur is absent. A transthoracic echocardiogram is recommended to confirm the diagnosis. Aortic sclerosis is a risk factor for adverse prognosis due to a higher incidence of atherosclerotic cardiovascular disease.

In patients with bicuspid aortic valve without aortic stenosis, a short ejection systolic murmur preceded by an ejection sound is frequently heard and an early diastolic murmur of trivial aortic regurgitation may also be present. The carotid pulse and S2 are normal. A transthoracic echocardiogram is recommended to confirm the diagnosis.

In dynamic left ventricular outflow tract obstruction due to Hypertrophic Obstructive Cardiomyopathy (HOCM), an ejection systolic murmur is always present. The murmur is best heard along the lower left sternal border or over cardiac apex. The murmur does not radiate to the neck. The intensity of the murmur varies with maneuvers (Table 14) due to changes in the severity of obstruction. Standing from squatting position is

TABLE 14

The influence of maneuvers on the intensity of the murmurs of hypertrophic obstructive cardiomyopathy, aortic valve stenosis and primary mitral regurgitation

Murmur	HOCM	AS	MR
Standing	++	-	-
Squatting	-	-	+
Handgrip	-/+	-/+	+
Valsalva	++	-	-
Amyl nitrite	++	+	-

Abbreviations: HOCM: Hypertrophic obstructive cardiomyopathy; AS: Fixed aortic valve stenosis; MR: Mitral regurgitation
++, markedly increased; -, decreased; +, increased; -/+, may decrease or increase

associated with increased obstruction and increased intensity of the murmur. In patients with fixed aortic valve stenosis or mitral regurgitation the intensity of the murmur decreases. During the phase II of Valsalva maneuver, the severity of obstruction is increased and the intensity of the murmur also increases. The carotid pulse volume either remains unchanged or decreases. During the phase II Valsalva maneuver, in fixed aortic stenosis or mitral regurgitation, the intensity of the murmurs decreases. With amyl nitrate inhalation, in HOCM, the intensity of the murmur increases along with the increase in the outflow gradient. In patients with fixed aortic stenosis the intensity of the murmur also increases. In mitral regurgitation the intensity of the murmur decreases as the severity of mitral regurgitation decreases because of reduction in systemic vascular resistance.

The murmur of dynamic left ventricular outflow obstruction has been rarely observed in patients with acute myocardial infarction or apical ballooning syndrome who can develop transient left ventricular outflow obstruction.[45]

Innocent Murmurs

The innocent murmurs are typical ejection systolic murmurs and are not associated with any other abnormal findings. The duration and intensity of innocent murmurs are variable. The innocent murmurs are related to increased flow across semilunar valves. The high cardiac output, such as with anemia, thyrotoxicosis and pregnancy, may be associated with flow murmurs. In over 80% of normal pregnant women, a pulmonary ejection systolic murmur can be heard.

The Still's murmur is a short, low-pitched vibrating murmur which is heard in children along the left lower sternal border in absence of any other abnormality. It is thought that it is caused by the vibrations of the attachments of the pulmonary valve leaflets.

In children another innocent ejection systolic murmur can be heard over the left second interspace which is thought to originate from the vibrations of the pulmonary trunk. The straight back syndrome may be associated with an innocent ejection systolic murmur.[47]

PULMONARY OUTFLOW OBSTRUCTION

An ejection systolic murmur is present in pulmonary valve, supravalvular or subvalvular stenosis. The pulmonary valve stenosis is associated with a harsh ejection systolic murmur which is best heard over the left second interspace. It is usually preceded by the pulmonary ejection sound. The intensity of the murmur increases during inspiration but that of the ejection sound decreases. The duration of the murmur correlates with the severity of stenosis. The longer the duration, more severe is the stenosis. The interval between A2 and P2 also correlates with the severity. The wider the interval, more severe is the stenosis. In pulmonary valve stenosis, the intensity of P2 is decreased as the pressure beyond the pulmonary valve is lower.

Occasionally the long ejection systolic murmur of pulmonary valve stenosis can be mistaken for the murmur of ventricular septal defect particularly when the intensity of P2 is decreased. The murmur of ventricular septal defect is a regurgitant murmur and starts with the first heart sound. It is best heard along the lower left sternal border. In ventricular septal defect the S2 is normal, while in pulmonary stenosis S2 is widely split. Inhalation of amyl nitrite is sometimes useful for the differential diagnosis. The intensity of the murmur of ventricular septal defect is decreased; the murmur of pulmonary valve stenosis is increased.

The idiopathic dilatation of the pulmonary artery is associated with a relatively short ejection systolic murmur, an ejection sound and a widely split S2 with normal intensity of P2. There is occasionally an early diastolic murmur of mild pulmonary regurgitation. The auscultatory findings are similar in pulmonary hypertension; however, in pulmonary arterial hypertension the intensity of P2 is increased and the splitting of S2 is narrower.

Regurgitant Murmurs

The systolic regurgitant murmurs start with S1 and may or may not extend to S2. When the murmur extends to S2 or beyond, it is called pansystolic or holosystolic murmur. It is caused when blood flows from a chamber whose pressure throughout the systole is higher than the pressure in the chamber receiving the flow. Mitral or tricuspid valve regurgitation and unrestricted ventricular septal defect are the major causes of holosystolic murmurs. When the murmur does not extend to S2, it is termed early systolic regurgitant murmur. Mitral or tricuspid valve regurgitation and ventricular septal defect may be associated with early systolic murmurs. When the murmur starts after S1 and extends to S2, it is termed late systolic murmur. The late systolic murmurs are auscultatory findings of relatively mild mitral or tricuspid regurgitation.

Mitral regurgitation: The murmurs of mitral regurgitation are high pitched and best appreciated with the diaphragm of the stethoscope over cardiac apex with the patient in partial left lateral decubitus position. The intensity of the murmur in part determines radiation. The direction of radiation is along the direction of regurgitation jet from left ventricle to left atrium. When the regurgitant jet is directed posterolaterally, the murmurs radiate toward the left axilla, inferior angle of left scapula and thoracic spine. In some patients this murmur radiates up the spine and can be heard over the top of the head.

When the regurgitant jet is directed anteromedially against the interatrial septum, the murmur radiates toward the base and root of the neck. This radiated murmur can be mistaken as the murmur of aortic stenosis. However, other findings of aortic stenosis or mitral regurgitation provide clues for the diagnosis. A transthoracic echocardiogram should be always performed for establishing the diagnosis.

The physical findings of acute severe mitral regurgitation are different than those of chronic severe mitral regurgitation. Acute severe mitral regurgitation, e.g. due to ruptured chordae, is associated with sudden onset of dyspnea due to pulmonary edema. The physical findings are characterized by an early systolic regurgitant murmur, evidence for pulmonary hypertension, and a hyperdynamic left ventricular apical impulse and normal left ventricular ejection fraction (Fig. 12). The murmur terminates in mid-systole or late systole when the left atrial pressure equalizes with left ventricular systolic pressure. The cardiomegaly and S3 are usually absent.

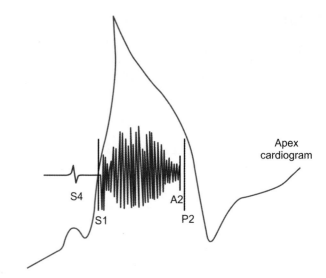

FIGURE 12: The schematic illustrations of physical findings of acute severe mitral regurgitation showing that the regurgitant murmur terminates before A2 because of equalization of left ventricular and left atrial pressures and cessation of regurgitation. Left ventricular apical impulse is hyperdynamic indicating normal ejection fraction. The intensity of P2 is increased indicating pulmonary hypertension

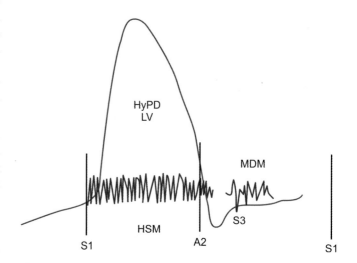

FIGURE 13: The schematic illustrations of physical findings of chronic severe mitral regurgitation showing that the high-pitched murmur is holosystolic (HSM) and extends beyond A2 as the left ventricular pressure remains higher than the left atrial pressure even after closure of the aortic valve. S3 is frequently present. Occasionally a low pitch mid-diastolic flow murmur (MDM) is heard. The left ventricular apical impulse is hyperdynamic (HyPD LV) indicating normal left ventricular ejection fraction

It should be appreciated that a short early systolic murmur may also be observed in patients with very mild mitral regurgitation such as due to mitral annular calcification.

The physical findings of chronic severe mitral regurgitation are characterized by a holosystolic murmur, a widely split S2 and an S3 (Fig. 13). The murmur frequently extends beyond A2 as the left ventricular pressure still remains higher than the left atrial pressure even after the closure of the aortic valve. The cardiac enlargement is also appreciated. The left ventricular apical impulse is hyperdynamic indicating normal ejection fraction. However, in patients with chronic severe primary mitral regurgitation with continued volume overload, the left ventricular ejection fraction declines. When left ventricular ejection fraction is substantially reduced, it cannot be distinguished from secondary mitral regurgitation such as in patients with dilated cardiomyopathy. Chronic severe primary mitral regurgitation may be associated with postcapillary pulmonary hypertension.

The most common cause of late systolic murmur is prolapse of the mitral valve. The late systolic murmur resulting from mitral valve prolapse is usually preceded by clicks. The commonest etiology of mitral valve prolapse is the redundancy of the valve tissue with respect to the valve ring. The valve appears "floppy" (Barlow's syndrome). The onset of the prolapse that causes the late systolic murmur is not only related to the severity of mitral valve prolapse but also to the changes in ventricular volume. Standing, sitting and Valsalva maneuver cause an earlier onset of the click and the murmur because these maneuvers decrease left ventricular end-diastolic volume and with the onset of systole the prolapse occurs earlier.

Elevation of legs, squatting and handgrip, which is associated with increased left ventricular volume, delays the onset of the prolapse and the late systolic murmur.

Late systolic murmur due to mitral regurgitation can also occur from papillary muscle displacement in patients with ischemic heart disease.

In patients with pseudohypertrophic muscular dystrophy or Becker's muscular dystrophy, mitral valve prolapse and late systolic murmur are indications of cardiac involvement and result from fibrosis of the posterior left ventricular wall. The electrocardiogram almost always reveals a taller R wave in leads V1 and V2.

Tricuspid regurgitation: The tricuspid regurgitation murmur can be holosystolic, early systolic or late systolic. The early and late systolic murmurs indicate mild tricuspid regurgitation. The holosystolic murmur is usually associated with more severe tricuspid regurgitation. The murmurs of tricuspid regurgitation are best heard over the lower left parasternal area and the intensity increases during inspiration (Carvallo's sign, sometimes spelled Carvello's). During inspiration there is increased systemic venous return, which is associated with more severe tricuspid regurgitation. Presence of a right ventricular S3 and a mid-diastolic flow murmur, which also increase in intensity during inspiration, indicates more severe tricuspid regurgitation. These auscultatory findings are frequently detected in patients with atrial septal defect and a large left-to-right shunt.

The murmur of severe regurgitation may radiate to the right lower parasternal area and to the epigastrium.

Tricuspid regurgitation is most frequently secondary to pulmonary hypertension, which can be diagnosed at the bedside by the presence of a loud (Fig. 14).

Primary tricuspid regurgitation without associated pulmonary hypertension is encountered much less frequently. It can occur in patients with right-sided bacterial endocarditis, carcinoid heart disease, Ebstein's anomaly, traumatic ruptured chordae or prior right ventricular myocardial infarction. Rarely, it occurs in Uhl's syndrome.

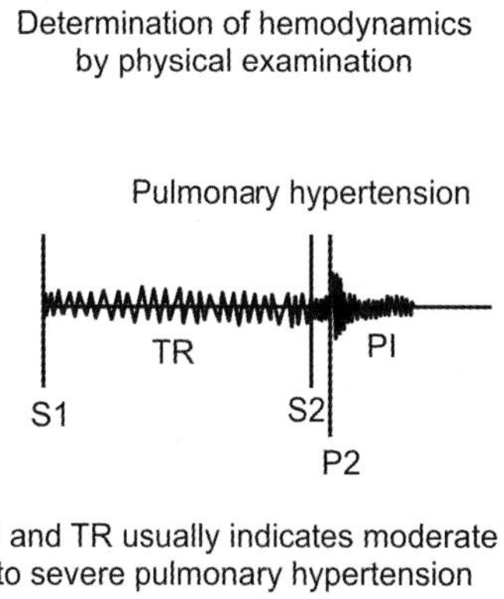

Determination of hemodynamics
by physical examination

Pulmonary hypertension

PI and TR usually indicates moderate
to severe pulmonary hypertension

FIGURE 14: Schematic auscultatory findings of secondary tricuspid regurgitation. (Abbreviations: TR: Tricuspid regurgitation murmur; P1: Pulmonary insufficiency murmur; S1: First heart sound; A2: Aortic component of the second heart sound; P2: Pulmonary component of the second heart sound which is increased in intensity which indicates pulmonary arterial hypertension

TABLE 15
Tricuspid regurgitation—physical findings
• Elevated jugular venous pressure with prominent "V" wave and "y" descent
• Pansystolic murmur which increases in intensity during inspiration
• Systolic hepatic pulsation

A more frequent cause of primary tricuspid regurgitation is related to the right ventricular pacing electrode, which prevents complete closure of the tricuspid valve. Severe tricuspid regurgitation occurs when the pacing electrode perforates the tricuspid valve leaflets.

Late systolic murmur due to tricuspid valve prolapse is uncommon in absence of mitral valve prolapse. It may be preceded by clicks. The intensity of the murmur increases during inspiration.

The unrestricted ventricular septal defect is associated with a holosystolic murmur and it is best heard over the lower left third and fourth interspace. It is frequently associated with a palpable thrill. The intensity of the murmur does not vary with respiration. The muscular ventricular septal defect causes an early systolic murmur. The physical findings of tricuspid regurgitation are summarized in Table 15.

DIASTOLIC MURMURS

Early Diastolic Murmurs

Early diastolic murmurs result most frequently, either from aortic or pulmonary regurgitation. The aortic and pulmonary regurgitation murmurs start with or shortly after A2 or P2, respectively. These murmurs are of relatively higher pitched and best heard with the use of the diaphragm of the stethoscope.

Aortic regurgitation: Auscultation is essential for the diagnosis of aortic regurgitation. The detection of an early diastolic murmur during auscultation has a positive likelihood ratio of 8.8 for the presence of aortic regurgitation. When the early

170 diastolic murmur is absent during auscultation, the negative likelihood ratio is 0.2:0.3.[48] These findings indicate that when an early diastolic murmur is heard, the likelihood of presence of aortic regurgitation is very high.

The murmur is best heard when a firm pressure is applied with the diaphragm of the stethoscope and the patient leaning forward and during held expiration. Auscultation should be performed over the right second interspace, along left sternal border and over the cardiac apex for the detection of the murmur. The radiation of aortic regurgitation murmur is toward cardiac apex. Occasionally radiation occurs along the right sternal border when aortic regurgitation occurs due to aortic root or aortic cusp abnormalities.

The high-pitched early diastolic murmur of aortic regurgitation has a decrescendo configuration and a "blowing" quality. Occasionally the murmur can have a musical quality (diastolic whoop), which appears to be due to flail everted aortic cusp.

The duration of the murmur is variable. A pandiastolic regurgitation murmur indicates a persistent gradient between aortic diastolic and left ventricular diastolic pressures. When the murmur is of brief duration, the severity of aortic regurgitation can be mild or very severe. Not only the anatomic changes causing aortic regurgitation determine the severity of regurgitation and hence the duration of the murmur, the hemodynamic consequences of aortic regurgitation also influence the duration of the murmur. In patients with acute severe aortic regurgitation, the murmur can be short because of a rapid increase in left ventricular diastolic pressure, which equalizes with aortic diastolic pressure soon after the onset of the diastole. Due to a marked rapid increase in left ventricular diastolic pressure, S1 may be absent due to premature closure of the mitral valve. In acute severe aortic regurgitation, S4 may be absent because of a marked increase in left ventricular diastolic pressure, which may prevent effective left ventricular filling. The intensity of P2 is increased due to postcapillary pulmonary hypertension. The carotid pulse volume is decreased because of reduced forward stroke volume. Left ventricular impulse is not displaced and maintains normal character indicating normal ejection fraction. In acute severe aortic regurgitation, there is no left ventricular adaptation to severe

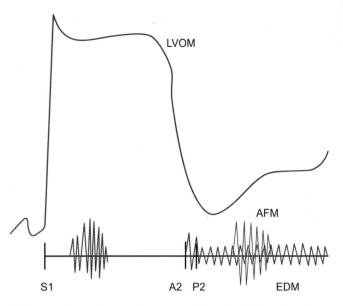

FIGURE 15: The schematic illustrations of physical findings in chronic severe aortic regurgitation showing a long early diastolic murmur, Austin Flint Murmur (AFM), reversed splitting of S2 and hyperdynamic left ventricular impulse. (Abbreviations: EDM: Early diastolic murmur; A2: Aortic component of second heart sound; P2: Pulmonic component of second heart sound; S1: First heart sound; LVOM: Left ventricular outward murmur)

volume overload and there is lack of left ventricular dilatation and hypertrophy.

The physical findings of chronic hemodynamically significant aortic regurgitation are illustrated in Figure 15 and Table 16. The early diastolic murmur is longer in duration and can be pandiastolic. A low-pitched mid-diastolic murmur, called "Austin Flint" murmur, may be heard. The intensity of A2 is usually decreased but it does not necessarily indicate severe aortic regurgitation. Reversed splitting of S2 in the absence of left bundle branch block results from a marked increase in left ventricular forward stroke volume and usually associated with significant aortic regurgitation. The increased flow may also be associated with an ejection systolic murmur. The decreased intensity of S1 indicates increased left ventricular end-diastolic pressure, which is more likely to occur in severe aortic regurgitation. Similarly presence of the physical findings of

TABLE 16

The differences in the physical findings in acute and chronic severe aortic regurgitation

	Acute	*Chronic*
Carotid pulse small volume	small volume	bisferiens quality, large volume, sharp upstroke
S1	decreased intensity or absent	decreased intensity or normal
S2	normal or decreased	normal or decreased
P2	increased	normal or increased
Apical impulse	normal and nondisplaced	displaced, normal or sustained
S4	absent	present
EDM	short	long or short
AFM	absent	present

Abbreviations: S1: First heart sound; S2: Second heart sound; P2: Pulmonic component of second heart sound; S4: Fourth heart sound; EDM: Early diastolic murmur; AFM: Austin Flint murmur pulmonary hypertension and right heart failure indirectly suggest severe aortic regurgitation. The carotid pulse upstroke is sharp and may have a bisferiens character. Presence of a normal character of left ventricular apical impulse indicates normal ejection fraction. However, a sustained apical impulse does not necessarily indicate reduced ejection fraction as severe hypertrophy may also be associated with a sustained apical impulse. The apical impulse is usually displaced laterally and downward due to dilatation of the left ventricle.

Occasionally aortic regurgitation murmur is heard in patients with hypertension, aortic aneurysm and bicuspid aortic valve. Aortic regurgitation is mild in these conditions.

A diastolic murmur similar to aortic regurgitation can be heard in some patients with stenosis of the left anterior descending coronary artery (Dock's murmur).[49] This murmur is very localized and usually heard over the left second or third interspace just lateral to the left sternal border. It is caused by turbulent flow across a moderately severe stenosis. The murmur is absent after angioplasty or bypass surgery. For practical purposes, in all patients with suspected Dock's murmur, an echocardiographic study should be performed to exclude other commoner causes of early diastolic murmur.

Pulmonic regurgitation: Very mild or trivial pulmonary valve regurgitation is detected in many normal subjects by echo-Doppler studies and do not have any clinical significance.

In the adult patients, the most common cause of pulmonic regurgitation is pulmonary hypertension (Graham-Steel murmur).[50] It is high pitched and starts with a loud P2 and has a "blowing" quality. The duration is variable. The murmur may increase in intensity during inspiration. An echocardiographic study is essential to exclude aortic regurgitation.

Pulmonary regurgitation is common after repair of Tetralogy of Fallot and after pulmonary valvulotomy for pulmonary valve stenosis. The murmur is of lower pitch. The intensity of P2 is reduced as the pulmonary artery pressure is normal or low.

Pulmonic regurgitation can occur in patients with idiopathic dilatation of the pulmonary artery, with right-sided endocarditis and congenital absence of the pulmonary valve. In congenital absence of pulmonary valve, P2 is absent and a loud to-and-fro murmur may be heard.

Mid-Diastolic Murmurs

The mid-diastolic murmurs are low- or medium-pitched murmurs and have rumbling quality and thus these murmurs are frequently called "rumbles". An anatomic or functional obstruction of the atrioventricular valves is associated with mid-diastolic murmurs.

Mitral Stenosis

The characteristic auscultatory findings of mitral stenosis are a loud S1, a mid-diastolic murmur with or without presystolic accentuation. It is best heard with the bell of the stethoscope over the cardiac apex with the patient in the left lateral decubitus. The murmur originates in the left ventricular cavity explaining why it is best heard over the cardiac apex. The presystolic component of the mid-diastolic murmur can be present even in presence of atrial fibrillation. The mid-diastolic murmur due to

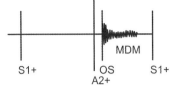

Best heard along lower left sternal border
increased intensity of MDM during inspiration

FIGURE 16: Schematic illustrations of auscultatory signs of tricuspid stenosis. Right sided opening snap (OS), mid-diastolic murmur (MDM) and increased intensity of the first heart sound (S1+). (Abbreviation: A2+: Aortic component of the second heart sound)

mitral stenosis is preceded by the opening snap until the mitral valve is heavily calcified and immobile. The duration of the murmur correlates with the severity of mitral stenosis. The longer the duration, more severe is mitral stenosis. It should be appreciated however that low cardiac output is associated with shorter duration of the murmur and the intensity of the murmur is decreased even in presence of severe mitral stenosis. The mitral regurgitation murmur is frequently heard because of the presence of obligatory mitral regurgitation. A loud P2 and the Graham-Steel murmur can be present if there is significant pulmonary hypertension.

Tricuspid Stenosis

The auscultatory findings of tricuspid stenosis are very similar to those of mitral stenosis (Fig. 16). However, in tricuspid stenosis, the intensity of the murmur increases during inspiration because of increased gradient across the tricuspid valve (Carvallo'sign). The mid-diastolic murmur can be associated with an opening snap.

Isolated tricuspid valve obstruction is uncommon and it occurs in association with mitral and aortic valve disease in rheumatic valvular heart disease. The physical findings of tricuspid valve stenosis are summarized in Table 17.

When isolated tricuspid stenosis is present, right atrial myxoma or carcinoid heart disease should be suspected. An echocardiographic study is mandatory for the differential diagnosis.

Left and right atrial myxomas can be associated with the auscultatory findings, similar to those of mitral and tricuspid valve stenosis. The "tumor plop" sounds can be similar to opening snaps.

TABLE 17

Tricuspid stenosis—physical findings

- Elevated jugular venous pressure with prominent "a" wave and slow "y" descent
- Mid diastolic rumble which increases in intensity during inspiration
- Right sided opening snap
- Right sided presystolic murmur
- Presystolic hepatic pulsation

The echocardiographic evaluation is essential for establishing the correct diagnosis.

Austin Flint Murmur

It is a low-pitched rumbling murmur associated with aortic regurgitation. Controversy exists about the genesis of the murmur. Fluttering of the mitral valve and relative mitral stenosis due to movement of the mitral valve leaflets to the semi-closed position has been proposed as the potential mechanisms. It is however present most frequently in patients with hemodynamically significant aortic regurgitation.

Carey-Coombs Murmur

Acute rheumatic mitral valvulitis can be associated with a mid-diastolic murmur, which is transient. It is caused by swelling of the mitral valve leaflets and other signs of rheumatic carditis are usually present.

Increased flow across the atrioventricular valves can be associated with mid-diastolic murmurs. Severe mitral regurgitation and ventricular septal defects with large left-to-right shunts can cause left-sided mid-diastolic flow murmurs. An atrial septal defect with a large left-to-right shunt can be associated with a right-sided mid-diastolic flow murmur.

In patients with complete atrioventricular block, with a slow ventricular rate, a late diastolic murmur can be heard. This murmur is also called *Rytand's murmur*. The mechanism of this murmur remains unclear and diastolic mitral regurgitation has been postulated.[51]

CONTINUOUS MURMURS

The continuous murmurs begin in systole and extend to diastole. These murmurs result from blood flow from a higher pressure chamber or vessel to a lower pressure chamber or vessel.

In the adult patient, a patent ductus arteriosus and a venous hum are the usual causes of continuous murmurs. The venous hum can be easily diagnosed at the bedside. The venous hum is not heard in supine position. Pressure at the root of the neck also causes disappearance of the venous hum. The "mammary soufflé" associated with pregnancy is another cause of benign continuous murmur. Congenital or acquired arteriovenous fistulas also cause continuous murmurs. Following cardiac catheterization, an arteriovenous communication can occur at the site of insertion of the intravascular catheters, and a continuous murmur can be heard.

In patients with coarctation of aorta, a continuous murmur can be heard in the back overlying the area of constriction. In these patients, continuous murmurs can be heard over large tortuous intercostal arteries which can also be visible (Suzman's sign).[52]

The pulmonary arteriovenous malformations are usually silent, but occasionally a continuous murmur can be heard. Peripheral pulmonary artery branch stenosis can cause a continuous murmur.

Fistulous communication between an internal mammary artery graft to the vein accompanying the left anterior descending coronary artery is another rare cause of continuous murmur.[53]

The continuous murmurs associated with aortopulmonary window and truncus arteriosus and coronary arteriovenous fistulas are rarely encountered in adult patients.

REFERENCES

1. Shy GM, Drager GA. A neurologic syndrome associated with orthostatic hypotension. A clinical-pathologic study. Arch Neurol. 1960;2:511-27.
2. Rich LL, Epinette WW, Nasser WK. Argyria presenting as cyanotic heart disease. Am J Cardiol. 1972;30:290-2.
3. Protonotarios N, Tsatsopoulou A. Naxos disease: cardiocutaneous syndrome due to cell adhesion defect. Orphanet J Rare Dis. 2006;1:4.
4. van Gent M WF, Post MC, Snijder, et al. Real prevalence of pulmonary right-to-left shunt accoding to genotype in patients with hereditary hemorrhagic telangiectasia: a transthoracic contrast echocardiography study. Chest. 2010;1378:1849.
5. Kalev I, Maru K, Teek R, et al. LEOPARD syndrome with recurrent PTPN11 mutation Y279C and different cutaneous manifestations: two case reports and a review of the literature. Eur J Pediatr. 2010;169:469-73.
6. Holdveen-Geronimus M, Merriam JC. Cholesterol embolization: from pathological curiosity to clinical entity. Circulation. 1967;35:946-53.
7. Rolan CA, Chavez J, Wiest PW, et al. Aortic root disease and valve disease associated with ankylosing spondylitis. J Am Coll Cardiol. 1998;32:1397-404.
8. Lane D, Beevers M, Barnes N, et al. Inter-arm differences in blood pressure: when are they clinically significant? J Hypertens. 2002;20:1089-95.
9. Masserli FH, Ventura HO, Amodeo C. Osler's maneuver and pseudohypertension. N Engl J Med. 1985;312:1548-51.
10. Vinyaak AG, Levitt J, Gehlbach AS, et al. Usefulness of the external jugular vein examination in detecting abnormal central venous pressure in critically ill patients. Arch Intern Med. 2006;166:2132-7.
11. Constant J. Using internal jugular pulsations as a manometer for right atrial pressure measurements. Cardiology. 2000;93:26-30.
12. Conn RD, O'Keefe JH. Cardiac physical diagnosis in the digital age: an important but increasingly neglected skill (from Stethoscopes to Microchips). Am J Cardiol. 2009;104:590-5.
13. Seth R, Magner P, Matzinger F, et al. How far is the sternal angle from the mid-right atrium? J Gen Intern Med. 2002;17:852-6.
14. Devine PJ, Sullenberger LE, Bellin DA, et al. Jugular venous pulse: window into the right heart. South Med J. 2007;100:1022-7.
15. McGee SR. Physical examination of venous pressure: a critical review. Am Heart J. 1998;136:10-18.
16. Drazner MH, Rame JE, Stevenson LW, et al. Prognostic importance of elevated jugular venous pressure and a third heart sound in patients with heart failure. N Engl J Med. 2001;345:574-81.
17. Kircher BJ, Himelman RB, Schiller NB. Noninvasive estimation of right atrial pressure from the inspiratory collapse of the inferior vena cava. Am J Cardiol. 1990;66:493-6.
18. Willems J, Roelandt J, Kesteloot H. The jugular venous pulse tracing. Proc Vth European Cong Cardiol. 1968. p. 433.
19. Lee CH, Xiao HB, Gibson DG. Jugular venous "a" wave in dilated cardiomyopathy: sign of abbreviated right ventricular filling time. Br Heart J. 1991;65:342-5.
20. Stojnic BB, Brecker SJD, Xiao HB, et al. Jugular venous "a" wave in pulmonary hypertension: new insights from a Doppler echocardiographic study. Br Heart J. 1992;68:187-91.
21. Manga P, Vythilingum S, Mitha AS. Pulsatile hepatomegaly in constrictive pericarditis. Br Heart J. 1984;52:465-7.
22. Cohn J, Hamosh P. Experimental observations on pulsus paradoxus and hepatojugular reflux. In: Reddy PS (Ed). Pericardial Disease. New York: Raven Press; 1982. p. 249.

23. Ewy GA. The abdominojugular test: technique hemodynamic correlates. Ann Intern Med. 1998;109:456-60.

24. Chizner MA. Cardiac auscultation: rediscovering the lost art. Current Probl Cardiol. 2008;33:326-408.

25. Armstong TG, Gotsman MS. The left parasternal lift in tricuspid incompetence. Am Heart J. 1974;88:183-90.

26. Tucker WT, Knowles JL, Eddelman EE. Mitral insufficiency: cardiac mechanics as studied with the kinetocardiogram and ballistocardiogram. Circulation. 1955;12:278-85.

27. el-Sherif A, el-Said G. Jugular, hepatic, and praecordial pulsations in constrictive pericarditis. Br Heart J. 1971;33:305-12.

28. Herman H, Raizner AE, Chahine RA, et al. Congenital absence of the left pericardium: an unusual palpation finding and echocardiographic demonstration of the defect. South Med J. 1976;69:1222-5.

29. Foster E, Lease, KE. New untwist on diastole: what goes around comes back. Circulation. 2006;113:2477-9.

30. Braunwald E, Lambrew CT, Rockoff SD, et al. Idiopathic hypertrophic subacute stenosis. A description of the disease based upon an analysis of 64 patients. Circulation. 1964;30:3-119.

31. O'Toole JD, Reddy PS, Curtiss EI, et al. The contribution of tricuspid valve closure to the first heart sound: an intracardiac micromanometer study. Circulation. 1976;53:752-8.

32. Luisada AA, MacCanon DM, Kumar S, et al. Changing views on the mechanism of the first and second heart sounds. Am Heart J. 1974;88:503-14.

33. Leatham A. Auscultation and phonocardiography: a personal view of the past 40 years. Br Heart J. 1987;57:397-403.

34. Oki T, Fukuda N, Tabata T, et al. The "sail sound" and tricuspid regurgitation in Ebstein's anomaly: the value of echocardiography in evaluating their mechanisms. J Heart Valve Dis. 1997;6:189-92.

35. Damore S, Murgo JP, Bloom KR, et al. Second heart sound dynamics in atrial septal defect. Circulation. 1981;64:IV28.

36. Marcus GM, Michaels AD, De Marco T, et al. Usefulness of the third heart sound in predicting an elevated level of B-type natriuretic peptide. Am J Cardiol. 2004;93:1312-3.

37. Marcus GM, Gerber IL, McKeown BH, et al. Association between phonocardiographic third and fourth heart sounds and objective measures of left ventricular function. JAMA. 2005;293:2238-44.

38. Drazner MH, Rame JE, Stevenson LW, et al. Prognostic importance of elevated jugular venous pressure and a third heart sound in patients with heart failure. N Engl J Med. 2001;345:574-81.

39. Sze KC, Shah PM. Pseudoejection sound in hypertrophic subaortic stenosis: an echocardiographic correlative study. Circulation. 1976;54:504-9.

40. Behar VS, Whalen RE, McIntosh HD. The ballooning mitral valve in patients with the "precordial honk" or "whoop". Am J Cardiol. 1967;20:789-95.

41. Leatham A, Gray I. Auscultatory and phonocardiographic signs of atrial septal defect. Br Heart J. 1956;18:193-208.

42. Wei J, Fortuin NJ. Diastolic sounds and murmurs associated with mitral valve prolapse. Circulation. 1981;63:559-64.

43. Spodick, DH. Hypertrophic obstructive cardiomyopathy of the left ventricle (idiopathic hypertrophic subaortic stenosis). In: Burch GE, Brest AN (Eds). Cardiovascular Clinics. Philadelphia: FA Davis; 1972. p. 156.

44. Goettlieb JD, Ericsson JA, Sweet RB. Venous air embolism: a review. Anesth Analg. 1965;44:773-9.

45. Mineo K, Cummings J, Josephson R, et al. Acquired left ventricular outflow tract obstruction during acute myocardial infarction: diagnosis of a new cardiac murmur. Am J Geriatr Cardiol. 2001;10:283-5.

46. Bonow RO, Carabello BA, Chatterjee K, et al. 2008 Focused update incorporated into the ACC/AHA 2006 guidelines for the management of patients with valvular heart disease: a report of the American College of Cardiology/American Heart Association Task Force on Practice Guidelines (Writing Committee to Revise the 1998 Guidelines for the Management of Patients with Valvular Heart Disease): endorsed by the Society of Cardiovascular Anesthesiologists, Society for Cardiovascular Angiography and Interventions, and Society of Thoracic Surgeons. Circulation. 2008;118:e523.

47. Deleon AC, Perloff JK, Twig H, et al. The straight back syndrome: clinical cardiovascular manifestations. Circulation. 1965;32:193-203.

48. Choudhry NK, Etchells EE. Does the patient have aortic regurgitation? JAMA. 1999;281:2231-8.

49. Dock W, Zoneraich SA. A diastolic murmur arising in a stenosed coronary artery. Am J Med. 1967;42:617-8.

50. Perloff JK. Auscultatory and phonocardiographic manifestations of pulmonary hypertension. Prog Cardiovasc Dis. 1967;9:303-40.

51. Rutishauser W, Wirz P, Gander M, et al. Atriogenic diastolic reflux in patients with atrioventricular block. Circulation. 1966;34:807-17.

52. Campbell M, Suzman SS. Coarctation of the aorta. Br Heart J. 1947;9:185-212.

53. Guray U, Guray Y, Ozbakir C, et al. Fistulous connection between internal mammary graft and pulmonary vasculature after coronary artery bypass grafting: a rare cause of continuous murmur. Int J Cardiol. 2004;96:489-92.

Chapter 11

Plain Film Imaging of Adult Cardiovascular Disease

Brad H Thompson, Edwin JR van Beek

Chapter Outline

INTRODUCTION

Plain film radiography of the chest offers valuable information about the cardiovascular system, and appropriately, should serve as the initial investigative test in patients suspected of having cardiovascular disease, especially those with presenting with chest pain. Furthermore, by analysis of cardiac morphology, pulmonary vasculature and the vascular pedicle, chest films can provide additional semi-quantitative information about heart function, pulmonary blood flow and circulating blood volume. As such, serial chest films ideally serve as a non-invasive, inexpensive modality to monitor the efficacy of treatment regimens for conditions, like heart failure, and provide useful surveillance of the cardiovascular system in post-surgical patients following coronary bypass or heart transplantation. This chapter will cover the salient features of a variety of those cardiovascular diseases and anomalies which are commonly encountered in adults.

CHEST FILM TECHNIQUE

Radiographic assessment of the thoracic cardiovascular structures ideally requires the acquisition of two projections of the chest. This is primarily due to the oblique position of the heart within the chest. Frontal chest radiographs can be obtained either with the ventral chest closest to the film (PA projection) or reversed (AP film). Conventionally, frontal radiographs of the chest obtained within the department are usually obtained in the PA projection while all portable films use an AP technique. Selection between these two options however is not entirely academic as there are significant changes relating to heart size between these two exams. Since the heart is located ventrally within the chest cavity, the divergence of the X-ray beam which occurs with AP films results in an undesirable artifactual magnification of the cardiac silhouette (Figs 1A and B). Furthermore, portable AP films usually compound this problem in large part to associated recumbency and diminished lung volumes, which tend to further magnify the apparent size of the heart.

Qualitative assessment of cardiac enlargement can be quickly established radiographically by measuring the cardiothoracic ratio (CTR). This ratio, as measured on upright PA chest radiographs, refers to the ratio of the transverse diameter of the cardiac silhouette (measured horizontally) compared to the transverse chest diameter (as measured horizontally from inner margins of the ribs at the level of the right diaphragm). A normal CTR measured by this method should be 0.5 or smaller, provided there is good inspiratory effort. Decreases in lung volumes will produce an artificial increase in the systolic time ratio (STR), due the more horizontal axis of the heart along the left diaphragm (Figs 2A and B). Due to magnification and diminished lung volumes commonly encountered with AP chest films, the calculation of the STR is unreliable and should not be performed, especially on portable films.

Due to the oblique orientation of the heart within the chest, single frontal radiographs generally do not provide sufficient qualitative information about cardiac morphology, and as such complementary lateral films are desirable whenever possible. Normal anatomy of the heart on both frontal and lateral chest radiographs will be discussed later.

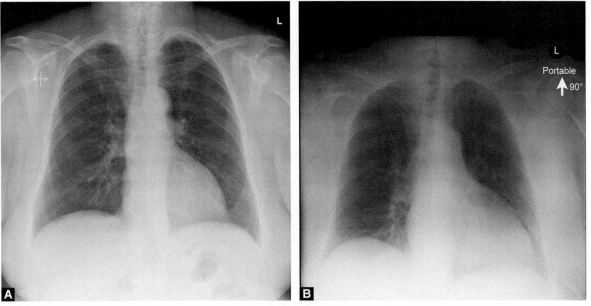

FIGURES 1A AND B: PA vs AP films: (A) PA film and (B) AP film on the same patient days apart. Note the significant increase in the size of the cardiac silhouette on the AP film due to magnification

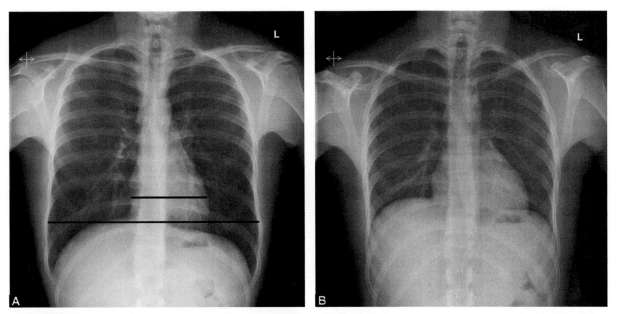

FIGURES 2A AND B: (A) Inspiratory vs (B) expiratory PA chest films. Horizontal lines reflect points of measurements for the cardio-thoracic ratio (TR). Note the apparent increase in the size of the heart with expiration (B)

OVERVIEW OF CARDIOMEDIASTINAL ANATOMY

Located centrally within the chest, the cardiomediastinal silhouette comprises the heart, the central large vessels (aorta, pulmonary artery, superior and inferior vena cava and azygos vein), the tracheobronchial, esophagus and the adipose tissue of the mediastinum (Figs 3A and B).

On either side of the central core structures are the hilar regions, which are composed of the central pulmonary arteries, mainstem bronchi, pulmonary veins and lymphatics. In general, the hila on chest films are largely composed of the pulmonary arterial shadows. The left hilum on the frontal radiographs is almost always higher in location than the right, reflecting the normal anatomical location of the left pulmonary artery as it courses superior to the left mainstem bronchus. This anatomical relationship is inverted on the right side, i.e. the right mainstem bronchus is hyparterial. These relationships are also substantiated on the lateral film as well.

The assessment of the pulmonary vasculature should be performed on review of every chest radiograph as changes either in the vessel size or border definition provides excellent physiologic information both about the volume status of the patient as well as the severity of congestive heart failure. Normally, the pulmonary arteries should be sharply defined and show a normal gravitationally dependent increase in lower lobe vascular conspicuity compared to the upper

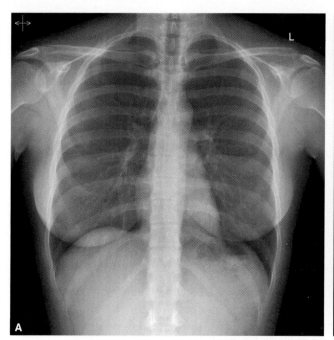

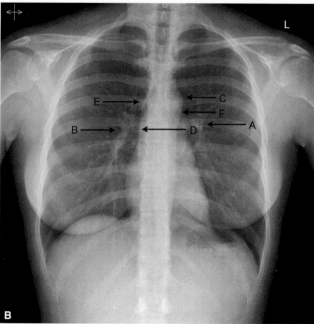

FIGURES 3A AND B: (A) Normal PA chest film with (B) annotations. (Abbreviations: A: Left hilum; B: Right hilum; C: Aortic knob; D: Superior vena cava (SVC); E: Azygous vein; F: AP window)

lobes (Fig. 3A). This phenomenon, reflecting the increase in blood flow to the lower portions of the lungs can be demonstrated to good advantage by viewing an inverted PA chest film. With this maneuver, the observer will quickly appreciate the disparity of blood flow, i.e. vessel size and conspicuity between the upper and lower regions of the lungs. Furthermore, the observer should always evaluate the caliber of the pulmonary arteries. The normal caliber of normal pulmonary arteries should approximate the caliber of the adjacent bronchus. Determination of this arterial-bronchial ratio (A:B ratio) (normal = 1:1) is most easily performed evaluating the central-most vessels in the perihilar regions (Fig. 4). An increase in the size of the upper lobe vessels indicating recruitment can be seen in left to right shunt lesions, high intravascular volumes/pregnancy and left heart failure or left heart obstructive lesions.

The thoracic aorta is visible in several regions on chest radiographs. Normally the ascending portion of the thoracic aorta is best demonstrated on the lateral projection residing in the retrosternal space. The ascending aorta is not usually apparent on frontal chest radiographs but with enlargement, the ascending aortic shadow may become visible along the right edge of the mediastinal silhouette above the right hilum. Conspicuous dilatation of the ascending aorta is seen in systemic hypertension, aneurysm, or aortic stenosis (Figs 5 and 23A). The transverse portion of the thoracic aorta creates the aortic knob which is visible at the top left portion of the mediastinum above the left hilar shadow (Fig. 3B). On well-penetrated films, the descending aorta may be visible as a tubular opacity running inferiorly, parallel to the thoracic spine.

On the lateral radiograph, the thoracic aorta will be seen as an arch, extending superiorly from the cardiac silhouette, arching backward and subsequently inferiorly along the ventral aspects of mid and lower portions of the thoracic spine. The descending thoracic aorta is usually poorly visualized on the lateral film, unless atherosclerotic calcifications exist.

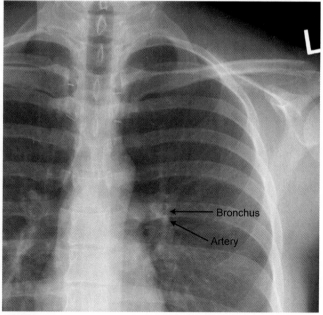

FIGURE 4: Normal arterial-bronchial relationship. Coned image from a PA chest film showing the normal 1:1 ratio of vessel size to adjacent bronchus (arterial-bronchus ratio). Also note the normal sharp definition of the arterial wall and thin bronchial wall

CARDIAC ANATOMY ON CHEST RADIOGRAPHS

On the frontal radiograph (Fig. 6), the heart is normally orientated slight to the left of midline with the inter-ventricular septum normally orientated 30 degrees left anterior oblique (LAO). This orientation results in superimpositioning of the right ventricle in front of the left ventricle. As such, the left heart border is composed entirely of the left ventricle. On the right side, the right atrium composes the right heart shadow (Fig. 3B). The shadow of the superior vena cava (SVC) comprises the vertical right paramedian shadow coursing

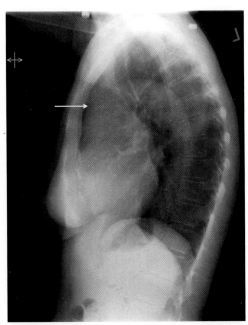

FIGURE 5: Patient with systemic hypertension. Lateral chest radiograph showing fusiform dilatation of the ascending thoracic aorta (arrow)

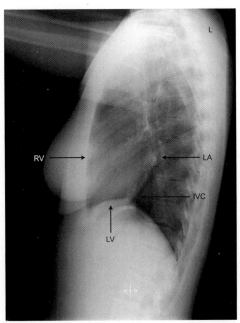

FIGURE 7: Normal cardiac anatomy on lateral radiograph. The right ventricle (RV) forms the ventral border of the cardiac silhouette while the inferoposterior border is composed of the left ventricle (LV). The left atrium (LA) composes the posterior-most border of the cardiac silhouette. The posterior border of the inferior vena cava (IVC) is also demonstrated to good advantage

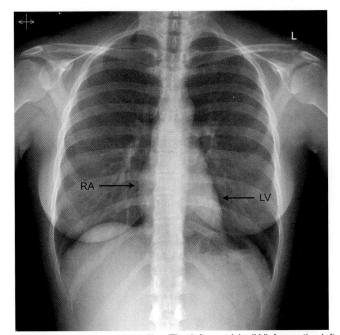

FIGURE 6: Normal PA chest film. The left ventricle (LV) forms the left heart border while the right heart border is composed of the lateral margin of the right atrium (RA)

the aortic knob. Inferiorly, the left hilum (pulmonary artery) comprises the second mogul. While not normally present, the third mogul arises when there is enlargement of the left atrial appendage. This enlargement produces a conspicuous convexity along the normally concave left heart border (Fig. 11A).

The aorticopulmonary window refers to the concave space which is located immediately inferior to the aortic knob and just above the left pulmonary artery. Filling in or convexity of this space usually reflects either adenopathy or a mediastinal mass (Fig. 3B).

On the lateral radiograph (Fig. 7), the cardiac silhouette occupies the retrosternal region with the apex directly inferiorly toward the xiphoid process. Anteriorly, the right ventricle creates the anterior cardiac border. The left atrium forms the superior portion of the posterior aspect of the cardiac silhouette, with the mainstem bronchi immediately superiorly. The left ventricle forms the lower portion of the posterior margin of the heart shadow, with the diaphragm immediately below it. With sufficiently good inspiration, the posterior border of the inferior vena cava (IVC) may be visualized on well positioned lateral films (Fig. 7).

CARDIAC CHAMBER ENLARGEMENT

LEFT VENTRICULAR ENLARGEMENT

Enlargement of the left ventricle will result in an enlargement of the cardiac silhouette, producing a bulbous left cardiac apex which is displaced down and out on the frontal radiograph (Fig. 8). On the lateral projection (Fig. 9), the left ventricular shadow will extend toward the thoracic spine away from the posterior border of the IVC. Normally, the posterior edge of the left ventricular shadow should reside within two centimeters of the posterior edge of the IVC at a point two centimeters above

inferiorly from the upper mediastinum to the right atrium. In the middle of the SVC, directly superior to the proximal right mainstem bronchus lies the azygous vein, which appears as a teardrop vascular shadow reflecting the anterior course of this vein as it empties into the SVC. The left atrium, which is the most posterior cardiac chamber, is not normally visualized on frontal chest films, unless it is enlarged. Normally, the left heart border in adults should be concave on frontal radiographs.

On frontal radiographs, the concept of the three cardiac mogul shadows comprising the left cardiomediastinal silhouette needs to addressed. The superior most mogul reflects

Diagnosis

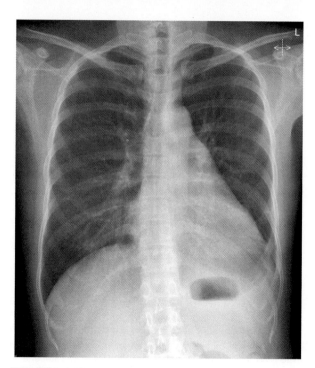

FIGURE 8: Left ventricular enlargement. PA chest film showing classic down and out configuration of the cardiac silhouette

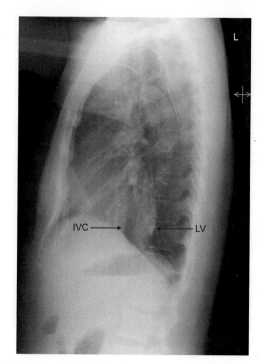

FIGURE 9: Left ventricular (LV) enlargement. Lateral film shows posterior displacement of the left ventricular shadow relative to the inferior vena cava (IVC) (arrows)

the diaphragm (Rigler's rule). With left ventricular hypertrophy, cardiac morphology is generally preserved with no apparent increase in the overall size or change in the configuration of the left ventricle.

RIGHT VENTRICULAR ENLARGEMENT

Right ventricular enlargement, although uncommon, is manifested by uplifting of the ventricular apex on frontal

projections producing the "boot-shaped" heart or *coer en sabot* configuration. On the lateral film there should be corresponding encroachment toward the sternum with "filling in" the retrosternal clear space (Figs 10A and B).

LEFT ATRIAL ENLARGEMENT

Left atrial/appendage enlargement will result in the formation of the third mogul as described above (Figs 11A and B).

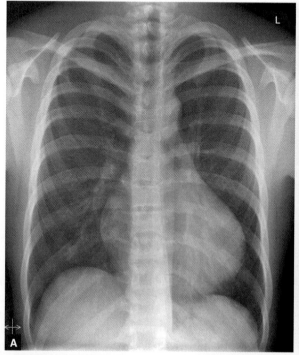

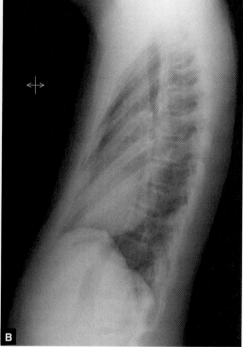

FIGURES 10A AND B: Right ventricular enlargement. PA and lateral films in patient with Tetralogy of Fallot. (A) The PA film shows the upturned ventricular shadow producing the "*coer en sabot*" or boot shaped heart. (B) The lateral film shows filling in of the retrosternal region by the enlarged right ventricle

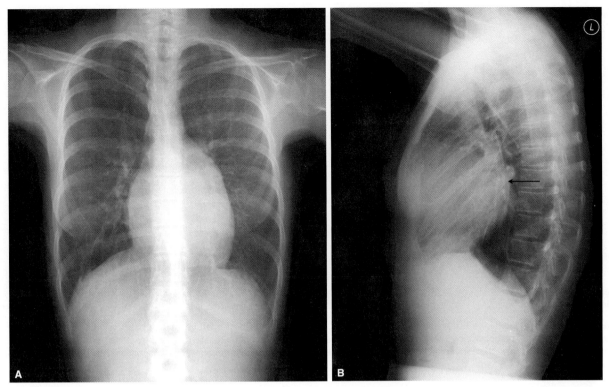

FIGURES 11A AND B: Left atrial enlargement. (A) PA and (B) lateral chest films showing classic cardiac silhouette of left atrial dilatation. On the PA film, there is bulging of the left cardiac border (third mogul). On the lateral film, note the conspicuous posterior displacement of the left atrial shadow (arrow). Also see Figure 25

With progressive atrial enlargement the left atrial shadow may extend across midline to produce a second shadow overlapping upon the right atrium (double density sign) (Figs 25A and B).

Soft tissue fullness in the subcarinal region which reflects enlarged atrial volume can occasionally produce uplifting of the left mainstem bronchus. On the lateral radiography, the posterior heart border will appear protruberant (Fig. 25B).

RIGHT ATRIAL ENLARGEMENT

Right atriual enlargement often goes relatively unnoticed, but will result in lateral displacement of the right cardiac border on the frontal radiograph (Fig. 12). A sausage shaped density may become more evident as the atrial appendage enlarges.

RADIOGRAPHIC MANIFESTATIONS OF CONGESTIVE HEART FAILURE

Plain film radiography of the chest is an excellent modality to diagnose and measure the effectiveness of therapy in patients with congestive heart failure. In fact, it has been established that the characteristic stages of radiographic features of congestive heart failure on chest films correlate very well with hemodynamic measurements obtained with left atrial wedge pressures as determined with Swan Ganz catheterization.

The radiographic stages of congestive heart failure are well known, and relate to the physiologic changes and hemodynamic perturbations occurring along the capillary and venous regions of the pulmonary circulation. The physiologic factors that determine the quantity of extravascular fluid depend on several factors namely: intravascular hydrostatic pressure (promoting

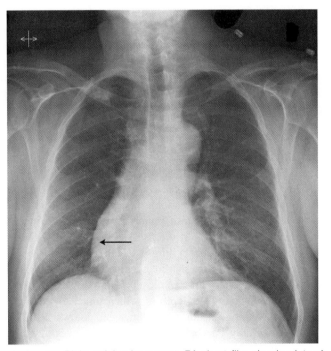

FIGURE 12: Right atrial enlargement. PA chest film showing lateral prominence of the right heart border (arrow) in patient with tricuspid insufficiency

fluid escape from the intravascular space); plasma oncotic pressure and interstitial hydrostatic pressures (which acts to keep intravascular fluid within vessels) and interstitial oncotic forces (acting to pull fluid out of the intravascular spaces). Normally, these opposing forces result in a net positive fluid escape from

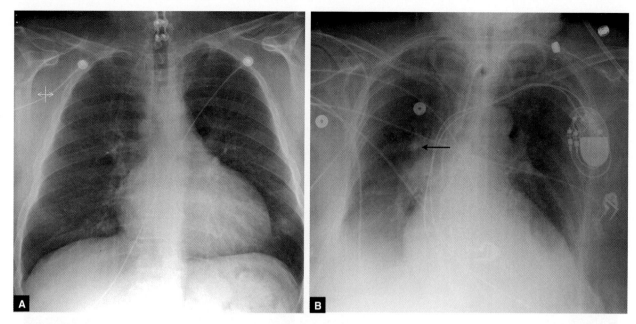

FIGURES 13A AND B: Cephalad redistribution of pulmonary blood flow in patient with mild left ventricular heart failure. (A) Note the increase in the size and conspicuity of the upper lobe vessels compared to normal. Also note the characteristic morphology of the heart reflecting left ventricular dilatation. (B) This figure shows the corresponding enlargement of the upper lobe arteries (arrow) with corresponding A:B ratio of 3:1. On both films, the vessel definition remains sharp

the intravascular spaces into the interstitum which is in turn returned to the central venous circulation via the lymphatics. In heart failure, as hydrostatic forces within the pulmonary arterial circulation increase, there are corresponding and predictable radiographic changes which reflect the increase of both increased pulmonary blood flow and eventual transudation of fluid out around the arterioles and capillaries into the perivascular interstitum and lymphatic spaces. The following discusses the characteristic radiographic manifestations of congestive heart failure as they correlate with capillary wedge pressures.

As was previously discussed, the normal pulmonary vascular pattern on upright chest radiographs exhibit the expected gravitational effects of increased blood flow to the lower lobes. Again, this can best be demonstrated by inverting the chest film upside down, which shows the conspicuous increase expected in the pulmonary vascular markings in the lower lobes compared to the upper lobes. It is also important to recognize that the pulmonary vessels should themselves be normally sharply defined throughout both lungs. Close inspection of the pulmonary arteries in the perihilar regions also reveal that the size of the pulmonary arteries closely approximate the caliber of the adjacent bronchus, both of which travel together in a common adventitial sheath. This relationship, known as the A:B ratio is essentially 1:1 (Fig. 4). In the earliest stages of cardiac decompensation where there is only a modest increase in left atrial wedge pressures above normal (16–18 mm Hg), chest radiographs will demonstrate an increase in the size of the pulmonary vessels in the upper lobes reflecting shunting of blood flow to the upper lobes (Fig. 13A). This recruitment phenomenon, known as cephalad redistribution, results in disruption of normal A:B ratio whereby the caliber of the vessel becomes larger than the adjacent bronchus (Fig. 13B).

Despite this redistribution, the pulmonary vessels should remain sharply defined as should the associated bronchus. This recruitment of upper lobes vessels is felt to reflect a physiologic attempt to improve gas O_2-CO_2 exchange, i.e. oxygenation.

In the second stage of congestive heart failure, corresponding to wedge pressures around 18 mm Hg, there is enough intravascular hydrostatic force at the venule side of the capillary to increase or drive fluid out into the interstitial spaces surrounding the artery and bronchus. When this occurs, the increase in interstitial fluid essential creates a partial masking or silhouetting of the vessels which is known as vascular congestion (Fig. 14).

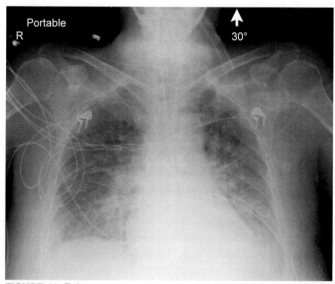

FIGURE 14: Pulmonary vascular congestion. AP radiograph of the chest showing indistinct margins of the pulmonary vasculature reflecting perivascular edema. Also note the fluid around the bronchi producing peribronchial cuffing

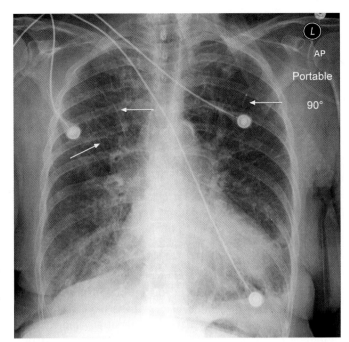

FIGURE 15: Interstitial edema. PA radiograph of patient in moderate congestive heart failure showing Kerley A (arrows) and parallel Kerley B lines in the lung bases reflecting interstitial edema

Similarly, the increase in interstitial fluid surrounding to the airways produces a blurring of central perihilar vessels, and with time, a collar of haze may develop resulting in bronchial cuffing. Both of these observations collectively indicate an increase in interstitial fluid. It should be pointed out that in itself, peribronchial cuffing can also occur with bronchial inflammation, so if observed alone, peribronchial cuffing is not specific for early heart failure.

With further increases in vascular hydrostatic pressures, and as progressively more fluid accumulates in the interstium of the lungs, fine linear shadows develop which are known as Kerley lines (Fig. 15). Radiographically, Kerley lines represent thickening (edema) of the intralobular septae that surround the secondary pulmonary lobule. Normally invisible on chest films, these septae histologically represent a part of the connective tissue supporting infrastructure of the lungs in which course the pulmonary veins and lymphatics. In congestive heart failure, the development of septal lines, which reflect both interstitial fluid and augmentation of lymphatic flow, become radiographically visible as either long linear shadows emanating out into the middle para-central regions of both lungs (Kerley A lines) (Fig. 15) or as parallel shorter subpleural lines (Kerley B lines) running perpendicular to the pleural surface (usually in the middle and lower lung zones regions). Kerley C lines, which are believed to represent summation of Kerley B lines, typically are found in the lower lung zone regions but are more central, slightly longer and much less common than B lines. When present, Kerley lines should be identified in both lungs and generally should be symmetric in distribution. Kerley lines develop with modest elevations of left atrial wedge pressures (20–22 mm Hg). One must also recognize that other etiologies capable of elevating the intravascular hydrostatic pressures will similarly produce interstitial edema separate from left heart failure, namely fluid overload, lymphatic blockage, left heart

obstructive lesions (mitral stenosis and atrial myxoma) and pulmonary embolic disease. Renal failure and hypervolemia may also produce interstitial edema both through an increase in hydrostatic pressure and decreases in plasma oncotic pressures.

With further increases in intravascular hydrostatic pressures, typically corresponding following the development of interstitial edema, accumulation of fluid in the pleural spaces bilaterally (pleural effusions) may occur, and depending on the degree of intravascular hydrostatic elevation, range from small to moderate in size.

In cases of significant elevations of hydrostatic pressures, (wedge pressures greater than 25 mm Hg), after the interstitial space is saturated and no longer capable of accommodating additional fluid, migration of fluid occurs into the lower pressure environment of the alveoli and airways. Once this occurs, chest radiographs will exhibit the classic perihilar haze or batwing airspace changes of pulmonary edema. Again, radiographically this phenomenon should be bilateral, and characteristically symmetric in distribution. In cases of severe heart failure, the edema may become generalized resulting in uniformly opaque lung tissue (Fig. 16). In cases when there is an abrupt massive rapid elevation of intravascular hydrostatic pressures, the chest radiograph may progress directly into frank pulmonary edema without a significant or appreciable interstitial phase. Pleural effusions are common at this stage due to significant accumulations of edema within the subpleural regions of the lungs.

The concept of the vascular pedicle needs to be addressed when evaluating radiographs for heart failure as it provides ancillary information regarding the circulating blood volume. The vascular pedicle essentially refers to the conglomerate radiographic shadows encompassing both the venous and arterial circulation within the mediastinum. Since the contour of the right paramedian mediastinal shadow is largely composed of large compliant mediastinal veins, i.e. SVC and azygous vein, widening or narrowing of this border effectively conveys changes in intravascular volume. The vascular pedicle width is determined on frontal radiographs by drawing a line across the

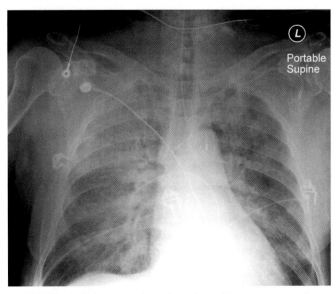

FIGURE 16: Pulmonary edema in patient with severe congestive heart failure due to acute myocardial infarction

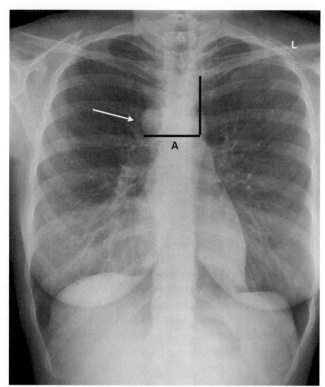

FIGURE 17: Vascular pedicle. The assessment of the vascular pedicle can easily be determined on PA chest radiographs by drawing a horizontal line from the junction of the SVC and right mainstem bronchus to a point drawn perpendicular from the left innominate artery. The horizontal line (A) represents the vascular pedicle which should be normally around 5 cm in length

mid portion of the mediastinum extending from where the right mainstem bronchus crosses the SVC, to a point intersecting a vertical line drawn the origin of the left brachiocephalic artery (Fig. 17). A normal vascular pedicle is around 5 cm. The actual measurement of the pedicle width is not as important as are *changes* in the width on serial radiographs. Widening of the vascular pedicle width between comparable radiographs (i.e. AP vs PA films) provides useful information indicating an increase in intravascular volume, and/or an increase in right atrial pressure. Similarly, decreases in the pedicle width are seen in patients with volume depletion, or those responding to diuretic therapy. In similar fashion, the width of the azygous vein (normal = 1 cm) as noted on frontal projections also provides clues as to changes in circulating blood volume, and right atrial pressures, similar to the vascular pedicle width. As such the serial changes or increases in both the vascular pedicle width and azygous venous diameter on radiographs provide diagnostic evidence of fluid balance (acute increase relating to hypervolemia, or elevated right heart pressures, i.e. right heart failure.

These observations hold important clues when evaluating radiographs in patients with heart failure. In patients with acute left heart decompensation (no predecedent heart disease) there is usually not a corresponding increase in the vascular pedicle width despite the presence of frank pulmonary edema. In contrast, those patients with chronic left heart failure, where there is usually an increase in intravascular volume due salt and water retention secondary to impaired renal perfusion. In patients with right heart decompensation, there is usually an increase in both the vascular pedicle width and azygous venous diameters without the corresponding pulmonary vascular changes of left heart failure. These changes reflect the increase in the volume of venous blood secondary to the failing right heart. In cases of acute biventricular failure, one should expect to see both the pulmonary manifestations of acute failure as well as concomitant widening of the pedicle and azygous venous diameter.

The interpretation of the radiographic changes characteristic of left sided heart failure can be further refined to assist in differentiating between acute and chronic left ventricular failure. In acute (rapid) heart failure, it is common not only to see a normal vascular pedicle width along with a normal cardiac silhouette despite the presence of frank pulmonary edema. In these cases, the normal or narrowed vascular pedicle reflects a diminished intravascular fluid balance due to the development of edema within the lungs. Additionally in cases of very rapid left ventricular decompensation (acute infarction), the distribution of edema within both lungs is often para-central (batwing edema), and may develop without any radiographic evidence of interstitial edema and peribroncial cuffing. Redistribution of pulmonary blood flow also is usually conspicuously absent in cases of rapid left heart failure. Pleural effusions generally are uncommon as well secondary to an absence of sup-pleural pulmonary edema. In cases of chronic left heart failure, cephalad redistribution is much more common, likely a physiologic response of regional impaired O_2-CO_2 exchange in the lower lobes due to microscopic edema along the capillary-alveolar interface as well as reflex vasoconstriction of the lower lobe pulmonary veins to augment left atrial stroke volume. The conspicuous absence of interstitial edema in patients with chronic compensated left ventricular dysfunction may also be explained by augmentation of pulmonary lymphatic drainage that develops over time to facilitate the removal of interstitial edema from the lungs.

CARDIAC CALCIFICATIONS

Evaluation of unusual of calcifications overlying the cardiac silhouette may provide important clues about specific disease processes which may not be clinically suspected. Most importantly, the identification of coronary calcium indicates severe, advance atherosclerosis, which in younger patients suggests possible abnormalities of blood lipid levels, i.e. hypercholesterolemia (Fig. 18). Due to the limitations of resolution of coronary calcium on chest radiographs, the identification of coronary calcium implies significant disease with an associated higher likelihood of significant stenosis, and portends even more significance when discovered in patients with acute chest pain syndromes. Linear myocardial calcifications may be encountered in patients with a history of prior myocardial infarction (Figs 19A and B), and if protuberant, may indicate associated formation of ventricular aneurysm (Figs 20A and B). Typically, the protuberant thin-walled calcified aneurysms at the apex of the left ventricle are true aneurysms, while those residing along the posterior aspect of the left ventricle are most commonly pseudoaneurysms.

Valvular calcifications when identified on chest films generally are associated with significant valvular stenosis.

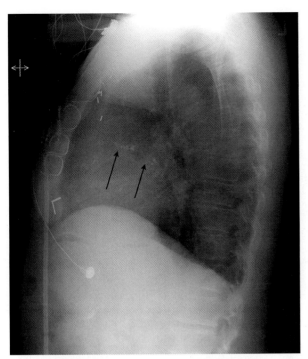

FIGURE 18: Calcification of the left anterior descending coronary artery (arrows)

Mitral annular calcifications are commonly demonstrated on radiographs occurring on 10% of adult patients, usually appearing as an incomplete ring of beaded appearing calcification (Figs 21A and B). Usually, mitral annular calcifications due to atherosclerosis in the elderly are incidental and of no clinical significance. Although there is little correlation with the extent of annular calcifications and likelihood of mitral valve disease, mitral annular calcifications are seen in 35–40% of patients with mitral stenosis. Generally, the more severe the annular calcification, the greater likelihood of associated mitral valve disease.

Pericardial calcifications (Figs 22A and B), usually stemming from either prior pericarditis or hemopericardium, may be associated with hemodynamic features of pericardial constriction, and as such may warrant further evaluation of cardiac function with echocardiography as well as ventricular compliance by assessment of diastolic filling. Conglomerate calcifications within the cardiac chamber can reflect either intracardiac thrombus, or rarely calcification within intracardiac tumors (fibroma, myxoma and teratoma).

ACQUIRED VALVULAR HEART DISEASE

Aortic and mitral valve disorders are the most commonly encountered forms of valvular heart disease in adults and both have characteristic radiographic manifestations. Characteristically, most of these disorders stem from either congenital structural valvular abnormalities or rheumatic heart disease. Tricuspid and pulmonary valve disorders in adults are overall less common and less commonly are associated with cardiovascular changes on radiographs.

AORTIC STENOSIS

The most common form of congenital heart disease is the biscuspid aortic valve, with a prevalence of 1–2% in the general population. Responsible for most all cases of aortic stenosis in adults, the severity of the hemodynamic derangements across the aortic valve coincide with the degree of associated thickening and/or calcification of the aortic valve leaflets. Other causes of aortic stenosis which include degenerative aortic valve disease and rheumatic heart disease are likewise are associated with similar valvular changes, although the presence of valve calcium is less common in these entities. The typical radiographic feature of aortic stenosis which is related to the severity of stenosis is poststenotic dilatation of the ascending thoracic aorta due to the jet effect of blood exiting the stenotic valve (Figs 23A and B).

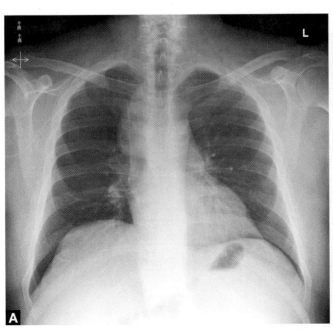

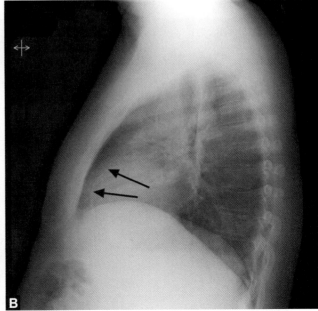

FIGURES 19A AND B: (A) Myocardial calcification in patient with prior myocardial infarction. (B) Note on the lateral projection a fine linear zone of calcification within the myocardium (arrows)

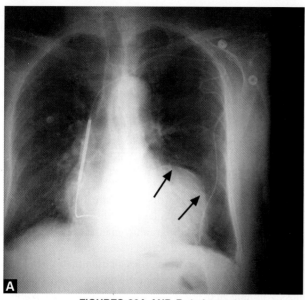
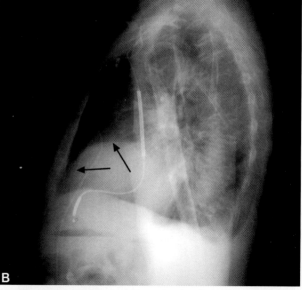

FIGURES 20A AND B: Left ventricular aneurysm. (A) PA and (B) lateral chest films showing linear calcification along the border of a large left ventricle aneurysm (arrows)

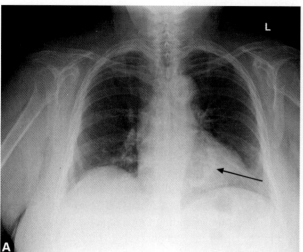
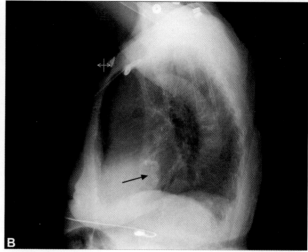

FIGURES 21A AND B: Mitral annular calcification. (A) PA and (B) lateral chest films showing the beaded calcium within the mitral valve annulus (arrows)

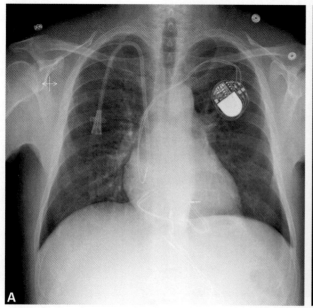
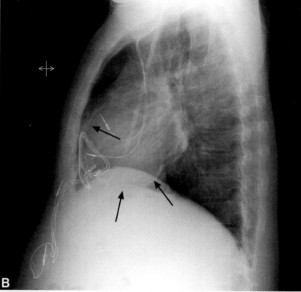

FIGURES 22A AND B: (A and B) Pericardial calcification. Lateral chest film shows heavy calcifications along the pericardial surface (arrows)

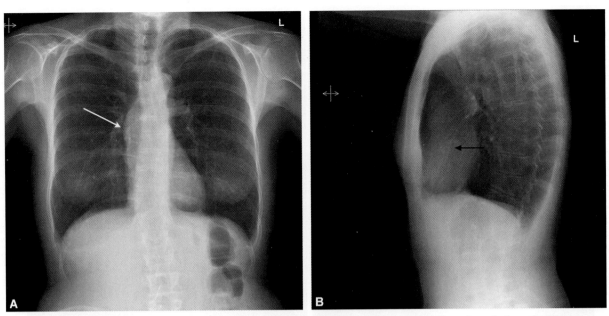

FIGURES 23A AND B: Aortic stenosis. (A) PA film shows dilatation of the ascending thoracic aorta (arrow) without associated left ventricular dilatation. (B) Lateral film shows calcification of the aortic valve (arrow)

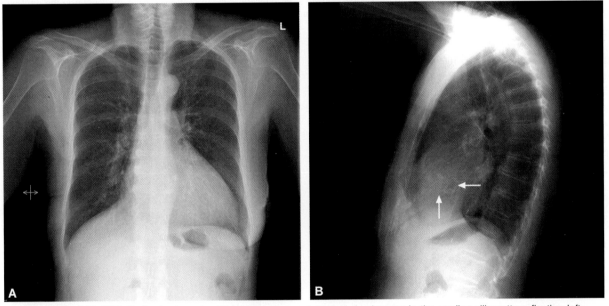

FIGURES 24A AND B: Aortic stenosis. (A) PA film shows characteristic changes in the cardiac silhouette reflecting left ventricular dilatation (failure). (B) Lateral film showing calcifications involving the aortic valve apparatus (arrows)

Usually the configuration of the heart appears normal. Not until left ventricular failure develops will there be radiographic changes in the heart shadow reflecting left ventricular enlargement which occurs late in the disease, if at all (Figs 24A and B). Left ventricular hypertrophy, in and by itself, is not associated with any morphologic changes of the cardiac silhouette on chest radiographs. When present, aortic valve calcifications, which are best identified on lateral radiographs, indicates significant valvular stenosis, and are most commonly seen in cases of biscuspid aortic stenosis (Figs 23A and B and 24A and B). The pulmonary vascular pattern in aortic stenosis is normal.

AORTIC INSUFFICIENCY

Aortic insufficiency in adults can be attributed to either aortic valve disease or disorders of the aortic root such as aneurysm or dissection. The radiographic manifestations of aortic insufficiency, like aortic stenosis, are related to both the severity and duration of the disease. Features of aortic insufficiency on chest films include both dilatation of the ascending thoracic aorta with associated left ventricular enlargement. Enlargement of the left atrium rarely occurs providing compentency of the mitral valve. In most cases the pulmonary circulation appears normal.

MITRAL STENOSIS

Most cases of mitral stenosis are a sequela of rheumatic fever. The radiographic manifestations of mitral stenosis coincide with the degree of the severity of the stenosis. Characteristically, radiographs will usually are diagnostic for this disease and demonstrate left atrial enlargement which can be marked in severe cases (Figs 25A and B). Severe stenosis at the mitral valve resulting in significant left heart obstruction may also

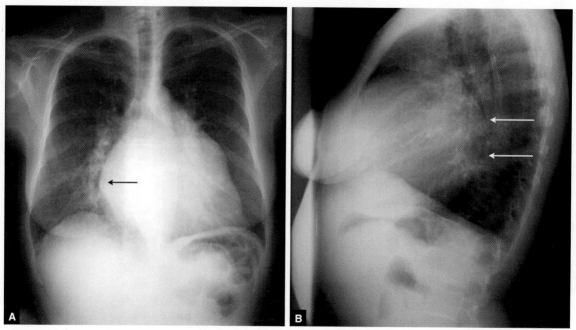

FIGURES 25A AND B: Mitral valve stenosis. (A) PA film shows radiographic findings of mitral valve stenosis including left atrial enlargement and pulmonary venous hypertension. The arrow points to the double density sign reflecting overlap of the left atrial shadow upon the right atrium. (B) The lateral film shows marked posterior bulging of the left atrial shadow (arrows)

produce radiographic changes of congestive heart failure as well as pulmonary arterial hypertension. Recurrent pulmonary edema in cases of long-standing mitral stenosis may result in deposition of hemosiderin with the lungs which radiographically appears as discrete punctate calcified pulmonary nodules, occasionally with associated areas of associated pulmonary fibrosis. Calcification of the mitral valve, annulus or the left atrium may also be detected on radiographs (Fig. 26).

MITRAL REGURGITATION

While associated with rheumatic heart disease, mitral valve insufficiency in adults is more commonly seen in mitral valve prolapse. Similar to mitral stenosis, chest films demonstrate marked left atrial enlargement with pulmonary venous hypertension. Frequently, there is a component of associated dilatation of the left ventricle as well, especially in long-standing cases. Occasionally in cases of severe mitral regurgitation, passive venous congestion with or without pulmonary edema may be encountered. Unilateral right upper lobe edema/hemorrhage secondary to the jet effect of regurgitant blood entering the right upper lobe pulmonary vein may also occasionally be encountered (Fig. 27). Patients, presenting with mitral insufficiency due to acute rupture of a papillary muscle, usually present with radiographic features of acute congestive heart failure without corresponding cardiomegaly.

PULMONARY VALVE STENOSIS

Pulmonary valve stenosis is generally a component of congenital heart disease and is an uncommon acquired valvular disorder in adult, resulting from fusion on the commissures. In any case, the typical radiographic feature of pulmonary stenosis is unilateral dilatation of the left pulmonary artery arising from

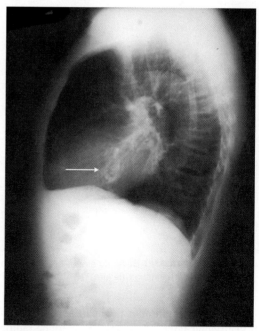

FIGURE 26: Mitral valve calcification. Lateral chest film showing extensive calcification of the mitral valve and annulus (arrow)

the poststenotic jet effect of blood exiting the pulmonary valve (Fig. 28). Long standing cases may show associated enlargement of the right ventricular shadow.

PULMONARY VALVE INSUFFICIENCY

Distinctly uncommon in adults, insufficiency of the pulmonary valve often is not associated with any specific morphologic changes of the cardiovascular structures on chest films other than occasional right heart enlargement.

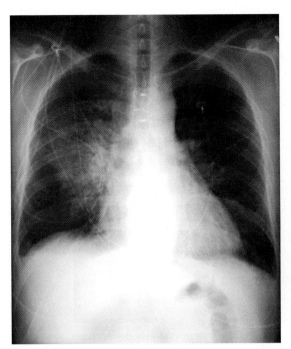

FIGURE 27: Mitral valve insufficiency. PA chest film showing unilateral right upper lobe edema from severe mitral regurgitation in patient with acute papillary muscle rupture

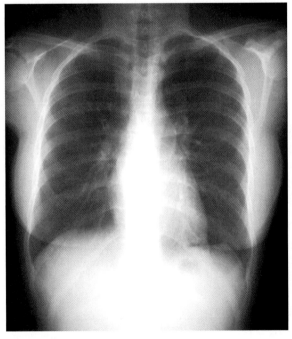

FIGURE 28: Pulmonary valve stenosis. PA film showing unilateral dilatation of the left pulmonary arterial trunk

TRICUSPID INSUFFICIENCY

In most cases of triscuspid insufficiency, there are no discernable radiographic changes suggestive of this disease. When severe, prominence of the right heart border reflecting right atrial enlargement occurs (Fig. 12). Associated widening of the vascular pedicle (especially SVC shadow) and dilatation of the azygous vein may also present indicating an increase in right atrial pressure.

PERICARDIAL EFFUSION

It is important to realize that the heart shadow as demonstrated on plain films is composed of both the heart and the surrounding pericardial sac. As such, an apparent increase in the heart shadow may be due to either intrinsic cardiac chamber(s) dilatation or alternatively reflect accumulation of fluid in the pericardial space. While small pericardial effusions usually will go undetected by chest films, large amounts will alter the overall shape of the heart shadow resulting in a globular relatively featureless cardiac silhouette (aka water bottle configuration) (Fig. 29). The lateral film may show an opaque line (fat pad sign) along the ventral surface of the heart reflecting separation of visceral and parietal pericardial fat by the effusion. The absence of ancillary findings of congestive heart failure, such as pulmonary venous hypertension, may help differentiate a pericardial effusion from dilated cardiomyopathic heart (Fig. 30). A sudden or significant enlargement of the size of the

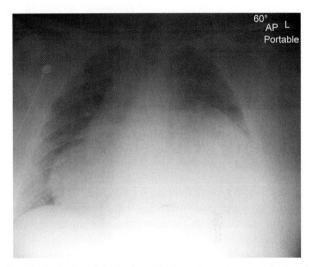

FIGURE 29: Pericardial effusion. PA chest films shows marked global enlargement (water bottle configuration) of the cardiac silhouette secondary to a large pericardial effusion

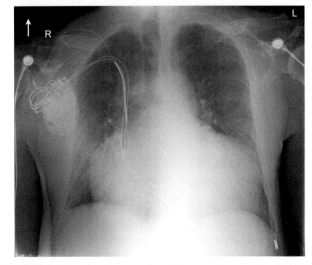

FIGURE 30: Dilated cardiomyopathy. PA chest radiograph showing global enlargement of the cardiac silhouette. Note the similar cardiac configuration to Figure 29

CHAPTER 11 Plain Film Imaging of Adult Cardiovascular Disease

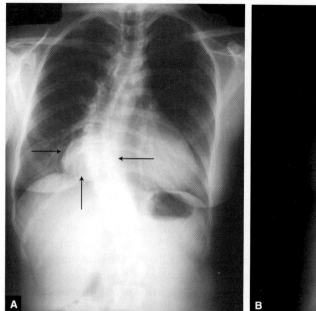

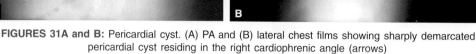

FIGURES 31A and B: Pericardial cyst. (A) PA and (B) lateral chest films showing sharply demarcated pericardial cyst residing in the right cardiophrenic angle (arrows)

heart shadow on serial chest films is an important radiographic observation that should suggest a pericardial effusion rather than intrinsic heart disease. Unfortunately, too many times patients' films have been erroneously interpreted as cardiomegaly (failing heart) only to discover on further evaluation that the heart was entirely normal but enveloped within a large pericardial effusion.

PERICARDIAL CYSTS

Pericardial cysts present radiographically as sharply demarcated mass-like opacities usually residing immediately adjacent to the heart, and are usually an incidental discovery in asymptomatic

patients. Most commonly residing in the region of cardiophrenic angles, more so on the right side, these cysts are usually several centimeters in diameter (Figs 31A and B). Once discovered, computed tomography or magnetic resonance imaging scans can provide confirmation of the diagnosis by demonstrating the characteristic morphologic features of these cysts.

CONGENITAL ABSENCE OF THE PERICARDIUM

Congenital defects of the pericardial sac, like pericardial cysts, are usually an incidental finding in either children or adults. The pericardial defect may be focal, partial or complete. Left-sided absence, the most common variety, occurs in 55% of the cases of congenital absence of the pericardium. Radiographically, these pericardial defects produce unusual changes in the shape of the cardiac silhouette, resulting in focal bulge-like contour changes reflecting herniation of cardiac structures such as the left atrial appendage (Fig. 32). Radiographic features of complete absence of the pericardium are leftward displacement of the cardiac silhouette without a corresponding shift of the mediastinum.

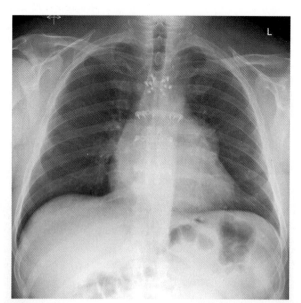

FIGURE 32: Absence of the pericardium. PA chest radiograph showing herniation of the left atrial appendage in patient who had recently undergone coronary bypass surgery. Note the focal bulge along the left heart border. Similar findings would be expected in congenital absence of the pericardium

BIBLIOGRAPHY

1. David J Skorton (Ed). Cardiac Imaging: A Companion to Braunwald's Heart Disease. Philadelphia: WB Saunders Company; 1996.
2. Eric NC Milne, Massimo Pistolesi. Reading the Chest Radiograph. A Physiologic Approach. St. Louis: Mosby; 1993.
3. Eugene Gedaudas, James H Moller, Wilfredo R. Castaneda-Zuniga, et al. Cardiovascular Radiology. Philadelphia: WB Saunders Company; 1985.
4. Michael E Jay. Plain Film in Heart Disease. London: Blackwell Scientific Publications; 1993.
5. Stephen Wilmot Miller. Cardiac Imaging. The Requisites. Philadelphia: Elsevier Mosby; 2005.
6. W Richard Webb, Charles B Higgins. Thoracic Imaging: Pulmonary and Cardiovascular Radiology. Philadelphia: Lippincott Williams and Wilkins; 2005.

Electrocardiogram

Donald Brown

Chapter Outline

INTRODUCTION

The electrocardiogram remains one of the most valuable, most readily available and relatively least expensive laboratory tools. Its accurate interpretation is absolutely critical to patient care. While computer assisted interpretation of the 12 lead electrocardiogram is almost universally available, the computer based interpretation should never be assumed to be accurate. In addition rhythm strips off of monitors do not usually have computer based interpretation. Therefore, the clinician's ability to interpret accurately a 12 lead electrocardiogram and a rhythm strip is absolutely crucial to patient care.

BASIS OF ELECTROCARDIOGRAPHY

The electrocardiogram in its most basic sense represents the recording of electrical potentials from the heart projected on to the body surface and fed into a galvanometer set up as a voltmeter. The electrical potentials are produced by depolarization and repolarization of the atrial and ventricular myocardial cells of the heart. The basic principle is that as a set of cells depolarize the negative charge of the interior of the cell relative to the exterior is reversed as channels open to allow ions to flow out of the cell to produce an interior now more positively charged relative to the exterior. As this process moves longitudinally along a line of cells in a direction toward the exploring electrode of a voltmeter, an upright or positive deflection is produced. As a repolarizing wave moves in the same direction along the same longitudinal path, a negative deflection is inscribed by the voltmeter.

As is well appreciated, the heart's activation normally begins with the discharge of the sinoatrial node located in the right atrium beginning just below the superior vena cava. This discharge is of such a tiny magnitude that the electrocardio-

gram cannot record it. Nevertheless this leads to the depolarization of the atrial musculature from the high right atrium, over the right atrium and over to the left atrium creating what has been designated as a p wave. Under normal circumstances, this depolarizing wave then moves from the atrial chambers and passes on to the discrete conduction pathways connecting the atrium to the ventricular musculature, specifically through the atrioventricular (AV) node, then through the common or His bundle, and then out simultaneously through the right and left bundle branches to activate the ventricular musculature. The AV node is located at the base of the atrial septum on its right atrial side. Specifically it is located at the apex of "Koch's triangle". The apex of this triangle is formed by the annulus of the tricuspid valve's septal leaflet and Todaro's tendon, a structure that runs from the rostral portion of the coronary sinus downward to the central fibrous body ("cardiac skeleton") of the heart. The base of the triangle is the orifice of the coronary sinus (Fig. 1). The depolarization then proceeds through the AV bundle (common bundle or bundle of His) that penetrates the dense connective tissue of the central fibrous body and runs down along the right ventricular side of the membranous interventricular septum. The common bundle then bifurcates into the right and left bundles. The right bundle runs as a quite discrete bundle along a particularly prominent trabecular band known as the moderator band across to the base of the anterior papillary muscle of the right ventricle. The left bundle passes beneath the membranous part of the interventricular septum to reach the left side of the septum where it eventually divides into two broad bands. The anterior division is relatively more discrete and activates the anterior superior portion of the left ventricle. The much broader band is the posterior division that activates the posterior inferior portion of the left ventricle. All three bundles fan out as the Purkinje fibers of the interior of

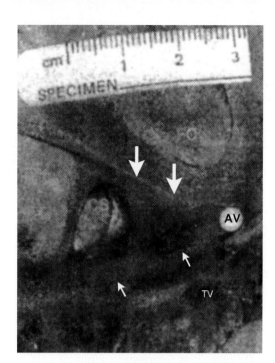

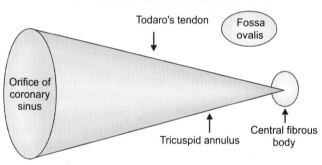

FIGURE 1: Illustration of Koch's triangle

The blood supply of the sinoatrial node and the portions of the conducting system noted above are important particularly from the standpoint of patients afflicted with ischemic heart disease and the electrocardiographic consequences of infarction. Estimates of the percentages of blood supply to portions of the conducting system vary from author to author and also vary according to the technique used, e.g. dissection, injection of the coronaries by various materials or by various modern imaging techniques. Percent estimates will also be affected by the numbers of heart examined, thus leading to variance based on sample size.

The supply to the sinoatrial node most commonly is from the right coronary artery, perhaps 60–70% of the time. Usually this arterial supply arises quite proximally from the right coronary artery, although occasionally distally. The supply is from the left coronary artery in about 10–30% of the cases. The artery supplying the sinoatrial node from the left coronary artery almost always arises from the proximal circumflex coronary artery, although it may rarely arises from the left main coronary artery or the quite distal circumflex artery. There appears to be a dual supply from both right and left coronary arteries about 5–10% of the time.

The blood supply to the AV node is almost always from an artery that arises at the U-turn of the artery that crosses the crux of the heart where the AV groove meets the proximal posterior interventricular groove. Relatively consistently the supply to this node is solely by the right coronary artery 80% of the time, solely from the circumflex artery in about 10% of the time and from both right coronary and left circumflex arterial sources about 10% of the time.

The His or common bundle most commonly has a dual blood supply from the AV nodal artery and a septal branch of the anterior descending coronary artery. The proximal portion of the right bundle may have a similar dual supply in perhaps 50% of the cases with most of the remainder of cases demonstrating supply only by the septal artery and in rare cases solely by the AV nodal artery. The portion of the right bundle along the moderator band appears to be supplied solely by a septal branch from the left anterior descending coronary artery. The supply to the proximal portion of the anterior half of the left bundle is similar to the right bundle in its blood supply, with about half of all individuals having a dual supply from the AV nodal artery and a septal branch of the left anterior descending, about half the individuals having a supply by just a septal branch only, and, uncommonly, an individual's supply by the AV nodal artery only. The posterior portion of the left bundle is supplied solely by the AV nodal artery about half the time with most of the remainder of the time by a dual supply from the AV nodal artery and a septal artery; occasionally the supply is solely by a septal artery.

Of importance to some of the nonischemic causes of conduction disturbances is the proximity of the His bundle and proximal bundles to the cardiac skeleton. This fibrous skeleton consists of the fibrous annuli of the four cardiac valves plus the membranous septum and the aortic intervalvular, right and left fibrous trigones. The dominant portion of the skeleton is the right fibrous trigone through which the His bundle passes. The left bundle as previously noted passes beneath the membranous septum.

the ventricles activating the ventricular musculature from the endocardial to epicardial surface.

The first portion of the ventricle to be activated is the ventricular septum. This begins via tiny fibers off of the left bundle spreading out as Purkinje fibers from about the midportion of the left side of the ventricular septum leading to depolarization of the septal musculature from its left ventricular side to its right ventricular side. Hence septal depolarization under normal circumstances accounts for a dominate portion of the initial portion of the depolarization of the ventricles recorded by the electrocardiogram and designated the QRS complex. Continued conduction in the right and left bundles is occurring simultaneously while this septal activation is occurring. The right and left bundles carry their impulse on to the interior of the free walls of the two ventricles as they spread out as cells identical to themselves known as Purkinje cells coating the endocardial surface of the two ventricles. This leads to depolarization of the entire ventricular muscles masses from endocardium to epicardium. Importantly these depolarizing waves spreads out in a spiral fashion that leads to excitation and thus contraction of the ventricular musculature from apex to base, thus wringing out the heart from apex to base toward the aortic and pulmonary valves.

COMPONENT PARTS OF THE ELECTROCARDIOGRAM

The depolarization of the atrial chambers produces waves called p waves. In a general any type of rhythm that involves depolarization of the atrial chambers could be called a p wave; however, certain waves typical of certain atrial rhythm disturbances have been given specific names such as flutter waves or fibrillatory waves. The repolarization of the atrial chambers is usually not evident on the surface ECG tracing. The summation of all the depolarizations of the ventricular chambers (a summation of phase 0 of all the action potentials of the ventricular myocardial cell depolarizations) is expressed as the QRS complex. By custom, a Q wave must be an initial deflection of a QRS complex and must be a negative or downward deflection. All upward or positive deflections are called R waves and negative deflections that are not the initial deflection of the QRS complex are called S waves. If there is more than one R or S wave in the complex, the second deflection is labeled R prime (R') or S prime (S'). Descriptively sometimes R or S waves may be represented by capital or lower case letters depending on the size of the deflection. The summation of the repolarization of the ventricular chambers (primarily the phase 3 of the action potentials of the ventricular myocardial cells) is represented on the ECG by the T wave. The deflection or direction of the T wave is generally in the same direction as the major direction of the QRS complex for most leads since the left ventricle, which by its mass dominates the formation of the QRS complex, depolarizes from the endocardium out to the epicardium but repolarizes from the epicardium inward to the endocardium. The T wave may be followed by a low voltage wave names the U wave. The origin of this wave remains in dispute.

LEAD SYSTEMS USED TO RECORD THE ELECTROCARDIOGRAM

As mentioned, the electrocardiogram is just the recording of cardiac electrical potentials from the body surface by a galvanometer set up as a voltmeter. The original system devised by Einthoven consists of the leads from the left arm, the right arm and left leg set up to compare the recordings from one extremity to a second extremity by feeding the recordings into the either side of the voltmeter. The three potential combinations have been designated as bipolar leads. As designed by Einthoven, lead I is the comparison of the left arm potentials versus the right arm potentials connected to the voltmeter so that an upright wave is recorded in lead I when the left arm's potential is positive relative to the right arm's electrical potential. Given the assumption that the Einthoven triangle for the three leads is an equilateral triangle, this means that lead I looks horizontally straight across from left to right (though the scalene triangle described by Burger and van Milaan more accurately depicts the geometry, Einthoven's triangle is so entrenched and so useful as to remain the conceptual framework for the limb lead system). Einthoven's second lead, lead II, consists of the comparison of the potentials on the left leg versus the right arm connected so that an upright deflection in lead II occurs when the left leg's potential is positive compared to the right arm's

potential. Lead III is a comparison of the potentials from the left leg versus the left arm connected to the voltmeter so that this lead registers an upright deflection when the left leg's potential is positive relative to the left arm's potential. Thus the three leads create a triangle with three points of view separated by 60 degrees (Fig. 2). Kirchhoff's second law based on the conservation of energy states that the algebraic sum of the potentials around a closed path must be zero. This means that the electrical potential recorded in lead II is equal to the sum of the potentials recorded in leads I and III. This can perhaps be better visualized and understood by collapsing the three leads points of view so they intersect at a central points and thinking in terms of vector forces (Fig. 2). Viewed in this manner, all the vector forces in lead II are predicted by leads I and II.

Frank Wilson and his colleagues developed a system of recording electrical potentials from a single extremity compared to an "indifferent electrode" whose recorded potentials are minimal. The purpose was to record just the potentials from a given extremity representing each of the apices of Einthoven's triangle. They created the indifferent electrode by fusing the connections of each into a single central terminal. A 5,000 ohm resistor was placed between each extremity electrode and the fusion at the central terminal. The potentials from the exploring electrode from the right arm, left arm or left leg are compared by the voltmeter with this minimal potential from the central terminal lead. Electrocardiographic leads using this system are indicated by the letter V, hence VR, VL and VF. The connections to the voltmeter are such that an upright wave is recorded in VR when its potentials are positive. Emanuel Goldberger modified this V lead system as it pertains to the extremity leads in such a way as to increase the amplitude of the potentials recorded. Goldberger removed the resistors between the extremity connections and the central terminal. Goldberger further modified the "central terminal" by removing the connection of an extremity's electrode to the "central terminal" when that extremity's electrical potential was to be compared to the central terminal's minimal potential. This augmentation of the potential recorded from a given extremity is indicated by the "a" preceding the name of that lead, i.e. aVR, aVL and aVF (Fig. 2). Traditionally these augmented leads have been called the "augmented unipolar leads", a phrase from Goldberger's original paper in 1942. In truth, the term "unipolar" is improper in an electrical sense. Thus aVR is really the comparison of the electrical potential recorded from the right arm versus the averaged potentials recorded from the left leg and left arm. Thus aVR is right arm potential minus (i.e. versus) [left arm potential + left leg potential/2]. By the same reasoning as used to state that lead II's recording is predicted by the potentials recorded in leads I and III, lead aVR's recording is entirely described by "minus" the recording in aVL and "minus" the recording in aVF. From the standpoint of vectors for each lead, the potential recorded in any given lead is already described by any two leads equidistant from that leads point of view. For instance, lead aVF is completely described by the sum of lead II and lead III divided by 2.

The formulae usually presented then are as follows:

$$II = I + III;$$
$$aVF = (II + III)/2.$$

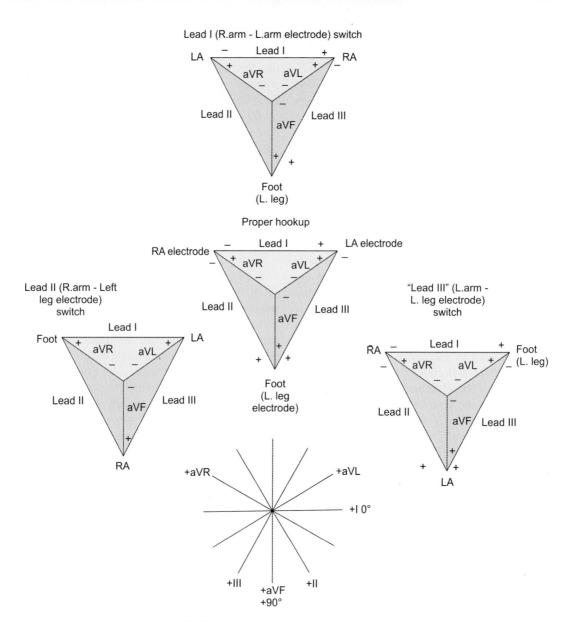

FIGURE 2: Leads orientation and vector forces

All other comparisons can be given by algebraic rearrangement of these two equations.

Later the precordial leads were developed using Wilson's central terminal versus the exploring electrode placed at various positions on the chest wall. For accuracy of electrocardiographic interpretations and especially in comparing serial recordings, the correct placement of the precordial leads is absolutely essential. Lead V1 must be placed in the 4th intercostal space just to the right of the sternal border; lead V2 in the 4th intercostal space just to the left of the sternal border; lead V4 at the left midclavicular line in the 5th intercostal space; lead V3 at the midpoint of a diagonal line connecting leads lead V2 and lead V4. Lead V5 is placed at the anterior axillary line at the anterior axillary line's intersection with a line extending out perpendicular to the rostral-caudal line of the body from the position of V4. Lead V6 is placed at the midaxillary line along the same line as V4 and V5. The midaxillary line is best defined in terms of lead placement as the mid or central plane of the thorax. There is a common misconception that V5 and V6 stay

in the same interspace as V4. If the anterior axillary line is not well defined, lead V5 should be placed midway between V4 and V6.

COMMON ELECTRODE MISPLACEMENTS

An experienced interpreter of the electrocardiogram should be able to recognize artifact produced by improper placement of the electrocardiographic electrodes. A distinct discrepancy of a current electrocardiogram compared to a previous one in terms of P, QRS and T wave axes or precordial leads showing tall R waves in V1 declining progressively in V2 and V3 and then abruptly becoming larger again in V4 provide clues that electrodes have been misplaced. Specific examples will now be discussed.

Misplacements of the left arm, right arm or left leg electrodes onto the wrong extremity (as a visual reference see Figure 2). Viewing Einthoven's triangle with the six frontal plane (extremity leads) properly connected predicts what would happen to the QRS complex when improperly connected.

A common extremity electrode misplacement involves placement of the right arm electrode on the left arm and the left arm electrode on the right arm. In terms of Einthoven's triangle the configuration now looks as depicted in Figure 2 under lead I switch. Recalling that a lead's point of view is from the positive looking toward the negative, lead I's point of view has been switched from looking left toward right and now looks right toward left. Thus, what should be the proper inscription of lead I is inscribed upside down. Further inspection of the diagram reveals that the inscription labeled lead II, normally a comparison of the electrical potentials of the left leg versus the right arm now is inscribing a comparison of the potentials of the left leg versus the left arm and thus is inscribing lead III. Similarly the inscription labeled as lead III is actually an inscription of lead II. Similarly, aVR should be a comparison of the potential from the right arm versus the input from the modified central terminal lead. With this electrode switch that inscribed as aVR is actually a comparison of the potential from the left arm versus the central terminal lead or lead aVL. The inscription of lead aVF is not changed.

A visual clue that this electrode switch has occurred is that not only is the QRS upside down but the p wave in lead I is also inverted. An additional clue comes from the precordial leads V1–V6. When properly placed, leads V5–V6 should have the same left to right point of view. When lead I appears to be the inversion of V5–V6, consideration should be given to a left arm-right arm electrode switch (a "lead I switch"). When the heart's anatomical position is truly "switched from left to right" as occurs in situs inversus, the standard proper hookup of the electrocardiogram will look like a left arm-right arm electrode switch in the frontal plane and the precordial V1 through V6 leads will show a progressive decrement of the amplitude of the R wave rather than the progressive increment expected in the amplitude of the R wave. In a patient with situs inversus the interpretation of the recording of the electrocardiogram using the usual criteria for QRS, ST and T abnormalities in the various leads can be facilitated by intentionally placing the right arm electrode on the left arm and the left arm electrode on the right arm, and placing the precordial electrodes in the usual interspaces but starting with V1 at the left sternal border and moving rightward so that V6 is at the right anterior axillary line.

LEFT ARM

A less common but not rare electrode switch involves placing the left arm electrode on the left leg and the left leg electrode on the left arm, a so-called lead III switch (Fig. 2). To correct for this electrode switch, the inscription of lead I, normally a comparison of left arm versus right arm is actually an inscription that compares left leg to right arm and thus is actually inscribing lead II; similarly lead II is not inscribing the comparison of left leg to right arm but rather left arm to right arm or lead I. By similar analysis lead III will be inscribed upside down (inverted). Similarly lead aVL is actually inscribing lead aVF, lead aVF is inscribing aVL. Lead aVR is not altered since the right arm electrode is in the proper location.

A quite uncommon extremity electrode switch involves placement of the left leg electrode on the right arm and the right arm electrode on the left leg, a so-called lead II switch (Fig. 2).

In this case, lead I is actually inscribing a comparison of left arm to left leg or the inversion of lead III; lead III is actually inscribing comparison of right arm to left arm or the inversion of what lead I should be and lead II is inscribing the comparison of right arm to left leg or the inversion of lead II. Lead aVR is now recording aVF, lead aVF is recording lead aVR, and lead aVL is properly recording lead aVL since the left arm electrode has not been moved.

From these descriptions, the electrocardiographer can appreciate what would happen to the main direction of the QRS forces in the frontal plane, called the mean QRS axis in the frontal plane, a concept to be further described subsequently. Normally the main direction of the QRS forces is about 60 degrees, i.e. forces pointing down and leftward. Visualize how a "lead I switch", the switch of the left arm and right arm electrodes, turns Einthoven's triangle by flipping it right to left along the axis of the point of view of lead aVF. Thus the mean QRS axis moves from about 60 degrees to about 150 degrees, i.e. now pointing down and rightward. A lead II switch or right arm-left leg electrode switch rotates the triangle around the axis of the point of view of lead aVR and thus flips a normal QRS axis upward and leftward. Such marked axis shifts help in recognizing these electrode switches compared to prior electrocardiograms. By recognizing around which augmented lead axis the rotation of the axis has occurred and realizing that this augmented lead axis will be perpendicular to the point of the lead that has been switched, e.g. lead aVL being perpendicular to lead II indicates a right arm-left leg electrode switch, i.e. a lead II switch. The lead III switch or left arm-left leg switch can be difficult to recognize since the rotation of the triangle is around the axis of lead aVR. This does not change the mean QRS since it is normally directed down and leftward and it will remain pointing down and to the left. Nevertheless noting that the prior electrocardiogram's lead III has been inverted in the present electrocardiogram will allow recognition. An extension of the above descriptors is the appreciation that the augmented "unipolar" lead that does not change in a frontal plane electrode switch compared to the prior electrocardiogram helps to identify the type of electrode switch. The augmented "unipolar" lead that does not change be the lead that is perpendicular to the line connecting the electrode switch, e.g. lead aVF point of view is perpendicular to the right arm-left arm (lead I) point of view in a right arm-left arm electrode switch.

RIGHT LEG ELECTRODE

This electrode acts as an electronic reference that serves to improve the rejection of unwanted noise. Misplacing the right leg electrode by switching it with the left leg electrode does not alter the electrocardiogram since the isopotential lines are identical for the two legs. However, misplacing it onto the arms, most commonly by switching it with the right arm electrode, completely distorts the electrocardiogram in such a way that no interpretation of the frontal plane leads can be done. This misplacement of the right leg electrode placed on the right arm and the right arm electrode placed on the right leg is most easily detected by noting that lead II is essentially a flat line with minimal QRS deflections. This is true because the "right arm electrode" placed on the right leg will feed into the "negative"

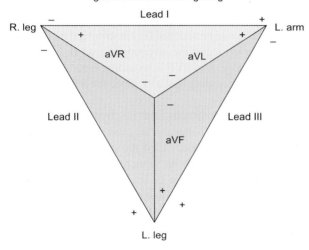

FIGURE 3: Leads inversion

SECTION 3

Diagnosis

side of the voltmeter an identical electrical potential to that fed into the positive side of the voltmeter from the electrode on the left leg when the machine is recording what "it" thinks is lead II. Thus the comparison between the two by the voltmeter renders a straight line. In addition lead I will be an exact inversion of lead III, and lead aVL and lead I will be identical (Fig. 3).

Under the bizarre circumstance that the right leg electrode is switched with the left arm electrode, lead III will be an essentially flat line with minimal QRS deflections.

Lead II now records Foot versus Foot and thus records a straight line.

The most bizarre of all the electrodes switches is when the right and left leg electrodes are moved to the right and left arms and the electrodes from the arms are moved to the legs. This produces a straight line in lead I.

A frequent technical error involving the precordial leads consists on switching V1 and V3 electrode placements creating a taller R in "V1" with a smaller R in V3 with then a suddenly taller R in V4.

Misplacements of the precordial leads an interspace to high often creates the impression of unusually small r waves or actual Q waves in the right precordial leads. Improper placement of leads V4, V5 and V6 often creates the impression that these leads are recording R waves that are still less than the S wave amplitudes in those leads.

OTHER LEAD SYSTEMS

For detection of p waves difficult to define on the surface electrocardiogram, bipolar esophageal lead systems that combine simultaneously recorded electrograms from an electrode positioned in the esophagus directly behind the left atrium and a surface lead, such as lead II, can be quite helpful. However, these systems are not routinely readily available. Routinely available is a "Lewis lead" for detection of sinus activity. To obtain a Lewis lead the right arm electrode is placed just to the right of the sternum in the second right intercostal space or just to the right of the manubrium and the left arm electrode is placed

in the fourth or fifth intercostal space just to the right of the sternum.

A SYSTEMATIC WAY OF LOOKING AT THE INTERPRETATION OF THE ELECTROCARDIOGRAM

A Systematic Way of Looking at the Rhythm

For the purposes of this discussion, the suggestions to follow are principally for interpretation of the electrocardiogram of adults.

IDENTIFICATION OF ATRIAL ACTIVITY

Proceeding in a systematic fashion helps to prevent omissions and leads to better conclusions. It is recommended that analysis should start with identification of the atrial activity including its name, e.g. sinus activity, atrial flutter, etc. Following identification of the atrial activity, attention should go on to determining the numerical relationship to the dominant atrial activity and the dominant (most frequent) QRS complexes. Basically this amounts to a decision as to whether there is a 1:1 relationship with a fixed PR or RP interval, or the dominant atrial activity is more frequent (going faster) than the dominant QRSs or the dominant QRSs outnumber the dominant atrial waves. While proceeding through the identification of the atrial activity and the relation of the atrial activity to the dominant QRSs, certain diagnoses or impressions will have occurred that indicate that the atrial activity is not responsible for producing the dominant QRSs, e.g. AV dissociation. At that point and only then the reader should proceed to the determination of what is creating the QRS complexes, a decision based primarily on the QRS duration and the rate of the QRS complexes.

In identifying the name of the atrial activity, the first question should be is the atrial activity "sinus activity". This is based on the rate (for adults perhaps as low as 40 per minute and up to 180 when at rest and faced with high output stresses such as fever, infection, etc. and up to about 200 with maximal exercise). The maximal heart rate for the adult with exercise can be roughly estimated by subtracting the person's age from 220. If the activity fits within these ranges, then sinus activity is a potential diagnosis. The next criterion is the morphology of the p waves, especially in lead II. At the slower rates, the p of sinus activity should be upright or flat but not inverted in lead II and at faster rates definitely upright in lead II. The p morphology generally remains constant in appearance, although at the slower rates associated with sinus arrhythmia the p wave in lead II may be more upright when the p to p interval is shorter and more flat when the p to p interval is longer. The third criterion on the electrocardiogram is that the p intervals are reasonably regular. With high vagal tone producing slower rates such as in athletes the p to p interval may expand and shorten in synchrony with inspiration and exhalation, a normal variant called sinus arrhythmia. Finally, at the bedside, activity thought to be sinus should make sense with the clinical presentation. For instance, a rhythm disturbance to be discussed later, focal ectopic atrial tachycardia, may present with upright p waves in lead II and a quite regular rate of 140 BPM or more, thus simulating sinus

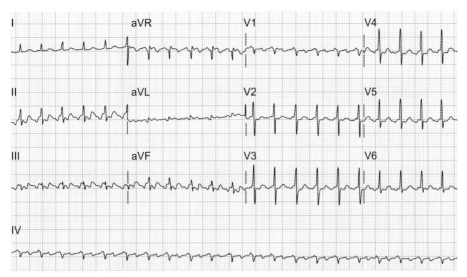

FIGURE 4: An example of atrial flutter with 2:1 conduction

tachycardia. One of the clues that the diagnosis probably is not sinus tachycardia but rather is a focal ectopic atrial tachycardia may be that the clinical situation does not seem to include any state, such as fever, volume depletion, etc., that would lead to a sinus tachycardia.

If the conclusion is that the atrial activity is not sinus, the observed atrial activity should be categorized into one of three groups: (1) "Organized": specifically that the atrial wave morphology in any given lead maintains a constant morphology and a constant atrial wave to atrial wave interval; (2) "Chaotic": specifically that the atrial morphology in any given lead is constantly varying in morphology and wave to wave interval or (3) The atrial activity cannot be found consistently.

If the conclusion is that the atrial activity is organized but not sinus, then the proper diagnosis can usually be based on the rate of the atrial waves and their morphology. Based on these considerations, usually the conclusion will be that the atrial activity represents atrial flutter (Fig. 4), an ectopic atrial tachycardia (re-entrant or focal ectopic) (Fig. 5) or retrograde p waves. For instance if the atrial rate is 220–360 inclusively and the atrial waves, especially in leads II, III and aVF, have the typical saw tooth or sine wave appearance, the diagnosis of atrial flutter is almost unequivocal. However, atrial flutter may present with slightly slower rates in the presence of antiarrhythmic drugs that slow conduction velocity in the atrial reentrant pathway. If the atrial rate is around 140 and up to a bit less than 220 and no flutter waves are discernible, then the diagnosis of one of the types of the ectopic supraventricular tachycardias (reentrant or focal ectopic) is appropriate. If there is a single p wave apparent as an inverted p waves in leads II and aVF immediately following each narrow QRS (duration of less than 120 msecs), then the diagnosis of a reentrant (usually AV nodal using) supraventricular tachycardia is secure. If the p waves, inverted in II or not, do not bear a fixed relation with one p following each QRS, then the diagnosis of a focal ectopic atrial tachycardia is appropriate. Since these p waves may be upright in lead II because they emanate from an ectopic focus near the sinus node, they will resemble sinus p waves. Due to the rapid rates of these p waves, these focal ectopic atrial tachycardia p waves often conduct with

variable degrees of second degree AV block whereas most sinus tachycardias at these rates will conduct 1:1. The lack of expected response to physiologic interventions such as vagal maneuvers and the lack of the presence of any clinically apparent reason for a sinus tachycardia also help to distinguish these focal ectopic tachycardias from sinus tachycardia. The third general category for organized atrial waves is the retrograde p wave, i.e. an inverted p wave in leads II and aVF indicative of depolarization of the atria from caudal to rostral. These can be of two varieties: the passive retrograde p wave that is the result of activation from some source distal to the atrium, e.g. from the AV node, the junctional tissue or ventricular rhythms. The hallmark of the passive retrograde p wave is that the p wave is found right after the QRS and is locked onto the QRS by a fixed interval, usually about 260 msecs from the beginning of the QRS complex to the end of the retrograde p wave. The other type of retrograde p wave is the active retrograde p wave, i.e. the atrial wave is derived directly from the atrium but its point of origin is low in the atrium. It is distinguished from the passive retrograde p wave because it is never in a one to one relation with the QRS complexes and attached just after the QRS complex. Note should be made of the fact that passive retrograde p waves may certainly be observed as part of the reentrant supraventricular rhythms but that passive retrograde p waves may also be seen due to other rhythms such as junctional or ventricular rhythms including ventricular tachycardia. The distinction among these potential sources of passive retrograde p waves is usually apparent based on the width of the QRS complexes and their rate. Note should be made again that focal ectopic atrial tachycardias may demonstrate active retrograde p waves when the focal source is low in the atrium; however, if that focal source is near the sinus node, the p waves will be similar to sinus p waves and will not be retrograde in appearance.

If the atrial activity is not organized but instead is chaotic, i.e. constantly varying in morphology and wave to wave interval, the two most likely rhythms are atrial fibrillation and multifocal atrial tachycardia. The former, of course, is characterized by rapidly undulating atrial wavelets at 400 or more beats per minute, and the ventricular response to uncomplicated atrial

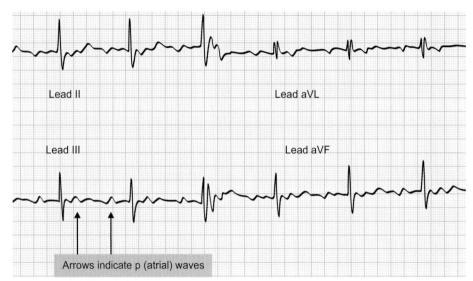

Lead II   Lead aVL

Lead III   Lead aVF

Arrows indicate p (atrial) waves

FIGURE 5: An example of focal ectopic atrial tachycardia with 2:1 atrio-ventricular block

fibrillation will manifest irregularly irregular R-to-R intervals. The ventricular response in those individuals with normal AV conduction pathways and on no rate controlling medications is usually about 130–180 beats per minute. A regular ventricular response in the presence of atrial fibrillation implies complete AV dissociation with a junctional escape rhythm or an accelerated junctional escape rhythm, the latter often reflecting digitalis toxicity. In contrast the atrial activity in multifocal atrial tachycardia consists of isolated p waves consistent with sinus activation plus three or more premature atrial complexes, each of different morphology, with an average heart rate of greater than 100 BPM. For the most part there will be one atrial wave per QRS, although an occasional premature atrial beat may not be conducted.

An atrial wave with consistent p wave morphology but an irregular p to p interval is retrograde activation of the atria from conduction from a source distal to the AV node, e.g. a ventricular tachycardia, but conducting retrograde back up through the AV node with a ventriculoatrial second degree block, e.g. with Mobitz I (Wenckebach) characteristics. However, this is a quite rare phenomenon and difficult to detect on the routing electrocardiogram. Theoretically junctional or ventricular rhythms could penetrate the AV node with 2 to 1 conduction ratios producing one retrograde p with a fixed R-P interval after every other QRS complex.

The third general observational possibility involving detection and characterization of the atrial activity is that the atrial activity either cannot be clearly found or is only detected for only one or two beats during the rhythm strip. Under these circumstances, characterizing the dominant QRS complexes into one of three general observational groups is helpful.

The first such group would be *regular* R-to-R intervals with "narrow" QRS complexes (arbitrarily defined by this author as being < 120 msecs wide). This breaks down into a slow variety and a fast variety. The slow variety would in general consist of a heart rate of 60 BPM or less with plenty of room between QRS complexes to allow for detection of atrial waves. If no such waves can be observed in any of the 12 leads, it is likely that this represents atrial asystole with the expected emergence

of a junctional escape rhythm. The more common situation is the "fast" variety in which there is rapid QRS rates of about 100–220 BPM) The likely candidates explaining this finding include sinus tachycardia where the sinus p waves have become difficult to identify, atrial flutter with 2 to 1 AV conduction and "paroxysmal supraventricular tachycardia" (usually AV nodal using reentrant supraventricular tachycardia) (Fig. 6). In general a first approximation of the likely diagnosis or diagnoses is to note the exact rate of the tachycardia. If the rate is greater than 180 it would be quite unlikely to be sinus tachycardia in an adult who is not exercising and equally unlikely that it would be atrial flutter with 2 to 1 AV conduction, since it would be quite unusual for the atrial rate in atrial flutter to exceed 360. At rates significantly less than 140 BPM, the paroxysmal supraventricular tachycardia becomes much less likely. Of course, at rates of about 140–180, all three possibilities are reasonably likely just based on the heart rate. Given these latter two rate possibilities, reexamine the electrocardiograph (EKG) and look more closely for the p wave on the downstroke of the T wave right before the next QRS complex and to assess the patient clinically to see if there is a clinical reason evident that would account for a sinus tachycardia. Given that none is found, it becomes reasonably unlikely that the rhythm is sinus. The next possibility to consider and the possible rhythm most likely to be present in the postoperative state is atrial flutter with 2 to 1 AV conduction. Multiple different observations often need to be used to unmask atrial flutter with 2 to 1 AV conduction. The first is to ignore the QRS complexes in leads II, III and aVF, and in doing so try to appreciate the sine wave or saw tooth pattern in those leads. Scrutiny for a potential atrial wave in leads V1 and V2 should be carried out. Often with atrial flutter, one of the two flutter waves will be evident in those leads and often the wave resembles a sinus generated atrial wave. Note the PR interval in those leads. If the PR interval is not reasonably short as would be expected with a sinus tachycardia, there is a high probability that the wave is not a sinus p wave. In addition, take the measured PR interval in those leads and apply it to lead II. Does a potential atrial wave there as identified by the PR interval look like a sinus p wave? Finally

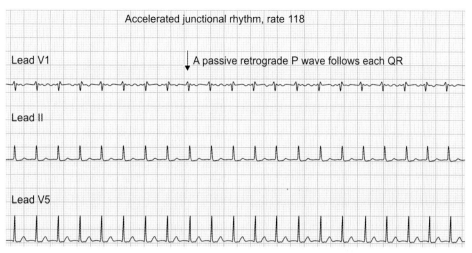

FIGURE 6: An example of atrio-ventricular reentratachycardia (AVNRT)

take the measured observed p to p interval or the measured R-to-R interval observed in lead V1 or V2 and cut that interval time in half, e.g. the measured interval will be about two large electrocardiogram boxes plus a couple of small electrocardiogram boxes. Simply reduce the caliper tip to tip distance to one big and one small EKG box. Place one tip of the caliper on the observed p wave in lead V1 or V2 and swing it forward and backward so that the second tip brings your visual attention to the second identical wave often merged to the beginning or end of the QRS complexes. In addition, using that same caliper distance, examine leads II, III and aVF to see if that will trace out a sine wave or saw tooth pattern. Failing to be able to dissect out flutter waves or identify definite sinus p waves leaves the paroxysmal supraventricular tachycardia as the likely diagnosis given that the ventricular rate is from about 140 up to about 220 BPM. Finally, at the bedside performing vagal maneuvers or giving intravenous adenosine may clarify the diagnosis substantially. Sinus activity should slow and then reaccelerate gradually; atrial flutter waves will continue unabated but the conduction numbers through the AV node should diminish substantially creating long R-to-R intervals and exposing obvious flutter waves; and, if done effectively, the reentrant supraventricular tachycardias should cease abruptly.

The next possibility under the "can't find the atrial activity section", is that the dominant QRS intervals are varying in an irregularly irregular way, i.e. a completely unpredictable and unpatterned R-to-R variation. A reasonable assumption under the circumstance when no atrial activity can be discerned is that the rhythm is "fine" (very low amplitude) atrial fibrillation.

The final observational set under "can't find the atrial activity" is that the above two steps did not lead to a reasonable diagnosis or, more commonly, that there are regular but wide (≥ 120 msec) regular QRSs. Under this circumstance, moving to the ventricular analysis to be described subsequently is useful in choosing whether the QRSs reflect a ventricular rhythm versus a rhythm that is not of ventricular origin and is not from an atrial source.

Given that an atrial activity has been identified, the next step is to identify in a general way what the numerical relationship is between the dominant atrial waves and the dominant QRSs. Simplistically, the first possibility is that the dominant atrial activity and the dominant QRSs exist in a one to one relationship. Thus one atrial wave would need to be observed for each dominant QRS complexes with either a fixed PR length or a fixed RP length. The fixation of the timing implies that that which occurs first gives rise to the following event. With a fixed PR, the atrial wave (most commonly a sinus p wave) proceeds antegrade to give rise to the QRS. In situations where the atrial wave is found at the end of the QRS complex or shortly thereafter in the ST segment with a fixed interval between the QRS and a p wave that is inverted in leads II and aVF, almost always this represents a passive retrograde activation of the atria from a source distal to the atrial chambers. This source can be a reentrant focus using the AV node, a junctional mechanism or a ventricular mechanism.

When the rate of the dominant atrial waves is consistently always greater than the dominant QRS rate, almost invariably this indicates a second or third degree AV block. This block could be pathological, i.e. given that at the atrial rate discerned, atrial waves would be expected to conduct one to one to the ventricles. On the other hand, this block could be physiologic in that the atrial rate is so rapid that it would not be likely to conduct one to one in the presence of healthy conducting pathways, e.g. atrial flutter conducting with a 2 to 1 conduction ratio. Regardless, the name of the type of block can be most easily and quickly discerned by first looking at the PR intervals, although not assuming that a p followed by a QRS necessarily indicates that the p gives rise to the QRS. If the PR interval does not vary, then describing the numerical relation between the number of p waves and the number of the dominant QRS complexes will produce an appropriate name for the block. If there are two waves for each QRS with a fixed PR, the appropriate name is 2 to 1 second degree AV block. If there is a fixed ratio of 3 or more p waves per QRS with a fixed PR, the appropriate name would be advanced second degree AV block. All others fitting the description of more dominant p waves than dominant QRS complexes but with a fixed PR can be appropriately diagnosed as Mobitz II second degree AV block. If the PR does vary, the two possibilities are Mobitz type I second degree AV block (essentially synonymous with Wenckebach second degree AV block) and third degree or complete AV block. Given that Mobitz I second degree AV block intermittently manifests as a p wave that does not produce a QRS, the other hallmark of this type of block besides the varying PR interval is the intermittent production of a significantly longer R-to-R interval. On the other hand, with the third degree AV block junctional or ventricular escape rhythms should emerge and these rhythms are regular and do not demonstrate intermittent, patently obvious, R-to-R pauses. Thus if the PR varies and the R-to-R distinctly and obviously varies, the diagnosis is Mobitz type I or Wenckebach second degree AV block. If the R-to-R interval does not grossly vary, then the diagnosis becomes third degree (complete) AV block. There may be caliper detectable, subtle variations in the R-to-R interval with third degree AV block with a junctional escape rhythm since the junctional mechanism is under the influence of vagal tone, which is likely to vary under this circumstance with variable atrial filling of the ventricles as well as with inhalation and exhalation.

There is one final caveat relative to the appropriate diagnosis of third degree AV block when atrial rate exceeds ventricular rate. When electronic pacing of the ventricle is occurring in the now less common circumstance where there is no sequential atrial pacing, confirmation of the presence of third degree AV block should include inspection of the rhythm strip to be sure that no p waves occurring after the T wave of the preceding QRS are producing an early QRS complex, i.e. an atrial capture of the ventricle. If such capture is observed then the situation is not truly complete AV block.

The third possibility for the numerical relationship of the dominant atrial activity and the dominant ventricular activity is more frequent, more rapid dominant QRS complexes than dominant atrial waves. This usually constitutes another and different form of AV dissociation than third degree AV block. This usually represents interference AV dissociation created by a slowing of the sinus rate below the rate of normal physiologic escape pacemakers, usually junctional escape pacemakers, and/or development of a pathological ectopic tachycardia, from a source distal to the AV node, regardless if that is junctional or ventricular (Fig. 7). The explanation for the dissociation is that impulses are arriving at the top and the bottom of the AV node almost simultaneously, with conduction into the AV node antegrade and retrograde almost simultaneously. Thus there is collision of the impulses nearly head on or at least within the refractory periods caused by each one. The key point is that the AV dissociation here is not a matter of pathology in the AV

conducting pathways. The AV pathway is the innocent bystander of the effect of inappropriately slow sinus activity and/or pathological ectopic focus distal to the AV node. Clinically the distinction is important. Under this circumstance attention should be directed to increasing the rate of sinus activity or suppressing the pathological ectopic focus and not trying to improve AV conduction.

There is one other potential circumstance when AV dissociation may occur. This is when there is a slow sinus arrhythmia whose rate gradually slows and gradually quickens to rates just above and below that of a junctional escape rhythm. Under this circumstance the atrial rate may not ever accelerate enough to place a p wave far enough ahead of the next QRS emanating from the junctional focus and thus is never able to capture the ventricle. This circumstance is called isorhythmic AV dissociation.

Having clarified the AV numerical relationship as best as possible, the next step is only necessary if some impression or diagnosis has come about in the preceding step that implies that the dominant atrial mechanism is not producing the dominant QRS complexes. In general the descriptors or diagnoses that would indicate this would be: (1) passive retrograde p waves (inverted p waves in II and aVF following the QRS with a fixed interval from onset of QRS to completion of the p wave); (2) AV dissociation (whether it be due to complete AV block or interference dissociation) and (3) the final step three under "can't find the atrial activity". Specifically this last situation means that the first two steps under "can't find the atrial activity" didn't work or there are regular wide QRSs without discernible atrial waves. Given the findings noted for steps 1, 2 and 3 as just stated, the QRS complexes are likely the result of a ventricular rhythm or a nonventricular rhythm that is not of atrial origin. The next step in sorting out the possibilities is to note if the dominant QRS complexes are unusually wide, specifically 120 msecs or greater. In making this determination, the measurement should take into account the inscription of the QRS in all 12 leads, using the widest inscription found for the dominant QRS. If the QRS is less than 120 msecs, it is quite likely that the rhythm producing the QRS complexes is not of ventricular origin. Thus the likely possibilities become a junctional escape rhythm recognized by its rate of about 60 BPM or less, an accelerated junctional rhythm recognized by its rate of greater than 70 BPM but less than 130 BPM (Fig. 6), or the paroxysmal (usually AV nodal using reentrant) supraventricular

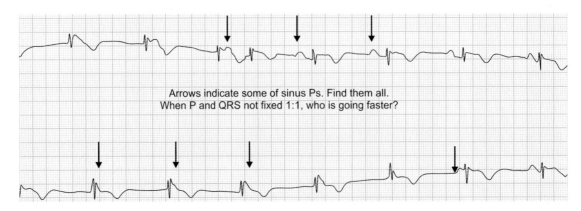

FIGURE 7: An example of sinus bradycardia with junctional escape rhythm creating interference atrio-ventricular dissociation

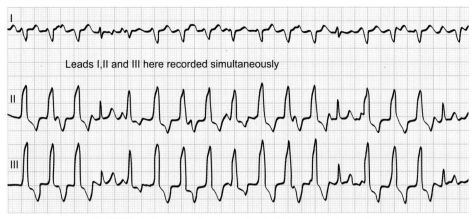

FIGURE 8: An example of accelerated idioventricular rhythm

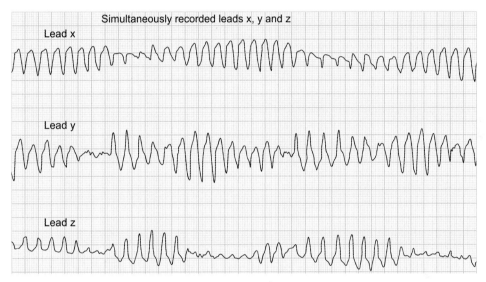

FIGURE 9: An example of torsades de pointes

tachycardia recognized by its rate of about 140 BPM or more. If the QRS duration is 120 msecs or greater, knowledge of the morphology of the QRS complexes prior to the onset of the rhythm disturbance can be critical. For instance, if the QRS prior to the onset of a pathological tachycardia happened to be a left bundle branch block and the patient then developed a paroxysmal supraventricular tachycardia, it would be likely that the QRS complexes under this circumstance would be identical to those prior to the tachycardia and thus would simulate a ventricular tachycardia. Therefore, if the QRS complexes after the onset of a rhythm disturbance are identical to those prior to its onset, the analysis should proceed as though the QRS complexes during the dysrhythmia are narrow and the diagnosis made on the basis of the rates given for the narrow QRS complexes discussed above. If the QRS complexes are wide and not identical to those prior to the onset of the rhythm disturbance, the correct diagnosis can usually be made by noting the QRS rate. If the rate is less than 40 BPM, the diagnosis is ventricular escape rhythm. If the rate is about 55–110, the diagnosis is accelerated idioventricular rhythm (Fig. 8). If the rate is above 120 BPM, the diagnosis is ventricular tachycardia. The rate in this circumstance is usually 140 or more. Ventricular tachycardias, especially those due to ischemic heart disease

maintain the same QRS morphology in any given lead and are appropriately called monomorphic ventricular tachycardia. In contrast, some ventricular tachycardias display QRS morphologies that gradually change their shape as though the depolarization and repolarization of the ventricle was turning on a point. When associated with factors that prolong the QT interval, the ventricular tachycardia is called torsades de pointes (Fig. 9). When the ventricular tachycardia has this same appearance but has not been provoked by factors causing prolongation of the QT interval, the tachycardia is called polymorphous ventricular tachycardia.

There is one peculiar circumstance where a pathological tachycardia of supraventricular origin, such as paroxysmal supraventricular tachycardia, may conduct to the ventricles with a new bundle branch block morphology not present prior to the pathological tachycardia. This usually indicates the presence of a conduction phenomenon known as aberrancy. The phenomenon is created by the arrival of a premature supraventricular impulse at just the precise moment that the AV node and one of the bundle branches is beyond their absolute refractory periods but the opposite bundle is still within its refractory period. Thus the supraventricular impulse is conducted with a new bundle branch block morphology. The situation is made more likely to occur if the premature supraventricular impulse occurs after a preceding R-to-R interval that is longer than usual. When only a single premature beat is involved it is relatively easy to discern a premature atrial contraction from a premature ventricular contraction by identifying the premature p wave in front of the premature QRS. However, when there is a sustained ectopic tachycardia, the situation is significantly more difficult in discriminating between supraventricular reentrant tachycardia conducted aberrantly and ventricular tachycardia. The actual rate of the tachycardia is of no value in the discrimination and the presence of various symptoms in reaction to the tachycardia is equally of no value. The finding of AV dissociation due to interference with sinus p waves beating completely independently from the regular QRS complexes is almost diagnostic that the tachycardia under this circumstance is ventricular tachycardia. Finding AV association with one passive retrograde p wave discernible following each wide QRS is of no value in the discrimination since almost all the paroxysmal supraventricular tachycardias and perhaps a third of the ventricular tachycardias will also demonstrates one QRS to one passive retrograde p wave relationship. Other more subtle points have been developed by Brugada and his coworkers and by other research groups. However, too much time spent trying to make this distinction following the onset of the dysrhythmia can have disastrous results for the patient presenting in an emergency situation. Discriminating between ventricular tachycardia on the basis of the heart rate itself or the presence versus the absence of symptoms and hypotension is completely unreliable. Quickly looking for a single p wave in front of the QRS complexes is reasonable. Taking an undue amount of time trying to discern if there are sinus p waves walking through the QRS complexes (i.e. defining that there is AV interference dissociation) will only use up precious time and, if found, will only confirm that the diagnosis is what was believed in the first place, namely ventricular tachycardia. A practical approach in the emergency situation is to assume that a rapid, quite regular, wide QRS tachycardia of rate 120, usually 140 or higher, is ventricular tachycardia until proven otherwise and not to waste too much time trying to prove otherwise.

Having completed the analysis to this point, the next step is to look for unexpected early QRS complexes and to look for unexpected long R-to-R pauses, given that the dominant QRS complexes have been otherwise characterized by regular R-to-R intervals. Except in the presence of interference AV dissociation, unexpected early QRS complexes would represent ectopic premature beats of atrial, junctional or ventricular origin. If the premature complex (whether identical to or different than the dominant QRS complexes in morphology) is preceded by a premature p wave, then it is reasonably to presume that the premature beat is an atrial premature beat, usually associated with a noncompensatory pause (the R-to-R interval encompassing the premature beat being less than the R-to-R interval preceding or following the premature beat). If the premature beat is distinctly different than the prior QRSs and does not have a premature p in front of it, then it is reasonable to presume that the beat is a ventricular premature beat, which will usually produce a fully compensatory pause (the R-to-R interval encompassing the premature beat being essentially twice the R-to-R interval preceding or following the premature beat).

Junctional premature complexes tend not to be preceded by a premature p wave and tend to be identical to the morphology of the dominant QRSs and tend to be associated with a completely compensatory pause.

There is one circumstance when an unexpected early QRS does not represent a premature ectopic beat. The circumstance is the presence of interference AV dissociation. An early QRS complex with the dominant atrial activity in front of it terminating the AV interference dissocation will represent an atrial capture of the ventricle.

Attention should then turn to identifying any long R-to-R intervals (unexpected pauses) interrupting otherwise regular R-to-R intervals. Since the usual reason that a QRS complex is created is that an atrial impulse has traveled via the conduction pathways to activate the ventricles, the usual general reason that a QRS complex does not appear on time and thus creates a long R-to-R interval is that no atrial impulse arrived at the ventricles. This could occur if no on time atrial activity occurred, which would represent sinoatrial arrest or block. A second reason is that the dominant atrial activity, usually sinus, failed to conduct, thus the appearance of a Mobitz I or Mobitz II second degree AV block. The final possibility is that a premature atrial beat occurred so premature that it ran into the refractory period of some portion of the conducting network, usually the AV node. Thus, to define the reason for an unexpectedly long pause, observe what has occurred during the pause. An early p represents a nonconducted atrial premature beat; an on time p represents the appearance of Mobitz I or II second degree AV block and the absence of either a premature p or an on time p represents sinoatrial arrest or sinoatrial block. The distinction between SA arrest and block may be difficult, but if the p-to-p interval of the pause seems to represent a mathematical relationship to the preceding or following p-to-p intervals (e.g. twice the dominant p-to-p interval), then sinoatrial block may be more likely.

One final commentary is necessary with regard to rhythm analysis. This involves the presence of atrial and/or ventricular electronic pacing. Pacing spikes are vertical slashes occurring during the rhythm. What they are pacing is given by the wave that follows them, i.e. an atrial wave for atrial pacing, a QRS for ventricular pacing, or neither if the pacing fails to capture. Most commonly in the current era, pacing electrodes will be placed, usually transvenously, to stimulate the right atrium and one or both ventricles in sequential fashion. In the presence of chronic atrial fibrillation, an atrial pacing wire may not be placed. The electronics of the generator system will be adjusted so that the atrial or ventricular pacing will not occur if there is spontaneous atrial or ventricular activity respectively of a given rate, i.e. they are set in a demand mode. Inspection of the QRS complexes associated with transvenous pacing will usually indicate the pacing site. With ventricular pacing from the right ventricular apex, the site most commonly used the QRS complex in lead V1 will have a left bundle branch block appearance, i.e. mainly a negative deflection, and will have a left axis deviation. Under the unusual circumstance of pacing from near the outflow tract of the right ventricle, the QRS will have the same left bundle branch appearance but will have a normal axis. In the modern era, usually in patients with poor left ventricular systolic function and a wide QRS other than a right bundle branch block, biventricular pacing of the right ventricle and of the left ventricle via the coronary sinus is often used. This produces a greater initial r wave in lead V1 than with the right ventricular pacing and a QRS axis that is either rightward or is in the northwest quadrant between 180 and minus 90 degrees.

CHARACTERIZATION OF QRS COMPLEX

Having characterized the rhythm fully, the next step is to characterize the QRS complexes as to whether they are normal or represent some deformity indicative of a bundle branch block, myocardial hypertrophy, myocardial infarction, etc. However, if the dominant QRS complexes represent a ventricular rhythm (ventricular escape, accelerated idioventricular rhythm or ventricular tachycardia), such an analysis is not reasonable since that QRS has already been deformed by the rhythm and the QRS diagnoses to follow cannot be made with accuracy. Given that the QRS complexes concerned do not represent a ventricular rhythm, e.g. a ventricular escape rhythm, then the clinician can reasonably proceed with the QRS analysis. Starting with the determination as to whether the QRS complexes are wider than normal ($\geq$ 120 msecs) is important since several of the conditions producing this widening render further QRS diagnoses relatively difficult and inaccurate. Having determined that the QRSs in question are unusually wide, attention should shift to determine if the PR interval is unusually short, usually less than 120 msecs. Visually this may be best appreciated by looking for the PR segment (end of p to onset of QRS) where the QRS inscription is the widest in the 12 leads. The absence of any PR segment associated with the wide QRS complexes almost always indicates the diagnosis of the Wolff-Parkinson-White anomaly (preexcitation sydrome) due to the presence of an anomalous or accessory conducting pathway from atrium to ventricle (Fig. 10). In general, any further QRS diagnoses are very difficult to make. A practical approach under the circumstance is always to obtain a transthoracic echocardiogram to look for any further structural heart disease that might be associated with this anomaly. In fact, for all causes of an unusually wide QRS, obtaining a transthoracic echocardiogram would be quite justifiable.

If the QRS is wide, a very practical next step is to look in lead V1. The reason is that this will almost always allow the interpreter to determine if there is a right bundle branch block (Fig. 11). This conduction disturbance produces a delayed and prolonged depolarization of the right ventricle causing R waves to be found as the terminal portion of the QRS with these depolarizing forces directed anteriorly and rightward toward lead V1. It does not matter in this circumstance if the pattern is the traditional rSR' pattern or a qR pattern or even just a tall, although fractured R wave. All are indicative at this point in the analysis of a right bundle branch block. While the additional presence of left anterior hemiblock usually does not obscure the presence of this diagnostic R wave in V1, rarely the presence of left anterior hemiblock accompanying a wide QRS will obscure the characteristic pattern of an associated right bundle branch block in lead V1. The presence of the characteristic R in V1 can be demonstrated by placing the V1 lead in a higher intercostal space and also by recording right-sided chest leads.

If the diagnosis of right bundle branch block has been established, this implies that the conduction disturbance by itself has not distorted left ventricular depolarization. Therefore, having made the diagnosis of right bundle branch block, the interpreter can proceed on to the next two steps, specifically determination of the QRS axis and the search for pathological Q waves indicative of the presence of a myocardial infarction.

If inspection of the EKG does not confirm the presence of a right bundle branch block, but rather shows a tiny r-large S wave or a QS pattern in lead V1, left bundle branch block then needs consideration. Classic left bundle branch block is best confirmed by finding notching or fracturing in the middle of the QRS complex with a QRS duration of at least 120 msecs (Fig. 12). This notching is usually best seen in the leads with tall R waves, although it may be observed in those with deep S waves. Since a left bundle branch block implies a completely distorted activation of the left ventricle, attempting to make other diagnoses, such as left ventricular hypertrophy or myocardial infarction, cannot be done with a great deal of accuracy. Thus, further QRS analysis as given below is probably not of significant value. Pursuit of such further diagnoses is probably best done by utilization of echocardiography, perfusion scans

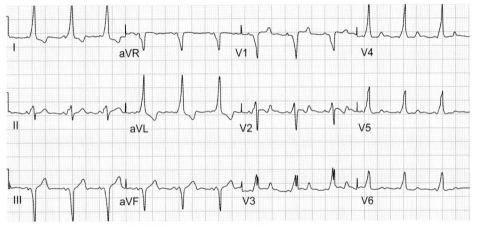

FIGURE 10: An example of accessory pathway

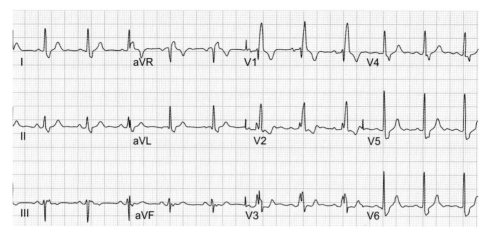

FIGURE 11: An example of right bundle branch block

and/or angiography. In addition, due to the complete distortion of left ventricular depolarization, marked ST and T wave abnormalities called secondary STT changes are to be expected in the presence of a left bundle branch block. However, these STT abnormalities are relatively predictable in any given EKG lead in that the ST and T waves should be directed in the opposite direction of the direction of the QRS complex in that lead. Finding ST and T waves and QRS complexes headed in the same direction usually indicates that some other process over and beyond the left bundle branch block is present, for instance some type of ischemia. However, it is well to remember that not finding such inappropriately directed ST and T does not mean that there is not some other process such as ischemia going on. The QRS axis, to be discussed next, is almost always either a normal axis or a left axis. While those with normal versus left axis differ generally in their clinical presentation, the axis itself does not seem to have relevance to the conduction disturbance itself. In very rare instances a left bundle branch block will demonstrate a right axis deviation.

If the wide QRS of 120 msecs or more is not due to Wolff-Parkinson-White anomaly, right bundle branch block or left bundle block, then the descriptive term of nonspecific intraventricular conduction defect is appropriate and the QRS analysis can proceed as outlined next.

If the analysis given above allows the interpreted to proceed on, attention should be directed to the mean QRS axis. The range of the normal mean frontal plane QRS axis is dependent on the age group of the individuals, shifting leftward with increasing age. For adults the normal axis is from about positive 90 degrees up and leftward to minus 30 degrees. In normal young people in their early teenage years it is not unusual to find an axis as far rightward as positive 120 degrees. In normal persons in their later teenage years and early twenties, an axis as rightward as 105 degrees is not surprising. Arbitrarily moderate left axis deviation is between minus 30 and minus 45 degrees and marked left axis deviation is from minus 45 to minus 90 degrees. When marked left axis deviation is present (i.e. an axis of minus 45 degrees to minus 90 degrees), a diagnosis of left anterior hemiblock is appropriate. Right axis deviation in adults has been divided into moderated right axis deviation when the axis is from plus 90 to plus 120 degrees and marked right axis deviation when the axis is between plus 120 and plus 180 degrees. When right axis deviation is present, three general considerations should come to mind: (1) right ventricular hypertrophy and/or emphysema; (2) high lateral myocardial infarction and (3) left posterior hemiblock. Often other electrocardio-graphic features and other clinical information will need to be assessed in order to choose among these three. If other

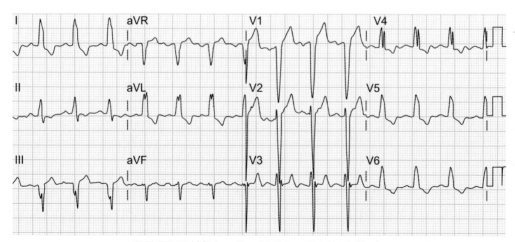

FIGURE 12: An example of left bundle branch block

electrocardiographic evidence of right ventricular hypertrophy, such as an unusually tall R or R prime wave is present in lead V1, then the diagnosis of right ventricular hypertrophy is the most likely correct choice. However, the absence of a prominent R wave in lead V1 does not mean that right ventricular hypertrophy is not the correct interpretation. The lack of a pathologically large Q wave in lead I speaks against the choice a "high lateral" infarct as the cause of the right axis deviation. However, the presence of such a Q wave merely allows infarction as a reasonable choice but still allows other possibilities such as right ventricular hypertrophy. Left posterior hemiblock is statistically the least common abnormality present. When left posterior hemiblock is present, often extreme right axis deviation is present. The presence of other conduction defects, such as right bundle branch block or Mobitz type II second degree AV block, would tend to favor left posterior hemiblock as the correct explanation of the right axis deviation.

Occasionally all of the leads in the frontal plane appear to be essentially isoelectric and then the term "indeterminate axis" is appropriate.

One final comment about the calculation of the mean QRS axis is necessary. Technically the determination of the axis by the electrocardiographer uses the area inscribed the Q, R and S waves. This is the manner in which the axis is determined by most computer-assisted electrocardiographic interpretations. This works well when the individual deflections in a given lead are of about the same width. However, in the presence of a right bundle branch block, it would be advisable to ignore the contribution of the wide terminal deflection to the QRS when estimating the axis, especially when trying to suggest the additional presence of left anterior or left posterior hemiblock.

Having dealt with the mean QRS axis, attention can then be given to the presence of Q waves indicative of the presence of a myocardial infarction. What constitutes a pathological Q wave indicative of the presence of a myocardial infarction, previously termed a "transmural" infarction and now defined simply as a Q wave infarction has been based on studies of autopsy series and patient records and expert consensus documents reflecting the combined expertise of such organizations as the American Heart Association, the American College of Cardiology and the European Society of Cardiology and the World Heart Federation. With no prior electrocardiogram with

which to compare, the presence of a prior myocardial infarction has been defined as probably present if the Q waves meet certain standards of width and of depth. Currently, Q waves of equal to or greater than 0.3 s width and equal to or greater than 0.1 mV depth (1 mm depth on the usual electrocardiographic recording) when found in leads I or II or aVF or one of the precordial leads V2 through V6 correlate well with the diagnosis of myocardial infarction. Large Q waves in lead III or lead aVL or lead V1 unsupported by large Q waves in spatially adjacent leads (aVF or I or V2 respectively) have little or no diagnostic import. In addition smaller q waves in V2 of 0.02 s duration should be considered abnormal and suggestive of a prior myocardial infarction. As a practical matter, judgments based on q waves in lead aVF are traditionally problematic. Frequently, the q in this lead on one day may be quite unimpressive in width, and an electrocardiogram done shortly thereafter may show Q waves that appear to meet width criteria for infarction, and an electrocardiogram done subsequently may record QRS complexes in that lead some of which look quite nondiagnostic and some look quite diagnostic. In addition, there is variation from one interpreter to the next as to the width of the q wave.

These criteria discussed above should not discourage the diagnosis of a Q wave infarction when new but small q waves develop on serial electrocardiograms accompanied by associated evolving ST elevations and T wave changes.

The naming of the infarction as to site has been based upon the leads in which the Q waves developed. This may vary from author to author. Pathological Q waves in lead I might be termed a high lateral myocardial infarction. Pathological Q waves in aVF may be termed inferior (or diaphragmatic) wall myocardial infarction (Fig. 13). Pathological Q waves in lead II are usually accompanied by pathological Q waves in lead aVF as part of an inferior wall myocardial infarction, but, if not, might be referred to as an apical infarction. Pathological Q waves in V2 and/or V3 might be termed anterior, anteroseptal or septal myocardial infarcts. Discriminating as to whether the anterior wall or the septum or both are involved cannot be done with great accuracy. Pathological Q waves in leads V5 and/or V6 might be termed a lateral wall infarction. Pathological Q waves in lead V4 may be considered to be part of either anterior wall or lateral wall infarctions. As will be discussed, with normal QRS widths a tall R wave in lead V1 (indicative of a large Q

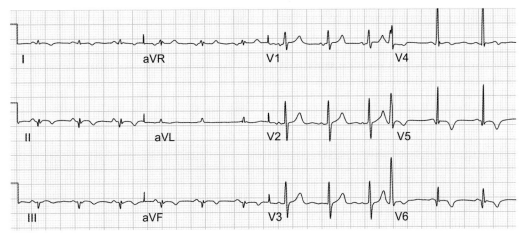

FIGURE 13: An example of inferior, posterior and lateral myocardial infarction

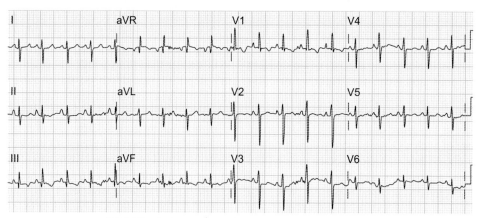

FIGURE 14: An example of right ventricular hypertrophy

wave posteriorly) may represent a posterior wall myocardial infarction.

Having completed analysis for the presence of pathological Q waves, attention can turn to the relative amplitudes of the negative and positive QRS deflections in the precordial leads. This starts with an analysis of the relative amplitudes of R waves in lead V1. Given that a right bundle branch block will produce prominence of R waves in lead V1, it would be reasonable to stop further analysis of the electrocardiogram manifesting a right bundle branch block following the search for pathological Q waves and not proceed on to this section. Reasonable screening criteria for unusually prominent R waves in lead V1 would include an R or R prime that is greater than 0.5 mV (5 mm height) and also is greater than the amplitude of any negative deflection in lead V1. This would reflect unusually prominent anteriorly directed forces which could be explained by addition of electromotive forces anteriorly, i.e. right ventricular hypertrophy (Fig. 14) or destruction of equivalent forces posteriorly, i.e. a posterior myocardial infarction (in truth probably a posterolateral infarction). The choice between the two possibilities is based on accompanying electrocardiographic features. The presence of Q waves indicative of an inferior wall infarction or of a lateral wall infarction would lead to the diagnosis of posterior wall infarction (Fig. 13). The presence of right axis deviation (in the absence of a high lateral wall infarction) would lead to the diagnosis of right ventricular hypertrophy as the explanation of the prominent R or R prime in V1.

The above conclusions are based on the observations that the R or R prime in V1 is taller than 5 mm and bigger than any negative deflection in V1 and that the QRS is not abnormally wide. In discussing this possibility, it is useful to think of the variations in V1 from normal to definitely abnormal. The normal variants in lead V1 include the most common pattern of a small r followed by a deeper S wave. A QS pattern in V1 is a normal finding. A variation found in about 5% of the population is the rSr' pattern where neither r is bigger than 5 mm tall or bigger than the S wave in V1. As defined above, a distinctly abnormal pattern would be an R or R prime greater than 5 mm tall and bigger than any negative deflection. If the R or R prime is bigger than 5 mm tall or taller than the depth of any negative wave in V1 but not both the possibilities would be: (1) possibly still a normal variant; (2) right ventricular hypertrophy; (3) a posterior

infarction and (4) a right bundle branch block that is not quite as wide as usual, an "incomplete" right bundle branch block (Flow chart 1). If right axis deviation is present, this would favor either incomplete right bundle branch block or right ventricular hypertrophy. If other evidence of conduction disturbance exists, e.g. Mobitz type 2 second degree AV block, then the former would be favored. If not, right ventricular hypertrophy would be favored. Volume overload leading to right ventricular hypertrophy more often presents with prominence of the R prime whereas pressure overload leading to right ventricular hypertrophy more commonly produces just a prominent R wave. Presence of infarction in a wall adjacent to the posterior wall favors posterior infarction. Since this is really the reciprocal of a large posterior Q wave, the pattern here will be that of a prominent initial R wave rather than a prominent R prime.

Observation then proceeds to assessment of unusually deep negative waves in the right precordial leads and unusually tall R waves in lateral leads. Using the voltages recorded in these leads has been used to suggest the presence of left ventricular hypertrophy (Fig. 15). The problem with the electrocardiographic diagnosis of left ventricular hypertrophy based solely on voltage criteria is that the sensitivity of such criteria using precordial leads is only about 50% and about 10–15% of normal people will be labeled as having left ventricular hypertrophy when they do not have it. Using voltage criteria from the limb leads, such as lead I or lead aVL, eliminates much of the inaccuracy related to people without left ventricular hypertrophy but only identifies about 15% of those who do have left ventricular hypertrophy. An additional problem with voltage criteria is normal young people tend to have larger negative deflections in the right precordial leads and taller R waves in the lateral precordial leads apparently related to their more slender chest walls and due to the fact that many of them have physiologic hypertrophy related to endurance training. The presence of the typical ST and T abnormality accompanying left ventricular hypertrophy (called by some a "strain pattern") and found in the tall R wave leads as so beautifully demonstrated by Romhilt and Estes only reduces the false positives but still leaves the sensitivity at about 50%. Finally, newer imaging modalities, such as magnetic resonance imaging, are now beginning to help sort out the relative values of various voltage criteria. For the time being, using a combined sum of the largest negative wave in

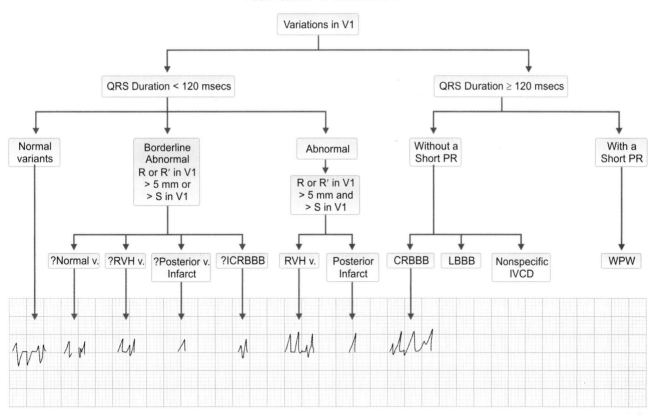

(Abbreviations: +: Consider possible; RVH: Right ventricular hypertrophy; ICRBBB: Incomplete right bundle branch block; CRBBB: Complete right bundle branch block; LBBB: Left bundle branch block; IVCD: Intraventricular conduction defect; WPW: Wolff-Parkinson-White anomaly)

V1 or V2 plus the tallest R wave in V5 or V6 of more than 35 mm in an individual over 35 years of age as an electrocardiographic screening to suggest possible left ventricular hypertrophy would seem reasonable. Unless the voltages are extreme, perhaps the best interpretation might be to apply the term "possible left ventricular hypertrophy" and label the electrocardiogram as perhaps borderline abnormal. R waves of greater than 15 mm in lead I or in lead aVL of greater than 11 mm in the absence of moderate to marked left axis deviation might be more forcefully labeled as representing true left ventricular hypertrophy. For those electrocardiograms with high precordial voltages in those less than 35 years old, one should be cautious about being dogmatic about the diagnosis of left ventricular hypertrophy. Of course, the presence of the typical STT "strain pattern" should be respected as relatively quite diagnostic of the diagnosis of left ventricular hypertrophy, especially when accompanied by voltage criteria. Currently, the most readily available and reasonably accurate method to follow-up on the possibility of left ventricular hypertrophy is the transthoracic echocardiogram.

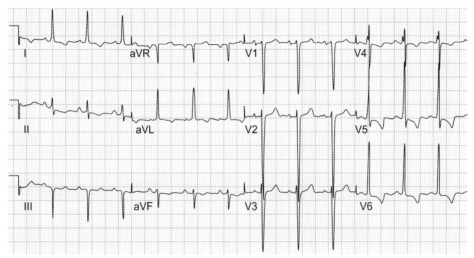

FIGURE 15: An example of left ventricular hypertrophy with secondary repolarization abnormality

CHAPTER 12

Electrocardiogram

Completion of the inspection of the precordial leads involves looking for "poor r wave progression" and/or "late precordial transition". These are purely descriptive terms and should not be viewed as necessarily reflecting any true pathology of the heart. Descriptively "poor r wave progression" is meant to mean that there is an unusually small initial r wave in lead V2 and/or that the r wave in V3 is not larger than the r wave in V2. Late precordial transition means that the transition across the precordial leads from right to left to the lead where the R wave has become larger than the S wave has not occurred by at least lead V5. Transition before that in the right precordial leads including lead V2 is usually a normal finding. Unfortunately these aberrations described may be produced by improper electrode placement such as placement of the right precordial leads an interspace too rostral or by improper placement of leads V5 or V6. Even without improper lead placement, the significance of these findings is not substantial. The interpreter might suggest the possibility of right ventricular hypertrophy and/or emphysema, the possibility of an anterior wall myocardial infarction, the possibility that the finding simply reflects conditions causing right or left axis deviation, or the possibility that the poor r progression might be due to left ventricular hypertrophy. In the absence of electrocardiographic or other clinical abnormalities, it would be more than reasonable to deemphasize this finding.

ST-T WAVE ABNORMALITIES

Having completed, the observation for QRS abnormalities, attention can be given to T wave abnormalities. In the adult with no prior electrocardiogram for comparison, the leads that are the most critical are the same leads as suggested for identification of pathological Q waves indicative of a myocardial infarction. Specifically this would exclude leads aVR, III, aVL and V1. Consistently in the adult the T waves in leads I and II should be upright and should be isoelectric or upright in lead aVF. In the precordial leads, T waves should be isoelectric or upright in lead V2 and always upright in leads V3 through V6. In the pediatric age group, inverted T waves extending further leftward than lead V2 are often present. By the teenage years and in some individuals in their early twenties, T wave inversion in V2 and sometimes V3 may represent normal variants. If prior electrocardiograms are available, then new T wave changes in any lead may have clinical relevance.

Having identified definite T wave abnormalities always requires clinical correlation without assuming that the changes represent serious cardiac abnormality. Certainly they could reflect a relatively benign condition such as hyperventilation. In some young people, T wave inversions have been observed following meals and are absent when the electrocardiogram is recorded in the fasting state. Such T changes following a meal revert to normal following the administration of oral potassium. They usually do not represent serious cardiac abnormality. Other conditions such as low serum potassium or the presence of a drug affecting cardiac ion channels may be responsible for T wave changes. Subarachnoid hemorrhage may produce profound and diffuse T wave abnormalities and in some cases produce changes of an acute evolving ST elevation myocardial infarction. Certainly T wave changes may also reflect serious myocardial abnormality from chronic or new ischemia to injury to non-Q wave myocardial infarction.

Perhaps the most difficult judgments have to do with ST segment deviations. In general observable ST depressions other than in lead aVR should be considered abnormalities. While many of these ST depressions are quite nonspecific, the ST segments manifesting as a straight line that is horizontal or downsloping in two spatially adjacent leads should suggest serious cardiac ischemia as a highly likely possibility. The greatest difficulty can be the discrimination between ST elevations that might represent a normal variant and those that represent acute transmural ischemic injury. Standards have been published that state that ST elevations with a J point elevation of equal to or greater than 0.2 mV (2 mm) in men and equal to or greater than 0.15 mV in women in leads V2-V3 and equal to or greater than 0.1 in any other two contiguous leads should be considered as indicative of acute myocardial ischemia in the absence of left bundle branch block or left ventricular hypertrophy. As opposed to these more focal ST elevations in leads "overlying" specific ventricular wall segments served by a specific coronary artery, more diffuse ST elevations have a different interpretation. Diffuse ST elevations may be defined as ST elevation in leads I, II, aVF and usually III plus leads V2 through V6. Usually lead aVL is not involved while lead V1 does not show significant ST elevation, although it may. The finding of this diffuse ST elevation should strongly suggest the presence of acute pericarditis (Fig. 16). The additional finding of PR depression can be a helpful confirmatory finding. Nevertheless, for both localized ST elevations and diffuse ST elevations, the overlap with ST elevations representing such normal variants as "early repolarization" is quite real. Prior electrocardiograms are most helpful in making this discrimination. In addition ST elevations that are greater with faster heart rates than those elevations recorded on prior electrocardiograms with slower heart rates favors epicardial injury from pericarditis over early repolarization.

Following the schema outline above with practice and experience should lead to rapid and reasonably accurate interpretations of electrocardiograms. Once the rhythm is determined, then, when appropriate, moving on to the QRS-ST-T analysis. A quick determination of QRS width and QRS axis leads to the implications and diagnoses described above. A sweep of the eye of leads I, II and aVF plus leads V2 through V6 for pathological Q waves, ST and T waves, plus looking at the precordial leads V1 through V6 for indications of right and left ventricular hypertrophy (plus observing leads I and aVL for voltages suggesting left ventricular hypertrophy) almost completes the process. As mentioned observing the precordial leads for the nebulous terms "poor r wave progression and/or late precordial transition" would be included as the eye sweeps across leads V2 through V6.

THE "U" WAVE

The U wave is a low amplitude wave of about 0.3 mV (0.3 mm) following the T wave. It is most likely to be observed in leads V2 and V3. Under normal circumstances, it most commonly observed at heart rates of 65 or less and uncommonly

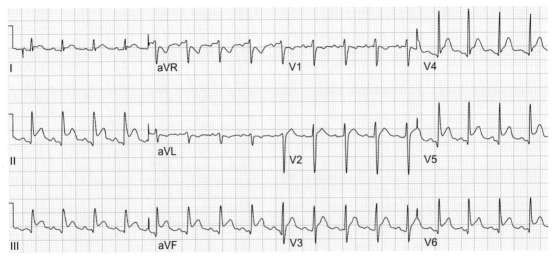

FIGURE 16: An example of acute pericarditis

with heart rates above. Under these circumstances, it is a normal finding. Its physiologic explanation is still debated. Exaggeration of the amplitude of the U wave may exist by itself without accompanying ST or T wave abnormality. More commonly exaggerated amplitude of the U wave may be associated with ST depression and/or diminished T wave amplitude. In some instances the u wave may fuse with the T wave. Under these circumstances, search for causative factors is critical, including hypokalemia as well as cardioactive and other medications that lead to a prolonged QT interval as well congenital varieties of the long QT syndrome.

THE QT INTERVAL

The QT interval is derived by the measurement from the onset of the QRS complex representing the onset of ventricular depolarization to the end of the T wave representing the latest indication of ventricular repolarization. There are major problems with defining the normal QT interval because of variations on a gender and age basis, because of difficulties in determining the end of the T wave, because of lack of consensus as the best way to correct for the normal variation in the QT interval based on heart rate, and because of unified opinion as to which lead or leads should be used to measure the QT interval. Further compounding the problem is potential fusion of the u wave with the T wave. Furthermore, the initial estimates of the normal QT interval were done using single channel machines with leads recorded sequentially. Most electrocardiograms today are done using digital automated machines recording all leads simultaneously. In the latter instance, the true initial onset of the QRS and the true completion of the T wave can be derived. Relative to correction of the QT interval for heart rate, the most commonly used method is the Bazett's formula in which the measured QT is divided by the square root of the R-to-R interval in seconds. For instance, a measured QT derived at a heart rate of 60 beats per minute would be the corrected the corrected QT interval or QTc. However, the validity of this correction especially at elevated heart rates is open to serious question. More recent population studies have used correction of the QT based on a linear or power function of the R-to-R interval.

Attempting to define a QT interval when there is substantial variation in the R-to-R intervals as occurs with atrial fibrillation or when the defining the end of the T wave is unreliable is discouraged.

Current recommendations defining an abnormally prolonged adjusted QT interval are equal to or greater than 460 msecs in women and equal to or greater than 450 msecs in men. Current recommendation defines a short rate adjusted QT as equal to or less than 390 msecs. The FDA has recommended that rate corrected QT intervals should be subdivided into three severities when considering QT prolonging properties of drugs: greater than 450 msecs, greater than 480 msecs and greater than 500 msecs.

Adjustment of the QT interval in situations where the QRS duration is prolonged can be done by using the QT interval minus the QRS duration and applying established standards for this JT interval.

Finally, all QT prolongations generated by computer-assisted automated electrocardiographic machines should be confirmed by visual inspection by the interpreter.

ABNORMALITIES SUGGESTING RIGHT OR LEFT ATRIAL ENLARGEMENT, DILATATION OR HYPERTROPHY

Perhaps better terms would be right or left atrial abnormality. Tall p waves in lead II, e.g. 3 mm or greater in amplitude, might suggest right atrial abnormality related to emphysema or congenital heart disease. However, sinus tachycardia by itself may also cause this. Tall p waves in the right precordial leads reasonably correlate with right abnormality in congenital heart disease. Left atrial abnormality may manifest as broadened and double humped p waves in lead II and/or as a prominent terminal downward deflection of the p wave in lead V1. A similar finding may occur with sinus tachycardia. Since the validation of the right atrial and left atrial abnormalities with both pressure and volume changes in the respective chambers has been somewhat lacking, sparing and judicious use of these terms is to be recommended, and dogmatic use of these diagnoses in the absence of clinical correlates is to be avoided.

1. Hancock WE, Deal BJ, Mirvis DM, et al. AHA/ACCF/HRS recommendation and interpretation of the electrocardiogram: Part V: electrocardiogram changes associated with cardiac chamber hypertrophy: a scientific statement from the American Heart Association Electrocardiography and Arrhythmias Committee, Council on Clinical Cardiology; the American College of Cardiology Foundation; and the Heart Rhythm Society: Endorsed by the International Society for Computerized Electrcardiology. Circulation. 2009;119:e251-61.

2. Kliigfield P, Getets LS, Bailley JJ, et al. Recommendations for the standardization of the electrocardiogram: Part I: the electrocardiogram and its technology: a scientific statement from the American Heart Association Electrocardiography and Arrythmias Committee, Council on Clinical Cardiology; the American College of Cardiology Foundation; and Heart Rhythm Society Endorsed by the International Society for Computerized Electrocardiology. Circulation. 2007;115:1306-24.

3. Mason JW, Hancock WE, Gettes LS. Recommendations for the standardization and interpretation of the electrocardiogram: Part II: electrocardiography diagnostic stetement list; a scientific statement from the American Heart Association Electrocardiography and Arrythmias Committee, Council on Clinical Cardiology; the American College of Cardiology Foundation; and the Heart Rhythm Society; Endorsed by the International Society for Computerized Electrocardiology. Circulation. 2007;115:1325-32.

4. Rautaharju PM, Surawicz B, Gettes LS. AHA/ACCF/HRS recommendations for the standardization and interpretation of the electrocardiogram: Part IV: the ST segment, T and U waves, and the QT interval: a scientific statement from the American Heart Association Electrocardiography and Arrythmias Committee, Council on Clinical cardiology; the American College of Cardiology Foundation; and the Heart Rhythm Society: Endorsed by the International Society for Computerized Electrocardiology. Circulation. 2009;119:e241-50.

5. Surawicz B, Childers R, Deal B, et al. AHA/ACCF/HRS Recommendations for the standardization and interpretation of the electrocardiogram: Part III: intraventricular conduction disturbances: a scientific statement from the American Heart Association Electrocardiography and Arrythmias Committee, Council on Clinical Cardiology; the American College of Cardiology Foundation; and the Heart Rhythm Society; Endorsed by the International Society for Computerized Electrocardiology. Circulation. 2009;119:e235-40.

6. Thygesen K, Alpert JS, White HD. On behalf of the Joint ESC/ACCF/AHA/WHF. Universal definition of myocardial infarction. Circulation. 2007;116:2634-53.

7. Wagner GS, Macfarlane P, Wellens, et al. AHA/ACCF/HRS recommendations for the standardization and interpretation of the electrocardiogram: Part VI: Acute Ischemia/Infarction: a scientific statement from the American Heart Association Electrcardiography and Arrhythmias Committee, Council on Clinical cardiology; the American College of Cardiology Foundation; and the Heart Rhythm Society: Endorsed by the International Society for Computerized Electrocardiology. Circulation. 2009;119:e262-70.

SECTION 3

Diagnosis

ECG Exercise Testing

Abhimanyu (Manu) Uberoi, Victor F Froelicher

Chapter Outline

INTRODUCTION

Exercise testing is a noninvasive tool to evaluate the cardiovascular system's response to exercise under carefully controlled conditions. Exercise is the body's most common physiologic stress, and it places major demands on the cardiopulmonary system. Thus, exercise can be considered the most practical test of cardiac perfusion and function. The exercise test, alone and in combination with other noninvasive modalities, remains an important testing method due to its high yield of diagnostic, prognostic and functional information.

In short, the adaptations that occur during an exercise test allow the body to increase its metabolic rate to greater than 20 times that of rest, during which time cardiac output can increase as much as sixfold. The magnitude of these responses is dependent on a multitude of factors including age, gender, body size, type of exercise, fitness and the presence or absence of heart disease. The major central and peripheral changes that occur from rest to maximal exercise will be described in the proceeding pages of this chapter. The interpretation of the exercise test requires understanding exercise physiology and pathophysiology as well as expertise in electrocardiography. Certification for those who conduct the exams is extremely important because this technology has spread beyond the subspecialty of cardiology. For this reason, the American College of Physicians (ACP) and American College of Cardiology (ACC) and the American Heart Association (AHA) have published clinical competence guidelines for physicians performing exercise testing (www.acc.org/qualityandscience/clinical/statements.htm, www.cardiology.org)[1,2]

The exercise test plays a critical role in the diagnosis and management of heart disease patients because the equipment and personnel for performing it are readily available, the testing equipment is relatively inexpensive, it can be performed in the doctor's office, and it does not require injections or exposure to radiation. Furthermore, it can determine the degree of disability and impairment to quality of life as well as be the first step in rehabilitation and altering a major risk factor (physical inactivity).

BEFORE THE TEST

INDICATIONS FOR EXERCISE TESTING (PATIENT SELECTION)

The indications for an exercise test according to the guidelines are now presented and will be discussed later.

EXERCISE TESTING FOR DIAGNOSIS

The ACC/AHA guidelines for the diagnostic use of the standard exercise test have stated that it is appropriate for testing of adult male or female patients (including those with complete right bundle-branch block or with less than one millimeter of resting ST depression) with an *intermediate pretest probability* of

Pretest probability of coronary artery disease by symptoms, gender and age

Age[a]	Gender	Typical/angina[b]	Atypical/probable angina	Nonanginal chest pain	Asymptomatic
30–39	Men	Intermediate	Intermediate	Low	Very low
	Women	Intermediate	Very low	Very low	Very low
40–49	Men	High	Intermediate	Intermediate	Low
	Women	Intermediate	Low	Very low	Very low
50–59	Men	High	Intermediate	Intermediate	Low
	Women	Intermediate	Intermediate	Low	Very low
60–69	Men	High	Intermediate	Intermediate	Low
	Women	High	Intermediate	Intermediate	Low

[a]There are no data for patients younger than 30 or older than 69, but it can be assumed that the prevalence of CAD is low for those less than 30 years of age and higher for those over 69 years of age.
[b]High = > 90%, intermediate = 10–90%, low = < 10%, very low = < 5%.

coronary artery disease (CAD) based on gender, age and symptoms (Table 1).

EXERCISE TESTING FOR PROGNOSIS

Indications for exercise testing to assess risk and prognosis in patients with symptoms or with a prior history of CAD:

Class I (Definitely Appropriate)

Conditions for which there is evidence and/or general agreement that the standard exercise test is useful and helpful to assess risk and prognosis in patients with symptoms or a prior history of CAD who:
- are undergoing initial evaluation with suspected or known CAD. Specific exceptions are noted below in Class IIb.
- have suspected or known CAD previously evaluated with significant change in clinical status.

Class IIb (May Be Appropriate)

Conditions for which there is conflicting evidence and/or a divergence of opinion that the standard exercise test is useful and helpful to assess risk and prognosis in patients with symptoms or a prior history of CAD but the usefulness/efficacy is less well established.
- Patients who demonstrate the following ECG abnormalities:
  — Pre-excitation (Wolff-Parkinson-White) syndrome
  — Electronically paced ventricular rhythm
  — More than one millimeter of resting ST depression
  — Complete left bundle branch block.
- Patients with a stable clinical course who undergo periodic monitoring to guide management.

EXERCISE TESTING PATIENTS PRESENTING WITH ACUTE CORONARY SYNDROMES

The CNR Cardiology Research group in Italy has reviewed the literature to evaluate whether evidence still supports the use of ECG as first-choice stress-testing modality for acute coronary syndromes (ACS).[3] They concluded that a large body of evidence still supports the use of the exercise ECG as the most cost-effective tool for prognostic purposes as well as for quality of life assessment following ACS. This is consistent with the ACC/AHA guidelines, which state that patients who are pain free, have either a normal or non-diagnostic ECG or one that is unchanged from previous tracings, and have a normal set of initial cardiac enzymes are appropriate candidates for further evaluation with exercise ECG stress testing. If the patient is low risk and does not experience any further ischemic discomfort has a low risk follow-up 12-lead ECG after 6–8 hours of observation, the patient may be considered for an early exercise test. Ideally, this test is performed before discharge and is supervised by an experienced physician. In the conservative arm of the Treat Angina with aggrastat and determine Cost of Therapy with an Invasive or Conservative Strategy—Thrombolysis In Myocardial Infarction (TACTICS-TIMI) 18 trial, patients with appropriate medical therapy could safely endure exercise or pharmacologic stress testing within 48–72 hours of admission, as only one death occurred following stress testing in 847 patients with unstable angina or non-ST elevation myocardial infarction (NSTEMI).[4] Alternatively, a patient can be discharged and return for the test as an outpatient within 3 days. A recent study randomizing patients with ACS and negative troponins to either stress echocardiography or symptom-limited ECG treadmill testing, however, suggested that the incorporation of the imaging modality resulted in better risk stratification. Furthermore, there was significant cost benefit as fewer patients were classified as intermediate risk which would elicit further testing.[5]

EXERCISE TESTING PATIENTS WITH HEART FAILURE

Traditionally, exercise tests were thought to only be a tool to diagnose coronary disease; however, it is now recognized to have major applications for assessing functional capabilities, therapeutic interventions, and estimating prognosis in heart failure. Numerous hemodynamic abnormalities underlie the reduced exercise capacity commonly observed in chronic heart failure, including:
- impaired heart rate responses;
- inability to distribute cardiac output normally;

- abnormal arterial vasodilatory capacity;
- abnormal cellular metabolism in skeletal muscle;
- higher than normal systemic vascular resistance;
- higher than normal pulmonary pressures;
- ventilatory abnormalities that increase the work of breathing and cause exertional dyspnea.[6]

Intervention with angiotensin-converting enzyme (ACE)-inhibition, β blockade, cardiac resynchronization therapy (CRT) or exercise training can improve many of these abnormalities. Over the last 20 years, exercise testing with ventilatory gas exchange responses has been shown to have a critical role in the risk paradigm in heart failure.

EXERCISE TESTING PATIENTS AFTER MYOCARDIAL INFARCTION

The benefits of performing an exercise test in post-MI patients are listed in Table 2. Evaluation of patients with exercise testing can expedite and optimize their discharge from the hospital. Patients' responses to exercise, their work capacity and limiting factors (pulmonary, cardiovascular, or mechanical) at the time of discharge can be assessed by the exercise test. An exercise test prior to discharge is helpful in providing patients with guidelines for exercise at home, reassuring them of their physical status, advising them to resume or increase their activity level, advising them on timing of return to work and in determining the risk of complications. Psychologically, it can improve the patient's self-confidence by making the patient less anxious about daily physical activities and help them to rehabilitate themselves, which is an unquantifiable benefit. The test has been helpful in reassuring spouses of post-MI patients of their physical capabilities as well.

Exercise testing is also an important tool in exercise training as part of comprehensive cardiac rehabilitation. It can be used to develop and modify an exercise prescription, assist in providing activity counseling and assess the patient's progress by comparing physiologic response at the initiation of the exercise training program to response after weeks or months of training.

TABLE 2

Benefits of exercise testing post-MI

Predischarge submaximal test
• Optimizing discharge
• Altering medical therapy
• Triaging for intensity of follow-up
• First step in rehabilitation—assurance, encouragement
• Reassuring spouse
• Recognizing exercise-induced ischemia and dysrhythmias
Maximal test for return to normal activities
• Determining limitations
• Prognostication
• Reassuring employers
• Determining level of disability
• Triaging for invasive studies
• Deciding on medications
• Exercise prescription
• Continued rehabilitation

TABLE 3

Contraindications to exercise testing

Absolute
• High-risk unstable angina
• Uncontrolled cardiac arrhythmias causing symptoms or hemodynamic compromise
• Symptomatic severe aortic stenosis
• Uncontrolled symptomatic heart failure
• Acute pulmonary embolus or pulmonary infarction
• Acute myocarditis or pericarditis
• Acute aortic dissection
Relative[a]
• Left main coronary stenosis
• Moderate stenotic valvular heart disease
• Electrolyte abnormalities
• Severe arterial hypertension[b]
• Tachyarrhythmias or bradyarrhythmias
• Hypertrophic cardiomyopathy and other forms of outflow tract obstruction
• Mental or physical impairment leading to inability to exercise adequately
• High-degree atrioventricular block

[a]Relative contraindications can be superseded if the benefits of exercise outweigh the risks.
[b]In the absence of definitive evidence, the committee suggested systolic blood pressure (SBP) of greater than 200 mm Hg and/or diastolic blood pressure of greater than 110 mm Hg.
(*Source:* Gibbons, Balady, Bricker, et al.[9])

One consistent finding in the review of the post-MI exercise test literature that included a follow-up for cardiac end points, is that patients who achieved whatever criteria set forth for exercise testing were at lower risk than patients not tested. From meta-analyses of multiple studies, only an abnormal SBP response or a low exercise capacity were consistently associated with a poor outcome and were more predictive of adverse cardiac events after MI than measures of exercise-induced ischemia.[7,8]

CONTRAINDICATIONS TO EXERCISE TESTING

Table 3 lists some of the absolute and relative contraindications to exercise testing that must be considered prior to prescribing a test for a patient.

METHODOLOGY OF EXERCISE TESTING

Use of proper methodology is critical for patient safety and accurate results. Updated guidelines are available from the AHA/ACC that are based on a multitude of research studies over the last 20 years and have led to greater uniformity in methods.[9,10]

SAFETY PRECAUTIONS AND EQUIPMENT

The safety precautions outlined in the guidelines are very explicit with regard to the requirements for exercise testing. Perhaps due to an expanded knowledge concerning indications, contraindications and endpoints, maximal exercise testing appears safer today (< 1 untoward event per 10,000 tests) than it did two decades ago.

Besides emergency equipment, the safety and accuracy of the testing equipment must be considered. The treadmill should have front and side rails to help subjects steady themselves and should be calibrated monthly. Although numerous clever devices have been developed to automate blood pressure measurement during exercise, none can be recommended except those that allow audible monitoring of the Korotkoff sounds with operator validation. The time-proven method of holding the subject's arm with a stethoscope placed over the brachial artery remains the most reliable.

PRETEST PREPARATIONS

When the test is scheduled, the patient should be instructed not to eat, drink or smoke at least 2 hours prior to the test and to come dressed for exercise, including proper footwear.

During the pretest evaluation, the patient's usual level of exercise activity should be established to help determine a baseline and an appropriate target workload for testing. The physician should also review the patient's medical history, considering any conditions that can increase the risk of testing. The Table 3 lists the absolute and relative contraindications to exercise testing. Testing patients with aortic stenosis should be done with great care because they can develop severe cardiovascular complications. *Thus, a physical examination—including assessment of systolic murmurs—should be performed before all exercise tests.* If a loud systolic murmur is heard and/or the carotid pulse exhibits a slow upstroke, an echocardiogram is recommended prior to testing.

Pretest standard 12-lead ECGs are necessary in both the supine and the standing positions. Good skin preparation is necessary for appropriate conductance to avoid artifacts and is especially important for elderly patients who have a higher skin resistance with tendency toward contact noise. The electrical perturbations and artifact caused by exercise can be minimized by appropriate electrode placement, keeping the arm electrodes off the chest and placing them on the shoulders, placing the ground (right leg) electrode on the back, outside of the cardiac field, placing the left leg electrodes below the umbilicus and recording the baseline ECG supine. The supine baseline ECG in this modified exercise limb-lead placement can serve as the reference resting ECG prior to the onset of exercise.

Hyperventilation should be avoided before testing. Subjects with or without disease can exhibit ST-segment changes with hyperventilation; thus, hyperventilation to identify false-positive responders is no longer considered useful. The next important methodological issue is when to terminate for safety reasons and these indications are summarized in the Table 4.

EXERCISE TEST MODALITIES

Three types of exercise can be used to stress the cardiovascular system: (1) isometric; (2) dynamic or (3) a combination of the two. *Isometric exercise,* defined as constant muscular contraction without movement (such as handgrip), imposes a disproportionate pressure load on the left ventricle relative to the body's ability to supply oxygen. *Dynamic exercise* is defined as rhythmic muscular activity resulting in movement, and it initiates a more appropriate increase in cardiac output and oxygen exchange. This chapter considers only dynamic exercise testing, because a delivered workload can be calibrated accurately and

SECTION 3 · Diagnosis

TABLE 4

Indications for terminating exercise testing

Absolute indications

- Moderate to severe angina
- Increasing nervous system symptoms (e.g. ataxia, dizziness or near-syncope)
- Signs of poor perfusion (cyanosis or pallor)
- Technical difficulties in monitoring ECG or SBP
- Subject's desire to stop
- Sustained ventricular tachycardia
- ST-segment elevation (≥ 1.0 mm) in leads without diagnostic Q waves (other than V_1 or aVR)

Relative indications

- Drop in SBP of ≥ 10 mm Hg from baseline blood pressure despite an increase in workload in the absence of other evidence of ischemia
- ST or QRS changes such as excessive ST-segment depression (> 2 mm of horizontal or down-sloping ST-segment depression) or marked axis shift
- Arrhythmias other than sustained ventricular tachycardia, including multifocal PVCs, triplets of PVCs, supraventricular tachycardia, heart block or bradyarrhythmias
- Fatigue, shortness of breath, wheezing, leg cramps or claudication
- Development of bundle branch block or intraventricular conduction delay that cannot be distinguished from ventricular tachycardia
- Increasing chest pain
- Hypertensive response[a]

(Abbreviation: PVCs: Premature ventricular contractions)
[a]In the absence of definitive evidence, the committee suggests SBP of > 250 mm Hg and/or a diastolic blood pressure of > 115 mm Hg.
(*Source:* Gibbons, Balady, Bricker, et al.[9])

the physiologic response measured easily. Isometric exercise is not recommended for routine exercise testing.

Bicycle Ergometer versus Treadmill

The bicycle ergometer usually costs less, takes up less space and makes less noise than a treadmill. Although bicycling is a dynamic exercise, most individuals perform more work on a treadmill because a greater muscle mass is involved, and most subjects are more familiar with walking than cycling. These factors create considerable variability in test results, which is reflected in most studies comparing exercise on an upright cycle ergometer versus a treadmill exercise. Specifically, while maximal heart rate values have been demonstrated to be roughly similar, maximal oxygen uptake has been shown to be up to 25% greater during treadmill exercise.

Exercise Protocols

The most common protocols, their stages and the predicted oxygen cost of each stage are illustrated in Figure 1. The exercise protocol should be progressive with even increments in speed and grade whenever possible. Smaller, even, and more frequent work increments are preferred over larger, uneven, and less frequent increases, because the former yield a more accurate estimation of exercise capacity. Recent guidelines suggest that protocols should be individualized for each subject such that test duration is approximately 8–12 minutes. Because ramp testing uses small and even increments, it permits a more

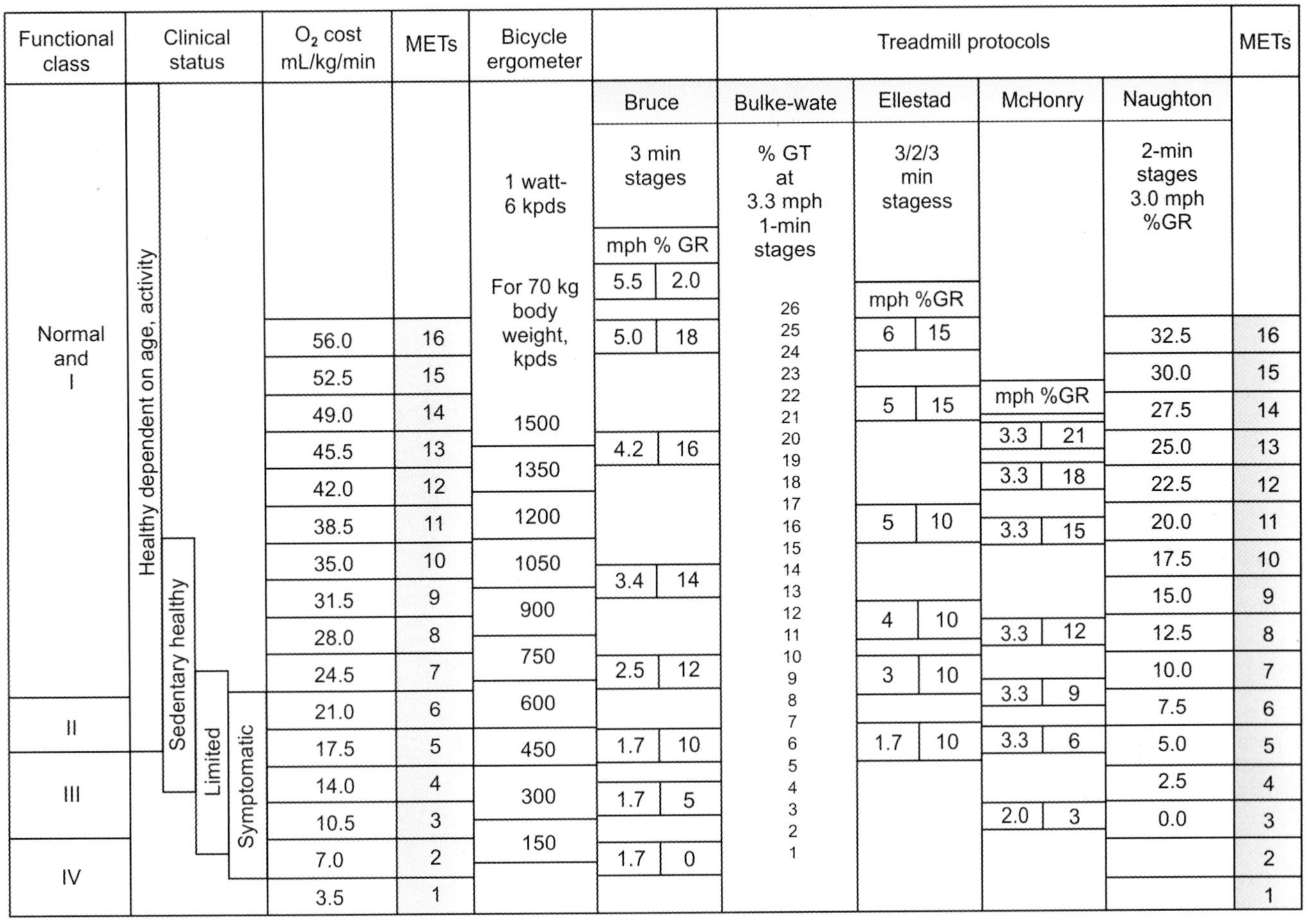

Functional class	Clinical status	O₂ cost mL/kg/min	METs	Bicycle ergometer	Bruce mph	Bruce % GR	Bulke-ware % GT at 3.3 mph 1-min stages	Ellestad mph	Ellestad %GR	McHonry mph	McHonry %GR	Naughton 2-min stages 3.0 mph %GR	METs
				1 watt-6 kpds	5.5	2.0	26						
Normal and I		56.0	16	For 70 kg body weight, kpds	5.0	18	25 / 24	6	15			32.5	16
		52.5	15				23					30.0	15
		49.0	14	1500			22 / 21	5	15			27.5	14
		45.5	13	1350	4.2	16	20 / 19			3.3	21	25.0	13
		42.0	12				18 / 17			3.3	18	22.5	12
		38.5	11	1200			16	5	10	3.3	15	20.0	11
	Sedentary healthy	35.0	10	1050	3.4	14	15 / 14					17.5	10
		31.5	9	900			13 / 12					15.0	9
		28.0	8	750			11	4	10	3.3	12	12.5	8
		24.5	7		2.5	12	10 / 9	3	10	3.3	9	10.0	7
II	Limited	21.0	6	600			8 / 7					7.5	6
	Symptomatic	17.5	5	450	1.7	10	6 / 5	1.7	10	3.3	6	5.0	5
III		14.0	4	300	1.7	5	4					2.5	4
		10.5	3	150			3 / 2			2.0	3	0.0	3
IV		7.0	2		1.7	0	1						2
		3.5	1										1

(Left vertical labels: *Healthy dependent on age, activity*)

FIGURE 1: The most common protocols, their stages and the predicted oxygen cost of each stage
(Abbreviations: GR: Grade; METs: Metabolic equivalents)

accurate estimation of exercise capacity and can be individualized to yield targeted test duration.

Add-Ons to the Exercise Test

Some of the newer add-ons or substitutes for the exercise test have the advantage of being able to localize ischemia as well as diagnose coronary disease when the baseline ECG negates ST analysis (more than one millimeter ST depression, left bundle-branch block, WPW). Stress echocardiograms, stress nuclear perfusion scans and cardiac MRIs also provide an estimation of ventricular function as well as tissue viability information. Non-exercise stress techniques also permit diagnostic assessment of patients unable to exercise. Although the newer technologies appear to have better diagnostic characteristics, this is not always the case. When used, diagnostic scores that incorporate other variables in addition to the ST-segment yield results similar to imaging procedures.

DURING THE TEST

PHYSIOLOGY REVIEW

This would be a good time to do a quick review of some of the basic principles of physiology that are pertinent to understanding the mechanisms behind the body's response to exercise. For brief overviews of the major central and peripheral adaptations that occur from rest to maximal exercise see Figures 2A and B.

Oxygen Consumption

Two basic principles of exercise physiology are important to understand in regard to exercise testing. The first is a *physiologic principle*: total body oxygen uptake and myocardial oxygen uptake are distinct in their determinants and in the way they are measured or estimated (Table 5).

TABLE 5

Two basic principles of exercise physiology

Myocardial oxygen consumption	=	Heart rate × SBP (determinants include wall tension = left ventricular pressure × volume; contractility; and heart rate)
Ventilatory oxygen consumption (VO_2)	=	External work performed, or cardiac output[a] × A-VO_2 difference

(Abbreviations: A-VO_2: Arteriovenous oxygen difference; VO_2: Volume oxygen consumption; vol%: Volume percent).
[a]The arteriovenous O_2 difference is approximately 15–17 vol% at maximal exercise in most individuals; therefore, VO_{2max} generally reflects the extent to which cardiac output increases.

(Right margin: **CHAPTER 13** ECG Exercise Testing)

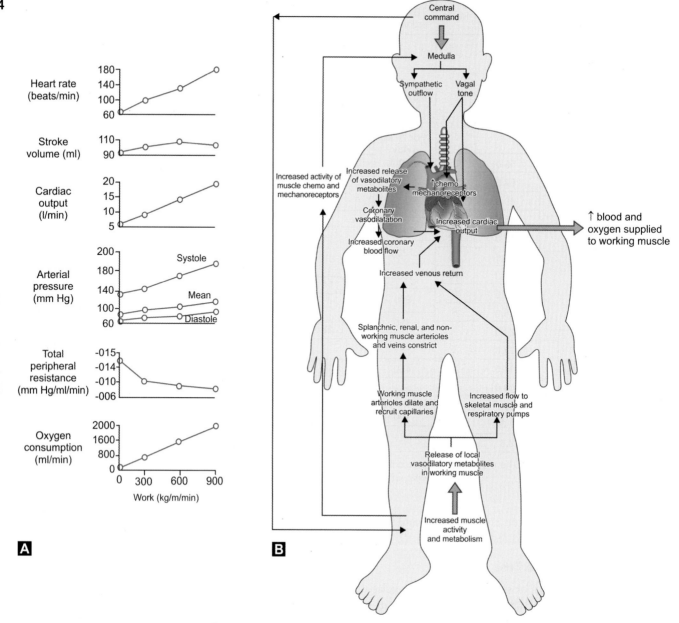

FIGURES 2A AND B: (A) Graphs of the hemodynamic responses to dynamic exercise. (B) Sequence of physiological responses to dynamic exercise (*Source*: Modified from Cardiovascular Physiology at a Glance, Blackwell Publishers, 2004)

Total body or ventilatory oxygen uptake [volume oxygen consumption (VO_2)] is the amount of oxygen extracted from inspired air (Flow charts 1 and 2). The determinants of VO_2 are cardiac output and the peripheral arteriovenous oxygen difference. Maximal arteriovenous difference is physiologically limited to roughly 15–17 ml/dL. Thus maximal arteriovenous difference behaves more or less as a constant, making maximal oxygen uptake an indirect estimate of maximal cardiac output.

Myocardial oxygen uptake is the amount of oxygen consumed by the heart muscle. The determinants of myocardial oxygen uptake include intramyocardial wall tension (left ventricular pressure and end-diastolic volume), contractility, and heart rate. It has been shown that myocardial oxygen uptake can be estimated by the product of heart rate and SBP, or double product. This information is valuable clinically because exercise-induced angina often occurs at the same myocardial oxygen demand (double product), and the higher the double product achieved, the better is myocardial perfusion and prognosis. When such is not the case, the influence of other factors should be suspected, such as a recent meal, abnormal ambient temperature or coronary artery spasm. Thus, it is not surprising that the double product during exercise testing has long been known to be a significant independent predictor of myocardial ischemia severity[11] and prognosis.[12,13]

The second principle is one of *pathophysiology*: considerable interaction takes place between the exercise test manifestations of abnormalities in myocardial perfusion and function. The electrocardiographic response and angina are closely related to myocardial ischemia (usually secondary to CAD), whereas exercise capacity, SBP and heart rate responses to exercise can

FLOW CHART 1: Central determinants of maximal oxygen uptake

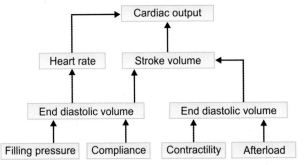

(*Source*: Myers J, Froelicher VF. Hemodynamic determinants of exercise capacity in chronic heart failure. Ann Intern Med. 1991;115:377-86)

FLOW CHART 2: Peripheral determinants of maximal oxygen uptake. The A-VO$_2$ difference is the difference between arterial and venous oxygen

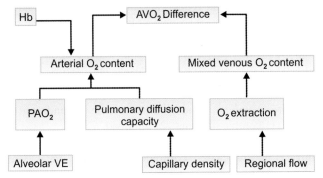

(Abbreviations: A-VO$_2$: Arteriovenous oxygen difference; Hb: Hemoglobin; PAO$_2$: Partial pressure of alveolar oxygen; VE: Minute ventilation). (*Source*: Myers J, Froelicher VF. Hemodynamic determinants of exercise capacity in chronic heart failure. Ann Intern Med. 1991;115:377-86)

be determined by the presence of myocardial ischemia, myocardial dysfunction or responses in the periphery. Exercise-induced ischemia can cause cardiac dysfunction which results in exercise impairment and an abnormal SBP response.

Metabolic Equivalents Term (MET)

Since exercise testing fundamentally involves the measurement of work, there are several concepts regarding work that are important to understand. The common biologic measure of total body work is the oxygen uptake, which is usually expressed as a rate (making it a measure of power) in liters per minute. The MET is the term commonly used to express the oxygen requirement of work during an exercise test on a treadmill or cycle ergometer. One MET is equated with the resting metabolic rate (approximately 3.5 mL of O$_2$/kg/min), and a MET value achieved from an exercise test is a multiple of the resting metabolic rate, either measured directly (as oxygen uptake) or estimated from the maximal workload achieved using standardized equations.[14] Table 6 lists clinically meaningful METs for exercise, prognosis and maximal performance, and Figure 3 depicts exercise capacity and the relationship between age and METs.

Exercise capacity
(% of normal in referral males)

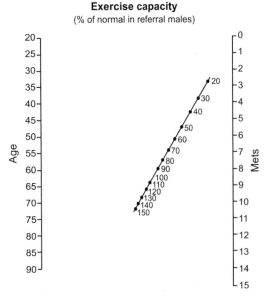

FIGURE 3: The exercise capacity nomogram, providing a relative estimate of normal for age, with 100% being as expected for age in a clinical population. (Abbreviation: METs: Metabolic equivalents)

TABLE 6

Clinically significant metabolic equivalents for maximum exercise

1 MET	Resting
2 METs	Level walking at 2 mph
4 METs	Level walking at 4 mph
< 5 METs	Poor prognosis; peak cost of basic activities of daily living
10 METs	Prognosis with medical therapy as good as coronary artery bypass surgery; unlikely to exhibit significant nuclear perfusion defect
13 METs	Excellent prognosis regardless of other exercise responses
18 METs	Elite endurance athletes
20 METs	World-class athletes

(Abbreviations: MET: metabolic equivalent, or a unit of sitting resting oxygen uptake; 1 MET: 3.5 mL/kg/min oxygen uptake; mph: Miles per hour)

Acute Cardiopulmonary Response to Exercise

The intact cardiovascular system responds to acute exercise with a series of adjustments that assure the following (Fig. 2):
• Active muscles receive blood supply according to their metabolic demands
• Heat generated by the muscles is dissipated
• Blood supply to the brain and heart are maintained

This response requires a major redistribution of cardiac output along with a number of local metabolic changes. The usual measure of the capacity of the body to deliver and use oxygen is the maximal oxygen consumption (VO$_{2max}$). Thus, the limits of the cardiopulmonary system are defined by VO$_{2max}$, which can be expressed by the Fick principle:

$$VO_{2max} = \text{maximal cardiac output} \times \text{maximal arteriovenous oxygen difference}$$

Cardiac output must closely match ventilation in the lung to deliver oxygen to the working muscle. The VO$_{2max}$ is determined by the maximal amount of ventilation [volume of expired gas (V_E)] moving into and out of the lung and by the fraction of this ventilation that is extracted by the tissues:

$$VO_2 = V_E \times (FiO_2 - FeO_2)$$

where V_E is minute ventilation, and FiO_2 and FeO_2 are the fractional concentration of oxygen in the inspired and expired air respectively. To measure VO_2 accurately, CO_2 in the expired air [carbon dioxide elimination (VCO_2)] must also be measured; the major purpose of VCO_2 in this equation is to correct for the difference in ventilation between inspired and expired air. The VCO_2 is also a valuable measurement clinically for chronic heart failure patients because the rate of increase in VCO_2 relative to the work rate or ventilation parallels the severity of heart failure and is a powerful prognostic marker.

The cardiopulmonary limits (VO_{2max}) are therefore defined by the following:

- A central component (cardiac output) describes the capacity of the heart to function as a pump.
- Peripheral factors (arteriovenous oxygen difference) describe the capacity of the lung to oxygenate the blood delivered to it as well as the capacity of the working muscle to extract this oxygen from the blood.

Central Factors

Heart rate: Sympathetic and parasympathetic nervous system influences are responsible for the cardiovascular system's first response to exercise, which is an increase in heart rate. Vagal withdrawal is responsible for the initial 10–30 beats per minute change, whereas the remainder is thought to be largely caused by increased sympathetic outflow. Of the two major components of cardiac output, heart rate and stroke volume, heart rate is responsible for most of the increase in cardiac output during exercise, particularly at higher levels. Heart rate increases linearly with workload and oxygen uptake.

The heart rate response to exercise is influenced by several factors including age, type of activity, body position, fitness, the presence of heart disease, medication use, blood volume and environment. Of these, the most important factor is age, as a significant decline in maximal heart rate occurs with increasing age. This attenuation is thought to be a result of intrinsic cardiac changes rather than neural influences. It should be noted that there is a great deal of variability around the regression line between maximal heart rate and age, thus, age-related maximal heart rate estimates are a relatively poor index of maximal effort. Since prediction of maximal heart rate is inaccurate, exercise should be symptom-limited and not targeted on achieving a certain heart rate. Therefore, diagnostic information can be obtained even if a certain target heart rate (i.e. 85% of age-predicted maximal heart rate) is not achieved. Interestingly, of all heart rate measurements during exercise and recovery, the heart rate increase at peak exercise in 1,959 patients referred for clinical treadmill testing was the most powerful predictor of cardiovascular prognosis after adjustments for potential confounders.[15] Maximal heart rate is unchanged or can be slightly reduced after a program of training whereas resting heart rate is frequently reduced after training as a result of enhanced parasympathetic tone.

Stroke volume: The product of stroke volume, which is the volume of blood ejected per heartbeat, and heart rate determines cardiac output. Stroke volume is equal to the difference between end-diastolic and end-systolic volume. Thus, a greater diastolic filling (preload) will increase stroke volume. Alternatively, factors that increase arterial blood pressure will resist ventricular outflow (afterload) and result in a reduced stroke volume. During exercise, stroke volume increases up to approximately 50–60% of maximal capacity, after which increases in cardiac output are caused by further increases in heart rate. The extent to which increases in stroke volume during exercise reflect an increase in end-diastolic volume or a decrease in end-systolic volume, or both, is not entirely clear but appears to depend on ventricular function, body position and intensity of exercise. In healthy subjects, after a period of exercise training, stroke volume increases at rest and during exercise. Although the mechanisms have been debated, evidence suggests that this adaptation is caused more by increases in preload, and possibly local adaptations that reduce peripheral vascular resistance, rather than by increases in myocardial contractility. The end-diastolic and end-systolic responses to acute exercise have varied greatly in the literature, but are certainly dependent on presence and type of disease, exercise intensity and exercise position (supine vs upright).

End-systolic volume: End-systolic volume depends on two factors: (1) contractility and (2) afterload.

Contractility describes the forcefulness of the heart's contraction. Increasing contractility reduces end-systolic volume, which results in a greater stroke volume and thus greater cardiac output. Contractility is commonly quantified by the ejection fraction, the percentage of blood ejected from the ventricle during systole (traditionally measured using echo-cardiographic, radionuclide or angiographic techniques).

Afterload is a measure of the force resisting the ejection of blood by the heart. Increased afterload (or aortic pressure, as is observed with chronic hypertension) results in a reduced ejection fraction and increased end-diastolic and end-systolic volumes. During dynamic exercise, the force resisting ejection in the periphery (total peripheral resistance) is reduced by vasodilation, owing to the effect of local metabolites on the skeletal muscle vasculature. Thus, despite even a fivefold increase in cardiac output among normal subjects during exercise, mean arterial pressure increases only moderately.

Peripheral Factors
(Arteriovenous Oxygen Difference)

Oxygen extraction by the tissues during exercise reflects the difference between the oxygen content of the arteries (generally 18–20 ml O_2/100 ml at rest) and the oxygen content in the veins (generally 13–15 ml O_2/100 ml at rest, yielding a typical arteriovenous oxygen difference (A-VO_2) at rest of 4–6 ml O_2/100 ml, approximately 23% extraction). During exercise, this difference widens as the working tissues extract greater amounts of oxygen; venous oxygen content reaches very low levels and A-VO_2 can be as high as 16–18 ml O_2/100 ml with exhaustive exercise. Some oxygenated blood always returns to the heart; however, as smaller amounts of blood continue to flow through, metabolically less active tissues do not fully extract oxygen. The A-VO$_2$ is generally considered to widen by a relatively *fixed* amount during exercise, and differences in VO$_{2max}$ are predominantly explained by differences in cardiac output. Some patients with cardiovascular or pulmonary disease, however, exhibit reduced VO$_{2max}$ values that can be attributed to a combination of both central and peripheral factors.

Determinants of arterial oxygen content: Arterial oxygen content is related to the partial pressure of arterial oxygen, which is determined in the lung by alveolar ventilation and pulmonary diffusion capacity, as well as hemoglobin content of the blood. In the absence of pulmonary disease, arterial oxygen content and saturation are usually normal throughout exercise. Patients with symptomatic pulmonary disease often neither ventilate the alveoli adequately nor diffuse oxygen from the lung into the bloodstream normally, resulting in a decrease in arterial oxygen saturation during exercise. Arterial hemoglobin content is also usually normal throughout exercise.

Determinants of venous oxygen content: Venous oxygen content reflects the capacity to extract oxygen from the blood as it flows through the muscle and capillary beds. Extraction is effected by the volume of regional flow through the muscle and capillary density. Muscle blood flow increases in proportion to increased oxygen requirement, which is determined by increased work rate. The increase in blood flow is brought about not only by the increase in cardiac output but also by a preferential redistribution of the cardiac output to the exercising muscle. Locally produced vasodilatory mechanisms along with possible neurogenic dilatation resulting from higher sympathetic activity reduce local vascular resistance and mediate the greater skeletal muscle blood flow. A marked increase in the number of open capillaries reduces diffusion distances, increases capillary blood volume and increases mean transit time, facilitating oxygen delivery to the muscle.

AUTONOMIC CONTROL

Neural Control Mechanisms

The neural control mechanisms responsible for the cardiovascular response to exercise occur through two processes that initiate and maintain this response:

1. *Central command*: Neural impulses, arising from the central nervous system, recruit motor units, excite medullary and spinal neuronal circuits and cause the cardiovascular changes during exercise.
2. *Muscle afferents*: Muscle contraction stimulates afferent endings within the skeletal muscle, which in turn, reflexively evoke the cardiovascular changes.

The latter mechanism called *exercise pressor reflex*, comprises all of the cardiovascular responses reflexively induced from contracting skeletal muscle that cause changes in the efferent sympathetic and parasympathetic outputs to the cardiovascular system. This is ultimately responsible for increases in arterial blood pressure, heart rate, myocardial contractility, cardiac output and blood flow distribution. A specific subset of muscle afferents serve as ergo-receptors activated by either mechanical or metabolic perturbations.

As the demand for cardiac output increases, parasympathetic activity becomes attenuated, while sympathetic activity increases. The sympathetic system releases norepinephrine directly through the sympathetic trunk to the sinus node and myocardium. In addition, norepinephrine and epinephrine from the adrenal medulla act to increase heart rate and increase myocardial contractility, as well as to shunt blood flow to working muscle. By mediating peripheral vasoconstriction in relatively inactive tissues (e.g. kidney and gut), the sympathetic system increases venous return, and vasodilatory metabolites maintain local increased flow to active skeletal muscle. Actively contracting skeletal muscle also increases preload by acting as a venous pump and stimulating sympathetic afferent fibers within the muscle itself.

Pharmacologic blockade studies have helped to elucidate the differential contributions of the two autonomic branches during exercise. Blockade of parasympathetic control with atropine reveals that most of the initial response to exercise, up to a heart rate of 100–120 beats per minute [i.e. a delta heart rate (HR) of 30–40 beats per minute (bpm)], is attributable to the withdrawal of tonic vagal activity. Vagal withdrawal induces a rapid increase in heart rate and cardiac output. Conversely, blockade of sympathetic control with propranolol reveals the importance of augmented sympathetic activity during moderate and heavy exercise. During light exercise, with work loads of 25–40% of VO$_{2max}$ or while heart rate remains within 30 beats per minute over baseline, plasma norepinephrine levels do not significantly increase, confirming that the sympathetic nervous system is more important with higher levels of exercise.

AUTONOMIC MODULATION DURING IMMEDIATE RECOVERY FROM EXERCISE

Autonomic physiology during recovery from acute bouts of exercise involves reactivation of the parasympathetic system and deactivation of sympathetic activity. The decline of heart rate after cessation of exercise is the variable most commonly analyzed to assess the underlying mechanisms. A delay in heart rate recovery has been used as a marker of autonomic dysfunction and/or failure of the cardiovascular system to respond to the normal autonomic responses to exercise. This delay has been shown to be a powerful prognostic marker.[16,17] Time constants have been calculated by fitting heart rate decay data to a number of mathematical models, but the simple change in heart rate from peak exercise to minute 1 or 2 of recovery appears to distinguish and prognosticate survival as well. Early recovery after acute bouts of exercise appears to be dominated by parasympathetic reactivation, with sympathetic withdrawal becoming more important later in recovery. In a pharmacologic blockade study, Imai and his colleagues[18] computed HR recovery decay curves using beat-to-beat data and concluded that short-term and moderate-term HR recovery curves are vagally mediated, because HR decay 30 seconds and 2 minutes into recovery was prolonged with atropine and dual blockade; however, the HR decay for 2 minutes was more prolonged with dual blockade than with atropine alone, indicating that later recovery also depends on sympathetic modulation. Rather than declining, plasma norepinephrine concentrations during the first minute of recovery remain constant or even increase immediately after exercise.

The above principles explain the mechanisms of change during exercise, and now we will explain the clinical correlations that you may expect to see in the patient and how the parameters we follow for diagnostic and prognostic indicators change.

Hemodynamics

The increased demand for myocardial oxygen required by dynamic exercise is the key to the use of exercise testing as a diagnostic tool for CAD. Myocardial oxygen consumption cannot be directly measured in a practical manner, but its relative demand can be estimated from its determinants, such as heart rate, wall tension (left ventricular pressure and diastolic volume), contractility and cardiac work. Although all of these factors increase during exercise, increased heart rate is particularly important in patients who have obstructive CAD. An increase in heart rate results in a shortening of the diastolic filling period, the time during which coronary blood flow is the greatest. In normal coronary arteries, dilation occurs. In obstructed vessels, however, dilation is limited and flow can be decreased by the shortening of the diastolic filling period. This causes inadequate blood flow and therefore insufficient oxygen supply.

Hemodynamic data, including heart rate, blood pressure, and exercise capacity, are important features of the exercise test. Since it can objectively quantify exercise capacity, exercise testing is now commonly used for disability evaluation rather than reliance on functional classifications. No questionnaire or submaximal test can provide as reliable a result as a symptom-limited exercise test.

Heart Rate

Age-predicted maximal heart rate targets are relatively useless for clinical purposes, and they should not be used for exercise testing endpoints. It is surprising how much steeper the age-related decline in maximal heart rate is in clinically referred populations as compared with age-matched normal subjects or volunteers.

Exercise Capacity

When expressing exercise capacity as a relative percentage of what is deemed normal, careful consideration should be given to population characteristics. Exercise capacity is influenced by many factors other than age and gender, including health, activity level, body composition and the exercise mode and protocol used. Exercise capacity should not be reported in total time, rather as the oxygen uptake or MET equivalent of the workload achieved. This method permits the comparison of the results of many different exercise testing protocols. In a recent study of 974 patients who underwent quantitative exercise myocardial perfusion imaging, only 2 of 473 (0.4%) patients achieved greater than or equal to 10 METs demonstrated nuclear perfusion defects consistent with ischemia while 7.1% of patients who achieved fewer than 7 METs had nuclear defects consistent with ischemia.[19] Thus, myocardial perfusion imaging is of little value in patients with predicted exercise capacity greater than 10 METs and simple referral for ECG exercise testing will provide substantial cost-savings.

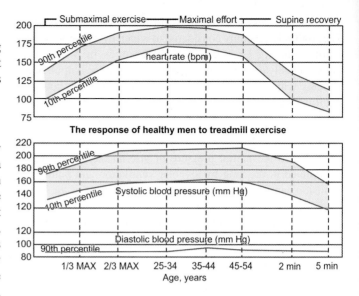

FIGURE 4: The results of a large number of normal individuals who underwent a progressive treadmill test show the response of heart rate and blood pressure according to age (Abbreviation: bpm: Beats per minute)

Blood pressure: The SBP should rise with increasing treadmill workload, whereas diastolic blood pressure usually remains approximately the same or drops (Fig. 4). Although exertional hypotension has been described in many different ways, it has been shown to predict severe angiographic CAD and is associated with a poor prognosis.[20] A drop in SBP below pre-exercise values is the most ominous criterion. A failure of SBP to adequately increase is particularly worrisome in patients who have sustained an MI, have valvular heart disease or have heart failure.

Possible complications: Most complications of the exercise stress test can be avoided by measuring blood pressure, monitoring the ECG, questioning the patient about symptoms and levels of fatigue and assessing appearance during the test. Subjects should be reminded not to grasp the front or side rails because this decreases the work performed and creates noise in the ECG. The subject can rest his or her hands on the rails for balance but should not hang on. Hanging on the rails results in an overestimation of exercise capacity.

As previously mentioned, target heart rates based on age should not be used because the relationship between maximal heart rate and age is poor, and a wide scatter exists around the many different recommended regression lines. Such heart-rate targets result in a submaximal test for some individuals, a maximal test for some, and an unrealistic goal for others. The absolute and relative indications for test termination are listed in Table 4. If none of these endpoints are met, the test should be symptom-limited. The Borg scales are an excellent means of quantifying an individual's effort. Subjects should be monitored for perceived effort level by using the 6–20 Borg scale at 2-minute intervals.

To ensure the safety of exercise testing, the following list of the most dangerous circumstances in the exercise testing laboratory should be recognized:

- When patients exhibit ST-segment elevation (without baseline diagnostic Q waves), this can be associated with dangerous arrhythmias and infarction. The prevalence is approximately 1 in 1,000 clinical tests and usually occurs in V_2 or aVF rather than V_5.

- When a patient with an ischemic cardiomyopathy exhibits severe chest pain due to ischemia (angina pectoris), a cool-down walk is advisable.
- When a patient develops exertional hypotension accompanied by ischemia (angina or ST-segment depression) or when it occurs in a patient with a history of congestive heart failure (CHF), cardiomyopathy or recent myocardial infarction (MI), safety is a serious issue.
- When a patient with a history of sudden death or collapse during exercise develops premature ventricular depolarizations that become frequent, a cool-down walk is advisable.

Recovery after Exercise

If maximal sensitivity is to be achieved with an exercise test, patients should return to a supine as soon as possible during the post-exercise period (maximal wall stress). It is advisable to record approximately 10 seconds of ECG data while the patient is standing motionless but still at near-maximal heart rate and then have the patient lie down. Having the patient perform a cool-down walk after the test can delay or eliminate the appearance of ST-segment depression, while having patients lie down enhances ST-segment abnormalities in recovery.[21]

Monitoring should continue for at least 5 minutes after exercise or until changes stabilize. An abnormal response occurring only in the recovery period is neither unusual nor necessarily suggestive of a false-positive result. The recovery period, particularly the third minute is critical for ST analysis. Noise should not be a problem, and ST depression at that time has important implications regarding the presence and severity of CAD.[22,23]

A cool-down walk can be helpful in performing tests on patients with an established diagnosis undergoing testing for other than diagnostic reasons, as in testing athletes or patients with CHF, valvular heart disease or a recent MI.

Beta blockers: In our most recent study of the effects of β blockade and heart rate response, we found the sensitivity and predictive accuracy of standard ST criteria for exercise-induced ST-depression significantly decreased in male patients taking β blockers and not reaching an adequate heart rate. In those who fail to reach target heart rate and are not β blocked, sensitivity and predictive accuracy were maintained. The only way to maintain sensitivity with the standard exercise test in the β blocker group who failed to reach target heart rate was to use a treadmill score or 0.5-mm ST-depression as the criterion for abnormal.[24] Due to a greater potential for cardiac events with the cessation of β blockers, they should not be automatically stopped prior to testing. If a patient is to be tested off β blockers, they should not be stopped abruptly but tapered off gradually under physician guidance.

Women

The summary from the guidelines are clearly stated regarding testing women: concern about false-positive ST responses can be addressed by careful assessment of pretest probability and selective use of a stress imaging test before proceeding to

angiography. The optimal strategy for circumventing false-positive test results for the diagnosis of coronary disease in women requires the use of scores. There is insufficient data to justify routine stress imaging tests as the initial test for women.

Diagnostic Scores

Studies considering non-ECG data consistently demonstrate that the multivariable equations outperform simple ST diagnostic criteria. These equations generally provide a predictive accuracy of 80% (ROC area of 0.80). To obtain the best diagnostic characteristics with the exercise test, clinical and non-ECG test responses should be considered. We have validated simple scores for both men and women. Calculation of a *simple* exercise test score can be done using Figure 5[25] for men and Figure 6[26]

Variable	Circle response	Sum	Men
Maximal heart rate	Less than 100 bpm = 30		
	100 to 129 bpm = 24		
	130 to 159 bpm = 18		
	160 to 189 bpm = 12		
Exercise ST depression	190 to 200 bpm = 6		< 40 = Low probability
	1-2 mm = 15		
Age	>2 mm = 25		
	>55 yrs = 20		40-60 = Intermediate probability
Angina history	40 to 55 yrs = 12		
	Definite/typical = 5		
	Probable/atypical = 3		
	Non-cardiac pain =1		> 60 = High probability
Hypercholesterolemia?	Yes = 5		
Diabetes?	Yes = 5		
Exercise test induced angina?	Occurred = 3		
	Reason for stopping = 5		
Total Score :			

FIGURE 5: Calculation of the simple score for angiographic coronary disease in men. Choose only one per group. (Abbreviation: bpm: Beats per minute)

Variable	Circle response	Sum	Women
Maximal heart rate	Less than 100 bpm = 20		
	100 to 129 bpm = 16		
	130 to 159 bpm = 12		
	160 to 189 bpm = 8		
	190 to 220 bpm = 4		< 37 = Low probability
Exercise ST depression	1-2 mm = 6		
Age	> 2 mm =10		
	> 65 yrs = 25		37-57 = Intermediate probability
Angina history	50 to 65 yrs =15		
	Definite/typical = 10		
	Probable/atypical = 6		
	Non-cardiac pain = 2		> 57= High probability
Hypercholesterolemia?	Yes = 10		
Diabetes?	Yes = 10		
Exercise test induced angina?	Occurred = 9		
	Reason for stopping = 15		
Estrogen status	Positive = -5, Negative = 5		
Total Score :			

FIGURE 6: Calculation of the simple score for angiographic coronary disease in women. Choose only one per group

CHAPTER 13 — ECG Exercise Testing

for women. Diagnostic scores should be applied during every exercise test because they are easy to use and significantly improve the prediction of angiographic CAD.[27]

AFTER THE TEST

ECG INTERPRETATION: FACTORS DETERMINING PROGNOSIS

ST-Segment Analysis

ST-segment depression represents global subendocardial ischemia, with a direction determined largely by the placement of the heart in the chest. ST-depression does not localize coronary artery lesions. ST-depression in the inferior leads (II, AVF) is most often caused by the atrial repolarization wave, which begins in the PR segment and can often extend into the beginning of the ST-segment. Severe transmural ischemia, resulting in wall motion abnormalities, causes a shift of the vector in the direction of the wall motion abnormality. Preexisting areas of wall motion abnormality (i.e. scar), however, usually indicated by a Q wave are also capable of causing such shifts resulting in ST elevation without the presence of ischemia. While the resting ECG exhibits Q waves from an old MI, ST elevations are caused by ischemia, wall-motion abnormalities, or both, whereas accompanying ST-depression can be caused by a second area of ischemia or reciprocal changes. When the resting ECG is normal, however, ST elevation is a result of severe ischemia (spasm or a critical lesion), although accompanying ST-depression is reciprocal. Such ST elevation is uncommon, very arrhythmogenic, and it is localizing. Exercise-induced ST-depression loses its diagnostic power in patients with left bundle-branch block, Wolff-Parkinson-White (WPW) syndrome, electronic pacemakers, intraventricular conduction defects (IVCDs) with inverted T-waves and in patients with more than one millimeter of resting ST-depression. ST-segment changes isolated to the inferior leads are more likely to be false-positive responses unless profound (i.e. > 1 mm). The various patterns of ST segment changes are illustrated in Figure 7.

Precordial lead V_5 alone consistently outperforms the inferior leads or the combination of leads V_5 with II, because lead II has been shown to have a high false-positive rate.[28] Exercise-induced ST-segment depression in inferior limb leads is a poor marker for CAD in and of itself.[29] In patients without prior MI and normal resting electrocardiograms, ST-depression in precordial lead V_5 along with V_4 and V_6 are reliable markers for CAD, and the monitoring of inferior limb leads adds little additional diagnostic information. This said, however, elevation inferiorly should not be ignored.

Exercise-induced R-wave and S-wave amplitude changes are not associated with the changes in left ventricular volume, ejection fraction or ischemia. Many studies suggest that such changes do not have diagnostic value. ST-segment depression limited to the recovery period does not generally represent a "false-positive" response. Inclusion of analysis during this time period increases the diagnostic yield of the exercise test. Other criteria including down-sloping ST changes in recovery and prolongation of depression can improve test performance.

Computerized ST measurements should be used cautiously and require physician over-reading. Errors can be made both in the choice of isoelectric line and the beginning of the ST segment. Filtering and averaging can cause false ST depression due to distortion of the raw data.

SILENT ISCHEMIA

There is minimal evidence in the literature for exaggerated concern with silent ischemia. Patients with silent ischemia (painless ST-depression) usually have milder forms of coronary disease and consequently, a better prognosis. The evidence base for silent ischemia being more prevalent in diabetics is not as convincing as one would think given its widespread clinical acceptance. Many physicians feel that treadmill testing should be used for routine screening of diabetics but has yet to be adopted as it is not evidence based.[30]

EXERCISE INDUCED ARRHYTHMIAS

As with resting ventricular arrhythmias, exercise-induced ventricular arrhythmias have an independent association with

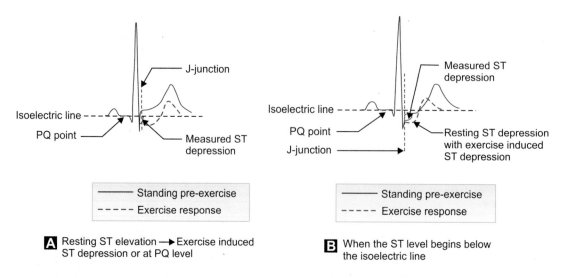

FIGURES 7A AND B: The various patterns of ST-segment shift. The standard criterion for abnormal is 1 mm of horizontal or downsloping ST-segment depression below the PR isoelectric line or 1 mm further depression if there is baseline depression

death in most patients with coronary disease and in asymptomatic individuals.[31] The risk can be more delayed (> 6 years) than that associated with ST-depression. Nonsustained ventricular tachycardia is uncommon during routine clinical treadmill testing but is usually well-tolerated if exhibited. In patients with a history of syncope, sudden death, physical examination with a large heart, murmurs, ECG showing prolonged QT, pre-excitation, Q waves and heart failure, then exercise-testing-induced ventricular arrhythmias are more worrisome. When healthy individuals exhibit premature ventricular contractions (PVCs) during testing, there is no need for immediate concern. However, in patients referred for exercise stress testing, frequent PVCs during recovery have been demonstrated to be associated with increased mortality during follow-up, while PVCs during exercise were related to heart rate increase with exercise.[32,33] Exercise-testing-induced supraventricular arrhythmias are relatively rare compared to ventricular arrhythmias and appear to be benign except for their association with the development of atrial fibrillation in the future.

PROGNOSTIC UTILIZATION OF EXERCISE TESTING

The two principal reasons for estimating prognosis are to:
- Provide accurate answers to patients' questions regarding the probable outcome of their illnesses
- Identify those patients in whom interventions might improve outcome and which measures to take to achieve such benefits.

Exercise capacity is the primary predictor of prognosis in all categories of patients. With each decrease in the MET value achieved there is a 10–20% increase in overall mortality.[34] Exercise capacity interacts with age such that even after accounting for age and gender, exercise capacity is a weaker predictor of death in elderly individuals than younger individuals undergoing exercise stress testing.[35] To further validate the continued use of exercise testing, a recent meta-analysis of 33 studies with over 100,000 healthy subjects undergoing exercise stress testing demonstrated the prognostic importance of exercise capacity and value in predicting the presence of CAD.[36]

Recent studies of prognosis have provided important information focused on endpoints specific to cardiovascular causes, such as death of cardiovascular etiology. In current society, this data is relatively easy to obtain from death certificates, whereas previously investigators had to follow the patients, contact their survivors, or review their medical records. While death certificates have their limitations, in general, they classify those with accidental, gastrointestinal (GI), pulmonary and cancer deaths so that those remaining are most likely to have died of cardiovascular causes. Although all-cause mortality is a more important endpoint for intervention studies, cardiovascular mortality is more appropriate for evaluating a cardiovascular test (i.e. the exercise test).

The mathematical models for determining prognosis are usually more complex than those used for identifying severe angiographic disease. Diagnostic testing can use multivariate discriminant function analysis to determine the probability of severe angiographic disease being present or not. Prognostic

TABLE 7

Prognostic scores: the Duke Treadmill Score and the VA Treadmill Score

Duke score	= METs − 5 × (mm E-I ST depression) − 4 × (TMAP index)
VA score	= 5 × (CHF/Dig) + mm E-I ST depression + change in SBP score − METs

(Abbreviations: CHF: Congestive heart failure; METs: Metabolic equivalents; SBP: Systolic blood pressure; TMAP: Treadmill angina pectoris).
TMAP score: 0 if no angina, 1 if angina occurred during test, 2 if angina was the reason for stopping.
Change in SBP score: from 0 for rise greater than 40 mm Hg to 5 for drop below rest.

testing, however, must use survival analysis, which includes censoring for patients with uneven follow-up due to "lost to follow-up" or other cardiac events [i.e. coronary artery bypass surgery or percutaneous coronary intervention (PCI)] and must account for time-person units of exposure.

There is ample data supporting the use of exercise testing as the first noninvasive step after the history, physical examination and resting ECG in the prognostic evaluation of CAD patients. It accomplishes both of the purposes of prognostic testing to provide information regarding the patient's status and to help make recommendations for optimal management. This assessment should always include calculation of a properly designed score such as the Duke Treadmill Score or the VA Treadmill Score (Table 7).

Recently, we have added to the Duke nomogram to improve its prognostic value (Fig. 8).[37,38]

Recent studies have considered other exercise test responses including heart rate recovery[39] and ectopy[40] and found both to have independent prognostic power in patients with heart failure. These exercise test responses have not yet been combined or compared to expired gas analysis results and could improve risk stratification. Interestingly, heart rate recovery has been shown to improve following exercise training in patients with heart failure.[41,42]

In summary, VO_{2max} or other related measures should not be used as the only prognostic markers in heart failure. The combination of cardiopulmonary exercise data and other clinical and hemodynamic responses in multivariate scores has been shown to more powerfully stratify risk.

SCREENING

Screening for asymptomatic CAD has become a topic of increased interest as some recent data suggest efficacy of the statins in reducing the risk of cardiac events even in asymptomatic individuals. Global risk factor equations, such as the Framingham score, should be the first step in screening asymptomatic individuals for preclinical coronary. These are available as nomograms that can easily applied by health care professionals, or be calculated as part of a computerized patient record. Several additional testing procedures that have promise for screening include the simple ankle-brachial index (particularly in the elderly), C-reactive protein and other emerging biomarkers, carotid ultrasound measurements of intimal medial

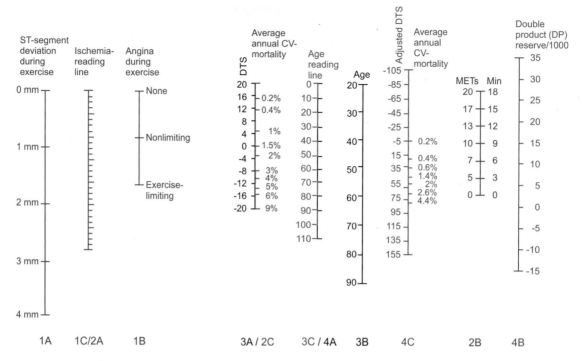

FIGURE 8: Age and double product (DP) adjusted Duke Treadmill Score (DTS) nomogram. Determination of average annual CV mortality adjusted for age and DP reserve proceeds as follows: at first, DTS will be obtained as described before; briefly, the marks for the observed amount of exercise-induced ST-segment deviation (1A) and degree of angina (1B) on their respective lines are connected with a straight edge. The point where this line intersects the ischemia-reading line (1C) is noted. Then, the mark for ischemia (2A) is connected with that for exercise duration in minutes or the equivalent in METs (2B). The point at which this line intersects the DTS line indicates the amount of DTS and the average annual CV mortality (2C). Subsequently, the point at which the drawing line from the marks for DTS (3A) to the corresponding value for age (3B) intersects age—DTS line indicates average annual CV mortality adjusted for age (3C). Finally, the point where the modified DTS line intersects the line drawn from the age—DTS line (4A) to the corresponding value for DP reserve/1,000 (4B) indicates average annual CV mortality adjusted for age and DP reserve (4C) (*Source:* Modified from Sadrzadeh Rafie AH, et al. Age and double product (SBP x heart rate) reserve-adjusted modification of the Duke Treadmill Score nomogram in men. Am J Cardiol. 2008;102:1407-12

thickness, and the resting ECG (particularly spatial QRS-T wave angle). Despite the promotional concept of atherosclerotic burden, electron-beam computed tomography (EBCT) has not been shown to have test characteristics superior to the standard exercise test.

Screening tests are controversial because they often generate a high rate of false positives, which can lead to unnecessary follow-up procedures and unquantifiable negative consequences like emotional repercussions. Ultimately, the overall cost-benefit to society is unclear.

This is further highlighted by the uncertainty of what to do with the information obtained from the screening test. In other words, it is unclear whether asymptomatic patients with silent ischemia detected on exercise treadmill testing have improved outcomes with revascularization compared with medical therapy. Given the findings of the Clinical Outcomes Utilizing Revascularization and Aggressive Drug Evaluation (COURAGE) trial in which patients with stable angina had similar major adverse cardiovascular events with either medical therapy or revascularization,[43] it seems unlikely that patients with silent ischemia demonstrated during exercise testing would benefit from revascularization unless they have left main or three-vessel CAD. However, the Asymptomatic Cardiac Ischemia Pilot (ACIP) study demonstrated that patients randomized to revascularization had significantly lower major adverse cardiovascular events at 2-year follow-up compared with those

randomized to antianginal therapy.[44] Therefore, given these seemingly contradictory reports and the lack of clarity involving the data, it seems reasonable that patients with CAD risk factors should simply be initiated on aspirin, statin therapy and other medications with proven cardioprotective benefits rather than proceeding with CAD screening tests unless the findings will truly change management.

Several well-designed follow-up studies have improved our understanding of the application of exercise testing as a screening tool. The predictive value of the abnormal maximal exercise electrocardiogram ranges 5–46%. The first prospective studies of exercise testing in asymptomatic individuals included angina as a cardiac disease end point. As this is a soft or subjective endpoint, there was a bias for individuals with abnormal tests to subsequently report angina or to be diagnosed as having angina resulting in a high predictive value being reported for the test. When only hard end points (death or MI) were used, the results were less encouraging. The test could only identify one-third of the patients with hard events, and only 5% of the abnormal responders developed coronary heart disease over the follow-up period. Therefore, greater than 90% of the abnormal responders were false positives. Overall, the exercise test's characteristics as a screening test probably lie in between the results of studies using hard or soft endpoints because some of the subjects who develop chest pain really have angina and coronary disease. The sensitivity is probably between

30% and 50% (at a specificity of 90%), but the critical limitation is the predictive value (and risk ratio), which depends on the prevalence of disease (which is low in the asymptomatic population).

The iatrogenic problems resulting from screening (i.e. morbidity from subsequent procedures, employment and insurance issues) would make using a test with a high false-positive rate unreasonable. The recent US Preventive Services Task Force statement states that "false positive tests are common among asymptomatic adults, especially women, and can lead to unnecessary diagnostic testing, over treatment and labeling" (www.preventiveservices.ahrq.gov or www. guideline.gov).[45] In the majority of asymptomatic people, screening with any test or test add-on is more likely to yield false positives than true positives. This is the mathematical reality associated with all of the available tests.

If the exercise treadmill test is to be used to screen, it should be done in groups with a higher estimated prevalence of disease using the Framingham score or another predictive model. Additionally, a positive test result should not immediately lead to invasive testing. In most circumstances an add-on imaging modality (echo or nuclear) should be the first choice in evaluating asymptomatic individuals with an abnormal exercise test. The Detection of Ischemia in Asymptomatic Diabetics (DIAD) study highlights the challenges of screening an asymptomatic population.[30] The study randomized 1,123 subjects with type 2 diabetes mellitus and no symptoms of CAD to either undergo adenosine-stress radionuclide myocardial perfusion imaging or no screening. During the mean follow-up of 4.8 years, there was no difference in cardiovascular death or non-fatal MI between the two groups (2.7% vs 3%, p = 0.73). Interestingly, the primary medical prevention appropriately increased equally in both groups, suggesting that the results of screening did little to change medical management. While pharmacologic stress imaging has obvious differences from ECG exercise testing, this study highlights the potential pitfalls of screening asymptomatic patients, and how careful physician discretion should be applied to only screen asymptomatic high-risk patients such as sedentary diabetics with other risk factors prior to engaging in an exercise program (class IIa recommendation[9]).

Three recent studies lead to the logical conclusion that exercise testing should be part of the preventive health recommendations for screening healthy, asymptomatic individuals along with risk-factor assessment. The data from Norway (2,000 men, 26-year follow-up),[46] the Cooper Clinic (26,000 men, 8-year follow-up),[47] and Framingham (3,000 men, 18-year follow-up)[48] provide additional risk classification power and demonstrate incremental risk ratios for the synergistic combination of the standard exercise test and risk factors.

There are several other reasons why the exercise test should be promoted for screening. Most tests currently being promoted for screening do not have the documented favorable test characteristics of the exercise test. In addition, physical inactivity has reached epidemic proportions and what better way to make our patients conscious of their deconditioning than having them do an exercise test that can also "clear them" for exercise? Including the exercise test in the screening process sends a strong message to our patients that we consider their exercise status as important. Each 1 MET increase in exercise capacity equates with to a 10–25% improvement in survival in all populations studied[49] as well a 5% decline in health care costs.[50]

If screening could be performed in a logical way with test results helping to make decisions regarding therapies rather than leading to invasive interventions, insurance or occupational problems, then the recent results summarized above should be applied to preventive medicine policy. There may still be enough evidence, however, to consider recommending a routine exercise test every five years for men older than 40 and women older than 50 years of age, especially if one of the potential benefits is the adoption of an active lifestyle.[51]

CONCLUSION

The exercise test complements the medical history and the physical examination, and it remains the second most commonly performed cardiologic procedure next to the routine ECG. The addition of echocardiography or myocardial perfusion imaging does not negate the importance of the ECG or clinical and hemodynamic responses to exercise. The renewed efforts to control costs undoubtedly will support the role of the exercise test. Convincing evidence that treadmill scores enhance the diagnostic and prognostic power of the exercise test certainly has cost-efficacy implications.

Use of proper methodology is paramount for safety and obtaining accurate and comparable results. The use of specific criteria for exclusion and termination, interaction with the subject and appropriate emergency equipment is essential.

Table 8 lists important rules to follow for getting the most information from the standard exercise test.

TABLE 8

Exercise testing rules to maximize information obtained

- The exercise protocol should be progressive, with even increments in speed and grade whenever possible.
- The treadmill protocol should be adjusted to the patient, and one protocol is not appropriate for all patients; consider using a manual or automated ramp protocol.
- Report exercise capacity in METs, not minutes of exercise.
- Hyperventilation prior to testing is not indicated.
- ST-segment measurements should be made at ST0 (J-junction), and ST-segment depression should be considered abnormal only if horizontal or downsloping.
- Raw ECG waveforms should be considered first and then supplemented by computer-enhanced (filtered and averaged) waveforms when the raw data are acceptable.
- In testing for diagnostic purposes, patients should be placed supine as soon as possible after exercise, with a cool-down walk avoided.
- The 3-minutes recovery period is critical to include in analysis of the ST-segment response.
- Measurement of SBP during exercise is extremely important and exertional hypotension is ominous; manual blood pressure measurement techniques are preferred.
- Age-predicted heart rate targets are largely useless due to the wide scatter for any age; exercise tests should be symptom limited.
- A treadmill score should be calculated for every patient; use of multiple scores or a computerized consensus score should be considered as part of the treadmill report.

(Abbreviaition: METs: Metabolic equivalents).

The ACC/AHA guidelines for exercise testing clearly indicate the correct uses of exercise testing. Since the last guidelines, exercise testing has been extended as the first diagnostic test in women and in individuals with right bundle-branch block and resting ST-segment depression. The use of diagnostic scores and prognostic scores, such as the Duke Treadmill Score, increases the value of the exercise test. In fact, the use of scores results in test characteristics that approach the nuclear and echocardiographic add-ons to the exercise test.

MODIFIED SUMMARY OF GUIDELINES
AAA/AHA 2002 Guideline Update for Exercise Testing: Summary Article: A Report of the American College of Cardiology/American Heart Association Task Force on Practice Guidelines (Committee to Update the 1997 Exercise Testing Guidelines) Circulation 2002;106:1883-92

Modified by Kanu Chatterjee

Class I: Conditions for which there is evidence and/or general agreement that a given procedure/therapy is useful and effective

Class II: Conditions for which there is conflicting evidence and/or a divergence of opinion about the usefulness/efficacy of performing the procedure/therapy

Class IIa: Weight of evidence/opinion is in favor of usefulness/efficacy

Class IIb: Usefulness/efficacy is less well established by evidence/opinion

Class III: Conditions for which there is evidence and/or general agreement that a procedure/therapy is not useful/effective and in some cases may be harmful

Level A (highest): Derived from multiple randomized clinical trials

Level B (intermediate): Data are on the basis of a limited number of randomized trials, nonrandomized studies or observational registries

Level C (lowest): Primary basis for the recommendation was expert opinion

Exercise Testing Guideline Recommendation

Class I:

1. Patients undergoing initial evaluation with suspected or known CAD including patients with complete right bundle branch block or less that 1 mm ST depression (Level of Evidence B)
2. Patients with known or suspected CAD previously evaluated presenting with new or changing symptoms (Level of Evidence B)
3. Low-risk unstable angina patients (Level of Evidence B)
4. Intermediate-risk unstable angina patients 2-3 days after presentation and without evidence active ischemia or heart failure (Level of Evidence B)

Class IIa: Intermediate-risk unstable angina patients with negative cardiac markers and without significant change in ECG (Level of Evidence B)

Class IIb:

1. Patients with ECG abnormalities of pre-excitation, electronically paced ventricular rhythm, 1 mm or more resting ST depression, patients with LBBB or QRS duration of > 120 ms.
2. Patients with a stable clinical course who undergo periodic monitoring to guide treatment (Level of Evidence B)

Class III:

1. Patients with severe comorbidity likely to limit the expectancy and/or candidacy for revascularization
2. High-risk unstable angina patients (Level of Evidence C)

Patients With Acute Coronary Syndrome

Class I:

1. Submaximal exercise at about 4 to 6 days before discharge for assessment of prognosis, activity prescription or for evaluation of medical therapy
2. Symptom limited exercise test about 14 to 21 days after discharge for assessment of prognosis, activity prescription, or evaluation medical therapy if predischarge exercise test has not been done.
3. Symptom limited exercise test at 3 to 6 weeks after discharge to assess prognosis, activity prescription or evaluation of medical therapy if early exercise test was submaximal

Class IIa: After discharge for activity counseling and/or exercise training as part of cardiac rehabilitation in patients who have undergone reavascularization

Class IIb:
1. In patients with ECG abnormalities of LBBB, pre-excitation syndrome, left ventricular hypertrophy, digoxin therapy, greater than 1 mm resting ST depression electronically paced ventricular rhythm
2. Periodic monitoring in patients who continue to participate in exercise training or cardiac rehabilitation

Class III:
1. Severe comorbidity likely to limit life expectancy and/or candidacy for revascularization.
2. To evaluate patients with acute myocardial infarction with uncompensated heart failure, cardiac arrythmia or noncardiac conditions that limit the ability to exercise (Level of Evidence C)
3. Predischarge exercise test in patients who had already cardiac catheterization (Level of Evidence C)

Asymptomatic Diabetic Patients

Class IIa: Evaluation of asymptomatic patients with diabetes who plan to do vigorous exercise
(Level of Evidence C)

Class IIb:
1. Evaluation of patients with multiple risk factors as guide to risk-reduction therapy
2. Evaluation of asymptomatic men older than 45 years or women older than 55 years who plan to do vigorous exercise or who are involved in an occupation in which exercise impairment may impact public safety or who are at high risk for CAD

Class III: Routine screening of asymptomatic men or women.

Patients with Valvular Heart Disease

Class I: In patients with chronic aortic regurgitation for assessment of symptoms and functional capacity in whom it is difficult assess symptoms

Class IIa:
1. In patients with chronic aortic regurgitation for evaluation of symptoms and functional capacity before participation in athletic activity
2. In patients with chronic aortic regurgitation for assessment of prognosis before aortic valve replacement in asymptomatic or minimally symptomatic patients with left ventricular dysfunction

Class IIb: Evaluation of patients with valvular heart disease (see guidelines in valvular heart disease)

Class III: For diagnosis of CAD in patients with moderate to severe valvular heart disease or with LBBB, electronically paced rhythm, pre-excitation syndrome or greater than 1 mm ST depression in the rest ECG.

Patients with Rhythm Disorders

Class I:
1. For identification of appropriate settings in patients with rate-adaptive pacemakers
2. For evaluation of congenital complete heart block in patients considering increased physical activity or participation in competitive sports (Level of Evidence C)

Class IIa:
1. Evaluation of patients with known or suspected exercise-induced arrhythmias
2. Evaluation medical, surgical or ablation therapy in patients with exercise-induced arrhythmias (including atrial fibrillation)

Class IIb:
1. Investigation of isolated ventricular ectopic beats in middle aged patients without other evidence of CAD
2. For investigation of prolonged first degree atrioventricular block or type I second degree Wenckebach, left bundle-branch block, right bundle-branch block or isolated ectopic beats in young persons considering participation in competitive sports (Level of Evidence C).

Class III: Routine investigations of isolated ectopic beats in young patients.

1. COCATS Guidelines. Guidelines for Training in Adult Cardiovascular Medicine, Core Cardiology Training Symposium. June 27-28, 1994. American College of Cardiology. J Am Coll Cardiol. 1995;25:1-34.

2. Schlant RC, Friesinger GC 2nd, Leonard JJ. Clinical competence in exercise testing. A statement for physicians from the ACP/ACC/AHA Task Force on Clinical Privileges in Cardiology. J Am Coll Cardiol. 1990;16:1061-5.

3. Bigi R, Cortigiani L, Desideri A. Exercise electrocardiography after acute coronary syndromes: still the first testing modality? Clin Cardiol. 2003;26:390-5.

4. Karha J, et al. Safety of stress testing during the evolution of unstable angina pectoris or non-ST-elevation myocardial infarction. Am J Cardiol. 2004;94:1537-9.

5. Jeetley P, et al. Clinical and economic impact of stress echocardiography compared with exercise electrocardiography in patients with suspected acute coronary syndrome but negative troponin: a prospective randomized controlled study. Eur Heart J. 2007;28:204-11.

6. Pina IL, et al. Exercise and heart failure: a statement from the American Heart Association Committee on exercise, rehabilitation, and prevention. Circulation. 2003;107:1210-25.

7. Froelicher VF, et al. Application of meta-analysis using an electronic spread sheet to exercise testing in patients after myocardial infarction. Am J Med. 1987;83:1045-54.

8. Shaw LJ, et al. A metaanalysis of predischarge risk stratification after acute myocardial infarction with stress electrocardiographic, myocardial perfusion, and ventricular function imaging. Am J Cardiol. 1996;78:1327-37.

9. Gibbons RJ, et al. ACC/AHA 2002 guideline update for exercise testing: summary article: a report of the American College of Cardiology/American Heart Association Task Force on Practice Guidelines (Committee to Update the 1997 Exercise Testing Guidelines). Circulation. 2002;106:1883-92.

10. Fletcher GF, et al. Exercise standards for testing and training: a statement for healthcare professionals from the American Heart Association. Circulation. 2001;104:1694-740.

11. Berman JL, Wynne J, Cohn PF. A multivariate approach for interpreting treadmill exercise tests in coronary artery disease. Circulation. 1978;58:505-12.

12. Villella M, et al. Prognostic significance of double product and inadequate double product response to maximal symptom-limited exercise stress testing after myocardial infarction in 6296 patients treated with thrombolytic agents. GISSI-2 Investigators. Grupo Italiano per lo Studio della Sopravvivenza nell-Infarto Miocardico. Am Heart J. 1999;137:443-52.

13. Sadrzadeh Rafie AH, et al. Prognostic value of double product reserve. Eur J Cardiovasc Prev Rehabil. 2008;15:541-7.

14. American College of Sports Medicine. Guidelines for Exercise Testing and Prescription, 6th edition. Baltimore: Lippincott, Williams and Wilkins; 2000.

15. Leeper NJ, et al. Prognostic value of heart rate increase at onset of exercise testing. Circulation. 2007;115:468-74.

16. Nishime EO, et al. Heart rate recovery and treadmill exercise score as predictors of mortality in patients referred for exercise ECG. JAMA. 2000;284:1392-8.

17. Shetler K, et al. Heart rate recovery: validation and methodologic issues. J Am Coll Cardiol. 2001;38:1980-7.

18. Imai K, et al. Vagally mediated heart rate recovery after exercise is accelerated in athletes but blunted in patients with chronic heart failure. J Am Coll Cardiol. 1994;24:1529-35.

19. Bourque JM, et al. Achieving an exercise workload of e" 10 metabolic equivalents predicts a very low risk of inducible ischemia: does myocardial perfusion imaging have a role? J Am Coll Cardiol. 2009;54:538-45.

20. Le VV, et al. The blood pressure response to dynamic exercise testing: a systematic review. Prog Cardiovasc Dis. 2008;51:135-60.

21. Gutman RA, et al. Delay of ST depression after maximal exercise by walking for 2 minutes. Circulation. 1970;42:229-33.

22. Savage MP, et al. Usefulness of ST-segment depression as a sign of coronary artery disease when confined to the postexercise recovery period. Am J Cardiol. 1987;60:1405-6.

23. Froelicher VF, et al. Value of exercise testing for screening asymptomatic men for latent coronary artery disease. Prog Cardiovasc Dis. 1976;18:265-76.

24. Gauri AJ, et al. Effects of chronotropic incompetence and beta-blocker use on the exercise treadmill test in men. Am Heart J. 2001;142:136-41.

25. Raxwal V, et al. Simple treadmill score to diagnose coronary disease. Chest. 2001;119:1933-40.

26. Morise AP, Lauer MS, Froelicher VF. Development and validation of a simple exercise test score for use in women with symptoms of suspected coronary artery disease. Am Heart J. 2002;144:818-25.

27. Lipinski M, et al. Comparison of exercise test scores and physician estimation in determining disease probability. Arch Intern Med. 2001;161:2239-44.

28. Viik J, et al. Correct utilization of exercise electrocardiographic leads in differentiation of men with coronary artery disease from patients with a low likelihood of coronary artery disease using peak exercise ST-segment depression. Am J Cardiol. 1998;81:964-9.

29. Miranda CP, et al. Usefulness of exercise-induced ST-segment depression in the inferior leads during exercise testing as a marker for coronary artery disease. Am J Cardiol. 1992;69:303-7.

30. Young LH, et al. Cardiac outcomes after screening for asymptomatic coronary artery disease in patients with type 2 diabetes: the DIAD study: a randomized controlled trial. JAMA. 2009;301:1547-55.

31. Beckerman J, et al. Exercise test-induced arrhythmias. Prog Cardiovasc Dis. 2005;47:285-305.

32. Frolkis JP, et al. Frequent ventricular ectopy after exercise as a predictor of death. N Engl J Med. 2003;348:781-90.

33. Dewey FE, et al. Ventricular arrhythmias during clinical treadmill testing and prognosis. Arch Intern Med. 2008;168:225-34.

34. Myers J, et al. Exercise capacity and mortality among men referred for exercise testing. N Engl J Med. 2002;346:793-801.

35. Kim ES, et al. External prognostic validations and comparisons of age- and gender-adjusted exercise capacity predictions. J Am Coll Cardiol. 2007;50:1867-75.

36. Kodama S, et al. Cardiorespiratory fitness as a quantitative predictor of all-cause mortality and cardiovascular events in healthy men and women: a meta-analysis. JAMA. 2009;301:2024-35.

37. Sadrzadeh Rafie AH, et al. Age and double product (systolic blood pressure x heart rate) reserve-adjusted modification of the Duke Treadmill Score nomogram in men. Am J Cardiol. 2008;102:1407-12.

38. Rafie AH, et al. Age-adjusted modification of the Duke Treadmill Score nomogram. Am Heart J. 2008;155:1033-8.

39. Lipinski MJ, et al. The importance of heart rate recovery in patients with heart failure or left ventricular systolic dysfunction. J Card Fail. 2005;11:624-30.

40. O'Neill JO, et al. Severe frequent ventricular ectopy after exercise as a predictor of death in patients with heart failure. J Am Coll Cardiol. 2004;44:820-6.

41. Streuber SD, Amsterdam EA, Stebbins CL. Heart rate recovery in heart failure patients after a 12-week cardiac rehabilitation program. Am J Cardiol. 2006;97:694-8.

42. Myers J, et al. Effects of exercise training on heart rate recovery in patients with chronic heart failure. Am Heart J. 2007;153:1056-63.

43. Boden WE, et al. Optimal medical therapy with or without PCI for stable coronary disease. N Engl J Med. 2007;356:1503-16.

44. Davies RF, et al. Asymptomatic Cardiac Ischemia Pilot (ACIP) study two-year follow-up: outcomes of patients randomized to initial

SECTION 3

Diagnosis

strategies of medical therapy versus revascularization. Circulation. 1997;95:2037-43.

45. Screening for coronary heart disease: recommendation statement. Ann Intern Med. 2004;140:569-72.

46. Erikssen G, et al. Exercise testing of healthy men in a new perspective: from diagnosis to prognosis. Eur Heart J. 2004;25:978-86.

47. Gibbons LW, et al. Maximal exercise test as a predictor of risk for mortality from coronary heart disease in asymptomatic men. Am J Cardiol. 2000;86:53-8.

48. Balady GJ, et al. Usefulness of exercise testing in the prediction of coronary disease risk among asymptomatic persons as a function of the Framingham risk score. Circulation. 2004;110: 1920-5.

49. Myers J, et al. Fitness versus physical activity patterns in predicting mortality in men. Am J Med. 2004;117:912-8.

50. Weiss JP, et al. Health-care costs and exercise capacity. Chest. 2004;126:608-13.

51. DiPietro L, et al. Improvements in cardiorespiratory fitness attenuate age-related weight gain in healthy men and women: the Aerobics Center Longitudinal Study. Int J Obes Relat Metab Disord. 1998;22:55-62.

CHAPTER 13

ECG Exercise Testing

Chapter 14

The Left Ventricle

Rakesh K Mishra, Nelson B Schiller

Chapter Outline

INTRODUCTION

Echocardiography is the most commonly used clinical diagnostic tool for the evaluation of left ventricular (LV) systolic and diastolic function. In addition to measuring LV ejection fraction (EF), echocardiography provides clinically useful information about various aspects of LV structure and function. For instance, the anatomy of the LV may be altered in several pathologically significant ways and can be accurately measured and expressed by measuring cross-sectional segments of the LV from sets of echocardiographic images. The LV may dilate in diastole and remains so in systole and this enlargement may change both its global shape and regional geometry. There may be hypertrophy of the LV walls in several distinct patterns (some are uniform and some are not), each of which has its own implications. The systolic function of the LV may be normal (or not) while its filling or diastolic function is greatly impaired. Thrombi and tumors may form within the walls or cavity and the interstitium of the myocardium may become glycosylated, infiltrated with fibrous tissue, infused with protein deposits or invaded with tumor cells. Most, if not all, of these processes are recognized by echocardiography, their severity quantified, their rate of progression documented and their recovery appreciated. Finally, impressions of LV function gained by quantitation are verified by observing the beating heart in real time as images are being acquired or at anytime thereafter on archived digital loops. Echocardiography, after all, is the only imaging modality that permits continuous acquisition and visualization of highly resolved real time images.

SYSTOLIC FUNCTION

The reliable, precise, cost effective and expeditious characterization of regional and global systolic LV function is best accomplished by echocardiography. Quantitative expressions of global LV function may be obtained directly by calculation of left ventricular ejection fraction (LVEF) from its components, end systolic volume (ESV) and end diastolic volume (EDV), by determination of rate of pressure rise in the left ventricle from spectral Doppler flow signals, by low velocity tissue Doppler signals from annular and myocardial motion and by determination of global strain and strain rate using either tissue Doppler or speckle tracking. An initial impression of LV systolic function may be accomplished by visual evaluation of LV contraction. The standard views from the apical and parasternal windows are sufficient for this purpose. One usually starts with parasternal long and short axis views of the LV. From the apical window, the LV should be examined in standard 4-chamber, 2-chamber and long axis views. The LV may also be evaluated from the subcostal window in both short and long axis views.

LEFT VENTRICULAR EJECTION FRACTION

The most commonly applied measure of the global LV systolic function in the clinical setting is the EF of the left ventricle (LVEF), or the fraction of the LV diastolic volume ejected with each contraction. It is determined as:

$$LVEF = (EDV - ESV)/EDV \times 100\%$$

where EDV is end diastolic volume and ESV is end systolic volume.

However, because EF is highly sensitive to loading conditions and varies widely, it is a rough estimate of myocardial contractile state. Moreover, despite its clinical importance, and despite recommendations from the American Society of Echocardiography (ASE) of 20 years' standing[1,2] to the opposite, EF is still frequently estimated visually from real time two-dimensional (2D) images and not *measured* quantitatively.

There are a number of reasons for the universality of LVEF: it expresses the complex motion of a three-dimensional (3D) structure with a simple number; it is easy to measure or estimate; it is interchangeable when determined by different methods; it parallels LV contractility; its prognostic significance and clinical utility for treatment stratification are considered established.

These advantages notwithstanding, EF has significant limitations, and these should be considered in each clinical setting. Besides LV contractility, LVEF, as with most other indices, depends on the loading conditions under which the ventricle operates. These conditions include the *preload* (filling pressure and EDV) and *afterload or wall stress* (blood pressure, chamber volume, wall mass and aortic valve resistance). For example, in valvular insufficiency, the EDV or preload of the left ventricle may increase; as a result, LVEF may appear depressed despite normal LV contractility. Conversely, in mitral regurgitation, the low resistance pathway offered by back flow into the low pressure left atrium may mask diminished contractility by augmenting EF. In hypertrophy, wall stress (the ultimate expression of afterload) is reduced and a normal value may mask an inherent deficiency in contractility. The nature of indices of contractility necessitates consideration of other data to characterize LV function. For example, ESV is frequently used as an index of LV contractility that is *relatively* load independent. Finally, small changes in EDV (either through measurement variability or minimal preload fluctuations) may raise or lower EF without there having been any clinically meaningful change in systolic function.

The universal practice of "eyeball" estimation of EF and the few studies that support its accuracy among experienced observers notwithstanding, other studies and our own cumulative experience[3] show they are inferior to calculated LVEF; we recommend *routine* quantitation unreservedly. This recommendation has been reinforced by improvements in imaging that have resulted from engineering improvements such as harmonic imaging, contrast-enhanced border detection and improved electronic focusing and beam formation. It is expected that with refinements in the emerging technique of 3D imaging, the accuracy of the component measurements of EF will improve to the point where they will be automated.

We therefore recommend calculation of LV volumes in all patients both for their own inherent value and as the sole means

of calculating EF. There are several reasons for this recommendation:

- When performed properly from technically adequate images, quantitatively acquired volume and EF are more accurate than the visual estimation and the gap in accuracy continues to widen with improvement of imaging techniques.
- Quantitation provides additional valuable informations—LV volume and mass—which are superior in outcome prediction to linear dimensions.[4,5]
- Continuous feedback to the echocardiographer allows maintenance of skill in visual estimation of LV global function; the ability of the physician to perform accurate visual estimation further increases the reliability of calculations, allowing the reader to identify those studies, in which calculations were performed poorly, and repeat or correct those measurements. In the final analysis, visual estimation, however skillful the observer, is less reliable than quantification by a skilled sonographer.[3]

There are multiple methods for the calculation of LV volumes from the 2D echocardiographic images. Most of these formulae are based on certain geometric assumptions regarding the shape of the LV. Consequently, these formulae are less reliable when the shape of LV is distorted. The authors have not discussed most of these methods.

The method of disk summation, or modified Simpson's rule, is the only biplane algorithm without geometric assumptions and is the standard method for LV volume calculations.[1,2] In this method, the left ventricle is modeled as stacked disks or coins (usually 20), and the volume of each disk is calculated from its orthogonal diameters. The sum of the volumes of each of these disks represents chamber volume. Once the endocardial border is traced or planimetered manually in two orthogonal imaging planes of equal length (usually, the apical 2- and 4-chamber views), software bundled with contemporary echocardiography instruments automatically performs these calculations. These measurements are from tracings obtained at end diastole and end systole.

Figure 1 demonstrates two orthogonal views of the LV for volume calculations by the method of disk summation. The endocardial border should be traced covering the inner contour; papillary muscles are excluded from measurements. Care must be taken to avoid mistaking trabeculations for the endocardium along the lateral free wall, especially in the apical half of the ventricle. Trabeculations mimic the endocardial border when sonographers foreshorten the image to improve resolution of the lateral wall. A clue that this error has been committed is observing that the myocardial tracing creates an inner apical border where the underlying myocardium appears to be thicker than the base rather than its usual thinner dimension. Proper imaging and tracing of the lateral endocardium is best learned by using left sided contrast to improve endocardial border detection. Normal values of the end diastolic volume and index of the left ventricle are provided in the Table 1.

Accurate measurements of the LV volumes require that:

- Imaging plane transects the true apex of the left ventricle. 3D echocardiography facilitates avoidance of foreshortening the left ventricle; however, with 2D echocardiography this mistake can be avoided by maximizing the image of the cavity and by using pulmonary crossing left sided

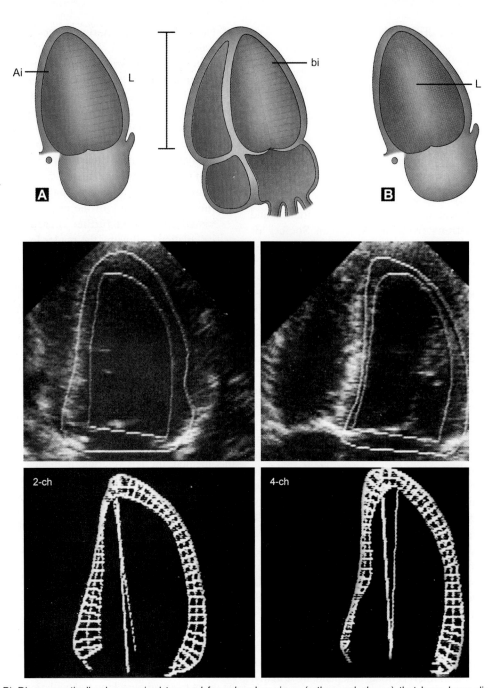

FIGURE 1: (A and B) Diagrammatically shows paired two and four chamber views (orthogonal planes) that have been divided into slices for analysis by the biplane method of discs. A single plane view (two chamber view on B) is a usable but less accurate alternative to biplane volume analysis.

Computer processing of the left ventricular images. (Above) Superimposition of systolic and diastolic left ventricular contours in 2- and 4-chamber views. (Below) Diastolic and systolic contours are combined for quantitative analysis of regional left ventricular function. In this case, the center of the left ventricle, rather than the long axis, was combined for systolic and diastolic images. Automatic methods for evaluation of regional left ventricular function should be used with caution, as their reliability has not been sufficiently documented. In the example above, the left ventricular mass has been calculated using the formula for truncated ellipsoid, and left ventricular ejection fraction was calculated both by the method of disk summation and by the area-length formula in each of the views. Left ventricular mass turned out to be elevated at 220 gm. Values for left ventricular ejection fraction were markedly different for different views (61% for 2-chamber and 46% for 4-chamber). These differences are explained by the hypokinesis of the interventricular septum. The more exact method of disk summation provides left ventricular ejection fraction of 55%. End diastolic volume of the left ventricle is increased at 147 mL; however, the body surface area is 1.93 m^2, and the end diastolic volume index of the left ventricle (76 mL/m^2) is within normal[9]

contrast in poor images to enhance endocardial borders. To image the apex, the transducer should be initially placed just posterior to the apical impulse location and moved gradually anteriorly until maximized full length images are obtained.

- Record images during suspended respiration.
- Exclude papillary muscles and trabeculations from the tracings.
- Doppler echocardiography adds to the information provided by 2D imaging. Accuracy of Doppler methods in the

TABLE 1

Normal left ventricular end-diastolic volume and index in adults

	End diastolic volume (ml)	End diastolic volume index (ml/m²)
Method of disks in orthogonal planes:		
Males	111 ± 22 (62–170)	55 ± 10 (36–82)
Females	80 ± 12 (55–101)	

Note: Average values and standard deviations are listed. Limits of normal are provided in brackets.

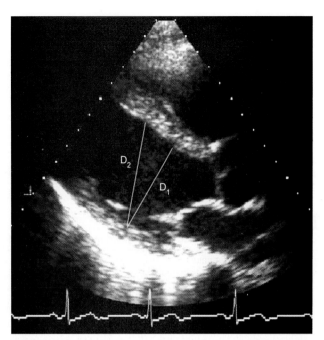

FIGURE 2: Anterior-posterior dimension of the left ventricle is easier to determine from the 2D images, than from the m-mode. M-mode measurements frequently lead to exaggeration of the true size, due to oblique direction of the ultrasound beam that results from either an angulated (sigmoid) septum of a low interspace. End systolic dimension of the left ventricle here by 2D examination (D1) is 46 mm and by unguided m-mode (D2) is 55 mm. The complexity of the "endoarchitecture" of the endocardial surface is another source of error that arises from using discrete loci as line anchors

determination of the stroke volume has been demonstrated, and may be used for quality control of LV volume measurements. In the absence of significant mitral or aortic regurgitation, stroke volume obtained by volume calculations may be compared with the Doppler stroke volume, and in case of significant discrepancy, calculations ought to be repeated.

Linear Measurements in the Assessment of LV Function

Linear dimensions (so-called m-mode) should be performed under 2D guidance, and only if the beam can be directed perpendicular to the transected LV walls and cavity long axis. Linear dimensions are not routinely performed in our laboratory but relegated to a confirmatory role; as discussed above, the authors prefer to use 2D volumetric and Doppler quantitative flow data instead because they have demonstrated superiority in predicting outcomes and because they are interchangeable with MRI and CT derived volume data. The use of linear dimensions may lead to two types of errors: the first is from the incorrect positioning of the ultrasound beam (Fig. 2) that may be corrected by meticulous use of 2D echo guidance. The second is that linear dimensions sample only a limited area near the LV base; assumptions regarding the geometric shape and symmetry of the left ventricle must be made to derive indices of global LV function. In patients with CAD and segmental wall motion abnormalities, these assumptions cannot be made. Consequently, linear measurements are not representative of global function and are thus misleading. Single dimensional derivations of LVEF are only reliable in patients with completely symmetric LV function in a LV having a ratio of its long axis twice that of the short.

Despite our reservations regarding the use of linear dimensions, the authors are mindful of the widespread use of these measurements and provide herein a table with normal linear measurements (Tables 2A and B). Figure 3 demonstrates the nomogram, used for body surface area (BSA) calculations; these are needed for calculation of indexes of both volumetric and linear measurements. Although some laboratories recommend correcting linear and volumetric measurements by height or body mass index (BMI), our research has shown no advantage (or particular disadvantage) of any method over that of correcting measurements by BSA.[6] The authors therefore continue to recommend the universally used BSA correction for normalization of echocardiographic data.

Diameters of the left ventricular outflow tract (LVOT) and of aortic root are also measured more correctly from the 2D images.

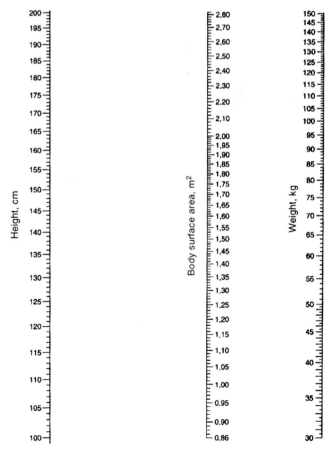

FIGURE 3: Nomogram for determination of the body surface area in adults. A straight line should connect patient's weight and height; its intersection with the middle scale will indicate the body surface area

TABLE 2A

Normal dimensions of left heart in normal adults

• Short axis left ventricle, diastole (end diastolic dimension of the left ventricle)	3.5–6.0 cm (2.3 ± 3.1 cm/m²)
• Short axis left ventricle, systole (end systolic dimension of the left ventricle)	2.1–4.0 cm (1.4 ± 2.1 cm/m²)
• Long axis of the left ventricle, diastole	6.3–10.3 cm (4.1 ± 5.7 cm/m²)
• Long axis of the left ventricle, systole	4.6–8.4 cm
• Thickness of the interventricular septum and posterior wall of left ventricle	0.6–1.1 cm
• Anterior-posterior dimension of the left atrium	2.3–3.5 cm (1.6–2.4 cm/m²)
• Medial-lateral dimension of the left atrium (from apical 4-chamber view)	2.5–4.5 cm (1.6–2.4 cm/m²)
• Superior-inferior dimension of the left atrium (from apical 4-chamber view)	3.4–6.1 cm (2.3–3.5 cm/m²)
Note: The indexes of dimension (normalized to BSA) are provided in brackets.	

TABLE 2B

Normal dimensions of cardiac chambers and major vessels in adults

• Diameter of aortic annulus	1.4–1.6 cm (1.3 ± 0.1 cm/m², up to 1.6 cm/m²)
• Diameter of aortic root (at the aortic cusps)	2.2–3.6 cm (1.7 ± 0.2 cm/m², up to 2.1 cm/m²)
• Diameter of ascending aorta	2.1–3.4 cm (1.5 ± 0.2 cm/m²)
• Diameter of aortic arch	2.0–3.6 cm
• Short axis left ventricle, diastole (end diastolic dimension of the left ventricle)	3.5–6.0 cm (2.3 ± 3.1 cm/m²)
• Short axis left ventricle, systole (end systolic dimension of the left ventricle)	2.1–4.0 cm (1.4 ± 2.1 cm/m²)
• Long axis of the left ventricle, diastole	6.3–10.3 cm (4.1 ± 5.7 cm/m²)
• Long axis of the left ventricle, systole	4.6–8.4 cm
• Thickness of the interventricular septum and posterior wall of left ventricle	0.6–1.1 cm
• Anterior-posterior dimension of the left atrium	2.3–4.5 cm (1.6–2.4 cm/m²)
• Medial-lateral dimension of the left atrium (from apical 4-chamber view)	2.5–4.5 cm (1.6–2.4 cm/m²)
• Superior-inferior dimension of the left atrium (from apical 4-chamber view)	3.4–6.1 cm (2.3–3.5 cm/m²)
• Thickness of the anterior wall of the right ventricle	0.2–0.5 cm (0.2 ± 0.05 cm/m²)
• Anterior-posterior dimension of the outflow tract of the right ventricle	2.2–4.4 cm (1.0–2.8 cm/m²)
• End diastolic dimension of the right ventricle (long axis)	5.5–9.5 cm (3.8–5.3 cm/m²)
• End systolic dimension of the right ventricle (long axis)	4.2–8.1 cm
• Diameter of the annulus of the pulmonary valve	1.0–2.2 cm
• Diameter of the main pulmonary artery	0.9–2.9 cm
• Diameter of the inferior vena cava (at insertion into the right atrium)	1.2–2.3 cm
Note: The indexes of dimension (normalized to BSA) are provided in brackets.	

The derived functional indices from single dimensional measurements include: fractional shortening of the left ventricle, E-point to septal separation (EPSS) and the amplitude of the aortic root motion.

Fractional shortening is a single dimensional analog of LVEF and is the ratio of the difference of the diastolic and systolic short axis diameters of the left ventricle to the diastolic short axis diameter [left ventricular end-diastolic dimension (LVEDD)-left ventricular end-systolic dimension (LVESD)/ LVEDD]. Normal fractional shortening is 30% or more.

E-point to septal separation is the distance between the tip of the anterior mitral leaflet at the time of its widest opening in the early diastole and the most posterior systolic excursion of the interventricular septum. Normally this distance is less than 7 mm.[7] With decreasing global LV contractility, the size of the chamber at end systole and its residual volume increase; concurrently, with decline of the cardiac output, the mitral valve open orifice has to accommodate smaller stroke volume, with resultant decrease of the amplitude of its opening. As LV contractility declines, the EPSS continues to increase. In their current practice, the authors use EPSS to divide patients into those with EFs above or below 45%.

Amplitude of the aortic root motion[8] has mostly qualitative significance. It is roughly proportionate to the stroke volume. Aortic root motion is determined by the filling of the left atrium relative to its smallest volume. Normally, aortic root moves anteriorly in systole by more than 10 mm.

COMPONENTS OF EJECTION FRACTION

End Systolic Volume

Left ventricular end systolic volume indexed (ESVI) to BSA is a simple yet powerful stand-alone marker of ventricular remodeling[9] that can and should be measured routinely in the clinical practice of echocardiography. It is the opinion of the authors that, among all other measures of systolic function, this single parameter is the most informative and load independent. From clinical experience and outcomes research,[10] the authors recommend first considering ESVI when judging systolic function. An example of a common situation where ESVI is particularly helpful include a borderline or low normal EF (i.e. between 50% and 60%); in this setting, only a minimally increased ESVI indicates that systolic function may be reduced to a degree sufficient to adversely influence major outcomes.[4]

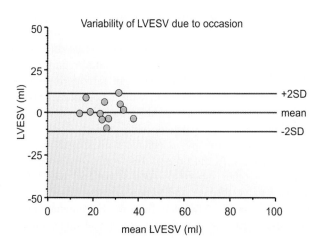

FIGURE 4: Variability of LVESV due to occasion

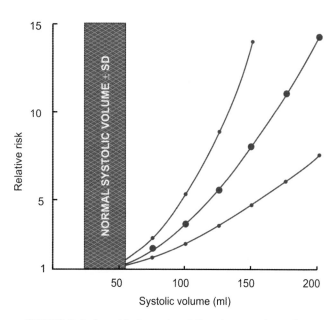

FIGURE 5: Left ventricular end systolic volume as the major determinant of survival after recovery from myocardial infarction[9]

Figure 1 demonstrates manual digitization of the orthogonal apical 2- and 4-chamber views. From these planimetric images, frozen at end diastole and end systole, systolic and diastolic volumes are computed by an algorithm that models the LV cavity as a stack of coins (formally called the method of disks and often incorrectly called modified Simpson's rule). By summation of the volume of each coin in the stack, a close approximation of volume is achieved. This disk summation method is more commonly but incorrectly referred to as Simpson's rule. Although single plane measurements from either 2-chamber or 4-chamber view suffice in some settings, biplane measurements are the method of choice and recommended by the ASE. A technical note for the physician or sonographer about the proper and simplest method for choosing precise frames that represents the largest cavity (end diastole) and the smallest (end systole). The authors have found that the most logical and most reproducible marker of these events is the position of the mitral valve. The digital frame preceding the initial opening motion of the mitral valve identifies end systole while the initial moment of coaptation after the A wave, end diastole. Tantamount to frame selection is the selection of tomographic views that avoid foreshortening and that display at least 75% of the endocardium. Similarly critical, tracing the endocardium and not the epicardium will foster accuracy. Automated tracing (always with manual adjustment of tracking) and 3D volume sets promise to speed the quantitative process—if not automate it and provide stronger reproducibility. ESV is more reproducible than EDV because the endocardium is most visible during this phase of the cardiac cycle.

When properly measured, ESV is the most reproducible volumetric parameter of systolic function. Figure 4 shows a Bland Altman plot of the variability from examining the same hemodynamically stable subject on two occasions. Variability also arises from using different sonographers and different readers. These sources of variability were explored in a study from authors' laboratory.[11,12]

Invasively determined LV end systolic volume has been shown to be an important determinant of survival after myocardial infarction[9] (Fig. 5).

Physiologic Basis of Left Ventricular End Systolic Volume

Physiologically, ESV is a direct window on a key property of the heart, elastance. Elastance is defined as the quality of recoiling without disruption on removal of pressure, or an expression of the measure of the ability to do so in terms of unit of volume change per unit of pressure change and is the reciprocal of compliance. Figure 6 (courtesy of Dr. Sanjiv J. Shah of Northwestern University) shows the location of ESV at the intersection of the lines defining arterial and end systolic elastance at fixed contractility and varying loading conditions.

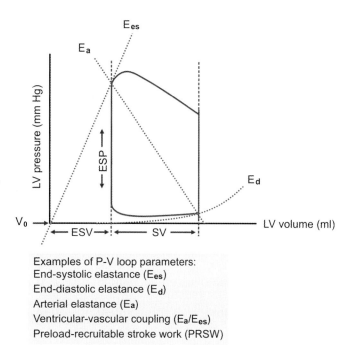

Examples of P-V loop parameters:
End-systolic elastance (E_{es})
End-diastolic elastance (E_d)
Arterial elastance (E_a)
Ventricular-vascular coupling (E_a/E_{es})
Preload-recruitable stroke work (PRSW)

FIGURE 6: Pressure volume loop

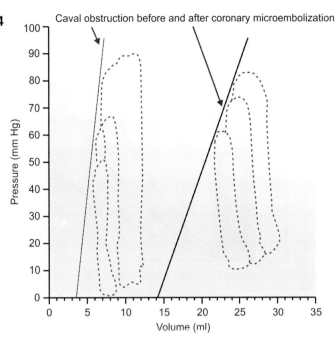

FIGURE 7: Caval obstruction before and after coronary microembolization[13]

In physiologic experiments, embolization of the myocardium increases the ESV and decreases the elastance slope. This effect can be seen when the response of the normal myocardium to changes in loading conditions (degrees of caval obstruction) to that of post-embolic myocardium[13] (Fig. 7).

Left Ventricular End Systolic Volume and Clinical Outcomes

A decrease in ESV with angiotensin converting enzyme inhibitor therapy has been associated with a reduction in cardiac events in patients with moderately decreased LV systolic function. Using LV contrast ventriculography, end systolic volume has been shown to be an important predictor of both postoperative ventricular function and survival after coronary artery bypass grafting in patients with decreased LV function.[9] The aforementioned studies have consistently shown that large increases in ESV predict adverse cardiovascular outcomes in participants with LV systolic dysfunction. In aortic regurgitation, a 10-year outcome study[10] (Mayo) has shown that ESV is a powerful predictor of outcome whereas systolic dimension is not predictive. The degree of elevation in ESVI has also been shown to most closely reflect BNP elevation in mitral regurgitation.[14]

Normal values for ESVI are given in Table 3. It points out that there is disagreement with where the abnormal range begins. Orginally, values as high as 33 mL/m² were considered within normal limits. However, in patients with coronary disease, values higher than 25 mL/m² are associated with sharply increased adverse outcomes. At the time of this writing, the upper range of normal for other subgroups such as patients with varying degrees of valve disease and young athletes have yet to be established. Note that MRI data from the Framingham normal cohort have smaller values for the lower and upper limits of normal than authors' data at UCSF and the ASE recommended value. Authors' outcomes research in coronary disease strongly suggests that at least in older individuals with that condition, the Framingham data is more likely to be correct.

In developing outcome data for ESV, the authors examined the association of ESVI with hospitalization for heart failure (HF) and mortality in a prospective cohort study of ambulatory patients with CHD.[4] The authors divided the study population into quartiles of ESVI and used a Cox proportional-hazards analysis to compare events among quartiles. The authors adjusted for potential confounders, including known cardiovascular risk factors, medication use and echocardiographic variables. Of 989 participants, 110 (11%) were hospitalized for HF during 3.6 ± 1.1 years of follow-up. Among participants in the highest ESVI quartile (> 25 mL/m²), 67 of 248 (27%) developed HF, compared with 8 of 248 (3%) among those in the lowest quartile. The association of ESVI with HF hospitalization persisted after adjustment for potential confounders (HR 4.6, 95% CI 1.3–16.2; p = 0.02). When compared to other echocardiographic measures of LV remodeling using area under ROC curve analysis, ESVI was a superior predictor of hospitalization for HF. In this prospective cohort study of ambulatory patients with CHD, LV ESVI greater than 25 mL/m² was independently associated with a 4.6 fold increased rate of HF hospitalization (Fig. 8). Our findings suggest that even small increases in ESVI independently predict increased HF in patients with CHD.

Figure 9 demonstrates the incremental predictive value of ESV on combined end point of HF or mortality. Here systolic

TABLE 3

Normal values for end systolic volume index for men and women from three sources

	Men				Women			
LVESV/BSA	*Reference range*	*Mild Incr.*	*Moderate Incr.*	*Severe Incr.*	*Reference range*	*Mild Incr.*	*Moderate Incr.*	*Severe Incr.*
ASE 2005	12-30	31-36	37-42	> 42	12-30	31-36	37-42	> 43
F'ham MRI	Mean 15-24 (.9UCB)	24-31*	32-41	> 42	18-31 (.9UCB)	32-45	46-59	> 60
UCSF	Mean 18-32 (.9UCB)	33-47*	47-61	> 61	18-30 (.9UCB)	31-43	44-56	> 57

*mild, moderate, severe defined in increments of +2SD
(*Source:* American Society of Echocardiography 2005[2] recommendations, Framingham normal cohort by MRI[15] and University of California San Francisco (UCSF) published normal values.[16-18] Note that the abnormal range for MRI begins above 24 ml/m² (circled column). Authors' outcome data discussed above is in agreement with a lower estimate of where the abnormal range begins.

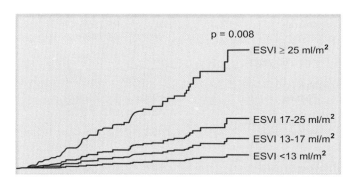

FIGURE 8: Cumulative risk of heart failure by quartile of end systolic volume index

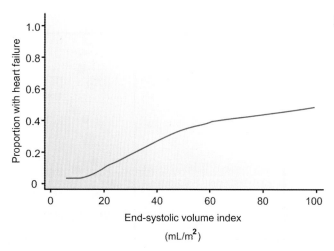

FIGURE 10: Lowess plot of the proportion of patients hospitalized with heart failure during follow-up according to baseline left ventricular end systolic volume index (Lowess = smooth locally-weighted scatterplot)

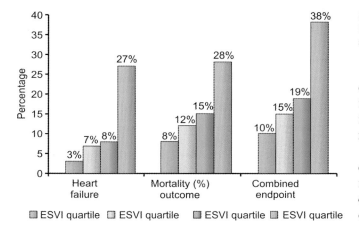

*Combined endpoint = heart failure or mortality

FIGURE 9: Percentage of participants with adverse cardiovascular outcomes by end systolic volume index (EVSI) quartile[4]

disease who develop HF in 5 years of follow-up. Note that even in the upper normal range (as defined by previous series) there is an increased risk of HF that continues to rise throughout the range of values.

Figure 8 shows that the cumulative risk of HF increases even within the normal range and that it rises sharply above 25 mL/m². The finding that ESVs that seemed only minimally elevated carried such strong predictive value for risk supports our contention that ESVI is among the most powerful parameters of outcome in cardiology.

Figure 11 compares the receiver operator curves for predicting CHF hospitalization of single end systolic linear dimension (so-called m-mode) with ESVI. Since the majority of laboratories continue to cling to linear dimensions as their central LV measurements, these data offer compelling reasons for abandoning this practice in favor of volumetric measurements. Hazard ratio plot for risk of hospitalization for heart failure associated with an ESVI greater than or equal to 25 mL/m² in specified subgroups described in Figure 12.

volumes are grouped by quartiles. Note that any increase of ESVI is associated with an increase in adverse outcomes.

Figure 10 is a Lowess plot of the magnitude of ESV and its association with the proportion of patients with stable coronary

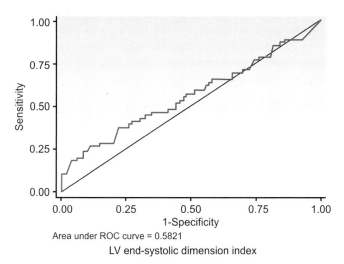

Area under ROC curve = 0.5821

LV end-systolic dimension index

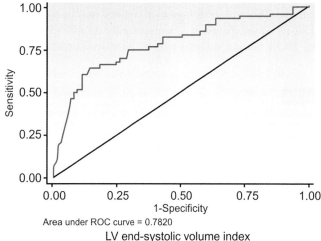

Area under ROC curve = 0.7820

LV end-systolic volume index

FIGURE 11: Receiver-operating characteristic curves for left ventricular end systolic dimension index and end-systolic volume index as predictors of hospitalization for heart failure (p < 0.0001)

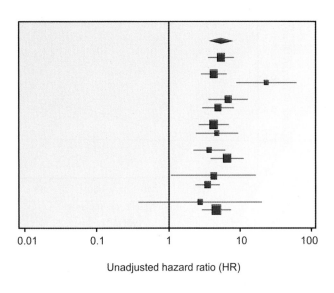

Overall	N	HR (95% CI)
	989	5.6 (3.8-8.2)
Age < 65 years	413	5.7 (2.6-12.3)
Age ≥ 65 years	576	5.4 (3.5-8.4)
Male	804	4.4 (2.9-6.6)
Female	184	23.4 (8.8-62)
No history of MI	452	6.8 (3.6-12.8)
History of MI	530	5.0 (3.0-8.2)
No history of HF	809	4.3 (2.6-7.1)
History of HF	174	4.8 (2.4-9.6)
CrCl < 60 ml/min	227	3.7 (2.2-6.3)
CrCl ≥ 60 ml/min	706	6.6 (3.9-11.3)
NT-proBNP < 173 pg/ml	477	4.3 (1.1-16.8)
Nt-ProBNP ≥ 173 pg/ml	476	3.5 (2.4-5.3)
EF < 50%	112	2.8 (0.4-20.5)
EF ≥ 50%	876	4.6 (2.9-7.4)

FIGURE 12: Hazard ratio plot for risk of hospitalization for heart failure associated with an ESVI ≥ 25 mL/m^2 in specified subgroups

End Diastolic Volume

End diastole is the moment in the cardiac cycle when the left ventricle completes filling and reaches its largest volume. A healthy heart has the property of increasing diastolic volume in response to a spectrum of preloads without altering its elliptical shape and with only small increases in filling pressure. In cardiomyopathic states, the left ventricle remodels so that as volume increases it assumes a more spherical shape and filling pressure rises sharply with small increments in volume. In normality, ESV changes are small so that changes in stroke volume are mainly mediated by increases in EDV. Due to relative preload dependence, EDV changes and degrees of enlargement are less reliable indicators of myocardial contractility. Table 4 presents normal values for end diastolic volume index (EDVI) from three sources: ASE recommended values, Framingham MRI data and UCSF data. In unpublished data, the authors have found that adverse outcomes in an older coronary disease population begin to appear when left ventricle end diastolic volume index (LVEDVI) reaches 64 mL/m^2. Thus values as high as 80 mL/m^2 may be too liberal and based on the inclusion of younger persons with slow heart rates. Older normal subjects tend to have smaller hearts than their younger counterparts and thus dilation may be considered to begin at a small volume.

CONTRAST-ENHANCED ECHOCARDIOGRAPHY

Suboptimal endocardial border definition limits the accurate measurement of LV volumes by echocardiography. In the authors' experience, unenhanced 2D echocardiography underestimates LV volumes by 30–40% and LVEF by 3–6%. In addition, up to 11% of unenhanced scans are deemed uninterpretable for the assessment of LV function. Endocardial border definition is particularly challenging in the setting of obesity, chronic lung disease, ventilator support and chest wall deformities. Contrast echocardiography, by increasing the mismatch between the acoustic impedance of blood and that of myocardium enhances the discrimination between myocardial tissue and the blood pool and improves the accuracy of echocardiography to quantitate LV volumes. These advantages are particularly apparent in large spherical hearts in which the lateral and anterior walls are situated in the portion of the image with the poorest resolution. In the authors' experience, sonographers are likely to foreshorten the image of a spherically dilated ventricle in order to image the lateral wall and confuse

TABLE 4

Normal values for end diastolic volume index from three sources

LVEDV/BSA	Men				Women			
	Reference range	Mild Incr.	Moderate Incr.	Severe Incr.	Reference range	Mild Incr.	Moderate Incr.	Severe Incr.
ASE 2005	35-75	76-86	87-96	> 97	35-75	76-86	87-96	> 97
F'ham MRI	Mean 58-80 (.9UCB)	81-103*	104-126	> 127	50-66 (.9UCB)	67-83	84-100	> 101
UCSF	Mean 58-80 (.9UCB)	81-103*	104-126	> 127	53-66 (.9UCB)	67-80	80-93	> 94
*mild, moderate, severe defined in increments of +2SD								

trabeculations along the lateral wall with the true endocardium. These technical problems may underestimate ventricular volume by as much as 100 cc in the largest hearts imaged without contrast. The LV cavity is effectively opacified by the intravenous administration of engineered microbubbles that consist of a gas contained by an outer shell. Recent studies indicate that contrast-enhanced 2D echocardiography has excellent correlation with radionuclide, magnetic resonance and computed tomographic measurements of LV volumes and LVEF, with improved interobserver agreement and physician interpretation confidence. The 2008 ASE consensus statement recommends the use of contrast agents in difficult-to-image patients with reduced image quality, where greater than or equal to 2 contiguous segments are not seen on unenhanced images and in patients requiring accurate quantification of LVEF regardless of image quality, with the intention of increasing the confidence of the interpreting physician in assessing LV volumes and systolic function.[19,20]

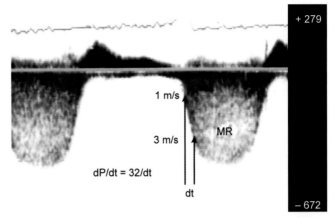

FIGURE 13: Calculation of dP/dt of the left ventricle, CW Doppler of mitral regurgitation (MR). Interval between velocities of mitral regurgitation of 1 and 3 m/sec here is 40 m/sec. Pressure difference is 32 mm Hg: according to Bernoulli equation $dP = 4(V_1^2 - V_2^2) = 4(3^2 - 1^2) = 32$. Thus dP/dt = 32/0.04 = 800 mm Hg/sec (normal > 1300)[23]

OTHER ECHO-DERIVED INDICES OF LV SYSTOLIC FUNCTION

Left ventricular stroke volume is routinely calculated by multiplication of the velocity-time integral (VTI) of the pulsed wave Doppler flow signal from the LVOT, by the cross-sectional area of the LVOT calculated from its radius [Area = pi × (radius)^2]. VTI of forward blood flow is the length of the column of blood in centimeter, passing through the LVOT during systole. Multiplication of this value by the cross-sectional area, through which this column is moving, provides an expression of stroke volume. The product of stroke volume and heart rate is cardiac output in l/min. Since the size of the LVOT is usually a function of BSA,[21,22] in our practice, the authors prefer to use VTI and minute distance (VTI × heart rate) as analogs of stroke volume. Normal VTI from LVOT pulsed wave Doppler is between 18 cm and 23 cm and normal minute distance between10 m/min and 20 m/min.

Another index of global LV systolic function is the velocity of pressure increase in the left ventricle at the initial part of ejection period (dP/dt).[23] Echocardiographic calculation of dP/dt is possible only in the presence of a complete mitral regurgitation continuous wave Doppler envelope during its initial acceleration (Fig. 13). Measurement of the time required for the mitral regurgitant jet to increase its velocity from 1 m/sec to 3 m/sec is obtained. Assuming that the left atrial pressure remains constant, pressure change in the left ventricle between velocities of 1 m/sec and 3 m/sec by modified Bernoulli equation is 32 mm Hg. This value is divided by the time, measured from the acceleration of the mitral regurgitant envelope, to accelerate from 1 m/sec to 3 m/sec to yield dP/dt, which normally is above 1,350 mm Hg/sec.

STRAIN-DERIVED INDICES

In mechanics, strain is the change in the metric properties of a *continuous* body in the displacement from an initial placement to a final placement in response to a *stress* field induced by applied *forces*. In echocardiography parlance, strain is defined as myocardial deformation relative to its baseline dimension

due to a stress.[24,25] The rate of deformation over time is termed strain rate. Both strain and strain rates can be measured using tissue pulsed Doppler and speckle tracking. The former technique uses gated tissue Doppler to compare the myocardial motion of two points, usually 1 cm apart, along a single beam of interrogation; this method is angle dependent. The newer strain measurement technique that uses the gray scale speckle pattern of myocardial images is angle-independent. Strain and strain rate can be used to evaluate both regional and global LV systolic and diastolic function. Moreover, these deformation indices can quantify myocardial function in various planes, including longitudinal, circumferential and radial. These measures may be useful in determining early systolic dysfunction (regional and global) in the setting of normal EF. In a study comparing patients with hypertrophic cardiomyopathy (HCM) and a normal control group, both with normal LVEF, Richand and colleagues found that the patients with HCM had significantly reduced longitudinal, transverse, radial and circumferential strain as assessed by speckle tracking.[26] In another recent study, Ng and colleagues used speckle tracking to demonstrate impaired LV systolic and diastolic longitudinal strain and strain rate in patients with type 2 diabetes mellitus.[27] Interestingly, both circumferential and radial function was preserved in these patients. In addition to the utility of the amplitudes of systolic strain and strain rates, differences in time to peak systolic strain and strain rate among myocardial segments have been used extensively to quantitate electro-mechanical dyssynchrony, a potentially significant predictor of clinical outcomes in HF and response to cardiac resynchronization therapy.[28] In summary, strain and strain rate, especially, as quantified by speckle tracking, are emerging approaches to a more quantifiable understanding of myocardial systolic and diastolic function.

RECOGNIZING THE ETIOLOGY OF CARDIAC DYSFUNCTION

According to the report of the World Health Organization/ International Society and Federation of Cardiology Task Force on the definition and classification of cardiomyopathies,[29] there are five major types of cardiomyopathy (i.e. diseases of the myocardium associated with cardiac dysfunction) that can be appreciated by echocardiography. These conditions can affect either ventricle, but are most often recognized when they involve the left chamber.

1. Dilated cardiomyopathy arising as primary myocardial disease of unknown etiology or as disorders of ischemic, toxic, familial or infective origin.
2. Hypertrophic cardiomyopathy, arising as a primary condition or secondary process to conditions such as aortic stenosis or hypertension.
3. Restrictive or infiltrative cardiomyopathies such as cardiac amyloidosis.
4. Arrhythmogenic right ventricular dysplasia or cardiomyopathy (not discussed here).
5. Unclassified cardiomyopathy including endomyocardial fibroelastosis and ventricular noncompaction.

DILATED CARDIOMYOPATHY

Dilated cardiomyopathy is readily identified by echocardiography when it is fully developed but is more difficult to detect in its early stages. Without clinical history, patient examination and other diagnostic test results, echocardiography alone is often unable to establish the cause of myocardial disease.

ECHOCARDIOGRAPHIC FINDINGS

The most distinctive 2D echocardiographic findings in a dilated cardiomyopathy are LV spherical dilatation, normal or reduced wall thickness, poor systolic wall thickening and/or reduced inward endocardial systolic motion. All of the systolic indices are reduced, including fractional shortening, fractional area change and EF. Four-chamber cardiac enlargement is often present. On m-mode echocardiography, additional features related to systolic dysfunction are increased separation of the mitral leaflet E-point from the septum,[7] poor mitral valve opening, poor aortic valve opening[30] and early closure from a reduced stroke volume, and poor systolic aortic root motion.[8] In patients with dilated cardiomyopathy, the LVEDVI often exceeds 100 mL/m^2 (upper normal is approximately 75 mL/m^2). The EF, derived from the ESV and EDV determinations can, at times, fall below 20%, but is usually between 20% and 40% (normal > 55%). Despite the reduced EF, cardiac output calculations (stroke volume times heart rate) are frequently normal. There are two reasons for this finding. First, patients with cardiomyopathy frequently have elevated heart rates. Second, since the stroke volume is equal to the product of the LVEDV and EF, the effect of a low EF can be counter balanced by an elevation in EDV. As an example, a patient with an EDV of 300 mL, an EF of 30% and a heart rate of 100 beats per minute has a cardiac output of 9 l/min. In patients with ischemic cardiomyopathy who have global dysfunction with segmental evidence of infarction, an ESVI of 45 mL/m^2 identifies patients with a poor outcome.[9]

ISCHEMIC CARDIOMYOPATHY

Ischemic cardiomyopathy is a common cause of HF that can be difficult to differentiate from idiopathic or primary dilated cardiomyopathy. In both ischemic and primary forms, LV wall motion abnormalities and the intensity of scarring can be segmentally variable or heterogeneous. In most patients, ischemic cardiomyopathy is associated with regional remodeling, which is characterized by local segments that have their own radius of curvature. Ischemic cardiomyopathy also tends to have areas of endocardial brightening or scarring that occurs in the areas where infarctions are most common: the inferior base and the apex.

Patients with ischemic cardiomyopathy tend to have calcification of the aortic annulus, aortic valve, sinotubular junction, mitral annulus, papillary muscle and proximal coronaries. They may also have visible plaque in the aortic arch and abdominal aorta.

HYPERTROPHIC CARDIOMYOPATHY

Hypertrophic cardiomyopathy is characterized by increased LV mass, which is quantitated by determining the mean wall thickness and the volume of the cavity. When these findings are present without apparent etiology, it is considered to be a primary HCM that is likely to be genetic in origin. HCM is considered secondary when due to an identifiable disorder such as hypertension or aortic stenosis. The hypertrophy is often asymmetric in primary HCM, and symmetric in secondary disease.

PRIMARY HYPERTROPHIC CARDIOMYOPATHY

Primary HCM characteristically shows asymmetric septal hypertrophy (ASH); the increased wall thickness is localized or most intense in the basal septum. ASH is recognized by a septal to posterior wall ratio of 1.3 to 1; high-risk ASH is recognized by a ratio of 3 to 1. The patterns of distribution of this hypertrophic state are not well understood because they follow an unpredictable pattern. A puzzling aspect of this condition is that the patterns of involvement differ among affected family members.[31] In an unusual variant of ASH, the apex is the site of the most intensive hypertrophy.[32]

In our experience, apical hypertrophy is more difficult to identify by echocardiography because the apical myocardium is more difficult to image. When this condition is suspected (e.g. by finding deeply inverted precordial T waves on ECG), it is helpful to use an echocardiographic contrast agent to confirm the diagnosis.

ECHOCARDIOGRAPHIC FEATURES

The echocardiogram with Doppler is the most reliable means for diagnosing HCM, particularly when the condition is fully developed and outflow tract obstruction accompanies ASH. Since the outflow obstruction portends a poorer prognosis, identifying the presence of obstruction is critical. However, when the obstruction is dynamic, i.e. provocable but mild or absent at rest, the task of the echocardiographic laboratory is more difficult. Use of Doppler techniques, particularly continuous wave, is mandatory. This modality is typically used to measure the systolic flow velocity in the LVOT and mid cavity at rest and during provocative maneuvers (normal 0.9 m/sec). Doppler in this setting will also enable the recognition of dynamic mitral regurgitation that often appears in concert with outflow tract obstruction.

The echocardiographic diagnosis of HCM is based upon the finding of a hypertrophied, nondilated left ventricle and maximal wall thickness greater than or equal to 15 mm that is not associated with systemic hypertension.

Fully developed HCM consists of the following features:

- Asymmetric septal hypertrophy
- Systolic anterior motion (SAM) of the mitral valve
- Crowding of the mitral apparatus by the LVOT
- Partial mid systolic closure or notching of the aortic valve
- Calcification of the mitral annulus frequently accompanies HCM, and, in some patients, this finding is the only clue to the potential for dynamic outflow tract obstruction
- Mitral regurgitation often accompanies obstruction and may be difficult to distinguish from one another
- Left atrial enlargement
- Diastolic dysfunction as manifested to delayed relaxation pattern occurring at an earlier age

SECONDARY HYPERTROPHIC CARDIOMYOPATHY

Secondary left ventricular hypertrophy (LVH) is most commonly encountered as a complication of hypertension or aortic stenosis. The presence of LVH in hypertensive subjects increases the likelihood of cardiovascular morbidity and mortality.

ECHOCARDIOGRAPHIC FEATURES

Echocardiography is the procedure of choice for identifying secondary HCM since the sensitivity of the different ECG criteria may be as low as 7–35% with mild LVH and only 10–50% with moderate to severe disease. Historically, echocardiographic criteria for the diagnosis of LVH were largely based on m-mode echocardiography and included a LV mass index greater than or equal to 134 g/m^2 in men and greater than or equal to 110 g/m^2 BSA in women.

Most of the echocardiographic studies of LVH have relied on m-mode echocardiography. However m-mode echocardiography may not be ideally suited for this task due to a relatively low yield in older patients, suboptimal reproducibility, possible erroneous results in distorted ventricles, and use of a geometric algorithm that tends to overestimate mass. 2D echocardiography increases the precision and produces estimates of LV mass that more closely approximate values derived from pathology, MRI and CT.

The most commonly used 2D methods for measure LV mass are area-length and truncated ellipse. Both methods have been previously validated and endorsed by the ASE.[1,2] The most recent ASE published guidelines for diagnosis of LVH included criteria for mild, moderate and severe LVH for men as 103–116, 117–130 and greater than 130 g/m^2, and for women as 89–100, 101–112 and greater than 112 g/m^2 respectively. Based on our outcome data,[33] the authors consider LV mass index greater than 95 g/m^2 indicative of mass in the abnormal range.

RESTRICTIVE CARDIOMYOPATHY

Restrictive cardiomyopathies are more difficult to diagnose with echocardiography than dilated or hypertrophic cardiomyopathies, and may be challenging to distinguish from constrictive pericarditis. Echocardiography, including Doppler interrogation, is the most effective noninvasive means for the recognition of this group of conditions. Restrictive cardiomyopathy is characterized by a low or normal diastolic volume, normal or only mildly reduced LVEF, atrial enlargement, normal pericardium and abnormal diastolic function. Diastolic dysfunction is frequently restrictive, with an elevated peak mitral inflow velocity, rapid early mitral inflow deceleration and reduced Doppler tissue imaging (DTI) early annular velocity.

DIABETES MELLITUS

Perhaps the most common restrictive cardiomyopathy is the small, stiff heart of diabetes arising from glycosylation of the myocardium, in which diastolic dysfunction is the predominant functional abnormality.[34] In the majority of diabetics, this condition is clinically unapparent. Quantitation of LV function reveals a normal EF and LV volumes that are lower than expected. Due to this form of diastolic dysfunction, diabetics with critical coronary artery stenosis and normal LV systolic function are highly prone to rapid onset of pulmonary congestion (flash pulmonary edema) in association with angina or acute myocardial infarction.

AMYLOID INFILTRATIVE CARDIOMYOPATHY[35]

Amyloid heart disease is an uncommon disorder that can occur as a part of systemic primary (AL) or secondary (AA) amyloidosis or as an isolated cardiac condition in patients with senile amyloidosis.[36] The last condition is more common in blacks apparently due to a higher frequency of a predisposing variant in the transthyretin gene. When the amyloid precursor protein is produced by the liver, liver transplantation may halt the process. The prognosis is poor, especially in those who exhibit restrictive diastolic filling patterns by Doppler. Diastolic dysfunction is the most common, earliest and most important echocardiographic abnormality in cardiac amyloidosis. Echocardiography in patients with overt cardiac amyloidosis frequently demonstrates symmetric LV wall thickening, typically involving the interventricular septum, small ventricular chambers, thickening of the atrial septum, pericardial effusion and dilated atria. Increased right ventricular wall thickness, when present, may be associated with right ventricular diastolic dysfunction, which can be demonstrated by Doppler examination. Disproportionate right ventricular enlargement may also occur.

Another common echocardiographic finding in cardiac amyloidosis is a granular, "sparkling" appearance of the myocardium, resulting from the presence of amyloid and collagen nodules in the heart. This finding alone is relatively nonspecific but the combination of these refractile echoes and atrial septum thickening are highly suggestive of cardiac amyloid.

Apparent preservation or exaggeration of contractile function in a subgroup of patients with amyloid cardiomyopathy is explained by very low wall stress, which is the ultimate expression of afterload and is greatly reduced by the combination of thickened walls, very small cavity and low generated systolic pressure (arterial hypotension). When contractile function is preserved, amyloid cardiomyopathy can be mistaken for HCM and diagnosis can be delayed.

ENDOMYOCARDIAL FIBROSIS

Endomyocardial fibrosis (now designated by WHO as "unclassified cardiomyopathy") is a cause of restrictive cardiomyopathy in North Africa and South America. The condition is associated with eosinophilia in about 50% of those afflicted, and is also known as Loeffler's or Davies disease when encountered in North Africa.

The recognition of endomyocardial fibrosis[37,38] depends on a high level of clinical suspicion and characteristic echocardiographic appearance. There are mass-like apical lesions in the left ventricle resulting from a thrombotic fibrocalcific process. These lesions are associated with restriction of LV and right ventricular filling due to obliteration of one or both cardiac apices. In addition to the unique appearance of the apices, the atria are strikingly enlarged, and mitral and tricuspid regurgitation are often present. As the condition progresses, more and more of the LV cavity is obliterated, leading to a progressively restrictive physiology.

LEFT VENTRICULAR NONCOMPACTION

Left ventricular noncompaction,[39] also called LV hypertrabeculation or spongy myocardium, is an uncommon cause of dilated cardiomyopathy that results from intrauterine arrest of compaction of the loose interwoven meshwork that makes up the fetal myocardial primordium. This disorder should be suspected when unexpectedly heavy LV trabeculation is noted, particularly toward the lateral apex. Noncompaction has recently been reassigned to the "unclassified" category of cardiomyopathy, which also includes endomyocardial fibrosis, fibroelastosis, systolic dysfunction with minimal dilatation and mitochondrial diseases.

VISUAL QUALITATIVE INDICATORS OF SYSTOLIC DYSFUNCTION

Earlier in this chapter the authors discussed their recommendations concerning the visual estimation of EF. Foremost among these was that visual estimation be used as confirmatory evidence of quantitation rather than for primary evaluation. The authors believe that among the more useful qualitative findings associated with all stages of systolic dysfunction are *sphericity*[40] and *descent of the cardiac base*.[41]

The shape of the healthy left ventricle is elliptical and the ratio of its long axis to its short axis is approximately 2:1. In decompensated states, particularly those with volume overload, its shape becomes spherical with the ratio of the axes approaching unity (1:1). Although this ratio has been correlated with EF,[41] the concept of sphericity is most useful when appreciated visually (Fig. 14).

The descent of the cardiac base is the normal movement of the mitral annular plane toward the fixed location of the LV apex. This movement represents the longitudinal function of the LV that in three dimensions is seen to be a twisting, wringing or torsion of the myocardium around the cavity. This movement is most easily appreciated in the apical long axis 2- and

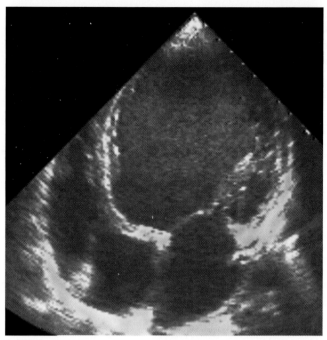

FIGURE 14: Four-chamber view of peripartum cardiomyopathy in a 25-year-old woman. Note the marked spherical remodeling of the LV such that the long and short axis dimensions approach a ratio of 1:1. Compare the shape with the LV shown in Figure 15. Note that the RV is relatively normal

4-chamber views and to a lesser extent in the precordial long axis. Despite seemingly normal inward motion of the endocardium, blunting of basal descent should be treated as an early sign of myocardial dysfunction.

LEFT VENTRICULAR MASS

Left ventricular hypertrophy is universal as an early compensatory change in LV disease and is commonly encountered in patients with ischemic heart disease, congestive HF and advanced age. Concentric LVH, in which LV mass is increased with preserved size and function, may occur in response to chronically increased afterload. Eccentric LVH is seen with ventricular remodeling and chamber enlargement in response to acute or progressive decline in systolic function and typically accompanies a dilated cardiomyopathy. Concentric remodeling is seen as an early stage of LVH[42] and is manifested by increased wall thickness but normal LV mass. All stages of hypertrophy have been associated with adverse outcomes, including sudden death and HF.[43]

The wall thickness of the LV has long been an informative m-mode echocardiographic measurement. Taken by itself, the linear thickness of the septum or of the posterior wall, or both, has been used as an index of LVH (> 1.1 cm). The ratio of posterior wall thickness to septal thickness is used as an index of asymmetric hypertrophy (> 1.3:1). As in the case of LV cavitary dimension, many laboratories use the simple linear measurement of wall thickness to assess LV mass indirectly and some extrapolate LV mass indirectly by an algorithm that extrapolates wall thickness from linear dimensions of opposing walls and subtended cavity. With the disappearance of stand-alone m-mode echocardiographs and the availability of 2D instruments, the use of wall thickness as an index of

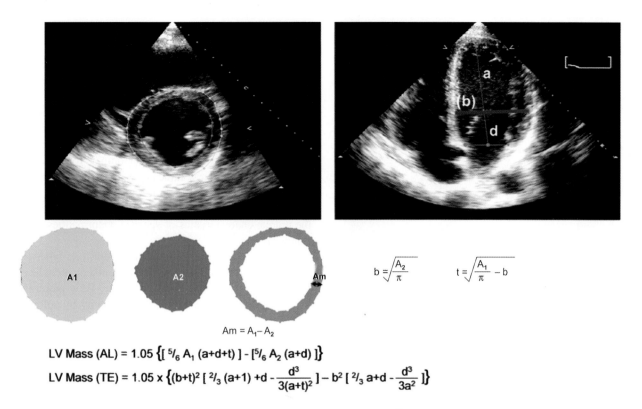

$$b = \sqrt{\frac{A_2}{\pi}} \qquad t = \sqrt{\frac{A_1}{\pi}} - b$$

$$A_m = A_1 - A_2$$

$$\text{LV Mass (AL)} = 1.05 \left\{ \left[\tfrac{5}{6} A_1 (a+d+t) \right] - \left[\tfrac{5}{6} A_2 (a+d) \right] \right\}$$

$$\text{LV Mass (TE)} = 1.05 \times \left\{ (b+t)^2 \left[\tfrac{2}{3} (a+1) + d - \frac{d^3}{3(a+t)^2} \right] - b^2 \left[\tfrac{2}{3} a + d - \frac{d^3}{3a^2} \right] \right\}$$

FIGURE 15: Truncated ellipsoid and area length methods of 2D LV mass measurement.[44] The mean wall thickness is estimated by tracing the epicardial and endocardial areas at the papillary muscle tip level of the short axis LV view. The areas are treated as circles and their mutual radii subtracted to yield an expression of mean wall thickness. This method decreases the potential error of relying on two isolated measurements of wall thickness by averaging many points. As a rule, if the epicardial (outer area) is less than 40 cm^2, the mass is usually normal

hypertrophy has been questioned. The central point of this issue is that wall thickness is being used as an indirect expression of LV mass or weight. If, for example, the weight of the left ventricle is normal, but the preload or filling volume is greatly reduced, the wall will appear to be thickened in diastole. Similarly, if the cavity is dilated the wall will appear to be thin, in spite of normal or even increased mass. For these reasons the authors prefer to measure LV mass as an expression of LVH. There are a number of methods that have been proposed to measure LV mass from m-mode echocardiography. Unfortunately, they suffer the same theoretical limitation as the cube method of estimating LV volume from the minor axis dimension. This limitation is imposed in this case by the inability to extrapolate the volume of the myocardium from a linear dimension. This limitation is most keenly felt in attempting to deal with asymmetric hearts. Working with more uniform hearts

and in large populations where individual variations become unimportant, a number of studies have used m-mode methods and have given us valuable insight into the implications of ventricular hypertrophy, and sensitivity and specificity of electrocardiographic criteria for hypertrophy in the hypertensive population.[45]

Based on their own outcomes research, the authors feel that LV mass should be measured directly from 2D images. The ASE recommended method for estimating LV mass is illustrated in Figure 15. See figure legend for details of methods.

Values of two dimensionally calculated mass are given in Table 5.

Note that the ASE values recommended in the 2005 standards document are larger than those from the Framingham MRI and UCSF 2D echocardiography studies. In coronary disease, the authors have found that increased adverse outcomes

TABLE 5

Normal values for LV mass from three sources

LVMass g/BSA	Men				Women			
	Reference range	Mild Incr.	Moderate Incr.	Severe Incr.	Reference range	Mild Incr.	Moderate Incr.	Severe Incr.
ASE 2005	50-102	103-116	117-130	> 131	44-88	89-100	101-112	> 113
F'ham MRI	Mean 78-95 (.95UCB)	96-113*	114-131	> 132	61-75 (.95UCB)	76-90	91-105	> 106
UCSF	Mean 71-95 (.9UCB)	96-120*	121-135	> 136	62-89 (.95UCB)	90-117	118-135	> 136
*mild, moderate, severe defined in increments of +2SD								

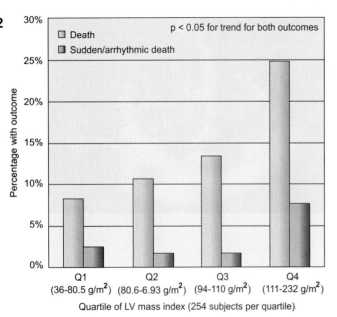

FIGURE 16: Rates of all-cause mortality and sudden death through the end of follow-up, stratified by quartile of left ventricular mass index

in males begin when LV mass exceeds 90 g/m^2 and in females 85 g/m^2.

In the Heart and Soul study, the authors have found that increased LV mass predicts adverse outcomes such as sudden death and HF.[33] In developing an index to predict HF hospitalization, the authors found that mass was the most powerful predictor of subsequent events.[46]

Relationship of death and sudden death to quartile of LV mass in a population of 1,000 patients with coronary heart disease follows for 5 years (Fig. 16).

DIASTOLIC FUNCTION

Echocardiography allows detailed investigation and integration of the complex array of flow related events that occur during LV filling. Whereas systolic function or the process of ejection is known as *inotropy*, diastolic function or the process of filling is termed *lusitropy*. As befits its complexity, multiple measurements and indices have been created to study "diastolic function" and many of these are now standard components of routine echocardiographic examinations. There are several reasons for emphasizing diastolic function:

1. At least one-third of patients with congestive HF have normal or minimally reduced LV systolic function[47] and, among these, congestive HF is mainly a consequence of diastolic dysfunction. In patients with clinical HF and normal systolic function, echocardiographic diastolic parameters confirm the presence and severity of diastolic dysfunction, and guide the type and intensity of treatment and follow-up.

2. Importantly, diastolic parameters are noninvasive surrogates of LV filling pressures in situations of both normal and abnormal LV systolic function. Lowering filling pressures is a goal of treatment and can be confirmed by documenting improvement in echocardiographic indices. Whether diastolic dysfunction is improved or merely masked by

lowering filling pressure is a question that is neither easy to answer nor to fathom.

Diastolic function of the left ventricle is determined by interaction of an active, energy-consuming process of myocardial relaxation, defining the early phases of diastole—isovolumic relaxation and early filling—and by mechanical (elastic) properties of the myocardium, which influence all of diastole. Mechanical properties of the myocardium are described as elasticity (change of length per unit of force), compliance (change of ventricular volume per unit of pressure) and stiffness, which is the inverse of compliance. The filling portion of pressure-volume loops (Figs 17A and B) graphically illustrate the unique characteristics of specific abnormalities of diastolic function.

Echocardiographic analysis of the diastolic function of the left ventricle is based on multiple parameters, including pulsed wave Doppler of the transmitral flow, flow patterns in the pulmonary veins, flow propagation velocity by color m-mode of the LV inflow tract and tissue Doppler studies of motion of the LV base in diastole. In addition, left atrial volume provides a measure of the chronicity of abnormal LV filling conditions. Each of these parameters is determined by multiple physiologic processes, and when taken together, they permit a reasonable understanding of the diastolic state of the left ventricle.

TECHNICAL ASPECTS OF RECORDING AND MEASUREMENT OF DIASTOLIC PARAMETERS

Transmitral Flow

The measurement of transmitral flow velocities by the pulse wave Doppler is the starting point and central component of the classification of LV diastolic function by Doppler echocardiography (Figs 18A to D). However, it is important to understand that the recorded transmitral flow velocities are a result of complex interaction of the "pull" by the left ventricle (active suction which occurs in the early diastole) and the "push" from left atrial passive and active pressure. The pattern on the Doppler signal of transmitral flow created by cyclical rising and falling of transmitral velocity is highly sensitive to and influenced by relatively minor shifts in LV relaxation rate, as well as changes in left atrial pressure due to preload, force of contraction and left atrial compliance. Stand-alone recordings of transmitral flow do not usually provide sufficient information for conclusions about diastolic function and must be supplemented by other information.

Transmitral flow for analysis of intervals, velocities and patterns is recorded with the pulse wave sample volume placed in the inflow tract of the left ventricle at the level of the tips of opened mitral valve leaflets. Routine measurements obtained from transmitral flow recordings include maximal velocities of early and late diastolic LV filling (E and A), and deceleration time of the early LV filling (DT). Atrial fibrillation, mitral stenosis, prosthetic valves, severe aortic insufficiency, A-V block or rapid heart rate (above 90–100/min) leading to the fusion of E and A waves limit the use of transmitral flow for the classification of LV diastolic function.

The 2009 ASE recommendations for measurement of diastolic function list the following measurements to be made

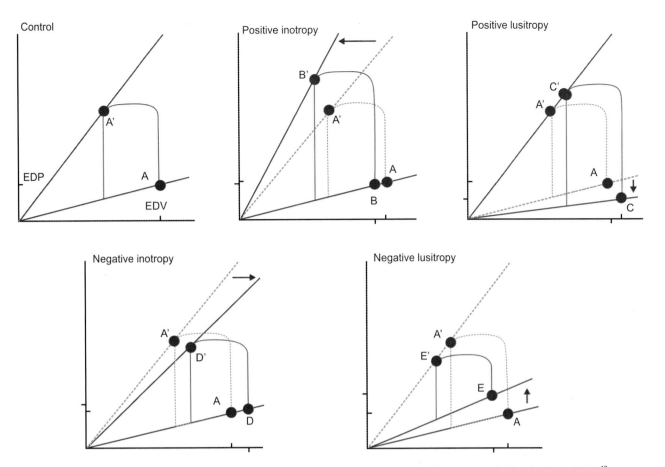

FIGURE 17A: Pressure-volume loops illustrating the result of pure changes in either inotropy (left) or lusitropy (right)[48]

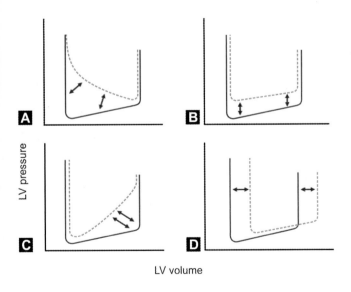

FIGURE 17B: Volume-pressure loops in abnormalities of diastolic function of the left ventricle, caused by different pathologic processes. Only lower parts of the loops, reflecting diastolic function, are shown. The uninterrupted line demonstrates normal diastolic function. (A) Abnormal relaxation of the left ventricle. (B) Restricted filling of the left ventricle in constrictive pericarditis or cardiac tamponade. (C) Decreased compliance of the left ventricle, commonly seen in left ventricular hypertrophy, cardiac amyloidosis, endomyocardial fibrosis or myocardial ischemia. (D) Increased filling pressure of the left ventricle (i.e. in volume overload of the left ventricle). (*Source:* Zile MR. Diastolic dysfunction: detection, consequences, and treatment: II diagnosis and treatment of diastolic function. Mod Concepts Cardiovasc Dis. 1990;59:1-6, Copyright 1990 American Heart Association)

from the mitral inflow signal: isovolumic relaxation time (IVRT), E/A ratio, DT (deceleration time or time required for deceleration of peak early diastolic inflow to baseline), A duration. Normal ranges are given in Table 6.[49]

Measurement of the IVRT, the time interval between cessation of flow in LVOT and the onset of flow in LV inflow tract is obtained from a continuous or pulse wave recording, with the sample volume in a position intermediate between those used for recording of the LV inflow and outflow (Fig. 19). If mitral inflow is used for flow quantitation, the sample volume is placed in the annulus so that its cross-sectional area can be measured from annular diameter and used for calculating volumetric flow.

Propagation Velocity of the Early Diastolic Flow in the Left Ventricle

Normal diastolic filling, enhanced by forceful suction by the left ventricle, produces rapid flow propagation; Figure 20 demonstrates color Doppler recording of normal diastolic filling with simultaneous unidirectional flow rapidly reaching uniform maximum velocity from the starting point of the pulmonary veins and continuing in an unbroken line into the apex of the left ventricle. Because the column of inflow blood accelerates to its maximum so rapidly, the authors believe that the initial acceleration occurs simultaneously in all parts (i.e. from base to apex) of the end systolic blood pool and is an expression of coordinated global active relaxation rather than the migration

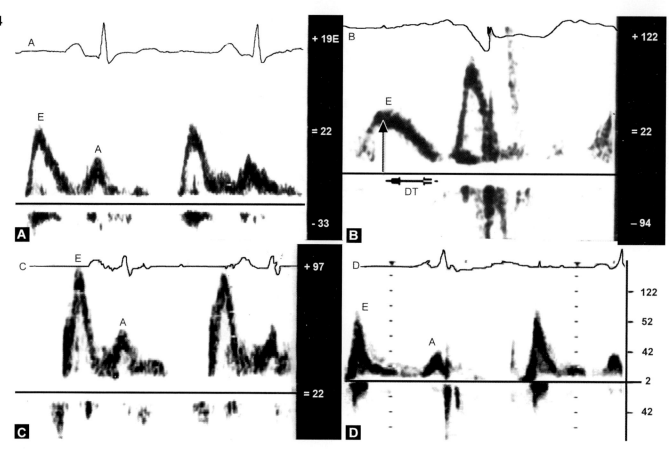

FIGURES 18A TO D: PW Doppler recording of transmitral flow patterns commonly encountered. Types of transmitral flow are shown: normal (A) delayed relaxation with dominant left ventricular filling in atrial systole (B), pseudonormal (C) and restrictive (D)

of a bolus of blood from the pulmonary veins to apex. Measurement of the propagation velocity (Vp) of early diastolic flow in the left ventricle uses color m-mode (Fig. 21). For proper measurement, the Nyquist limit is decreased to achieve aliasing in the early diastolic flow. Propagation velocity is the rate at which the wave front of the fastest red cells appear to migrate from base to apex and is represented by the slope of the border between normal and aliased spectrum of the flow signal. Normal values for Vp are greater than 55 cm/sec (45 cm/sec in the elderly). Since Vp is a relatively preload (LA pressure) independent index of LV relaxation, it may be used in the differentiation of normal from pseudonormal mitral flow pattern.

Limitations of Vp include loss of reliability in small ventricular chambers and poor reproducibility due to the

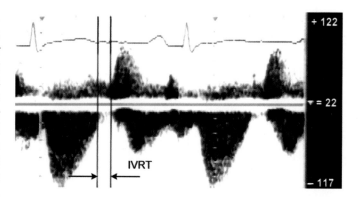

FIGURE 19: Measurement of isovolumic relaxation time is done from a position, intermediate between those used for recording of left ventricular inflow and outflow; both aortic and mitral flow are seen in this tracing; IVRT is the time interval between cessation of aortic flow and onset of mitral flow

TABLE 6

Normal values for Doppler-derived diastolic measurements

	Age group (y)			
Measurement	16-20	21-40	41-60	>60
IVRT (ms)	50 ± 9 (32-68)	67 ± 8 (51-83)	74 ± 7 (60-88)	87 ± 7 (73-101)
E/A ratio	1.88 ± 0.45 (0.98-2.78)	1.53 ± 0.40 (0.73-2.33)	1.28 ± 0.25 (0.78-1.78)	0.96 ± 0.18 (0.6-1.32)
DT (ms)	142 ± 19 (104-180)	166 ± 14 (138-194)	181 ± 19 (143-219)	200 + 29 (142-258)
A duration (ms)	113 ± (79-147)	127 ± 13 (101-153)	133 ± 13 (107-159)	138 ± 19 (100-176)

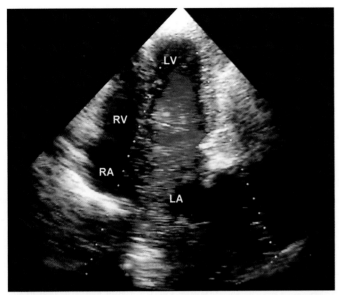

FIGURE 20: Color Doppler study of early diastolic filling of the left ventricle from apical 4-chamber view. Unidirectional flow is seen from pulmonary veins into the left atrium and deep into left ventricle, almost all the way to the apex. (Abbreviations: LA: Left atrium; LV: Left ventricle; RA: Right atrium; RV: Right ventricle)

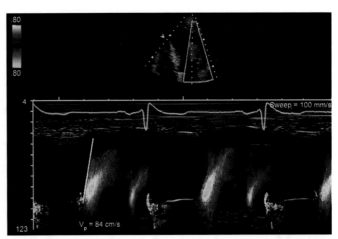

FIGURE 21: Color m-mode study of transmitral flow from apical window: propagation velocity (Vp) of early diastolic left ventricular filling is determined as the slope of aliased flow in the early filling spectrum. Normal Vp exceeds 55 cm/sec, in elderly—45 cm/sec

frequently curvilinear shape of early diastolic flow slope, which can make measurement of Vp somewhat arbitrary.

Pulmonary Venous Flow

The recording of pulsed wave Doppler signal from the pulmonary venous flow is an integral part of each echocardiographic study. Transthoracic echocardiography allows accurate recording of blood flow in pulmonary veins in nearly 90% of patients. Examples of flow signals recorded in pulmonary veins are shown in Figure 22 and diagrammatically in Figure 23. Systolic flow from the veins into the left atrium consists of two components, the first generated by suction from left atrial relaxation (SE) and the second by suction provided by the piston-like descent of the base of the heart toward apex while the mitral valve is closed (SL).[50] Diastolic flow is influenced by left atrial and ventricular filling pressures, and is concurrent with the E wave of transmitral flow. The impetus for early pulmonary vein flow (directly from vein to ventricle) is provided simultaneously by both atrial preload and by active ventricular relaxation. The former provides a push while the latter provides suction into the ventricle. At slow heart rates, the interval between the early rapid flow into the ventricle and the reverse flow retrograde into the pulmonary vein is called the conduit phase. During this phase, flow is slower but continues antegrade. Although both VTIs and peak velocities of the systolic and diastolic components of pulmonary venous flow are measured, the literature correlating pulmonary vein flow with LV filling pressure is based on comparing the integral of the systolic component with the diastolic forward component.[51] Normally the VTI of systolic flow is at least 60% of the total forward flow.

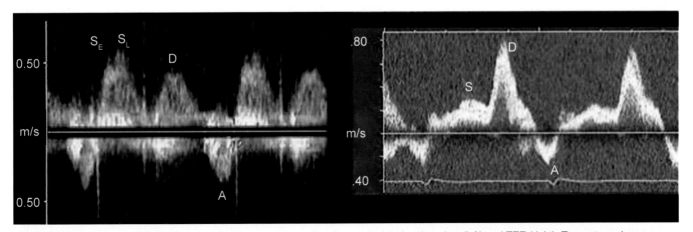

FIGURE 22: Recording of the PW Doppler of pulmonary venous flow from apical 4-chamber view (left) and TEE (right). Two antegrade waves are seen—systolic (S) and diastolic (D)—and a small retrograde wave during atrial systole (A). Sometimes (as in this case in transthoracic study) two systolic antegrade waves are present—early (SE) and late (SL). SE is considered to result from left atrial relaxation, SL—from the movement of the base of the left ventricle toward apex. Diastolic wave D corresponds to early diastolic filling of the left ventricle, although it starts approximately 50 msec later. In rapid heart rates, systolic and diastolic waves merge. Thus antegrade flow in pulmonary veins may be monophasic, biphasic or triphasic. It is important to note that dominance of systolic or diastolic flow should be determined from velocity-time integrals, and not from maximal flow velocities

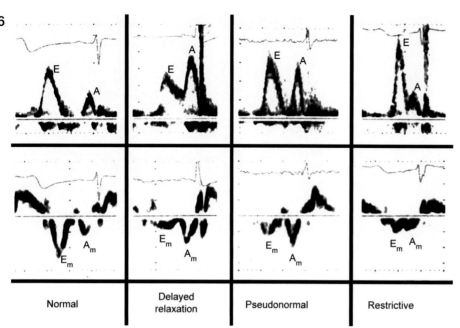

| Normal | Delayed relaxation | Pseudonormal | Restrictive |

FIGURE 23: The mitral inflow at rest in the subgroups of diastolic dysfunction

In healthy subjects greater than 30 years old, systolic flow usually is dominant (as is true for all central veins). When the patient is younger than 30 and/or when the heart rate is slow, systolic flow remains robust but peak velocity of diastolic flow may be slightly higher. In hypovolemia, diastolic flow in pulmonary veins decreases and may disappear, while systolic component increases. In atrial fibrillation most of the flow in pulmonary veins occurs in diastole, and systolic flow appears blunted. Some research suggests that systolic dominance may be maintained in hypertrophic cardiomyopathies despite elevated LVEDP.[52] In this study and in the ASE guidelines on diastolic function, pulmonary vein measurements are limited to peak systolic and diastolic velocities despite direct experimental hemodynamic data that supports the use of the VTI ratio of systolic and diastolic components and not peak velocity.[50,53] For this reason and for others, the authors remain unconvinced that the recognition of normal LV filling pressure by systolic dominance is vitiated in hypertrophy; the authors have noted that, in unstable conditions where LVEDP is rising from low levels to elevated, the change in pulmonary vein in flow pattern from systolic to diastolic dominant may lag behind the hemodynamics. On the other hand, in the OR, the pulmonary vein Doppler pattern tracks hemodyamic changes accurately.[53]

It should also be noted that with appearance of atrial fibrillation, systolic components of PV flow either become attenuated without necessarily connoting elevated filling pressure. Failure to recognize atrial fibrillation may lead to a false assumption that filling pressure is elevated.

Additional attention should be directed to measurement of duration of the wave of atrial systolic reversal of pulmonary flow (A in Figure 22). With left atrial contraction, blood can move either antegrade into the left ventricle, or flow retrograde into the pulmonary veins. Comparison of flow duration from atrial contraction retrograde from the left atrium into the pulmonary veins (atrial systolic reversal) with antegrade flow into the left ventricle (A wave of transmitral flow) allows another expression of end diastolic LV pressure. Increase of end diastolic

pressure in the left ventricle causes longer duration of retrograde flow into the pulmonary veins during atrial contraction than duration of forward transmitral flow. Normally, the duration of atrial reversal should not exceed the forward A wave of transmitral flow by more than 30 msec.[54]

The deceleration of the diastolic component of pulmonary vein inflow is also a useful index of diastolic dysfunction.[55] When the deceleration time of this wave form is less than 150 msec, elevated LV filling pressure is suspected. The validity of this measurement is retained in atrial fibrillation.

Doppler Tissue Imaging of Mitral Annular Motion in Diastole

Recording of mitral annular diastolic ascent (reflective of timing and amount of filling volume) and systolic descent (reflective of quantity and timing of LV emptying) (Fig. 24 lower panel) is accomplished from the apical acoustic window by imaging the 4-chamber view and placing the pulse wave Doppler sample volume on the lateral mitral annulus (preferred) or the intersection of the interventricular septum and the medial annulus (second choice). Filters are set to allow only very low frequencies (< 20 cm/s) to eliminate high-velocity blood flow signals and allow only the slower motion of the annulus to form the signal. Annular motion is proportional to the quantity of blood flow that leaves and enters the ventricle and provides a vehicle to compare with cavitary Doppler flow signals that represent velocity of blood but not its amount. Three main waives can be identified on the Doppler tracing of mitral annular motion (as conventionally displayed): (1) a positive wave reflects systolic motion of the annulus toward the apex (Sm); (2) two negative diastolic waves resulting from motion of the annulus away from apex in early diastole (Em) and (3) with atrial systole (Am). Normally, Em is of greater amplitude than Am.

Tissue Doppler early diastolic velocity mitral annular motion (e'), when combined with mitral inflow peak diastolic

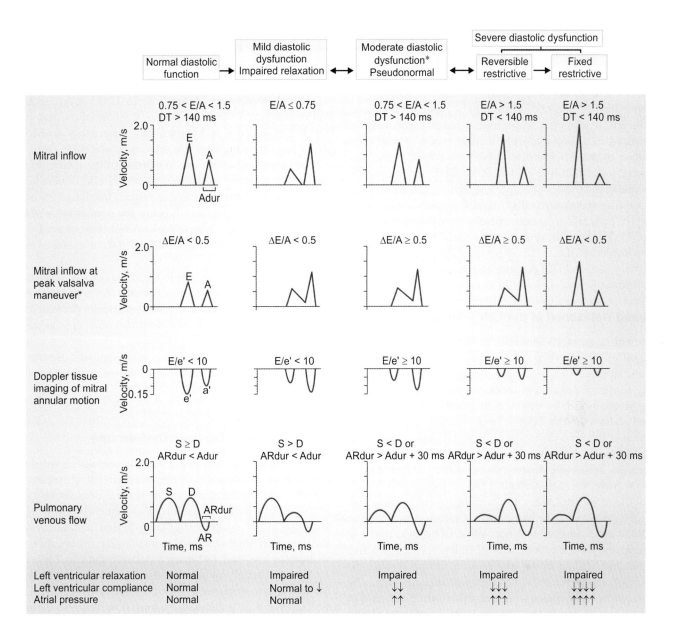

FIGURE 24: Types of transmitral flow (upper row) and corresponding types of tissue Doppler interrogation of the mitral annular motion (lower row). Sample volume is placed on the interventricular septal part of the mitral annulus from the apical 4-chamber view. Tissue Doppler recording allows discrimination of normal and pseudonormal flow. (Abbreviations: A: Transmitral flow during atrial systole; Am: Mitral annular motion during atrial systole; E: Early diastolic transmitral flow; Em: Early diastolic motion of the mitral annulus[56])

velocity (E) as a ratio (E/é), provides an independent measure of LV diastolic performance and can reliably differentiate normal from patterns that arise from elevated filling pressure. In practice, |E/é ratios that are less than 8 or more than 16 have a high sensitivity for normal and elevated filling pressure respectively and can help to avoid misinterpretation of pseudonormal Doppler flow pattern from one that is normal (Fig. 23). However, this method, like most others, has drawbacks. Principally, the E/e' ratio presents a rather wide gray area between the ratios of 8 and 16 where there is poor correlation between this ratio and filling pressure.[52]

Left Atrial Volume and Index

Left atrial volume can be considered tantamount to "the hemoglobin A1c of LV diastolic function", because it seems to reflect the historic average of the filling pressure of the left ventricle; it should be viewed as an important part of the complete evaluation of LV diastolic function. The left atrial volume index (left atrial volume indexed to BSA) predicts risk of cardiac death in patients after myocardial infarction. In addition, in ambulatory patients with stable coronary artery disease, left atrial volume index predicted both HF and death. Left atrial function may also be calculated so as to differentiate from abnormal those atria that are considered enlarged but have become so as a result of elevated stroke volume rather than diastolic dysfunction. It is also a useful in measuring the degree of dysfunction and noting recovery. The formula is:

LA fractional change × LVOT VTI/LAESVI = LAFI

Where fractional change is = LA end systolic volume – LA end diastolic volume/LA end systolic volume; LAESVI is LA end systolic volume corrected for BSA and LVOT VTI is the VTI of the systolic flow signal obtained from the LVOT.[57]

TYPES OF DIASTOLIC DYSFUNCTION

Abnormalities of diastolic function exist along a continuum, which, based on echocardiographic parameters, may be categorized into four relatively distinct types: (1) impaired relaxation of the left ventricle (type 1 diastolic dysfunction); (2) pseudonormal filling (type 2 diastolic dysfunction); (3) restrictive filling (type 3 diastolic dysfunction) that is reversible with Valsalva maneuver and (4) type 4 diastolic dysfunction-restrictive pattern that is irreversible with Valsalva maneuver. Figure 24 diagrammatically shows the mitral inflow at rest and its response to Valsalva in the subgroups of diastolic dysfunction. Pulmonary vein and DTI patterns are also depicted for each of the subgroups.

Impaired Relaxation of the Left Ventricle

The initial stage of LV diastolic dysfunction is manifest by impaired or slowed relaxation of the left ventricle (type 1 diastolic dysfunction). It is characterized by slowing of the energy-consuming process governing ventricular relaxation; the filling pressures usually remain normal, with brief elevation at the end of diastole at the time of atrial contraction. Because the elevation of the presystolic a wave at end diastole is brief, the mean diastolic pressure remains low. However, when tachycardia intervenes, diastole shortens and the contribution of the A wave to mean diastolic pressure increases; in many patients, exercise intolerance results. Furthermore, patients with type 1 dysfunction may be intolerant to atrial fibrillation because the loss of atrial contraction causes left atrial pressure to rise in compensation for the loss of 60% of filling volume by active transport and refilling atrium with an equal amount through the suction of active relaxation.[49] Delayed relaxation can be recognized by examination of mitral inflow where the ratio of the E and A waves is less than1, IVRT is prolonged and deceleration time (pre-A wave deceleration of inflow) (DT) lengthened. Pulmonary venous flow demonstrates pronounced systolic dominance associated with augmented atrial relaxation and decreased VTI of the diastolic wave, and slowed propagation velocity (Vp). The Em velocity on the tissue Doppler recording of mitral annular motion is also reduced. This filling pattern is consistent with essentially normal mean LV and LA diastolic pressures and does not impart a worsened prognosis in coronary disease.

Pseudonormal Filling

The next stage, stage 2, in the decline in diastolic function that follows impaired LV diastolic function (stage 1) is associated with elevation of the LV and left atrial diastolic pressure. Although LV relaxation remains slowed, higher left atrial pressure leads to an increase in early transmitral filling (E wave) velocity and impaired LV compliance leads to rapid termination of filling when ventricular capacity is prematurely achieved. The abrupt termination of filling shortens the deceleration time toward normal. The increase in left atrial pressure also causes mitral valve to open sooner with consequent shortening of the

IVRT. The elevation of LV filling pressures is a direct consequence of decreased chamber compliance which sees the pressure in the left ventricle rise more rapidly during filling. These changes "pseudonormalize" transmitral flow, and make it difficult to distinguish from normal. However, with the Valsalva maneuver, preload decreases, left atrial pressure drops and the "pseudonormal" pattern may temporarily revert back to the pattern of impaired LV relaxation (stage 1).

Other features of the pseudonormal filling pattern include loss of or decrease in the degree of systolic dominance of pulmonary flow; the proportion or systolic fraction of PV inflow to the atria during systole falls below the normal value of 60% of the total of systole plus diastole. Atrial flow reversal in the pulmonary veins is prolonged relative to the duration of mitral A wave inflow.[54]

Color m-mode of inflow velocity reveals slowed acceleration of the propagation velocity. Em velocity on the tissue Doppler recording of mitral annular motion is markedly decreased, and becomes confirmatory evidence that differentiates pseudonormal from normal transmitral flow pattern.

Pseudonormal filling pattern is consistent with elevated LV and left atrial pressures and imparts a worsened prognosis in patients with CHF or CAD.[47]

Restrictive Filling
(Grades 3 and 4 Diastolic Dysfunction)

Further increase in LV filling pressure results in worsening effective LV compliance. During diastolic filling, pressure in the left ventricle rises exponentially, and exceeds left atrial pressure very early in diastole. Consequently, most of the diastolic filling occurs early, contribution of late filling is minimal, E to A ratio becomes more than 2:1, deceleration time shortens to less than 140 msec and IVRT shortens further.

By the time of mitral valve closure at the end of diastole, the left atrium does not empty completely. Due to this, the systolic wave of pulmonary venous flow becomes severely blunted and most of pulmonary venous flow occurs in diastole. Moreover, left atrial systolic reversal is prolonged and increased in amplitude. Also, color m-mode reveals further slowing of the propagation velocity and Em velocity on the tissue Doppler recording of mitral annular motion is also markedly decreased. Restrictive LV filling is a poor prognostic sign in various disease states, including patients with low LVEF and in patients with infiltrative cardiomyopathies. Patients who continue to exhibit restrictive filling pattern despite Valsalva (stage 4) or following aggressive medical treatment are at especially high risk.

EVALUATION OF LEFT VENTRICULAR FILLING PRESSURES

The ultimate significance of diastolic parameters is due to their ability to noninvasively evaluate LV filling pressure (Fig. 25). Identification of the diastolic filling pattern provides an approximate understanding of the level of LV filling pressure. Typically, delayed relaxation pattern is associated with normal filling pressures, pseudonormal pattern with mild to moderate elevation of pressures and restrictive pattern with markedly elevated filling pressures. In addition, deceleration time of early diastolic filling may be an accurate indicator of LV filling

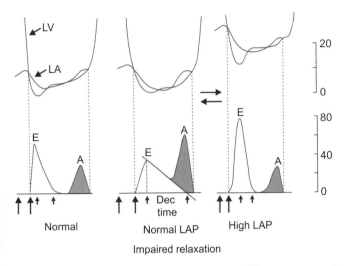

FIGURE 25: Diagrammatic relationship between filling pressure and mitral inflow pattern[49]

pressure in patients with low LVEF, in whom a deceleration time less than 150 msec nearly always indicates mean left atrial pressure above 25 mm Hg.[58]

However patterns of mitral inflow as predictors of filling pressure are vulnerable to confounding. Heart rate, preload, afterload, contractility, valvular regurgitation and the position of the sample volume may influence transmitral flow independently of diastolic function. In certain diseases, mitral inflow pattern has been found unreliable by some investigators: in patients with hypertrophic obstructive cardiomyopathy or

severe LVH, transmitral pattern frequently remains consistent with delayed relaxation despite elevated filling pressures (Figs 26A and B). Even in these patients, however, serial studies will reveal changes within these patterns as filling pressure changes.

FORMULAE THAT ATTEMPT TO PROVIDE QUANTITATION OF LV FILLING PRESSURE

More quantitative estimations of LV filling pressure may be calculated from Doppler-derived parameters. The following methods illustrate attempts at more precise determination of LV filling pressures:

1. Systolic fraction of the pulmonary venous flow is a simple and reliable way of identifying patients with elevated left atrial pressures. Separate measurement of systolic and diastolic wave VTIs allows calculation of the systolic fraction of pulmonary venous flow:

$$\text{Systolic fraction} = \text{SVTI}/(\text{SVTI} + \text{DVTI}) \times 100\%$$

where SVTI is velocity-time integral of systolic, and DVTI is velocity-time integral of diastolic pulmonary venous flow. Normal systolic fraction of pulmonary venous flow exceeds 55%. Investigation conducted by Kuecherer and colleagues[53] demonstrated a correlation of systolic fraction with mean pressure in the left atrium, and diastolic pressure in the left ventricle. The following formula allows noninvasive calculation of this pressure:

$$\text{Pressure in the left atrium (mm Hg)} = 35-0.39 \, [\text{systolic fraction (\%)}]$$

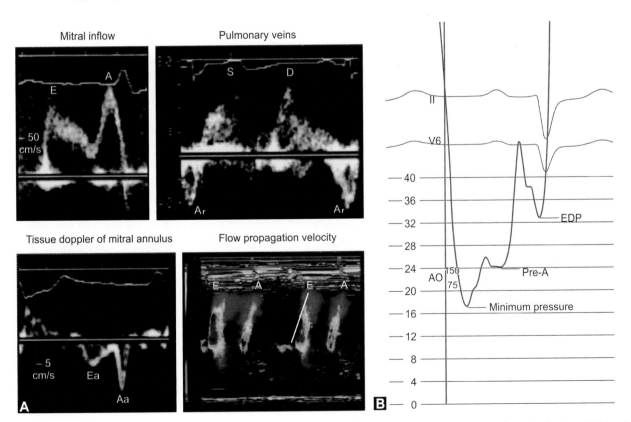

FIGURES 26A AND B: (A) Transmitral velocities, PV velocities, mitral annular velocities by TD and flow propagation velocity in an HCM patient. Time lines represent 200 ms. Notice that E velocity is (almost equal to) 1 m/s and lower than A velocity. DT = 400 ms. Systolic (S) PV flow is almost equal to the diastolic (D) flow. Ea = 6 cm/s, flow propagation velocity = 37 cm/s. (B) LV diastolic pressures from the same patient. LVEDP = 33 mm Hg, preA pressure = 24 mm Hg and minimal pressure = 17 mm Hg. EDP indicates LVEDP; Pre-A indicates preA[59]

In practice, it is sufficient to calculate systolic fraction; if it is less than 40%, end diastolic pressure in the left ventricle is likely to be above 18 mm Hg, and frequently coincides with either pseudonormal or restrictive types of LV filling.

2. Tissue Doppler evaluation of mitral annular motion in early diastole (E') provides a relatively preload in dependent measure of LV relaxation. Since the E wave of transmitral filling is determined by an interaction of left atrial pressure and LV relaxation, the ratio of E/E', which corrects E for the volume of inflow (ascent of the base) that resulted in the E' velocity; E/E' relates well to mean left atrial pressure or pulmonary capillary wedge pressure (PCWP).

Nagueh and colleagues (JACC 1997;30(6):1527-33) showed that the following formula allows noninvasive estimation of PCWP:

$$PCWP \ (mm \ Hg) = 1.24 \ [E/Ea] + 1.9$$

Subsequently E/Em index was demonstrated to retain its utility in patients with sinus tachycardia and fused E and A waves, and in patients with atrial fibrillation. Moreover, it seems valid in both low and normal LVEF.

E/Em greater than or equal to 15, where Em is measured in the septal part of annulus, is specific for elevated LVEDP, whereas E/E' less than or equal to 8 is specific for normal to low filling pressures.[60] The method has a problematic weakness in that the values between an E/e' 8 and 15 correlated poorly with LVEDP and weaker correlation in HCM.[52]

3. Propagation velocity of early diastolic filling also correlates with LV relaxation, and is relatively independent of left atrial pressure. The propagation of flow into the LV is due to a complex interaction of events but in health it occurs very rapidly (see above discussion). Garcia and colleagues[61] established this correlation, and suggested the following formula:

$$PCWP \ (mm \ Hg) = 5.27 \times (E/Vp) + 4.6$$

CONCLUSION

Left ventricular systolic and diastolic parameters can be comprehensively measured by echocardiography/Doppler and provide a wealth of information about ejection and filling functions and have strong prognostic significance. However they are best utilized when interpreted together in an expertly performed comprehensive echocardiographic study in the light of the pertinent clinical questions and context.

REFERENCES

1. Schiller NB, Shah PM, Crawford M, et al. Recommendations for quantitation of the left ventricle by two-dimensional echocardiography. American Society of Echocardiography Committee on Standards, Subcommittee on Quantitation of Two-Dimensional Echocardiograms. J Am Soc Echocardiogr. 1989;2:358-67.
2. Lang RM, Bierig M, Devereux RB, et al. Recommendations for chamber quantification: a report from the American Society of Echocardiography's Guidelines and Standards Committee and the Chamber Quantification Writing Group, developed in conjunction with the European Association of Echocardiography, a branch of the European Society of Cardiology. J Am Soc Echocardiogr. 2005;18:1440-63.
3. Schiller NB, Foster E. Analysis of left ventricular systolic function. Heart. 1996;75:17-26.
4. McManus DD, Shah SJ, Fabi MR, et al. Prognostic value of left ventricular end systolic volume index as a predictor of heart failure hospitalization in stable coronary artery disease: data from the Heart and Soul Study. J Am Soc Echocardiogr. 2009;22:190-7.
5. Pflugfelder PW, Landzberg JS, Cassidy MM, et al. Comparison of cine MR imaging with Doppler echocardiography for the evaluation of aortic regurgitation. AJR Am J Roentgenol. 1989;152:729-35.
6. Ristow B, Ali S, Na B, et al. Predicting heart failure hospitalization and mortality by quantitative echocardiography: is body surface area the indexing method of choice? The Heart and Soul Study. J Am Soc Echocardiogr. 2010;23:406-13.
7. Massie BM, Schiller NB, Ratshin RA, et al. Mitral-septal separation: new echocardiographic index of left ventricular function. Am J Cardiol. 1977;39:1008-16.
8. Pratt RC, Parisi AF, Harrington JJ, et al. The influence of left ventricular stroke volume on aortic root motion: an echocardiographic study. Circulation. 1976;53:947-53.
9. White HD, Norris RM, Brown MA, et al. Left ventricular end systolic volume as the major determinant of survival after recovery from myocardial infarction. Circulation. 1987;76:44-51.
10. Detaint D, Messika-Zeitoun D, Maalouf J, et al. Quantitative echocardiographic determinants of clinical outcome in asymptomatic patients with aortic regurgitation: a prospective study. JACC Cardiovasc Imaging. 2008;1:1-11.
11. Kuecherer HF, Kusumoto F, Muhiudeen IA, et al. Pulmonary venous flow patterns by transesophageal pulsed Doppler echocardiography: relation to parameters of left ventricular systolic and diastolic function. Am Heart J. 1991;122:1683-93.
12. Kuecherer HF, Kee LL, Modin G, et al. Echocardiography in serial evaluation of left ventricular systolic and diastolic function: importance of image acquisition, quantitation, and physiologic variability in clinical and investigational applications. J Am Soc Echocardiogr. 1991;4:203-14.
13. Steine K, Stugaard M, Smiseth OA. Mechanisms of retarded apical filling in acute ischemic left ventricular failure. Circulation. 1999;99:2048-54.
14. St John Sutton M, Pfeffer MA, Plappert T, et a.. Quantitative two-dimensional echocardiographic measurements are major predictors of adverse cardiovascular events after acute myocardial infarction. The protective effects of captopril. Circulation. 1994;89:68-75.
15. Salton CJ, Chuang ML, O'Donnell CJ, et al. Gender differences and normal left ventricular anatomy in an adult population free of hypertension. A cardiovascular magnetic resonance study of the Framingham Heart Study Offspring cohort. J Am Coll Cardiol. 2002;39:1055-60.
16. Wahr DW, Wang YS, Schiller NB. Left ventricular volumes determined by two-dimensional echocardiography in a normal adult population. J Am Coll Cardiol. 1983;1:863-8.
17. Byrd BF 3rd, Wahr D, Wang YS, et al. Left ventricular mass and volume/mass ratio determined by two-dimensional echocardiography in normal adults. J Am Coll Cardiol. 1985;6:1021-5.
18. Byrd BF 3rd, Schiller NB, Botvinick EH, et al. Normal cardiac dimensions by magnetic resonance imaging. Am J Cardiol. 1985;55:1440-2.
19. Wei K. Contrast echocardiography: what have we learned from the new guidelines? Curr Cardiol Rep. 2010;12:237-42.
20. Mulvagh SL, Rakowski H, Vannan MA, et al. American Society of Echocardiography Consensus Statement on the clinical applications of ultrasonic contrast agents in echocardiography. J Am Soc Echocardiogr. 2008;21:1179-201.
21. Haites NE, McLennan FM, Mowat DH, et al. Assessment of cardiac output by the Doppler ultrasound technique alone. Br Heart J. 1985;53:123-9.
22. Goldman JH, Schiller NB, Lim DC, et al. Usefulness of stroke distance by echocardiography as a surrogate marker of cardiac output that is independent of gender and size in a normal population. Am J Cardiol. 2001;87:499-502.

23. Kolias TJ, Aaronson KD, Armstrong WF. Doppler-derived dP/dt and -dP/dt predict survival in congestive heart failure. J Am Coll Cardiol. 2000;36:1594-9.

24. Abraham TP, Nishimura RA. Myocardial strain: can we finally measure contractility? J Am Coll Cardiol. 2001;37:731-4.

25. Abraham TP, Nishimura RA, Holmes DR Jr, et al. Strain rate imaging for assessment of regional myocardial function: results from a clinical model of septal ablation. Circulation. 2002;105:1403-6.

26. Richand V, Lafitte S, Reant P, et al. An ultrasound speckle tracking (two-dimensional strain) analysis of myocardial deformation in professional soccer players compared with healthy subjects and hypertrophic cardiomyopathy. Am J Cardiol. 2007;100:128-32.

27. Ng AC, Delgado V, Bertini M, et al. Myocardial steatosis and biventricular strain and strain rate imaging in patients with type 2 diabetes mellitus. Circulation. 2010;122:2538-44.

28. Lamia B, Tanabe M, Kim HK, et al. Quantifying the role of regional dyssynchrony on global left ventricular performance. JACC Cardiovasc Imaging. 2009;2:1350-6.

29. Richardson P, McKenna W, Bristow M, et al. Report of the 1995 World Health Organization/International Society and Federation of Cardiology Task Force on the definition and classification of cardiomyopathies. Circulation. 1996;93:841-2.

30. Gardin JM, Tommaso CL, Talano JV. Echographic early systolic partial closure (notching) of the aortic valve in congestive cardiomyopathy. Am Heart J.1984;107:135-42.

31. Maron BJ, Nichols PF 3rd, Pickle LW, et al. Patterns of inheritance in hypertrophic cardiomyopathy: assessment by m-mode and two-dimensional echocardiography. Am J Cardiol. 1984;53:1087-94.

32. Maron BJ, Bonow RO, Seshagiri TN, et al. Hypertrophic cardiomyopathy with ventricular septal hypertrophy localized to the apical region of the left ventricle (apical hypertrophic cardiomyopathy). Am J Cardiol. 1982;49:1838-48.

33. Turakhia MP, Schiller NB, Whooley MA. Prognostic significance of increased left ventricular mass index to mortality and sudden death in patients with stable coronary heart disease (from the Heart and Soul study). Am J Cardiol. 2008;102:1131-5.

34. Bouchard A, Sanz N, Botvinick EH, et al. Noninvasive assessment of cardiomyopathy in normotensive diabetic patients between 20 and 50 years old. Am J Med. 1989;87:160-6.

35. Roberts WC. Cardiomyopathy and myocarditis: morphologic features. Adv Cardiol. 1978;22:184-98.

36. Shah KB, Inoue Y, Mehra MR. Amyloidosis and the heart: a comprehensive review. Arch Intern Med. 2006;166:1805-13.

37. Acquatella H, Schiller NB. Echocardiographic recognition of Chagas' disease and endomyocardial fibrosis. J Am Soc Echocardiogr. 1988;1:60-8.

38. Acquatella H, Schiller NB, Puigbó JJ, et al. Value of two-dimensional echocardiography in endomyocardial disease with and without eosinophilia. A clinical and pathologic study. Circulation. 1983;67:1219-26.

39. Paterick TE, Gerber TC, Pradhan SR, et al. Left ventricular noncompaction cardiomyopathy: what do we know? Rev Cardiovasc Med. 2010;11:92-9.

40. Mendes LA, Picard MH, Dec GW, et al. Ventricular remodeling in active myocarditis. Myocarditis treatment trial. Am Heart J. 1999;138:303-8.

41. Simonson JS, Schiller NB. Descent of the base of the left ventricle: an echocardiographic index of left ventricular function. J Am Soc Echocardiogr. 1989;2:25-35.

42. Berger J, Ren X, Na B, et al. Relation of concentric remodeling to adverse outcomes in patients with stable coronary artery disease (from the Heart and Soul Study). Am J Cardiol. 2011;107:1579-84. Epub 2011.

43. Gardin JM, McClelland R, Kitzman D, et al. M-mode echocardiographic predictors of six- to seven-year incidence of coronary heart disease, stroke, congestive heart failure, and mortality in an elderly cohort (the Cardiovascular Health Study). Am J Cardiol. 2001;87:1051-7.

44. Schiller NB, Skiôldebrand CG, Schiller EJ, et al. Canine left ventricular mass estimation by two-dimensional echocardiography. Circulation. 1983;68:210-6.

45. Okin PM, Roman MJ, Lee ET, et al. Combined echocardiographic left ventricular hypertrophy and electrocardiographic ST depression improve prediction of mortality in American Indians: the Strong Heart Study. Hypertension. 2004;43:769-74. Epub 2004.

46. Stevens SM, Farzaneh-Far R, Na B, et al. Development of an echocardiographic risk-stratification index to predict heart failure in patients with stable coronary artery disease: the Heart and Soul study. JACC Cardiovasc Imaging. 2009;2:11-20.

47. Ren X, Ristow B, Na B, et al. Prevalence and prognosis of asymptomatic left ventricular diastolic dysfunction in ambulatory patients with coronary heart disease. Am J Cardiol. 2007;99:1643-7.

48. Katz AM. Influence of altered inotropy and lusitropy on ventricular pressure-volume loops. J Am Coll Cardiol. 1988;11:438-45.

49. Nagueh SF, Appleton CP, Gillebert TC, et al. Recommendations for the evaluation of left ventricular diastolic function by echocardiography. J Am Soc Echocardiogr. 2009;22:107-33.

50. Barbier P, Solomon S, Schiller NB, et al. Determinants of forward pulmonary vein flow: an open pericardium pig model. J Am Coll Cardiol. 2000;35:1947-59.

51. Kuecherer HF, Muhiudeen IA, Kusumoto FM, et al. Estimation of mean left atrial pressure from transesophageal pulsed Doppler echocardiography of pulmonary venous flow. Circulation. 1990;82:1127-39.

52. Ommen SR, Nishimura RA, Appleton CP, et al. Clinical utility of Doppler echocardiography and tissue Doppler imaging in the estimation of left ventricular filling pressures: a comparative simultaneous Doppler-catheterization study. Circulation. 2000;102:1788-94.

53. Kuecherer HF, Muhiudeen IA, Kusumoto FM, et al. Estimation of mean left atrial pressure from transesophageal pulsed Doppler echocardiography of pulmonary venous flow. Circulation. 1990;82:1127-39.

54. Rossvoll O, Hatle LK. Pulmonary venous flow velocities recorded by transthoracic Doppler ultrasound: relation to left ventricular diastolic pressures. J Am Coll Cardiol. 1993;21:1687-96.

55. Hunderi JO, Thompson CR, Smiseth OA. Deceleration time of systolic pulmonary venous flow: a new clinical marker of left atrial pressure and compliance. J Appl Physiol. 2006;100:685-9. Epub 2005.

56. Sohn DW, Chai IH, Lee DJ, et al. Assessment of mitral annulus velocity by Doppler tissue imaging in the evaluation of left ventricular diastolic function. J Am Coll Cardiol. 1997;30:474-80.

57. Thomas L, Hoy M, Byth K, et al. The left atrial function index: a rhythm independent marker of atrial function. Eur J Echocardiogr. 2008;9:356-62.

58. Giampaolo Cerisano, Leonardo Bolognese, Nazario Carrabba, et al. Clinical investigation and reports Doppler-derived mitral deceleration time an early strong predictor of left ventricular remodeling after reperfused anterior acute myocardial infarction. Circulation. 1999;99:230-236. doi: 10.1161/01.CIR.99.2.230. © 1999 American Heart Association, Inc.

59. Nagueh SF, Lakkis NM, Middleton KJ, et al. Doppler estimation of left ventricular filling pressures in patients with hypertrophic cardiomyopathy. Circulation. 1999;99:254-61.

60. Wang J, Nagueh SF. Echocardiographic assessment of left ventricular filling pressures. Heart Fail Clin. 2008;4:57-70. Review.

61. Garcia MJ, Ares MA, Asher C, et al. An index of early left ventricular filling that combined with pulsed Doppler peak E velocity may estimate capillary wedge pressure. J Am Coll Cardiol. 1997;29:448-54.

Chapter 15

Ventricular Function—Assessment and Clinical Application

Kanu Chatterjee, Wassef Karrowni, William Parmley

Chapter Outline

INTRODUCTION

Assessment of ventricular mechanical function is essential in clinical cardiology not only for understanding of the pathophysiologic mechanisms of various cardiovascular disorders but also for appropriate management of the dysfunctions and for assessment of prognosis.

The ability to shorten and develop force is the fundamental functional characteristic of cardiac muscle. The performance of the cardiac muscle is influenced by the change in initial muscle length (Frank-Starling mechanism) and in contractility. The determinants of performance of cardiac muscle are initial muscle length (preload), the load against which the muscle shortens (afterload), the contractile state and heart rate.

The same principles and the determinants regulate the performance of the intact ventricles.

Since left ventricle delivers cardiac output to maintain organ perfusion and systemic arterial pressure, more studies have been done to assess left ventricular (LV) function. However right ventricle also plays an important role to maintain appropriate pulmonary blood flow, adequate LV filling and systemic output.

In this chapter, assessments of both right and left ventricular function and clinical implications have been discussed.

DETERMINANTS OF LEFT VENTRICULAR PERFORMANCE

The major determinants of LV performance are preload, afterload, contractile state and heart rate.

PRELOAD

In the isolated muscle the initial muscle length before shortening represents preload. In the intact heart, ventricular wall stress before ejection is regarded as its preload.[1] Wall stress in clinical practice is calculated as follows:

$$\text{Wall stress} = \frac{\text{Ventricular pressure} \times \text{Radius of curvature (volume)}}{2 \times \text{Wall thickness}}$$

It is apparent that wall stress is increased with an increase in intraventricular pressure and ventricular volume and a decrease in wall thickness. In the intact heart preload is represented by the end-diastolic wall stress. The calculation of wall stress is difficult in clinical practice. Frequently ventricular end-diastolic volume or end-diastolic pressure is used to represent its preload. It should be appreciated that LV diastolic pressure can be used as filling pressure only when pressures opposing distention of the ventricles during filling is normal. The transmural pressure is also used as the filling pressure and is calculated as follows:

Transmural pressure = LV diastolic pressure – pericardial and mediastinal pressure. It is apparent that in presence of normal pericardial and mediastinal pressures, LV diastolic pressure can be used as its preload. When intrapericardial pressure is increased as in cardiac tamponade, LV diastolic pressure cannot be used to represent its transmural and filling pressures.

The LV end-diastolic volume can be determined by contrast ventriculography during cardiac catheterization. However, in clinical practice, it is assessed noninvasively by echocardiography, radionuclide angiography, contrast computerized tomography or cardiac magnetic resonance (CMR) imaging. Transthoracic echocardiography is the most frequently employed noninvasive imaging modality to determine LV end-diastolic volume. In the critical care units, it is difficult to use transthoracic echocardiography to measure LV end-diastolic volume frequently. With the advent of balloon floatation catheters, pulmonary capillary wedge pressure (balloon occluded pressure) is frequently used to represent LV end-diastolic pressure and preload.[2] It should be appreciated that pulmonary capillary wedge pressure represents LV end-diastolic pressure only in the absence of mitral valve obstruction.

In patients with normal LV function and in the absence of obstruction to flow between pulmonary artery and left ventricle, pulmonary artery end-diastolic or pulmonary capillary wedge pressures maintain a constant relationship to left atrial and LV diastolic pressure. At end-diastole, pulmonary capillary wedge, left atrial and LV diastolic pressures are equal.[3-6]

The LV diastolic and pulmonary capillary wedge pressures correlates well with LV end-diastolic volume in presence of normal LV compliance.[7,8] When LV compliance is decreased, there is a poor correlation between LV end-diastolic volume and end-diastolic pressure.[7,8]

AFTERLOAD

In the isolated heart muscle, the afterload is defined as the additional load that the muscle faced as it develops force and attempt to shorten. In the intact heart, wall stress during LV isovolumic systole and ejection phases represents its afterload. It should be appreciated that LV wall stress constantly changes during systolic phases as the volume, pressure and wall thickness change. Although peak systolic wall stress can be used to represent LV afterload, it appears that some more integrated measure of overall wall stress during systole is more appropriate and desirable.

The measurement of changing systolic wall stress is thus difficult in clinical practice and the alternative measures of afterload are frequently used. Aortic instantaneous impedance is another index of LV afterload, which is less dependent on preload. Aortic impedance comprises of pulsatile reactive component and a static resistive (mean) component of the vascular loads. The dominant component of the impedance is systemic vascular resistance. However, the compliance of the aorta and the larger arteries and the branching characteristics of the arterial system which generates reflected waves contribute substantially to aortic input impedance, also difficult to measure in routine clinical practice.[9-12] Aortic input impedance can be estimated from LV pressure-volume loop. The end-systolic pressure/stroke volume (Pes/SV) ratio which is termed effective arterial elastance (Ea) has been used as an estimate of aortic impedance.[13]

Aortic pressure can be used as LV afterload as the left ventricle has to eject its stroke volume against aortic systolic pressure. Another measure of LV afterload is systemic vascular resistance which is calculated as follows:

$$\text{Systemic vascular resistance} = \frac{\text{Mean arterial pressure (mm Hg)} - \text{Mean right atrial pressure (mm Hg)}}{\text{Cardiac output (l/min)}}$$

In patients with systemic hypertension, systemic vascular resistance is increased primarily due to increased arterial pressure. In patients with systolic heart failure, however, systemic vascular resistance may increase even without hypertension primarily due to peripheral arterial vasoconstriction. It should be appreciated that these indices are only indirect measures of afterload and the true afterload is LV wall stress.

VENTRICULAR-ARTERIAL COUPLING

The matching of systolic force generated by the heart to the vascular load during each ejection is termed "ventricular-arterial coupling". The interactions of these two components influence several hemodynamic functions such as cardiac output, arterial pressure, ejection fraction, and mechanical work and efficiency. Left ventricular-arterial coupling also influences LV systolic and diastolic function. Changes in arterial stiffening is associated with changes in LV end-systolic chamber stiffness.[14,15] Increased arterial stiffening increases LV end-systolic stress which can occur irrespective of LV hypertrophy.[14,15] Ventricular-arterial coupling also influences the adaptation of the cardiovascular system in response to stress such as exercise.

Ventricular-arterial coupling is often determined from LV pressure-volume loops. The pressure-volume loops are constructed by relating ventricular pressure and volume throughout the cardiac cycle (Fig. 1). Several loops can be constructed during transient reduction of preload, for example by venacaval inflow obstruction by balloon catheter. The end-systolic pressure volume relation (ESPVR) and its slope are determined. The ventricular-arterial coupling is expressed as the ratio of the Ea/ESPVR slope. The optimal ventricular arterial performance is observed when the ratio is 1.0 or close to 1.0.[16,17]

CONTRACTILE STATE

In the isolated cardiac myocyte, the contractile state refers to the rate of actin myosin interaction with fixed preload and afterload. In the intact heart it is difficult to measure contractility and various indices have been proposed; however, none of these indices have been proven to be entirely satisfactory. In clinical practice it is easier to measure indices of pump function which appears to have a greater clinical applicability.

MEASURES OF MAXIMUM RATE OF PRESSURE DEVELOPMENT

The maximum rate of force development (dF/dt) has been documented as a useful index of cardiac muscle contractility. With a constant preload, dF/dt reflects a reliable measurement of contractility.

Extrapolation of this concept to measure contractile state of the left ventricle, the maximum rate of pressure development (dP/dt) has been used.[18] It should be appreciated that there are a number of limitations for the use of dP/dt to assess contractile state of left ventricle. The maximal dP/dt is influenced by changes in LV end-diastolic pressure and the level of the arterial pressure at the time of the opening of the aortic valve. The maximal dP/dt is also influenced by the heart rate.

However, the maximal dP/dt can be used as an index of contractility if the heart rate, LV end-diastolic pressure and aortic pressure remain unchanged.

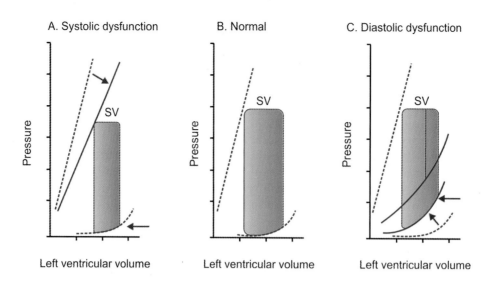

FIGURE 1: Left ventricular pressure-volume relation. Diastolic filling starts with the opening of the mitral valve. At the end of diastole the mitral valve closes and the isovolumic systole begins. During this phase there is an increase in left ventricular pressure without any change in volume. At the end of isovolumic systole, the aortic valve opens and left ventricle ejects its stroke volume into aorta. At the end of ejection the aortic valve closes and the isovolumic relaxation phase begins. During this phase, left ventricular pressure falls without any change in its volume. At the end of isovolumic relaxation phase, the mitral valve opens and the cardiac cycle is repeated. At the end of ejection, the end-systolic pressure terminates on the isovolumic pressure line. With increased contractility, the end-systolic pressure-volume line shifts to the left and upward. With decreased contractile function it shifts downward and to the right. In diastolic heart failure the diastolic pressure-volume curve shifts upward and to the left. This is associated with an increase in left ventricular diastolic pressure and patients may experience of symptoms of pulmonary venous congestion. With a further upward and leftward shift of the diastolic pressure-volume curve, there is also restriction of ventricular filling which is associated with decreased stroke volume

The LV dP/dt is usually measured invasively in the cardiac catheterization laboratory during diagnostic or interventional cardiac catheterization; however, it can be measured non-invasively by echocardiography.[19] Echocardiographic and Doppler studies were performed simultaneously with cardiac catheterization. The maximal LV dP/dt was determined both invasively and noninvasively. In this study, 30 patients undergoing clinically indicated LV catheterization were investigated. Between invasive and noninvasive techniques there was a statistically significant correlation between the measured maximal dP/dt. The noninvasively determined maximal dP/dt was found to be independent of preload and afterload and correlated well to the changes in contractility. The mitral regurgitant velocity spectrum can be used to measure LV maximal dP/dt and the relaxation time constant.[20] In 12 patients with mitral regurgitation, the Doppler mitral regurgitant velocity spectrum was recorded concurrently with LV pressure pulse with the use of micromanometer catheter. The correlation coefficient between the catheter derived and the Doppler derived maximal dP/dt was excellent (r = 0.91). There was also an excellent correlation between the catheter derived and the Doppler derived relaxation time constant (r = 0.93).

Doppler myocardial imaging has been employed to assess LV contractile reserve during dobutamine infusion.[21] In this study, 25 patients with non-ischemic dilated cardiomyopathy with left ventricular ejection fraction (LVEF) of less than 30% were investigated. The peak systolic velocity was measured in the basal segment of the septum and the inferior wall, and LVEF was measured concurrently. The peak systolic velocity and LVEF increased during dobutamine infusion. There was a significant and linear correlation between the changes in peak systolic velocity and ejection fraction. The results of this study

suggest that Doppler myocardial imaging can be used to assess LV contractile reserve.

It has been suggested that the isovolumic acceleration measured by tissue Doppler echocardiography can be used to assess LV global contractile function and it appears not to be influenced by changes in preload.[22]

Systolic time intervals, such as pre-ejection period (PEP) and left ventricular ejection time (LVET) and the ratio of PEP/LVET, have been used to assess LV contractile function. Systolic time intervals can be measured by echocardiographic techniques. In a multicenter study, LVEF, maximal dP/dt, LV stroke volume, PEP, LVET and PEP/LVET ratio were measured prospectively in 134 consecutive patients with systolic heart failure and 43 normal control subjects by pulsed Doppler echocardiography.[21] The PEP/LVET ratio increased with increased LVEF and there was a significant positive correlation. Using the receiver operating curve analyses, for PEP/LVET ratio, the area under the curve was 0.91 which allowed detection of LVEF of less than 35% with a specificity of 84% and sensitivity of 87%. Thus, measurement of systolic time intervals may be useful for assessment of LV contractile function. It should be appreciated however that PEP is influenced by developed pressure. In patients with severe heart failure, the developed pressure may be very low, causing disproportionate changes in PEP, LVET and the PEP/LVET ratio.[23] Furthermore, in the most echo-cardiographic laboratories, this index of contractile function with measurement of systolic intervals is not routinely measured.

VELOCITY OF CONTRACTILE ELEMENT

In the isolated myocyte or papillary muscle studies, velocity of the contractile element reflects a reliable index of contractility.

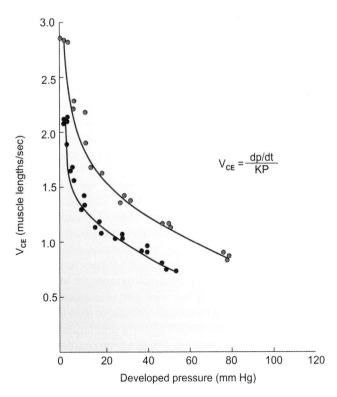

$$V_{CE} = \frac{dp/dt}{KP}$$

FIGURE 2: Calculated pressure-velocity relation (VCE) in relation to developed pressure and before or after coronary artery bypass surgery demonstrating an upward and rightward shift after coronary artery bypass surgery indicating improved contractile function

In the intact human left ventricle, overall mean contractile element velocity (VCE) can be measured from the simultaneously recorded LV pressure pulse and its first derivative (dP/dt) using the formula VCE = dP/dt/KP (where P is the developed pressure and K is the series elastic constant). It should be appreciated that the measurement of VCE in the intact beating human heart is not precise. Usually the VCE at 5 mm Hg developed pressure is used to measure as an approximation of maximal velocity of contraction. Myocardial ischemia is a potent cause of depressed contractile function. Relief of ischemia following coronary artery bypass graft surgery is associated with a right and upward shift of the pressure velocity curves (Fig. 2).[24] These findings suggest that it is feasible to measure LV contractile function in the cardiac catheterization laboratory applying the three-element mechanical model used in the isolated papillary muscles.[25,26] Other indices of contractility have been developed from the measurements of rate of rise of LV pressure and the developed pressure.[27] It has been suggested that (dP/dt)/P at different levels of developed pressure can be used to assess LV contractility.[27] It should be appreciated that for measurements of these contractile indices, in the intact heart, high-fidelity micromanometer tip catheters should be used.

In the intact heart, LV contractility can be measured by determining the maximum rate of flow velocity (acceleration) in the ascending aorta.[28]

Aortic flow during systole is LV stroke volume which is influenced by changes in preload and afterload. Any index of contractility dependent on measurement of stroke volume is also influenced by changes in preload and afterload. In the modern echocardiographic laboratories, Doppler echocardiography can

be employed to measure aortic flow. Transthoracic echocardiography and simultaneous measurement of blood pressure allows normalization of aortic flow for preload and afterload.

The LV ejection rate normalized for end-diastolic volume (EDV) can be used to assess LV contractile state.[29,30] The LVEF is calculated from the ratio of LV total stroke volume (TSV) and EDV. To calculate normalized ejection rate, LVEF is divided by left ventricular end-diastolic volume (LVEDV). Normalized ejection rate is best calculated from a volume-time curve. The normalized ejection rate is decreased in patients with systolic heart failure compared to normal subjects. The ejection rate can be measured invasively by contrast ventriculography or noninvasively such as radionuclide ventriculography.

LEFT VENTRICULAR PUMP FUNCTION

VENTRICULAR FUNCTION CURVE

The construction of ventricular function curve provides useful information about ventricular performance. In clinical practice, stroke volume or stroke work (vertical axis) is plotted against a measure of preload such as EDV or end-diastolic pressure (horizontal axis) (Fig. 3). In the critical care units, pulmonary capillary wedge pressure (pulmonary artery occluded pressure) is frequently used as LV preload. When LV volume or pressure is increased, as during volume expansion therapy, the stroke volume increases by the Frank-Starling mechanism. When right ventricular function is assessed, right atrial pressure is used as its preload. The optimal LV filling pressure is usually 15–20 mm Hg.[31] The optimal filling pressure of the right ventricle is 3–8 mm Hg. As discussed earlier right atrial or pulmonary capillary wedge pressures can be used as their filling pressures only in presence of normal pericardial and mediastinal pressures.

The ventricular function curve shifts upward and to the left with the improvement of ventricular function, and downward and to the right, when it is depressed. In many clinical situations there is a disparity between changes in right and left ventricular function. For example, in patients with acute or chronic isolated

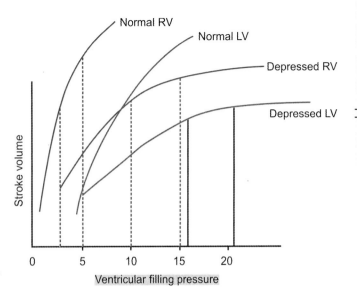

FIGURE 3: Ventricular function curves constructed relating stroke volume (vertical axis) to the ventricular filling pressures (horizontal axis) (Abbreviations: RV: Right ventricle; LV: Left ventricle)

right ventricular failure (right ventricular myocardial infarction or pre-capillary pulmonary hypertension), right ventricular filling pressure is elevated and right ventricular function curve shifts downward and to the right; however, LF filling pressure and function curve remain unchanged. In contrast, in patients with isolated acute or chronic LV failure (LV myocardial infarction or dilated cardiomyopathy), LV filling pressure is elevated and its function curve shifts downward and to the right.[32] When the changes in the right and left ventricular functions are not parallel, treatments to improve right or left ventricular function may be associated with worsening function of the contralateral ventricle. For example, in patients with depressed LV function with normal right ventricular function, volume loading to correct hypotension may precipitate pulmonary edema. In presence of depressed LV function with a flat LV function curve, the pulmonary capillary wedge pressure is already elevated and during volume loading, there is an excessive increase in pulmonary capillary wedge pressure which induces pulmonary edema. It should also be appreciated that in presence of very depressed LV systolic function the magnitude of increase in stroke volume is relatively small with an increase in end-diastolic volume during volume loading therapy compared to when LV systolic function is preserved. For example, in patients with systolic heart failure, when LV end-diastolic volume is increased by timed atrial contraction, stroke volume increases only slightly compared to the patients with normal ejection fraction, when there is a substantial increase in stroke volume with a similar increase in EDV.[33]

EJECTION FRACTION

In clinical practice, ejection fraction is most commonly used index to assess LV pump function. As discussed earlier, ejection fraction is the ratio of left ventricular total stroke volume (LVSV) and end-diastolic volume (EDV) and it can be measured by various invasive and noninvasive methods. The normal ejection fraction has not been clearly defined and it varies with age, gender and the loading conditions. For clinical purposes, 55% ejection fraction is used to distinguish between diastolic and systolic heart failure. In many clinical studies, an ejection fraction of 45% has been used to separate between heart failure with preserved and reduced ejection fraction.

It should be appreciated that ejection fraction is load dependent. Thus, at the time of measurement of ejection fraction, the loading conditions should be considered. For example, if the blood pressure is high, the ejection fraction will be lower when the blood pressure is reduced.

The LV stroke volume may remain normal not only at rest but also during exercise even when the ejection fraction is markedly reduced. This is accomplished by a markedly increased LVEDV.

TECHNIQUES FOR ASSESSMENT OF LEFT VENTRICULAR EJECTION FRACTION

Echocardiography

Two-dimensional (2D) echocardiography is the most frequently used technique for measurement of LVEF. The visual assessment of LVEF has poor reproducibility. Also, there is a wide variation in the reproducibility of the quantitative measurements of LV global and regional function.[34] In ten healthy subjects, two experienced echocardiographers performed 20 complete echo-Doppler studies. The inter-observer reproducibility was better in the measurements of systolic M-mode annulus excursion than other traditional and newer indices of LV systolic and diastolic function. The quantitative measurements by 2D transthoracic echocardiography using biplane methods can introduce errors in estimation of ejection fraction due to underestimation of LVEVD.[35] To reduce the errors, echocardiography with the use of ultrasound contrast agents have been introduced.[36,37] The use of contrast agent allows a clearer delineation of the LV endocardium. Measurements of LV volumes and ejection fraction by 2D transthoracic echocardiography with contrast agents have a better agreement with other imaging modalities such as CMR imaging and radionuclide ventriculography.[38] Myocardial contrast echocardiography has been used to assess hibernating myocardium and has been compared to single photon emission computed tomography (SPECT).[39] In a preliminary study of 39 patients with ischemic heart disease, myocardial contrast echocardiography was found to be superior in predicting the recovery of LV function. It should be appreciated that the use of ultrasound contrast agents are contra indicated in patients with intra-cardiac shunts.

Three-dimensional real time echocardiography (3DE) with or without the use of ultrasound contrast agents are being increasingly used to measure LV volumes and ejection fraction. The determination of LV volumes by 3DE does not require any geometric assumption. The determinations of LV volumes by 3DE have a low intra- and inter-observer variability and good agreements with other imaging modalities, such as CMR, have been observed.[40] Three-dimensional speckle tracking echocardiographic technique has been used to assess regional LV function.[41] In 32 subjects with or without LV dysfunction, 3DE and 2DE speckle tracking echocardiography was performed concurrently. In this study, 3DE speckle tracking was superior to 2DE speckle tracking echocardiography to measure regional wall motion indices (please see the chapter "Three Dimensional Echocardiography").

Cardiac Computed Tomography

Cardiac computed tomography (CCT) can be used for measurement of LV volumes and ejection fraction. Most frequently multislice multiphase CCT with the use of contrast agent is employed to assess LV volumes and ejection fraction. The measurement of LV volumes by CCT does not require geometric assumption. There is also a good agreement between CCT, CMR, echocardiography and contrast ventriculography for the measurements of LV volumes and ejection fraction.[42]

Assessment of LV volumes and ejection fraction with 320-row multidetector computed tomography has been performed and compared to 2D echocardiographic imaging.[43] In this study, the 320-row multidetector CCT and 2D echocardiography were performed in 114 patients concurrently. There was an excellent correlation between the two imaging techniques. Thus, an accurate assessment of LV function is feasible with a single cardiac cycle 320-row multidetector CCT.

The contrast CCT can be used to assess right ventricular volumes and function. It can also be used for the diagnosis of coronary artery anomalies and to assess the severity of coronary artery obstruction.

It should be appreciated that CCT is associated with radiation exposure and, when contrast agent is used, it can induce contrast nephropathy (please see the chapter "Cardiac Computed Tomography").

Nuclear Scintigraphy

A number of radionuclide scintigraphic techniques can be employed for the measurement of ventricular volumes and ejection fraction.

The gated equilibrium radionuclide angiography and first-pass radionuclide angiography can be used for assessment of both right and left ventricular volumes and ejection fraction. These nuclear scintigraphic techniques do not require geometric assumptions.[44,45]

In clinical practice, however, LV volumes and ejection fraction are determined more frequently, during gated SPECT and positron emission tomography (PET) usually used for detection of presence and the severity of myocardial ischemia and viability.[46] The PET appears to have advantages over SPECT due to better spatial and temporal resolution. The gated blood-pool SPECT has been compared to CMR in assessing LV volumes and ejection fraction.[47] In this study, 55 consecutive patients were investigated. The correlation coefficients between these two techniques in measuring LV end-diastolic and end-systolic volumes were r = 96 and 92 respectively. For determination of LVEF it was 0.84.[47] It should be appreciated that nuclear imaging techniques are associated with radiation exposure.

Cardiac Magnetic Resonance Imaging

The CMR imaging can be used to measure LV volumes and ejection fraction. The measurement of LVEF by CMR has several advantages. It is not associated with radiation exposure. It has also high temporal and spatial resolution. The measurement of LV volume by CMR does not depend on geometric assumptions. The CMR is used as the reference technique for measurement of ventricular volumes and ejection fraction[48] (please see the chapter "Magnetic Resonance Imaging").

Left ventricular volumes and ejection fraction measured by CMR were compared to those measured by monoplane cine ventriculography and unenhanced echocardiography.[48a]

There were good agreements between these three techniques are discussed in Table 1.

TABLE 1

LV volumes and EF determined by the different imaging techniques

	Cine	Echo	MRI
EDV (ml)	184.78 ± 69.77	159.90 ± 54.00	177.10 ± 73.50
ESV (ml)	53.53 ± 50.62	71.97 ± 44.74	73.82 ± 54.93
EF (%)	73.28 ± 17.22	57.49 ± 12.41	61.43 ± 14.34
(Source: Published with permission from Reference 48a)			

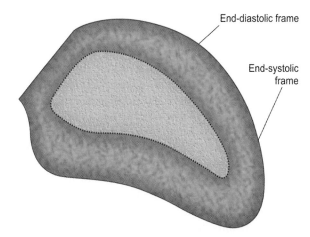

FIGURE 4: Schematic illustration of contrast ventriculography to determine left ventricular ejection fraction. The EDV is determined by outlining the end-diastolic frame. The end-systolic volume is determined by outlining the end-systolic frame

Contrast Ventriculography

Contrast ventriculography is usually performed during cardiac catheterization. The injection of contrast agent into the cavity of left ventricle allows measurement of LV volumes and ejection fraction. Most frequently biplane methods are used. The LV cineangiograms are obtained at a high speed (30–60 frames/sec). The endocardial edge detection and calculation of LV volumes and ejection fraction are done by automated computerized techniques (Fig. 4).

PRESSURE-VOLUME RELATIONS

The pressure-volume relation is one of the precise methods for the assessment of LV systolic and diastolic functions in the intact heart as illustrated in the Figure 1. During diastole with the opening of the mitral valve, LV filling begins. Most of the ventricular filling occurs during the early rapid filling phase. During atrial contraction, there is further ventricular filling. At the end of diastole, the isovolumic phase of ventricular systole begins and during this phase the LV pressure rises without any change in its volume. Following opening of the aortic valve, the ejection phase starts. Initially the ejection is rapid and then it is slower till the aortic valve closes. Following closure of the aortic valve, the isovolumic relaxation phase begins. During this phase LV pressure declines without any change in its volume till the mitral valve opens and the rapid filling phase begins. The pressure-volume loop is counterclockwise. The area inside the pressure-volume loop represents LV stroke work. Stroke work is calculated by the formula:

Stroke work = Stroke volume × (Mean LV systolic ejection pressure – Mean LV diastolic pressure)

In clinical practice, mean arterial pressure is used instead of mean LV systolic ejection pressure, and mean pulmonary capillary wedge pressure is used to represent mean LV diastolic pressure, for calculation of stroke work. The stroke work index is calculated by dividing the stroke work by the body surface area to normalize for the size of the patients. In critical care units, LV function is assessed by relating stroke work index to the pulmonary capillary wedge pressure.

The construction of the pressure-volume loops allows a more precise load independent measurement of LV contractile function. When a number of pressure-volume loops are constructed by increasing or decreasing LV volumes the endpoint of systolic contraction of each loop tends to fall on the same line which is termed the isovolumic pressure line. In the intact heart, the endpoint of systolic contraction is recognized by the crossing point of dicrotic notch pressure and end-systolic volume. The isovolumic pressure line does not appear to be influenced by changes in afterload or preload.[49] With changes in contractile state however there is shifts of the isovolumic pressure-volume line; with increased contractility the isovolumic pressure line shifts upward and to the left and with decreased contractility, it shifts downward and to the right. It should be appreciated that there are a few limitations in using the isovolumic pressure-volume line as a totally load independent index of contractility. The isovolumic pressure-volume line may shift upward and to the left without any changes in intrinsic contractility, when the LV systolic pressure is higher than normal as in patients with hypertension or aortic stenosis. In these patients, end-systolic volumes may also be lower than normal; thus the end-systolic pressure/volume ratio is increased as occurs when the contractility is increased. In patients with relatively lower end-systolic pressures as following use of vasodilators or in patients with severe chronic aortic regurgitation, the isovolumic pressure-volume line may shift downward and to the right as when intrinsic contractility is decreased. In these clinical circumstances, the end-systolic pressure/volume ratio may also decrease without any change in intrinsic contractility. In presence of significant mitral regurgitation, there is no isovolumic systole and thus the isovolumic pressure-volume index cannot be used to assess contractility. However, despite these limitations, the uses of pressure-volume loops remain an important method of determining LV contractility. In some studies, peak systolic pressure/end-systolic volume ratio has been used to assess contractility and appears that it is practical and can be determined noninvasively.[50] The peak systolic pressure can be measured by measuring cuff blood pressure, and end-systolic volume can be measured by noninvasive imaging techniques such as transthoracic echocardiography.

HEART RATE

Heart rate is a major determinant for cardiac performance. Cardiac output is the product of the heart rate and stroke volume, and the higher the heart rate, higher is the cardiac output. However, an excessive increase in heart rate may compromise ventricular filling and decrease stroke volume. It should also be appreciated that left ventricle is perfused during diastole. Thus a marked increase in heart rate is associated with decreased LV perfusion time. Heart rate is also a major determinant of myocardial oxygen demand, and faster heart rate increases myocardial oxygen demand.[51] Impaired LV perfusion and a concomitant increase in myocardial oxygen demand may induce myocardial ischemia and decrease contractile function.

Normally an increase in heart rate is associated with an increased force of contraction.[51] This phenomenon is defined as a positive force-frequency relation. Noninvasive techniques, such as tissue Doppler imaging, have been used to assess changes in contractility with changes in heart rate.[52] Myocardial acceleration during isovolumic systole was used to measure contractility. The LV maximal dP/dt was also measured by micromanometer catheter. In this study, there was a positive correlation between heart rate and myocardial acceleration during isovolumic systole and maximal dP/dt. As heart rate increased, both indices of contractility increased. In other studies using maximal dP/dt as a measure of contractility, the positive force-frequency relation has been demonstrated.[53]

Effects of changes in heart rate have been investigated in failing and non-failing explanted human hearts.[54] In the non-failing hearts, contractility increased with increased heart rates. In the failing hearts, however, increasing heart rate was associated with a decrease in force of contraction which is termed inverse force-frequency relation. The alterations of the force frequency relation in failing heart are more pronounced in patients with more severe heart failure.[54a] In the study by Schmidt et al., myocardium from explanted human heart of patients with end stage systolic heart failure (NYHA IV) (ejection fraction 24 ± 2%), patients with mitral valve disease with mild to moderately severe heart failure (NYHA II-III), (ejection fraction 55.9 ± 2.9%) and normal non-failing heart from donor hearts were studied. There were 22 patients in NYHA IV group; 10 patients in the NYHA II-III group and 5 patients in the non-failing group. Myocardial biopsy specimens in patients with mitral valve disease were obtained during mitral valve replacements surgery. Myocardial force generation during increasing frequency of stimulation was markedly reduced in NYHA IV patients compared to control. It was mildly reduced in the myocardium of patients NYHA II-III heart failure (Table 2). There was also downregulation of the beta-adreno-receptors in the myocardium of the failing hearts. It has been reported in patients with non-ischemic or ischemic dilated cardiomyopathy, that during increased heart rate left ventricular maximal dP/dt declines and it has been thought to be due to myocardial beta-adrenergic dysfunction.[54b] Altered handling of intracellular calcium has been demonstrated as the potential mechanism of the inverse force-frequency relation in human dilated cardiomyopathy.[55] In patients with severe systolic heart failure, a reduction in heart rate may be associated with an increase in force development and contractile state. This might be a contributory mechanism for the beneficial effect of beta blocker therapy in patients with systolic heart failure.

In patients with diastolic heart failure the force-frequency relation remains normal but the relaxation-frequency relation

TABLE 2

Force-frequency relation in human left ventricular papillary muscle strips from non-failing heart (12 preparations), NYHA II-III (18 preparations) and NYHA IV (39 preparations) are summarized

Frequency (HZ)	Non-failing (FOC mN)	NYHA II-III (FOC mN)	NYHA IV (FOC mN)
0.5	1.7 ± 0.2	2.3 ± 0.1	2.4 ± 0.2
1.5	2.7 ± 0.3	2.6 ± 0.1	2.0 ± 0.1
3	3.0 ± 0.2	2.0 ± 0.1	1.4 ± 0.1

(Abbreviation: FOC: Force of contraction). (*Source:* Modified from Reference. 54a and published with permission from Schmidt U et al. AM J Cardiol. 1994;74:1066-8)

is impaired.[55a,55b] The time constant of left ventricular relaxation (minimal negative dP/dt) is decreased.

DIASTOLIC FUNCTION

Diastolic function is an important determinant of hemodynamic abnormalities of heart failure. Diastolic function can be assessed from studies of the pressure-volume relations during diastole (Fig. 1). The diastolic pressure-volume curve is exponential which indicates that, when the patient is on the flat portion of the curve, there is less change in pressure with a given change in volume. When the patient is on the steep portion of curve, there is much greater increase in pressure for the same change in volume.

The LV compliance or distensibility is altered in many pathologic conditions. Decreased compliance (increased stiffness) is associated with an upward and leftward shift of the diastolic pressure-volume relation. For a given increase in diastolic volume, there is a disproportionate increase in LV diastolic pressure. There is a passive increase in left atrial and pulmonary venous pressure which may precipitate pulmonary edema. If ventricular filling is also compromised due to a marked upward shift of the diastolic pressure-volume relation, stroke volume decreases and cardiac output may also decline. Along with increase in pulmonary venous pressure, pulmonary artery pressure increases which may cause right heart failure due to increased right ventricular afterload.

Increased diastolic stiffness may be caused by LV hypertrophy. In patients with hypertension, there is not only increase in LV mass but also in myocyte thickness. There is also myocardial fibrosis. Increased fibrosis occurs not only in hypertensive hearts but also in the hearts of patients with diastolic and systolic heart failure. Diastolic dysfunction contributes to the hemodynamic abnormalities in both systolic and diastolic heart failure. Decreased LV diastolic compliance may occur both acutely and chronically.

An acute increase in LV afterload causes an upward and leftward shift of the diastolic pressure-volume curve.[56] Acute changes in the diastolic pressure-volume relation can also occur in patients with ischemia during angina.[57]

Pericardial constraining effect also decreases LV compliance. In patients with acute right ventricular infarction, right ventricular dilatation is associated with increased intra-pericardial pressure as the pericardium cannot stretch acutely. The pericardial constraining effect impairs ventricular filling and cardiac output declines. During acute volume expansion, pericardial constraining effect causes upward and leftward shift of the LV diastolic pressure-volume curve.[58] In constrictive pericarditis also, pericardial constraining effect shifts diastolic pressure-volume curve upward and produces similar hemodynamic abnormalities. It should be appreciated that increased myocardial stiffness is a major mechanism of diastolic dysfunction independent of pericardial constraining effect.

The interaction between the intracardiac chambers also alters diastolic function.[59] In patients with pre-capillary pulmonary hypertension and enlarged right atrium and right ventricle, inter-atrial and inter-ventricular septum shift toward the left atrium and left ventricle and left atrial and LV volumes are decreased with a concomitant increase in their diastolic pressures. In patients with severe LV systolic heart failure with markedly enlarged left ventricle, right ventricular volume decreases due to the rightward shift of the inter-ventricular septum with consequent decrease in right ventricular compliance.

In certain clinical conditions LV diastolic compliance is increased. The diastolic pressure-volume curve shifts to the right as in patients with chronic aortic regurgitation and primary mitral regurgitation. In these conditions, even with a substantial increase in LV diastolic volume there is very little increase in diastolic pressure and these patients remain asymptomatic even during exercise.

TECHNIQUES OF MEASUREMENT OF DIASTOLIC FUNCTION

Conventionally assessment of LV compliance by measurements of LV pressure-volume relation has been performed by invasive techniques during cardiac catheterization. During cardiac catheterization it is also possible to determine the negative dP/dt and the time constant of the LV pressure decay (tau). With decreased compliance the values of negative dP/dt and tau are decreased. The LV diastolic function however can be assessed by noninvasive techniques.[60]

Echocardiography

Echo-Doppler methods are most frequently employed to assess LV diastolic function. Determination of isovolumic relaxation time provides insight about diastolic functional properties. In patients with impaired LV relaxation, the isovolumic relaxation time is prolonged. It should be appreciated that the isovolumic relaxation time is influenced by changes in preload.

The mitral inflow patterns are frequently employed to assess LV diastolic function by Doppler echocardiography. The early filling of left ventricle is termed "E" wave and filling during atrial systole is termed "A" wave. When LV compliance is decreased, the "E/A" ratio is decreased. Tissue Doppler mitral annular motion appears to be a more load independent index of diastolic function.[61] The mitral valve moves away from the apex in early diastole resulting in 'e' wave. During late diastole during atrial contraction there is an 'a' wave. When there is significant diastolic dysfunction, the 'E/e' ratio increases. The pulmonary vein flow patterns, the propagation velocity of the wave front of LV filling and other echocardiographic indices can be used to assess LV diastolic function (please see the chapter "Transthoracic Echocardiography").

Nuclear Scintigraphy

Radionuclide ventriculography and gated SPECT can be used to measure indices of diastolic function. The time-count curves or time-volume curves are constructed and time to peak filling rate and peak filling rates are calculated. Diastolic dysfunction is associated with increased time to peak filling and decreased peak filling[62,63] (please see the chapter "Nuclear Imaging").

Cardiac Magnetic Resonance Imaging

Similar to nuclear scintigraphy CMR can be used to construct LV time-volume curve and filling rate can be measured to assess

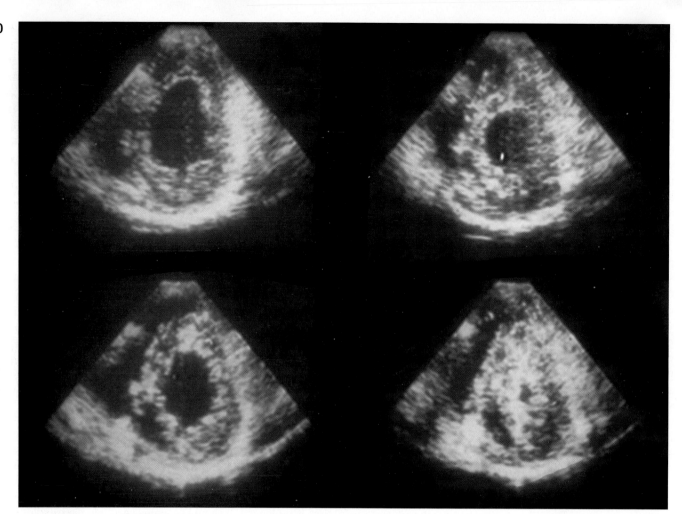

FIGURE 5: The transthoracic echocardiographic images in the short-axis view during exercise. During exercise left ventricular volumes decrease and calculated ejection fraction increases

diastolic function.[64,65] The CMR can also be used to measure diastolic flow across the mitral valve and pulmonary veins flow (please see the chapter "Cardiac Magnetic Resonance").

LEFT VENTRICULAR FUNCTIONAL ASSESSMENT DURING STRESS

Assessment of LV function during stress is useful to determine patient's functional capacity and LV reserve.[66] In clinical practice, noninvasive tests, such as treadmill exercise test with or without nuclear imaging, and exercise or dobutamine stress echocardiography (Fig. 5), are most commonly used. During stress tests the severity of symptoms and the level of exercise that induces symptoms are observed.

RIGHT VENTRICULAR FUNCTION

The right ventricle has complex geometry and anatomic features which are different from that of left ventricle. Normally it is a thin-walled structure and the thickness of the free wall of the right ventricle is less than 4 mm. It has a pyramidal shape and has three anatomic areas: (1) the inflow region formed by the tricuspid valve apparatus; (2) the trabeculated apical and the free wall and (3) the outflow region.[67] During right ventricular systole, the tricuspid valve annular descent is followed by contraction of apical, free wall and outflow tract segments. In the absence of tricuspid or mitral valve regurgitation and intracardiac shunts, right and left ventricular stroke volume is the same. Normally right ventricular afterload is lower than that of left ventricle primarily due to lower pulmonary artery pressure and pulmonary vascular resistance compared to systemic arterial pressure and systemic vascular resistance. Due to lower afterload, right ventricle can eject the same stroke volume as that of left ventricle but at a lower level of work.[67-69]

Right ventricular function can be assessed by both invasive and noninvasive techniques. In the critical care units, right ventricular function curve is constructed by correlating right ventricular stroke work to right ventricular filling pressure. Right ventricular filling pressure is determined by measuring right atrial pressure. Determination of right ventricular stroke work requires measurement of pulmonary artery pressure, pulmonary capillary wedge pressure and stroke volume. With the use of balloon floatation catheters, the determinants of the right ventricular stroke work can be estimated in the critical care units at the bedside. The right ventricular stroke work is calculated by the formula:

$$\frac{\text{Mean pulmonary artery pressure} - \text{Mean pulmonary capillary wedge pressure}}{\text{Right ventricular stroke volume}}$$

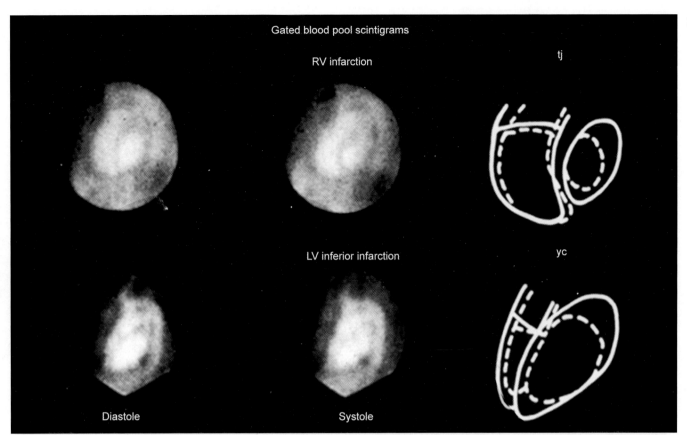

FIGURE 6: Gated blood pool scintigraphy in a patient with right ventricular infarction showing increased right ventricular end-diastolic and end-systolic volumes. Left ventricular volumes remain normal. In a patient with inferior wall myocardial infarction without right ventricular involvement, right and left ventricular volumes remain normal

With the improvement of right ventricular function the right ventricular function curve shifts upward and to the left. With the deterioration of right ventricular function, right ventricular stroke work declines even with an increase in right ventricular filling pressure (Fig. 3).

Right ventricular function can also be assessed by a number of noninvasive techniques. Different radionuclide techniques can be employed to evaluate right ventricular volumes and ejection fraction.[68,69]

Radionuclide ventriculography has been employed to assess right ventricular volumes and ejection fraction. The first pass, equilibrium and gated blood-pool SPECT can be used to estimate right ventricular volumes and ejection fraction. For example, in patients with acute right ventricular myocardial infarction, right ventricle is dilated and its ejection fraction is decreased (Fig. 6). In patients with inferior myocardial infarction, without involvement of the right ventricle, right ventricle is not dilated and its ejection fraction remains normal.

The equilibrium or first pass radionuclide ventriculography has been employed to assess right ventricular function.[70] The SPECT/PET techniques may also be used for determination of right ventricular volumes and ejection fraction.[71]

In clinical practice, echocardiography is most frequently used imaging technique to evaluate right ventricular function.[72] Two-dimensional transthoracic echocardiography allows qualitative assessment of right ventricular volumes and function. It is also useful for the diagnosis of the etiology of right ventricular dysfunction. For example, in patients with right ventricular failure due to severe precapillary pulmonary

hypertension right ventricle is dilated and right ventricular ejection fraction is reduced (Fig. 7). Doppler-echocardiography can be used concurrently to measure the severity of pulmonary hypertension.

Two-dimensional and Doppler-echocardiography can also be used for quantitative assessment of right ventricular volumes and ejection fraction. Measurement of right ventricular functional area and tricuspid annular plane systolic excursion provides a quantitative measure of right ventricular systolic function.[73] The measurement of right ventricular myocardial performance index by Doppler-echocardiography is also used for quantitative assessment of right ventricular systolic function.[74]

Right ventricular function can also be assessed non-invasively by measuring right ventricular myocardial acceleration during isovolumic systole, using tissue Doppler imaging.[75] Three-dimensional echocardiography is being increasingly employed for quantitative assessment of right ventricular volumes and function. Right ventricular volumes and ejection fraction measured by three-dimensional echocardiography correlate well with the values determined by CMR imaging.[76] In a study of 25 patients with postoperative severe pulmonary regurgitation, three-dimensional echocardiography and CMR imaging were performed. There was a significant positive correlation in right ventricular volumes and ejection fraction determined by the two techniques.[77]

The multidetector CCT has been used for assessment of right ventricular volumes and function. However, cardiac magnetic resonance (CMR) imaging is currently employed for accurate

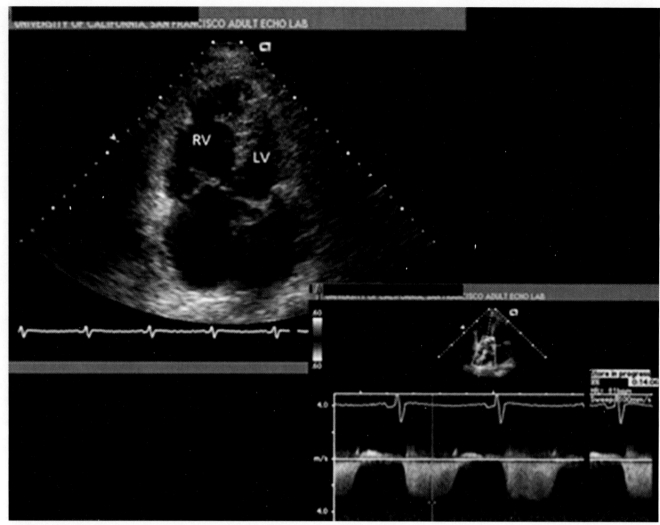

FIGURE 7: Transthoracic two-dimensional echocardiography in a patient with precapillary pulmonary hypertension is illustrated. Right ventricular volume is increased with a shift of the interventricular septum toward the left ventricle. Doppler echocardiographic studies reveal pulmonary arterial hypertension

quantitative assessment of right ventricular volumes and ejection fraction. The three imaging techniques—CMR imaging, multidetector CCT and three-dimensional echocardiography—were compared, and CMR imaging yielded the most accurate values for right ventricular volumes and ejection fraction.[78]

CONCLUSION

Assessment of left and right ventricular function is essential for understanding of the pathophysiologic mechanisms of various cardiac disorders. In clinical studies, LVEF is routinely employed to distinguish between systolic and diastolic heart failure. Assessment of left and right ventricular functions is also used to assess response to therapy. In critical care units, hemodynamic measurements of left and right ventricular functions are useful of selection of therapies and response to therapy.

REFERENCES

1. Mirsky I. Elastic properties of the myocardium: a quantitative approach with physiological and clinical applications. In: Berne RM, Sperelakis N, Geiger SR (Eds). Handbook of Physiology (Section 2—The Cardiovascular System). Bethesda, MD: American Physiological Society; 1979. pp. 497-531.

2. Swan HJC, Ganz W, Forrester J, et al. Catheterization of the heart in man with use of flow-directed balloon-tipped catheter. N Engl J Med. 1970;283:447-51.

3. Kaltman AJ, Herbert WH, Conroy RJ, et al. The gradient in pressure across the pulmonary vascular bed during diastole. Circulation. 1966;34:377-84.

4. Falicov RE, Resnekov L. Relationship of the pulmonary end-diastolic pressure to the left ventricular end-diastolic and mean filling pressures in patients with and without left ventricular dysfunction. Circulation. 1970;42:65-73.

5. Bouchard RJ, Gault JH, Ross J Jr. Evaluation of pulmonary arterial end-diastolic pressure as an estimate of left ventricular end-diastolic pressure in patients with normal and abnormal left ventricular performance. Circulation. 1971;44:1072-9.

6. Jenkins BS, Bradley RD, Branthwaite MA. Evaluation of pulmonary arterial end-diastolic pressure as an indirect estimate of left atrial mean pressure. Circulation. 1970;42: 75-8.

7. Broder MI, Rodriguera E, Cohn JN. Evolution of abnormalities in left ventricular function after myocardial infarction. (Abstr) Ann Intern Med. 1971;74:817-8.

8. Weisse AB, Saffa RS, Levinson GE, et al. Left ventricular function during early and later stages of scar formation following experimental myocardial infarction. Am Heart J. 1970;79:370-83.

9. O'Rourke MF. Vascular impedance in studies of arterial and cardiac function. Physiol Rev. 1982;62:570-623.

10. Murgo JP, Westerhof N, Giolma JP, et al. Aortic input impedance in normal man: relationship to pressure wave forms. Circulation. 1980;62:105-16.

11. Pollack GH, Reddy RV, Noordergraaf A. Input impedance, wave travel, and reflections in the human pulmonary arterial tree: studies using an electrical analog. IEEE Trans Biomed Eng. 1968;15:151-64.

12. Merillon JP, Fontenier GJ, Lerallut JF, et al. Aortic input impedance in normal man and arterial hypertension: its modification during changes in aortic pressure. Cardiovas Res. 1982;16:646-56.

13. Kelly RP, Ting CT, Yang TM, et al. Effective arterial elastance as an index of arterial vascular load in humans. Circulation. 1992;86:513-21.

14. Chen CH, Nakayama M, Nevo E, et al. Coupled systolic-ventricular and vascular stiffening with age: implications for pressure regulation and cardiac reserve in the elderly. J Am Coll Cardiol. 1998;32:1221-7.

15. Kass DA. Ventricular arterial stiffening; integrating the pathophysiology. Hypertension. 2005;46:185-93.

16. Sunagawa K, Maughan WL, Burkhoff D, et al. Left ventricular interaction with arterial load studied in isolated canine ventricle. Am J Physiol. 1983;245:H773-80.

17. Burkhoff D, Sagawa K. Ventricular efficiency predicted by an analytical model. Am J Physiol. 1986;250:R1021-7.

18. Gleason WL, Braunwald E. Studies on the first derivative of the ventricular pressure pulse in man. J Clin Invest. 1962;41:80-91.

19. Zhong L, Tan RS, Ghista DN, et al. Validation of a novel noninvasive cardiac index of left ventricular contractility in patients. Am J Physiol Heart Circ Physiol. 2007;292: H2764-72.

20. Chen C, Rodriguez L, Lethor JP, et al. Continuous wave Doppler echocardiography for noninvasive assessment of left ventricular dP/dt and relaxation time constant from mitral regurgitant spectra in patients. J Am Coll Cardiol. 1994;23:970-6.

21. Fülöp T, Hegedüs I, Edes I. Examination of left ventricular contractile reserve by Doppler myocardial imaging in patients with dilated cardiomyopathy. Congest Heart Fail. 2001;7:191-5.

22. Dalsgaard M, Snyder EM, Kjaegaard J, et al. Isovolumic acceleration measured by tissue Doppler echocardiography is preload independent in healthy subjects. Echocardiography. 2007;24:572-9.

23. Reant P, Dijos M, Donal E, et al. Systolic time intervals as simple echocardiographic parameters of left ventricular systolic performance: correlation with ejection fraction and longitudinal two-dimensional strain. Eur J Echocardiogr. 2010;11:834-44.

24. Diamond G, Forrester JS, Chatterjee K, et al. Mean electromechanical dP/dt: an indirect index of the peak rate of rise of left ventricular pressure. Am J Cardiol. 1972;30:338-42.

25. Chatterjee K, Swan HJC, Parmley WW, et al. Influence of direct myocardial revascularization on left ventricular asynergy and function in patients with coronary heart disease: with and without previous myocardial infarction. Circulation. 1973;47:276-86.

26. Parmley WW, Sonnenblick EH. Series elasticity in heart muscle: its relation to contractile element velocity and proposed muscle models. Circ Res. 1967;20:112-23.

27. Mason DT, Braunwald E, Covell JW, et al. Assessment of cardiac contractility. The relation between the rate of pressure rise and ventricular pressure during isovolumic systole. Circulation. 1971;44:47-58.

28. Mahler F, Ross J Jr, O'Rourke RA, et al. Effects of changes in preload, afterload and inotropic state on ejection and isovolumic phase measures of contractility in the conscious dog. Am J Cardiol. 1975;35:626-34.

29. Peterson KL, Uther JB, Shabeetai R, et al. Assessment of left ventricular performance in man. Instantaneous tension-velocity-length relations obtained with the aid of an electromagnetic velocity catheter in the ascending aorta. Circulation. 1973;47:924-35.

30. Hood WP, Rackley CE, Rolett EL. Ejection velocity and ejection fraction as indices of ventricular contractility in man. Circulation. 1968;38:101.

31. Chatterjee K, Sacoor M, Sutton GC, et al. Assessment of left ventricular function by single plane cineangiographic volume analysis. Brit Heart J. 1971;33:565-71.

32. Crexells C, Chatterjee K, Forrester JS, et al. Optimal level of filling pressure in the left side of the heart in acute myocardial infarction. N Engl J Med. 1973;289:1263-6.

33. Greenberg B, Chatterjee K, Parmley WW, et al. The influence of left ventricular filling pressure on atrial contribution to cardiac output. Am Heart J. 1979;98:742-51.

34. Thorstensen A, Dalen H, Amundsen BH, et al. Reproducibility in echocardiographic assessment of the left ventricular global and regional function, the HUNT study. Eur J Echocardiogr. 2010;11:149-56.

35. Chandra S, Skali H, Blankstein R. Novel techniques for assessment of left ventricular systolic function. Heart Fail Rev. 2010:14 (DOI: 10.1007/s10741-010-9219-x).

36. Thomson HL, Basmadjian AJ, Rainbird AJ, et al. Contrast echocardiography improves the accuracy and reproducibility of left ventricular remodeling measurements: a prospective randomly assigned, blinded study. J Am Coll Cardiol. 2001;38:867-75.

37. Malm S, Frigstad S, Sagberg E, et al. Accurate and reproducible measurement of left ventricular volume and ejection fraction by contrast echocardiography: a comparison with magnetic resonance imaging. J Am Coll Cardiol. 2004;44:1030-5.

38. Hoffmann R, von Bardeleben S, ten Cate F, et al. Assessment of systolic left ventricular function: a multi-centre comparison of cineventriculography, cardiac magnetic resonance imaging, unenhanced and contrast-enhanced echocardiography. Eur Heart J. 2005;26:607-16.

39. Mor-Avi V, Jenkins C, Kühl HP, et al. Real-time 3-dimensional echocardiographic quantification of left ventricular volumes: multicenter study for validation with magnetic resonance imaging and investigation of sources of error. JACC Cardiovasc Imaging. 2008;1:413-23.

40. Chelliah RK, Hickman M, Kinsey C, et al. Myocardial contrast echocardiography versus single photon emission computed tomography for assessment of hibernating myocardium in ischemic cardiomyopathy: preliminary qualitative and quantitative results. J Am Soc Echocardiogr. 2010;23:840-7.

41. Maffessanti F, Nesser HJ, Weinert L, et al. Quantitative evaluation of regional left ventricular function using three-dimensional speckle tracking echocardiography in patients with and without heart disease. Am J Cardiol. 2009;104:1755-62.

42. Wu YW, Tadamura E, Yamamuro M, et al. Estimation of global and regional cardiac function using 64-slice computed tomography: a comparison study with echocardiography, gated-SPECT and cardiovascular magnetic resonance. Int J Cardiol. 2008;128:69-76.

43. de Graaf FR, Schuijf JD, van Velzen JE, et al. Assessment of global left ventricular function and volumes with 320-row multidetector computed tomography: a comparison with 2D-echocardiography. J Nucl Cardiol. 2010;17:225-31.

44. Corbett JR, Akinboboye OO, Bacharach SL, et al. Equilibrium radionuclide angiocardiography. J Nucl Cardiol. 2006;13:e56-79.

45. Friedman JD, Berman DS, Borges-Neto S, et al. First-pass radionuclide angiography. J Nucl Cardiol. 2006;13:e42-55.

46. Harel F, Finnerty V, Grégoire J, et al. Gated blood-pool SPECT versus cardiac magnetic resonance imaging for the assessment of left ventricular volumes and ejection fraction. J Nucl Cardiol. 2010;17:427-34.

47. Stegger L, Lipke CS, Kies P, et al. Quantification of left ventricular volumes and ejection fraction from gated ^{99m}Tc-MIBI SPECT: validation of an elastic surface model approach in comparison to cardiac magnetic resonance imaging, 4D-MSPECT and QGS. Eur J Nucl Med Mol Imaging. 2007;34:900-9.

48. Alfakih K, Reid S, Jones T, et al. Assessment of ventricular function and mass by cardiac magnetic resonance imaging. Eur Radiol. 2004;14:1813-22.

CHAPTER 15

Ventricular Function—Assessment and Clinical Application

48a. Chunjian Li, Lossnitzer D, Katus HA, et al. Comparison of left ventricular volumes and ejection fraction by monoplane cine ventriculography, unenhanced echocardiography and cardiac magnetic resonance imaging. Int J Cardiovascular Imaging. 2011;10.1007/s10554-011-9924-0.

49. Suga H, Sagawa K, Shoukas AA. Load independence of the instantaneous pressure-volume ratio of the canine left ventricle and effects of epinephrine and heart rate on the ratio. Circ Res. 1973;32:314-22.

50. Slutsky R, Karliner J, Gerber K, et al. Peak systolic blood pressure/end-systolic volume ratio: assessment at rest and during exercise in normal subjects and patients with coronary heart disease. Am J Cardiol. 1980;46:813-20.

51. Boerth RC, Covell JW, Pool PE, et al. Increased myocardial oxygen consumption and contractile state associated with increased heart rate in dogs. Circ Res. 1969;24:725-34.

52. Vogel M, Cheung MM, Li J, et al. Noninvasive assessment of left ventricular force-frequency relationships using tissue Doppler-derived isovolumic acceleration. Circulation. 2003;107:1647-52.

53. Banerjee A, Mendelsohn AM, Knilans TK, et al. Effect of myocardial hypertrophy on systolic and diastolic function in children: insights from the force-frequency and relaxation-frequency relationships. J Am Coll Cardiol. 1998;32:1088-95.

54. Hasenfuss G, Holubarsch C, Hermann HP, et al. Influence of the force-frequency relationship on hemodynamics and left ventricular function in patients with non-failing hearts and in patients with dilated cardiomyopathy. Eur Heart J. 1994;15:164-70.

54a. Schmidt U, Schwinger RHG, Bohm M, et al. Alterations of the force-frequency relation depending on stages of heart failure in humans. AM J Cardiol. 1994;74:1066-8.

54b. Bhargava V, Shabetai R, Mathiasen RA, et al. Loss of adrenergic control of the force-frequency relation in heart failure secondary to idiopathic or ischemic cardiomyopathy. Am J Cardiol. 1998;81:1130-7.

55. Pieske B, Kretschmann B, Meyer M, et al. Alterations in intracellular calcium handling associated with the inverse force-frequency relation in human dilated cardiomyopathy. Circulation. 1995;92:1169-78.

55a. Yamanaka T, Onishi K, Tanabe M, et al. Force and relaxation relations in patients with diastolic heart failure. Am Heart J. 2006;152:966.e1-7.

55b. Wachter R, Schmidt-Schweda S, Westerman D, et al. Blunted frequency-dependent upregulation of cardiac output is related to impaired relaxation in diastolic heart failure. Eur Heart J. 2009;30:3027-36.

56. Alderman EL, Glantz SA. Acute hemodynamic interventions shift the diastolic pressure-volume curve in man. Circulation. 1976;54:662-71.

57. Mann T, Goldberg S, Mudge GH Jr, et al. Factors contributing to altered left ventricular diastolic properties during angina pectoris. Circulation. 1979;59:14-20.

58. Tyberg JV, Misbach GA, Glantz SA, et al. The mechanism for shifts in the diastolic, left ventricular, pressure-volume curve: the role of the pericardium. Eur J Cardiol. 1978;7:163-75.

59. Bemis CE, Serur JR, Borkenhagen D, et al. Influence of right ventricular filling pressure on left ventricular pressure and dimension. Circ Res. 1974;34:498-504.

60. Salerno M. Multi-modality imaging of diastolic function. J Nucl Cardiol. 2010;17:316-27.

61. Alnabhan N, Kerut EK, Geraci SA, et al. An approach to analysis of left ventricular diastolic function and loading conditions in the echocardiography laboratory. Echocardiography. 2008;25:105-16.

62. Muntinga HJ, van den Berg F, Knol HR, et al. Normal values and reproducibility of left ventricular filling parameters by radionuclide angiography. Int J Card Imaging. 1997;13:165-71.

63. Akincioglu C, Berman DS, Nishina H, et al. Assessment of diastolic function using 16-frame 99mTc-sestamibi gated myocardial perfusion SPECT: normal values. J Nucl Med. 2005;46:1102-8.

64. Feng W, Nagaraj H, Gupta H, et al. A dual propagation contours technique for semi-automated assessment of systolic and diastolic cardiac function by CMR. J Cardiovasc Magn Reson. 2009;11:30.

65. Kawaji K, Codella NC, Prince MR, et al. Automated segmentation of routine clinical cardiac magnetic resonance imaging for assessment of left ventricular diastolic dysfunction. Circ Cardiovasc Imaging. 2009;2:476-84.

66. Kivowitz C, Parmley WW, Donoso R, et al. Effects of isometric exercise on cardiac performance. The Grip Test. Circulation. 1971;44:994-1002.

67. Voelkel NF, Quaife RA, Leinwand LA, et al. Right ventricular function and failure: report of a National Heart, Lung, and Blood Institute working group on cellular and molecular mechanisms of right heart failure. Circulation. 2006;114:1883-91.

68. Dell'Italia LJ. The right ventricle: anatomy, physiology, and clinical importance. Curr Probl Cardiol. 1991;16:653-720.

69. Rich JD, Ward RP. Right-ventricular function by nuclear cardiology. Curr Opin Cardiol. 2010;25:445-50.

70. Ramani GV, Gurm G, Dilsizian V, et al. Noninvasive assessment of right ventricular function: will there be resurgence in radionuclide imaging techniques? Curr Cardiol Rep. 2010;12:162-9.

71. Slart RH, Poot L, Piers DA, et al. Evaluation of right ventricular function by NuSMUGA software: gated blood-pool SPECT vs first-pass radionuclide angiography. Int J Cardiovasc Imaging. 2003;19:401-7.

72. Mangion JR. Right ventricular imaging by two-dimensional and three-dimensional echocardiography. Curr Opin Cardiol. 2010;25:423-9.

73. López-Candales A, Dohi K, Rajagopalan N, et al. Defining normal variables of right ventricular size and function in pulmonary hypertension: an echocardiographic study. Postgrad Med J. 2008;84:40-5.

74. Tei C, Dujardin KS, Hodge DO, et al. Doppler echocardiographic index for assessment of global right ventricular function. J Am Soc Echocardiogr. 1996;9:838-47.

75. Vogel M, Schmidt MR, Kristiansen SB, et al. Validation of myocardial acceleration during isovolumic contraction as a novel noninvasive index of right ventricular contractility. Circulation. 2002;105:1693-9.

76. Gopal AS, Chukwu EO, Iwuchukwu CJ, et al. Normal values of right ventricular size and function by real-time 3-dimensional echocardiography: comparison with cardiac magnetic resonance imaging. J Am Soc Echocardiogr. 2007;20:445-55.

77. Grewal J, Majdalany D, Syed I, et al. Three-dimensional echocardiographic assessment of right ventricular volume and function in adult patients with congenital heart disease: comparison with magnetic resonance imaging. J Am Soc Echocardiogr. 2010;23:127-33.

78. Sugeng L, Mor-Avi V, Weinert L, et al. Multimodality comparison of quantitative volumetric analysis of the right ventricle. JACC Cardiovasc Imag. 2010;3:10-18.

SECTION 3

Diagnosis

Transthoracic Echocardiography

Byron F Vandenberg, Richard E Kerber

Chapter Outline

INTRODUCTION

Echocardiography is the examination of the heart using reflected sound waves. The early clinically applied technology was m-mode (i.e. motion-based mode). This provided a one dimensional view of the heart with motion recorded at a high frame rate of 1,000–2,000 frames per second. A variety of two-dimensional (2D) methods have become available for cross-sectional display of cardiac structures, but at a lower frame rate of 30–100 frames per second. Doppler techniques provide the recording of intracardiac blood flow, and with color Doppler, the Doppler signal is displayed as 2D imaging using color to denote the direction and character of flow.

Echocardiography is widely recognized as an appropriate imaging modality in evaluating patients with a variety of symptoms and signs of heart disease (Table 1). These indications include the assessment of chamber quantitation, left ventricular (LV) systolic and diastolic function, pulmonary hypertension, pericardial disease, valvular heart disease, intracardiac masses and congenital heart disease.[1]

CHAMBER QUANTITATION

Left ventricular linear dimensions are important measurements in the management of patients with heart disease, especially in patients with volume overload due to valvular heart disease.[2] LV internal dimensions at end-diastole (LVIDd) and at end-systole (LVIDs) are usually made from parasternal long axis images at the level of the minor axis (i.e. perpendicular to the long axis of the left ventricle), at the level of the mitral leaflet tips or chords with measurements obtained at the tissue-blood interface (Fig. 1). The normal reference range for LV end diastolic diameter varies with gender: women, less than or equal to 5.3 cm [≤ 3.2 cm/m^2 when indexed for body

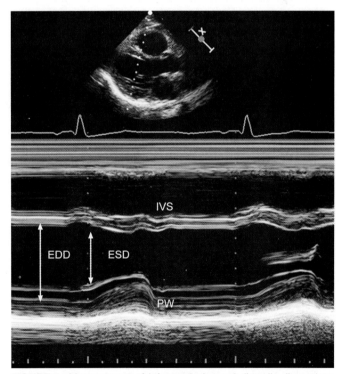

FIGURE 1: Measurement of left ventricular end diastolic dimensions (EDD) and end systolic dimensions (ESD) from m-mode of the LV using the parasternal long axis view (inset) for landmark identification. (Abbreviations: IVS: Interventricular septum; PW: Posterior wall)

surface area (BSA)] and men, less than or equal to 5.9 cm (≤ 3.1 cm/m^2 when indexed for BSA).[3]

The development of LV hypertrophy (Figs 2A and B) predicts increased risk of stroke, systolic heart failure and mortality; however, reduction in LV mass corresponds with improved outcomes.[4,5] Wall thickness is measured at end

TABLE 1

Appropriate indications for echocardiography

Symptoms:
• Dyspnea
• Chest pain with suspected myocardial ischemia in patients with nondiagnostic laboratory markers and ECG and in whom a resting echocardiogram can be performed during pain
• Lightheadedness or syncope
• TIA or cerebrovascular event
Prior testing that is concerning for heart disease (e.g. abnormal chest X-ray or electrocardiogram, elevated BNP)
Native valve disease:
• Murmur
• Suspected mitral valve prolapse
• Initial evaluation of known or suspected native valve stenosis or regurgitation
• Routine (yearly) re-evaluation of asymptomatic patient with severe native valvular stenosis or regurgitation
• Re-evaluation of patient with native valve stenosis or regurgitation with a change in clinical status
Prosthetic valve:
• Initial evaluation of prosthetic valve for establishment of baseline after placement
• Re-evaluation due to suspected dysfunction or thrombosis or a change in clinical status
Infective endocarditis:
• Initial evaluation of suspected infective endocarditis with positive blood culture or new murmur
• Re-evaluation of infective endocarditis in patients with virulent organism, severe hemodynamic lesion, aortic involvement, persistent bacteremia, a change in clinical status or symptomatic deterioration.
Known or suspected adult congenital heart disease
Sustained or nonsustained ventricular tachycardia
Evaluation of intracardiac and extracardiac structures and chambers
• Cardiovascular source of embolus
• Evaluation for cardiac mass due to suspected tumor or thrombus
• Evaluation of pericardial conditions such as effusion, constrictive pericarditis and tamponade
Known or suspected Marfan disease for evaluation of proximal aortic root and/or mitral valve
Heart failure:
• Initial evaluation of known or suspected heart failure (systolic or diastolic)
• Re-evaluation to guide therapy in a patient with a change in clinical status
Pacing device evaluation:
• Evaluation for dyssynchrony in patient being considered for cardiac resynchronization therapy
• Known implanted pacing device with symptoms possibly due to suboptimal pacing device settings to re-evaluate for dyssynchrony and/or revision of pacing device setting
Hypertrophic cardiomyopathy:
• Initial evaluation of known or suspected hypertrophic cardiomyopathy
• Re-evaluation of known hypertrophic cardiomyopathy in a patient with a change in clinical status to guide or evaluate therapy
Cardiomyopathy:
• Evaluation of suspected restrictive, infiltrative or genetic cardiomyopathy
• Screening for structure and function in first-degree relatives of patients with inherited cardiomyopathy
Cardiotoxic agents:
• Baseline and serial re-evaluation in patients undergoing therapy with cardiotoxic agents
Myocardial infarction:
• Initial evaluation of LV function after acute MI
• Re-evaluation of LV function following MI during recovery when results will guide therapy
• Evaluation of suspected complication of myocardial ischemia/infarction such as acute mitral regurgitation, ventricular septal defect, heart failure, thrombus and RV involvement
Pulmonary:
• Respiratory failure with suspected cardiac etiology
• Known or suspected pulmonary embolism to guide therapy (i.e. thrombectomy and thrombolytics)
• Evaluation of known or suspected pulmonary hypertension including evaluation of RV function and estimated pulmonary artery pressure
Hemodynamic instability of uncertain or suspected cardiac etiology
(*Source:* Reference 1)

diastole with normal thickness less than or equal to 0.9 cm.[3] Formulas are available for the calculation of LV mass. The American Society of Echocardiography (ASE) recommended formula for estimation of LV mass from LV linear dimensions is:

$$LV\ mass = 0.8 \times \{1.04\ [(LVIDd + PWTd + SWTd)^3 - (LVIDd)^3]\} + 0.6\ gm$$

where PWTd and SWTd are posterior wall thickness and septal wall thicknesses at end diastole respectively. The normal

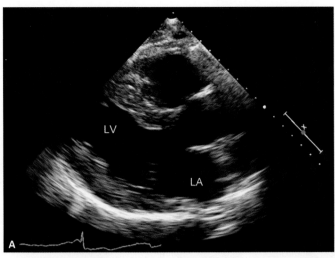

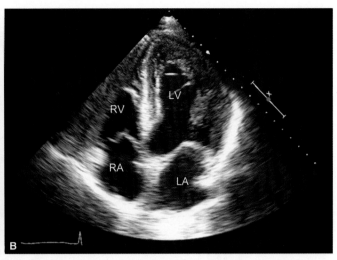

FIGURES 2A AND B: Increased LV wall thickness consistent with LV hypertrophy due to hypertension. (A) Parasternal long axis view. (B) Apical 4-chamber view. (Abbreviations: LV: Left ventricle; LA: Left atrium; RV: Right ventricle; RA: Right atrium)

reference range varies with gender: men, 88–224 gm and women, 67–162 gm. LV mass can also be calculated from measurement of myocardial area at the mid-papillary muscle level 2D echo with long axis linear dimensions.[3]

Left ventricular ejection fraction (LVEF) predicts mortality and is proportional to survival (i.e. the lower the LVEF, the lower the individual patient's survival). In addition, LVEF guides therapeutic decision-making, helping to identify patients for drug therapy initiation (e.g. angiotensin converting enzyme inhibitors and beta-blockers in patients with LVEF $\leq$ 40%) and for implantation of internal cardiac defibrillators.[4] Left ventricular

ejection fraction is calculated from the end diastolic volume (EDV) and end systolic volume (ESV) from the formula: EF = (EDV – ESV)/EDV. The normal LVEF is greater than or equal to 55%.[3] Left ventricular ejection fraction is frequently visually estimated but it can be estimated using quantitative methods. LV volume assessment is commonly obtained from 2D measurement using the biplane method of disks (also known as the modified Simpson's rule). Total volume is calculated as the sum of the volumes of a stack of elliptical disks (Fig. 3). If two orthogonal planes are not available, a single plane can be used, assuming the each disk has the area of a circle. When

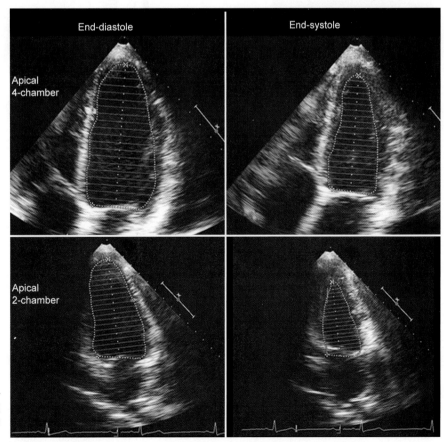

FIGURE 3: Two-dimensional measurements for LV volume calculation using the biplane method of disks in apical 4-chamber and 2-chamber views at end-diastole and end-systole

CHAPTER 16

Transthoracic Echocardiography

Diagnosis

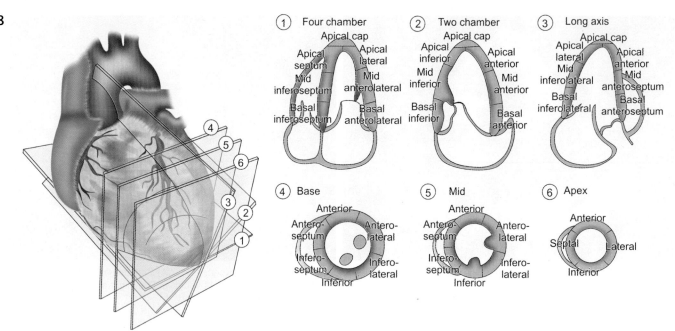

FIGURE 4: Seventeen segment model of left ventricular regional wall analysis based on apical and parasternal short axis views. (*Source:* Modified from Lang RM, Bierig M, Devereux RB, et al. Recommendations for chamber quantification: a report from the American Society of Echocardiography's guidelines and standards committee and the chamber quantification writing group, developed in conjunction with the European Association of Echocardiography, a branch of the European Society of Cardiology. J Am Soc Echo. 2005:18:1440-63, with permission)

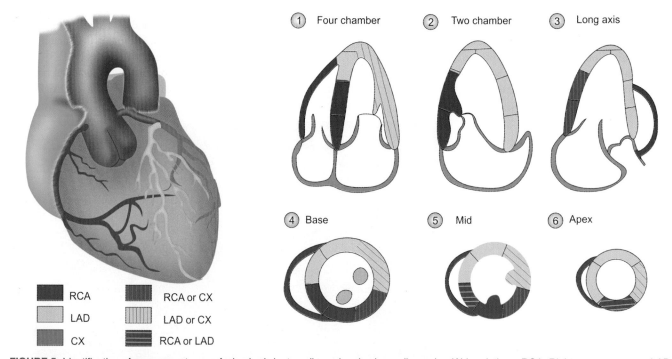

FIGURE 5: Identification of coronary artery perfusion beds by two-dimensional echocardiography. (Abbreviations: RCA: Right coronary artery; LAD: Left anterior descending artery; CX: Circumflex coronary artery). (*Source:* Lang RM, Bierig M, Devereux RB, et al. Recommendations for chamber quantification: a report from the American Society of Echocardiography's guidelines and standards committee and the chamber quantification writing group, developed in conjunction with the European Association of Echocardiography, a branch of the European Society of Cardiology. J Am Soc Echo. 2005:18:1440-63, with permission)

endocardial definition is not adequate for tracing, area-length methods using the major length and a short axis LV cross-sectional area have been validated as alternative methods for volume estimation. The upper limit of normal for the LV end diastolic volume varies with gender: women, less than or equal to 104 ml (≤ 75 ml/m^2 when indexed for BSA) and men, less than or equal to 155 ml (≤ 75 ml/m^2 when indexed for BSA).[3]

Regional wall motion of the left ventricle can be assessed with 2D echocardiography. A standard model of analysis involves dividing the left ventricle into 17 segments (Fig. 4). The identification of segments is useful for the identification of coronary perfusion territories (Fig. 5). In the presence of a functionally significant stenosis, segmental wall motion (usually assessed as endocardial excursion and/or myocardial thickening)

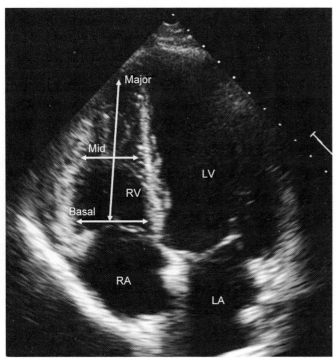

FIGURE 6: Right ventricular diameters measured in apical 4-chamber view. (Basal) Minor diameter measured at the base of the RV. (Mid) Minor diameter measured at mid level of RV. (Major) Major length diameter measured from RV apex to RV base. (Abbreviations: RV: Right ventricle; LV: Left ventricle; RA: Right atrium)

may become abnormal at rest in the presence of supply ischemia, or under stress conditions that provoke demand ischemia. Regional wall motion can be quantitated [e.g. normal or hyperkinesis = 1, hypokinesis (i.e. decreased motion) = 2, akinesis (i.e. no motion) = 3, dyskinesis (i.e. paradoxical motion = 4 and aneurysmal = 5] and an index derived as the sum of the scores divided by the number of segments scored.[3]

Right ventricular (RV) size is influenced by afterload and pressure changes as well as diseases such as myocardial infarction and RV dysplasia. In the apical 4-chamber view, the RV area or midcavity diameter should be smaller that the LV, otherwise RV dilation is present. Right ventricular (RV) diameter is measure at end diastole and dilation is present with basal minor diameter greater than 4.2 cm, mid level diameter greater

than 3.5 cm or major length greater than 8.6 cm (Fig. 6). The RV is composed of three distinct portions: the smooth muscular inflow (i.e. the body), the outflow region and the trabecular apical region. Volumetric quantitation of RV function is challenging due to many geometric assumptions. A simple method of quantitating RV systolic function involves measurements of area at end diastole and end systole and calculating the fractional area change with abnormal less than 35% (Figs 7A to C). Right ventricular (RV) wall thickness greater than 5 mm indicates RV hypertrophy.[6]

Left atrial (LA) enlargement as determined by echocardiography is a predictor of cardiovascular outcomes.[7] Left artrial (LA) size is measured at ventricular end systole, when the LA chamber is at its largest dimension. The standard measurement previously used in clinical practice was the m-mode or 2D anteroposterior (AP) linear dimension obtained from the parasternal long axis view. However, LA volume provides a more accurate measure of LA size since expansion of the LA may occur in directions other than the AP dimension. LA volumes are usually calculated using either an area length or method of disks model (Fig. 8). The normal LA volume indexed for BSA is 22 ± 6 ml/m^2.[3]

Right atrial (RA) enlargement has adverse prognostic implications in patients with pulmonary hypertension and is discussed later in this chapter. Compared to the LA, there is less data available on quantitation of the RA. However, RA enlargement is considered to be a minor dimension greater than 4.4 cm or a major dimension greater than 5.3 cm.[6]

DOPPLER ECHO

When ultrasound is reflected from moving red blood cells, there is a change in ultrasound frequency (ΔF), which is related to velocity (V) according to the equation:

$$\Delta F = (V \times 2F_o \times \cos \theta)/c$$

where F_o is the transducer frequency, θ is the angle between the direction of flow and insonifying beam and c is the speed of sound in tissue (i.e. 1,540 m/sec). When solving the Doppler equation, an angle between flow and beam of 0 or 180° (i.e. cosine θ = 1.0) is assumed for cardiac applications.[8] However, as the angle increases beyond 20°, the change in frequency is

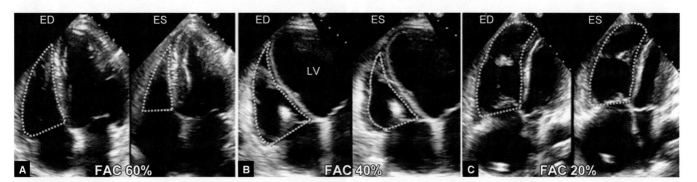

FIGURES 7A TO C: Examples of right ventricular fractional area change (FAC). Percentage FAC = 100 × (end diastolic area − end systolic area)/ end diastolic area. The endocardial border is traced in apical 4-chamber views from the tricuspid annulus along the free wall to the apex, then back to the annulus, along the interventricular septum at end diastole (ED) and end systole (ES). Trabeculation, tricuspid leaflets and chords are included in the chamber. (A) Normal subject, FAC 60%. (B) Moderately dilated right ventricle (RV), FAC 40% and a markedly dilated left ventricle (LV). (C) Dilated RV, FAC 20% and the LV is foreshortened as a result of optimizing the view for the right ventricular chamber. (*Source:* Rudski LG, Lai WW, Afilalo J, et al. Guidelines for the echocardiographic assessment of the right heart in adults: a report from the American Society of Echocardiography. J Am Soc Echocardiogr. 2010;23:685-713)

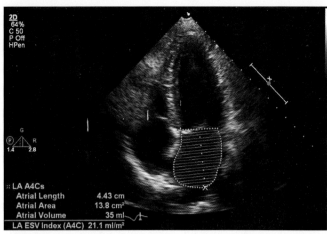

FIGURE 8: Measurement of the end systolic left atrial (LA) volume from the apical 4-chamber view using the method of disks

underestimated. Thus beam orientation is important for accurate measurements.

There are three modalities: (1) pulsed wave; (2) continuous wave and (3) color Doppler. Pulsed wave Doppler measures flow velocity within a specific site (i.e. range gate) but is limited in the measurement of high velocities. Continuous wave Doppler can record high velocities but cannot localize the site of origin of the velocity. Color Doppler estimates flow velocities within regions of interest with the 2D image. Color Doppler provides a rapid assessment of flow with a spatial and directional (color-coded) display of velocities on a 2D echo (Figs 9A and B). Pulsed and continuous wave Doppler provide quantitation of flow velocity and pressure gradient. Using the modified Bernoulli equation (i.e. pressure gradient = $4v^2$), velocity can be converted to pressure gradient and this permits estimation of hemodynamic variables such as valve stenosis and pulmonary hypertension severity. Flow is derived as the product of the cross-sectional area (CSA) of an orifice [e.g. the LV outflow tract (LVOT)] and the average velocity of the blood cells passing through the orifice. The calculation of flow can be used to estimate the CSA of the aortic valve (AV) using the continuity

equation (Fig. 10) and is discussed in the section on valvular heart disease.[8]

DIASTOLIC FUNCTION

Approximately one half of patients with a new diagnosis of heart failure have normal or near normal LV systolic function and these patients frequently have abnormalities of diastolic function. Morphologic abnormalities include LV hypertrophy. Wall thickness and LV mass can be assessed as described above and with increased filling pressures, LA volume increases which can also be assessed with 2D echocardiography.[9]

Doppler measurement of mitral inflow velocities, pulmonary vein velocities and LV myocardial tissue velocities are used to provide additional assessment of LV diastolic dysfunction (Figs 11A to C). These are obtained from the apical 4-chamber view which allows proper alignment of the Doppler beam. The major mitral inflow velocity parameters are: peak early filling (E) and late diastolic filling (A) velocities, the E/A ratio and deceleration time (DT) of early filling velocity. In addition, the isovolumic relaxation period can be determined by placing continuous wave Doppler beam in the LVOT to simultaneously display the end of aortic ejection and the onset of mitral inflow.[9]

The mitral E velocity primarily reflects the LA-LV pressure gradient during early diastole and is affected by preload and alterations in LV relaxation. The mitral A velocity reflects the LA-LV pressure gradient during late diastole, which is affected by LV compliance and LA contractile function. The DT of the E wave is influenced by LV relaxation, LV diastolic pressures after mitral valve opening and LV compliance (Fig. 12).[9]

The four mitral inflow patterns are: (1) normal (i.e. the mitral E velocity is dominant); (2) impaired LV relaxation (i.e. the mitral A velocity is dominant); (3) restrictive filling (i.e. elevated mitral E velocity with shortened DT) and (4) pseudonormal (i.e. normal mitral E velocity dominance) (Figs 13 and 14). A pseudonormal pattern is caused by a mild to moderate increase in LA pressure (and therefore an increase in the LA-LV gradient), in the setting of delayed myocardial relaxation and

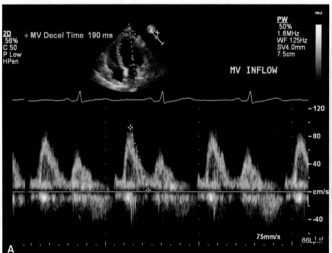

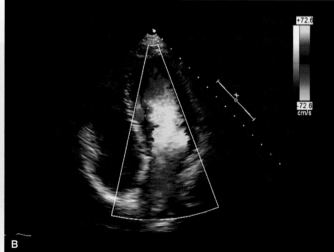

FIGURES 9A AND B: Comparison of pulsed wave and color Doppler imaging. (A) Pulsed Doppler with sample volume placed in mitral inflow to measure velocities in this location for diastolic function assessment. (B) Color Doppler of diastolic inflow into left ventricle (LV) demonstrates spatial display of filling the LV. This display does not allow quantitation of velocities

Continuity equation

Flow(Q) = CSA x Velocity

$$Q_1 = Q_2$$

$$Q_1 = A_1 \times V_1 = A_2 \times V_2$$

$$A_2 = Q_1/V_2$$

FIGURE 10: Diagrammatic representation of the continuity equation. When laminar flow encounters a small discrete stenosis, it must accelerate rapidly to pass through small orifice. Flow proximal to stenosis is same as flow passing through stenosis. Because flow equals velocity times cross-sectional area of stenotic orifice can be derived if velocity through orifice and flow is known (*Source:* Modified from Quinones MA, Otto CM, Stoddard M, et al. Recommendations for quantification of Doppler echocardiography: a report from the Doppler Quantification Task Force of the Nomenclature and Standards Committee of the American Society of Echocardiography. J Am Soc Echocardiogr. 2002;15:167-84, with permission)

the mitral inflow velocity pattern therefore appears normal. Additional Doppler measurements of pulmonary venous flow and myocardial velocities may be helpful to distinguish a normal pattern from a pseudonormal one.[9] For example, as LV relaxation is delayed, the LV myocardial velocity (e') is reduced.[10,11]

Impaired LV relaxation may occur with advancing age and LV hypertrophy. As the LV diastolic pressure increases, the LA-LV pressure gradient decreases and the contribution of atrial filling increases.[10] A restrictive filling pattern is seen in restrictive cardiomyopathies, such as amyloidosis, and is related to rapid early filling. Typically there is blunting of the normal respiratory variation in early filling velocity with restrictive physiology. Patients with a restrictive pattern and dilated cardiomyopathy have increased risk for poor prognosis.[12]

A Doppler beam placed into a pulmonary vein will provide a recording of the systolic (S) and diastolic (D) velocities. The S velocity is influenced by changes in LA pressure, contraction and relaxation. The D velocity is influenced by changes in LV filling and compliance. With an increase in LA pressure, the S velocity is expected to decrease and the D velocity increases (similar to the E velocity increase on mitral inflow Doppler). However, with increasing age, the S/D ratio will also increase as LV relaxation becomes impaired (Table 2).

CHAPTER 16

Transthoracic Echocardiography

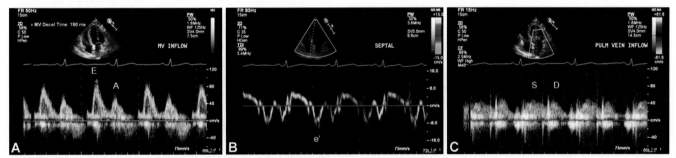

FIGURES 11A TO C: Diastolic function assessment with Doppler echocardiography. (A) Mitral inflow Doppler velocity profiles of early (E) and late atrial (A) filling. (B) Septal wall tissue Doppler imaging for assessment of e'. (C) Pulmonary vein Doppler velocity profiles for measurement of systolic (S) and diastolic (D) velocities

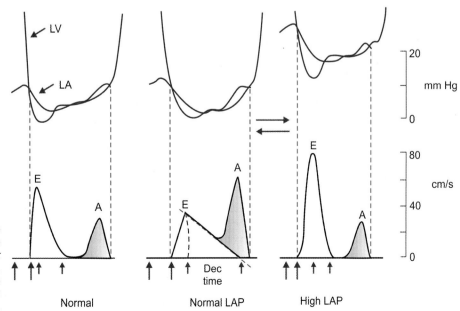

FIGURE 12: Schematic diagram of the changes in mitral inflow in response to the transmitral pressure gradient. (*Source:* Modified from Nagueh SF, Appleton CP, Gillebert TC, et al. Recommendations for the evaluation of left ventricular diastolic function by echocardiography. J Am Soc Echocardiogr. 2009;22:107-33, with permission)

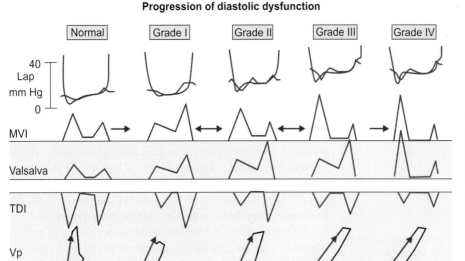

FIGURE 13: The progression of left ventricular diastolic dysfunction can be readily assessed using a combination of Doppler echocardiographic variables. Each successive grade represents a worsening state of diastolic dysfunction: Grade I—impaired relaxation; Grade II—pseudonormalization; Grade III/IV—restrictive. (Abbreviations: MVI: Mitral valve inflow; TDI: Tissue Doppler imaging; Valsalva: Response of mitral valve inflow to Valsalva maneuver; Vp: Mitral inflow propagation velocity). (*Source:* Modified from Ommen SR, Nishimura RA. A clinical approach to the assessment of left ventricular diastolic function by Doppler echocardiography: update 2003. *Heart.* 2003;89:iii18-23, with permission)

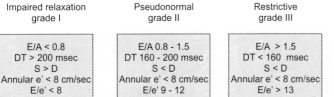

Impaired relaxation grade I	Pseudonormal grade II	Restrictive grade III
E/A < 0.8 DT > 200 msec S > D Annular e' < 8 cm/sec E/e' < 8	E/A 0.8 - 1.5 DT 160 - 200 msec S < D Annular e' < 8 cm/sec E/e' 9 - 12	E/A > 1.5 DT < 160 msec S < D Annular e' < 8 cm/sec E/e' > 13

FIGURE 14: Grading diastolic dysfunction: integrating measurements from mitral inflow velocity, pulmonary vein and myocardial tissue velocities (Abbreviations: E/A: Mitral E/A velocity ratio; DT: Deceleration time of the mitral early filling velocity; S, D: Pulmonary vein systolic (S) and diastolic (D) velocities; Annular e': Tissue Doppler derived myocardial velocity averaged from septal and lateral tissue Doppler velocities). (*Source:* Modified from Nagueh SF, Appleton CP, Gillebert TC, et al. Recommendations for the evaluation of left ventricular diastolic function by echocardiography. J Am Soc Echocardiogr. 2009;22:107-33, with permission)

TABLE 2

Age related changes in Doppler indices of diastolic function

	Age		
	21–40 yr	*41–60 yr*	*> 60 yr*
E/A ratio	1.5 ± 0.4	1.3 ± 0.2	1.0 ± 0.2
DT (msec)	166 ± 14	181 ± 19	200 ± 29
PV S/D ratio	1.0 ± 0.3	1.2 ± 0.2	1.4 ± 0.5
Septal e' (cm/s)	16 ± 3	12 ± 2	10 ± 2
Lateral e' (cm/s)	20 ± 3	16 ± 2	13 ± 3
(*Source:* Reference 9)			

Pulsed Doppler measurement of myocardial velocities provides an additional method for assessing LV diastolic filling. The primary measurement is the early diastolic (e') velocity, which is influenced by LV relaxation, preload, systolic pressure and LV minimal pressure. Tissue Doppler signals are acquired at the septal and lateral sides of the mitral annulus and the e' velocities are averaged for the calculation of the E/e' ratio, a measure of LV filling pressure.[9] With impaired LV relaxation, the e' velocity is reduced. A ratio greater than 15 is associated with increased LV filling pressure and a ratio less than 8 is associated with normal LV filling pressure. A value between 8 and 15 is indeterminate for predicting LV filling pressure.[13] As is the case with mitral and pulmonary vein Doppler measurements, the normal value for e' velocity changes with age.[9]

PULMONARY HYPERTENSION

Pulmonary arterial (PA) hypertension results from restricted flow through the PA circulation, increased pulmonary vascular resistance and ultimately in right heart failure. Pulmonary arterial hypertension is defined as mean PA pressure greater than 25 mm Hg at rest, PA wedge pressure less than 15 mm Hg and pulmonary vascular resistance greater than 3 Wood Units. Pulmonary hypertension can also result from disorders associated with elevated LV filling pressures such as LV dysfunction (either systolic or diastolic) and valvular heart disease.[14]

Transthoracic echocardiography (TTE) may identify conditions that predispose to PH or suggest a specific disease entity (Table 3).[14] A complete 2D and Doppler echo study can provide an estimate of RV systolic pressure or cardiac sequelae of PH (Figs 15A to D). Right ventricular (RV) systolic pressure greater than 40 mm Hg generally warrants further evaluation in the patient with unexplained dyspnea. Other findings of PH are RA or RV enlargement or interventricular septal flattening (Figs 16A and B). The presence of any degree of pericardial effusion, RA enlargement and RV enlargement or dysfunction is predictor of poor prognosis.

When tricuspid regurgitation is present, the application of the modified Bernoulli equation to the peak tricuspid regurgitation velocity provides a close estimate of the peak pressure gradient between RV and RA. Then, RV systolic pressure can be derived by adding an estimate of mean RA pressure to the

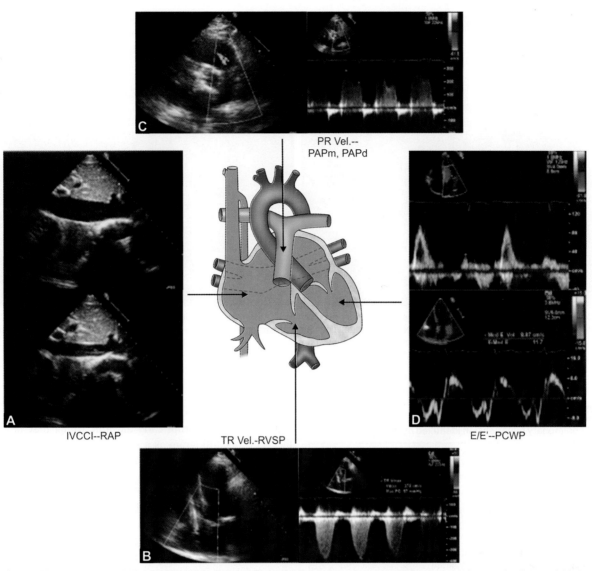

FIGURES 15A TO D: Illustration of "Echo Right Heart Catheterization". (A) Inferior vena caval (IVC) size and degree of collapse yields an estimate of right atrial pressure (RAP). (B) The tricuspid regurgitant velocity (TR Vel) is used to estimate the systolic right ventricle—right atrium gradient (and the pulmonary artery systolic pressure, in the absence of pulmonic stenosis). (C) The maximal pulmonic valve regurgitant velocity is used to estimate the mean pulmonary artery pressure (PAPm). The end diastolic pulmonic regurgitant velocity is used to estimate diastolic pulmonary artery pressure (PAPd). (D) The early mitral inflow (E wave)/early diastolic mitral valve annular motion (E' wave) ratio is used to assess pulmonary capillary wedge pressure (PCWP). (Abbreviations: E/E': Ratio of early diastolic mitral inflow velocity to early diastolic velocity of the mitral valve annulus; IVCCI: Inferior vena cava collapsibility index; PR Vel: Pulmonic valve regurgitant velocity; RVSP: Right ventricular systolic pressure). (*Source:* Kirkpatrick JN, Vannan MA, Narula J, et al. Echocardiography in heart failure: application, utility, and new horizons. J Am Coll Cardiol. 2007;50:381-96)

peak RV-RA gradient.[6,15] In the absence of pulmonic stenosis, the peak RV pressure is equivalent to the PA systolic pressure.[8]

The RA pressure can be estimated by the inferior vena cava appearance. A normal RA pressure of 0–5 mm Hg is predicted by an inferior vena cava diameter of less than 2.1 cm with collapse greater than 50% with a sniff. An elevated RA pressure of 10–20 mm Hg is suggested by inferior vena cava diameter greater than 2.1 cm with collapse less than 50% with a sniff.[6]

PERICARDIAL DISEASE

Echocardiography can be useful in detecting a variety of conditions that affect the pericardium including: (1) effusion; (2) tamponade; (3) constriction; (4) partial or complete absence of the pericardium and (5) pericardial cysts or tumors.[16]

Pericardial effusion is recognized as an echo-free space between the visceral and the parietal pericardium surrounding the heart. Small effusions are generally limited to the posterior atrioventricular groove. As the effusion increases, fluid extends laterally and with large effusion, fluid surrounds the heart.[16]

When the ability of the pericardium to stretch is exceeded by fluid accumulation, pericardial sac pressure increases and may exceed intracardiac pressures during the cycle, resulting in tamponade physiology. The signs of tamponade include RA wall inversion and diastolic compression of the RV free wall. Plethora of the inferior vena cava is a useful indicator of elevated RA pressure. Tamponade produces reciprocal respiration-related changes in diastolic filling of the LV and the RV, and exaggerated respiratory changes in mitral and tricuspid inflow velocities can be demonstrated by pulsed Doppler (Figs 17A and B).[16,17]

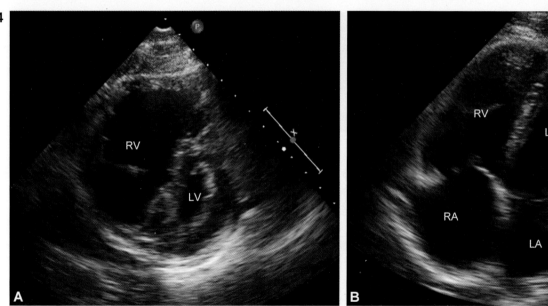

FIGURES 16A AND B: Echocardiographic features of pulmonary hypertension. (A) Parasternal short axis view. (B) Apical 4-chamber view. Common echocardiographic findings in pulmonary hypertension include: right atrial enlargement; right ventricular enlargement; abnormal contour of the interventricular septum and underfilled left heart chambers. (Abbreviations: LA: Left atrium; LV: Left ventricle; RA: Right atrium; RV: Right ventricle)

TABLE 3

Causes of pulmonary hypertension identified by echocardiography

Conditions that predispose to pulmonary hypertension:
- Congenital or acquired valvular disease (mitral regurgitation, mitral stenosis, aortic stenosis and prosthetic valve dysfunction)
- Left ventricular systolic dysfunction
- Impaired left ventricular diastolic function (hypertensive heart disease, hypertrophic cardiomyopathy, Fabry's disease and infiltrative cardiomyopathy)
- Other obstructive lesions (coarctation, supravalvular aortic stenosis, subaortic membrane and cor triatriatum)
- Congenital disease with shunt (atrial septal defect, ventricular septal defect, coronary fistula, patent ductus arteriosus and anomalous pulmonary venous return)
- Pulmonary embolus (thrombus in inferior vena cava, right-sided cardiac chamber or pulmonary artery; tricuspid or pulmonic valve vegetation)
- Pulmonary vein thrombosis/stenosis

Findings that suggest specific disease entity:
- Left-sided valve changes (systemic lupus erythematosus and anorexigen use)
- Intra-pulmonary shunts (hereditary hemorrhagic telangiectasia)
- Pericardial effusion (idiopathic pulmonary artery hypertension, systemic lupus erythematosus and systemic sclerosis)

(*Source:* Reference 14)

Constrictive pericarditis is characterized by impaired diastolic cardiac filling and elevated ventricular filling pressures due to a rigid pericardium with fusion of the visceral and parietal layers. While increased pericardial thickness may be visualized with TTE, sensitivity and correlation with pathologic measurement are suboptimal.[18] Constrictive pericarditis is usually associated with elevated and equal pressures in all four cardiac chambers. At the onset of diastole, the rate of ventricular filling is increased but is rapidly halted by pericardial constraint.[16] The abrupt early diastolic filling may be seen on the 2D echocardiogram as a septal "bounce". Mitral inflow as assessed by Doppler echocardiography demonstrates an increased early diastolic filling velocity and shortened DT (i.e. < 160 msec).[16,18] Increased filling of one ventricle occurs at the expense of the other and this results in a respiratory shift in the position of the interventricular septum (Fig. 18) and exaggeration of normal respiratory changes in mitral and tricuspid flow (Figs 19A to E).[19] In constrictive pericarditis, tricuspid flow increases greater than 25% and mitral flow decreases greater than 25% with inspiration.[16,18]

Constriction can be distinguished from restrictive cardiomyopathy since marked respiratory changes in intracardiac velocities are not present with the latter (Fig. 20, Table 4).[19] Hepatic vein Doppler profiles differ between the two disorders as well. In patients with constriction, during expiration there is a decrease in RV filling resulting in a decrease in tricuspid valve velocity and an augmentation of diastolic flow reversal in the hepatic vein. Patients with restrictive cardiomyopathy exhibit diastolic flow reversal in inspiration.[18,19] Analysis of mitral annular velocities can also help in the differentiation. Patients with restrictive cardiomyopathy have impaired myocardial relaxation, leading to reductions in myocardial velocity. On the other hand, with constriction, annular vertical velocity is usually preserved. Furthermore, the septal myocardial velocity is usually increased due to preserved LV longitudinal expansion compensating for limited lateral and AP expansion.[8]

VALVULAR HEART DISEASE

AORTIC STENOSIS

The most common cause of aortic stenosis in adults is calcification of a normal trileaflet or a congenital bicuspid

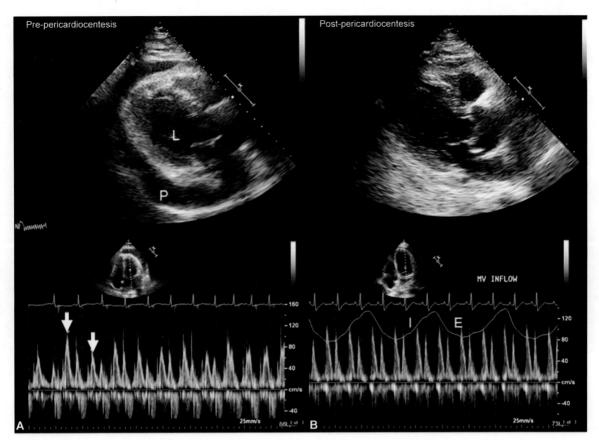

FIGURES 17A AND B: (A) Large pericardial effusion (PE) demonstrated on 2D echo and with respiratory variation > 25% of early filling velocity on mitral inflow Doppler (arrows) consistent with cardiac tamponade. (B) After pericardiocentesis, there is resolution of pericardial effusion and respiratory variation of early filling velocity. (Abbreviations: I: Inspiration; E: Expiration)

FIGURE 18: Schematic of respiratory variation in transvalvular and central venous flow velocities in constrictive pericarditis. With inspiration, the driving pressure gradient from the pulmonary capillaries to the left cardiac chambers decreases, resulting in a decrease in mitral inflow and diastolic pulmonary venous (PV) flow velocity. The decreased left ventricular filling results in ventricular septal shift to the left (small arrow), allowing augmented flow to the right-sided chambers shown as increased tricuspid inflow and diastolic hepatic venous (HV) flow velocity because the cardiac volume is relatively fixed as a result of the thickened shell of pericardium. The opposite changes occur during expiration. (Abbreviations: LA: Left atrium; LV: Left ventricle; RA: Right atrium; RV: Right ventricle; D: Diastole; S: Systole). (*Source:* Modified from Oh JK, Hatle LK, Seward JB, et al. Diagnostic role of Doppler echocardiography in constrictive pericarditis. J Am Coll Cardiol. 1994;23:154-62, with permission)

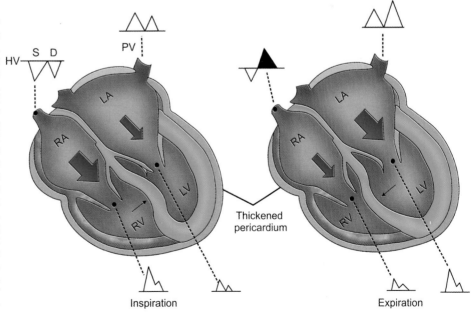

CHAPTER 16

Transthoracic Echocardiography

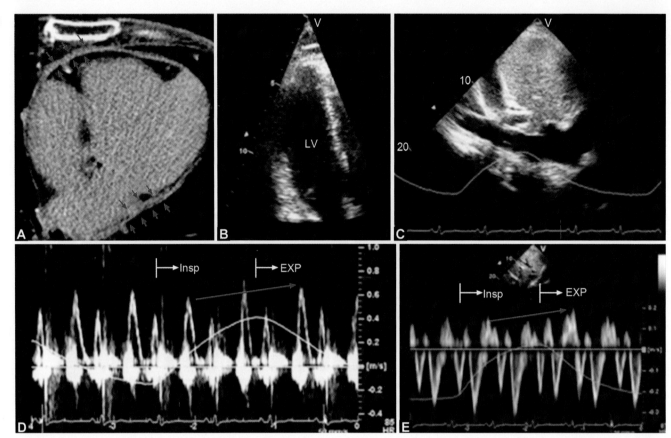

FIGURES 19A TO E: Findings in patients with constrictive pericarditis (CP). (A) Computed tomography in a patient with CP shows the extent of pericardial thickening (red arrows). Apical 4-chamber view of the left ventricle (LV) (B) and dilated inferior vena cava (C) with increased respiratory variations in transmitral early diastolic flow (D) and hepatic venous Doppler flow (E) are shown for the same patient with CP (red arrows in D and E indicate respiratory-dependent change in Doppler flow). (Abbreviations: Exp: Expiration; Insp: Inspiration). (*Source:* Dal-Bianco JP, Sengupta PP, Mookadam F, et al. Role of echocardiography in the diagnosis of constrictive pericarditis. J Am Soc Echocardiogr. 2009;22:24-33)

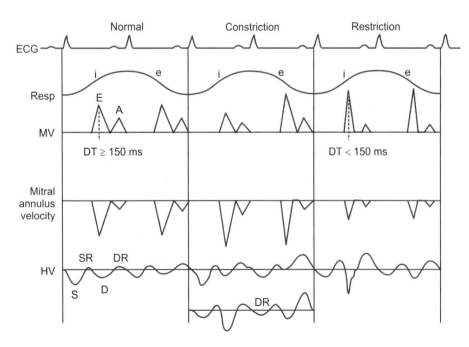

FIGURE 20: Schematic diagram of Doppler echocardiographic features in constrictive pericarditis versus restrictive cardiomyopathy. Schematic illustration of Doppler velocities from mitral inflow (MV), mitral annulus velocity and hepatic vein (HV). Electrocardiographic (ECG) and respirometer (Resp) recordings indicating inspiration (i) and expiration (e) are also shown. (Abbreviations: A: Atrial filling; D: Diastolic flow; DR: Diastolic flow reversal; DT: Deceleration time; E: Early diastolic filling; S: Systolic flow; SR: systolic flow reversal) (*Source:* Modified from Oh JK, Hatle LK, Seward JB, et al. Diagnostic role of Doppler echocardiography in constrictive pericarditis. J Am Coll Cardiol. 1994;23:154-62, with permission)

TABLE 4

Differentiation of constrictive pericarditis from restrictive cardio-myopathy

	Constriction	Restriction
Septal motion	Respiratory shift ("septal bounce")	Normal
Mitral E/A ratio	> 1.5	> 1.5
Mitral DT (msec)	< 160	< 160
Mitral inflow respiratory variation	Usually present	Absent
Hepatic vein Doppler	Expiratory diastolic flow reversal	Inspiratory diastolic flow reversal
Mitral septal annulus e'	> 7 cm/sec	< 7 cm/sec
Mitral lateral annulus e'	Lower than septal e'	Higher than septal e'
(Source: Reference 9)		

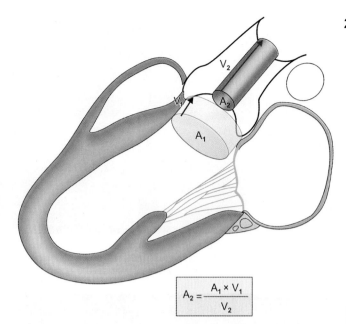

$$A_2 = \frac{A_1 \times V_1}{V_2}$$

FIGURE 21: Schematic diagram of continuity equation. Since the stroke volume in the LV outflow tract ($A_1 V_1$) is the same as the stroke volume at the aortic valve ($A_2 V_2$), A_2 (the aortic valve area) can be solved if A_1, V_1 and V_2 are known. (Source: Modified from Baumgartner H, Hung J, Bermejo J, et al. Echocardiographic assessment of valve stenosis: EAE/ASE recommendations for clinical practice. J Am Soc Echocardiogr. 2009;22:1-23, with permission)

valve.[2] Anatomic evaluation of the AV with 2D echo is based on a combination of short and long axis images to identify the number of leaflets, and to describe leaflet mobility, thickness and calcification. Unfortunately, the accuracy of direct planimetry of the valve area is limited by artifacts from calcification. Doppler echocardiography allows the determination of the level of obstruction and the quantitation of the pressure gradient (Table 5). The primary hemodynamic parameters for the clinical evaluation of aortic stenosis severity are jet velocity, mean transaortic gradient and valve area by the continuity equation.[20]

Jet velocity is measured across the narrowed AV using continuous wave Doppler ultrasound. Multiple acoustic windows are interrogated and the highest velocity is used. The pressure gradient (ΔP) between the left ventricle and the aorta in systole is calculated from the velocity (v) using the modified Bernoulli equation (i.e. $\Delta P = 4v^2$). The mean gradient is determined by averaging the instantaneous gradients over the ejection period. The modified Bernoulli equation assumes that the LV outflow velocity is negligible but if the proximal velocity is more than 1.5 m/sec, it should be included in the equation (i.e. $\Delta P = 4 (v^2_{max} - v^2_{proximal})$).[20]

Calculation of the stenotic orifice area or valve area is helpful when flow rates are very low or very high since the velocity

and pressure gradient are flow-dependent. According to the continuity equation, the stroke volume (SV) across the AV is equal to the SV in the LVOT. Since SV = CSA × flow velocity over the ejection period [or the velocity-time integral (VTI)], according to the continuity equation, $CSA_{AV} \times VTI_{AV} = CSA_{LVOT} \times VTI_{CSA}$. Solving for CSA_{AV}, the AV area = ($CSA_{LVOT} \times VTI_{CSA}$) ÷ VTI_{AV} (Figs 21 and 22A to C, Video 1).[20,21]

The CSA measurement may introduce error in the area calculation if images are not optimal for the LVOT diameter measurement. However, the Doppler velocity ratio (i.e. $V_{LVOT} \div V_{AV}$) provides an alternative assessment of valve stenosis severity if the CSA cannot be accurately determined. Severe stenosis is present when the ratio is less than or equal to 0.25.[19]

When low LV systolic function accompanies severe aortic stenosis, the transvalvular velocity and gradient may be low due to the low-flow state. Low-flow, low-gradient aortic stenosis generally refers to the presence of: (1) valve area less than 1.0 cm^2; (2) LVEF less than 40% and (3) mean pressure gradient less than 30–40 mm Hg. In cases when the stenosis severity is ambiguous, assessment of changes in gradient and area with increasing flow associated with dobutamine infusion may be helpful. An increase in valve area to a final valve area greater than 1.0 cm^2 suggests that the stenosis is not severe.[20]

Obstruction to LV ejection can occur at several levels: subaortic (LVOT), aortic (valvular) and supravalvular. Hypertrophic cardiomyopathy is characterized by inappropriate hypertrophy, interstitial fibrosis, myocardial disarray and impaired LV performance (Figs 23A to D). Asymmetric LV hypertrophy typically involves the septum, but almost any myocardial segment can be involved. Systolic anterior motion of the anterior mitral leaflet with or without a pressure gradient across the LVOT is related to the hydrodynamic

TABLE 5

Classification of aortic stenosis severity

	Mild	Moderate	Severe
Aortic jet velocity (m/s)	2.6–2.9	3.0–4.0	> 4.0
Mean gradient (mm Hg)	< 20 < 30*	20–40 30–50*	> 40 > 50*
Aortic valve area (cm^2)	> 1.5	1.0–1.5	< 1.0
Indexed aortic valve area (cm^2/m^2)	> 0.85	0.60–0.85	< 0.6
Doppler velocity ratio	> 0.50	0.25–0.50	< 0.25

*European Society of Cardiology Guidelines
(Source: Reference 20)

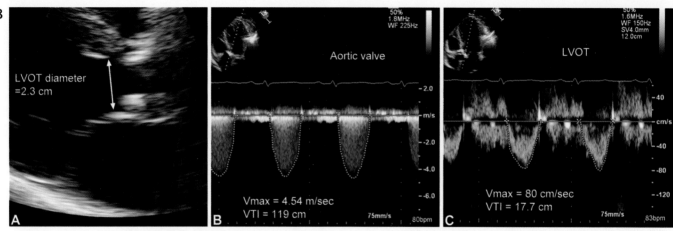

FIGURES 22A TO C: Calculation of the aortic valve area with the continuity equation includes: (A) an estimate of the left ventricular (LV) outflow tract area calculated from the diameter; (B) the velocity time integral (VTI) obtained across the valve and (C) the VTI in the LV outflow tract. Valve area was calculated as 0.62 cm² consistent with severe aortic stenosis

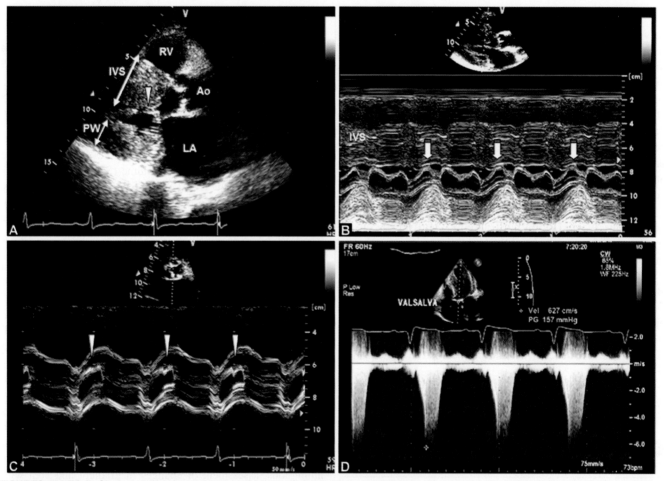

FIGURES 23A TO D: Characteristic echocardiographic features of obstructive hypertrophic cardiomyopathy: (A) parasternal long axis view depicting severe asymmetric septal hypertrophy and systolic anterior mitral valve motion (arrowhead); (B) m-mode across the mitral leaflets depicting prominent systolic anterior motion (thick arrows) of the anterior mitral leaflet; (C) m-mode tracing across the aortic valve demonstrating partial closure of aortic leaflets (arrowheads) and (D) accentuation of late-peaking dynamic left ventricular outflow tract obstruction after the Valsalva maneuver. (Abbreviations: Ao: Aorta; IVS: Interventricular septum; LA: Left atrium; PW: Posterior wall). (*Source:* Afonso LC, Bernel J, Bax JJ, et al. Echocardiography in hypertrophic cardiomyopathy: the role of conventional and emerging technologies. JACC Cardiovasc Imaging. 2008;1:787-800)

forces on the leaflet. The shape of the velocity profile may assist in identifying the level of obstruction as well as the severity. A dynamic LVOT obstruction in patients with hypertrophic cardiomyopathy shows a characteristic late-peaking velocity curve. A resting LVOT obstruction greater than 30 mm Hg is a strong predictor of death and progression to heart failure. In symptomatic patients with a resting gradient less than 30 mm Hg, obstruction may be provoked by amyl nitrite inhalation or the Valsalva maneuver. LV systolic function is typically normal, but diastolic

TABLE 6

Classification of aortic regurgitation severity

	Mild	Moderate	Severe
Jet width/LVOT width (%) - Color Doppler	< 25	25–64	≥ 65
Jet cross-sectional area/LVOT cross-sectional area (%) - Color Doppler	< 5	5–59	≥ 60
Vena contracta width (cm) - Color Doppler	< 0.3	0.3–0.6	> 0.6
Effective regurgitant orifice area (cm^2) - Color Doppler	< 0.10	0.10–0.29	≥ 0.30
Jet deceleration rate [Pressure half-time (msec)] - Continuous wave Doppler	> 500	500–200	< 200
Diastolic flow reversal in descending aorta - Pulsed wave Doppler	Early diastolic reversal	Intermediate	Prominent holodiastolic reversal

(*Source:* Reference 23)

dysfunction is common and characterized by Doppler echocardiography as impaired relaxation.[22]

AORTIC REGURGITATION

Chronic aortic regurgitation is a condition of combined volume and pressure overload. While the LV may compensate for the increased load, eventually depressed contractility may occur, sometimes while the patient remains asymptomatic. LV dysfunction is initially reversible with recovery after valve replacement but eventually this recovery may not be achievable. Thus echocardiography is useful not only in the assessment of aortic regurgitation etiology and severity but also for LV size and function.[2]

Color Doppler evaluation of aortic regurgitation includes the measurement of the regurgitant jet size, the vena contracta through the orifice, and the flow convergence toward the regurgitant orifice area[23] (Table 6). The proximal regurgitant jet width or CSA is measured in the LVOT, within 1 cm of the valve, usually from the parasternal view and then compared to the 2D echocardiographic measurement of LV outflow diameter or CSA. The vena contracta is measured as the width of diastolic flow at the AV. The flow convergence or proximal isovelocity surface area (PISA) method is discussed in detail in the section on mitral regurgitation (MR) since there is relatively less experience with the method in aortic regurgitation compared to MR.[23]

Continuous and pulsed wave Doppler methods for quantitation of aortic regurgitation are based on velocity measurements from systolic and diastolic velocity profiles. The rate of deceleration of the diastolic regurgitant jet (i.e. deceleration slope) reflects the equalization of pressures between the aorta and the left ventricle. As aortic regurgitation severity increases, the deceleration slope increases. In severe aortic regurgitation, the deceleration pressure half-time (i.e. the time required to decrease the diastolic pressure gradient between the aorta and the LV by one half) is under 200 msec. Reversal of aortic flow in the descending aorta suggests at least moderate regurgitation (Fig. 24, Video 2).[23]

Quantitation of forward and total SV can be determined flow by pulsed Doppler methods. In addition, total SV can be determined from quantitation of LV volumes by 2D echocardio-graphy. However, these methods are for the most part limited to research.[23]

Transesophageal echocardiography (TEE) provides an alternative to evaluation of aortic regurgitation and is described in chapter "Transesophageal Echocardiography".

MITRAL STENOSIS

The principle cause of mitral stenosis is rheumatic heart disease and despite a decrease in the prevalence of rheumatic fever, mitral stenosis remains a significant problem, particularly due to immigration from developing countries. The evaluation of mitral stenosis with echocardiography is directed at determining severity of stenosis and suitability for balloon valvuloplasty.[24]

Direct measurement of the valve area is possible by tracing the valve orifice area from the parasternal short axis view (Figs 25A to D). However careful attention to gain settings is needed since excessive setting may lead to underestimation of area. In addition, scanning should be performed from the apex to base of the LV to assure that the area is measured at the level of the leaflet tips (i.e. the smallest measurable orifice).[20,24]

The estimation of the diastolic pressure gradient across the mitral valve in mitral stenosis uses the modified Bernoulli equation ($\Delta P = 4v^2$). For accurate measurement, the Doppler ultrasound beam must be oriented parallel to flow, so the apical 4-chamber view is preferred for imaging. Doppler ultrasound provides an alternative method to direct planimetry for assessing valve area. The decline in velocity of diastolic transmitral blood flow is inversely proportional to valve area according to the formula:

$$\text{Mitral valve area} = 220/T_{1/2}$$

where $T_{1/2}$ is the time (in msec) between the maximum mitral gradient in early diastole and the point at which the gradient is half the maximum initial value. $T_{1/2}$ can be measured directly from the velocity profile as the time from maximum velocity to the velocity corresponding to maximum velocity ÷ $\sqrt{2}$. In the valve area equation, 220 is an empirically derived constant (Fig. 26, Videos 3 and 4).[20]

Recommendations for classification of mitral stenosis severity (Table 7) are based on Doppler assessment of the mitral

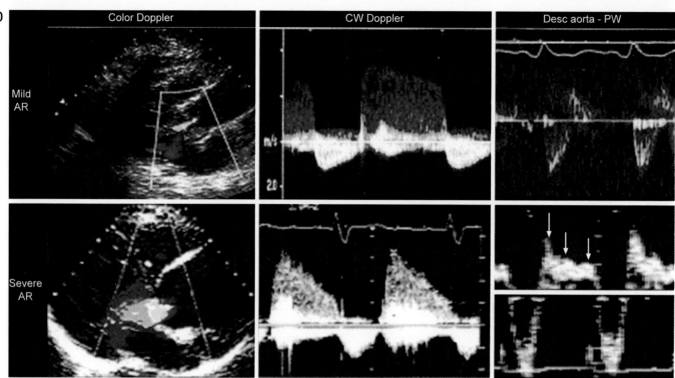

Color Doppler	CW Doppler	Desc aorta - PW

Mild AR

Severe AR

FIGURE 24: Color Doppler and continuous wave (CW) Doppler recordings of the regurgitant jet as well as pulsed wave (PW) Doppler recording of flow in the descending thoracic aorta in examples of mild and severe aortic regurgitation (AR). Compared to mild AR, severe AR has a larger jet width in the left ventricular outflow, a steep deceleration rate of the AR velocity by CW Doppler and a holo-diastolic flow reversal in the descending (desc) aorta (arrows). (*Source:* Zoghbi WA, Enriguez-Sarano M, Foster E, et al. Recommendations for evaluation of the severity of native valvular regurgitation with two-dimensional and Doppler echocardiography. J Am Soc Echocardiogr. 2003;16:777-802)

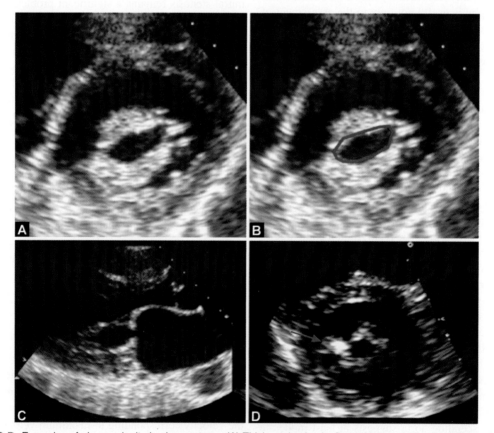

FIGURES 25A TO D: Examples of abnormal mitral valve anatomy. (A) Thickened valve leaflets without calcification. (B) Planimetry of mitral valve area in parasternal short axis view. (C) Rheumatic mitral valve in parasternal long axis view demonstrating "doming" of the anterior leaflet and failure of the mitral commissures to separate (i.e. commissural fusion). (D) Calcification localized at the level of the medial commissures (small red arrow). (*Source:* Messika-Zeitoun D, Lung B, Brochet E, et al. Evaluation of mitral stenosis in 2008. Arch Cardiovasc Dis. 2008;101:653-63)

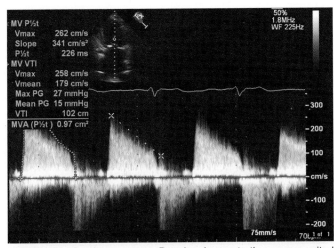

FIGURE 26: Continuous wave Doppler demonstrating severe mitral stenosis. The pressure half-time ($P_{1/2}t$) is 226 ms, predicting a valve area of 0.97 cm^2

TABLE 7

Classification of mitral stenosis severity

	Mild	Moderate	Severe
Valve area (cm^2)	> 1.5	1.0–1.5	< 1.0
Mean gradient (mm Hg)	< 5	5–10	> 10
Pulmonary artery systolic pressure (mm Hg)	< 30	30–50	> 50
(*Source:* Reference 20)			

stenosis as well as secondary findings of pulmonary hypertension severity.

Percutaneous mitral balloon valvulotomy is effective treatment for patients with symptomatic moderate or severe mitral stenosis and favorable valve morphology, in the absence of LA thrombus or moderate to severe MR. Patients with

valvular calcification, thickened fibrotic leaflets with decreased mobility and subvalvular fusion have a higher incidence of acute complications and a higher rate of recurrent stenosis on follow-up.[2]

MITRAL REGURGITATION

An initial comprehensive TTE in a patient with suspected MR provides a baseline assessment left-sided chamber size and LVEF. In addition, TTE provides an approximation of MR severity, anatomic information regarding mechanism and PA pressure. Changes from baseline values are useful in guiding the timing of mitral valve surgery.[2]

The echocardiographic exam of the mitral valve begins with a 2D echo evaluation since the etiology of regurgitation may be visualized. Examples include underlying mitral valve prolapse[25] (Figs 27A and B, Video 5) and annular dilatation due to LV enlargement. The natural history of mitral valve prolapse is variable and the most frequent predictor of cardiovascular mortality is MR severity.[2] With chronic MR, enlargement of the LA and LV are common. Pulsed wave, continuous wave and color Doppler evaluation complement 2D echocardiography in the evaluation of MR (Table 8).[23]

Color flow Doppler evaluation includes visualization of the origin of the regurgitant jet and its width (i.e. the vena contracta), as well as spatial orientation in the left atrium. Visualization of the regurgitant jet area in the receiving chamber can provide screening for the presence and direction of the regurgitant jet as well as a semiquantitative assessment of severity. Jet area measurements are influenced by technical factors such as transducer frequency, gain settings, output power and Nyquist limit [i.e. aliasing velocity (Va)]. Planimetry of the jet area in the LA provides a quantitative parameter for assessing MR, but the jet area may underestimate severity if regurgitation is eccentric (Figs 28A to C, Videos 6 and 7).[23]

The vena contracta is the narrowest portion of a jet that occurs at or just downstream from the orifice and represents a

CHAPTER 16

Transthoracic Echocardiography

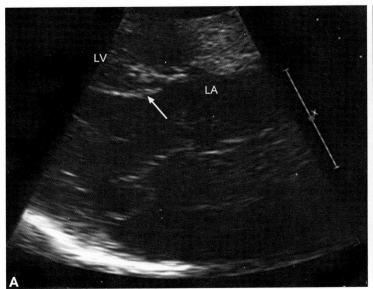

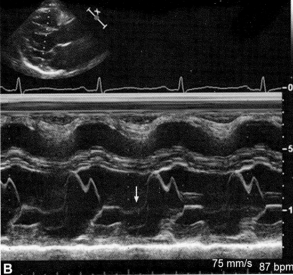

FIGURES 27A AND B: Parasternal long axis view 2D (A) and m-mode (B) echocardiograms demonstrating prolapse of the mitral valve posterior leaflet (arrow). (Abbreviations: LA: Left atrium; LV: Left ventricle)

TABLE 8

Classification of mitral regurgitation severity

	Mild	Moderate	Severe
Jet area - Color Doppler	< 4 cm² or < 20% of LA area	Variable	> 10 cm² or > 40% of LA area
Vena contracta width (cm) - Color Doppler	< 0.3	0.3–0.69	≥ 0.7
EROA (cm²) - Color Doppler	< 0.20	0.20–0.39	≥ 0.40
Mitral inflow - Pulsed Doppler	A wave dominant	Variable	E wave dominant (usually ≥ 1.2 m/sec)
Mitral jet contour - Continuous wave	Parabolic	Usually parabolic	Early peaking
Mitral jet density - Continuous wave	Incomplete or faint	Dense	Dense
Pulmonary vein flow	Systolic dominance	Systolic blunting	Systolic flow reversal

(*Source:* Reference 23)

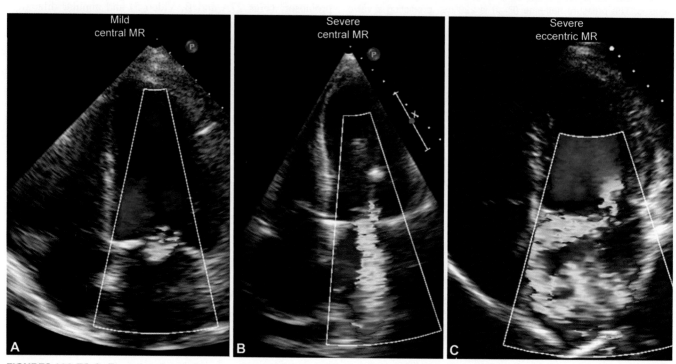

FIGURES 28A TO C: Examples of color flow recordings of different mitral regurgitation (MR) lesions from the apical window. (A) The case of mild regurgitation has a small regurgitant jet area, in contrast to that of severe central MR (B), which shows a larger regurgitant jet area. (C) Example with severe eccentric MR has a jet area impinging on the wall of the left atrium

measure of the effective regurgitant orifice area. The size of the vena contracta is independent of flow rate and driving force.[23]

Flow convergence into the regurgitant orifice area is a useful indicator of regurgitation severity. The PISA or flow convergence method is derived from the principle that blood velocity increases at a regurgitant orifice area as hemispheric shells of increasing velocity and decreasing surface area. The Va is determined by setting the Nyquist limit to visualize the hemisphere. The flow rate through the orifice area is the product of the hemisphere surface area ($2 \pi r^2$) and Va. The effective regurgitant orifice area is then calculated using the flow rate and the peak regurgitant velocity (i.e. effective regurgitant orifice area = flow rate/peak regurgitant velocity) (Fig. 29)[23,26]

Continuous wave Doppler signal of the regurgitant jet measures maximum velocity which does not provide quantitation of jet severity. However, the contour of the profile and its density are useful. Pulsed Doppler evaluation of the mitral inflow velocity at the mitral leaflet tips provides measurement of the early and late filling velocities. As regurgitation severity increases there is loss of relative contribution of atrial filling and an increase in early filling. Pulmonary vein flow into the LA demonstrates a progressive decrease in systolic velocity with increasing severity of MR, and reversal of flow in the presence of severe MR (Figs 30A and B).[23]

Estimates of regurgitant volume and fraction are possible with pulsed Doppler assessment of volumetric flow and 2D echocardiographic measurement of LV volumes for SV; however, these parameters have limited general clinical application due to the time constraints of these measurements.

Transesophageal echocardiography (TEE) provides improved visualization of the mitral valve and quantitation of regurgitation and is discussed in chapter "Transesophageal Echocardiography".

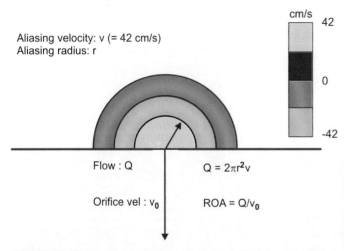

Aliasing velocity: v (= 42 cm/s)
Aliasing radius: r

Flow : Q $Q = 2\pi r^2 v$

Orifice vel : v_0 $ROA = Q/v_0$

FIGURE 29: The proximal convergence method. By using the aliasing velocity of the color Doppler display, it is possible to measure the radius to an isovelocity shell as blood converges on the regurgitant orifice. Assuming a hemispheric shape to the shell, flow rate is given as $Q = 2\pi r^2 v$. Dividing this flow rate by the maximal velocity through the orifice (given by continuous wave Doppler) yields an estimation for the regurgitant orifice area (ROA). (*Source:* Modified from Thomas JD. Doppler echocardiographic assessment of valvar regurgitation. Heart. 2002;88:651-7, with permission)

TRICUSPID STENOSIS

Isolated tricuspid stenosis is uncommon and the same principles as for mitral stenosis apply. However, an empiric constant of 190 has been proposed and the mean gradient in significant tricuspid stenosis is lower than for mitral stenosis. Hemodynamically significant stenosis is defined as: a mean pressure gradient greater than 5 mm Hg, and $T_{1/2}$ greater than 190 msec (corresponding to a valve area less than 1.0 cm² and assuming an empiric constant of 190). Additional supportive findings on 2D echocardiography include enlargement of the RA and dilatation of the inferior vena cava (Figs 31A and B).[20]

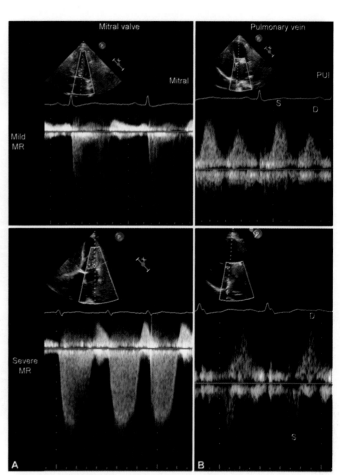

FIGURES 30A AND B: Mitral valve continuous wave Doppler and pulmonary vein flow pulsed Doppler recordings in mild and severe mitral regurgitation (MR). In mild MR (A), continuous wave Doppler has a soft density with a parabolic, rounded contour of the regurgitant velocity whereas in severe MR (B), the jet is dense with a triangular, early peaking of the velocity. Pulmonary vein flow is normal in mild MR with predominance of systolic flow (S). In contrast, with severe MR systolic flow reversal may occur. (Abbreviation: D: Diastolic flow velocity)

CHAPTER 16 — Transthoracic Echocardiography

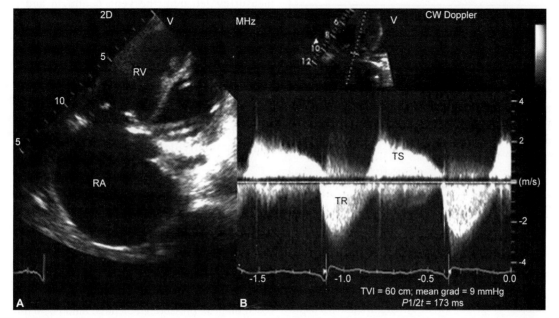

FIGURES 31A AND B: (A) 2D echocardiographic image of a stenotic tricuspid valve obtained in a modified apical 4-chamber view during diastole. Note the thickening and diastolic doming of the valve and the marked enlargement of the right atrium (RA). (B) Continuous wave (CW) Doppler recording through the tricuspid valve. Note the elevated peak diastolic velocity of 2 m/s and the systolic tricuspid regurgitation (TR) recording. The diastolic time-velocity integral (TVI), mean gradient (Grad) and pressure half-time ($T_{1/2}$) values are listed. (*Source:* Baumgartner H, Hung J, Bermejo J, et al. Echocardiographic assessment of valve stenosis: EAE/ASE recommendations for clinical practice. J Am Soc Echocardiogr. 2009;22:1-23)

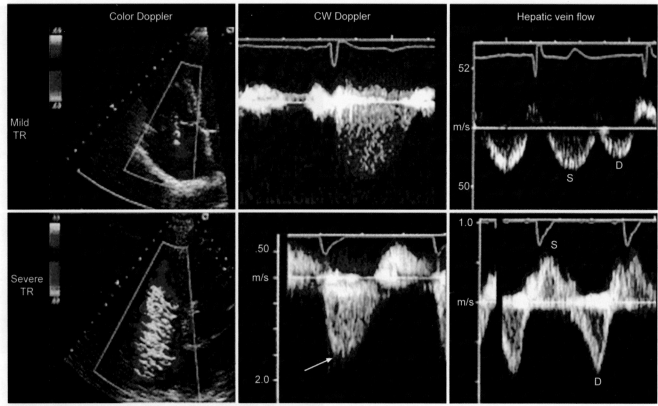

FIGURE 32: Examples of jet recordings by color Doppler, continuous wave (CW) Doppler, and hepatic vein flow by pulsed Doppler in mild and severe tricuspid regurgitation (TR). The case of mild TR shows a small central color jet with minimal flow convergence in contrast to the severe TR with a very large flow convergence and jet area in the right atrium. CW Doppler recording shows a parabolic spectral display in mild TR whereas in severe TR, early peaking and triangular shape of the velocity is seen (arrow). Hepatic vein flow pattern in mild TR is normal whereas in severe TR, hepatic venous flow reversal in systole (S) is seen. (Abbreviation: D: Diastolic hepatic venous flow). (*Source:* Zoghbi WA, Enriguez-Sarano M, Foster E, et al. Recommendations for evaluation of the severity of native valvular regurgitation with two-dimensional and Doppler echocardiography. J Am Soc Echocardiogr. 2003;16(7):777-802)

TABLE 9

Classification of tricuspid regurgitation severity

	Mild	Moderate	Severe
Jet area (cm²) - Color Doppler	< 5	5–10	> 10
Vena contracta width (cm) - Color Doppler		< 0.7	> 0.7
PISA radius (cm) - Color Doppler	≤ 0.5	0.6–0.9	> 0.9
Tricuspid jet density - Continuous wave Doppler	Faint	Dense	Dense
Tricuspid jet contour - Continuous wave Doppler	Parabolic	Variable	Early peaking
Hepatic vein flow - Pulsed wave Doppler	Systolic dominance	Systolic blunting	Systolic flow reversal
(*Source:* Reference 23)			

TRICUSPID REGURGITATION

Similar to MR, tricuspid regurgitation is assessed by integrating information on right-sided chamber size, septal motion and Doppler parameters (Fig. 32, Table 9). Significant tricuspid regurgitation is often associated with RA and RV enlargement and in the presence of significant volume overload of the RV, there may be paradoxical septal motion. Right atrial (RA)

pressure estimation can be appreciated by the size and respiratory variation of the inferior vena cava.[23]

Color Doppler methods for assessing severity include measuring jet area, the vena contracta and the effective regurgitant orifice area using methods described above for MR. Continuous wave Doppler methods are also similar to those described for MR and include signal intensity and the contour of the velocity curve. Pulsed Doppler can measure the RV filling velocities and with severe tricuspid regurgitation, early filling velocities are elevated and can be greater than 1.0 m/sec. The hepatic vein velocity profile, in similar fashion to the pulmonary vein velocity profile in significant MR, demonstrates blunting of the normally dominant systolic wave with increasing regurgitation systolic flow reversal with severe regurgitation.[23]

PULMONIC STENOSIS

Isolated pulmonic stenosis is usually congenital in origin. In addition to valvular lesions, congenital subvalvular and supravalvular location of stenosis are possible and may be difficult to differentiate from valvular stenosis. The severity of stenosis is determined by the pressure gradient as calculated from the modified Bernoulli equation. The grading of severity based on peak pressure gradient is: mild [< 36 mm Hg (corresponding to peak velocity < 3 m/sec)]; moderate [36–64 mm Hg (or a peak velocity of 3–4 m/sec)] and severe [> 64 mm Hg (or a peak velocity of > 4 m/sec)].[20] Evaluation of the valve's anatomy with 2D echo may provide additional information. For example, a domed shape of the leaflets suggests stenosis due to fusion of the leaflets.[2] In addition, RV hypertrophy and enlargement as well as RA enlargement may be present if there is significant pressure overload of these chambers.[20]

PULMONIC REGURGITATION

Mild pulmonic regurgitation may be present in normal subjects; however, significant regurgitation suggests the presence of underlying structural heart disease. In the adult, acquired pulmonic regurgitation is most often seen in patients with PH and related to dilation of the PA and/or RV, but is rarely severe. Pulmonic regurgitation of severe nature is usually observed in patients with anatomic abnormalities of the pulmonic valve or after valvotomy.[23]

Color Doppler flow mapping is the most widely used method for detection and regurgitation. The jet or vena contracta widths are common measurements in the assessment of regurgitation severity.[8] As severity of regurgitation increases, continuous wave Doppler demonstrates a rapid deceleration of diastolic flow as diastolic pressure in PA and RV equalize.[23]

INFECTIVE ENDOCARDITIS

Echocardiography is central to the diagnosis and management of patients with infective endocarditis. Transesophageal echocardiography (TTE) is an appropriate test for the detection of valvular vegetation, with or without positive blood cultures for the diagnosis of infective endocarditis (Fig. 33), although TEE is considered more sensitive than TTE in detecting vegetations. In addition, TTE can characterize the hemodynamic severity of valvular lesions and potential complications of endocarditis (e.g. abscess, valve perforation, shunt). Transesophageal echocardiography is also recommended for reassessment of high-risk patients (e.g. those with a virulent organism, clinical deterioration, persistent or recurrent fever, new murmur or persistent bacteremia).[2]

Echocardiographic evidence of endocardial involvement is considered the major criteria for the diagnosis of infective endocarditis according to the modified von Reyn criteria. Positive echocardiographic evidence of infective endocarditis

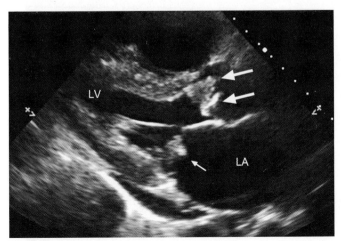

FIGURE 33: Parasternal long axis view of transthoracic echo showing large vegetations on the aortic valve (large arrows) and on the mitral valve (small arrow). (Abbreviations: LA: Left atrium; LV: Left ventricle)

is defined as an "oscillating intracardiac mass on valve or supporting structures, in the path of regurgitant jets, or on implanted material in the absence of an alternative anatomic explanation; or abscess; or new partial dehiscence of prosthetic valve; or new valvular regurgitation".[27] Transesophageal echocardiography has a sensitivity of 60–65% and specificity of 94–96% in the detection of vegetations. In contrast, improved sensitivity of 85–98% is reported for TEE. False negative TTE studies are more frequent with small vegetations, presence of prosthetic material or technically deficient studies.[28]

Current recommendations for the use of TEE in patients with endocarditis include: (1) symptomatic patients with infective endocarditis if TTE is nondiagnostic (to assess hemodynamic severity of a valve lesion); (2) patients with valvular heart disease and positive blood culture if TTE is nondiagnostic; (3) patients with possible complications of infective endocarditis and (4) patients with suspected prosthetic valve endocarditis.[2] The role of TEE in the evaluation of endocarditis is discussed further in chapter "Transesophageal Echocardiography".

Echocardiographic features that suggest potential need for surgical intervention include: perivalvular extension with abscess formation, valve perforation, acute valve regurgitation and increasing vegetation size despite appropriate antibiotic therapy.[27,29] A vegetation size greater than 10 mm is associated with increased embolic risk and this risk appears higher in patients with mitral valve endocarditis.[2]

INTRACARDIAC MASSES

Abnormal intracardiac masses are typically echodensities that represent thrombus or tumor. However, there are normal variants that can be confused with mass lesions. For example, prominent papillary muscles, dense mitral annular calcification, a prominent moderator band in the RV, a prominent Chiari network in the RA and lipomatous hypertrophy of the interatrial septum can mimic abnormal pathology.[30]

Primary tumors are uncommon and about 75% are benign, usually representing myxoma in the adult and rhabdomyoma in children under 15 years. About 75–90% of myxomas are found in the LA, pedunculated and attached to the interatrial septum, in or adjacent to the fossa ovalis (Figs 34A and B). The remainder occurs in the RA, or infrequently in the ventricles. About one-fourth of primary cardiac tumors are malignant and the majority are sarcomas. Angiosarcoma is the most common sarcoma and has a propensity to occur on the right side of the heart, especially in the RA. Rhabdomyosarcoma can occur in any cardiac chamber, grow rapidly and have usually invaded the pericardium by the time of diagnosis. Leiomyosarcomas are very rare and are usually found in the LA.[30,31]

Metastatic tumors are up to 40 times more common than primary tumors, and are typically encountered in patients with widespread systemic tumor dissemination. Metastatic tumors are most commonly lung, breast, ovarian, kidney, leukemia, lymphoma and esophageal. However malignant melanoma appears to have a preference for metastasizing to the heart, with metastases occurring in up to 50% of patients.[30,32] Metastases to the pericardium are more common than to the myocardium.[30]

In patients presenting with unexplained stroke, attention is usually directed at identifying clinically inapparent sources of

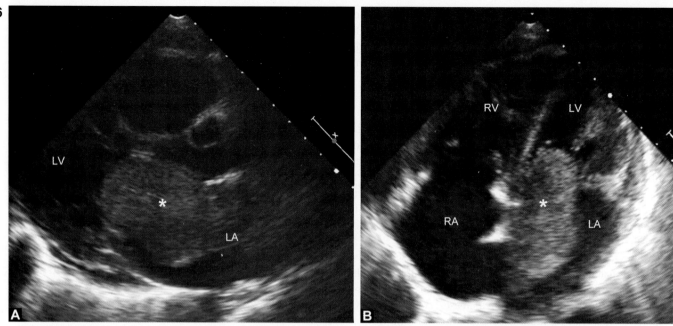

FIGURES 34A AND B: Transthoracic parasternal long axis (A) and apical 4-chamber (B) views demonstrating left atrial myxoma (asterisk). (Abbreviations: LV: Left ventricle; RV: Right ventricle; LA: Left atrium; RA: Right atrium)

embolism. Transesophageal echocardiography can usually exclude some of the high-risk abnormalities (e.g. LV akinesis/ dyskinesis, dilated cardiomyopathy, LV thrombus and mitral stenosis). However, TEE is superior to TTE in the detection of LA thrombus, complex thoracic aorta atheromas, valve vegetations, interatrial septal aneurysm and small tumors.[33]

CONTRAST ECHOCARDIOGRAPHY

Echo contrast agents used in contrast echocardiography include agitated saline for the assessment of right-to-left intracardiac shunts and manufactured microbubbles with shell composition of lipid, human albumin or phospholipid and gas (e.g. air, perfluoropropane, sulfur hexafluoride, etc.). The manufactured microbubbles are very small (i.e. < 5 μ in diameter), able to traverse the pulmonary circulation and then opacify the left heart chambers.[34]

In the presence of a patent foramen ovale, there may be only intermittent right-to-left shunting of the microbubbles produced by IV injection of agitated saline since the flap of the patent foramen ovale may be functionally closed during part of the respiratory cycle, when LA pressure exceeds RA pressure. A cough or Valsalva maneuver release may be needed to provoke a transient increase in RA pressure relative to LA pressure and allow the flap of the foramen to open and allow microbubble passage from the RA to the LA. However late appearance (i.e. more than three cycles after appearance in the RA) of microbubbles into the LA may be related to trans-pulmonary passage of the microbubbles. When a right-to-left shunt is seen by saline contrast, the distinction between a patent foramen ovale and an atrial septal defect can be made by assessing the size of the RA and the RV, which are usually enlarged due to an atrial septal defect, but normal when a

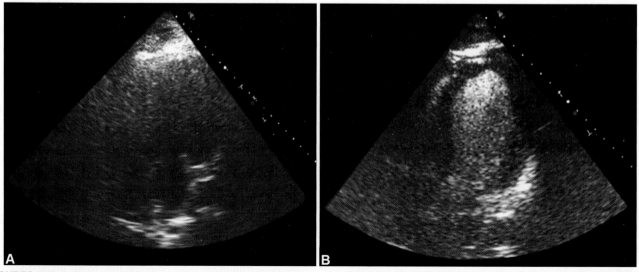

FIGURES 35A AND B: Contrast opacification of the left ventricular cavity. (A) Apical 4-chamber views with poor endocardial definition. (B) The same view with improved endocardial definition after echocardiographic contrast administration. (*Source:* Echocardiography in heart failure: application, utility, and new horizons. J Am Coll Cardiol. 2007;50:381-96r)

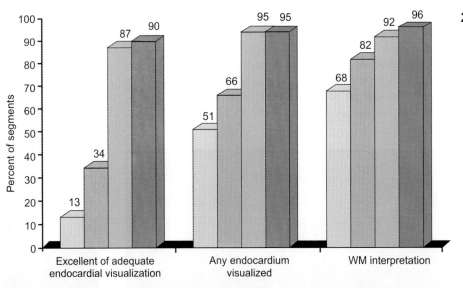

FIGURE 36: Percent of segments visualized and interpreted for wall motion (WM) using fundamental imaging (open bars), harmonics (dotted bars) and contrast echo (slashed bars) with harmonics from the transthoracic approach and with TEE (filled bars). (*Source:* Modified from Yong Y, Wu D, Fernandes V, et al. Diagnostic accuracy and cost-effectiveness of contrast echocardiography on evaluation of cardiac function in technically very difficult patients in the intensive care unit. Am J Cardiol. 2002;89:711-8, with permission)

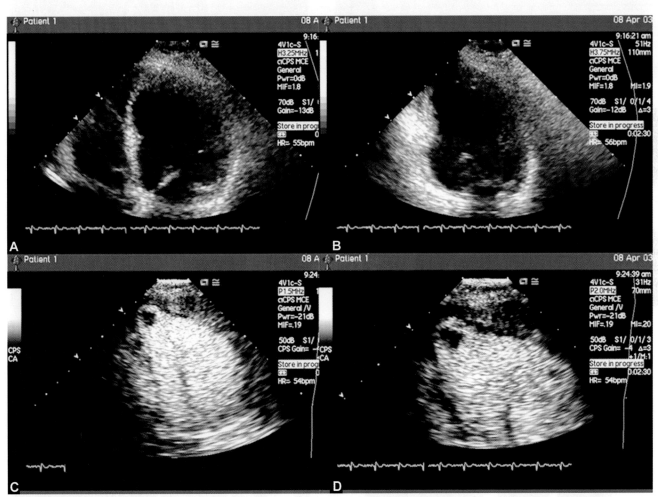

FIGURES 37A TO D: Apical 4- and 2-chamber views in a patient post stroke (A and B). With contrast, an apical thrombus is visualized as a contrast defect in the cavity (C) 2-chamber view, (D) Zoomed apex). (*Source:* Kirkpatrick JN, Vannan MA, Narula J, et al. Echocardiography in heart failure: application, utility, and new horizons. J Am Coll Cardiol. 2007;50:381-96)

patent foramen ovale is present. Contrast echo is also useful in the detection of a residual shunt after device closure of an atrial septal defect.[35]

Manufactured contrast agents may be useful in improving the accuracy and reproducibility of the assessment of LV structure and function at rest and during stress. Suboptimal echocardiograms can be converted to diagnostic examinations in 75–90% of patients due to improved endocardial definition (Figs 35A and B). This is especially helpful in patients who are obese, have lung disease or are on ventilators (Fig. 36).[36-38]

Echocardiographic contrast agents may be particularly useful in improving the visualization of the apex. In addition, apical thrombi may be difficult to visualize in non-contrast images due to the uncertainty of proper beam orientation and potential shortening of the major length of the left ventricle due to poor endocardial definition of the apex (Figs 37A to D).

Patients with pulmonary hypertension or unstable cardiopulmonary conditions should be monitored for 30 minutes after contrast agents administration. In addition, these products should not be administered to patients with right-to-left, bidirectional or transient right-to-left cardiac shunts;

hypersensitivity to perfluorocarbon; or hypersensitivity to blood, blood products or albumin (which applies to those agents with an albumin shell).[36]

Finally, there is experimental work in the assessment of myocardial perfusion using contrast agents. The initial studies demonstrated definition of risk area during acute coronary occlusion and progressed to evaluation of the success of tissue reperfusion and residual infarct size. More recent studies have shown the ability of myocardial contrast echocardiography to detect coronary stenosis during stress. However the application of myocardial contrast echocardiography as a clinical tool awaits approval of the contrast agents for this indication.[34]

FIGURE 38: M-mode echocardiogram at midventricular level of left ventricle (LV) demonstrating septal to posterior wall delay of 190 msec, consistent with significant dyssynchrony

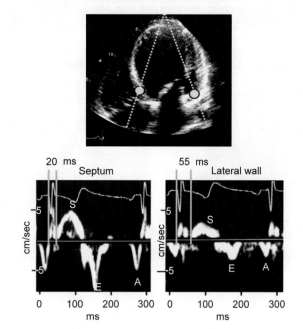

FIGURE 39: Pulsed tissue Doppler demonstrating dyssynchrony with delayed time to onset of systolic velocity in lateral wall, as compared with septum in a patient with left bundle branch block before resynchronization therapy. (Abbreviations: S: Systolic velocity; E: Early filling velocity; A: Atrial filling velocity). (*Source:* Gorcsan J 3rd, Abraham T, Agler DA, et al. Echocardiography for cardiac resynchronization therapy: recommendations for performance and reporting—a report from the American Society of Echocardiography dyssynchrony writing group. J Am Soc Echocardiogr. 2008;21:191-213)

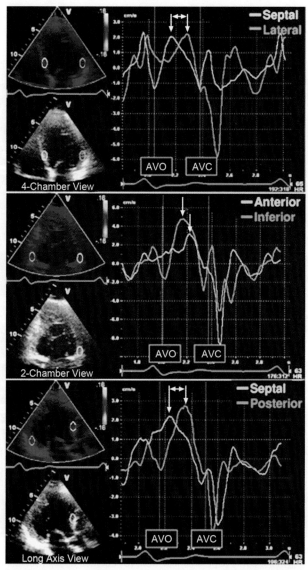

FIGURE 40: Color-coded tissue Doppler study from three standard apical views of a patient who responded to resynchronization therapy. Time-velocity curves from representative basal or mid levels are shown. Maximum opposing wall delay was seen in apical long axis view of 140 milliseconds between septum and posterior wall, consistent with significant dyssynchrony (≥ 65 milliseconds). (Abbreviations: AVO: Aortic valve opening; AVC: Aortic valve closure). (*Source:* Gorcsan J 3rd, Abraham T, Agler DA, et al. Echocardiography for cardiac resynchronization therapy: recommendations for performance and reporting—a report from the American Society of Echocardiography dyssynchrony writing group. J Am Soc Echocardiogr. 2008;21:191-213)

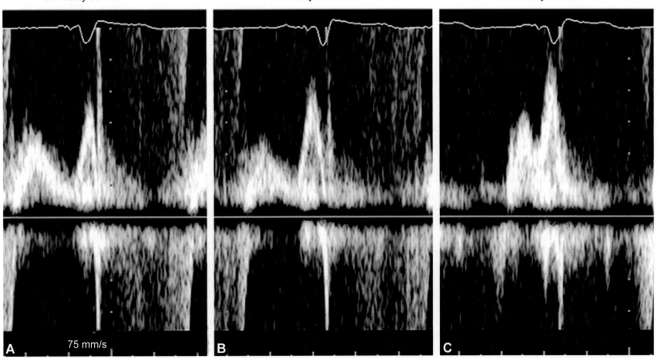

AV delay 80 ms | AV delay 120 ms | AV delay 180 ms

A   75 mm/s   B   C

FIGURES 41A TO C: The iterative method for atrioventricular optimization. (C) The sequence starts at a long atrioventricular (AV) delay (180 ms, shorter than intrinsic PR interval to ensure capture) and then shortening by 20 ms increments, until (A) A wave truncation appears (80 ms). Then atrioventricular delay is lengthened by 10 ms increments until A wave truncation disappears and maximum E and A wave separation is provided (B). (*Source:* Abraham T, Kass D, Tonti G, et al. Imaging cardiac resynchronization therapy. JACC Cardiovasc Imaging. 2009;2:486-97)

CARDIAC RESYNCHRONIZATION THERAPY

Echocardiography has been used to improve patient selection for chronic resynchronization therapy (CRT), also referred to as biventricular pacing, and to optimize device settings after implantation. Current recommendations for CRT include New York Heart Association functional class III or IV, widened QRS interval greater than or equal to 120 msec and LVEF less than or equal to 35%.[39]

Unfortunately, approximately 25–35% of patients undergoing CRT do not have an appropriate response. While a number of explanations have been proposed for the suboptimal response, the absence of dyssynchrony (i.e. regions of early and late contraction within the left ventricle) is a likely factor and can potentially be identified by echocardiography. A number of measurements have been proposed and evaluated, but there is no parameter that would justify withholding CRT therapy. Rather, a dyssynchrony study may be of potential benefit when evaluating patients with borderline QRS duration, borderline ejection fraction or ambiguous clinical history for NYHA functional class.[39]

M-mode echo provides excellent temporal resolution due to a sampling rate 1,000/sec. A delay from septal wall peak inward motion to posterior wall peak inward motion of greater than or equal to 130 msec has been proposed as a marker of dyssynchrony (Fig. 38). However follow-up studies have found the reproducibility of this technique to be suboptimal and the method should be used only to supplement other methods. The parameter may be difficult to obtain due to inaccuracy in determining the maximal septal deflection in patients with ischemic cardiomyopathy.[39,40]

Tissue Doppler imaging (TDI) measures the velocity of myocardium in relationship to the cardiac cycle and parameters such as peak systolic velocity, time to onset of systolic velocity and time to peak systolic velocity can be measured. With pulsed wave TDI, only one region can be interrogated at a time which increases procedure time and precludes simultaneous comparison of segments (Fig. 39). Color-coded TDI acquires velocity data from the entire sector and allows multiple simultaneous interrogations (Fig. 40).[40]

The majority of studies have used color-coded tissue Doppler to assess LV dyssynchrony and predict outcomes. The delay between segmental motion is measured and delay greater than 65 msec is predictive of clinic response to CRT. Speckle tracking is a more recent advance in assessing dyssynchrony. Tracking at the midventricular short axis level measures radial strain and a difference greater than or equal to 130 msec in peak strain between anterior septal and posterior wall has been used to identify responders.[39,40]

Since the ventricles are paced with CRT, the AV delay is programmed. The optimal AV delay is the time that allows completion of the atrial contribution to diastolic filling. This can be determined by optimizing the pulsed Doppler mitral inflow velocity: the E and A waves should be separated and the A wave termination should occur before the QRS onset (Figs 41A to C).[41] In addition, optimization of interventricular delay (i.e. V-V delay) is possible. V-V optimization is generally performed by changing the V-V sequence, starting with the LV being activated before the RV and then stepwise lengthening or shortening the V-V interval by 20 msec intervals.[39]

Video 1   Aortic regurgitation, severe parasternal long axis
Video 2   Aortic stenosis (parasternal long axis and parasternal short axis)
Video 3   Mitral regurgitation parasternal long axis
Video 4   Severe mitral regurgitation apical 4 chamber
Vidoe 5   Mitral stenosis (parasternal long axis and parasternal short axis)
Video 6   Mitral stenosis apical 4 chamber
Video 7   Mitral valve prolapse parasternal long axis

REFERENCES

1. Douglas PS, Khandheria B, Stainback RF, et al. ACCF/ASE/ACEP/ASNC/SCAI/SCCT/SCMR 2007 appropriateness criteria for transthoracic and transesophageal echocardiography. J Am Coll Cardiol. 2007;50:187-204.
2. Bonow RO, Carabello BA, Chatterjee K, et al. ACC/AHA 2006 guidelines for the management of patients with valvular heart disease. Executive Summary. Circulation. 2006;114:450-527.
3. Lang RM, Bierig M, Devereux RB, et al. Recommendations for chamber quantification: a report from the American Society of Echocardiography's guidelines and standards committee and the chamber quantification writing group, developed in conjunction with the European Association of Echocardiography, a branch of the European Society of Cardiology. J Am Soc Echo. 2005;18:1440-63.
4. Dittoe N, Stultz D, Schwartz BP, et al. Quantitative left ventricular systolic function: from chamber to myocardium. Crit Care Med. 2007;35:S330-9.
5. Verdecchia P, Angeli F, Achilli P, et al. Echocardiographic left ventricular hypertrophy in hypertension: marker for future events or mediator of events? Curr Opin Cardiol. 2007;22:329-34.
6. Rudski LG, Lai WW, Afilalo J, et al. Guidelines for the echocardiographic assessment of the right heart in adults: a report from the American Society of Echocardiography. J Am Soc Echocardiogr. 2010;23:685-713.
7. Abhayaratna WP, Seward JB, Appleton CP, et al. Left atrial size: physiologic determinants and clinical applications. J Am Coll Cardiol. 2006;47:2357-63.
8. Quinones MA, Otto CM, Stoddard M, et al. Recommendations for quantification of Doppler echocardiography: a report from the Doppler Quantification Task Force of the Nomenclature and Standards Committee of the American Society of Echocardiography. J Am Soc Echocardiogr. 2002;15:167-84.
9. Nagueh SF, Appleton CP, Gillebert TC, et al. Recommendations for the evaluation of left ventricular diastolic function by echocardiography. J Am Soc Echocardiogr. 2009;22:107-33.
10. Little WC, Oh JK. Echocardiographic evaluation of diastolic function can be used to guide clinical care. Circulation. 2009;120:802-9.
11. Ommen SR, Nishimura RA. A clinical approach to the assessment of left ventricular diastolic function by Doppler echocardiography: update 2003. Heart. 2003;89:18-23.
12. Kirkpatrick JN, Vannan MA, Narula J, et al. Echocardiography in heart failure: application, utility, and new horizons. J Am Coll Cardiol. 2007;50:381-96.
13. Ommen SR, Nishimura RA, Appleton CP, et al. Clinical utility of Doppler echocardiography and tissue Doppler imaging in the estimation of left ventricular filling pressures: a comparative simultaneous Doppler catheterization study. Circulation. 2000;102:1788-94.
14. McLaughlin VV, Archer SL, Badasch DB, et al. ACCF/AHA 2009 expert consensus document on pulmonary hypertension. Circulation. 2009;119:2250-94.
15. Milan A, Magnino C, Veglio F. Echocardiographic indexes for the non-invasive evaluation of pulmonary hemodynamics. J Am Soc Echocardiogr. 2010;23:225-39.
16. Wann S, Passen E. Echocardiography in pericardial disease. J Am Soc Echocardiogr. 2008;21:7-13.
17. Burstow DJ, Oh JK, Bailey KR, et al. Cardiac tamponade: characteristic Doppler observations. Mayo Clin Proc. 1989;64:312-24.
18. Dal-Bianco JP, Sengupta PP, Mookadam F, et al. Role of echocardiography in the diagnosis of constrictive pericarditis. J Am Soc Echocardiogr. 2009;22:24-33.
19. Oh JK, Hatle LK, Seward JB, et al. Diagnostic role of Doppler echocardiography in constrictive pericarditis. J Am Coll Cardiol. 1994;23:154-62.
20. Baumgartner H, Hung J, Bermejo J, et al. Echocardiographic assessment of valve stenosis: EAE/ASE recommendations for clinical practice. J Am Soc Echocardiogr. 2009;22:1-23.
21. Nistri S, Galderisi M, Faggiano P, et al. Practical echocardiography in aortic valve stenosis. J Cardiovasc Med. 2008;9:653-65.
22. Afonso LC, Bernel J, Bax JJ, et al. Echocardiography in hypertrophic cardiomyopathy: the role of conventional and emerging technologies. JACC Cardiovasc Imaging. 2008;1:787-800.
23. Zoghbi WA, Enriquez-Sarano M, Foster E, et al. Recommendations for evaluation of the severity of native valvular regurgitation with two-dimensional and Doppler echocardiography. J Am Soc Echocardiogr. 2003;16:777-802.
24. Messika-Zeitoun D, Iung B, Brochet E, et al. Evaluation of mitral stenosis in 2008. Arch Cardiovasc Dis. 2008;101:653-63.
25. Kerber RE, Isaeff DM, Hancock EW. Echocardiographic patterns in patients with the syndrome of systolic click and late systolic murmur. N Engl J Med. 1971;284:691-3.
26. Thomas JD. Doppler echocardiographic assessment of valvar regurgitation. Heart. 2002;88:651-7.
27. Baddour LM, Wilson WR, Bayer AS, et al. Infective endocarditis: diagnosis, antimicrobial therapy, and management of complications. Circulation. 2005;111:e394-434.
28. Cecchi E, Imazio M, Trinchero R. Infective endocarditis: diagnostic issues and practical clinical approach based on echocardiography. J Cardiovasc Med. 2008;9:414-8.
29. Zakkar M, Chan KM, Amirak E, et al. Infective endocarditis of the mitral valve: optimal management. Prog Cardiovasc Dis. 2009;51:472-7.
30. Peters PJ, Reinhardt S. The echocardiographic evaluation of intracardiac masses: a review. J Am Soc Echocardiogr. 2006;19:230-40.
31. Maraj S, Pressman GS, Figueredo VM. Primary cardiac tumors. Int J Cardiol. 2009;133:152-6.
32. Neragi-Miandoab S, Kim J, Vlahakes GJ. Malignant tumors of the heart: a review of tumor type, diagnosis and therapy. Clin Oncol. 2007;19:748-56.
33. Kizer JR. Evaluation of the patient with unexplained stroke. Coron Artery Dis. 2008;19:535-40.
34. Kaul S. Myocardial contrast echocardiography: a 25-year retrospective. Circulation. 2008;118:291-308.
35. Soliman OI, Geleijnse ML, Meijboom FJ, et al. The use of contrast echocardiography for the detection of cardiac shunts. Eur J Echocardiogr. 2007;8:S2-12.
36. Mulvagh SL, Rakowski H, Vannan MA, et al. American Society of Echocardiography Consensus Statement on the clinical applications of ultrasonic contrast agents in echocardiography. J Am Soc Echocardiogr. 2008;21:1179-201.
37. Olszewski R, Timperley J, Szmigielski C, et al. The clinical applications of contrast echocardiography. Eur J Echocardiogr. 2007;8:S13-23.
38. Yong Y, Wu D, Fernandes V, et al. Diagnostic accuracy and cost-effectiveness of contrast echocardiography on evaluation of cardiac function in technically very difficult patients in the intensive care unit. Am J Cardiol. 2002;89:711-8.
39. Gorcsan J 3rd, Abraham T, Agler DA, et al. Echocardiography for cardiac resynchronization therapy: recommendations for performance and reporting—a report from the American Society of Echocardiography dyssynchrony writing group. J Am Soc Echocardiogr. 2008;21:191-213.
40. Mazur W, Chung ES. The role of echocardiography in cardiac resynchronization therapy. Curr Heart Fail Rep. 2009;6:37-43.
41. Abraham T, Kass D, Tonti G, et al. Imaging cardiac resynchronization therapy. JACC Cardiovasc Imaging. 2009;2:486-97.

SECTION 3

Diagnosis

Chapter 17

Stress Echocardiography

Ellen El Gordon, Richard E Kerber

Chapter Outline

A. INTRODUCTION

Coronary artery disease (CAD) has been the number one killer in Western society since the turn of the century. Identifying those at risk and preventing the sequelae of ischemic disease is thus a major goal of current day practice. Stress echocardiography (SE) has been used in this regard for over a quarter of a century. This chapter has explored the clinical uses of SE. Given the rapid escalation in use,[1,2] and the associated costs associated with SE, it is necessary for both cardiologists and non-cardiologists alike to have an in-depth understanding of all clinical uses.

Over three-fourth of a century ago, Tennant and Wiggers (1935)[3] occluded a coronary artery and demonstrated the resulting wall motion abnormality. The stage was set for measurement of the functional significance of a coronary stenosis but it would take 40 more years before the resulting wall motion abnormality could be seen by ultrasound.

In 1975, Kerber et al.[4] reported the characteristic of echo detectable wall motion abnormality following an experimental decrease in coronary blood flow.

In 1986, advances in computer technology allowed for ultrasound visualization of a functional myocardial blood flow mismatch. The resulting echo images, however, were viewed little more than a "complement" to standard electrocardiogram (EKG) exercise testing.[5]

Today, SE is far more than a complement to exercise testing. Indications for stress testing have expanded far beyond the initial role in diagnosing ischemic disease. Exercise and pharmacologic stress protocols have been developed to estimate prognosis and evaluate the hemodynamic effects of valvular heart disease.

In this chapter, the authors have focused on the clinical uses of echocardiographic stress testing. Sections have been organized by clinical questions. In the first section, the authors have reviewed the pathophysiology involved in SE imaging. This is followed by a review of the role of SE in diagnosing ischemic disease. Subsequent sections have focused on assessing prognosis in ischemic disease, and assessing myocardial viability. The final section has briefly listed the use of SE in other disease states. Within each section imaging protocols for the specific procedures have been provided, and pros and cons of the various SE modalities have been reviewed. Finally, speculation about what the future holds of SE imaging has been discussed.

B. USING STRESS ECHOCARDIOGRAPHY IN CLINICAL DECISIONS

1. PATHOPHYSIOLOGY INVOLVED IN STRESS ECHO

The major uses of SE have been in (1) diagnosing and (2) estimating risk in patients with suspected or known ischemic disease. An understanding of several factors involved in the disease pathophysiology and in the pathophysiology of the various forms of stress testing is critical to the appropriate use of SE. In order to establish a diagnosis of ischemic disease, SE must show a functional mismatch between myocardial oxygen supply and demand. The "gold standard", however, is not a functional test, but rather an anatomic measurement of coronary stenosis. In addition, the decrease in blood flow necessary to produce ischemia and, hence, a wall motion abnormality has been variably defined in the literature. Both 50% and 70% stenoses of a major epicardial artery (as defined by coronary angiography) have been used to derive sensitivity or specificity of SE. These distinctions are important in understanding the limitations of SE and have resulted in some variation in the reported test characteristics.

The increase in myocardial oxygen demand achieved by stress testing can occur by various mechanisms. Three general modalities are commonly used: (1) an exercise stress which produces a dynamic increase in myocardial oxygen demand;

(2) a pharmacologic stress (dobutamine) which increases in myocardial oxygen demand and (3) a vasodilator stress which produces a coronary "steal".

Exercise stress increases myocardial demand by increase in both chronotropy and inotropy. Due to the important prognostic implications associated with exercise tolerance, use of exercise as a stressor is almost always preferred.

In the United States, dobutamine is the predominant pharmacologic agent used to increase myocardial oxygen demand. It acts by both an increase in inotropy followed by an increase in chronotropy, both of which can be easily confirmed during the stress test. Atropine, added at the end of the protocol if heart rate (HR) response is inadequate, works via anti-cholinergic effects.

Dipyridamole (and adenosine) has been used more commonly in Europe in SE. The drug works as a vasodilator by setting up a coronary artery steal. An advantage of vasodilators includes the extremely short half-life of these drugs. Disadvantages include the lack of a physiologic endpoint (i.e. wall motion abnormality) as study conclusion is often based on completion of dipyridamole protocol.

2. STRESS ECHOCARDIOGRAPHY AND THE DIAGNOSIS OF CORONARY ARTERY DISEASE

a. Exercise Stress Echo (ESE)

(1) Assessment prior to an exercise stress echo: All stress testing begins with a review of the indication(s) for the stress test in particular, and contraindications for stress testing in general (Table 1).

Indications for SE have been outlined by several groups with the most recent being the appropriateness criteria endorsed by the major cardiac societies.[6] In the area of diagnosis of ischemic disease, the most common appropriate indications include the following: (1) diagnosis of chest pain syndromes in patients with intermediate probability of disease; (2) diagnosis of chest pain syndrome in patients with abnormal baseline EKG and (3) diagnosis in patients with prior equivocal stress testing. A more complete listing of appropriate indications can be found in Table 2. For a more detailed review of all SE indications (congestive heart failure, arrhythmias etc.), the reader is referred to the referenced article.

Inappropriate indications generally include patients in low-risk categories but can include both symptomatic and asymptomatic populations. Inappropriate conditions include: (1) use of SE in *symptomatic* patient with a low pretest probability of disease with an interpretable EKG and the ability to exercise and (2) use in *asymptomatic* patients with low or intermediate probability of CAD with an interpretable EKG.[6]

The recent literature suggests that there is room for improvement in the appropriate use of SE testing.[7] Using the 2008 appropriateness criteria, McCully et al. reviewed 298 consecutive stress echocardiograms and classified them as appropriate, inappropriate, uncertain or not classifiable. Of the 298, 54% were classified as appropriate, 8% as uncertain, 19% were not classifiable and 19% were inappropriate. The largest number of appropriate studies was in use of SE for diagnosis in

symptomatic patients (94% appropriate). In contrast, the largest number of inappropriate studies involved use of SE in asymptomatic individuals (72% inappropriate and 26% uncertain).

Contraindications to exercise stress echocardiography (ESE) are similar to those outlined for exercise testing in general. They are listed in Table 3.[8-11]

If there are no absolute or relative contraindications to testing, assessing the patient's ability to exercise should be the next clinical question. Use of the Duke activity status index (DASI) can be helpful in this regard. Initially developed in 1989 by Hlatky et al.,[12] it has recently been validated in women.[13,14] DASI consists of 12 questions about daily activity. The patient is instructed to circle all activities that they can do with "no difficulty". Answers such as "I don't do this" or "I can do this with some difficulty" do not count in the final assessment (Table 4). Positive answers are summed using the scores listed in the far right column under metabolic equivalent (MET) value. The total sum has been correlated with MET level achieved on the Bruce protocol and is, therefore, helpful in choosing the appropriate test protocol. Finally musculoskeletal limitations that may influence the patient's ability to exercise should be reviewed by asking what typically limits exercise.

If it is established that the patient can exercise, an exercise protocol is almost always recommended due to the added information gained about prognosis. If the patient cannot exercise or if exercise is limited, then a pharmacologic stress protocol should be considered.

Regardless of the type of study to be used, clinical symptoms should then be reviewed in order to assess pretest risk. Traditional definitions of angina outlined by the coronary artery surgery study (CASS) registry and later validated by Diamond et al. can provide a good start for estimating pretest probability. Definitions are shown in Table 5.

An additional scoring system published by Morise is shown in Table 6. This pretest score has been validated in both men and women and can also be used to assess pretest probability.[15-18]

TABLE 1

Checklist for patient assessment prior to exercise stress echocardiography

Appropriate clinical indications (Table 2)
No contraindications to exercise (Table 3)
Ability to exercise—DASI score (Table 4)
• Exercise limitations
• Musculoskeletal limitations
Clinical symptom review
• Pretest probability (Table 5)
• Pretest score (Morise) (Table 6)
Baseline EKG review
• Normal
• Baseline abnormalities
Current medications
• Beta blocker (held for 48 Hrs)
• Diltiazem or Verapamil
• Long acting nitrates
• Digoxin

TABLE 2

Selected appropriate indications for stress testing—detection of CAD in chest pain syndromes, CHF or abnormal testing[6]

Indication	Evaluation of chest pain syndrome or anginal equivalent	Appropriateness score (1–9)
1.	• Low pre-test probability of CAD • ECG interpretable and able to exerccise	1 (3)
2.	• Low pre-test probability of CAD • ECG uninterpretable or unable to exercise	A (7)
3.	• Intermediate pre-test probability of CAD • ECG interpretable and able to exercise	A (7)
4.	• Intermediate pre-test probability of CAD • ECG uninterpretable or unable to exercise	A (9)
5.	• High pre-test probability of CAD • Regardless of ECG interpretability and ability to exercise	A (7)
6.	• Prior stress ECG test is uninterpretable or equivocal	A (8)
Acute Chest Pain		
7.	• Intermediate pre-test probability of CAD • ECG no dynamic ST changes and serial cardiac enzyme negative	A (8)
8.	• High pre-test probability of CAD • ECG-ST elevation	I (1)
New-Onset/Diagnosed Heart Failure with Chest Pain Syndrome or Anginal Equivalent		
9.	• Intermediate pre-test probability • Normal LV systolic function	A (8)
10.	• LV systolic function	U (5)

(*Source:* Douglas PS, Khandheria B, Stainback RF, et al. ACCF/ASE/ACEP/AHA/ASNC/SCAI/SCCT/SCMR 2008 appropriateness criteria for stress echocardiography. J Am Coll Cardiol. 2008;51:1127-47)

TABLE 3

Contraindications to exercise testing

- Acute myocardial infarction, recent
- Unstable angina (not stabilized by medical therapy or recent pain at rest)
- Uncontrolled heart failure
- Uncontrolled symptomatic arrhythmias
- Symptomatic severe aortic stenosis
- Acute pulmonary embolus or pulmonary infarction
- Deep vein thrombosis
- Acute myocarditis or pericarditis
- Acute aortic dissection (or recent aortic surgery)
- Uncontrolled hypertension (> 220/120 mm Hg)
- Significant left main coronary stenosis
- Significant electrolyte abnormalities (particularly hyper or hypokalemia)
- Severe hypertrophic cardiomyopathy
- High-degree atrioventricular block
- Inability to exercise adequately due to physical or mental limitation

(*Source:* References 9–11)

Both of these measures provide an estimate of the pretest probability, necessary for correctly interpreting any exercise result.

The next clinical decision will be based on the patient's EKG. A normal EKG with no ST segment abnormalities in a low-risk patient would not require the use of or added expense of imaging testing and is in keeping with current guidelines.[6] However with any baseline ST segment abnormality, a stress imaging protocol using imaging should be considered.

The final clinical decision to be made before starting an exercise test is to review the medication list for medications which may interfere with testing or with test interpretation. Concomitant use of beta blockers may result in an inability to achieve 85% of maximum predicted HR, and as a result, has been reported to lower the sensitivity of testing. Therefore, if beta blockers can be discontinued safely prior to testing, then it is recommended that they be discontinued for approximately 4–5 half lives or 48 hours prior to testing. Similarly, other drugs which slow HR response (diltiazem and verapamil) or alter the ischemic response (nitrates) should be reviewed and discontinued if clinically appropriate. If the question is not diagnostic in nature but rather one of adequacy of treatment, then beta blockers may be continued in certain clinical circumstances. Use of digoxin, a known cause of baseline ST changes on EKG, is also another appropriate indication for the addition of imaging to exercise testing.[6]

(2) Choosing an exercise protocol: The choice of the type of exercise is often made by what is available at one's own institution. In the United States, exercise treadmill is the most common form of stress exercise. Outside of the United States, exercise using a bicycle ergometer is performed more frequently. There are advantages and disadvantages to both. Exercise treadmill has the advantage in that walking is familiar to all, whereas patients may not be as familiar with use of a bike. From an SE standpoint, however, imaging must be performed after

TABLE 4

The Duke Activity Status Index (in METs)[12,14]

Can you.......		Score only for answers: "Yes, with No difficulty"	MET value
1.	Take care of yourself, that is, eating, dressing, bathing, and using the toilet?		0.8
2.	Walk indoors, such as around your house?		0.5
3.	Walk a block or two on level ground?		0.8
4.	Climb a flight of stairs or walk up a hill?		1.6
5.	Run a short distance?		2.3
6.	Do light work around the house like dusting or washing dishes?		0.8
7.	Do moderate work around the house like vacuuming, sweeping floors, carrying in groceries?		1.0
8.	Do heavy work around the house like scrubbing floors, or lifting or moving heavy furniture?		2.3
9.	Do yard work like raking leaves, weeding or pushing a power mower?		1.3
10.	Have sexual relations?		1.5
11.	Participate in moderate recreational activities, like golf, bowling dancing, doubles tennis, or throwing baseball or football?		1.7
12.	Participate in strenuous sports like swimming, singles tennis, football, basketball or skiing?		2.1
		Total score:	

(*Source:* Shaw LJ, Olson MB, Kip K, et al. The value of estimated functional capacity in estimating outcome: results from the NHBLI-sponsored Women's Ischemia Syndrome Evaluation (WISE) Study. J Am Coll Cardiol. 2006;47:S36-43)

SECTION 3

Diagnosis

TABLE 5

Pretest probability of coronary artery disease (defined as >70% stenosis) in men and women according to chest pain description and age

Age (yrs)	Non-anginal		Atypical angina		Typical angina	
	Men	Women	Men	Women	Men	Women
30–39	5	1	22	4	70	26
40–49	14	3	46	13	87	55
50–59	22	8	59	32	92	79
60–69	28	19	67	54	94	91
Overall	21	5	70	40	90	62

(*Source:* Adapted overall data from Reference 111 and Age data from Reference 112)

TABLE 6

Pretest score[16]

Variable			Choose response	Sum
Age	Men	Women		
	< 40	< 50	3	
	40–54	50–64	6	
	≥ 55	≥ 65	9	
Estrogen status			Positive = − 3	
	Women only		Negative = +3	
Angina history			Typical = 5	
	Diamond method		Atypical = 3	
			Non-anginal = 1	
Diabetes?			2	
Hyperlipidemia?			1	
Hypertension			1	
Smoking? (Any)			1	
Family Hx CAD? 1°			1	
Obesity? BMI > 27			1	
			Total score:	

(Abbreviation: BMI: Body mass index). (*Source:* Morise AP, Olson MB, Merz CN, et al. Validation of the accuracy of pretest and exercise test scores in women with a low prevalence of coronary disease: the NHLBI-sponsored Women's Ischemia Syndrome Evaluation (WISE) study. Am Heart J. 2004;147:1085–92)

the completion of treadmill exercise and carries the risk that ischemic wall motion abnormalities will have resolved before imaging can be completed. In contrast, imaging is performed continuously during bicycle exercise, although image degradation due to motion artifact can be troublesome. It is therefore, not surprising that there is a lower sensitivity for SE performed with treadmill versus bike ergometry.[19-21] Most recently, Peteiro et al. have reported success with imaging during peak treadmill exercise. While technically more difficult, the technique appears promising with potentially higher sensitivities.[22]

The most common protocol used in exercise treadmill testing is the Bruce protocol. This protocol has the advantage of widespread use and literature validation. However, the large MET increase between stages is not optimal for all patients.

For example, patients with musculoskeletal disorders may do better with a protocol such as the Naughton, with a 1 MET workload increase between each stage. This compares with the 4.7, 7 and 10 MET levels attained at the end of Bruce stages I, II and III respectively. Often a modification to the Bruce protocol is used which involves starting exercise at a lower level. The workload at the end of the two additional stages is equal to 2.9

and 3.7 METs, for Stages 0 and 1/2 respectively. Finally, if an exercise prescription for rehabilitation is to be given based on the stress testing results, a protocol, such as the Naughton or Balke-Ware, is recommended.[8,9]

Overall, complication rates are low with ESE. Marwick has estimated a rate of approximately 3:1,000 serious complications.[23] The risk of death or myocardial infarction (MI) with exercise testing has been reported to occur in approximately 1/2,500 patients.[8,9] Earlier data involving exercise testing alone suggested a serious complication rate (MI, serious arrhythmia or death) of approximately 1/10,000.[24]

(3) Conducting the exercise stress echo: A detailed account of the technique required to conduct treadmill exercise testing is beyond the scope of this chapter. The reader is referred to the references provided on exercise testing[8,9] and to the chapter on Treadmill Exercise Testing (see Chapter 13). Comments about the protocol will be limited to the additional considerations associated with echo imaging.

Baseline echo images should be reviewed prior to the start of exercise. Secondary harmonic imaging should always be used. Images should be checked to ensure that they are centered within the chamber and not foreshortened. Segments within all coronary distributions should be visualized prior to starting exercise. If two or more segments cannot be visualized, then use of a contrast agent should be considered.[25] Given the US food and drug administration (FDA) black box warning associated with the use of contrast agents, use of perflutren contrast agents cannot be used in many situations. Originally, the FDA issued a black box warning which restricted the use of perflutrens and required that all patients be monitored for 30 minutes following use (Table 7). Recently, however, Kusnetzky et al. reported a retrospective review of all deaths that occurred with 24 hours of an echo study.[26] No statistically significant difference was found in death rates between patients who received a contrast agent versus those who did not. Patients who did receive the contrast agent were found to have an increased number of comorbidities. The FDA black box warning has subsequently been revised and is shown in Table 7.

In the majority of cases, a symptom limited exercise study is recommended unless a study endpoint is reached. Exercise endpoints have been outlined by the ACC and AHA in guidelines published in 2002.[8,9] Exercise endpoints are listed in Table 8.

TABLE 7

FDA black box warning reuse of an ultrasound contrast agents

A. Original black box warning:
• Unstable angina
• Acute heart attacks
• Unstable cardiopulmonary disease
ECG monitoring of all patients for 30 minutes after completion of the study.
B. Revised Black Box Warning:
• Known or suspected right-to-left, bidirectional or transient right-to-left cardiac shunts
• Hypersensitivity to perflutren
ECG monitoring in only patients with pulmonary hypertension or unstable cardiopulmonary conditions
Do not administer definity by intra-arterial injection

(Abbreviation: FDA: US food and drug administration)

TABLE 8

Endpoints for stress echocardiography

• Achievement of target heart rate
• Symptom limitation
• Protocol completion (i.e. maximal dobutamine or dipyridamole dose)
• Significant wall motion abnormality (see text)
• Ischemic EKG response (i.e. ≥ 2 mm ST depression or ST elevation > 1 mm in non-Q wave lead)
• Severe ischemic symptoms (i.e. chest discomfort or exertional dyspnea)
• Severe hypertension (systolic BP > 220 mm Hg or diastolic BP > 120 mm Hg)
• Hypotension or fall in BP > 20 mm Hg with exercise
• Arrhythmias (SVT, VT, heart block, BBB)
• CNS symptoms

(*Source:* Reference 8)

(4) Interpretation of exercise stress echo: Final interpretation of the ESE should consider all components of the study: symptoms, EKG changes, blood pressure (BP) response, echo imaging and exercise tolerance. Reports should contain all of the information that is standard in exercise treadmill studies. This would include information about limiting symptoms, BP response to exercise, EKG changes with exercise, HR achieved and percentage of maximum predicted HR, rate pressure product and exercise tolerance as a percent of predicted.

The most widely used method of echo interpretation is visual. Function in each myocardial segment is evaluated at rest and then compared at peak exercise. Contraction in each segment is graded as normal or hyperdynamic, hypokinetic, akinetic or dyskinetic. Both the timing of wall motion and thickening should be considered as ischemia results in both delayed contraction and relaxation (Videos 1 to 4). A wall motion scoring system can be used in a semiquantitative way to report the findings. The overall ventricular cavity size in systole should also be reviewed. Lack of a decrease in cavity size (or failure to develop hyperdynamic function) would be indicative of significant CAD.[27] For a review of the recommended left ventricular (LV) segments see chapter "Transthoracic Echocardiography", Figure 4, ASE 16 or 17 segment model.

Final interpretation of the stress echocardiogram should include a review of factors known to reduce the sensitivity of exercise stress echocardiograms: inadequate HR response (< 85%), concomitant antianginal treatment, poor image quality and delayed imaging post exercise. To avoid problems with the latter, HR for both maximal exercise and image acquisition should be reviewed.[23] Finally, mild CAD, particularly involving the left circumflex distribution can result in falsely negative studies. In contrast, false positive studies can be seen with pre-existing disease, in particular baseline abnormal septal motion (commonly seen following cardiothoracic surgery or in LBBB) or with a hypertensive response to stress. Overinterpretation has been documented. Interobserver agreement is lowest for isolated basal inferior wall motion abnormalities and highest for basal anterior wall segments.[28]

(1) Assessing the patient prior to pharmacologic stress testing: Similar to the ESE, pharmacologic SE starts with a review of the indication(s) for the stress test and contraindications for stress agent to be used (Table 9). As with ESE, the reader is referred to the appropriateness criteria for SE for a review of the indications.[6] Appropriate indications for use of dobutamine stress echocardiography (DSE) for diagnosis are similar to those listed for use of ESE (Table 1).

Contraindications to DSE differ considerably from ESE. Contraindications for both dobutamine use and atropine use should be reviewed.[28-30] A detailed list can be found in Table 10. Because beta blockers are potent inhibitors of the increase in HR and contractility seen with dobutamine and may be frequently needed to reverse ischemic signs or symptoms, contraindications to their use should also be considered. In our laboratory, we use an intravenous dose of the beta blocker, esmolol, to immediately slow the HR response and decrease contractility in the setting of any significant ischemic response.

Contraindications for dipyridamole stress echocardiography (DiSE) include severe conduction disease or advanced asthma. Vasodilator stress should be avoided in these patients, particularly given the other options for testing.

Similar to ESE, clinical symptoms are next reviewed to assess pretest risk (Table 5). As DSE is being performed in higher risk patients, it is incumbent that clinical stability of the patient be confirmed prior to initiating the study. Baseline EKGs should be reviewed and compared with previous tracings whenever possible. When performed in the setting of acute chest pain, serial cardiac enzymes should also be documented to be normal before proceeding with the test.

The final clinical decision before starting a DSE is a review of the medications. Not only should medications that slow the HR response be considered, but review should include medications which interact with either dobutamine or atropine. Beta

---

TABLE 9

Checklist for patient assessment prior to pharmacologic stress testing/echocardiography

- Appropriate clinical indications (Table 2)
- No Contraindications to:
  Dobutamine:
     Contraindications (Table 10)
     Precautions due to known side effects of dobutamine (Table 10)
     Other considerations (Table 10)
  Atropine:
     Contraindications (Table 10)
     Precautions due to known side effects of atropine (Table 10)
     Beta blockers (if needed to reverse ischemic response)
     Dipyridamole
- Clinical symptoms:
     Pretest probability (Table 4)
     Clinically stable
- Baseline EKG
     Baseline abnormalities
     Previous EKG available for comparison
- Current medication use:
     Beta blocker held?
     Diltiazem or verapamil held? (particularly if high dose)
     Xanthine containing medications or caffeine (if using dipyridamole)

TABLE 10

Contraindications and precautions with use of dobutamine and atropine[28-30]

Contraindications to dobutamine:
- Symptomatic severe aortic stenosis
- Acute aortic dissection
- Recent or unstable coronary syndrome
- Obstructive hypertrophic cardiomyopathy
- Hypersensitivity

Conditions which may worsen due to dobutamine side effects:
- Uncontrolled atrial fibrillation or PSVT
- Uncontrolled hypertension
- Known ventricular arrhythmias

Precautions with other conditions:
- Electrolyte abnormalities (particularly hypokalemia)
- Intraventricular thrombus
- Arterial aneurysms
- High degree AV block
- Significant asthma and high risk patients (higher need for use of beta blockers as reversal agent)

Contraindications to atropine:
- Narrow angle glaucoma
- Obstructive GI disease
- Myasthenia gravis
- Hypersensitivity to atropine or anticholinergics
- Significant BPH or obstructive uropathy

Conditions which may worsen because of atropine side effects:
- Uncontrolled atrial fibrillation or PSVT
- Uncontrolled hypertension
- Known ventricular arrhythmias

---

blockers are routinely stopped 48 hours (4–5 half lives) before the study if the question is one of diagnosis. If dipyridamole stress is being considered, all xanthine containing medications should be stopped for 72 hours or caffeine containing substances should be stopped 24 hours prior to testing.

(2) Pharmacologic stress echo protocols:

(i) Dobutamine stress protocol: In early studies, dobutamine protocols started with 5 mcg/kg per minute and increased every 3 minutes to a maximum dose of 40 mcg/kg per minute.[5,10,20,30] If the maximum HR was less than 85% of the target HR, atropine was then added in 0.5 mg doses up to a dose of 1–2 mg. Today, protocols have routinely become more aggressive. They begin at 10 μg/kg per minute and now increase to a maximum dose of 50 mcg/kg per minute.[31] Atropine is added at the doses listed above. Use of atropine at the end of the protocol also allows additional time for dobutamine to reach steady state. If there is a vagal response to dobutamine with manifest bradycardia and relative hypotension, atropine may be added prior to the end of the dobutamine protocol. This is not uncommonly seen at dobutamine doses of 40 mcg/kg per minute or greater. In settings where atropine will not be used or is contraindicated, an additional 3 minutes may be added to protocol to ensure that dobutamine reaches steady state.

(ii) Dipyridamole stress protocol: Dipyridamole continues to be widely used in Europe.[32,33] Protocols vary but generally can be divided into two types. The first standard, longer protocol consists of dipyridamole intravenously at a total dose of 0.84 mg/kg over 10 minutes. The initial infusion rate is

0.56 mg/kg for 4 minutes, followed by a 4 minute period of no infusion. A second infusion follows at a lower dose of 0.28 mg/kg. If no endpoint is reached, atropine can be added in doses of 0.25 mg up to a maximal dose of 1 mg. The second, shorter protocol consists of dipyridamole infusion at the 0.84 mg/kg over 6 minutes.

With the use of either protocol, aminophylline 240 mg IV should be readily available for immediate use with any adverse events and is often routinely infused at the end of the protocol (120 mg in 1 minute up to a total of 240 mg in 2 minutes).

Other protocols have been described in the literature include infusion of adenosine, use of atrial pacing[34] and hand grip exercise.[35] These protocols are less commonly used in the routine clinical setting. The reader is referred to the listed references for additional details.

(3) Complications of pharmacologic stress echo:

(i) Dobutamine: As familiarity with use of dobutamine has grown, sicker patients are now being referred for DSE testing. Given the increase in dosing and increased severity of illness, concern has been raised about the safety of the DSE. Geleijnse et al. have recently reviewed the complications associated with DSE testing.[31] In their review of over 55,000 patients in 26 studies, they report a complication rate of potentially life-threatening complications of approximately 1/475 cases. Marwick reports a serious complication rate of 3:1,000.[23] A list of the complications and incidence reported by Geleijnse is provided in Table 11.

An additional complication of dobutamine infusion reported by Pellikka et al. is that of left ventricular outflow tract (LVOT) obstruction with associated hypotension.[36] Pellikka described an average increase in velocity of 2.3 m/sec (21 mm Hg gradient) at peak dose. Peak dose velocities ranged from 2 m/sec to 5 m/sec. The associated change in BP ranged from a drop of 15 mm Hg to an increase of 4 mm Hg. In our experience, this complication is most often seen in patients with

small LV cavities, hyperdynamic LV function at baseline or significant left ventricular hypertrophy (LVH) at baseline. In this setting, we routinely measure the LVOT Doppler at baseline and intermittently throughout the procedure. This complication can be rapidly reversed by saline infusion and reversal of the effects of dobutamine with beta blocker.

(ii) Dipyridamole: Varga et al. have recently reported complications associated with the use of dipyridamole as a stress agent in over 24,000 cases. Serious, life-threatening complications were reported in 19 patients for an event rate of 1 in 1,294 cases. This compared to dobutamine event rate of 1 in 557 and exercise event rate of 1 in 6,574 cases. There was 1 reported death following dipyridamole stress testing. The authors concluded that exercise was the safest testing modality with dipyridamole stress second. However they noted that selection bias could account for the latter. As outlined, most complications due to dipyridamole can be rapidly reversed with the use of IV aminophylline. For a more complete review, the reader is referred to the listed reference.[37]

(4) Conducting the pharmacologic stress test: As with ESE, baseline echo images should be reviewed prior to the start of the DSE. Secondary harmonic imaging should always be used.[38] Images should be checked to ensure that they are centered within the chamber and not foreshortened. An off-center baseline image may result in a "smaller" LV cavity. When compared to peak stress imaging, this may result in the false conclusion that there was no hypercontractile response.

Segments within all coronary distributions should be visualized prior to starting dobutamine infusion. If two or more segments cannot be visualized, then use of a contrast agent should be considered.[25] Contraindications to the use of contrast agents and a more extensive discussion of their use has been previously outlined and can be found in Table 7.[26]

Throughout the DSE, the patient is monitored by 12 lead EKG. Blood pressure (BP) is checked at the end of every stage (every 3 minutes) and as clinically indicated. Echo imaging may be screened for all stages but is recorded at low dose (20 mcg/kg per minute) and at peak dose. Recovery images are also recorded at the end of the protocol when the HR was returned to baseline and clinical symptoms have resolved. Today's SE software allows additional image acquisition at anytime during the study. For example, we routinely record additional echo images with any ischemic symptoms or EKG changes.

During infusion of dobutamine, a flow sheet listing the dobutamine dose, use of atropine, patient's symptoms, HR response and BP response is recommended. Unlike ESE, the DSE protocol may be terminated due to imaging endpoints. This would include the development of a new wall motion abnormality or worsening of a baseline abnormality.

(5) Interpretating the pharmacologic stress echo: The most widely used method of echo imaging interpretation is visual. Like ESE, function in each myocardial segment is evaluated at baseline, and then compared at peak dobutamine or dipyridamole dose (Videos 5 to 8). With use of dobutamine, however, comparison with low dose must be considered. An ischemic biphasic response may occur in which an increase in contractility is seen at low dose, followed by no further change

TABLE 11

Complications associated with use of dobutamine and atropine

Complication	Incidence (%)
Mortality	< 0.01
Cardiac rupture	< 0.01
Myocardial infarction incidence	0.02
Cardiovascular accident	< 0.01
Cardiac asystole	< 0.01
Sustained ventricular tachycardia	0.15
Premature atrial complexes	7.9
Supraventricular tachycardia	1.3
A fib	0.9
AV block	0.23
Coronary spasm	0.14
Hypotension	1.7
Hypertension	1.3
Atropine intoxication	0.03
Dobutamine extravasation	one in two cases
Dobutamine hypersensitivity	1 patient

298 or a decrease at peak dose. As with ESE, contraction in each segment is graded as normal or hyperdynamic, hypokinetic, akinetic or dyskinetic. Both the timing of wall motion and thickening are evaluated. A wall motion scoring system, such as the ASE 16 segment model or the 17 segment model, can be used in a semiquantitative way to report the findings. (see chapter 16 "Transthoracic Echocardiography" Figure 39) The overall change in ventricular cavity size in systole should also be reviewed. A progressive decrease in chamber size reflecting the progressive increase in contractility is expected. A lack of a decrease in cavity size in systole would be indicative of severe CAD.

The definition of an abnormal DSE has varied in the literature. In many studies, either a stress-induced wall motion abnormality or a fixed wall motion abnormality has been used as the definition of an ischemic response. In other studies, only stress-induced wall motion abnormalities are felt to represent ischemia. In studies which included patients with prior MIs (and presumably an increase in resting wall motion abnormalities), sensitivities are generally reported higher with lower specificities. This has resulted in considerable variation in the reported test characteristics. Sensitivities have ranged from 54% to 96% and specificities have ranged from 62% to 93%.[39]

In a meta-analysis summarizing 45 studies which included patients with prior MI and 17 studies which excluded prior MI, Geleijnse et al. have reported the test characteristics for DSE (Table 12). The factor found to have the largest effect on test characteristics was the inclusion or exclusion of baseline wall motion abnormalities. Defining cases with resting wall

TABLE 13

Summary of test characteristics for dipyridamole stress echocardiography[33]

Overall sensitivity (%)	Sensitivity (single vessel CAD) (%)	Sensitivity (mutivessel CAD) (%)	Specificity (%)
87	81	90	90

motion abnormalities as positive raised sensitivity. Specificity, however, was lower when referral bias was present.[39] Test characteristics for DiSE are similar and can be found in Table 13.

The inclusion of patients with resting wall motion abnormalities likely affects study validity in multiple ways. By including patients with previous MI, spectrum bias and inclusion of sicker patients may falsely increase study sensitivity, just as including resting wall motion abnormality in the definitions of abnormal would be expected to increase sensitivity. Other factors which have been reported to affect sensitivity and specificity include referral bias (Table 14). The varying definition of the gold standard between 50% and 70% stenosis should theoretically affect test characteristics but was not found to be a significant factor in Geleijnse's review.[39] The authors theorized that few patients actually had stenoses between 50% and 70% as the reason for this finding. Surprisingly, neither use of beta blockers nor use of atropine was found to affect outcome. Addition of atropine has been reported by others to affect test characteristics.[40]

In addition to interpretation of imaging results, a complete SE report, should include information about symptoms, BP response to dobutamine, EKG changes or arrhythmias noted during infusion or in recovery, HR achieved in beats per minute and as a percentage of the maximum predicted HR and rate pressure product.

Final interpretation of the pharmacologic stress echocardiogram (dobutamine or dipyridamole) should include a review of factors known to reduce the sensitivity of stress echocardiograms: inadequate HR response (< 85%), concomitant antianginal treatment, poor image quality. Finally, mild CAD, particularly involving the left circumflex distribution can result in falsely negative studies. In contrast, false positive studies can be seen with pre-existing disease, in particular baseline abnormal septal motion (commonly seen following cardiothoracic surgery or in LBBB) or with a hypertensive response

TABLE 12

Summary of test characteristics for DSE: (A) Test characteristics for studies without resting wall motion abnormalities; (B) Test characteristics for studies with resting wall motion abnormalities; (C) Sensitivities for studies which allowed calculation of single versus multivessel disease

A. Studies without resting wall motion abnormalities (17 studies)	
Sensitivity (weighted mean)	Specificity (weighted mean)
74%	85%
LR(+)	LR (−)
2.84	0.35
B. Studies with resting wall motion abnormality (45 studies)	
Sensitivity (weighted mean)	Specificity (weighted mean)
83%	81%
LR (+)	LR (−)
4.37	0.21
C. Studies which allowed calculation of sensitivity for single vs multivessel disease (n–48)	
Degree of CAD	Sensitivity (%)
Overall	81
Single vessel CAD	73
Multivessel CAD	88
(Source: Reference 39)	

TABLE 14

Factors which alter test characteristics of stress echocardiography[39]

Factors associated with increased sensitivity of stress echocardiography
• Clinical spectrum of coronary disease in study population
• Inclusion of resting wall motion abnormality in definition of abnormal response
Factors associated with decreased specificity of stress echocardiography
• Referral bias

to stress. As with ESE, interpretation has varied the most with wall motion changes involving the basal inferior wall.[28]

In summary, diagnosis of ischemic disease can be assessed with either exercise or pharmacologic SE. The choice of the testing modality should be based on the ability of the patient to exercise, the presence or absence of baseline EKG abnormalities, and the experience of the echocardiography lab. A compilation of studies which directly compare the various echo modalities can be found in the consensus statement by the European Association of Echocardiography.[33] When used in patients with appropriate indications, both study types have been shown to identify patients at risk of ischemic disease with a high degree of accuracy.[28]

3. STRESS ECHOCARDIOGRAPHY AND ESTIMATING RISK OR PROGNOSIS IN CORONARY ARTERY DISEASE

a. Assessing Prognosis—Introduction

Stress echocardiography has been used to answer questions about diagnosis and can also be used to estimate ischemic risk and prognosis. For example, SE has been used to predict severity and risk of coronary disease, and assess risk of mortality. This section will first review caveats regarding the design of studies about prognosis, and will be followed by a review of the use of ESE and pharmacologic SE in assessing prognosis of ischemic disease. A summary of prognostic implications of SE in special populations will be provided.

(1) Caveats for the busy clinician regarding studies about prognosis: In a perfect world, testing for ischemic disease would identify those patients who not only have obstructive CAD but also those who have an unstable plaque (diagnosis). Prognostic studies would then tell us which unstable plaque is likely to rupture or cause thrombosis (prognosis). The reader is reminded that, because stress testing is often correlated with an anatomic diagnosis (coronary angiography), SE is best used in the setting of obstructive disease. Our ability to predict the future ischemic events that often result from non-flow limiting atherosclerotic plaque is, therefore, limited.

Study design represents another limitation of prognostic studies. Study populations are rarely randomized to various workups with measurements of patient outcome, although the need for such studies has recently been outlined.[41-43] In the worst case, studies are designed based on retrospective reviews of cases and controls with their inherent selection bias. In better studies, non-randomized cohorts of consecutive patients are followed prospectively. The study population should consist of a well-defined population who are at a similar point in the course of disease.[44] Due to this, prognostic studies are, therefore, highly dependent on the make-up of the selected patient population and have a high potential for both selection bias and referral filter bias.

The definition of outcome is another important factor in determining quality of a prognostic study. Due to the expense of conducting long-term studies, investigators often use a combination of events (composite outcome) as their primary endpoint. This can result in a decrease in time of study design but can introduce significant problems in clinical application.

By definition, a composite endpoint represents a combination of multiple endpoints. Montori et al. have developed three questions designed to help interpret composite endpoints:[45]
1. "Are the component outcomes of similar importance to patients?"
2. "Did the more and less important outcomes occur with similar frequency?"
3. "Are the component outcomes likely to have similar relative risk reductions (RRRs)?"

To illustrate further assume that a statistically significant decrease in a composite endpoint of angina and cardiac death is reported. This may not mean that a significant decrease in both events has occurred. By applying Montori's questions, an appropriate interpretation can be made. For example, in answering the first question, it becomes obvious that the importance of angina and cardiac death may differ. The second question reveals that the outcomes will likely occur at differing frequencies. Finally, by quickly looking at the RRR and confidence intervals for the individual events, a final interpretation can be made. In the example provided, it is conceivable that a statistically significant composite outcome could be based predominantly on the change in frequency of angina.

b. Exercise Stress Echo (ESE) and Prognosis in Coronary Artery Disease

(1) Prognostic variables in ESE: Exercise SE has been used to assess prognosis in ischemic disease for many years. The advantages of ESE include the additional clinical information found from the exercise portion of the study. In reviewing ESE studies and prognosis, both exercise, imaging and combination variables have been shown to be helpful in predicting prognosis and will be subsequently reviewed. ESE variables which have been used to predict prognosis are listed in Table 15.

TABLE 15

Exercise stress echocardiography—summary of prognostic variables

Variable	Poor prognostic indicators
Summary	Effort-induced or limiting angina
EKG	• ST segment depression or elevation • Arrhythmias
Hemodynamics—BP	• No rise in BP with exercise • Fall in BP with exercise
Hemodynamics—HR	< 85% of maximum predicted heart rate
Echo imaging	• New or worsening regional wall motion abnormality • Lack of decrease in LV systolic dimension with exercise
Workload	• < 5 METs in women • < 7 METs in men
Combination variables	• Duke treadmill score ($\leq$ 11 points) • Exercise score (men > 60; women > 57)

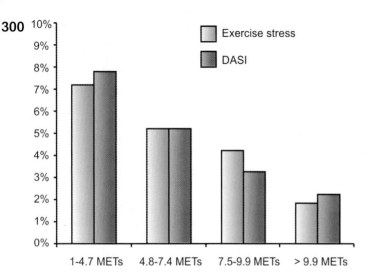

FIGURE 1: Mortality and exercise capacity in the WISE study.[14] Annual mortality is predicted by exercise treadmill stage (blue bars) or estimated exercise capacity using the Duke activity status index (DASI) (brown bars) (*Source:* Shaw LJ, Olson MB, Kip K, et al. The value of estimated functional capacity in estimating outcome: results from the NHBLI-sponsored Women's Ischemia Syndrome Evaluation (WISE) Study. J Am Coll Cardiol. 2006;47:S36-43)

(i) Exercise variables: Despite years of technical progress, one of the most powerful predictors of outcomes remains exercise tolerance. Arruda-Olson et al. confirmed this with exercise echo in 2002.[46] The authors followed 5,798 consecutive patients who had an exercise echo for known or suspected CAD for an average of 3.5 years. Outcomes were defined as non-cardiac death and nonfatal MI. Of all of the exercise EKG predictors, workload was the only one predicted by multivariate analysis. Other authors have reported similar findings.[47] Additional predictive variables have included a fall (or lack of rise) in systolic BP with exercise which has also correlated with a poorer prognosis.[48] Exercise-induced angina was originally found to predict a poorer prognosis[49] but has been shown to be less predictive when exercise tolerance is included.[48-50]

The importance of exercise tolerance as a predictor of mortality is not new as it has been shown to be important in non-imaging stress testing. In the WISE study, exercise tolerance in women, whether measured by treadmill stage or estimated by DASI score, correlated inversely with mortality and was shown to be one of the strongest predictors of mortality (Fig. 1).

Nomograms for predicted exercise capacity have been published for both men and women. Myers et al. followed 6,213 men with cardiovascular risk factors who had undergone exercise testing. They found that exercise tolerance was the most powerful predictor of death. For every 1 MET increase in exercise tolerance, there was a 12% decrease in mortality.[51] Gulati et al. found that the risk of death in women with exercise tolerance less than 85% of that predicted for age was twice that of women whose exercise tolerance was greater than 85% of predicted. This was found in both symptomatic and asymptomatic women.[52]

Achievement of greater than 85% of maximal predicted HR has been a standard component of exercise testing. Failure to achieve this threshold has reported as a poor prognostic indicator

TABLE 16

Duke treadmill score[59]

Duke Treadmill Score:
- low risk: $\geq$ +5 points,
- intermediate risk: −10 to +4 points,
- high risk: $\leq$ −11 points (9).

Duke Treadmill Score Equation:
Duration of exercise in minutes − (5 × the maximal ST segment deviation during or after exercise, in millimeters) − (4 × the treadmill angina index)

even after adjustment for echo indicators of myocardial ischemia.[53]

(ii) Imaging variables: Echo imaging abnormalities have been found to be highly predictive and have been reported to add incremental value to the exercise variables. Abnormal responses have variably been defined by the following ways:
- New or worsening regional wall motion abnormality
- No decrease in LV end systolic size with exercise
- Abnormal resting LV wall motion.

The most commonly agreed upon definitions include the first two. The reader is again cautioned as inclusion of resting LV wall motion abnormalities as part of the abnormal response can have significant effects on reported sensitivity and specificity. Numerous authors have reported that the severity and extent of wall motion abnormalities was predictive of cardiac death and major adverse cardiac events (MACEs), most often defined as cardiac death, nonfatal MI and unstable angina.[22,46,54-56]

(iii) Combining clinical variables: Adding clinical information to the data obtained from an ESE has been reported to show further increases in predictive accuracy. In 2001, Marwick et al. reported that the use of the Duke treadmill score added to the prognostic ability of ESE, particularly when applied to intermediate risk patients.[57] Previously shown to improve clinical prediction in men, the Duke treadmill score[12] has recently been validated in women.[13,58] The scoring system outlined in Table 16. Duke treadmill score can be quickly calculated following any exercise test using the Bruce protocol.

Morise et al. have also combined clinical factors with ESE results and published an exercise score for both men (Table 17A) and women (Table 17B). In patients undergoing exercise testing for suspicion of CAD, clinical factors and ESE results are scored as outlined. The total exercise score correlates with probability of outcome and has shown an improved prediction of all-cause mortality when compared with the Duke treadmill score.[16]

Both scores can be used to complement ESE interpretation as they provide a way to incorporate clinical factors which have been shown to independently predict risk in ESE studies.

(2) ESE in ischemic disease: Exercise SE has been used in many populations. Most commonly it has been used to assess chest pain in patients with known or suspected CAD. Because the interpretation of any study is highly dependent on the extent and severity of ischemic disease in the study population, studies will be reviewed according to clinical presentation. This section will review early prognostic studies, followed by a review of

TABLE 17A

Exercise score—men[16]

Variable	Choose response		Sum
Maximal heart rate	Less than 100 bpm	=	30
	100 to 129 bpm	=	24
	130 to 159 bpm	=	18
	160 to 189 bpm	=	12
	190 to 220 bpm	=	6
Exercise ST depression	1–2 mm	=	15
	> 2 mm	=	25
Age	> 55 years	=	20
	40 to 55 years	=	12
Angina history	Definite/typical	=	5
	Probable/atypical	=	3
	Non-cardiac pain	=	1
Hypercholesterolemia?	Yes	=	5
Diabetes?	Yes	=	5
Exercise test induced angina	Occurred	=	3
	Reason for stopping	=	5
	Total Score:		

(*Source:* Morise AP, Olson MB, Merz CN, et al. Validation of the accuracy of pretest and exercise test scores in women with a low prevalence of coronary disease: the NHLBI-sponsored Women's Ischemia Syndrome Evaluation (WISE) study. Am Heart J. 2004;147: 1085-92)

TABLE 17B

Exercise score—women[18]

Variable	Choose response		Sum
Maximal heart rate	Less than 100 bpm	=	20
	100 to 129 bpm	=	16
	130 to 159 bpm	=	12
	160 to 189 bpm	=	8
	190 to 220 bpm	=	4
Exercise ST depression	1–2 mm	=	6
	> 2 mm	=	10
Age	> 65 years	=	25
	50 to 65 years	=	15
Angina history	Definite/typical	=	10
	Probable/atypical	=	6
	Non-cardiac pain	=	2
Smoking?	Yes	=	10
Diabetes?	Yes	=	10
Exercise test induced angina	Occurred	=	9
	Reason for stopping	=	15
Estrogen status	Positive = –5, Negative	=	5

(*Source:* Morise AP, Olson MB, Merz CN, et al. Validation of the accuracy of pretest and exercise test scores in women with a low prevalence of coronary disease: the NHLBI-sponsored Women's Ischemia Syndrome Evaluation (WISE) study. Am Heart J. 2004;147:1085-92)

studies in patients with chest pain, with known CAD and in patients undergoing coronary interventions.

(i) Early studies of ESE and prognosis: Early studies confirmed the increased prognostic ability of ESE over exercise treadmill testing.[60] In 1998, McCully et al.[47] reviewed the outcome of 1,325 patients who had a normal exercise echocardiogram. Regardless of pretest risk, patients with negative ESE were shown to be free of cardiac death, MI or revascularization over the ensuing year. At 1 year, 2 years and 3 years, event-free survival was reported as 99.2%, 97.8% and 97.4% respectively.

Predictors of increased risk included low exercise tolerance, angina during exercise, echocardiographic LVH and increased age. In their meta-analysis, Metz et al.[61] confirmed the low event rate following a normal ESE. They reported 98.4% of those with a negative ESE to be free of cardiac death and MI over 33 months follow-up.

(ii) Patients presenting with atypical chest pain or as outpatients: Exercise stress echocardiography studies in patients with suspected ischemic symptoms are limited, as most include patients with known underlying CAD. Colon et al. reported an early retrospective analysis of patients presenting with atypical chest pain without known disease. The event-free survival at 30 months was found to be 93% when patients had a normal stress EKG and 97% following a normal stress echocardiogram. In contrast, an abnormal stress echocardiogram predicted an event-free rate of major cardiac events of only 74% when wall motion abnormalities were noted.[55]

Leischik et al. studied 3,329 outpatients with ESE. Patients were followed for 5 years for the occurrence of cardiac death, MI and revascularization. Patients with abnormal SE had a 61.9% event rate compared with a 6.3% event rate in patients who had negative stress echocardiographies.[56]

In order to evaluate the additive role of echo imaging, Bouzas-Mosquera et al. reported 4.5 years f/u on 4,004 pts (29% with history of CAD) who underwent ESE and had no chest pain or EKG changes with exercise.[54] Patients were stratified by development of an ischemic response, defined as development of new of worsening wall motion abnormality. In patients with ischemic response, death and MACE occurred at a rate of 12.1% and 10.1% respectively. In comparison, event rates in patients with no ischemic response were 6.4% and 4.2% respectively. The authors argued that ESE imaging provides prognostic information above that obtained by a normal exercise stress test.

In 2007, Metz et al. published a meta-analysis in which the prognostic value of a normal exercise echocardiogram was evaluated in patients with suspected CAD. The primary outcome was defined as MI and cardiac death. A normal ESE conferred a 98.4% negative event rate over 33 months or an annualized rate of 0.54% per year for primary events.[61]

Most recently, researchers have begun to evaluate the outcomes in patients with "false positive" SE, where patients, with an abnormal SE (exercise or dobutamine stress), are found to have less than 50% coronary artery stenosis by angiogram.

To answer this question, From et al. reported a retrospective analysis of 1,477 patients who had both a SE and a coronary angiogram within 30 days (patients represented a subset of 7,352 with abnormal stress echocardiographies). All had previously undergone coronary angiography within 30 days. Around 67.5% were found to have obstructive CAD defined as greater than or equal to 50% stenosis and 32.5% were categorized as "false positives" given the absence of significant coronary stenosis. Analysis of a subset with "markedly positive" stress echocardiographies (defined as an abnormal left ventricular end systolic size response to stress and > 5 segments abnormal at peak stress) and less than 50% stenosis by coronary angiogram revealed 140 deaths during 2.4 years follow-up. The death rate of this subgroup was reported to be similar to the death rate of those with significant coronary stenosis.

In an editorial response, Labovitz reviews the limitations of the study but argues for the prognostic power of an abnormal stress echocardiogram.[62] Regardless of whether or not the mechanism for the poor outcome is due to vasomotor changes, endothelial dysfunction, small vessel disease or microvascular abnormalities, one is reminded that the culprit is the unstable plaque, which is not always obstructive. Clearly additional studies are needed to more fully understand the meaning of a "false positive" SE. In the interim, the literature includes increasing support for medical treatment of this population and aggressive risk factor modification.[62,63]

(iii) Patients with known or suspected CAD: A negative ESE also confers an excellent prognosis on patients with known CAD. In 2001, Marwick et al. reported 10 years follow-up following SE in over 5,000 patients with known or suspected ischemic disease. During the study period, 649 deaths were reported. In this setting, a normal ESE predicted an overall mortality rate of 1% per year.[57]

Similarly, in a study of over 3,000 outpatients who were undergoing evaluation for chest pain, patients with known CAD and a negative SE were reported to have cardiac death rates of less than 1% during the subsequent year.[56]

An abnormal ESE confers a significantly higher risk of death and MI. Patients who developed a new or worsening wall motion abnormality with ESE had a 5-year mortality rate of 12.1% and 5-year MACE rates of 10.1%.[54] Peteiro looked at peak and post-exercise imaging and also reported high rates for patients with abnormal wall motion score indexing (5-year mortality rate 15.3% at peak exercise, and 14% post exercise).[22]

Once again, the importance of exercise tolerance is found to be an important clinical predictor. In patients with suspected or known CAD who had an abnormal ESE and good exercise tolerance (women > 5 METs and men > 7 METs), McCully et al. reported a low event rate for cardiac death and nonfatal MI per person year of follow-up (1.6% for patients with a decrease in LV systolic size with exercise; 1.2% for patients without regional wall motion abnormalities).[64] However, in patients with an abnormal ESE and poor exercise tolerance, the event rate increased (4.4% risk per person year of follow-up).[65]

Finally, ESE is predictive in various age groups, including the elderly. In 2001, Arruda et al. reported the results of ESE in 2,632 patients over the age of 65 years. Fifty-six percent of the population were male and 44% female. All underwent clinically indicated ESE testing and were followed for an average of 2.9 ± 1.7 years. Thirty-six percent had baseline wall motion abnormalities. Both clinical exercise and echo variables were recorded. An exercise-induced wall motion abnormality was seen in 1,082, or 41% of the population. Follow-up revealed 68 cardiac deaths and 89 fatal MIs. Multivariate analysis revealed that predictors of cardiac death included workload achieved and exercise EF. When exercise EF was excluded, the regional wall motion score was highly predictive. The presence of angina during testing or ST segment changes did not add to the predictor. An increase in or lack of decrease in exercise left ventricular end systolic volume (LVESV) correlated with an increase in cardiac events.

In summary, a negative ESE in patients with good exercise tolerance appears to confer a good prognosis regardless of the presence or absence of CAD, whereas a positive ESE appears to carry a poorer prognosis regardless of the presence or absence of obstructive CAD. Good exercise tolerance may provide additional risk stratification in those with abnormal studies.

(iv) Prognosis following ESE—patients undergoing percutaneous coronary intervention (PCI): Another major use of ESE has been in the evaluation of patients undergoing PCI. Identifying an ischemic region has been shown to help plan coronary interventions, particularly in patients with known underlying disease. Consequently, current guidelines recognize PCI in patients with class I or II angina and a "moderate to severe degree of ischemia on noninvasive testing" as a class IIa indication (level of evidence B) and PCI in patients "no evidence of myocardial injury or ischemia on objective testing" as a class III indication.[66]

It would, therefore, be assumed that ESE would play a large role in the planning of coronary interventions. However recent medicare data suggests that noninvasive testing is rarely used in this setting. Less than 50% of patients undergoing PCI had any type of noninvasive testing prior to PCI.[67] Whether or not this practice will change given the current emphasis of optimal utilization of resources remains to be seen.[68]

(3) ESE in special populations: Exercise stress echocardiography has been successfully studied in many populations. It has been shown to be predictive in women,[46,52,58,69-75] patients with hypertension or LVH,[76] diabetics,[77,78] patients with atrial fibrillation[79] and patients with ESRD.[80] Detailed review of all of these studies is beyond to scope of this chapter. The reader is referred to references provided in the reference section. ESE, however, is not routinely recommended for use in patients with LBBB. Guidelines suggest use of pharmacologic stress[81] in this setting.

In summary, a normal ESE with good exercise tolerance appears to correlate with a good prognosis regardless of the presence or absence of known CAD (not necessarily angiographically negative). Use of a clinical prediction score appears to improve clinical assessment. Exercise tolerance and LVESV response to exercise (or wall motion score, if LVESV response not analyzed) are powerful predictors of hard cardiac endpoints.

In contrast, an abnormal ESE appears to predict a poorer prognosis. In the presence of underlying obstructive CAD, the event rates are significant. However, even in the presence of underlying nonobstructive CAD, events rates are significantly higher, particularly when studies are markedly abnormal.

c. Dobutamine Stress Echo (DSE) and Prognosis in Coronary Artery Disease

Like ESE, many articles have been published regarding the use of DSE in predicting risk and prognosis. Like ESE, imaging variables have been shown to be highly predictive. This section is, therefore, reviewed the general prognostic factors associated with DSE, evaluate prognostic implications of both normal and abnormal DSE in ischemic disease, and finally review the use of DSE in predicting preoperative risk.

Unlike ESE, DSE has the disadvantage of not providing the additional prognostic value associated with exercise variables. While this will vary considerably with the severity of disease in the study of population, the reader is reminded that, in general, prognosis is poorer in patients who cannot exercise.

This was well-illustrated by Shaw et al. when they studied 5-year mortality in 4,234 women and 6,898 men who had undergone either ESE or DSE.[75] Women with no ischemia on DSE had a similar risk adjusted 5-year mortality as women with either 2 or 3 vessel ischemia on ESE (95% and 95% respectively). This finding was also seen in men with no ischemia on DSE compared with men with 2 or 3 vessel ischemic response on ESE (5-year mortality was 92% and 94% respectively).

(1) Prognostic variables in DSE: One of the earliest DSE studies by Chuah et al. followed 860 patients with known or suspected CAD for 52 months.[82] In this population they found that multivariate predictors of cardiac events included a history of congestive heart failure, an abnormal LVESV response to stress, and the number of abnormal segments at peak stress. A new wall motion abnormality was also found to be a powerful predictor in studies by Poldermans[83] and Elhendy.[84] Poldermans' study included patients with resting wall motion abnormalities while Elhendy's study included only patients with normal baseline LV systolic function. In the former study, 5-year probability of an abnormal cardiac outcome (cardiac death, MI or revascularization) following a normal DSE was 14%. In the latter, only an ischemic wall motion abnormality was predictive of hard cardiac endpoints.

(2) Dobutamine stress echo and prognosis in ischemic disease: In evaluating patients with ischemic disease, Marwick et al. reported a low risk of death following a normal DSE.[85] In this study, he evaluated 3,156 patients who had undergone DSE (1,073 of whom had coronary angiography). These patients were then followed for 9 years. A normal DSE was associated with a total mortality of 8% per year and a cardiac mortality of 1% per year. Similar outcomes were reported by Sozzi (2% mortality in first 2 years, 2.4% in years 4 and 5)[86] and Yao (0.9% per year event rate).[87] In one of the larger studies, Chaowalit reported a 95% survival at 1 year.[88] In this study, 3,014 patients were studied following a normal DSE. Cardiac event-free rates were 98% at 1 year, 93% at 5 years and 89% at 10 years.

In contrast, both mortality and cardiac event rates increase in the setting of an abnormal DSE. Whereas a negative DSE resulted in 1.1% annual rate, an ischemic response increased the event rate fivefold (5% annual event rate)[84] in patients with normal resting LV systolic function.

In reviewing DSE in men and women, Shaw et al. reported risk adjusted 5-year survival rates of 95% in women with no ischemia and 86% in patients with ischemia consistent with multivessel disease. Men with no ischemic response on DSE had a 92% survival at 5 years compared to 84% survival in the setting of an ischemic response.[75] There was no statistically significant difference between men and women who had a nonischemic response. There was, however, felt to be a significant difference in survival between men and women who exhibited an ischemic response. This was attributed to a greater extent of ischemic disease in men.

Recently, From et al. retrospectively analyzed markedly abnormal stress tests in patients who were found to have nonobstructive coronary disease.[89] An about 1,477 consecutive patients who had both an abnormal SE and coronary angiography were analyzed. Around 67.5% were found to be true positives, whereas 32.5% were considered false positives (coronary stenosis < 50% by angiography). In this latter population, 605 patients were felt to have a markedly abnormal response, defined as greater than 5 segments abnormal at peak stress or an abnormal LV in systolic size response to stress. After 2.4 years of follow-up the investigators found no difference in death rates between those with obstructive disease and those with nonobstructive disease. In other words, the outcome of patients with markedly abnormal "false positive" studies was similar to that seen in patients with obstructive coronary disease.

In summary, prognosis following a normal DSE is generally good whereas prognosis following a markedly abnormal DSE is not good, irrespective of the presence or absence of underlying obstructive disease.

(3) Dobutamine stress echo and prognosis in special settings: Like ESE, DSE has been used in special settings. These include risk assessment prior to and following PCI, and risk prediction prior to noncardiac surgery. Special populations have also been studied using DSE and include women, diabetics, patients with peripheral vascular disease and patients found to have LVOT gradients.

Stress testing has been studied prior to and following PCI. In patients with stable CAD, stress testing has been recommended as a gateway to invasive procedures. Updated guidelines recommend use of PCI in patients with stable angina who meet the following conditions:[66]

Percutaneous coronary intervention (PCI) is reasonable in patients with asymptomatic ischemia or CCS class I or II angina and with 1 or more lesions in 1 or 2 coronary arteries suitable for PCI with a high likelihood of success and a low risk of morbidity and mortality. The vessels to be dilated must subtend a moderate to large area of viable myocardium or be associated with a moderate to severe degree of ischemia on noninvasive testing (level of evidence B).

As indicated, stress testing would be expected to help define the severity and degree of ischemia and therefore justify the need for invasive procedures, particularly given the problems with visual estimates of coronary lesions, the risks of dual antiplatelet therapy, and the lack of a decrease of stroke, MI or death in patients with stable symptoms.[90] Early studies found SE testing prior to PCI did just this and described testing as a clinically useful, cost effective strategy in patients with stable angina[91] and in women with suspected CAD.[92]

As previously noted, recent medicare data suggests that stress testing is not frequently used prior to the planning of PCI in patients with stable angina.[67] In a randomized trial, Sharples et al. reported that in 20–25% of cases, the results of the stress test resulted in a change in management plan (i.e. patients were not referred for angiography).[93] This data, in combination with the results of the recent COURAGE trial,[94] suggests that stress testing may be an underused modality in patients with stable angina.

Yao et al. recently confirmed the value of SE in predicting cardiac events in a retrospective analysis of 3,121 consecutive patients. They found SE to be an effective gatekeeper and that an abnormal SE positively influenced the need for revascularization.[95]

Cortigiani et al. have studied the use of exercise, dipyridamole and dobutamine stress tests in 1,063 patients following PCI.[96] Ischemia during stress was associated with higher 5-year mortality and a higher instance of heart cardiac endpoints.

A large literature has also addressed the use of SE in evaluating perioperative risk. Guidelines currently recommend use of stress testing in patients with active cardiac symptoms, and in patients with significant risk factors and a low functional capacity (< 4 METs) prior to undergoing either vascular surgery or intermediate risk surgery (for detailed list of the recommendations, the reader is referred to the reference by Fleisher et al.[97]). DSE has been shown in several studies to add to the predictive ability of clinical data.[98,99] Labib et al. found that a negative DSE predicted a similar perioperative event rate in patients regardless of whether or not they achieved their maximum predicted HR with stress. In the authors' hands, the presence of a resting wall motion abnormality predicted increased risk even in the absence of provacable ischemia.

As previously described, SE has been found studied in both women and men and found to be equally predictive of ischemia.[75,100]

In a study of 2,349 patients with diabetes followed for an average of 5.4 years, SE variables added to the clinical and resting echo prediction model.[101] Significant predictors of mortality derived from SE testing included failure to achieve target HR and percentage of ischemic segments.

Similarly, when DSE was studied in patients with peripheral arterial disease, Chaowalit et al. found that both the failure to achieve 85% maximum predicted HR in response to dobutamine and the ischemic response seen with imaging was predictive of mortality and morbidity.[102]

Left ventricular outflow tract obstruction is a finding not commonly seen with SE. In order to evaluate its prognostic significance, Dawn et al.[103] studied 237 patients with LVOT documented by continuous wave Doppler. They then followed a subset with no DSE provocable ischemia for 31 months. The presence of dobutamine-induced or resting LVOT obstruction predicted an increased incidence of chest pain and syncope or near syncope.

Finally, Sicari et al. reviewed the implications of concomitant antianginal treatment in the setting of DSE testing. Antianginal therapy was defined as use of nitrates, calcium channel blockers or beta blockers. The best overall survival was found in untreated patients who had a negative DSE. In contrast, the worst overall survival was found in treated patients with abnormal stress testing response. Survival rates at 2.6 years were 95% versus 81% respectively.[104] There was no statistically significant difference between treated patients with a negative test (88% survival) and untreated patients with a positive test (84% survival).

(4) Dipyridamole stress echo (DiSE) and prognosis in coronary artery disease: As previously noted, DiSE is used more frequently in Europe. Studies using this modality have confirmed its use in assessing prognosis in patients with CAD. As with DSE, a negative DiSE confers a good prognosis. As with dobutamine, dipyridamole has been tested to be useful in ambulatory patients,[105] in planning PCI[96] and in perioperative risk assessment.[106]

In summary, the major predictor of mortality following a pharmacologic SE is extent of ischemic response. In general, prognosis following a normal study is generally good. This contrasts significantly with the outcomes in patients who exhibit an ischemic response.

4. STRESS ECHO AND MYOCARDIAL VIABILITY

In addition to use in diagnosis and prognosis of ischemic disease, SE has also been used to determine myocardial viability. In patients with resting wall motion abnormalities, viable myocardium is felt to be present when an increase in contractility or increase in endocardial motion can be demonstrated in response to stress. Given that revascularization may benefit up to 50% of patients with chronic "hibernating" myocardial (myocardium that is chronically ischemic and, therefore, dysfunctional), determination of viability may have a significant impact on management decisions.[107-109]

Due to the need to assess serial response to an increase in stress, DSE is the preferred testing modality and has been reported to be the most specific test.[109] The assessment prior to the start of the procedure is similar to that described under diagnostic testing. The protocol, however, varies slightly and is much less aggressive. Dobutamine infusion starts at 5 µg/kg per minute for 3 minutes and increases to 10 µg/kg per minute for an additional 3 minutes. In patients with critical coronary disease, some have advocated starting at an even lower dose— 2.5 µg/kg per minute. The endpoints include the following: (1) a lack of increase in baseline contractility suggesting myocardial necrosis; (2) an increase in myocardial contractility suggesting myocardial stunning or hibernation or (3) a biphasic response in which an increase in contractility is seen at the lower dose but regional wall motion worsens at the higher dose as ischemia is induced.

In order to assess the prognosis of patients following revascularization, Rizzello et al. performed dobutamine viability studies in 128 consecutive patients with ischemic cardiomyopathy prior to revascularization.[110] The best multivariate predictors of cardiac death included the presence of multivessel disease, the wall motion score index at low dose dobutamine, and echo evidence of an increase in contractility (or viability) in greater than or equal to 25% of the dysfunctional segments. Patients with viable myocardium were found to have a good prognosis following revascularization. This compared with a much poorer outcome in patients with viable myocardium who were treated medically.[111]

Schinkel et al. have recently reported a comparison of dobutamine echo with Thallium-201, and with technetium-99m scintigraphy.[108] Dobutamine viability studies compared favorably with other modalities and were found to have the highest specificity.[108] A recent review by the European Association of Echocardiography also recommended low dose dobutamine as the best test for viability.[33] For additional details regarding comparisons of the various testing modalities, the reader is referred to references provided in the reference section.

5. STRESS ECHO AND THE ASSESSMENT OF HEMODYNAMICS OF VALVULAR DISEASE

Because both cardiac structure and valvular hemodynamics can be assessed, SE is increasingly being used to assess valvular heart disease. The most common uses of SE have included assessment of patients with valvular stenosis. ACC/AHA guidelines support use of SE in the assessment of asymptomatic patients with severe aortic stenosis (AS) (class IIb), patients with AS and LV dysfunction, and in patients with mitral stenosis who are either asymptomatic with severe mitral stenosis, or who are symptomatic with mild to moderate mitral stenosis at rest (class I recommendation, level of evidence C). The role of SE in patients with mitral regurgitation or aortic regurgitation is less clear. For a detailed review, the reader is referred to the listed references[112] provided in the reference section and to the textbook chapters on the Specific Valves.

C. THE FUTURE OF STRESS ECHO

In summary, SE has been proven to be vital resource in evaluation of CAD. Future advances with a focus on 3-dimensional SE, tissue Doppler and contrast perfusion scoring will likely further enhance its usefulness. Given the lack of radiation exposure and cost effectiveness,[113] it will likely to be used for many years to come. Future studies of comparative effectiveness research will likely help to refine its use as a diagnostic and prognostic tool in cardiovascular disease.[9]

VIDEO LEGENDS

Video 1   Abnormal exercise stress (parasternal long axis view)

Video 2   Abnormal exercise stress (parasternal short axis view)

Video 3   Abnormal exercise stress (apical 4 chamber view)

Video 4   Abnormal exercise stress (apical 2 chamber view)

Video 5   Normal dobutamine stress (parasternal long axis view)

Video 6   Normal dobutamine stress (parasternal short axis view)

Video 7   Normal dobutamine stress (apical 4 chamber view)

Video 8   Normal dobutamine stress (apical 2 chamber view).

REFERENCES

1. Office GA. Medicare: trends in fees, utilization, and expenditures for imaging services before and after implementation of the Deficit Reduction Act of 2005 (GAO-08-1102R). 2008. Available at: http://www.gao.gov/new.items/d081102r.pdf. [Accessed August, 2010]

2. Lucas FL, DeLorenzo MA, Siewers AE, et al. Temporal trends in the utilization of diagnostic testing and treatments for cardiovascular disease in the United States, 1993-2001. Circulation. 2006;113: 374-9.

3. Tennant R, Wiggers CJ. The effects of coronary occlusion on myocardial contraction. Am J Physiol. 1935;112:351-61.

4. Kerber RE, Marcus ML, Ehrhardt J, et al. Correlation between echocardiographically demonstrated segmental dyskinesis and regional myocardial perfusion. Circulation. 1975;52:1097-104.

5. Armstrong WF, O'Donnell J, Dillon JC, et al. Complementary value of two-dimensional exercise echocardiography to routine treadmill exercise testing. Ann Intern Med. 1986;105:829-35.

6. Douglas PS, Khandheria B, Stainback RF, et al. ACCF/ASE/ACEP/AHA/ASNC/SCAI/SCCT/SCMR 2008 appropriateness criteria for stress echocardiography: a report of the American College of Cardiology Foundation Appropriateness Criteria Task Force, American Society of Echocardiography, American College of Emergency Physicians, American Heart Association, American Society of Nuclear Cardiology, Society for Cardiovascular Angiography and Interventions, Society of Cardiovascular Computed Tomography, and Society for Cardiovascular Magnetic Resonance endorsed by the Heart Rhythm Society and the Society of Critical Care Medicine. J Am Coll Cardiol. 2008;51:1127-47.

7. McCully RB, Pellikka PA, Hodge DO, et al. Applicability of appropriateness criteria for stress imaging: similarities and differences between stress echocardiography and single photon emission computed tomography myocardial perfusion imaging criteria. Circ Cardiovasc Imaging. 2009;2:213-8.

8. Gibbons RJ, Balady GJ, Bricker JT, et al. ACC/AHA 2002 guideline update for exercise testing: summary article. A report of the American College of Cardiology/American Heart Association Task Force on Practice Guidelines. J Am Coll Cardiol. 2002;40:1531-40.

9. Gibbons RJ, Balady GJ, Beasley JW, et al. ACC/AHA Guidelines for Exercise Testing. A report of the American College of Cardiology/American Heart Association Task Force on Practice Guidelines (Committee on Exercise Testing). J Am Coll Cardiol. 1997;30:260-311.

10. Hill J, Timmis A. Exercise tolerance testing. BMJ. 2002;324:1084-7.

11. Lear SA, Brozic A, Myers JN, et al. Exercise stress testing. An overview of current guidelines. Sports Med. 1999;27:285-312.

12. Hlatky MA, Boineau RE, Higginbotham MB, et al. A brief self-administered questionnaire to determine functional capacity (the Duke Activity Status Index). Am J Cardiol. 1989;64:651-4.

13. Bairey Merz CN, Olson MB, McGorray S, et al. Physical activity and functional capacity measurement in women: a report from the NHLBI-sponsored WISE study. J Womens Health Gend Based Med. 2000;9:769-77.

14. Shaw LJ, Olson MB, Kip K, et al. The value of estimated functional capacity in estimating outcome: results from the NHBLI-sponsored Women's Ischemia Syndrome Evaluation (WISE) Study. J Am Coll Cardiol. 2006;47:S36-43.

15. Morise AP. Simplifying prognostication and decision making using exercise testing. J Cardiopulm Rehabil. 2002;22:408-9.

16. Morise AP, Jalisi F. Evaluation of pretest and exercise test scores to assess all-cause mortality in unselected patients presenting for exercise testing with symptoms of suspected coronary artery disease. J Am Coll Cardiol. 2003;42:842-50.

17. Morise AP, Lauer MS, Froelicher VF. Development and validation of a simple exercise test score for use in women with symptoms of suspected coronary artery disease. Am Heart J. 2002;144:818-25.

18. Morise AP, Olson MB, Merz CN, et al. Validation of the accuracy of pretest and exercise test scores in women with a low prevalence of coronary disease: the NHLBI-sponsored Women's Ischemia Syndrome Evaluation (WISE) study. Am Heart J. 2004;147:1085-92.

19. Hecht HS, DeBord L, Shaw R, et al. Usefulness of supine bicycle stress echocardiography for detection of restenosis after percutaneous transluminal coronary angioplasty. Am J Cardiol. 1993;71:293-6.

20. Hecht HS, DeBord L, Sotomayor N, et al. Supine bicycle stress echocardiography: peak exercise imaging is superior to postexercise imaging. J Am Soc Echocardiogr. 1993;6:265-71.

21. Hecht HS, DeBord L, Shaw R, et al. Digital supine bicycle stress echocardiography: a new technique for evaluating coronary artery disease. J Am Coll Cardiol. 1993;21:950-6.

22. Peteiro J, Bouzas-Mosquera A, Broullón FJ, et al. Prognostic value of peak and postexercise treadmill exercise echocardiography in patients with known or suspected coronary artery disease. Eur Heart J. 2010;31:187-95.

23. Marwick TH. Stress echocardiography. Heart. 2003;89:113-8.

24. Stuart RJ, Ellestad MH. National survey of exercise stress testing facilities. Chest. 1980;77:94-7.

25. Pellikka PA, Nagueh SF, Elhendy AA, et al. American Society of Echocardiography recommendations for performance, interpretation, and application of stress echocardiography. J Am Soc Echocardiogr. 2007;20:1021-41.

26. Kusnetzky LL, Khalid A, Khumri TM, et al. Acute mortality in hospitalized patients undergoing echocardiography with and without an ultrasound contrast agent: results in 18,671 consecutive studies. J Am Coll Cardiol. 2008;51:1704-6.

27. Attenhofer CH, Pellikka PA, Oh JK, et al. Comparison of ischemic response during exercise and dobutamine echocardiography in patients with left main coronary artery disease. J Am Coll Cardiol. 1996;27:1171-7.

28. Geleijnse ML, Fioretti PM, Roelandt JR. Methodology, feasibility, safety and diagnostic accuracy of dobutamine stress echocardiography. J Am Coll Cardiol. 1997;30:595-606.

29. Dobutamine. DRUGDEX® System. 2011. Available from http://www.thomsonhc.com/micromedex2. [Accessed March, 2011].

30. Atropine. DRUGDEX® System. 2011. Available from http://www.thomsonhc.com/micromedex2. [Accessed March, 2011].

31. Geleijnse ML, Krenning B, Nemes A, et al. Incidence, pathophysiology, and treatment of complications during dobutamine-atropine stress echocardiography. Circulation. 2010;121:1756-67.

32. Cortigiani L, Picano E, Landi P, et al. Value of pharmacologic stress echocardiography in risk stratification of patients with single vessel disease: a report from the Echo-Persantine and Echo-Dobutamine International Cooperative Studies. J Am Coll Cardiol. 1998;32:69-74.

33. Sicari R, Nihoyannopoulos P, Evangelista A, et al. Stress echocardiography expert consensus statement: European Association of Echocardiography (EAE) (a registered branch of the ESC). Eur J Echocardiogr. 2008;9:415-37.

34. Atar S, Nagai T, Cercek B, et al. Pacing stress echocardiography: an alternative to pharmacologic stress testing. J Am Coll Cardiol. 2000;36:1935-41.

35. Strizik B, Chiu S, Ilercil A, et al. Usefulness of isometric handgrip during treadmill exercise stress echocardiography. Am J Cardiol. 2002;90:420-2.

36. Pellikka PA, Oh JK, Bailey KR, et al. Dynamic intraventricular obstruction during dobutamine stress echocardiography. A new observation. Circulation. 1992;86:1429-32.

37. Varga A, Garcia MA, Picano E, et al. Safety of stress echocardiography (from the International Stress Echo Complication Registry). Am J Cardiol. 2006;98:541-3.

38. Sozzi FB, Poldermans D, Bax JJ, et al. Second harmonic imaging improves sensitivity of dobutamine stress echocardiography for the diagnosis of coronary artery disease. Am Heart J. 2001;142:153-9.

39. Geleijnse ML, Krenning BJ, Van Dalen B, et al. Factors affecting sensitivity and specificity of diagnostic testing: dobutamine stress echocardiography. J Am Soc Echocardiogr. 2009;22:1199-208.

40. McNeill AJ, Fioretti PM, el-Said SM, et al. Enhanced sensitivity for detection of coronary artery disease by addition of atropine to dobutamine stress echocardiography. Am J Cardiol. 1992;70:41-6.

41. Shaw LJ, Min J, Hachamovitch R, et al. Cardiovascular imaging research at the crossroads. JACC Cardiovasc Imaging. 2010;3:316-24.

42. VanLare JM, Conway PH, Sox HC. Five next steps for a new national program for comparative-effectiveness research. N Engl J Med. 2010;362:970-3.

43. Spertus JA, Bonow RO, Chan P, et al. ACCF/AHA new insights into the methodology of performance measurement. J Am Coll Cardiol. 2010;56:1767-82.

44. Laupacis A, Wells G, Richardson WS, et al. Users' guides to the medical literature. V. How to use an article about prognosis. Evidence-Based Medicine Working Group. JAMA. 1994;272:234-7.

45. Montori VM, Busse JW, Permanyer-Miralda G, et al. How should clinicians interpret results reflecting the effect of an intervention on composite endpoints: should I dump this lump? ACP J Club. 2005;143:A8.

46. Arruda-Olson AM, Juracan EM, Mahoney DW, et al. Prognostic value of exercise echocardiography in 5,798 patients: is there a gender difference? J Am Coll Cardiol. 2002;39:625-31.

47. McCully RB, Roger VL, Mahoney DW, et al. Outcome after normal exercise echocardiography and predictors of subsequent cardiac events: follow-up of 1,325 patients. J Am Coll Cardiol. 1998;31:144-9.

48. Morrow K, Morris CK, Froelicher VF, et al. Prediction of cardiovascular death in men undergoing noninvasive evaluation for coronary artery disease. Ann Intern Med. 1993;118:689-95.

49. Mark DB, Hlatky MA, Harrell FE, et al. Exercise treadmill score for predicting prognosis in coronary artery disease. Ann Intern Med. 1987;106:793-800.

50. Weiner DA, Ryan TJ, McCabe CH, et al. Prognostic importance of a clinical profile and exercise test in medically treated patients with coronary artery disease. J Am Coll Cardiol. 1984;3:772-9.

51. Myers J, Prakash M, Froelicher V, et al. Exercise capacity and mortality among men referred for exercise testing. N Engl J Med. 2002;346:793-801.

52. Gulati M, Black HR, Shaw LJ, et al. The prognostic value of a nomogram for exercise capacity in women. N Engl J Med. 2005;353:468-75.

53. Lauer MS, Mehta R, Pashkow FJ, et al. Association of chronotropic incompetence with echocardiographic ischemia and prognosis. J Am Coll Cardiol. 1998;32:1280-6.

54. Bouzas-Mosquera A, Peteiro J, Alvarez-García N, et al. Prediction of mortality and major cardiac events by exercise echocardiography in patients with normal exercise electrocardiographic testing. J Am Coll Cardiol. 2009;53:1981-90.

55. Colon PJ, Mobarek SK, Milani RV, et al. Prognostic value of stress echocardiography in the evaluation of atypical chest pain patients without known coronary artery disease. Am J Cardiol. 1998;81:545-51.

56. Leischik R, Dworrak B, Littwitz H, et al. Prognostic significance of exercise stress echocardiography in 3,329 outpatients (5-year longitudinal study). Int J Cardiol. 2007;119:297-305.

57. Marwick TH, Case C, Vasey C, et al. Prediction of mortality by exercise echocardiography: a strategy for combination with the duke treadmill score. Circulation. 2001;103:2566-71.

58. Alexander KP, Shaw LJ, Shaw LK, et al. Value of exercise treadmill testing in women. J Am Coll Cardiol. 1998;32:1657-64.

59. Mark DB, Shaw LJ, Harrell FE, et al. Prognostic value of a treadmill exercise score in outpatients with suspected coronary artery disease. N Engl J Med. 1991;325:849-53.

60. Marwick TH, Mehta R, Arheart K, et al. Use of exercise echocardiography for prognostic evaluation of patients with known or suspected coronary artery disease. J Am Coll Cardiol. 1997;30:83-90.

61. Metz LD, Beattie M, Hom R, et al. The prognostic value of normal exercise myocardial perfusion imaging and exercise echocardiography: a meta-analysis. J Am Coll Cardiol. 2007;49:227-37.

62. Labovitz AJ. The "myth" of the false positive stress echo. J Am Soc Echocardiogr. 2010;23:215-6.

63. Shaw LJ, Bairey Merz CN, Pepine CJ, et al. Insights from the NHLBI-Sponsored Women's Ischemia Syndrome Evaluation (WISE) Study: Part I: gender differences in traditional and novel risk factors, symptom evaluation, and gender-optimized diagnostic strategies. J Am Coll Cardiol. 2006;47:S4-20.

64. McCully RB, Roger VL, Mahoney DW, et al. Outcome after abnormal exercise echocardiography for patients with good exercise capacity: prognostic importance of the extent and severity of exercise-related left ventricular dysfunction. J Am Coll Cardiol. 2002;39:1345-52.

SECTION 3

Diagnosis

65. McCully RB, Roger VL, Ommen SR, et al. Outcomes of patients with reduced exercise capacity at time of exercise echocardiography. Mayo Clin Proc. 2004;79:750-7.

66. Smith SC, Feldman TE, Hirshfeld JW, et al. ACC/AHA/SCAI 2005 Guideline Update for Percutaneous Coronary Intervention—summary article: a report of the American College of Cardiology/American Heart Association Task Force on Practice Guidelines (ACC/AHA/SCAI Writing Committee to Update the 2001 Guidelines for Percutaneous Coronary Intervention). Circulation. 2006;113:156-75.

67. Lin GA, Dudley RA, Lucas FL, et al. Frequency of stress testing to document ischemia prior to elective percutaneous coronary intervention. JAMA. 2008;300:1765-73.

68. Diamond GA, Kaul S. The disconnect between practice guidelines and clinical practice—stressed out. JAMA. 2008;300:1817-9.

69. Bigi R, Cortigiani L. Stress testing in women: sexual discrimination or equal opportunity? Eur Heart J. 2005;26:423-5.

70. Geleijnse ML, Krenning BJ, Soliman OI, et al. Dobutamine stress echocardiography for the detection of coronary artery disease in women. Am J Cardiol. 2007;99:714-7.

71. Makaryus AN, Shaw LJ, Mieres JH. Diagnostic strategies for heart disease in women: an update on imaging techniques for optimal management. Cardiol Rev. 2007;15:279-87.

72. Marwick TH, Anderson T, Williams MJ, et al. Exercise echocardiography is an accurate and cost-efficient technique for detection of coronary artery disease in women. J Am Coll Cardiol. 1995;26:335-41.

73. Marwick TH, Shaw LJ, Lauer MS, et al. The noninvasive prediction of cardiac mortality in men and women with known or suspected coronary artery disease. Economics of Noninvasive Diagnosis (END) Study Group. Am J Med. 1999;106:172-8.

74. Merz NB, Johnson BD, Kelsey PSF, et al. Diagnostic, prognostic, and cost assessment of coronary artery disease in women. Am J Manag Care. 2001;7:959-65.

75. Shaw LJ, Vasey C, Sawada SG, et al. Impact of gender on risk stratification by exercise and dobutamine stress echocardiography: long-term mortality in 4,234 women and 6,898 men. Eur Heart J. 2005;26:447-56.

76. Bangalore S, Yao SS, Chaudhry FA. Usefulness of stress echocardiography for risk stratification and prognosis of patients with left ventricular hypertrophy. Am J Cardiol. 2007;100:536-43.

77. Anand DV, Lim E, Lahiri A, et al. The role of noninvasive imaging in the risk stratification of asymptomatic diabetic subjects. Eur Heart J. 2006;27:905-12.

78. Young LH, Wackers FJ, Chyun DA, et al. Cardiac outcomes after screening for asymptomatic coronary artery disease in patients with type 2 diabetes: the DIAD study: a randomized controlled trial. JAMA. 2009;301:1547-55.

79. Bouzas-Mosquera A, Peteiro J, Broullón FJ, et al. Prognostic value of exercise echocardiography in patients with atrial fibrillation. Eur J Echocardiogr. 2010;11:346-51.

80. Sharma R, Mehta RL, Brecker SJ, et al. The diagnostic and prognostic value of tissue Doppler imaging during dobutamine stress echocardiography in end-stage renal disease. Coron Artery Dis. 2009;20:230-7.

81. Geleijnse ML, Vigna C, Kasprzak JD, et al. Usefulness and limitations of dobutamine-atropine stress echocardiography for the diagnosis of coronary artery disease in patients with left bundle branch block. A multicentre study. Eur Heart J. 2000;21:1666-73.

82. Chuah SC, Pellikka PA, Roger VL, et al. Role of dobutamine stress echocardiography in predicting outcome in 860 patients with known or suspected coronary artery disease. Circulation. 1998;97:1474-80.

83. Poldermans D, Fioretti PM, Boersma E, et al. Long-term prognostic value of dobutamine-atropine stress echocardiography in 1,737 patients with known or suspected coronary artery disease: a single-center experience. Circulation. 1999;99:757-62.

84. Elhendy A, Schinkel AF, Bax JJ, et al. Prognostic value of dobutamine stress echocardiography in patients with normal left ventricular systolic function. J Am Soc Echocardiogr. 2004;17:739-43.

85. Marwick TH, Case C, Sawada S, et al. Prediction of mortality using dobutamine echocardiography. J Am Coll Cardiol. 2001;37:754-60.

86. Sozzi FB, Elhendy A, Roelandt JR, et al. Long-term prognosis after normal dobutamine stress echocardiography. Am J Cardiol. 2003;92:1267-70.

87. Yao SS, Qureshi E, Sherrid MV, et al. Practical applications in stress echocardiography: risk stratification and prognosis in patients with known or suspected ischemic heart disease. J Am Coll Cardiol. 2003;42:1084-90.

88. Chaowalit N, McCully RB, Callahan MJ, et al. Outcomes after normal dobutamine stress echocardiography and predictors of adverse events: long-term follow-up of 3,014 patients. Eur Heart J. 2006;27: 3039-44.

89. From A, Kane G, Bruce C, et al. Characteristics and outcomes of patients with abnormal stress echocardiograms and angiographically mild coronary artery disease (< 50% stenoses) or normal coronary arteries. J Am Soc Echocardiogr. 2010;23:207-14.

90. Lin GA, Redberg RF. Use of stress testing prior to percutaneous coronary intervention in patients with stable coronary artery disease. Expert Rev Cardiovasc Ther. 2009;7:1061-6.

91. Shaw LJ, Hachamovitch R, Berman DS, et al. The economic consequences of available diagnostic and prognostic strategies for the evaluation of stable angina patients: an observational assessment of the value of precatheterization ischemia. Economics of Non-invasive Diagnosis (END) Multicenter Study Group. J Am Coll Cardiol. 1999;33:661-9.

92. Kim C, Kwok YS, Saha S, et al. Diagnosis of suspected coronary artery disease in women: a cost-effectiveness analysis. Am Heart J. 1999;137:1019-27.

93. Sharples L, Hughes V, Crean A, et al. Cost-effectiveness of functional cardiac testing in the diagnosis and management of coronary artery disease: a randomised controlled trial. The CECaT trial. Health Technol Assess. 2007;11:iii-iv, ix-115.

94. Shaw LJ, Berman DS, Maron DJ, et al. Optimal medical therapy with or without percutaneous coronary intervention to reduce ischemic burden: results from the Clinical Outcomes Utilizing Revascularization and Aggressive Drug Evaluation (COURAGE) trial nuclear substudy. Circulation. 2008;117:1283-91.

95. Yao SS, Bangalore S, Chaudhry FA. Prognostic Implications of Stress Echocardiography and Impact on Patient Outcomes: an Effective Gatekeeper for Coronary Angiography and Revascularization. J Am Soc Echocardiogr. 2010;23: 832-9.

96. Cortigiani L, Sicari R, Bigi R, et al. Usefulness of stress echocardiography for risk stratification of patients after percutaneous coronary intervention. Am J Cardiol. 2008;102:1170-4.

97. Fleisher LA, Beckman JA, Brown KA, et al. ACC/AHA 2007 Guidelines on Perioperative Cardiovascular Evaluation and Care for Noncardiac Surgery: Executive Summary: a Report of the American College of Cardiology/American Heart Association Task Force on Practice Guidelines (Writing Committee to Revise the 2002 Guidelines on Perioperative Cardiovascular Evaluation for Noncardiac Surgery) Developed in Collaboration with the American Society of Echocardiography, American Society of Nuclear Cardiology, Heart Rhythm Society, Society of Cardiovascular Anesthesiologists, Society for Cardiovascular Angiography and Interventions, Society for Vascular Medicine and Biology, and Society for Vascular Surgery. J Am Coll Cardiol. 2007;50:1707-32.

98. Poldermans D, Bax JJ, Thomson IR, et al. Role of dobutamine stress echocardiography for preoperative cardiac risk assessment before major vascular surgery: a diagnostic tool comes of age. Echocardiography. 2000;17:79-91.

99. Labib SB, Goldstein M, Kinnunen PM, et al. Cardiac events in patients with negative maximal versus negative submaximal dobutamine echocardiograms undergoing noncardiac surgery: importance of resting wall motion abnormalities. J Am Coll Cardiol. 2004;44: 82-7.

100. McKeogh JR. The diagnostic role of stress echocardiography in women with coronary artery disease: evidence based review. Curr Opin Cardiol. 2007;22:429-33.

101. Chaowalit N, Arruda AL, McCully RB, et al. Dobutamine stress echocardiography in patients with diabetes mellitus: enhanced prognostic prediction using a simple risk score. J Am Coll Cardiol. 2006;47:1029-36.

102. Chaowalit N, Maalouf JF, Rooke TW, et al. Prognostic significance of chronotropic response to dobutamine stress echocardiography in patients with peripheral arterial disease. Am J Cardiol. 2004;94:1523-8.

103. Dawn B, Paliwal VS, Raza ST, et al. Left ventricular outflow tract obstruction provoked during dobutamine stress echocardiography predicts future chest pain, syncope, and near syncope. Am Heart J. 2005;149:908-16.

104. Sicari R, Cortigiani L, Bigi R, et al. Prognostic value of pharmacological stress echocardiography is affected by concomitant antiischemic therapy at the time of testing. Circulation. 2004;109:2428-31.

105. Sicari R, Pasanisi E, Venneri L, et al. Stress echo results predict mortality: a large-scale multicenter prospective international study. J Am Coll Cardiol. 2003;41:589-95.

106. Kertai MD, Boersma E, Sicari R, et al. Which stress test is superior for perioperative cardiac risk stratification in patients undergoing major vascular surgery? Eur J Vasc Endovasc Surg. 2002;24:222-9.

107. Schinkel AF, Poldermans D, Elhendy A, et al. Prognostic role of dobutamine stress echocardiography in myocardial viability. Curr Opin Cardiol. 2006;21:443-9.

108. Schinkel AF, Bax JJ, Poldermans D, et al. Hibernating myocardium: diagnosis and patient outcomes. Curr Probl Cardiol. 2007;32:375-410.

109. Schinkel AF, Bax JJ, Delgado V, et al. Clinical relevance of hibernating myocardium in ischemic left ventricular dysfunction. Am J Med. 2010;123:978-86.

110. Rizzello V, Poldermans D, Schinkel AF, et al. Long-term prognostic value of myocardial viability and ischemia during dobutamine stress echocardiography in patients with ischemic cardiomyopathy undergoing coronary revascularization. Heart. 2006;92:239-44.

111. Picano E, Pibarot P, Lancellotti P, et al. The emerging role of exercise testing and stress echocardiography in valvular heart disease. J Am Coll Cardiol. 2009;54:2251-60.

112. Picano E. Economic and biological costs of cardiac imaging. Cardiovasc Ultrasound. 2005;3:13.

113. Redberg RF. The appropriateness imperative. Am Heart J. 2007;154:201-2.

Transesophageal Echocardiography

Seyed M Hashemi, Paul Lindower, Richard E Kerber

Chapter Outline

INTRODUCTION

Over the past few decades, transesophageal echocardiography (TEE) has become a commonly performed imaging modality that is complementary to transthoracic echocardiography (TTE).[1-3] It is widely available, portable, provides real time imaging, and may be performed in a variety of clinical settings. These settings range from the ambulatory echocardiography laboratory to the cardiac catheterization laboratory as well as the intensive care unit. The use of the esophagus as an acoustic window has permitted the use of higher frequency transducers than those used in TTE studies. This results in improved spatial resolution allowing for visualization of small structures such as small vegetations and thrombi. In addition, the esophagus provides a unique window to posterior cardiac structures that are not well seen from the chest surface. These structures include the left atrial appendage, the interatrial septum, the mitral valve and the thoracic aorta.

HISTORY

Doppler TEE was initially reported by Side and Gosling in 1971 who performed continuous wave Doppler velocity measurements in the thoracic aorta using a dual element transducer mounted on a standard gastroscope.[4] In 1976, Frazin and his colleagues performed m-mode TEE imaging with a crystal mounted on a modified endoscopic probe (Fig. 1).[5] Hisanaga and his colleagues then reported the first two-dimensional (2D) TEE imaging in 1977 using a single rotating element enclosed in an inflatable oil bag to ensure contact with the esophageal wall.[6] More recently, TEE technology has significantly evolved and it currently permits all major echocardiographic capabilities. These include multiplane 2D imaging, color Doppler, pulse wave Doppler, continuous wave Doppler as well as three-dimensional (3D) volume acquisitions.

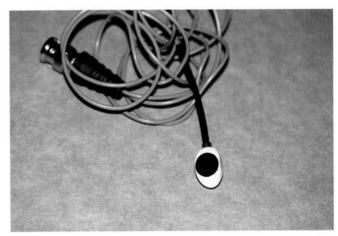

FIGURE 1: Frazin m-mode transesophageal echocardiography probe

GUIDELINES

Transesophageal echocardiography is a minimally invasive procedure that is being increasingly performed by cardiologists as well as anesthesiologists, surgeons and intensive care specialists. Guidelines for TEE competence have been published by the American College of Cardiology and American Heart Association.[7] Training requirements endorse attainment of at least Level 2 experience in TTE as well as the performance of 25 esophageal intubations with a TEE probe and further performance of approximately 50 TEE studies under the supervision of an experienced (Level 3 trained) echocardiographer.

PERFORMANCE

Transesophageal echocardiography should be performed in a laboratory equipped with appropriate tools as well as trained personnel. In addition to the ultrasound machine and multiplane imaging probe, the laboratory must possess the necessary sanitizing equipment to disinfect the TEE probes and transducers. Since performing TEE requires conscious sedation, it necessitates the assistance of a nurse or another qualified assistant who monitors the patient's vital signs, arterial saturation and level of consciousness throughout the procedure. The patient's airway is also monitored with suctioning of oral secretions as necessary to reduce the risk of aspiration. Prior to esophageal intubation, a careful history is obtained from the patient to exclude significant laryngeal or gastroesophageal pathology. If necessary, the assistance of an anesthesiologist or gastroenterologist may be obtained to facilitate the intubation part of the procedure. The patient is kept fasting for at least 6 hours, and peripheral IV access is obtained to provide moderate conscious sedation with low doses of an IV benzodiazepine and a narcotic. The oropharynx is anesthetized by asking the patient to gargle and swallow a lidocaine solution. Additionally, topical benzocaine spray may be utilized if there is a significant residual gag reflex. Since topical benzocaine products carry risk of methemoglobinemia, we do not recommend using benzocaine spray routinely or as the first choice. The patient is then placed in the left lateral decubitus position with the neck flexed. The TEE probe is positioned in the posterior oropharynx. The esophagus is then intubated as the patient initiates a swallow.

SAFETY

The procedural risks of TEE are relatively small but may include: transient throat pain, laryngospasm, aspiration, hypoxemia, hypotension, dysrhythmia, bleeding, esophageal rupture or even death. In a large European multicenter study analyzing 10,419 TEE examinations, premature termination was necessary in 90 procedures (0.88%).[8] Most of these were due to patient intolerance to the probe. There were also 18 patients who had pulmonary, cardiac, bleeding related or other complications. One of the bleeding related complications resulted in a death (0.01%). In general, bleeding complications are rare and usually mild in the face of therapeutic levels of anticoagulation. The risk of bacteremia with TEE is very low and most operators do not routinely treat with prophylactic antibiotics. Methemoglobinemia is a potentially life-threatening complication of topical benzocaine use. It is suspected clinically in the presence of cyanosis with normal arterial oxygen saturation and may be treated with methylene blue and supportive measures. Contraindications to TEE include esophageal stricture, diverticulum, tumor and recent esophageal or gastric surgery. Relative contraindications include prior mediastinal irradiation, esophageal varices and coagulopathy. Patients should always be questioned about a history of dysphagia, esophageal varices and/or liver disease before attempting intubation.

VIEWS

Using a multiplane transesophageal echoscope, standard echocardiographic views of the heart may be obtained.[9] The American Society of Echocardiography (ASE) recommends twenty cross-sectional views composing a comprehensive TEE examination (Figs 2A to T). The probe is initially advanced into the proximal esophagus, and images are taken from four general positions: (1) the basal esophagus; (2) mid esophagus or

4-chamber view; (3) transgastric and (4) aortic positions. In addition, the plane of the scan may be rotated through an arc of 180°. At 0°, the plane of interrogation is horizontal or transverse to the heart. More vertical orientation of the crystal provides longitudinal sectioning of the heart. The probe may also be manipulated anteriorly or posteriorly by flexing or extending the probe respectively in the coronal plane.

MAJOR CLINICAL APPLICATIONS

SOURCE OF EMBOLISM

According to the 2011 ASE appropriateness criteria, TEE evaluation for cardiovascular source of embolic event in a stroke patient with no identified non-cardiac source is considered highly appropriate (score 7/9). Up to 15–20% of ischemic strokes may be on the basis of an intracardiac source.[10] Transesophageal echocardiography (TEE) has been found to be superior to TTE in detecting cardiac sources of embolism[11,12] and may also be a more cost effective approach in their detection.[13] The yield of TEE is higher in patients with clinical cardiac disease including atrial fibrillation, rheumatic mitral stenosis, prosthetic valves, atherosclerosis, left ventricular aneurysm and infective endocarditis.[14] Potential cardiac sources of embolism may be categorized as: (1) masses (thrombus, atherosclerotic plaque, vegetation or tumor); (2) passageways for paradoxic embolization (patent foramen ovale and atrial septal aneurysm) and (3) propensity for thrombus formation (left atrial spontaneous echo contrast, mitral annular calcification).

Masses

Left atrial thrombus is commonly associated with atrial fibrillation and rheumatic mitral stenosis. It may be seen in up to 27% of patients with chronic atrial fibrillation (Fig. 3).[15] It is only present in 1% of patients in sinus rhythm and no mitral valve disease or left atrial dysfunction.[16] Left ventricular thrombus occurs in approximately 5% of patients with acute myocardial infarction, particularly when the infarct is anterior in location.[17] It is also seen in about 4% of patients with dilated cardiomyopathy. These same cardiomyopathy patients also have an even greater risk of developing left atrial thrombus.[18] Prosthetic valves may develop thrombus, especially mechanical valves in the atrioventricular position, in the setting of subtherapeutic anticoagulation.[19] Thrombi may display high-risk characteristics for embolization which include large size, protruding appearance, high mobility and central echolucency.

Aortic atherosclerotic plaques are associated with hypertension and are more common in elderly patients. Plaques may be categorized as simple or complex with the latter being more prone to thromboembolization. Features of complex atheromas include a wall thickness greater than 4 mm, ulceration, mobility, pedunculation and echolucency (Fig. 4).[20]

Vegetative lesions are readily identified in patients with clinical features of infective endocarditis (Fig. 5). Vegetation size greater than 1 cm, vegetation mobility and mitral location are all risk factors for systemic embolization.[21] Additionally, TEE permits visualization of perivalvular abscess in patients with infective endocarditis (Fig. 6).

Primary cardiac tumors commonly include myxomas and papillary fibroelastomas. Myxomas are usually benign tumors

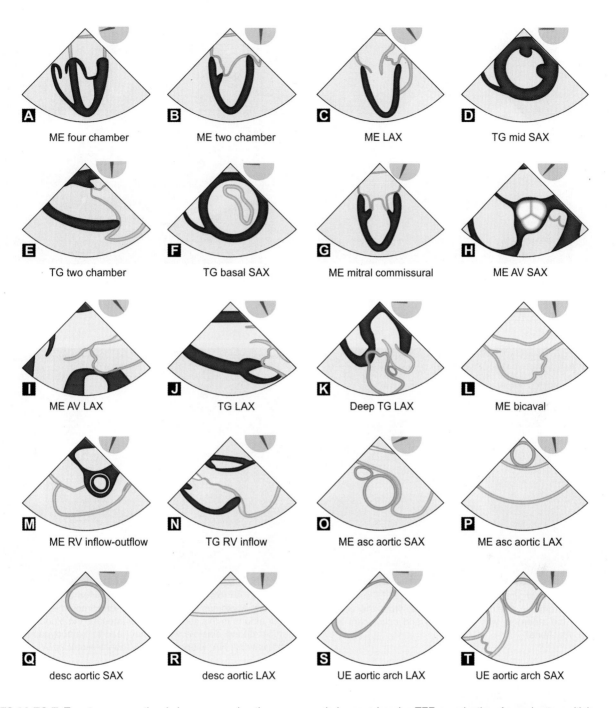

FIGURES 2A TO T: Twenty cross-sectional views composing the recommended comprehensive TEE examination. Approximate multiplane angle is indicated by the icon adjacent to each view. (Abbreviations: ME: Mid esophageal; LAX: Long axis; TG: Transgastric; SAX: Short axis; AV: Aortic valve; RV: Right ventricle; Asc: Ascending; Desc: Descending; UE: Upper esophageal). (*Source:* Reproduced with permission from Shanewise JS et al. ASE/SCA guidelines for performing a comprehensive intraoperative multiplane TEE. J Am Soc Echocardiogr. 1999;12:884-900)

found in the left atrium attached to the interatrial septum in the region of the fossa ovale (Fig. 7). They may present with embolization greater than 50% of the time.[22] Papillary fibroelastomas generally are pedunculated and commonly located on the aortic or mitral valve, although they are also found on the endocardial surface.[23]

Passageways for Paradoxic Embolization

Interatrial septal abnormalities are associated with thromboembolic events. These include atrial septal defect as well as patent foramen ovale with or without an atrial septal aneurysm.[24] Patients with an interatrial shunt may have intermittent right-to-left shunting particularly if there is a transient increase in right-sided pressure as occurs with coughing or performing a Valsalva maneuver. In this setting, venous thrombi may potentially enter the systemic circulation resulting in paradoxical embolism. Right-to-left shunting may be demonstrated by the administration of intravenous agitated saline contrast. Approximately 25% of normal hearts are found to have a patent foramen ovale at the time of autopsy.[25] A patent foramen ovale

Transesophageal Echocardiography

CHAPTER 18

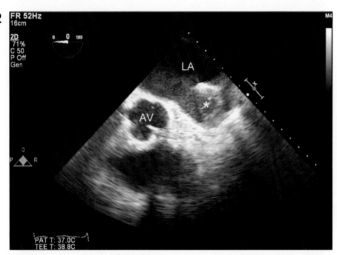

FIGURE 3: Transesophageal echocardiography (TEE) showing a left atrial appendage thrombus (depicted by the asterisk) in a patient with chronic atrial fibrillation. Note the presence of smoke in the left atrium. (Abbreviations: LA: Left atrium; AV: Aortic vlave)

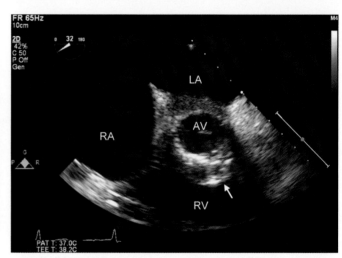

FIGURE 6: Short axis view through aortic valve demonstrating a bioprosthetic aortic valve with an aortic root abscess (arrow). (Abbreviations: LA: Left atrium; RA: Right atrium; RV: Right ventricle; AV: Aortic valve)

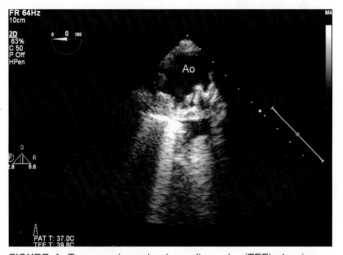

FIGURE 4: Transesophageal echocardiography (TEE) showing an example of atheroma in the descending aorta. Note the complex appearance of the atheroma with echodense and echolucent areas. (Abbreviation: Ao: Aorta)

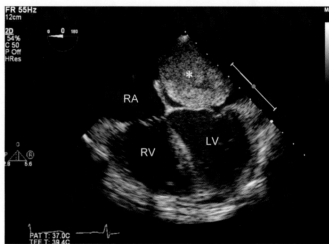

FIGURE 7: An example of a myxoma (depicted by the asterisk) in the left atrium. Myxomas vary in size and sometimes may occupy most of the left atrium. In this case, the tumor impedes the blood flow to the left ventricle during diastole which may lead to hemodynamic instability. (Abbreviations: RA: Right atrium; RV: Right ventricle; LV: Left ventricle)

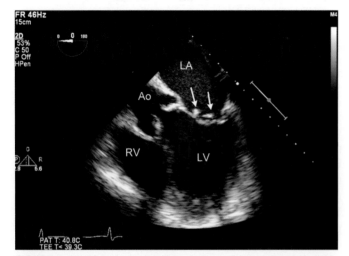

FIGURE 5: An example of vegetations (indicated by the arrows) involving the mitral valve in a patient with infective endocarditis. (Abbreviations: LA: Left atrium; Ao: Aorta; RV: Right ventricle; LV: Left ventricle)

alone is not associated with an increased risk of recurrent stroke or death in patients with a cryptogenic stroke. An atrial septal aneurysm is a congenital variant with redundant, mobile, interatrial septal tissue in the region of the fossa with a base measuring 15 mm and an excursion of at least 10 mm during the cardiorespiratory cycle.[26] Atrial septal aneurysms are associated with patent foramen ovale (Fig. 8). There is conflicting data as to whether the combination of a patent foramen ovale and an atrial septal aneurysm confers additional risk for recurrent stroke or death among patients with a cryptogenic stroke.[24,27]

Propensity for Thrombus Formation

Spontaneous echo contrast or smoke-like echoes are strongly associated with left atrial thrombi. This occurs in the setting of erythrocyte aggregation in low shear rate conditions and is

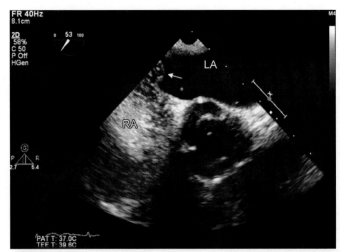

FIGURE 8: Interatrial septal aneurysm (denoted by the arrow) is often associated with a patent foramen ovale demonstrated by a positive bubble study in this patient. (Abbreviations: LA: Left atrium; RA: Right atrium)

mediated by plasma proteins such as fibrinogen.[28,29] These proteins reduce electrostatic forces on the surface of red blood cells which are usually repulsive, thus promoting rouleaux formation. Mitral annular calcification is commonly associated with the elderly, left atrial enlargement and atrial fibrillation. It is unclear whether this may also act as a nidus for thrombus formation.[30]

Transesophageal echocardiography is warranted when the history and physical examination is suggestive of a cardiac source of embolism and the treatment plan would be modified based upon its results.

ATRIAL FIBRILLATION

Atrial fibrillation is associated with a 4–6 fold increased risk of thromboembolism presumably from left atrial appendage thrombi.[31] Thrombi in the left atrial appendage have been demonstrated in up to 14% of patients with new onset atrial fibrillation and up to 27% of those in chronic atrial fibrillation (Fig. 3).[15] The conversion of atrial fibrillation to sinus rhythm involves a small risk of thromboembolism from blood clots that may form in the left atrial appendage during or shortly after sinus rhythm restoration. A conventional approach to cardioversion involves providing anticoagulation for at least 3 weeks before the procedure and continuing anticoagulation therapy for an additional 4 weeks afterward. With the advent of TEE, the left atrial appendage can be assessed for the presence of thrombus. This is the basis of a TEE guided strategy for cardioversion. If a thrombus is not detected, cardioversion may be expedited and performed immediately after TEE. If a thrombus is detected, anticoagulation may be intensified and then the TEE should be repeated before further cardioversion attempts are made. The ACUTE trial was a large, multicenter randomized study that compared the performance of a TEE guided strategy with a conventional strategy in patients with new onset atrial fibrillation.[31] Its major finding was that the TEE guided strategy afforded a shorter period of anticoagulation with a shorter time to cardioversion and fewer bleeding events when compared to the conventional strategy. There were

no differences in embolization rate, death, maintenance of sinus rhythm or functional status between the two groups. It was felt by the authors that patients best suited for the TEE guided strategy are those who are hospitalized with new onset atrial fibrillation, or who have subtherapeutic or undetermined anticoagulation status, or who may be at a higher-risk for bleeding or thromboembolism.

ENDOCARDITIS

Transesophageal echocardiography has greatly facilitated the diagnosis of endocarditis. It permits improved detection of small vegetations and the identification of coexisting paravalvular abnormalities. Although the procedure is minimally invasive and entails added expense, it has been shown to have higher sensitivity and specificity than TTE and is also better able to assess complications of endocarditis than TTE.[32] These complications include abscess formation, valve perforation, fistulous communication or valvular regurgitation. The modified Duke criteria for endocarditis include four major criteria on the basis of echocardiography findings.[33] These are the presence of an oscillating mass (vegetation), abscess, partial dehiscence of a prosthetic valve and new valvular regurgitation. Vegetation characteristics by echocardiography may also indicate embolic potential. Larger vegetations are greater than 1 cm, increased mobility and mitral valve involvement are associated with increased embolic risk.[21] This risk of embolization is reduced with the duration of antibiotic therapy.[34] Right-sided valve lesions are not necessarily better demonstrated by TEE as they are in the far field of view; except in the transgastric position where the tricuspid valve is optimally imaged. In addition, prosthetic valve endocarditis may be confounded by impaired visualization of the valves from shadowing and reverberations associated with the prosthetic material. However, in the case of mitral valve prosthesis, the TEE probe is positioned behind the prosthetic valve and assessment is not confounded by these issues.[35] A negative TEE study in a patient with an intermediate likelihood of endocarditis effectively rules out endocarditis. A repeat TEE study would be warranted in high likelihood patients in approximately 7–10 days; however, as smaller vegetations may not be initially detected.[36]

STRUCTURAL VALVE ASSESSMENT

Transesophageal echocardiography is an ideal technique for visualization of the mitral valve apparatus owing to the proximity of the TEE probe to the left atrium. Mitral valve prolapse (Fig. 9, Videos 1 and 2) and flail mitral valve (Fig. 10, Video 3) are readily assessed by TEE. Another use of TEE is to identify the mechanism and severity of mitral valve regurgitation (Figs 11 and 12, Video 4). In patients with mitral stenosis in whom a high quality transthoracic echo can be obtained, TEE may not necessarily provide additional information. However TEE is capable of demonstrating high-resolution images of mitral stenosis (Fig. 13, Video 5).

Transesophageal echocardiography allows for highly accurate diagnosis of structural valvular abnormalities in aortic positions. Higher image resolution produces sharper images of aortic valve cusps and clear visualization of bicuspid aortic valve (Fig. 14, Video 8). Transesophageal echocardiography is also a

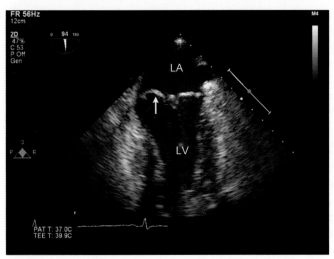

FIGURE 9: A 2-chamber view shows prolapse of the mitral valve posterior leaflet (arrow). (Abbreviations: LA: Left atrium; LV: Left ventricle)

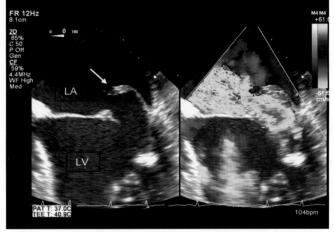

FIGURE 10: Close-up view of mitral valve showing flail posterior leaflet (arrow). The right-sided image demonstrates a regurgitant jet directed anteriorly. (Abbreviations: LA: Left atrium; LV: Left ventricle)

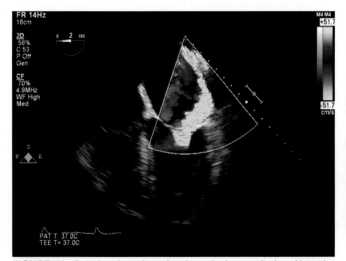

FIGURE 11: A 4-chamber view showing mitral regurgitation. Note the eccentric posteriorly directed MR jet indicating anterior MV pathology

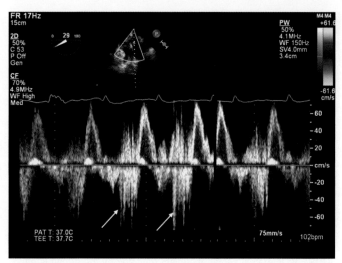

FIGURE 12: Pulmonary vein pulse Doppler imaging recorded from transesophageal echocardiography (TEE) in a patient with mitral regurgitation. Note the systolic flow reversal through the pulmonary vein indicating severe mitral regurgitation

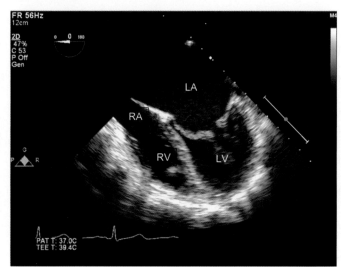

FIGURE 13: A 4-chamber view transesophageal echocardiography (TEE) showing rheumatic mitral stenosis. Note the thickened mitral valve leaflets with restricted mobility. (Abbreviations: LA: Left atrium; RA: Right atrium; RV: Right ventricle; LV: Left ventricle)

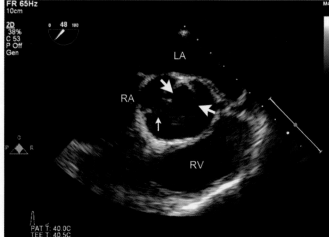

FIGURE 14: A short axis view of TEE through aortic valve showing an example of bicuspid aortic valve (thick arrows indicate the two leaflets and the thin arrow points to the raphe). (Abbreviations: LA: Left atrium; RA: Right atrium; RV: Right ventricle)

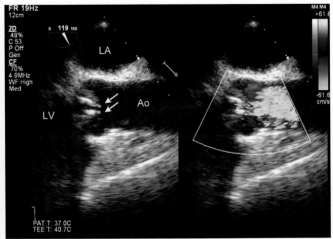

FIGURE 15: A long axis view transesophageal echocardiography (TEE) through the aortic valve from a patient with aortic stenosis. Note the severely restricted aortic valve leaflet mobility (arrows) causing turbulent flow (depicted by color Doppler on the right sided image). (Abbreviations: LA: Left atrium; LV: Left ventricle; Ao: Aorta)

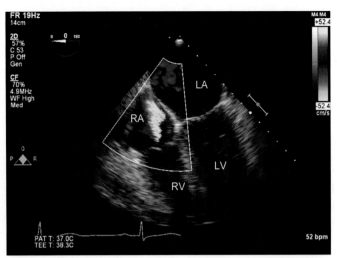

FIGURE 18: A 4-chamber view TEE showing tricuspid regurgitation. (Abbreviations: LA: Left atrium; RA: Right atrium; RV: Right ventricle; LV: Left ventricle)

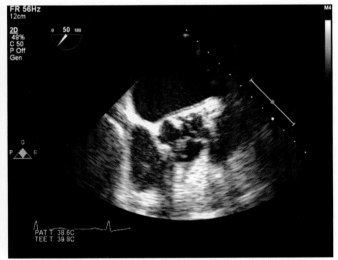

FIGURE 16: A short axis view of aortic valve in a patient with aortic stenosis showing restricted aortic valve leaflet mobility

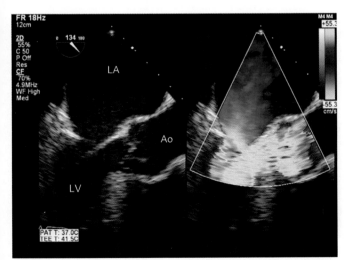

FIGURE 17: A 3-chamber view transesophageal echocardiography (TEE) showing long axis of the aortic valve with severe aortic insufficiency. (Abbreviations: LA: Left atrium; LV: Left ventricle; Ao: Aorta)

valuable tool for assessment of aortic stenosis (Figs 15 and 16, Videos 6 and 7) and aortic regurgitation (Fig. 17, Video 8).

The valvular structures on the right side of the heart being positioned anteriorly (in the far field of view from the TEE probe) are less conducive to assessment by TEE. However the tricuspid valve in most cases can be assessed fairly accurately in transgastric view (Video 9). Four-chamber view is suitable for diagnosis of tricuspid regurgitation (Fig. 18, Video 10). Pulmonary valvular abnormalities are relatively rare and not necessarily easier evaluated by transesophageal echocardiography.

Prosthetic valves present several limitations to echocardiographic techniques due to artifacts that are created from shadowing and reverberation of ultrasound by the non-biologic material in the valve. Transthoracic Doppler echocardiography provides very reliable hemodynamic information regarding prosthetic valve function. Assessment of prosthetic mitral valve function by TTE, however, is difficult due to its posterior location. TEE is indicated when there is a high clinical suspicion of valvular dysfunction, there are difficulties surrounding poor acoustic transthoracic windows, or there is concern regarding prosthetic mitral valve function. Transesophageal echocardiography offers significant advantages over TTE, although the combination of both studies allows for a complete assessment of prosthetic valve function. All mechanical prosthetic valves demonstrate a small amount of transvalvular regurgitation due to the closure volume of the prosthesis with movement of the occluder disk.[37] In some prosthetic valves, gaps between the valve posts or holes in the valve disk result in small amounts of prosthetic valve regurgitation. This normal regurgitation varies depending on the type of prosthesis and must be distinguished from pathologic regurgitation. Paravalvular regurgitation is always pathologic and bioprosthetic valves generally display only trace or no regurgitation. An increased transvalvular pressure gradient compared with baseline or established normal values will be observed in patients with an obstructed prosthetic valve. The etiology of obstruction includes: pannus ingrowth, thrombus or vegetation. The most common etiology of prosthetic valve obstruction is thrombus formation. This may be further suggested in the setting of a short duration of symptoms, subtherapeutic anticoagulation, and demonstration of a soft, mobile echodensity attached to the valve occluder.[38] Thrombolytic therapy may be an effective alternative to surgery in such patients although it is associated with modest morbidity and mortality.[39]

ACUTE AORTIC DISSECTION

Transesophageal echocardiography has significant advantages over magnetic resonance imaging (MRI) or computed tomography (CT) in the assessment of acute aortic dissection.[40] It may be rapidly performed at the bedside of patients who are unstable for transport to MRI or CT suites. It may also be performed in the operating room as patients are being prepared for surgery. The characteristic finding in patients with an aortic dissection is the identification of an intimal flap (Figs 19 and 20). Furthermore, the location and extent of the flap as well as entry and exit points may be well delineated by TEE. Additional pertinent findings on TEE would include the aortic diameter, presence of thrombus in the false lumen, presence of a pericardial effusion, presence of aortic regurgitation, or involvement of branch vessels or coronary arteries. An aortic intramural hematoma is characterized by thickening of the aortic wall greater than 7 mm and may be either crescentic or circular in nature with evidence of an intramural accumulation of blood.[41] A penetrating atherosclerotic ulcer may be identified as an ulcer-like projection into an aortic intramural hematoma, usually in the descending aorta.[42] These entities may coexist with an aortic dissection and they are managed in a similar fashion. Acute aortic dissection patients with proximal involvement of the aorta are considered for emergent surgery. Patients with isolated distal aortic involvement are initially managed medically, but may require surgery if propagation, leak or ischemic complications develop. The sensitivity of TEE to detect aortic dissection is approximately 98%. The specificity is somewhat lower at 95% due to false positive findings in the ascending aorta.[40] Reverberation artifacts may be differentiated from dissection by using m-mode echocardiography.[43] The upper portion of the ascending aorta and arch is difficult to visualize due to the interposition of the air-filled trachea between the esophagus and the aorta.

PROCEDURAL ADJUNCT OR INTRAOPERATIVE TEE

Transesophageal echocardiography is commonly used as an adjunct to fluoroscopic imaging during interventional procedures in the cardiac catheterization laboratory. In patients with significant right-to-left shunting, percutaneous closure of an atrial septal defect or patent foramen ovale is an attractive alternative to open surgical repair. Transesophageal echocardiography offers the advantage of real time imaging of the interatrial septum as well as the surrounding structures, the closure device and catheters.[44] The atrial septal defect size may be measured by TEE for selection of the appropriate closure device (Fig. 21). The position and deployment of the device is also guided by TEE. Further, the adequacy of closure of the defect and the detection of potential complications may be determined with TEE. Transesophageal echocardiography is also used to guide many aspects of mitral balloon valvuloplasty.[45] It may be used for patient selection, guidance of transseptal puncture, exclusion of left atrial appendage thrombus, and wire and balloon positioning. It is also used to assess for potential complications of the procedure including atrial septal defect,

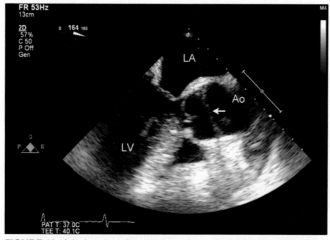

FIGURE 19: A 3-chamber view transesophageal echocardiography (TEE) demonstrating type A aortic dissection. The arrow denotes the dissection flap. (Abbreviations: LA: Left atrium; Ao: Aorta; LV: Left ventricle)

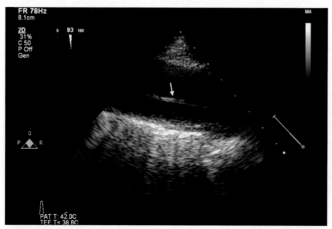

FIGURE 20: Longitudinal view of the descending aorta demonstrating type B aortic dissection. The arrow indicates the dissection flap

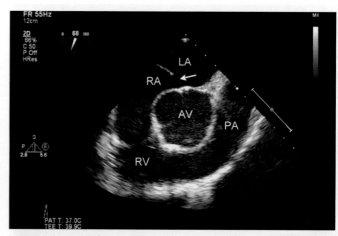

FIGURE 21: Short axis view through aortic valve demonstrating a defect in interatrial septum (depicted by the arrow) which represents an example of secundum atrial septal defect. (Abbreviations: LA: Left atrium; RA: Right atrium; RV: Right ventricle; PA: Pulmonary artery; AV: Aortic valve)

worsening mitral regurgitation or cardiac tamponade and may shorten procedural and fluoroscopic times.[46] Intraoperative TEE is increasingly performed for the evaluation of the mitral valve during surgical repair. A comprehensive examination of the mitral valve can accurately guide the surgeon.[47] Assessment of leaflet length, thickness, mobility and calcification is obtained. Leaflet motion may be characterized as excessive, restrictive or normal, and specific scallop involvement can be identified. In addition, annular dimension and calcification, left ventricular function, and the degree and direction of regurgitant jets are all noted. The anatomy most conducive to surgical repair is isolated posterior mitral leaflet prolapse. This is approached with quadrangular resection and placement of an annuloplasty ring.

CONCLUSION

Transesophageal echocardiography provides significant complementary information to TTE. Although semi-invasive in nature, it is generally safe when performed by appropriately trained operators. It may be rapidly performed at the bedside of critically ill patients. In some clinical applications, it is superior to TTE such as the detection of left atrial appendage thrombus, vegetations, aortic dissection and prosthetic mitral valve function. Transesophageal echocardiography will likely continue to expand in its application with future technologic advancements including 3D echocardiography which is discussed in a separate chapter "Real Time Three-Dimensional Echocardiography".

VIDEO LEGENDS

Video 1	Mitral valve prolapse
Video 2	Mitral valve flial with mitral regurgitation
Video 3	Mitral regurgitation with eccentric jet
Video 4	Mitral stenosis
Video 5	Aortic stenosis long axis
Video 6	Aortic stenosis short axis
Video 7	Aortic regurgitation
Video 8	Tricuspid valve (transgastric view)
Video 9	Tricuspid regurgitation.

REFERENCES

1. Sengupta PP, Khandheria BK. Transesophageal echocardiography. Heart. 2005;91(4):541-7.
2. Peterson GE, Brickner E, Reimold SC. Transesophageal echocardiography. Clinical indications and applications. Circulation. 2003;107:2398-402.
3. Daniel WG, Mugge A. Transesophageal echocardiography. N Engl J Med. 1995;332:1268-79.
4. Side CD, Gosling RG. Non-surgical assessment of cardiac function. Nature. 1971;232:335-6.
5. Frazin L, Talano JV, Stephanides L, et al. Esophageal echocardiography. Circulation. 1976;54:102-8.
6. Hisinaga KHA, Nagata K, Yoshida S. A new transesophageal real time two-dimensional echocardiographic system using a flexible tube and its clinical application. Pro Jpn Soc Ultrasonics Med. 1977;32:43-4.
7. Quinones MA, Douglas PS, Foster E, et al. ACC/AHA clinical competence statement on echocardiography: a report of the American College of Cardiology/American Heart Association/American College of Physicians-American Society of Internal Medicine Task Force on Clinical Competence. J Am Coll Cardiol. 2003;41:687-708.
8. Daniel WG, Erbel R, Kasper W, et al. Safety of transesophageal echocardiography: a multicenter survey of 10,419 examinations. Circulation. 1991;83:817-21.
9. Seward JB, Khandheria BK, Freeman WK, et al. Multiplane transesohageal echocardiography: image orientation, examination technique, anatomic correlations, and clinical applications. Mayo Clinic Proc. 1993;68:523-51.
10. Cerebral Embolism Task Force. The second report of the cerebral embolism task force. Arch Neurol. 1989;46:727-43.
11. Pearson AC, Labovitz AJ, Tatineni S, et al. Superiority of transesophageal echocardiography in detecting cardiac source of embolism in patients with cerebral ischemia of uncertain etiology. J Am Coll Cardiol. 1991;17:66-72.
12. DeRook FA, Comess KA, Albers GW, et al. Transesophageal echocardiography in the evaluation of stroke. Ann Intern Med. 1992;117:922-32.
13. McNamara RL, Lima JAC, Whelton PK, et al. Echocardiographic identification of cardiovascular sources of emboli to guide clinical management of stroke: a cost effective analysis. Ann Intern Med. 1997;127:775-87.
14. Come PC, Riley MF, Bivas NK. Roles of echocardiography and arrhythmia monitoring in the evaluation of patients with suspected systemic embolization. Ann Neurol. 1983;13:527-31.
15. Stoddard MF, Dawkins PR, Prince CR, et al. Left atrial appendage thrombus is not uncommon in patients with acute atrial fibrillation and a recent embolic event: a transesophageal echocardiographic study. J Am Coll Cardiol. 1995;25:452-9.
16. Omran H, Rang B, Schmidt H, et al. Incidence of left atrial thrombi in patients in sinus rhythm and with a recent neurologic deficit. Am Heart J. 2000;140:658-62.
17. Lapeyre AC, Steele PM, Kazimier FJ, et al. Systemic embolization in chronic left ventricular aneurysm: incidence and the role of anticoagulation. J Am Coll Cardiol. 1985;6:534-8.
18. Vigna C, Russo A, De Rito V, et al. Frequency of left atrial thrombi by transesophageal echocardiography in idiopathic and ischemic dilated cardiomyopathy. Am J Cardiol. 1992;70:1500-1.
19. Cannegieter SC, Rosendaal FR, Wintzen AR, et al. Optimal oral anticoagulation therapy in patients with mechanical heart valves. N Engl J Med. 1995;33:11-7.
20. Ferrari E, Vidal R, Chevallier J, et al. Atherosclerosis of the thoracic aorta and aortic debris as a marker of poor prognosis: benefit of oral anticoagulants. J Am Coll Cardiol. 1999;33:1317-22.
21. Mugge A, Daniel WG, Frank G, et al. Echocardiography in infective endocarditis: reassessment of prognostic implications of vegetation size determined by transthoracic and the transesophageal approach. J Am Coll Cardiol. 1989;14:631-8.
22. Wold LE, Lie JT. Cardiac myxomas: a clinicopathologic profile. Am J Pathology. 1980;101:219-40.
23. Sun JP, Asher CR, Yang XS, et al. Clinical and echocardiographic characteristics of papillary fibroelastomas: a retrospective and prospective study in 162 patients. Circulation. 2001;103:2687-93.
24. Lamy C, Giannesini C, Zuber M, et al. Clinical and imaging findings in cryptogenic stroke patients with and without patent foramen ovale: the PFO-ASA study. Stroke. 2002;33:706-11.
25. Hagen PT, Scholtz DG, Edwards WD. Incidence and size of patent foramen ovale during the first 10 decades of life: an autopsy study of 965 normal hearts. Mayo Clin Proc. 1984;59:17-20.
26. Cabanes L, Mas JL, Cohen A, et al. Atrial septal aneurysm and patent foramen ovale as risk factors for cryptogenic stroke in patients less than 55 years of age: a study using transesophageal echocardiography. Stroke. 1993;24:1865-73.
27. Homma S, Sacco RL, Di Tullio MR, et al. Effect of medical treatment in stroke patients with patent foramen ovale; patent foramen ovale in cryptogenic stroke study. Circulation. 2002;105:2625-31.
28. Black IW, Hopkins AP, Lee LC, et al. Left atrial spontaneous echo contrast: a clinical and echocardiographic analysis. J Am Coll Cardiol. 1991;18:398-404.

29. Fatkin D, Loupas T, Low J, et al. Inhibition of red cell aggregation prevents spontaneous echocardiographic contrast formation in human blood. Circulation. 1997;96:889-96.

30. Stein JH, Soble JS. Thrombus associated with mitral valve calcification. A possible mechanism for embolic stroke. Stroke. 1995;26: 1697-9.

31. Klein AJ, Grimm RA, Murray RD, et al. Use of transesophageal echocardiography to guide cardioversion in patients with atrial fibrillation. N Engl J Med. 2001;344:1411-20.

32. Bayer AS, Bolger AF, Taubert KA, et al. Diagnosis and management of infective endocarditis and its complications. Circulation. 1998;98: 2936-48.

33. Li JS, Sexton DJ, Mick N, et al. Proposed modifications to the Duke criteria for the diagnosis of infective endocarditis. Clin Infect Dis. 2000;30:633-8.

34. Vilacosta I, Graupner C, San Roman JA, et al. Risk of embolization after institution of antibiotic therapy for infective endocarditis. J Am Coll Cardiol. 2002;39:1489-95.

35. Khandheria BK, Seward JB, Oh JK, et al. Value and limitations of transesophageal echocardiography in assessment of mitral valve prostheses. Circulation. 1991;83:1956-68.

36. Sochowski RA, Chan KL. Implication of negative results on a monoplane transesophageal echocardiographic study in patients with suspected infective endocarditis. J Am Coll Cardiol. 1994;21:216-21.

37. Flachskampf FA, O'Shea JP, Griffin BP, et al. Patterns of transvalvular regurgitation in normal mechanical prosthetic valves. J Am Coll Cardiol. 1991;18:1493-8.

38. Barbetseas J, Nagueh SF, Pitsavos C, et al. Differentiating thrombus from pannus formation in obstructed mechanical prosthetic valves: an evaluation of clinical transthoracic and transesophageal echocardiographic parameters. J Am Coll Cardiol. 1998;32: 1410-7.

39. Tong AT, Roudaut R, Ozkan M, et al. Transesophageal echocardiography improves risk assessment of thrombolysis of prosthetic valve thrombosis: results of the international PRO-TEE registry. J Am Coll Cardiol. 2004;43:77-84.

40. Keren A, Kim CB, Hu BS, et al. Accuracy of biplane and multiplane tranesophageal echocardiography in diagnosis of typical acute aortic dissection and intramural hematoma. J Am Coll Cardiol. 1996;28: 627-36.

41. Vilacosta I, San Roman JA, Ferreiros J, et al. Natural history and serial morphology of aortic intramural hematoma: a novel variant of aortic dissection. Am Heart J. 1997;134:495-507.

42. Vilacosta I, San Roman JA, Aragoncillo P, et al. Penetrating atherosclerotic ulcer: documentation by transesophageal echocardiography. J Am Coll Cardiol. 1998;32:83-9.

43. Evangelista A, del Castillo HG, Gonzalez-Alujas T, et al. Diagnosis of ascending aortic dissection by transesophageal echocardiography: utility of m-mode in recognizing artifacts. J Am Coll Cardiol. 1996;27:102-7.

44. Butera G, Chessa M, Bossone E, et al. Transcatheter closure of atrial septal defect under combined transesophageal and intracardiac echocardiography. Echocardiography. 2003;20:389-90.

45. Goldstein SA, Campbell AN. Mitral stenosis: evaluation and guidance of valvuloplasty by transesophageal echocardiography. Cardiol Clin. 1993;11:409-25.

46. Park SH, Kim MA, Hyon MS. The advantages of online transesophageal echocardiography guide during percutaneous balloon mitral valvuloplasty. J Am Soc Echocardiogr. 2000;13:26-34.

47. Agricola E et al. Multiplane tranesophageal echocardiography performed according to the guidelines of the American Society of Echocardiography in patients with mitral valve prolapse, flail, and endocarditis: diagnostic accuracy in the identification of mitral regurgitant defects by correlation with surgical findings. J Am Soc Echocardiogr. 2003;16:61.

Chapter 19

Real Time Three-dimensional Echocardiography

Manjula V Burri, Richard E Kerber

Chapter Outline

INTRODUCTION

The heart is a three-dimensional structure with complex asymmetric anatomy and sophisticated functional mechanisms. Two-dimensional echocardiography (2DE) is a thin slice sector imaging technique that requires mental reconstruction and geometrical assumptions, and any slight error in image plane positioning will cause substantial errors in both qualitative and quantitative interpretation. This created the need and niche for three-dimensional echocardiography (3DE), the most preliminary of which was performed by Dekker and his colleagues in 1974.[1] They used a long mechanical arm to locate the position of the transducer in space, and allow alignment of multiple 2D images to generate a 3D image. Regrettably, they found the images to be primitive and the equipment to be impractical for clinical use. Subsequently, Raab and his colleagues[2] developed an electromagnetic locator that ultimately led to free-hand scanning, but this relatively advanced technique of those times was not put to much clinical use due to the complexity of equipment and time needed.

Drastically changing clinical practice, in the early 1990s transesophageal 3DE (3D TEE) was introduced; this used a special transesophageal transducer that allowed moving a phased-array transducer element parallel within the esophagus. The movement of this transducer was controlled by a stepper motor gated to the patient's Electrocardiograph (EKG) and respiratory cycle, monitored on a separate machine. One of the first 3D reconstructions using a multiplane TEE acquisition was performed by Nanda in 1992.[3] Subsequently, a mechanical device was used to advance a standard 2DE transducer over a region of interest and applied transthoracic 3DE (3D TTE) acquisition methods. Researchers then evaluated several different acquisition devices like parallel scan device, fan-like scan motion and rotational acquisition devices (Figs 1A to C) and digital reconstruction of spatially recorded images.[4] Mostly, rotational type devices achieved the greatest popularity, with others rarely used. Of note, all such techniques required laborious offline reconstruction to render 3D volumes, to permit further analysis and hence were not readily embraced.

The revolutionary technique of real time three-dimensional echocardiography (RT3DE) was originally developed by von Ram at Duke University during the last decade of the 20th century.[5] However, due to the limitations posed by lack of high speed computer processing and memory, true real time 3D imaging was impractical. Instead, multiple 2D slices derived from 3D imaging were available online but 3D volume rendering was possible only offline at a separate workstation.

Live or real time 3DE, that is in practice now, made all the above forms of reconstructive 3DE obsolete. This was made possible by enhanced computer processing speed and memory, and the invention of a micro-beamformer. The micro-beamformer has capabilities to fully sample more than 3,000 elements in a 10,000 channel dense matrix array transducer and generate a pyramidal burst of ultrasound. Initially limited to transthoracic capabilities, RT3DE is now also available in the transesophageal mode of image acquisition.

The newer generation RT3DE transducers available, depending on the vendor and model, are varyingly capable of providing instantaneous, dense, EKG gated, stitched 3D volumes with and without color Doppler within a single breath hold, or non-stitched sparse images even within a single heart beat. The latter increases the speed of acquisition, eliminates not only the need for inconvenient breath holding but also the stitch artifacts associated with the former. In addition, most new transducers have 2D, M-mode, biplane imaging, color and spectral Doppler; and harmonic generation capabilities. The footprint of the most

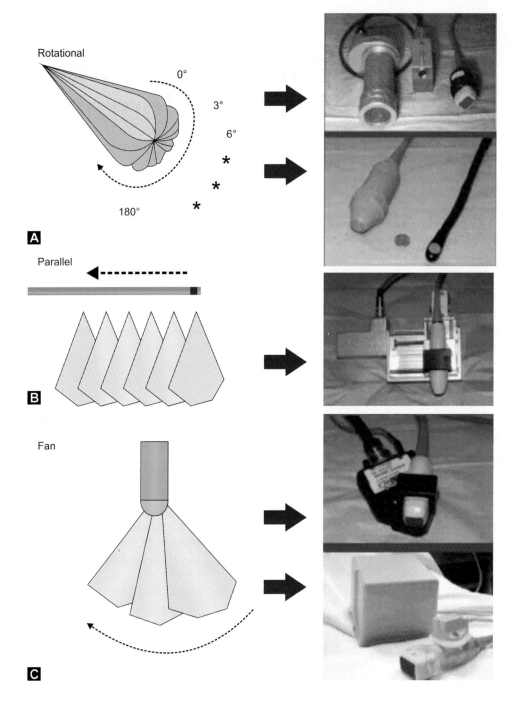

FIGURES 1A TO C: (A) Rotational methods of data collection used commercially available probes attached to an external device that mechanically rotated the probe (A, top) at defined angle increments or (A, bottom) internally electronically driven imaging planes using a transthoracic or transesophageal probe; (B) Parallel acquisition mode using a motorized device is illustrated; (C) Fanlike acquisition using a probe attached to either a motor-driven device (C, top) or a magnetic sensor (C, bottom). (*Source:* Modified from Sugeng L, Weinert L, Thiele K, et al. Real time three-dimensional echocardiography using a novel matrix array transducer. Echocardiography. 2003;20:623-35)

recent probes is small enough to image even pediatric patients. They also conveniently display, after volume rendering, 2–3 orthogonal 2D imaging planes if chosen besides several transverse planes. The full volume datasets or the real time images can be further processed as described below to extract more information. The authors focus on this latest RT3DE technique in this chapter for all practical purposes unless specified.

TECHNIQUE

Obtaining the best quality 2DE images is of paramount importance to acquiring interpretable 3D datasets. The Flow chart 1 shows the general overview, capabilities and commonly used pathways of RT3DE. The 3D capable matrix array transducer should be positioned to obtain the 2D view desired, the echocardiographic, color and time gain and compression should be

FLOW CHART 1: The general overview, capabilities and commonly used pathways of live/real time three-dimensional echocardiography

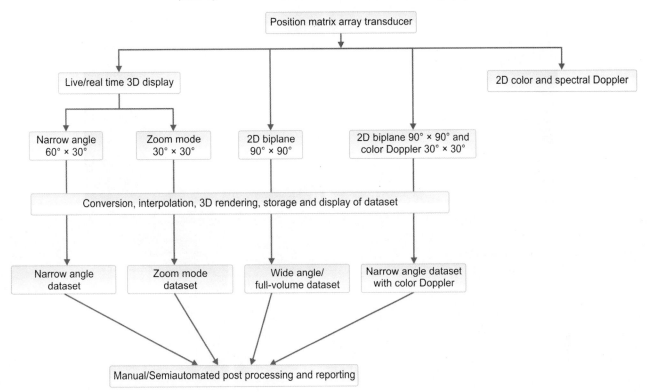

optimized to maximize the quality, and the depth should be decreased to the least required to increase the frame rate and temporal resolution of the 3D dataset to be acquired. Then, one can choose among various available modes of imaging, to display or acquire the 3D pyramidal datasets needed. Narrow angle real time 3D imaging (Fig. 2A, Video 1A) is commonly used for guiding interventional or electrophysiological procedures or to acquire a narrow angle pyramidal dataset in a single heartbeat to examine smaller structures of the heart, such as the valves, that are expected to fit within the 60° x 30° sector. The Zoom mode (Fig. 2B) can also be used for similar purposes but is popularly used to acquire and assess even smaller structures such as small vegetations or mass lesions. Biplane imaging (Fig. 2C) is the most commonly used standard modality to acquire a full volume dataset (Fig. 2D, Video 1B, wide angle, 90° × 90°) usually over 4 cardiac cycles, especially useful for chamber quantitation purposes. Biplane imaging with color Doppler (Fig. 2E) is used to acquire a pyramidal dataset with color (Fig. 2F), usually over 7 cardiac cycles, to commonly assess valvular or paravalvular regurgitation, atrial and ventricular septal defects and fistulae. This wide-angle mode requires ECG gating and is ideally performed during a single breath hold while the patient is lying still, as the full volume or color Doppler dataset is compiled by stitching 4 or 7 narrower pyramidal subvolumes obtained over 4 or 7 consecutive heartbeats respectively.

Most of the 3,000 element dense matrix array transducers used for RT3DE imaging have a bigger foot print than their 2DE counterparts, making it a difficult task to scan thin or pediatric patients with small windows. The rate of sampling of the 3DE system is less due to the magnitude of information it has to process. The decreased frame rate of the dataset leads to decreased temporal resolution compared to a 2D study. The line density which determines the spatial resolution of the image is directly proportional to the number of the subvolumes used to render the full volume 3D dataset and is inversely proportional to the sector width when it is altered. Hence, the more the number of subvolumes acquired, the narrower the sector width of each subvolume and higher the spatial resolution. One caveat is the ability of the patient to remain still without breathing for the entire duration of acquisition, limiting the process to 4–7 cardiac cycles. The Zoom mode has the highest number of individual images obtained within a narrow sector width over a single cardiac cycle and has the best spatial resolution. Various modes of RT3DE acquisition and their salient features are shown in Table 1.

In simple terms, the diagnostic value and the esthetic quality of RT3DE volume, rendering or displaying in addition to the above mentioned, depend on one or more of the following factors:
- The quality of the 2D images—the 2D image obtained with the 3D transducer must be optimized for gain, depth, sector width and focus. Too low a gain can not only fails to visualize certain structures with low echo density but also introduces artifacts in the cavities of the chambers that could be mistaken for thrombi or masses. Too high a gain may mask small structures of clinical significance. Effort should be made to make the gain uniform along the entire depth of the image. An uncompensated high gain in an area resulting in increased density of that structure could be erroneously interpreted as increased thickness or calcification. The depth and sector width should be decreased to the minimum needed if possible to increase the line density and the frame rate of the image.

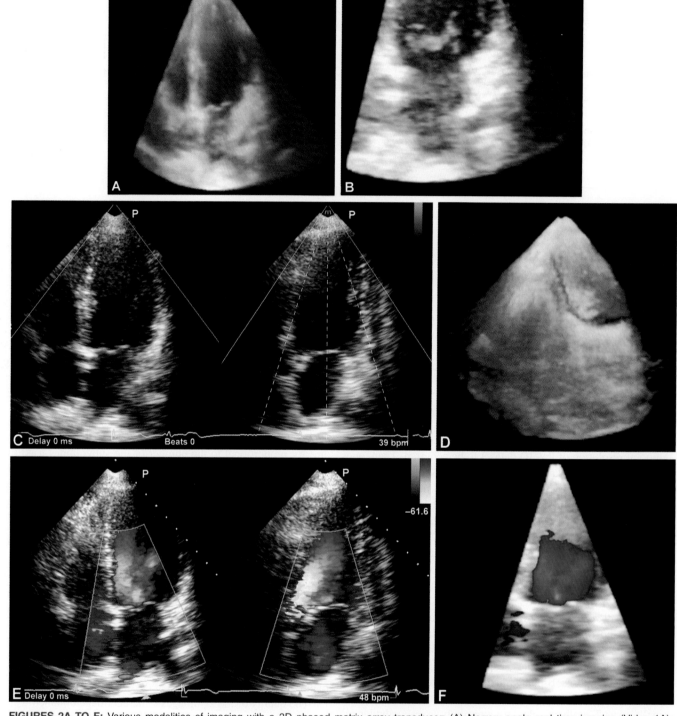

FIGURES 2A TO F: Various modalities of imaging with a 3D phased matrix array transducer: (A) Narrow angle real time imaging (Video 1A); (B) Zoom mode real time imaging; (C) Biplane imaging without color, real time imaging used to acquire full volume datasets; (D) Wide angle or full volume acquisition (Video 1B); (E) Biplane imaging with color Doppler, real time imaging used to acquire color Doppler datasets; (F) the color Doppler acquisition

• A regular non-rapid heart rate—as the images acquired within a limited number of cardiac cycles are stitched on top of another, it is essential for them to be in synchrony with respect to the cardiac cycle or the subvolumes within the dataset would appear disjointed in time. However, if the heart rate is irregular or if the EKG signal is not detectable, 3D volume datasets can still be obtained by switching the EKG trigger mode to the user-defined time trigger mode, accepting the imperfect nature of same.

• The ability of the patient to lay still and hold his or her breath—as the subvolumes acquired over 4–7 cardiac cycles are stitched in time to obtain the volumetric dataset, any amount of movement or breathing will introduce artifacts

TABLE 1

Common modes of imaging: features and applications

	Wide angle/full volume acquisition	Color Doppler acquisition	Real time display/ acquisition	Zoom mode display/ acquisition
Real time	No	No	Yes	Yes
Time taken to acquire	4–7 cardiac cycles for dense acquisition 1 cardiac cycle for sparse acquisition	4–14 cardiac cycles	1 cardiac cycle	Usually 1, can be up to 6 cardiac cycles if the sector is wide
Temporal resolution	Good (40–50 Hz)	Low (up to 20 Hz)	Moderate (20–30 Hz)	Lowest (up to 10 Hz)
Spatial resolution	Moderate (good for dense acquisitions with multiple subvolumes)	Moderate	Moderate	High
Applications	Volumetric analysis of various chambers, LV dyssynchrony, ASD, VSD, thrombi, tumors, pericardial pathology, mitral and tricuspid valve pathology, congenital heart disease	Valvular/paravalvular regurgitation, ASD, VSD, abscess, fistulae	Guidance of interventional and electrophysiologic procedures	Valvular pathology, vegetations, LAA

(Abbreviations: ASD: Atrial septal defects; VSD: Ventricular septal defects; LAA: Left atrial appendage; LV: Left ventricular)

along the axis perpendicular to the axis of imaging (Figs 3A and B, Videos 2A and B) leading to a dataset that appears disjointed in space.

Using the latest generation 3D transducers that have a true real time volume rendering capabilities, patients with arrhythmias and those who cannot hold their breath for more than a few seconds should still be optimally imaged. Right and left ventricular contrast agents have been used with success similar to 2DE.

A good quality pyramidal 3D dataset thus acquired is stored usually after digital compression into smaller files for archiving purposes. The dataset may be retrieved from storage and cropped or cropped online to make visible the cardiac structures of interest and define their intricate anatomic relationships or function. Cropping can be performed in any of the three predetermined cropping planes (x, the green; y, the blue and z, the red) either individually or simultaneously, or in any single slice plane that is manually adjustable (purple) as shown in Figure 4A. Manually adjustable planar cropping may be repeated any number of times, one after another in different planes if needed (Fig. 4B). Alternatively, the 2D images derived from this dataset can be displayed in 3 or more user adjustable planes (Fig. 4C) by using commercially available software in addition to performing volumetric chamber analyses as described below.

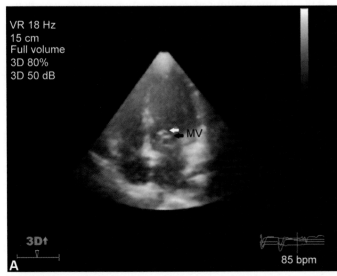
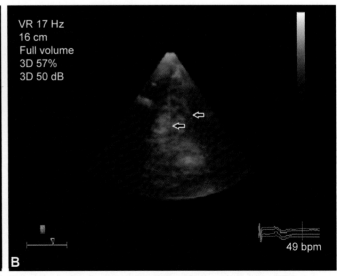

FIGURES 3A AND B: Common artifacts during full volume acquisition in three-dimensional echocardiography: (A) the mitral valve (MV) appears double; part of it that belongs to one subvolume (black arrow) is lagging behind in time compared to the part of it from another subvolume (white arrow) due to a PVC or irregular heart rhythm causing a temporal stitch artifact (Video 2A); (B) respiratory motion causing stitch artifacts (arrows) in space, seen perpendicular to the axis of imaging between the subvolumes (Video 2B)

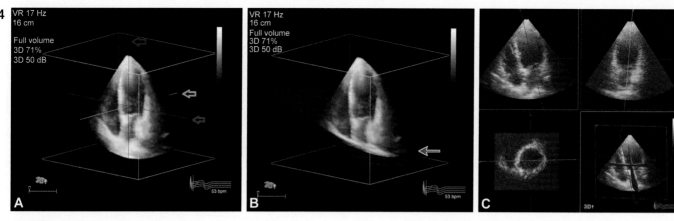

FIGURES 4A TO C: (A) Crop box display of a full volume dataset displaying three orthogonal axes (red, green and blue arrows) for convenient cropping; (B) Crop plane display showing a user adjustable cropping plane (purple arrow); (C) 2D display in three orthogonal user adjustable planes from a full volume 3D dataset

Some preliminary cropping of the datasets online is recommended to ensure their adequacy prior to ending the examination for post-processing. The reporting of findings should include two descriptors, the axis of imaging used to acquire the dataset and the viewing perspective in relation to the cropping plane as shown in Figures 5A to E.[6] The reader should note that the nomenclature of the axes refers to the heart as an organ and not the body of the person. There will be times when this classic nomenclature may not be applicable, especially when user defined adjustable potentially oblique plane or planes of cropping are used, in which case the pathology should be described as best possible using well known intra-cardiac structures as reference or vantage points.

Endocardial segmentation of full volume datasets of the ventricles using various commercialized software may be performed to render wire frame, surface and quantitative data display. Segmentation is a technique used to extract anatomic information from the volumetric data using either difference in texture of the image that is dynamically changing or by level setting. Shape and time information have also been incorporated in some of these models. Dimensions, volumes, ejection fraction (EF), time to peak contraction or time to minimal volume can be synthesized from the volume rendering (Figs 6A and B, Videos 3A and B). Wire frame and surface rendering can be color coded to show time to peak contraction which identifies the dyssynchronous myocardium. Epicardial segmentation is more challenging due to lack of significant contrast between myocardium and the background, compared to that between the endocardium and the blood pool.

Some of the commercial systems provide epicardial and endocardial speckle or wall motion tracking methods (Fig. 7) allowing estimation of myocardial deformation which facilitates determination of velocity, volumes; transmural or radial, longitudinal and circumferential global and regional strain or strain rate; twist and torsion.

The color Doppler datasets may be cropped to obtain regurgitant orifice area (ROA) which in combination with spectral Doppler derived velocity time integral (VTI) can aid in calculation of regurgitant volume using the formula ROA × VTI.

TABLE 2

A complete 3D echocardiographic protocol

- Wide-angle acquisition, parasternal long-axis window: 3D color interrogation of the aortic and mitral valves; 3D color interrogation of the tricuspid and pulmonic valves
- Wide-angle acquisition, apical 4-chamber window: 3D color interrogation of the mitral, aortic and tricuspid valves
- Wide-angle acquisition, subcostal window: 3D color interrogation of the atrial and ventricular septa
- Wide-angle acquisition, suprasternal notch: 3D color interrogation of the descending aorta

(*Source:* Hung J, Lang R, Flachskampf F, et al. 3D echocardiography: a review of the current status and future directions. J Am Soc Echocardiogr. 2007;20:213-33)

The views needed to perform an RT3DE are dependent on the indication of the study. The American Society of Echocardiography position paper on 3DE, published in 2007 tabulates a protocol for complete study as shown in Table 2.[7] Frequently, RT3DE is added to a 2D study when the findings of the 2D study call for more information regarding a particular clinical issue; the authors encourage customizing the views to answer the question.

CLINICAL APPLICATIONS

DETERMINATION OF LEFT VENTRICULAR VOLUMES AND FUNCTION

Determination of left ventricular (LV) global and regional function and EF is crucial to decision-making in several clinical situations in the management of an adult cardiac patient and hence is the most common indication for echocardiography; as it is a versatile, real time and noninvasive technique with no risk. This assessment is commonly accomplished by a very subjective "eye-balling" method based on 2DE; a challenging technique for the inexperienced eyes. The other commonly used methods for EF quantification not only require accurate image plane positioning to avoid foreshortening but also make several geometric assumptions. The geometric assumptions are fraught

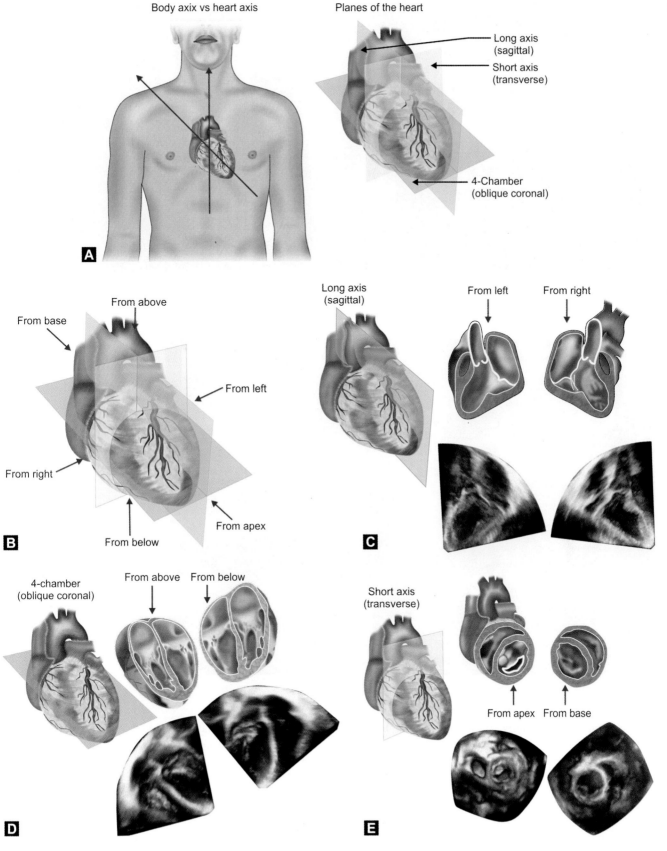

FIGURES 5A TO E: (A) The long axis of the heart is at an angle to the body axis. The planes of the heart are in reference to the heart itself and not the body axis; (B) The heart may be described using two descriptive terms, the plane and the viewing perspective; (C) Sagittal (long axis or longitudinal) section—viewed from left side or right side; (D) Oblique coronal (frontal) section—viewed from above and below; (E) Transverse (short axis) section—viewed from base or apex. (*Source:* Reproduced with permission from Nanda, et al[6])

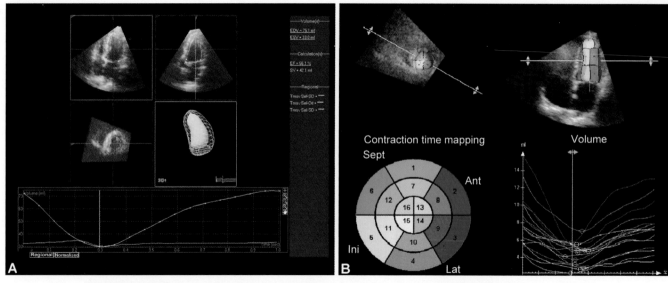

FIGURES 6A AND B: (A) Semiautomated quantification of global and regional (Video 3A). (B) Left ventricular function showing the user adjustable contours and time volume curves (Video 3B)

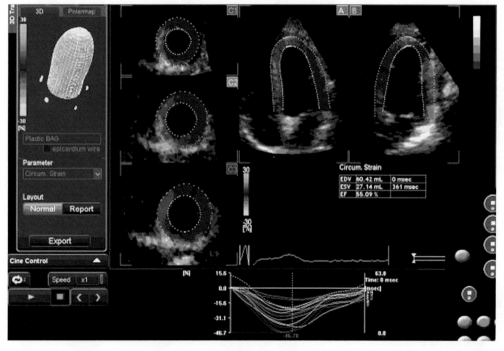

FIGURE 7: Three-dimensional wall motion tracking (WMT) of a left ventricle with normal ejection fraction and without segment dysfunction (*Source:* Modified from Pérez de Isla L, Balcones DV, Fernández-Golfín C, et al. Three-dimensional-wall motion tracking: a new and faster tool for myocardial strain assessment: comparison with two-dimensional-wall motion tracking. J Am Soc Echocardiogr. 2009;22:325-30)

with inaccuracies especially in diseased hearts. Hence, EF determination based on 2DE has significant interobserver and intraobserver variability.[8,9]

Contrary to this, RT3DE analysis of LV volumes and function (Figs 6A and B) is based on user adjustable direct endocardial surface detection by segmentation techniques for every single frame of the cardiac cycle, and therefore obviates the need for geometric assumptions. This method is also not hampered by foreshortened views or oblique plane positioning. The volumes obtained by RT3DE are more reproducible than 2DE,[10] accurate compared to cardiac magnetic resonance imaging (CMR)[11,12] or quantitative gated single-photon emission computed tomography (SPECT)[13] and can be performed rapidly online or offline using commercially available software.

Several studies have reported that the LV volumes derived from RT3DE were significantly underestimated.[14-21] However, a recent multicenter study validated RT3DE determined LV volumes compared to *magnetic resonance imaging* (MRI), although with a small underestimation bias (end diastolic volume, EDV and end systolic volume, ESV were 26% and 29% lower by RT3DE in one study) which could be easily remedied by including the trabeculae in the endocardial border tracing.[14] RT3DE has also been shown to be accurate in assessing LV volumes in aneurysmal and remodeled ventricles following myocardial infarction (MI)[13,16,22] and is of value if sequential volumes are used to guide management.[12] In addition, the use of contrast to enhance LV endocardial border detection has been shown to help quantify both global and regional LV function in patients with poor acoustic windows.[20,23] However, acquisition of contrast images has been recommended by selective dual triggering at end-systole and end-diastole instead of during continuous imaging. This is to avoid microbubble destruction by continuous imaging which could then lead to under-opacification of the chambers and thereby underestimation of volumes.[24] The fusion imaging combining the 3DE images from various cardiac cycles has been shown to be of value in enhancing the image quality, aiding endocardial border detection and procuring complete datasets.[25]

DETERMINATION OF REGIONAL WALL MOTION AND DYSSYNCHRONY

Assessment of regional wall motion is crucial in evaluation of a patient with chest pain, ischemic heart disease or systolic dysfunction. Visual assessment for identification of regional wall motion abnormalities results in high-interobserver variability. As the RT3DE volumetric data comprises the information of all the segments in entirety, quantitative analysis of regional volumes and function by semi-automated segmentation

techniques is feasible. The various segments are color coded and displayed either as a surface rendering or as a parametric map as shown in Figure 8A and Video 4A.

Segmental volumes and regional function based on time volume curves can be obtained in a quantitative manner (Fig. 8B, Video 4B).

RT3DE can also obtain information on time from R wave on ECG to regional endocardial contraction and hence, can identify differences in time to peak regional contraction and thus identify dyssynchrony. Color coded parametric maps, including deformation front mapping based on time to peak regional deformation can also be obtained. A 3D LV systolic dyssynchrony index (SDI), standard deviation of time to minimal regional volume, peak contraction or ejection expressed as a percentage of cardiac cycle, has been popularly used as an index of LV dyssynchrony (Figs 8C and D).[26] This has been validated against gated myocardial perfusion single photon emission computed tomography with phase analysis, with good correlation.[26] We lack large randomized controlled trials to show the usefulness of LVSDI in predicting favorable LV remodeling to cardiac resynchronization therapy (CRT) at this time.

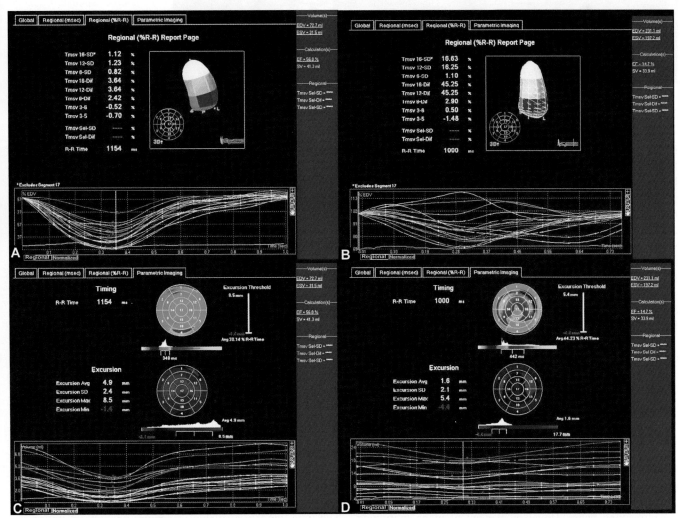

FIGURES 8A TO D: Semiautomated quantitation of regional left ventricular (LV) volumes, function and dyssynchrony. Color-coded display of the 16 LV segments depicted in the cast display and as a graph between time and regional volumes in a normal (A) (Video 4A) and a heart failure (B) (Video 4B) patient. Also depicted is the standard deviation of time to minimal systolic volume (Tmsv) of the 16 LV segments expressed as a percentage of R-R interval (systolic dyssynchrony index or SDI) is elevated in the heart failure patient. Parametric imaging showing uniform excursion in the normal patient (C), which is disturbed in the patient with heart failure (D) as cued by the color coding on the Bull's eye display of the LV segments

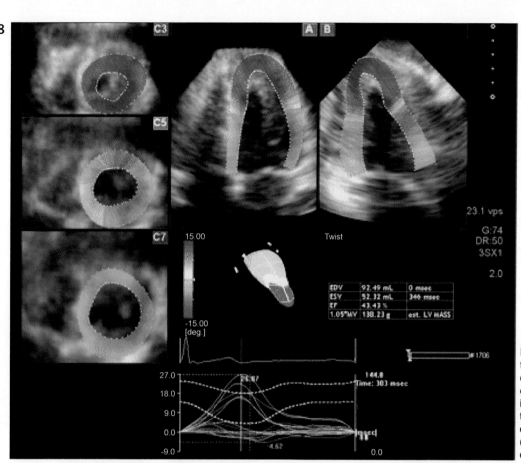

FIGURE 9: Global left ventricular twist values detected by three-dimensional speckle-tracking echocardiography and also shown in color overlays superimposed on the gray-scale images and color-coded three-dimensional cast (*Source:* Modified from Andrade, et al[39])

However, RT3DE is potentially superior to conventional tissue Doppler imaging (TDI) for dyssynchrony assessment, as the latter strictly evaluates the longitudinal or radial endomyocardial velocity or strain while RT3DE derives the regional function from segmental volumes which encompass overall endomyocardial contraction.[27,28] Reports of single center small observational studies studying the utility of LVSDI over TDI show that the presence of dyssynchrony by LVSDI correlated with favorable LV remodeling, regardless of the QRS duration. One study proposed a cut-off of 6.4% for SDI with a sensitivity of 88% and a specificity of 85% to predict response to CRT.[29-31] Further work is needed to determine the prognostic value of 3D echocardiography in potential CRT candidates, especially as its 4D applications and segmentations undergo technical improvements. The use of RT3DE in the electrophysiology laboratory can aid in accurate lead placement at the site of latest mechanical activation.

Strain imaging has the advantage of differentiating actual active deformation of normal myocardium from traction or translational motion of the scar tissue. 2D Speckle Tracking Echocardiography (2DSTE) has been favored to obtain angle independent measures of multidirectional myocardial strain in contrast to TDI which is dependent on the insonation angle of the ultrasound beam. However, the out of plane motion of speckles results in noise and suboptimal tracking. In addition due to the geometric assumptions needed, the LV volumes were underestimated by 2DSTE. RT3DE has been synergized with speckle tracking to take advantage of the utility of each modality.

This allows insonation angle independent extraction of global and segmental parameters such as displacement and strain in longitudinal, radial and circumferential axes (Fig. 7).[32] This could either be displayed as numerical values on an excel spread sheet from the onset of the cardiac cycle, or as a graphical depiction over time, for all the frames of a cineloop. Color coded parametric mapping of any of these parameters provides a quick visual cue to the identification of the abnormal segment(s). In addition, regional and global volumes, function, rotation, twist (Fig. 9) and torsion can also be quantified using this technique. The decrease in the magnitude of displacement, contraction or strain and the temporal dispersion of the peak value of any of these parameters can give an indication of segmental LV dysfunction or dyssynchrony respectively (Figs 10A and B).

The clinical applications of such complex and time consuming techniques, which require advanced expertise in the field, are yet to be defined in a convincing fashion, although there are some promising preliminary reports of potential utility.[33-38] Based on the above techniques, one can also assess diastolic function from the diastolic velocity, displacement and strain.

APPLICATIONS TO STRESS IMAGING

The time window available to acquire peak stress images is brief. Conventional 2DE can only visualize a limited number of segments at a time. Hence, 2DE is very much dependent on the skill of the sonographer to acquire standard views in a rapid manner before heart rate recovery following peak

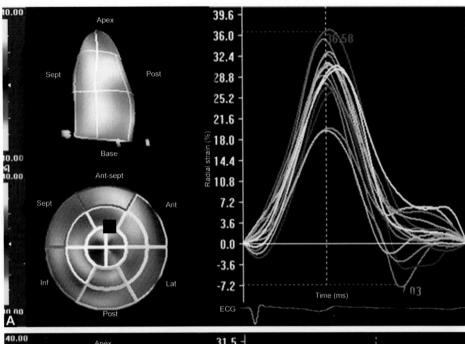

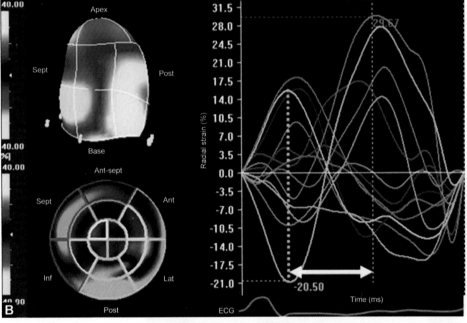

FIGURES 10A AND B: (A) Color-coded 3-D LV display (top left) and bull's-eye plot image (bottom left) and corresponding time-to-strain curves from 16 LV sites (right) from a normal control subject, demonstrating synchronous time-to-peak-strain curves represented by homogenous coloring at end-systole. (B) Color-coded 3-D LV display (top left) and bull's-eye plot image (bottom left) and corresponding time-to-strain curves from 16 LV sites (right) from a patient with HF and left bundle branch block, demonstrating dys-synchronous time-to-peak-strain curves represented by heterogeneous coloring at end-systole, with early peak strain in septal segments and delayed peak strain in posterior lateral segments (arrow). (Abbreviations: Ant: Anterior; Ant-sept: Anterior-septum; HF: Heart failure; Inf: inferior; Lat: Lateral; LV: Left ventricle; Post: Posterior; Sept: septal). (*Source:* Modified from Tanaka, et al[33])

exercise or dobutamine infusion. Imaging at lower heart rates decreases the sensitivity of the test and hence makes it essentially nondiagnostic. The ability to acquire a full volume dataset containing all the 17 segments of the LV within a few seconds or even within one heartbeat, using RT3DE makes this an interesting area of its application. Thus acquired dataset can be cropped in any plane desired, to obtain standard comparable views for rest and stress phases, to allow accurate interpretation. It has been shown that RT3DE decreases the study time, improves its sensitivity and diagnostic value compared to 2DE. There was also a trend toward increased sensitivity in 3DE group where coronary angiograms were available for correlation in one study.[39,40] The two limitations with the 3D technique are suboptimal spatial and temporal resolution. While the former can be overcome by using a

contrast agent, the latter is of particular concern especially with higher heart rates at peak stress. This can cause under-sampling of cardiac phases leading to potential misinterpretation from the available frames.

The 3D full volume dataset can also be fed into 4D analysis software for further segmentation and analysis of regional ventricular function over time as described above at rest and stress. Speckle tracking may be performed on the 3D datasets to obtain 3D strain, strain rate, twist and torsion during rest and stress phases of the study. Stress induced diastolic dysfunction can be assessed from the diastolic velocity, displacement and strain parameters.

Multimodality stress imaging combining RT3DE and SPECT has been shown to be more accurate than any one of them, when angiography was used as the gold standard.[41]

Quantification of myocardium at risk, dependent on the presence or absence of collaterals in the distribution of a stenotic epicardial artery is of prognostic significance. The development of gas filled microbubbles that reflect ultrasound beam as they pass through the coronary circulation led to the potential application of echocardiography in identifying the ischemic myocardium at risk. However, 2DE is limited due to the number of views required to image all the LV segments. In some applications it requires repeated injections of contrast to obtain comprehensive information. Quantification of myocardium at risk was difficult, requiring mental 3D reconstruction based on 2D images, obtained at times in off-axis planes. RT3DE through its volume rendering capabilities can encompass the entire LV in 1 or 2 datasets and hence does not need repeat contrast administration. Several animal studies have indicated the feasibility, rapidity and accuracy of RT3DE in quantification of myocardial perfusion (Figs 11A to D)[42-45], while it remains in its infancy for clinical use at this time.[46,47]

DETERMINATION OF LEFT VENTRICULAR MASS

It has been established that left ventricular hypertrophy (LVH) or increased LV mass is an independent marker of cardiovascular disease and is of tremendous prognostic importance. Cardiologists follow LV mass to assess response to pharmacologic therapy in various cardiac conditions such as hypertension and other treatable causes of hypertrophic cardiomyopathy. M-mode

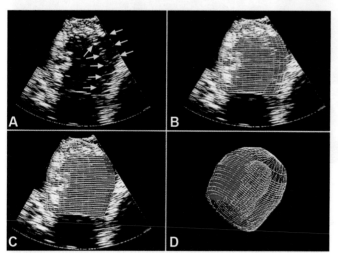

FIGURES 11A TO D: Representative example of methodology used to quantitatively assess mass of underperfused myocardium from RT3D images in sheep with acute occlusion of circumflex coronary artery: (A) tomographic view derived from volumetric image showing area of myocardium devoid of contrast opacification (arrows); (B) three-dimensional rendering of left ventricular (LV) endocardial (in green) and epicardial (in yellow) surfaces generated by computer, based on operator's tracing. Area between both surfaces corresponds to myocardial volume, which is used to calculate myocardial mass; (C) rendering of LV region without contrast opacification generated by computer, based on operator's tracing of corresponding endocardial surface. Red area represents volume used to calculate mass of underperfused myocardium; (D) after tracing is completed, volumetric image can be freely rotated to examine three-dimensional appearance of LV endocardial and epicardial surfaces and underperfused myocardium. (*Source:* Modified from Camarano, et al[42])

and 2DE methods of determination of LV mass are fraught with limitations, similar to volume determination, due to inability to align the cursor perpendicular to the ventricular axis with the former, geometric assumptions and foreshortening associated with the latter. RT3DE by semiautomated tracking of endocardium and epicardium, directly quantifies LV myocardial volume (epicardial volume-endocardial volume), which then is multiplied by the myocardial tissue density (1.05 gm/ml) to derive the LV mass. LV mass derived from RT3DE has been validated by cardiac MRI and is more accurate than other echocardiographic methods with good reproducibility.[48]

ASSESSMENT OF RIGHT VENTRICULAR VOLUMES AND FUNCTION

The right ventricle (RV) is a complex structure with no standard geometric shape and hence 2DE, requiring geometric assumptions, is at a disadvantage in estimating the RV volumes and function. Currently MRI remains the gold standard, as both the area-length and the disc summation methods introduce a significant underestimation bias and hence are not recommended for clinical use.[49]

As with any chamber, the acquisition of an accurate 3D full volume dataset is dependent on the adequacy of the acoustic window and the experience and skill of the sonographer. A modified apical 4-chamber view to maximize visualization of RV with further anterior angulation to capture the RVOT or subcostal transducer locations has been commonly used. Contrast administration may be necessitated for endocardial delineation.

RT3DE by directly measuring RV volumes without the need for geometrical assumptions can reliably quantify RV size, stroke volumes and EF. The RV full volume dataset encompasses the RV 3D including the RV outflow tract. The commercially available 4D RV analysis software allows for semiautomated detection of the RV endocardial borders in axial, sagittal and coronal planes during various phases of the cardiac cycle (Figs 12A and B, Videos 5A and B). This method has been validated by several in-vitro and in-vivo models either by direct methods in the lab or the operating suite; or with radionuclide ventriculography and CMR. RT3DE analysis of RV was determined to be fast, feasible, accurate and reproducible not only in in-vitro models but also in normals and in a variety of disease states such as RV infarction, congenital heart disease and pulmonary arterial hypertension.[50-57]

RT3DE does seem to hold promise as a less expensive alternative to CMR in providing reliable estimation of RV volumes and EF in patients with adequate acoustic windows. Recently, there has been much interest in utility of RT3DE in the assessment of advanced pulmonary hypertension treatment effects. This is being addressed in an ongoing prospective study.[58]

ASSESSMENT OF LEFT AND RIGHT ATRIA

Left atrial enlargement is generally considered a marker for adverse clinical outcomes in conditions such as atrial fibrillation, MI, stroke, heart failure, hypertrophic obstructive cardiomyopathy, aortic and mitral valvular disease. Whether reversing this remodeling improves clinical outcomes remains

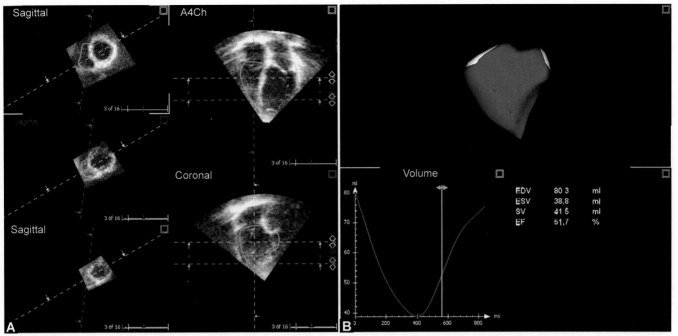

FIGURES 12A AND B: (A) Semiautomated right ventricular (RV) endocardial tracing in axial, sagittal and coronal planes of a full volume dataset acquired from the RV directed apical 4-chamber view (Video 5A). (B) 3D cast representation of the RV inclusive of outflow tract, based on above tracings obtained over various phases of the cardiac cycle providing RV volume and ejection fraction (Video 5B)

to be demonstrated. Assessment of left atrial volume is best accomplished by 3D imaging as the enlargement can happen asymmetrically in anteroposterior, transverse or superoinferior dimensions and geometric assumptions required by 2D techniques will be flawed. RT3DE has not only been shown to be feasible, more accurate and reproducible compared to 2DE but also been validated against CMR (Fig. 13). In addition to obtaining the volumes at the maximal and minimal atrial expansion, the pre-A (atrial contraction) volume can also be obtained. Indices of left atrial contractile and reservoir function, such as passive atrial emptying fraction, active atrial emptying fraction and atrial expansion index, can be calculated from the above.[59-64]

A common indication for TEE is to scrutinize the left atrial appendage (LAA) for thrombus or to ascertain the LAA orifice area for accurate sizing of the occluder device placement. RT3D TEE is instrumental in providing elaborate views of the LAA including *en face* views of the orifice and cross sectional views of the appendage at multiple levels that is just not feasible by 2DTEE. The sizing of LAA orifice area by RT3D TEE has been validated against 64 slice CT with narrow limits of agreement compared to 2DTEE (Figs 14A and B).[65] RT3D TTE also seems to be of diagnostic importance in patients with excellent acoustic views and may obviate the need for TEE to exclude an LAA thrombus especially as the spatial resolution of this technique gets enhanced in the future.[66]

There is limited experience with right atrial volume assessment by RT3DE.[67] RT3D TEE, due to high imaging quality also enables visualization of complex anatomic structures of the right atrium that might be of importance to the electrophysiologist.[68] Right atrial vegetations or thrombi potentially associated with pacemaker wires can be clearly visualized by RT3D TEE.

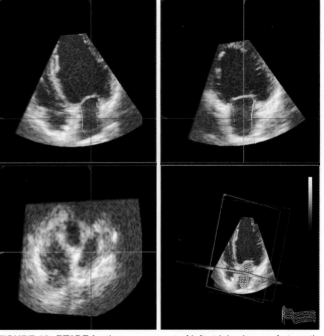

FIGURE 13: RT3DE for the assessment of left atrial volumes. Automatic border detection can be applied to the apical 4-chamber and 2-chamber view (upper panels) for quantification of left atrial volumes. (*Source:* Modified from Tops KF, Schalij MJ, Bax JJ, et al. Imaging and atrial fibrillation: the role of multimodality imaging in patient evaluation and management of atrial fibrillation. Eur Heart J. 2010;31:542-51.)

ASSESSMENT OF VALVULAR DISORDERS

Mitral Valve

The mitral valve is a complex structure and RT3D epicardial, transthoracic or TEE is instrumental in providing volume

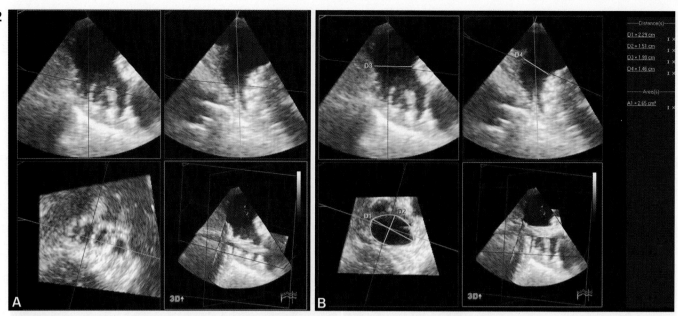

FIGURES 14A AND B: (A) RT3D TEE of the left atrial appendage (LAA) cropping down into the appendage reveals pectinate muscles traversing the LAA from wall to wall. (B) The cropping needed to size the LAA occluder device and the position of its placement is shown by lines D$^{1-4}$

rendered images of the mitral valve, thus enabling the demonstration and quantification of the complex saddle shape of the mitral annulus, the commissural length, the coaptation area, the surface area of the leaflets and the scallops, the billowing height in MV prolapse, the aorto-mitral angle (the angle between the mitral valve plane at the highest saddle point and the aortic valve plane), the tenting volumes and the tethering distance to the papillary muscle using commercially available software.[69,70] Figure 15 illustrates several of these measurements.

RT3DE provides important insights into the pathophysiology of functional and ischemic mitral regurgitation which results from distortion of the spatial relationships between the LV and the mitral valve apparatus.[71-74] There is displacement of the papillary muscle along with tethering of the leaflets in ischemic mitral regurgitation.[74] Evolving new approaches for treatment of ischemic mitral regurgitation are based on the above mentioned information aiming at the chordal or papillary muscle level.[75,76] In contrast, the decrease in mitral valve coaptation surface area, possibly due to apical displacement of the coaptation or increase in tenting volume due to annular dilation, is thought to be the underlying mechanism of mitral regurgitation in dilated cardiomyopathy (DCM). The RT3DE derived coaptation index, the index of the difference in 3D tenting surface area at the onset of mitral valve closure and at maximal closure over that at the onset of mitral valve closure" this represents the proportion of the valve surface that engages in coaptation. This has been proposed as a quantitative measure of the extent of leaflet coaptation, which is shown to be significantly smaller in DCM patients compared to normals.[77] This could be used to follow these patients after optimal medical management to determine if there is favorable remodeling with improvement in mitral regurgitation.

RT3DE has been used to characterize the mitral valve (Figs 16A to D and 17) and its pathologies such as prolapse or flail,[78] native and prosthetic valve endocarditis,[79,80] and congenital abnormalities.[81,82] The identification and quantification of the prolapsed or flail segment is more accurate by RT3DE (Figs 18A to D) compared to 2DTTE and TEE.[69,83,84] The parasternal window acquisition has been shown to be superior in visualization of the posterior mitral leaflet[85] among the 3D transthoracic methods. Mitral valve repair is preferable to replacement for degenerative mitral regurgitation as it is more likely to preserve LV function and obviates the need for long-term anticoagulation and eliminates the risk of prosthetic valve complications. The success of the mitral valve repair depends upon proper understanding of anatomy under physiological conditions of a beating heart. 3D TEE assessment of native and prosthetic mitral valves (Figs 19A and B) has been validated against surgical pathology with 96% agreement in 87 patients.[86] The ability to maneuver the images to obtain the surgeon's view (Fig. 17) increases the surgeon's confidence in the diagnosis and helps with surgical planning. The degree of mitral regurgitation can be determined by RT3DE with more confidence compared to other methods and has been validated against velocity encoded CMR.[84,87,88] The regurgitant volume calculated by RT3DE is more accurate than that determined by 2DE and strongly correlated with that assessed by CMR with no significant bias, especially in the presence of an asymmetric regurgitant orifice.[88] The RT3DE derived ROA of the mitral valve is irregular (Figs 20A to D) and correlates with the recommended 2DE derived cut-offs for effective ROA for grading of mitral regurgitation severity, except in those with small orifices.[89] RT3DE is being used increasingly to assess the adequacy of surgical mitral valve repair and variably to guide percutaneous edge to edge mitral valve repair in a beating heart. For all the aforementioned causes, this would also be a good tool to follow patients with native or prosthetic mitral valve conditions either before or after percutaneous and surgical procedures.[90,91]

2D planimetry and Doppler methods (pressure half time, proximal isovelocity surface area) have several limitations in assessment of mitral stenosis. RT3DE allows identification of

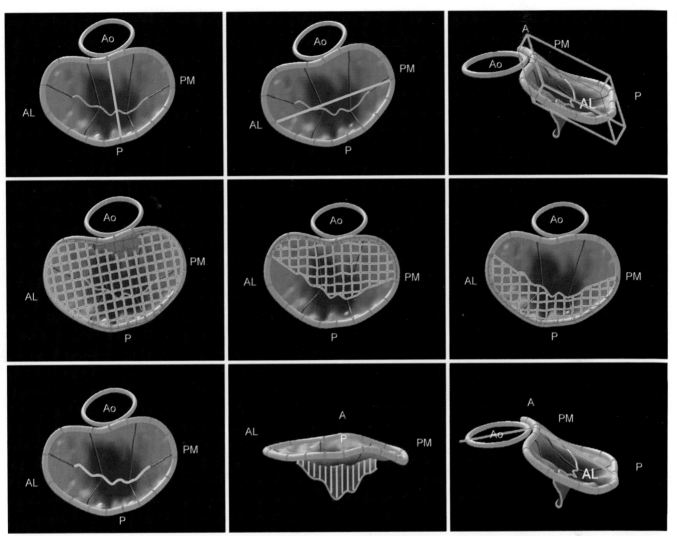

FIGURE 15: Three-dimensional reconstruction of the MV, from which several parameters were automatically calculated. From top to bottom, left to right: anteroposterior diameter of the mitral annulus; mitral annular anterolateral (AL)–posteromedial (PM) diameter; mitral annular height, defined as the height of the bounding box of the MV in the atrial-ventricular direction; mitral annular area, as the area of the minimal surface spanning the annulus; exposed area of the anterior (A) leaflet; exposed area of the posterior (P) leaflet; coaptation length, as the length of the coaptation line projected to approximate leaflet surface; coaptation area, as the area of the region where the leaflets are overlapped, and coaptation height as the mean height of the same region; the aortic (AO) to mitral plane angle. (*Source:* Modified from Maffessanti, et al[69])

the *en face* plane with the narrowest mitral valve orifice, by serial cropping of the full volume dataset from the ventricular perspective. 3D guided planimetry of the mitral valve orifice area for quantification of mitral stenosis is considered a first line recommendation by experienced users.[7,92] In addition, 3DE best agreed with invasive mitral orifice area calculations derived using the Gorlin formula in rheumatic heart disease patients (Figs 21A to C, Videos 6A to C).[93] Intraobserver and interobserver variabilities were also low compared to other echocardiographic modalities. RT3DE is accurate in determination of mitral stenosis severity in calcific mitral stenosis, by planimetry of the orifice at the most restrictive portion. The narrowest orifice is not necessarily at the tips of the leaflets in contrast to that of rheumatic mitral stenosis.[94] Data acquisition for assessment of mitral stenosis can be performed either from apical or parasternal windows of a TTE or mid-esophageal or transgastric long axis views of a TEE for this purpose.

The realistic *en face* views obtained by RT3DE also enable accurate assessment of leaflet thickness, calcification and extent of commissural fusion in rheumatic mitral stenosis. The subvalvular apparatus can be evaluated especially from the transgastric long axis views. Information regarding chordal length, thickness, calcification and fusion can all be obtained. A score akin to Wilkins score has been proposed based on detailed 3D analysis of the mitral valve and subvalvular apparatus;[95] its utility beyond the traditional Wilkins score is yet to be investigated at this time. RT3D TEE in addition also increases the spatial resolution and ease of acquisitions and, in combination with live imaging, makes possible the immediate assessment of mitral valve structure and function. The ability to evaluate commissural splitting (Figs 22A to C), mitral valve area and mitral regurgitation online in the cardiac catheterization laboratory makes this a desirable technique for intra-procedural monitoring during percutaneous balloon mitral valvuloplasty.[91,96]

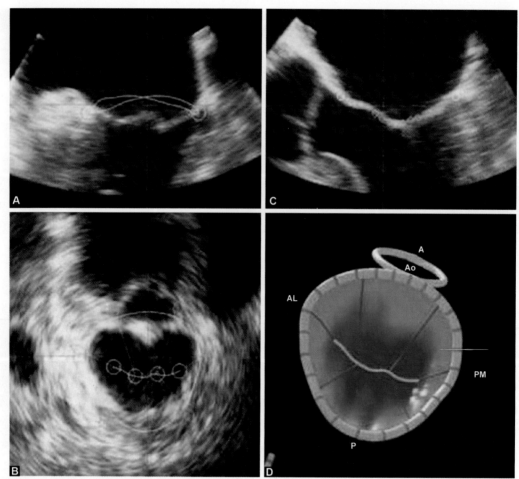

FIGURES 16A TO D: (A) Morphological 3D analysis of a normal mitral valve. Mitral annulus is manually initialized in one plane. (B) Then repeated in multiple rotated planes and interpolated. (C) MV leaflets are manually traced from commissure to commissure in multiple parallel planes. (D) The resultant surface is displayed as a color-coded 3D rendered valve surface. (*Source:* Modified from Chandra, et al[70])

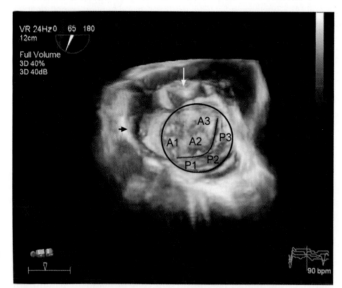

FIGURE 17: Real time three-dimensional echocardiography of the mitral valve (MV) viewed from the left atrium oriented to surgeon's view with the aortic valve (arrow) at 12 O'clock position and the left atrial appendage (arrowhead) at 9 O'clock position. The curved line overlies the MV commissure and the circle overlies the MV annulus. (Abbreviations: A1: Lateral; A2: Middle; A3: Medial scallops of the anterior mitral leaflet; P1: Lateral; P2: Middle; P3: Medial scallops of the posterior mitral leaflet)

Aortic Valve

Planimetry of the aortic valve at peak systole by 3D TEE has been shown to be superior to 2DE in calculating the severity of aortic valve stenosis (Fig. 23).[97] RT3DE similarly is a promising tool from the initial experience in the assessment of aortic valve stenosis mainly due to its ability to identify the perpendicular plane at which the area is the narrowest.[98-100] It has been shown to complement 2DE in identifying other aortic valve and root pathologies (Figs 24A to D, Video 7) including regurgitant lesions.

Other Valves

Due to its unique ability to visualize the complex tricuspid valve *en face* (Figs 25A and B), RT3DE has incremental value over 2DE in delineating complex tricuspid valve pathologies including carcinoid disease, Ebstein's anomaly, rheumatic disease (Figs 26A to D), prolapse, chordae rupture and regurgitation.[101,102]

RT3DE makes possible the visualization of pulmonic valve *en face* (Fig. 27)[103] and merits further exploration for its use especially in congenital conditions.[104]

Prosthetic Valves

In the hands of the experienced, RT3DE is superior to conventional 2D and Doppler echocardiography in assessing St Jude

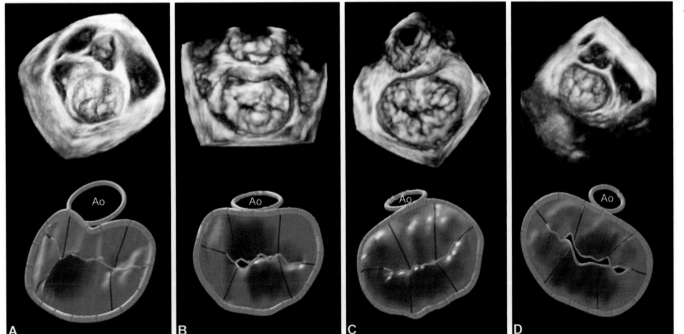

FIGURES 18A TO D: Example of volume-rendered mitral valve (MV) (top) as seen from the left atrium in patients with varying distribution, severity and extent of MV prolapse. The 3D representations (bottom) clearly show the morphology of the MV and the region and severity of prolapse in red: isolated P2 scallop (A and B) versus diffuse prolapse with redundant tissue (C and D). (Abbreviation: Ao: Aorta). (*Source:* Modified from Maffessanti, et al[69])

mechanical prosthetic valve structure and function. The presence of concurrent, brisk motion of both the leaflets (Figs 28A and B, Video 8), at times difficult to demonstrate on a single plane 2DE, can be made possible by diligent cropping of the RT3DE datasets. This takes away the reliance on Doppler gradients, which at times are misleading.[105] Its application to other prosthetic valves remains to be assessed better but preliminary experience is promising.[106]

Prosthetic valve complications such as fracture, dehiscence, paravalvular leak (Figs 29A to D, Videos 9A to C), pannus, thrombosis, vegetation, abscess, fistulae can all be better assessed with a 3D technique especially RT3D TEE.[107-112]

MISCELLANEOUS CONDITIONS

Mass lesions such as thrombi or tumors occurring in the heart can undoubtedly be better imaged by RT3DE compared to 2DE, due to its volume rendering abilities. It helps define the origin, size, structure (brightness indicative of fibrosis;[113] echolucency characteristic of clot lysis (Figs 30A and B),[114] vascularity[115] and cysts[116]) it can demonstrate the extent, volume, mobility and attachments of a mass,[117] along with hemodynamic significance that can result from obstruction to flow. These observations based on RT3DE can possibly translate into better treatment decisions.

Evaluation of the interatrial septum is a common indication for TEE. RT3D TEE in a literal sense has multiplied the magnitude of information echocardiography can provide in accurate assessment of anatomy, treatment planning, guidance and post-procedural or surgical evaluation of atrial septal defects (ASD). The determination of the location, extent, adequacy of the aortic rim is crucial in planning appropriate therapeutic strategy in

these patients. The TUPLE, tilt-up-then-left (rotate-left-in-Z-axis), maneuver when acquiring 3D TEE datasets at 0° from mid-esophageal view (Figs 31A to C); tilt up, rotate counter-clockwise in Z-axis till superior vena cava (SVC) at 12 O'clock (ROLZ) and then turn left to see the left atrial aspect maneuver when acquiring at higher angles has been proposed as a standard maneuver to facilitate accurate diagnosis and description purposes to ensure meaningful communication between imagers, interventionalists and the surgeons.[118] Figure 32 illustrates the effect of higher angles on the orientation of SVC and hence the need for integration of ROLZ maneuvers into TUPLE while imaging at higher angles. RT3DE has not been studied as a tool for shunt quantification across the ASD.

Likewise, RT3DE can also evaluate the size, location and complexity of the ventricular septal defect (VSD) in addition to displaying it *en face* and guide corrective procedures as described below.[119]

RT3DE can be used to identify any structure that is in the vicinity of the ultrasound beam by examining its 3D relations and meticulous cropping (Figs 33A to C).[120] This technique is also of evolving importance in the evaluation of congenital heart diseases and is beyond the scope of this chapter.

GUIDANCE OF PERCUTANEOUS PROCEDURES

As the technology and the skill of operators evolve, more and more complex percutaneous procedures are being performed on the beating heart. Although these procedures are routinely performed under fluoroscopy, real time 2DTEE and intracardiac echocardiography (ICE) are commonly used to provide important visualization of soft tissue structures of the heart; these cannot usually be otherwise obtained in a cardiac catheterization

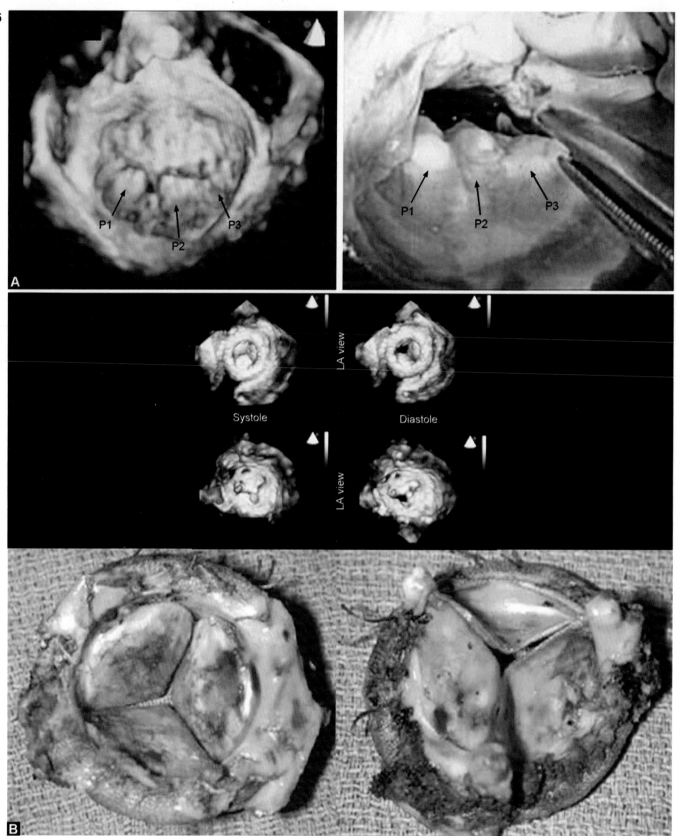

FIGURES 19A AND B: (A) Example of a patient with multiscallop mitral valve prolapse of the posterior leaflet (as usually seen in Barlow's syndrome) visualized using three-dimensional matrix transesophageal echocardiographic imaging (left) and a corresponding surgical view (right) (P1—Lateral; P2—middle; P3—medial). (B) Example of systolic and diastolic still frames of three-dimensional (3D) matrix transesophageal real time volume renderings of a bioprosthetic mitral valve (MV) as visualized from the left atrial (LA) (top) and left ventricular (LV) (bottom) perspectives. Note the well-visualized struts in the LV views of the valve. (Right) Explanted stenotic bioprosthetic MV, confirming the 3D matrix transesophageal echocardiographic findings. (*Source:* Modified from Sugeng, et al[86])

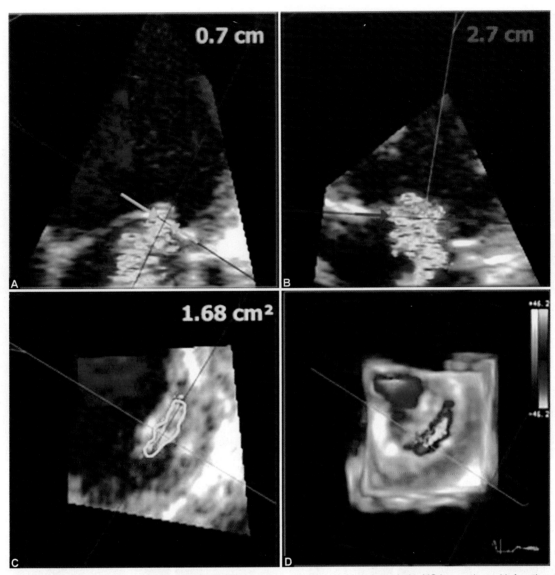

FIGURES 20A TO D: Example of measurement of VC dimensions in a cross-sectional plane through the VC in a patient with functional MR caused by leaflet tethering using onboard 3D analysis software (QLAB, Philips Medical Systems, Andover, MA): (A) 4CH view with measurement of narrow 3D VCW-4CH; (B) 2CH view with measurement of broad 3D VCW-2CH; (C) Cross-sectional plane through the VC with direct planimetry of VCA. The green and the red line indicate the orientation of the 4CH plane (panel 1A, green frame) and the 2CH plane (panel B, red frame); (D) 3D *en face* view of VCA. (Abbreviations: CH: Chamber; MR: Mitral regurgitation; VC: Vena contracta; VCA: Vena contracta area; VCW: Vena contracta width). (*Source:* Modified from Kahlert, et al[87])

suite. In the past, however, the echocardiographer was limited in the views obtained by 2D single plane technique to guide a procedure that is occurring in 3D. With the advent of RT3DE, especially TEE, easily comprehensible views can be obtained in real time that guide precise wire, catheter or instrument positioning, making the procedure safe and successful. While additional venous access is not needed as with ICE, general anesthesia may be required for prolonged RT3D TEE guidance. Several studies have shown the incremental value of RT3DE during device deployments for patent foramen ovale, ASD (Figs 34A to F), VSD, paravalvular leaks, LAA occlusion (Figs 35A and B), balloon mitral valvuloplasty, percutaneous edge to edge mitral valve repair (Figs 36A to C), aortic valvuloplasty, percutaneous (Figs 37A to C) and transapical aortic valve implantation.[91,121-123]

Endomyocardial biopsy can also be safely performed under RT3DE guidance not only to ensure avoidance of injury to the valvular apparatus but also to monitor for complications as with other procedures. It has been shown to be of incremental value in proper bioptome positioning.[124] Transatrial septal puncture and pulmonary vein isolation procedures have been successfully guided by RT3DE.[91]

Catheter positioning in the first proximal septal perforator is crucial to the success of alcohol septal ablation. If the operator is not diligent, an alternative coronary branch can be mistaken for the first septal perforator, which may lead to inadvertent iatrogenic MI of innocent myocardium. RT3DE can localize the complete extent and distribution of contrast better, clearly delineating the area intended for controlled infarction by alcohol injection.[91]

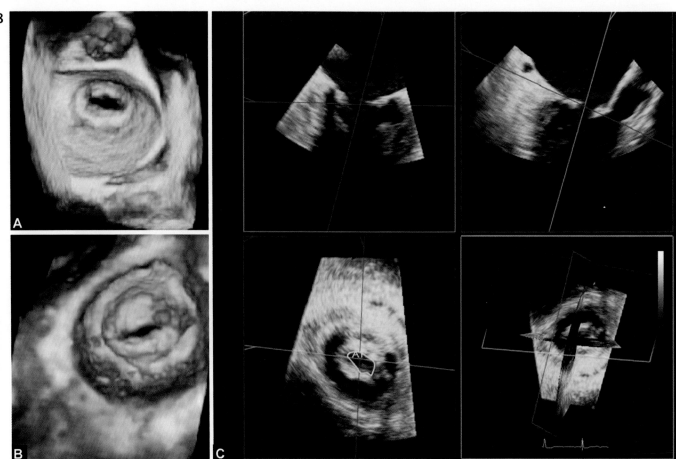

FIGURES 21A TO C: Rheumatic mitral stenosis by RT3D TEE: (A) zoom mode acquisition obtained from the mid esophageal transducer position cropped transversely viewed from the left atrium and left ventricle (Video 6A); (B) shows the stenotic mitral valve orifice (Video 6B); (C) the cropping in 3D needed to obtain *en face* view of the limiting mitral valve orifice and planimetry of its area labeled A1 in the left lower panel (Video 6C)

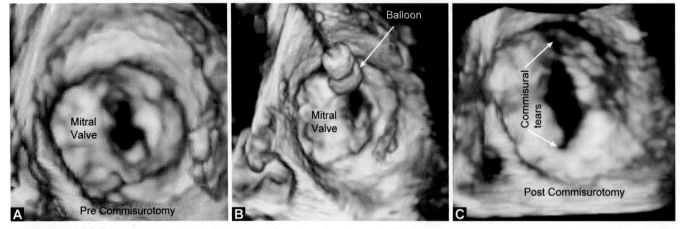

FIGURES 22A TO C: Mitral balloon valvuloplasty: (A) *en face* view of a stenosed mitral valve, with restricted opening, as seen from the left atrial perspective (3D zoom mode acquisition); (B) guiding catheter with a balloon placed across the mitral valve commissures, as seen from the left atrium (3D zoom mode acquisition); (C) *en face* view of the mitral valve after commissural tears have been created as seen from the left atrial side. The mitral valve orifice is visibly larger than it was before commissurotomy (3D zoom mode acquisition). (*Source:* Modified from Perk, etal[91])

Procedural guidance is an actively evolving advanced application of RT3DE and is yet to be validated well on a larger scale. RT3DE is currently underutilized due to several factors including the potential need for general anesthesia, lack of standardization of 3D echocardiographic views, prolongation of the procedure time (but less radiation/contrast exposure), the

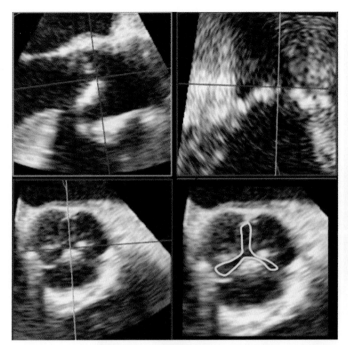

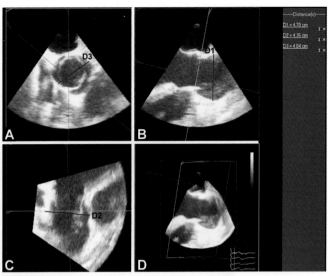

FIGURES 24A TO D: Measurement of the size of aortic enlargement in multiple axes by 3D TEE in a patient with ascending aortic aneurysm and bicuspid aortic valve (Video 7)

FIGURE 23: Measurement of aortic valve anatomic area (AVA) by volumetric three-dimensional transoesophageal echocardiography. Two orthogonal long-axis views of the aortic valve (green quadrant; anterior-posterior projection, red quadrant; medial-lateral projection) were extracted using multiplanar reconstruction mode. Third plane perpendicular to the other two long-axis planes was the cross-sectional view of the aortic valve for the correct tracing of aortic valve area. Aortic valve area was traced when the optimal cross-section of the valve is achieved during its maximal systolic opening. (*Source:* Modified from Nakai H, Takeuchi M, Yoshitani H, et al. Pitfalls of anatomical aortic valve area measurements using two-dimensional transoesophageal echocardiography and the potential of three-dimensional transoesophageal echocardiography. Eur J Echocardiogr. 2010;11:369-76)

FUTURE DIRECTIONS

Since its advent in 2002, RT3DE has plunged forward holding interest of the advanced imagers, and now with the integration of the miniaturized matrix probe with the TEE probe, the indications for its use in valvular and procedural applications are exploding. Further advances in this technology will allow for a probe with smaller footprints, better spatiotemporal resolution, wider acoustic angle, single beat wide angle and color flow acquisition capabilities, eliminating artifacts and patient discomfort to a large extent. Undersampling issues will be resolved with higher frame rates. A comprehensive echocardiogram can potentially be completed in a fraction of a time needed now, as one can eliminate the different 2D views currently acquired, thereby improving the workflow in the echocardiographic laboratory. Stress echocardiograms may possibly be performed solely in a 3D format or in combination with single photon emission computerized tomography, as the

interventional or electrophysiologist's need to integrate continuously the multimodality visual feedback to catheter manipulation, lack of adequate trained operators in advanced echocardiography and the lack of standard nomenclature conventions to describe the position of the device in space, that could lead to potential harm.

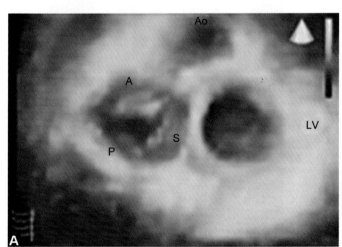

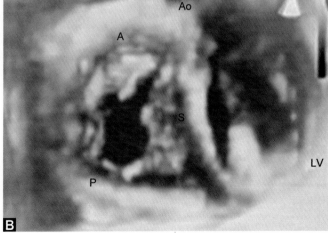

FIGURES 25A AND B: Live or real time three-dimensional transthoracic echocardiography. Three leaflets of the tricuspid valve. (A and B) *En face* views in two different patients showing all three tricuspid valve leaflets in the open position. (Abbreviations: A: Anterior leaflet; Ao: Aorta; LV: Left ventricle; P: Posterior leaflet; S: Septal leaflet). (*Source:* Reproduced with permission from Pothineni, et al[101])

Diagnosis

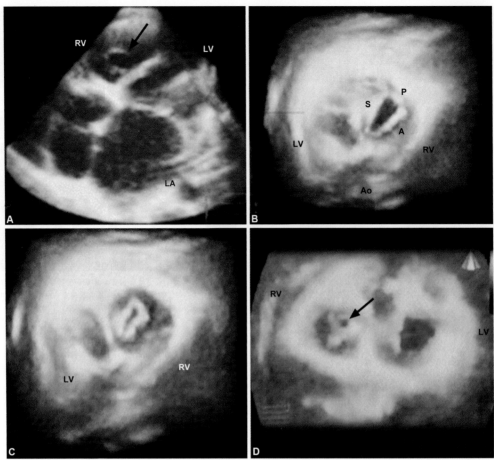

FIGURES 26A TO D: Live or real time three-dimensional transthoracic echocardiography. Rheumatic tricuspid valve stenosis or tricuspid regurgitation. (A) The arrow points to the tricuspid orifice in a patient with tricuspid valve stenosis. The orifice area measured 2.02 cm² in diastole. (B and C) *En face* views in another patient with mild tricuspid stenosis but severe tricuspid regurgitation. The tricuspid orifice area measured 2.4 cm² in diastole (B). Systolic frame (C) shows non-coaptation of tricuspid valve leaflets. This measured 0.4 cm² in area and resulted in severe tricuspid regurgitation as assessed by two-dimensional color Doppler. (D) *En face* view from the ventricular aspect showing systolic non-coaptation (arrow) of the tricuspid valve in a third patient with rheumatic heart disease. (Abbreviations: A: Anterior leaflet; Ao: Aorta; LA: Left atrium; LV: Left ventricle; P: Posterior leaflet; RV: Right ventricle; S: Septal leaflet). (*Source:* Reproduced with permission from Pothineni, et al[101])

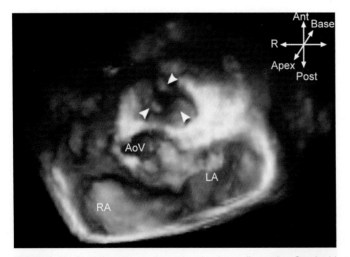

FIGURE 27: Real time three-dimensional echocardiography. Carcinoid syndrome: *en face* view from right ventricular perspective showed thickened and retracted annulus and cusps of pulmonary valve (arrowheads). (Abbreviations: Ant: Anterior; AoV: Aortic valve; L: Left; LA: Left atrium; Post: Posterior; R: Right; RA: Right atrium). (*Source:* Modified from Lee, et al[103])

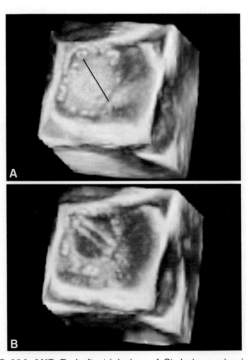

FIGURES 28A AND B: Left atrial view of St Jude mechanical mitral prosthesis in (A) systole and (B) diastole by RT3D TEE (Video 8). The black line overlies the central closure line

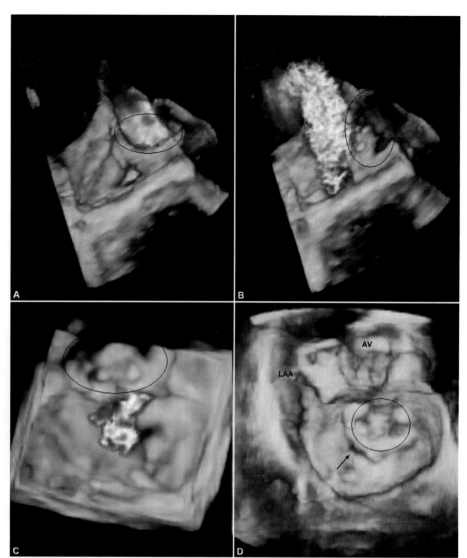

FIGURES 29A TO D: Paravalvular leak in a patient with bioprosthetic mitral valve replacement (MVR) imaged by real time three-dimensional transesophageal echocardiography. Color Doppler datasets viewed from left atrium (LA) in (A) diastole; (B) systole (Videos 9A and B) *en face*; (C) the diastolic mitral inflow occurs through the MVR ring as in A (overlaid with a black circle,) while the systolic mitral regurgitation as in B and C occurs primarily through the posteriorly located paravalvular perforation (arrow in D) Full volume dataset without color oriented to surgeon's view, viewed from LA (Video 9C) (Abbreviations: AV: Aortic valve; LAA: Left atrial appendage)

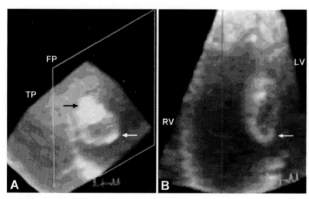

FIGURES 30A AND B: Cropped 3D dataset obtained from apical 4-chamber view with a left ventricular (LV) thrombus attached to the LV apex. Cropping with the transverse plane (TP) shows the absence of echolucency indicative of clot lysis in the stalk (arrow) (A) cropping with frontal plane (FP) shows the presence of echolucency within the body of the thrombus indicative of clot lysis or potential therapeutic efficacy. (Abbreviation: RV: Right ventricle). (*Source:* Modified from Sinha, et al[114])

temporal resolution improves. Myocardial perfusion echocardiography applications should emerge with this 3D technique as further evidence gathers. RT3DE will discover its applications

and limitations in determining regional RV volumes in various conditions affecting the RV.

3D speckle or strain imaging, making possible the extension of robust strain derived information to three dimensions will find its applications in a variety of conditions. Similar integration to contraction front mapping in electrophysiological procedures would allow for RT3DE guided ablation procedures, along with RT3DE guided placement of the LV lead to obtain an optimal response to CRT.

The user interface will be further refined and made user friendly with ability to crop in a more intuitive fashion. The advent of real time triplane imaging will eliminate the cropping time while retaining the advantage of imaging in three dimensions that may be adequate for evaluation of certain conditions such as aortic stenosis and stress imaging. As more operators are trained in RT3DE, this modality has the potential to become the standard of care especially in the interventional laboratory and the operating room.

Further advances in technology may make possible stereoscopic vision display (3D display as opposed to the current 2D display of 3D images) of RT3DE to better guide intracardiac beating-heart procedures or surgery.

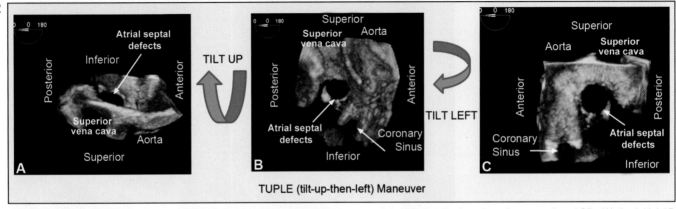

TUPLE (tilt-up-then-left) Maneuver

FIGURES 31A TO C: Imaging of a secundum ASD at 0°. The TUPLE maneuver is applied to the imaging of a secundum ASD: (A) the initial 3D TEE image (opening scene); (B) the right atrial aspect of the ASD; (C) the left atrial aspect of the ASD. (Abbreviations: ASD: Atrial septal defects; SVC: Superior vena cava). (*Source:* Modified from Saric, et al[114])

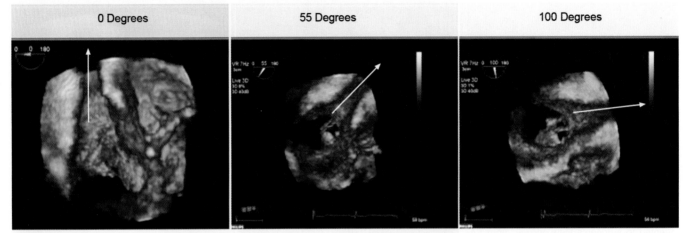

FIGURE 32: Imaging at intermediate angles. The impact of various acquisition angles on the 3D images of the interatrial septum is demonstrated. Each image demonstrates the right atrial aspect of the interatrial septum. Note that as the angle of image acquisition increases, the position of the SVC rotates progressively in the clockwise rotation (see text). (*Source:* Modified from Saric, et al[114])

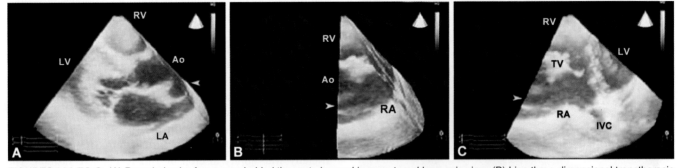

FIGURES 33A TO C: (A) Bounded echo-free space behind the aorta imaged in parasternal long-axis view. (B) Live three-dimensional transthoracic echocardiography. (C) Tilting of the full volume 3D dataset shows the bounded echo-free space (arrowhead) to be continuous with the RA. This is consistent with SVC. (Abbreviations: Ao: Aorta; IVC: Inferior vena cava; LA: Left atrium; LV: Left ventricle; RA: Right atrium; RV: Right ventricle; SVC: Superior vena cava; TV: Tricuspid valve). (*Source:* Modified from Burri, et al[120])

LIMITATIONS

The main limitation of RT3DE is the need for advanced expertise of the operator which calls for independent judgment and problem solving skills similar to that demanded by 2DE. As with any newly developed technique, there is a substantial learning curve. At this time, not all institutions offer training in RT3DE. Guidelines for training requirements are yet to be established.

Quality of the 2DE image dictates the quality of the 3D dataset. Most of the currently used 3D probes have compromised spatial and temporal resolution (especially with color Doppler)

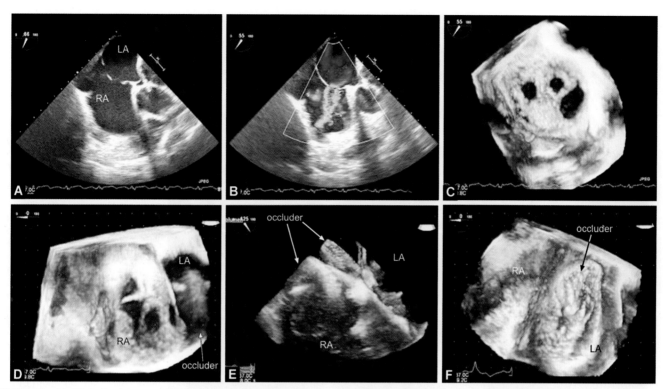

FIGURES 34A TO F: Real time 3D TEE guided closure of three atrial septal defects: (A) 2D imaging suggested more than 1 defect of a mobile interatrial septum with; (B) left-to-right shunt obtained by color Doppler; (C) a 3D left atrial view more detailed demonstrated three separated defects; (D) the septum was crossed under 3D guidance and a 34 mm Amplatzer occluder (occluder) was advanced from the left atrium (LA); (E and F) online 3D imaging allowed positioning the left-sided disc so that it covered all defects and assuring secure placement of the right sided disc (Abbreviation: RA: Right atrium). (*Source:* Modifie from Dodos, et al[123])

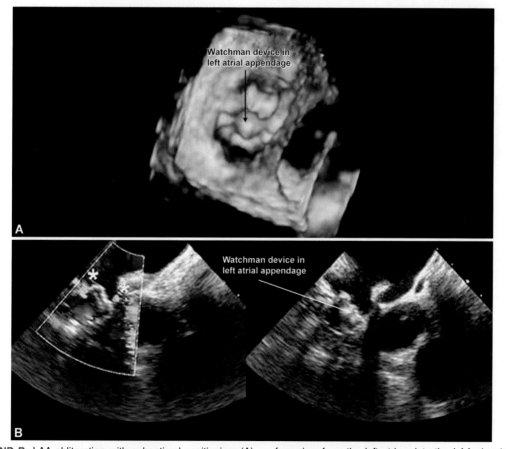

FIGURES 35A AND B: LAA obliteration with suboptimal positioning: (A) *en face* view from the left atrium into the LAA showing off-angle LAA occlusion device. The device is not perpendicular to the opening of the LAA, and a residual potential communication between the LAA and the main left atrium is still noticeable (3D zoom mode acquisition); (B) two-dimensional imaging of the off-angle closure device with color Doppler (asterisk) demonstrating residual flow between the LAA and the main left atrium. (*Source:* Modified from Perk, et al[69])

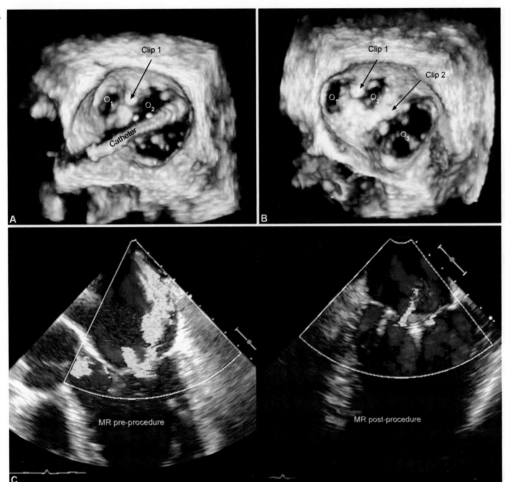

FIGURES 36A TO C: Mitral valve clipping with two clips: (A) mitral valve with the first clip in place seen from the left atrium. A double orifice mitral valve has been created (O_1 and O_2). However, color Doppler interrogation demonstrated significant residual mitral regurgitation (MR), so a second clip was deemed necessary. The guiding catheter is seen directed toward the larger part of the mitral valve orifice (O_2) to place another clip in the mitral valve (3D zoom mode acquisition); (B) two clips have been deployed in the mitral valve, resulting in a three-orifice mitral valve. The image shows an *en face* view of the mitral view, as seen from the left atrium. The three orifices (O_1, O_2 and O_3) are noted (3D zoom mode acquisition); (C) color Doppler demonstration of the result of the procedure. (Left) Before the procedure, severe MR is clearly demonstrated. (Right) After the procedure, only mild MR can be seen (*Source:* Modified from Perk, et al[69])

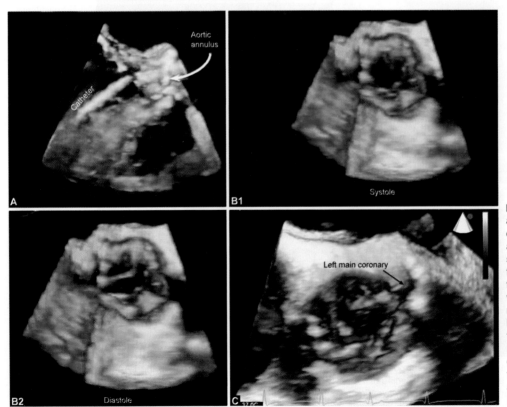

FIGURES 37A TO C: Percutaneous aortic valve replacement: (A) guiding catheter seen passing through the aortic valve (3D zoom mode acquisition); (B_1) systolic and (B_2) diastolic frames of a percutaneously implanted aortic valve as seen from the left ventricular perspective (3D zoom mode acquisition); (C) the proximal left main coronary artery, as seen from the left ventricular perspective. Patency of the ostium of the left main coronary artery is confirmed after valve implantation (3D zoom mode acquisition). (*Source:* Modified from Perk, et al[69])

compared to their 2D counterparts. The 3D dataset is displayed in 2D and hence the depth perception is limited during procedural guidance. Novel displays provide differential color hues with respect to depth of the image; however, unless one performs carefully calibrated depth measurements by manipulating the image to display the Z-axis (depth) parallel to the screen, certainty of depth perception is questionable. The analysis of the volumetric data can be time consuming.

Artifacts that are seen with 2DE are all common to 3DE as well. In addition, stitch artifacts in space or time, as alluded to previously, can be seen due to respiratory motion or due to irregular heart rates respectively, during the acquisition of pyramidal subvolumes of a full volume dataset.

VIDEO LEGENDS

Videos 1A and B   Modalities of live/real time three dimensional echocardiographic imaging: narrow angle real time imaging (A) and wide angle/full volume acquisition (B)

Videos 2A and B   Common artifacts during full volume acquisition in live/real time three dimensional echocardiography: a temporal (A) and a spatial stitch artifact (B)

Videos 3A and B   Semiautomated quatification of global (A) and regional (B) left ventricular function and corresponding time volume curves for all the phases of cardiac cycle

Videos 4A and B   Color-coded display of 16 left ventricular segments depicted in a cast display, in a normal (A) and a heart failure (B) patient

Videos 5A and B   Semiautomated right ventricular endocardial tracing in axial, sagittal and coronal planes of a full volume dataset (A) Three dimensional cast representation of the right ventricle (RV) providing RV volumes and ejection fraction (B)

Videos 6A and B   Zoom mode RT 3DTEE acquisition cropped transversely and viewed from left atrium (A) and left ventricle (B) in a patient with rheumatic mitral stenosis

Video 6C   The cropping in 3D needed to obtain the limiting mitral valve orifice area on an *en face* view (left lower panel) in rheumatic mitral stenosis

Video 7   RT 3DTEE in a patient with bicuspid aortic valve

Video 8   Left atrial view of St Jude mechanical mitral prosthesis by RT 3DTEE

Videos 9A to C   (A and B) Color Doppler RT 3DTEE of paravalvular regurgitation in a patient with a bioprosthetic mitral valve. (C) The relationship of the paravalvular regurgitation (posterior) to the valve is shown. The aortic valve is seen anteriorly.

REFERENCES

1. Dekker DL, Piziali RL, Dong E. A system for ultrasonically imaging the human heart in three dimensions. Comput Biomed Res. 1974;7:544-53.

2. Raab FH, Blood EB, Steiner TO, et al. Magnetic position and orientation tracking system. IEEE Trans Aerosp Electron Syst. 1979;AES-15:709-18.

3. Nanda N, Pinheiro L, Sanyal R, et al. Multiplane transesophageal echocardiographic imaging and three-dimensional reconstruction. Echocardiography. 1992;9:667-76.

4. Nikravesh PE, Skorton DJ, Chandran KB, et al. Computerized three-dimensional finite element reconstruction of the left ventricle from cross-sectional echocardiograms. Ultrason Imaging. 1984;6:48-59.

5. von Ramm OT, Smith SW. Real time volumetric ultrasound imaging system. J Digit Imaging. 1990;3:261-6.

6. Nanda NC, Kisslo J, Lang R, et al. Examination protocol for three dimensional echocardiography. Echocardiography. 2004;21:763-8.

7. Hung J, Lang R, Flaschskampf F, et al. 3D echocardiography: a review of the current status and future directions. J Am Soc Echocardiogr. 2007;20:213-33.

8. Lang RM, Bierig M, Devereux RB, et al. Recommendations for chamber quantification: a report from the American Society of Echocardiography's guidelines and standards committee and the chamber quantification writing group, developed in conjunction with the Europian Association of Echocardiography, a branch of Europian Society of Cardiology. J AM Soc Echocardiogr. 2005;18:1440-63.

9. Gordon EP, Schnittger I, Fitzgerald PJ, et al. Reproducibility of left ventricular volumes by two-dimensional echocardiography. J Am Coll Cardiol. 1983;2:506-13.

10. Jenkins C, Bricknell K, Hanekom L, et al. Reproducibility and accuracy of echocardiographic measurements of left ventricular parameters using real-time three-dimensional echocardiography. J Am Coll Cardiol. 2004;44:878-86.

11. Nikitin NP, Constantin C, Loh PH, et al. New generation 3-dimensional echocardiography for left ventricular volumetric and functional measurements: comparison with cardiac magnetic resonance. Eur J Echocardiogr. 2006;7:365-72.

12. Pouleur AC, le Polain de, Waroux JB, et al. Assessment of left ventricular mass and volumes by three-dimensional echocardiography in patients with or without wall motion abnormalities: comparison against cine magnetic resonance imaging. Heart. 2008;94:1050-7.

13. Arai K, Hozumi T, Matsumura Y, et al. Accuracy of measurement of left ventricular volume and ejection fraction by new real-time three-dimensional echocardiography in patients with wall motion abnormalities secondary to myocardial infarction. Am J Cardiol. 2004;94:552-8.

14. Mor-Avi V, Jenkins C, Kühl HP, et al. Real-time 3-dimensional echocardiographic quantification of left ventricular volumes: multicenter study for validation with magnetic resonance imaging and investigation of sources of error. J Am Coll Cardiol Img. 2008;1:413-23.

15. Jacobs LD, Salgo IS, Goonewardena S, et al. Rapid online quantification of left ventricular volume from real-time three-dimensional echocardiographic data. Eur Heart J. 2006;27:460-8.

16. Jenkins C, Bricknell K, Chan J, et al. Comparison of two- and three-dimensional echocardiography with sequential magnetic resonance imaging for evaluating left ventricular volume and ejection fraction over time in patients with healed myocardial infarction. Am J Cardiol. 2007;99:300-6.

17. Kuhl HP, Schreckenberg M, Rulands D, et al. High-resolution transthoracic real-time three-dimensional echocardiography: quantitation of cardiac volumes and function using semi-automatic border detection and comparison with cardiac magnetic resonance imaging. J Am Coll Cardiol. 2004;43:2083-90.

18. Sugeng L, Mor-Avi V, Weinert L, et al. Quantitative assessment of left ventricular size and function: side-by-side comparison of real-time three dimensional echocardiography and computed tomography with magnetic resonance reference. Circulation. 2006;114:654-61.

19. Jenkins C, Chan J, Hanekom L, et al. Accuracy and feasibility of online 3-dimensional echocardiography for measurement of left ventricular parameters. J Am Soc Echocardiogr. 2006;19:1119-28.

20. Krenning BJ, Kirschbaum SW, Soliman OI, et al. Comparison of contrast agent-enhanced versus non-contrast agent-enhanced real-time three-dimensional echocardiography for analysis of left ventricular systolic function. Am J Cardiol. 2007;100:1485-9.

21. Soliman OI, Krenning BJ, Geleijnse ML, et al. Quantification of left ventricular volumes and function in patients with cardiomyopathies by real-time three dimensional echocardiography: a head-to-head comparison between two different semiautomated endocardial border detection algorithms. J Am Soc Echocardiogr. 2007;20:1042-9.

22. Qin JX, Jones M, Shiota T, et al. validation of real-time three-dimensional echocardiography for quantifying left ventricular volumes in the presence of a left ventricular aneurysm: in vitro and in vivo studies. J Am Coll Cardiol. 2000;36:900-7.

23. Corsi C, Coon P, Goonewardena S, et al. Quantification of regional left ventricular wall motion from real-time 3-dimensional echocardiography in patients with poor acoustic windows: effects of contrast enhancement tested against cardiac magnetic resonance. J Am Soc Echocardiogr. 2006;19:886-93.

24. Caiani EG, Coon P, Corsi C, et al. Dual triggering improves the accuracy of left ventricular volume measurements by contrast-enhanced real-time 3-dimensional echocardiography. J Am Soc Echocardiogr. 2005;18:1292-8.

25. Szmigielski C, Rajpoot K, Grau V, et al. Real-time 3D fusion echocardiography. JACC Cardiovasc Imaging. 2010;3:682-90.

26. Kapetanakis S, Kearney MT, Siva A, et al. Real-time three-dimensional echocardiography: a novel technique to quantify global left ventricular mechanical dyssynchrony. Circulation. 2005;112:992-1000.

27. Marsan NA, Henneman MM, Chen J, et al. Real-time three-dimensional echocardiography as a novel approach to quantify left ventricular dyssynchrony: a comparison study with phase analysis of gated myocardial perfusion single photon emission computed tomography. J Am Soc Echocardiogr. 2008;21:801-7.

28. Burgess MI, Jenkins C, Chan J, et al. Measurement of left ventricular dyssynchrony in patients with ischaemic cardiomyopathy: a comparison of real-time three dimensional and tissue Doppler echocardiography. Heart. 2007;93:1191-6.

29. Kleijn SA, van Dijk J, de Cock CC, et al. Assessment of intra-ventricular mechanical dyssynchrony and prediction of response to cardiac resynchronization therapy: comparison between tissue Doppler imaging and real-time three-dimensional echocardiography. J Am Soc Echocardiogr. 2009;22:1047-54.

30. Marsan NA, Bleeker GB, Ypenburg C, et al. Real-time three-dimensional echocardiography permits quantification of left ventricular mechanical dyssynchrony and predicts acute response to cardiac resynchronization therapy. J Cardiovasc Electrophysiol. 2008;19:392-9.

31. Marsan NA, Bleeker GB, Ypenburg C, et al. Real-time three-dimensional echocardiography as a novel approach to assess left ventricular and left atrium reverse remodeling and to predict response to cardiac resynchronization therapy. Heart Rhythm. 2008;5:1257-64.

32. Kawagishi T. Speckle tracking for assessment of cardiac motion and dyssynchrony. Echocardiography. 2008;25:1167-71.

33. Tanaka H, Hara H, Saba S, et al. Usefulness of three-dimensional speckle tracking strain to quantify dyssynchrony and the site of latest mechanical activation. Am J Cardiol. 2010;105:235-42.

34. Li CH, Carreras F, Leta R, et al. Mechanical left ventricular dyssynchrony detection by endocardium displacement analysis with 3D speckle tracking technology. Int J Cardiovasc Imaging. 2010;26:867-70.

35. Nesser HJ, Mor-Avi, V, Gorissen W, et al. Quantification of left ventricular volumes using three-dimensional echocardiographic speckle tracking: comparison with MRI. Eur Heart J. 2009;30:1565-73.

36. Tanaka H, Hara H, Adelstein EC, et al. Comparative mechanical activation mapping of RV pacing to LBBB by 2D and 3D speckle tracking and association with response to resynchronization therapy. JACC Cardiovasc Imaging. 2010;3:461-71.

37. Flu WJ, Kuijk JP, Bax JJ. Three-dimensional speckle tracking echocardiography: a novel approach in the assessment of left ventricular volume and function? Eur Heart J. 2009;30:2304-7.

38. Andrade J, Cortez LD, Campos O, et al. Left ventricular twist: comparison between two- and three-dimensional speckle-tracking echocardiography in healthy volunteers. Eur J Echocardiogr. 2011;12:76-9.

39. Ahmad M, Xie T, McCulloch M, et al. Real-time three-dimensional dobutamine stress echocardiography in assessment of ischemia: comparison with two-dimensional dobutamine stress echocardiography. J Am Coll Cardiol. 2001;37:1303-9.

40. Matsumura Y, Hozumi T, Arai K, et al. Non-invasive assessment of myocardial ischaemia using new real-time three-dimensional dobutamine stress echocardiography: comparison with conventional two-dimensional methods. Eur Heart J. 2005;26:1625-32.

41. Walimbe V, Jaber WA, Garcia MJ, et al. Multimodality cardiac stress testing: combining real-time 3-dimensional echocardiography and myocardial perfusion SPECT. Nucl Med. 2009;50:226-30.

42. Camarano G, Jones M, Freidlin RZ, et al. Quantitative assessment of left ventricular perfusion defects using real-time three-dimensional myocardial contrast echocardiography. J Am Soc Echocardiogr. 2002;15:206-13.

43. Yao J, De Castro S, Delabays A, et al. Bulls-eye display and quantitation of myocardial perfusion defects using three-dimensional contrast echocardiography. Echocardiography. 2001;18:581-8.

44. Chen LX, Wang XF, Nanda NC, et al. Real-time three-dimensional myocardial contrast echocardiography in assessment of myocardial perfusion defects. Chin Med J (Engl). 2004;117:337-41.

45. Pemberton J, Li X, Hickey E, et al. Live real-time three-dimensional echocardiography for the visualization of myocardial perfusion—a pilot study in open-chest pigs. J Am Soc Echocardiogr. 2005;18:956-8.

46. Bhan A, Kapetanakis S, Rana BS, et al. Real-time three-dimensional myocardial contrast echocardiography: is it clinically feasible? Eur J Echocardiogr. 2008;9:761-5.

47. Toledo E, Lang RM, Collins KA, et al. Imaging and quantification of myocardial perfusion using real-time three-dimensional echocardiography. J Am Coll Cardiol. 2006;47:146.

48. Yap SC, van Geuns RJ, Nemes A. Rapid and accurate measurement of LV mass by biplane real-time 3D echocardiography in patients with concentric LV hypertrophy: comparison to CMR. Eur J of Echocardiogr. 2008;9:255-60.

49. Rudski LG, Lai WW, Afilalo J, et al. Guidelines for the Echocardiographic Assessment of the Right Heart in Adults: a Report from the American Society of Echocardiography Endorsed by the European Association of Echocardiography, a registered branch of the European Society of Cardiology, and the Canadian Society of Echocardiography. J Am Soc Echocardiogr. 2010;23:685-713.

50. Gopal AS, Chukwu EO, Iwuchukwu CJ, et al. Normal values of right ventricular size and function by real-time 3-dimensional echocardiography: comparison with cardiac magnetic resonance imaging. J Am Soc Echocardiogr. 2007;20:445-55.

51. Hoch M, Vasilyev NV, Soriano B, et al. Variables influencing the accuracy of right ventricular volume assessment by real-time 3-dimensional echocardiography: an in vitro validation study. J Am Soc Echocardiogr. 2007;20:456-61.

52. Schindera ST, Mehwald PS, Sahn DJ, et al. Accuracy of real-time three-dimensional echocardiography for quantifying right ventricular volume: static and pulsatile flow studies in an anatomic in vitro model. J Ultrasound Med. 2002;21:1069-75.

53. Niemann PS, Pinho L, Balbach T, et al. Anatomically oriented right ventricular volume measurements with dynamic three-dimensional echocardiography validated by 3-Tesla magnetic resonance imaging. J Am Coll Cardiol. 2007;50:1668-76.

54. Nesser HJ, Tkalec W, Patel AR, et al. Quantitation of right ventricular volumes and ejection fraction by three-dimensional echocardiography in patients: comparison with magnetic resonance imaging and radionuclide ventriculography. Echocardiography. 2006;23:666-80.

55. Jenkins C, Chan J, Bricknell K, et al. Reproducibility of right ventricular volumes and ejection fraction using real-time three-dimensional echocardiography comparison with cardiac MRI. Chest. 2007;131:1844-51.

56. Leibundgut G, Rohner A, Grize L, et al. Dynamic assessment of right ventricular volumes and function by real-time three-dimensional echocardiography: a comparison study with magnetic resonance imaging in 100 adult patients. J Am Soc Echocardiogr. 2010;23:116-26.

57. van der Zwaan HB, Helbing WA, McGhie JS, et al. Clinical value of real-time three-dimensional echocardiography for right ventricular quantification in congenital heart disease: validation with cardiac magnetic resonance imaging. J Am Soc Echocardiogr. 2010;23:134-40.

58. Badano LP, Ginghina C, Easaw J, et al. Right ventricle in pulmonary arterial hypertension: haemodynamics, structural changes, imaging, and proposal of a study protocol aimed to assess remodelling and treatment effects. Eur J Echocardiogr. 2010;11:27-37.

59. Rossi M, Cicoira L, Zanolla L, et al. Determinants and prognostic value of left atrial volume in patients with dilated cardiomyopathy. J Am Coll Cardiol. 2002;40:1425.

60. Hage FG, Karakus G, Luke WD, et al. Effect of alcohol-induced septal ablation on left atrial volume and ejection fraction assessed by real time three-dimensional transthoracic echocardiography in patients with hypertrophic cardiomyopathy. Echocardiography. 2008;25:784-9.

61. Abhayaratna WP, Seward JB, Appleton CP, et al. Left atrial size: physiologic determinants and clinical applications. J Am Coll Cardiol. 2006;47:2357-63.

62. Anwar AM, Soliman OI, Geleijnse ML, et al. Assessment of left atrial volume and function by real-time three-dimensional echocardiography. Int J Cardiol. 2008;123:155-61.

63. Pritchett AM, Jacobsen SJ, Mahoney DW, et al. Left atrial volume as an index of left atrial size: a population-based study. J Am Coll Cardiol. 2003;41:1036-43.

64. Jenkins C, Bricknell K, Marwick TH. Use of real-time three-dimensional echocardiography to measure left atrial volume: comparison with other echocardiographic techniques. J Am Soc Echocardiogr. 2005;18:991-7.

65. Shah SJ, Bardo DM, Sugeng L, et al. Real-time three-dimensional transesophageal echocardiography of the left atrial appendage: initial experience in the clinical setting. J Am Soc Echocardiogr. 2008;21:1362-8.

66. Karakus G, Kodali V, Inamdar V, et al. Comparative assessment of left atrial appendage by transesophageal and combined two- and three-dimensional transthoracic echocardiography. Echocardiography. 2008;25:918-24.

67. Müller H, Noble S, Keller PF, et al. Biatrial anatomical reverse remodelling after radiofrequency catheter ablation for atrial fibrillation: evidence from real-time three-dimensional echocardiography. Europace. 2008;10:1073-8.

68. Faletra FF, Ho SY, Auricchio A. Anatomy of right atrial structures by real-time 3D transesophageal echocardiography. JACC Cardiovasc Imaging. 2010;3:966-75.

69. Maffessanti F, Marsan NA, Tamborini G, et al. Quantitative analysis of mitral valve apparatus in mitral valve prolapse before and after annuloplasty: a three-dimensional intraoperative transesophageal study. J Am Soc Echocardiogr. 2011;24:405-13.

70. Chandra S, Salgo IS, Sugeng L, et al. Characterization of degenerative mitral valve disease using morphologic analysis of real-time three-dimensional echocardiographic images: objective insight into complexity and planning of mitral valve repair. Circ Cardiovasc Imaging. 2011;4:24-32.

71. Watanabe N, Ogasawara Y, Yamaura Y, et al. Mitral annulus flattens in ischemic mitral regurgitation: geometric differences between inferior and anterior myocardial infarction: a real-time 3-dimensional echocardiographic study. Circulation. 2005;112:1458-62.

72. Ahmad RM, Gillinov AM, McCarthy PM, et al. Annular geometry and motion in human ischemic mitral regurgitation: novel assessment with three-dimensional echocardiography and computer reconstruction. Ann Thorac Surg. 2004;78:2063-8.

73. Kwan J, Shiota T, Agler DA, et al. Geometric differences of the mitral apparatus between ischemic and dilated cardiomyopathy with significant mitral regurgitation: real-time three-dimensional echocardiography study. Circulation. 2003;107:1135-40.

74. Otsuji Y, Handschumacher MD, Liel-Cohen N, et al. Mechanism of ischemic mitral regurgitation with segmental left ventricular dysfunction: three-dimensional echocardiographic studies in models of acute and chronic progressive regurgitation. J Am Coll Cardiol. 2001;37:641-8.

75. Hung J, Guerrero JL, Handschumacher MD, et al. Reverse ventricular remodeling reduces ischemic mitral regurgitation: echo-guided device application in the beating heart. Circulation 2002;106:2594-600.

76. Langer F, Rodriguez F, Ortiz S, et al. Subvalvular repair: the key to repairing ischemic mitral regurgitation? Circulation. 2005;112:1383-9.

77. Tsukiji M, Watanabe N, Yamaura Y, et al. Three-dimensional quantitation of mitral valve coaptation by a novel software system with transthoracic real-time three-dimensional echocardiography. J Am Soc Echocardiogr. 2008;21:43-6.

78. Grewal J, Suri R, Mankad S, et al. Mitral annular dynamics in myxomatous valve disease: new insights with real-time 3-dimensional echocardiography. Circulation. 2010;121:1423-31.

79. Schwalm SA, Sugeng L, Raman J, et al. Assessment of mitral valve leaflet perforation as a result of infective endocarditis by 3-dimensional real-time echocardiography. J Am Soc Echocardiogr. 2004;17:919-22.

80. Hansalia S, Biswas M, Dutta R, et al. The value of live/real time three-dimensional transesophageal echocardiography in the assessment of valvular vegetations. Echocardiography. 2009;26:1264-73.

81. Aggarwal G, Schlosshan D, Arronis C, et al. Images in cardiovascular medicine. Real-time 3-dimensional transesophageal echocardiography in the evaluation of a patient with concomitant double-orifice mitral valve, bicuspid aortic valve, and coarctation of the aorta. Circulation. 2009;120:e277-9.

82. Biaggi P, Greutmann M, Crean A. Utility of three-dimensional transesophageal echocardiography: anatomy, mechanism, and severity of regurgitation in a patient with an isolated cleft posterior mitral valve. J Am Soc Echocardiogr. 2010;23:1114.e1-4.

83. Pepi M, Tamborini G, Maltagliati A, et al. Head-to-head comparison of two- and three-dimensional transthoracic and transesophageal echocardiography in the localization of mitral valve prolapse. J Am Coll Cardiol. 2006;48:2524-30.

84. Miller AP, Nanda NC. Live/real-time three-dimensional transthoracic assessment of mitral regurgitation and mitral valve prolapse. Cardiol Clin. 2007;25:319-25.

85. Sugeng L, Coon P, Weinert L, et al. Use of real-time 3-dimensional transthoracic echocardiography in the evaluation of mitral valve disease. J Am Soc Echocardiogr. 2006;19:413-21.

86. Sugeng L, Shernan SK, Weinert L, et al. Real-time three-dimensional transesophageal echocardiography in valve disease: comparison with surgical findings and evaluation of prosthetic valves. J Am Soc Echocardiogr. 2008;21:1347-54.

87. Kahlert P, Plicht B, Schenk IM, et al. Direct assessment of size and shape of noncircular vena contracta area in functional versus organic mitral regurgitation using real-time three dimensional echocardiography. J Am Soc Echocardiogr. 2008;21:912-21.

88. Marsan NA, Westenberg JJ, Ypenburg C, et al. Quantification of functional mitral regurgitation by real-time 3D echocardiography: comparison with 3D velocity-encoded cardiac magnetic resonance. JACC Cardiovasc Imaging. 2009;2:1245-52.

89. Little SH, Pirat B, Kumar R, et al. Three-dimensional color Doppler echocardiography for direct measurement of vena contracta area in

mitral regurgitation: in vitro validation and clinical experience. JACC Cardiovasc Imaging. 2008;1:695-704.

90. Grewal J, Mankad S, Freeman WK, et al. Real-time three-dimensional transesophageal echocardiography in the intraoperative assessment of mitral valve disease. J Am Soc Echocardiogr. 2009; 22:34-41.

91. Perk G, Lang RM, Garcia-Fernandez MA, et al. Use of real time three-dimensional transesophageal echocardiography in intracardiac catheter based interventions. J Am Soc Echocardiogr. 2009;22:865-82.

92. Mannaerts HFJ, Kamp O, Visser CA. Should mitral valve area assessment in patients with mitral stenosis be based on anatomical or on functional evaluation? A plea for 3D echocardiography as the new clinical standard. Eur Heart J. 2004;25:2073-4.

93. Zamorano J, Cordeiro P, Sugeng L, et al. Real-time three-dimensional echocardiography for rheumatic mitral valve stenosis evaluation: an accurate and novel approach. J Am Coll Cardiol. 2004;43:2091-6.

94. Chu JW, Levine RA, Chua S, et al. Assessing mitral valve area and orifice geometry in calcific mitral stenosis: a new solution by real-time three-dimensional echocardiography. J Am Soc Echocardiogr. 2008;21:1006-9.

95. Anwar AM, Attia WM, Nosir YF, et al. Validation of a new score for the assessment of mitral stenosis using real-time three-dimensional echocardiography. J Am Soc Echocardiogr. 2010;23:13-22.

96. Zamorano J, Perez de Isla L, Sugeng L, et al. Non-invasive assessment of mitral valve area during percutaneous balloon mitral valvuloplasty: role of real-time 3D echocardiography. Eur Heart J. 2004;25:2086-91.

97. Ge S, Warner JG, Abraham TP, et al. Three-dimensional surface area of the aortic valve orifice by three-dimensional echocardiography: clinical validation of a novel index for assessment of aortic stenosis. Am Heart J. 1998;136:1042-50.

98. Suradi H, Byers S, Green-Hess D, et al. Feasibility of using real time "Live 3D" echocardiography to visualize the stenotic aortic valve. Echocardiography. 2010;27:1011-20.

99. Vengala S, Nanda NC, Dod SH, et al. Images in geriatric cardiology. Usefulness of live three-dimensional transthoracic echocardiography in aortic valve stenosis evaluation. Am J Geriatr Cardiol. 2004;13: 279-84.

100. Mallavarapu RK, Nanda NC. Three-dimensional transthoracic echocardiographic assessment of aortic stenosis and regurgitation. Cardiol Clin. 2007;25:327-34.

101. Pothineni KR, Duncan K, Yelamanchili P, et al. Live/real time three-dimensional transthoracic echocardiographic assessment of tricuspid valve pathology: incremental value over the two-dimensional technique. Echocardiography. 2007;24:541-52.

102. Sugeng L, Weinert L, Lang RM. Real-time 3-dimensional color Doppler flow of mitral and tricuspid regurgitation: feasibility and initial quantitative comparison with 2-dimensional methods. J Am Soc Echocardiogr. 2007;20:1050-7.

103. Lee KJ, Connolly HM, Pellikka PA. Carcinoid pulmonary valvulopathy evaluated by real-time 3-dimensional transthoracic echocardiography. J Am Soc Echocardiogr. 2008;21:407.e1-2.

104. Anwar AM, Soliman O, van den Bosch AE, et al. Assessment of pulmonary valve and right ventricular outflow tract with real-time three-dimensional echocardiography. Int J Cardiovasc Imaging. 2007;23:167-75.

105. Singh P, Inamdar V, Hage FG, et al. Usefulness of live/real time three dimensional transthoracic echocardiography in evaluation of prosthetic valve function. Echocardiography. 2009;26:1236-49.

106. Keenan NG, Cueff C, Cimadevilla C, et al. Diagnosis of early dysfunction of a tissue mitral valve replacement by three-dimensional transoesophageal echocardiography. Eur J Echocardiogr. 2010;11: E33.

107. Kronzon I, Sugeng L, Perk G, et al. Real-time 3-dimensional transesophageal echocardiography in the evaluation of post-operative mitral annuloplasty ring and prosthetic valve dehiscence. J Am Coll Cardiol. 2009;53:1543-7.

108. Singh P, Manda J, Hsiung MC, et al. Live/real time three-dimensional transesophageal echocardiographic evaluation of mitral and aortic valve prosthetic paravalvular regurgitation. Echocardiography. 2009;26:980-7.

109. Paul B, Minocha A. Thrombosis of a bileaflet prosthetic mitral valve: a real-time three-dimensional transesophageal echocardiography perspective. Int J Cardiovasc Imaging. 2010;26:367-8.

110. Ozkan M, Gündüz S, Yildiz M, et al. Diagnosis of the prosthetic heart valve pannus formation with real-time three-dimensional trans-oesophageal echocardiography. Eur J Echocardiogr. 2010;11: E17.

111. Naqvi TZ, Rafie R, Ghalichi M. Real-time 3D TEE for the diagnosis of right-sided endocarditis in patients with prosthetic devices. JACC Cardiovasc Imaging. 2010;3:325-7.

112. Kort S. Real-time 3-dimensional echocardiography for prosthetic valve endocarditis: initial experience. J Am Soc Echocardiogr. 2006;19:130-9.

113. Pothineni KR, Nanda NC, Burri MV, et al. Live/real time three-dimensional transthoracic echocardiographic description of chordoma metastatic to the heart. Echocardiography. 2008;25:440-2.

114. Sinha A, Nanda NC, Khanna D, et al. Morphological assessment of left ventricular thrombus by live three-dimensional transthoracic echocardiography. Echocardiography. 2004;21:649-55.

115. Dod HS, Burri MV, Hooda D, et al. Two- and three-dimensional transthoracic and transesophageal echocardiographic findings in epithelioid hemangioma involving the mitral valve. Echocardiography. 2008;25:443-5.

116. Sinha A, Nanda NC, Panwar RB, et al. Live three-dimensional transthoracic echocardiographic assessment of left ventricular hydatid cyst. Echocardiography. 2004;21:699-705.

117. Thuny F, Avierinos JF, Jop B, et al. Images in cardiovascular medicine. Massive biventricular thrombosis as a consequence of myocarditis: findings from 2-dimensional and real-time 3-dimensional echocardiography. Circulation. 2006;113:e932-3.

118. Saric M, Perk G, Purgess JR, et al. Imaging atrial septal defects by real-time three-dimensional transesophageal echocardiography: step-by-step approach. J Am Soc Echocardiogr. 2010;23:1128-35.

119. Halpern DG, Perk G, Ruiz C, et al. Percutaneous closure of a post-myocardial infarction ventricular septal defect guided by real-time three-dimensional echocardiography. Eur J Echocardiogr. 2009;10: 569-71.

120. Burri MV, Mahan EF, Nanda NC, et al. Superior vena cava, right pulmonary artery or both: real time two- and three-dimensional transthoracic contrast echocardiographic identification of the echo-free space posterior to the ascending aorta. Echocardiography. 2007;24:875-82.

121. Pedrazzini GB, Klimusina J, Pasotti E, et al. Complications of percutaneous edge-to-edge mitralvalve repair: the role of real-time three-dimensional transesophageal echocardiography. J Am Soc Echocardiogr. 2011;24:706.e5-7.

122. Silvestry FE, Kerber RE, Brook MM, et al. Echocardiography-guided interventions. J Am Soc Echocardiogr. 2009;22: 213-31.

123. Dodos F, Hoppe UC. Percutaneous closure of complex atrial septum defect guided by real-time 3D transesophageal echocardiography. Clin Res Cardiol. 2009;98:455-6.

124. Amitai ME, Schnittger I, Popp RL, et al. Comparison of three-dimensional echocardiography to two-dimensional echocardiography and fluoroscopy for monitoring of endomyocardial biopsy. Am J Cardiol. 2007;99:864-6.

Chapter 20

Intravascular Coronary Ultrasound and Beyond

Teruyoshi Kume, Yasuhiro Honda, Peter J Fitzgerald

Chapter Outline

INTRODUCTION

Intravascular ultrasound (IVUS) is widely used as a major diagnostic and assessment technique that provides detailed cross-sectional imaging of blood vessels in the cardiac catheterization laboratory. The first ultrasound imaging catheter system was developed by Bom and his colleagues in Rotterdam, the Netherland, in 1971.[1] By the late 1980s, the first images of human vessels were recorded by Yock and his colleagues.[2] Since then, IVUS has become a pivotal catheter-based imaging technology that can provide scientific insights into vascular biology and practical guidance for percutaneous coronary interventions (PCIs) in clinical settings. In this chapter, IVUS and the other catheter-based imaging devices—optical coherence tomography (OCT), angioscopy and spectroscopy—are described. These newly developed imaging technologies provide supplemental and unique insights into vascular biology as well.

INTRAVASCULAR ULTRASOUND

BASICS OF IVUS AND PROCEDURES

The IVUS imaging systems use reflected sound waves to visualize the vessel wall in a two-dimensional format analogous to a histologic cross-section. In general, higher frequencies of ultrasound limit the scanning depth but improve the axial resolution, and current IVUS catheters used in the coronary arteries have center frequencies ranging 20–45 MHz. There are two different types of IVUS transducer systems: (1) the solid-state dynamic aperture system (the electronically switched multi-element array system) and (2) the mechanically rotating single-transducer system (Table 1 and Figs 1A and B). Several types of artifacts can be observed common or unique to each system (Figs 2A to D). With both systems, still frames and video images can be digitally archived on local storage memory or a remote server using digital imaging and communications in medicine (DICOM) Standard 3.0. Regardless of IVUS system used in the patient, both require preprocedural administration of intravenous heparin (5,000–10,000 U), or equivalent anticoagulation along with intracoronary nitroglycerin (100–300 μg), to reduce the potential for coronary spasm.

NORMAL VESSEL MORPHOLOGY

The interpretation of IVUS images is possible as the layers of a diseased arterial wall can be identified separately. Particularly in muscular arteries, such as the coronary tree, the media of the

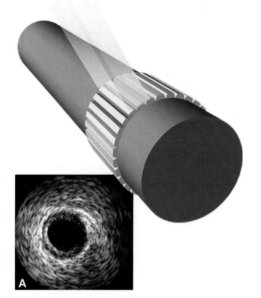

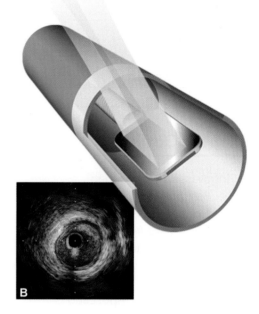

FIGURES 1A AND B: Diagrams of two basic imaging catheter designs: (A) solid state and (B) mechanical. (A: bottom) an Image obtained using a solid-state catheter imaging system. (B: bottom) an image obtained using a mechanical catheter imaging system

TABLE 1

Comparison of two IVUS designs

	Solid-state dynamic aperture system	*Mechanically rotating single-transducer system*
Basics	An electronic solid state catheter system with multiple imaging elements at its distal tip, providing cross-sectional imaging by sequentially activating the imaging elements in a circular way	A mechanical system that contains a flexible imaging cable which rotates a single transducer at its tip inside an echolucent distal sheath
Products	One system is commercially available (Volcano Corporation, Inc., Rancho Cordova, CA)	Several systems are commercially available (Boston Scientific Corporation, Natick, MA; Volcano Corporation, Inc., Rancho Cordova, CA; Terumo Corporation, Tokyo, Japan)
Features	The imaging catheter has 64 transducer elements arranged around the catheter tip and uses a center frequency of 20 MHz The outer shaft diameter of IVUS catheters in a rapid-exchange configuration is 2.9 Fr and thus compatible with a 5 Fr guide catheter	The imaging catheter uses a 40- or 45 MHz transducer with a distal crossing profile of 3.2 Fr (compatible with 6 Fr guide catheters)
Image quality	This imaging catheter has better scanning depth but poorer axial resolution compared with the mechanical systems	Higher frequencies improve the axial resolution. Therefore, mechanical transducers have traditionally offered advantages in image quality compared with the solid-state systems
Artifacts	The guidewire runs inside the IVUS catheter thereby preventing guidewire artifact This system does not require flushing with saline	The guidewire runs outside the IVUS catheter, parallel to the imaging segment, resulting in guidewire artifact This system requires flushing with saline before insertion to eliminate any air in the path of the beam. Incomplete flushing artifact may result in poor image quality
	This system eliminates nonuniform rotational distortion (NURD)	The NURD can occur when bending of the drive cable interferes with uniform transducer rotation, causing a wedge-shaped, smeared image to appear in one or more segments of the image
	Since the solid-state transducer has a zone of "ring-down artifact" encircling the catheter, an extra step is required to form a mask of the artifact and subtract this from the image	The imaging catheters have excellent near-field resolution and do not require the subtraction of a mask
Others	Short transducer-to-tip distance (10.5 mm) facilitates visualization of distal coronary anatomy	The pullback trajectory is stabilized and it reduces the risk of a nonuniform speed in a continuous pullback

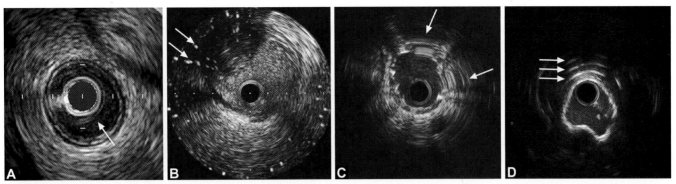

FIGURES 2A TO D: Common IVUS image artifacts: (A) A "halo" or a series of bright rings immediately around the mechanical IVUS catheter is usually caused by air bubbles that need to be flushed out. (B) Radiofrequency noise appears as alternating radial spokes or random white dots in the far-field. The interference is usually caused by other electrical equipment in the cardiac catheterization laboratory. (C) Nonuniform rotational distortion (NURD) results in a wedge-shaped, smeared appearance in one or more segments of the image (between 12 O'clock and 3 O'clock in this example). This may be corrected by straightening the catheter and motor drive assembly, lessening tension on the guide catheter, or loosening the hemostatic valve of the Y-adapter. (D) Circumferential calcification causes reverberation artifact between 10 O'clock and 1 O'clock

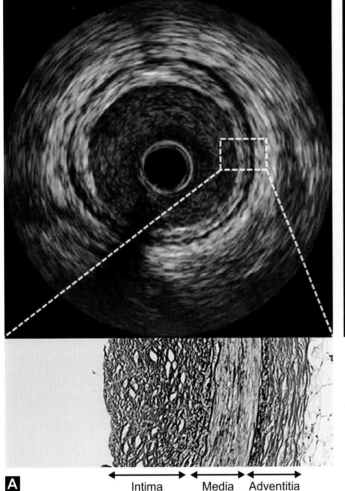

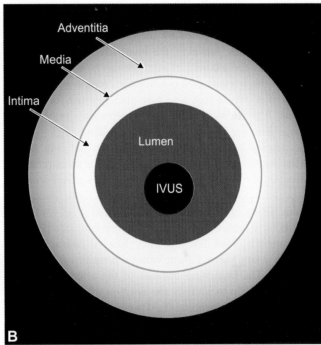

FIGURES 3A AND B: Cross-sectional format of a representative IVUS image. The bright-dark-bright, three-layered appearance is seen in the image with corresponding anatomy as defined. The "IVUS" represents the imaging catheter in the vessel lumen. Histologic correlation with intima, media and adventitia are shown. The media has lower ultrasound reflectance owing to less collagen and elastin compared with neighboring layers. Since the intimal layer reflects ultrasound more strongly than the media, there is a spillover in the image, resulting in slight overestimation of the thickness of the intima and a corresponding underestimation of the medial thickness

vessel is characterized by a dark band compared with the intima and adventitia (Figs 3A and B). Differentiation of the layers of elastic arteries, such as the aorta and carotid, can be problematic because media are less distinctly seen by IVUS. However, most of the vessels currently treated by catheter techniques are muscular or transitional arteries. These include the coronary, iliofemoral, renal and popliteal systems. Therefore, it is usually easy to identify the medial layer.

The relative echolucency of media compared with intima and adventitia gives rise to a three-layered appearance (bright-dark-bright), first described in vitro by Meyer and his colleagues.[3] Due to the lack of collagen and elastin compared to neighboring layers, the media displays lower ultrasound reflection. "Blooming", a spillover effect, is seen in the IVUS image because the intimal layer reflects ultrasound more strongly than the media. This results in a slight overestimation of the thickness of the intima and a corresponding underestimation of the medial thickness. On the other hand, the media/adventitia border is accurately rendered, because a step-up in echo reflectivity occurs at this boundary and no blooming appears. The adventitial and periadventitial tissues are similar enough in echoreflectivity that a clear outer adventitial border cannot be defined.

Several deviations from the classic three-layered appearance are encountered in clinical practice. The echoreflectivity of the intima and internal lamina may not be sufficient to resolve a clear inner layer in truly normal coronary arteries from young patients. This is particularly true when the media has a relatively high content of elastin. However, most adults seen in the cardiac catheterization laboratory have enough intimal thickening to show a three-layered appearance, even in angiographically normal segments. At the other extreme, patients with a significant plaque burden have thinning of the media underlying the plaque. As a result, the media is often indistinct or undetectable in at least some part of the IVUS cross-section. This problem is exacerbated by the blooming phenomenon. Even in these cases, however, the inner adventitial boundary (at the level of the external elastic lamina) is always clearly defined. For this reason, most IVUS studies measure and report the plaque-plus-media area as a surrogate measure for plaque area alone. The addition of the media represents only a tiny percentage increase in the total area of the plaque.

The determination of the position of the imaging plane within the artery is one important aspect of image interpretation. For example, an IVUS beam penetrates beyond the coronary artery, providing images of perivascular structures, including the cardiac veins, myocardium and pericardium (Figs 4A to C). These structures provide useful landmarks regarding the position of the imaging plane because they have a characteristic appearance when viewed from various positions within the arterial tree. The branching patterns of the arteries are also distinctive and help to identify the position of the transducer. In the left anterior descending (LAD) coronary artery system, for example, the septal perforators usually branch at a wider

angle than the diagonals. On the IVUS scan, the septals appear to bud away from the LAD much more abruptly than the diagonals (Figs 5A to D). The branching pattern and perivascular landmarks, once understood, can provide a reference to the actual orientation of the image in space.

IVUS MEASUREMENTS

The IVUS images have an intrinsic distance calibration, which is usually displayed as a grid in the image. Electronic caliper (diameter) and tracing (area) measurements can be performed at the tightest cross-section, as well as at reference segments located proximal and distal to the lesion.

In everyday clinical practice, where accurate sizing of devices is needed, vessel and lumen diameter measurements are important. The maximum and minimum diameters (i.e. the major and minor axes of an elliptical cross-section) are the most widely used dimensions. The ratio of maximum to minimum diameter defines a measure of symmetry. Area measurements are performed with computer planimetry; lumen area is determined by tracing the leading edge of the blood/intima border, whereas vessel or external elastic membrane (EEM) area is defined as the area enclosed by the outermost interface between media and adventitia. Plaque area or plaque-plus-media area is calculated as the difference between the vessel and lumen areas; the ratio of plaque to vessel area is termed percent plaque area, plaque burden or percent cross-sectional narrowing. Area measurements can be added to calculate volumes using Simpson's rule with the use of motorized pullback. In general, the investigator selects the most normal-looking cross-section (i.e. largest lumen with smallest plaque burden) occurring within 10 mm of the lesion with no intervening major side branches as the reference segment.[4]

TISSUE CHARACTERIZATION

The IVUS can provide detailed information about plaque composition. Regions of calcification are very brightly echo-reflective and create a dense shadow more peripherally from

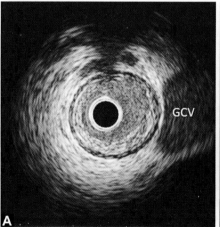
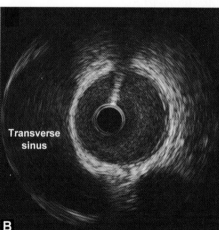
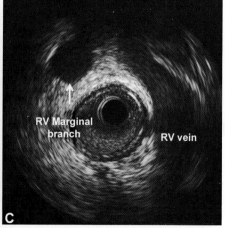

FIGURES 4A TO C: Perivascular landmarks: (A) The great cardiac vein (GCV), running superiorly to the left circumflex coronary artery (LCx), appears as a large, low-echoic structure with fine blood speckle. Recurrent atrial branches emerge from the LCx in an orientation directed toward the GCV, whereas the obtuse marginal branches emerge opposite the GCV and course inferiorly to cover the lateral myocardial wall. (B) In the proximal portion of the left main coronary artery, a clear echo-free space filled with pericardial fluid, called the transverse sinus, is found adjacent to the artery, immediately outside of the left lateral aspect of the aortic root. (C) At the level of the middle right coronary artery, the veins arc over the artery, typically at a position just adjacent to the right ventricular marginal branches

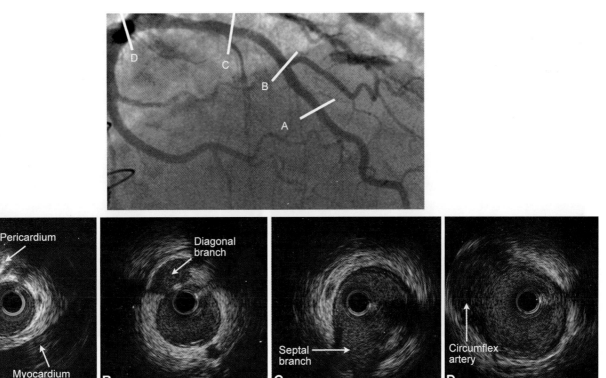

FIGURES 5A TO D: Pullback imaging sequence from mid to proximal portion of the left anterior descending (LAD) artery: (A) The mid and distal portions of the LAD often lie deeper in the sulcus than the proximal LAD and myocardium may be observed. The pericardium is seen at the opposite site of myocardium. (B and C) The septal branches emerge opposite to the pericardium, but the diagonal branches take off more superiorly. The angle between the septal and the diagonal branches usually increases to as much as 180 degrees. (D) The left circumflex artery emerges on the same side as the emergence of the diagonal branches

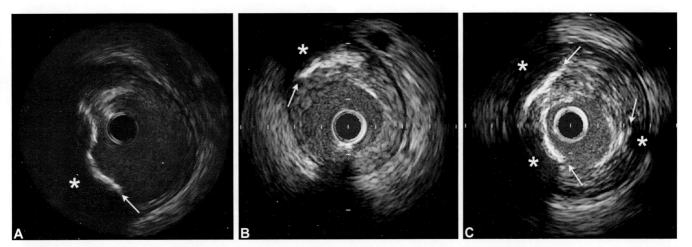

FIGURES 6A TO C: Examples of coronary calcification: (A) Superficial calcification is seen between 6 O'clock and 10 O'clock. The deeper vessel structure is obscured by the shadowing of the calcium layer (acoustic shadowing: asterisk). (B) Deep deposit of calcium is seen in a rim of fibrous plaque. (C) There are superficial and deep calcium deposits with acoustic shadowing

the catheter, a phenomenon known as "acoustic shadowing" (Figs 6A to C). Shadowing prevents determination of the true thickness of a calcific deposit and precludes visualization of structures in the tissue beyond the calcium. Reverberation is another characteristic finding with calcification. It causes the appearance of multiple ghost images of the leading calcium interface, spaced at regular intervals radially (Fig. 2D). Like calcium, densely fibrotic tissue appears bright on the ultrasound scan. Fatty plaque is less echogenic than fibrous plaque. The brightness of the adventitia can be used as a gauge to

discriminate between predominantly fatty from fibrous plaque. Therefore, an area of plaque that appears darker than the adventitia is fatty. In an image of extremely good quality, the presence of a lipid pool can be inferred from the appearance of a dark region within the plaque (Figs 7A and B). Furthermore, the "hot" lesions like ruptured plaques responsible for unstable angina or acute coronary syndromes can be observed by IVUS (Figs 8A and B).

Recently, the clinical impact of attenuated plaques characterized as hypoechoic plaque with ultrasound attenuation

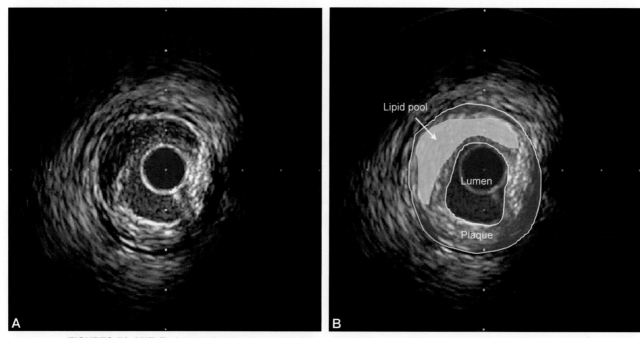

FIGURES 7A AND B: Atherosclerotic plaque with lipid pool. Lipid pool is defined as an echolucent area within the plaque and observed at 8-2 O'clock in this IVUS image

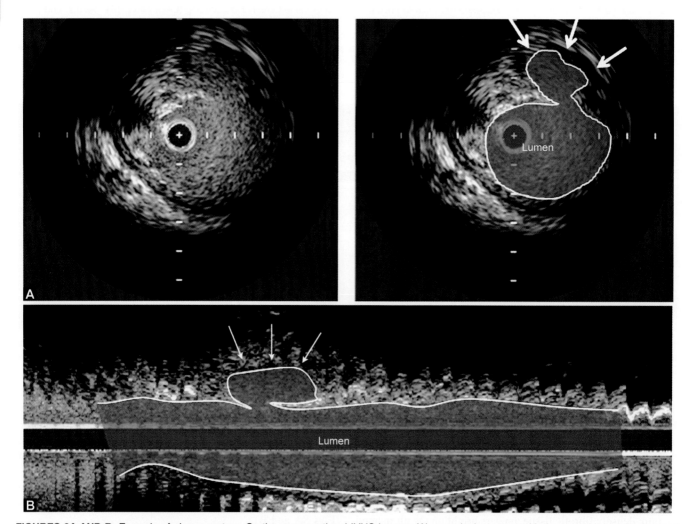

FIGURES 8A AND B: Example of plaque rupture. On the cross-sectional IVUS images (A), a cavity in contact with the vessel lumen is observed. The longitudinal IVUS image (B) shows a spatial representation of the plaque rupture. The rupture occurs in an eccentric plaque and has a residual thin flap that probably corresponds to a thin fibrous cap

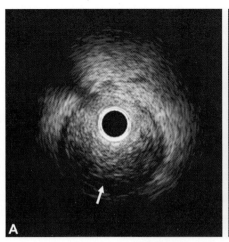 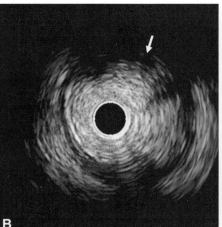 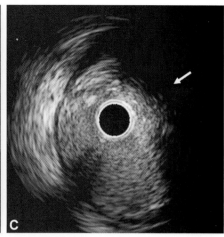

FIGURES 9A TO C: Examples of attenuated plaques. Attenuated plaque was defined as plaque with deep ultrasonic attenuation despite absence of bright calcium

despite little evidence of calcium has been reported (Figs 9A to C). These specific plaques are more often seen in patients with acute coronary syndromes than in those with stable angina and are characterized by positive remodeling and nearby calcification.[5] Clinical studies have indicated that attenuated plaques are associated with no reflow and creatine kinase-MB elevation after PCI because of distal embolization.[6,7] This novel defined plaque may contain microcalcification, thrombus or cholesterol crystals.[8]

Visual interpretation of conventional grayscale IVUS images is limited in the detection and quantification of specific plaque components. Therefore, computer-assisted analysis of raw radiofrequency (RF) signals in the reflected ultrasound beam has recently been developed (Figs 10A to C). Virtual Histology™ (VH) IVUS (Volcano Corporation, Rancho Cordova, California,) is recognized as the first commercialized RF analysis technology. A classification algorithm developed from ex vivo human coronary data sets can generate color-mapped images of the vessel wall with a distinct color for each category: fibrous, necrotic, calcific and fibro-fatty.[9] Another mathematical technique used in RF ultrasound backscatter analysis is Integrated Backscatter (IB) IVUS (YD Corporation, Nara, Japan). This method utilizes IB values, calculated as the average power of the backscattered ultrasound signal from a sample tissue volume. The IB-IVUS system constructs color-coded tissue maps, providing a quantitative visual readout as four types of plaque composition: calcification, fibrosis, dense fibrosis and lipid pool.[10] Similar to these RF-based tissue characterization techniques, iMap™ (Boston Scientific Inc, Natick, Massachusetts) has recently been introduced as an up-to-date tissue characterization method that is compatible with the latest 40-MHz mechanical IVUS imaging system (as opposed to VH-IVUS with 20-MHz solid-state IVUS system). The iMap allows identification and quantification of four different types of atherosclerotic plaque components: fibrotic, necrotic, lipidic and calcified tissues with accuracies at the high level of confidence (95%, 97%, 98% and 98% for fibrotic, necrotic, lipidic and calcified tissues, respectively).[11] Recently, multiple investigators have been trying to elucidate the clinical utility of RF analysis technology, particularly for prediction of future adverse coronary events. Providing regional

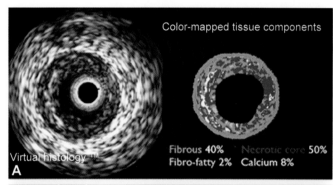

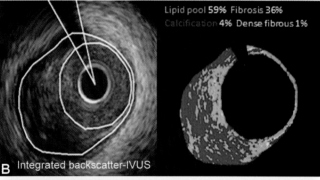

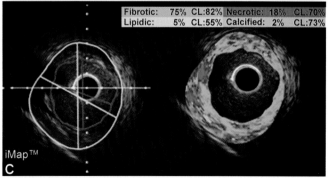

FIGURES 10A TO C: Color-mapped images of the coronary plaque. Conventional grayscale IVUS images (left). (A) Virtual Histology ™ shows a distinct color for each of the fibrous, necrotic, calcific and fibro-fatty. (B) Integrated Backscatter-IVUS can provide a quantitative visual readout as four types of plaque composition: calcification, fibrous, dense fibrosis and lipid pool. (C) iMap™ allows identification of four different types of plaque components (fibrotic, necrotic, lipidic and calcified tissue) with a confidence level assessment of each plaque component. (*Source:* Figure A Dr Kenji Sakata)

CHAPTER 20

Intravascular Coronary Ultrasound and Beyond

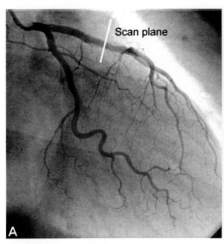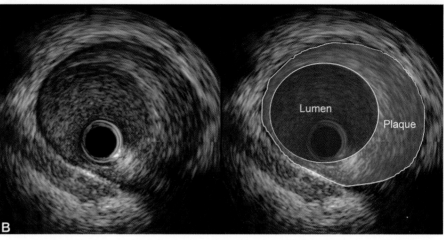

FIGURES 11A AND B: Angiographically silent disease: (A) An angiogram of the left coronary artery suggests minimal disease. (B) IVUS images show significant eccentric plaque. The lumen is well preserved, round and regular, accounting for the benign angiographic appearance

observations to study predictors of events in the coronary tree (PROSPECT) trial is one of the largest natural history trials to employ three-vessel imaging with VH-IVUS in 700 acute coronary syndrome patients. Multivariate analysis identified VH-IVUS determined thin-cap fibroatheroma (TCFA) (common type of vulnerable plaque defined as the presence of a confluent, necrotic core greater than 10% of plaque in contact with lumen at more than 30 degrees) at baseline as one of the independent predictors of future cardiac events (cardiac death, cardiac arrest, myocardial infarction, unstable angina or increasing angina) (HR = 3.35, P <0.001).[12]

INSIGHTS INTO PLAQUE FORMATION AND DISTRIBUTION

Some of the classic pathologic findings in arterial disease have been "rediscovered" *in vivo* by IVUS. In a vessel that appears to have a discrete stenosis by angiography, IVUS almost invariably shows considerable plaque burden throughout the entire length of the vessel (Figs 11A and B). In fact, IVUS studies have shown that the reference segment for an intervention which by definition is normal or nearly normal angiographically has, on average, 35–51% of its cross-sectional area occupied by plaque.

The phenomenon of remodeling, first described in human coronary specimens by the pathologist Glagov, is well illustrated *in vivo* by IVUS (Figs 12A and B).[13,14] The IVUS studies have also added to the original descriptions in the pathology literature by demonstrating that the remodeling response is in fact bidirectional, with some segments showing the positive remodeling of the typical Glagov paradigm and others showing negative remodeling, or constriction, in the area of lumen stenosis (Figs 12A and B).[14] One important issue in evaluating this heterogeneous process by IVUS is the methodology used to quantify and categorize arterial remodeling. Although remodeling was originally conceptualized as a change in vessel size in response to plaque accumulation over time, most histomorphometric or IVUS studies have relied on measurements of reference sites as a surrogate for the size of the vessel before it became diseased. Therefore, results can vary distinctly according to the choice of reference site as well as the manner of addressing vessel tapering.[15] Theoretically, the use of the

proximal reference, rather than the distal reference or the average of proximal and distal references, should preclude the potential influence of distal flow and pressure disturbance due to the presence of the IVUS catheter in the stenotic site. A remodeling index (the ration of vessel area at the lesion site to that at the reference site) as a continuous variable may also be preferable to categorical classifications, because arterial remodeling is considered to be a continuous biologic process. In fact, this remodeling index has been shown to conform to the normal frequency distribution in patients with chronic stable angina.[16] The assessment of remodeling is clinically important, not only for optimal therapeutic device sizing but also for risk stratification regarding plaque rupture or evaluating procedural and long-term outcomes of intervention. The vulnerable lesions responsible for acute coronary syndromes have usually undergone extensive positive remodeling. A histopathologic study by Pasterkamp and his colleagues supported these clinical IVUS observations by demonstrating that positive remodeling is frequently associated with large, soft, lipid-rich plaques with increased inflammatory cell infiltrate.[17] One IVUS study reported an association between preinterventional positive remodeling and creatine kinase elevation after intervention—a marker of distal embolization and future adverse cardiac events.[18] Furthermore, other investigators directly showed that preinterventional positive remodeling assessed by IVUS predicts target lesion revascularization after coronary interventions.[19] Although the predictive values of these parameters in the context of stenting have not been established with certainty, preinterventional IVUS may identify lesions with significant positive remodeling, providing triage information for increased risk of unfavorable outcomes and possible need of adjunctive biologic modalities for antirestenosis therapy in specific patients.

INTERVENTIONAL APPLICATIONS

According to the 2005 American College of Cardiology/ American Heart Association/Society for Cardiovascular Angiography and Interventions (ACC/AHA/SCAI) 2005 Guideline Update for PCI, it is reasonable to use IVUS: (a) to assess the adequacy of coronary stent deployment, including the extent of apposition and minimum luminal diameter within the stent; (b) to determine the cause of stent restenosis and guide

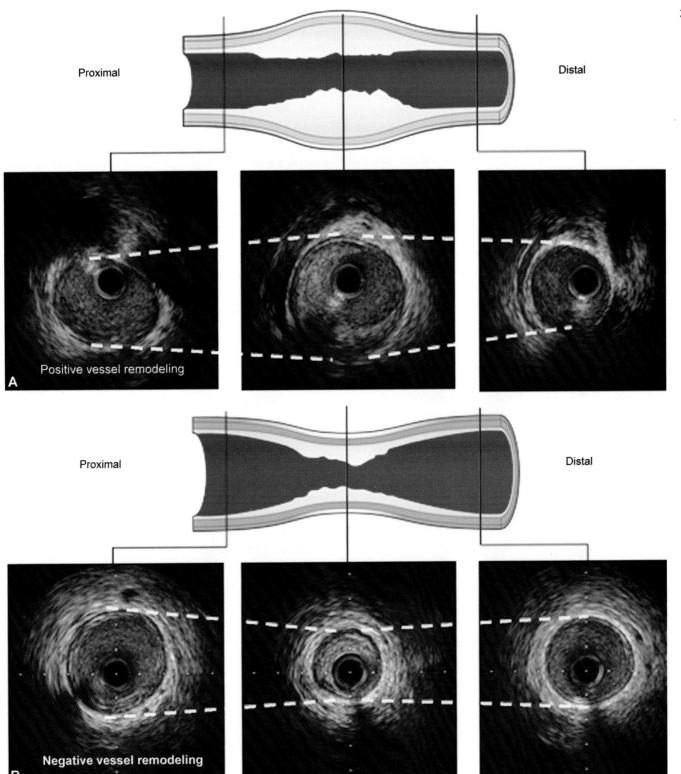

FIGURES 12A AND B: IVUS images showing remodeling: (A) Positive remodeling with localized expansion of the vessel in the area of plaque accumulation. (B) Negative remodeling or shrinkage where the lesion has a smaller media-to-media diameter than the adjacent less diseased sites

selection of appropriate therapy; (c) to evaluate coronary obstruction in a patient with a suspected flow-limiting stenosis when angiography is difficult because of location and (d) to assess a suboptimal angiographic result after PCI.[20] In addition, not only after PCI but also before PCI, IVUS is a useful application to assess lesion characteristics.

PREINTERVENTIONAL IMAGING

Preinterventional IVUS has been used to clarify situations in which angiography is equivocal or difficult to interpret (especially in ostial lesions or tortuous segments in which the angiogram may not lay out the vessel well for interpretation).

CHAPTER 20

Intravascular Coronary Ultrasound and Beyond

In addition, intermediate coronary lesions identified by angiography (40–70% angiographic stenosis) represent a challenge for revascularization decision-making. Although anatomic evaluation does not provide direct estimation of hemodynamic significance of a given coronary lesion, minimum lumen area (MLA) measured by IVUS demonstrated good correlation with results from physiologic assessment. The ischemic MLA threshold is 3.0–4.0 mm^2 for major epicardial coronary arteries,[21,22] and 5.5–6.0 mm^2 for the left main coronary artery,[23] based on physiologic assessment with coronary flow reserve, fractional flow reserve or stress scintigraphy.

Validated fractional flow reserve data have shown that deferring interventions in lesions with intermediate severity that are not considered hemodynamically significant (> 0.8 mm^2) have a favorable clinical prognosis.[24] Similarly, patients with intermediate coronary lesions in whom intervention was deferred based on IVUS findings (MLA >4.0 mm^2) showed that the rate of the composite endpoint was only 4.4% and target lesion revascularization 2.8%.[25] As a result, IVUS imaging appears to be an acceptable alternative to physiological assessment in patients presenting with intermediate coronary lesions.

Preinterventional IVUS imaging is also useful in determining the appropriate catheter-based intervention strategy. With current IVUS catheters, most of the significant stenoses can be safely imaged before intervention providing detailed information about the circumferential and longitudinal extent of plaque as well as the character of the tissue involved. This can lead to a change in interventional strategy in 20–40% of cases.[26,27] In particular, the presence, location and extent of calcium can significantly affect the results of balloon angioplasty, atherectomy and stent deployment. The amount and distribution of plaque can be accurately determined and may favor atheroablative procedures as primary or adjunctive

treatment. Precise measurements of lesion length and vessel size can guide the optimal sizing of devices to be employed. Detailed assessment of target lesion anatomy in the coronary tree is also useful to prevent major side branch encroachment by intervention.

BALLOON ANGIOPLASTY

The IVUS imaging of percutaneous transluminal coronary angioplasty (PTCA) sites demonstrates plaque disruption or dissection more often than angiography does (40–70% of cases versus 20–40% by angiography).[28,29] The IVUS is able to characterize the depth and extent of dissections created by balloon inflation with relatively high accuracy. Although the extent of dissections is relatively unpredictable, it is frequently possible to predict where tears will occur, based on certain morphologic features shown by IVUS. If a plaque deposit is eccentric, tears usually occur at the junction between the plaque and the normal wall (Figs 13A and B). This is presumably because the non-diseased wall is more elastic than the plaque, and, with balloon inflation, it stretches away from the plaque, creating a cleavage plane running either within the media or within the plaque substance, close to the media. Another important factor in determining the location of tears is the presence of localized calcium deposits. During balloon inflation, shear forces are highest at the junction between the calcium and the softer, surrounding plaque. This creates an "epicenter" for the start of a tear, which then extends out to the lumen. In lesions with localized calcification, cutting balloon angioplasty may be preferable, owing to its controlled tearing, to avoid the risk of unfavorable large dissections. Creating dissections in a controlled manner may also be beneficial to lessen acute elastic recoil after balloon angioplasty. Data from phase I of the GUIDE trial showed that lesions with tears had less recoil than lesions that had not torn, suggesting that plaque tearing may effectively

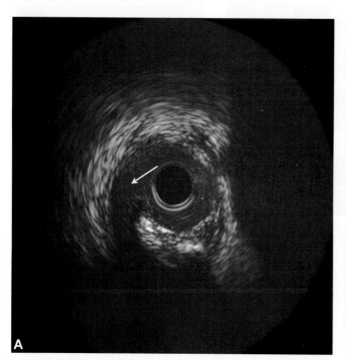
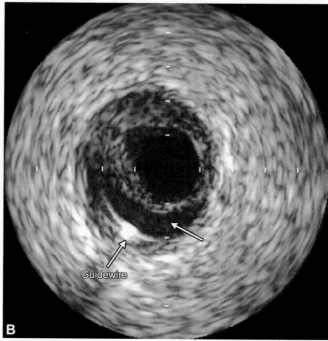

FIGURES 13A AND B: Examples of dissections: (A) A superficial dissection starts at 8 O'clock and extends counterclockwise. (B) Eccentric plaque with deeper dissection is seen between 4 O'clock and 9 O'clock. A guidewire is seen inside the cavity of dissection

act to release the diseased segment from the mechanical constriction process caused by the plaque.[28]

Guidance of Procedures

A direct approach to balloon sizing, based on IVUS images, was pursued by the Clinical Outcomes with Ultrasound Trial (CLOUT) investigators, who reasoned that more aggressive balloon sizing might be more safely accomplished using the "true" vessel size and plaque characteristics as determined by IVUS.[30] In this prospective, nonrandomized study, balloon sizes were chosen to equal the average of the reference lumen and media-to-media diameters for cases in which the plaques were not extensively calcified. This led to an average 0.5 mm "oversizing" of the balloon compared with sizing based on standard angiographic criteria, and resulted in a significant decrease in post-procedure residual stenosis (from 28% to 18%). Importantly, there was no increase in clinically significant complications from this aggressive balloon sizing approach. One-year follow-up of this trial showed a late adverse event rate (death, myocardial infarction or target lesion revascularization) of 22%.[31] This IVUS-guided aggressive PTCA strategy was expanded and confirmed by two single-center studies of provisional stenting, wherein balloon sizing was performed based on IVUS measurements of media-to-media diameter at the lesion site.[32,33] Angiographic or clinical follow-up of these studies also showed long-term outcomes equivalent to those of elective stenting.

BARE METAL STENT IMPLANTATION

The IVUS clearly visualizes stent struts as bright, distinct echoes. Stents essentially provide a rigid scaffold against the force of vessel recoil. During stent implantation, axial extrusion of noncalcified plaque into the adjacent reference zones can occur.[34] However, commensurate with the ability of the stent to enlarge and hold open the treated segment, the extrusion effect in stenting may be more prominent than for balloon angioplasty. Extrusion of plaque may also contribute to the step-up/step-down appearance on angiography, as well as some of the side branch encroachment seen after stent deployment.

Guidance of Procedures

The IVUS has identified several stent deployment issues, including incomplete expansion and incomplete apposition (Figs 14A to C). Incomplete expansion occurs when a portion of the stent is inadequately expanded compared with the distal and proximal reference dimensions, as may occur where dense fibrocalcific plaque is present. Incomplete apposition (seen in 3–15% of stent cases) occurs when part of the stent structure is not fully in contact with the vessel wall, possible increasing local flow disturbances and the potential risk for subacute thrombosis in certain clinical settings. Tobis and Colombo developed the current high-pressure stent deployment technique after their collaboration in the early 1990s revealed an unexpectedly high percentage of these stent deployment issues.[35,36]

After stent implantation, tears at the edge of the stent (marginal tears or pocket flaps) occur in 10–15% of cases (Figs 13A and B).[37] These tears have been attributed to the shear forces created at the junction between the metal edge of the stent and the adjacent, more compliant tissue or to the effect of balloon expansion beyond the edge of the stent (the "dog-bone" phenomenon). Although minor nonflow-limiting edge

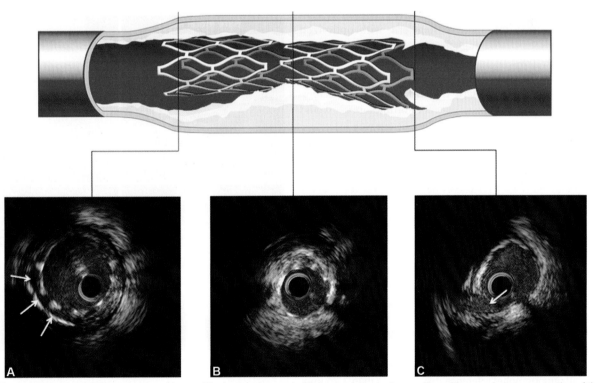

FIGURES 14A TO C: The IVUS-detected problems with stent deployment: (A) Incomplete stent apposition with a gap between a portion of the stent and the vessel wall between 6 O'clock and 10 O'clock. (B) Incomplete stent expansion relative to the ends of the stent and the reference segments. (C) An edge tear or "pocket flap" with plaque disruption at the stent margin

dissections may not be associated with late angiographic in-stent restenosis, significant residual dissections can lead to an increased risk of early major adverse cardiac events.[38] The current practice in our laboratory is to determine from the IVUS image whether the tear appears to be flow-limiting (i.e. whether there is an extensive tissue arm projecting into the lumen), and, if so, an additional stent is placed to cover this region.

Over the past decade, a number of studies have shown that IVUS-guided stent placement improves the clinical outcome of bare metal stents.[39–44] In the landmark trial, Multicenter Ultrasound-guided Stent Implantation in Coronaries (MUSIC) trial, three main IVUS variables were considered for assessing optimal stent deployment: (1) complete stent apposition over the entire stent length; (2) in-stent minimum stent area (MSA) greater than or equal to 90% of the average of the reference areas or 100% of the smallest reference area and (3) symmetric stent expansion with the minimum/maximum lumen diameter ratio greater than or equal to 0.7.[45] This study highlights that appropriate evaluation of stent deployment by IVUS impacts restenosis rate.

A subacute thrombosis rate of less than 2% was believed to represent a reduction compared with nonguided deployment, although, with current antiplatelet regimens, similar results can usually be achieved by high-pressure postdilation without IVUS confirmation. Nevertheless, a number of studies have suggested a link between suboptimal stent implantation and stent thrombosis, including the predictors and outcomes of stent thrombosis (POST) registry, which demonstrated that 90% of thrombosis patients had suboptimal IVUS results (incomplete apposition, 47%; incomplete expansion, 52% and evidence of thrombus, 24%), even though only 25% of patients had abnormalities on angiography.[46] In a more recent study by Cheneau and his colleagues, these observations were replicated suggesting that mechanical factors continue to contribute to stent thrombosis, even in this modern stent era, with optimized antiplatelet regimens.[47] Although the use of IVUS in all patients for the sole purpose of reducing thrombosis is clearly not warranted given the costs, IVUS imaging should be considered in patients who are at particularly high risk for thrombosis (e.g. slow flow) or in whom the consequences of thrombosis would be severe (e.g. left main coronary artery or equivalent).

The MSA, as measured by IVUS, is one of the strongest predictors for both angiographic and clinical restenosis after bare metal stenting.[48–50] Kasaoka and his colleagues indicated that the predicted risk of restenosis decreases 19% for every 1 mm^2 increase in MSA and suggested that stents with MSA greater than 9 mm^2 have a greatly reduced risk of restenosis.[49] In the can routine ultrasound improve stent expansion (CRUISE) trial, IVUS guidance by operator preferences increased MSA from 6.25 mm^2 to 7.14 mm^2, leading to a 44% relative reduction in target vessel revascularization at 9 months, compared with angiographic guidance alone.[42] In the angiography versus IVUS-directed stent placement (AVID) trial, IVUS-guided stent implantation resulted in larger acute dimensions (7.54 mm^2) than angiography (6.94 mm^2), without an increase in complications, and lower 12-month target lesion revascularization rates for vessels with angiographic reference diameter less than 3.25 mm, severe stenosis at preintervention (> 70% angiographic diameter stenosis), and vein grafts.[51] However, some IVUS-guided stent

trials produced controversial results,[52,53] presumably due to differing procedural end points for IVUS-guided stenting, and the various adjunctive treatment strategies that were used in these trials in response to suboptimal results. Overall, a meta-analysis of nine clinical studies (2,972 patients) demonstrated that IVUS-guided stenting significantly lowers 6-month angiographic restenosis [odds ratio = 0.75, 95% confidence interval (CI), 0.60–0.94; P = 0.01] and target vessel revascularization (OR = 0.62; 95% CI, 0.49–0.78; P = 0.00003), with a neutral effect on death and nonfatal myocardial infarction, compared to an angiographic optimization.[54]

Insights into Long-Term Outcomes

Intimal proliferation rather than chronic stent recoil primarily causes in-stent restenosis. Growth of neointima is usually greatest in areas with the largest plaque burden,[55] and the intimal growth process seems to be more aggressive in diabetic patients.[56] The IVUS can be helpful to differentiate pure intimal ingrowth from poor stent expansion in the treatment of in-stent restenosis (Figs 15A and B). Using serial IVUS immediately before and after balloon angioplasty for in-stent restenosis, Castagna and his colleagues[57] demonstrated in 1,090 consecutive in-stent restenosis lesions that 38% of lesions had an MSA of less than 6.0 mm^2. Even with minimal neointimal hyperplasia, stent underexpansion can result in clinically significant lumen compromise. For this type of in-stent restenosis, mechanical optimization is appropriate in most cases.

The IVUS can also track the response to treatment, with evidence that angioplasty of in-stent restenosis is followed by early lumen loss due to decompression and/or reintrusion of tissue immediately after intervention. This phenomenon was more prominent in longer lesions and in those with greater

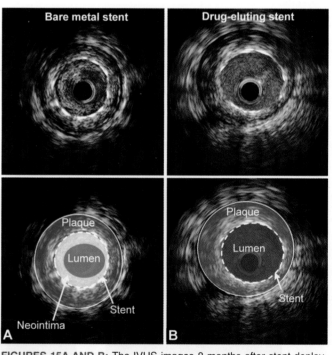

FIGURES 15A AND B: The IVUS images 8 months after stent deployment: (A) A conventional bare metal stent shows a considerable amount of neointima inside the stent. (B) In contrast, significant suppression of instent neointimal proliferation is observed when a drug-eluting stent was used

in-stent tissue burden, perhaps accounting for the worse long-term outcomes in diffuse versus focal in-stent restenosis. Direct tissue removal, rather than tissue compression/extrusion through the stent struts, may help minimize early lumen loss due to this phenomenon. Several investigators have reported a considerable reduction in angiographic and/or clinical recurrence of in-stent restenosis in patients with diffuse in-stent restenosis treated with ablative therapies (directional coronary atherectomy, rotational atherectomy or laser angioplasty) compared with PTCA alone.[58–60]

DRUG-ELUTING STENT IMPLANTATION

In current clinical experience, IVUS observations of antiproliferative drug-eluting stents (DES) have shown a striking inhibition of in-stent neointimal hyperplasia (Fig. 15). Thus, it comes as no surprise that since the introduction of DES, both the rate of restenosis and need for repeat revascularization have been dramatically reduced. Moreover, both statistical and geographic distributions of neointimal hyperplasia can be significantly different between biologic (DES) and mechanical (bare metal) stents, despite mechanical performances of DES being similar to those of conventional bare metal stents.[61] In general, neointimal volume (as a percentage of stent volume) within bare metal stents follows a near-Gaussian or normal frequency distribution, with a mean value of 30–35%. The standard deviation of this statistical distribution represents biologic variability in vascular response to acute and/or chronic vessel injury as a result of interventions. In contrast, biologic modifications through DES often result in a non-Gaussian frequency distribution, with variable degrees of the tail ends. Since restenosis corresponds to the right tail at the end of the distribution curve, a discrepancy between mean neointimal volume and binary or clinical restenosis can occur in DES trials. Similarly, bare metal stents show a wide individual variation in geographic distribution of neointima along the stented segment, whereas some types of DES demonstrate predilection of in-stent neointimal hyperplasia for specific locations (e.g. proximal stent edge). In serial IVUS studies with multiple long-term follow-ups, neointima within nonrestenotic bare metal stents showed mild regression after 6 months.[62] In contrast, both sirolimus- and paclitaxel-eluting stents showed a slight but continuous increase in neointimal hyperplasia for up to 4 years.[63–65]

Guidance of Procedures

The value of MSA remains as a powerful predictor for in-stent restenosis in the DES era.[66,67] A recent IVUS work by Sonoda and his colleagues demonstrated that sirolimus-eluting stents showed a stronger positive relation, with a greater correlation coefficient between baseline MSA and 8-month MLA, compared to control bare metal stents (0.8 vs 0.65 and 0.92 vs 0.59, respectively).[66] The utility of IVUS to ensure adequate stent expansion cannot be overemphasized, particularly if there are clinical risk factors for DES failure (e.g. diabetes, renal failure). In this context, preinterventional IVUS can provide useful information about plaque composition. In particular, calcified plaque is important to identify, because the presence, degree and location of calcium within the target vessel can substantially affect the delivery and subsequent deployment of coronary stents

(Fig. 6). One important advantage of online IVUS guidance is the ability to assess the extent and distance from the lumen of calcium deposits within a plaque. For example, lesions with extensive superficial calcium may require rotational atherectomy before stenting. Conversely, apparently significant calcification on fluoroscopy may subsequently be found by IVUS to be distributed in a deep portion of the vessel wall or to have a lower degree of calcification (calcium arc < 180 degrees). In these cases, stand-alone stenting is usually adequate to achieve a lumen expansion large enough for DES deployment.

The stent deployment techniques on clinical outcomes of patients treated with the cypher stent (STLLR) trial demonstrated that geographic miss (defined as the length of injured or stenotic segment not fully covered by DES) had a significant negative impact on both clinical efficacy (target vessel and lesion revascularization) and safety (myocardial infarction) at 1 year after sirolimus-eluting stent implantation.[68] These findings suggest that less aggressive stent dilation and complete coverage of reference disease may be beneficial, as long as significant underexpansion and incomplete strut apposition are avoided. Another single center study showed optimal stent longitudinal positioning of sirolimus-eluting stents using unique stepwise IVUS criteria (mainly targeting the sites with plaque burden < 50%). In this study, plaque burden in the reference lesion was the strongest predictor of stent margin restenosis.[69] Online IVUS guidance can facilitate both the determination of appropriate stent size and length and the achievement of optimal procedural end points, with the goal being to cover significant pathology with reasonable stent expansion while anchoring the stent ends in relatively plaque-free vessel segments. The efficacy of DES is related not only to the pharmacological (drug and polymer) kinetics but also to how well the stent is deployed within the coronary artery.

Insights into Long-Term Outcomes

Several large studies have assessed the impact of IVUS guidance during DES implantation on long-term clinical outcomes. In a single-center study of IVUS-guided DES implantation versus propensity score matched control population with angiographic guidance alone, a higher rate of definite stent thrombosis was seen in the angiography-guided group at both 30 days (0.5% vs 1.4%, P = 0.046) and 12 months (0.7% vs 2.0%, P = 0.014).[70] In addition, a trend was seen in favor of IVUS guidance in 12-month target lesion revascularization (5.1% vs 7.2%, P = 0.07). In addition, recent results of the revascularization for unprotected left main coronary artery stenosis: comparison of percutaneous coronary angioplasty versus surgical revascularization (MAIN-COMPARE) registry showed significantly lower 3-year mortality in the IVUS-guidance group as compared with the conventional angiography-guidance group (4.7% vs 16.0%, log-rank P = 0.048) in patients treated with DES.[71] Despite the growing evidence of the benefits of IVUS-guided DES implantation, few multicenter studies have been conducted to prove this hypothesis in a randomized controlled fashion. The Angiographic versus IVUS Optimization (AVIO) study was the first randomized trial designed to establish modern, universal criteria for IVUS optimization of DES implantation in complex coronary lesions.[72,73] This study proposed unique optimization criteria in which the target stent area was determined according to the size of a post-dilation, noncompliant balloon chosen on the basis of IVUS-measured media-to-media diameters at multiple different sites within the stented segment. Post-procedure minimum lumen diameter, as the primary endpoint of this study, was significantly larger in the IVUS-guided group, particularly when optimal IVUS criteria were met, with no increased complication as compared to the angiography-guided group (target IVUS criteria met: 2.86 mm, target IVUS criteria not met: 2.6 mm, angiography alone: 2.51 mm). Further studies with a larger population are required to determine whether this acute benefit in complex lesions can translate into improved long-term clinical outcomes.

Due to the low incidence of DES failure, clarification of its exact mechanisms awaits the cumulative analysis of large clinical studies. Nevertheless, suboptimal deployment or mechanical problems appear to contribute to the development of both restenosis and thrombosis. Particularly, the most common mechanism is stent underexpansion, the incidence of which has been reported as 60–80% in DES failures. In a study of 670 native coronary lesions treated with sirolimus-eluting stents, the only independent predictors of angiographic restenosis were postprocedural final MSA and IVUS-measured stent length (OR = 0.586 and 1.029, respectively).[67]

Recurrent restenosis after DES implantation for bare metal stent restenosis was also recently investigated using IVUS. In a series of 48 in-stent restenosis lesions treated with sirolimus-eluting stents, 82% of recurrent lesions had an MSA of less than 5.0 mm^2, compared with only 26% of nonrecurrent lesions (P = 0.003).[74] In addition, a gap between sirolimus-eluting stents was identified in 27% of recurrent lesions versus 5% of nonrecurrent lesions. These observations emphasize the importance of procedural optimization at DES implantation for both *de novo* and in-stent restenosis lesions.

Although published data on DES thrombosis are further limited, one single-center IVUS study reported stent underexpansion (P = 0.03) and a significant residual reference segment stenosis (P = 0.02) as independent multivariate predictors of sirolimus-eluting stent thrombosis (median time, 14 days after implantation).[75] The IVUS features of stent thrombosis from another single-center IVUS study appear analogous to the previous observations.[76]

For very late DES thrombosis (> 12 months), another investigator group has suggested incomplete stent apposition as a possible risk factor.[77] Late-acquired incomplete stent apposition with DES has been reported in both experimental (paclitaxel)[78] and clinical (sirolimus and paclitaxel) studies (Fig. 16).[79–82] Several IVUS studies have indicated that the main mechanism is focal, positive vessel remodeling (Figs 17A and B).[79,81] In addition, there is strong suggestion that incompletely apposed struts are seen primarily in eccentric plaques, and that gaps develop mainly on the disease-free side of the vessel wall. Thus, the combination of mechanical vessel injury during stent implantation and biologic vessel injury with pharmacologic agents or polymer in the setting of little underlying plaque may predispose the vessel wall to chronic, pathologic dilation (Figs 18A and B). Despite a recent meta-analysis suggesting an increased risk of late/very late stent thrombosis in patients with late-acquired incomplete stent apposition,[83] it remains

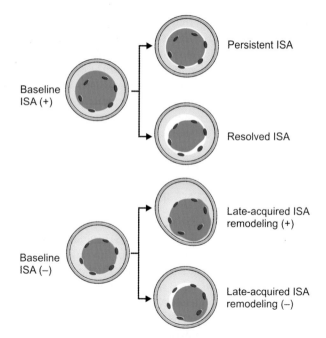

FIGURE 16: Classification of incomplete stent apposition (ISA). The ISA observed at follow-up is either persistent from baseline or late acquired. Late-acquired ISA without vessel remodeling is typically seen in thrombus-containing lesions, whereas late-acquired ISA with focal, positive vessel remodeling is more characteristic to drug-eluting stents

controversial whether this morphologic abnormality independently contributes to the occurrence of stent thrombosis.[84–86]

Other IVUS-detected conditions that may be of importance in DES include nonuniform stent strut distribution and stent fractures after implantation (Figs 19A and B). Theoretically, both abnormalities can reduce the local drug dose delivered to the arterial wall, as well as affecting the mechanical scaffolding of the treated lesion segment. By IVUS, strut fracture is defined as longitudinal strut discontinuity and can be categorized based upon its morphological characteristics: (1) strut separation; (2) strut subluxation or (3) strut intussusceptions (Fig. 20).[87] A recent IVUS study of 24 sirolimus-eluting stent restenosis cases identified the number of visualized struts (normalized for the number of stent cells) and the maximum interstrut angle as independent multivariate IVUS predictors of both neointimal hyperplasia and MLA.[88] In addition, angiographic or IVUS studies have reported the incidence of DES fracture as 0.8–7.7%, wherein in-stent restenosis or stent thrombosis occurred at 22–88%.[89] The exact incidence and clinical implications of strut fractures remain to be investigated in large clinical studies.

SAFETY

As with other interventional procedures, the possibility of spasm, dissection and thrombosis exists when intravascular imaging catheters are used. In a retrospective study of 2,207 patients, Hausmann and his colleagues identified spasm in 2.9% of patients, and other complications, including dissection, thrombosis and abrupt closure with "certain relation" to IVUS, in 0.4%.[90] Another multicenter European registry revealed 1.1% complications were reported (spasm, vessel dissection or guidewire entrapment) in a total of 718 examinations.[91] These studies were performed with first-generation catheters in the 1990s, and it is likely (although not documented) that the

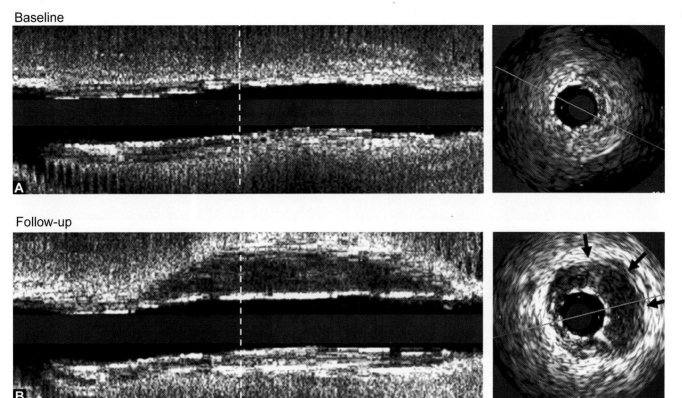

FIGURES 17A AND B: Serial IVUS images of late-acquired incomplete stent apposition: (A) Baseline IVUS shows excellent post-procedure results of a mid-left anterior descending coronary artery lesion treated with a drug-eluting stent. (B) At 6 months, focal increase in vessel size is observed in the longitudinal IVUS image (left). On the cross-sectional IVUS images (right), stent struts are separated from the vessel wall which was not seen at stent implantation

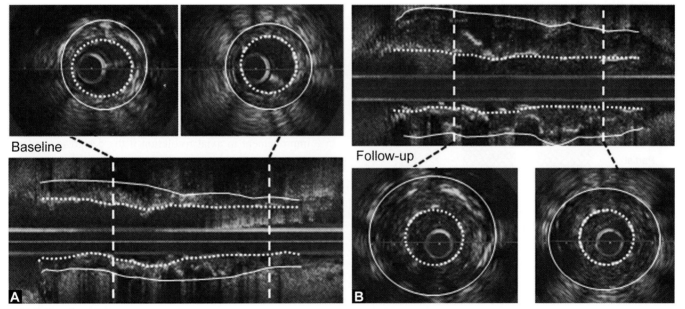

FIGURES 18A AND B: Positive vessel remodeling associated with very late stent thrombosis. Serial IVUS examination shows a significant increase in vessel size 3 years after stent deployment (dotted line: stent contour; solid line: vessel contour)

incidence of spasm and other complications is substantially lower with the current generation of catheters.

FUTURE DIRECTIONS

An interesting approach would be to combine IVUS with a therapeutic device, such as balloon catheter. In 2010, one angioplasty balloon catheter to integrate IVUS imaging (Vibe™

RX, Volcano Corporation, Rancho Cordova, California) gained CE-mark clearance in Europe. This new device can provide precise IVUS-guided balloon dilatation with immediate confirmation of interventional results without additional catheters or catheter exchanges.

Another interesting device iteration is "forward-looking" IVUS which can visualize the vessel wall in front of the imaging

Baseline

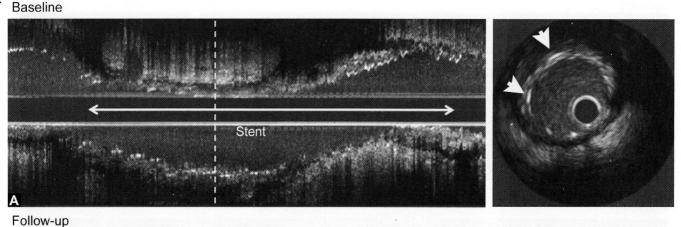

Follow-up

FIGURES 19A AND B: Stent strut discontinuity (fracture) observed 8 months after deployment. On the cross-sectional IVUS images (B, right), partial separation of the stent, not seen at implantation (A, right), is detected at a portion of the mid stent. The longitudinal IVUS image (left) shows an acute-angled bend at follow-up

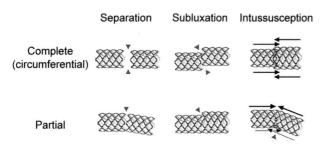

FIGURE 20: Classification of stent strut fracture. By IVUS, strut fracture is defined as longitudinal strut discontinuity and can be categorized based on morphological characteristics

catheter thereby having the potential to visualize the true and false lumens in chronic total occlusion (CTO) lesions. This enhanced visualization could be used to improve CTO crossing by continually maintaining and directing the catheter or wire toward the true lumen.[92]

Currently, commercially available IVUS catheters used in the coronary arteries have center frequencies ranging from 20 MHz to 45 MHz with the highest frequency IVUS being the 45 MHz Revolution™ IVUS catheter (Volcano Corporation, Inc., Rancho Cordova, California). In general, higher frequencies of ultrasound improve the axial resolution. On the other hand, higher frequency IVUS may result in stronger scattering echoes from the blood, hampering visualization of the vessel

lumen and thereby limiting the scanning depth. Therefore, IVUS frequencies higher than the current 45 MHz range IVUS may have inherent limitations. By overcoming these limitations, the next generation higher frequency IVUS catheter will enable better axial resolution (Figs 21A to C). Theoretically, an increase of center frequency from 40 MHz to 50 MHz corresponds to a 25% improvement in axial resolution if the design is similar.

OPTICAL COHERENCE TOMOGRAPHY

The principal technology was developed and first described by researchers at the Massachusetts Institute of Technology in 1991.[93] Since then, optical coherence tomography (OCT) has been applied clinically in ophthalmology, dermatology, gastroenterology and urology. Currently, intracoronary OCT has emerged as an *in vivo* optical microscopic imaging technology, as it generates real-time tomographic images from backscattered reflections of infrared light. Thus, the use of optical echoes by OCT can be regarded as an optical analog of IVUS, with its greatest advantage being its significantly higher resolution (10 times or greater) compared to conventional pulse-echo and other ultrasound-based approaches.

IMAGING SYSTEMS AND PROCEDURES

The imaging catheter includes a fiberoptic core with a microlens and prism at the distal tip to generate a focused scanning beam perpendicular to the catheter axis, thereby providing circumferential imaging of the arterial wall. In standard OCT systems,

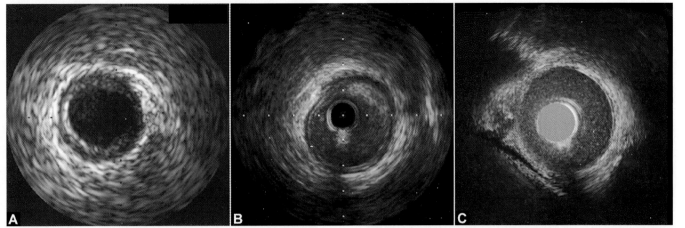

| 20 MHz | 40 MHz | 60 MHz |

FIGURES 21A TO C: Comparing variable frequency IVUS images. Higher frequency IVUS can produce improved image quality due to higher resolution (60 MHz IVUS image). (*Source:* Silicon Valley Medical Instrument, Inc., CA)

the optical engine includes a superluminescent diode as a source of low coherent, infrared light, typically with a wavelength around 1300 nm. The first commercialized intravascular OCT device (St. Jude Medical, Inc. St. Paul, Minnesota) consisted of a guidewire-based imaging catheter with a profile of 0.014 inches, a proximal low-pressure occlusion balloon catheter, and a system console containing the optical imaging engine and computer for signal acquisition, analysis and image reconstruction. The imaging procedure of intravascular OCT is similar to that of IVUS except that blood must be displaced by saline or contrast medium while imaging. Technically, this is because the dominant mode of signal attenuation in OCT is multiple scattering, so that additional scattering by red blood cells results in very large signal loss (Fig 22B). During OCT image acquisition, blood flow is interrupted by inflating the balloon with a modest amount of liquid flush from the distal flush exit ports of the occlusion catheter. The balloon inflation is performed at a low pressure to avoid unnecessary vessel stretching. Although this first generation intravascular OCT system was not approved by the United States Food and Drug Administration, the Fourier-domain OCT system (the so-called second generation OCT system) (St. Jude Medical, Inc.) was approved in 2010. Other companies have been developing similar rapid-scan OCT systems, referred to as optical frequency-domain imaging (OFDI). This technique measures

optical echo time delay using a light source whose light output can be rapidly swept over a range of wavelengths (e.g. 1,260–1,360 nm). Fourier transform techniques enable conversion of the frequency-domain (or wave length dependent) data to be converted to a time-domain representation. While first generation OCT (time-domain OCT) systems have a frame rate of 4–20 frames/sec, the Fourier/frequency-domain OCT achieves 80–110 frames/sec acquisition, allowing comprehensive scanning of long arterial segments during one bolus flush through the guide catheter without the need for occlusion. Since the OCT catheter has a short guidewire lumen at the distal portion of the catheter tip, the guidewire can be seen as a point artifact with shadowing (Figs 22A to D).

IMAGE INTERPRETATION

The higher resolution of OCT can often provide superior delineation of each structure compared with IVUS. The OCT can reliably visualize the microstructure (i.e. 10–50 μm, vs 150–200 μm for IVUS) of normal and pathologic arteries. Typically, the media of the vessel appears as a lower signal intensity band than the intima and adventitia, providing a three-layered appearance similar to that seen by IVUS (Figs 23A and B). Atheromatous lesions and fibrous plaques exhibit homogeneous, signal-rich (highly backscattering)

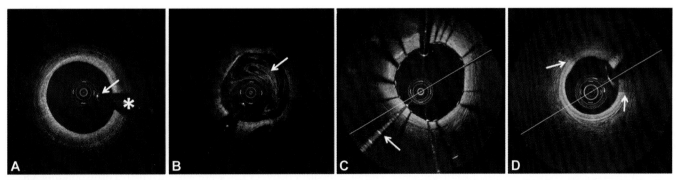

FIGURES 22A TO D: Common image artifacts: (A) A guidewire (arrow) produces a radial invisible part formed in the circumferential direction (asterisk). (B) Residual blood inside the vessel lumen causes deterioration of OCT image quality. (C) Highly reflective objects, like stent struts, can produce a series of ghost reflections that appear as a replica at a fixed distance away from the primary image of an object. (D) The silicone fluid gap inside the OCT catheter causes scatter of the light beam, casting a shadow in OCT image

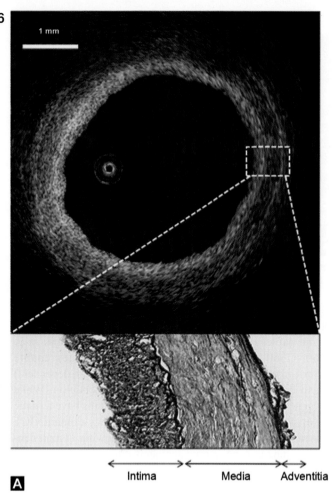

A

Intima | Media | Adventitia

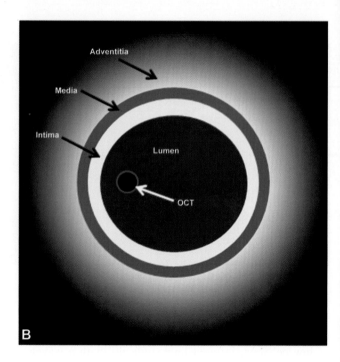

B

FIGURES 23A AND B: Example of cross-sectional image format of OCT. The bright-dark-bright, three-layered appearance is seen in the image with corresponding anatomy as defined. Histologic correlation with intima, media and adventitia are shown. The OCT shows the three layer appearance of normal vessel wall, with the muscular media being revealed as a low signal layer comprised between intima and adventitia

regions; lipid-rich plaques exhibit signal-poor regions (lipid pools) with poorly defined borders and overlying signal-rich bands (corresponding to fibrous caps); and calcified plaques exhibit signal-poor regions with sharply delineated borders (Figs 24A to C). The OCT has the advantage of being able to image through calcium without shadowing, as would be seen with IVUS. On the other hand, signal penetration through the diseased arterial wall is generally more limited (no more than 2 mm with current OCT devices), making it difficult to investigate deeper portions of the artery or to track the entire circumference of the media-adventitia interface. Plaque characteristics of OCT versus IVUS are listed in Table 2.

The diagnostic accuracy of OCT for the above plaque characterization criteria was confirmed by an ex vivo study of 307 human atherosclerotic specimens including aorta, carotid, and coronary arteries.[94] Independent evaluations by two OCT analysts demonstrated a sensitivity and specificity of 71–79% and 97–98% for fibrous plaques; 90–94% and 90–92% for lipid-rich plaques and 95–96% and 97% for fibrocalcific plaques, respectively (overall agreement vs histopathology, κ values of 0.88–0.84). The interobserver and intraobserver reproducibility of OCT assessment was also high (κ values of 0.88 and 0.91, respectively).

CLINICAL EXPERIENCE

In the first coronary OCT study in humans reported by Jang and his colleagues, 17 coronary segments in 10 patients were imaged with 3.2F OCT catheters (modified IVUS catheters) during intermittent saline flushes through the guide catheter.[95] The maximum penetration depth of OCT imaging measured 1.25 mm versus 5 mm for IVUS. *In vivo* axial resolutions, determined by measuring the full-width half-maximum of the first derivative of a single axial reflectance scan at the surface of the tissue, were 13 ± 3 μm with OCT versus 98 ± 19 μm with IVUS. All fibrous plaques, macrocalcifications and echolucent regions identified by IVUS were visualized in corresponding OCT images. Intimal hyperplasia and echolucent regions, which may correspond to lipid pools, were identified more frequently by OCT than by IVUS.

TABLE 2

Plaque characteristics of OCT versus IVUS

Tissue type	OCT	IVUS
Fibrous	Homogeneous	Homogeneous
	Signal-rich (highly backscattering)	High echogenicity
Calcium	Sharply delineated borders	Very high echogenicity
	Signal-poor	Shadowing
Lipid	Poorly defined borders Signal-poor	Low echogenicity

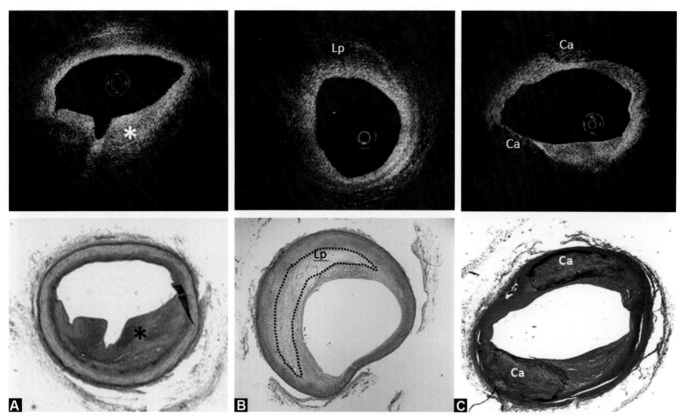

FIGURES 24A TO C: The OCT images (top) and corresponding histology (bottom) for (A) lipid-rich, (B) fibrous and (C) calcific plaques. In fibrous plaques, the OCT signal is observed to be strong and homogenous (asterisk). In comparison, both lipid-rich (Lp) and calcific (Ca) regions appear as a signal-poor region within the vessel wall. Lipid-rich plaques have diffuse or poorly demarcated borders, whereas the borders of calcific nodules are sharply delineated (Histologic stainings: elastica van Gieson for left, hematoxylin and eosin for middle and right, respectively)

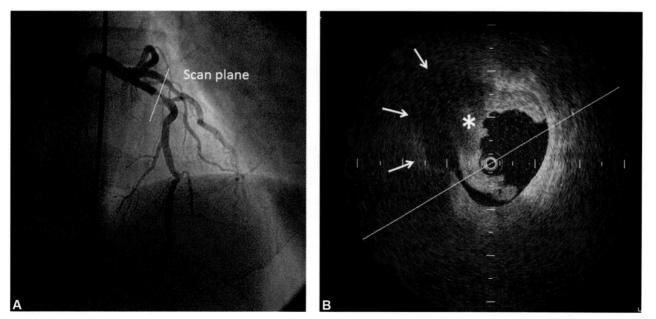

FIGURES 25A AND B: Culprit lesion in the left anterior descending (LAD) artery in a patient with unstable angina: (A) Coronary angiogram shows significant lumen narrowing at the proximal portion of LAD. (B) OCT clearly visualizes the protruded thrombus (asterisk) attached to the plaque rupture site (arrow)

In addition, recent clinical reports by the same investigator group showed that intravascular OCT detected lipid-rich plaques and thrombus more frequently in acute myocardial infarction or unstable angina than in stable angina lesions.[96] In a recent study using the first commercialized OCT system, Kubo and his colleagues reported that the plaque rupture and thrombus in patients with acute myocardial infarction were identified more frequently by OCT than by IVUS (73% vs 40%, P = 0.009, and 100% vs 33%, P < 0.001) (Figs 25A and B).[97]

Intravascular Coronary Ultrasound and Beyond

CHAPTER 20

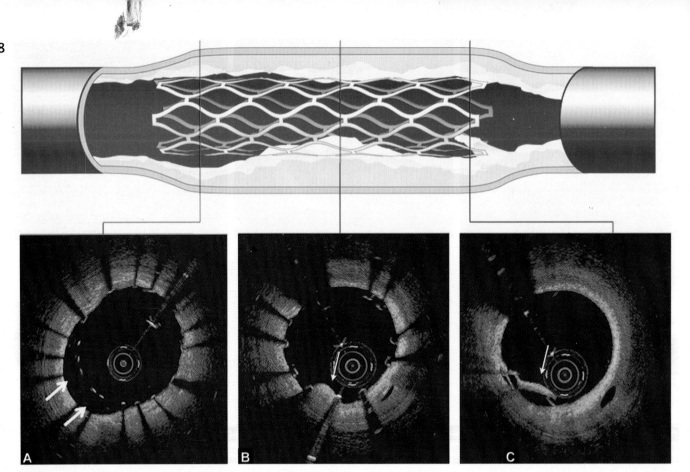

FIGURES 26A TO C: Stent deployment problems detected by OCT: (A) Incomplete stent apposition, in which there is a gap between a portion of the stent and the vessel wall between 6 O'clock and 10 O'clock. (B) Tissue prolapse between the stent struts at 6 to 7 O'clock. (C) An edge tear or "pocket flap" with a disruption of plaque at the stent margin

Encouraging preliminary results have been reported in the assessment of coronary interventions as well. Bouma and his colleagues successfully imaged 42 coronary lesions before and immediately after stenting.[98] In this series, OCT detected dissections, instent tissue prolapse and incomplete stent apposition more often than IVUS (Figs 26A to C). With a dedicated OCT catheter, Grube and his colleagues reported a follow-up OCT examination 6 months after drug-eluting stent implantation for the treatment of instent restenosis.[99] The high resolution of OCT allowed clear visualization of the overlapped stents (stent-in-stent), distinctly identifying each stent strut as well as a very thin neointimal layer covering the drug-eluting stent struts (Figs 27A and B). More recently, some investigator groups have reported that OCT images can visualize the thin neointima on each stent strut and quantify its thickness after drug-eluting stent implantation.[100,101] The OCT revealed the majority of stent struts were covered by a thin neointima layer less than 100 μm thick, which is beyond IVUS resolution capabilities, 6 months after sirolimus-eluting stent implantation.[100] In addition, Otake and his colleagues reported that subclinical thrombus after sirolimus-eluting stenting was significantly associated with longer stents, a larger number of uncovered struts, and greater average of neointimal unevenness score (maximum neointimal thickness in the cross section/average neointimal thickness of the same cross section).[102] Although the exact clinical impact of intravascular OCT findings requires systematic evaluation, these preliminary reports have confirmed

that this new imaging technology has the potential to provide a new level of anatomic detail, not only as a research technique but also as a clinical tool (Figs 28A to C). In fact, OCT has been used as a tool for evaluating neointimal proliferation after commercially available stents or newly developed stents in some multicenter trials.[103–106] OCT for DES SAfety (ODESSA) reported the frequency of uncovered stent struts at 6 months in overlapped segments (sirolimus-eluting stent, 8.7 ± 13.3%; paclitaxel-eluting stent, 8.3 ± 20.9%; zotarolimus-eluting stent, 0.05 ± 0.19%; bare metal stents, 1.8 ± 4.0%) and in non-overlapped segments (sirolimus-eluting stent, 7.9 ± 11.3%; paclitaxel-eluting stent, 2.3 ± 4.1%; zotarolimus-eluting stent, 0.01 ± 0.05%; bare metal stents, 0.5 ± 2.2%).[103] In the OCT in acute myocardial infarction (OCTAMI) study, uncovered stent struts were reported in 0.00% of zotarolimus-eluting stent and in 1.98% of bare metal stents (P = 0.13) 6 months after stent implantation in patients with ST-segment elevation myocardial infarction.[106]

DETECTION OF VULNERABLE PLAQUE

One of the most valuable challenges for OCT is its role in the detection of vulnerable plaque. OCT is often able to identify a thin fibrous cap of vulnerable plaque, the thickness of which (< 65 μm) is technically below the image resolution of IVUS (~ 150 μm). The TCFA, that is the primary plaque type at the site of plaque rupture, exists in nonculprit lesions and is

Bare metal stent

Drug-eluting stent

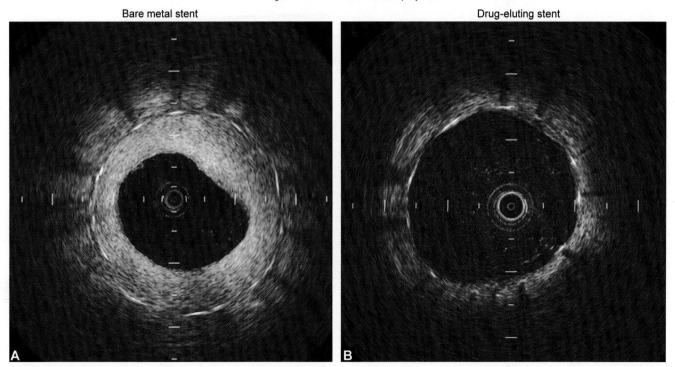

FIGURES 27A AND B: OCT images 8 months after stent deployment: (A) OCT visualizes the stent struts covered by a thick neointima that appeared as a bright luminal layer surrounding the stent struts after bare metal stent implantation. (B) The OCT shows stent struts and thin, bright reflective tissue coverage after drug-eluting stent implantation

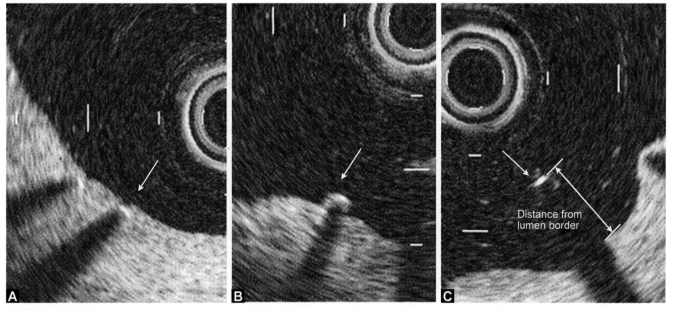

Distance from lumen border

FIGURES 28A TO C: Strut assessment by OCT in relation to the vessel wall. Due to a blooming effect of metal struts, the highest intensity point within the strut image should be used for the measurement. Strut apposition to the vessel wall is determined by measuring the distance from the stent strut surface to the vessel wall as compared to the nominal strut thickness (Nominal strut thickness; Cypher®, Cordis, Johnson and Johnson Co, Miami, FL; 154 µm, TAXUS Liberté®, Boston Scientific Inc, Natick, MA; 115 µm, Endeavor®, Medtronic, Santa Rosa, CA; 96 µm, Xience™V, Abbott Vascular, Santa Clara, CA; 89 µm)

distributed in all three coronary arteries. Fujii and his colleagues performed three-vessel OCT examination in patients with ischemic heart disease and showed that TCFAs tend to cluster in predictable spots within the proximal segment of the LAD artery yet develop relatively evenly in the left circumflex and right coronary artery.[107] These data were similar to prior histologic data indicating that TCFAs were concentrated in the proximal portions of the LAD artery and more uniformly distributed in the right coronary artery.[108] The unique capabilities of OCT as an investigational tool for high-risk lesions will serve the cardiology community well, as it advances us toward a better understanding and identification of vulnerable plaque

CHAPTER 20

Intravascular Coronary Ultrasound and Beyond

thereby improving our ability to more precisely treat our patients, both acutely and for the long term.

SAFETY AND LIMITATIONS

Since the biologic safety of applied energies in OCT has been well established in other medical fields, potential issues predominantly derive from the mechanical designs of intravascular devices (imaging catheters and flush delivery system) and transient ischemia during coronary imaging.

Preliminary experiences of first generation OCT system with both occlusive and nonocclusive images acquisition showed the technique to be safe. No major complications or arrhythmias were reported in a study of 60 patients examined using the non-occlusive technique.[109] Ischemic ECG changes were transient and occurred in 21 patients (35%), with ST depression in 17 (28%) and ST elevation in 4 (7%). Another multicenter study reported on the safety of the occlusive image acquisition technique in 76 patients with coronary artery disease. There were no significant procedural complications including ventricular tachycardia or ventricular fibrillation, acute vessel occlusion, dissection, thrombus formation, or vasospasm.[110] Second generation OCT systems have faster frame rates and can obtain a scan of up to 50 mm of a vessel within 3 seconds. Therefore, OCT images can be acquired with the smaller volume of flush in shorter pullback acquisition time without blood flow occlusion. A preliminary study reported the Fourier-domain OCT system had better safety results than the first generation time-domain OCT system.[111]

Although OCT has a higher image resolution than IVUS, OCT is not capable of studying tissue at a cellular level. Therefore, OCT cannot discriminate the different kinds of tissues covering stent strut (i.e. endothelium, smooth muscle cells, fibrin, etc.) after stent implantation.

FUTURE DIRECTIONS

One interesting aspect of OCT regarding in-depth plaque characterization is macrophage quantification in the fibrous cap of atherosclerotic plaques. This signal-processing technique is based on the hypothesis that macrophage-infiltrated caps may have a higher heterogeneity of optical refraction index, exhibiting stronger optical scattering with a higher signal variance than less infiltrated fibrous caps (Figs 29A and B). In an *ex vivo* study of 26 lipid-rich atherosclerotic arterial segments, Tearney and his colleagues compared the standard deviation of the OCT signal intensity with cap macrophage density quantified by immunohistochemistry.[112] Prior to analysis, the computation background and speckle noises were filtered out and the standard deviation was normalized by the maximum and minimum OCT signals in the image. There was a high degree of positive correlation between OCT and histologic measurements of fibrous cap macrophage density (r = 0.84, p < 0.0001). A range of OCT signal standard deviation thresholds (6.15–6.35%) yielded 100% sensitivity and specificity for identifying caps containing more than 10% CD68 staining. Based on this signal-processing technique, several clinical studies reported that macrophage density was significantly higher in vulnerable plaque features such as rupture sites or positive vessel

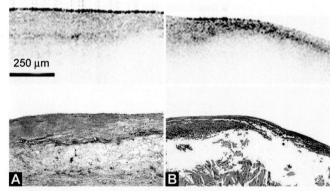

FIGURES 29A AND B: The OCT images (top) and corresponding histology (CD68 immunoperoxidase; original magnification 100X, bottom) of (A) a fibroatheroma with a low macrophage density within the fibrous cap and (B) a fibroatheroma with a high macrophage density within the fibrous cap. (*Source:* Tearney GJ, et al. Quantification of macrophage content in atherosclerotic plaques by optical coherence tomography. Circulation. 2003;107:113-9, with permission)

remodeling sites.[113,114] Despite direct visualization of individual mononuclear macrophages being limited with current intra-vascular OCT devices, advanced image-processing algorithms, as shown in these studies, may be of great utility in the assessment of plaque instability.

Spectroscopic analysis is another interesting assessment tool. It uses a spectrum of infrared light reflected from the structures to color code the information on tomographic images providing insights into the biochemical contents of the tissue. Polarization analysis, measuring the degree of birefringence in the tissue, may also be helpful in plaque component discrimination, since regions with highly oriented fibrous or smooth muscle cell components are more sensitive to the polarity of the imaging light than degenerated atheromatous regions with randomly oriented cells. The OCT Doppler and elastography are analogous to those of ultrasound-based approaches but may offer improved sensitivity, owing to higher resolution and contrast. In addition, viscoelasticity of the structure may be accurately assessed based on its intrinsic properties using laser speckle analysis.

ANGIOSCOPY

Intracoronary angioscopy is an endoscopic technology that allows direct visualization of the surface color and superficial morphology of atherosclerotic plaque, thrombus, neointima, or stent struts. In 1985, the first clinical experience of intracoronary angioscopy was reported[115] and since then, technical improvements have occurred resulting in image quality enhancement, catheter miniaturization and development of subselective catheterization systems. Although the Food and Drug Administration has not yet approved any coronary angioscopy system for use in the United States, clinical investigators worldwide have been using this unique diagnostic modality to provide considerable information in the pathophysiology of coronary lesions, particularly in the field of acute coronary syndromes.

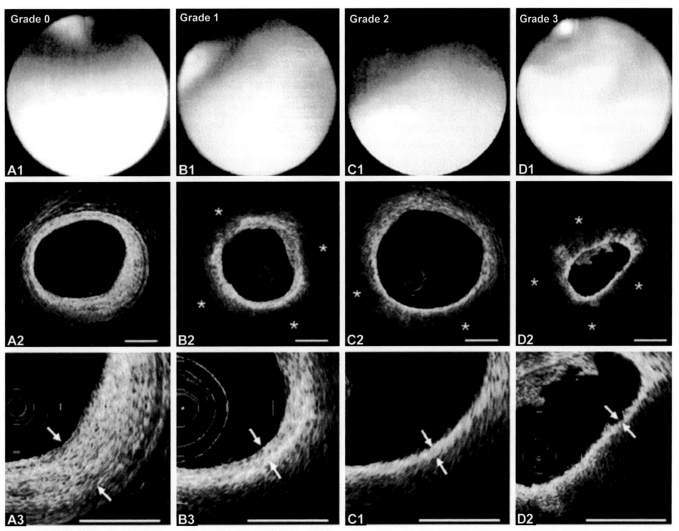

FIGURES 30A TO D: An example of yellow plaque grading by angioscopy and corresponding optical coherence tomography images. The surface color represents a lipid-rich core seen through a fibrous cap, and its intensity rises as the fibrous cap thins and becomes increasingly transparent (Top, grade 0 to 3). OCT has demonstrated that the fibrous cap is thinner in the more intensively yellow plaques (Bottom; enlarged images, scale bar; 1 mm). Thickness of the fibrous cap is indicated by the two arrows. (*Source:* Kubo T, et al. Implication of plaque color classification for assessing plaque vulnerability: a coronary angioscopy and optical coherence tomography investigation. JACC Cardiovasc Interv. 2008;1:74-80, with permission)

IMAGING SYSTEMS AND PROCEDURES

In general, intracoronary angioscopy consists of an external optical engine incorporating a light source and a charge coupled device (CCD) camera; a fiberoptic catheter for illumination and imaging; a subselective delivery catheter system and a video monitor with an image recording system. The light source emits a high-intensity white light to illuminate the target object through the fiberoptic catheter. The imaging catheter contains a flexible fiber optic bundle of several thousand pixels; the latest-generation catheter, which incorporates 6,000 fibers, is 0.75 mm in outer diameter with a microlens that provides a 70° field of view and a focused depth that ranges from 1 mm to 5 mm. Although conventional delivery systems are equipped with a distal balloon to create a blood-free field for optical imaging, an alternative system uses a smaller catheter to continuously flush an optically clear liquid in front of the angioscope tip for transient blood displacement.

IMAGE INTERPRETATION

Similar to gastrointestinal angioscopy, coronary angioscopic images are interpreted based on the surface color and endoluminal morphology of vessel walls or structures. The normal coronary artery surface appears as grayish white and smooth in contour without any protruding structure whereas atherosclerotic plaques can show varying degrees of yellowish color (Figs 30A to D) with or without visible irregularities of the luminal surface. The yellow plaque surface signifies a lipid-rich core seen through a fibrous cap, and the yellow intensity rises as the fibrous cap thins and becomes increasingly transparent. Dissections are characterized as visible cracks or fissures on the luminal surface and/or sail-like white protruding structures that can be loose or immobile inside the lumen. Intimal flaps are visualized as thin, faint, highly mobile fronds of white tissue. Both structures are generally contiguous and of similar appearance to the adjacent vessel wall. Thrombi are recognized as masses that are red, white or mixed in color, which adhere to the intima or protrude into the lumen. Red masses, not dislodged by flushing, are considered as fibrin/erythrocyte-rich thrombi, whereas white granular cotton-like appearances are characteristics of platelet-rich thrombi. Subintimal hemorrhage may be detected as distinct, demarcated patches of red coloration that are clearly within the vessel wall. To circumvent subjectivity of color interpretation, quantitative colorimetric methods have been proposed. The Ermenonville classification was established by a European coronary angioscopy working group, featuring several parameters, such as image quality, lumen diameter, surface color, atheroma, dissection and thrombus, graded in 3–5 categories.[116] In addition, κ values for chance-corrected intraobserver and interobserver agreement of diagnostic items were low at 0.51–0.67 and 0.13–0.29, respectively. On the other hand, the important items, such as red thrombus and dissection, were shown to have a good intraobserver and acceptable interobserver agreement when recorded more simply as either present or absent. Similarly, relatively simple classifications by other investigators resulted in good reproducibility.[117]

CLINICAL EXPERIENCE

Angioscopy has contributed valuable information of the underlying mechanisms of acute coronary syndromes. Angioscopically, most culprit lesions show occlusive or mural thrombi frequently overlying disrupted yellow plaque. The thrombi are predominantly white, but can turn into red or mixed once they become occlusive. On the other hand, the majority of ruptured plaques at the angiographically mild to moderate stenosis may remain subclinical.

The detailed healing process of infarct-related, disrupted plaques has also been evaluated in vivo by serial angioscopy. In a study by Ueda and his colleagues,[118] culprit lesions were examined immediately after PCI and/or thrombolysis and at 1, 6 and 18-month follow-up. Thrombus was detected in 93% at baseline and in 64% even 1 month after the onset of acute myocardial infarction, suggesting prolonged and persistent thrombogenicity at the culprit lesion. The prevalence of thrombus, however, markedly decreased at the following time points, accompanied by a significant reduction in visually graded yellow color intensity of the plaque. Interestingly, these stabilization processes were significantly impaired in patients with diabetes mellitus or hyperlipidemia.

Assessment of lesions before or after coronary intervention represents another commonly reported application of coronary angioscopy. One early study, for example, evaluated 122 patients undergoing conventional PCI and revealed that angioscopic thrombus was strongly associated with in-hospital adverse outcomes (either a major complication or a recurrent ischemic event) after PCI (relative risk, 3.11; 95% CI, 1.28–7.60; P = 0.01).[119]

Coronary angioscopy may significantly contribute to our understanding of new interventional devices or pharmacologic interventions as well. In coronary stenting, for example, several investigators have evaluated *in vivo* vessel response to bare metal stent implantation by serial angioscopy. Unlike animal models, these human studies suggested that, in some cases, several months may be required for visible completion of neointimal coverage over the metal struts. In-stent neointima became thick and nontransparent up to 6 months but completely disappeared by 3 years, indicating that functional neointimal maturation may require several months following stent implantation. A more recent study investigated the effect of stenting on infarct-related lesions as well.[120] At baseline, most lesions had complex morphology (96%) and yellow plaque color (96%), most of which still being observed even 1 month after stenting. At 6-month follow-up, the plaque shape and color mostly turned into smooth (97%) and white (93%), suggesting that stent implantation may lead to a sealing of unstable plaque with neointimal proliferation. Similar changes in plaque color have also been reported with lipid-lowering interventions.[121] As for drug-eluting stents, angioscopy revealed a difference in neointimal formation pattern between sirolimus- and paclitaxel-eluting stents.[122] In this study, paclitaxel-eluting stents showed more heterogeneous neointimal coverage and higher incidence of thrombus formation (70% vs 11%, P < 0.001) as compared with sirolimus-eluting stents at 18 months after stent implantation. The same investigator group reported similar results in a comparison to bare metal stents: paclitaxel-eluting stents showed the most heterogeneous neointimal formation and the highest incidence of thrombus formation at 6 months after stent implantation (50% in paclitaxel-eluting stent, 12% in sirolimus-eluting stent and 3% in bare metal stent, p < 0.001).[123]

Another investigator group reported that serial angioscopic examination immediately after the 10 months of sirolimus-eluting stent implantation (n = 57) showed significant increase in the yellow color grade of the stented lesion from baseline to follow-up.[124] Lesions with yellow color grade had significantly higher prevalence of thrombus than with white color grade (25% vs 5%, P < 0.01). These data may suggest that sirolimus-eluting stents promote formation of yellow plaque and is associated with an increased incidence of mural thrombus in stented lesions at 10 months follow-up.

DETECTION OF VULNERABLE PLAQUE

To date, a number of angioscopic studies have suggested that intensive yellow surface color of plaque is associated with unstable lesion morphology or clinical presentations. An early clinical study showed that yellow plaques were more common in patients with acute coronary disorders (50%) than in those with stable angina (15%) or old myocardial infarction (8%).[125] In a more recent study of 843 patients who underwent cardiac catheterization for suspected coronary disease, 1,253 yellow plaques were detected at nonstenotic (diameter stenosis < 50%) segments and were graded as 1–3 (from light to intensive yellow) using prespecified color samples.[126]

Pathophysiologic mechanisms for this association may be partly explained by structural and mechanical characteristics of yellow plaques. An experimental study using a bovine model of lipid-rich plaque showed an inverse correlation between angioscopic percent yellow saturation and histologic plaque cap thickness.[127] A similar correlation was also reported in a clinical study by comparing angioscopic surface colors and plaque cap thickness measured by OCT (Figs 31A to E).[128]

On the other hand, yellow surface color of individual plaques alone may not have a sufficiently high predictive value for future

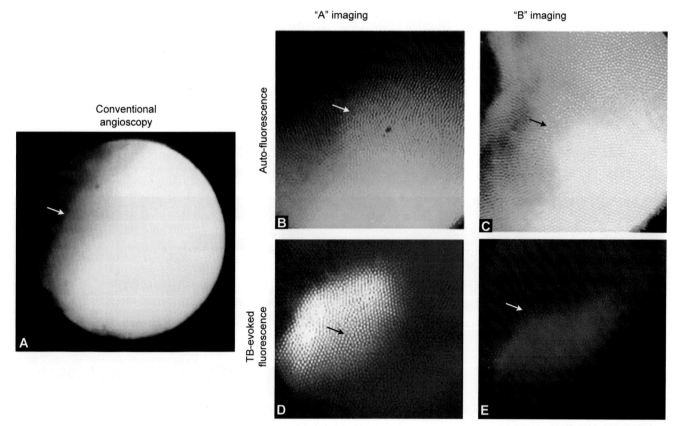

"A" imaging "B" imaging

FIGURES 31A TO E: Lysophosphatidylcholine in a coronary plaque imaged by a color fluorescence angioscopy system (CFA). (A) Yellow plaque imaged by conventional angioscopy. (B and C) The CFA image of the same plaque before administration of Trypan blue dye (TB). (D and E) The CFA images after administration of TB. The plaque showed red fluorescence by both "A" and "B" imaging, indicating the existence of lysophosphatidylcholine. (*Source:* Uchida Y, et al. Imaging of lysophosphatidylcholine in human coronary plaques by color fluorescence angioscopy. Int Heart J. 2010;51:129-33)

clinical events, presumably owing to the presence of "silent" plaque rupture as well as the need of additional factors for triggering the events. Uchida and his colleagues reported the first prospective 12-month follow-up study and found that acute coronary syndromes occurred more frequently in patients with yellow plaques than in those with white plaques.[129] Moreover, the syndromes occurred more frequently in patients with glistening yellow plaques than in those with nonglistening yellow plaques, but the positive predictive values of overall yellow and glistening yellow plaques were only 28% and 69%, respectively. More recently, Asakura and his colleagues performed extensive angioscopic examination of all three major coronary arteries in patients undergoing follow-up cardiac catheterization 1 month after myocardial infarction.[130] Both infarct-related and non-infarct related coronary arteries showed equally prevalent, multiple yellow plaques (3.7 ± 1.6 vs 3.4 ± 1.8 plaques per artery, respectively), indicating a pan-coronary process of vulnerable plaque development. Clinical follow-up (931 ± 107 days) of the enrolled patients showed a secondary event rate of only 20%. On this basis, the same investigator group proposed a plaque index (number of yellow plaques multiplied by maximum color grade) and found that patients who suffered another acute event during 5-year follow-up had a higher index at baseline than patients who did not (9.5 ± 6.8 vs 4.4 ± 4.0, P = 0.02). Although angioscopic examination of

the entire coronary tree is not practical in clinical settings, angioscopic plaque characterization has the potential to offer unique complementary information in the field of vulnerable plaque/patient investigation and risk stratification.

SAFETY AND LIMITATIONS

The light source of angioscopy provides a high intensity but "cold" light (low infrared content) to avoid thermal damage to the illuminated vessel wall. On the other hand, mechanical designs of the angioscope and its delivery catheter can significantly affect the safety profile of this invasive imaging tool. To date, several complications have been reported related to the occlusion cuff of the delivery catheter or transient ischemia owing to flow obstruction during imaging. Another complication is so-called wire-trapping caused by a loop formation of the guidewire between the two monorail wire channels of a particular angioscopy system. With the new over-the-wire system with no occlusion cuff, one experienced group reported a complication rate less than 1% during 1,200 procedures, but no comprehensive report of a large multicenter experience currently exists.

Despite recent technical advances, angioscopy is still limited in evaluating small vessel segments or imaging across tight stenoses. Other technical limitations include its limited

CHAPTER 20

Intravascular Coronary Ultrasound and Beyond

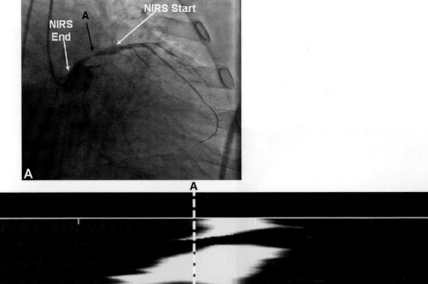

FIGURES 32A AND B: Near-infrared spectroscopy scan of a patient and corresponding angiogram. (A) Coronary angiogram of the left coronary artery of a 71-year-old man with post-infarct angina. There is a severe culprit stenosis (A) in the proximal left anterior descending artery. (B) the corresponding chemogram reveals a prominent, circumferential lipid core-containing coronary plaque signal between 8 mm and 18 mm in the area of the culprit lesion. The narrowest area of luminal stenosis is approximately 14 mm and demarcated in the chemogram (A). The block chemogram shows that the strongest lipid core-containing coronary plaque signals extended from 9–17 mm. (*Source:* Waxman S, et al. In vivo validation of a catheter-based near-infrared spectroscopy system for detection of lipid core coronary plaques. J Am Coll Cardiol Imag. 2009;2:858-68, with permission)

capability to assess inner tissue structures and the subjectivity of qualitative interpretation that potentially results in relatively large intraobserver and/or interobserver variability.

FUTURE DIRECTIONS

One technical solution to the subjective color interpretation is a quantitative colorimetric analysis of angioscopic images. In addition to the variability of lumen color perception, hardware-induced chromatic distortions can occur depending on angioscopic systems, individual catheters, illuminating light settings and spatial location of the object within the view field. Quantitative colorimetric methods measuring coronary plaque color after proper adjustment for brightness can overcome these limitations, and excellent measurement reproducibility with this technique has been reported in preliminary clinical studies.[131,132]

Molecular imaging of coronary plaques by fluorescence angioscopy is another interesting challenge. Fluorescence 'excited' through a specific band pass filter can visualize lysophosphatidylcholine, which is a major component of oxidized low-density lipoprotein and acts as a proatherogenic agent in the presence of trypan blue dye (Figs 32A and B).[133] If these molecular substances are visualized *in vivo* by using fluorescence angioscopy, more information can be acquired about the exact mechanisms of the progression of athero-sclerosis.

SPECTROSCOPY

Spectroscopy determines the chemical composition of plaque substances based on the analysis of spectra induced by interaction of electromagnetic radiation, or light, with the tissue materials. To date, several forms of photonic spectroscopy have been adapted for characterization of atherosclerotic plaques, including diffuse reflectance near-infrared (NIR), Raman and fluorescence spectroscopy. When tissues are exposed to a light beam containing a broad mixture (spectrum) of wavelengths, those wavelengths absorbed by the illuminated molecules will be missing from the spectrum of the original light after it has traversed the tissue. Diffuse reflectance NIR spectroscopy analyzes the amount of this absorbance as a function of wavelengths within the NIR window (700–2,500 nm). On the other hand, Raman spectroscopy uses a light beam of a single wavelength and monitors shifts in wavelength as some of the incident photons interact with the molecules so as to gain or lose energy (i.e. shift in wavelength). Raman spectroscopy measures this inelastic scattering, or so-called Raman scattering, since it contains unique information on the substance with which the photons interacted. Under certain conditions, the photons can excite molecules to a higher energy level, the decay from which releases the energy difference in the form of light. The Raman shift is more specific for individual chemicals than is diffuse NIR reflectance, but the signal is much weaker and therefore more difficult to detect in vivo.

Fluorescence spectroscopy uses photoluminescence or luminescent emission to identify the properties of the tissue being illuminated. Each technique has shown promising ex vivo results and is under active investigation for in vivo coronary applications.

IMAGING SYSTEMS AND PROCEDURES

Development of a catheter-based spectroscopy system for percutaneous coronary applications has faced several technical challenges. First, NIR light must be delivered to the artery and collected with minimal risk to the patient. Second, the undesirable effect of blood on the signal must be overcome. Third, the effect of coronary motion on spectra must be managed. Fourth, a scan of all major coronary arteries is needed for clinical use. One coronary catheter system overcame these problems and was approved by the United States Food and Drug Administration in 2008 (Intravascular Chemogram™, InfraReDx, Inc., Cambridge, Massachusetts). The 3.2F NIR catheter contains fiberoptic bundles for delivery and collection of light within a protective outer sheath. The rapid-exchange platform of the catheter enables advancement to the coronary segment of interest using a standard interventional technique, and can direct light to the vessel wall with a mirror, located at the tip, to acquire spectra within 20 milliseconds through flowing blood. This configuration allows not only circumferential data collection but also a complete longitudinal scan of the target segment using controlled pullback of the probe. The collected light is analyzed by a spectrometer; using a diagnostic algorithm, the processed data are color coded and displayed in a grid pattern with the spatial (circumferential and longitudinal) information. Signal acquisition is performed through a 6F guide catheter without the need for artery occlusion or blood displacement, and the process is similar in use to IVUS.

Although further improvement is still required prior to clinical testing, a miniaturized fiberoptic probe with a real-time analysis system has been developed for future intravascular application of Raman spectroscopy as well. The probe (Visionex, Atlanta, Georgia) consists of a central fiber (core diameter: 400 μm) for laser delivery and seven collection fibers (core diameter: 300 μm) around the central fiber. Both fibers have a dielectric filter to block the Raman signal generated by the fiber material. The system uses an 830 nm diode laser (Process Instruments Diode Laser, Salt Lake City, Utah) as a light source, and spectra acquisition times were reported to be 3–5 seconds for reliable detection of cholesterol and 1 second for calcium in an ex vivo setting. Although this prototype is a forward-viewing system, other investigators are also developing side-viewing catheter probes suitable for intravascular Raman scattering or fluorescence measurements.

EXPERIMENTAL DATA

Over the past decade, a number of experimental studies have reported the ability of biospectroscopy (reflectance, Raman and fluorescence) to identify the basic chemical components of atherosclerotic plaques in animal models or human arterial samples. Particularly, intensive efforts are now focused on the characterization of the specific features of plaque vulnerability. Using diffuse reflectance NIR spectroscopy, Moreno and his colleagues examined 199 human aortic samples and compared the findings with corresponding histology.[134] A diagnostic algorithm was constructed with 50% of the samples used as a reference set; blinded predictions of plaque composition were then performed on the remaining samples. The sensitivity and specificity of NIR spectroscopy for histologic plaque vulnerability were 90% and 93% for lipid pool, 77% and 93% for thin fibrous cap (< 65 μm), and 84% and 89% for inflammatory cell infiltration, respectively. Similar promising results of NIR spectroscopy to identify lipid-rich plaques have been reported in human carotid endoatherectomy[135] and coronary autopsy specimens[136] as well. Whereas these ex vivo studies were performed in a blood-free laboratory setup, a recent in vivo study using a 1.5 mm fiber-bundle NIR catheter system also showed the feasibility of intravascular NIR spectroscopy through blood.[137] In this rabbit aortic model, the catheter-based system identified lipid areas greater than 0.75 mm^2 with 78% sensitivity and 75% specificity.

Although Raman spectroscopy has a theoretical advantage in direct quantification of individual plaque components, only a small percentage of photons are recruited into the Raman shift, resulting in a low signal-to-noise ratio and poor tissue penetration. However, recent exclusive use of the NIR wavelength laser (750–850 μm), coupled with enhanced CCD array cameras, may significantly improve the signal-to-noise ratio. In addition, mathematical tools have been developed to separate the contribution of background fluorescence in the Raman spectrum. In an ex vivo study of human coronary specimens, Romer and his colleagues also demonstrated that a tissue layer of 300 μm attenuates the Raman cholesterol signals by 50% at 850 nm excitation,[138] indicating that a lipid core up to 1–1.5 mm from the lumen could still be detected with this technique. Accordingly, the first in vivo application of catheter-based, intravascular Raman spectroscopy was demonstrated by Buschman and his colleagues.[139] This experimental study showed that the in vivo intravascular Raman signal obtained from an aorta was a simple summation of signal contributions of the vessel wall and blood. More recently, a compact fiberoptic-based Raman system for in vivo applications has been developed.[140] In autopsy studies of human coronary arteries and aortas, the system detected cholesterol and calcification, indicating that Raman spectroscopy has the potential to perform plaque characterization in patients if problems of in vivo measurement can be overcome.

On the other hand, the strong fluorescence of arterial tissue is a potential advantage of fluorescence spectroscopy over Raman analysis, permitting good signal-to-noise ratio with rapid spectra acquisition. Nevertheless, the encouraging ex vivo studies with fluorescence spectroscopy has not been translated into successful in vivo applications of this technique. This is in part owing to the significant spectra attenuation and distortion by the interplay of absorption and scattering at the presence of hemoglobin. Recently, a combined approach using fluorescence and diffuse reflectance spectroscopy has been proposed to minimize this technical limitation.

TABLE 3

Characteristics of catheter-based imaging devices

	IVUS	OCT	Angioscopy	Spectroscopy
Resolution	100–250 μm	10–20 μm	N/A	1 mm
Penetration depth	4–8 mm	1.5–2 mm	Surface only	Several millimeter
Vessel occlusion	No	No/Yes	No/Yes	No
Morphological information	Yes	Yes	Yes	No
Remodeling/plaque distribution	+++	+	-	-
Lipid identification	+	++	+	+++
Inflammation	-	+	-	+
Thrombus	+	++	+++	-
Stent struts distribution	++	+++	+	-
Stent struts apposition	+	+++	-	-

CLINICAL EXPERIENCE

Clinical experience has been collected since a prototype device of intravascular NIR spectroscopy was developed in 2001.[141] In the preliminary study, however, substantial motion artifact was present. In 2006, the new NIR catheter system was used in patients with stable coronary artery disease at the time of PCI and showed that signals obtained in the artery differ from those obtained in blood alone.[142] This system (Intravascular Chemogram™) developed and manufactured by InfraReDx is the only commercially available NIR spectroscopy system for coronary imaging at present.[143] Initial results of the SPECTroscopic Assessment of Coronary Lipid (SPECTACL) study were reported in 2009.[144] This study was the first multicenter study designed to demonstrate the applicability of the lipid core-containing plaques detection algorithm in patients with stable coronary artery disease or acute coronary syndrome. SPECTACL trial showed spectral similarity between acquired spectra in vivo and those from autopsy data sets in 40 of 48 spectrally adequate scans (83% success rate, 95% confidence interval: 70–93%, median spectral similarity/pullback: 96%, interquartile range 10%) (Fig. 32). These findings suggest the feasibility of invasive detection of coronary lipid core-containing plaques with this NIR spectroscopy system. Although the current NIR spectroscopy system can provide compositional information but not structural information like IVUS, intravascular investigation of chemical composition of a coronary plaque has the possibility to offer useful insights into risk stratification and clinical management of vulnerable plaques/patients. Table 3 shows characteristics of NIR spectroscopy and in comparison with other light-based diagnostic techniques.

SAFETY AND LIMITATIONS

The preliminary study of the NIR spectroscopy system confirmed that clinical outcomes did not differ from those expected with stenting and IVUS usage.[144] No device-related adverse events occurred. However, the safety of NIR spectroscopy has not been well established in a large number of patients. In addition, unacceptably high rates of failure to obtain adequate data were seen in early clinical experience.

FUTURE DIRECTIONS

A catheter-based spectroscopy device combined with another structural imaging modality, such as IVUS or OCT, may allow comprehensive plaque evaluation by providing both chemical and anatomical information. In fact, one combined coronary catheter system (NIR spectroscopy combined with IVUS) has been developed and is under clinical evaluation (LipiScan IVUS system™, InfraReDx, Inc).[145]

Another interesting concept is to use diffuse reflectance NIR spectroscopy for in situ measurement of tissue pH or lactate concentration in atherosclerotic plaques. These metabolic parameters may indicate the activity of macrophages and other inflammatory cells, offering additional functional measures of plaque vulnerability. The feasibility of this technique has been demonstrated in an ex vivo study using human carotid endoatherectomy specimens,[146] and further technical refinements are awaited for future clinical applications.

REFERENCES

1. Bom N, Lancee CT, Van Egmond FC. An ultrasonic intracardiac scanner. Ultrasonics. 1972;10:72-6.
2. Yock PG, Linker DT, Angelsen BA. Two-dimensional intravascular ultrasound: technical development and initial clinical experience. J Am Soc Echocardiogr. 1989;2:296-304.
3. Meyer CR, Chiang EH, Fechner KP, et al. Feasibility of high-resolution, intravascular ultrasonic imaging catheters. Radiology. 1988;168:113-6.
4. Mintz GS, Nissen SE, Anderson WD, et al. American College of Cardiology Clinical Expert Consensus Document on Standards for Acquisition, Measurement and Reporting of Intravascular Ultrasound Studies (IVUS). A report of the American College of Cardiology Task Force on Clinical Expert Consensus Documents. J Am Coll Cardiol. 2001;37:1478-92.
5. Hara H, Tsunoda T, Yamamoto M. The ultrasound attenuation behind coronary atheroma predicts embolic complication during percutaneous intervention (abstract). J Am Coll Cardiol. 2005;45:58A-59A.
6. Okura H, Taguchi H, Kubo T, et al. Atherosclerotic plaque with ultrasonic attenuation affects coronary reflow and infarct size in patients with acute coronary syndrome: an intravascular ultrasound study. Circ J. 2007;71:648-53.
7. Lee SY, Mintz GS, Kim SY, et al. Attenuated plaque detected by intravascular ultrasound: clinical, angiographic, and morphologic

features and post-percutaneous coronary intervention complications in patients with acute coronary syndromes. JACC Cardiovasc Interv. 2009;2:65-72.

8. Yamada R, Okura H, Kume T, et al. Histological characteristics of plaque with ultrasonic attenuation: a comparison between intravascular ultrasound and histology. J Cardiol. 2007;50:223-8.

9. Nair RS, Fuchs RL, Schuette SA. Current methods for assessing safety of genetically modified crops as exemplified by data on roundup ready soybeans. Toxicol Pathol. 2002;30:117-25.

10. Kawasaki M, Takatsu H, Noda T, et al. Noninvasive quantitative tissue characterization and two-dimensional color-coded map of human atherosclerotic lesions using ultrasound integrated backscatter: comparison between histology and integrated backscatter images. J Am Coll Cardiol. 2001;38:486-92.

11. Sathyanarayana S, Carlier S, Li W, et al. Characterisation of atherosclerotic plaque by spectral similarity of radiofrequency intravascular ultrasound signals. EuroIntervention. 2009;5:133-9.

12. Stone GW, Maehara A, Lansky AJ, et al. A prospective natural-history study of coronary atherosclerosis. N Engl J Med. 2011;364:226-235.

13. Glagov S, Weisenberg E, Zarins CK, et al. Compensatory enlargement of human atherosclerotic coronary arteries. N Engl J Med. 1987;316:1371-5.

14. Schoenhagen P, Ziada KM, Vince DG, et al. Arterial remodeling and coronary artery disease: the concept of "dilated" versus "obstructive" coronary atherosclerosis. J Am Coll Cardiol. 2001;38:297-306.

15. Hibi K, Ward MR, Honda Y, et al. Impact of different definitions on the interpretation of coronary remodeling determined by intravascular ultrasound. Catheter Cardiovasc Interv. 2005;65:233-9.

16. Mintz GS, Kent KM, Pichard AD, et al. Contribution of inadequate arterial remodeling to the development of focal coronary artery stenoses. An intravascular ultrasound study. Circulation. 1997;95:1791-8.

17. Pasterkamp G, Schoneveld AH, van der Wal AC, et al. Relation of arterial geometry to luminal narrowing and histologic markers for plaque vulnerability: the remodeling paradox. J Am Coll Cardiol. 1998;32:655-62.

18. Mehran R, Dangas G, Mintz GS, et al. Atherosclerotic plaque burden and CK-MB enzyme elevation after coronary interventions: intravascular ultrasound study of 2256 patients. Circulation. 2000;101:604-10.

19. Okura H, Hayase M, Shimodozono S, et al. Impact of pre-interventional arterial remodeling on subsequent vessel behavior after balloon angioplasty: a serial intravascular ultrasound study. J Am Coll Cardiol. 2001;38:2001-5.

20. Smith SC Jr., Feldman TE, Hirshfeld JW, et al. ACC/AHA/SCAI 2005 guideline update for percutaneous coronary intervention: a report of the American College of Cardiology/American Heart Association Task Force on Practice Guidelines (ACC/AHA/SCAI Writing Committee to Update 2001 Guidelines for Percutaneous Coronary Intervention). Circulation. 2006;113:e166-e286.

21. Takagi A, Tsurumi Y, Ishii Y, et al. Clinical potential of intravascular ultrasound for physiological assessment of coronary stenosis: relationship between quantitative ultrasound tomography and pressure-derived fractional flow reserve. Circulation. 1999;100:250-5.

22. Briguori C, Anzuini A, Airoldi F, et al. Intravascular ultrasound criteria for the assessment of the functional significance of intermediate coronary artery stenoses and comparison with fractional flow reserve. Am J Cardiol. 2001;87:136-41.

23. Jasti V, Ivan E, Yalamanchili V, et al. Correlations between fractional flow reserve and intravascular ultrasound in patients with an ambiguous left main coronary artery stenosis. Circulation. 2004;110:2831-6.

24. Tonino PA, De Bruyne B, Pijls NH, et al. Fractional flow reserve versus angiography for guiding percutaneous coronary intervention. N Engl J Med. 2009;360:213-24.

25. Abizaid AS, Mintz GS, Mehran R, et al. Long-term follow-up after percutaneous transluminal coronary angioplasty was not performed based on intravascular ultrasound findings: importance of lumen dimensions. Circulation. 1999;100:256-61.

26. Mintz GS, Pichard AD, Kovach JA, et al. Impact of preintervention intravascular ultrasound imaging on transcatheter treatment strategies in coronary artery disease. Am J Cardiol. 1994;73:423-30.

27. Gorge G, Ge J, Erbel R. Role of intravascular ultrasound in the evaluation of mechanisms of coronary interventions and restenosis. Am J Cardiol. 1998;81:91G-95G.

28. Fitzgerald PJ, Yock PG. Mechanisms and outcomes of angioplasty and atherectomy assessed by intravascular ultrasound imaging. J Clin Ultrasound. 1993;21:579-88.

29. Baptista J, di Mario C, Ozaki Y, et al. Impact of plaque morphology and composition on the mechanisms of lumen enlargement using intracoronary ultrasound and quantitative angiography after balloon angioplasty. Am J Cardiol. 1996;77:115-21.

30. Stone GW, Hodgson JM, St Goar FG, et al. Improved procedural results of coronary angioplasty with intravascular ultrasound-guided balloon sizing: the CLOUT Pilot Trial. Clinical Outcomes With Ultrasound Trial (CLOUT) Investigators. Circulation. 1997;95:2044-52.

31. Stone GW, Frey A, Linnemeier TJ. 2.5 year follow-up of the CLOUT study: long-term implications for an aggressive IVUS guided balloon angioplasty strategy. J Am Coll Cardiol. 1999;33:81A.

32. Schroeder S, Baumbach A, Haase KK, et al. Reduction of restenosis by vessel size adapted percutaneous transluminal coronary angioplasty using intravascular ultrasound. Am J Cardiol. 1999;83:875-9.

33. Abizaid A, Pichard AD, Mintz GS, et al. Acute and long-term results of an intravascular ultrasound-guided percutaneous transluminal coronary angioplasty/provisional stent implantation strategy. Am J Cardiol. 1999;84:1298-303.

34. Honda Y, et al. Longitudinal redistribution of plaque is an imprtant mechanism for lumen expansion in stenting (abstract). J Am Coll Cardiol. 1997;29:281A.

35. Nakamura S, Colombo A, Gaglione A, et al. Intracoronary ultrasound observations during stent implantation. Circulation. 1994;89:2026-34.

36. Colombo A, Hall P, Nakamura S, et al. Intracoronary stenting without anticoagulation accomplished with intravascular ultrasound guidance. Circulation. 1995;91:1676-88.

37. Goldberg SL, Colombo A, Nakamura S, et al. Benefit of intracoronary ultrasound in the deployment of Palmaz-Schatz stents. J Am Coll Cardiol. 1994;24:996-1003.

38. Nishida T, Colombo A, Briguori C, et al. Outcome of nonobstructive residual dissections detected by intravascular ultrasound following percutaneous coronary intervention. Am J Cardiol. 2002;89:1257-62.

39. Albiero R, Rau T, Schluter M, et al. Comparison of immediate and intermediate-term results of intravascular ultrasound versus angiography-guided Palmaz-Schatz stent implantation in matched lesions. Circulation. 1997;96:2997-3005.

40. Blasini R, Neumann FJ, Schmitt C, et al. Restenosis rate after intravascular ultrasound-guided coronary stent implantation. Cathet Cardiovasc Diagn. 1998;44:380-6.

41. Gaster AL, Slothuus Skjoldborg U, Larsen J, et al. Continued improvement of clinical outcome and cost effectiveness following intravascular ultrasound guided PCI: insights from a prospective, randomised study. Heart. 2003;89:1043-9.

42. Fitzgerald PJ, Oshima A, Hayase M, et al. Final results of the can routine ultrasound influence stent expansion (CRUISE) study. Circulation. 2000;102:523-30.

43. Frey AW, Hodgson JM, Muller C, et al. Ultrasound-guided strategy for provisional stenting with focal balloon combination catheter: results from the randomized strategy for intracoronary ultrasound-guided PTCA and stenting (SIPS) trial. Circulation. 2000;102:2497-502.

44. Oemrawsingh PV, Mintz GS, Schalij MJ, et al. Intravascular ultrasound guidance improves angiographic and clinical outcome of stent implantation for long coronary artery stenoses: final results of a randomized comparison with angiographic guidance (TULIP Study). Circulation. 2003;107:62-7.

45. de Jaegere P, Mudra H, Figulla H, et al. Intravascular ultrasound-guided optimized stent deployment. Immediate and 6 months clinical and angiographic results from the multicenter ultrasound stenting in coronaries study (MUSIC Study). Eur Heart J. 1998;19:1214-23.

46. Uren NG, Schwarzacher SP, Metz JA, et al. Predictors and outcomes of stent thrombosis: an intravascular ultrasound registry. Eur Heart J. 2002;23:124-32.

47. Cheneau E, Leborgne L, Mintz GS, et al. Predictors of subacute stent thrombosis: results of a systematic intravascular ultrasound study. Circulation. 2003;108:43-7.

48. Hoffmann R, Mintz GS, Mehran R, et al. Intravascular ultrasound predictors of angiographic restenosis in lesions treated with Palmaz-Schatz stents. J Am Coll Cardiol. 1998;31:43-9.

49. Kasaoka S, Tobis JM, Akiyama T, et al. Angiographic and intravascular ultrasound predictors of in-stent restenosis. J Am Coll Cardiol. 1998;32:1630-5.

50. Morino Y, Honda Y, Okura H, et al. An optimal diagnostic threshold for minimal stent area to predict target lesion revascularization following stent implantation in native coronary lesions. Am J Cardiol. 2001;88:301-3.

51. Russo RJ, Silva PD, Teirstein PS, et al. A randomized controlled trial of angiography versus intravascular ultrasound-directed bare-metal coronary stent placement (the AVID Trial). Circ Cardiovasc Interv. 2009;2:113-23.

52. Mudra H, di Mario C, de Jaegere P, et al. Randomized comparison of coronary stent implantation under ultrasound or angiographic guidance to reduce stent restenosis (OPTICUS Study). Circulation. 2001;104:1343-9.

53. Orford JL, Denktas AE, Williams BA, et al. Routine intravascular ultrasound scanning guidance of coronary stenting is not associated with improved clinical outcomes. Am Heart J. 2004;148:501-6.

54. Casella G, Klauss V, Ottani F, et al. Impact of intravascular ultrasound-guided stenting on long-term clinical outcome: a meta-analysis of available studies comparing intravascular ultrasound-guided and angiographically guided stenting. Catheter Cardiovasc Interv. 2003;59:314-21.

55. Hibi K, Suzuki T, Honda Y, et al. Quantitative and spatial relation of baseline atherosclerotic plaque burden and subsequent in-stent neointimal proliferation as determined by intravascular ultrasound. Am J Cardiol. 2002;90:1164-7.

56. Kornowski R, Mintz GS, Kent KM, et al. Increased restenosis in diabetes mellitus after coronary interventions is due to exaggerated intimal hyperplasia. A serial intravascular ultrasound study. Circulation. 1997;95:1366-9.

57. Castagna MT, Mintz GS, Leiboff BO, et al. The contribution of "mechanical" problems to in-stent restenosis: an intravascular ultrasonographic analysis of 1090 consecutive in-stent restenosis lesions. Am Heart J. 2001;142:970-4.

58. Mehran R, Mintz GS, Satler LF, et al. Treatment of in-stent restenosis with excimer laser coronary angioplasty: mechanisms and results compared with PTCA alone. Circulation. 1997;96:2183-9.

59. Sharma SK, Kini A, Mehran R, et al. Randomized trial of rotational atherectomy versus balloon angioplasty for diffuse in-stent restenosis (ROSTER). Am Heart J. 2004;147:16-22.

60. Dahm JB, Kuon E. High-energy eccentric excimer laser angioplasty for debulking diffuse in-stent restenosis leads to better acute- and 6-month follow-up results. J Invasive Cardiol. 2000;12:335-42.

61. de Ribamar Costa J Jr., Mintz GS, Carlier SG, et al. Intravascular ultrasound assessment of drug-eluting stent expansion. Am Heart J. 2007;153:297-303.

62. Kuroda N, Kobayashi Y, Nameki M, et al. Intimal hyperplasia regression from 6 to 12 months after stenting. Am J Cardiol. 2002;89:869-72.

63. Sousa JE, Costa MA, Abizaid A, et al. Four-year angiographic and intravascular ultrasound follow-up of patients treated with sirolimus-eluting stents. Circulation. 2005;111:2326-9.

64. Sousa JE, Costa MA, Sousa AG, et al. Two-year angiographic and intravascular ultrasound follow-up after implantation of sirolimus-eluting stents in human coronary arteries. Circulation. 2003;107:381-3.

65. Aoki J, Colombo A, Dudek D, Banning AP, et al. Peristent remodeling and neointimal suppression 2 years after polymer-based, paclitaxel-eluting stent implantation: insights from serial intravascular ultrasound analysis in the TAXUS II study. Circulation. 2005;112:3876-83.

66. Sonoda S, Morino Y, Ako J, et al. Impact of final stent dimensions on long-term results following sirolimus-eluting stent implantation: serial intravascular ultrasound analysis from the sirius trial. J Am Coll Cardiol. 2004;43:1959-63.

67. Hong MK, Mintz GS, Lee CW, et al. Intravascular ultrasound predictors of angiographic restenosis after sirolimus-eluting stent implantation. Eur Heart J. 2006;27: 1305-10.

68. Costa MA. Impact of stent deployment techniques on long-term clinical outcomes of patients treated with sirolimus-eluting stents: results of the multicenter prospective S.T.L.L.R. trial. Transcatheter Cardiovascular Therapeutics Convention. Washington, DC; 2006.

69. Morino Y, Tamiya S, Masuda N, et al. Intravascular ultrasound criteria for determination of optimal longitudinal positioning of sirolimus-eluting stents. Circ J.74:1609-16.

70. Roy P, Steinberg DH, Sushinsky SJ, et al. The potential clinical utility of intravascular ultrasound guidance in patients undergoing percutaneous coronary intervention with drug-eluting stents. Eur Heart J. 2008;29:1851-7.

71. Park SJ, Kim YH, Park DW, et al. Impact of intravascular ultrasound guidance on long-term mortality in stenting for unprotected left main coronary artery stenosis. Circ Cardiovasc Interv. 2009;2:167-77.

72. Rogacka R, Latib A, Colombo A. IVUS-guided stent implantation to improve outcome: a promise waiting to be fulfilled. Curr Cardiol Rev. 2009;5:78-86.

73. Colombo A, Caussin C, Presbitero P, et al. AVIO: a prospective, randomized trial of intravascular ultrasound guided compared to angiography guided stent implantation in complex coronary lesions (abstract). J Am Coll Cardiol. 2010;56:Suppl. B.

74. Fujii K, Mintz GS, Kobayashi Y, et al. Contribution of stent underexpansion to recurrence after sirolimus-eluting stent implantation for in-stent restenosis. Circulation. 2004;109:1085-8.

75. Fujii K, Carlier SG, Mintz GS, et al. Stent underexpansion and residual reference segment stenosis are related to stent thrombosis after sirolimus-eluting stent implantation: an intravascular ultrasound study. J Am Coll Cardiol. 2005;45:995-8.

76. Okabe T, Mintz GS, Buch AN, et al. Intravascular ultrasound parameters associated with stent thrombosis after drug-eluting stent deployment. Am J Cardiol. 2007;100:615-20.

77. Cook S, Wenaweser P, Togni M, et al. Incomplete stent apposition and very late stent thrombosis after drug-eluting stent implantation. Circulation. 2007;115:2426-34.

78. Drachman DE, Edelman ER, Seifert P, et al. Neointimal thickening after stent delivery of paclitaxel: change in composition and arrest of growth over six months. J Am Coll Cardiol. 2000;36:2325-32.

79. Serruys PW, Degertekin M, Tanabe K, et al. Intravascular ultrasound findings in the multicenter, randomized, double-blind RAVEL (Randomized study with the sirolimus-eluting velocity balloon-expandable stent in the treatment of patients with de novo native coronary artery Lesions) trial. Circulation. 2002;106:798-803.

80. Weissman NJ, Koglin J, Cox DA, et al. Polymer-based paclitaxel-eluting stents reduce in-stent neointimal tissue proliferation: a serial volumetric intravascular ultrasound analysis from the TAXUS-IV trial. J Am Coll Cardiol. 2005;45:1201-5.

81. Ako J, Morino Y, Honda Y, et al. Late incomplete stent apposition after sirolimus-eluting stent implantation: a serial intravascular ultrasound analysis. J Am Coll Cardiol. 2005;46:1002-5.

82. Tanabe K, Serruys PW, Degertekin M, et al. Incomplete stent apposition after implantation of paclitaxel-eluting stents or bare metal stents: insights from the randomized TAXUS II trial. Circulation. 2005;111:900-5.

83. Hassan AK, Bergheanu SC, Stijnen T, et al. Late stent malapposition risk is higher after drug-eluting stent compared with bare-metal stent implantation and associates with late stent thrombosis. Eur Heart J. 2010;31:1172-80.

84. Hong MK, Mintz GS, Lee CW, et al. Late stent malapposition after drug-eluting stent implantation: an intravascular ultrasound analysis with long-term follow-up. Circulation. 2006;113:414-9.

85. Bavry AA, Kumbhani DJ, Helton TJ, et al. What is the risk of stent thrombosis associated with the use of paclitaxel-eluting stents for percutaneous coronary intervention?: a meta-analysis. J Am Coll Cardiol. 2005;45:941-6.

86. Hoffmann R, Morice MC, Moses JW, et al. Impact of late incomplete stent apposition after sirolimus-eluting stent implantation on 4-year clinical events: intravascular ultrasound analysis from the multicentre, randomised, RAVEL, E-SIRIUS and SIRIUS trials. Heart. 2008;94:322-8.

87. Honda Y. Drug-eluting stents. Insights from invasive imaging technologies. Circ J. 2009;73:1371-80.

88. Takebayashi H, Mintz GS, Carlier SG, et al. Nonuniform strut distribution correlates with more neointimal hyperplasia after sirolimus-eluting stent implantation. Circulation. 2004;110:3430-4.

89. Doi H, Maehara A, Mintz GS, et al. Classification and potential mechanisms of intravascular ultrasound patterns of stent fracture. Am J Cardiol. 2009;103:818-23.

90. Hausmann D, Erbel R, Alibelli-Chemarin MJ, et al. The safety of intracoronary ultrasound. A multicenter survey of 2207 examinations. Circulation. 1995;91:623-30.

91. Batkoff BW, Linker DT. Safety of intracoronary ultrasound: data from a Multicenter European Registry. Cathet Cardiovasc Diagn. 1996;38:238-41.

92. Degertekin FL, Guldiken RO, Karaman M. Annular-ring CMUT arrays for forward-looking IVUS: transducer characterization and imaging. IEEE Trans Ultrason Ferroelectr Freq Control. 2006;53:474-82.

93. Huang D, Swanson EA, Lin CP, et al. Optical coherence tomography. Science. 1991;254:1178-81.

94. Yabushita H, Bouma BE, Houser SL, et al. Characterization of human atherosclerosis by optical coherence tomography. Circulation. 2002;106:1640-5.

95. Jang IK, Bouma BE, Kang DH, et al. Visualization of coronary atherosclerotic plaques in patients using optical coherence tomography: comparison with intravascular ultrasound. J Am Coll Cardiol. 2002;39:604-9.

96. Jang IK, Tearney GJ, MacNeill B, et al. In vivo characterization of coronary atherosclerotic plaque by use of optical coherence tomography. Circulation. 2005;111:1551-5.

97. Kubo T, Imanishi T, Takarada S, et al. Assessment of culprit lesion morphology in acute myocardial infarction: ability of optical coherence tomography compared with intravascular ultrasound and coronary angioscopy. J Am Coll Cardiol. 2007;50:933-9.

98. Bouma BE, Tearney GJ, Yabushita H, et al. Evaluation of intracoronary stenting by intravascular optical coherence tomography. Heart. 2003;89:317-20.

99. Grube E, Gerckens U, Buellesfeld L, et al. Images in cardiovascular medicine. Intracoronary imaging with optical coherence tomography: a new high-resolution technology providing striking visualization in the coronary artery. Circulation. 2002;106:2409-10.

100. Matsumoto D, Shite J, Shinke T, et al. Neointimal coverage of sirolimus-eluting stents at 6-month follow-up: evaluated by optical coherence tomography. Eur Heart J. 2007;28:961-7.

101. Kim JS, Jang IK, Kim TH, et al. Optical coherence tomography evaluation of zotarolimus-eluting stents at 9-month follow-up: comparison with sirolimus-eluting stents. Heart. 2009;95:1907-12.

102. Otake H, Shite J, Ako J, et al. Local determinants of thrombus formation following sirolimus-eluting stent implantation assessed by optical coherence tomography. JACC Cardiovasc Interv. 2009;2:459-66.

103. Guagliumi G, Musumeci G, Sirbu V, et al. Optical coherence tomography assessment of in vivo vascular response after implantation of overlapping bare-metal and drug-eluting stents. JACC Cardiovasc Interv. 2010;3:531-9.

104. Iaccarino D, Politi L, Rossi R, et al. Rationale and study design of the OISTER trial: optical coherence tomography evaluation of stent struts re-endothelialization in patients with non-ST-elevation acute coronary syndromes—a comparison of the intrEpide tRapidil eluting stent vs. taxus drug-eluting stent implantation. J Cardiovasc Med (Hagerstown). 2010;11:536-43.

105. Serruys PW, Ormiston JA, Onuma Y, et al. A bioabsorbable everoli-mus-eluting coronary stent system (ABSORB): 2-year outcomes and results from multiple imaging methods. Lancet. 2009;373:897-910.

106. Guagliumi G, Sirbu V, Bezerra HG, et al. Strut coverage and vessel wall response to zotarolimus-eluting and bare-metal stents implanted in patients With ST-segment elevation myocardial infarction. J Am Coll Cardiol Intv. 2010;3:680-7.

107. Fujii K, Kawasaki D, Masutani M, et al. OCT assessment of thin-cap fibroatheroma distribution in native coronary arteries. JACC Cardiovasc Imaging. 2010;3:168-75.

108. Cheruvu PK, Finn AV, Gardner C, et al. Frequency and distribution of thin-cap fibroatheroma and ruptured plaques in human coronary arteries: a pathologic study. J Am Coll Cardiol. 2007;50:940-9.

109. Prati F, Cera M, Ramazzotti V, et al. Safety and feasibility of a new non-occlusive technique for facilitated intracoronary optical coherence tomography (OCT) acquisition in various clinical and anatomical scenarios. EuroIntervention. 2007;3:365-70.

110. Yamaguchi T, Terashima M, Akasaka T, et al. Safety and feasibility of an intravascular optical coherence tomography image wire system in the clinical setting. Am J Cardiol. 2008;101:562-7.

111. Takarada S, Imanishi T, Liu Y, et al. Advantage of next-generation frequency-domain optical coherence tomography compared with conventional time-domain system in the assessment of coronary lesion. Catheter Cardiovasc Interv. 2010;75:202-6.

112. Tearney GJ, Yabushita H, Houser SL, et al. Quantification of macrophage content in atherosclerotic plaques by optical coherence tomography. Circulation. 2003;107:113-9.

113. MacNeill BD, Jang IK, Bouma BE, et al. Focal and multi-focal plaque macrophage distributions in patients with acute and stable presentations of coronary artery disease. J Am Coll Cardiol. 2004;44:972-9.

114. Raffel OC, Merchant FM, Tearney GJ, et al. In vivo association between positive coronary artery remodelling and coronary plaque characteristics assessed by intravascular optical coherence tomography. Eur Heart J. 2008;29:1721-8.

115. Spears JR, Spokojny AM, Marais HJ. Coronary angioscopy during cardiac catheterization. J Am Coll Cardiol. 1985;6:93-7.

116. den Heijer P, Foley DP, Hillege HL, et al. The 'Ermenonville' classification of observations at coronary angioscopy—evaluation of intra- and inter-observer agreement. European Working Group on Coronary Angioscopy. Eur Heart J. 1994;15:815-22.

117. de Feyter PJ, Ozaki Y, Baptista J, et al. Ischemia-related lesion characteristics in patients with stable or unstable angina. A study with intracoronary angioscopy and ultrasound. Circulation. 1995;92:1408-13.

118. Ueda Y, Asakura M, Yamaguchi O, et al. The healing process of infarct-related plaques. Insights from 18 months of serial angioscopic follow-up. J Am Coll Cardiol. 2001;38:1916-22.

119. White CJ, Ramee SR, Collins TJ, et al. Coronary thrombi increase PTCA risk. Angioscopy as a clinical tool. Circulation. 1996;93:253-8.

120. Sakai S, Mizuno K, Yokoyama S, et al. Morphologic changes in infarct-related plaque after coronary stent placement: a serial angioscopy study. J Am Coll Cardiol. 2003;42:1558-65.

121. Takano M, Mizuno K, Yokoyama S, et al. Changes in coronary plaque color and morphology by lipid-lowering therapy with atorvastatin: serial evaluation by coronary angioscopy. J Am Coll Cardiol. 2003;42:680-6.

122. Hara M, Nishino M, Taniike M, et al. High incidence of thrombus formation at 18 months after paclitaxel-eluting stent implantation: angioscopic comparison with sirolimus-eluting stent. Am Heart J. 2010;159:905-10.

123. Hara M, Nishino M, Taniike M, et al. Difference of neointimal formational pattern and incidence of thrombus formation among 3 kinds of stents: an angioscopic study. JACC Cardiovasc Interv. 2010;3:215-20.

124. Higo T, Ueda Y, Oyabu J, et al. Atherosclerotic and thrombogenic neointima formed over sirolimus drug-eluting stent: an angioscopic study. JACC Cardiovasc Imaging. 2009;2:616-24.

125. Mizuno K, Miyamoto A, Satomura K, et al. Angioscopic coronary macromorphology in patients with acute coronary disorders. Lancet. 1991;337:809-12.

126. Ueda Y, Ohtani T, Shimizu M, et al. Assessment of plaque vulnerability by angioscopic classification of plaque color. Am Heart J. 2004;148:333-5.

127. Miyamoto A, Prieto AR, Friedl SE, et al. Atheromatous plaque cap thickness can be determined by quantitative color analysis during angioscopy: implications for identifying the vulnerable plaque. Clin Cardiol. 2004;27:9-15.

128. Kubo T, Imanishi T, Takarada S, et al. Implication of plaque color classification for assessing plaque vulnerability: a coronary angioscopy and optical coherence tomography investigation. JACC Cardiovasc Interv. 2008;1:74-80.

129. Uchida Y, Nakamura F, Tomaru T, et al. Prediction of acute coronary syndromes by percutaneous coronary angioscopy in patients with stable angina. Am Heart J. 1995;130:195-203.

130. Asakura M, Ueda Y, Yamaguchi O, et al. Extensive development of vulnerable plaques as a pan-coronary process in patients with myocardial infarction: an angioscopic study. J Am Coll Cardiol. 2001;37:1284-8.

131. Ishibashi F, Mizuno K, Kawamura A, et al. High yellow color intensity by angioscopy with quantitative colorimetry to identify high-risk features in culprit lesions of patients with acute coronary syndromes. Am J Cardiol. 2007;100:1207-11.

132. Inami S, Ishibashi F, Waxman S, et al. Multiple yellow plaques assessed by angioscopy with quantitative colorimetry in patients with myocardial infarction. Circ J. 2008;72:399-403.

133. Uchida Y, Kawai S, Kanamaru R, et al. Imaging of lysophosphatidylcholine in human coronary plaques by color fluorescence angioscopy. Int Heart J. 2010;51:129-33.

134. Moreno PR, Lodder RA, Purushothaman KR, et al. Detection of lipid pool, thin fibrous cap, and inflammatory cells in human aortic atherosclerotic plaques by near-infrared spectroscopy. Circulation. 2002;105:923-7.

135. Wang J, Geng YJ, Guo B, et al. Near-infrared spectroscopic characterization of human advanced atherosclerotic plaques. J Am Coll Cardiol. 2002;39:1305-13.

136. Gardner CM, Tan H, Hull EL, et al. Detection of lipid core coronary plaques in autopsy specimens with a novel catheter-based near-infrared spectroscopy system. JACC Cardiovasc Imaging. 2008;1: 638-48.

137. Moreno P, Ryan S, Hopkins Dea. Identification of lipid-rich aortic atherosclerotic plaques in living rabbits with a near infrared spectroscopy catheter (abstract). J Am Coll Cardiol. 2001;37:3A.

138. Romer TJ, Brennan JF 3rd, Schut TC, et al. Raman spectroscopy for quantifying cholesterol in intact coronary artery wall. Atherosclerosis. 1998;141:117-24.

139. Buschman HP, Marple ET, Wach ML, et al. In vivo determination of the molecular composition of artery wall by intravascular Raman spectroscopy. Anal Chem. 2000;72:3771-5.

140. van de Poll SW, Kastelijn K, Bakker Schut TC, et al. On-line detection of cholesterol and calcification by catheter based Raman spectroscopy in human atherosclerotic plaque ex vivo. Heart. 2003;89:1078-82.

141. Moreno PR, Muller JE. Identification of high-risk atherosclerotic plaques: a survey of spectroscopic methods. Curr Opin Cardiol. 2002;17:638-47.

142. Waxman S, L'Allier P, Tardif JC, et al. Scanning near-infrared (NIR) spectroscopy of coronary arteries for detection of lipid-rich plaque in patients undergoing PCI-early results of the SPECTACL study (abstract). Circulation. 2006;114:II-647.

143. Maini B. Clinical coronary chemograms and lipid core containing coronary plaques. JACC Cardiovasc Imaging. 2008;1:689-90.

144. Waxman S, Dixon SR, L'Allier P, et al. In vivo validation of a catheter-based near-infrared spectroscopy system for detection of lipid core coronary plaques: initial results of the SPECTACL study. JACC Cardiovasc Imaging. 2009;2:858-68.

145. Hull EL, Doucet CM, Gardner CM. Improved characterization of coronary plaques by the use of both near-infrared spectroscopy and grayscale intravascular ultrasound. The Society for Cardiovascular Angiography and Interventions Meeting; 2009.

146. Naghavi M, John R, Naguib S, et al. pH Heterogeneity of human and rabbit atherosclerotic plaques: a new insight into detection of vulnerable plaque. Atherosclerosis. 2002;164:27-35.

Chapter 21

Cardiovascular Nuclear Medicine— Nuclear Cardiology

Elias H Botvinick

Chapter Outline

INTRODUCTION

The primary advantage of nuclear medicine methods is their ability to image physiology.[1] Nowhere is this more apparent and valued then in their cardiac applications. Approximately 8,000,000–10,000,000 nuclear cardiology studies are performed each year in the USA. Most of these are stress single photon emission computed tomography (SPECT) perfusion studies performed for the diagnosis, localization and risk stratification of coronary artery disease (CAD). With its growing availability of positron emission tomography (PET) myocardial perfusion studies are increasingly applied. Positron emission tomography, with its added resolution, accuracy and quantitative ability, competes with SPECT studies and the increasingly diverse choice of noninvasive imaging methods in CAD. These and other scintigraphic methods used to evaluate ventricular function, myocardial synchrony, metabolism, innervation and necrosis are evolving. The field is invigorated by new instrumentation, new acquisition, processing and display hardware and software, new stress testing (ST) and imaging agents and the

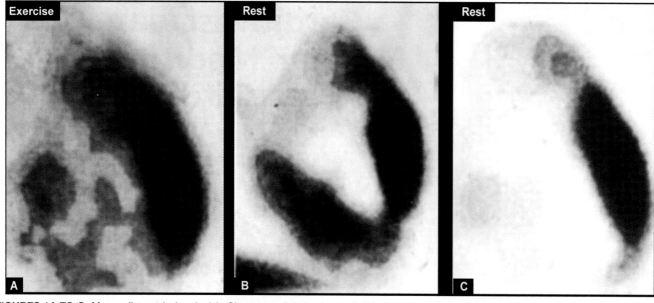

FIGURES 1A TO C: Myocardium at ischemic risk. Shown are digital enhanced, (A) planar exercise and (B) rest myocardial perfusion scintigrams from a patient with right coronary artery (RCA) stenosis estimated to be 40%. Although somewhat contoured by the processing, the scintigrams clearly reveal evidence of reversible inferior ischemia. (C) Subsequently, the patient had a spontaneous infarction of the same region, as shown on the rest image. This study illustrates the difference between angiographic anatomy and scintigraphic pathophysiology, and provides one form of evidence for the ability of scintigraphy to identify myocardium at ischemic risk. (*Source:* Goris M, MD, Stanford University, Palo Alto, CA)

integration of computed tomographic methods. Scintigraphic methods are finding new applications in acute coronary syndromes (ACSs), heart failure and electrophysiologic conditions. This review will consider these methods in their current and potential clinical roles, with reflection on the principles of cardiac and coronary physiology in which they are based.

PATHOPHYSIOLOGIC CONSIDERATIONS

LESION SEVERITY

(See Chapter "Changing focus in global burden of cardiovascular diseases") Some studies support the assumed relationship between lesion severity and events, and directly relate the presence of a severely stenotic lesion to regional ischemic risk[2] (Figs 1A to C). However, several angiographic studies demonstrate that acute coronary occlusion and resultant myocardial infarction (MI), not uncommonly relate to vessels which may not have "significant" coronary lesions when assessed a variable time before that event.[3,4] Many of these studies are biased by their retrospective nature, the lack of coronary evaluation shortly prior to the event and the exclusion of patients with the most severe lesions and prior revascularization. When analyzed quantitatively, on a vessel-by-vessel basis, since severely stenotic vessels are far less frequent than those with modest narrowing, the likelihood of an event precipitated by occlusion of a tightly stenotic vessel far exceeds the likelihood of an event related to occlusion of any insignificantly stenotic vessel, even when most events occur in relation to less stenotic vessels.[5] Nonetheless, coronary occlusion may, not uncommonly, involve vessels which are not significantly stenotic and in such cases, coronary occlusion and related

prognosis is determined by some condition other than the degree of coronary stenosis. Yet clinically, coronary related risk is clearly correlated with the extent and severity angiographic stenosis as revealed by myocardial perfusion imaging (MPI) defect extent and severity, the timing, severity and extent of stress induced ST changes and wall motion abnormalities. The prognostic value of methods based on lesion severity is well established and strongly relied upon in clinical decision making. So how can these apparently mutually exclusive observations be reconciled? How can coronary events be predicted based on findings which relate directly to the severity and extent of CAD when these events do not necessarily relate to even flow limiting lesions?

The conclusion that coronary occlusion may occur in vessels with stenosis of varying significance is unavoidable and may relate to factors regulating the stability of atheromata. Perhaps the relationship of ischemic parameters to prognosis and events is due to the fact that severe ischemic disease identified by these methods, also likely occurs in the presence of numerous lesser lesions, which occur in some proportion to lesion severity. All contribute to the "total ischemic burden"[6] and it is this factor linking events to lesion severity.[7]

In any given patient, the likelihood of a coronary occlusion varies directly with the "ischemic (or plaque) burden", the full extent of myocardium subtended by all atherosclerotic vessels and presumably representing all myocardium which may be involved with an acute coronary occlusion and event. It appears that cardiac risk is directly, or indirectly, related to the "ischemic burden", the extent and pathophysiologic, but not necessarily anatomic, severity of coronary lesions. A more physiologic index, the "ischemic burden" generally correlates well with the magnitude of the vascular hyperemic response, the coronary

TABLE 1

Scintigraphic evidence of extensive myocardium at ischemic risk and related poor prognosis based on gated single-photon perfusion imaging

- Extensive, severe, reversible defects
- Modest or severe defects at a low level of stress or accompanied by extensive fixed defects
- Perfusion defects outside the infarct zone in patients with prior MI
- Stress related lung uptake or cavitary dilation
- Extensive, stress induced wall motion abnormalities or a reduced LVEF or increased LV end-diastolic volume with stress, especially with stress induced perfusion defects
- Reduced rest LVEF with extensive, severe CAD with limited fixed or reversible defects

flow reserve (CFR). As a measure of CFR, MPI is a noninvasive measure of the presence of flow limiting coronary lesions, of the extent of myocardium at ischemic risk[8] and, indirectly, of the "ischemic burden". Studies which reveal a relationship between the severity of coronary stenosis, a measure of the extent of "myocardium at ischemic risk", and events, may reflect their ability to image the "ischemic burden". However neither the quantitative measure of coronary stenosis nor its effect on CFR permits the prediction of plaque rupture and an acute coronary event.[9]

OWING TO STRESS TESTING DEFICIENCIES

(See Chapter "Electrocardiogram") MPI is being increasingly applied to identify and monitor high risk CAD patients (Table 1), and assess the varied benefits of medical versus revascularization therapy.[10] It presents the possibility of differentiating those at risk for death versus acute MI, with their different preventive and treatment measures. This differentiation presents a basis for management decisions among high risk CAD patients.[11-12a]

THE ISCHEMIC CASCADE

(See Chapter "Evaluation of chest pain") The high resistance of the coronary bed at rest normally permits vigorous flow augmentation of three to five times rest levels, with stress induced dilation. This augmentation represents the CFR. Compensatory vasodilation in the presence of significant stenoses, supports normal flow at rest until stenosis becomes subtotal and compensation fails.[14] The dilated resistance bed of the stenotic vessel has reduced or blunted flow reserve compared with that of the patent vessel, which maintains its full vasodilator reserve. A reduced hyperemic response with stress or reduced CFR is the primary abnormality exposed with ST and relates to myocardial ischemia with the increased flow demands of exercise testing and to flow heterogeneity, generally without ischemia, when imposed by direct coronary dilation. When ischemia is induced with exercise or with occasional vasodilator related "coronary steal", the ischemic indicators of reduced perfusion, diastolic dysfunction, systolic dysfunction, electrocardiographic (ECG) changes and pain, will appear in this sequence as described by the "ischemic cascade". This sequence can be seen during percutaneous intervention (PCI) and provides

an explanation for: breathlessness as an early ischemic indicator; the occurrence of "silent ischemia"; and the fact that the perfusion ischemic indicator on ST, the earliest ischemic change, has proven to be the most diagnostic and prognostic parameter for clinical decision making.

STRESS TESTING

Dynamic Exercise Testing

(See Chapter "Electrocardiogram")[12] Image findings must be interpreted in the light of the findings on related stress test. Exercise testing seeks to incrementally augment exercise workload and related myocardial oxygen demands, heart rate and afterload, or its surrogate, systolic blood pressure. These then increase flow demands, and so tests the CFR. Tests are generally *maximal*, that is performed to a symptom or safety limited endpoint. An *adequate* or *inadequate* exercise test simply indicates that the test did or did not adequately address the clinical question for which it was indicated and ordered. An *optimal* or *suboptimal* exercise test indicates that the test did or did not fully test the CFR, stimulating maximal coronary vasodilation by reaching a high level of myocardial oxygen and flow demand. This optimal level generally requires the attainment of 85% of predicted heart rate for age or a double (rate x pressure) product in the range of 20,000–25,000. Maximal tests, especially when negative, may yet be inadequate and suboptimal. In such cases and others, where patients cannot perform exercise stress adequately for the clinical need, pharmacologic ST is indicated.

Pharmacologic Stress Testing

The direct coronary vasodilators adenosine, regadenoson, an adenosine analog and dipyridamole[12,13] (Figs 2 and 3) act directly on the coronary resistance vessels to augment coronary flow and test the CFR (Tables 2 and 3). They uncommonly cause myocardial ischemia by a "coronary steal" mechanism, where reduced resistance in the normal bed, eliminates the pressure gradient driving collateral flow, resulting in ischemia in beds perfused by severely stenotic vessels. Ischemic ST changes, induced with "steal" in the setting of vasodilator stress are very

TABLE 2

The mechanism of stress testing (testing the CFR—the hyperemic flow response

Direct tests of CFR (Vasodilator stress agents)
- Seeks to provoke flow heterogeneity
- Best suited for the perfusion ischemic endpoint
- Less likely influenced by beta blockers
- Strongest, most reproducible tests of CFR

Indirect tests of CFR (Exercise/dobutamine)
- Seek to provoke ischemia (perfusion or wall motion abnormality)
- Suites either perfusion of function ischemic endpoint
- Vary in ability to augment flow demands and test CFR
- Permit serial function analysis

Source: Botvinick EH. Stress imaging: Current clinical options for the diagnosis, localization and evaluation of coronary artery disease. Med Clin N Amer. 1995;79:1025-61

SECTION 3

Diagnosis

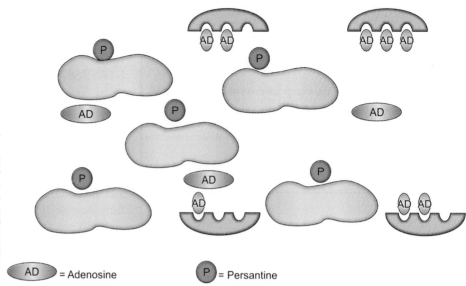

FIGURE 2: Dipyridamole effect. The elevated blood adenosine levels produced by dipyridamole (persantine, P) induced inhibition of adenosine degradation, find coronary endothelial binding sites and cause vigorous coronary dilation (*Source:* Modified from Self Study Program III; Nuclear Medicine: Cardiology Topic 2-Pharmacologic Stress and Associated Topics. Soc Nucl Med Publ. 1998)

AD = Adenosine   P = Persantine

Persantine: Mechanism of Action

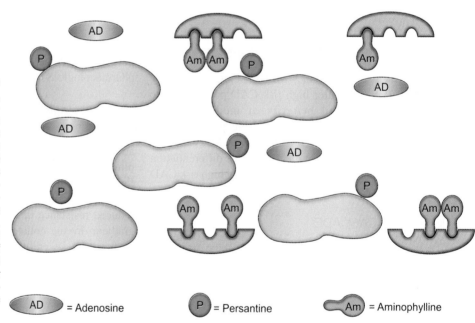

FIGURE 3: Vasodilator antidote. The effects of adenosine can be terminated, and the effects of vasodilation and pharmacologic stress ended by the administration of aminophylline which preferentially binds the adenosine binding site. Dipyridamole continues active for an additional 30–60 minutes, however, and adenosine levels remain elevated for 30–60 minutes theoretically, vasodilation can recur if aminophylline effects subside while dipyridamole persists and before adenosine levels fall. Such a prolonged effect can be avoided with direct adenosine infusion or use of Regadenoson, Lexiscan (*Source:* Modified from Self Study Program III; Nuclear Medicine: Cardiology Topic 2-Pharmacologic Stress and Associated Topics. Soc Nucl Med Publ. 1998)

AD = Adenosine   P = Persantine   Am = Aminophylline

specific for ischemia.[14] More typically the method produces heterogeneous coronary flow augmentation with related abnormalities on MPI in the absence of induced ischemia. Regardless of the mechanism, the diagnostic and prognostic value of vasodilator stress imaging is equal to that of maximal and optimal exercise stress imaging, well able to induce abnormalities of the CFR generally without inducing ischemia. These vasodilators are the most widely applied pharmacologic stress agents in the nuclear medicine laboratory (Tables 2 and 3). Dobutamine, an ischemic stress agent, is widely applied for pharmacologic stress in the echocardiography laboratory but less frequently in the nuclear lab due to the presence of better and safer agents. It is prohibited in the setting of a variety of ischemic, hypertensive and other conditions which are aggravated by its effects. The 3 minute "stages" of the incremental titration dobutamine stress protocol are a poor match for its 2.4 minutes half time, bringing a delayed, poorly controlled and sometimes dangerous response. Even with these inclusions, the mortality and morbidity of dobutamine stress has been shown to be about tenfold greater than that of vasodilator or exercise stress.[15] Although some European investigators advocate its use, vasodilator agents are not generally applied with echocardiography which seeks a decremental wall motion response, a marker for true ischemia

TABLE 3

Pharmacologic stress agents

	Dipyridamole	Adenosine	Regodenoson	Dobutamine
Source	Synthetic	Natural	Synthetic	Synthetic
Mechanism	Tests CFR	Tests CFR	Tests CFR	Ischemic stress
Action of CFR	Indirect	Direct	Indirect	Indirect
Administration	IV infusion	IV infusion	Bolus	IV infusion
Agent preparation	Mix mg/kg dose	Mix mg/kg dose	Single dose ampule	Mix mg/kg dose
Agent duration	Prolonged	Very short	Short	Short
Stress test duration (uncomplicated)	7 min	< 6 min	5 min	> 15 min
Prognostic value	High	High	NA	Modest
Patient exclusions	Rare	Rare	Rare	Common
Patient tolerance	High	High	Very high	Modest
Arrhythmia	Rare	Rare	Rare	Not infrequent
Safety	Like ETT	Like ETT	Like ETT	Less than ETT (many patient exclusions)
End test/Antidote	Aminophylline	Discontinue/ Aminophylline	Aminophylline	Beta blocker
Speed of reversal	Minutes	Seconds	Seconds	Minutes
Diagnostic indicator	Perfusion	Perfusion	Perfusion	Perfusion/wall motion

which is rarely induced by these agents. In the absence of a reliable perfusion marker and any other alternative stress method, dobutamine is applied widely by those who seek to use echocardiography as the stress imaging modality, but used rarely in the nuclear lab in selected patients when the risk of vasodilators is prohibitive. Many of the prohibitions of vasodilator stress which serve as justification for some to apply dobutamine relate to the potential for bronchospasm and can be overcome with an incrementally titrated infusion of adenosine or the new agent regadenoson. Of course dobutamine perfusion scintigraphy, while less desirable than vasodilator pharmacologic stress imaging, has demonstrated greater sensitivity for CAD detection than dobutamine stress echo-cardiography.[16]

MYOCARDIAL PERFUSION IMAGING

IMAGE ACQUISITION PROTOCOLS

Protocols for ST with exercise, regadenoson, adenosine, dipyridamole and dobutamine have been established. The imaging protocols, whether one or two day, applying ^{99m}Tc-based sestamibi or tetrofosmin or combined radiotracers, performed in the sequence of rest versus stress or the reverse, are varied and may be individualized to the patient and laboratory[17] (Figs 4A to D). Adding low level exercise to vasodilator stress appears to reduce background image activity, but adds nothing to diagnostic accuracy. Although there are differences in linearity with flow, excretion pattern and target to background ratio,[18] (Figs 5 and 6) ^{99m}Tc sestamibi and ^{99m}Tc tetrofosmin have similar diagnostic sensitivity and clinical utility. Each protocol has its advantages and disadvantages. However ^{201}Tl has fallen from use due to its low emission energy, long half-life and related poor image resolution and relatively high radiation exposure. Regardless of the protocol employed, the scintigraphic method, as all, remains imperfect.

IMAGE DISPLAY

The perfusion image display divides the left ventricular (LV) myocardium into 17 or 20 segments which may be grouped to represent the distribution of the three coronary arteries on a polar map of regional LV activity[19] (Figs 7 to 10). An objective 5-point semi-quantitative scoring system is applied in each segment to grade the severity and together, the extent, of regional and global myocardial perfusion defects. The resultant summed stress scores (SSS), summed rest scores (SRS) and summed difference or reversibility scores (SDS) have established prognostic value. Here a score of 9–13 relates to an increased infarct risk in the year after testing and scores greater than 13 relate to an increased incidence of death, generally recommending selective coronary angiography (SCA) and, where appropriate, coronary revascularization. A standard image formatting method for nuclear medicine, cardiology, radiology and all of medicine, digital imaging and communications in medicine (DICOM), has been established and is compatible with other imaging modalities, display devices and data storage systems.[20]

GATED—MYOCARDIAL PERFUSION IMAGING

[99m]Tc-based perfusion tracers permit a high injected dose and allow acquisition of gated studies with adequate count statistics in each of 8 or 16 frames. Gated studies and their assessment of LV systolic function add to the ability of the perfusion method to risk stratify CAD where decremental left ventricular ejection fraction (LVEF) with stress, raises dramatically the prognostic risk related to any image perfusion defect.[21] The "partial volume effect"[22] produces intensity changes linearly related to myocardial wall thickening, the basis for accuracy in the measurement of percent wall thickening on gated perfusion images (Figs 11 and 12). The intensity variation accompanying myocardial thickening closely correlates with percentage wall thickening. Calculation of diastolic dysfunction is possible, but beset with pitfalls. Gating aids the differentiation of perfusion

Stress ^{201}Tl Myocardial Perfusion Imaging (MPI) Protocols

Dynamic or
pharmacologic
stress ^{201}Tl
(3-4 mCi)

/→ 20 min → SPECT → 4 hours → SPECT → reinject → SPECT

1 mCi ^{201}Tl
(if needed)

Dynamic or
pharmacologic
stress ^{201}Tl
(3-4 mCi)

/→ 20 min → SPECT → 4 hours → reinject → SPECT → 24 hours → SPECT

1 mCi ^{201}Tl
(if needed)

A

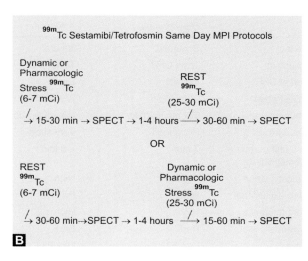

^{99m}Tc Sestamibi/Tetrofosmin Same Day MPI Protocols

Dynamic or
Pharmacologic
Stress ^{99m}Tc   REST
(6-7 mCi) ^{99m}Tc
(25-30 mCi)

/→ 15-30 min → SPECT → 1-4 hours —/→ 30-60 min → SPECT

OR

REST   Dynamic or
^{99m}Tc   Pharmacologic
(6-7 mCi)   Stress ^{99m}Tc
(25-30 mCi)

/→ 30-60 min → SPECT → 1-4 hours —/→ 15-60 min → SPECT

B

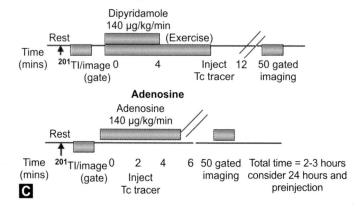

Infusion Protocols
Dipyridamole

Dipyridamole
140 μg/kg/min   (Exercise)

Rest

Time
(mins) ^{201}Tl/image 0   4   Inject   12   50 gated
         (gate)   Tc tracer   imaging

Adenosine

Adenosine
140 μg/kg/min

Rest

Time
(mins) ^{201}Tl/image 0   2   4   6   50 gated   Total time = 2-3 hours
         (gate)   Inject   imaging   consider 24 hours and
                        Tc tracer   preinjection

C

Example CardioGen-82 PET Protocol
(approximately 45 minutes)

^{82}Rb ^{82}Rb
(40-60 mCi)   (40-60 mCi)

Transmission	90-120 sec	Gated Rest	Lexiscan	90-120 sec	Gated Stress	Transmission

D 4-10 minutes   5 minutes   4-5 minutes   5 minutes   4-10 minutes
                                         (10 sec bolus)

FIGURES 4A TO D: (A) ^{201}Tl based protocols—shown diagrammatically is the sequence of stress-rest ^{201}Tl perfusion imaging protocol. A number of permutations may be applied for delayed redistribution and reinjection in order to capture the full extent of myocardial viability. Two such possibilities are illustrated; (B) ^{99m}Tc based protocols—shown diagrammatically is the sequence of the stress-rest and rest-stress 1 day protocols. The latter is preferred since it provides an uncontaminated rest image and gives the highest dose of the imaging agent during stress, where image resolution is most required and gating most beneficial. Each of these is aided by the higher radionuclide dose. Radiation exposure may best be limited in relatively low likelihood patients by performing a stress only study. Rest imaging may be performed subsequently only if needed; (C) Dual isotope sequential perfusion imaging protocol—shown diagrammatically is the sequence of the dual isotope sequential perfusion imaging protocol. With expectation of image abnormality at rest, prior infarction or known abnormal left ventricular wall motion and patient access, ^{201}Tl can be injected the day before stress imaging. The subsequent rest ^{201}Tl image will have been "preinjected". Imaged 24 hours later, before stress ^{99m}Tc administration, these delayed ^{201}Tl images will provide the ultimate for viability evaluation. The protocol is quick and cost-effective in busy labs. Until recently, this was the most popular, most widely applied protocol. Some have now raised concerns regarding the related radiation exposure when compared with other, ^{99m}Tc based protocols (see radiation concerns in the text); (D) ^{82}Rb PET MPI protocol—shown diagrammatically is the ^{82}Rb PET MPI protocol with Regadenoson, Lexiscan as the pharmacologic stress agent. The method employs the CardioGen Rb-82 generator. Owing to the short half-life of the radionuclide, it can be used only for pharmacologic stress evaluation (*Source:* (4A to C) Botvinick EH, MD, UCSF, San Francisco, CA; (4D) Modified from DiCarli MF. Major achievements in nuclear cardiology XI. Advances in positron emission tomography. J Nucl Cardiol. 2004;11:719-32)

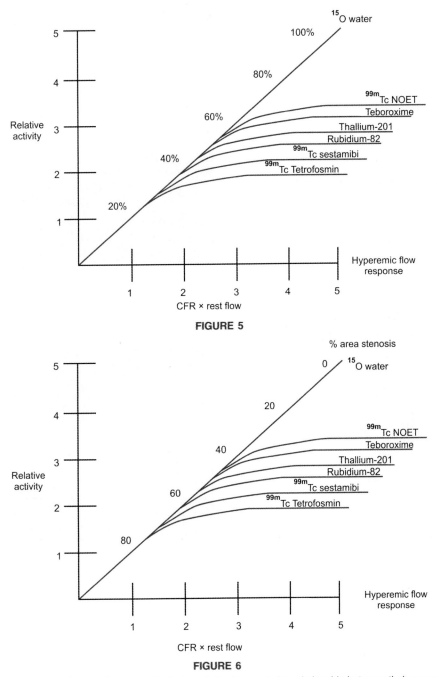

FIGURE 5

FIGURE 6

FIGURES 5 AND 6: Linearity with flow. Shown diagrammatically in both the figures is the relationship between their myocardial uptake and regional myocardial blood flow or coronary flow reserve, measured in multiples of resting flow (CFR x Rest Flow), for a variety of the available and proposed perfusion agents. Each agent departs from the diagonal line of identity or complete flow linearity, at the approximate limit of their specific linearity with flow. In Figure 5, the line of linearity is labeled with the percentage of the CFR reflecting a linear flow relationship at any given level. In Figure 6, the perfusion agents are similarly plotted, but now the range of percent stenosis related to the CFR is approximated. All agents have a high sensitivity for tight, severely stenotic, lesions. However, less severe, less flow limiting agents will be best identified by agents with greater flow linearity. As is evident here, agents with better linearity with flow are needed. While ^{15}O water demonstrates absolute linearity with flow, it is not used clinically owing to its short half-life and other unfavorable properties. The preservation of radionuclide distribution in a linear relationship to flow is an important indicator of its success as a marker of the regional myocardial perfusion. When the blunted hyperemic flow response related to a given level of stenosis exceeds the level of tracer linearity with flow, the tracer concentration and image intensity matches that of the normal flow response and so cannot be identified as abnormal. The greater the tracer flow linearity the higher it can track the blunted hyperemic response. Greater obstruction brings greater abnormalities of the hyperemic response and greater compatibility with the linearity of the agents, making the identification of tighter lesions more successful. Differences in flow linearity relate to the ability of the tracer to identify abnormal responses related to less stenotic vessels in the higher range of the abnormal flow response. Thus, all other factors being equal, the greater the linearity with flow the greater the ability of the agent to identify less severe, but significant lesions, and the higher its expected sensitivity. This data again indicates the fact that the high prognostic value of the method appears to relate to the fact that most events do, in fact, relate to the presence of a severe stenosis, somewhere in the coronary bed. ^{99m}Tc Teboroxime is an FDA approved perfusion imaging agent which has been withdrawn from the market when its rapid extraction feature was found to be incompatible with the slower rate of SPECT acquisition. However it seems quite optimal for rapid dynamic methods of SPECT acquisition now being studied to gain quantitation of regional perfusion. ^{99m}Tc NOET (bis (N-ethoxy, N-ethyl dithiocarbamato) nitrido ^{99m}Tc (V)) (TcN-NOET) is a member of a new group of cardiac imaging agents with a technetium nitido core. It is a neutral lipophilic cardiac perfusion imaging agent with the highest linear relationship to flow among all agents so far evaluated. Not yet FDA approved, it promises to be a "hot spot" label for ischemic and viable myocardium with traits similar to ^{201}Tl including redistribution, and the additional advantages of its ^{99m}Tc label (*Source:* Botvinick EH, MD, UCSF, San Francisco, CA)

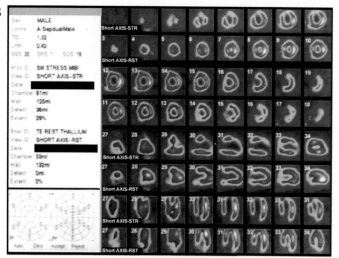

FIGURE 7

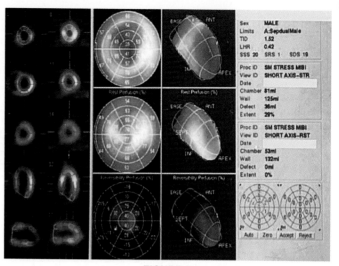

FIGURE 8

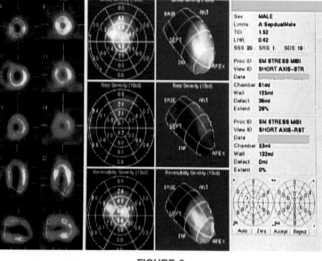

FIGURE 9

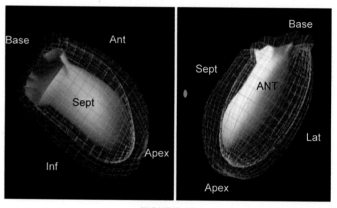

FIGURE 10

FIGURES 7 TO 10: Gated perfusion imaging identification of critical coronary disease and a high prognostic risk. AutoQuant (Cedars Sinai Medical Center, LA) is one of the several commercially available software packages for quality assurance, analysis, quantitation and display of myocardial perfusion images and related data.

Shown in Figure 7 in the first 4 rows according to the standard AutoQuant formatted display are: short axis slices from apex (left) to base (right), vertical long axis slices from septum (left) to lateral wall (right) in the next 2 rows, and horizontal long axis slices, from inferior wall (left) to anterior wall (right), in the bottom 4 rows, in a 49-year-old man with atypical chest pain and no other apparent coronary risk factors. In each image set exercise stress related ^{99m}Tc sestamibi images are above, while the rest ^{201}Tl images are below, in this study acquired by the dual isotope sequential rest ^{201}Tl /^{99m}Tc sestamibi gated SPECT protocol. The patient exercised 10 minutes of a standard Bruce protocol, stopping with shortness of breath, with ST changes suggesting ischemia. Unlike the stress test, here the image gives a clear reading and sets a clinical management approach. A large, clear reversible defect in the distribution of the left anterior descending coronary artery is suggested with accompanying cavitary dilation. A review of associated images and materials suggested no technical issues in this man of normal size. The polar map summed stress score (SSS) of 20 (*Source:* Reproduced from Botvinick EH, MD, UCSF, San Francisco, CA)

Figure 8 demonstrates the AutoQuant display of regional perfusion related activity data, QPS, and the method of quantitation and standardization of perfusion defect size. Sample rest and stress slices are shown in the left 2 panels. Here, in the third panel, a 20 segment polar map is used. In the top frame, relative activity is painted on the stress polar map, with a similar map for the rest study below. At bottom, the difference map is shown. These values are painted on a model left ventricle at right and patient related and study generated information is shown at far right. Chamber, defect and wall volumes are presented, as is the polar map scores for rest and stress images at lower right where the SSS = 20 and SRS (summed rest score) = 1 or normal. Also shown at upper right are the lung-heart ratio (LHR) and the transient ischemic dilation ratio (TID). With the dual isotope protocol, this ratio could be as high as 1.30 owing to the different scatter and resolution of the tracers and the apparent differences in resultant wall thickness and cavitary size. This figure presents regional polar data in segmental standard deviations (SD) from the normal values generated by application of the protocol to gender matched normal subjects. These SD values are translated by an established table to the polar map scores at lower right (*Source:* Botvinick EH, MD, UCSF, San Francisco, CA)

Figure 9 presents regional polar data in segmental standard deviations (SD) from the normal values generated by application of the specific protocol to gender matched normal subjects. These SD values are translated by an established table to the polar map scores at lower right (*Source:* Botvinick EH, MD, UCSF, San Francisco, CA)

Figure 10 illustrates the left ventricular contour derived from the epicardial (orange mesh), and endocardial contours at end diastole (yellow mesh) and end systole (solid orange region) derived from the gated stress perfusion images in the patient illustrated in Figures 7 to 10. A clear septal wall motion abnormality is seen. Rest wall motion was normal here and this stress induced wall motion abnormality at once confirms the perfusion defect and the presence of coronary disease and also adds to its prognostic risk (Abbreviations: ANT: Anterior wall; INF: Inferior wall; SEPT: Septal wall; LAT: Lateral wall) (*Source:* Botvinick EH, MD, UCSF, San Francisco, CA)

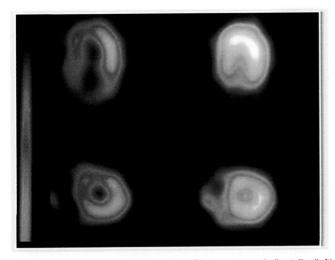

FIGURE 11: Gated sestamibi imaging. Shown are end diastolic (left) and end systolic (right) gated ^{99m}Tc sestamibi perfusion images in a normal heart in selected short (above) and horizontal long axis (below) SPECT slices. Inward systolic motion is evident as well as brightening, or increased intensity during systole. The latter, a result of partial volume effect, is well correlated with myocardial thickening (*Source:* Modified from Botvinick EH, Dae M, O'Connell JW, et al. The scintigraphic evaluation of the cardiovascular system. In: Parmley WW, Chatterjee K (Eds). Cardiology. Philadelphia: JB Lippincott; 1991)

defects and attenuation artifacts, where preserved regional motion in areas of "fixed" defects suggests attenuation; coronary and noncoronary cardiomyopathies, where segmental defects suggest the former; and the identification of the postpericardiotomy patient,[23] where an anterior LV "swing", paradoxical septal motion with preserved thickening indicates intrinsically normal septal contraction and suggests the unrestricted ventricular motion of the condition. Recently, there has been an outburst of new acquisition and analysis technology focused on the field of nuclear cardiology.[24]

Myocardial perfusion imaging presents a map of regional myocardial perfusion. Normal images are rarely the result of artifacts, but abnormal images are not uncommonly, based in artifact.[25] The polar map objectively identifies and compares areas of reduced activity to a normal gender matched normal control set (Figs 7 and 10). However areas of reduced activity unrelated to perfusion may relate to patient motion, attenuation by the breast, chest wall or diaphragm and must be clarified. SPECT attenuation correction (AC)[26] and prone imaging[27] have been used to distinguish such effects and improve diagnostic accuracy. AC methods aid viability evaluation, help overcome ambiguities related to high background activity, aid security in the evaluation of stress only studies and improve the accuracy of quantitative image parameters. AC is optional for SPECT image acquisition but is mandatory for PET which requires AC to fix the errors introduced by the gross loss of data intrinsic to its 360° acquisition.

Several commercial AC methods are approved and applied in routine practice. While each improves image specificity, AC methods vary and differ in their accuracy. Prone imaging has also been shown to improve the specificity of CAD diagnosis as it eliminates attenuation effects of the diaphragm and the breast, while often resolving motion artifacts with a second acquisition in a more stable position. ECG-gated SPECT imaging permits identification of wall motion abnormalities which help to identify true perfusion defects and allows the measurement of LVEF. Additionally, specific image patterns support a technical cause of the finding including: a normal polar map; defects worse at rest than stress; nonsegmental, shifting defects or those which improve on AC or prone imaging; and the findings on raw data. Expert readers use these tools, their relationships and their experience in image interpretation.

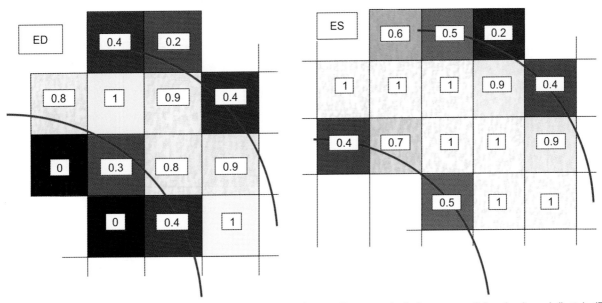

FIGURE 12: Brightening, wall thickening and the partial volume effect. Shown diagrammatically is a myocardial region in end diastole (ED) and end systole (ES). The squares represent pixels which are color coded for and labeled with the percentage of the pixel occupied by the myocardium. Thickening brings more pixels fully or more fully filled by the myocardium and related to a brighter (lighter) intensity response (*Source:* Modified from Botvinick EH, Ratzlaff N, Hoffman JIE, et al. Self Study Program III; Nuclear Medicine: Cardiology Topic 5-Myocardial Perfusion Scintigraphy by Single Photon Radionuclides-Planar and Tomographic (SPECT)-Technical Aspects. Soc Nucl Med Publ. 2003)

390 PET and SPECT may be combined with CT for both increased anatomic resolution and AC.

Raw images, the processed SPECT "splash" slice display, polar maps, gated images with thickening and quantitative data including cavitary and wall volumes, LVEF, AC or prone image findings should all be included in the study evaluation.

DIAGNOSTIC ACCURACY AND COST EFFECTIVENESS

No other stress imaging method has been so thoroughly studied for its CAD diagnostic and prognostic value in a variety of clinical subgroups. MPI plays an integral role in the evaluation of CAD in all its clinical variations. As with all such tests, apparent MPI accuracy and clinical value will vary with the pretest CAD probability. The test accuracy and choice will vary as well with the interpretability for ischemia of the baseline ECG, and the ability of the ST method to test the CFR (Figs 13 and 14). MPI sensitivity to CAD increases with disease extent, severity, the vigor of the stress test and other factors. Stress MPI has been well established to have a very high negative predictive diagnostic value in thousands of study patients, in those with a high pretest probability (> 85%), where the CAD diagnosis is known or highly likely. For those with a low pretest probability of CAD (< 15%), an interpretable ECG, and the ability to exercise adequately, an exercise test alone is all needed for diagnostic purposes. MPI is of greatest diagnostic value in those with an intermediate pretest CAD likelihood (between 15% and 85%) and of greatest prognostic value, rivaling that of SCA. Applied in this way, MPI is a cost-effective method

TABLE 4

When is perfusion imaging cost-effective for CAD diagnosis and prognosis

Extensive population studies indicate that myocardial perfusion scintigraphy is generally of clinical value and cost-effective
• *For CAD diagnosis:*
  In the presence of an intermediate pre-test CAD likelihood
  With an abnormal baseline electrocardiogram
 	
• *For CAD prognosis:*
  In the presence of an intermediate or high pre-test CAD likelihood
  In association with pharmacologic stress

Source: Botvinick EH, Maddahi J, Hachamovitch R, et al. Self-study program III; Nuclear medicine: Cardiology, topic 6: myocardial perfusion scintigraphy by single photon radionuclides–planar and tomographic (SPECT), clinical aspects. With permission of the Soc Nuc Med Publcns, 2004.

associated with a reduced length of hospital stay and decreased number of cardiac catheterizations performed (Table 4).

Stress test results interact strongly with image findings to determine CAD prognosis. The event rate related to a given MPI defect size varies inversely with the achieved heart rate and imposed myocardial flow demands (Fig. 15). Event rate is further increased in relation to any defect size in diabetics and other high risk populations. A normal stress MPI has a high predictive value of a benign course (< 1% annual risk of cardiac death or MI) in the general population. The high predictive prognostic value of an optimally performed negative stress MPI reduces the likelihood of coronary events among symptomatic patients with no known CAD to that of the general asymptomatic

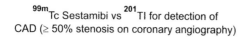

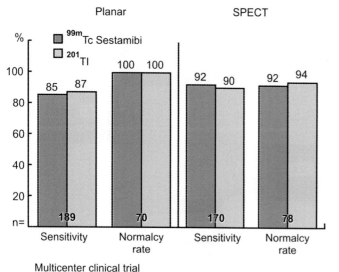

FIGURE 13

FIGURE 14

FIGURES 13 AND 14: Accuracy of ⁹⁹ᵐTc based perfusion imaging. Shown in Figure 13 are the results of an early multicenter trial evaluating the diagnostic sensitivity and normalcy of planar and SPECT ²⁰¹Tl and ⁹⁹ᵐTc sestamibi stress perfusion images. SPECT sensitivity was significantly higher than planar while preserving specificity. In the same way, Figure 14 compares sensitivity and specificity of ²⁰¹Tl and sestamibi planar and SPECT imaging for the identification of disease according to its extent. Unlike planar imaging, SPECT was equally sensitive to 1, 2 and 3 vessel coronary artery disease. Surprisingly, in this study, there was no difference in diagnostic accuracy between ²⁰¹Tl and ⁹⁹ᵐTc studies. However ⁹⁹ᵐTc agents provide best image quality and improved sensitivity and specificity, especially in large patients and women (*Source:* Modified from Taillefer R, Lambert R, Dupras G, et al. Clinical comparison between thallium-201 and technetium-99m methoxyisobutyl isonitrile (hexamibi) myocardial perfusion imaging for detection of coronary artery disease. Eur J Nucl Med. 1989;15(6):280-6)

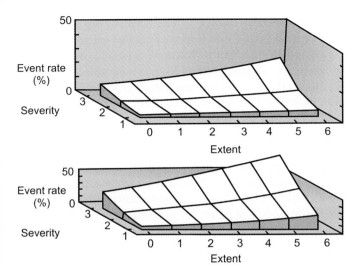

FIGURE 15: Relationship to prognosis. Shown in this 3-dimensional plot drawn from results generated in a large patient population, is the relationship between induced perfusion image defect extent (size, on the abscissa), severity (density, on the ordinate) and event rate (prognosis, on the vertical axis). Note the almost exponential relationship. The data are divided into two plots, above in patients who achieved 85% of predicted heart rate for age, and below, in those who failed to reach that level. The suggestion is that defects of similar conformation have a much higher event rate and relate to a graver prognosis when acquired in association with a lesser stress and test of the coronary flow reserve. The impact of image data must be related to the associated stress (*Source:* Modified from Ladenheim ML, Pollock BH, Rozanski A, et al. Extent and severity of myocardial hypoperfusion as predictors of prognosis in patients with suspected coronary artery disease. J Am Coll Cardiol. 1986;7:464-71)

population and generally permits a conservative approach to management. However, the predictive value of a normal stress MPI varies with the pretest CAD likelihood (Fig. 15). For the same reason, the high predictive value of a negative test has a varying warranty period with retesting required at intervals of 1–3 years to maintain appropriate surveillance depending on pretest CAD likelihood.

Myocardial perfusion imaging is also of value with a low pretest probability in the presence of a baseline ECG uninterpretable for ischemia as with ventricular pacing, left bundle branch block (LBBB), LV hypertrophy with "strain" or baseline ST abnormalities, an initial stress test with unexpected or ambiguous ST changes or an inadequate stress test. When the stress test is suboptimal and the patient cannot exercise adequately to gain the rate and pressure response needed to test the CFR and so address the clinical question, vasodilator pharmacologic stress would be helpful. While relatively uncommon, the likelihood of a coronary event rises to clinical concern when a markedly positive stress ECG, with greater than or equal to 2 mm within the first 6 minutes of a standard Bruce protocol, or the equivalent, accompanies a normal MPI.

INDICATORS OF MULTIVESSEL CORONARY ARTERY DISEASE AND RELATED RISK

Although greater than 90% of those with high risk, multivessel or left main CAD present with abnormal stress MPI, only 40–60% of these are identified by a reversible perfusion defect subtending over 15% of the LV or a total defect greater than 30%. Although superior to stress imaging with other modalities,

the sensitivity of SPECT MPI for the specific identification of those at highest coronary risk based only on the extent, severity and distribution of defects, is suboptimal. While the method can identify some ischemic abnormality in more than 90% of those with extensive CAD, stress MPI may underestimate disease involvement, and in only about 2 of 3 patients with left main or three vessel disease, at most, will an image pattern of extensive, high risk, multivessel disease be demonstrated.[28] Exceeded by PET methods, the sensitivity of SPECT MPI to high risk CAD benefits from findings unrelated to the character of the perfusion defect. These "nonperfusion" indicators of coronary risk include increased post-stress lung uptake of ^{201}Tl or less commonly ^{99m}Tc sestamibi or tetrofosmin with an increased lung/heart ratio (LHR), transient ischemic dilation (TID) of the LV and induced cavitary photopenia. Owing to their difference in physical characteristics, resolution and resultant apparent wall thickness, the cavity size may normally appear more than 30% greater on ^{99m}Tc stress than on ^{201}Tl rest images. A relative augmentation of activity at the usually deficient ventricular base, basal uptake or augmented right ventricular (RV) uptake in the absence of RV hypertrophy, suggest an extensive relative deficiency of activity and perfusion elsewhere in the LV consistent with extensive, high risk CAD. In conjunction with the defect score, the LHR, TID and induced cavitary photopenia further enhance the diagnostic accuracy and predictive value of SPECT MPI for the specific identification of severe, high risk CAD to a sensitivity of roughly 65–70%. The findings of induced wall motion abnormalities or falling LVEF with gated stress SPECT MPI, yields a further increment in diagnosis certainty and prognostic risk.

The extent of perfusion defect, regardless of its distribution or relationship to multivessel disease, provides the most reliable measure of the myocardium at ischemic risk which relates well to CAD risk. Quantitative stress MPI objectifies the severity and risk related to functionally significant CAD in those with chronic stable angina and other clinical CAD subgroups.[29] The SSS, introduced above, presents a quantitative measure of stress image defect extent and intensity, the amount of infarcted, ischemic or jeopardized myocardium, with proven abilities to identify risk of infarction or death. Hachamovitch R and his coworkers have presented retrospective and prospective studies demonstrating the value of stress related defect size, not only for prognosis but also for guidance in patient management. Defect size is greater than or equal to 12% of LV mass related to an unacceptably high risk of death in the year following the study and was related to improved survival with revascularization in comparison with medical management. Patients of both sexes with such image findings, but not necessarily those with smaller defects, would benefit from intervention and aggressive management.[30] Other multicenter studies which evaluate CAD prognosis with varying forms of treatment also indicate a benefit from scintigraphic analysis.[31] Stress induced dysfunction adds to this risk.[12,24,32]

NONPERFUSION INDICATORS OF CAD-RELATED RISK—LUNG/HEART RATIO

Increased LHR is due to prolonged pulmonary transit with increased radionuclide extraction. In the presence of known or suspected CAD, this finding suggests extensive stress-induced

LV dysfunction and multivessel CAD. It has been most thoroughly studied with ^{201}Tl where an increased LHR greater than 0.4 appears to correlate with more extensive CAD and lower LVEF at rest, with exercise, as well as vasodilator pharmacologic stress. The relationship has been studied with ^{99m}Tc-based perfusion agents where lung uptake occurs less frequently. However, with these agents as well, an increased LHR has been associated with more severe and extensive CAD than in the presence of a normal LHR and reduced LV function.

TRANSIENT ISCHEMIC DILATION

Transient ischemic dilation (TID), LV dilation with stress greater than 1.2 in single and greater than 1.4 in dual isotope protocols, is determined on the basis of calculated LV volumes, but supplemented by visual assessment. The measure correlates with extensive multivessel disease or severe high-grade coronary stenosis. TID with stress suggests stress induced LV dysfunction and has been found to be an independent predictor of total cardiac events. Its presence aids in the identification of those with reversible ischemia and who are most likely to benefit from revascularization. The finding has a high sensitivity, specificity and accuracy (91%, 77% and 84% respectively) regardless of the stress method.[33] In the presence of lung uptake or cavitary photopenia, the CAD risk related to any stress induced defect is increased.[34]

Left ventricular (LV) cavitary dilation may be global, consistent with functional compensation for a severe, presumably ischemic, reduction in ventricular function or local and associated with an apparent regional "thinning" of the LV wall. The local condition often presents a resultant apparent visual shift of the cavity from the LV center toward the perfusion abnormality in an "arrowhead" configuration with the tip pointing to the defect.

DENSE CAVITARY PHOTOPENIA

Although the perfusion agent is almost completely extracted from the blood pool, the LV cavity is rarely without intensity in a SPECT MPI. This relates to the incomplete tomographic nature of the SPECT study and the fact that slices are contaminated by the intense activity of the contracting perfused overlying and adjacent walls. Dense cavitary photopenia then relates to massive LV dilation, reduced wall motion or and/or severe regional underperfusion, each of which reduces the potential "contamination" of the cavity by the overlying myocardial wall and promotes cavitary photopenia. When seen only at stress it is yet another indicator of extensive myocardium at ischemic risk.

CLINICAL APPLICATIONS OF MYOCARDIAL PERFUSION IMAGING IN THE EMERGENCY DEPARTMENT—WITH ACUTE CHEST PAIN SYNDROMES

(See Chapter "Coronary syndrome I: unstable angina and non-ST segment elevation myocardial infarction diagnosis and early treatment")[35,36] Standard methods of clinical evaluation have been found to be unsatisfactory as a triage tool of the 8 million patients presenting each year to the emergency department (ED) with chest pain (CP) of suspected cardiac origin. There are 5 million patients admitted with acute or possible MI, 3 million of which are eventually shown to have noncardiac pain, while 3 million other patients are sent home, erroneously discharged with an ongoing ACS and 40,000 with a heart attack (MI)!

^{99m}Tc-based MPI is a useful tool in the triage and evaluation of patients in the acute ED setting. Rest MPI has been shown to be as accurate as serum enzyme analysis for MI diagnosis and has the advantage of speed, where two troponin determinations over 6 hours after CP onset are required to exclude an event. Rest MPI has a high negative predictive value, 99–100%, for the exclusion of acute MI or subsequent cardiac events. Acute rest MPI is especially useful in patients with acute CP and normal or nonspecific rest ECGs. Of course, the full extent of myocardium at ischemic risk is most certainly determined with subsequent stress MPI. The study may remain diagnostic with radionuclide injection as long as 6 hours after cessation of symptoms. However, the delay between the cessation of symptoms and the time of radionuclide injection may result in a missed diagnosis of ischemia and so injection should optimally be made no more than 2 hours after symptoms have abated. The method appears cost effective as well with accelerated triage time, reduced admissions and duration of hospital stay. As in other clinical settings, the method appears useful in diabetics, the elderly and in women presenting to the ED. Recently, Cancer Treatment Centers of America (CTCA), a diagnostic method based in anatomy, has taken a pivotal role in the ED triage of CP patients. However its superiority has yet to be established. An editorial considers the varied imaging options in the ED setting. Guidelines are available for the application of both planar and SPECT MPI.

Myocardial perfusion imaging (MPI) can be done safely 2–5 days post-MI with submaximal exercise or, most completely, with vasodilator pharmacologic agents to determine the amount of myocardium at risk prior to or early after discharge. This is a safe and valuable method of predischarge risk stratification in those where cardiac catheterization is not planned.

UNSTABLE ANGINA/NON-ST ELEVATION MYOCARDIAL INFARCTION

(See Chapter "Acute coronary syndrome II: ST-elevation myocardial infarction and postmyocardial infarction complications and care") The presence and extent of reversible perfusion defects on MPI is a useful tool in predicting future cardiac events.[35] If no recurrent ischemia or signs of congestive heart failure (CHF) are evident, vasodilator pharmacological stress MPI may be recommended in those patients with unstable angina/non-ST elevation myocardial infarction (UA/NSTEMI) to assess inducible ischemia and help to decide whether an early invasive strategy is warranted. For ACS (UA/NSTEMI, STEMI or CP syndrome) with coronary angiogram and stenosis of uncertain significance, MPI can again be helpful in determining the significance of the lesion. Unlike the rest ECG which may be quite benign in the setting of even an extensive infarction or with a large amount of myocardium at ischemic risk, the rest MPI is often demonstrative of the area involved.

FOLLOW-UP AFTER INITIAL ACS EVALUATION STRATEGY

The initial goal of evaluating patients with suspected ACS and nonischemic ECG results in the ED, through use of either resting MPI or serial cardiac serum markers, is to determine the likelihood of ACS and to stratify patient risk. Subsequent assessment of symptoms and risk usually requires some form of ST. Decisions about the type of stress used (treadmill exercise or pharmacologic stress) and the type of analysis performed (ECG testing alone or ECG testing in conjunction with gated MPI) can be made based on well-established clinical protocols such as those outlined in the American College of Cardiology (ACC)/American Heart Association (AHA) Stable Angina Guidelines. It is recommended either that such ST is performed in the ED before the patient is discharged or that the patient is discharged with an appointment for an outpatient stress test within 1 week. A thorough review of this subject was written by Kontos and his coworkers.[37]

RISK ASSESSMENT OF GENERAL AND SPECIFIC PATIENT POPULATIONS

GENERAL PRINCIPLES

The appropriateness of MPI in the general population is highly dependent upon the patient's likelihood for CAD based on the Framingham risk criteria and as outlined above. The time frame recommended for repeat study varies with the initial findings and clinical condition (See "warranty period" above). CT coronary calcium score may provide further guidance. However, studies have shown that stress MPI and CT may provide complementary rather than duplicate data. Criteria of test appropriateness have been formulated.

PREOPERATIVE EVALUATION FOR NONCARDIAC SURGERY

Identification and preoperative management of high risk CAD patients is best accomplished with the teamwork of the primary care physician, the surgeon, anesthesiologist and, where needed, a cardiologist. Noninvasive testing should only be done where results could influence management and outcome. Indications for coronary angiography are generally those as in the nonoperative setting with timing dependent on the urgency of noncardiac surgery, patient risk as evidenced by the history, physical examination and related testing, and the risk of the surgery to be done. The consultant should plan management for both the short (upcoming surgery) and the long term. The clinical predictors of increased cardiovascular risk, MI, CHF and death are presented in the ACC/AHA guideline update for perioperative cardiovascular evaluation for noncardiac surgery.[38,39] In these guidelines, noncardiac surgical procedures are risk stratified, a stepwise approach to perioperative cardiac risk assessment is presented, and a summary of long-term survival after vascular surgery is reviewed. The guidelines present the results of studies assessing the perioperative risk by ST as well as by stress MPI and the factors governing the choice of the stress test in perioperative cardiac risk stratification.

Appropriate use criteria for cardiac radionuclide imaging in the perioperative and in all clinical settings have been developed and updated.[40,41] These and other guidelines discussed below, further address the application of stress MPI. Almanaseer and his coworkers, from this same group, demonstrated that "Implementation of the ACC/AHA guidelines for cardiac risk assessment prior to noncardiac surgery in an internal medicine preoperative assessment clinic led to a more appropriate use of preoperative ST and beta-blocker therapy while preserving a low rate of cardiac complications".

THE EVALUATION OF CAD IN WOMEN

Special consideration for women and CAD detection has long been acknowledged. As presented above, stress MPI has incremental benefit in detecting and risk stratifying CAD in women.[30,42-44] With enhanced interpretive skills, ^{99m}Tc-based perfusion agents, tomographic, prone, attenuation corrected and gated images, SPECT MPI has demonstrated diagnostic and prognostic equality and even superiority to its application in men. Consensus statements on the role of MPI in the detection of CAD in women are available. The clinical role of stress MPI in the management of women with suspected CAD has been reviewed extensively, as well as its role in women with diabetes and CHF.

DIABETICS

Type 2 diabetics is considered a coronary disease equivalent. Such diabetics have a 2–4-fold increased risk of coronary events compared to the nondiabetic population and the MI risk in a diabetic patient is equal to the risk of reinfarction in a non-diabetic with a prior MI. Silent angina and MI is more common among diabetics and diabetics are more likely to die from their MI than those without diabetes. Coronary disease is the leading cause of death in type 2 diabetics. This risk is compounded and exaggerated by the epidemic of obesity worldwide. The need to identify early atherosclerosis and coronary disease in such people is well recognized and stress MPS can contribute to this end. Work has highlighted the high risk of even asymptomatic diabetic patients.[45] Noninvasive cardiac imaging with exercise or pharmacologic stress is cost effective in many categories applicable to large populations of diabetic patients.

MYOCARDIAL PERFUSION IMAGING IN THE ELDERLY

Left ventricular functional data assessed during myocardial gated SPECT provide independent and incremental information above clinical and perfusion SPECT data for the prediction of cardiac and all-cause death in patients aged 75 years or older referred for myocardial SPECT imaging.[46] Vasodilator pharmacologic stress SPECT MPI is safe and most useful for evaluating myocardial ischemia in this group.

POSTREVASCULARIZATION

Regardless of the time frame, MPI is recommended for those who are symptomatic postrevascularization, either by PCI or by coronary artery bypass graft (CABG). Guidelines[39,40] suggest that routine MPI is not indicated prior to hospital discharge postrevascularization if asymptomatic nor if asymptomatic within 1 year post-PCI or within 5 years post-CABG. However, MPI is recommended even if the patient is asymptomatic greater than 5 years after CABG. It is more a matter of individual judgment, whether MPI should be routinely performed in asymptomatic patients greater than 2 years after PCI. After bypass surgery or with any pericardiectomy, the unrestrained heart "swings" anteriorly in the chest giving the appearance of a septal wall motion abnormality. However, septal thickening and systolic function is preserved.[23]

HEART FAILURE

(See Chapter "Systolic heart failure and diastolic heart failure—epidemiology, risk factors, evaluation, diagnosis and management)[47] Patients with newly diagnosed CHF, whether in the setting of CP syndrome or not, should undergo MPI to determine the likelihood of CAD and assess for potential reversible ischemia.[48] The combination of reversible perfusion abnormalities and regional wall motion provides a 94% accuracy for the differentiation of ischemic from nonischemic cardiomyopathy.[49] Those with ischemic cardiomyopathy who are eligible for revascularization with known CAD on SCA should have assessment of myocardial viability. Additionally, those who are receiving potentially cardiotoxic therapy (i.e. doxorubicin) should undergo baseline and serial measurements of ventricular function.

APPROPRIATENESS CRITERIA FOR PERFUSION IMAGING

An appropriateness review was conducted for gated SPECT MPI[40,41] under the auspices of the American College of Cardiology Foundation (ACCF) and the ASNC. The review assessed the risks and benefits of SPECT MPI for 52 selected indications or clinical scenarios grading them as a reasonable approach, a generally reasonable approach and not a reasonable approach. The 52% of indications rated as appropriate, were derived more often, 89% of the time, from existing clinical practice guidelines than was the case for the 23% of uncertain indications, or for the 25% of inappropriate indications. The findings here confirmed and consolidated earlier findings. The guidelines text categorizes the appropriateness of SPECT MPI for the detection of CAD in the presence of an intermediate pretest CAD likelihood and for prognostic value in the setting of an intermediate or high risk pretest CAD likelihood. There is a wide and appropriate MPI application in the presence of CP, especially with an uninterpretable ECG except when CAD was very unlikely or, very likely. It also is quite applicable, especially with pharmacologic stress, in the setting of LBBB. In the absence of CP, the study was found to be appropriate for risk stratification with a high pretest CAD likelihood or a moderate likelihood in the setting of new onset arrhythmia, heart failure or valvular disease, with other worsening symptoms, with long-standing high CAD likelihood or known CAD, an ambiguous stress test, ACS with stenosis of unclear significance and after thrombolytic therapy. Ambiguous results of stress ECG, ST and CTCA, as well as a high coronary calcium score may also be appropriately resolved by MPI. MPI is of value after incomplete or remote revascularization, in the presence of silent ischemia and for the evaluation of myocardial viability.

POSITRON EMISSION TOMOGRAPHY PERFUSION AND METABOLISM

PET AND SPECT TECHNOLOGY

Compared with SPECT, PET has superior image resolution.[50] A number of factors make it most accurate for CAD diagnosis and prognosis and the index imaging method for assessment of myocardial viability. Major advances in PET technology add to its intrinsic physical advantages over SPECT and have contributed to its rapid growth and current application. Crystal options and camera design have moved from laboratory to the bedside and present a growing list of equipment options now available. Combined PET/CT instruments have proliferated widely for use in oncology making the instrumentation more available and the application of PET MPI possible. Reimbursement makes it practical. PET MPI combined with calcium scoring and CTCA add to its interest among practitioners. PET quantitation of flow reserve adds advantages beyond other methods and raises excitement for the future. High energy, 511 keV, PET studies require no extrinsic collimation where AC is performed in all studies generally using X-ray sources making PET quite advantageous in large patients.

Compared with SPECT, PET suffers a sparsity of commercial PET software to assess and correct for motion, alignment of emission and transmission images and perform a host of other tasks to assure quality control and aid acquisition and display. PET tracers are plentiful but suffer from their generally short half-life and their generation in cyclotrons rather than generators. Among PET perfusion agents, only ^{82}Rb is generator produced and available to institutions without a cyclotron. However its short half-life makes only vasodilator pharmacologic stress possible and relatively untested for flow reserve quantitation. ^{13}N ammonia is cyclotron produced and well applied for flow quantitation. Each has physical, kinetic and flow related advantages beyond ^{99m}Tc-based radiotracers. While PET technology remains more expensive, its greater clinical advantages, rapid throughput and extracardiac applications make it cost effective in specific applications, even now.

Single photon emission computed tomography (SPECT) technology is moving rapidly, seeking to equal or surpass the advantages of PET. New instruments, imaging methods and computer software provide new solid state detectors with rapid camera rotation and list mode acquisition. New detector materials provide increased sensitivity with improved energy resolution and reduced scatter. With these methods SPECT perfusion image acquisition may be accelerated to as brief as two minutes with high sensitivity, improved energy resolution and the potential for quantitation and simultaneous dual ^{99m}Tc stress/^{201}Tl rest imaging. Recent methods seek to measure the CFR by SPECT MPI.[51]

With approximately 10 million myocardial perfusion scans, 1.35 million PET scans and 100 million CT scans done each year in the USA, radiation dosage delivered by all methods is again under careful scrutiny (see below—radiation concerns).

TABLE 5

Spectrum of myocardial pathophysiology and viability

Myocardial state	Rest wall motion	Rest/stress perfusion	Metabolism
Normal	Normal	Normal	Normal
Scar	Abnormal	Abnormal—fixed defect	Abnormal
Ischemia	Normal	Abnormal—reversible defect	Normal
Stunned (Transient, post-ischemic dysfunction)	Abnormal	Normal	Normal
Hibernating (dysfunction due to marginal blood supply, serial stunning)	Abnormal	Reversible or fixed defects	Preserved

However, while studies must be performed only with proper indications[40,41] and all must be done to minimize radiation dosage, the tests are safe and should be applied when indicated. The linear extrapolation of risk from highest to lowest radiation exposure now suddenly popular is still not proven and, in some publications, suggests that (cancer) risk from a stress perfusion imaging study rivals that of the stress test. Yet we only request patient's permission for the latter and the benefits of low dose radiation (hormesis) is well established.[52]

IMAGING MYOCARDIAL VIABILITY

THE PRINCIPLES

When myocardium demonstrates systolic dysfunction, the question of myocardial viability arises. Dysfunctional myocardium may be scarred and beyond salvage, or it may be viable in one of several forms. Viable but dysfunctional myocardium may be ischemic, even in the absence of overt ischemic symptoms or signs, or "stunned" or "hibernating". Dysfunctional but viable myocardium is salvageable and may be restored to function with revascularization; a non inconsequential consideration in patients with systolic dysfunction and severe CHF (Tables 5 to 7). Here, with failure of medical treatment, reversal of dysfunction in extensive "hibernating" areas could be life saving and present an important and preferred choice to heart transplantation, which too often is not an available option.

"Stunning" represents transient postischemic dysfunction, generally requiring nothing more than recognition, patience and supportive care, after the ischemic episode passes. After bypass surgery "stunned" myocardium may persist for weeks (Figs 16 and 17). It may last minutes to hours after a positive exercise

TABLE 7

Scintigraphic evidence of myocardial viability and functional reversibility (in the presence of rest wall motion abnormalities and related coronary disease)

- Evidence of preserved perfusion in a dysfunctional segment
- Extensive reversible perfusion abnormalities in a region of abnormal wall motion
- Delayed redistribution of ^{201}Tl in a region with abnormal wall motion
- Post-reinjection ^{201}Tl uptake
- Modest fixed defect in a region with extensive wall motion abnormalities
- PET perfusion-metabolism mismatch
- Evidence of fatty acid uptake (metabolism)

TABLE 6

The basis for imaging myocardial viability

Viatility method	Principles
[201]Tl perfusion imaging/ MR contrast enhancement	Membrane integrity
MIBI/Tetrafosmin perfusion imaging	Mitochondrial integrity
Low dose dobutamine/ MR imaging	Inotropic contractile response
PET	Preserved metabolism

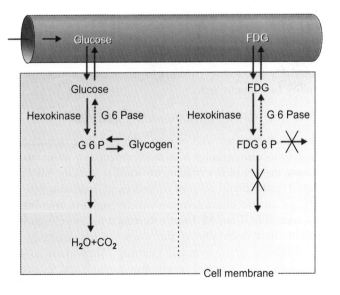

FIGURE 16: Mechanism of FDG localization. Shown diagrammatically is the action of FDG. Transported actively across the cell membrane as is glucose, it is not a substrate for hexokinase and so is not phosphorylated to FDG 6 phosphate (FDG 6 P), as is glucose to glucose 6 phosphate (G 6 P) (Abbreviation: FDG: ^{18}F-deoxyglucose G 6 Pase: enzyme glucose 6 phosphatase). Trapped in the cell it serves as a marker of membrane and energy metabolism integrity and cell viability (*Source:* Modified from Botvinick EH, Dae M, O'Connell JW, et al. The scintigraphic evaluation of the cardiovascular system. In: Parmley WW, Chatterjee K (Eds). Cardiology. Philadelphia: JB Lippincott; 1991)

PET Patterns of myocardial viability
(When Glucose loaded)

^{13}N ammonia ^{18}F-deoxyglucose

Transmural
match

Nontransmural
match

Mismatch

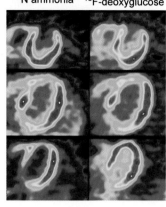

FIGURE 17: Patterns of FDG uptake. Shown on perfusion (left) and FDG metabolism images are matching patterns of varying intensity and the classic, perfusion-metabolism mismatch, suggesting viability. The severe matched defect suggests scar. The matched area with modest uptake on both perfusion and metabolism images suggest potential viability which varies directly with the intensity of FDG and perfusion uptake (*Source:* Reproduced from Maddahi J, UCLA, Los Angeles, CA, with permission)

test, and forms the basis for exercise stress echocardiography. It is characterized by preserved perfusion and metabolism with normal pathology on light microscopy. The cause of related post-ischemic dysfunction is unclear, but has been related to altered energy metabolism.

"Hibernation" has been called "chronic ischemia", a condition hard to imagine and difficult to produce in an animal model. Yet clinically, it may occur at any time and in any clinical setting in the absence of overt ischemia. It must be recognized, differentiated from other causes of systolic dysfunction, and the ischemic cause reversed. It may come and go and is thought to relate to repetitive "stunning". This is the form of occult, potentially reversible ischemic dysfunction, which image viability assessment seeks.

NONSCINTIGRAPHIC IMAGING OPTIONS

The improvement of wall motion with low dose dobutamine stress echocardiography is a more subjective noninvasive alternate manner of determining myocardial viability. MRI and delayed (gadolinium) contrast enhancement, indicating scar on MRI, are another alternative methods for viability assessment. However, SPECT and PET methods remain the most frequently applied, best documented and most trusted methods for determination of myocardial viability. They stand as the comparative gold standard for all other methods and the one to which they aspire.

SCINTIGRAPHIC IMAGING OPTIONS— PERFUSION RELATED

Most prominent among scintigraphic indicators of viability is the maintenance of regional perfusion. The presence of ^{201}Tl or ^{82}Rb, potassium analogs which enter the cell by energy requiring active transport, or any of the ^{99m}Tc perfusion tracers, which

enter viable cells by diffusion, indicates viability. Here, the level of radiotracer uptake is directly proportional to the likelihood of viability and restoration of function after revascularization. ^{201}Tl is initially distributed to the myocardium in proportion to regional flow. With time the intracellular ^{201}Tl distribution parallels intracellular space or viability. These distributions are generally the same, but if viable cells are ischemic at rest, an initial rest related perfusion defect may "fill in" or normalize with time. Delayed ^{201}Tl imaging at 4 and 24 hours or the delayed "reinjection" of a small dose of the radionuclide may normalize perfusion, an indicator of viability. The time to redistribution is directly proportional to the severity of the stenosis and related flow abnormality. Reinjection and related viability detection appear to be augmented with nitroglycerin. Reinjection of the radionuclide too close to the time of redistribution imaging may re-establish an already resolved defect and result in an underestimation of viability. Administration of nitrates has been advocated to increase radiotracer uptake and optimize the evaluation of viability with single photon perfusion agents.

SCINTIGRAPHIC IMAGING OPTIONS— METABOLISM BASED

With fasting or with ischemia, myocardial metabolism shifts from its primary metabolite, fatty acids, to glucose. Imaging a radiolabeled analog of glucose, ^{18}F-deoxyglucose (FDG), which is trapped in the myocyte but not metabolized, remains the noninvasive imaging standard for myocardial viability. Scintigraphically, the density of a perfusion defect at rest has been found proportional to the likelihood of viability. However, even severe PET perfusion defects are roughly divided between those which are and those which are not, viable (Figs 16 and 17). Here, viability is determined by evidence of ^{18}F-FDG uptake, revealing a perfusion-metabolism mismatch and indicating active metabolism in the area of underperfusion[53] (Figs 16 and 17). When present in a major mass of dysfunctional myo-cardium, the "mismatch" pattern is highly predictive of functional and symptomatic improvement and reduced mortality after revascularization where a failure to revascularize such ventricles relate to increased mortality. However, the smaller the extent of mismatch, the larger the "matched", scarred area, the more prolonged the dysfunction, the more delayed is revascularization, or a baseline LVEF too low, less than 30%, end diastolic volume (LVEDV) too high with LVED diameter greater than or equal to 6 cm each has an adverse effect on the outcome and relates to an increased risk with revascularization, particularly CABG. The complexity of predicting postrevas-cularization functional improvement has been reviewed.[54] The advantages of viability evaluation by PET perfusion with ^{13}N-ammonia compared with ^{99m}Tc-based perfusion tracers were analyzed.[55] Most recently, the identification of infarcted myocardium on a contrast MRI study has engendered excitement as a more direct manner of determining regional myocardial viability, although with only modest ability to assess myo-cardium at ischemic risk. Guidelines have been published for application of cardiac PET studies as well as for qualifications to practice cardiac PET.[53]

RUBIDIUM (^{82}Rb) CHLORIDE

Strontium generator produced ^{82}Rb (T 1/2 = 75 sec) is being applied with increasing frequency for pharmacologic stress MPI.[56-59] Compared with current ^{99m}Tc-based agents it has improved imaging characteristics and better spatial resolution, superior flow linearity, shorter acquisition time with imaging begun at the time of radionuclide administration and completed within 1 hour, more rigorous AC and ready availability. The review of ^{82}Rb PET MPI presented in the PET guidelines[53] notes an overall diagnostic sensitivity of 89% and specificity of 86% for CAD, superior to SPECT MPI. The method is clearly advantageous for use in heavy patients and women where issues of attenuation often cloud interpretation. SPECT ^{99m}Tc sestamibi and PET ^{82}Rb MPS gated rest/pharmacologic stress studies have been compared in patient populations matched by gender, body mass index, and presence and extent of CAD PET demonstrated higher image quality, diagnostic accuracy and interpretive confidence in both men and women, in obese and nonobese patients, and for correct identification of multivessel CAD. Similar to SPECT perfusion imaging, the PET method also gains significant prognostic value with added functional information with gated acquisition. As opposed to stress SPECT, where gated images are acquired post-stress, the PET ^{82}Rb method acquires true peak stress gated images, with evaluation of LV wall motion and ejection fraction (EF). This can be compared with rest images for a better diagnosis and prognosis of induced ischemia and CAD, where lack of stress induced LVEF augmentation could indicate occult evidence of an ischemic response. Dynamic image acquisition could permit quantification of the regional stress related augmentation of perfusion and CFR. An editorial considers the clinical roles of SPECT and PET perfusion imaging. The method is highly cost effective in high volume laboratories which can utilize the continuous and endless availability of the ^{82}Rb generator at a cost of $28,000 monthly. Unlike SPECT studies, there is a dearth of commercial PET software to assess and correct for motion, compare with a normal database, score defects or provide other analytic tools. Nonetheless, the potential benefits of PET compared to SPECT are extensive. While a dedicated PET cardiac camera is not practical in most imaging practices, cardiac cases can be well integrated with oncology demands to fill spaces in PET camera schedules with collaboration between referring internists and cardiologists and imaging radiologists and nuclear physicians.

NITROGEN (^{13}N) AMMONIA

With cyclotron produced ^{13}N (T 1/2 = 75 sec) ammonia, the longer agent half-life permits the performance of gated exercise MPI. However excellent coordination with an on-site cyclotron is needed. These considerations may favor the choice and more widespread application of ^{82}Rb in spite of the better imaging characteristics of ^{13}N ammonia. The availability of either agent will provide PET rather than SPECT perfusion to compare with FDG metabolism, an important for the evaluation of myocardial viability.

Guidelines have been developed for patient preparation for data acquisition, interpretation and reporting of both ^{18}F-FDG cardiac PET for myocardial viability and for PET perfusion imaging performed with generator produced ^{82}Rb as well as with cyclotron produced ^{13}N ammonia. Future applications with PET/CT scanners could find PET perfusion and CT coronary anatomy fused noninvasively into an image with optimal information content.

The reimbursement of PET stress MPI appears well justified by its accuracy, better localizing value with a clearer roadmap of CAD involvement, relative ease of performance, its added speed and reduced radioactivity exposure compared to ^{99m}Tc-based perfusion agents. Then should PET MPI replace SPECT? This may not necessarily be the case as SPECT methods have also gained accuracy. However, those with equivocal SPECT studies, obese subjects, those with more complicated coronary anatomy and high likelihood or known CAD post-MI, PCI or CABG, those with a known cardiomyopathy of ischemic or unknown cause are likely to benefit most from PET perfusion evaluation.

However, if exercise is needed, in the absence of a cyclotron, SPECT MPI is required even in an obese patient weighing over 250 lbs. If SPECT images are suboptimal then ^{82}Rb PET MPI with vasodilator stress becomes an option. The ready availability of generator produced ^{82}Rb, its rapid throughput and the safety of vasodilator stress make it appropriate for ED evaluation.

QUANTITATION OF REGIONAL CORONARY FLOW AND FLOW RESERVE

Currently, perfusion imaging is evaluated as a "heterogeneity map" and read as abnormal based on the degree and extent of intensity or counts heterogeneity. The ability to accurately and reproducibly quantitate absolute regional myocardial stress induced hyperemia would increase diagnostic sensitivity beyond the relative visual method of perfusion imaging.[60-62] Calculation of the exact regional flow at rest and stress in absolute ml/min/g of tissue could evaluate each region independently but presents greater technical obstacles and imaging challenges which are not currently in the realm of standard clinical imaging. However, flow quantitation with identification of regional CFR and the increase in hyperemic compared to normal flow is a relative yet superior value, which is likely within the technical abilities of most well-disciplined clinical imaging labs. CFR quantitation would free regional sampling from the insensitivity resulting when abnormal regions are best perfused, yet underperfused. The grossest example of this problem relates to the occurrence of the oft-noted but rarely observed example of "balanced ischemia", where all regions may be similarly underperfused and so could appear homogeneous and normal on standard relative perfusion imaging. This could result in normal scans in the setting of triple vessel disease. To a lesser degree this relative intensity comparison is a reason for underestimating the full extent of disease by such relative regional analysis. It should be noted, however, that MPI sensitivity increases with the severity and extent of CAD and the strong prognostic value of the method also argues against the frequent error in the diagnosis of multivessel, high risk CAD. Even with balanced ischemia, the scintigraphic method would be expected to reveal heterogeneity in long axis slices where regions proximal to the stenoses are more intense than those distal. Of course, even with misleading balanced intensities, the nonperfusion indicators of extensive disease including cavitary dilation and lung uptake, induced cavitary photopenia in addition to ischemic symptoms and ECG changes could present clues to the severity of the condition and the reader must always consider the image in the overall context of stress test findings. Of course, MPI sensitivity directly parallels the level of stress applied as a test of the CFR. While not common, there is a higher incidence of reported normal images with adequate stress and extensive CAD in selected studies. Of course, any level of such error is unacceptable and anything which can practically be done to increase the diagnostic and prognostic yield, even in relation to "suboptimal" stress tests, should be applied. PET perfusion quantitation presents the best noninvasive hope. Some advocate CTCA to identify this group and even suggest its application to asymptomatic subjects. Those who do, assume a high specificity of the CTCA method, not supported to date, set aside copious data supporting the high predictive value of a negative stress perfusion image over the spectrum of clinical presentations and overlook the already documented high prognostic value and superior cost effectiveness of the physiologic compared with the anatomic evaluation of coronary disease. In other settings, such measures of CFR may help identify an altered coronary vasoreactivity in the absence of flow limiting stenoses, in those with advanced atherosclerosis or other condition and provide insight into disease pathophysiology and symptoms in a variety of vascular diseases and cardiomyopathies. For these reasons quantitation of perfusion is important. With the clinical proliferation of PET perfusion imaging, quantitation is sure to follow as a widely or selectively applied method.

BLOOD POOL IMAGING—EQUILIBRIUM RADIONUCLIDE ANGIOGRAPHY AND FIRST PASS RADIONUCLIDE ANGIOGRAPHY

GUIDELINES

Guidelines have been formulated for the acquisition and clinical application of first pass radionuclide angiography (FPRNA) and equilibrium radionuclide angiography (ERNA).[63,64] Although in recent years these methods have often been relegated to a supportive or confirmatory role, they are highly quantitative and reproducible for the evaluation of biventricular wall motion and EF. With greater effort absolute volumes can be calculated. Popular clinical applications relate to those scenarios where accuracy and reproducibility in serial measurements are required as for the monitoring of chemotherapy induced cardiotoxicity.[65] Here starting from a normal LVEF, greater than or equal to 55%, a fall in LVEF of 10% or to less than or equal to 50% is significant and requires ERNA monitoring before subsequent doses. Chemotherapy should be interrupted for a period of recovery if LVEF falls a further 10% or to lesser than 40% with careful monitoring thereafter or the patient risks a permanent loss of LV systolic function. Exercise LVEF can also help identify cardiotoxicity when the LVEF at rest is normal but there are no specific guidelines.

The method now seems to be gaining increased importance in the serial evaluation of patients with CHF due to systolic dysfunction and particularly to evaluate ventricular synchrony as cardiac resynchronization therapy (CRT) is applied to improve severe systolic dysfunction, CHF symptoms and outcomes.[66]

INTRODUCTION

Two radionuclide based techniques have been used to measure ventricular function for over three decades.[67] One method employs tracers that label the myocardial walls (e.g. ^{99m}Tc-MIBI, ^{18}F-FDG, etc.) and examines wall thickening and motion throughout the cardiac cycle. Here, wall thickening is proportional to cyclical intensity changes while volumes and LVEF are based in calculations based geometric chamber analysis. This is the principle applied to gain functional information in perfusion imaging, as discussed above. Alternatively, the blood can be labeled and imaged in two ways, by first pass or equilibrium methods. In the FPRNA, ventricular volumes and function are assessed from the passage of the radionuclide through the chamber, while in ERNA, calculations are based on the fact that counts are proportional to volume. In both methods, geometric analysis may be applied or more appropriately and more accurately, volumes and EF can be calculated from chamber counts and systolic wall motion and sequence can be determined by an examination of the changes in the intensity and configuration of the ventricular blood pool through the cardiac cycle. The latter method has been discussed below.

LABELING THE BLOOD POOL

This method has the advantage of providing a direct measure of ventricular volumes. In the ideal circumstance with truly quantitative imaging, measurement of absolute volume can be obtained directly from the images, where:

$$\text{LV volume} = \text{Total cavitary radioactivity}/\text{Activity in the blood.}$$

The ability to make accurate quantitative measurements from images of cavitary activity is currently limited to PET. SPECT blood pool techniques have greater inaccuracies of attenuation and scatter, and cannot currently be used to quantitate ventricular volumes from image data alone. PET and SPECT volumetric methods are most arduous, require blood sampling and counting, and are not done clinically. However, nearly all clinical applications, simply seek to make relative measurements of ventricular function and LVEF which depend only on the relative accuracy of the imaging modality. Planar imaging methods can do this quite well, whereas SPECT offers some advantages for regional function evaluation. The most commonly used tracer for ERNA is ^{99m}Tc labeled red blood cells but any tracer which passes through the lungs may be used for FPRNA.[63] Thus one can obtain LV function data from FPRNA data acquired with a study done for some other purpose, as bone scans. Commercial kits are available and generally applied. PET is not used for clinical blood pool imaging where LVEF is readily generated with perfusion imaging by analysis of the myocardial label.

FIRST PASS CURVE ANALYSIS

VENTRICULAR FUNCTION

First pass radionuclide angiography (FPRNA) can be accurately performed with as little as 1–2 mCi of any agent which stays in

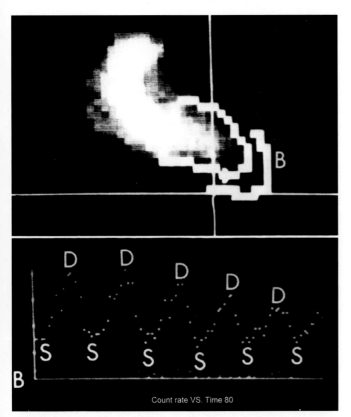

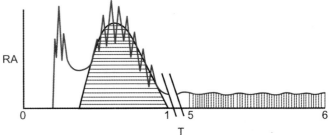

FIGURE 19: First pass analysis. The figure presents a sketch of a first pass time (T), versus radioactivity (RA) curve. The area under the left ventricular component (horizontal lines) is proportional to cardiac output and is calibrated for volume by dividing it into the integrated area under one minute of the equilibrium time versus radioactivity curve (vertical lines), acquired when the radiotracer is thoroughly mixed in the blood. Alternatively, volumes may be calculated from ventricular outlines using geometric considerations (*Source:* Modified from FA Davis Co. Botvinick EH, Glazer HB, Shosa DW. What is the reliability and utility of scintigraphic methods for the assessment of ventricular function? Cardiovasc Clin. 1983;13:65-78. Legend adapted with permission from Botvinick EH (Ed). Radionuclide angiography: equilibrium and first pass methods. Self-Study Program III; Nuclear Medicine: Cardiology, Soc Nucl Med Publ.)

FIGURE 18: First pass analysis of the levophase. An irregular region of interest is drawn (top) on the levophase of the first pass ventriculogram. High temporal sampling of the left ventricular data produces the curve shown below. Correcting for background activity, the diastolic peaks (D) and systolic valleys (S) are compared to calculate the LVEF (*Source:* Modified from Botvinick EH (Ed). Radionuclide angiography: equilibrium and first pass methods. Self-Study Program III; Nuclear Medicine: Cardiology, Soc Nucl Med.)

the blood pool for the first circulation, but, with this low dose, images are not available (Figs 18 and 19).

"First pass" imaging presents an alternative method of blood pool acquisition with imaging the subject while injecting the tracer as a bolus. Nearly all the considerations discussed for standard gating of MPI, above, can be applied to this first pass methodology. Regardless of its ultimate disposition, during its brief first transit through the heart, most tracers stay in the arterial blood for seconds to minutes, before they are taken up by the myocardium or other tissues. During that brief transit time, the tracer behaves as though it were a blood pool tracer. When the tracer is injected as a bolus, gating is necessary in order to capture the EF. For first pass studies only a few beats of data need be added together. In addition, it is possible to position the gamma camera in an RAO view and obtain early gated images during the passage of the radioisotope through the RV, prior to contamination by counts from the LV. One of the disadvantages of the first transit is that one usually must obtain all the LV function information from only a small number of beats. This means a rapid bolus injection must be given, resulting in very high count rates during passage of the tracer through the cardiac chambers. Such high count rates require state of the art cameras. Additionally, the EF, calculated from the average values based on the magnitude of the peak counts, proportional to ED volume, and the valleys, proportional to ES volume, correcting for background activity, is based on few

samples and so is prone to greater variability. Fewer samples relate to right ventricular ejection fraction (RVEF) evaluation and so require a tight RV bolus passage.

First pass radionuclide angiography (FPRNA), like ERNA, may be applied to evaluate the effects of exercise on ventricular function and were earlier applied with great frequency to evaluate the functional reserve in aortic valvular disease and for the diagnosis of CAD. These applications have been largely replaced by the echo-Doppler evaluation of valve disease and by MPI.

LEFT-TO-RIGHT SHUNT ANALYSIS

First pass radionuclide angiography (FPRNA) remains a method for the quantitation of left-to-right intracardiac shunts (Figs 20A and B). It demonstrates the calculation of the pulmonic to systemic (Qp/Qs) flow ratio; the left-to-right shunt magnitude in a patient with an atrial septal defect according to the method of Maltz and Treves. Here, by the principles of "dye dilution" analysis, the area under the first fitted curve, Area 1, is proportionate to systemic flow while the area under the second passage curve, Area 2, is proportional to the shunt flow. As shown diagrammatically in the following Figure, Area 1 = Qs (systemic) and Area 2 = Qsh (shunt). Thus, Qp = Qs - Qsh and

$$Qp/Qs = \frac{Qp}{Qs - Qsh} = \frac{Area\ 1}{Area\ 2 - Area\ 1}$$

The method is not a diagnostic tool but one meant for accurate quantitation of such shunts between Qp/Qs of 1.2–3, and so is useful in prognosis and management. It is another scintigraphic method which is underutilized owing to the widespread availability and capabilities of echo-Doppler examination.

EQUILIBRIUM GATED IMAGING—ERNA

The method of equilibrium gated blood pool image acquisition is demonstrated here, often called ERNA.[63] ERNA requires a

CHAPTER 21

Cardiovascular Nuclear Medicine—Nuclear Cardiology

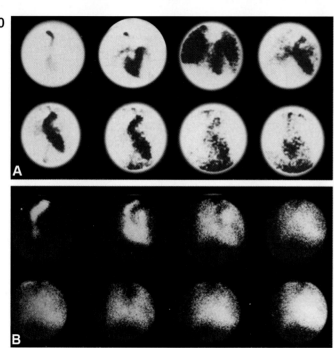

FIGURES 20A AND B: First pass images in normal patient and in a patient with left to right shunt. Shown in panel (A) are serial images acquired during the first passage of the radioactive bolus through the central circulation with a normal heart. Note lung clearance in frame 4 and the teardrop shape of the left ventricle in frames 4–6. In panel (B) are similar images taken in a patient with a significant left to right shunt. The lungs never clear due to continued recirculation of the bolus. As a result, the left ventricle teardrop and the levophase are not seen. This "smudge sign" generally relates to a left to right shunt with "Qp/Qs e" 1.5 (*Source:* Modified from Botvinick EH (Ed). Physical and technical aspects of nuclear cardiology. Self-Study Program III; Nuclear Medicine: Cardiology, Soc Nucl Med Publ. 2009)

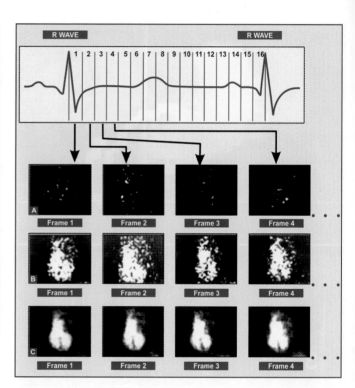

FIGURE 21: Computer acquisition of the equilibrium study (see text) (*Source:* Modified from Parker DA, Karvelis KC, Thrall JH, et al. Radio-nuclide ventriculography: methods. In: Gerson MC (Ed). Cardiac Nuclear Medicine, 2nd edn. Legend adapted with permission from Botvinick EH (Ed). Physical and technical aspects of nuclear cardiology. Self-Study Program III; Nuclear Medicine: Cardiology, Soc Nucl Med Publ.)

blood pool agent, typically labeled red blood cells, which are injected, and then allowed to mix with the 5–6 liters of blood in a typical subject. After 3 or 4 minutes of mixing, the tracer will be uniformly distributed, and the tracer is then said to be "in equilibrium". If a single heart beat were 960 msec long (i.e. a heart rate of about 63 bpm), we could divide that single beat into 16 images, each 60 msec long. The first image would be acquired for 60 msec and then the second would acquire all the data in the next 60 msec, etc. Each image would reflect a different portion of the cardiac cycle, from end diastole through systole, and back again. Unfortunately, an acquisition that was only 60 msec long would have too few counts to make an interpretable image. With the typical activities injected in a patient (10–30 mCi, or 370–1,110 MBq for either blood pool or myocardial imaging), one would need to acquire each image many 100s of times longer—perhaps 10–20 seconds or longer. To solve this problem, we use the technique of ECG gating. Here, an ECG is connected to the patient, and its output is put through a "trigger" device which generates a "gating" signal at each R wave peak, for example. For the first 60 msec after the first R wave, all the photons are sorted into the first image. After 60 msec have elapsed, all data are then sorted into the second image, and so on. Finally, at the next R wave, signifying the beginning of the next cardiac cycle, the process is repeated, and the next 60 msec of data are again added to the first image (called image 1 in the Figure), and similarly for all the

subsequent images. If this process continues for 300 beats, then each image is acquired for (60 msec/beat)*300 sec = 18 seconds. Note that the total acquisition time for collecting data is not determined directly by the imaging time, but rather by the number of beats times the duration of each frame. At high heart rates, then, this time builds up more quickly than at low heart rates. Computer acquisition of the ERNA is illustrated in Figure 21. Shown is the relationship between the cardiac cycle or R-R interval acquired over 16 separate frames or intervals and the related images in each frame over the course of the acquisition. The counts acquired during the frame 2 are stored in frame 2; those acquired during frame 3 are stored in frame 3 and so on. Only data accumulated over the first four frames is illustrated here. Owing to the low count rate in this study, 750 counts per frame, there is little to see after acquisition over a single cycle (A). However, after the accumulation and addition of the counts from 20 R-R cycles, now with 15,000 counts per frame, the cardiac chambers are taking from (B). With the addition of counts acquired over 400 cycles and 300,000 counts per frame, image quality is excellent and the acquisition is over (C). A typical but relatively high frequency ERNA time versus radioactivity curve is shown in Figure 22.

A RV region of interest can be applied to an end diastole and end systole region of interest in an equilibrium blood pool study to calculate RVEF. Overlap of the right atrium reduces accuracy of RVEF calculation but the method compares well with other methods for RVEF measurement, a difficult task by all methods due to the position and shape of the chamber.

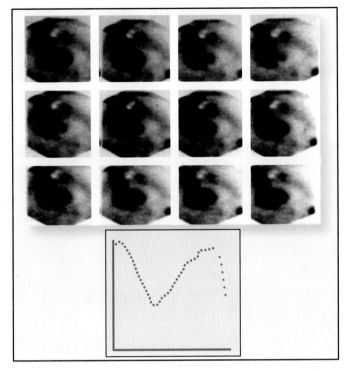

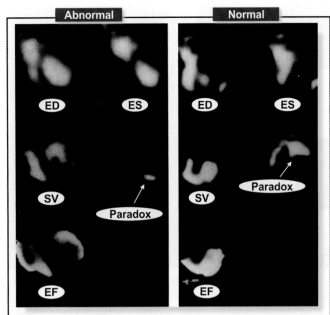

FIGURE 22: Equilibrium radionuclide angiography images and time versus radioactivity curve. Shown above, in the "best septal" projection are 12 selected frames from a multiple-gated equilibrium study. End diastole is shown at upper left, with contraction progressing left to right and top to bottom. End systole is in frame 5, below end diastole. A clear halo around the left ventricular images here relates to the myocardial boundaries, suggesting hypertrophy in this case. The area of reduced radioactivity in the region of the septum is of normal thickness, as may be seen with pericardial effusion. However the halo does not extend to the pericardial reflections, as is commonly seen with a large, nonloculated effusion. Below is the time versus radioactivity curve derived from counts in the left ventricular region in this study where peak counts are proportional to end diastolic volume and lower counts are proportional to end systolic volume. Terminal count fall-off relates to irregularity of the cardiac rhythm and R-R interval over the acquisition period, where short cycles do not add data to the terminal frames (*Source:* Modified from Green MV, Ostrow HG, Douglas MA, et al. High temporal resolution ECG-gated scintigraphic angiocardiography. J Nucl Med. 1975;16:95-8. Legend adapted with permission from Botvinick EH (Ed). Physical and technical aspects of nuclear cardiology. Self-Study Program III; Nuclear Medicine: Cardiology, Soc Nucl Med Publ.)

FIGURE 23: Functional or parametric images. Shown in the left panel above are end diastolic (ED) and end systolic (ES) frames from a normal equilibrium blood pool study. In the center row are stroke volume (SV) and paradox images. The former represents the pixel-by-pixel representation of the difference in ED and ES counts, while the latter represents the converse. Since ES-ED represents a positive value in the atrial regions, they are evident in the paradox but not in the SV image. Conversely, ventricular regions are well seen in the SV image but present negative values in the paradox image and are absent. Unlike SV and paradox images, amplitude images are sign neutral and will proportionately present any region that changes counts (volume) with the cardiac cycle, regardless of its phase. The bottom row shows the ejection fraction (EF) image, where each pixel of the SV image has been divided by per pixel ED counts, yielding an image comprised of pixel-by-pixel, intensity coded EF. At right are the same parametric images derived from a patient with a left ventricular apical aneurysm (*Source:* Modified from Botvinick EH (Ed). Radionuclide angiography: equilibrium and first pass methods. Self-Study Program III; Nuclear Medicine: Cardiology, Soc Nucl Med Publ.)

THE VALUE OF FUNCTIONAL IMAGING

There are many useful clinical parameters which can be extracted from the LV volume curve shown in the previous figures. The most useful measure is EF, defined as stroke volume (SV)/ED volume = (ED counts - ES counts)/ED counts, where the counts are corrected for background. Many other parameters can be extracted from this curve including the peak ejection rate and its time of occurrence, the time to end systole and the peak filling rate. A variety of functional images are illustrated in Figure 23.

Equilibrium radionuclide angiography (ERNA) functional or parametric images are of value in adding objectivity to the interpretation of studies to evaluate exercise evaluation of possible coronary disease (Figs 24A to C), the pathophysiologic significance of aortic regurgitation or other valve lesion (Figs 25 and 26). A regurgitant index, quantitating the relative regurgitant volume can be accurately calculated.[68]

PHASE ANALYSIS

Phase image analysis is based on functional images derived from the gated ERNA. They have been successfully applied to characterize the sequence of ventricular contraction. While ERNA is a long established method, this application promises added clinical value in the assessment of the newest treatment of advanced heart failure, CRT. The basis for the method and some applications are illustrated in Figures 27 and 28.

IMAGING MYOCARDIAL SYMPATHETIC INNERVATION

Metaiodobenzylguanidine (MIBG) is an analog of norepinephrine and can be radiolabeled to reveal a map of the scattered presynaptic terminals throughout the rich myocardial sympathetic innervation. Autonomic abnormalities may be a common final pathway for sudden cardiac death, taking 300,000–400,000 yearly. Normal values have been established.[69-72] Extensive studies have demonstrated that scintigraphic evaluation of ^{123}I labeled MIBG intensity and distribution can aid risk stratification and therapy in patients with heart failure of any cause.[73-77] The agent is now completing Phase III evaluation and will, pending

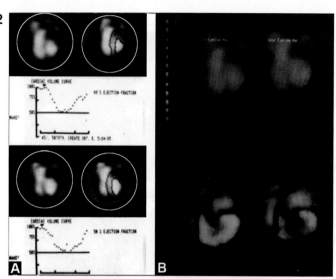

Rest		Exercise
127	EDV(cc)	158
65	ESV(cc)	79
62	SV(cc)	79
49	LVEF(%)	50
65	HR(bpm)	126
4	CO(1/min)	10
	Workload 400 kpm	

C

FIGURES 24A TO C: The value of functional imaging. In (A), at left shows the automated left ventricular edge fit to the equilibrium blood pool image of a patient with coronary disease, above, at rest, and below during peak reclining bicycle exercise. The LVEF showed no significant change. However induced wall motion abnormalities are clearly seen in (B), with a loss of septal intensity at stress, right, compared to rest, left, in the color ejection images, with a break in the "ejection shell" above, and with reduced amplitude, an analog of regional stroke volume, the red color in the septum of the stress image, right, compared to rest, left, in the color amplitude images, below. Shown in (C) are the volumes calculated from this blood pool data at rest and stress, where end diastolic (EDV) and end systolic volume (ESV) increased. Note the blunted LVEF response with a rise in ESV with exercise (Abbreviations: CO: Cardiac output; HR: Heart rate; LVEF: Left ventricular ejection fraction; SV: Stroke volume) (*Source:* Modified from Botvinick EH, Dae MW, O'Connell JW. Blood pool scintigraphy. Cardiol Clin. 1989;7:537-63. Legend adapted with permission from Botvinick EH (Ed). Radionuclide angiography: equilibrium and first pass methods. Self-Study Program III; Nuclear Medicine: Cardiology, Soc Nucl Med Publ.)

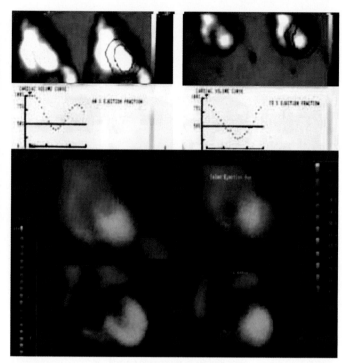

FIGURE 25: Equilibrium blood pool assessment of aortic regurgitation. Shown are left ventricular time versus activity curves derived from a left ventricular region of interest (top panel); ejection fraction images, color-coded for regional ejection fraction (middle panel); and phase-amplitude images (bottom panel), at rest (left) and with maximal exercise (right) in a young patient with severe aortic regurgitation. Here, the left ventricular edge is derived between the limits of the edges drawn, and background is taken within these geometric boundaries. Dual color and intensity coded images, shown here, permit the integration of multiple parameters in a single image and are an example of the analytic and display potential of the scintigraphic modality. The LVEF increases with exercise. This is supported by the increased area covered by yellow and green and high ejection fraction values in the ejection fraction image. Although colors shift to later phase angles as heart rate increases, amplitude, intensity, is maintained and apparent ventricular size decreases in all images, consistent with a normal response to exercise. The uniform phase shift, related to increased symmetry of the time versus radioactivity curve with increased heart rate and shortening of end diastole, represents a normal finding, as do all the image results shown here (*Source:* Modified from Botvinick EH, Dae MW, O'Connell JW. Blood pool scintigraphy. Cardiol Clin. 1989;7:537-63. Legend adapted with permission from Botvinick EH (Ed). Radionuclide angiography: equilibrium and first pass methods. Self-Study Program III; Nuclear Medicine: Cardiology, Soc Nucl Med Publ.)

likely early FDA approval, soon be available. A large prognostic multicenter trial including 55 in the United States and 25 in the European medical centers, studies New York Heart Association Class II–III CHF patients with LVEF less than 35% by SPECT MIBG. In heart failure, a low heart/mediastinal (H/M) MIBG ratio less than 1.2 or a slow myocardial washout less than 27% per hour indicates a poor prognosis, even in the absence of CAD. Diabetics are at an increased risk since the condition appears to effect autonomic innervation in an independent manner. In some studies, the H/M was a more significant predictor of death than the LVEF. Improvement in this ratio could serve to demonstrate the beneficial effects of heart failure therapy (Figs 29 and 30). Evidence suggests that denervated regions with preserved perfusion, an MIBG/perfusion mismatch, place the patient at greatest risk. The combination of heart rate variability, another

reflection of autonomic innervation, and MIBG washout appears to reflect survival and varies with treatment in CHF patients. This combination of heart rate variability and MIBG distribution differentiated between those with implanted defibrillators who did or did not receive a shock on follow-up evaluation. PET imaging of perfusion and the norepinephrine analog 11C-HED could add yet greater resolution and quantitation to this evaluation, but would require an on-site cyclotron. The potential role for MIBG in the clinical evaluation of the heart failure patient is presented above (Figs 29 and 30). MIBG image findings may well impact too on the state of chemotherapy induced cardiotoxicity.

RADIATION CONCERNS

When taken in the context of natural background radiation, man-made radiation represents 18% of that delivered. Yet, this is primarily medical in origin and, of course, may be controlled

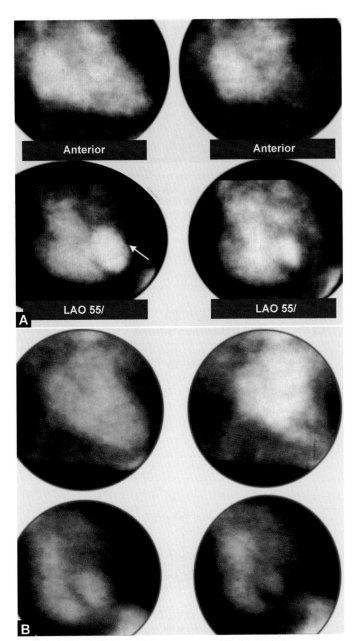

FIGURES 26A AND B: Gated blood pool studies pre- and post-repair of mitral regurgitation. Panel (A) illustrates end diastolic (left) and end systolic (right) images in the anterior (top) and "best septal" (bottom) projections in the equilibrium blood pool study in a patient with a systolic murmur, breathlessness and fatigability. The arrow points to the enlarged left ventricle in this patient presenting with severe mitral regurgitation. Panel (B) illustrates the study post-mitral valve replacement, in the same format. The size and relative intensity, indicators of volume, of the left ventricle, are dramatically reduced. The obvious visual difference between right and left ventricular stroke volume present on the preoperative study is no longer evident after surgery (*Source:* Modified from Botvinick EH, Dae MW, O'Connell JW. Blood pool scintigraphy. Cardiol Clin. 1989;7:537-63. Legend adapted with permission from Botvinick EH (Ed). Radionuclide angiography: equilibrium and first pass methods. Self-Study Program III; Nuclear Medicine: Cardiology, Soc Nucl Med Publ.)

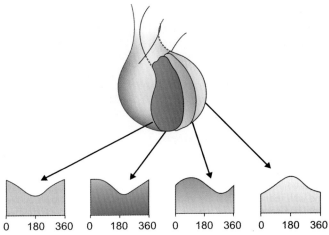

FIGURE 27: Phase analysis. This diagram presents a ventricle that is gray scale coded for increasing delay in contraction sequence from septum to lateral wall. The resultant cosine curves, fitted to the regional time-versus-radioactivity curve, are shown below. The septum and its corresponding curve begin contraction at the R wave. The region has a phase angle of 0° and is coded dark gray. The lateral wall and its related cosine curve fill when the ventricle should empty. This wall would demonstrate paradoxical motion and the curve would have a phase angle of 180° (*Source:* Modified from Exerpta Medica, Inc. from Frais MA, Botvinick EH, Shosa DW, et al. Phase image characterization of ventricular contraction in left and right bundle branch block. Am J Cardiol. 1982;50:95-105)

development of solid and hematologic cancers in humans. Absorbed radiation dose refers to the amount of energy deposited by exposure to the ionizing radiation per patient unit mass. Units of absorbed radiation dose are rads or milliards in conventional units or gray in international system of units (SI). The effective dose is expressed in conventional units of rem or millirem or the SI units of sievert (Sv) or millisievert (mSv). Since the effects of low dose radiation, from 0 to 100 mSv (millisieverts), are small and so difficult to measure, a linear response is extrapolated from high dose effects. Although such extrapolation and these related effects are controversial, they are not inconsequential and must be considered in ordering and performing any test with such potential effects. The full body effective dose is highest for MPI performed with ^{201}Tl or with the dual isotope ^{201}Tl rest-^{99m}Tc stress protocol and less when performed exclusively with ^{99m}Tc-based agents or [82]Rb. Of course, stress only ^{99m}Tc or [82]Rb studies present lowest dose (Tables 8 and 9). A 64 slice modified discrete cosine transform (MDCT) without ECG pulsing but with retrospective gating

TABLE 8

Radiation dosage of selected exposures

Study	Total body effective dose (mSv)
Chest radiographs in 2 views	0.08
Mammogram	0.13
Average US background radiation	3.0/y
Smoking cigarettes	2.8/y
Air travel	0.01 per 1000 miles

Source: Thompson RC, Cullom SJ. Radiation dosage of cardiac nuclear and radiography procedures. J Nucl Cardiol. 2006;13:19-23.

by design and application of diagnostic and therapeutic methods. The seventh report of the National Research Council's Committee on the Biological Effects of Ionizing Radiation (BIER) on the medical effects of low dose ionizing radiation was released in 2005.[78] It assumes a linear dose response relationship between exposure to ionizing radiation and the

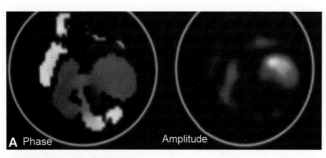 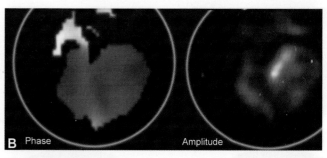

FIGURES 28A AND B: Phase image analysis of synchrony before and after biventricular pacing. Shown are examples of phase and amplitude images, left and right in each panel, respectively, derived from gated blood pool scintigrams in a patient with heart failure. Panel A shows images acquired from the patient at baseline, with evidence of gross regional dyssynchrony in the phase image at left (white color in the septum and apex) and with reduced amplitude in most of the distal LV, as shown by the low intensity regions of the amplitude images at right. In panel B, color is more homogeneous and phase is more synchronous, with much improvement in the intensity of the amplitude image following biventricular pacemaker insertion. Not surprisingly, the patient was much improved clinically after the procedure (*Source:* Modified from Rosenquist M, Botvinick EH, Dae M, et al. Left ventricular function during pacing: the relative importance of activation sequence compared to AV synchrony. J Nucl Med. 1990;31:752)

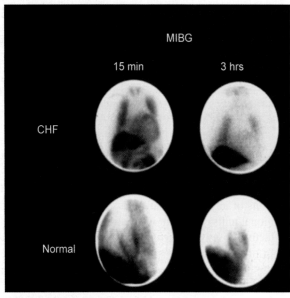

FIGURE 29: MIBG imaging in congestive heart failure (CHF). Shown in these anterior planar images is the distribution of ^{123}I MIBG in a patient with CHF and a normal patient. The CHF distribution is marked by the presence of a markedly enlarged heart with dense lung uptake on both early and late imaging, poor myocardial tracer localization on early imaging and near complete washout on late imaging. This stands in contrast to the normal cardiac contour, brisk myocardial localization and excellent target to lung background on the delayed images in the normal patient (*Source:* Courtesy of Dae M, MD, UCSF, San Francisco, CA)

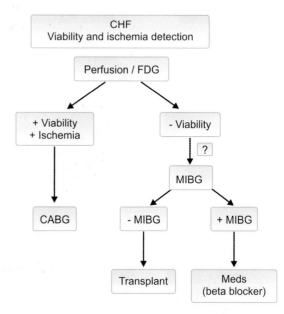

FIGURE 30: Possible role of MIBG in the management of severe congestive heart failure (CHF) with systolic dysfunction. First a determination must be made of the myocardial viability of abnormally contracting and poorly perfused segments. In those with coronary disease, evident ischemia, and "sufficient" viable myocardium, coronary artery bypass (CABG) or percutaneous catheter intervention, stent, may be performed. In those without viability or in the absence of coronary disease which may be revascularized, MIBG imaging may be performed. MIBG uptake indicates preserved neuronal binding sites and the potential for improvement and reduced risk with beta blockers and medical therapy. In the absence of MIBG uptake, heart transplantation would be the remaining option (*Source:* Courtesy of Dae M, MD, UCSF, San Francisco, CA)

optimizes the accuracy of the CTCA method but presents a much higher effective dosage, while CT applied only as a transmission source delivers a very low exposure. The radiation exposure from CT to females is much greater than to males and the CT exposure to the female breast, intervening between X-ray source and target and a focus of the delivered X-ray, is high and far exceeds that of scintigraphic methods, where the dose is delivered more uniformly body wide and to the target organ. While the risks are real, they are relatively small in patients in the coronary disease age range, increasing cancer mortality from 0.01 to 0.05%. Further, this increment is applied over the life of a patient and decreases in impact with increasing age at application. They are far less significant in the elderly. The

cardiovascular risk addressed by many such studies is much greater, and focused on a brief period of decision and management. Physicians working with these methods must be fully informed regarding the dosimetry and the technical aspects of the diagnostic test. The basic principle to keep dosage as low as possible must be observed. However, as clinicians, they must also weigh the clinical need and risks versus benefits, in order to apply to the patient the proper evaluation with greatest accuracy and least ambiguity. Preferably the test selected will make others (which give yet further radiation exposure)

TABLE 9

Radiation dosage of cardiovascular radionuclide studies

Study	Total body effective dose (mSv)
^{99m}Tc trofosmin rest-stress (10 mCi + 30 mCi)	10.6
^{99m}Tc sestamibi 1-day rest-stress (10 mCi + 30 mCi)	12
^{99m}Tc sestamibi-stress only (30 mCi)	8
^{99m}Tc sestamibi 2-day stress-rest (30 mCi + 30 mCi)	17.5
^{201}Tl stress and reinjection (3.0 mCi + 1.0 mCi)	25.1
Dual-isotope (3.0 mCi ^{201}Tl (30 mCi ^{99m}Tc)	27.3
^{82}Rb PET myocardial perfusion (45 mCi + 45 mCi)	16
Ge-68 or Gd-153 transmission for PET (approximate)	0.08
CT transmission source for PET (low-dose CT protocol)	0.8
Fluorine 18 FDG PET viability (10 mCi)	7
ERNA, ^{99m}Tc -labelled RBCs (20 mCi ^{99m}Tc)	5.2
Ventilation/perfusion lung (200 MBq ^{99m}Tc MAA + 70 MBq ^{99m}Tc aerosol)	2.8

unnecessary. A stimulating overview of this issue has recently been published.[79] Also to be considered and addressed is the general public phobia of all things radioactive. While the public attitudes toward nuclear power as a method of energy generation had recently been mellowed with realization of its benefits, an increased and almost certainly exaggerated concern has emerged with the recent events related to the natural disaster in Japan. This has reignited the ever present phobia which certainly extends to the medical use of nuclear methods and must be addressed through a rational consideration of events, alternatives and public education. The involved, informed physician advocate must take the educational lead. While concerns are not without basis, they must be kept in perspective. Patients must not be permitted to discard a useful and beneficial diagnostic or therapeutic method simply because it is "nuclear". Unfair and biased use of this public fear and prejudice by other physicians for their own benefit must not be permitted. The public must be made aware that radiation is a fact of life to which they are exposed constantly with increased exposure at altitude and even when sleeping with their partner. While all accept these as reasonable and even necessary exposures with an acceptable risk, so too are appropriately applied diagnostic nuclear imaging and radiographic methods.

REFERENCES

1. Hendel RC, Berman DS, Di Carli MF, et al. Cardiac radionuclide imaging: a report of the American College of Cardiology Foundation Appropriate Use Criteria Task Force, the American Society of Nuclear Cardiology, the American College of Radiology, the American Heart Association, the American Society of Echocardiography, the Society of Cardiovascular Computed Tomography, the Society for Cardiovascular Magnetic Resonance, and the Society of Nuclear Medicine Endorsed by the American College of Emergency Physicians published online May 18, 2009.

2. Galvin JM, Brown KA. The site of acute myocardial infarction is related to the coronary territory of transient defects on prior myocardial perfusion imaging. J Nucl Cardiol. 1996;3:382-8.

3. Wilson RF, Holida MD, White CW. Quantitative angiographic morphology of coronary stenoses leading to myocardial infarction or unstable angina. Circulation. 1986;73:286-93.

4. Little WC, Constantinescu M, Applegate RJ, et al. Can coronary angiography predict the site of a subsequent myocardial infarction in patients with mild to moderate coronary artery disease? Circulation. 1988;78:1157-66.

5. Alderman EL, Corley SD, Fisher LD, et al. Five-year angiographic follow-up of factors associated with progression of coronary artery disease in the Coronary Artery Surgery Study (CASS). J Amer Coll Cardiol. 1993;22:1141-54.

6. Farb A, Tang AL, Burke AP, et al. Sudden coronary death: frequency of active coronary lesions, inactive coronary lesions and myocardial infarction. Circulation. 1995;92:1701-9.

7. Nakakomi A, Celermajer DS, Lumley T, et al. Angiographic coronary narrowing is a surrogate marker for the extent of coronary atherosclerosis. Am J Cardiol. 1996;78:516-9.

8. Mahmarian JJ, Pratt CM, Boyce TM, et al. The variable extent of jeopardized myocardium in patients with single vessel coronary artery disease: quantification by thallium-201 single photon emission computed tomography. J Am Coll Cardiol. 1991;17:355-62.

9. Giroud D, Li JM, Urban P, et al. Relation of the site of acute myocardial infarction to the most severe coronary arterial stenosis at prior angiography. Am J Cardiol. 1992;69:729-32.

10. Udelson JE, Bonow RO, Allman KC, et al. Wintergreen panel summaries. Assessing myocardial viability in left ventricular dysfunction and heart failure. Udelson JE, Chair. J Nucl Cardiol. 1999;6:156-72.

11. Hachamovitch R, Berman DS, Shaw LJ, et al. Incremental prognostic value of myocardial perfusion single photon emission computed tomography for the prediction of cardiac death: differential stratification for risk of cardiac death and myocardial infarction. Circulation. 1998;97:535-43.

12. Sharir T, Germano G, Kang X, et al. Prediction of myocardial infarction versus cardiac death by gated myocardial perfusion SPECT: risk stratification by the amount of stress-induced ischemia and the poststress ejection fraction. J Nucl Med. 2001;42:831-7.

12a. Self Study Program III. Nuclear Medicine: Cardiology topic 2: pharmacologic stress and associated topics. Soc Nucl Med Publ. 1998.

13. Henzlova MJ, Cerqueira MD, Hansen CL, et al. ASNC imaging guidelines for nuclear cardiology procedures, stress protocols and tracers. J Nucl Cardiol [online]. Available from www. onlinejnc. Com [Accessed 1/09].

14. Cosmai EM, Heller GV. The clinical importance of electrocardiographic changes during pharmacologic stress testing with radionuclide myocardial perfusion imaging. J Nucl Cardiol. 2005;12:466-72.

15. Lattanzi F, Picano E, Adamo E, et al. Dobutamine stress echocardiography: safety in diagnosing coronary artery disease. Drug Saf. 2000;22:251-62.

16. Geleijnse ML, Elhendy A, Fioretti PM, et al. Dobutamine stress myocardial perfusion imaging. J Am Coll Cardiol. 2000;36:2017-27.

17. Holly TA, Abbott BG, Al-Mallah M, et al. ASNC imaging guidelines for nuclear cardiology procedures. Single photon-emission computed tomography. J Nucl Cardiol. Published on-line 6/15/10 by the American Society of Nuclear Cardiology available at www.onlinejnc.com. J Am Coll Cardiol. 2003;42:1318-33.

18. Soman P, Taillefer R, DePuey EG, et al. Enhanced detection of reversible perfusion defects by ^{99m}Tc sestamibi compared to Tc-99m tetrofosmin during vasodilator stress SPECT imaging in mild-to-moderate coronary artery disease. J Am Coll Cardiol. 2001;37:458-62.

19. Berman DS, Abidov A, Kang X, et al. Prognostic validation of a 17-segment score derived from a 20 segment score for myocardial perfusion SPECT interpretation. J Nucl Cardiol. 2004;11:414-23.

20. DICOM and Interconectivity Update-Information statement, approved 9/05. www.asnc.org.

21. Sharir T, Germano G, Kavanagh PB, et al. Incremental prognostic value of poststress left ventricular ejection fraction and volume by

gated myocardial perfusion single photon emission computed tomography. Circulation. 1999;100:1035-42.

22. Soret M, Bacharach SL, Buvat I. Partial-volume effect in PET tumor imaging. J Nucl Med. 2007;48:932-45.

23. Yun JH, Block M, Botvinick EH. Unique contraction pattern in patients after coronary bypass graft surgery by gated SPECT myocardial perfusion imaging. Clin Nucl Med. 2003;28:18-24.

24. Garcia EV, Faber TL, Esteves FP. Cardiac dedicated ultrafast SPECT cameras: new designs and clinical implications. J Nucl Med. 2011;52:210-7.

25. Tilkemeier PL, Cooke CD, Grossman GB, et al. ASNC imaging guidelines for nuclear cardiology procedures. Standardized reporting of radionuclide myocardial perfusion and function. J Nucl Card [online]. Available from www.onlinejnc.com [Accessed 6/09].

26. Botvinick EH, Ratzlaff N, Hoffman JIE, et al. Self Study Program III-Nucl Med Cardiol. Topic 5-Myocardial Perfusion Scintigraphy by Single Photon Radionuclides-Planar and Tomographic(SPECT)-Technical Aspects, Soc Nucl Med Publ, 2003.

27. Nishina H, Slomka PJ, Abidov A, et al. Combined supine and prone quantitative myocardial perfusion SPECT: method development and clinical validation in patients with no known coronary artery disease. J Nucl Med. 2006;47:51-8.

28. Iskandrian AS, Heo J, Lemlek J, et al. Identification of high risk patients with left main and three vessel coronary disease using stepwise descriminant analysis of clinical, exercise and tomographic thallium data. Am Heart J. 1993;125:221-5.

29. Fraker TD Jr, Fihn SD. 2007 chronic angina focused update of the ACC/AHA 2002 guidelines for the management of patients with chronic stable angina. J Am Coll Cardiol. 2007;50:2264-74.

30. Mieres JH, Shaw LJ, Hendel RC, et al. The women study: what is the optimal method for ischemia evaluation in women? A multi-center, prospective, randomized study to establish the optimal method for detection of coronary artery disease (CAD) risk in women at an intermediate-high pretest likelihood of CAD: study design. Am Soc Nucl Cardiol. 2008;10:105-12.

31. Shaw LJ, Heller GV, Casperson P, et al. Gated myocardial perfusion single photon emission computed tomography in the clinical outcomes utilizing revascularization and aggressive drug evaluation (COURAGE) trial, Veterans Administration Cooperative Study no. 424. J Nucl Cardiol. 2006;13:685-98.

32. Matsumoto N, Sato Y, Suzuki Y, et al. Incremental prognostic value of cardiac function assessed by ECG-gated myocardial perfusion SPECT for the prediction of future acute coronary syndrome. Circ J. 2008;72:2035-9.

33. Abidov A, Bax JJ, Hayes SW, et al. Transient ischemic dilation ratio of the left ventricle is a significant predictor of future cardiac events in patients with otherwise normal myocardial perfusion SPECT. J Am Coll Cardiol. 2003;42:1818-25.

34. Canhasi B, Dae M, Botvinick E, et al. Interaction of "supplementary" scintigraphic indicators of ischemia and stress electrocardiography in the diagnosis of multivessel coronary disease. J Am Coll Cardiol. 1985;6:581-8.

35. Kushner FG, Hand M, Smith SC Jr, et al. 2009 focused updates: ACC/AHA guidelines for the management of patients with ST-elevation myocardial infarction and ACC/AHA/SCAI guidelines on percutaneous coronary intervention. Circulation. 2009;120:2271-306.

36. Anderson JL, Adams CD, Antman EM, et al. ACC/AHA 2007 guidelines for the management of patients with unstable angina/non ST-elevation myocardial infarction. Circulation. 2007;116:e148-304.

37. Kontos MC, Tatum JL. Imaging in the evaluation of the patient with suspected acute coronary syndrome. Semin Nucl Med. 2003;33:246-58.

38. Eagle KA, Berger PB, Calkins H, et al. ACC/AHA guideline update for perioperative cardiovascular evaluation for noncardiac surgery. J Am Coll Cardiol. 2002;39:542-53.

39. Fleisher LA, Beckman JA, Brown KA, et al. ACC/AHA 2007 guidelines on perioperative cardiovascular evaluation and care for noncardiac surgery. Circulation. 2007;116:1971-96.

40. Hendel RC, Berman DS, Di Carli MF, et al. ACCF/ASNC/ACR/AHA/ASE/SCCT/SCMR/SNM 2009 appropriate use criteria for cardiac radionuclide imaging: a report of the American College of Cardiology Foundation appropriate use criteria Task Force, the American Society of Nuclear Cardiology, the American College of Radiology, the American Heart Association, the American Society of Echocardiography, the Society of Cardiovascular Computed Tomography, the Society for Cardiovascular Magnetic Resonance, and the Society of Nuclear Medicine. J Am Coll Cardiol. 2009;53:2201-29.

41. Brindis RG, Douglas PS, Hendel RC, et al. ACCF/ASNC appropriateness criteria for single photon emission computed tomography myocardial perfusion imaging (SPECT MPI). J Am Coll Cardiol. 2005;46:1587-605.

42. Mosca L, Banka CL, Benjamin EJ, et al. Evidence-based guidelines for cardiovascular disease prevention in women: 2007 update. J Am Coll Cardiol. 2007;49:1230-50.

43. America YG, Bax JJ, Boersma E, et al. The additive prognostic value of perfusion and functional data assessed by quantitative gated SPECT in women. Circulation. 2008;72:2035-9.

44. Taillefer R, DePuey EG, Udelson JE, et al. Comparative diagnostic accuracy of Tl-201 and Tc-99m sestamibi SPECT imaging (perfusion and ECG-gated SPECT) in detecting coronary disease in women. J Am Coll Cardiol. 1997;29:69-77.

45. Berman DS, Kang X, Hayes SW, et al. Adenosine myocardial perfusion single photon emission computed tomography in women compared with men. Impact of diabetes mellitus on incremental prognostic value and effect on patient management. J Am Coll Cardiol. 2003;41:1125-33.

46. De Winter O, Velghe A, Van de Veire N, et al. Incremental prognostic value of combined perfusion and function assessment during myocardial gated SPECT in patients aged 75 years or older. J Nucl Cardiol. 2005;12:662-70.

47. Hunt SA, Abraham WT, Chin MH. 2009 focused update incorporated into the ACC/AHA 2005 guidelines for the diagnosis and management of heart failure in adults. Circulation. 2009;119:1330-52.

48. Sugura T, Takase H, Toriyama T, et al. Usefulness of Tc-99m methoxyisobutylisonitrile scintigraphy for evaluating congestive heart failure. J Nucl Cardiol. 2006;13:50-64.

49. Danias PG, Papaioannou GI, Ahlberg AW, et al. Usefulness of electrocardiographic-gated stress technetium-99m sestamibi single photon emission computed tomography to differentiate ischemic from nonischemic cardiomyopathy. Am J Cardiol. 2004;94:14-9.

50. Vasken Dilsizian V, Bacharach SL, Beanlands RL, et al. ASNC imaging guidelines for nuclear cardiology procedures. PET myocardial perfusion and metabolism clinical imaging. J Nucl Cardiol [online]. Available from www.onlinejnc.Com [Accessed 1/09].

51. Petretta M, Soricelli A, Storto G, et al. Assessment of coronary flow reserve using single photon emission computed tomography with technetium 99m-labeled tracers. J Nucl Cardiol. 2008;15:456-65.

52. Javad SM, Mortazavi M, Bruce M. An introduction to radiation, radiation hormesis after 85 years. Health Physics Society Newsletter. 1987.

53. Schelbert HR, Beanlands R, Bengel F, et al. PET myocardial perfusion and glucose metabolism imaging: Part 2-Guidelines for interpretation and reporting. J Nucl Cardiol. 2003;10:557-71.

54. Di Carli MF, Hachamovitch R, Berman DS. The art and science of predicting postrevascularization improvement in left ventricular (LV) function in patients with severely depressed LV function. J Am Coll Cardiol. 2002;40:1744-7.

55. Schinkel AF, Bax JJ, Biagini E, et al. Myocardial technetium-99m-tetrofosmin single photon emission computed tomography compared with ^{18}F-fluorodeoxyglucose imaging to assess myocardial viability. Am J Cardiol. 2005;95:1223-5.

56. Bateman TM, Heller GV, McGhie AI, et al. Diagnostic accuracy of rest/stress ECG-gated [82]Rb myocardial perfusion PET: comparison with ECG-gated ^{99m}Tc sestamibi SPECT. J Nucl Cardiol. 2006;13:24-33.

57. Dorbala S, Hachamovitch R, Curillova Z, et al. Incremental prognostic value of gated [82]Rb positron emission tomography myocardial perfusion imaging over clinical variables and rest LVEF. JACC Cardiovasc Imaging. 2009;2:846-54.

58. Al-Mallah MH, Sitek A, Moore SC, et al. Assessment of myocardial perfusion and function with PET and PET/CT. J Nucl Cardiol. 2010;17:498-513.

59. Naya M, Di Carli MF. Myocardial perfusion PET/CT to evaluate known and suspected coronary artery disease. Q J Nucl Med Mol Imaging. 2010;54:145-56.

60. Parkash R, deKemp RA, Ruddy TD, et al. Potential utility of rubidium 82 PET quantification in patients with 3-vessel coronary artery disease. J Nucl Cardiol. 2004;11:440-9.

61. El Fakhri G, Kardan A, Sitek A, et al. Reproducibility and accuracy of quantitative myocardial blood flow assessment with [82]Rb PET: comparison with (13)N-ammonia PET. J Nucl Med. 2009;50:1062-71.

62. Anagnostopoulos C, Almonacid A, El Fakhri G, et al. Quantitative relationship between coronary vasodilator reserve assessed by [82]Rb PET imaging and coronary artery stenosis severity. Eur J Nucl Med Mol Imaging. 2008;35:1593-601.

63. Friedman JD, Berman DS, Borges-Neto S, et al. ASNC imaging guidelines for nuclear cardiology procedures first-pass radionuclide angiography. J Nucl Cardiol [online]. Available from www.onlinejnc.com [Accessed 1/09].

64. Corbett JR, Akinboboye OO, Bacharach SL, et al. ASNC imaging guidelines for nuclear cardiology procedures. Equilibrium radionuclide angiocardiography. J Nucl Cardiol [online]. Available from www.onlinejnc.com [Accessed 1/08].

65. Schwartz RG, McKenzie WB, Alexander J, et al. Congestive heart failure and left ventricular dysfunction complicating doxorubicin therapy. Seven-year experience using serial radionuclide angiocardiography. Am J Med. 1987;82:1109-18.

66. Botvinick EH. Scintigraphic blood pool and phase image analysis: the optimal tool for the evaluation of resynchronization therapy. J Nucl Cardiol. 2003;10:424-8.

67. Botvinick E, Bacharach S. Blood pool imaging. In: Narula J, Dilsizian V (Eds). Atlas of Nuclear Cardiology, 2nd edition. Springer; 2009.

68. Dae M, Botvinick E, O'Connell JW, et al. Atrial corrected fourier amplitude ratios for the scintigraphic quantitation of valvular regurgitation. Am J Noninvas Card. 1987;1:155-62.

69. Giubbini R, Milan E, Bertagna F, et al. Nuclear cardiology and heart failure. Eur J Nucl Med Mol Imaging. 2009;36:2068-80.

70. Ji SY, Travin MI. Radionuclide imaging of cardiac autonomic innervation. J Nucl Cardiol. 2010;17:655-66.

71. Carrió I, Cowie MR, Yamazaki J, et al. Cardiac sympathetic imaging with MIBG in heart failure. JACC Cardiovasc Imaging. 2010;3:92-100.

72. Agostini D, Carrio I, Verberne HJ. How to use myocardial 123I-MIBG scintigraphy in chronic heart failure. Eur J Nucl Med Mol Imaging. 2009;36:555-9.

73. Kasama S, Toyama T, Sumino H, et al. Prognostic value of serial cardiac 123I-MIBG imaging in patients with stabilized chronic heart failure and reduced left ventricular ejection fraction. J Nucl Med. 2008;49:907-14.

74. Tamaki S, Yamada T, Okuyama Y, et al. Cardiac iodine-123 metaiodobenzylguanidine imaging predicts sudden cardiac death independently of left ventricular ejection fraction in patients with chronic heart failure and left ventricular systolic dysfunction: results from a comparative study with signal-averaged electrocardiogram, heart rate variability, and QT dispersion. J Am Coll Cardiol. 2009;53:426-35.

75. Jacobson AF, Senior R, Cerqueira MD, et al. Myocardial iodine-123 meta-iodobenzylguanidine imaging and cardiac events in heart failure. Results of the prospective ADMIRE-HF (AdreView Myocardial Imaging for Risk Evaluation in Heart Failure) study. J Am Coll Cardiol. 2010;55:2212-21.

76. Gallego-Page JC. Re: Improvement in cardiac sympathetic nerve activity in responders to resynchronization therapy. Europace. 2008;10:892-3.

77. Boogers MJ, Borleffs CJ, Henneman MM, et al. Cardiac sympathetic denervation assessed with 123-iodine metaiodobenzylguanidine imaging predicts ventricular arrhythmias in implantable cardioverter-defibrillator patients. J Am Coll Cardiol. 2010;55:2769-77.

78. The seventh report of the National Research Council's Committee on the Biological Effects of Ionizing Radiation (BIER) on the medical effects of low dose ionizing radiation released in 2005: BIER VII:Health risks from exposure to low levels of ionizing radiation. Sponsored by US Department of Energy, US Nuclear Regulatory Commission, US Environmental Protection Agency and US Department of Homeland Security. Available from the National Academies Press, 500 Fifth Street, NW, Washington, DC 20001.

79. Thompson RC, Cullom SJ. Issues regarding radiation dosage of cardiac nuclear and radiography procedures. J Nucl Cardiol. 2006;13:19-23.

Chapter 22

Cardiac Computed Tomography

Isidore C Okere, Gardar Sigurdsson

Chapter Outline

INTRODUCTION

Soon after Sir Godfrey Hounsfield first developed his prototype computed tomography (CT) scanner in the early 1970s,[1]-there was interest in imaging the heart. The first scientific report of CT of the heart was in 1976.[2] Reports of EKG gated image acquisition[3] and the concept of "stop-action" heart imaging occurred in 1977.[4] The first scanners acquired data over several minutes, and image analysis was done overnight by assistance of primitive computer technology. The initial CT scanners were affected by low temporal and spatial resolution. Ultrafast CT, also called electron beam CT, was introduced in the 1980s and allowed for temporal resolution that was a fraction of a second. This allowed for reliable imaging of the heart but spatial resolution was suffering. Its greatest strength was detection of coronary calcifications and coronary stenosis analysis was less reliable. Greater spatial resolution was obtained by helical multidetector row CT technology.[5] Multidetector row technology allowed for subsecond temporal resolution and submillimeter spatial resolution. First multicenter trial was done in 2004 with 16 detector row scanner[6] and following this a progressive increase in number of detector rows has currently peaked at 320 with spatial resolution of 0.4 mm and temporal resolution of 150–200 ms. Dual source CT has further improved temporal resolution to about 80 ms by adding a second set of generator and detector. With the advent of multidetector row technology the radiation exposure was initially increased but with progressive improvements in image acquisition protocols there has been dramatic reduction in radiation. Current top of the line scanners can acquire a single phase image of the whole heart within a fraction of a second with radiation dose that is 60–80% less than a standard abdominal or chest CT.[7,8]

Due to progressive improvement in CT technology, both hardware and software, the image acquisition can be done in a few seconds and computerized processing of raw data takes a few minutes resulting in thousands of images covering the whole heart from different parts of the cardiac cycle. With multiphase imaging the door has been open not only to evaluation of the coronary anatomy but also to comprehensive analysis of other heart structures including chamber sizes, biventricular systolic function, regional wall motion abnormalities, valve pathology, cardiac masses and congenital anomalies.

TECHNICAL ASPECTS

BASIC PRINCIPLES OF COMPUTED TOMOGRAPHY

Image acquisition during CT relies on catching X-ray beams as they travel through the body. This requires an X-ray generator and X-ray detector. To produce an axial image or a "slice" of the body, with minimal artifacts, the X-ray beam has to travel through the body at multiple angles, and images are produced from the attenuation pattern of X-rays as they reach the detectors.

X-ray beams are generated identically to X-rays during standard chest X-ray or invasive coronary angiography. X-ray generator will produce X-ray beams of differing *energy* [kilovoltage (kV)] profiles and *current* [milliamperes (mA)]. Most commonly used energy profile is 100 or 120 kV based on patient size. Imaging acquisition done simultaneously with multiple energy profiles (ranging 80–140 kV) can allow for better tissue discrimination (e.g. dual energy imaging).

The X-ray detectors generate images by the assistance of complex mathematical models calculated by computer, hence the prior nomenclature of computer assisted tomography or "CAT" scanning. Current high-end CT detectors have multiple rows of detectors that can capture 64–320 slices or images during partial rotation. Collimation typically used during cardiac images aims at smallest possible slice thickness of about 0.5–0.75 mm. In combination with standard reconstruction algorithm using 50% overlapping, the *spatial resolution* can be as low as 0.4 mm.

Gantry of the CT scanner refers to the circular or doughnut shaped structure that holds the X-ray generator and detectors. The gantry rotates around the patient and current high--end CT systems will complete a full rotation of 360° in 270–500 ms. The patient is placed within the middle of the gantry on a table that will move in a longitudinal plane most often referred to as the *Z-axis*. Longitudinal movement of the scan table in *Z-axis* in relationship to the detector size is referred to as *pitch*. Formula for pitch is table movement during image acquisition divided by detector length.

In most scanners the detector length or combined coverage of all detector rows is less than the longitudinal length of the heart in *Z-axis*. Two modes of scanning exist to allow for this shortcoming. One called *helical* (or *spiral*) *scanning* where continuous radiation is generated with continuous image acquisition. Typically this is done with very slow motion of the CT table in *Z-axis* (low pitch of 0.2–0.5). Slow motion of the scan table makes for low pitch and redundant data collection with an increased radiation. This allows for flexibility in postprocessing reconstruction algorithms where, if the patient has an ectopic beat, the EKG editing tool can give an option to remove the raw data related to the ectopic beat. This can improve image quality substantially and allows for greater reliability of acquiring diagnostic images. More recently dual source scanners have allowed for a unique high pitch mode of 3.4 ("FLASH" mode, Siemens) where there is a minimal redundancy of raw data and considerable lowering of radiation with image acquisition time for the whole heart of about 280 ms.

Second mode is *axial scanning*. During this mode, the CT table does not move during image acquisition and images are acquired in axial mode only. No spiral scanning is done. While moving to the next position the radiation is turned off. When the CT table has reached the next segment it will stop and wait until the correct portion of the EKG is reached. When the predetermined cardiac cycle is reached, axial images are acquired again. This sequence of events is frequently referred to as "step and shoot" as the scanner first steps and then shoots the radiation. This mode is used primarily when heart rate is less than 65 bpm as diastasis is then long enough to allow for motion free image acquisition.

To produce an image with minimal artifacts most scanners will need to cover more than 180° or half rotation plus the detector fan beam angle. *Temporal resolution* is dependent on gantry rotational speed that is limited by centrifugal forces and rotational time of about 300–400 ms. As such single source CT scanners (single set of generator and detector) will have temporal resolution of greater than 150 ms during axial imaging. Dual source CT scanners have two sets of generator/detector. This allows for rapid image acquisition and temporal resolution of 83 ms during axial imaging.

Single source CT scanners can attempt to improve temporal resolution by a postprocessing method called *multi-segment* or *multi-cycle reconstruction*. This requires use of continuous helical (spiral) scanning mode at low pitch (< 0.5) and post-processing methods which include partial data from several cardiac cycles and at different adjacent angles but within near identical phase of the cardiac cycle. This method can lower temporal resolution 2–3 fold but this requires minimal heart rate variability that is typically only seen with heavy beta-blockage, in transplanted hearts or in patients with severe cardiomyopathy.

Due to cardiac motion it is essential to have EKG gating during image acquisition and reconstruction. As images are always acquired with EKG data present and reconstruction of raw data is always done based on the corresponding EKG, it could be stated that all cardiac CT is done with retrospective gating (Table 1). But in general, when referring to prospective or retrospective EKG gating a reference is made to how the X-ray generation is controlled. Early CT protocols would not allow for prospective EKG-gated radiation modulation and continuous radiation was produced and protocol called only

TABLE 1

CT protocol terms

General protocol terms	Scan mode	Pitch	Prospective EKG gated X-ray generation	EKG editing	Image reconstruction	When used	Radiation
Retrospective	Helical mode	0.2–0.5	No	Yes	Retrospective	Irregular heart rhythm, e.g. Atrial fibrillation	Highest
Dose modulated	Helical mode	0.2–0.5	Yes—Prospective modulation of current (mA)	Yes	Retrospective	Coronary and ventricular function analysis	Intermediate
FLASH or high pitch	Helical mode	3.4	Yes—Prospective during diastole only	No	Retrospective	Coronary analysis when heart rate is below 65 bpm	Lowest
Prospective or Step and Shoot	Axial mode	1	Yes—Prospective interrupted mode (on and off)	If padding (window) is increased	Retrospective	Coronary analysis when heart rate is below 65 bpm	Lowest
Sequential adaptive	Axial mode	1	Yes—Mix of modulation and interrupted mode	Limited	Retrospective	Coronary analysis when heart rate is below 65 bpm	Low— Intermediate

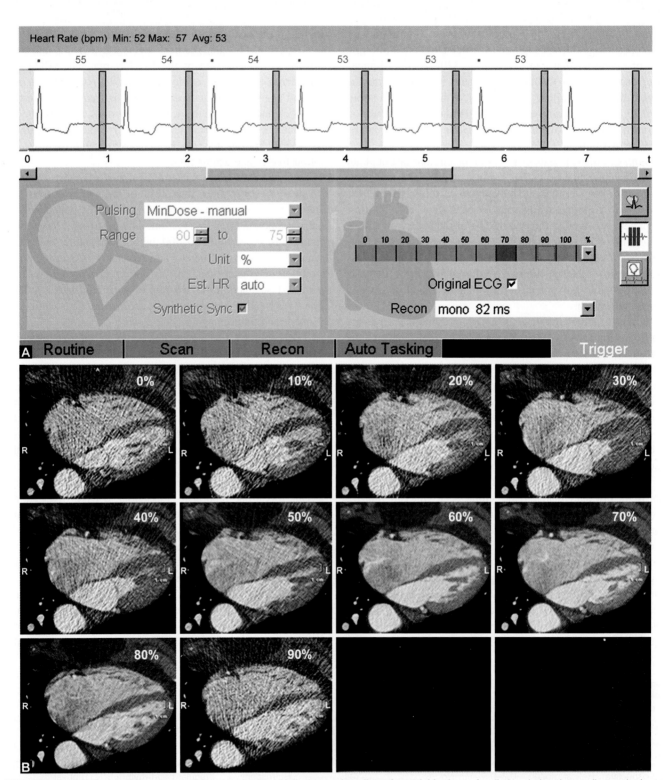

FIGURES 1A AND B: (A) EKG gating and dose modulation. Helical scanning allows for variable dose of radiation during the cardiac cycle, hence radiation dose modulation. The pictures show an example of dose modulation where full dose of radiation is only administered during diastolic phases (light blue 60–90%). In this example, the 70% phase (dark blue) is selected for reconstruction. (B) Phase selection. Sample of image from 10 equally spaced phases. Dose modulation with radiation reduction is caused for granular images in several phases. The 70% phase shows the least motion of the RCA and was selected for coronary analysis

"*retrospective*". This protocol is currently used only for patients with very irregular rhythm, such as atrial fibrillation, where EKG editing is frequently required.

Other image acquisition protocols utilize EKG gating to decrease radiation in a prospective manner. EKG from prior cardiac cycles is used to predict when it is optimal to generate

radiation. The common protocols are "dose modulation" and axial scanning. The "*dose modulation*" protocol (Figs 1A and B) is done with helical scanning, and during image acquisition the scanner will prospectively lower the current (mA) by 80–96% during a selective portion of the cardiac cycle (frequently late diastole and early systole) and allow full dose during the motion less part of the cardiac cycle, late systole (isovolemic relaxation) and/or mid-diastole (diastasis). The *axial* protocol frequently termed "*prospective*" "*axial-sequential*" or "*step and shoot*" protocol are based on EKG of prior beats and the X-rays are only generated during specific portion of the cardiac cycle (e.g. diastasis) where X-ray generation is done with table/patient stationary and, while X-ray generation is turned off, the table moves patient to allow imaging of another portion of the heart. In the new table position, the X-ray generation is not started until the quiescent portion of the EKG is reached. Newer protocols with novel features are "FLASH" and "sequential adaptive". The "FLASH" mode has been described earlier and the sequential adaptive protocol is an example of a mixed protocol that does both axial imaging and dose modulation without spiral scanning. The last two protocols are specific to Siemens equipment.

RADIATION

Utilization of medical imaging with ionizing radiation is rapidly growing. Radiation with each modality alone is considered low (< 50–100 mSv) but serial imaging and cumulative exposure is of concern. Medical personnel exposed to radiation are limited to an exposure of 50 mSv per year. Calculation of risk for cancer with ionizing radiation is based on data from World War II atomic bombing, with substantially higher radiation doses than are seen in medical imaging. The assumption of a linear relationship between very low level radiation exposure and cancer risk are not accepted by all societies.[9]

Technical advancements have allowed for considerable lowering of radiation with cardiac CT. The most advanced scanners are able to perform cardiac CT with an equal or lower dose than annual background radiation (2–4 mSv). Less advanced CT scanners are now able to use protocols with radiation that is comparable or lower than invasive angiography, nuclear studies or standard CT of chest or abdomen[10,11] (Table 2).

When considering the use of cardiac CT the risk-benefit ratio with radiation and contrast need to be weighed against the benefit of correct diagnosis. For example, the risk of missing the diagnosis of acute coronary syndrome in an emergency room patient is 2.1% and theoretical estimated lifetime risk of cancer following dose modulated cardiac CT is less than 0.5%.[12]

IMAGE ANALYSIS

Current multidetector technology gives isotropic image reconstruction where each pixel in an image can be viewed as a voxel with equal resolution in x-, y- and z-axis. This isotropic image resolution allows for image analysis from any view (axial/sagittal/coronal) without distortion. This was not possible with prior electron beam technology. Each image pixel has designated CT value or density value also named Houndsfield unit (HU). In routine imaging of the body (at 120 kV) these density values can differentiate accurately between soft tissue and bone where bone will have density value from 130 to more than 1,000. Fat tissue has negative HUs (–20 to –150). Muscle and blood will have similar density 30–70 HU. Intravenous contrast administration allows for differentiation of blood and muscle. Contrast administration will increase density of blood pool to 100–500 HU depending on contrast type, rate of administration and mixture. Contrast administration will also increase density of soft tissue depending on vasculature of the tissue.

Energy level (kV) during image acquisition will affect density values of contrast, soft tissue and bone. Lower energy level to 80–100 kV will make for denser images where contrast enhanced blood will have higher density (HU) and calcium or bone will have density above 150–200 HU. The effect of differing density with differing energy levels can be used to differentiate between tissues and extract contrast ("iodine mapping") or to differentiate better between contrast and calcium.

Viewing of raw images is done in gray scale. This scale can be manipulated to allow for better tissue characterization. Density value range of lung tissue and the heart is very different and requires different gray scale range for evaluation. Center (or level) of image density (HU) and window width (or range) determine image brightness and ease of differentiation and analysis of differing tissues. In coronary analysis where there are very dense objects, such as metallic stents or calcium, it is important to increase the window width further (Figs 2A to C). This reduces somewhat the blooming artifact related to dense objects but at the same time decreases

TABLE 2

Radiation with CT and other modalities[10,11]

Examination	Representative Effective dose value (mSv)	Range of reported Effective dose value (mSv)
Chest X-ray PA and lateral	0.1	0.05–0.24
CT chest	7	4–18
CT abdominal	8	4–25
CT pelvis	6	3–10
Coronary calcium CT*	3	1–12
Coronary CT angiogram	16	5–32
64-Slice coronary CTA		
without tube current modulation	15	12–18
with tube current modulation	9	8–18
with lower energy—100 kV	8.4	—
Dual-source coronary CTA		
with tube current modulation	13	6–17
Prospectively triggered coronary CTA	3	2–4
Diagnostic invasive coronary angiogram	7	2–16
Percutaneous coronary intervention or radiofrequency ablation	15	7–57
Myocardial perfusion study		
Sestamibi (1-day) stress/rest	9	—
Thallium stress/rest	41	—
F-18 FDG	14	—
Rubidium-82	5	—

412 the ability to evaluate softer density structures such as non-calcified atherosclerotic plaque or clot.

Raw images of the heart are typically around 300 and reconstructed in axial plane. The most simple viewing software allows for evaluation of these images in only the axial plane but more sophisticated viewing software will combine images to allow for evaluation of thicker images in any plane. Thickening of the image slice will reduce image noise but can also result in loss of information. There are three basic modes of thickening images—(1) MIP, (2) MinIP and (3) Average.

Maximum intensity projection (MIP) will display only the highest density value within a thickened image. *Minimum intensity projection* (MinIP) will display the lowest density value within the thickened image. *Average* will display the average of all values seen within the designated image thickness. MIP view is frequently used for coronary stenosis analysis with image thickness of 5 mm (Figs 2A to C). Higher or lower image thickness can also be used depending on the software. MIP view allows the contrast-filled vessel to be viewed in single frame and can simplify stenosis analysis and images will represent more of an angiographic view. The downside of MIP analysis is underestimation of non-calcified plaque and overestimation of calcium related stenosis. Calcified coronary plaque in MIP images can also give artificial appearance of calcium within the mid lumen of a vessel (Figs 2A to C). MinIP projection is primarily used for evaluation of thinner low density structures that are surrounded by higher density contrast-filled structures such as valves. Thickening images and averaging the density within the thickened images are primarily used in analysis of the myocardium and for assessment of the contrast density of the myocardium. Myocardium also be assessed by MinIP to increase sensitivity for detection of scars on first pass images and MIP to emphasize the contrast enhancement within the myocardium in delayed contrast enhancement analysis.

A stack of axial images (typically around 300) can be combined to make a 3D model of the heart (Figs 3A and B). This type of representation has limited benefit when analyzing coronary stenosis but can sometimes allow for better understanding of relationship between the adjacent structures such as in complex congenital heart disease or for analyzing anomalous coronary vessels.

The basic viewing planes (axial/sagittal/coronal) can be sufficient to analyze the heart but to allow for displaying a coronary vessel in a single image (Fig. 4), an oblique view is necessary. Multi planar reconstruction (MPR) is a compilation of oblique views that allow for depicting of an entire vessel through its whole length in orthogonal views.

Image reconstruction of a single data set is typically done by reconstruction of a phase within the cardiac cycle. The phases are defined based on dividing the cardiac cycle into relative lengths (percents between the R waves) where the full cardiac cycle is 100% and the middle of cardiac cycle is 50% into the cardiac cycle (Figs 1A and B). This type of reconstruction requires minimal heart rate variability where length of each cardiac cycle during image acquisition is mostly constant. Low heart rate (below 65 bpm) allows for reconstruction within diastasis (phase 65–75%). Of note the definition of phases varies between image vendors where some define the phase based on

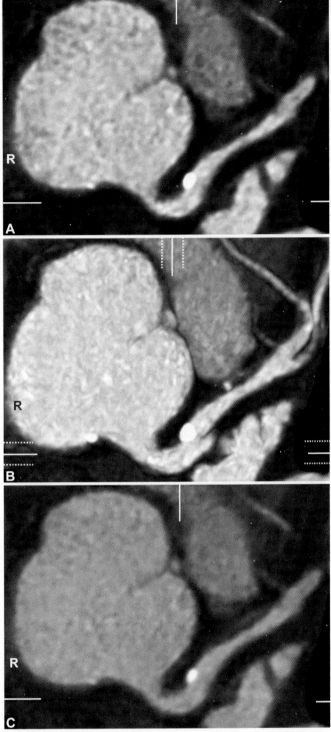

FIGURES 2A TO C: Single plane image of the left main coronary artery and proximal left anterior descending artery (LAD). LAD with ostial calcium and mixed plaque (calcified and noncalcified) in the proximal segment. (A) Thin slice image (0.75 mm) with narrow window (W750/C250). (B) Thick slice (5 mm) maximum intensity projection (MIP) image with narrow window (W750/C250). Calcium becomes prominent and artifically appears to occlude vessel. Minor calcium within soft plaque is noted. (C) Thin slice image with wide window (W1800/C400). Calcium smaller and plaque less prominent

the beginning of the reconstruction interval and other based on the middle of the reconstruction interval. If there is increased heart rate variability, such as in atrial fibrillation, a fixed interval from the R wave will allow for better image assessment.

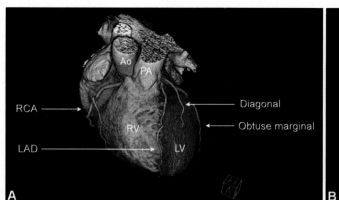

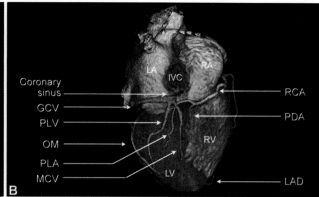

FIGURES 3A AND B: Volume-rendering technique. Normal 3D anatomy. (A) Anterior view shows left ventricle (LV), right ventricle (RV), pulmonary artery (PA) and aorta (Ao). Coronary arteries visualized are left anterior descending (LAD), diagonal artery, obtuse marginal artery and right coronary artery (RCA). (B) Inferior/Posterior view shows left ventricle (LV), right ventricle (RV), inferior vena cava (IVC), right atrium (RA) and left atrium (LA). Coronary arteries visualized are left anterior descending (LAD), obtuse marginal (OM) artery, right coronary artery (RCA), posterior descending coronary artery (PDA) and posterolateral artery (PLA). Cardiac veins are coronary sinus, great cardiac vein (GCV), middle cardiac vein (MCV) and posterolateral vein (PLV)

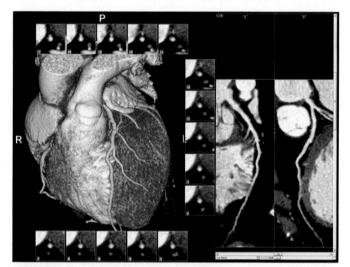

FIGURE 4: Volume-rendering technique (VRT) and curved multi-planar reconstruction (cMPR) for coronary analysis. Sample of how VRT in combination with cMPR allows for orthogonal views of the LAD and short axis views of the coronary lumen and vessel wall

IMAGE QUALITY AND ARTIFACTS

The image quality is determined by multiple factors—scanner type, protocol selection, patient size, contrast protocol, patient co-operation and heart rhythm. Currently the community standard for multidetector CT scanners is 64 detector row scanners with sub-millimeter collimation and gantry speed less than half a second (< 500 ms) where spatial resolution is 0.5–0.8 mm and temporal resolution 75–190 ms. Optimal scanners are also required to have high current output to allow imaging of larger patients and avoid photon starvation. Selection of acquisition protocol takes into consideration patient's heart rate and the clinical question. Contrast rate and amount is also individualized and suboptimal contrast opacification will lead to low signal to noise ratio with decreased diagnostic quality. High heart rate and arrhythmia can lead to motion artifacts and misalignment artifacts that can sometimes be corrected or reduced with postprocessing and EKG editing.

Patient preparation always involves selection of patients that can comply with breath holding and patients where use of radiation and contrast is justified based on the clinical question. Ideally patient could be consented prior to scanning but at this time it is not common practice. Knowledge of patient's size, renal function and history of contrast allergy is important for all studies irrespective of scanner type and protocol. Patients with higher heart rate and irregular heart rhythm might be better assessed in scanners with high temporal resolution.

Common practice is to use beta-blockers to lower heart rate prior to image acquisition as this allows for better image quality through longer diastasis, less motion of the vessel and lower heart rate variability. It also allows the use of imaging protocols with very low radiation when heart rate is less than 60–65 bpm (Table 1). Oral administration of beta-blocker is done an hour or sometimes several hours prior to scanning and intravenous administration is done a few minutes prior to scanning while patient is on the CT table or in adjacent patient care area. In patients who do not tolerate a beta-blocker, a nondihydro-pyridine calcium channel blocker can work as an alternative.

Nitroglycerin is also commonly administered just prior to scanning. It is thought to allow for better visualization of the whole coronary tree including smaller vessels (around 1.5 mm).

All patients are required to have intravenous access for contrast administration. Ideally patients have large bore needle, such as 18G in anticubital vein, to allow for contrast administration rate up to 6–7 ml/min but in smaller patients (BMI < 40) a rate of 4–5 ml/min is sufficient and this requires only 20G access.

CONTRAST

Contrast is required to assess the chambers and vessels of the heart. Without contrast it is not possible to assess coronary artery obstruction or chamber sizes. Allergic reaction to contrast and renal failure are the most common side effects of contrast administration.

High iodine concentration of the contrast is important to allow for less contrast dose and improve signal to noise ratio during vessel or chamber opacification. In the United States iopamidol (Isovue-370) has the highest concentration (370 mg/ml) and in Europe even higher concentrations are used. Iso-osmolar contrast with lower iodine concentration (i.e.

iodixanol) is also used when concerns are for increased risk of renal failure such as in diabetic patients.

Timing of contrast injection is critical to image quality. The contrast transit time varies between subjects based on location of IV catheter, injection rate and patient's hemodynamic state. Some institutions use test bolus method where a single test bolus is given and density curve done to guide timing of the main imaging. A simpler contrast protocol is bolus tracking where a region of interest is drawn within the descending or ascending aorta and when the density has increased by 100 HU the scanning starts.

Contrast protocols are dependant on the clinical question. When the clinical question relates primarily to the coronaries and possible left ventricular systolic function a biphasic protocol where saline is administered during second phase can be sufficient. Tri-phasic protocol can allow for assessment of right ventricle and pulmonary arteries. In this tri-phasic mode additional 30 ml of contrast in mixture with 30 ml of water (50% mix) can be sufficient to allow diagnosis of pulmonary embolism or volumetric assessment of right ventricular systolic function.

When ordering a noncontrast CT to assess for coronary calcium, it is important to know that it is currently not covered by insurance companies in many states and patients frequently pay out of pocket to have this performed. Noncontrast CT is frequently performed prior to contrast enhanced CT to determine feasibility of contrast enhanced CT. The practice of cancelling contrast injection based the quantity of coronary calcium (Agatston score 400–1000) varies between clinical facilities and also depends on the clinical question.

Contrast enhanced CT can be divided into comprehensive versus coronary analysis alone. During imaging of the coronaries alone information is also gained of adjacent structures. Axial scanning only gives a single cardiac phase and does not allow for analysis of left ventricular ejection fraction. Multiphase imaging opens the door for *comprehensive cardiac CT* that allows for assessment of left and right ventricular systolic function in addition to coronaries, cardiac veins, valves and pericardium.

"Triple rule out CT" refers to contrast enhanced CT where imaging is done of the aortic arch, pulmonary vasculature and the heart in a single scan.

CORONARY ARTERY DISEASE

The coronary arteries can be evaluated by CT both with and without contrast. Noncontrast CT is best suited for assessment of coronary calcifications in primary prevention. Contrast CT angiography is reserved for symptomatic patients primarily to exclude presence of obstructive disease. Patients with previously known coronary disease have less benefit from contrast CT due to blooming artifacts from coronary calcifications.

NONCONTRAST CT AND CORONARY CALCIFICATIONS

Noncontrast CT can estimate atherosclerotic burden but has limited value in predicting coronary stenosis. The magnitude of coronary calcifications correlates well with atherosclerotic

burden in histologic studies[13,14] but not as well with stenosis analysis.[14] Assessment of coronary calcium by CT was first done in the late 1980s[15] and proposal for a quantification method was presented by Agatston et al. in 1990.[16] The Agatston scoring method is a weighted sum score based on plaque area and density. This can be done with semi-automated software that is widely available. The Agatston score is generally referred to as "calcium scoring". Other methods to quantify the coronary calcifications are based on volume and mass[17] but these are not used in clinical practice.

Multiple retrospective and prospective studies have consistently shown that calcium scoring is an independent predictor of future cardiovascular events. These studies have also shown that its power of prediction exceeds current standard Framingham risk scoring.[18,19]

The greatest clinical value of calcium scoring is in patients at intermediate Framingham risk for future cardiovascular events where reclassification by Agatston scoring might allow for better determination of which patients might benefit from more intense medical therapy.[20,21] Current primary prevention guidelines support the use of calcium scoring in patients at intermediate risk for coronary events.[22]

In general, Agatston score less than 100 is considered to convey low risk and greater than 300–400 high risk. In patients at intermediate Framingham risk, a calcium score above 400 is associated with 2.4% annual risk for cardiac death or myocardial infarction.[18] Serial calcium scans to monitor the effect of medical therapy is thought to have limited value.

CONTRAST CT AND CORONARY ANGIOGRAPHY

EKG gated contrast enhanced CT is primarily used to exclude the presence of obstructive coronary disease in patients with chest discomfort. Patients with known coronary disease are generally not considered good candidates for CT due to blooming artifacts from coronary calcium that can limit stenosis analysis. Contrast enhanced CT differs from invasive angiography since it not only determines stenosis but also assesses the presence of atherosclerotic plaque and type of plaque similar to intravascular ultrasound (IVUS).

Careful selection of patients for coronary CT is very important to minimize risk to the patient and optimize appropriate use. Due to high sensitivity and high negative predictive value, CT is best suited for symptomatic patients with intermediate or low risk for obstructive coronary disease.[23]

Limitations in spatial resolution affect the overall accuracy of CT in stenosis analysis. Currently the spatial resolution is 0.4–0.8 mm. This makes evaluation of coronary branches (i.e. diagonal and obtuse marginal) less accurate as these vessels are frequently less than 2 mm in diameter.[24] In patients with low prevalence of coronary disease, CT has high sensitivity and specificity for stenosis detection (Table 3) but in patient with increased prevalence of coronary disease the specificity of stenosis analysis is decreased and false positive rate is increased.[25-28] Ratio between false positives and false negatives can be 6:1 or greater, and the most common reason for false positive findings are artifacts from calcium or motion.[27]

Temporal resolution is also an important factor for accuracy of CT. Coronary vessels within the atrioventricular grooves [right coronary artery (RCA) and left circumflex (LCX)]

TABLE 3

Patient-based analysis for detection of greater than 50% stenosis in (a) multicenter trials with 64 detector row scanners, (b) meta-analysis using 12 detector row or greater scanners published in 2010 and (c) meta-analysis of low dose scanning methods published in 2011

		N	Sens	Spec	NPV	PPV	Prev	Uneval
(a)	Accuracy[26]	230	95%	83%	99%	64%	24%	1.3%
	Core 64[25]	291	85%	90%	83%	91%	56%	1.7%
	Meijboom[27]	360	99%	64%	97%	86%	68%	0%
(b)	Meta-analysis[23]	7516	97%	87%				
(c)	Low dose[28]	960	100%	89%				9.5%

(Abbreviations: N: Number; Sens: Sensitivity; Spec: Spacificity; NPV: Negative predictive value; PPV: Positive predictive value; Prev: Prevalence; Uneval: Unevaluable)

experience considerable motion during the cardiac cycle and slowing heart rate with beta-blockers allows for near motion free imaging. Dual source CT scanners with temporal resolution of 70–90 ms allow for reliable imaging without beta-blockers.

Left main coronary artery evaluation with CT is considered highly accurate. This is due to the combination of large diameter of the vessel and limited motion.

In general, CT is highly sensitive for detection of coronary disease and has the ability to detect disease before a vessel has hemodynamically significant stenosis. This might allow earlier preventive measures, an advantage not shared by stress testing or other noninvasive functional imaging. Data from the CONFIRM registry shows that patients with nonobstructive coronary disease by CT angiography are at increased mortality risk.[29]

CT is able to characterize coronary plaque into—calcified, noncalcified and mixed plaque (mixture of calcified and non-calcified plaque elements). Reliable differentiation of soft and fibrous plaque has not yet materialized and this is due to limitations in spatial resolution. Additionally there appears to be systemic underestimation of noncalcified plaque size due to partial volume effect.[30,31] Despite this, the number of segments with atherosclerotic plaque is associated with future prognosis.[32,33] Current CT technology does not allow for direct visualization of thin fibrous plaque but it can detect positive remodeling and low attenuation plaque that in a single cohort study have been associated with the increased risk of acute coronary syndrome.[34]

The greatest strength of CT is the low event rate of 0.17–0.37%[29,35] in patients with a normal coronary CT. This is comparable to the background event rate among healthy low-risk individuals (< 1%). In patients with coronary stenosis (> 50%) the number of vessels and location of stenosis predict future cardiac events.[29,32,33,35]

Appropriate Indications

Correct selection of patients for contrast enhanced coronary CT is very important and requires a physician's evaluation to minimize risk to patients and optimize appropriate use. Due to high sensitivity and very high negative predictive value, CT is best suited for symptomatic patients with intermediate or low risk for obstructive coronary disease.[36] Patients with atypical chest pain and no increase in cardiac enzymes in the ER setting are also good candidates as performing of CT can be done earlier than traditional tests. Studies comparing CT to standard stress testing in the emergency room showed significant shortening of hospital stay and subsequent reduction in cost.[37-40]

Patients with left bundle branch block are good candidates for CT[41] as they frequently have false positive imaging stress tests and are not suitable for stress testing with EKG alone. This might also be the case for patients with WPW but it has not yet been investigated. Other clinical scenarios are patients with new onset heart failure[42] and preoperative evaluation including patients planned for valve surgery.[43]

Currently published appropriateness criteria[36] suggest that patient with known coronary disease, chronic stable angina or history of myocardial infarction are not good candidates for CT.

Two large randomized multicenter comparative effectiveness trials, the PROMISE and the RESCUE trial, will assess the clinical value of cardiac CT in comparison to stress testing in symptomatic patients.

CORONARY STENT

Coronary stent evaluation by CT is limited by blooming artifacts. The stent size, design and metal type will have varying effect on artifacts. Stents with diameter greater than 3–3.5 mm[44] are better suited than smaller stents. Asymptomatic patients with stents are not appropriate for cardiac CT but selected symptomatic patients with adequate stent size and possible equivocal stress test results, combined with peripheral vascular disease or history of stroke might be candidates for CT to avoid higher risk invasive angiography.

CORONARY BYPASS GRAFTS

Coronary bypass grafts can be evaluated by contrast CT with good results due to large diameter of the grafts and lack of motion. Metal clip artifacts and severe native coronary disease with diffuse coronary calcifications have limited the clinical applicability. As such cardiac CT has limited clinical use in routine evaluation of bypass graft patency.

CT is considered appropriate in presurgical planning prior to redothoracic or cardiac surgery where it can accurately account for location of prior bypass grafts in relationship to sternum and sternal wires. Additionally it will assess the distance of the right ventricular free wall from the sternum. Routine use of CT has been shown to decrease surgical complications, transfusion and hospital stay.[45] Additionally, in patients with

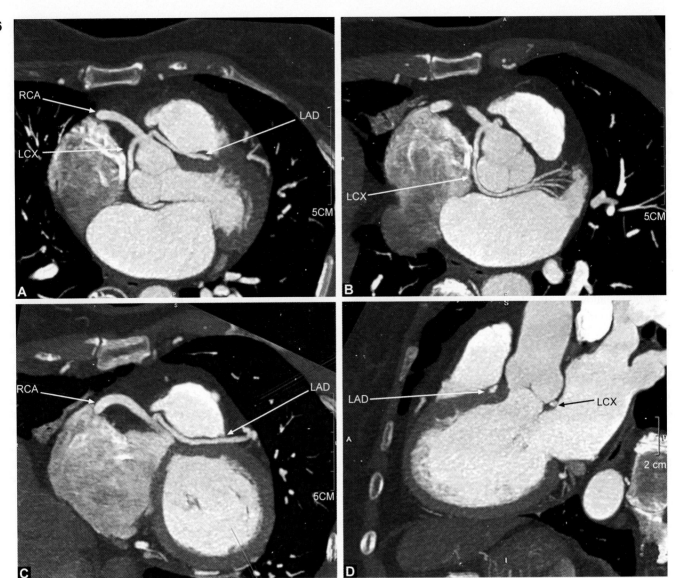

FIGURES 5A TO D: Anomalous coronary arteries. (A) Oblique planar images with anomalous left anterior descending (LAD) and left circumflex (LCX) arising from the right coronary sinus of Valsalva adjacent to the right coronary artery (RCA). (B) LCX travels posterior to the aorta. (C) LAD travels below the pulmonic valve within the left ventricular myocardium. (D) LAD with intramyocardial course. LCX travels posterior to the aorta

history of stroke where there can be concerns for engaging the left internal mammary artery (LIMA) with coronary catheter or there is clinical concern for left subclavian stenosis, a CT scan can evaluate the origin of the LIMA graft and assess the subclavian artery at the same time.

ANOMALOUS CORONARY ARTERIES

Screening for anomalous coronary vessels with EKG gated contrast CT is considered Class I indication.[46] CT allows for more accurate evaluation of the course of the vessels where exclusion of inter-arterial course is paramount.[47,48] The anomalous vessels are of great variety and the course of the proximal portion of each vessel determines the clinical significance. A course anterior to the pulmonary artery, or posterior to the aortic root, is benign where as an inter-arterial course, between the aorta and the pulmonary artery, is frequently considered malignant.[49] Left main coronary anomaly arising from right sinus of Valsalva and traveling between the

pulmonary artery and the aortic root is considered malignant but when the vessel travels below the pulmonic valve and is within the myocardium (Figs 5A to D) it is considered a benign finding.[48] RCA with inter-arterial course[50] is considered an indication for surgery when ischemia is present.[46] LCX arising from the right sinus of Valsalva and traveling posterior to the aortic root is considered a benign variant (Figs 5A to D).

OTHER CORONARY FINDINGS

Coronary aneurysms are well characterized by CT and can be found in association with atherosclerosis, Kawasaki disease, Takayasu arteritis and cocaine use.[51]

Myocardial bridging of the coronary arteries is a common finding on CT, and more commonly detected by CT compared to invasive angiography.[52] Clinical importance of myocardial bridging is under debate.[53] Noncalcified plaques at the site of the myocardial bridge could theoretically be missed on CT as noncalcified plaque could have similar density as the adjacent myocardium.

Coronary fistulas can be evaluated by CT.[54] Small fistulas are of limited clinical significance but larger fistulas benefit from characterization prior to surgical interventions. Coronary fistula to low pressure chambers such as atrium or cardiac veins are frequently dilated due to increased flow. During invasive angiography, it is sometimes difficult to determine the course, due to lack of selective contrast filling but with high resolution CT a detailed evaluation is possible.

MYOCARDIUM AND CHAMBERS

The first report of CT of the heart in 1976 involved imaging of myocardial contrast perfusion defects in an animal model of myocardial infarction.[2] Since then there has been progressive improvement in spatial and temporal resolution that now allows for accurate assessment of ventricular ejection fraction plus regional systolic wall thickening.[55] Due to radiation involved with CT, other techniques, such as echocardiography and magnetic resonance imaging (MRI), are considered first line imaging techniques for assessing the myocardium and chambers. Temporal resolution with *single source* CT has been considered suboptimal leading to concern that it was unable to accurately capture the end-systolic phase thus underestimating the stroke volume and left ventricular ejection fraction.[56] *Dual source* CT scanners have been able to show excellent image quality irrespective of heart rate and during phantom imaging able to assess global function with greater accuracy than MRI.[57] Right ventricular systolic function can also be assessed by CT with equal or better interobserver and intraobserver variability than MRI.[58,59] Low radiation (equal to MUGA) and low contrast protocols exist for analyzing simultaneously left and right ventricular systolic function but due to general availability of alternative modalities there has been limited adoption of this.[60] Left ventricular ejection fraction measured by CT has prognostic value that can supplement clinical history and coronary findings.[33]

Qualitative and quantitative myocardial perfusion analysis can be performed by CT.[61] Research dating back to the 1980s suggested that despite significant diffusion of contrast into the interstitial space there was still a fairly linear relationship between myocardial contrast enhancement and myocardial perfusion.[62] Artifacts affected the myocardial analysis by electron beam CT.[62] Multidetector CT has less artifacts and this has renewed interest in myocardial perfusion analysis by CT. Radiation with myocardial perfusion imaging is expected to be similar or less than radiation with nuclear perfusion studies.[61] Technology exists to acquire analysis of myocardial blood flow with reasonable radiation burden but at this time most research is focused on qualitative evaluation of myocardial contrast enhancement.[61] Combining coronary analysis with myocardial contrast enhancement and wall motion analysis improves accuracy of coronary analysis[63] and is expected to be a cost effective way of analyzing ischemic heart disease in the future. Extensive research including multicenter trial, underway for analysis of myocardial contrast enhancement during adenosine infusion.[61]

For image evaluation of myocardial perfusion defects the image settings are different than during coronary evaluation (center ~100 and width of 150–200). Additionally increased

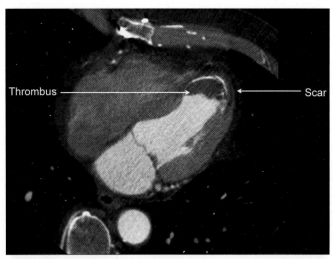

FIGURE 6: Myocardial scaring of the apex with thinning, calcification, fatty transformation and large thrombus

images thickness (5–10 mm) with average or MinIP has superior contrast to noise ratio compared to MIP and thin slices images.[64]

Assessment of myocardial scaring can be done by CT. Wall thinning and fatty transformation of scar (Fig. 6) can be readily detected by CT where the fatty tissue will have negative CT density (HU –30 to –60).[65] More subtle signs of myocardial scaring without wall thinning can also be detected by CT and delayed contrast enhancement imaging.[66] Animal studies of recent myocardial infarction suggest that good correlation exist between delayed enhancement detect by CT and MRI. Limitations of CT are contrast to noise ratio between areas of delayed enhancement and normal myocardium.

Currently evaluation of myocardial contrast enhancement is not part of established clinical care as there is not yet consensus for ideal protocol and clinical research is still limited. During the comprehensive evaluation of the myocardium, there is a general agreement for using the "stress" adenosine infusion and, during the initial image acquisition, and this is then followed by "non-stress" contrast imaging and later by delayed enhancement imaging.

Current clinical use for detection of myocardial scar by CT is aimed at patients who are not able to undergo MRI due to presence of an ICD. These are typically patients with reoccurring ventricular tachycardia awaiting catheter ablation therapy.[67] In these cases, CT can possibly detect the location of scar by hypoenhancement during the first pass imaging, wall thinning, delayed enhancement and exclude mural thrombus. Additionally the CT images can be used for anatomic mapping for the ablation procedure, similar to common practice of mapping left atrium during ablation of atrial fibrillation.

Another indication for delayed enhancement with cardiac CT could be perimyocarditis where young individuals with clinical diagnosis for pericarditis and elevated troponin could get cardiac CT to rule out the coronary anomaly or disease in addition to analyzing left ventricular function and detection of delayed enhancement.[68]

Left ventricular thrombus can be easily accessed by CT and apical thrombus is frequently detected on non-gated contrast enhanced CT of the chest.[69] Due to high spatial and temporal resolution of cardiac CT, it is congenial for detection of left

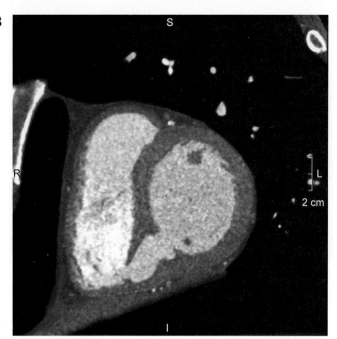

FIGURE 7: Postinfarction ventricular septal defect

ventricular thrombus. High contrast to noise ratio between the thrombus (HU density 30–60) and contrast mixed blood (HU density of 200–500) allows for detection of small clots that can be missed by echocardiography.

Due to high affinity of CT for detection of fatty tissue and high spatial resolution, cardiac CT might be ideal for assessing the right ventricular dysplasia.[70] Few publications exist on this matter and this will require dedicated contrast bolus timing for the right ventricle that is frequently avoided during the coronary imaging. Additionally software for analyzing the right ventricular systolic function is currently limited.

Ventricular (Fig. 7) and atrial (Figs 8A and B) septal defects can be detected by CT.[71] Other reported findings on cardiac CT are hypertrophic cardiomyopathy, noncompaction, congenital heart disease and ventricular aneurysm.[72,73]

PULMONARY VEINS

With the advent of radiofrequency ablation for atrial fibrillation, there is an increased need for visualization of the left atrium, left atrial appendage and pulmonary veins. Other imaging modalities, such as transesophageal echocardiography, intracardiac echocardiography and MRI can also delineate these structures. CT is frequently the test of choice due to its widespread availability and the ease of performance. The excellent contrast to noise ratio of CT images makes them well-suited for developing a 3D map of the highly variable anatomy of the left atrium, appendage and pulmonary veins prior to the ablation procedure (Fig. 9). Integration of the 3D map with electroanatomic mapping and real-time location of ablation catheters is thought to increase safety and efficacy of the procedure in addition to facilitating shorter periprocedural fluoroscopic time.[74,75] CT can exclude the presence of the left atrial appendage thrombus (Fig. 10) and determine the relationship between the atrium and the esophagus, as ablation adjacent to the esophagus can result in catastrophic perforation with atrial-esophageal fistula. Additionally a detailed EKG gated CT is able to detect accessory atrial appendages and other possible recesses that could be sites for an increased risk of catheter induced perforation.[76] Following the ablation procedure, a patient can undergo repeat imaging to exclude pulmonary vein stenosis and CT is considered the optimal modality.[77]

CT prior to ablation can be done both with and without EKG gating.[78,79] EKG gating of CT in patients in atrial fibrillation does currently not allow for radiation reduction protocols such as prospective dose modulation or sequential scanning.[79] This might change in the future with more sophisticated EKG detection software. By using the "retrospective EKG gating", the postprocessing allows for motion free end-systolic (atrial diastolic) visualization of the

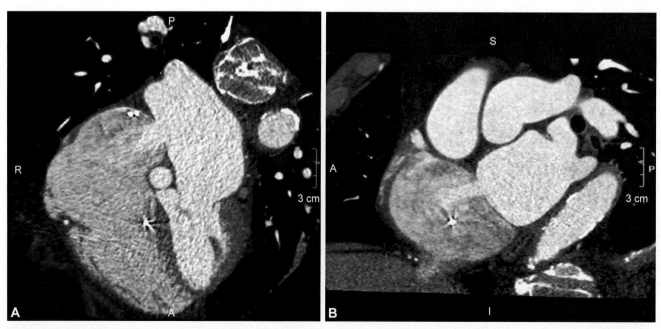

FIGURES 8A AND B: Atrial septal defect with contrast traveling from left atrium to right atrium. Enlargement of right ventricle and both atria

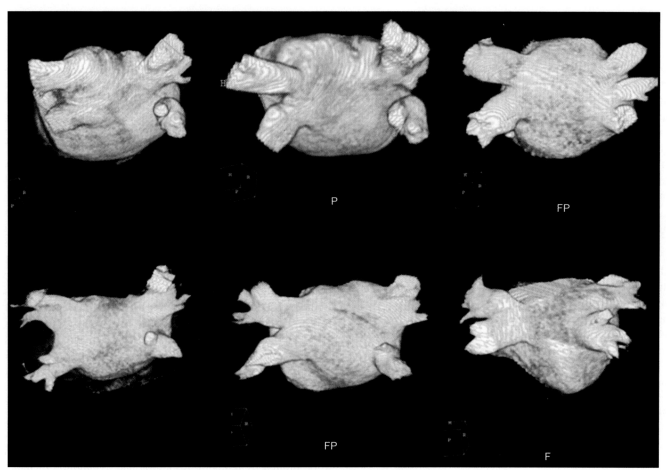

FIGURE 9: Left atrial and pulmonary venous anatomy is highly variable as is demonstrated in these six examples

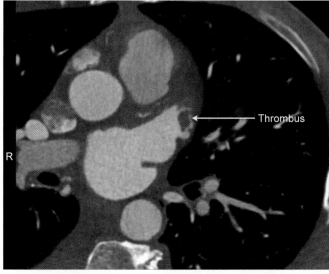

FIGURE 10: Thrombus within the left atrial appendage

left atrium by reconstruction of images 275–350 ms following the R-wave.[80] This type of reconstruction has also been termed "absolute delay reconstruction". Radiation associated with nongated CT is less but motion artifacts affecting the left atrial appendage would make exclusion of thrombus less reliable. Nongated CT might be sufficient in patients with CHADS[2] score less than 1.[79] Patients with

left ventricular systolic dysfunction, dilatation of the left atrium and low blood flow frequently have partial contrast filling of the left atrial appendage during the first pass imaging.[81] This often necessitates repeat scanning within 60–90 seconds of the first scan to exclude pseudothrombus.[82] On review of the delayed images, the density ratio between the left atrial appendage and the ascending aorta can be used to quantitatively assess for thrombus.[82] Additionally it has been proposed that prone imaging might also facilitate contrast filling of appendage and prevent the problem of partial filling.[83]

CARDIAC VEINS

Cardiac venous anatomy is readily assessed by CT. This requires slight delay of image acquisition time to allow adequate levophase maturation. Cardiac venous anatomy is highly variable and theoretically it could be assessed prior to placement of the left ventricular pacemaker lead. The anterior cardiac vein originates in the anterior interventricular groove parallel to the left anterior descending coronary and empties into the great cardiac vein in the atrioventricular groove which empties into the coronary sinus and finally the right atrium. Middle cardiac vein runs within the posterior interventricular groove and also joins the coronary sinus prior to emptying into the right atrium. The posterolateral cardiac vein

CHAPTER 22 Cardiac Computed Tomography

(Figs 3A and B), which is frequently used for resynchronization therapy is frequently absent in ischemic heart disease.[84]

Combining assessment of left ventricular dyssynchrony and cardiac venous anatomy prior to insertion of a biventricular pacemaker has been proposed[85,86] with favorable results in smaller studies. Large randomized prospective trials have not been completed. Assessment of cardiac venous anatomy is more commonly done following failure to place a left ventricular lead as this can both explain the cause for a failed procedure and aid in planning for epicardial lead placement. Additionally CT can be used prior to consideration of resynchronization therapy in patients with complex congenital heart disease.[87]

VALVULAR DISEASE

Evaluation of valves by CT is, in general, done as a byproduct of coronary analysis. Echocardiography remains the gold standard for valvular assessment due to safety, lack of radiation, higher temporal resolution and ability to assess the functional significance of valvular lesions. CT is considered appropriate when the significant valvular dysfunction is suspected and other noninvasive methods are inadequate.[36]

Imaging protocol for valvular assessment requires higher radiation as data from most of the cardiac cycle is needed and dose modulation can be detrimental. Imaging with prospective single phase protocol limits the valvular analysis substantially. Contrast opacification of the right ventricle can also be helpful for functional assessment and this will lead to overall increased contrast dose. Image analysis benefits from thicker image slabs (3–10 mm) with MinIP. This allows for better evaluation of thin leaflets both for stenotic and regurgitant orifice area measurements. Three- and four-dimensional image analysis with so-called blood pool inversion volume-rendering technique can allow for easier morphologic evaluation but thin leaflets are not always well visualized.[88]

Left-sided valves are better visualized than right-sided valves and stenotic orifice areas are better measured than regurgitant lesions.[89] CT can readily detect the number of aortic valve leaflets, aortic valve stenosis, mitral valve stenosis (Figs 11A and B) and mitral valve prolapse. Aortic valve area during mid-systole and mitral valve area during early diastole can be assessed with fairly good accuracy. Assessment of aortic valve stenosis has been validated by multiple studies and some studies suggest that valve area is systematically larger by CT than with echocardiography and this could be due to erroneous systematic underestimation of left ventricular outflow tract (LVOT) area by echocardiography.[90,91]

CT imaging can quantify valvular calcifications better than other imaging modalities and this can be valuable prior to percutaneous valvuloplasty.[92] In patients with mitral valve stenosis, during preprocedural planning, CT can also detect left atrial appendage thrombus, valvular, subvalvular thickening and calcifications. Right-sided valve analysis is limited by spatial resolution, thin leaflet structures and contrast mixing artifacts. Procedural planning for percutaneous interventional treatment of mitral valve with a coronary sinus device can be done by cardiac CT. The contrast enhanced EKG gated images can assess the location of target vein and adjacent LCX and thus assess the risk of circumflex compression injury.

Assessment of valves by CT is primarily done by morphologic evaluation, and functional assessment is limited. Estimations of flow by combination of volume and area measurements over time are still investigational and expected to be limited by temporal resolution and assumption of intact integrity of other valves.[91] Estimation of regurgitant volume and regurgitant fraction can be done by analyzing right and left ventricular volumes in patients with single valve disease.[93]

Mechanical valves can be visualized by contrast and non-contrast enhanced CT (Figs 11A and B). Evaluation of metallic valves by echocardiography and MRI suffers from metal

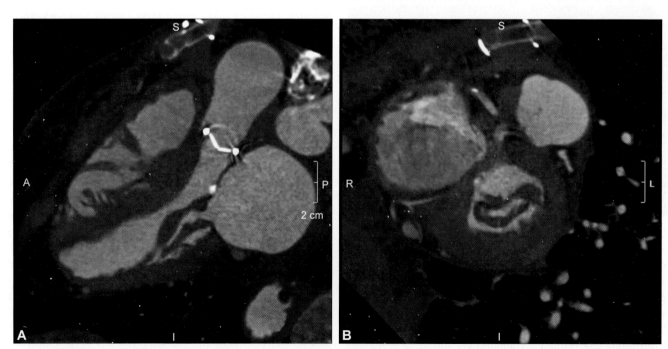

FIGURES 11A AND B: Mitral valve disease with bileaflet thickening and calcification of anterior leaflet. Prosthetic mechanical bileaflet aortic valve. Right ventricle dilated with hypertrophy

artifacts making image analysis frequently inadequate. Artifacts during CT are less prominent. Similar to simple fluoroscopy a cardiac CT without contrast has the potential to show mechanical leaflet motion with great accuracy. Contrast enhanced CT allows for detection of thrombus formation and pannus in addition to assessment of leaflet immobility. Additionally CT can delineate pseudoaneurysm, quantify dehiscence of a prosthesis and rocking motion.[94]

A limited number of publications exist on assessment of endocarditis by CT.[95] Size and possible contrast opacification of the vegetation will limit detectability. Additionally vegetative lesions are highly mobile and conventional assessment of mid-diastolic or end-systolic phases might not be sufficient. Small perforation of thin valve leaflets can also be difficult to appreciate by CT. At this time, it is unclear what additional information can be obtained over standard echocardiography.

The future role of cardiac CT in evaluation of valvular disease appears to be more as a complimentary tool to echocardiography. The areas where it would be expected to give the greatest benefit would be during procedural planning of valvular surgery or transcatheter interventions.

PERICARDIUM

Superior spatial resolution of CT allows for excellent visualization and characterization of pericardial pathology. Initial imaging modality for pericardial disease is echocardiography but CT offers advantages over echocardiography in regards to superior spatial resolution, detection of calcification (Fig. 12) and characterization of adjacent intrathoracic structures.[96] High spatial resolution and separation of myocardium from pericardium by epicardial fat allows for accurate measurements of pericardial thickness. Normal pericardial thickness is less than 2–4 mm.[97] Assessment of the pericardium is best adjacent to the right ventricular free wall and can be difficult over the left ventricular free wall due to the lack of epicardial fat. Selection of systolic phases

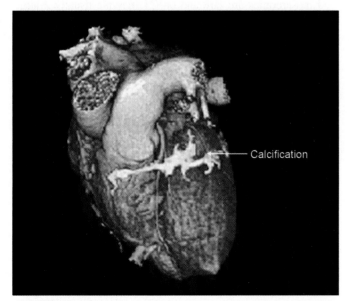

FIGURE 12: Pericardial calcification visualized by volume rendering technique

can allow for better separation of pericardium from myocardium. CT is highly sensitive for detection of pericardial effusion and multiphase cine imaging allows for assessment of dynamic changes during the cardiac cycle.

Constrictive cardiomyopathy with thickening of the pericardium can be easily diagnosed by CT. Contrast administration is not necessary but it can facilitate better separation between pericardium and adjacent structures. Thickness greater than 4 mm is suggestive for constriction, and greater than 6 mm thickness would be considered highly specific. Calcification of the pericardium is also a very specific finding strongly associated with constrictive physiology. Constriction caused by thin pericardium has been described and invariably is associated with deformation of the cardiac chambers that is best seen with contrast administration.[98,99] Additional signs of constrictions could be dilatation of the IVC, ascites and pleural effusion.

In patients with established diagnosis of constrictive cardiomyopathy CT can assist in preoperative planning by accurately delineating the extent of pericardial calcification. It also allows for assessment of the relationship between the pericardium and the sternum or coronaries.

Pericardial effusion can be easily detected by CT and quantified volumetrically if necessary. Characterization of the fluid can be done by CT image density (HU). Serous, transudative, fluid has density between 0–30 HU and exudative 30–70 HU. Hemorrhagic effusion can have variable density ranges from 32–70 HU. Hemopericardium complicating aortic dissection can be readily diagnosed by CT and thus prevent impending catastrophe with pericardiocentesis. Chylous effusion might have negative HU due to fatty content but a mix of chylous fluid with high protein content or exudative fluid could give measurements in the normal range.[100,101] Diagnosis of tamponade is primarily a clinical diagnosis but some features of tamponade physiology can be detected by CT such as right-sided chamber collapse. Reflux of contrast into the inferior vena cava has been considered a sign of tamponade but specificity of this finding is low.

Enhancement of the pericardial layers can be seen in pericarditis. Sensitivity and specificity of this finding is unknown. Small amount of pericardial fluid can make this finding more prominent. The inflammatory enhancement of the pericardial layers is also seen in effusion secondary to malignancies. Both pyogenic and malignant effusion would be expected to have signal density of 30–70 HU.

Pericardial tumors such as metastatic disease or primary cardiac tumors will enhance during contrast administration.[102] Nonenhancing tumor may be a pericardial cyst. Typical features of pericardial cysts are thin walls without septation and signal density of 0–30 HU. The most common pericardial tumors are metastatic disease from breast and lung cancer.

Congenital absence of pericardium is rare. Findings, such as interposition of lung tissue between the ascending aorta and the pulmonary artery or left ward displacement of the heart, are features that depend on the degree of absence. Partial or complete absence of pericardium is associated with other congenital defects such as atrial septal defect, patent ductus arteriosus and tetralogy of Fallot.

Echocardiography is the most widely used modality for evaluating or detecting a cardiac mass but it is limited by poor acoustic windows, operator dependency and limited tissue characterization ability. Additionally it is limited in assessing extracardiac extent of lesions. Some of the limitations of poor acoustic windowing can be overcome by transesophageal echocardiography. Magnetic resonance imaging (MRI) has been the imaging modality of choice for tissue characterization of the majority of cardiac tumors due to better spatial resolution in addition to high contrast resolution and multi planar image reconstruction capacity.

Cardiac computer tomography is highly rated in the ACCF/SCCT/ACR/AHA/ASE/ASNC/NASCI/SCAI/SCMR 2010 appropriateness criteria for evaluation of cardiac mass, in patients with technically limited echocardiography or MRI, due to high spatial and temporal resolution and complete coverage of the heart and adjacent organs.[36]

EKG gated CT scanning improves soft tissue characterization similar to MRI and can better identify fatty content, and calcification compared to echocardiography. Additionally it can aid in evaluating the vascular supply of tumors.[103]

Image acquisition protocols for evaluation of a cardiac mass might be best done in three phases; noncontrast scanning, "first-pass" contrast imaging and delayed enhancement imaging. The noncontrast and delayed enhancement imaging can be done with axial protocols to lower overall radiation dose.[104] The non-contrast images are ideal for detection of calcium within the tumor. The "first-pass" contrast images allow assessment of blood supply and possible tumor necrosis. The delayed images allow for assessment of inflammation and low flow state within the tumor or adjacent structures. Large field of view reconstructions are well suited for assessment of extracardiac metastatic disease.

Myxomas are the most common benign cardiac tumor and can be detected by CT based on a common location within the left atrium with attachment to the atrial septum adjacent to the fossa ovale. Occasionally calcifications are seen within the myxoma. More "gelatinous", friable, poorly defined and mobile myxomas are associated with embolism, fever and weight loss.

Lipomas are the second most common benign primary cardiac tumors with variable location within the heart. On CT, they are characteristically with negative signal density and may be located in the cardiac chamber, the myocardium or the pericardium.

Fibromas are a common primary benign cardiac neoplasm in children with calcifications and they usually arise in the interventricular septum or the anterior ventricular wall.

Hemangiomas are vascular tumors that mostly occur in the lateral wall of the left ventricle. On noncontrasted CT, it is usually a well-defined, round or oval mass with heterogeneous attenuation and interspersed fat. A common characteristic of hemangiomas are calcified thrombi.

Fibroelastomas are the most common valvular tumors (Fig. 13). The differential diagnosis for valvular tumor would include vegetation, thrombus or myxoma. Most patients are asymptomatic and when symptoms occur, they are likely due to thromboembolic event.

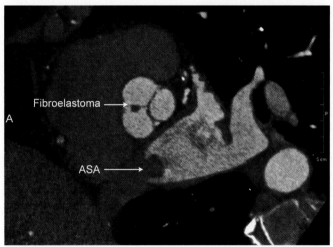

FIGURE 13: Fibroelastoma of the aortic valve attached to the non-coronary sinus of Valsalva. (Abbreviation: ASA: Atrial septal aneurysm).

MALIGNANT CARDIAC NEOPLASM

Angiosarcomas are malignant and usually arise from the right atrium with associated pericardial or pleural effusions, metastatic lung lesions and right-sided heart failure. On CT, it is often broad-based with heterogeneous enhancement or a low-attenuated mass which might be nodular or irregular.

Myxosarcomas are a rare form of a primary malignant cardiac tumor and very difficult to differentiate from a myxoma on CT. It is characterized by local recurrence and has been shown to involve the pulmonary artery, pericardium, pleura or distant metastasis, especially to the brain.

Primary cardiac lymphoma is rare and commonly affects the subepicardial fat, the right atrium, pericardium, and AV groove. Pericardial effusion is sometimes the only finding. When visualized, it may present as a large focal mass, multiple nodules or diffuse soft tissue infiltration with heterogeneous enhancement. Extracardiac findings may include mediastinal lymphadenopathy.[103]

Liposarcomas are rare and on CT they are usually a large solitary mass with mostly fatty and soft tissue components, infiltrating cardiac chambers and pericardium with mild contrast enhancement.

Metastatic cardiac tumors make up the bulk of malignant cardiac tumors. Most of the tumors originate through direct or transvenous invasion from the lungs, breasts, esophagus or other mediastinal tumors. Transvenous spread may also occur through the inferior vena cava from an adrenal or kidney tumor. Bronchogenic carcinoma can spread through the pulmonary vein to the left atrium. CT findings of metastatic malignant tumors are usually nonspecific and PET scanning can help to determine the extent of tumor spread or even localize the primary tumor.

NONCANCEROUS MASSES

Intracardiac thrombus is the most common intracardiac mass.[105] Most intracardiac thrombi occur in the setting of hypercoagulable state which can be as a result of left ventricular wall motion abnormality, presence of artificial devices (like mechanical valves) or atrial fibrillation. The major concern about an intracardiac thrombus is the propensity for embolization with a 15% risk of embolic stroke. Thrombus is most commonly found in the left side of the heart.

CT can be used in patients with suspected left-sided thrombus who are not candidates for transesophageal echocardiogram. On CT, left atrial thrombus usually appears as a round or oval filling defect commonly found in the atrial appendage. The draw back of CT for left atrial thrombus differentiation is the phenomenon of "pseudo-filling" defect or mixing artifact. The pseudo-filling defects occur in cases with circulatory stasis, as can be seen with atrial fibrillation, and is due to incomplete mixing of blood with contrast. The problem of pseudo-filling defect can be overcome by delayed imaging, that is done in 60–90 seconds after the initial contrast scan because thrombus persist in both early and late phases, while pseudo-filling defect does not.[106]

Ventricular Thrombus

These are seen as crescent shaped filling defects close to infarcted or dyskinetic areas. Attenuation is usually less than that of the myocardium, but greater than fatty tissue. Chronic or long-standing thrombus may appear laminated or become calcified (Fig. 6). Thrombus can be differentiated from myxoma based on the location and also most thrombi are immobile.

Hiatal Hernia

This can be identified by the presence of gastric folds.

Lipomatous Hypertrophy of Intra-Atrial Septum

This occurs frequently in older and obese individuals. Patients are usually asymptomatic, but a few may develop arrhythmias. This is characterized by the accumulation of mature fat cells in the intra-atrial septum. CT findings are bilobed, dumb-bell shaped intra-atrial septum that is usually greater than 2 cm in transverse diameter. Attenuation is usually in the range of fatty tissue (–110 HU). The fossa ovale is characteristically spared.

INCIDENTAL FINDINGS

Integral part of cardiac CT is the evaluation of the adjacent organs to the heart. Multiple studies have assessed the incidental noncardiac findings and the reported incidence varies greatly ranging from 3% to 40%.[107] The most important incidental findings, such as aortic dissection, pulmonary embolism and cancer, are rare. Additionally findings of esophageal hiatal hernia and lung nodules are more common. Granulomatous disease with nodular calcifications is considered benign, but other noncalcified lung nodules, especially in patients with history of smoking are of concern. Patients with lung nodules are advised to undergo follow-up scans based on the Fleischner criteria that determine frequency and number of the follow-up studies.[108] Until recently,

incidental lung nodule findings were, by some, considered a nuisance with limited clinical benefit,[109] but a randomized prospective study on smokers suggests there is a mortality benefit in the use of screening CT[110] and this might translate into benefit to patients who undergo a cardiac CT. Of note, a standard cardiac CT does not cover the whole lung field, and a half of incidental lung cancer findings could be missed.[111,112] At this time, it is not a common practice to offer full chest CT as an additional radiation would be expected with EKG gating and low pitch protocols.

FUTURE

The future of cardiac CT is very promising. The fast pace of technology has allowed a progressive improvement in CT scanning methods. Moore's law for annual increase in transistor computational power appears to apply for the CT technology. In the last decade, we have reached sub-millimeter spatial resolution and sub-second temporal resolution. At current time, we are able to acquire an image of the whole heart within a third of a second and with considerably less radiation than is used by other standard tests such as SPECT, CT chest, CT abdomen and CT of the head.

Cardiac CT has reached a state where its image quality is competitive with other imaging modalities such as SPECT, PET, echocardiography and MRI. Two randomized multicenter trials are in progress that will compare the anatomic assessment by CT with functional tests in patients with chest discomfort. These trials, the PROMISE and the RESCUE, are expected to solidify the clinical usefulness of Cardiac CT.

Research with myocardial perfusion CT is very promising and likely to be highly successful. Cardiac CT already allows for comprehensive evaluation of the heart by simultaneous anatomic assessment of the coronary arteries, cardiac chambers and valves. With successful myocardial perfusion imaging CT could become the primary test for evaluation of patients with chest pain.

With progression of technology, we can expect to see better spatial resolution, lower radiation and better tissue characterization. Multi-energy detectors with photon counting are under development and could allow for better detection of vulnerable plaque and discrimination between calcium and contrast within the coronary arteries. This would allow for more accurate stenosis analysis and improve prognostication of future cardiac events.

Cardiac CT has been embraced by cardiologist worldwide but due to concerns for overuse and presence of competing imaging modalities, the insurance companies have aggressively regulated and prevented the current use within the United States. Comparative effectiveness studies are expected to give the evidence based platform for future use of cardiac CT within the United States.

GUIDIELINES
2010 ACCF/AHA GUIDELINES FOR ASSESSMENT OF CARDIOVASCULAR RISK IN ASYMPTOMATIC ADULTS

Recommendations for Calcium Scoring Methods

Class IIa level of evidence: B	Measurement of coronary artery calcium (CAC) is reasonable for cardiovascular risk assessment in asymptomatic adults at intermediate risk (10–20% 10-year risk).
Class IIb level of evidence: B	Measurement of CAC may be reasonable for cardiovascular risk assessment in persons at low to intermediate risk (6–10% 10-year risk).
Class III level of evidence B	Person at low risk (< 6% 10 year risk) should not undergo CAC measurements for cardiovascular risk assessment

Recommendation for Coronary Computed Tomography Angiography

Class III Level of evidence: C	Coronary computed tomography angiography is not recommended for cardiovascular risk assessment in asymptomatic adults

Source: Greenland P, Alpert JS, Beller GA, et al. American College of Cardiology Foundation; American Heart Association. 2010 ACCF/AHA guidelines for assessment of cardiovascular risk in asymptomatic adults: a report of the American College of Cardiology Foundation/American Heart Association Task Force on Practice Guidelines. J Am Coll Cardiol. 2010;56(25):e50-103.

AHA SCIENTIFIC STATEMENT 2006
ASSESSMENT OF CORONARY ARTERY DISEASE BY CARDIAC COMPUTED TOMOGRAPHY

Coronary Calcium Assessment

Class IIb Level of evidence: B	Coronary artery calcium (CAC) assessment may be reasonable for the assessment of symptomatic patients, especially in the setting of equivocal treadmill or functional testing
	Patients with chest pain with equivocal or normal EKGs and negative cardiac enzyme studies may be considered for CAC assessment
	There are other situations when CAC assessment might be reasonable. CAC measurement may be considered in the symptomatic patient to determine the cause of cardiomyopathy
Class III Level of evidence: C	Serial imaging for assessment of progression of coronary calcification is not indicated at this time

CT Coronary Angiography

Class IIa Level of evidence: B	CT coronary angiography is reasonable for the assessment of obstructive disease in symptomatic patients
Class IIa Level of evidence: C	CT coronary angiography reasonable to use CT as one of the first-choice imaging modalities in the workup of known and suspected coronary anomalies
Class IIb Level of evidence: C	Clinically, however, it might be reasonable in most cases not only to assess the patency of the bypass graft but also the presence of coronary stenoses in the course of the bypass graft or at the anastomotic site as well as in the native coronary artery system
Class III Level of evidence: C	Several small studies have assessed the value of EBCT and MDCT for detecting restenosis after stent placement. At this time, however, imaging of patients to follow-up stent placement cannot be recommended
	The use of both CT modalities to evaluate noncalcified plaque (NCP) is promising but premature. There are limited data on variability but none on the prognostic implications of CT angiography for NCP assessment or on the utility of these measures to track atherosclerosis or stenosis over time; therefore, their use for these purposes is not recommended
	CT coronary angiography is not recommended in asymptomatic persons for the assessment of occult CAD

Hybrid Nuclear/CT Imaging

Class III Level of evidence: C	The incremental benefit of hybrid imaging strategies will need to be demonstrated before clinical implementation, as radiation exposure may be significant with dual nuclear/CT imaging. Therefore, hybrid nuclear/CT imaging is not recommended

Source: Budoff MJ, Achenbach S, Blumenthal RS, et al. Assessment of coronary artery disease by cardiac computed tomography: a scientific statement from the American Heart Association Committee on Cardiovascular Imaging and Intervention, Council on Cardiovascular Radiology and Intervention, and Committee on Cardiac Imaging, Council on Clinical Cardiology. Circulation. 2006;114:1761-79.

ACCF/SCCT/ACR/AHA/ASE/ASNC/NASCI/SCAI/SCMR 2010 APPROPRIATE USE CRITERIA FOR CARDIAC COMPUTED TOMOGRAPHY

Detection of CAD in Symptomatic Patients without Known Heart Disease Symptomatic—Non-acute Symptoms Possibly Representing an Ischemic Equivalent

- Intermediate pretest probability of CAD

OR

- Low pretest probability of CAD
- EKG uninterpretable or unable to exercise

Detection of CAD in Symptomatic Patients without Known Heart Disease Symptomatic—Acute Symptoms with Suspicion of ACS (Urgent Presentation)

- Normal EKG and cardiac biomarkers
- Low pretest probability of CAD

OR

- Nondiagnostic EKG or equivocal cardiac biomarkers
- Intermediate pretest probability of CAD

Detection of CAD in Other Clinical Scenarios—New-Onset or Newly Diagnosed Clinical HF and No Prior CAD

- Reduced left ventricular ejection fraction
- Low pretest probability of CAD

OR

- Reduced left ventricular ejection fraction
- Intermediate pretest probability of CAD

Detection of CAD in Other Clinical Scenarios—Preoperative Coronary Assessment Prior to Non-coronary Cardiac Surgery

- Coronary evaluation before non-coronary cardiac surgery
- Intermediate pretest probability of CAD

Use of CTA in the Setting of Prior Test Results—Prior EKG Exercise Testing

- Normal EKG exercise test
- Continued symptoms

OR

- Prior EKG exercise testing
- Duke Treadmill Score—intermediate risk findings

Use of CTA in the Setting of Prior Test Results—Sequential Testing after Stress Imaging Procedures

- Discordant EKG exercise and imaging results

OR

- Stress imaging results: equivocal

Use of CTA in the Setting of Prior Test Results—Prior Coronary Calcium Score (CCS)

- Diagnostic impact of coronary calcium on the decision to perform contrast CTA in symptomatic patients
- CCS < 100

OR

- Diagnostic impact of coronary calcium on the decision to perform contrast CTA in symptomatic patients
- CCS 100–400

Use of CTA in the Setting of Prior Test Results—Evaluation of New or Worsening Symptoms in the Setting of Past Stress Imaging Study

- Previous stress imaging study normal

Risk Assessment Postrevascularization (PCI or CABG)—Symptomatic (Ischemic Equivalent)

- Evaluation of graft patency after CABG

Risk Assessment Postrevascularization (PCI or CABG)—Asymptomatic—Prior Coronary Stenting

- Prior left main coronary stent with stent diameter 3 mm

Evaluation of Cardiac Structure and Function—Adult Congenital Heart Disease

- Assessment of anomalies of coronary arterial and other thoracic arteriovenous vessels

OR

- Assessment of complex adult congenital heart disease

Evaluation of Cardiac Structure and Function—Evaluation of Ventricular Morphology and Systolic Function

- Inadequate images from other noninvasive methods
- Evaluation of left ventricular function
- Following acute MI or in HF patients

OR

- Quantitative evaluation of right ventricular function

OR

- Assessment of right ventricular morphology
- Suspected arrhythmogenic right ventricular dysplasia

Evaluation of Cardiac Structure and Function—Evaluation of Intracardiac and Extracardiac Structures

- Characterization of native cardiac valves
- Suspected clinically significant valvular dysfunction
- Inadequate images from other noninvasive methods

OR

- Characterization of prosthetic cardiac valves
- Suspected clinically significant valvular dysfunction
- Inadequate images from other noninvasive methods

OR

- Evaluation of cardiac mass (suspected tumor or thrombus)
- Inadequate images from other noninvasive methods

OR

- Evaluation of pericardial anatomy

OR

- Evaluation of pulmonary vein anatomy
- Prior to radiofrequency ablation for atrial fibrillation

OR

- Noninvasive coronary vein mapping
- Prior to placement of biventricular pacemaker

OR

- Localization of coronary bypass grafts and other retrosternal anatomy
- Prior to reoperative chest or cardiac surgery

Source: Taylor AJ, Cerqueira M, Hodgson JM, et al. ACCF/SCCT/ACR/AHA/ASE/ASNC/NASCI/SCAI/SCMR 2010 Appropriate use criteria for cardiac computed tomography: a report of the American College of Cardiology Foundation Appropriate Use Criteria Task Force, the Society of Cardiovascular Computed Tomography, the American College of Radiology, the American Heart Association, the American Society of Echocardiography, the American Society of Nuclear Cardiology, the North American Society for Cardiovascular Imaging, the Society for Cardiovascular Angiography and Interventions, and the Society for Cardiovascular Magnetic Resonance. J Am Coll Cardiol. 2010;56:1864-94.

1. Beckmann EC. CT scanning the early days. Br J Radiol. 2006;79:5-8.

2. Adams DF, Hessel SJ, Judy PF, et al. Differing attenuation coefficients of normal and infarcted myocardium. Science. 1976;192:467-9.

3. Sagel SS, Weiss ES, Gillard RG, et al. Gated computed tomography of the human heart. Invest Radiol. 1977;12:563-6.

4. Harell GS, Guthaner DF, Breiman RS, et al. Stop-action cardiac computed tomography. Radiology. 1977;123:515-7.

5. Hurlock GS, Higashino H, Mochizuki T. History of cardiac computed tomography: single to 320-detector row multislice computed tomography. Int J Cardiovasc Imaging. 2009;25:31-42.

6. Garcia MJ, Lessick J, Hoffmann MH, et al. Accuracy of 16-row multidetector computed tomography for the assessment of coronary artery stenosis. JAMA. 2006;296:403-11.

7. Raff GL. Radiation dose from coronary CT angiography: five years of progress. J Cardiovasc Comput Tomogr. 2010;4:365-74.

8. Pantos I, Thalassinou S, Argentos S, et al. Adult patient radiation doses from noncardiac CT examinations: a review of published results. Br J Radiol. 2011;84:293-303.

9. Cohen BL. The linear no-threshold theory of radiation carcinogenesis should be rejected. Journal of American Physicians and Surgeons. 2008;13:70-6.

10. Gerber TC, Carr JJ, Arai AE, et al. Ionizing radiation in cardiac imaging: a science advisory from the American Heart Association Committee on Cardiac Imaging of the Council on Clinical Cardiology and Committee on Cardiovascular Imaging and Intervention of the Council on Cardiovascular Radiology and Intervention. Circulation. 2009;119:1056-65.

11. Hausleiter J, Martinoff S, Hadamitzky M, et al. Image quality and radiation exposure with a low-tube voltage protocol for coronary CT angiography results of the PROTECTION II Trial. JACC Cardiovasc Imaging. 2010;3:1113-23.

12. Einstein AJ, Henzlova MJ, Rajagopalan S. Estimating risk of cancer associated with radiation exposure from 64-slice computed tomography coronary angiography. JAMA. 2007;298:317-23.

13. Rumberger JA, Simons DB, Fitzpatrick LA, et al. Coronary artery calcium area by electron-beam computed tomography and coronary atherosclerotic plaque area. A histopathologic correlative study. Circulation. 1995;92:2157-62.

14. Sangiorgi G, Rumberger JA, Severson A, et al. Arterial calcification and not lumen stenosis is highly correlated with atherosclerotic plaque burden in humans: a histologic study of 723 coronary artery segments using nondecalcifying methodology. J Am Coll Cardiol. 1998;31:126-33.

15. Tanenbaum SR, Kondos GT, Veselik KE, et al. Detection of calcific deposits in coronary arteries by ultrafast computed tomography and correlation with angiography. Am J Cardiol. 1989;63:870-2.

16. Agatston AS, Janowitz WR, Hildner FJ, et al. Quantification of coronary artery calcium using ultrafast computed tomography. J Am Coll Cardiol. 1990;15:827-32.

17. Ghadri JR, Goetti R, Fiechter M, et al. Inter-scan variability of coronary artery calcium scoring assessed on 64-multidetector computed tomography vs. dual-source computed tomography: a head-to-head comparison. Eur Heart J. 2011.

18. Greenland P, Bonow RO, Brundage BH, et al. American College of Cardiology Foundation Clinical Expert Consensus Task Force (ACCF/AHA Writing Committee to Update the 2000 Expert Consensus Document on Electron Beam Computed Tomography); Society of Atherosclerosis Imaging and Prevention; Society of Cardiovascular Computed Tomography. ACCF/AHA 2007 clinical expert consensus document on coronary artery calcium scoring by computed tomography in global cardiovascular risk assessment and in evaluation of patients with chest pain: a report of the American College of Cardiology Foundation Clinical Expert Consensus Task Force (ACCF/AHA Writing Committee to Update the 2000 Expert Consensus Document on Electron Beam Computed Tomography) developed in collaboration with the Society of Atherosclerosis Imaging and Prevention and the Society of Cardiovascular Computed Tomography. J Am Coll Cardiol. 2007;49:378-402.

19. Detrano R, Guerci AD, Carr JJ, et al. Coronary calcium as a predictor of coronary events in four racial or ethnic groups. N Engl J Med. 2008;358:1336-45.

20. Elias-Smale SE, Proença RV, Koller MT, et al. Coronary calcium score improves classification of coronary heart disease risk in the elderly: the Rotterdam study. J Am Coll Cardiol. 2010;56:1407-14.

21. Polonsky TS, McClelland RL, Jorgensen NW, et al. Coronary artery calcium score and risk classification for coronary heart disease prediction. JAMA. 2010;303:1610-6.

22. Greenland P, Alpert JS, Beller GA, et al. American College of Cardiology Foundation/American Heart Association Task Force on Practice Guidelines. 2010 ACCF/AHA guideline for assessment of cardiovascular risk in asymptomatic adults: a report of the American College of Cardiology Foundation/American Heart Association Task Force on Practice Guidelines. Circulation. 2010;122:e584-636.

23. Schuetz GM, Zacharopoulou NM, Schlattmann P, et al. Meta-analysis: noninvasive coronary angiography using computed tomography versus magnetic resonance imaging. Ann Intern Med. 2010;152:167-77.

24. Cheng V, Gutstein A, Wolak A, et al. Moving beyond binary grading of coronary arterial stenoses on coronary computed tomographic angiography: insights for the imager and referring clinician. JACC Cardiovasc Imaging. 2008;1:460-71.

25. Miller JM, Rochitte CE, Dewey M, et al. Diagnostic performance of coronary angiography by 64-row CT. N Engl J Med. 2008;359:2324-36.

26. Budoff MJ, Dowe D, Jollis JG, et al. Diagnostic performance of 64-multidetector row coronary computed tomographic angiography for evaluation of coronary artery stenosis in individuals without known coronary artery disease: results from the prospective multicenter ACCURACY (Assessment by Coronary Computed Tomographic Angiography of Individuals Undergoing Invasive Coronary Angiography) trial. J Am Coll Cardiol. 2008;52:1724-32.

27. Meijboom WB, Meijs MF, Schuijf JD, et al. Diagnostic accuracy of 64-slice computed tomography coronary angiography: a prospective, multicenter, multivendor study. J Am Coll Cardiol. 2008;52:2135-44.

28. von Ballmoos MW, Haring B, Juillerat P, et al. Meta-analysis: diagnostic performance of low-radiation-dose coronary computed tomography angiography. Ann Intern Med. 2011;154:413-20.

29. James K Min, Dunning A, Achenbach S, et al. Abstract 14571: Prognostic Value of 64-Detector Row Coronary CT Angiography for the Prediction of All-Cause Mortality: results from 21,062 Patients in the Prospective Multinational CONFIRM Registry (Coronary CT Angiography Evaluation For Clinical Outcomes: An International Multicenter Registry). Circulation. 2010;122:A14571.

30. Achenbach S, Moselewski F, Ropers D, et al. Detection of calcified and noncalcified coronary atherosclerotic plaque by contrast-enhanced, submillimeter multidetector spiral computed tomography: a segment-based comparison with intravascular ultrasound. Circulation. 2004;109:14-7.

31. Leber AW, Knez A, Becker A, et al. Accuracy of multidetector spiral computed tomography in identifying and differentiating the composition of coronary atherosclerotic plaques: a comparative study with intracoronary ultrasound. J Am Coll Cardiol. 2004;43:1241-7.

32. Min JK, Shaw LJ, Devereux RB, et al. Prognostic value of multi-detector coronary computed tomographic angiography for prediction of all-cause mortality. J Am Coll Cardiol. 2007;50:1161-70.

33. Chow BJ, Wells GA, Chen L, et al. Prognostic value of 64-slice cardiac computed tomography severity of coronary artery disease, coronary atherosclerosis, and left ventricular ejection fraction. J Am Coll Cardiol. 2010;55:1017-28.

34. Motoyama S, Sarai M, Harigaya H, et al. Computed tomographic angiography characteristics of atherosclerotic plaques subsequently resulting in acute coronary syndrome. J Am Coll Cardiol. 2009;54:49-57.

35. Hulten EA, Carbonaro S, Petrillo SP, et al. Prognostic value of cardiac computed tomography angiography: a systematic review and meta-analysis. J Am Coll Cardiol. 2011;57:1237-47.

36. Taylor AJ, Cerqueira M, Hodgson JM, et al. ACCF/SCCT/ACR/AHA/ASE/ASNC/NASCI/SCAI/SCMR 2010 appropriate use criteria for cardiac computed tomography: a report of the American College of Cardiology Foundation Appropriate Use Criteria Task Force, the Society of Cardiovascular Computed Tomography, the American College of Radiology, the American Heart Association, the American Society of Echocardiography, the American Society of Nuclear Cardiology, the North American Society for Cardiovascular Imaging, the Society for Cardiovascular Angiography and Interventions, and the Society for Cardiovascular Magnetic Resonance. J Am Coll Cardiol. 2010;56:1864-94.

37. Hoffmann U, Nagurney JT, Moselewski F, et al. Coronary multidetector computed tomography in the assessment of patients with acute chest pain. Circulation. 2006;114:2251-60.

38. Goldstein JA, Gallagher MJ, O'Neill WW, et al. A randomized controlled trial of multi-slice coronary computed tomography for evaluation of acute chest pain. J Am Coll Cardiol. 2007;49:863-71.

39. Rubinshtein R, Halon DA, Gaspar T, et al. Usefulness of 64-slice cardiac computed tomographic angiography for diagnosing acute coronary syndromes and predicting clinical outcome in emergency department patients with chest pain of uncertain origin. Circulation. 2007;115:1762-8.

40. Hollander JE, Chang AM, Shofer FS, et al. One-year outcomes following coronary computerized tomographic angiography for evaluation of emergency department patients with potential acute coronary syndrome. Acad Emerg Med. 2009;16:693-8.

41. Ghostine S, Caussin C, Daoud B, et al. Non-invasive detection of coronary artery disease in patients with left bundle branch block using 64-slice computed tomography. J Am Coll Cardiol. 2006;48:1929-34.

42. Andreini D, Pontone G, Bartorelli AL, et al. Sixty-four-slice multi-detector computed tomography: an accurate imaging modality for the evaluation of coronary arteries in dilated cardiomyopathy of unknown etiology. Circ Cardiovasc Imaging. 2009;2:199-205.

43. Meijboom WB, Mollet NR, Van Mieghem CA, et al. Pre-operative computed tomography coronary angiography to detect significant coronary artery disease in patients referred for cardiac valve surgery. J Am Coll Cardiol. 2006;48:1658-65.

44. Rixe J, Achenbach S, Ropers D, et al. Assessment of coronary artery stent restenosis by 64-slice multi-detector computed tomography. Eur Heart J. 2006;27:2567-72.

45. Khan NU, Yonan N. Does preoperative computed tomography reduce the risks associated with re-do cardiac surgery? Interact Cardiovasc Thorac Surg. 2009;9:119-23.

46. Warnes CA, Williams RG, Bashore TM, et al. ACC/AHA 2008 Guidelines for the Management of Adults with Congenital Heart Disease: Executive Summary: a report of the American College of Cardiology/American Heart Association Task Force on Practice Guidelines (writing committee to develop guidelines for the management of adults with congenital heart disease). Circulation. 2008; 118:2395-451.

47. Zeina AR, Blinder J, Sharif D, et al. Congenital coronary artery anomalies in adults: non-invasive assessment with multidetector CT. Br J Radiol. 2009;82:254-61.

48. Torres FS, Nguyen ET, Dennie CJ, et al. Role of MDCT coronary angiography in the evaluation of septal vs interarterial course of anomalous left coronary arteries. J Cardiovasc Comput Tomogr. 2010;4:246-54.

49. Taylor AJ, Rogan KM, Virmani R. Sudden cardiac death associated with isolated congenital coronary artery anomalies. J Am Coll Cardiol. 1992;20:640-7.

50. Zhang LJ, Wu SY, Huang W, et al. Anomalous origin of the right coronary artery originating from the left coronary sinus of valsalva with an interarterial course: diagnosis and dynamic evaluation using dual-source computed tomography. J Comput Assist Tomogr. 2009;33:348-53.

51. Johnson PT, Fishman EK. CT angiography of coronary artery aneurysms: detection, definition, causes, and treatment. AJR Am J Roentgenol. 2010;195:928-34.

52. Kim PJ, Hur G, Kim SY, et al. Frequency of myocardial bridges and dynamic compression of epicardial coronary arteries: a comparison between computed tomography and invasive coronary angiography. Circulation. 2009;119:1408-16.

53. Ishikawa Y, Akasaka Y, Suzuki K, et al. Anatomic properties of myocardial bridge predisposing to myocardial infarction. Circulation. 2009;120:376-83.

54. Dodd JD, Ferencik M, Liberthson RR, et al. Evaluation of efficacy of 64-slice multidetector computed tomography in patients with congenital coronary fistulas. J Comput Assist Tomogr. 2008;32:265-70.

55. Mahnken AH, Bruners P, Schmidt B, et al. Left ventricular function can reliably be assessed from dual-source CT using ECG-gated tube current modulation. Invest Radiol. 2009;44:384-9.

56. Sigurdsson G. CT for assessing ventricular remodeling: is it ready for prime time? Curr Heart Fail Rep. 2008;5:16-22.

57. Groen JM, van der Vleuten PA, Greuter MJ, et al. Comparison of MRI, 64-slice MDCT and DSCT in assessing functional cardiac parameters of a moving heart phantom. Eur Radiol. 2009;19:577-83.

58. Müller M, Teige F, Schnapauff D, et al. Evaluation of right ventricular function with multidetector computed tomography: comparison with magnetic resonance imaging and analysis of inter- and intraobserver variability. Eur Radiol. 2009;19:278-89.

59. Sugeng L, Mor-Avi V, Weinert L, et al. Multimodality comparison of quantitative volumetric analysis of the right ventricle. JACC Cardiovasc Imaging. 2010;3:10-8.

60. Salem R, Remy-Jardin M, Delhaye D, et al. Integrated cardio-thoracic imaging with ECG-gated 64-slice multidetector-row CT: initial findings in 133 patients. Eur Radiol. 2006;16:1973-81.

61. Ambrose MS, Valdiviezo C, Mehra V, et al. CT perfusion: ready for prime time. Curr Cardiol Rep. 2011;13:57-66.

62. Bell MR, Lerman LO, Rumberger JA. Validation of minimally invasive measurement of myocardial perfusion using electron beam computed tomography and application in human volunteers. Heart. 1999;81:628-35.

63. Cury RC, Nieman K, Shapiro MD, et al. Comprehensive assessment of myocardial perfusion defects, regional wall motion, and left ventricular function by using 64-section multidetector CT. Radiology. 2008;248:466-75.

64. Rogers IS, Cury RC, Blankstein R, et al. Comparison of postprocessing techniques for the detection of perfusion defects by cardiac computed tomography in patients presenting with acute ST-segment elevation myocardial infarction. J Cardiovasc Comput Tomogr. 2010;4:258-66.

SECTION 3

Diagnosis

65. Ichikawa Y, Kitagawa K, Chino S, et al. Adipose tissue detected by multislice computed tomography in patients after myocardial infarction. JACC Cardiovasc Imaging. 2009;2:548-55.

66. Mendoza DD, Joshi SB, Weissman G, et al. Viability imaging by cardiac computed tomography. J Cardiovasc Comput Tomogr. 2010;4:83-91.

67. Tian J, Jeudy J, Smith MF, et al. Three-dimensional contrast-enhanced multidetector CT for anatomic, dynamic, and perfusion characterization of abnormal myocardium to guide ventricular tachycardia ablations. Circ Arrhythm Electrophysiol. 2010;3:496-504.

68. Dambrin G, Laissy JP, Serfaty JM, et al. Diagnostic value of ECG-gated multidetector computed tomography in the early phase of suspected acute myocarditis. A preliminary comparative study with cardiac MRI. Eur Radiol. 2007;17:331-8.

69. Foster CJ, Sekiya T, Love HG, et al. Identification of intracardiac thrombus: comparison of computed tomography and cross-sectional echocardiography. Br J Radiol. 1987;60:327-31.

70. Kimura F, Sakai F, Sakomura Y, et al. Helical CT features of arrhythmogenic right ventricular cardiomyopathy. Radiographics. 2002;22:1111-24.

71. Rajiah P, Kanne JP. Computed tomography of septal defects. J Cardiovasc Comput Tomogr. 2010;4:231-45.

72. Knickelbine T, Lesser JR, Haas TS, et al. Identification of unexpected nonatherosclerotic cardiovascular disease with coronary CT angiography. JACC Cardiovasc Imaging. 2009;2:1085-92.

73. Yavari A, Sriskandan N, Khawaja MZ, et al. Computed tomography of a broken heart: chronic left ventricular pseudoaneurysm. J Cardiovasc Comput Tomogr. 2008;2:120-2.

74. Bertaglia E, Bella PD, Tondo C, et al. Image integration increases efficacy of paroxysmal atrial fibrillation catheter ablation: results from the CartoMerge Italian Registry. Europace. 2009;11:1004-10.

75. Powell BD, Packer DL. Does image integration improve atrial fibrillation ablation outcomes, or are other aspects of the ablation the key to success? Europace. 2009;11:973-4.

76. Abbara S, Mundo-Sagardia JA, Hoffmann U, et al. Cardiac CT assessment of left atrial accessory appendages and diverticula. AJR Am J Roentgenol. 2009;193:807-12.

77. Holmes DR Jr, Monahan KH, Packer D. Pulmonary vein stenosis complicating ablation for atrial fibrillation: clinical spectrum and interventional considerations. JACC Cardiovasc Interv. 2009;2:267-76.

78. Wagner M, Butler C, Rief M, et al. Comparison of non-gated vs. electrocardiogram-gated 64-detector-row computed tomography for integrated electroanatomic mapping in patients undergoing pulmonary vein isolation. Europace. 2010;12:1090-7.

79. Martinez MW, Kirsch J, Williamson EE, et al. Utility of non-gated multidetector computed tomography for detection of left atrial thrombus in patients undergoing catheter ablation of atrial fibrillation. JACC Cardiovasc Imaging. 2009;2:69-76.

80. Wolak A, Gutstein A, Cheng VY, et al. Dual-source coronary computed tomography angiography in patients with atrial fibrillation: initial experience. J Cardiovasc Comput Tomogr. 2008;2:172-80.

81. Saremi F, Channual S, Gurudevan SV, et al. Prevalence of left atrial appendage pseudothrombus filling defects in patients with atrial fibrillation undergoing coronary computed tomography angiography. J Cardiovasc Comput Tomogr. 2008;2:164-71.

82. Hur J, Kim YJ, Lee HJ, et al. Left atrial appendage thrombi in stroke patients: detection with two-phase cardiac CT angiography versus transesophageal echocardiography. Radiology. 2009;251:683-90.

83. Tani T, Yamakami S, Matsushita T, et al. Usefulness of electron beam tomography in the prone position for detecting atrial thrombi in chronic atrial fibrillation. J Comput Assist Tomogr. 2003;27:78-84.

84. Van de Veire NR, Schuijf JD, De Sutter J, et al. Non-invasive visualization of the cardiac venous system in coronary artery disease patients using 64-slice computed tomography. J Am Coll Cardiol. 2006;48:1832-8.

85. Knackstedt C, Mühlenbruch G, Mischke K, et al. Registration of coronary venous anatomy to the site of the latest mechanical contraction. Acta Cardiol. 2010;65:161-70.

86. Van de Veire NR, Marsan NA, Schuijf JD, et al. Non-invasive imaging of cardiac venous anatomy with 64-slice multi-slice computed tomography and noninvasive assessment of left ventricular dyssynchrony by 3-dimensional tissue synchronization imaging in patients with heart failure scheduled for cardiac resynchronization therapy. Am J Cardiol. 2008;101:1023-9.

87. Al Fagih A, Al Najashi K, Dagriri K, et al. Feasibility of cardiac resynchronization therapy in a patient with complex congenital heart disease and dextrocardia, facilitated by cardiac computed tomography and coronary sinus venography. Hellenic J Cardiol. 2010;51:178-82.

88. Entrikin DW, Carr JJ. Blood pool inversion volume-rendering technique for visualization of the aortic valve. J Cardiovasc Comput Tomogr. 2008;2:366-71.

89. LaBounty TM, Glasofer S, Devereux RB, et al. Comparison of cardiac computed tomographic angiography to transesophageal echocardiography for evaluation of patients with native valvular heart disease. Am J Cardiol. 2009;104:1421-8.

90. Abdulla J, Sivertsen J, Kofoed KF, et al. Evaluation of aortic valve stenosis by cardiac multislice computed tomography compared with echocardiography: a systematic review and meta-analysis. J Heart Valve Dis. 2009;18:634-43.

91. Schultz CJ, Papadopoulou SL, Moelker A, et al. Transaortic flow velocity from dual-source MDCT for the diagnosis of aortic stenosis severity. Catheter Cardiovasc Interv. 2011;78:127-35.

92. Vahanian A, Himbert D, Brochet E. Transcatheter valve implantation for patients with aortic stenosis. Heart. 2010;96:1849-56.

93. Reiter SJ, Rumberger JA, Stanford W, et al. Quantitative determination of aortic regurgitant volumes in dogs by ultrafast computed tomography. Circulation. 1987;76:728-35.

94. Tsai WL, Tsai IC, Chen MC, et al. Comprehensive evaluation of patients with suspected prosthetic heart valve disorders using MDCT. AJR Am J Roentgenol. 2011;196:353-60.

95. Feuchtner GM, Stolzmann P, Dichtl W, et al. Multislice computed tomography in infective endocarditis: comparison with transesophageal echocardiography and intraoperative findings. J Am Coll Cardiol. 2009;53:436-44.

96. Verhaert D, Gabriel RS, Johnston D, et al. The role of multimodality imaging in the management of pericardial disease. Circ Cardiovasc Imaging. 2010;3:333-43.

97. Bull RK, Edwards PD, Dixon AK. CT dimensions of the normal pericardium. Br J Radiol. 1998;71:923-5.

98. Talreja DR, Edwards WD, Danielson GK, et al. Constrictive pericarditis in 26 patients with histologically normal pericardial thickness. Circulation. 2003;108:1852-7.

99. Maisch B, Seferovic PM, Ristic AD, et al. Guidelines on the diagnosis and management of pericardial diseases executive summary; The Task Force on the Diagnosis and Management of Pericardial Diseases of the European Society of Cardiology. Eur Heart J. 2004;25:587-610.

100. Lavis RA, Barrett JA, Kinsella DC, et al. Recurrent dysphagia after oesophagectomy caused by chylomediastinum. Interact Cardiovasc Thorac Surg. 2004;3:68-70.

101. Ossiani MH, McCauley RG, Patel HT. Primary idiopathic chylopericardium. Pediatr Radiol. 2003;33:357-9.

102. Rajiah P, Kanne JP. Computed tomography of the pericardium and pericardial disease. J Cardiovasc Comput Tomogr. 2010;4:3-18.

103. Rajiah P, Kanne JP, Kalahasti V, et al. Computed tomography of cardiac and pericardiac masses. J Cardiovasc Comput Tomogr. 2011;5:16-29.

104. Krauser DG, Cham MD, Tortolani AJ, et al. Clinical utility of delayed-contrast computed tomography for tissue characterization of cardiac thrombus. J Cardiovasc Comput Tomogr. 2007;1:114-8.

105. Schvartzman PR, White RD. Imaging of cardiac and paracardiac masses. J Thorac Imaging. 2000;15:265-73.

106. Hur J, Kim YJ, Lee HJ, et al. Left atrial appendage thrombi in stroke patients: detection with two-phase cardiac CT angiography versus transesophageal echocardiography. Radiology. 2009;251:683-90.

107. Jacobs PC, Mali WP, Grobbee DE, et al. Prevalence of incidental findings in computed tomographic screening of the chest: a systematic review. J Comput Assist Tomogr. 2008;32:214-21.

108. MacMahon H, Austin JH, Gamsu G, et al. Guidelines for management of small pulmonary nodules detected on CT scans: a statement from the Fleischner Society. Radiology. 2005;237:395-400.

109. Budoff MJ, Fischer H, Gopal A. Incidental findings with cardiac CT evaluation: should we read beyond the heart? Catheter Cardiovasc Interv. 2006;68:965-73.

110. The National Lung Screening Trial Research Team. Reduced lung-cancer mortality with low-dose computed tomographic screening. N Engl J Med. 2011 [Epub ahead of print].

111. Kim TJ, Han DH, Jin KN, et al. Lung cancer detected at cardiac CT: prevalence, clinicoradiologic features, and importance of full-field-of-view images. Radiology. 2010;255:369-76.

112. Johnson KM, Dennis JM, Dowe DA. Extracardiac findings on coronary CT angiograms: limited versus complete image review. AJR Am J Roentgenol. 2010;195:143-8.

Cardiovascular Magnetic Resonance

Robert M Weiss

Chapter Outline

INTRODUCTION

The history of magnetic resonance imaging (MRI) for characterization of cardiovascular morphology and function has been one of continuous innovation and refinement for over 25 years. Advancements in device design, image acquisition methodology and image analysis are rapidly translated into standardized methods for broad application in clinical cardiovascular medicine and cardiovascular research.

The fundamental principles of MRI are described in exquisite detail elsewhere.[1] The purpose of this chapter is to acquaint clinicians and clinical researchers with the ways that cardiovascular magnetic resonance (CMR) can solve problems in cardiovascular medicine.

INFORMATION PROVIDED BY CARDIOVASCULAR MAGNETIC RESONANCE

Morphology, kinematics and tissue characterization together form the crux of cardiovascular assessment with CMR. Assessments of left and right ventricular volumes and mass are highly reproducible and, when indexed for body habitus, are able to report relatively narrow reference ranges[2-4] (Table 1). It is important to note, however, that reference ranges depend somewhat upon the specific CMR image acquisition method,[5] and vary by sex and ethnic lineage.[4]

TABLE 1

Normal values for CMR using true-FISP acquisition

	Males*	Females*
LVEDV (ml)	168.5 ± 33.4	134.9 ± 19.3
LVESV (ml)	60.8 ± 16.0	48.9 ± 10.7
LVSV (ml)	107.7 ± 20.7	86.0 ± 12.3
LVEF (%)	64.2 ± 4.6	64.0 ± 4.9
LV Mass (g)	133.2 ± 23.9	90.2 ± 12.0
LV EDV/BSA (ml/m²)	82.3 ± 14.7	77.7 ± 10.8
LV Mass/BSA (g/m²)	64.7 ± 9.3	52.0 ± 7.4
LV EDV/HT (ml/m)	95.0 ± 17.3	82.6 ± 10.9
LV Mass/HT (g/m)	75.1 ± 12.3	55.3 ± 7.0
RVEDV (ml)	176.5 ± 33.0	130.6 ± 23.7
RVESV (ml)	79.3 ± 16.2	52.3 ± 9.9
RVSV (ml)	97.8 ± 18.7	78.3 ± 16.9
RVEF (%)	55.1 ± 3.7	59.8 ± 5.0
RV EDV/BSA (ml/m²)	86.2 ± 14.1	75.2 ± 13.8
RV EDV/HT (ml/m)	99.5 ± 16.9	80.0 ± 14.2

*mean ± SD
(Abbreviations: LV: Left ventricle; RV: Right ventricle; EDV: End-diastolic volume; ESV: End-systolic volume; SV: Stroke volume; EF: Ejection fraction; BSA: Body surface area; HT: Height; true-FISP: True fast imaging with steady-state precession). (*Source:* Alfakih, Plein S, Thiele H, et al. Normal human left and right ventricular dimensions for MRI as assessed by turbo gradient echo and steady-state free precession imaging sequences. J Magn Reson Imaging. 2003;17:329-9, with permission)

The superior quantitative accuracy of CMR characterization of ventricular anatomy and function does not depend on any assumptions regarding chamber geometry, a distinct advantage over purely planar techniques. The CMR has emerged as a reference standard against which the accuracy of newer applications using conventional methods (e.g. 3-dimensional echocardiography) can be compared.[6] The high reproducibility and narrow reference ranges of CMR ventriculographic data have been utilized in clinical trials for about 20 years.[7] The CMR offers increased statistical power and drastically reduces the necessary sample size in clinical trials, compared to echocardiography.[8] A search of a public database using the terms "heart and magnetic resonance" returns 436 ongoing or recently completed clinical trials.[9]

DIAGNOSIS OF EPICARDIAL CORONARY ARTERY STENOSIS

Myocardial infarction caused by flow limitation in epicardial coronary arteries [coronary artery stenosis (CAS)] is responsible for about one-sixth of all deaths in the United States.[10] Since myocardial infarction and sudden cardiac death (SCD) are often not preceded by intractable symptoms, a diagnostic armamentarium has been developed for the purpose of detecting disease in the epicardial coronary arteries. The CMR techniques for CAS detection, by and large, recapitulate established approaches using other techniques: functional evaluation at rest and during inotropic stress; perfusion assessment during vasodilator stress and coronary angiography.

ASSESSMENT OF GLOBAL AND REGIONAL LEFT VENTRICULAR FUNCTION AT REST AND DURING INOTROPIC STRESS

Ischemia is detected when the increased myocardial oxygen demand induced by inotrope infusion exceeds its supply, resulting in a wall motion abnormality (Figs 1A and B). In the twenty years following a small demonstration-of-principle study,[11] assessment of global and regional left ventricular systolic function during stepped infusion of the inotrope dobutamine has emerged as the CMR method most widely employed for detection of CAS. Subsequent series, involving thousands of patients, consistently report diagnostic performance and safety record that compares favorably to other noninvasive methods for detection of CAS.[12,13] Optimal diagnostic sensitivity is achieved when heart rate is raised to greater than or equal to 85% of predicted maximum, which often requires coadministration of the muscarinic blocker atropine.

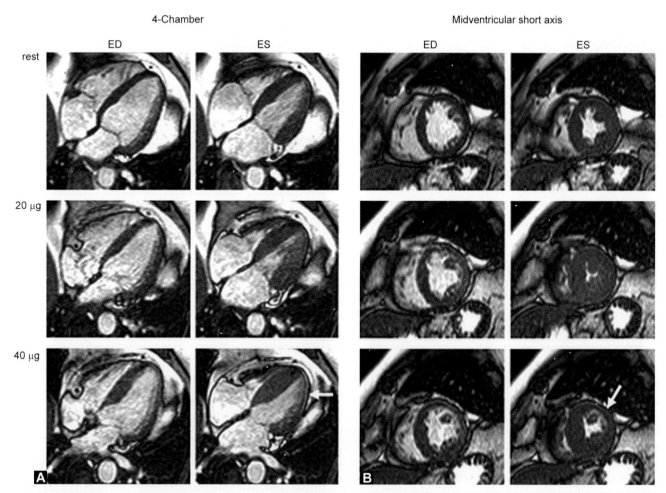

FIGURES 1A AND B: End-diastolic (ED) and End-systolic (ES) SSFP images at rest and during stepped infusion of dobutamine in an individual with flow-limiting stenosis of the left circumflex coronary artery. During high-dose infusion (40 µg/kg/min), a wall motion abnormality appears in the mid- and apical lateral wall (arrows) (*Source:* Wahl A, Paetsch I, Gollesch A, et al. Safety and feasibility of high-dose dobutamine-atropine stress cardiovascular magnetic resonance for diagnosis of myocardial ischemia: Experience in 1000 consecutive cases. Eur Heart J 2004;25:1230-6, with permission)

At centers with significant expertise, CMR can be particularly useful for stress studies in patients with suboptimal acoustic access for echocardiography.[14] Unsuitability for an echocardiographic stress study can be ascertained at rest—avoiding the need to subject a patient to the repetitive risks and discomfort of inotropic stress. Use of echocardiography for assessment of the presence of residual CAS in patients with resting wall motion abnormalities is challenging. In that setting CMR can provide higher diagnostic yield for CAS.[15] The diagnostic accuracy of stress CMR can be incrementally improved when myocardial tagging is employed.[16] The incremental prognostic power of stress CMR has been established. Subjects who complete an inotropic stress protocol without CMR evidence of inducible ischemia have an excellent prognosis, whereas subjects with inducible ischemia are at greater risk of major adverse cardiac events.[17]

Since the intent of inotropic stress is to provoke and recognize myocardial ischemia, personnel and equipment must be available to manage its consequences, including myocardial infarction, malignant arrhythmia and shock.[18] Identification and treatment of complications can be more challenging in a CMR environment than in others, due to restricted patient contact. Recognition of ischemia requires frequent sampling and prompt assessment of left ventricular wall motion. Convenient access to emergency drugs and resuscitation equipment by experienced personnel is critically important in the CMR setting.[13]

MYOCARDIAL PERFUSION IMAGING

Adenosinergic drugs cause vasodilation in coronary resistance vessels. In the presence of flow-limiting epicardial coronary stenosis, resistance arteries will be at least partially dilated at rest, in order to maintain normal myocardial perfusion. During vasodilator stress, then, the incremental increase in tissue perfusion will be diminished in regions subserved by a stenotic epicardial vessel, compared to regions subserved by nonstenotic epicardial vessels, forming the basis for recognition of CAS.

In experienced centers, adequate diagnostic accuracy for CAS has been achieved using CMR to assess regional myocardial perfusion and perfusion reserve, during adenosine infusion.[19,20] A comprehensive CMR evaluation which includes perfusion assessment during adenosine stress provides incremental prognostic information, over and above consideration of routine clinical variables.[21]

As with inotrope stress, vasodilator stress can result in intractable ischemia, malignant arrhythmia and shock. Thus, similar precautions for recognition and management apply.[18] In addition, there is concern that recognition of ischemia during vasodilator stress may require computation of regional myocardial perfusion, which could delay remedial measures to a greater degree than visual recognition of ischemic wall motion abnormalities during inotrope stress.

CARDIOVASCULAR MAGNETIC RESONANCE CORONARY ANGIOGRAPHY

The CMR is useful to identify the origin and proximal course of the coronary arteries for the purpose of confirming or rejecting the presence of anomalies[22,23] (Figs 2A and B). The CMR has been employed to identify the presence of coronary

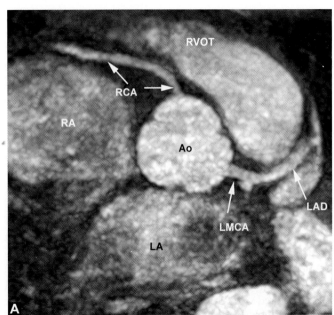

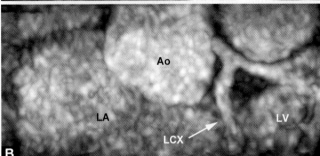

FIGURES 2A AND B: Free-breathing True-FISP 3-D coronary angiogram from a young man with chest pain, dyspnea, abnormal ECG, and elevated serum cardiac troponin-T. The origins and courses of the proximal coronary arteries are normal, effectively ruling out coronary anomaly as the etiology of the patient's clinical findings (Abbreviations: Ao: Aorta; RA: Right atrium; LA: Left atrium; RVOT: Right ventricular outflow tract; LV: Left ventricle; LMCA: Left main coronary artery; LAD: Left anterior descending coronary artery; LCX: Left circumflex coronary artery; RCA: Right coronary artery) (*Source:* Alan H. Stolpen, MD, PhD, Department of Radiology, University of Iowa Carver College of Medicine)

aneurysms in patients with Kawasaki disease.[24,25] Coronary artery bypass graft patency can be ascertained with high diagnostic accuracy.[26]

Detection of stenoses in native coronary arteries generally requires specialized 3-D methods.[23,27] Discrimination between clinically significant gradations in the severity of stenoses can be problematic, possibly rendering CMR coronary angiography more of a "screening tool", identifying patients who may benefit from evaluation of the physiological significance of identified lesions. However, in some highly specialized centers, CMR coronary angiography attains diagnostic yield comparable to other noninvasive methods for detecting CAS.[28]

UNRECOGNIZED MYOCARDIAL INFARCTION

At least 20% of incident myocardial infarctions occur in the absence of recognizable symptoms.[10] The condition often comes to a clinician's attention by virtue the appearance of pathological Q-waves on an elective electrocardiogram. More recently, it has become clear that a significant number of prior silent infarctions do not produce such findings and are only detected by characteristic findings on CMR-late gadolinium enhancement (LGE) with subendocardial predominance, in a typical distribution of a major coronary artery branch. That finding contributes significantly to the overall diagnostic sensitivity of CMR for detection of CAS.[29] Furthermore, the finding is a powerful independent predictor of future major adverse cardiac events, even in patients with known CAD.[30,31]

DILATED CARDIOMYOPATHY

Despite advances in prevention and treatment, the prevalence and impact of heart failure are increasing in Western Societies.[10] Dilated cardiomyopathy (DCM) is the most common cause of heart failure, and the most frequent reason for referral for heart transplantation or mechanical cardiac assist device implantation.[32,33]

Although management strategies for patients with DCM have matured over the past decade, clinicians continue to be presented with significant challenges for the management of individual patients.[34] Applications of established CMR methods can be useful in decision-making in selected patients with DCM.

ETIOLOGY

The DCM can arise from diverse processes—genetic or environmental—and can be a presenting feature of systemic diseases such as atherosclerosis, hypertension or endocrine imbalance. The CMR is useful for directing therapy designed to treat the underlying cause of DCM in a number of instances where generic treatment of "heart failure" would be expected to yield a suboptimal outcome.

Coronary Artery Stenoses

In patients presenting with systolic heart failure due to DCM, it is incumbent upon the clinician to ascertain the presence or absence of flow-limiting coronary artery stenoses (CAS). As noted above, CMR can be useful for identifying patients with DCM due to CAS. Equally important, CMR confers the ability to precisely define the extent and severity of ischemic myocardial fibrosis in patients with DCM.[35,36]

Several decades ago, a landmark clinical trial reported that patients with DCM and symptomatic stenoses of the three major epicardial coronary branches, and those with flow-limiting stenosis of the left main coronary artery, fared better with revascularization than with medical therapy alone.[37] More recently, this longstanding paradigm has been refined so as to suggest that the benefits of revascularization are most likely for patients who demonstrate a limited extent of ischemic scar in regions with systolic dysfunction (viable myocardium). The unique ability of CMR to depict the transmural extent of ischemic scar allows accurate prediction of functional recovery after successful revascularization,[38-40] and directly influences prognosis in patients with ischemic DCM.[41,42] Some experts advise consideration of performing assessment of myocardial viability in patients with heart failure, with an eye toward revascularization, even when angina pectoris is not present.[43] The surgical treatment for ischemic heart failure (STICH) study is a multicenter clinical trial designed to determine whether the potential benefit of surgical revascularization in patients with DCM and CAS is dependent on the presence of viable myocardium.[44] Early results indicate that echocardiographic or scintigraphic confirmation of myocardial viability did not forecast improved outcome in patients who underwent surgical revascularization for CAS with DCM, compared to patients without viable myocardium. At this time it is not known whether the superior quantitative precision of CMR for identification of ischemic scar would result in improved identification of patients who would derive the most benefit from surgical revascularization for ischemic DCM.

Myocarditis

The actual incidence of myocarditis is not known. The clinical manifestations of the disease can be nonspecific—fever, myalgias, exercise intolerance—and its course is usually mild and self-limited. However, patients with fulminant disease, and those with chronic indolent myocarditis, can present with incident heart failure, and require special attention.

Patients with incident heart failure due to fulminant myocarditis require admission to the hospital, continuous ECG-monitoring and aggressive supportive care. Although early mortality is relatively high (~ 10%), those surviving to hospital discharge have an excellent prognosis[45] findings which emphasize the importance of early diagnosis. Patients with giant cell myocarditis often develop fulminant progression of disease with very poor prognosis, if untreated.[46] The CMR can facilitate diagnosis of giant cell myocarditis by identifying sentinel features of inflammation—edema and expansion of the extracellular space (Figs 3A and B).

Indolent myocarditis is characterized by subacute or chronic cardiac dysfunction and poor long-term prognosis.[45] No broadly applied treatment regimen has demonstrated efficacy for the treatment of all patients with indolent myocarditis.[48] However, emerging evidence suggests that confirmation of the diagnosis of myocarditis and subsequent etiology-specific treatment can favorably influence the prognosis for some patients.

In a nonrandomized prospective study of patients with chronic lymphocytic myocarditis, those for whom infectious etiologies were identified fared worse with immunosuppressive therapy than those for whom infectious etiologies were excluded.[49] A subsequent randomized study in patients with non-viral lymphocytic myocarditis demonstrated improved left ventricular systolic function in patients treated with an immunosuppression regimen, compared to patients who received placebo.[50]

The diagnosis of myocarditis itself can be problematic. Electrocardiographic and echocardiographic findings may be nonspecific or absent, and blood enzymology is not sufficiently sensitive.[51] Referral for endomyocardial biopsy requires a very high level of clinical suspicion, and that procedure can be subject to low diagnostic yield, presumably due to the patchy nature of the disease in many cases.[52]

In addition to providing quantitatively precise assessment of global and regional ventricular function, CMR findings point to a diagnosis of myocarditis by virtue of visualizing expansion of the myocardial extravascular space, reflecting edema, inflammation or fibrosis. T2-weighted (black blood) imaging

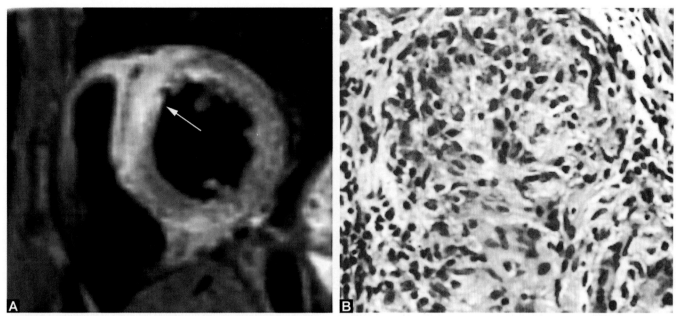

FIGURES 3A AND B: Giant cell myocarditis. (A) Short-axis double inversion-recovery image from a young man with acute heart failure. Bright signal in the anterior interventricular septum indicates myocardial edema (arrow). (B) Hematoxyllin and eosin stain of endomyocardial biopsy specimen shows abundant inflammation and several multi-nucleated giant cells (*Source:* Berry CJ, Johnson FL, Cabuay BM, et al. Evanescent asymmetrical septal hypertrophy and rapidly progressive heart failure in a 32-year-old man. Circulation. 2008;118:e126-8, with permission)

produces increased signal intensity in regions with unrestrained extravascular water (Figs 3A and B). Exclusion of other causes of myocardial edema—ischemic injury, trauma, toxin exposure—guides the clinician toward a diagnosis of myocarditis. The CMR techniques which utilize LGE also produce increased signal intensity in regions with expansion of the extracellular extravascular space (Figs 4A and B), and are preferred in some settings, due to greater signal-to-noise ratio than T2-weighted imaging.

The CMR is emerging as the diagnostic procedure of choice for identification of myocarditis in patients presenting with incident left ventricular dysfunction. In relatively small series, CMR has demonstrated very high sensitivity and specificity for

detection of myocardial inflammation.[53,54] The CMR localization of myocardial inflammation has been found to improve the diagnostic yield of endomyocardial biopsy in some,[55] but not all,[56] studies.

PROGNOSIS

Ischemic Dilated Cardiomyopathy

In patients with DCM due to CAS, the extent of irreversibly injured myocardium (scar) varies widely (Figs 5A and B). Prognosis is directly related to the extent of ischemic scar, independent of the severity of left ventricular systolic dysfunction, or the decision to undergo revascularization.[57,58]

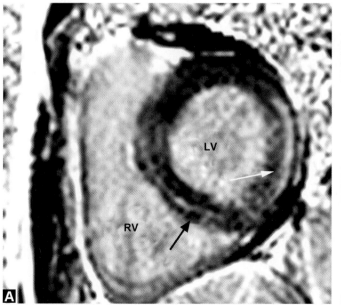
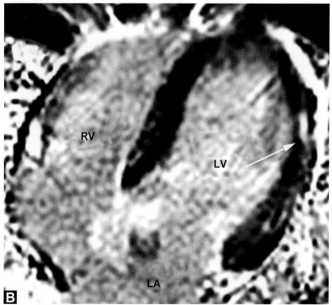

FIGURES 4A AND B: Indolent myocarditis. A young male presented with chest pain, abnormal ECG and troponinemia one week following a viral prodrome. (A) Short-axis and (B) Four-chamber phase-sensitive inversion recovery images acquired 10 minutes following administration of Gd-DTPA. Dense LGE with epicardial predominance appears in the lateral LV wall, with streaky midmyocardial LGE in the septum (arrows)

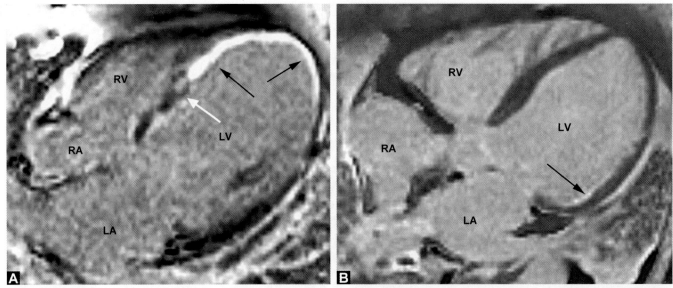

FIGURES 5A AND B: Four-chamber phase-sensitive inversion recovery images 10 minutes after administration of Gd-DTPA from two patients, each with 3-vessel CAS, LV dilation and LVEF < 0.30. (A) In Patient A there is transmural infarction (black arrows) in the septum and apex, including microvascular obstruction in the basal septum (white arrow). The findings forecast little benefit of revascularization in those regions. (B) In Patient B there is only subendocardial infarction in the basal lateral wall (black arrow), indicating a high likelihood of functional improvement following successful revascularization

Patients with ischemic DCM and extensive ischemic scar are more likely to incur ventricular tachycardia during programmed electrical stimulation, than patients with little or no LGE.[59] Preliminary studies indicate that the extent of LGE in patients with ischemic DCM may have independent utility for identifying patients at risk of SCD. A study designed to determine whether CMR assessment of scar burden is an appropriate indication for implantation of a cardioverter-defibrillator is in progress.[60]

Prognosis in Idiopathic Dilated Cardiomyopathy

In patients with DCM that is not associated with CAS, CMR provides powerful prognostic information. Morphology and systolic function of the right ventricle (RV) are not optimally characterized by planar techniques, but exert a strong influence on prognosis in patients with DCM.[61] The superior quantitation of right ventricular abnormalities of CMR thus provides improved prognostic power, compared to conventional methods.

Although idiopathic DCM was previously thought to invariably entail abundant myocardial fibrosis, recent evidence indicates substantial variability in the degree of fibrosis among patients with DCM—an attribute linked to prognosis and the likelihood of therapeutic response to therapeutic intervention.[62] Myocardial fibrosis in idiopathic DCM is often visualized as midmyocardial LGE (Figs 6A and B). The CMR depiction of LGE, representing myocardial fibrosis, is associated with increased risk of death or hospitalization in patients with DCM, compared to patients with DCM without LGE, and the association is more pronounced in patients with abundant scar.[63]

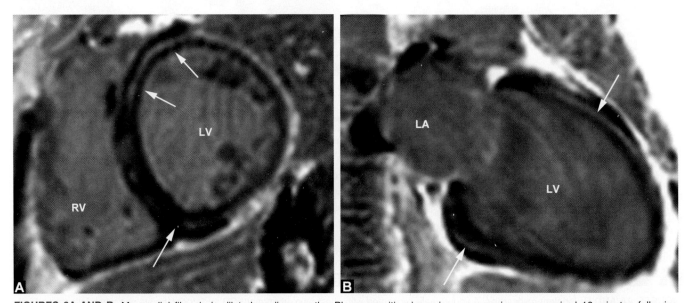

FIGURES 6A AND B: Myocardial fibrosis in dilated cardiomyopathy. Phase-sensitive inversion recovery images acquired 10 minutes following administration of Gd-DTPA in a 31-year-old man with idiopathic DCM. (A) Short-axis, and (B) Two-chamber long-axis views demonstrate midmyocardial LGE in the anterior and inferior LV walls (arrows)

In patients with systolic heart failure due to non-ischemic DCM, SCD or appropriate intervention by an implantable cardiac defibrillator (ICD) are fourfold more likely in patients with LGE than in patients without LGE.[64]

Although these studies in patients with DCM strongly support the prognostic power of CMR in patients with DCM, the role of CMR in clinical decision-making, e.g. whether or not to refer an individual patient for ICD placement, has not been definitively determined.

HYPERTROPHIC CARDIOMYOPATHY

Hypertrophic cardiomyopathy (HCM) is a leading cause of sudden death in young people and in competitive athletes.[65] The disease is usually characterized by morphologic left ventricular hypertrophy (LVH) in the absence of pressure-overload or volume-overload or systemic conditions associated with cardiac hypertrophy. Genetic testing reveals cardiac sarcomere-related mutations in about 50% of cases.[66,67] Cellular hypertrophy with myocyte disarray and increased interstitial collagen are histo-pathologic hallmarks of the disease.[68] Clinical manifestations include diastolic heart failure, arrhythmic and neurogenic syncope and SCD.[69] The diagnosis is most often suspected based on clinical and family history, physical examination and electro-cardiography, and is most often confirmed by echocardiography. Since sudden death commonly occurs in the absence of intractable symptoms, risk stratification algorithms have been proposed and are in continuous evolution.

DIAGNOSIS

The CMR can offer higher diagnostic sensitivity for HCM than echocardiography. This is more often the case when the left ventricular region of hypertrophy occurs in a location other than the basal interventricular septum,[70] or when visualization of the heart with echocardiography is suboptimal.[71] Echo-cardiographic visualization of the left ventricular apex with sufficient clarity to ascertain wall thickness can be problematic in some patients with suboptimal acoustic windows. The CMR can provide diagnostic certainty in such cases, where the clinical suspicion of apical HCM is high.[72] In some cases, CMR can be useful to definitively discriminate between apical HCM and left ventricular noncompaction (LVNC) (Figs 7A and B). In patients with HCM, there is frequently involvement of the RV,[73] a finding of uncertain clinical significance.

The clinical course of carriers of HCM-associated gene mutations who do not manifest morphologic HCM can be unclear. Strijack et al. report a case of a gene-positive carrier with a family history of sudden death, with multiple morpho-logy-positive first-degree relatives, whose echocardiogram showed normal wall thickness and left ventricular mass.[74] On CMR examination, the individual demonstrated abundant LGE, indicating ongoing disease in the absence of morphologic LVH (Figs 8A and B). However, in a later series, CMR was found to be nondiagnostic in gene-positive morphology-negative patients who demonstrated biochemical evidence of myocardial collagen turnover.[75]

PROGNOSIS

Established risk factors for SCD in patients with HCM include: prior arrhythmic cardiac arrest, spontaneous sustained or nonsustained ventricular tachycardia, family history of unexplained SCD, regional diastolic left ventricular wall thickness greater than 3 cm and abnormal blood pressure response to exercise. The presence of multiple SCD risk factors is associated with incremental risk.[76]

The CMR can be helpful in elucidating the risk profile in individual patients. In addition to higher diagnostic sensitivity for the disease itself, Rickers et al. reported that CMR identified patients with wall thickness greater than 3 cm in 10% of cases where echocardiography did not.[70] In patients

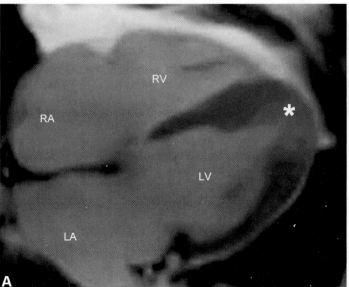
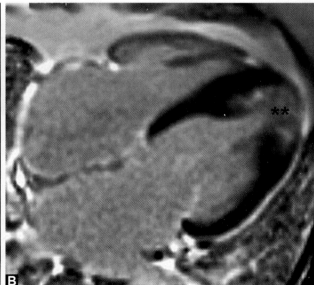

FIGURES 7A AND B: Apical HCM. A 57-year-old man complained of chest pain and dyspnea on exertion. Coronary angiography revealed no CAS. Echocardiography raised the question of apical HCM vs LVNC. (A) Four-chamber true-FISP image at end-diastole reveals grossly thickened apical myocardium (*). (B) Phase-sensitive inversion recovery image acquired 10 minutes after administration of Gd-DTPA reveals abundant LGE in apical myocardium (**). Endomyocardial biopsy from the LV apex revealed myocyte hypertrophy and disarray with profound interstitial fibrosis, in the absence of inflammation or infiltration—confirming the diagnosis of apical HCM

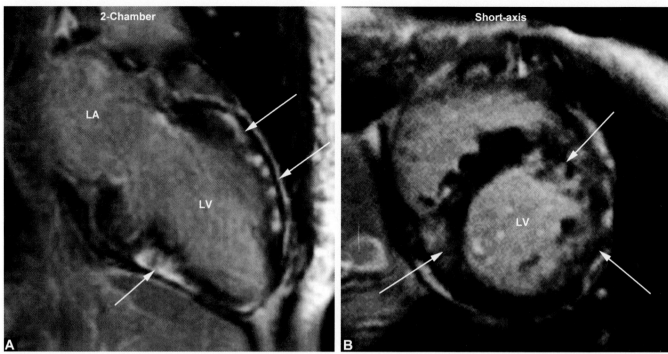

FIGURES 8A AND B: Inversion recovery images late after administration of Gd-DTPA from a patient who is gene-positive, but morphology negative for HCM. Arrows indicate abundant LGE within LV myocardium (arrows) [Images reprinted with permission from the Society of Cardiovascular Magnetic Resonance (Strijack, et al[73])]

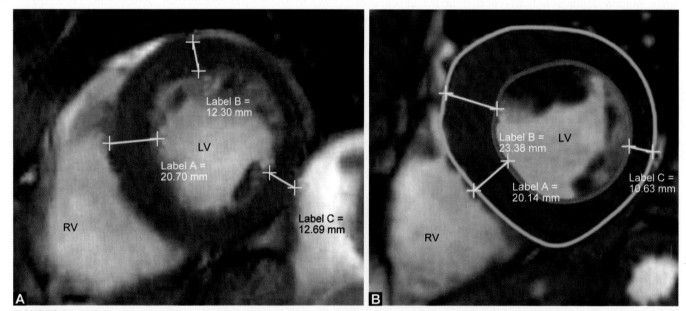

FIGURES 9A AND B: Differing extent of regional left ventricular hypertrophy in two patients with HCM. Mid-septal wall thicknesses are similar in both patients, ~ 20–21 mm. However, profound hypertrophy extends into the anterolateral LV wall in Patient B, a finding occasionally not appreciated on echocardiography.[70] In addition, LV mass index is > 4 SD above the normal mean, a finding which has been linked to worse prognosis[77]

with HCM, CMR-derived total left ventricular mass demonstrates greater than twofold greater sensitivity for prediction of SCD, compared to echo-derived maximum wall thickness, and there is a relatively weak correlation between the two parameters[77] (Figs 9A and B).

The presence and extent of LGE varies widely among patients with HCM (Figs 10A and B). The presence of LGE is associated with the occurrence of malignant arrhythmias.[78] The extent of myocardial LGE is positively correlated with the

likelihood of a composite "adverse outcome" (heart failure progression or SCD).[79-82]

CORRELATIVE FINDINGS

The CMR provides dynamic evidence of left ventricular outflow obstruction (Figs 11A and B), which may be useful for planning ablative or surgical procedures, and can provide follow-up confirmation of the efficacy of the procedure.[83] Mitral valve regurgitation frequently complicates the course of patients with

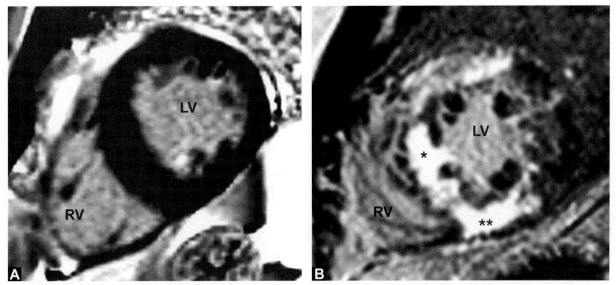

FIGURES 10A AND B: Late gadolinium enhancement in HCM. Phase-sensitive inversion recovery imaging 10 minutes after administration of Gd-DTPA. Two patients with similar magnitude of septal hypertrophy. In Patient A, no myocardial LGE is detected, while in Patient B, there is extensive LGE in the septum (*) and posterior wall (**)

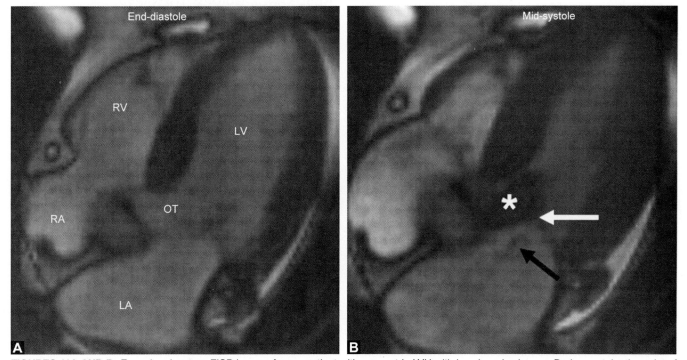

FIGURES 11A AND B: Four-chamber true-FISP images from a patient with concentric LVH with basal predominance. During systole, the point of mitral leaflet coaptation is drawn toward the septum (white arrow). Flow acceleration in the outflow tract (OT) results in dephasing of the blood signal (*), and a trace of mitral regurgitation occurs (black arrow)

HCM, and can be quantitated using CMR, thus assisting in the decision to refer for mitral valve replacement or repair (Figs 12A and B).

HCM is associated with functional abnormalities of the microcirculation, which may correlate with its clinical course.[84,85] Abnormalities of myocardial energetics can be ascertained in patients with HCM, and often precede onset of symptoms.[86]

RESTRICTIVE CARDIOMYOPATHY

Restrictive cardiomyopathy (RCM) comprises a diverse set of conditions which often entail a long period of clinical latency, followed by progressive cardiac dysfunction and death due to refractory heart failure or SCD. Symptoms consist of pulmonary and systemic venous congestion and inability to raise cardiac output during exertion, all of which can be ascribed to decreased compliance of one or both ventricles.

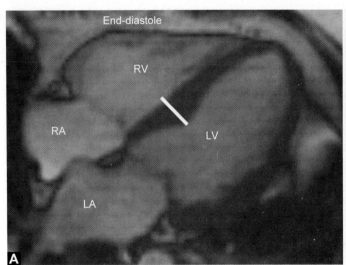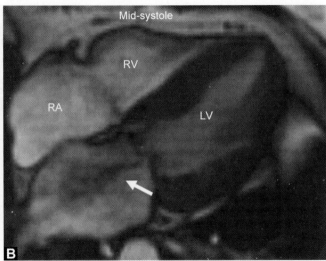

FIGURES 12A AND B: Four-chamber true-FISP images from a young woman with focal septal hypertrophy (white bar = 1.7 cm). During systole there is mitral regurgitation demonstrated by dephasing of the blood signal (arrow)

DIAGNOSIS

Symptoms, signs and hemodynamic findings of restrictive cardiomyopathies often mimic those which occur with constrictive pericarditis.[87] The CMR can be useful for discriminating between the two conditions. Constrictive pericarditis is readily identified using methods described below. In a patient with a clinical diagnosis of heart failure, CMR provides quantitative corroboration of the salient features of restrictive cardiomyopathy early in the course of disease—normal or decreased left ventricular end-diastolic volume, normal or increased left ventricular mass, preserved or only mildly decreased left ventricular ejection fraction.

ETIOLOGY

Although disease-specific treatment is not available for many patients with RCM, effective treatments have been developed for some disease etiologies—forming a justification for a rigorous diagnostic strategy. In addition to morphologic and functional data, CMR can identify expansion of the extracellular space—a common finding in restrictive cardiomyopathy caused by amyloidosis,[88] Fabry's disease,[89] sarcoidosis[90] and hypereosinophilic syndromes.[91] The CMR methods for RCM assessment resemble those for detection of myocarditis (which can also manifest as restrictive cardiomyopathy). Double inversion-recovery ("black blood") techniques identify myocardial edema. Phase-sensitive inversion-recovery (PSIR) imaging is used to depict LGE, in a manner similar to methods employed to detect myocardial infarction (Figs 13A to F).

Iron overload states represent a special case for the diagnosis of restrictive cardiomyopathy. Clinically important levels of iron deposited in myocardium can sufficiently alter the local CMR signal so as to be diagnostic. Special techniques have been developed which compare T2*-weighted signal intensity to routine T2*-weighted signal. When tissue iron is abundant, local effects serve to diminish T2 intensity, rendering myocardium darker in areas of infiltration.[92]

CARDIOVASCULAR MAGNETIC RESONANCE-GUIDED THERAPY

In some cases, e.g. hypereosinophilia, therapeutic decisions are guided by routine clinical assessments and laboratory testing. In other cases, longitudinal CMR studies can help optimize management of chronic conditions responsible for restrictive cardiomyopathy.

Immunosuppressive therapy for sarcoidosis may result in sustained disease quiescence or, in some cases, may convert active granulomatous inflammation to interstitial fibrosis—a process which could hypothetically increase or decrease susceptibility to malignant arrhythmia. For that reason, Mehta et al. have proposed a stepped diagnostic regimen which utilizes CMR to triage patients for invasive electrophysiologic studies.[93] The algorithm demonstrated high predictive power for identifying patients who subsequently received appropriate ICD shocks.

Plasma cell dyscrasias can cause restrictive cardiomyopathy via deposition of immunoglobulin components in myocardium—a form of amyloidosis. Available treatments entail a significant risk of systemic and cardiac toxicity. The CMR can identify the extent of cardiac amyloidosis in such patients, along with critical cardiac function data, which guide therapy. Tissue iron overload is a frequent complication of chronic anemias that require periodic transfusion, and is the most common cause of death in thalassemia major.[94] The CMR is useful for identification of patients at risk of heart failure due to iron overload, and longitudinal CMR studies are useful to determine efficacy of chelation therapy.[95]

VALVULAR HEART DISEASE

Echocardiography, via transthoracic or transesophageal approaches, is most often the procedure of choice for assessment of the morphology of the cardiac valves. The CMR studies usually require compilation of image data over multiple cardiac cycles, in order to achieve sufficient signal-to-noise ratios—a

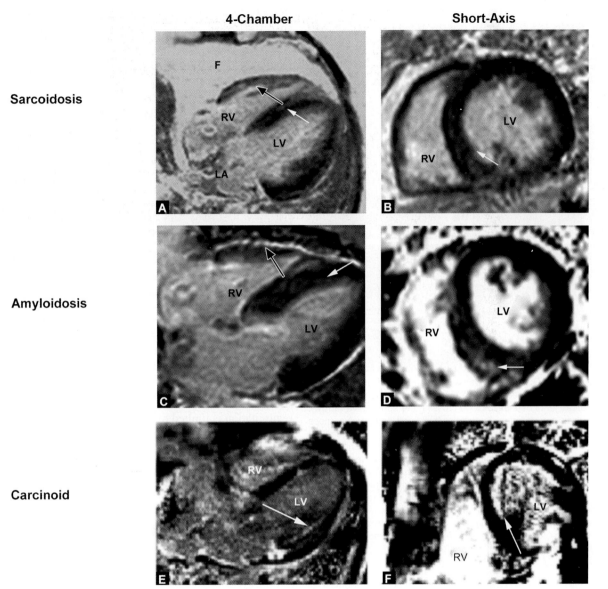

4-Chamber

Short-Axis

Sarcoidosis

Amyloidosis

Carcinoid

FIGURES 13A TO F: Restrictive cardiomyopathy. Phase-sensitive inversion recovery images in four-chamber view (left) and short-axis (right) planes 10 minutes after administration of Gd-DTPA. (A and B) sarcoidosis, (C and D) amyloidosis, (E and F) carcinoid tumor. There is late gadolinium enhancement in left ventricular myocardium (white arrows) and in the right ventricular free wall (dark arrow). Abundant epicardial fat (F) is present in the patient with sarcoidosis, a common finding in patients receiving long-term corticosteroid therapy

requirement not ideally suited to visualization of thin structures exhibiting complex motion during the cardiac cycle. "real-time" CMR techniques have been applied, but do not generally offer improved valve visualization compared to best-quality echocardiographic images.

The CMR can be useful for assessment of valve morphology and function when echocardiographic images are suboptimal, but is more often utilized to characterize the impact of valve disease upon cardiac chamber morphology and function. In patients with mitral or aortic regurgitation, left ventricular size and systolic function are key determinants of the timing of valve surgery.[96] In cases where the left ventricle (LV) demonstrates pathological remodeling and/or impaired systolic function, the contribution of valve regurgitation to those processes can be quantitatively ascertained using CMR methods[97] (See below). In cases where there is regurgitation of multiple valves, complementary CMR techniques can be employed to discern the relative contributions of the individual valve lesions.

VALVE STENOSIS

The CMR assessment of valve stenosis is preliminarily approached by visualization of valve leaflet motion during the cardiac cycle, best accomplished using multiple planes. Limitation of leaflet excursion and high velocity blood dephasing, identify a stenotic valve[98] (Figs 14A to D). More advanced methods have been introduced, which utilize velocity encoding in a manner similar to established Doppler echocardiography methods, in order to estimate transvalvular gradients.[99] In general, these CMR methods do not yield greater accuracy for assessment of stenosis severity than Doppler techniques, except in cases where echocardiography is technically suboptimal.

VALVULAR REGURGITATION

Regurgitant flow across a cardiac valve causes turbulent dephasing in "white blood" CMR images, facilitating qualitative or semi-quantitative assessment of the magnitude of back

Diastole | Systole

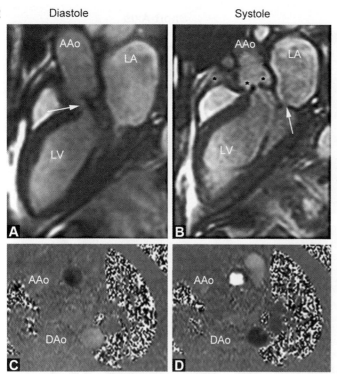

FIGURES 14A TO D: Complex Valve Disease: (A and B) True-FISP images from a middle-aged man with dyspnea on exertion. In diastole, there is a broad jet of dephased blood crossing the aortic valve (arrow), indicating aortic regurgitation. In systole, thickened aortic valve cusps with restricted excursion are evident (*). There is also a small regurgitant jet across the mitral valve (arrow). (C and D) Velocity encoding, where cephalad flow is depicted in white and caudal flow is depicted in black. Antegrade flow in the ascending aorta (AAo) was 116 ml/cycle, and retrograde AAo flow was 46 ml, yielding a regurgitant fraction of 40%. Confirmation of the hemodynamic significance of aortic regurgitation is supported by observation of faint cephalad (retrograde) flow in the descending aorta (DAo) during diastole. Subsequent comparison of net ventriculographic stroke volumes from the LV (70 ml) and from the RV (63 ml) yielded a mitral regurgitant fraction of 10%

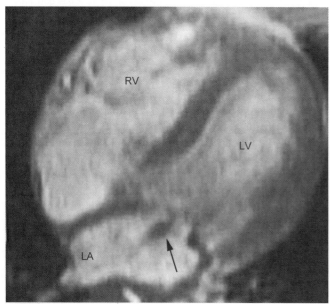

FIGURE 15: Four-chamber cine-FLASH image in mid-systole from a patient with DCM. Dephasing of blood crossing the mitral valve (arrow) indicates mild mitral regurgitation

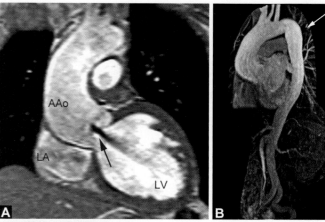

FIGURES 16A AND B: (A) Coronal oblique true-FISP image during mid-diastole from a patient with ascending aortic (AAo) aneurysm. Dephasing of blood crossing the aortic valve indicates moderate-severe aortic valve regurgitation (black arrow). In this patient with univalvular regurgitation, stroke volume analysis revealed a regurgitant volume of 96 ml, and a regurgitant fraction of 52%. (B) Gadolinium enhanced aortagram, after 3-D rendering, reveals extent of aortic dilation, including the proximal descending thoracic aorta (white arrow) (*Source:* Alan H. Stolpen, MD, PhD, Department of Radiology, University of Iowa Carver College of Medicine)

flow[100] (Figs 14 to 16). In cases where clinically significant regurgitation is limited to one valve and no shunts are present, quantitation of regurgitant volume is most readily achieved by comparing left and right ventricular stroke volumes (Figs 16A and B).

Velocity mapping studies in the proximal pulmonary artery and in the aortic root can be used to produce measurements of net forward stroke volume for each ventricle. The findings can be used to corroborate findings in cases of univalvular regurgitation. When multivalvular regurgitation is present, velocity mapping can be used in combination with ventriculographic data to parse regurgitant flow measurements among the individual valves (Figs 14A to D).

Integration of CMR into decision-making paradigms for patients with valvular heart disease depends largely upon local expertise and practice patterns. Consensus about its utility arises when echocardiographic evaluation is technically suboptimal or inconclusive.[101] The CMR can provide clinically useful additions to more conventional assessments in patients with valve disease that is associated with pathology of the aorta (Figs 16A and B). Advocacy of CMR for longitudinal clinical evaluations in patients with valvular heart disease is based on its superior quantitative accuracy, whereas the requirement for CMR in such cases is not yet firmly established.[101]

DISEASES WITH RIGHT VENTRICULAR PREDOMINANCE

Right ventricular morphology and function are often altered in patients with left ventricular disease. In addition, a number of conditions exert preferential effects on the RV, with relative sparing of the LV. The superior quantitative accuracy of CMR characterizations of right ventricular volumes and mass facilitate evaluation with a high degree of confidence. In addition, techniques capable of quantitating through plane blood velocity

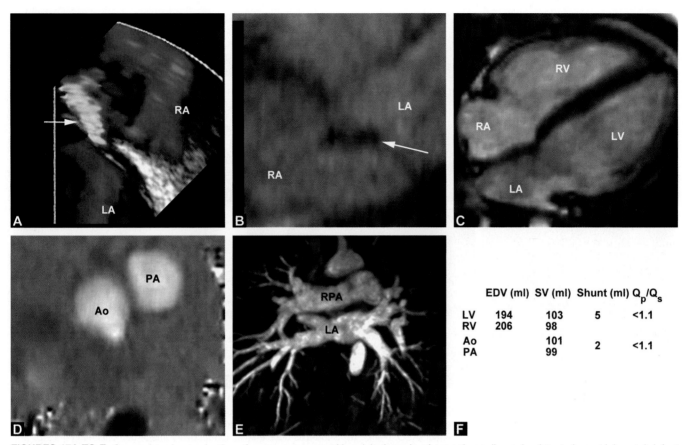

FIGURES 17A TO F: Comprehensive evaluation of a young woman with palpitations, in whom echocardiography detected an atrial septal defect (ASD) and possible RV enlargement. (A) Transesophageal echocardiogram demonstrating left-to-right flow across the ASD (arrow). (B) Cine-FLASH four-chamber CMR image with dephasing (black) of ASD flow (arrow). (C) End-diastolic four-chamber true-FISP image showing near-equal sizes of right and left heart chambers, respectively. When normalized for body surface area, all four cardiac chamber volumes are within normal limits. (D) Velocity-encoded images used for calculation of right- and left-heart flows (Q_p and Q_s, respectively). (E) Pulmonary venous angiogram demonstrating normal locations of the ostia of all four pulmonary veins—effectively excluding anomalous venous return. (F) Volumetric flow calculations showing very good agreement between methods, and effectively excluding simple left-to-right intracardiac shunting as an explanation for the patient's symptoms (Abbreviations: RPA: Right pulmonary artery; LA: Left atrium)

The table within Figure F:

	EDV (ml)	SV (ml)	Shunt (ml)	Q_p/Q_s
LV	194	103	5	<1.1
RV	206	98		
Ao		101	2	<1.1
PA		99		

(velocity encoding) provide useful information in cases where left and right ventricular stroke volumes are unequal, and where there is significant valvular regurgitation.

INTRACARDIAC SHUNT

In adults with intracardiac shunting of blood, clinical decision-making and prognosis depend critically upon right ventricular morphology and function. Clinical decision-making is also strongly influenced by the magnitude and direction of shunting. The shape of the RV defies simple characterization, which creates difficulty in obtaining quantitative assessments with techniques, such as echocardiography, which acquire images on only a few planes.

The CMR provides quantitative evaluation of intracardiac shunting utilizing three complementary and corroborative methods: (1) ventriculographic comparison of left and right ventricular stroke volumes, (2) calculation of stroke volumes in the main pulmonary artery and ascending aorta by means of velocity encoding techniques and (3) calculation of volumetric flow in the shunt itself using velocity encoding techniques (Figs 17 and 18).

PULMONARY ARTERY HYPERTENSION

Primary pulmonary hypertension is a progressive disease of resistance arteries in the lungs, in the absence of a systemic disease known to affect pulmonary artery pressure. Secondary pulmonary hypertension can develop as a complication of diverse disease processes—collagen vascular disorders,[102] pulmonary embolism, congenital malformations of the heart or great vessels, cor pulmonale or mass effects.

Historically, treatment and prognosis were guided by measurement of pulmonary artery pressure itself; along with determination of cardiac output.[103] Subsequently, echo Doppler methods have replaced the need for repetitive invasive measurement of pulmonary artery systolic pressure. More recently, with the introduction of reliable methods, assessments of right ventricular morphology and systolic function have emerged as critical tools for management.[104,105]

Although advanced 3-D echocardiographic techniques are under development to address this need, CMR methods continue to serve as the reference standard for such methods, and CMR yields superior reproducibility with lower interobserver bias.[106]

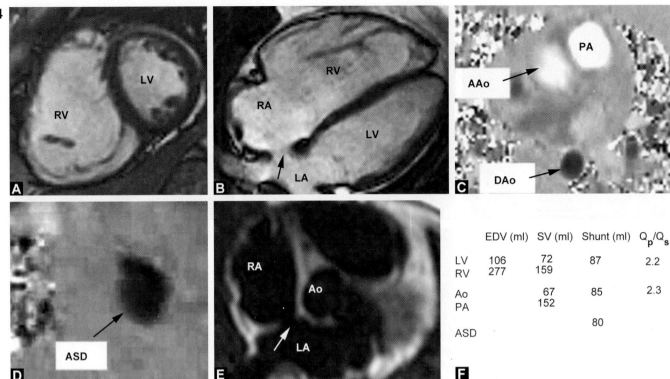

FIGURES 18A TO F: Comprehensive CMR studies from a young man with exertional dyspnea. (A) Short-axis end-diastolic true-FISP image showing RV enlargement. (B) Four-chamber end-diastolic true-FISP image showing RV and RA enlargement and an interatrial communication (arrow). (C) Short-axis velocity-encoded image where cephalad flow is depicted in white and caudal flow is depicted in black. (D) Velocity-encoded image of left-to-right flow across the atrial septal defect (ASD, black). (E) Short-axis double inversion-recovery image demonstrating the size and location of the ASD (arrow). (F) Volumetric flow calculations, demonstrating very good agreement between the three methods for shunt quantitation (Abbreviations: RA: Right atrium; LA: Left atrium; AAo: Ascending aorta; PA: Pulmonary artery; DAo: Descending aorta)

	EDV (ml)	SV (ml)	Shunt (ml)	Q_p/Q_s
LV	106	72	87	2.2
RV	277	159		
Ao		67	85	2.3
PA		152		
ASD			80	

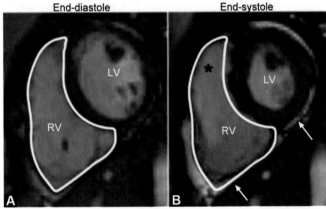

FIGURES 19A AND B: Short-axis true-FISP images from a young woman with recurrent syncope due to ventricular tachycardia. The RV end-diastolic silhouette is shown in both end-diastolic and end-systolic frames, in order to accentuate akinesis/dyskinesis in the more anterior region of the RV (*). RVEF = 0.29 and RVEDV index = 120 ml/m^2, fulfilling a major criterion for the diagnosis of arrhythmogenic right ventricular cardiomyopathy.[109] Epicardial fat abuts the myocardium of both ventricles (arrows)— a nonspecific finding not useful in making the diagnosis of ARVC[110]

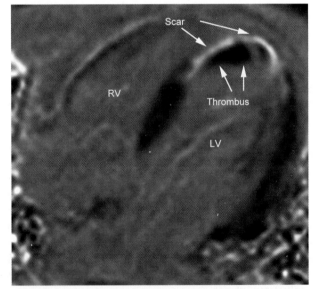

FIGURE 20: Four-chamber phase-sensitive inversion-recovery image acquired 10 minutes after administration of Gd-DTPA. There is a mural thrombus overlying a zone of transmural infarction (scar)

ARRHYTHMOGENIC RIGHT VENTRICULAR CARDIOMYOPATHY

Arrhythmogenic right ventricular cardiomyopathy (ARVC) is a genetically determined disorder characterized by myocyte loss and fibrofatty replacement in right ventricular myocardium.[107]

Left ventricular involvement ranges from negligible to predominant.[108] The disease is manifest by symptomatic arrhythmias, including SCD, often not preceded by progressive heart failure. The diagnosis, or its exclusion, requires a careful search for characteristic abnormalities of the electrocardiogram

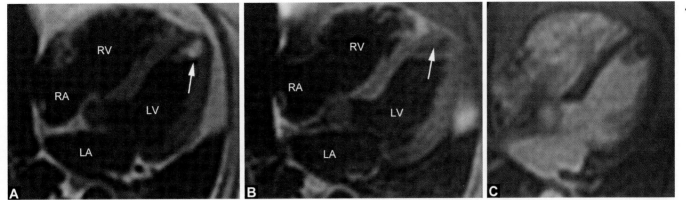

FIGURES 21A TO C: Four-chamber views from a middle-aged woman with an apical mass discovered incidentally by echocardiography. (A) Double inversion (IR) recovery sequence reveals a mass in the LV apex exhibiting high signal intensity (arrow). (B) Double IR with a "fat saturation" pulse completely attenuates the mass signal, indicating a high lipid content. (C) Image acquired during first-pass of Gd-DTPA reveals absence of enhancement of the mass—indicating low vascularity. The findings support a diagnosis of benign lipoma, and the patient was managed conservatively

during sinus rhythm and during episodes of ventricular tachycardia, right ventricular morphology and function and right ventricular histology, along with a definitive family history and/or genetic testing.[109] Unfortunately, absence of any one feature is not sufficient to exclude the disease, nor to support a benign prognosis over the long-term.

The CMR is useful to define the presence or absence of morphologic and functional features of the disease[110] (Figs 19A and B), and can provide a basis for more intensive subsequent investigation. Since arrhythmias can precede overt morphologic changes in ARVC, CMR can be useful for longitudinal studies when the initial evaluation is negative or inconclusive.[111]

MISCELLANEOUS CONDITIONS

CARDIAC THROMBI

The diagnosis of LV mural thrombus is usually based on clinical suspicion and confirmation of characteristic findings on echocardiography; echogenic mass protruding into the LV cavity from a myocardial region after ischemic insult. More recently, CMR has been shown to provide increased diagnostic accuracy in patients at high-risk for mural thrombus and consequent systemic embolization[112] (Fig. 20). The CMR has diagnostic accuracy similar to transesophageal echocardiography for detection of left atrial appendage mural thrombi, and is less invasive.[113]

CARDIAC MASSES

The CMR can be useful to discriminate between solid-tissue cardiac masses and mural thrombi. Information regarding tissue character and vascularity augment decisions about treatment and prognosis (Figs 21A to C).

LEFT VENTRICLE TRABECULATIONS AND NONCOMPACTION

The LVNC is a genetic disorder characterized by failure of coalescence of myocardium during fetal development.[114] Improvements in imaging technology have facilitated its

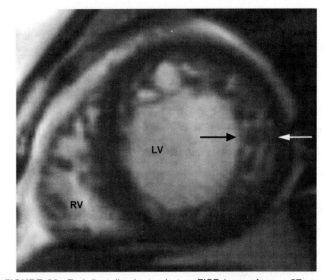

FIGURE 22: End-diastolic short-axis true-FISP image from a 27-year-old man with heart failure. There is abundant trabeculation and thinning of the compacted myocardium, most prominent in the lateral LV wall (arrows)

diagnosis, and the morphologic phenotype appears to be far more common than the sum of known genetic abnormalities, raising the question of whether LVNC can be acquired postnatally.[115,116]

In some cases, the echocardiographic diagnosis is unclear, and CMR can provide confirmation or rejection of its presence[117] (Fig. 22).

PERICARDIAL DISEASE

The CMR is a useful adjunct for assessment of pericardial disease and its functional consequences[118] (Figs 23A and B). The CMR can estimate pericardial effusion. However echocardiography is the imaging technique of choice and clinical application of CMR for the diagnosis and management of pericardial effusion is limited. However, CMR can be used to assess pericardial thickness in patients with suspected constrictive pericarditis.

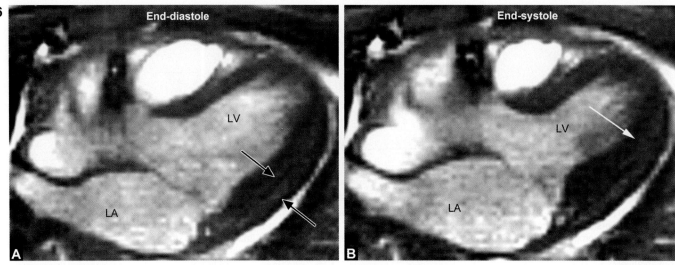

FIGURES 23A AND B: Axial true-FISP images from a patient with lower extremity edema and ascites. Visceral and parietal pericardial layers are thickened (maximum = 8 mm; black arrows), and are fused along the apical lateral wall (white arrow)

ABBREVIATIONS

ARVC: Arrhythmogenic right ventricular cardiomyopathy

CAS: Coronary artery stenosis

CMR: Cardiovascular magnetic resonance

DCM: Dilated cardiomyopathy

HCM: Hypertrophic cardiomyopathy

LGE: Late gadolinium enhancement

LV: Left ventricle

PSIR: Phase-sensitive inversion-recovery

RCM: Restrictive cardiomyopathy

RV: Right ventricle

SCD: Sudden cardiac death

SSFP: Steady-state free precession

True-FISP: True fast imaging with steady-state precession.

REFERENCES

1. Ridgway JP. Cardiovascular magnetic resonance physics for clinicians. J Cardiovasc Magn Reson. 2010;12:71.
2. Sandstede J, Lipke C, Beer M, et al. Age- and gender-specific differences in left and right ventricular cardiac function and mass determined by cine magnetic resonance imaging. Eur Radiol. 2000;10:438-42.
3. Salton CJ, Chuang ML, O'Donnell CJ, et al. Gender differences and normal left ventricular anatomy in an adult population free of hypertension. A cardiovascular magnetic resonance study of the Framingham Heart Study Offspring cohort. J Am Coll Cardiol. 2002;39:1055-60.
4. Tandri H, Daya SK, Nasir K, et al. Normal reference values for the adult right ventricle by magnetic resonance imaging. Am J Cardiol. 2006;98:1660-4.
5. Alfakih K, Plein S, Thiele H, et al. Normal human left and right ventricular dimensions for MRI as assessed by turbo gradient echo and steady-state free precession imaging sequences. J Magn Reson Imaging. 2003;17:323-9.
6. Malm S, Frigstad S, Sagberg E, et al. Real-time simultaneous triplane contrast echocardiography gives rapid, accurate, and reproducible assessment of left ventricular volumes and ejection fraction: a comparison with magnetic resonance imaging. J Am Soc Echocardiogr. 2006;19:1494-501.
7. Doherty III NE, Seelos KC, Suzuki J-I, et al. Application of cine nuclear magnetic resonance imaging for sequential evaluation of response to angiotensin-converting enzyme inhibitor therapy in dilated cardiomyopathy. J Am Coll Cardiol. 1992;19:1294-302.
8. Grothues F, Smith GC, Moon JC, et al. Comparison of interstudy reproducibility of cardiovascular magnetic resonance with two-dimensional echocardiography in normal subjects and in patients with heart failure or left ventricular hypertrophy. Am J Cardiol. 2002;90:29-34.
9. www.clinicaltrials.gov
10. Roger V, Turner MB. Heart Disease and Stroke Statistics—2011 Update. Circulation. 2011;123:e18-209.
11. Pennell DJ, Underwood SR, Manzara CC, et al. Magnetic resonance imaging during dobutamine stress in coronary artery disease. Am J Cardiol. 1992;70:34-40.
12. Wahl A, Paetsch I, Gollesch A, et al. Safety and feasibility of high-dose dobutamine-atropine stress cardiovascular magnetic resonance for diagnosis of myocardial ischemia: Experience in 1000 consecutive cases. Eur Heart J. 2004;25:1230-6.
13. Charoenpanichkit C, Hundley WG. The 20 year evolution of dobutamine stress cardiovascular magnetic resonance. J Cardiovasc Magn Reson. 2010;12:59.
14. Hundley WG, Hamilton CA, Thomas MS, et al. Utility of fast cine magnetic resonance imaging and display for the detection of myocardial ischemia in patients not well suited for second harmonic stress echocardiography. Circulation. 1999;100:1697-702.
15. Wahl A, Paetsch I, Roethemeyer S, et al. High-dose dobutamine atropine stress cardiovascular MR imaging after coronary revascularization in patients with wall motion abnormalities at rest. Radiology. 2004;233:210-6.
16. Kuijpers D, Ho KY, van Dijkman PR, et al. Dobutamine cardio-vascular magnetic resonance for the detection of myocardial ischemia with the use of myocardial tagging. Circulation. 2003;107:1592-7.
17. Hundley WG, Morgan TM, Neagle CM, et al. Magnetic resonance imaging determination of cardiac prognosis. Circulation. 2002;106:2328-33.
18. Rodgers GP, Ayanian JZ, Balady G, et al. American College of Cardiology/American Heart Association Clinical Competence Statement on Stress Testing. A Report of the American College of Cardiology/American Heart Association/American College of Physicians-American Society of Internal Medicine Task Force on Clinical Competence. Circulation. 2000;102:1726-38.

19. Doyle M, Fuisz A, Kortright E, et al. The impact of myocardial flow reserve on the detection of coronary artery disease by perfusion imaging methods: an NHLBI WISE study. J Cardiovasc Magn Reson. 2003;5:475-85.

20. Ishida N, Sakuma H, Motoyasu M, et al. Noninfarcted myocardium: correlation between dynamic first-pass contrast-enhanced myocardial MR imaging and quantitative coronary angiography. Radiology. 2003;229:209-16.

21. Bingham SE, Hachamovitch R. Incremental Prognostic Significance of Combined Cardiac Magnetic Resonance Imaging, Adenosine Stress Perfusion, Delayed Enhancement, and Left Ventricular Function Over Preimaging Information for the Prediction of Adverse Events. Circulation. 2011; doi:10.1161/CIRCULATIONAHA. 109.907659 [in press].

22. Post JC, van Rossum AC, Bronzwaer JG, et al. Magnetic resonance angiography of anomalous coronary arteries. A new gold standard for delineating the proximal course? Circulation. 1995;92: 3163-71.

23. Bunce NH, Lorenz CH, Keegan J, et al. Coronary artery anomalies: assessment with free-breathing three-dimensional coronary MR angiography. Radiology. 2003;227:201-8.

24. Greil GF, Stuber M, Botnar RM, et al. Coronary magnetic resonance angiography in adolescents and young adults with Kawasaki disease. Circulation. 2002;105:908-11.

25. Mavrogeni S, Papadopoulos G, Douskou M, et al. Magnetic resonance angiography is equivalent to X-ray coronary angiography for the evaluation of coronary arteries in Kawasaki disease. J Am Coll Cardiol. 2004;43:649-52.

26. Galjee MA, van Rossum AC, Doesburg T, et al. Value of magnetic resonance imaging in assessing patency and function of coronary artery bypass grafts. An angiographically controlled study. Circulation. 1996;93:660-6.

27. Kim WY, Danias PG, Stuber M, et al. Coronary magnetic resonance angiography for the detection of coronary stenoses. N Engl J Med. 2001;345:1863-9.

28. Liu X, Zhao X, Huang J, et al. Comparison of 3-D free-breathing coronary MR angiography and 64-MDCT angiography for detection of coronary stenosis in patients with high calcium scores. Am J Roentgenol. 2007;189:1326-32.

29. Steel K, Broderick R, Gandla V, et al. Complementary prognostic values of stress myocardial perfusion and late gadolinium enhancement imaging by cardiac magnetic resonance in patients with known or suspected coronary artery disease. Circulation. 2009;120:1390-400.

30. Kwong RY, Sattar H, Wu H, et al. Incidence and prognostic implication of unrecognized myocardial scar characterized by cardiac magnetic resonance in diabetic patients without clinical evidence of myocardial infarction. Circulation. 2008;118:1011-20.

31. Kwong RY, Chan AK, Brown KA, et al. Impact of unrecognized myocardial scar detected by cardiac magnetic resonance imaging on event-free survival in patients presenting with signs or symptoms of coronary artery disease. Circulation. 2006;113:2733-43.

32. Taylor DO, Stehlik J, Edwards LB, et al. Registry of the International Society for Heart and Lung Transplantation: Twenty-sixth Official Adult Heart Transplant Report—2009. J Heart Lung Transplant. 2009;28:1007-22.

33. Slaughter MS, Rogers JG, Milano CA, et al. for the HeartMate II investigators. Advanced heart failure treated with continuous-flow left ventricular assist device. N Engl J Med. 2009;361:2241-51.

34. Hunt SA, Abraham WT, Chin MH, et al. 2009 focused update incorporated into the ACC/AHA 2005 Guidelines for the Diagnosis and Management of Heart Failure in Adults: a report of the American College of Cardiology Foundation/American Heart Association Task Force on Practice Guidelines: developed in collaboration with the International Society for Heart and Lung Transplantation. Circulation. 2009;119:e391-479.

35. Kim RJ, Fieno DS, Parrish TB, et al. Relationship of MRI delayed contrast enhancement to irreversible injury, infarct age, and contractile function. Circulation. 1999;100:1992-2002.

36. Ingkanisorn WP, Rhoads KL, Aletras AH, et al. Gadolinium delayed enhancement cardiovascular magnetic resonance correlates with clinical measures of myocardial infarction. J Am Coll Cardiol. 2004;43:2253-9.

37. Passamani E, Davis KB, Gillespie MJ, et al. A randomized trial of coronary artery bypass surgery. Survival of patients with a low ejection fraction. New Engl J Med. 1985;312:1665-71.

38. Kim RJ, Wu E, Rafael A, et al. The use of contrast-enhanced magnetic resonance imaging to identify reversible myocardial dysfunction. N Engl J Med. 2000;343:1445-53.

39. Selvanayagam JB, Kardos A, Francis JM, et al. Value of delayed-enhancement cardiovascular magnetic resonance imaging in predicting myocardial viability after surgical revascularization. Circulation. 2004;110:1535-41.

40. Carluccio E, Biagioli P, Alunni G, et al. Patients with hibernating myocardium show altered left ventricular volumes and shape, which revert after revascularization: evidence that dyssynergy might directly induce cardiac remodeling. J Am Coll Cardiol. 2006;47:969-77.

41. Allman KC, Shaw LJ, Hachamovitch R, et al. Myocardial viability testing and impact of revascularization on prognosis in patients with coronary artery disease and left ventricular dysfunction: a meta-analysis. J Am Coll Cardiol. 2002;39:1151-8.

42. Camici PG, Prasad SK, Rimoldi OE. Stunning, hibernation, and assessment of myocardial viability. Circulation. 2008;117:103-14.

43. ACC/AHA 2005 Guideline Update for the Diagnosis and Management of Chronic Heart Failure in the Adult—Summary Article. A Report of the American College of Cardiology/American Heart Association Task Force on Practice Guidelines. Circulation. 2005;112:1825-52.

44. Bonow RO, Maurer G, Lee KL, et al. the STICH Trial Investigators. Myocardial viability and survival in ischemic left ventricular dysfunction. N Engl J Med. 2011 (in press), PMID: 21463153.

45. McCarthy RE, Boehmer JP, Hruban RH, et al. Long-term outcome of fulminant myocarditis as compared with acute (nonfulminant) myocarditis. N Engl J Med. 2000;342:690-5.

46. Cooper LT, Berry GJ, Shabetai R for the Multicenter Giant Cell Myocarditis Study Group Investigators. Idiopathic Giant-Cell Myocarditis—Natural History and Treatment. N Engl J Med. 1997;336:1860-6.

47. Berry CJ, Johnson FL, Cabuay BM, et al. Evanescent asymmetrical septal hypertrophy and rapidly progressive heart failure in a 32-year-old man. Circulation. 2008;118:e126-8.

48. Mason JW, O'Connell JB, Herskowitz A, et al. A clinical trial of immunosuppressive therapy for myocarditis. The Myocarditis Treatment Trial Investigators. N Engl J Med. 1995;333:269-75.

49. Frustaci A, Chimenti C, Calabrese F, et al. Immunosuppressive therapy for active lymphocytic myocarditis: virological and immunologic profile of responders versus nonresponders. Circulation. 2003;107:857-63.

50. Frustaci A, Russo MA, Chimenti C. Randomized study on the efficacy of immunosuppressive therapy in patients with virus-negative inflammatory cardiomyopathy: the TIMIC study. Eur Heart J. 2009;16:1995-2002.

51. Magnani JW, Dec GW. Myocarditis: current trends in diagnosis and treatment. Circulation. 2006;113:876-90.

52. Hauck AJ, Kearney DL, Edwards WD. Evaluation of postmortem endomyocardial biopsy specimens from 38 patients with lymphocytic myocarditis: implications for role of sampling error. Mayo Clin Proc. 1989;64:1235-45.

53. Gagliardi MG, Polletta B. MRI for the diagnosis and follow-up of myocarditis. Circulation. 1999;99:457-60.

54. Laissy JP, Messin B, Varenne O, et al. MRI of acute myocarditis: a comprehensive approach based on various imaging sequences. Chest. 2002;122:1638-48.

CHAPTER 23 Cardiovascular Magnetic Resonance

55. Mahrholdt H, Goedecke C, Wagner A, et al. Cardiovascular magnetic resonance assessment of human myocarditis: a comparison to histology and molecular pathology. Circulation. 2004;109:1250-8.

56. Yilmaz A, Kindermann I, Kindermann M, et al. Comparative evaluation of left and right ventricular endomyocardial biopsy: differences in complication rate and diagnostic performance. Circulation. 2010;122:900-9.

57. Kwon DH, Halley CM, Carrigan TP, et al. Extent of left ventricular scar predicts outcomes in ischemic cardiomyopathy patients with significantly reduced systolic function: a delayed hyperenhancement cardiac magnetic resonance study. JACC Cardiovasc Imaging. 2009;2:34-44.

58. Krittayaphong R, Saiviroonporn P, Boonyasirinant T, et al. Prevalence and prognosis of myocardial scar in patients with known or suspected coronary artery disease and normal wall motion. Journal of Cardiovascular Magnetic Resonance. 2011;13:2.

59. Bello D, Fieno DS, Kim RJ, et al. Infarct morphology identifies patients with substrate for sustained ventricular tachycardia. J Am Coll Cardiol. 2005;45:1104-8.

60. www.clinicaltrials.gov Identifier # NCT00487279.

61. Ghio S, Gavazzi A, Campana C, et al. Independent and additive prognostic value of right ventricular systolic function and pulmonary artery pressure in patients with chronic heart failure. J Am Coll Cardiol. 2001;37:183-8.

62. Zannad F, Alla F, Dousset B, et al. Limitation of excessive extra-cellular matrix turnover may contribute to survival benefit of spironolactone therapy in patients with congestive heart failure: insights from the randomized aldactone evaluation study (RALES). Rales Investigators. Circulation. 2000;102:2700-6.

63. Assomull RG, Prasad SK, Lyne J, et al. Cardiovascular magnetic resonance, fibrosis, and prognosis in dilated cardiomyopathy. J Am Coll Cardiol. 2006;48:1977-85.

64. Wu KC, Weiss RG, Thiemann DR, et al. Late gadolinium enhancement by cardiovascular magnetic resonance heralds an adverse prognosis in nonischemic cardiomyopathy. J Am Coll Cardiol. 2008;51:2414-21.

65. Maron BJ. Sudden death in young athletes. N Engl J Med. 2003;349: 1064-75.

66. van Driest SL, Ellsworth EG, Ommen SR, et al. Prevalence and spectrum of thin filament mutations in an outpatient referral population with hypertrophic cardiomyopathy. Circulation. 2003;108:445-51.

67. Richard P, Charron P, Carrier L, et al. Hypertrophic cardiomyopathy: distribution of disease genes, spectrum of mutations, and implications for a molecular diagnosis strategy. Circulation. 2003;107:2227-32.

68. Ho CY, Seidman CE. A contemporary approach to hypertrophic cardiomyopathy. Circulation. 2006;113:e858-62.

69. Maron BJ. Hypertrophic cardiomyopathy: a systematic review. JAMA. 2002;287:1308-20.

70. Rickers C, Wilke NM, Jerosch-Herold M, et al. Utility of cardiac magnetic resonance imaging in the diagnosis of hypertrophic cardiomyopathy. Circulation. 2005;112:855-61.

71. Pons-Lladó G, Carreras F, Borrás X, et al. Comparison of morphologic assessment of hypertrophic cardiomyopathy by magnetic resonance versus echocardiographic imaging. Am J Cardiol. 1997;79:1651-6.

72. Moon JC, Fisher NG, McKenna WJ, et al. Detection of apical hypertrophic cardiomyopathy by cardiovascular magnetic resonance in patients with non-diagnostic echocardiography. Heart. 2004;90:645-9.

73. Maron MS, Hauser TH, Dubrow E, et al. Right ventricular involvement in hypertrophic cardiomyopathy. Am J Cardiol. 2007;100:1293-8.

74. Strijack B, Ariyarajah V, Soni R, et al. Late gadolinium enhance-ment cardiovascular magnetic resonance in genotyped hypertrophic cardiomyopathy with normal phenotype. J Cardiovasc Magn Reson. 2008;10:58.

75. Ho CY, López B, Coelho-Filho OR, et al. Myocardial fibrosis as an early manifestation of hypertrophic cardiomyopathy. N Engl J Med. 2010;363:552-63.

76. Elliott PM, Poloniecki J, Dickie S, et al. Sudden death in hypertrophic cardiomyopathy: identification of high risk patients. J Am Coll Cardiol. 2000;36:2212-8.

77. Olivotto I, Maron MS, Autore C, et al. Assessment and significance of left ventricular mass by cardiovascular magnetic resonance in hypertrophic cardiomyopathy. J Am Coll Cardiol. 2008;52:559-66.

78. Iles L, Pfluger H, Lefkovits L, et al. Myocardial fibrosis predicts appropriate device therapy in patients with implantable cardioverter-defibrillators for primary prevention of sudden cardiac death. J Am Coll Cardiol. 2011;57:821-8.

79. Moon JC, McKenna WJ, McCrohon JA, et al. Toward clinical risk assessment in hypertrophic cardiomyopathy with gadolinium cardiovascular magnetic resonance. J Am Coll Cardiol. 2003;41:1561-7.

80. O'Hanlon R, Grasso A, Roughton M, et al. Prognostic significance of myocardial fibrosis in hypertrophic cardiomyopathy. J Am Coll Cardiol. 2010;56:867-74.

81. Bruder O, Wagner A, Jensen CJ, et al. Myocardial scar visualized by cardiovascular magnetic resonance imaging predicts major adverse events in patients with hypertrophic cardiomyopathy. J Am Coll Cardiol. 2010;56:875-87.

82. Lehrke S, Lossnitzer D, Schöb M, et al. Use of cardiovascular magnetic resonance for risk stratification in chronic heart failure: prognostic value of late gadolinium enhancement in patients with nonischemic dilated cardiomyopathy. Heart. 2011;97:727-32, Epub 2010.

83. van Dockum WG, Beek AM, ten Cate FJ, et al. Early onset and progression of left ventricular remodeling after alcohol septal ablation in hypertrophic obstructive cardiomyopathy. Circulation. 2005;111:2503-8.

84. Petersen SE, Jerosch-Herold M, Hudsmith LE, et al. Evidence for microvascular dysfunction in hypertrophic cardiomyopathy: new insights from multiparametric magnetic resonance imaging. Circulation. 2007;115:2418-25.

85. Knaapen P, Germans T, Camici PG, et al. Determinants of coronary microvascular dysfunction in symptomatic hypertrophic cardiomyopathy. Am J Physiol Heart Circ Physiol. 2008;294:H986-93.

86. Jung WI, Sieverding L, Breuer J, et al. 31P NMR spectroscopy detects metabolic abnormalities in asymptomatic patients with hypertrophic cardiomyopathy. Circulation. 1998;97:2536-42.

87. Nihoyannopoulos P, Dawson D. Restrictive cardiomyopathies. Eur J Echocardiogr. 2009;10:iii23-33.

88. Maceira AM, Joshi J, Prasad SK, et al. Cardiovascular magnetic resonance in cardiac amyloidosis. Circulation. 2005;111:186-93.

89. Hughes DA, Elliott PM, Shah J, et al. Effects of enzyme replacement therapy on the cardiomyopathy of Anderson-Fabry disease: a randomised, double-blind, placebo-controlled clinical trial of agalsidase alfa. Heart. 2008;94:153-8.

90. Patel MR, Cawely PJ, Heitner JF. Improved diagnostic sensitivity of contrast enhanced cardiac MRI for cardiac sarcoidosis. Circulation. 2004;108:645.

91. Debl K, Djavidani B, Buchner S, et al. Time course of eosinophilic myocarditis visualized by CMR. J Cardiovasc Magn Reson. 2008;10:21.

92. Kirk P, Roughton M, Porter JB, et al. Cardiac T2 magnetic resonance for prediction of cardiac complications in thalassemia major. Circulation. 2009;120:1961-8.

93. Mehta D, Mori N, Goldbarg SH, et al. Primary prevention of sudden cardiac death in silent cardiac sarcoidosis: role of programmed ventricular stimulation. Circ Arrhythm Electrophysiol. 2011;4: 43-8.

94. Modell B, Khan M, Darlison M, et al. Improved survival of thalassaemia major in the UK and relation to T2 cardiovascular

magnetic resonance. J Cardiovasc Magn Reson. 2008;10:42.

95. Anderson LJ, Westwood MA, Holden S, et al. Myocardial iron clearance during reversal of sideriotic cardiomyopathy with intravenous desferrioxamine: a prospective study using T2 cardiovascular magnetic resonance. Br J Haematol. 2004;127:348-55.

96. Bonow RO, Carabello BA, Kanu C, et al. ACC/AHA 2006 guidelines for the management of patients with valvular heart disease: a report of the American College of Cardiology/American Heart Association Task Force on Practice Guidelines (writing committee to revise the 1998 Guidelines for the Management of Patients With Valvular Heart Disease): developed in collaboration with the Society of Cardiovascular Anesthesiologists: endorsed by the Society for Cardiovascular Angiography and Interventions and the Society of Thoracic Surgeons. Circulation. 2006;114:e84-231.

97. Chan KM, Wage R, Symmonds K, et al. Towards comprehensive assessment of mitral regurgitation using cardiovascular magnetic resonance. J Cardiovasc Magn Reson. 2008;10:61.

98. Djavidani B, Debl K, Lenhart M, et al. Planimetry of mitral valve stenosis by magnetic resonance imaging. J Am Coll Cardiol. 2005;45:2048-53.

99. Yap SC, van Geuns RJ, Meijboom FJ, et al. A simplified continuity equation approach to the quantification of stenotic bicuspid aortic valves using velocity-encoded cardiovascular magnetic resonance. J Cardiovasc Magn Reson. 2007;9:899-906.

100. Buchner S, Debl K, Poschenrieder F, et al. Cardiovascular magnetic resonance for direct assessment of anatomic regurgitant orifice in mitral regurgitation. Circ Cardiovasc Imaging. 2008;1:148-55.

101. Hundley WG, Bluemke DA, Finn JP, et al. ACCF/ACR/AHA/NASCI/SCMR 2010 expert consensus document on cardiovascular magnetic resonance: a report of the American College of Cardiology Foundation Task Force on Expert Consensus Documents. Circulation. 2010;121:2462-508.

102. Galiè N, Manes A, Farahani KV, et al. Pulmonary arterial hypertension associated to connective tissue diseases. Lupus. 2005;14:713-7.

103. D'Alonzo GE, Barst RJ, Ayres SM, et al. Survival in patients with primary pulmonary hypertension. Results from a national prospective registry. Ann Intern Med. 1991;115:343-9.

104. Gavazzi A, Ghio S, Scelsi L, et al. Response of the right ventricle to acute pulmonary vasodilation predicts the outcome in patients with advanced heart failure and pulmonary hypertension. Am Heart J. 2003;145:310-6.

105. Badano LP, Ginghina C, Easaw J, et al. Right ventricle in pulmonary arterial hypertension: haemodynamics, structural changes, imaging, and proposal of a study protocol aimed to assess remodelling and treatment effects. Eur J Echocardiogr. 2010;11:27-37.

106. Grapsa J, O'Regan DP, Pavlopoulos H, et al. Right ventricular remodelling in pulmonary arterial hypertension with three-dimensional echocardiography: comparison with cardiac magnetic resonance imaging. Eur J Echocardiogr. 2010;11:64-73.

107. Basso C, Corrado D, Marcus FI, et al. Arrhythmogenic right ventricular cardiomyopathy. Lancet. 2009;373:1289-300.

108. Norman M, Simpson N, Mogensen J, et al. Novel mutation in desmoplakin causes arrhythmogenic left ventricular cardiomyopathy. Circulation. 2005;112:636-42.

109. Marcus FI, McKenna WJ, Sherrill D, et al. Diagnosis of arrhythmogenic right ventricular cardiomyopathy/dysplasia: proposed modification of the task force criteria. Circulation. 2010;121:1533-41.

110. Tandri H, Castillo E, Ferrari VA, et al. Magnetic resonance imaging of arrhythmogenic right ventricular dysplasia: sensitivity, specificity, and observer variability of fat detection versus functional analysis of the right ventricle. J Am Coll Cardiol. 2006;48:2277-84.

111. Kiès P, Bootsma M, Bax JJ, et al. Serial reevaluation for ARVD/C is indicated in patients presenting with left bundle branch block ventricular tachycardia and minor ECG abnormalities. J Cardiovasc Electrophysiol. 2006;17:586-93.

112. Srichai MB, Junor C, Rodriguez LL, et al. Clinical, imaging, and pathological characteristics of left ventricular thrombus: a comparison of contrast-enhanced magnetic resonance imaging, transthoracic echocardiography, and transesophageal echocardiography with surgical or pathological validation. Am Heart J. 2006;152:75-84.

113. Ohyama H, Hosomi N, Takahashi T, et al. Comparison of magnetic resonance imaging and transesophageal echocardiography in detection of thrombus in the left atrial appendage. Stroke. 2003;34:2436-9.

114. Jenni R, Oechslin E, Schneider J, et al. Echocardiographic and pathoanatomical characteristics of isolated left ventricular non-compaction: a step towards classification as a distinct cardiomyopathy. Heart. 2001;86(6):666-71.

115. Sen-Chowdhry S, McKenna WJ. Left ventricular noncompaction and cardiomyopathy: cause, contributor, or epiphenomenon? Curr Opin Cardiol. 2008;23:171-5.

116. Finsterer J, Stöllberger C, Bonner E. Acquired noncompaction associated with coronary heart disease and myopathy. Heart Lung. 2010;39:240-1.

117. Petersen SE, Selvanayagam JB, Wiesmann F, et al. Left ventricular non-compaction: insights from cardiovascular magnetic resonance imaging. J Am Coll Cardiol. 2005;46:101-5.

118. Axel L. Assessment of pericardial disease by magnetic resonance and computed tomorgraphy. J Magn Reson Imaging. 2004;19:816-26.

Chapter 24

Molecular Imaging of Vascular Disease

Eric A Osborn, Jagat Narula, Farouc A Jaffer

Chapter Outline

INTRODUCTION

With the discovery of new molecular targets and pathways that both expand our knowledge base and refine classical teachings, there is an ongoing role for technological advances to illuminate these areas by offering improved diagnostic and therapeutic clinical tools. Molecular imaging aims to capitalize on these advances by employing small molecules and nanoparticles, which are coupled with imaging agents to visualize cellular and molecular events in living subjects, complementing clinical, anatomical and physiological imaging modalities. Clinical applications of molecular imaging in cardiovascular disease can provide novel insight into disease mechanisms, risk stratification, prognosis and the in vivo efficacy of biotherapeutics. In addition, molecular imaging is poised to alter the landscape of cardiovascular disease by offering targeted, personalized therapy and facilitating small scale clinical trials that can readily feedback important biological parameters that mark treatment response or disease progression. In this chapter, we focus on promising translational and clinical advances in molecular imaging of vascular disease.

MOLECULAR IMAGING FUNDAMENTALS

The specific detection and reporting of in vivo biological targets is the underlying goal of all molecular imaging strategies.[1,2] In order to achieve this goal, certain fundamental issues require attention by the investigator. First, an appropriate cellular or molecular target must be identified that can delineate the desired process and be targeted with a specific high-affinity ligand. Second, an imaging agent with advantageous biopharmacokinetic properties must be chosen that can be linked to and report on the target. Finally, an imaging system with appropriate resolution and sensitivity to detect the imaging target is needed.

As the range of potential cellular and molecular targets available for detection is vast, appropriate determination of the desired target is of critical importance. Ideal targets are those that reported on important biological processes and possess a unique biological signature that can be exploited, and abundant enough to enable in vivo detection. In certain cases, amplification schemes can be employed to boost a low-level signal, such as with internalizing receptors, enzymes or reporter gene approaches; however, other less easily accessed targets on DNA, RNA or proteins, expressed at low concentrations, can be more challenging. While both intracellular and extracellular targets are possible to sense, extracellular targets are generally more accessible as they avoid charge, size and solubility issues that limit intracellular targeting agents traversing the plasma membrane. Examples of cellular targets successfully identified in vascular disease include macrophages, lymphocytes and stem cells in atherosclerosis. Molecular targets are predominantly investigated and include cell surface receptors, neovessel epitopes and tissue enzymatic processes. Table 1 provides a list of explored molecular and cellular targets in vascular diseases that are either currently FDA-approved for clinical use or hold significant promise for clinical translation in the coming years.

Just as the numbers of potential cellular and molecular targets are large, there are even greater numbers of smaller molecules that can be employed in molecular imaging strategies as high-affinity ligands to detect the desired target. As with a lock and key, these small molecules should bind specifically to the cell or molecule of interest, in most cases, without disrupting its function, although there are certain instances where alteration or frank disruption of function may be an advantageous property. They must interact in such a fashion as to specifically identify the biological process in question and minimize nonspecific binding that reduces the signal-to-noise ratio (SNR). The most well-known example of binding partners are antibody-antigen combinations; however, antibodies have several suboptimal properties that make their use in molecular imaging strategies less desirable, such as relatively large size leading to steric hindrance and poor conjugation density when coupled to the imaging agent.

TABLE 1

451

Promising molecular imaging agents in vascular disease

Application	Agent	Modality*	Multi-channel	Primary target	Primary use	Clinical
Atherosclerosis	^{18}FDG (18-fluoro-deoxygulcose)	PET	No	Glucose transporter-1, hexokinase	Metabolism	Yes
	^{111}In-oxine (indium-111-oxyquinolone)	SPECT	No	Monocytes/macrophages	Inflammation	Yes
	USPIOs (Ferumoxtran)	MRI	No	Monocytes/macrophages	Inflammation	Yes
	^{99m}Tc-annexin A5	SPECT	No	Annexin-A5/macrophages	Apoptosis	Yes
	^{18}F-Galakto-RGD	PET	No	Integrins/endothelial cells	Neovascularization	Yes
	$\alpha_V\beta_3$ magnetic nanoparticles	MRI	No	$\alpha_V\beta_3$ integrins/ endothelial cells	Neovascularization	Promising
	^{99m}Tc-interleukin-2	SPECT	No	Interleukin-2/lymphocytes	Inflammation	Yes
	ProSense	NIRF, IVM	Yes	Cysteine protease activity	Inflammation	Promising
	MMPsense	NIRF, IVM	Yes	Matrix metallo-proteinase activity	Inflammation	Promising
	OsteoSense	NIRF	Yes	Hydroxyapatite	Calcification	Promising
	N1177	CT	No	Monocytes/macrophages	Inflammation	Promising
	Gadofluorine-M	MRI	No	Monocytes/macrophages	Inflammation	Promising
	P947	MRI	No	Matrix metalloproteinase activity	Inflammation	Promising
	VCAM-1 microbubbles	CEU	No	VCAM-1	Inflammation	Promising
	Tri-modality nanoparticle	MRI, PET, NIRF	Yes	Monocytes/macrophages	Inflammation	Promising
	Bis-5HT-DTPA (Gd)	MRI	No	Myeloperoxidase activity	Inflammation	Promising
	^{99m}Tc-RP805	SPECT	No	Matrix metalloproteinase activity	Inflammation	Promising
Thrombosis	^{99m}Tc-apcitide (AcuTect)	SPECT	No	GPIIb/IIIa receptor	Platelet activity	Yes
	EP-2104R	MRI	No	Fibrin	Coagulation factors	Yes
	Activated factor XIII (FXIIIa)	MRI, SPECT, NIRF	Yes	FXIIIa activity	Coagulation factors	Promising
Aneurysm	^{18}FDG (18-fluoro-deoxygulcose)	PET	No	Glucose transporter-1, hexokinase	Metabolism	Yes
	di-5-hydroxytryp-tamide of gado-pentetate dimeglumine	MRI	No	Myeloperoxidase activity	Inflammation	Promising
Vascular Injury	^{111}In-RP782	SPECT	No	Matrix metalloproteinase activity	Inflammation	Promising
Myocardial infarction	^{99m}Tc-NC100692	SPECT	No	$\alpha_V\beta_3$ integrins/ endothelial cells	Angiogenesis	Yes
	^{18}F-Galakto-RGD	PET	No	Integrins/endothelial cells	Angiogenesis	Yes
	^{99m}Tc-CRIP	SPECT	No	Collagen	Fibrosis	Promising
	^{99m}Tc-collagelin	SPECT	No	Collagen (type I and III)	Fibrosis	Promising
	EP-3533	MRI	No	Collagen (type I)	Fibrosis	Promising
	AnxCLIO-Cy5.5	MRI, fluorescence	No	Annexin/myocardial cells	Apoptosis	Promising
	^{19}F perfluorocarbons	MRI	No	Monocytes/macrophages	Inflammation	Promising
Cardiomyopathy	AnxCLIO-Cy5.5	MRI, fluorescence	No	Annexin/myocardial cells	Apoptosis	Promising
Transplant rejection	USPIOs (Ferumoxtran)	MRI	No	Monocytes/macrophages	Inflammation	Yes
Cardiac regeneration	Firefly luciferase	BLI	Yes	Luciferin gene expression	Reporter gene construct	Promising
	Sodium-iodide symporter (NIS)	PET	No	NIS gene expression	Reporter gene construct	Promising
	Herpes simplex virus thymidine kinase (HSV-tk)	SPECT	No	HSV-tk gene expression	Reporter gene construct	Promising
	USPIOs (Ferumoxtran)	MRI	No	Monocytes/macrophages	Inflammation	Yes
	^{18}FDG (18-fluoro-deoxygulcose)	PET	No	Glucose transporter-1, hexokinase	Metabolism	Yes
	Gadofluorine-M-Cy3	MRI, fluorescence	No	Monocytes/macrophages	Inflammation	Promising

(* for modality abbreviations, see Table 2)

TABLE 2

Comparison of small animal molecular imaging modalities

Technique	Resolution	Depth	Sensitivity	Scan time	Multi-channel	Agents	Clinical
Computed tomography (CT)	50 μm	Unlimited	+	Seconds to minutes	Yes	Iodine moieties	Yes
Magnetic resonance imaging (MRI)	10–100 μm	Unlimited	++	Minutes to hours	Yes	Paramagnetic and magnetic particles	Yes
Contrast-enhanced ultrasound (CEU)	50 μm	Centimeters	++	Seconds to minutes	No	Microbubbles	Yes
Single photon emission computed tomography (SPECT)	0.3–1 mm	Unlimited	+++	Minutes	Dual	Radiolabeled compounds (^{99m}Tc, ^{111}In, ^{131}I, ^{67}Ga, ^{201}Tl)	Yes
Positron emission tomography (PET)	1–2 mm	Unlimited	+++	Seconds to minutes	No	Radiolabeled compounds (^{18}F, ^{64}Cu, ^{11}C, ^{68}Ga)	Yes
Bioluminescence imaging (BLI)	3–5 mm	Millimeters	+++	Seconds to minutes	Multiple	Luciferase, luminol	Potential
Fluorescence reflectance imaging (FRI)	1 mm	Millimeters	+++	Seconds to minutes	Multiple	Fluorophores, photoproteins	Yes
Fluorescence mediated tomography (FMT)	1 mm	Centimeters	++	Minutes	Multiple	Near-infrared fluorophores	Developing
Intravital microscopy	1 μm	Micrometers	++	Seconds to hours	Multiple	Fluorophores, photoproteins	Developing

+ millimolar or less; ++ micromolar; +++ nanomolar or greater

More often, bioengineered nanoparticles or oligopeptides with superior pharmacokinetics are utilized that deliver specific target identification and allow higher probe-coating densities due to their smaller physical size.

Once a molecular or cellular target has been identified, a corresponding imaging agent must be selected. The choice of imaging agent must consider the various advantages and disadvantages of each imaging detection modality, as well as the characteristics of the imaging platform that will be used for detection (Table 2). Tradeoffs between spatial resolution, sensitivity and tissue penetration among other factors must be considered carefully for each biological application. Signal amplification strategies to boost the detection capability of certain probes are also possible, such as sequestration/cellular trapping and "activatable" probes that report on biologically functional enzymes.[3] Ever more frequently, investigators are creating flexible chemical backbones that can incorporate two or even three different imaging agents on a single molecular probe for multimodality imaging.[4] These multimodality agents thus harness the strengths of the complementary imaging technologies in a single probe and also offer the attractive possibility of multifunction "theranostic" probes that can deliver a therapeutic drug or other payload in concert with diagnostic imaging, all packaged in a single injectable agent.[5]

MOLECULAR IMAGING MODALITIES

A wealth of different imaging modalities have been utilized for cardiovascular molecular imaging, each of which offers certain advantages and limitations as outlined in (Table 2). Factors of importance include sensitivity, spatial and temporal resolution, depth penetration, scan time, radiation exposure and cost among others. Compared to other applications, such as cancer detection, cardiovascular molecular imaging also poses significant additional difficulties due to cardiac and respiratory motion artifacts for myocardial imaging, small vessel size for coronary plaque detection and competing signals from adjacent blood flow. Nevertheless, through improvements in newer generation imaging systems including faster scan times and gating of cardiac and respiratory motion, as well as enhancements of software packages and motion detection or correction strategies, these barriers continue to be overcome.

Of the imaging strategies in current clinical practice, superparamagnetic nanoparticles for magnetic resonance imaging (MRI) and ^{18}F-fluorodeoxyglucose (FDG) for positron emission tomography (PET) provide illustrative examples of the technical tradeoffs inherent to all of the different modalities. Imaging strategies, such as ^{18}FDG-PET, offer high sensitivity of detection but relatively poor spatial resolution, whereas MRI provides high spatial resolution and soft tissue contrast but relatively poor sensitivity of probe detection.

Combinatory use of multiple imaging modalities into hybrid imaging strategies is frequently utilized to overcome the limitations of a single imaging platform, such as with the commonly used hybrid SPECT-CT sequence or more recently with the advent of simultaneous PET-MRI following the development of solid-state photodetectors that are not affected by magnetic field variations.[6] Other molecular imaging modalities include contrast-enhanced ultrasound imaging with ligand-coated microbubbles and optical imaging strategies that utilize fluorescence (intravital microscopy, fluorescence molecular tomography, intravascular catheter-based imaging) and bioluminescence reporter gene imaging.

MOLECULAR IMAGING OF VASCULAR DISEASE PROCESSES

With an ever growing armamentarium of molecular imaging probes available for use and in development, there has been extensive growth of molecular imaging applications in vascular disease. High-priority areas include atherosclerosis, thrombosis, aneurysmal disease and vascular injury. While most molecular imaging probes are in preclinical testing and development phases, and only a few agents that are FDA approved are present, this balance is likely to shift significantly in the coming years with the translation of these new emerging agents into the clinical arena.

ATHEROSCLEROSIS

Atherosclerotic vascular disease, fueled by lipid deposition, endovascular inflammation and leukocytic infiltration of the vessel wall, is an important and well-studied focus of molecular imaging studies. Histopathologically, atherosclerosis represents the end result of a potent combination of lipid, chronic inflammation, cellular proliferation, apoptosis and necrosis, leading to progressive plaque expansion within the vessel wall that may encroach on the vessel lumen, obstructing blood flow or acutely rupturing and exposing thrombogenic elements that cause abrupt vessel occlusion. Atherosclerosis is a top priority within molecular imaging, with the goal of early detection and preventative treatment of lipid-rich "vulnerable" plaques that have the highest likelihood to rupture, resulting in an acute coronary syndrome, peripheral arterial occlusion or cerebrovascular accident. High-risk features of vulnerable atheroma include necrotic lipid cores, neovascularization, apoptosis and inflammation, and each of these components has been successfully targeted by molecular imaging strategies. Molecular imaging of atherosclerosis thus has the potential to offer high-yield complementary clinical information to that of current anatomic and physiologic imaging methods such as coronary angiography and exercise stress testing. Following detection, serial noninvasive molecular imaging has the potential to directly monitor atherosclerotic plaque evolution over time in an individual patient during pharmaceutical therapy.

From a clinical perspective, there are presently two major platforms for atherosclerosis detection, [18]FDG-PET imaging and ultrasmall superparamagnetic iron oxide (USPIO) nanoparticle-enhanced MRI, both of which can identify inflammatory foci in larger caliber arteries such as the carotid, aorta and femoral beds. Coronary artery atheroma, however, are less easily imaged

due to their small size but emerging technologies that also detect inflammation such as an intravascular catheter for near-infrared fluorochrome detection[3] and new [18]FDG-PET protocols to suppress obscuring background myocardial tissue uptake,[7] hold promise. Finally, there exist multiple new emerging atherosclerosis molecular imaging agents (Table 1) that with further testing hold significant potential for translation to clinical practice.

Inflammation

Large arteries (e.g. carotid, aorta and iliofemoral): Infiltration of the vessel wall with leukocytes in atherosclerosis predominantly composed of the key effector cells monocytes and macrophages, represent tissue sites of active inflammation and vessel remodeling.[8] In patients experiencing sudden cardiac death, the culprit ruptured plaque often contains an abundant monocyte/macrophage burden,[9] thus making these sites excellent targets for clinical imaging agents of vulnerable plaques.

Ultrasmall superparamagnetic iron oxide: Clinical ultrasmall superparamagnetic iron oxide (USPIO) are magnetic nanoparticles composed of a 3 nm superparamagnetic iron oxide core that induce MRI tissue contrast by strongly influencing local signals in T2- and T2*-weighted images. An external dextran-coating over the iron oxide core promotes phagocytosis of the agent, primarily by mononuclear cells, (monocytes and macrophages) allowing USPIO to hone to sites where these cells accumulate such as atherosclerotic plaques.[10-14] To allow sufficient tissue accumulation and blood pool washout of nonspecific circulating signal, MRI is performed 24–36 hours following USPIO injection and the images are collected over 1–2 hours. Due to its T2 relaxation effects, USPIO are detected as dark "negative" reductions in MRI signal. While a negative-contrast agent can be more challenging in low SNR environments such as in vessel wall MRI, in many cases, the dark lumen and brighter soft tissue components in the vessel wall offer sufficient contrast density differences to facilitate adequate detection. However, while USPIO-based MRI has advantages in spatial resolution, it has relatively lower sensitivity, limiting its ability to detect smaller inflammatory foci in the carotid arteries or aorta. This limitation is particularly problematic in the much smaller coronary arteries, but may be addressable with intravascular MRI catheters.[15]

Effects of pharmacotherapy: Several noninvasive molecular imaging studies have demonstrated changes in plaque biology in response to pharmacotherapy treatment and, in particular, statins. Statin treatment promotes atherosclerotic plaque stabilization via lipid depleting and anti-inflammatory effects, and has the potential to halt or perhaps even cause regression of atheroma burden. Molecular imaging approaches can identify inflammatory components that define high-risk plaques. Although plaque inflammation represents a surrogate clinical marker, changes in inflammation may guide future outcome studies and provide valuable in vivo insights into the mechanisms of action of putative anti-inflammatory agents.

Of note, the utility of clinical USPIOs to evaluate carotid plaque inflammation following dose-modulated stain therapy was examined in the "atorvastatin therapy: effects on reduction of macrophage activity" (ATHEROMA) trial.[16] In this study, 47 patients were randomized to 80 mg (high-dose) or 10 mg (low-dose) atorvastatin. Treatment with high-dose atorvastatin decreased USPIO-MRI detectable carotid plaque inflammation after only 12 weeks of statin pharmacotherapy (Figs 1A to G). Importantly, decreased inflammation correlated with fewer carotid emboli measured by transcutaneous Doppler.

[18]F-Fluorodeoxyglucose: The other major clinical atherosclerosis molecular imaging platform features [18]FDG-PET. [18]FDG is a glucose analog that becomes concentrated within metabolically active cells where it emits positrons (110 minute half life) for detection by clinical PET scanners. Intracellular concentration of [18]FDG occurs following active transport of the agent into the cytosol through normal glucose transport pathways where it becomes trapped upon phosphorylation by the enzyme hexokinase. Studies with [18]FDG have particularly become more prominent in recent years with the widespread availability of clinical [18]FDG-PET systems spurred by the growth of cancer imaging studies and the development of a broad radiopharmaceutical delivery network. Compared to USPIO-enhanced MRI, [18]FDG-PET is significantly more sensitive but must be coupled with coregistered CT (or other anatomical modality) to provide the high degree of spatial resolution required to enable precise tissue localization, which exposes the patient to additional ionizing radiation.

[18]FDG has been shown to be upregulated at inflammatory foci in the carotid and other larger arterial beds and correlates with monocyte/macrophage plaque content on histopathology.[17-21] Patients with the metabolic syndrome also

SECTION 3

Diagnosis

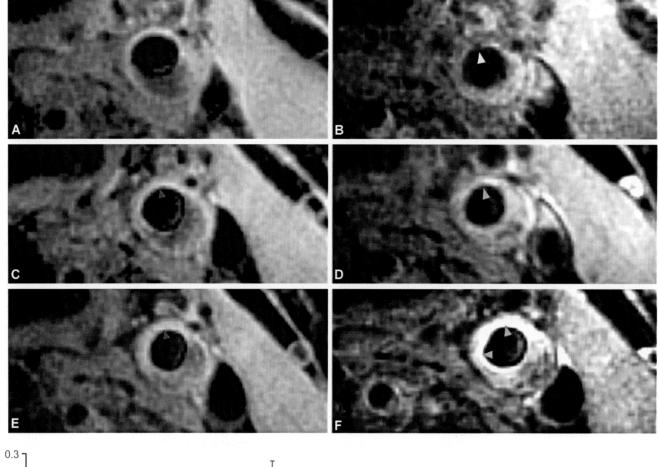

FIGURES 1A TO G: Clinical molecular MRI of low dose versus high dose statin effects on plaque inflammation. Representative T2-weighted images of the left common carotid artery during high-dose atorvastatin therapy before and after USPIO infusion at 0 week (A and B), 6 weeks (C and D) and 12 weeks (E and F). (B) Baseline USPIO signal (yellow arrowhead). (C and E) Pre-injection USPIO signal is similar across time points, signifying minimal tissue retention prior to each imaging session (red arrowhead). (D) By 6 weeks, there is enhancement of the atherosclerotic plaque (blue arrowhead) from a predominant T1 effect that suggests low-level USPIO deposition representing scant inflammation. (F) Following USPIO administration, plaque enhancement was observed without major signal voids (blue arrowheads). (G) Change in signal intensity (ΔSI) between low-dose (red line) and high-dose (dashed blue line) atorvastatin at baseline, 6 and 12 weeks with 95% confidence intervals (*Source:* Reference 16)

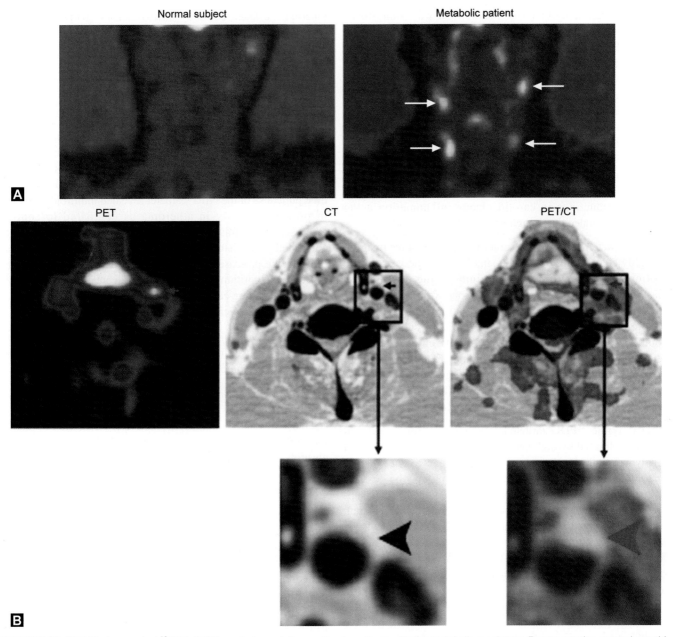

FIGURES 2A AND B: Augmented ^{18}FDG-PET-based plaque inflammation in patients with the metabolic syndrome. Representative coronal carotid artery ^{18}FDG-PET images from a patient with the metabolic syndrome and a control subject: (A) Red arrows identify areas of focal ^{18}FDG uptake; (B) Transaxial PET, contrast-enhanced CT and co-registered PET/CT images show ^{18}FDG signal (red arrowhead) in the carotid artery vessel wall (black arrowhead) of the metabolic syndrome patient. (*Source:* Reference 22)

demonstrate elevated ^{18}FDG signals in carotid atheroma (Figs 2A and B).[22] The prevalence of ^{18}FDG-identified carotid inflammation was further assessed in a series of 100 consecutive asymptomatic patients undergoing screening carotid ultrasonography. In patients with evidence of atherosclerosis (41%), approximately one-third had elevated ^{18}FDG uptake on PET/CT imaging, possibly identifying patients with inflamed plaques at a higher risk of future events.[23] Importantly for future application to clinical practice and trials, ^{18}FDG-PET/CT has demonstrated excellent reproducibility at least over the short term in a small series of high-risk patients.[24]

Pathophysiologically, human ^{18}FDG-PET imaging studies demonstrate greater uptake in patients with known vascular disease and primarily colocalize with non calcified, inflam-

matory loci.[25] Furthermore, not only upregulated expression of proinflammatory mRNA, particularly CD68, but also cathepsin K, matrix metalloproteinase (MMP-9) and interleukin (IL-18) are correlated with ^{18}FDG plaque uptake in ten carotid endarterectomy patients.[26] In multimodal carotid plaque studies, a report with ^{18}FDG-PET/MRI revealed that lipid-containing atheroma had greater ^{18}FDG uptake than collagen-rich fibromuscular or calcified plaques;[27] however, a separate investigation had only provided weak correlation between ^{18}FDG-PET signal and CT or MRI-guided plaque tissue composition.[28]

Recent clinical data has correlated ^{18}FDG plaque signals and future vascular events. In a retrospective 200 patient trial, the ^{18}FDG positive plaque number was correlated with the

CHAPTER 24 Molecular Imaging of Vascular Disease

number of cardiovascular risk factors, and was found to be inversely related to statin pharmacotherapy.[29] An observational [18]FDG-PET/CT trial in 932 asymptomatic cancer patients demonstrated that averaged [18]FDG signal uptake from the aorta, iliac and carotid arteries was the strongest indicator of a future vascular event over 29 months, notably being fourfold more predictive than atherosclerotic plaque calcification on co-registered CT images.[30] In a pharmacotherapeutic study, [18]FDG signal in human carotid plaques lessened over time with moderate dose simvastatin therapy, compared to dietary changes alone (Figs 3A to C).[31] Similar to the ATHEROMA study utilizing USPIOs, this study demonstrates the potential to assess reductions in carotid plaque inflammation using noninvasive molecular imaging.

Coronary arteries: Coronary atherosclerotic plaque imaging is highly challenging due to the small size of the vessels, the motion of surrounding myocardium during systole and diastole, as well as respirophasic variations. To overcome these challenges, imaging modalities must have both high spatial and temporal resolution, as well as high sensitivity, a combination not easily found in a single entity. However, several emerging technologies, including[18]FDG-PET/CT with myocardial suppression, macrophage-targeted molecular CT imaging and intravascular near infrared fluorescence (NIRF) imaging show promise for clinical investigation.

[18]FDG: While [18]FDG targeted imaging of coronary arterial plaques is limited by high background signal from the adjacent highly metabolically active myocardium, there is recent evidence that noninvasive coronary molecular imaging may be possible with [18]FDG-PET/CT utilizing a specialized myocardial suppression protocol.[7,32] To suppress the myocardial [18]FDG signal, patients consumed a high fat and low carbohydrate meal, the night before the study, and then drank a vegetable oil formulation on the morning of the study. While not all subjects obtained optimal myocardial suppression; however, in those with a good response, [18]FDG uptake was successfully observed in coronary artery segments. Patients with angiographically confirmed coronary artery disease tended to have more positive [18]FDG segments. Given the limitations of cardiac motion and lower resolution, it is envisioned that [18]FDG-PET imaging will assess the left main coronary artery and possibly the very proximal coronary arterial beds.

Molecular CT imaging: Macrophages can be targeted with N1177, an iodinated nanoparticle CT contrast agent dispersed with surfactant.[33,34] Atherosclerotic-prone rabbits subjected to aortic balloon-mediated injury demonstrated N1177 contrast enhancement within the injured aortic wall 2 hours after intravenous injection (Figs 4A to G). Comparison of N1177 signal with both [18]FDG-PET uptake in the same animals imaged one week later and histopathologic macrophage density showed general quantitative agreement. Given the excellent spatiotemporal resolution of modern multidetector CT imaging systems, already in clinical use for coronary artery imaging and the potential to discriminate atherosclerotic plaque constituents such as calcium versus fibrous tissue or lipid,[35,36] the addition of molecular targeted imaging agents, such as N1177 to coronary CT assessment, offers heightened ability to identify high-risk

macrophage-laden coronary atherosclerotic plaques that may prove future use in preventing ischemic events.

NIRF imaging: Intravascular molecular imaging technologies are also being advanced, exemplified by the development of a prototype intravascular catheter that allows real time, high resolution in vivo NIRF sensing of atherosclerotic plaque through flowing blood (Figs 5A to G).[3] Evaluation in atherosclerosis-laden rabbit iliac arteries, of similar size to human coronary vessels, was performed after intravenous administration of a cysteine protease-activatable NIRF imaging agent (ProSense750) that can detect vascular inflammation. Real time pullbacks of the NIRF catheter revealed multifold increases in protease activity in atheroma as compared to control atherosclerotic animals injected with saline. In vivo NIRF results correlated with histopathological macrophage infiltration and the cysteine protease cathepsin B. New detection and imaging processing algorithms[37], as well as the advent of novel 2D NIRF rotational imaging catheters[38] are likely to continue to improve the yield of this technique.

Additional promising preclinical molecular imaging strategies: Newer high sensitivity and novel agents are being developed at a rapid pace in preclinical studies.

Macrophages: A lipid-based gadolinium MRI probe shows strong affinity for the macrophage scavenger receptor-B (CD36), to enable noninvasive positive contrast MRI of plaque macrophages.[39] Agents with multimodality detection capabilities are becoming more prevalent, such as the trimodality nanoparticle for MRI, PET and NIRF detection of macrophages (Figs 6A to L).[4]

Proteases: There is also a particular focus on detecting enzymatic activity as a marker of active inflammatory changes and tissue destruction. In addition to cathepsin protease imaging, MMPs are frequently pursued targets on multiple platforms including an NIRF protease activity sensor,[40] a positive-contrast gadolinium chelate p947 for MRI[41,42] and the radionuclide SPECT tracers ^{111}In-RP782[43] and ^{99m}Tc-MMP.[44,45] Not only can MMP inflammatory activity be detected with these agents, but can also be measured over time following an intervention, such as that observed in hypercholesterolemic rabbits[44] and transgenic mice[45] where MMP-derived inflammation measured by ^{99m}Tc-MMP SPECT decreased with fluvastatin therapy or dietary modification. Customized enzymatic protease nanosensors (5–40 nm diameter) for optical molecular imaging have also been developed.[46]

Adhesion molecules: Endothelial surface glycoprotein receptors upregulated during inflammation, such as VCAM-1, E-selectin and P-selectin, have also been targeted using phage-display derived VCAM-1 specific nanoparticles (Figs 7A to H),[47] coated microbubbles for contrast-enhanced ultrasound,[48] iodine-containing liposomes conjugated to a receptor binding peptide with CT,[49] microparticles of iron oxide[50] and ^{18}F-labeled small affinity ligand.[51]

Cell tracking: Using adoptively transferred monocytes tagged with the clinical FDA-approved radionucleide tracer indium-111-oxyquinolone (^{111}In-oxine) and co-registered SPECT/CT

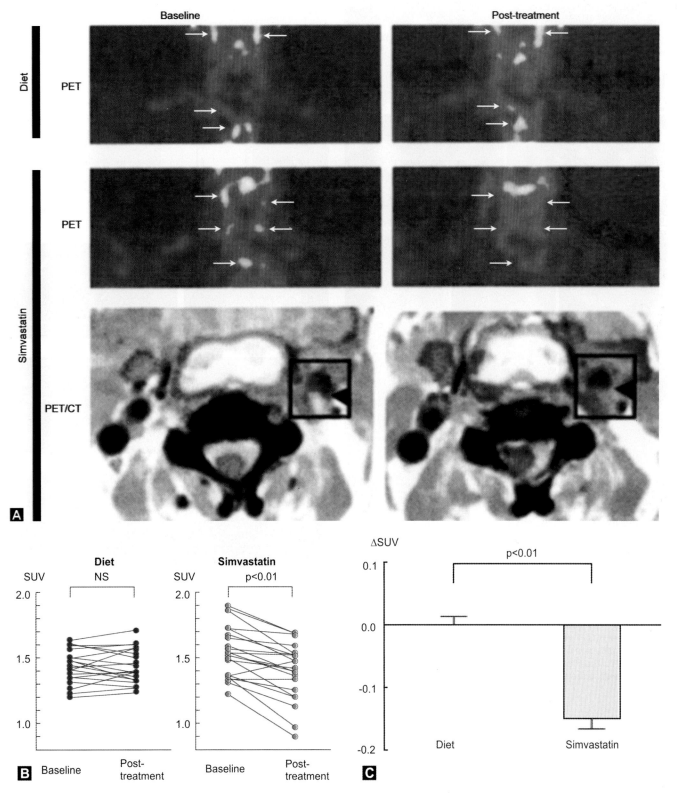

FIGURES 3A TO C: The effects of simvastatin therapy on atherosclerotic plaque inflammation assessed by serial [18]FDG-PET imaging. (A) Representative baseline images compared to post-treatment (3 months) showed no effect of altered diet alone on [18]FDG uptake (arrows, top images); however, simvastatin therapy diminished [18]FDG-detected plaque inflammation (middle images). Co-registered PET/CT identified areas of plaque [18]FDG disappearance after 3 months of simvastatin therapy (arrowheads, bottom images). (B) Quantitative anaylsis of [18]FDG plaque signal (average maximum standardized uptake values, SUVs) in individual subjects at baseline and after 3 months of simvastatin treatment. (C) Comparative change in plaque SUV from baseline demonstrated significant reductions with simvastatin therapy but not dietary modification alone. Bar = 1 SD (*Source:* Reference 31)

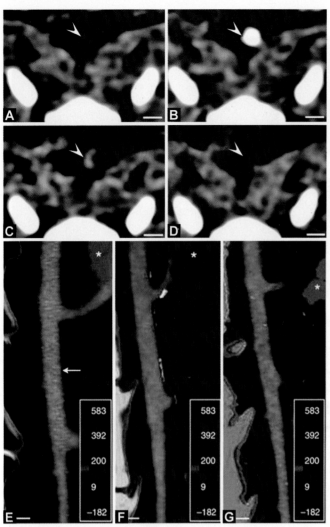

FIGURES 4A TO G: Molecular CT imaging of plaque inflammation in rabbits. Axial images of an aortic atherosclerotic plaque (white arrowheads) (A) before, (B) during and 2 hours following (C) N1177 nanoparticle administration or (D) a conventional contrast agent. Prior to contrast injection, the unvisualized atherosclerotic plaque becomes apparent once N1177 enhancement occurs, but is not seen with the conventional contrast agent. Color fusion image overlays onto the aortic plaques representing the density of vessel wall contrast enhancement demonstrated (E) focal regions of high signal intensity in atherosclerotic plaques after N1177 injection that was not observed with (F) a conventional contrast agent or (G) a non atherosclerotic control rabbit administered N1177. The insert shows the density color scale in HU. White asterisk identifies the spleen. Scale bar, 5 mm. (*Source:* Reference 33)

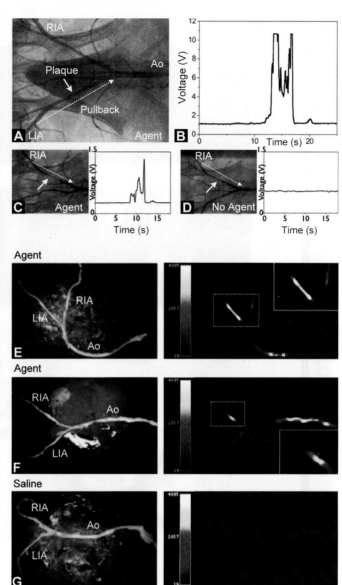

FIGURES 5A TO G: Atherosclerosis inflammation detected with in vivo real time NIR fluorescence intravascular sensing catheter. (A) Manual NIRF catheter pullback (trajectory defined by dotted arrow) in rabbit iliac arteries. (B and C) Protease-activatable NIRF activity following injection 24 hours before imaging, demonstrated significant fluorescence reporter activity (average TBR 6.8) at angiographically identified atheroma. (D) Saline injected control rabbits, exhibited significantly lower amplitude of NIRF signal. (E and F) Ex vivo arterial transmitted light and NIRF images revealed enhanced plaque protease fluorescence activity that was absent in (G) control animals that were administered saline (Abbreviations: RIA: Right iliac artery; LIA: Left iliac artery; Ao: Aorta). (*Source:* Reference 3)

molecular imaging, less monocyte trafficking to aortic plaques was observed in mice were treated with acute statin therapy.[52]

Oxidative Stress

The oxidation of phospholipids in atheroma contributes to the activation and recruitment of monocyte/macrophages and the production of enzymes, such as MMP, that degrade local tissue strength thus destabilizing plaque constituents. Detection of proinflammatory oxidative products by noninvasive molecular imaging may provide prospective information on the risk of individual plaques for future events or on the efficacy of therapeutics. Enzymatic detection agents for myeloperoxidase (MPO), a macrophage-derived product, have been evaluated by blue light bioluminescence using a small molecule luminol that activates fluorescence when oxidizing species are present,[53] as well as by MRI with the gadolinium agent bis-5HT-DTPA(Gd).[54] Another example of an oxidative species detection agent is gadolinium-retaining nanomicelles (20 nm diameter) with surface monoclonal antibodies that detect specific configurations of oxidized lipoproteins in atheroma.[55] Although presently untested, in the future combining information from oxidative stress imaging, in concert with more traditional macrophage or monocyte molecular imaging strategies, may bolster understanding of the underlying inflammatory state.

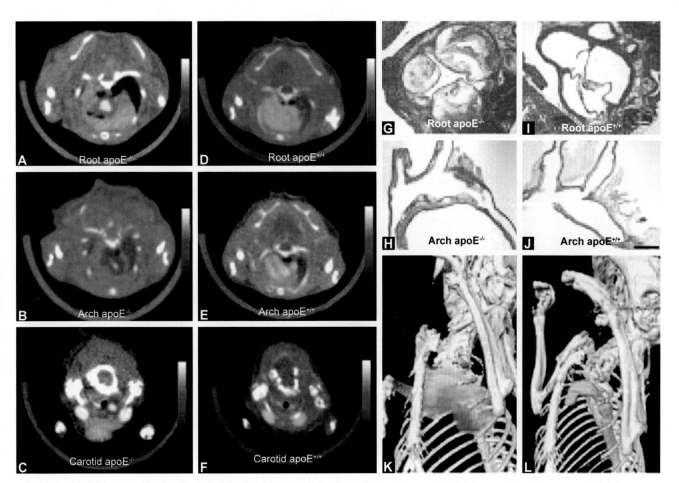

FIGURES 6A TO L: PET imaging of atherosclerotic plaque inflammation with a trimodality nanoparticle, ^{64}Cu-TNP. In atherosclerotic-prone ApoE$^{-/-}$ mice, ^{64}Cu-TNP PET imaging demonstrates enhancement in the (A) aortic root, (B) aortic arch and (C) carotid artery on co-registered CT fusion images identifying loci of inflammatory plaques. (D to F) On the contrary, wild type mice without atherosclerosis show no significant ^{64}Cu-TNP PET uptake. Hematoxylin and eosin histologic staining of excised aortas reveal advanced plaque burden in (G and H) ApoE$^{-/-}$ mice that is absent in (I and J) wild type controls (400 x magnification for G and I; 200 x magnification for H and J; bar 0.4 mm). Rendered three dimensional maximum intensity fused data set reconstructions show (K) proximal thoracic aorta (blue) focal ^{64}Cu-TNP PET signal (red) in ApoE$^{-/-}$ mice that is not seen in (L) control wild type mice. (*Source:* Reference 4)

Neovascularization

New vessel formation occurs during states where growth factors, such as vascular endothelial growth factor (VEGF) and others, are released stimulating endothelial and other supporting cells to create new blood channels. Endothelial cells organizing into interconnected vascular tubes and networks are anchored to extracellular matrix proteins in part through expression of the $\alpha_V\beta_3$ integrin surface receptor, a common target for neovascularization molecular imaging studies. While in certain clinical scenarios angiogenesis can be beneficial, such as myocardial preconditioning from ischemia-reperfusion injury, in atherosclerotic disease, neovascularization highlights underlying plaque instability where it may promote intraplaque hemorrhage. Although clinical neovascularization studies have not been performed, a number of promising agents have been preclinically tested, including many agents for integrin $\alpha_V\beta_3$, which can be detected by the peptide sequence RGD or RGD mimetics. Noninvasive plaque angiogenesis imaging was initially shown with paramagnetic integrin $\alpha_V\beta_3$-targeted agents for MRI.[56] Other approaches include PET imaging with ^{18}F labeling[57] or ^{76}Br on a degradable nanoparticle shell.[58]

Other, novel agents, such as gadofluorine-M for MRI, have been developed.[59]

Plaque neovascularization is one area within cardiovascular molecular imaging in which investigators have formulated agents that have the capability for both diagnostic detection and therapeutic purposes, a strategy termed "theranostics". One such agent was created by combining the endothelial mycotoxin fumagillin with an angiogenesis-specific magnetic nanoparticle, $\alpha_V\beta_3$-MNP that targets the $\alpha_V\beta_3$ integrin receptor and contains gadolinium for MRI detection.[5,56] In an atherosclerosis rabbit study,[60] administration of the fumagillin theranostic nanoparticle followed by serial MR imaging over 4 weeks with the diagnostic $\alpha_V\beta_3$-MNP demonstrated significantly diminished neovascularization in the animals treated with the theranostic agent compared to controls. In comparison, atorvastatin pharmacotherapy without administration of the fumagillin theranostic nanoparticle did not reduce angiogenesis, but in combination helped sustain the fumagillin effect. The ability to diagnose, monitor and treat a diseased state with a single injectable agent demonstrates the potential power of a theranostic molecular imaging approach, a strategy that will undoubtedly gain increased attention with the

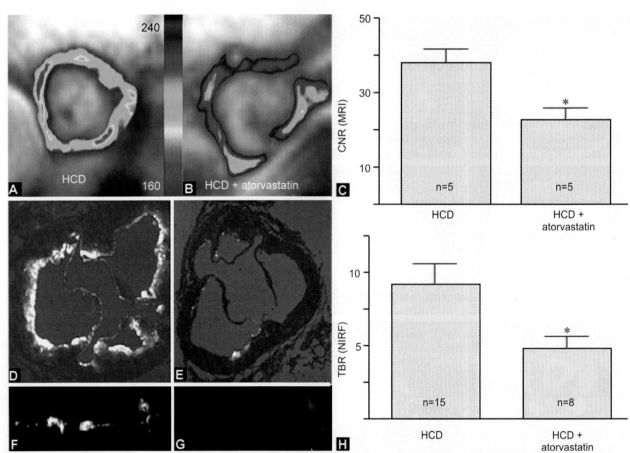

FIGURES 7A TO H: MRI detection of VCAM-1 expression on activated endothelial cells and the effects of statin therapy. VINP-28 injection, which targets endothelial VCAM-1 expression, revealed enhancement (color scale: red maximum and blue minimum signal) in the aortic root (short axis images) of (A) hypercholesterolemic ApoE$^{-/-}$ mice that was lessened in (B) an atorvastatin treated cohort. (C) Quantitative contrast-to-noise ratio (CNR) comparison demonstrated a significant reduction in atorvastatin treated mice compared to untreated controls (mean ± SD; P < 0.05 vs HCD). (D and E) Aortic root NIRF microscopy of the sections depicted in panels A and B show circumferential plaque VINP-28 fluorescence that was greater in non-atorvastatin fed mice. Fluorescence reflectance imaging in excised aortic specimens of (F) controls demonstrated greater NIRF signal than (G) atorvastatin treated mice, which correlated with (H) target-to-background ratios (TBR; mean ± SD; P < 0.05 vs HCD). (*Source:* Reference 47)

development of next generation clinical agents. Furthermore, theranostic strategies have the potential to locally deliver drugs at a fraction of the required systemic dose, limiting nonspecific tissue toxicity.

Apoptosis

Programmed cell death or apoptosis contributes to weakening of the fibrous cap via smooth muscle cell loss and facilitates expansion of the unstable lipid-filled necrotic core. Molecular signaling markers can identify cells destined for apoptotic demise, via annexin protein binding to exposed phosphatidylserine residues or via components of the caspase enzyme family that activate and execute the apoptotic cascade. The most widely utilized annexin-based imaging agents for apoptosis detection are high sensitivity SPECT-based tracers, such as ^{99m}Tc-annexin and ^{111}In-annexin, and can be combined with other readouts such as [18]FDG-derived inflammation[61] or MMP presence.[62] Inhibition studies with caspase blocking agents in atherosclerotic rabbits that diminish histologic plaque apoptosis have demonstrated the ability of ^{99m}Tc-annexin A5 SPECT imaging to discriminate between regions of different apoptotic activity.[63] Imaging of apoptosis has yielded insights into the

salutary benefit of statin therapy in atherosclerosis (Figs 8A and B).[62] Optical imaging with fluorescently labeled caspases have been developed with the opportunity for NIRF or preclinical FMT imaging applications.[64]

In a limited number of patients with transient ischemic attacks scheduled for carotid endarterectomy, ^{99m}Tc-annexin A5 SPECT imaging has illuminated the relationship between apoptotic activity and carotid plaque instability (Figs 9A to D).[65] ^{99m}Tc-annexin A5 SPECT signal was detectable only in those patients with recent clinical events (within 4 days), where it localized to the culprit lesion. In comparison, subjects with remote transient ischemic attacks had no significant carotid ^{99m}Tc-annexin A5 uptake, nor did the non-cuprit stenotic contralateral carotid lesions in patients with recent events. Postoperative immunohistopathologic specimens confirmed increased tissue macrophage content and hemorrhage associated with enhanced macrophage annexin A5-binding suggesting accelerated local apoptosis.

Calcification

Vascular calcification is increasingly linked to chronic vascular inflammation, likely representing the terminal phase of

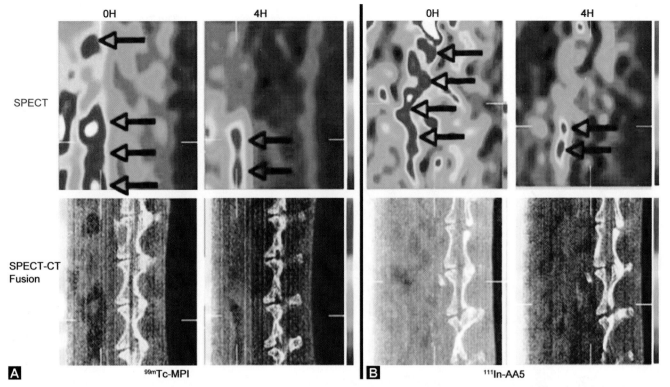

FIGURES 8A AND B: SPECT radionuclide imaging of atherosclerotic plaque MMP activity and apoptosis. Serial dual-target micro-SPECT radionuclide imaging of (A) matrix metalloproteinase (MMP) activity via the tracer ^{99m}Tc-MPI and (B) apoptosis with ^{111}In-Annexin (AA5) in atherosclerotic prone rabbits demonstrated aortic plaque target localization at 4 hours (arrows, right panels) following blood pool agent washout (left panels). The top panels show SPECT radiotracer uptake and the bottom panels SPECT-CT fusion images. (*Source:* Reference 62)

inflammatory lesions. In atherosclerosis, microcalcifications within plaques portend a greater risk for rupture and on a larger scale global coronary calcium scoring correlates with risk of future cardiovascular events. Another commonly encountered clinical scenario is calcification of the heart valves and supporting structures, such as aortic stenosis, which has many histopathological similarities to atherosclerosis and results in considerable cardiovascular morbidity and mortality particularly in an aging global population. The mechanisms of calcification in these disease states remain poorly understood as evidenced by the lack of effective nonsurgical management options, offering excellent opportunities for further research with in vivo molecular imaging. Currently available probes include optical agents such as fluorescently labeled enzymes substrates that identify the bone mineral component hydroxyapatite.[66]

The mechanism of bone mineral deposition in atherosclerotic calcification has been explored in molecular imaging studies of hypercholesterolemic mice with surgically induced renal failure to accelerate osteogenesis.[67] Using multichannel intravital fluorescence molecular imaging with a fluorescent quenched substrate for cathepsin S (CatS) and an optical bone mineral targeting agent (osteosense), the time course of enzymatic protease activity and bone deposition in arterial vascular and aortic valvular calcification was evaluated. Optical molecular imaging signals were then correlated with coinjected fluorescent USPIO nanoparticles that identified plaque macrophages. Results have demonstrated that the extent of calcification correspond to CatS activity. Mice deficient in CatS had less calcification but similar atherosclerotic plaque size, suggesting

that CatS mediated tissue elastin peptide degradation contributed to local mineralization. A similar intravital microscopic study in the carotid plaques of atherosclerotic prone mice coinjected with NIRF, USPIOs and osteosense illustrated that macrophage infiltration and subsequent local inflammatory changes occurred prior to tissue osteogenesis and that bone mineral activity could be detected prior to histological or CT evidence of calcification (Figs 10A and B).[68]

THROMBOSIS

While the activation of circulating plasma clotting factors and platelets is key to vascular hemostasis and repair following tissue injury, arterial and venous thrombosis syndromes are worldwide leading causes of cardiovascular morbidity and mortality. Molecular imaging of key thrombus-associated molecules and cells has the potential to biologically refine anatomical imaging methods such as ultrasound or CT. Moreover, molecular imaging strategies may provide additional guidance into optimal therapeutic strategies to treat fibrin-rich or platelet-rich thrombi. Other advantages include the ability to replace invasive thrombosis imaging strategies with noninvasive options. For example, intracardiac thrombus formation, as may occur in the atrial appendage from atrial fibrillation, often requires transesophageal echocardiography for diagnosis. Another clinical arena of importance is arteriolar thrombosis syndromes, where flow-based diagnostic methods may be limited due to spatial resolution and possibly nephrotoxic contrast material and radiation exposure. The diagnosis

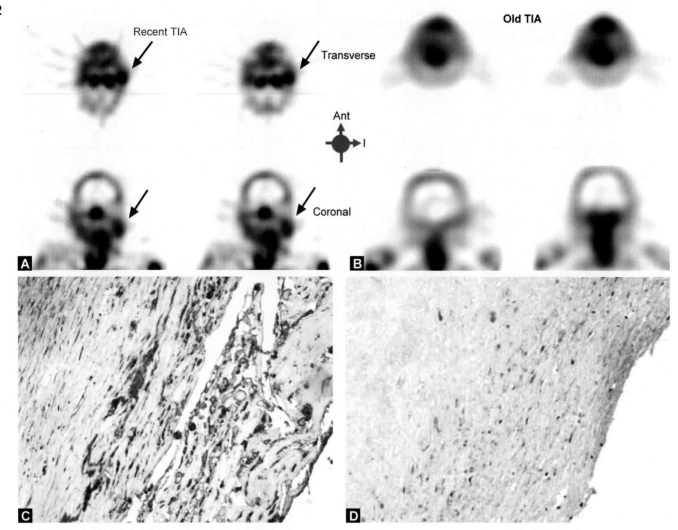

FIGURES 9A TO D: Clinical SPECT imaging of carotid plaque apoptosis in four patients with recent or remote TIA. (A) The apoptosis-targeted sensor ⁹⁹ᵐTc-annexin A5 was injected and was found to accumulate in the carotid lesion of a patient with recent TIA. (B) Immunohistochemical annexin A5 staining was pronounced in the surgically resected plaques (400 x magnification). A patient with remote TIA, in contrast had (C) minimal ⁹⁹ᵐTc-annexin A5 carotid plaque uptake and (D) annexin A5 immunochemical signal that was similar to background nonspecific staining. (Abbreviations: Ant: Anterior; L: Left). (*Source:* Reference 91)

of new thrombi over prior existing thrombi is also challenging for anatomic imaging methods and represents another opportunity for molecular imaging of thorombosis. Furthermore, subclinical arterial thrombi which may be present in unstable carotid or aortic plaques following recent non occlusive rupture or intraplaque hemorrhage can be difficult to detect due to small size and surrounding complex plaque constituents such as calcium-related artifact in CT scans that obscures local tissue contrast. The development of specific molecular imaging markers of arterial and venous thrombosis has the potential to improve detection characteristics in each of these categories and diminish patient-specific risks, facilitating serial imaging studies that can visually document thrombus resolution following definitive therapy.

Clinical Imaging of Fibrin-Rich Thrombi

Of the molecular imaging thrombosis detection agents in development, the fibrin-targeted peptide EP-2104R has completed a multicenter phase II human clinical trial.[69,70] The EP-2104R peptide has been derivatized with four gadolinium molecules per peptide, providing signal amplification necessary for MRI detection. Prior to clinical studies, the EP-2104R agent underwent extensive preclinical evaluation, and showed a high degree of specificity and robustness for fibrin imaging.[71-75] In patients with recently identified venous (n = 14) or arterial (n = 38) thrombi, the administration of EP-2104R followed by a 2–6 hour imaging agent blood pool washout delay prior to MRI resulted in increased thrombus detection at areas of gadolinium enhancement that were not apparent on non-contrast imaging studies. While there were very few reported adverse reactions to EP-2104R and the total gadolinium dose was significantly less than typical clinical MRI studies, a majority of venous (71%) and many arterial (16%) thrombi were undetected by EP-2104R, possibly secondary to impaired penetration of the agent into more organized and contracted thrombi. With additional optimization of dose and imaging parameters, EP-2104R has clinical potential to detect thrombi

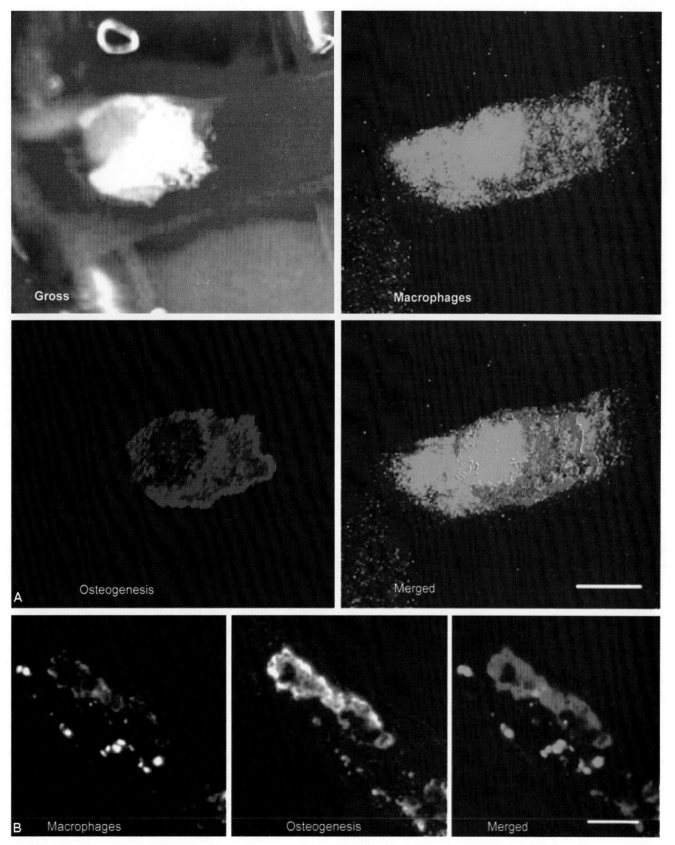

FIGURES 10A AND B: Multichannel NIRF image of macrophages and osteogenesis in murine atherosclerosis. (A and B) ApoE$^{-/-}$ mice with heavily calcified carotid artery atherosclerotic plaques demonstrated correlative gross morphology with intravital fluorescence microscopy of calcification (red) and macrophages (green). Merged fluorescence images show exclusion of macrophages from calcified regions and vice versa. Scale bar, 200 μm. (*Source:* Reference 68)

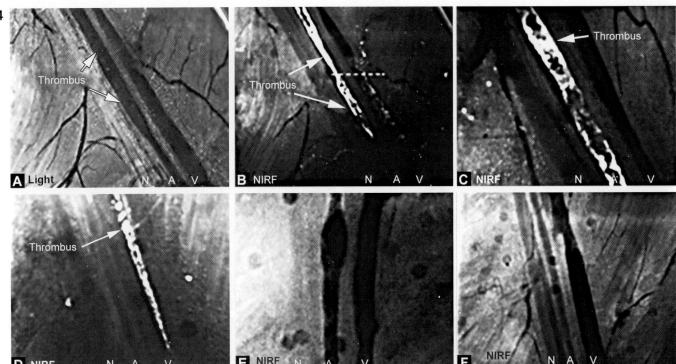

FIGURES 11A TO F: In vivo molecular imaging of activated transglutaminase FXIII (FXIIIa) via intravital epifluorescence microscopy. (A) Light image reveals dark clots (arrows) within the murine femoral vessels following ferric chloride chemical injury. (B) The FXIIIa targeted optical agent A15 was injected into mice harboring femoral thrombi. NIRF imaging at 82 minutes postinjection shows high TBRs in the arterial and venous vessels (arrows). The dashed line identifies a tissue region used for immunohistopathology (not shown). (C) On higher magnification of another A15-enhanced arterial thrombus (62 minute after injection), greater NIRF signal was observed at the thrombus margins and interface with the vessel wall. (D) A15 NIRF signal was also detected in venous thrombi (83 minute postinjection), but (E) not in older clots (72 minute after injection but 28 hours after thrombus induction), consistent with a time-dependent decrease in FXIIIa activity. (F) NIRF imaging of thrombi after administration of a control agent (AF680 fluorochrome) had minimal thrombus enhancement. (Abbreviations: N: Nerve; A: Artery; V: Vein). (*Source:* Reference 76)

through molecular MRI of fibrin, providing a more specific molecular alternative to current flow-based thrombosis diagnostic imaging methods such as ultrasound and contrast-enhanced CT and MRI.

Preclinical Thrombus Imaging Strategies

Additional preclinical thrombus detection agents targeting both blood clotting factors and platelet receptors are in development for a range of imaging platforms including optical, radionuclide imaging and MRI. Activated transglutaminase factor XIII (FXIIIa) is one example; a circulating clotting factor found within acute thrombi, where it protects against fibrinolysis by cross-linking fibrin strands and α2-antiplasmin into the growing clot. Intravital fluorescence microscopy (IVFM) studies demonstrated the ability of an NIRF FXIIIa-targeted agent to distinguish acute from subacute thrombi (Figs 11A to F)[76] and to evaluate cerebral sinus vein thrombosis.[77] By linking gadolinium and the fluorophore rhodamine to an oligopeptide sequence based on the amino terminus of α2-antiplasmin, a dual platform MRI and optical FXIIIa targeted agent was developed and then validated in a murine chemically induced carotid arterial thrombosis model to identify acute thrombi (90 min after induction), but not more established clots (24–48 hour old).[78] Platelet imaging, which preferentially identifies arterial clots that are relatively platelet-

rich compared to venous thrombi, has been established through binding to the surface glycoprotein IIb/IIIa receptor in its activated state with 1 μm diameter microparticles of iron oxide for MRI linked to a single chain monoclonal antibody (Figs 12A to C),[79] as well as by direct fluorescence labeling for NIRF imaging.[80] Serial MRI after non occlusive arterial thrombus formation demonstrated the feasibility of noninvasive monitoring of thrombolysis with this platelet-sensitive agent. Lastly, an optical sensor for thrombin activity imaging in acute thrombi has been evaluated using NIRF imaging.[81]

ANEURYSM

While aneurysms affect multiple arterial beds of varying size and wall thickness, including small intracranial vessels and the large thoracoabdominal aorta, they are similarly characterized by vessel wall weakening and lumen expansion driven by local inflammatory changes and its subsequent byproducts, with the potential for acute rupture and blood content extravasation. Often aneurysmal disease shares many of the same hallmark pathological features as atherosclerosis, which from a molecular imaging standpoint enables significant overlap in the available probes and detection strategies. In particular, inflammation and neovascularization, two important local processes that potentiate aneurysm formation, have been tested with molecular imaging strategies providing useful insight into this vascular disease process.

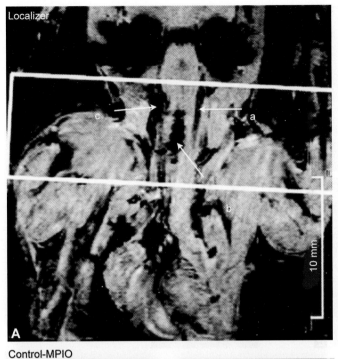

FIGURES 12A TO C: Molecular MRI of activated platelets in acute arterial thrombi. (A) Scout image for localizing imaging planes and anatomic landmarks including the (a) non injured left carotid artery, (b) trachea and (c) injured right carotid artery. (B and C) Transverse preinjection MR images show the injured right carotid artery (red circle) with non-occlusive thrombosis adherent to the vessel wall. The noninjured left carotid artery (green circle) serves as a negative control in all images. Sequential image sequences taken at 12, 48 and 72 minutes following injection of either control or activated platelet glycoprotein IIb/IIIa receptor targeted (LIBS) microparticles of iron oxide (MPIO) demonstrates an increasing signal void at the injured carotid site indicating LIBS MPIO binding and the induction of T2-weighted susceptibility artifact. (*Source:* Reference 79)

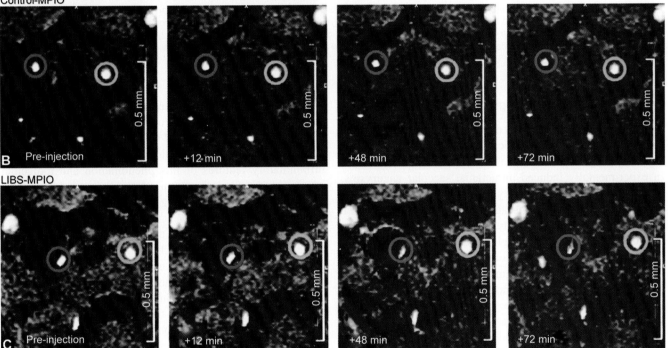

Clinical Aneurysm Inflammation Imaging

The use of [18]FDG-PET is an attractive clinical approach to investigate inflammation in aneurysms.[82] Inflammation as a predictor of aneursymal expansion has been evaluated in small-sized human trials. One recent study on 14 male patients with advanced infrarenal abdominal aortic aneurysms (AAA) undergoing surveillance imaging had demonstrated that [18]FDG uptake was highest in those that also had CT evidence of inflammatory changes, although there was no correlation with vessel diameter or recent expansion.[83] However, a case report of an asymptomatic patient with an incidentally discovered but rapidly expanding AAA had demonstrated areas of markedly increased [18]FDG uptake on serial PET/CT hybrid imaging studies (Figs 13A to E). At surgery, these areas were associated with microscopic collagen and elastin degradation, enhanced MMP expression and increased macrophage number.[84] Conversely, areas of low [18]FDG uptake had less histologic tissue inflammation and remodeling, suggesting that there may be AAA subsets that demonstrate detectable increases in [18]FDG-derived inflammatory signal as the aneurysms progress clinically. Given its clinical availability, [18]FDG-PET readouts of inflammation are well positioned to inform the risk of AAA expansion and rupture.

CHAPTER 24

Molecular Imaging of Vascular Disease

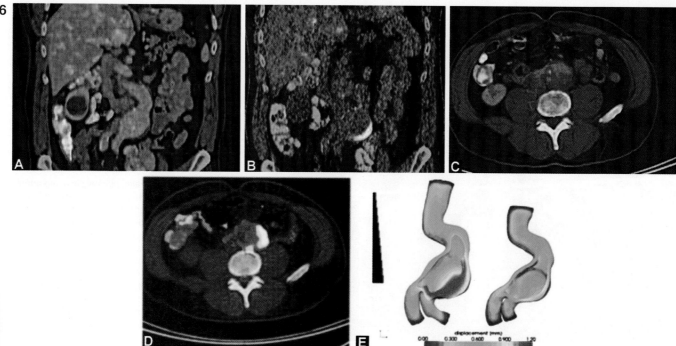

FIGURES 13A TO E: [18]FDG-PET imaging of metabolism/inflammation in a patient with an expanding abdominal aortic aneurysm. (A and C) [18]FDG-PET/CT images in the coronal and axial planes of the aneurysm at (A and C) baseline and (B and D) 6 months later. The red arrow indicates maximal glycolytic activity. (E) Three dimensional reconstruction with wall displacement of the smaller baseline aneurysm (left) and larger aneurysm observed at follow-up (right). The color scale identifies high (red) or low (blue) vessel wall displacement. (*Source:* Reference 84)

Preclinical Aneurysm Imaging Investigations

Preclinical studies have utilized many similar imaging strategies also examined for atherosclerotic disease in experimental animal models of large vessel inflammation and aneurysm formation. In experimentally induced intracranial saccular aneurysms, gadolinium-based MPO enzymatic activity representing oxidative stress has been visualized on a clinical strength 3T MRI scanner.[85] In another study, aneurysm neovascularization was assessed using optical imaging and a VEGF-specific probe labeled with an NIR fluorochrome. The VEGF tissue fluorescence in aneurysmal segments correlated positively with AAA diameter measured by ultrasound.[86] Recently endovascular imaging of inflammation in aneurysm disease was performed using NIRF imaging of MMP activity.[87] Additional translation of these and similar agents adopted from atherosclerosis studies will continue to aid in understanding of markers of aneurysm progression that can be utilized clinically to risk stratify those patients who may benefit from more aggressive early surgical or endovascular intervention.

VASCULAR INJURY

Injury of the vessel wall results in a local inflammatory response and smooth muscle cell hyperproliferation similar to atherosclerosis, leading to the formation of a pronounced neointima that progressively impacts oxygenated blood passage. In severe cases, the obstruction to blood movement becomes flow-limiting and causes downstream tissue ischemia and the development of associated symptoms. Diseases such as graft arteriosclerosis, in-stent restenosis and diabetic vasculopathies are characterized by this type of exaggerated neointimal expansion. Vascular injury models typically employing mechanical arterial wall insult with metal catheter guidewires or angioplasty balloons recapitulate many of the inflammatory features of this phenomenon and molecular imaging technologies are poised to allow tracking of the inflammatory and remodeling response over time as these lesions mature.

Due to the dependence of the vascular injury response on tissue remodeling, enzymes, such as MMPs, are prime molecular imaging targets, as they hasten extracellular matrix degradation to promote enhanced fibromuscular cell migration into the developing neointima. SPECT imaging of broad-spectrum MMP activity with ^{111}In-RP782 in the injured carotid arteries of atherosclerotic mice had demonstrated increased MMP signal within weeks of the insult, which correlated positively with the degree of hyperplastic neointimal expansion.[43] Importantly, the contralateral, sham-treated carotid artery showed no significant ^{111}In-RP782 signal uptake. Another ^{111}In labeled-probe, RP748 can identify activated $\alpha_V\beta_3$ integrin expression as a marker of neointimal vascular cell proliferation and has tracked angiogenesis within the expanding vessel wall.[88-91] The development of real-time intravascular catheters for optical NIRF probe detection of fluorescent enzymatic reporters that mark tissue injury and remodeling holds significant promise for clinical translation,[3,38] which in concert with advances in imaging processing protocols, such as normalization algorithms that reduce confounding blood pool fluorescence attenuation,[37] should accelerate the capability of this technology toward imaging of coronary stent-induced vascular injury.

OUTLOOK

Molecular imaging studies are yielding unparalleled in vivo insight into clinical aspects of vascular disease, including atherosclerosis, thrombosis, aneurysm formation and vascular injury. Clinical development of high-yield molecular imaging agents and the development of coronary-artery targeted imaging systems remain top priorities for the field. Preclinically, the emphasis remains on developing new highly sensitive, multifunctional/multimodal imaging agents with excellent safety and pharmacokinetic profiles. For molecular imaging to integrate into routine clinical practice, clear utility beyond functional and anatomical imaging will need to be established. In the near term, molecular imaging will likely assess the biological effects of new pharmacotherapies aimed to mitigate vascular disease. Thereafter, molecular imaging should improve the risk stratification and the clinical management of many vascular disease states.

ACKNOWLEDGMENT

NIH R01 HL 108229, American Heart Association Scientist Development Grant #0830352N, Howard Hughes Medical Institute Career Development Award.

REFERENCES

1. Jaffer FA, Libby P, Weissleder R. Molecular imaging of cardiovascular disease. Circulation. 2007;116:1052-61.
2. Sanz J, Fayad ZA. Imaging of atherosclerotic cardiovascular disease. Nature. 2008;451:953-7.
3. Jaffer FA, Vinegoni C, John MC, et al. Real-time catheter molecular sensing of inflammation in proteolytically active atherosclerosis. Circulation. 2008;118:1802-9.
4. Nahrendorf M, Zhang H, Hembrador S, et al. Nanoparticle PET-CT imaging of macrophages in inflammatory atherosclerosis. Circulation. 2008;117:379-87.
5. Winter PM, Neubauer AM, Caruthers SD, et al. Endothelial alpha(v)beta3 integrin-targeted fumagillin nanoparticles inhibit angiogenesis in atherosclerosis. Arteriosclerosis, Thrombosis, and Vascular Biology. 2006;26:2103-9.
6. Judenhofer MS, Wehrl HF, Newport DF, et al. Simultaneous PET-MRI: a new approach for functional and morphological imaging. Nat Med. 2008;14:459-65.
7. Wykrzykowska J, Lehman S, Williams G, et al. Imaging of inflamed and vulnerable plaque in coronary arteries with 18F-FDG PET/CT in patients with suppression of myocardial uptake using a low-carbohydrate, high-fat preparation. Journal of Nuclear Medicine. 2009;50:563-8.
8. Libby P. Inflammation in atherosclerosis. Nature. 2002;420:868-74.
9. Burke AP, Farb A, Malcom GT, et al. Coronary risk factors and plaque morphology in men with coronary disease who died suddenly. N Engl J Med. 1997;336:1276-82.
10. Kooi ME, Cappendijk VC, Cleutjens KBJM, et al. Accumulation of ultrasmall superparamagnetic particles of iron oxide in human atherosclerotic plaques can be detected by in vivo magnetic resonance imaging. Circulation. 2003;107:2453-8.
11. Trivedi RA, U-King-Im J-M, Graves MJ, et al. In vivo detection of macrophages in human carotid atheroma: temporal dependence of ultrasmall superparamagnetic particles of iron oxide-enhanced MRI. Stroke. 2004;35:1631-5.
12. Trivedi RA, Mallawarachi C, U-King-Im J-M, et al. Identifying inflamed carotid plaques using in vivo USPIO-enhanced MR imaging to label plaque macrophages. Arteriosclerosis, Thrombosis, and Vascular Biology. 2006;26:1601-6.
13. Tang T, Howarth SP, Miller SR, et al. Assessment of inflammatory burden contralateral to the symptomatic carotid stenosis using high-resolution ultrasmall, superparamagnetic iron oxide-enhanced MRI. Stroke. 2006;37:2266-70.
14. Tang TY, Howarth SP, Miller SR, et al. Correlation of carotid atheromatous plaque inflammation using USPIO-enhanced MR imaging with degree of luminal stenosis. Stroke. 2008;39:2144-7.
15. Larose E, Yeghiazarians Y, Libby P, et al. Characterization of human atherosclerotic plaques by intravascular magnetic resonance imaging. Circulation. 2005;112:2324-31.
16. Tang TY, Howarth SPS, Miller SR, et al. The ATHEROMA (Atorvastatin Therapy: Effects on Reduction of Macrophage Activity) Study. Evaluation using ultrasmall superparamagnetic iron oxide-enhanced magnetic resonance imaging in carotid disease. Journal of the American College of Cardiology. 2009;53:2039-50.
17. Rudd JHF, Warburton EA, Fryer TD, et al. Imaging atherosclerotic plaque inflammation with [18F]-fluorodeoxyglucose positron emission tomography. Circulation. 2002;105:2708-11.
18. Yun M, Jang S, Cucchiara A, et al. 18F FDG uptake in the large arteries: a correlation study with the atherogenic risk factors. Semin Nucl Med. 2002;32:70-6.
19. Tatsumi M, Cohade C, Nakamoto Y, et al. Fluorodeoxyglucose uptake in the aortic wall at PET/CT: possible finding for active atherosclerosis. Radiology. 2003;229:831-7.
20. Davies JR, Rudd JHF, Fryer TD, et al. Identification of culprit lesions after transient ischemic attack by combined 18F fluorodeoxyglucose positron-emission tomography and high-resolution magnetic resonance imaging. Stroke. 2005;36:2642-7.
21. Tawakol A, Migrino RQ, Bashian GG, et al. In vivo 18F-fluorodeoxyglucose positron emission tomography imaging provides a noninvasive measure of carotid plaque inflammation in patients. J Am Coll Cardiol. 2006;48:1818-24.
22. Tahara N, Kai H, Yamagishi S, et al. Vascular inflammation evaluated by [18F]-fluorodeoxyglucose positron emission tomography is associated with the metabolic syndrome. J Am Coll Cardiol. 2007;49:1533-9.
23. Tahara N, Kai H, Nakaura H, et al. The prevalence of inflammation in carotid atherosclerosis: analysis with fluorodeoxyglucose-positron emission tomography. Eur Heart J. 2007;28:2243-8.
24. Rudd J, Myers K, Bansilal S, et al. 18 Fluorodeoxyglucose positron emission tomography imaging of atherosclerotic plaque inflammation is highly reproducible implications for atherosclerosis therapy trials. Journal of the American College of Cardiology. 2007;50:892-6.
25. Rudd JHF, Myers KS, Bansilal S, et al. Relationships among regional arterial inflammation, calcification, risk factors, and biomarkers: a prospective fluorodeoxyglucose positron-emission tomography/computed tomography imaging study. Circulation: Cardiovascular Imaging. 2009;2:107-15.
26. Graebe M, Pedersen SF, Borgwardt L, et al. Molecular pathology in vulnerable carotid plaques: correlation with [18]-fluorodeoxyglucose positron emission tomography (FDG-PET). Eur J Vasc Endovasc Surg. 2009;37:714-21.
27. Silvera SS, Aidi He, Rudd JHF, et al. Multimodality imaging of atherosclerotic plaque activity and composition using FDG-PET/CT and MRI in carotid and femoral arteries. Atherosclerosis. 2009;207:139-43.
28. Kwee RM, Teule GJJ, van Oostenbrugge RJ, et al. Multimodality imaging of carotid artery plaques: 18 F-fluoro-2-deoxyglucose positron emission tomography, computed tomography, and magnetic resonance imaging. Stroke. 2009;40:3718-24.
29. Wasselius JA, Larsson SA, Jacobsson H. FDG-accumulating atherosclerotic plaques identified with 18F-FDG-PET/CT in 141 patients. Mol Imaging Biol. 2009;11:455-9.
30. Rominger A, Saam T, Wolpers S, et al. 18F-FDG PET/CT identifies patients at risk for future vascular events in an otherwise asymptomatic cohort with neoplastic disease. J Nucl Med. 2009;50:1611-20.

31. Tahara N, Kai H, Ishibashi M, et al. Simvastatin attenuates plaque inflammation: evaluation by fluorodeoxyglucose positron emission tomography. J Am Coll Cardiol. 2006;48:1825-31.

32. Rogers IS, Nasir K, Figueroa AL, et al. Feasibility of FDG imaging of the coronary arteries: comparison between acute coronary syndrome and stable angina. JACC Cardiovasc Imaging. 2010;3:388-97.

33. Hyafil F, Cornily J, Feig J, et al. Noninvasive detection of macrophages using a nanoparticulate contrast agent for computed tomography. Nat Med. 2007;13:636-41.

34. Hyafil F, Cornily J-C, Rudd JHF, et al. Quantification of inflammation within rabbit atherosclerotic plaques using the macrophage-specific CT contrast agent N1177: a comparison with 18F-FDG PET/CT and histology. Journal of Nuclear Medicine. 2009;50:959-65.

35. Miller JM, Rochitte CE, Dewey M, et al. Diagnostic performance of coronary angiography by 64-row CT. N Engl J Med. 2008;359:2324-36.

36. Brodoefel H, Burgstahler C, Sabir A, et al. Coronary plaque quantification by voxel analysis: dual-source MDCT angiography versus intravascular sonography. AJR Am J Roentgenol. 2009;192:W84-9.

37. Sheth RA, Tam JM, Maricevich MA, et al. Quantitative endovascular fluorescence-based molecular imaging through blood of arterial wall inflammation. Radiology. 2009;251:813-21.

38. Razansky RN, Rosenthal A, Mallas G, et al. Near-infrared fluorescence catheter system for two-dimensional intravascular imaging in vivo. Opt Express. 2010;18:11372-81.

39. Lipinski MJ, Frias JC, Amirbekian V, et al. Macrophage-specific lipid-based nanoparticles improve cardiac magnetic resonance detection and characterization of human atherosclerosis. JACC Cardiovasc Imaging. 2009;2:637-47.

40. Deguchi JO, Aikawa M, Tung C-H, et al. Inflammation in atherosclerosis: visualizing matrix metalloproteinase action in macrophages in vivo. Circulation. 2006;114:55-62.

41. Lancelot E, Amirbekian V, Brigger I, et al. Evaluation of matrix metalloproteinases in atherosclerosis using a novel noninvasive imaging approach. Arteriosclerosis, Thrombosis, and Vascular Biology. 2008;28:425-32.

42. Amirbekian V, Aguinaldo JGS, Amirbekian S, et al. Atherosclerosis and matrix metalloproteinases: experimental molecular MR imaging in vivo. Radiology. 2009;251:429-38.

43. Zhang J, Nie L, Razavian M, et al. Molecular imaging of activated matrix metalloproteinases in vascular remodeling. Circulation. 2008;118:1953-60.

44. Fujimoto S, Hartung D, Ohshima S, et al. Molecular imaging of matrix metalloproteinase in atherosclerotic lesions: resolution with dietary modification and statin therapy. Journal of the American College of Cardiology. 2008;52:1847-57.

45. Ohshima S, Petrov A, Fujimoto S, et al. Molecular imaging of matrix metalloproteinase expression in atherosclerotic plaques of mice deficient in apolipoprotein E or low-density-lipoprotein receptor. Journal of Nuclear Medicine. 2009;50:612-7.

46. Nahrendorf M, Waterman P, Thurber G, et al. Hybrid in vivo FMT-CT imaging of protease activity in atherosclerosis with customized nanosensors. Arterioscler Thromb Vasc Biol. 2009;29:1444-51.

47. Nahrendorf M, Jaffer F, Kelly K, et al. Noninvasive vascular cell adhesion molecule-1 imaging identifies inflammatory activation of cells in atherosclerosis. Circulation. 2006;114:1504-11.

48. Kaufmann BA, Carr CL, Belcik JT, et al. Molecular imaging of the initial inflammatory response in atherosclerosis: implications for early detection of disease. Arterioscler Thromb Vasc Biol. 2010;30:54-9.

49. Wyss C, Schaefer SC, Juillerat-Jeanneret L, et al. Molecular imaging by micro-CT: specific E-selectin imaging. Eur Radiol. 2009;19:2487-94.

50. McAteer MA, Schneider JE, Ali ZA, et al. Magnetic resonance imaging of endothelial adhesion molecules in mouse atherosclerosis using dual-targeted microparticles of iron oxide. Arterioscler Thromb Vasc Biol. 2008;28:77-83.

51. Nahrendorf M, Keliher E, Panizzi P, et al. 18F-4V for PET-CT imaging of VCAM-1 expression in atherosclerosis. JACC Cardiovasc Imaging. 2009;2:1213-22.

52. Kircher M, Grimm J, Swirski F, et al. Noninvasive in vivo imaging of monocyte trafficking to atherosclerotic lesions. Circulation. 2008;117:388-95.

53. Gross S, Gammon ST, Moss BL, et al. Bioluminescence imaging of myeloperoxidase activity in vivo. Nat Med. 2009;15:455-61.

54. Ronald JA, Chen JW, Chen Y, et al. Enzyme-sensitive magnetic resonance imaging targeting myeloperoxidase identifies active inflammation in experimental rabbit atherosclerotic plaques. Circulation. 2009;120:592-9.

55. Briley-Saebo K, Shaw P, Mulder W, et al. Targeted molecular probes for imaging atherosclerotic lesions with magnetic resonance using antibodies that recognize oxidation-specific epitopes. Circulation. 2008;117:3206-15.

56. Winter PM, Morawski AM, Caruthers SD, et al. Molecular imaging of angiogenesis in early-stage atherosclerosis with alpha(v)beta3-integrin-targeted nanoparticles. Circulation. 2003;108:2270-4.

57. Laitinen I, Saraste A, Weidl E, et al. Evaluation of αvβ3 integrin-targeted positron emission tomography tracer 18F-galacto-RGD for imaging of vascular inflammation in atherosclerotic mice. Circulation: Cardiovascular Imaging. 2009;2:331-8.

58. Almutairi A, Rossin R, Shokeen M, et al. Biodegradable dendritic positron-emitting nanoprobes for the noninvasive imaging of angiogenesis. Proc Natl Acad Sci USA. 2009;106: 685-90.

59. Sirol M, Moreno PR, Purushothaman K-R, et al. Increased neovascularization in advanced lipid-rich atherosclerotic lesions detected by gadofluorine-M-enhanced MRI: implications for plaque vulnerability. Circulation: Cardiovascular Imaging. 2009;2:391-6.

60. Winter P, Caruthers S, Zhang H, et al. Antiangiogenic synergism of integrin-targeted fumagillin nanoparticles and atorvastatin in atherosclerosis. JACC: Cardiovascular Imaging. 2008;1:624-34.

61. Zhao Y, Kuge Y, Zhao S, et al. Prolonged high-fat feeding enhances aortic 18F-FDG and 99mTc-annexin A5 uptake in apolipoprotein E-deficient and wild-type C57BL/6J mice. J Nucl Med. 2008;49:1707-14.

62. Haider N, Hartung D, Fujimoto S, et al. Dual molecular imaging for targeting metalloproteinase activity and apoptosis in atherosclerosis: molecular imaging facilitates understanding of pathogenesis. J Nucl Cardiol. 2009;16:753-62.

63. Sarai M, Hartung D, Petrov A, et al. Broad and specific caspase inhibitor-induced acute repression of apoptosis in atherosclerotic lesions evaluated by radiolabeled annexin A5 imaging. J Am Coll Cardiol. 2007;50:2305-12.

64. Edgington LE, Berger AB, Blum G, et al. Noninvasive optical imaging of apoptosis by caspase-targeted activity-based probes. Nat Med. 2009;15:967-73.

65. Kietselaer BLJH, Reutelingsperger CPM, Heidendal GAK, et al. Noninvasive detection of plaque instability with use of radiolabeled annexin A5 in patients with carotid-artery atherosclerosis. N Engl J Med. 2004;350:1472-3.

66. Zaheer A, Lenkinski RE, Mahmood A, et al. In vivo near-infrared fluorescence imaging of osteoblastic activity. Nat Biotechnol. 2001;19:1148-54.

67. Aikawa E, Aikawa M, Libby P, et al. Arterial and aortic valve calcification abolished by elastolytic cathepsin S deficiency in chronic renal disease. Circulation. 2009;119:1785-94.

68. Aikawa E, Nahrendorf M, Figueiredo J-L, et al. Osteogenesis associates with inflammation in early-stage atherosclerosis evaluated by molecular imaging in vivo. Circulation. 2007;116:2841-50.

69. Spuentrup E, Botnar RM, Wiethoff AJ, et al. MR imaging of thrombi using EP-2104R, a fibrin-specific contrast agent: initial results in patients. Eur Radiol. 2008;18:1995-2005.

70. Vymazal J, Spuentrup E, Cardenas-Molina G, et al. Thrombus imaging with fibrin-specific gadolinium-based MR contrast agent EP-2104R: results of a phase II clinical study of feasibility. Investigative Radiology. 2009;44:697-704.

71. Botnar RM, Buecker A, Wiethoff AJ, et al. In vivo magnetic resonance imaging of coronary thrombosis using a fibrin-binding molecular magnetic resonance contrast agent. Circulation. 2004;110: 1463-6.

72. Botnar RM, Perez AS, Witte S, et al. In vivo molecular imaging of acute and subacute thrombosis using a fibrin-binding magnetic resonance imaging contrast agent. Circulation. 2004;109:2023-9.

73. Sirol M, Fuster V, Badimon JJ, et al. Chronic thrombus detection with in vivo magnetic resonance imaging and a fibrin-targeted contrast agent. Circulation. 2005;112:1594-600.

74. Spuentrup E, Fausten B, Kinzel S, et al. Molecular magnetic resonance imaging of atrial clots in a swine model. Circulation. 2005;112:396-9.

75. Spuentrup E, Buecker A, Katoh M, et al. Molecular magnetic resonance imaging of coronary thrombosis and pulmonary emboli with a novel fibrin-targeted contrast agent. Circulation. 2005;111: 1377-82.

76. Jaffer FA, Tung C-H, Wykrzykowska JJ, et al. Molecular imaging of factor XIIIa activity in thrombosis using a novel, near-infrared fluorescent contrast agent that covalently links to thrombi. Circulation. 2004;110:170-6.

77. Kim DE, Schellingerhout D, Jaffer FA, et al. Near-infrared fluorescent imaging of cerebral thrombi and blood-brain barrier disruption in a mouse model of cerebral venous sinus thrombosis. J Cereb Blood Flow Metab. 2005;25:226-33.

78. Miserus R-JJHM, Herías MV, Prinzen L, et al. Molecular MRI of early thrombus formation using a bimodal alpha2-antiplasmin-based contrast agent. JACC Cardiovasc Imaging. 2009;2:987-96.

79. von zur Muhlen C, von Elverfeldt D, Moeller JA, et al. Magnetic resonance imaging contrast agent targeted toward activated platelets allows in vivo detection of thrombosis and monitoring of thrombolysis. Circulation. 2008;118:258-67.

80. Flaumenhaft R, Tanaka E, Graham GJ, et al. Localization and quantification of platelet-rich thrombi in large blood vessels with near-infrared fluorescence imaging. Circulation. 2006;115:84-93.

81. Jaffer FA, Tung C-H, Gerszten RE, et al. In vivo imaging of thrombin activity in experimental thrombi with thrombin-sensitive near-infrared molecular probe. Arteriosclerosis, Thrombosis, and Vascular Biology. 2002;22:1929-35.

82. Reeps C, Essler M, Pelisek J, et al. Increased 18F-fluorodeoxyglucose uptake in abdominal aortic aneurysms in positron emission/computed tomography is associated with inflammation, aortic wall instability, and acute symptoms. J Vasc Surg. 2008;48:417-23; discussion 424.

83. Kotze CW, Menezes LJ, Endozo R, et al. Increased metabolic activity in abdominal aortic aneurysm detected by 18F-fluorodeoxyglucose (18F-FDG) positron emission tomography/computed tomography (PET/CT). Eur J Vasc Endovasc Surg. 2009;38:93-9.

84. Reeps C, Gee MW, Maier A, et al. Glucose metabolism in the vessel wall correlates with mechanical instability and inflammatory changes in a patient with a growing aneurysm of the abdominal aorta. Circulation: Cardiovascular Imaging. 2009;2:507-9.

85. DeLeo MJ, Gounis MJ, Hong B, et al. Carotid artery brain aneurysm model: in vivo molecular enzyme-specific MR imaging of active inflammation in a pilot study. Radiology. 2009;252:696-703.

86. Tedesco MM, Terashima M, Blankenberg FG, et al. Analysis of in situ and ex vivo vascular endothelial growth factor receptor expression during experimental aortic aneurysm progression. Arteriosclerosis, Thrombosis, and Vascular Biology. 2009;29:1452-7.

87. Sheth RA, Maricevich M, Mahmood U. In vivo optical molecular imaging of matrix metalloproteinase activity in abdominal aortic aneurysms correlates with treatment effects on growth rate. Atherosclerosis. 2010;212:181-7.

88. Sadeghi MM, Krassilnikova S, Zhang J, et al. Detection of injury-induced vascular remodeling by targeting activated alphavbeta3 integrin in vivo. Circulation. 2004;110:84-90.

89. Trivedi RA, U-King-Im JM, Graves MJ, et al. Noninvasive imaging of carotid plaque inflammation. Neurology. 2004;63:187-8.

90. Kaufmann BA, Sanders JM, Davis C, et al. Molecular imaging of inflammation in atherosclerosis with targeted ultrasound detection of vascular cell adhesion molecule-1. Circulation. 2007;116:276-84.

91. Jaffer FA, Libby P, Weissleder R. Molecular and cellular imaging of atherosclerosis: emerging applications. J Am Coll Cardiol. 2006;47(7):1328-38.

Chapter 25

Cardiac Hemodynamics and Coronary Physiology

Amardeep K Singh, Andrew Boyle, Yerem Yeghiazarians

Chapter Outline

INTRODUCTION

The first living human cardiac catheterization was performed in 1929 by a German surgical resident physician, Werner Forssmann, when he inserted a urological catheter into his own antecubital vein, passed it to his right atrium, and then walked to the X-ray room to document the position of the catheter in his heart. Fired for his self-experimentation, Forssmann later won the Nobel Prize for his contributions to physiology and medicine.[1,2] This important step in cardiology demonstrated that cardiac catheterization could safely be performed in humans and opened the door to a more direct understanding of cardiac disease states.

CARDIAC CATHETERIZATION—THE BASICS

Proper cardiac diagnosis and disease management relies on accurate hemodynamic data acquisition. Caution must be applied for adequate flushing of catheters, avoidance of bubbles and equipment calibration. Proper placement of the pressure transducer prevents inaccurate hemodynamic data acquisition. Traditionally, the transducer is placed at the mid-chest level by dividing the patient's anterior-posterior chest diameter by two. However, to avoid the effects of hydrostatic pressure by the fluid filled catheter, the transducer should be optimally aligned to the upper blood level of the cardiac chamber being assessed. Placing the transducer below this level subjects pressure

assessment to include the hydrostatic pressure of fluid in the catheter and overestimates cardiac pressure. To minimize this effect, the transducer should be 5 cm below the left sternal border at the level of the fourth intercostal space and secured to a stationary pole.[3] To optimize confidence in data, the clinician should be astute to recognize artifacts that affect data integrity. The catheter, loose equipment connections, transducer, or amplifier and gain settings may create artifacts in pressure waveforms.

Underdampening of pressure waveforms results when either vigorous catheter movement or air bubble oscillation produces artifacts in peaks and dips of the pressure waveform. This is best avoided by repositioning and proper flushing of the catheter, respectively. Catheter kink or blood, contrast media, or air in the catheter can result in reduced pressure transmission and overdampening of the pressure waveform (Figs 1A to C).

Cardiac catheterization is a relatively safe procedure, however, knowledge of the relative contraindications and possible complications of cardiac catheterization are important in assessing the risks and benefits of the procedure (Tables 1 and 2). Furthermore, risk assessment must be performed on an individual basis as the risks associated with each procedure will vary based on the patient's comorbidities.

A common hazard of the cardiac catheterization laboratory is exposure of ionizing radiation to both patients and staff. Stochastic effects of radiation are those whose probability increases with increasing dose of radiation, such as

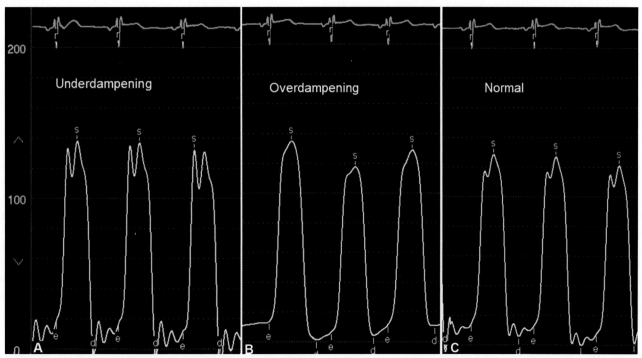

FIGURES 1A TO C: Left ventricle pressure waveform (A) Underdampening of pressure waveforms results when either excessive catheter movement or air bubble oscillations produce artifacts in peaks and dips of the pressure waveform, with falsely elevated systolic pressure and low diastolic pressure; (B) Catheter kink or blood, contrast media, or air in the catheter can result in reduced pressure transmission and overdampening of the pressure waveform, with smooth contour of the waveform; (C) Normal waveform. (Abbreviations: s: Systolic; d: Diastolic; e: End-diastolic pressure

CHAPTER 25 Cardiac Hemodynamics and Coronary Physiology

TABLE 1

Risks of cardiac catheterization and coronary angiography*

Complication	Risk (%)
Mortality	0.11
Myocardial infarction	0.05
Cerebrovascular accident	0.07
Arrhythmia	0.38
Vascular complications	0.43
Contrast reaction	0.37
Hemodynamic complication	0.26
Perforation of heart chamber	0.03
Other complications	0.28
Total of major complications	1.70
*Number of patients = 59,792	

Source: Scanlon PJ, Faxon DP, Audet AM, et al. ACC/AHA guidelines for coronary angiography: A report of the American College of Cardiology/American Heart Association Task Force on Practice Guidelines (Committee on Coronary Angiography). J Am Coll Cardiol. 1999; 33:1760.

TABLE 2

Relative contraindications to coronary angiography

- Acute renal failure
- Chronic renal failure secondary to diabetes
- Active gastrointestinal bleed
- Unexplained fever, that may be due to infection
- Untreated active infection
- Acute stroke
- Severe anemia
- Severe uncontrolled hypertension
- Severe symptomatic electrolyte imbalance
- Severe lack of patient cooperation, due to psychological or severe systemic illness
- Severe concomitant illness that drastically shortens life expectancy or increases risk of therapeutic intervention
- Patient refusal to consider definitive therapy such angioplasty or coronary artery bypass graft or valve surgery
- Digitalis intoxication
- Documented anaphylactoid reaction to angiographic contrast media
- Severe peripheral vascular disease limiting vascular access
- Decompensated congestive heart failure or acute pulmonary edema
- Severe coagulopathy
- Aortic valve endocarditis

Source: Scanlon PJ, Faxon DP, Audet AM, et al. ACC/AHA guidelines for coronary angiography: A report of the American College of Cardiology/American Heart Association Task Force on Practice Guidelines (Committee on Coronary Angiography). J Am Coll Cardiol. 1999; 33:1760-1.

carcinogenesis. Deterministic effects, such as skin injury, occur after a certain radiation dose threshold is reached. The purpose of radiation safety is to limit both stochastic and deterministic effects. Details of radiation safety are beyond the scope of this chapter, however, the operator must understand radiation physics and apply appropriate safety precautions that limit radiation exposure.

Right heart catheterization is performed for assessment of right-heart pressures, pulmonary arterial and pulmonary arterial wedge pressure (PAWP), which estimates left atrial pressure, and to calculate resistance of systemic and pulmonary vascular beds. This information is useful in studying conditions such as valvular heart disease, cardiac shunts, heart failure, pulmonary hypertension and to establish the etiology of shock.

Catheters are advanced under fluoroscopy through a sheath placed in a large vein, such as the femoral, internal jugular, subclavian or cephalic vein. Femoral venous access should not be used if an inferior vena cava filter is present. Venous systems with arteriovenous fistula (such as in dialysis patients) or suspected thrombus should also be avoided.

Classic woven Dacron catheters for right heart catheterization include the Cournard, which is a single end-hole catheter and the Goodale-Lubin, with two additional side holes. These catheters have excellent torquability, however, their stiffness makes them more traumatic catheters.[4] More commonly used are the flow-directed balloon floatation catheters such as the Swan-Ganz catheter, a balloon-tipped catheter with thermistor for measurement of cardiac output. Cardiac pressures are measured while advancing the catheter with the balloon tip inflated. When withdrawing the pulmonary artery catheter, it is important to keep balloon deflated to prevent trauma to cardiac or venous structures. Blood oxygen saturation sampled during right heart catheterization can be analyzed to assess for the presence of cardiac shunts.

CATHETERIZATION COMPUTATIONS

Assessment of cardiac output, vascular resistance and shunt severity are calculated from computations performed during right heart catheterization.

CARDIAC OUTPUT

Cardiac output is the volume of blood that circulates per unit time and is assessed using either the Fick method or the indicator dilution technique. Normal cardiac output is 5–6 l/min for males and 4–5 l/min for females. Cardiac index is cardiac output proportional to the body surface area.

FICK METHOD

Determination of the oxygen (O_2) content difference between arterial and venous (A-VO_2) blood is required for the Fick method. If no intracardiac shunt is present, pulmonary flow is equivalent to systemic flow and measurement of pulmonary A-VO_2 can be used. Simultaneous blood samples of the pulmonary artery and pulmonary vein (carefully obtained with balloon tip of catheter inflated) reflect venous and arterial content, respectively. In the absence of an intracardiac shunt, systemic arterial oxygen saturation may be used as a surrogate for pulmonary wedge oxygenation. Cardiac output using the Fick method is calculated using the following equation:

$$\text{Cardiac output (l/min)} = \frac{O_2 \text{ consumption (ml/min)}}{\text{Arterial } O_2 \text{ content} - \text{Mixed venous } O_2 \text{ content (ml/l)}}$$

where Oxygen content = 1.36 × Hemoglobin (g/dl) × SO_2 + (0.003 × PaO_2)

SO_2 is the percent oxygenation of arterial or venous blood.

PaO_2 is the arterial partial pressure of oxygen

Normal arterial oxygen content is 17–24 ml/dl and venous oxygen content is 12–17 ml/dl.

Oxygen consumption is measured during a graded exercise test during which the oxygen and carbon dioxide levels of inhaled and exhaled air are measured using a tight-fitting gas exchange mask. Because oxygen consumption determination using this method can be cumbersome, a nomogram is often used to estimate oxygen consumption using the patient's age, gender and heart rate.[5] However, accurate objective measurements of oxygen consumption are used to establish cardiac reserve and prognosis in patients with congestive heart failure, valvular heart disease, and hypertrophic cardiomyopathy, congenital heart disease, and coronary artery disease and risk stratify patients for cardiac transplant. Average oxygen consumption values for young males and females are 3.5 l/min and 2.0 l/min, respectively. The accuracy of the Fick method to determine cardiac output is compromised in the presence of intracardiac shunts due to mixing of oxygenated and deoxygenated blood.

INDICATOR DILUTION METHOD

The dilution of an indicator over time can be used to assess cardiac output. This method originally involved the injection of indocyanine green into one cardiac chamber and detection of its concentration in a downstream cardiac chamber. More commonly used is thermodilution, employing a thermal indicator of cold or room temperature saline. Using a catheter with a thermistor tip placed in the pulmonary artery, a temperature-time curve is generated after the injection of cold saline into the proximal port located in the right atrium. Using a computer model, the area under the thermodilution curve is converted to cardiac output and is inversely proportional to cardiac output. For example, in a low cardiac output state, the area under of the curve is greater as the thermistor senses a change in temperature over a longer period of time (Fig. 2). Conditions that prevent adequate forward flow, such as valve regurgitation, and intracardiac shunts or irregular heart rhythms, preclude the accurate measurement of cardiac output using the thermodilution technique. Hypothermia may also prevent assessment of cardiac output by thermodilution as the thermistor may not be able to detect a change in temperature

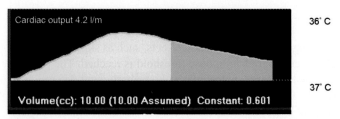

Cardiac output 4.2 l/m   36° C

                                                          37° C

Volume(cc): 10.00 (10.00 Assumed) Constant: 0.601

FIGURE 2: Temperature-time curve for cardiac output by thermodilution. A temperature-time curve is generated after the injection of cold saline into the proximal port located in the right atrium and thermistor tip placed in the pulmonary artery. Using a computer model, the area under the thermodilution curve is converted to cardiac output

of cooled normal saline depending on the degree of hypothermia.

VASCULAR RESISTANCE

The mean pressure gradient and flow across a vascular bed reflects the vascular resistance:

$$\text{Systemic Vascular Resistance (Woods units)} = \frac{\text{Mean arterial blood pressure — Right atrial pressure}}{\text{Cardiac Output (l/min)}}$$

$$\text{Pulmonary Vascular Resistance (Woods units)} = \frac{\text{Mean PA pressure — Mean PAWP}}{\text{Cardiac Output (l/min)}}$$

(PA = pulmonary artery, PAWP = pulmonary arterial wedge pressure)
1 Woods unit = 1 mm Hg x min/l = 8 MPascals.s/m^3 = 80 dynes.sec/cm^5

An indexed vascular resistance is calculated by multiplying vascular resistance by body surface area. In the presence of an intracardiac shunt, pulmonic and systemic cardiac outputs must be calculated separately when used to calculate PVR and SVR, respectively. See Table 3 for normal pulmonary and systemic vascular resistance.

INTRACARDIAC SHUNT RATIO

Flow across a vascular bed is defined as the oxygen consumption divided by the difference between the arterial and the venous oxygen content across a vascular bed.
Therefore,

$$\text{Pulmonary Flow (Qp)} = \frac{\text{O}_2 \text{ Consumption (ml/min)}}{\text{PvO}_2 - \text{PaO}_2 \times \text{Hemoglobin} \times 1.36 \times 10} = \text{l/min/m}^2$$

$$\text{Systemic Flow (Qs)} = \frac{\text{O}_2 \text{ Consumption (ml/min)}}{\text{SaO}_2 - \text{MvO}_2 \times \text{Hemoglobin} \times 1.36 \times 10} = \text{l/min/m}^2$$

SaO_2 = systemic arterial oxygen saturation, MvO_2 = mixed venous oxygen saturation, PvO_2 = pulmonary vein oxygen saturation, PaO_2 = pulmonary artery oxygen saturation.

The pulmonary to shunt flow ratio describes the magnitude and direction of an intracardiac shunt by the ratio of pulmonary to systemic blood flow using oximetry:

$$\text{Pulmonary Flow (Qp)} = \frac{\text{O}_2 \text{ Consumption}}{\text{PvO}_2 - \text{PaO}_2} = \text{SaO}_2 - \text{MvO}_2$$

$$\text{Systemic Flow (Qp)} = \frac{\text{O}_2 \text{ Consumption}}{\text{SaO}_2 - \text{MvO}_2} = \text{PvO}_2 - \text{PaO}_2$$

Venous blood from the superior vena cava has lower oxygen saturation than the inferior vena cava as more oxygen is extracted from the brain and upper extremities. Therefore, the Flamm formula allows for accurate MvO_2 using the oxygen saturation of the inferior and superior vena cava using the following equation:[6]

$$\text{MvO}_2 = \frac{3\,(\text{SVC O}_2) + \text{IVC O}_2}{4}$$

At rest, normal mixed venous oxygenation is approximately 75%.

In the absence of an intracardiac shunt, pulmonary and systemic flow are equivalent, Qp/Qs = 1. When a left-to-right shunt is present Qp/Qs > 1, with increased pulmonary flow. A Qp/Qs of > 1.5 suggests a more hemodynamically significant left-to-right shunt.

When a step up in blood oxygen saturation is noted from vena cava to the pulmonary artery of $\geq$ 8% and the systemic arterial oxygen saturation is less than pulmonic vein saturation, a bidirectional shunt should be suspected. To calculate the amount of blood flow shunted in each direction, the effective blood flow (EBF) must be calculated:

$$\text{EBF} = \frac{\text{O}_2 \text{ Consumption}}{(\text{Pulmonic vein O}_2 \text{ Saturation} - \text{Mixed venous O}_2 \text{ Saturation}) \times 10 \times 1.36 \times \text{Hemoglobin}}$$

The difference between the pulmonic blood flow and effective blood flow indicates flow shunted from left-to-right. The difference between the systemic blood flow and the effective blood flow indicates flow shunted from right-to-left.

The indicator dilution method using a dye curve over time also quantifies shunts. The curve of the concentration of dye over time is generated by injecting dye proximal to the shunt and sampling distal to the shunt. For a left-to-right shunt, a second peak occurs due to recirculation of the shunted dye. The area under the two curves is used to calculate the magnitude of the shunt. For a right-to-left shunt, the ascending limb of the curve has a single early peak.

CARDIAC CYCLE PRESSURE WAVEFORMS

ATRIAL PRESSURES

The right atrial pressure tracing exhibits "a" and "v" waves that reflect an increase in the atrial pressure with atrial contraction and filling during ventricular systole, respectively. The "a" wave is followed by a "c" deflection that results from closure of the tricuspid valve during isovolumetric ventricular contraction. During the x-descent, the atrium relaxes with a decline in pressure. The y-descent following the "v" wave reflects atrial emptying after opening of the tricuspid valve (Fig. 3).

Left atrial pressure waveform is similar to the right atrium but with increased amplitude of the "a" and "v" waves. Direct pressure assessment of the left atrium requires retrograde catheterization from the aorta or atrial transeptal puncture by an experienced operator. The PAWP provides an indirect yet reliable assessment of left atrial pressure, in the absence of mitral valve disease.

VENTRICULAR PRESSURES

In the absence of valve stenosis, systolic pressures of the right and left ventricle pressure equal those of the pulmonary artery

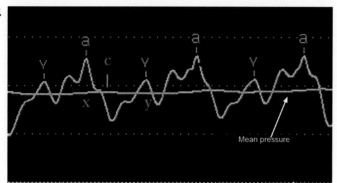

FIGURE 3: Right atrial pressure waveform. The "a" and "v" waves that reflect an increase in the atrial pressure with atrial contraction and filling during ventricular systole, respectively. The "c" deflection results from closure of the tricuspid valve during isovolumetric ventricular contraction. The atrium relaxes with a decline in pressure during the x-descent and the y-descent occurs during atrial emptying

and aorta, respectively. Ventricular diastolic pressures are dependent on myocardial compliance, which is inversely proportional to the slope of the pressure-volume curve. Wall thickness, volume, ischemia and medications affect myocardial compliance by altering the pressure-volume curve. Impaired myocardial compliance results in a "stiffer" chamber and elevation of ventricular end-diastolic pressure.

Left ventricle end-diastolic pressure (LVEDP) is approximately equal to left atrial and PAWP. During left heart catheterization, LVEDP is usually measured using a pigtail catheter placed in the left ventricle. However, if more accurate pressure recordings are required, a high-fidelity manometer can be used instead of a fluid-filled catheter. If a mid-cavity obstruction within the left ventricle is suspected, a straight or angled end-hole catheter should be used to assess left ventricular pressure.

LVEDP is measured on the left ventricular pressure tracing at a point just prior to isovolumetric contraction and immediately after the "a" wave of the PAWP tracing.[7] LVEDP also corresponds to the "R" wave of the electrocardiogram tracing (Fig. 4). If atrial fibrillation is present, the LVEDP of 10 cardiac cycles are averaged. Artifact of elevated diastolic pressure may occur when using a pigtail catheter with multiple holes if the holes are simultaneously partially present in the aorta and left ventricular cavity, producing a falsely elevated combined diastolic pressure. All holes of the pigtail catheter must be within the left ventricular cavity for accurate measurement of LVEDP. Normal cardiac pressures are listed in Table 3.

HEMODYNAMICS IN VALVULAR HEART DISEASE

AORTIC STENOSIS

Valvular AS is most often due to calcific degeneration of the valve seen in the elderly population. Young adults with AS often have a congenital malformation of the valve, such as a bicuspid aortic valve, that contributes to the development of AS. AS may also be supra-valvular or sub-vavular. Supra-valvular AS is usually congenital in etiology. Sub-valvular AS may be present due to basal septal hypertrophy or the presence of a subaortic membrane. Current guidelines discourage invasive hemodynamic evaluation of aortic stenosis when noninvasive findings regarding the severity of aortic stenosis by echocardiography are unequivocal. Invasive evaluation of AS is reserved for situations in which there is a discrepancy between echocardiographic findings and patient's symptoms.[8] Coronary angiography should be performed in patients referred

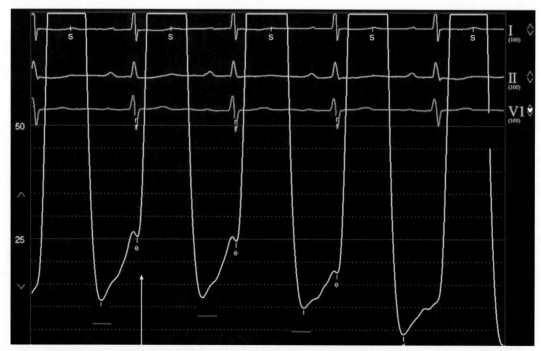

FIGURE 4: Identification of left-ventricle end diastolic pressure. Left ventricle pressure (yellow) and ECG leads tracing. LVEDP corresponds to the "R" wave of the electrocardiogram tracing. LVEDP may also be measured at a point just prior to isovolumetric contraction and immediately after the "a" wave of the PAWP tracing. (Abbreviation: e: end-diastolic pressure)

TABLE 3

Normal pressures and vascular resistance

	Pressure (mm Hg)
Right atrium	
a wave	6 (2–7)
v wave	5 (2–7)
Mean	3 (1–5)
Right ventricle	
Peak systolic	25 (15–30)
End-diastolic	4 (1–7)
Pulmonary artery	
Peak systolic	25 (15–30)
End-diastolic	9 (4–12)
Mean	15 (9–19)
Pulmonary artery wedge	9 (4–12)
Left atrium	
a wave	10 (4–16)
v wave	12 (6–21)
Mean	8 (2–12)
Left ventricle	
Peak systolic	130 (90–140)
End-diastolic	8 (5–12)
Aorta	
Peak systolic	130 (90–140)
End-diastolic	70 (60–90)
Mean	85 (70–105)
	Resistance (dyne-sec/cm^5)
Systemic vascular resistance	1100 (700–1600)
Pulmonary vascular resistance	70 (20–130)

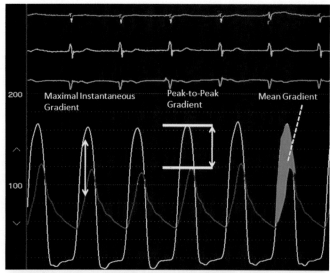

FIGURE 5: Aortic-Left ventricular systolic gradient in aortic stenosis. Maximal instantaneous gradient is the maximum pressure gradient between the aorta (red) and left ventricle (yellow) at a single point in time. Peak-to-peak gradient is the absolute difference between peak aortic systolic pressure and peak left ventricular systolic pressure. Mean gradient is defined by the area between the systolic left ventricular and aortic hemodynamic tracings (green shaded area)

for aortic valve surgery when a suspicion of coronary artery disease exists.

Hemodynamic measurements in AS reveal a gradient between the systolic aortic and the left ventricular pressures (Fig. 5). In severe aortic stenosis, the ascending limb of the aortic pressure waveform is delayed. One should be careful in using peripheral arterial pressure as a surrogate for central aortic pressure, as they may not always be equal. This is due to pressure waveform summation, different elasticity and size of the vessels, and peripheral vascular disease that often results in a differentiation in peripheral and aortic pressures. Therefore, two arterial catheters or a double lumen catheter may be used for catheterization of the left ventricle and aorta simultaneously. If a peripheral arterial pressure will be used as a surrogate for central aortic pressure, this should be calibrated with the central aortic pressure before crossing the valve. Use of a pigtail catheter with side-holes is discouraged due to pressure artifacts if holes are only partially present in one chamber. To avoid risk of thrombosis, anti-coagulation may be considered especially if measurements are to be taken with catheter placed in the left ventricle for sometime.

Peak aortic and left ventricular pressures are temporally separated. Thus, the gradient between the two can be described as peak-to-peak, peak instantaneous or mean gradient. Peak-to-peak gradient is the absolute difference between peak aortic systolic pressure and peak left ventricular systolic pressure. Peak instantaneous gradient is the maximum pressure gradient between the aorta and left ventricle at a single point in time. The area between the systolic left ventricular and aortic hemodynamic tracings defines the mean gradient and best quantifies the severity of aortic stenosis.

Aortic valve area (AVA) is calculated from hemodynamic data and cardiac output in ml/min using the Gorlin equation:[9]

$$\text{AVA (cm}^2) = \frac{\left(\text{Cardiac output [ml/min]/Systolic ejection period [sec]} \times \text{Heart rate [beats/minute]}\right)}{44.3 \times \sqrt{\text{mean gradient (mm Hg)}}}$$

The Hakki formula is a simplified version for AVA:[10]

$$\text{AVA (cm}^2) = \frac{\text{Cardiac output (l/min)}}{\sqrt{\text{Peak to peak gradient (mm Hg)}}}$$

AVA estimation using the Hakki formula is based on the finding that the product of systolic ejection period, heart rate, and the constant are close to 1000. Note that cardiac output in the Hakki formula is reported in liters per minute. If valve regurgitation is present, the Fick method for calculation of cardiac output is more accurate. AVA of lesser than 1 cm^2 and a mean gradient of greater than 40 mm Hg indicate severe AS. An AVA of greater than 1.5 cm^2 and a mean gradient of lesser than 20 mm Hg indicate mild aortic stenosis.

AORTIC REGURGITATION

Although, characterization of aortic regurgitation (AR) by echocardiography is often adequate, aortic angiography provides further information on aortic root size and qualitative information on regurgitation of blood across the aortic valve into the left ventricle. Aortic angiography is performed with a multi-side-hole catheter positioned just above the sinus of Valsalva in the left anterior oblique projection and a power injector is used to inject contrast; approximately 40 ml of

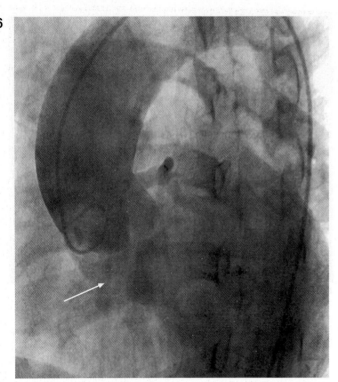

FIGURE 6: Aortic regurgitation on aortic angiography. Aortogram performed with pigtail catheter in the aorta demonstrating Grade 2 aortic regurgitation, with moderate opacification of the left ventricle

contrast at a rate of 20 ml/second. AR is graded on a scale of 1–4: Grade 1 (mild) minimal contrast opacifies the left ventricle; Grade 2 (moderate) opacification of entire left ventricular; Grade 3 (moderately severe) dense opacification of left ventricle over sequential cardiac cycles and Grade 4 (severe) dense opacification of entire left ventricle in one cardiac cycle[11] (Fig. 6). The pathophysiology and cardiac hemodynamics of acute and chronic AR are different. Recognizing the different patterns in the LVEDP and pulse pressure aid in making this distinction and are described below.

Chronic Aortic Regurgitation

As blood volume regurgitates from the aorta to the left ventricular chamber in diastole, arterial diastolic pressure falls. As the severity of AR worsens, the left ventricular end-diastolic volume also increases. An increased left ventricular ejection volume results in augmented arterial systolic pressure. Therefore, the pulse pressure increases as is evident on the aortic pressure waveform. Hemodynamically significant AR results in a bisferiens pulse, which is a double peak of the aortic systolic contour separated by a mid-systolic dip. The bisferiens pulse results from a rapid left ventricular ejection velocity and subsequent reflected wave from the periphery.

Increased wall stress from a chronically volume overloaded left ventricular chamber results in eccentric hypertrophy. The compliance of the left ventricular eventually begins to deteriorate and results in a modest rise in the LVEDP along with an increased slope of the ventricular diastolic waveform.

Acute Aortic Regurgitation

Acute AR may result from aortic dissection involving the aortic root, trauma or valve perforation from endocarditis. Regardless of the etiology, the unconditioned ventricular is suddenly exposed to a substantial increase in diastolic volume and a dramatic increase in LVEDP. Initially, premature closure of the mitral valve occurs. Eventually, the rise in volume and pressure transmits to the left atrium and pulmonary vasculature resulting in congestion and hypotension.

Unlike chronic AR, an increase in the aortic pulse pressure may not be as impressive acutely due to the absence of both an increased ventricular ejection velocity and decreased systemic vascular resistance. Pulsus alternans may be evident on the aortic pressure waveform with beat-to-beat variation in systolic amplitude due to variations in myocardial contraction strength.

MITRAL STENOSIS

Hemodynamic assessment of mitral stenosis (MS) requires simultaneous right and left cardiac catheterization. Mean gradients by doppler methods and valve area by planimetery, may be obtained by echocardiography. It must be emphasized that echocardiography plays a pivotal role in characterizing valvular and sub-valvular features, such as calcification, leaflet mobility and thickness, which help to determine suitability for percutaneous valvuloplasty.[12] During valvuloplasty, resolution of the mitral valve gradient and the undesirable development of mitral regurgitation are monitored by hemodynamics.

Measurement of the mean mitral valve gradient is made by the diastolic area difference between the left atrial and the left ventricular diastolic pressure waveforms (Fig. 7). PAWP approximates left atrial pressure and may be used as a surrogate to limit the risk associated with transeptal puncture. However, since the PAWP waveform is delayed 40–120 msec with respect to the left atrial pressure waveform, the tracing should be phase shifted so that the peak of the PAWP "v" wave is placed on the downslope of the left ventricular pressure tracing. With severe MS, the PAWP, pulmonary artery pressures and pulmonary vascular resistance increase.

Atrial fibrillation has a common association with MS. If atrial fibrillation is present, the mean mitral valve gradients of ten cardiac cycles should be averaged to increase accuracy. Alternatively, temporary pacing for a regular ventricular rhythm may be used to make more accurate measurements. A rapid heart rate also precludes the accurate assessment of the mean gradient as a short R-R interval abbreviates the diastolic period and prevents equilibration of left atrial and ventricular diastolic pressures, overestimating the mitral valve gradient.

Mitral valve area (MVA) is calculated using the Gorlin formula for the mitral valve:[13]

$$\text{MVA (cm}^2) = \frac{[\text{Cardiac output (ml/min)/Diastolic filling period (sec)} \times \text{Heart rate (beats/min)}]}{44.3 \times 0.85 \times \sqrt{\text{mean gradient (mm Hg)}}}$$

The diastolic filling period is measured at the start of diastole, where the pulmonary arterial wedge and left ventricular

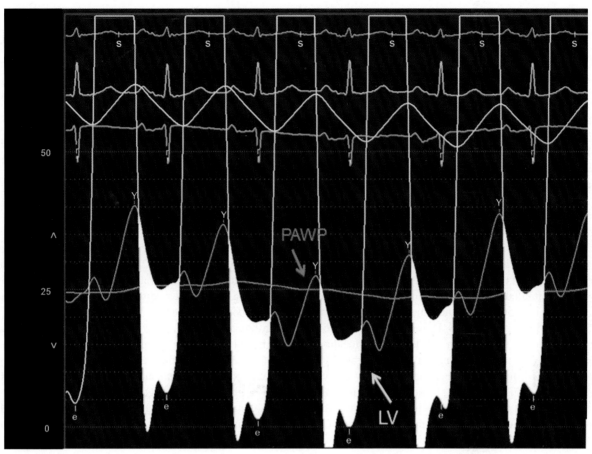

FIGURE 7: Mitral stenosis, diastolic gradient. Mean mitral valve gradient is determined by the diastolic area difference between the pulmonary arterial wedge pressure (PAWP) tracing in orange and left ventricle (LV) pressure tracing in yellow

pressure tracings cross, to end-diastole, identified as peak of the R wave on the electrocardiogram.[14]

MITRAL REGURGITATION

The mitral valve apparatus consists of an annulus and leaflets attached to papillary muscles via chordae tendinae. Disruption of any component of the mitral valve apparatus may result in regurgitation of blood from the left ventricle to the atrium during systole. 2D Echocardiography provides anatomical information on mitral valve structures and doppler calculations quantify mitral regurgitation (MR). Left ventriculography provides a qualitative assessment of mitral incompetence is performed using a pigtail catheter with side-holes in the 30 degrees right anterior oblique projection using 30 ml of contrast at a rate of 10 ml/second. Severity of MR on ventriculography is graded on a scale of 1–4: Grade 1 (mild) contrast partially opacifies the left atrium; Grade 2 (moderate) complete yet faint opacification of left atrium; Grade 3 (moderately severe) opacification of left atrium and left ventricle are comparable and Grade 4 (severely) dense opacification of complete left atrium in one beat[15] (Fig. 8).

Right and left heart catheterizations provide information on the hemodynamic effects of mitral competence. Increased "v" wave amplitude of the PAWP tracing is suggestive of significant MR. Recall that the "v" wave correlates with atrial filling during ventricular systole. Generation of "v" wave amplitude is not only dependent on regurgitant volume, but left atrial compliance

and size as well. Therefore, the absence of a tall "v" wave does not necessarily exclude the diagnosis of severe MR.

A comparison of the atrial and ventricular pressures in severe MR reveals the LVEDP to be lower than left atrial

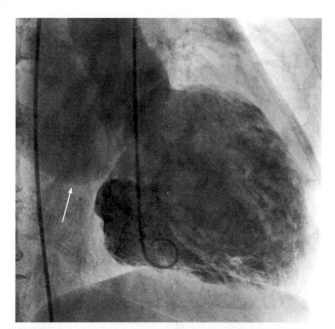

FIGURE 8: Mitral regurgitation, left ventriculography. Grade 3 (moderately severe) with equal opacification of left atrium (arrow) and the dilated left ventricle

pressure or mean PAWP. However, if left ventricular failure is present, the LVEDP may approach mean PAWP.

PULMONIC STENOSIS

Pulmonic stenosis (PS) is rare and most often congenital in etiology. PS may be valvular, supra- or sub-valvular. Echocardiography can be useful in identifying the location of the stenosis and quantifying the gradient. Right ventriculography to evaluate PS may be performed with a pigtail or Berman catheter. This often reveals the site of obstruction and, in valvular PS, may demonstrate the hallmark doming of the pulmonic valve, post-stenotic dilatation of the pulmonary artery, and hypertrophy of the right ventricle.

Catheter pullback from the pulmonary artery to the right ventricle quantifies and locates the obstruction. Quantification of the gradient may also be performed by a double lumen catheter or placement of catheters in the pulmonary artery and right ventricle simultaneously. A gradient across the pulmonary valve of greater than 50 mm Hg indicates severe PS and lesser than 25 mm Hg indicates mild PS. Diastolic pressures provide important diagnostic information to identify the location of the obstruction. Valvular PS reveals a systolic gradient and diastolic pressure difference between the pulmonary artery and the right ventricle (Figs 9A to C). If the obstruction is supra-valvular, the location of the gradient is in the pulmonary artery and thus the diastolic pressures are equal. Likewise, a sub-valvular or infundibular obstruction in the right ventricle would reveal a systolic pressure gradient from the obstruction but the same diastolic pressure of the right ventricle. Balloon valvuloplasty is the procedure of choice for PS.

PULMONIC REGURGITATION

Minimal pulmonic regurgitation (PR) is present in normal individuals. Significant PR may be due to processes involving the pulmonic valve or secondary to pulmonary hypertension. The hemodynamic interaction involving the right ventricle and pulmonary artery is similar to that of the left ventricle and aorta with AR. Significant PR results in a widened pulmonary arterial pulse pressure. A rapid rise in the right ventricular diastolic pressure is evidenced with an elevated RVEDP approaching pulmonary arterial diastolic pressure. However, other causes of elevated RVEDP, such as right ventricular diastolic dysfunction must also be considered.

Pulmonary arteriography is of limited value as a catheter across the pulmonic valve causes PR itself. Therefore, echocardiography has greater utility in defining the severity and characteristics of the PR jet.

TRICUSPID STENOSIS

Tricuspid Stenosis (TS) is rare, yet when present, may be congenital in etiology or secondary to rheumatic or carcinoid heart disease. Doppler and 2D echocardiography provide useful information on valve gradient and area, as well as other coexisting valvular heart disease; a finding not uncommon with TS. Hemodynamic tracings reveal elevated right atrial pressure with blunted y-descent due to impairment of right ventricular filling. Simultaneous catheters in the right atrium and right ventricle demonstrate the presence of a discrete diastolic gradient between the right atrium and ventricle. A mean gradient greater than or equal to 5 mm Hg across the tricuspid valve suggest hemodynamically significant TS. Varying degrees of tricuspid regurgitation almost always accompanies TS due to leaflet restriction and incomplete coaptation.

TRICUSPID REGURGITATION

Trace tricuspid regurgitation (TR) is present in normal patients without consequence due to the complex closure of the tricuspid valve leaflets. Primary TR includes processes that directly affect the tricuspid valve apparatus, such as endocarditis, right ventricular myocardial infarction, rheumatic or carcinoid heart disease. Congenital conditions that produce TR include tricuspid valve atresia and Ebstein's anomaly: a

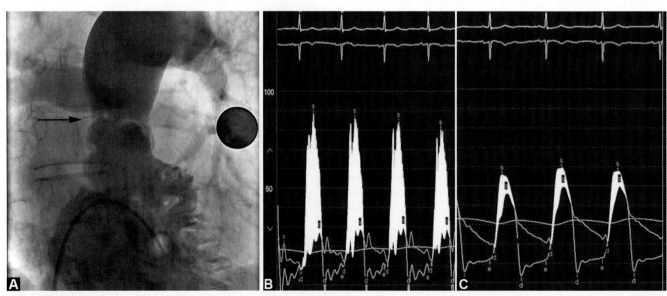

FIGURES 9A TO C: Pulmonic stenosis. (A) Right ventriculography revealing stenotic dilatation of the pulmonary artery. (B and C) Right ventricle and pulmonary artery pressure waveforms before and after balloon valvuloplasty of the stenotic pulmonic valve, respectively. The pulmonic valved peak to peak gradient is reduced from 65 mm Hg to 10 mm Hg after valvuloplasty

condition in which the septal and posterior leaflets are apically displaced. Functional TR may result from right ventricular and tricuspid annular dilatation from cardiomyopathy or pulmonary hypertension. With severe right ventricular dilatation or near complete failure of tricuspid valve leaflet coaptation, the right atrial pressure approaches right ventricular pressure.

Doppler and 2D-echocardiography provide information on jet severity and direction, hepatic vein systolic flow reversal, right ventricular size, valve morphology and the presence of pulmonary hypertension. A negative jet on right atrial angiography or contrast reflux across the tricuspid valve with right ventriculography provides a qualitative assessment of TR.

Hemodynamic tracing of right atrial pressure demonstrates a large "v" wave. However, it is important to note that the height of the "v" wave is also dependent on right atrial size and compliance. Thus, the absence of a tall "v" wave does not exclude the diagnosis of severe tricuspid regurgitation.

HEMODYNAMICS IN CARDIOMYOPATHY

Cardiomyopathy of any cause is usually associated with changes in cardiac hemodynamics, including elevation of end-diastolic pressures in the affected ventricle(s), reduced cardiac output, reduced mixed venous oxygen saturation and elevated atrial pressures. In more advanced cardiomyopathy, alternating higher and lower systolic pressures from one beat to the next can be seen in the affected ventricular tracing or in the aortic pressure wave. This is known as *pulsus alternans* and signifies ventricular dysfunction. In advanced heart failure, reduced aortic systolic pressures are also seen (cardiogenic shock). Hemodynamic tracings can help diagnose cardiomyopathy, assess severity, guide management and assess response to treatment. However, although some forms of cardiomyopathy may have distinct hemodynamic patters, hemodynamic assessment does not necessarily aid in establishing an etiology of the cardiomyopathy. However, some forms of cardiomyopathy may have distinct hemodynamic patterns.

HYPERTROPHIC OBSTRUCTIVE CARDIOMYOPATHY

Hemodynamics in left ventricular cavitary obstruction is amongst the most interesting in diagnostic catheterization. Variants of hypertrophic obstructive cardiomyopathy (HOCM) exist and not all patients with hypertrophic cardiomyopathy have an obstructive component. Likewise, not all patients with intracavitary obstruction have HOCM. For example, myocardial infarction or Takosubo's cardiomyopathy may alter myocardial contractility and generate an intracavitary gradient. When present, the intracavitary obstruction can be localized in the apex, mid-cavity or outflow tract of the left ventricle. Ventriculography provides a visual assessment of cavitary obliteration during systole.

Catheterization set-up for quantifying intracavitary obstruction is similar to that of aortic stenosis. Simultaneous catheters are placed in the aorta and left ventricular cavity. Pullback of a left ventricular end-hole catheter will identify the location as well as quantify the intracavitary gradient. Aortic and left ventricular systolic pressures will be equal in the area above cavitary obstruction. Pressure artifact may be produced if catheter entrapment occurs with the end-hole of the catheter embedded in the myocardium with transduction of intramyocardial pressure.

Intracavitary obstruction is dynamic and dependent on preload and myocardial contractility. Therefore, maneuvers or medications that alter these parameters may elicit an intracavitary gradient when not apparent at rest. An increase in the intracavitary gradient following a premature ventricular contraction (PVC) is seen in HOCM as a result of increased myocardial contractility, known as the Brokenbrough-Braunwald-Morrow sign.[16] In HOCM, the post-PVC beat is associated with a reduction in aortic systolic pressure and pulse pressure (Fig. 10). In comparison, the post-PVC beat in the case of fixed outflow obstruction, such as valvular aortic stenosis, is associated with an increase in the aortic pulse pressure. Furthermore, the upstroke of aortic pressure in systole is brisk in HOCM yet slow in severe aortic stenosis.

Further analysis of the aortic pressure tracing reveals a spike-and-dome contour during systole; generated by ventricular cavitary obstruction in mid-systole. The force generated by the hypertrophic myocardium results in a high velocity jet in the left ventricular outflow tract which generates a drag force on the anterior leaflet of the mitral valve, a phenomenon known as the Venturi effect. The result is a mid-systolic outflow tract obstruction that generates a spike-and-dome in the aortic systolic pressure tracing.

Alterations in preload affect the degree of intracavitary obstruction in HOCM. The Valsalva maneuver increases intrathoracic pressure and thus decreases venous return to the heart. The reduced preload causes further obstruction in the small cavity of the hypertrophied left ventricle and an increase in the intracavitary gradient.

Due to impaired myocardial compliance, left ventricular end-diastolic pressure (LVEDP) is elevated. The rate of diastolic pressure rise of the hypertrophied left ventricle is slow during the passive filling phase in early diastole due to diastolic dysfunction. Atrial systole then results in a prominent "a" wave and elevated LVEDP.[17]

A reduced or possibly abolished left ventricular outflow gradient is observed after percutaneous alcohol septal ablation therapy (Fig. 11). This procedure is a highly effective therapy that requires echocardiography and angiography to identify the septal artery perfusing the hypertrophied septal portion causing obstruction. Once identified, dehydrated alcohol is locally delivered in a controlled fashion through a balloon inflated in the target septal artery. Resolution of the outflow tract gradient is confirmed by the absence of postextrasystolic potentiation.[18,19]

RESTRICTIVE CARDIOMYOPATHY

Restrictive cardiomyopathy (RCM) results from infiltrative myocardial diseases such as amyloidosis, sarcoidosis, hemochromatosis as well as other rare conditions. Direct myocardial involvement of an infiltrative process results in reduced myocardial compliance and biventricular diastolic dysfunction, often with preserved systolic function. Secondary causes of diastolic dysfunction, such as coronary artery disease, must be ruled out prior to the making the diagnosis of restrictive cardiomyopathy.

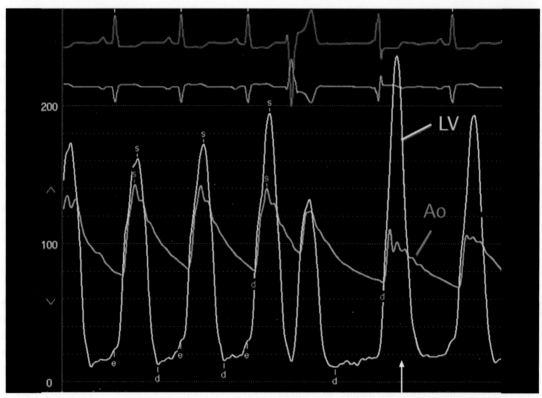

FIGURE 10: Post PVC potentiation in hypertrophic obstructive cardiomyopathy. An increase in the intra-cavitary gradient following a premature ventricular contraction (PVC) is seen in HOCM as a result of inceased myocardial contractility. The post PVC beat (arrow) is associated with a reduction in aortic systolic pressure and pulse pressure known as the Brokenbrough-Braunwald-Morrow sign.[16] (Abbreviations: LV: Left ventricle; Ao: Aorta)

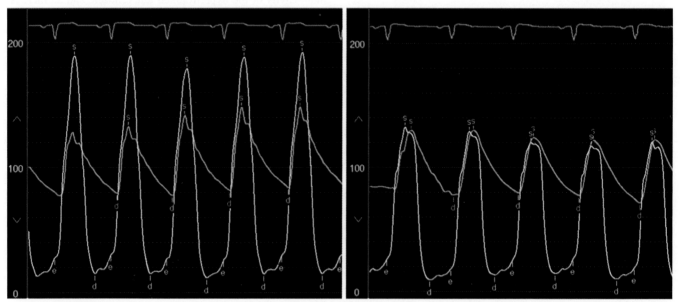

FIGURE 11: Left ventricle outflow gradient pre- and postalcohol septal ablation. Note resolution of the left ventricle-aortic gradient after alcohol administration in an isolated septal coronary artery

Evaluation of hemodynamics in RCM is performed by right heart catheterization to assess right atrial, right ventricular, pulmonary artery and PAWPs. Simultaneous catheters in the right and left ventricles allow analysis of the change in ventricular pressures during the respiratory cycle and help distinguish RCM from constrictive pericarditis; ventricular interdependence that occurs in constrictive pericarditis is not seen in RCM.

Reduced compliance and impedance to ventricular filling results in elevation of ventricular diastolic pressures for any given volume, accompanied by biatrial enlargement. Both right and left atrial pressures are elevated with prominent x- and y-

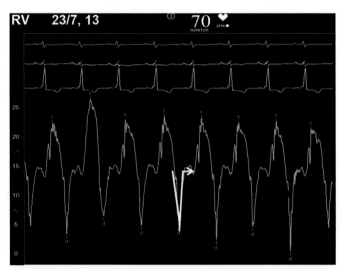

FIGURE 12: Dip-and-plateau configuration in restrictive or "square root sign" in restrictive cardiomyopathy and constrictive pericarditis. Note that the right ventricle end-diastolic pressure is >1/3 of the right ventricle systolic pressure

descents of the atrial pressure tracings. In the absence of valvular regurgitation, the prominent "v" wave reflects reduced atrial compliance.[20] When atrial fibrillation is present, only the "v" wave and y-descent are present due to the absence of atrial contraction.

Bi-ventricular diastolic pressures in RCM are elevated and often near equal within 5 mm Hg. However, since left ventricular involvement exceeds that of the right ventricle, LVEDP is greater than RVEDP. The ventricular diastolic tracing has a characteristic "dip-and-plateau" or "square-root sign" configuration due to abrupt cessation of ventricular filling followed by a restriction to further filling from impaired relaxation of the ventricle (Fig. 12). Pulmonary artery pressures in RCM are generally high and may exceed 55 mm Hg.

Restrictive cardiomyopathy (RCM) and constrictive pericarditis share many similar properties. However, distinguishing the two conditions is extremely important, as the treatment for the latter is surgical pericardiectomy. Several hemodynamic parameters to better distinguish these conditions have been evaluated (Table 4). Perhaps the most reliable is *respirophasic concordance* in RCM; left and right ventricular pressures follow normal physiologic properties with a decrease in systolic pressure during inspiration and increase in expiration. Respirophasic variation during the normal respiratory cycle occurs as intrathoracic pressures are transmitted to cardiac

chambers, a phenomenon that is uncoupled in constrictive pericarditis.[21,22]

Imaging modalities, such as computed tomography and magnetic resonance, may aid in diagnosis if a thick pericardium is present to suggest constrictive pericarditis. The absence of a thickened pericardium, however, does not rule out constrictive pericarditis. If diagnostic uncertainty remains, an endo-myocardial biopsy may aid in diagnosis.

HEMODYNAMICS IN PERICARDIAL DISEASE

The pericardium consists of visceral and parietal layers separated by a minimal amount of serous fluid, and extends to cover the heart and great vessels, excluding a portion of the left atrium and pulmonary veins. This anatomical relationship is important in understanding the physiology and hemodynamics of constrictive pericarditis.

Variations in intrathoracic pressures during the respiratory cycle are normally transmitted to the pericardial space and cardiac chambers. During inspiration, a decrease in the intrathoracic pressure is transmitted to the right heart, augmenting venous return. The increase in right ventricular diastolic pressure is transmitted across the intraventricular septum elevating left ventricular filling pressures. The gradient between the pulmonary veins and the left ventricle, the effective filling gradient, remains relatively constant throughout the respiratory cycle as the pericardial and pleural pressures follow intrathoracic pressure. The result is a decrease in left ventricular stroke volume with inspiration and reduced systemic systolic blood pressure.

CONSTRICTIVE PERICARDITIS

In constrictive pericarditis, a rigid thickened pericardium uncouples the pericardial and cardiac pressures from intrathoracic pressures; the variations in pressures with the respiratory cycle are no longer transmitted. Thus, producing an inspiratory increase in jugular venous pressure is also known as Kussmaul's sign. The right atrial pressure tracing reveals a steep y-descent due to rapid filling in early diastole. A prominent "a" wave during atrial contraction occurs due to elevated pressure, followed by a blunted x-descent secondary to impairment in ventricular filling; resulting in an "M" configuration of the right atrial pressure tracing.[21,22]

The rigid pericardium impairs the ventricular compliance and diastolic pressures are elevated and near equal. Intra-

TABLE 4

Sensitivity and specificity of hemodynamic parameters in constrictive pericarditis

	Constrictive pericarditis	Restrictive cardiomyopathy	Sensitivity (%)	Specificity (%)
LVEDP-RVEDP*	≤ 5 mm Hg	> 5 mm Hg	60	38
Pulmonary artery systolic pressure	< 55 mm Hg	> 55 mm Hg	93	24
Right ventricular systolic and EDP	> 1/3	≤ 1/3	93	38
Respiratory variation in mean right atrial pressure	Absent	Present	93	48
Left ventricular diastolic rapid filling wave	> 7 mm Hg	≤ 7 mm Hg	93	57
Ventricular interdependence	Present	Absent	100	95

(Abbreviations: *LV: Left ventricle; RV: Right ventricle; EDP: End-diastolic pressure). (*Source:* Hurrell DG, Nishimura RA, Higano ST, et al. Value of dynamic respiratory changes in left and right ventricular pressures for the diagnosis of constrictive pericarditis. Circulation. 1996; 93:2007-13)

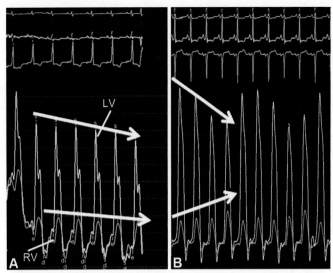

FIGURES 13A AND B: Respirophasic waveforms in (A) Restrictive cardiomyopathy with ventricular concordance of right and left ventricle pressures with a parallel change in right ventricle (RV) and left ventricle (LV) pressures (arrows). (B) Constrictive pericarditis demonstrating ventricular discordance of the right and left ventricle pressures

thoracic pressures are transmitted to the pulmonary veins and a portion of the left atrium not encased by the pericardium. However, the pressure of the pericardial bound left ventricle does not vary with intrathoracic pressure as a result of the dissociation from pericardial pressures in constrictive pericarditis. Thus, the effective filling gradient across the mitral valve is decreased in inspiration. With the reduced left ventricular volume and elevated right ventricular diastolic pressure, the interventricular septum shifts to the left. *Ventricular interdependence* or *discordance* during the respirophasic cycle is demonstrated by simultaneous catheters in the right and left ventricles (Figs 13A and B). An inspiratory decrease in left ventricular systolic pressure results in an increase in the right ventricular systolic pressure and the reverse occurs during expiration. If atrial fibrillation is present, evaluation with temporary ventricular pacing avoids the hemodynamic variation produced by an irregular rhythm.

Similar to restrictive cardiomyopathy, a "dip-and-plateau" configuration of the ventricular diastolic pressures occurs due to rapid early diastolic filling followed by an abrupt cessation to flow from impaired compliance (Fig. 12). The height of the early diastolic rapid filling wave is usually greater than 7 mm Hg in constrictive pericarditis. Table 4 lists hemodynamic criteria that exist to aid in the diagnosis of constrictive pericarditis with varying sensitivity and specificity.[23]

CARDIAC TAMPONADE

Between the visceral and parietal layers of the pericardium there is the pericardial space that normally contains less than 35 ml of plasma ultrafiltrate, or pericardial fluid. Normal pericardial pressure is between "5 to 5 mm Hg.[19] The pathologic accumulation of excess fluid in the pericardial space increases pericardial pressure and may comprise cardiac function if the pericardial pressure exceeds those of the cardiac chambers. The pericardium stretches to accommodate a higher volume when fluid accumulates chronically. However, rapid accumulation of fluid into the fixed pericardial space quickly compromises cardiac function.

The hemodynamics of cardiac tamponade shares similarities to constrictive pericarditis, with an elevation and near equalization of diastolic pressures. The fluid-filled pericardial space does not transmit intrathoracic pressures to the cardiac chambers. The dissociation of intrathoracic and intracardial pressures leads to ventricular discordance during the respirophasic cycle. The extrapericardial pulmonary veins follow intrathoracic pressure and the pulmonary venous pressure decreases in inspiration. This decreases the left sided effective filling gradient and left ventricular stroke volume. Thus pulsus paradoxsus, or a greater than normal (> 10 mm Hg) decrease in aortic blood pressure with inspiration occurs.[24]

Right atrial pressure is elevated, however, unlike constrictive pericarditis, a blunted y-descent is present on the right atrial pressure waveform in cardiac tamponade. The effect of the increased intrapericardial pressure on impairment atrial emptying is most present when the ventricle is filled in diastole, resulting in a blunted y-descent. The "a" wave is augmented due to elevated pressure in the right ventricle during atrial contraction. The x-descent following the "a" wave is sharp as the atrium relaxes from a higher pressure peak and the volume of the right ventricle decreases in systole, such that the effects of elevated intrapericardial pressure are less pronounced on the atrium.[24]

Unlike constrictive pericarditis, the dip-and-plateau configuration of the diastolic ventricular pressure tracing is not seen in cardiac tamponade. This is due to the lack of sudden restriction to filling.

CORONARY HEMODYNAMICS

Coronary angiography provides information on luminal contrast opacification and visual estimation of luminal diameter stenosis often dictates whether coronary intervention is performed. However, limitations of coronary angiography exist and are important to recognize prior to making clinical decisions regarding coronary intervention. Coronary angiography provides a 2-dimensional image of a 3-dimensional vascular lumen. Based on the angiographic views and plaque characteristics, such as eccentricity, angiography may not capture the area of maximal stenosis. Furthermore, assessment of certain anatomical locations, such as side branch ostial lesions, are often challenging with angiography due to vessel overlap and foreshortening with fluoroscopy. Assessing left main coronary lesions with standard angiography can be especially challenging. Indeed we extrapolate physiological reduction on blood supply based on anatomic measurement from coronary angiography. Knowledge of coronary physiology, using techniques such as fractional flow reserve (FFR) and coronary flow reserve (CFR), improves diagnostic accuracy of coronary lesions producing ischemia, particularly when angiography is limited in its ability to do.

FRACTIONAL FLOW RESERVE

FFR is a physiologic coronary study performed percutaneously at the time of coronary angiography to detect ischemia-producing stenoses. Ohm's law describes flow is equal to the change in pressure divided by resistance; the length of coronary stenosis is inversely proportional to coronary blood flow. Therefore, a lengthy intermediate coronary lesion of intermediate diameter stenosis may compromise coronary blood flow more than a short high-grade stenosis, a factor that would be difficult to assess using visual information alone. FFR is a comparison of pressure measured distal to the stenosis in question to that proximal to the stenosis. The procedure is performed using a pressure sensor guidewire that is calibrated and then advanced through a guide catheter across the coronary lesion in the target artery. FFR is calculated as the ratio of mean coronary artery pressure distal to the coronary lesion of interest at maximal hyperemia to the mean aortic pressure and is derived as such:[25-29]

$$FFR = \frac{1 - \text{Mean translesional pressure gradient}}{\text{Mean aortic pressure} - \text{Mean right atrial pressure}}$$

$$= \frac{\text{Mean pressure distal coronary pressure} - \text{Mean right atrial pressure}}{\text{Mean aortic pressure} - \text{Mean right atrial pressure}}$$

$$= \frac{\text{Mean pressure distal to coronary stenosis (Pd)}}{\text{Mean aortic pressure (Pa)}}$$

In order to assess the physiologic significance of coronary stenosis, maximal hyperemia with a vasodilator is required. If vasodilation is submaximal, stenosis severity may be underestimated. A vasodilator, such as adenosine, is administered intravenously 140 and 180 μg/kg/min (each dose administered for two minutes). If intracoronary adenosine is used to induce hyperemia then 15–40 μg is delivered to the left coronary system and 10–30 μg to the right coronary artery. Prior to the use of adenosine, the patient should be screened to ensure no contraindication to the use of adenosine exists such as reactive airway disease.

A FFR of lesser than 0.75 correlates with ischemia when compared to non-invasive stress testing with a sensitivity of 88% and specificity of 100%.[27] Interestingly, the largest study to date using FFR to guide percutaneous intervention in patients with multi-vessel disease, found that using FFR lesser than 0.8 to guide decision making reduced the primary endpoint of death, nonfatal myocardial infarction and repeat revascularization.[25] FFR has great utility for predicting ischemia where angiography is limited in doing so, particularly for intermediate-grade, left main, and ostial side branch stenosis. Figure 14 demonstrates hemodynamic assessment of coronary pressure during maximal hyperemia using FFR.

CORONARY FLOW RESERVE

Similar to FFR, coronary flow reserve (CFR) is a physiologic coronary study performed percutaneously at the time of coronary angiography for the detection of ischemia–producing stenoses. The technique of CFR involves use of a doppler tipped guidewire that transmits ultrasound doppler waves from which coronary flow can be assessed. CFR is the ratio of coronary flow distal to a stenosis at maximal hyperemia to basal coronary blood flow measured in a coronary artery without stenosis. A CFR of lesser than 2 identifies an ischemia-producing stenosis (Fig. 15).

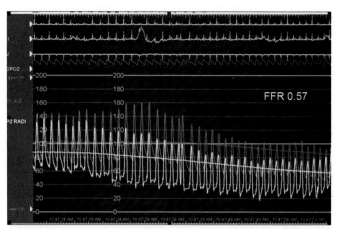

FIGURE 14: Fractional flow reserve. Aortic pressure (red) and coronary artery pressure (yellow) during adenosine infusion. Fractional flow reserve of mid left anterior descending coronary artery 70% angiographic luminal stenosis reveals positie physiological significance with value of 0.57

$$CFR = \frac{\text{Flow distal to stenosis}}{\text{Basal coronary flow}}$$

Alternatively, CFR may be derived from a coronary thermodilution curve with a pressor sensor wire with proximal and distal thermistors such that a thermodilution curve during the injection of saline is generated. The mean transit time is measured from the thermodilution curve. The ratio of the mean transit time at rest divided by the mean transit time at hyperemia reflects CFR.

Unlike FFR, CFR is influenced by conditions that affect vascular resistance such as microvascular disease and myocardial hypertrophy. Therefore, it has utility in the assessment of microvascular disease, and is an important research tool. Coronary flow is also influenced by hemodynamic variations

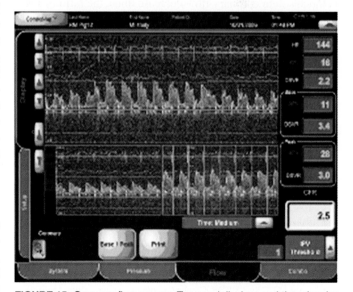

FIGURE 15: Coronary flow reserve. Top panel displays real-time doppler of coronary flow of the left anterior descending coronary artery. The bottom left panel demonstrates doppler at baseline and the bottom right panel is peak coronary doppler flow at maximal hyperemia during adenosine administration. The calculated coronary flow reserve is 2.5, with no significant physiologic impairment to coronary flow. (*Source:* Boyle, et al. Am J Cardiol. 2008;102:980-7, with permission)

such as tachycardia. Since CFR reflects both epicardial and microvascular flow, one must be aware of limitations with this technique in assessing the significance of coronary stenosis.

INDEX OF MICROCIRCULATORY RESISTANCE

Assessment of microcirculation is best performed by measuring the Index of microvascular resistance (IMR). This may be important in symptomatic patients with risk factors for epicardial coronary artery disease and yet no angiographic evidence of significant epicardial disease. Similar to FFR, IMR is performed by measuring the pressure distal to the coronary stenosis with a pressure sensor wire. A coronary thermodilution curve is generated using a pressor sensory wire with proximal and distal thermistor. The mean transit time is measured from the coronary thermodilution curve and the inverse of mean transit time is a surrogate of absolute flow. The product of the pressure distal to a coronary stenosis and the mean transit time at maximal hyperemia defines IMR:

$$Resistance = \frac{\Delta \text{ Pressure and Flow} \approx 1}{\text{Flow mean transit time}}$$

$$IMR = \frac{\text{Mean pressure distal to stenosis } - \text{ Right atrial pressure}}{1/\text{Mean transit time}}$$

Using the assumption that right atrial pressure is neglible:

$$IMR \text{ (mm Hg•s)} = \text{Mean transit time} \times \text{Pressure distal to stenosis}$$

Index of microcirculatory resistance (IMR) is measured at maximal hyperemia using a coronary vasodilator and reflects the resistance of the microcirculation, unaffected by the epicardial stenosis. In the presence of a stenosis or hemodynamic variations, both the pressure distal to the stenosis as well as the absolute coronary flow decrease, thus, the ratio of IMR will remain relatively unaffected.[30-32]

REFERENCES

1. Berry D. History of Cardiology: Werner Forssmann, MD. Circulation. 2006;113:f26-8.
2. Forsmann W. Die Sondierung des rechten Herzens. Klin Wochenschr. 1929;8:2085-7.
3. Courtois M, Fattal PG, Kovács SJ, et al. Anatomically and physiologically based reference level for measurement of intracardiac pressures. Circulation. 1995;92:1994-2000.
4. Grossman W. Percutaneous approach including trans-septal and apical puncture. In: Baim DS (Ed). Cardiac Catheterization, Angiography, and Intervention, 7th edition. Philadelphia: Lippincott; 2006. pp. 79-106.
5. Saksena FB. Nomogram to calculate oxygen consumption index based on age, sex, and heart rate. Pediatric Cardiology. 1983;4:1432-971.
6. Flamm MD, Cohn KE, Hancock EW. Measurement of systemic cardiac output at rest and exercise in patients with atrial septal defect. Am J Cardiol. 1969;23:258-65.
7. Kern MJ. The LVEDP. Cather Cardiovasc Diagn. 1998;44:70-4.
8. Bonow RO, Carabello BA, Chatterjee K, et al. ACC/AHA 2006 Practice guidelines for the management of patients with valvular heart disease: executive summary: a report of the American College of Cardiology/American Heart Association Task Force on practice guidelines. J Am Coll Cardiol. 2006;48:598-675.
9. Gorlin R, Gorlin G. Hydraulic formula for calculation of area of stenotic mitral valve, other cardiac valves and central circulatory shunts. Am Heart J. 1951;41:1-29.
10. Hakki AH, Iskandrian AS, Bemis CE, et al. A simplified valve formula for the calculation of stenotic cardiac valve areas. Circulation. 1981;63:1050-5.
11. Grossman W. Profiles in valvular heart disease. In: Baim DS (Ed). Cardiac Catheterization, Angiography and Intervention, 7th edition. Philadelphia: Lippincott; 2006. pp. 653-6.
12. Abascal VM, Wilkins GT, Choong CY, et al. Echocardiographic evaluation of mitral valve structure and function in patients followed for at least 6 months after percutaneous balloon mitral valvuloplasty. J Am Coll Cardiol. 1988;12:606-15.
13. Cohen MV, Gorlin R. Modified orifice equation for the calculation of mitral valve area. Am Heart J. 1972;84:839-40.
14. Grossman W. Calculation of stenotic valve orifice area. In: Baim DS (Ed). Cardiac Catheterization, Angiography and Intervention, 7th edition. Philadelphia: Lippincott; 2006. pp. 173-83.
15. Grossman W. Profiles in valvular heart disease. In: Baim DS (Ed). Cardiac Catheterization, Angiography and Intervention, 7th edition. Philadelphia: Lippincott; 2006. pp. 641-7.
16. Brockenbrough EC, Braunwald E, Morrow AG. A hemodynamic technique for the detection of hypertrophic subaortic stenosis. Circulation. 1961;23:189-94.
17. Kern MJ, Deligonui U. The left-sided v wave. Cathet Cardiovasc Diag. 1991;23:211-8.
18. Kern MJ, Deligonui U. Intraventricular pressure gradients. Cathet Cardiov Diagn. 1992;22:145-52.
19. Kern MJ, Rajjoub H, Bach R. Hemodynamic effects of alcohol-induced septal infarction for hypertrophic obstructive cardiomyopathy. Cathet Cardiov Diagn. 1999;47:221-8.
20. Fang JC, Eisenhauer AC. Profiles in cardiomyopathy and congestive heart failure. In: Baim DS (Ed). Grossman's Cardiac Catheterization, Angiography and Intervention, 7th edition. Philadelphia: Lippincott; 2006. pp. 711-6.
21. Higano ST, Azrak E, Tahirkheli NK, et al. Constrictive physiology. In: Kern MJ, Lim MJ, Goldstein JA (Eds). Hemodynamic Rounds, 3rd edition. New York: Wiley-Blackwell; 2009. pp. 231-45.
22. Golstein JA. Cardiac tamponade, constrictive pericarditis, and restrictive cardiomyopathy. Curr Probl Cardiol. 2004;503-67.
23. Robb JF, Laham RJ. Profiles in pericardial disease. In: Baim DS (Ed). Grossman's Cardiac Catheterization, Angiography and Intervention, 7th edition. Philadelphia: Lippincott; 2006. pp. 725-31.
24. Hurrell DG, Nishimura RA, Higano ST, et al. Value of dynamic respiratory changes in left and right ventricular pressures for the diagnosis of constrictive pericarditis. Circulation. 1996;93:2007-13.
25. Tonino PAL, Bruyne BD, Pijls NHJ, et al. Fractional flow reserve versus angiography for guiding percutaneous coronary intervention. N Eng J Med. 2009;360:213-24.
26. Kern MJ. Coronary hemodynamics. In: Kern MJ, Lim MJ, Goldstein JA (Eds). Hemodynamic Rounds, 3rd edition. New York: Wiley-Blackwell; 2009. pp. 339-66.
27. Pijls NHJ, DeBruyne, Peels K, et al. Measurement of fractional flow reserve to assess the functional severity of coronary artery stenoses. N Engl J Med. 1996;334:1703-8.
28. Kern MJ, Samady H. Current concepts of integrated coronary physiology in the catheterization laboratory. J Am Coll Cardiol. 2010;55:173-85.
29. Spaan JAE, Piek JJ, Hoofman JIE, et al. Physiological basis of clinically used coronary hemodynamic indices. Circulation. 2006;113:446-55.
30. Fearon WF, Balsam LB, Farouque O, et al. Novel index for invasively assessing the coronary microcirculation. Circulation. 2003;107:3129-32.
31. Ng MKC, Yeung AC, Fearon WF. Invasive assessment of the coronary microcirculation: superior reproducibility and less hemodynamic dependence of index of microcirculatory resistance compared with coronary flow reserve. Circulation. 2006;113:2054-61.
32. Fearon WF, Shah M, Ng M, et al. Predictive value of the index of microcirculatory resistance in patients with ST-segment elevation myocardial infarction. J Am Coll Cardiol. 2008;51:560-5.

Cardiac Biopsy

Vijay U Rao, Teresa De Marco

Chapter Outline

INTRODUCTION

The development and refinement of endomyocardial biopsy (EMB) has significantly advanced our understanding of many cardiac diseases which once confounded even the most astute clinicians. In fact, for several conditions, EMB is the only modality that provides a definitive diagnosis and, therefore, is the "gold standard" upon which other tests should be compared. The EMB has also helped to change the landscape of certain disease states. For example, EMB is partly responsible, in conjunction with the advent of immunosuppressive medications, for the dramatic reduction in mortality resulting from rejection in post heart transplant patients. Despite these benefits, there have been few, large, randomized controlled trials supporting the use of EMB in the clinical arena. In the face of our ever increasing knowledge about disease states, the clinician is faced not only with the onerous task of keeping pace but also making decisions about which diagnostic tools to employ. This chapter will attempt to highlight many of the salient features of EMB, including techniques, tissue processing as well as the characteristic pathological features for the most common diagnoses for which EMB is performed.

HISTORY AND DEVICES

The first transvenous EMB device was developed in Japan in 1962 and was called the Konno-Sakakibara bioptome (catheter-based biopsy system).[1] This device consisted of a 100 cm catheter shaft with two sharpened cusps at its tip. The catheter was introduced into the body by means of a cutdown of the saphenous or basilic vein (or the femoral or brachial artery) due to the large size of the catheter tip. The catheter was then advanced to the desired ventricle under fluoroscopic guidance and applied to the endocardial surface with the jaws closed. The catheter was then withdrawn a short distance, jaws opened, re-advanced into contact with the endocardium, jaws re-closed,

and withdrawn. With the exception of the cutdown, a similar technique is employed today. In 1972, the Konno-Sakakibara bioptome was redesigned to work specifically for right ventricular biopsy by way of the right internal jugular vein and was called the Caves-Schultz-Stanford bioptome (Fig. 1A).[2,3] The device consists of a somewhat flexible coil shaft made of stainless steel and coated by clear plastic tubing. The tip of the catheter has two hemispheric cutting jaws with a combined diameter of 3.0 mm (9 French). One jaw is opened and closed via stainless steel wire running through the center of the bioptome shaft, while the other jaw remains stationary. The control wire is attached to a ratcheting surgical mosquito clamp by a pair of spring-loaded adjustable nuts that allow the operator to set the amount of force that is applied during opening and closing of the surgical clamp.[4]

Current bioptomes come in several lengths depending upon whether a right internal jugular vein approach (short bioptome) or a femoral vein approach (long bioptome) is employed (Fig. 1B). The catheters come in multiple diameters (French) in order to fit inside standard sheaths. At the end of the catheter is a set of jaws that have been specially designed to allow precise cutting of endomyocardial tissue with preservation of myocardial architecture for pathological examination.

TECHNIQUES

A transvenous approach is taken for right ventricular EMB. Either the femoral vein or the internal jugular vein (either right or left) is cannulated with an introducer sheath via the modified Seldinger technique (Fig. 2).[5] Electrocardiographic rhythm, blood pressure and pulse oximetry should be monitored in all patients undergoing EMB. Ultrasound guidance can facilitate identification of the vein of interest for purposes of cannulation and has been shown to reduce procedure time and complications.[6,7] In addition, in patients with normal or low right atrial pressure, elevating the patient's legs, using the Trendelenburg

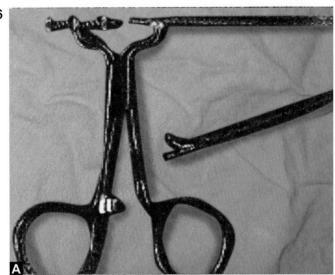

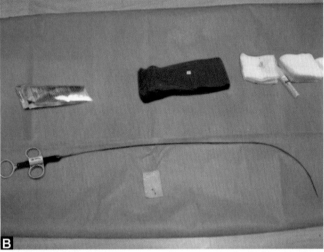

FIGURES 1A AND B: (A) Stanford (Caves-Schulz) bioptome; (B) Current generation short, disposable bioptome for use through the internal jugular vein (*Source:* Grossman's cardiac catheterization, angiography and intervention by LWW, 2000)

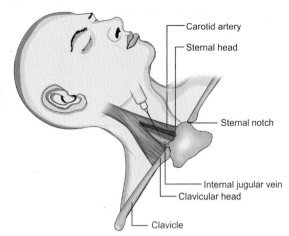

FIGURE 2: Regional anatomy for right internal jugular vein puncture. With the patient's head rotated to the left, the sternal notch, clavicle and the sternal and clavicular heads of the sternocleidomastoid muscle are identified. A skin nick is made between the two heads of the muscle, two fingerbreadths above the top of the clavicle, and the needle is inserted at an angle of 30–40° from vertical, and 20–30° right of sagittal. This approach leads to reliable puncture of the internal jugular vein and aims the needle away from the more medially located carotid artery (*Source:* Grossman's cardiac catheterization, angiography and intervention by LWW, 2000)

In Figure 2, the labels read: Carotid artery, Sternal head, Sternal notch, Internal jugular vein, Clavicular head, Clavicle

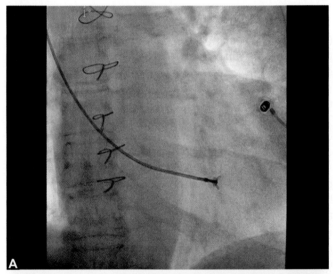

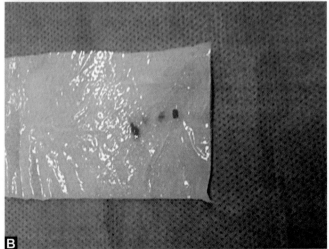

FIGURES 3A AND B: (A) Fluoroscopic image of bioptome in the right anterior oblique projection demonstrating open jaws just prior to right ventricular biopsy; (B) Right ventricular endomyocardial biopsy tissue specimens displayed on moistened filter paper

(head-down) position, or having the patient perform a Valsalva maneuver all elevate central venous pressure (CVP) which distends the internal jugular vein and allows for easier cannulation. Once the internal jugular vein has been cannulated, a 40 cm J guidewire is advanced into the right atrium. Then a sheath (7–9 French) with a side-arm and back-bleed valve (Cordis Corporation) is advanced over the guidewire. The CVP is then recorded via the side arm before the biopsy.

Next, the bioptome is inserted into the sheath with the tip pointed toward the lateral wall of the right atrium and advanced to the right atrium under either echocardiographic or fluoroscopic guidance. At the level of the mid-right atrium, the bioptome is rotated anteriorly in a clockwise direction approximately 180 degrees and is advanced through the tricuspid valve apparatus toward the right ventricle. The bioptome is then advanced to the interventricular septum. The bioptome position in the right ventricle should be confirmed with fluoroscopy (30 degree right anterior oblique and 60 degree left anterior oblique views). The bioptome should appear to lie across the spine and below the upper margin of the left hemidiaphragm (Fig. 3A). The goal of this step is to take proper precaution to avoid the thin, right ventricular free wall. Next, the jaws are opened and the bioptome is advanced to the right ventricular muscular septum. Proper localization of the bioptome is evidenced by lack of further advancement, the occurrence of premature ventricular contractions, and the transmission of ventricular impulses to the operator's hand. The jaws are then closed and allowed a brief delay to sever the tissue. The bioptome and enclosed sample are then slowly retracted all the way out of the sheath. Three to five separate biopsies should usually be obtained to account for sampling error. The samples are then placed in specific preservatives depending upon the diagnosis suspected. If a balloon-tipped pulmonary artery catheter was used to perform a right heart catheterization, such as during EMB for transplant rejection, it is our practice to advance the balloon-tipped pulmonary artery catheter to the right atrium for several minutes after completion of the EMB to ensure stable right atrial pressures and to screen for possible myocardial perforation which could lead to tamponade. Alternatively, repeat CVP measurement is obtained at conclusion of the biopsy through the side arm.

Left ventricular biopsy remains limited to individual cases in which the suspected disease is limited to the left ventricle.[8] The femoral artery is often used as the percutaneous access site for left ventricular biopsy.[9] In this approach, a preformed sheath is employed to maintain arterial patency. In addition, to avoid embolic events, the sheath must be maintained under constant pressurized infusion. Given the potential for serious consequences of left-sided embolization, aspirin or other antiplatelet agents are generally combined with heparin for left ventricular biopsy.

SAFETY AND COMPLICATIONS

Despite the invasive nature of the procedure and potential for severe complications, EMB is now considered a very safe technique. The EMB complications can be categorized as to those that occur in the acute setting and those that occur after a delayed period of time. Immediate periprocedural risks include perforation with pericardial tamponade, pneumothorax, pulmonary embolization, ventricular and supraventricular arrhythmias, heart block, recurrent laryngeal nerve paresis, damage to the tricuspid valve and creation of an arteriovenous fistula within the heart. Like any invasive procedure, degree of risk is heavily dependent upon operator's experience. In addition, baseline clinical features of the patient, access site and type of bioptome are also likely important. Delayed complications include access site bleeding, damage to the tricuspid valve, pericardial tamponade and deep vein thrombosis.

The precise risk of EMB is not known as the data are derived from several single-center experiences and registries. In one series of greater than 4,000 biopsies performed in transplantation and cardiomyopathy patients, complication rates were reported in less than 1%.[10] In addition, a worldwide survey of more than 6,000 cases of EMB reported a 1.17% complication rate with 28 perforations (0.42%) and 2 deaths (0.03%).[11]

Finally, a study by Deckers et al. from John's Hopkins hospital reported on complication rates in 546 consecutive biopsies in adults with cardiomyopathy.[12] There were 33 complications (6%) with 15 (2.7%) considered minor without sequelae and 18 (3.3%) serious with 2 (0.4%) deaths.

One of the most significant complications with EMB is cardiac perforation leading to tamponade. Several clinical features that have been associated with increased risk of perforation include: increased right ventricular systolic pressures, bleeding diathesis, recent receipt of heparin and right ventricular enlargement. Cardiac perforation should be suspected if the patient complains of chest pain with a biopsy pass, unexpected bradycardia or hypotension is encountered, or if the EMB samples float in 10% formalin (suggesting the presence of cardiac fat). In these circumstances, right atrial pressure, fluoroscopic appearance of the heart border and possibly bedside echocardiography should be used to monitor for hemopericardium. If confirmed, urgent pericardiocentesis should be performed. In most cases, in a patient with normal coagulation parameters, catheter drainage is sufficient to stabilize the patient. However, on occasion, it may be necessary to consult thoracic surgeons to evacuate the pericardial space. Of note, cardiac tamponade rarely occurs in patients after heart transplant or cardiac surgery as there is a layer of adhesive pericardium overlying the right ventricular free wall, although reported cases have occurred secondary to the pericardium being left open anteriorly.

Several additional approaches can be used to avoid EMB complications. In order to avoid pneumothoraces, a relatively high internal jugular vein approach should be employed which avoids the immediate supraclavicular location. Patients with pre-existing left bundle branch block can develop complete heart block when the catheter is placed into the right ventricle and pushes up against the interventricular septum. In this case, the catheter/bioptome should be withdrawn and, in most cases, the heart block will abate. However, in some patients, the heart block may persist and become permanent requiring temporary right ventricular pacing with eventual placement of a permanent pacemaker. Lidocaine injection into the jugular venous and carotid sheath can result in Horner's syndrome, vocal paresis and, occasionally, weakness of the diaphragm. These symptoms are usually transient and last only as long as it takes for the lidocaine to wear off.

ANALYSIS OF EMB TISSUE

The utility of EMB for diagnosis of suspected cardiac conditions is heavily dependent upon proper sampling technique, careful handling of the EMB sample and initial preparation of the sample in appropriate fixatives. In general, an attempt should be made to obtain samples from greater than 1 region of the right ventricular septum. In addition, between 5 and 10 samples of $1-2 \, mm^3$ in size should be obtained to minimize sampling errors. Biopsy samples should be removed gently from the jaws of the bioptome with a fine needle (not forceps) and placed on moistened filter paper (Fig. 3B).[13,14] Next, the samples should be transferred to a container with 10% neutral buffered formalin for light microscopy or 4% glutaraldehyde for transmission electron microscopy.[14] Contraction band artifacts may occur due to the specimen being torn away from the beating heart resulting in myocyte hypercontraction. These artifacts are accentuated with cold fixatives, but can be minimized by using fixatives at room temperature.[15] The EMB samples can also be snap frozen in OCT embedding medium and stored at −80°F for molecular studies, immunohistochemistry or immunofluorescence.

In general, flash freezing is appropriate for culture, polymerase chain reaction (PCR) or reverse transcriptase PCR (rtPCR) to identify viruses, but is not well-suited for standard histological preparations due to the development of ice crystal artifacts.

Diagnostic yield of EMB is also largely dependent upon sampling error. Many diseases with cardiac involvement are heterogeneously distributed in the heart. For example, in one study by Chow et al., right ventricular EMB was performed on 14 autopsy/post-transplant hearts with confirmed myocarditis and found that 5 biopsy samples had a combined sensitivity of only 43–57%. Sensitivity increased to 80% when combining all 17 samples, a number that is not practical for routine clinical use.[16]

LIGHT MICROSCOPY AND STAINS

Once the EMB samples have been fixed and transported from the catheterization laboratory to the pathology laboratory, they are then embedded in paraffin and serial 4 μm thick sections are cut and sequentially numbered. The specimens are then stained with hematoxylin and eosin (H&E) as well as Movat or elastic trichrome stain to visualize collagen and elastic tissue. It is a common practice for many laboratories to routinely stain one slide for iron on men and all postmenopausal women to screen for hemochromatosis. In addition, Congo red staining may be performed to screen for amyloidosis.

CARDIOTROPIC VIRUS DETECTION

The EMB samples can also be screened for cardiotropic viruses. Identification of viral genomes from EMB samples has recently become more feasible due to the development of rapid, quantitative (qPCR) and qualitative (nested PCR) molecular techniques. Several studies have reported a high incidence of viral genome detection in the myocardium of patients with suspected myocarditis and dilated cardiomyopathy (DCM).[17,18] The most common viruses detected in the myocardium include: enteroviruses, adenoviruses, parvovirus B19, cytomegalovirus (CMV), influenza, respiratory syncytial virus, herpes simplex virus, Epstein-Barr virus, human herpes 6, HIV and hepatitis C. Given the exquisitely sensitive nature of PCR, samples must be carefully handled to avoid possible contamination and degradation. Pathogen-free biopsy devices and storage vials should be employed. In addition, new fixatives, such as RNAlater (Ambion, Austin, Texas), allow for PCR and rtPCR to be performed on samples transported on dry ice at room temperature without losing sensitivity compared to frozen tissue. Despite the ability to detect viruses at very low copy numbers, the true sensitivity of these techniques with EMB samples is not known. As a result, a positive PCR result is diagnostic, whereas a negative PCR result does not rule out the presence of virus. At this time, however, given the heterogeneity in methods and interpretation of results across centers, routine screening of EMB samples for viruses is not recommended outside of established centers with experience in viral genome analysis.

INDICATIONS

Reports in the literature regarding the utility of EMB for the diagnosis of cardiovascular conditions are limited to case series and cohorts. As a result, one of the most difficult decisions facing the clinician is determining under what circumstances performing an EMB would lead to a clinically meaningful diagnosis or change in therapy while taking into account the risk of harm from the procedure itself. Recognizing the need for a comprehensive review of the literature and a unified set of recommendations, the American Heart Association (AHA), the American College of Cardiology Foundation (ACCF) and the European Society of Cardiology (ESC) convened a multidisciplinary group of experts, and recently released a joint scientific statement.[19] In this statement, the authors review 14 clinical case scenarios where EMB might be considered and provide Class I–III recommendations along with levels of evidence (Levels A–C) to support these recommendations (Table 1). The two Class I recommendations (conditions for which there is evidence or there is general agreement that a given procedure is beneficial, useful and effective) as well as the one Class III recommendation (conditions for which there is evidence and/or general agreement that a procedure/treatment is not useful/effective and in some cases may be harmful) are reviewed here. For further details regarding the other 11 clinical scenarios, the reader is referred to the article by Cooper et al.[19]

The two clinical scenarios that received a Class I indication for EMB were:

- In the setting of unexplained, new-onset heart failure of less than 2 weeks' duration associated with a normal-sized or dilated left ventricle in addition to hemodynamic compromise.
- In the setting of unexplained, new-onset heart failure of 2 weeks to 3 months duration associated with a dilated left ventricle and new ventricular arrhythmias, Mobitz type II second- or third-degree atrioventricular (AV) heart block, or failure to respond to usual care within 1–2 weeks.

The EMB should be performed in these two settings to identify three clinical entities: (1) lymphocytic myocarditis; (2) giant cell myocarditis (GCM) or (3) necrotizing eosinophilic myocarditis. Identification of these clinical entities is important both for prognostic as well as therapeutic purposes. Lymphocytic myocarditis is the most common type of myocarditis reported in the United States and Western Europe.[20] Adults and children presenting with severe left ventricular failure within two weeks of a distinct viral illness and have typical lymphocytic myocarditis on EMB have an excellent prognosis (Fig. 4A).[21,22] The left ventricular ejection fraction (EF) is often markedly depressed; however, the left ventricular volumes are generally normal.[23] Despite the benign long-term outcome in the acute setting, lymphocytic myocarditis often presents with cardiogenic shock requiring intravenous inotropic agents or mechanical assistance for circulatory support. Since lymphocytic myocarditis is still a relatively uncommon clinical entity, it is difficult to ascertain whether treatment with corticosteroids or intravenous immunoglobulin provides any significant clinical benefit. Necrotizing eosinophilic myocarditis is a rare condition that is characterized by an acute onset and rapid progression to hemodynamic compromise.[24] Histologically, there is a diffuse inflammatory infiltrate with predominant eosinophils associated with extensive myocyte necrosis (Fig. 4B). Therapy with a combination of immunosuppressive agents as well as biventricular assist device support has been associated with improved outcomes.[25]

TABLE 1

The role of endomyocardial biopsy in 14 clinical scenarios

Scenatio number	Clinical scenario	Class of recommendation (I, IIa, IIb, III)	Level of evidence (A, B, C)
1.	New-onset heart failure of < 2 weeks' duration associated with a normal-sized or dilated left ventricle and hemodynamic compromise	I	B
2.	New-onset heart failure of 2 weeks' to 3 months' duration associated with a dilated left ventricle and new ventricular arrhythmias, second- or third-degree heart block, or failure to respond to usual care within 1–2 weeks	I	B
3.	Heart failure of > 3 months' duration associated with a dilated left ventricle and new ventricular arrhythmias, second- or third-degree heart block, or failure to respond to usual care within 1–2 weeks	IIa	C
4.	Heart failure associated with a DCM of any duration associated with suspected allergic reaction and/or eosinophilia	IIa	C
5.	Heart failure associated with suspected anthracycline cardiomyopathy	IIa	C
6.	Heart failure associated with unexplained restrictive cardiomyopathy	IIa	C
7.	Suspected cardiac tumors	IIa	C
8.	Unexplained cardiomyopathy in children	IIa	C
9.	New-onset heart failure of 2 weeks' to 3 months' duration associated with a dilated left ventricle, without new ventricular arrhythmias or second- or third-degree heart block, that responds to usual care within 1–2 weeks	IIb	B
10.	Heart failure of > 3 months' duration assoicated with a dilated left ventricle, without new ventricular arrhythmias or second- or third-degree heart block, that responds to usual care within 1–2 weeks	IIb	C
11.	Heart failure associated with unexplained HCM	IIb	C
12.	Suspected ARVD/C	IIb	C
13.	Unexplained ventricular arrhythmias	IIb	C
14.	Unexplained atrial fibrillation	III	C

CHAPTER 26 Cardiac Biopsy

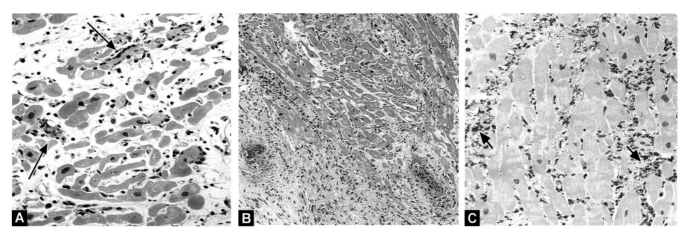

FIGURES 4A TO C: Myocarditis: (A) Lymphocytic myocarditis—sparse infiltrate of mononuclear cells is present in the interstitium surrounding individual damaged or dying myocytes (large arrows). (B) Giant cell myocarditis—there is extensive inflammation characterized by mononuclear cells and scattered giant cells (stars). The lower third of the field is comprised of granulation tissue due to extensive myocyte necrosis. (C) Hypersensitivity myocarditis—numerous interstitial eosinophils and very limited myocyte damage characterize the hypersensitivity reaction (small arrows). [H&E stains (400x magnification) (*Source:* Philip Ursell, UCSF pathology)]

The GCM, like necrotizing eosinophilic myocarditis and lymphocytic myocarditis, often presents with a fulminant picture. Both ventricular tachycardia (15%) and complete heart block (5%) can be complicating features of GCM. Presence of GCM in a patient with hemodynamic compromise should prompt consideration of biventricular mechanical circulatory device support as progressive right ventricular failure is often observed. However, most patients with GCM should be considered for early cardiac transplantation since this modality has been clearly shown to improve survival. The GCM is associated with a very high mortality; mean transplantation-free survival is only 5.5 months.[26] Therapy with cyclosporine has been shown to extend median transplantation-free survival to 12.3 months. Of note, GCM can recur in the transplanted heart with a 20–25% frequency.[27] Greater consideration to use of EMB to rule out GCM should also be given to patients presenting with a coexisting history of thymoma or drug hypersensitivity as there has been an association with both entities.[28,29] The sensitivity of EMB for GCM is 80–85% in patients who subsequently die or undergo heart transplantation.[30] The characteristic histologic feature of GCM is myocyte necrosis with a mixed inflammatory infiltrate composed of lymphocytes, plasma cells, histiocytes, eosinophils and multinucleated giant cells (Fig. 4C). Differentiation between GCM and granulomatous myocarditis due to sarcoidosis can be difficult. Helpful features that may point to a diagnosis of GCM include myocyte necrosis, poorly formed granulomas and eosinophils.

The diagnosis of myocarditis by EMB can be confidently ascertained when there is a highly abnormal inflammatory infiltrate such as eosinophilic, granulomatous, or giant cell inflammation. However, one of the key limitations of this technique is sampling error. In about 40% of cases, false negative results occur.[20,31] Therefore, it is recommended that between five and ten biopsy samples be examined, and cut at multiple levels. In 1987, the Dallas criteria were established to help standardize the reporting and diagnosis of myocarditis (Table 2).[32] Initial EMB results are categorized as either myocarditis, borderline myocarditis or no myocarditis. In order to diagnose myocarditis, two criteria must be met: (1) inflammation and (2) myocyte necrosis.

The only Class III recommendation from the 2007 joint scientific statement for EMB was: EMB should not be performed in the setting of unexplained atrial fibrillation. The Writing Group based on this recommendation on the lack of

SECTION 3

Diagnosis

TABLE 2

Clinical scenarios for the diagnosis of myocarditis

Clinical scenario	Duration of illness	Pathological correlates	Prognosis	Treatment
Acute myocardial infarction-like syndrome with normal coronary arteries	Several hours or days	Active lymphocytic myocarditis or, rarely, necrotizing eosinophilic myocarditis or giant-cell myocarditis	Good if lymphocytic myocarditis is present on biopsy	Supportive
Heart failure with normal-sized or dilated left ventricle and hemodynamic compromise	Less than 2 weeks	Active lymphocytic myocarditis or, less commonly, necrotizing eosinophilic myocarditis or giant-cell myocarditis	Good in fulminant lymphocytic myocarditis, but acute care often requires inotropic or mechanical circulatory support	Supportive; possible use of corticosteroids or IVIG* in children
Heart failure with dilated left ventricle and new ventricular arrhythmias, high-degree heart block, or lack of response to usual care within 1–2 weeks	A few weeks or months	Giant-cell myocarditis, eosinophilic myocarditis, or lymphocytic myocarditis	Poor, high likelihood or death or need for cardiac transplantation if giant-cell myocarditis is found on biopsy	Variable therapy according to histopathological results
Heart failure with dilated left ventricle without new ventricular arrhythmias or high-degree heart block	A few weeks or months	Nonspecific changes most likely, with the presence of viral genomes in 25–35% of patients and of lymphocytic myocarditis (Dallas criteria) in about 10%	Good in the first several years, but a risk of late disease progression with heart failure and cariomyopathy	Supportive; definition of genomic predictors of risk under investigation
Heart failure with eosinophilia	Any duration	Eosinophilic or hypersensitivity myocarditis, eosinophilic endomyocarditis	Poor	Supportive, including identification and treatment of underlying cause; possible use of corticosteroids for hypersensitivity myocarditis
Heart failure with dilated left ventricle and new ventricular arrhythmias, high-degree heart block, or lack of response to usual care in 1–2 weeks	More than several months	Cardiac sarcoidosis (idiopathic granulomatous myocarditis) or specific infection (e.g. *Trypanosoma cruzi* and *Borrelia burgdorfen*); nonspecific changes most likely	Increased risk of need for pacemaker or implantable cardioverter-defibrillator if sarcoidosis is confirmed on biopsy	Supportive; corticosteroids for biopsy-proven cardiac sarcoidosis
Heart failure with dilated left ventricle without new ventricular arrhythmias or high-degree heart block	More than several months	Nonspecific changes most likely; increased number of inflammatory cells shown by sensitive immunostaining in up to 40% of patients and the presence of viral genome in 25–35%	Depends on functional class ejection fraction and the presence or absence of inflammation and viral genomes on biopsy	Supportive; antiviral treatment and immunosuppression under investigation

*IVIG denotes intravenous immunoglobulin

significant evidence showing benefit of EMB in this setting. One small study was cited looking at EMB results in 14 "lone" atrial fibrillation patients unresponsive to traditional antiarrhythmic therapy.[33] In this study, all patients had some evidence of histologic abnormalities; however, 3 patients had EMB consistent with myocarditis and received steroid therapy with a reversion to sinus rhythm. Despite this apparent benefit of EMB diagnosis in lone atrial fibrillation, given the paucity of data, EMB was not felt to be appropriate in this setting.

DISEASE STATES

EMB IN CARDIOMYOPATHY

Dilated Cardiomyopathy

Dilated cardiomyopathy (DCM) is a common form of cardiomyopathy often observed in patients between the ages of 20 years and 60 years. Characteristic echocardiographic findings include 4-chamber dilatation with biventricular hypertrophy. Etiologies for DCM are numerous and include: end-stage hypertension, ischemic, valvular diseases, familial and secondary to specific heart muscle diseases. The EMB can be a useful adjunct to noninvasive modalities in defining the etiology of DCM. Often, EMB is more useful for excluding specific myocardial disorders than in diagnosing the etiology of DCM because it has nonspecific EMB findings such as myocyte hypertrophy and interstitial fibrosis (Fig. 5). In addition, the degree of interstitial fibrosis, myocyte diameters, and myofibril volume fraction have not been correlated with severity of clinical or hemodynamic data.[34,35] Other disorders that may be relevant to rule out in the patient with DCM include: iron deposition, amyloidosis, sarcoidosis, or lymphocytic myocarditis.

Hypertrophic Cardiomyopathy

Hypertrophic cardiomyopathy (HCM) is the most common congenital cardiomyopathy observed with an incidence of 1:500 of the general population.[36] Heart failure and sudden cardiac

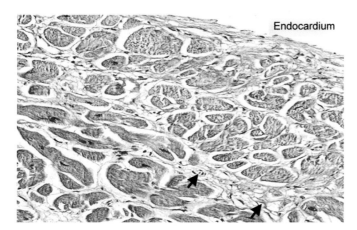

Endocardium

FIGURE 5: Dilated cardiomyopathy. In this subendocardial field, there is a delicate network of interstitial collagen (arrows) between hypertrophied myofibers; nonspecific histologic features of dilated cardiomyopathy [H&E stain (400x magnification) (*Source:* Philip Ursell, UCSF pathology)]

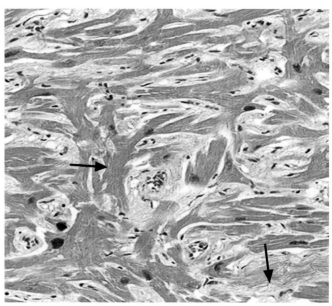

FIGURE 6: Hypertrophic cardiomyopathy. In the upper septum, disarray of hypertrophied myofibers and interstitial collagen (arrows) are hallmarks of hypertrophic cardiomyopathy [H&E stain (400x magnification). (*Source:* Philip Ursell, UCSF pathology)]

death are both severe manifestations of the disease which can occur at any age. The diagnosis of HCM is made in the setting of a hypertrophied left ventricle with normal to reduced volumes in a patient without other systemic cardiac diseases that result in left ventricular wall thickening (e.g. aortic stenosis or long-standing hypertension). Echocardiography and cardiac magnetic resonance imaging (MRI) are the main modalities used to diagnose HCM and new genetic tests have become available to screen for common mutations known to lead to the HCM phenotype.

The most common finding on EMB for HCM is myocyte nuclear enlargement (hypertrophy) and interstitial fibrosis. The specificity of EMB for HCM is low as many other cardio-myopathies and secondary myocardial diseases, such as diabetes, hypertension, valvular diseases and ischemic heart disease, have similar histopathologic features. Myocyte disarray (Fig. 6) is also thought to be a hallmark of HCM, but unfortunately, this finding may not be seen in the EMB sample as HCM often lies deep within the interventricular septum and also may be patchy. Importantly, additional variants of HCM exist, such as the apical form, which would not be detected with right ventricular EMB. As a result, EMB for HCM is often reserved only to rule out other conditions that may mimic HCM such as amyloidosis. Amyloid stains, such as Congo red, should routinely be used on EMB samples if HCM is a clinical consideration. Finally, storage diseases, such as Pompe's or Fabry's disease,[37] may mimic HCM. Interestingly, up to 12% of female patients with late-onset HCM have Fabry's (alpha-galactosidase deficiency) disease which responds to enzyme replacement therapy.[38]

Restrictive Cardiomyopathy

Restrictive cardiomyopathy encompasses a heterogeneous group of diseases that are characterized by the presence of restricted ventricular filling or advanced diastolic dysfunction. These diseases include idiopathic restrictive cardiomyopathy, Loffler's endocarditis, endomyocardial fibrosis and primary or secondary hypereosinophilic syndrome. Also in the differential include: amyloidosis, sarcoidosis, hemochromatosis and HCM with restrictive features. Early in these disease processes, the left ventricular volumes and systolic function are preserved, but there is evidence of atrial dilation and increased ventricular filling pressures.[39,40]

The restrictive cardiomyopathies can be divided into two groups based upon the presence or absence of eosinophilia. In the eosinophilic disorders, there is myocardial cell and microvascular damage thought to be due to the toxic metabolites (eosinophilic cationic protein and major basic protein) released from the infiltrating eosinophils. Early stages of these diseases are characterized by a necrotic stage which then progresses to a thrombotic stage with subsequent endomyocardial fibrosis.[41] The EMB can be useful for diagnostic purposes and reveals thrombus, eosinophils, myocyte necrosis and granulation-like tissue. In addition, EMB has been used to monitor response to steroid therapy.[42] In the non-eosinophilic disorders, EMB tends to be less useful as the findings are nonspecific and include myocyte hypertrophy and interstitial fibrosis.[40] In all cases where EMB samples are obtained for diagnosis of restrictive cardiomyopathies, amyloid stains should be utilized to rule out amyloidosis as this condition presents with similar hemodynamic findings.

Finally, in clinical cases where restrictive cardiomyopathy is being entertained as a diagnosis, the clinician should also consider a diagnosis of constrictive pericarditis. This is particularly important as pericardial surgery for constrictive pericarditis can be life-saving, and if a restrictive process is identified, the patient can be spared a pericardial biopsy. Generally, thickening or calcification of the pericardium should be visualized with either chest X-ray, MRI or CT. The EMB can help to differentiate between these two clinical entities as EMB samples from constrictive pericarditis reveals normal to slightly atrophic myocytes, whereas EMB samples from restrictive cardiomyopathy will reveal myocyte hypertrophy and interstitial fibrosis.[43]

Arrhythmogenic Right Ventricular Cardiomyopathy

Arrhythmogenic right ventricular cardiomyopathy (ARVC) is an autonomic dominant cardiomyopathy affecting young adults that is characterized by fibrofatty replacement of the right ventricular myocardium. Clinical manifestations of ARVC include ventricular arrhythmias, right heart failure and sudden cardiac death. Recently, a mutation has been found in the gene coding for the protein plakophilin-2 which is thought to be critical for the pathogenesis of this disease.[44]

Guidelines have been established for the diagnosis of ARVC. These include characteristic findings on electrocardiogram, transthoracic echocardiographic, cardiac MRI, right ventricular angiograms and EMB.[45] Anatomically, the most involved areas of the myocardium form the 'triangle of dysplasia', between the right ventricular infundibulum, the apex and the diaphragmatic surface of the right ventricle.[46,47] Left ventricular involvement is also seen in up to 47% of cases.[48] The sensitivity of EMB for detecting ARVC by itself is low since the disease process is often patchy and in most cases does not involve the septum. Sensitivity is improved if the right ventricular free wall is biopsied, but many groups are reluctant to biopsy the right ventricular free wall due to its limited thickness and increased risk of perforation with resultant cardiac tamponade. In addition, the diagnosis of ARVC by EMB is complicated by the fact that mature adipose tissue can be seen in many normal hearts. Histomorphologic criteria have been proposed to improve specificity and include more than 3% fat, more than 40% fibrous tissue and fewer than 45% myocytes.[49] On microscopic examination, the areas of involvement demonstrate severe infiltration of the myocardium with mature fat cells and surrounding fibrosis.[47,50] Interestingly, myocarditis, both active and borderline, has been noted in EMB specimens of ARVC, but it is unclear whether this merely represents a reactive process or whether this is critical to the pathogenesis of the disease.[51] Finally, if the clinical suspicion for ARVC is high and the patient is symptomatic, all means should be employed to confirm the diagnosis as implantable cardioverter defibrillators or transplantation could be life-saving.

EMB IN SPECIAL CARDIAC DISEASE STATES

Sarcoidosis

Sarcoidosis is a multi-system, granulomatous disease of unknown etiology. A predominant feature of the disease is the presence of noncaseating granulomas affecting the lungs and lymph nodes as well as the heart, liver, spleen, skin, eyes and parotid glands. The disease usually presents in young and middle-aged adults between the ages of 20 years and 40 years, and can be a benign, incidentally discovered condition or a life-threatening disorder. The estimated prevalence of sarcoidosis with cardiac involvement is approximately 25% based upon several autopsy studies.[52,53] A common cardiac manifestation is congestive heart failure due to either direct infiltration of the myocardium, valvular regurgitation secondary to papillary muscle dysfunction or secondary right ventricular failure due to pulmonary hypertension with pulmonary involvement.[54] In addition, patients can present with varying conduction abnormalities due to granuloma involvement of virtually any aspect of the conduction system. Complete heart block is the most common presenting conduction abnormality (23–30%) and most frequently presents as syncope.[55]

The diagnosis of cardiac sarcoidosis is often difficult to establish especially in patients without evidence of sarcoid in other organs. Many patients with cardiac sarcoidosis are often given a diagnosis of idiopathic DCM. Several features that can support a diagnosis of cardiac sarcoidosis over idiopathic DCM include: higher incidence of advanced AV block, abnormal wall thickness, uneven wall motion abnormalities and perfusion defects preferentially affecting the anteroseptal and apical regions of the left ventricle. While having a high specificity for cardiac sarcoidosis, EMB has been estimated to have a low sensitivity (20–63%) largely due to the heterogeneous, patchy, and often basal distribution of myocardial involvement.[56,57] Therefore, EMB is generally not recommended for routine screening of cardiac involvement of sarcoidosis; however, in clinical situations where suspicion is high and other noninvasive modalities are inconclusive, EMB may prove to be diagnostic.

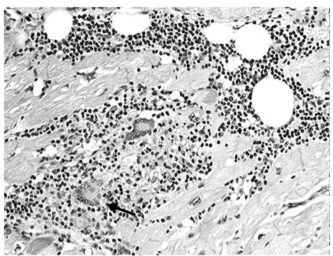

FIGURE 7: Cardiac sarcoidosis. In the central portion of the field, there are two myocardial granulomas characterized by clusters of mononuclear cells and giant cells (arrow) [H&E stain (400x magnification). (*Source:* Philip Ursell, UCSF pathology)]

The typical EMB findings include non-necrotizing granulomas which may also be associated with healed scars/fibrosis (Fig. 7). Of note, mycobacterial and fungal infections, hypersensitivity myocarditis and GCM may have overlapping features. In these instances, special stains and microbiological cultures may be useful. In Japan, where cardiac sarcoidosis has had an important clinical impact, the Ministry of Health and Welfare established specific guidelines for diagnosis based upon a combination of histological evidence, electrocardiographic, morphologic, scintigraphic or hemodynamic abnormalities (Table 3).[58] Unfortunately, these guidelines have not translated well to the international community. Finally, establishing a diagnosis of cardiac involvement with sarcoidosis is important as therapy with glucocorticoids, if initiated early, has been associated with improved five-year survival rates.[59]

Amyloidosis

Cardiac amyloidosis is classified by the protein precursor as primary, secondary (reactive), senile systemic, hereditary, isolated atrial and hemodialysis-associated. Patients with cardiac amyloidosis often present with clinical signs and symptoms of right heart failure including dyspnea and peripheral edema. One-important diagnostic clue to this diagnosis is observation

of low voltage on electrocardiography despite significant left ventricular wall thickness on echocardiography. This set of findings has a high sensitivity (72–79%) and specificity (91–100%) for cardiac involvement.[60,61] In addition, cardiac MRI with gadolinium enhancement has begun to play a larger role in the noninvasive assessment of amyloidosis with cardiac involvement. Two recent studies illustrate the utility of this approach with varying patterns of late gadolinium enhancement.[62,63] In patients with a known diagnosis of amyloidosis on biopsy (either fat pad, rectal or renal) and echocardiographic and/or cardiac MRI findings consistent with amyloid deposition in the myocardium, EMB may not be necessary. The type of amyloid can be confirmed by specific tissue stains, serum and urine immunofixation electrophoresis or genetic analysis. However, in many cases where the diagnosis is suspected, but the non-invasive imaging is equivocal and biopsy of other organs is non-contributory, EMB can be particularly useful.

Histopathology of amyloidosis on EMB is characterized by homogeneous, eosinophilic deposition in the interstitium, vessels, and subendocardium as nodular deposits (Fig. 8). A

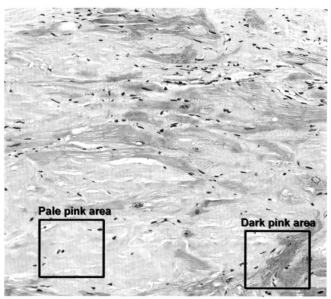

FIGURE 8: Cardiac amyloidosis. In this field there is abundant homogenous pale pink deposits of typical amyloid. The remaining viable myofibers (dark pink) are variably hypertrophied or atrophied [H&E stain (400x magnification). (*Source:* Philip Ursell, UCSF pathology)]

TABLE 3

Guidelines for diagnosing cardiac sarcoidosis (from the Japanese Ministry of Health and Welfare)

1. *Histologic diagnosis group*
   Cardiac sarcoidosis is confirmed when histologic analysis of operative or endomyocardial biopsy specimens demonstrates epithelioid granuloma without caseating granuloma

2. *Clinical diagnosis group*
   In patients with a histologic diagnosis of extracardiac sarcoidosis, cardiac sarcoidosis is suspected when item (a) and one or more of items (b) though (e) are present:

   a. Complete right bundle branch block, left axis deviation, atrioventricular block, VT, premature ventricular contraction (≥ Lown 2), or abnormal Q or ST-T change on the ECG or ambulatory ECG

   b. Abnormal wall motion, regional wall thinning, or dilatation of the left ventricle

   c. Perfusion defect by thallium-201 myocardial scintigraphy or abnormal accumulation by gallium-67 or technetium-99m myocardial scintigraphy

   d. Abnormal intracardiac pressure, low cardiac output or abnormal wall motion or depressed ejection fraction of the left ventricle

   e. Interstitial fibrosis or cellular infiltration over moderate grade even if the findings are nonspecific

Congo red stain reveals apple-green birefringence under polarized light. In cases of early amyloid deposition with minimal cardiac involvement, Congo red staining may not have high enough sensitivity. In these cases, addition of Congo red fluorescence may enhance the sensitivity in making the diagnosis.[64] Once cardiac amyloidosis is confirmed by EMB, it is important to type the amyloid as prognosis and treatment differs among the various forms. Immunohistochemical and immunogold staining can be used to help differentiate the type of amyloid fibril. If the EMB sample stains positive for transthyretin, additional analysis should include isoelectric focusing of the serum to help distinguish between senile (wild type transthyretin) and familial (mutated transthyretin) amyloidosis.

Hemochromatosis

Hemochromatosis is one of the most common inherited metabolic disorders with an estimated prevalence in the general population of 1:200 to 1:400 depending upon the specific genotype or phenotype analyzed.[65–67] Hemochromatosis can be subdivided into a primary hereditary form involving a point mutation (C282Y) in the HFE (transferring-receptor binding protein) gene or secondary due to chronic iron overload in conditions such as thalassemia major.[68] A common feature of this disease is iron deposition in multiple organs including the liver, heart, pituitary, pancreas, joints and skin. With respect to cardiovascular manifestations, one analysis of multiple-cause mortality showed that patients with hemochromatosis are five times more likely to have a cardiomyopathy than those without hemochromatosis (Yang 1998). In addition, patients can develop heart block due to iron deposition in the AV node as well as a dilated and/or restrictive cardiomyopathy leading to death or cardiac transplantation.[69–72]

In suspected clinical cases, initial laboratory analysis including a serum ferritin, transferrin saturation, and HFE gene mutations can have good positive predictive value.[73] If the initial screen is positive, patients often undergo liver biopsy to determine if hepatic iron overload is present which would then prompt therapeutic phlebotomy. Screening for cardiac iron overload is indicated in patients with systemic manifestations of iron overload in conjunction with conduction abnormalities or signs/symptoms of congestive heart failure. The EMB has traditionally been the gold standard for demonstration of myocardial iron deposition. Iron is typically localized to the perinuclear region of myocytes (Figs 9A and B). As a result of the progressive hemosiderin accumulation within the myocytes, progressive interstitial fibrosis and myocyte necrosis occurs. Serial EMB has also been utilized to monitor response to therapy (chelation and/or phlebotomy), although iron can still remain in the heart even after the patient develops microcytic anemia which is an indicator of adequate treatment.[74] Of note, there is a potential for EMB sampling error as iron deposition localizes predominantly to the subepicardium early in the disease process.[69,75]

A new technique called cardiac MRI T2* has been validated across centers as an initial screen for cardiac hemochromatosis[76,77] and is decreasing the need for EMB to make the diagnosis. This technique is based on the fact that iron overload

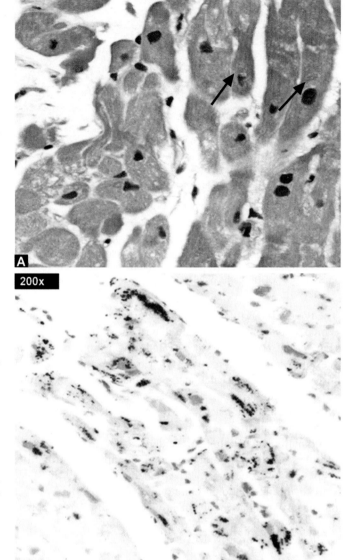

FIGURES 9A AND B: Hemochromatosis: (A) Multiple pigmented granules (arrows) are seen within myocytes consistent with iron [H&E stain (400x magnification)]. (B) A special stain discloses abundant bright blue iron in virtually every myofiber [Perl stain (200x magnification)]. (*Source:* Philip Ursell, UCSF pathology)

causes MRI signal loss in affected tissues because iron deposits become magnetized in the scanner leading to local irregularities in the magnetic field. The prognostic value of cardiac T2* was evaluated in a study of 652 thalassemia major patients who underwent 1,442 cardiac MRI scans at a single center in England.[78] The authors concluded that cardiac MRI T2* was a better predictor of high-risk heart failure and arrhythmia than serum ferritin and liver iron. While cardiac MRI T2* may eventually obviate the need for EMB to diagnose or monitor therapy in hemochromatosis, there remain a number of patients who are precluded from getting MRIs due to a history of an internal source of metal such as patients who have metallic valves, pacemaker/defibrillators, patent foramen ovale or atrial septal defect occluder devices, or aortic stents. In these cases,

EMB remains a useful modality for both the diagnosis and follow-up of cardiac hemochromatosis.

Storage Diseases and Myopathy

Glycogen storage diseases are rare autosomal recessive diseases that are characterized by glycogen deposition in one or more tissues throughout the body. Type II (Pompe disease), type III (Cori disease), and type IV (Andersen disease) glycogen storage diseases can all involve the heart. Pompe's disease, a deficiency in the enzyme α-1,4-glucosidase, can present with significant morbidity related to cardiomegaly and congestive heart failure due to restrictive physiology. The particular enzyme defect, and hence diagnosis, is best performed on tissue cultures derived from leukocytes, liver cells, skin fibroblasts or even dried blood spots on filter paper.[79] Nevertheless, EMB can be helpful in making the diagnosis. Importantly, if a glycogen storage disease is suspected, the EMB sample should be fixed in alcohol in order to prevent the glycogen from dissolving in aqueous solutions. In Pompe's disease, there is deposition of morphologically normal glycogen with marked vacuolization of the myocytes (Figs 10A and B). Vacuolization of myocytes can also be seen in mitochondrial myopathies, carnitine deficiency, as well as Fabry's disease. In Fabry's disease, a deficiency of α-galactosidase A, EMB samples should be fixed in glutaraldehyde as electron microscopy reveals characteristic lysosomal lamellar bodies. Making a diagnosis of Fabry's disease can have important clinical implications as enzyme replacement therapy is now available.[80]

The EMB can also be helpful in making the diagnosis of inherited myopathies such as myotonic dystrophy, Becker muscular dystrophy and Duchenne muscular dystrophy. Genetic studies and peripheral skeletal muscle biopsies are first-line in the diagnostic algorithm; however, in cases where these modalities are unable to establish the diagnosis and the patient presents with congestive heart failure or arrhythmia, EMB may provide the only means of detecting cardiac involvement. The EMB samples in Becker and Duchenne muscular dystrophy have characteristic immunohistochemical staining patterns for dystrophin.[81,82] In addition, EMB samples from myotonic dystrophy also have characteristic electron microscopic abnormalities.[83]

Drug Toxicity

Numerous chemotherapeutic drugs have been demonstrated to exert cardiotoxic effects. Anthracyclines, including daunorubicin and doxorubicin (adriamycin), are the best characterized of these agents and demonstrate dose-dependent cardiotoxic effects. Cardiotoxicity usually occurs within the first year of treatment, but delayed toxicity can also occur.[84,85] Several factors such as advanced age, prior mediastinal radiation, hypertension or pre-existing cardiovascular disease have also been shown to predispose to subsequent anthracycline cardiotoxicity.[86] Newer chemotherapeutic agents, such as trastuzumab (Herceptin) for HER2/neu positive breast cancer, have also been shown to lead to cardiotoxicity, especially in the setting of prior anthracycline chemotherapy.[87] Screening for drug-induced cardiotoxicity is now commonly performed using noninvasive imaging modalities such as transthoracic echocardiography and

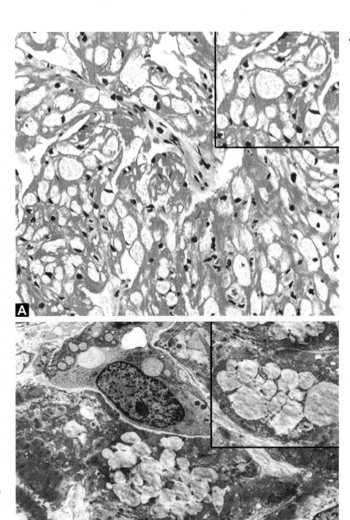

FIGURES 10A AND B: Pompe's disease: (A) At high magnification, light microscopy discloses large empty appearing vacuoles (inset) in virtually every myofiber. A special stain for glycogen (not shown) was markedly positive [H&E stain (400x magnification)]. (B) Electron microscopy shows that the vacuoles are membrane bound aggregates of glycogen (inset) [Uranyl acetate and lead citrate (5000x magnification)]. (*Source:* Philip Ursell, UCSF pathology)

radionuclide angiography (MUGA scan) focusing on left ventricular EF. A baseline scan is performed prior to the initiation of chemotherapy and scans are often performed every three months while on therapy.

Despite the ability of noninvasive means to detect myocardial dysfunction with chemotherapeutic agents, a tissue diagnosis made by EMB remains the gold standard.[88] Since chemotherapy-induced cardiotoxicity is best evaluated by electron microscopy, EMB samples should be specially processed. This includes analyzing both semi-thin and thin blocks of tissue.[88,89] While the primary lesion seen is myofibrillar loss, many of the changes seen can also be found in degenerative diseases such as DCM. Recognizing the need for a more comprehensive approach to detecting anthracycline

TABLE 4

Billingham anthracycline cardiotoxicity score

Grade	Billingham scoring system (morphologic characteristics)
0	Normal myocardial ultrastructural morphology
0.5	Not completely normal but no evidence of anthracycline-specific damage
1	Isolated myocytes affected and/or early myofibrillar loss; damage to < 5% of all cells
1.5	Changes similar to grade 1 except damage involves 6–15% of all cells
2	Clusters of myocytes affected by myofibrillar loss and/or vacuolization, with damage to 16–25% of all cells
2.5	Many myocytes (26–35% of all cells) affected by vacuolization and/or myofibrillar loss
3	Severe, diffuse myocyte damage (> 35% of all cells)

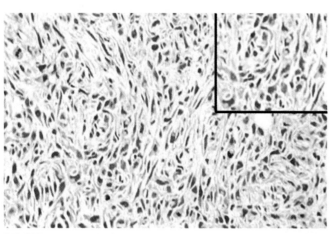

FIGURE 11: Anaplastic thyroid cancer. The entire tissue is comprised of poorly differentiated tumor (inset) consistent with anaplastic thyroid carcinoma [H&E stain of needle biopsy of right atrial mass (200x magnification)]. (*Source:* Philip Ursell, UCSF pathology)

cardiotoxicity, a grading scheme was developed in 1984 (Table 4) which takes into account the percentage of damage to myocardial cells.[89]

Neoplasms

Metastatic secondary tumors are the most common neoplasms affecting the heart and commonly infiltrate the pericardium. Renal cell carcinoma, lymphoma, leukemia, melanoma, breast cancer, lung cancer and anaplastic thyroid cancer can all metastasize to the heart (Fig. 11). Given the clinical necessity of obtaining a pathologic diagnosis to help direct treatment, transvenous biopsy plays a role in these settings. In addition, primary tumors (both benign and malignant) of the heart, such as atrial myxoma, angiosarcoma, leiomyosarcoma and undifferentiated sarcoma, have been detected by right and left heart biopsy.[90–93] If a tumor is suspected, it is appropriate to fix and freeze some of the biopsy specimens for immunohisto-chemistry, molecular studies and electron microscopy. While a majority of cardiac biopsies of tumors are made by cardio-thoracic surgeons, in certain cases, transesophageal echo-cardiography-guided transvenous biopsy may obviate the need for thoracotomy.

Cardiac Infections

Numerous systemic infections (viral, bacterial and protozoal) have been implicated in the pathogenesis of myocarditis. The role of EMB in these settings has been reviewed in the latest guideline statement from the ACC/AHA/ESC. Here it is worth mentioning several common infections with myocardial involvement and in which EMB may play a special role due to pathognomonic pathologic findings.

One of the leading causes of heart failure in South and Central America is infection with the tropical parasite *Trypanosoma cruzi* leading to Chagas disease. It is estimated that there are approximately 8–10 million infected people.[94] The disease is characterized by three phases: (1) an acute phase; (2) a latent phase and (3) a chronic phase. Cardiac involvement during the acute phase can be mild, but can also present with severe sequelae with a 3–5% mortality rate. The latent phase can last from up to 10–30 years and is often clinically silent. Eventually up to 30% of patients develop late manifestations, predominantly congestive heart failure, cardiac arrhythmias and sudden cardiac death. Historically, EMB has been widely performed in suspected Chagas cardiomyopathy and has led not only to a greater understanding of the pathophysiology, but also the clinical stages of the disease process.[95] *T. cruzi* parasites are rarely demonstrated in chronic Chagas cardiomyopathy, but are often demonstrated on histology in the acute phase. The PCR for *T. cruzi* DNA has been shown to be more sensitive and specific for detecting the organism.[96] In the acute phase, EMB histology can demonstrate myocarditis with inflammatory infiltrates around ruptured pseudocysts of parasites with associated myocyte necrosis and degeneration (Fig. 12).

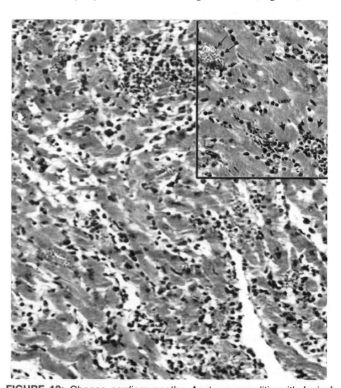

FIGURE 12: Chagas cardiomyopathy. Acute myocarditis with foci of myocytolytic necrosis and degeneration are seen with an intense inflammatory infiltrate around ruptured pseudocysts of parasite (short arrows), (in the inset). Intact intramyocyte parasite nest without inflammatory response (long arrows) (in the inset) [H&E staining]. (*Source:* Rossi et al. PLOS 2010)

Infectious complications, which can occur at any time after cardiac transplantation, remain a significant cause for concern among transplant physicians. The most common infections seen in the early post-transplant period include CMV and *Toxoplasma gondii*. Unlike bacterial and fungal infections which are often associated with predominantly neutrophilic inflammation, viral and protozoal infections can often mimic acute cellular rejection. In CMV infection and toxoplasmosis, the myocardium often contains a mixed inflammatory infiltrate with varying numbers of eosinophils. However, in the immunocompromised state, CMV inclusion bodies and *Toxoplasma* cysts can also be seen even in the absence of inflammation.

CARDIAC TRANSPLANTATION

Early experience with cardiac transplantation was limited by high rates of infection and allograft rejection. Before the advent of EMB, diagnosis of rejection relied upon noninvasive means such as electrocardiograms, echocardiography and nonspecific clinical signs/symptoms. As a result, identifying those patients who would benefit from rejection therapies had both low sensitivity and specificity. Over the past several decades there has been a remarkable improvement in outcomes for cardiac transplant patients driven largely by major advances in transplant immunology (such as the use of calcineurin inhibitors) as well as the widely accepted use of EMB to diagnose rejection.[97] Numerous studies have shown that EMB has both high sensitivity and specificity for detecting allograft dysfunction and is now the "gold standard" for monitoring of the cardiac allograft.[2] The EMB complication rates in experienced centers are low, and pathological diagnosis of rejection is more uniform secondary to newly established guidelines.[98,99]

In 2005, the International Society of Heart and Lung Transplantation (ISHLT) established criteria for defining and grading acute cardiac allograft rejection (Table 5).[99] In this classification scheme, grades 0–1 are considered low grade and often do not result in changes to therapy, particularly in asymptomatic individuals. Grade 2–3 lesions are significant and require augmentation of immunosuppressive therapy especially if there is evidence of allograft dysfunction. The histopathologic appearance/features of cellular and antibody-mediated rejection (AMR) are reviewed in Figures 13A to D. Confusion in grading may result from the presence of nodular infiltrates or "quilty" lesions which are thought to have a benign prognosis.[100,101]

Of note, false positive EMB results occur due to a number of histologic findings which may mimic grade 2 rejection. Specifically, this can occur due to biopsy sites being cut tangentially, identification of "quilty" lesions, ischemic injury, infection and post-transplant lymphoproliferative disorder. In addition, there are a number of patient cases of low-grade or no rejection who present with hemodynamic compromise.[102] Two explanations for these false negative EMB results have been posited. First, sampling error has been implicated as postmortem studies have confirmed that rejection and inflammatory lesions can be heterogeneous in nature and may be localized to the deep subendomyocardial regions not accessed by EMB. Second, acute AMR or humoral rejection may be the cause.

The AMR is thought to be responsible for a significant portion of chronic rejection and allograft vasculopathy. The

TABLE 5

IHSLT grading of cellular and antibody mediated allograft rejection

Cellular	
Grade 0 R[a]	*No rejection*
Grade 1 R, mild	Interstitial and/or perivascular infiltrate with up to 1 focus or myocyte damage
Grade 2 R, moderate	Two or more foci of infiltrate with associated myocyte damage
Grade 3 R, severe	Diffuse infiltrate with multifocal myocyte damage $\pm$ edema, $\pm$ hemorrhage $\pm$ vasculitis
Antibody	
AMR 0	Negative for acute antibody-mediate rejection No histologic or immunopathologic features of AMR
AMR 1	Positive for AMR Histologic features of AMR Positive immunofluorescence or immunoperoxidase staining for AMR (positive CD 68, C4d)

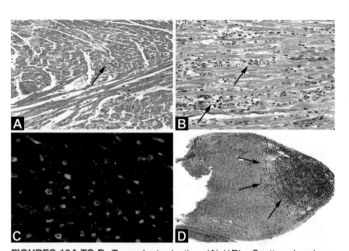

FIGURES 13A TO D: Transplant rejection: (A) (1R)—Scattered perivascular and interstitial infiltrates of mononuclear cells are present (arrow). No myocyte damage is identified. (B) (3R)—Diffuse interstitial infiltrates of mononuclear cells with scattered areas of myocyte damage (arrows) characterize cellular 3R rejection. (C) Immunofluorescence methods demonstrate abundant vascular deposits of C4d characteristic of acute antibody mediated rejection. (D) A localized endocardial nodule comprised of dense mononuclear cells identifies a "Quilty" nodule. The inflammatory process has invaded into the underlying myocardium (arrows). There were no signs of rejection in this biopsy.

recognition of AMR in the cardiac allograft has been facilitated by newer histological techniques. In particular, light microscopy and immunofluorescence demonstrate capillary endothelial swelling with capillary deposition of complement and immunoglobulin. These histological findings have been associated with a more aggressive clinical course and poorer responses to conventional anti-rejection therapies. As a result, the ISHLT recently revised their grading system to include assessments of AMR (Table 5).

While there is consensus regarding the necessity of EMB in allograft rejection surveillance, considerable variability still exists from center to center with regard to the frequency of biopsies required post-transplant. Most transplant centers utilize frequent EMB in the three month postoperative period (weekly for the first month, bi-weekly for the next two months, followed by every three months for the first year) as it is believed that the first three months represents the "critical window" for allograft rejection. The EMB frequency is also either maintained or decreased over time in relation to the incidence of rejection in preceding biopsies as well as the potency of the immuno-suppressive regimen. Routine use of surveillance EMB beyond one year from transplant has been questioned by several studies. One retrospective study of more than 13,000 biopsies performed over an 8-year period found positive biopsies for rejection in 19% over the first 3 months, 7% by the end of the first year, and 4.7%, 4.5%, 2.2% and less than 1% for postoperative years 2 through 5 respectively.[103] In another study of over 1,000 biopsies performed 1–12 years after transplantation, 99.3% demonstrated a rejection grade of 0–1. Of the 0.6% of biopsies with a rejection grade of 2 or higher (7 biopsies), six were diagnosed with grade 2 rejection and only one biopsy was diagnosed as grade 3A. As a result, the authors concluded that the routine use of surveillance biopsy beyond one year after transplantation does not affect patient treatment and that a selective approach to biopsy should be employed after this time point.[104]

Despite the fact that EMB complication rates have declined significantly with the advent of newer bioptomes and increased operator experience, there remains a risk of serious compli-cations, such as tricuspid valve dysfunction, pneumothorax and cardiac tamponade, not to mention the discomfort experienced by the patients themselves. As a result, there has been significant interest in developing strategies to reduce the number of biopsies without compromising care. Several new noninvasive approaches have been employed to detect allograft rejection including cardiac MRI, echocardiographic strain/strain rate analysis and serum blood tests identifying gene expression profiles consistent with rejection (AlloMap).[105–108] Two recent studies have highlighted the important clinical impact of molecular testing for transplant rejection. In a study by Starling et al.,[109] the amplification of 11 genes involved in cell-mediated rejection were analyzed from peripheral blood mononuclear cells of post heart transplant patients (AlloMap) by real-time PCR.

An AlloMap score of less than 34 was found to have a 100% negative predictive value for diagnosis of moderate/severe allograft rejection. In addition, in a study by Pham et al.[110] from the IMAGE study group, 602 cardiac allograft recipients were randomized to be screened for cellular transplant rejection either by conventional route of right ventricular EMB or by gene expression profiling. The authors found no significant difference in the risk of serious adverse outcomes between the two approaches. The authors concluded that after six months from transplant, patients can be safely followed by gene expression profiling obviating the need for routine invasive EMB. Many of these new approaches are already being implemented in transplant centers around the world and it is likely that many more innovative approaches will reach the clinical arena in the near future.

SUMMARY

The EMB has led to a greater understanding of many cardiac diseases and continues to provide useful diagnostic information to the clinician. While recommendations about the utility of EMB are limited by the lack of large, randomized trials, there appears to be consensus regarding the use of EMB in the clinical scenario of the acute onset of decompensated heart failure of less than 3 months duration as well as in monitoring of cardiac allograft rejection. The EMB is also recognized to play an important role in the diagnostic algorithms of many other cardiac disease states, although its practical use should be evaluated in the context of the diseases being considered (i.e. it is important to rule out diseases or identify diseases with specific therapies that influence outcome). With the advent of newer techniques and improved bioptomes, complication rates have declined significantly. As a result, the clinical burden of proving benefit over risk has lessened considerably. Nevertheless, research is actively being pursued to identify new modalities (e.g. imaging, serum markers and genetic tests) that may ultimately lead to significantly fewer EMB procedures, reduced costs and more convenience for patients.

MODIFIED SUMMARIES OF GUIDELINES
AHA/ACC/ESC SCIENTIFIC STATEMENT. THE ROLE OF ENDOMYOCARDIAL BIOPSY IN THE MANAGEMENT OF CARDIOVASCULAR DISEASE. CIRCULATION. 2007;116:2216-33

Kanu Chatterjee

Class I: Conditions for which there is evidence or there is general agreement that a given procedure is beneficial, useful and effective.

Class II: Conditions for which there is conflicting evidence and/or a divergence of opinion about the usefulness/efficacy of a procedure or treatment.

Class IIa: Conditions for which the weight of evidence/opinion is in favor of usefulness/efficacy.

Class IIb: Conditions for which usefulness/efficacy is less well established by evidence/opinion.

Class III: Conditions for which there is evidence and/or general agreement that a procedure/treatment is not useful and in some cases may be harmful.

THE LEVELS OF EVIDENCE

Level A (highest): Multiple randomized clinical trials.

Level B: (intermediate): Limited number of randomized trials, nonrandomized studies and registries.

Level C: Primarily expert consensus.

Class I

1. Unexplained, new-onset heart failure, 2 weeks duration with a normal or dilated left ventricle and hemodynamic compromise (level of evidence B).
2. Unexplained new-onset heart failure of 2 weeks to3 months' duration with a dilated left ventricle and new ventricular arrhythmias or advanced atrioventricular heart block or failure to respond to usual care in 1–2 weeks (level of evidence B).

Class IIa

1. Unexplained heart failure of greater than 3 months' duration with a dilated left ventricle and new ventricular arrhythmias or advanced atrio-ventricular heart block or failure to respond to usual care within 1–2 weeks. (level of evidence C).
2. Unexplained heart failure with a dilated cardiomyopathy of any duration and suspected allergic reaction and eosinophilia (level of evidence C).
3. Unexplained heart failure and suspected anthracycline cardiomyopathy (level of evidence C).
4. Heart failure with unexplained restrictive cardiomyopathy (level of evidence C).
5. With suspected (non-myxoma 0 cardiac tumors) (level of evidence C).
6. Unexplained cardiomyopathy in children (level of evidence C).

Class IIb

1. Unexplained new-onset heart failure of 2 weeks to 3 months' duration with a dilated left ventricle but without new ventricular arrhythmias or advanced atrioventricular heart block that responds to usual care within 1–2 weeks (level of evidence B).
2. Unexplained heart failure of greater than 3 months' duration with a dilated left ventricle without new ventricular arrhythmias or advanced atrioventricular heart block that responds to usual care within 1–2 weeks (level of evidence C).
3. Suspected arrhythmogenic right ventricular dysplasia/cardiomyopathy (level of evidence C).
4. Unexplained ventricular arrhythmias (level of evidence C).

Class III

Unexplained atrial fibrillation (level of evidence C).

CHAPTER 26 Cardiac Biopsy

1. Sakakibara S, Konno S. Endomyocardial biopsy. Jpn Heart J. 1962;3:537-43.

2. Caves PK, Stinson EB, Dong E Jr. New instrument for transvenous cardiac biopsy. Am J Cardiol. 1974;33:264-7.

3. Mason JW. Techniques for right and left ventricular endomyocardial biopsy. Am J Cardiol. 1978;41:887-92.

4. Baim D. Endomyocardial biopsy. Grossman's Cardiac Catheterization, Angiography, and Intervention. W. Philadelphia: Lippincott Williams & Wilkens; 2000. pp. 445-61.

5. Seldinger S. Catheter replacement of the needle in percutaneous arteriography: a new technique. Acta radiol. 1953;39:368-76.

6. Denys BG, Uretsky BF, Reddy PS, et al. An ultrasound method for safe and rapid central venous access. New England Journal of Medicine. 1991;324:566.

7. Denys BG, Uretsky BF, Reddy PS. Ultrasound-assisted cannulation of the internal jugular vein: a prospective comparison to the external landmark-guided technique. Circulation. 1993;87:1557-62.

8. Mahrholdt H, Smith GC, Wagner A, et al. Cardiovascular magnetic resonance assessment of human myocarditis: a comparison to histology and molecular pathology. Circulation. 2004;109:1250-8.

9. Brooksby IA, Jenkins BS, Coltart DJ, et al. Left-ventricular endomyocardial biopsy. Lancet. 1974;2:1222-5.

10. Fowles RE, Henzlova MJ. Endomyocardial biopsy. Ann Intern Med. 1982;97:885-94.

11. Sekiguchi M, Hiroe M, Take M, et al. Clinical and histopathological profile of sarcoidosis of the heart and acute idiopathic myocarditis. Concepts through a study employing endomyocardial biopsy. Jpn Circ J. 1980;44:249-63.

12. Deckers JW, Hare JM, Baughman KL. Complications of transvenous right ventricular endomyocardial biopsy in adult patients with cardiomyopathy: a seven-year survey of 546 consecutive diagnostic procedures in a tertiary referral center. J Am Coll Cardiol. 1992;19:43-7.

13. Veinot JP, Ghadially FN, Walley VM. Light microscopy and ultrastructure of the blood vessel and heart. In: Gotlieb AL, Silver MD, Schoen FJ (Eds). Cardiovascular Pathology, 3rd edition. New York: Churchill Livingstone Saunders; 2001. pp. 30-53.

14. Virmani R, Burke A, Farb A, et al. Cardiovascular Pathology. Philadelphia: Saunders; 2001. pp. 340-85.

15. Cunningham KS, Veinot JP, Butany J. An approach to endomyocardial biopsy interpretation. J Clin Pathol. 2006;59:121-9.

16. Chow LH, Cassling RS, Sears TD, et al. Insensitivity of right ventricular endomyocardial biopsy in the diagnosis of myocarditis. J Am Coll Cardiol. 1989;14:915-20.

17. Bowles NE, Ni J, Kearney DL, et al. Detection of viruses in myocardial tissues by polymerase chain reaction: evidence of adenovirus as a common cause of myocarditis in children and adults. J Am Coll Cardiol. 2003;42:466-72.

18. Kuhl U, Pauschinger M, Noutsias M, et al. High prevalence of viral genomes and multiple viral infections in the myocardium of adults with idiopathic left ventricular dysfunction. Circulation. 2005;111:887-93.

19. Cooper LT, Baughman KL, Feldman AM, et al. The role of endomyocardial biopsy in the management of cardiovascular disease. J Am Coll Cardiol. 2007;50:1914-31.

20. Mason JW, O'conelle JB, Herskowitz A, et al. A clinical trial of immunosuppressive therapy for myocarditis. The myocarditis treatment trial investigators. New England Journal of Medicine. 1995;333:269-75.

21. McCarthy RE, Boehmer JP, Hruban RH, et al. Long-term outcome of fulminant myocarditis as compared with acute (nonfulminant) myocarditis. New England Journal of Medicine. 2000;342:690-5.

22. Amabile N, Fraisse A, Bouvenot J, et al. Outcome of acute fulminant myocarditis in children. Heart. 2006;92:1269-73.

23. Felker GM, Boehmer JP, Hruban RH, et al. Echocardiographic findings in fulminant and acute myocarditis. J Am Coll Cardiol. 2000;36:227-32.

24. Herzog CA, Snover DC, Staley NA. Acute necrotizing eosinophilic myocarditis. Br Heart J. 1984;52:343-8.

25. Cooper LT. Giant cell and granulomatous myocarditis. Heart Fail Clin. 2005;1:431-7.

26. Cooper LT Jr, Berry GJ, Shabetai R. Idiopathic giant-cell myocarditis: natural history and treatment. Multicenter Giant Cell Myocarditis Study Group Investigators. New England Journal of Medicine. 1997;336:1860-6.

27. Cooper LT, Okura Y. Idiopathic giant cell myocarditis. Curr Treat Options Cardiovasc Med. 2001;3:463-7.

28. Kilgallen CM, Jacsonk E, Bankoff M, et al. A case of giant cell myocarditis and malignant thymoma: a postmortem diagnosis by needle biopsy. Clin Cardiol. 1998;21:48-51.

29. Daniels PR, Berry GJ, Tazelaar HD, et al. Giant cell myocarditis as a manifestation of drug hypersensitivity. Cardiovasc Pathol. 2000;9:287-91.

30. Shields RC, Tazelaar H, Berry GJ, et al. The role of right ventricular endomyocardial biopsy for idiopathic giant cell myocarditis. J Card Fail. 2002;8:74-8.

31. Edwards WD. Current problems in establishing quantitative histopathologic criteria for the diagnosis of lymphocytic myocarditis by endomyocardial biopsy. Heart Vessels. 1985;1:138-42.

32. Aretz HT. Myocarditis: the Dallas criteria. Hum Pathol. 1987;18:619-24.

33. Frustaci A, Caldarulo M, Buffon A, et al. Cardiac biopsy in patients with primary atrial fibrillation: histologic evidence of occult myocardial diseases. Chest. 1991;100:303-6.

34. Baandrup U, Florio RA, Rehahn M, et al. Critical analysis of endomyocardial biopsies from patients suspected of having cardiomyopathy II: comparison of histology and clinical/haemodynamic information. Br Heart J. 1981;45:487-93.

35. Grimm W, Rudolph S, Christ M, et al. Prognostic significance of morphometric endomyocardial biopsy analysis in patients with idiopathic dilated cardiomyopathy. Am Heart J. 2003;146:372-6.

36. Maron BJ, Towbin JA, Thiene G, et al. Contemporary definitions and classification of the cardiomyopathies: an American Heart Association Scientific Statement from the Council on Clinical Cardiology; Heart Failure and Transplantation Committee; Quality of Care and Outcomes Research and Functional Genomics and Translational Biology Interdisciplinary. Working Groups and Council on Epidemiology and Prevention. Circulation. 2006;113:1807-16.

37. Nippoldt TB, Edwards WD, Holmes DR, et al. Right ventricular endomyocardial biopsy: clinicopathologic correlates in 100 consecutive patients. Mayo Clin Proc. 1982;57:407-18.

38. Chimenti C, Pieroni M, Morgante E, et al. Prevalence of fabry disease in female patients with late-onset hypertrophic cardiomyopathy. Circulation. 2004;10:1047-53.

39. Lewis AB. Clinical profile and outcome of restrictive cardiomyopathy in children. Am Heart J. 1992;123:1589-93.

40. Ammash NM, Seward JB, Bailey K, et al. Clinical profile and outcome of idiopathic restrictive cardiomyopathy. Circulation. 2000;101:2490-6.

41. Hayashi S, Okamoto F, Terasaki F, et al. Ultrastructural and immunohistochemical studies on myocardial biopsies from a patient with eosinophilic endomyocarditis. Cardiovasc Pathol. 1996;5:105-12.

42. Hayashi S, Isobe M, Okubo Y, et al. Improvement of eosinophilic heart disease after steroid therapy: successful demonstration by endomyocardial biopsy specimens. Heart Vessels. 1999;14:104-8.

43. Edwards WD, Hauck AD. Histologic examination of tissues obtained by endomyocardial biopsy. In: Fowles RE (Ed). Cardiac Biopsy. Mount Kisco, NY: Futura; 1992. pp. 95-153.

44. Gerull B, Heuser A, Wichter T, et al. Mutations in the desmosomal protein plakophilin-2 are common in arrhythmogenic right ventricular cardiomyopathy. Nat Genet. 2004;36:1162-4.

45. McKenna WJ, Thiene G, Nava A, et al. Diagnosis of arrhythmogenic right ventricular dysplasia/cardiomyopathy. Br Heart J. 1994;71:215-8.

46. Marcus FI, Fontaine GH, Guiraudon G, et al. Right ventricular dysplasia: a report of 24 adult cases. Circulation. 1982;65:384-98.

47. Lobo FV, Heggtveit HA, Butany J, et al. Right ventricular dysplasia: morphological findings in 13 cases. Can J Cardiol. 1992;8:261-8.

48. Pinamonti B, Sinagra G, Salvi A, et al. Left ventricular involvement in right ventricular dysplasia. Am Heart J. 1992;123:711-24.

49. Angelini A, Basso C, Nava A, et al. Endomyocardial biopsy in arrhythmogenic right ventricular cardiomyopathy. Am Heart J. 1996;132:203-6.

50. Kullo IJ, Edwards WD, Seward JB. Right ventricular dysplasia: the Mayo Clinic experience. Mayo Clin Proc. 1995;70:541-8.

51. Sugrue DD, Edwards WD, Olney BA. Histolgoical abnormalities of the left ventricle in a patient with arrhythmogenic right ventricular dysplasia. Heart Vessels. 1985;1:179-81.

52. Iwai K, Sekiguti M, Hosoda Y, et al. Racial differences in cardiac sarcoidosis incidence observed at autopsy. Sarcoidosis. 1994;11:26-31.

53. Perry A, Vuitch F. Causes of death in patients with sarcoidosis. A morphologic study of 38 autopsies with clinicopathologic correlations. Arch Pathol Lab Med. 1995;119:167-72.

54. Cooper LT, Zehr KJ. Biventricular assist device placement and immunosuppression as therapy for necrotizing eosinophilic myocarditis. Nat Clin Pract Cardiovasc Med. 2005;2:544-8.

55. Roberts WC, McAllister H, Ferrans VJ. Sarcoidosis of the heart: a clinicopathologic study of 35 necropsy patients and review of 78 previously described necropsy patients. Am J Med. 1977;63:86-108.

56. Silverman KJ, Hutchine GM, Bulkley BH. Cardiac sarcoid: a clinicopathologic study of 84 unselected patients with systemic sarcoidosis. Circulation. 1978;58:1204-11.

57. Sekiguchi M, Take M. World survey of catheter biopsy of the heart. In: Olsen EG, Sekiguchi M (Eds). Cardiomyopathy: Clinical, Pathological, and Theoretical Aspects. Baltimore: University Park Press; 1980. pp. 217-25.

58. Hiraga H, Yuwai K, Hiroe M, et al. Guideline for the diagnosis of cardiac sarcoidosis study report on diffuse pulmonary diseases. Tokyo: The Japanese Ministry of Health and Welfare; 1993. pp. 23-24.

59. Yazaki Y, Isobe M, Hiroe M, et al. Prognostic determinants of long-term survival in Japanese patients with cardiac sarcoidosis treated with prednisone. Am J Cardiol. 2001;88:1006-10.

60. Carroll JD, Gaasch WH, McAdam KP. Amyloid cardiomyopathy: characterization by a distinctive voltage/mass relation. Am J Cardiol. 1982;49:9-13.

61. Rahman JE, Helox EF, Gelzer-Bell R, et al. Noninvasive diagnosis of biopsy-proven cardiac amyloidosis. J Am Coll Cardiol. 2004;43:410-5.

62. Maceira Am, Joshi J, Prasad SK, et al. Cardiovascular magnetic resonance in cardiac amyloidosis. Circulation. 2005;111:186-93.

63. Perugini E, Rapezzi C, Piva T, et al. Non-invasive evaluation of the myocardial substrate of cardiac amyloidosis by gadolinium cardiac magnetic resonance. Heart. 2006;92:343-9.

64. Linke RP. Highly sensitive diagnosis of amyloid and various amyloid syndromes using Congo red fluorescence. Virchows Arch. 2000;436:439-48.

65. Edwards CQ, Grittin LM, Goldgar D. Prevalence of hemochromatosis among 11,065 presumably healthy blood donors. New England Journal of Medicine. 1988;318:1355-62.

66. Leggett BA, Halliday J, Brown NN, et al. Prevalence of hemo-chromatosis amongst asymptomatic Australians. Br J Haematol. 1990;74:525-30.

67. Adams PC, McLaren KA, Barr RCE, et al. Population screening for hemochromatosis: a comparison of unbound iron-binding capacity, transferrin saturation, and C282Y genotyping in 5,211 voluntary blood donors. Hepatology. 2000;31:1160-4.

68. Lombardo T, Tamburino C, Bartoloni G, et al. Cardiac iron overload in thalassemic patients: an endomyocardial biopsy study. Ann Hematol. 1995;71:135-41.

69. Fitchett DH, Coltart DJ, Littler WA, et al. Cardiac involvement in secondary hemochromatosis: a catheter biopsy study and analysis of myocardium. Cardiovasc Res. 1980;14:719-24.

70. Dabestani A, Child JS, Perloff JK, et al. Cardiac abnormalities in primary hemochromatosis. Ann NY Acad Sci. 1988;526:234-44.

71. Surakomol S, Olson LJ, Rastogi A, et al. Combined orthotopic heart and liver transplantation for genetic hemochromatosis. J Heart Lung Transplant. 1997;16:573-5.

72. Schofield RS, Aranda JM Jr, Hill JA. Cardiac transplanation in a patient with hereditary hemochromatosis: role of adjunctive phlebotomy and erythropoietin. J Heart Lung Transplant. 2001;20:696-8.

73. Niederau C, Niederau CM, Lange S, et al. Screening for hemo-chromatosis and iron deficiency in employees and primary care patients in Western Germany. Ann Intern Med. 1998;128:337-45.

74. Short EM, Winkle RA, Billingham ME. Myocardial involvement in idiopathic hemochromatosis. Morphologic and clinical improvement following venesection. Am J Med. 1981;70:1275-9.

75. Olson LJ, Edwards WD, McCall JT, et al. Cardiac iron deposition in idiopathic hemochromatosis: histologic and analytic assessment of 14 hearts from autopsy. J Am Coll Cardiol. 1987;10:1239-43.

76. Anderson LJ, Holden S, Davis B, et al. Cardiovascular T2 star (T2*) magnetic resonance for the early diagnosis of myocardial iron overload. Eur Heart Journal. 2001;22:2171-9.

77. Tanner MA, He T, Westwood MA, et al. Multi-center validation of the transferability of the magnetic resonance T2* technique for the quantitation of tissue iron. Haematologica. 2006;91:1388-91.

78. Kirk P, Roughton M, Porter JB, et al. Cardiac T2* magnetic resonance for prediction of cardiac complications in thalassemia major. Circulation. 2009;120:1961-8.

79. Chamoles NA, Niizawa G, Blanco M, et al. Glycogen storage disease type II: enzymatic screening in dried blood spots. Clin Chim Acta. 2004;347:97-102.

80. Frustaci A, Chimenti C, Ricci R, et al. Improvement in cardiac function in the cardiac variant of Fabry's disease with galactose-infusion therapy. New England Journal of Medicine. 2001;345:25-32.

81. Melacini P, Fanin M, Danieli GA, et al. Cardiac involvement in Becker muscular dystrophy. J Am Coll Cardiol. 1993;22:1927-34.

82. Maeda M, Nakoo S, Miyazato H, et al. Cardiac dystrophin abnor-malities in Becker muscular dystrophy assessed by endomyocardial biopsy. Am Heart J. 1995;129:702-7.

83. Rakocevic-Stojanovic V, Pavlovic S, Seferovic P, et al. Pathologic changes in endomyocardial biopsy specimens in patients with myotonic dystrophy. Panminerva Med. 1999;41:27-30.

84. Bristow MR, Mason JW, Billingham ME, et al. Doxorubicin cardiomyopathy: evaluation by phonocardiography, endomyocardial biopsy, and cardiac catheterization. Ann Intern Med. 1978;88:168-75.

85. Shan K, Lincoff M, Young JB. Anthracycline-induced cardiotoxicity. Ann Intern Med. 1996;125:47-58.

86. Billingham ME, Bristow MR, Glatstein E, et al. Adriamycin cardiotoxicity: endomyocardial biopsy evidence of enhancement by irradiation. Am J Surg Pathol. 1977;1:17-23.

87. Slamon DJ, Leyland-Jones B, Shak S, et al. Use of chemotherapy plus a monoclonal antibody against HER2 for metastatic breast cancer that overexpresses HER2. New England Journal of Medicine. 2001;344:783-92.

88. Mackay B, Ewer MS, Carrasco CH, et al. Assessment of anthracycline chemotherapy by endomyocardial biopsy. Ultrastruct Pathol. 1994;18:203-11.

89. Billingham ME, Bristow MR. Evaluation of anthracycline cardiotoxicity: predictive ability and functional correlation of endomyocardial biopsy. Cancer Treatment Symposia. 1984;3:71-6.

502

90. Flipse TR, Tazelaar HD. Diagnosis of malignant cardiac disease by endomyocardial biopsy. Mayo Clin Proc. 1990;65:1415-22.

91. Poletti A, Cocco P, Valente M, et al. In vivo diagnosis of cardiac angiosarcoma by endomyocardial biopsy. Cardiovasc Pathol. 1993;12:89-91.

92. Amory J, Chou TM, Redberg RF, et al. Diagnosis of primary cardiac leiomyosarcoma by endomyocardial biopsy. Cardiovasc Pathol. 1996;5:113-7.

93. Chan KL, Veinot J, Leach A, et al. Diagnosis of left atrial sarcoma by transvenous endomyocardial biopsy. Can J Cardiol. 2001;17:206-8.

94. WHO Centers for Disease Control and Prevention. A new global effort to eliminate chagas disease. Wkly Epidemiol Rec. 2007;82:259-60.

95. Milei J, Storino R, Fernandez Alonso G, et al. Endomyocardial biopsies in chronic chagasic cardiomyopathy. Immunohistochemical and ultrastructural findings. Cardiology. 1992;80:424-37.

96. Benvenuti LA, Roggério A, Mansur AJ, et al. Chronic American trypanosomiasis: parasite persistence in endomyocardial biopsies is associated with high-grade myocarditis. Ann Trop Med Parasitol. 2008;102:481-7.

97. Patel JK, Kobashigawa JA. Cardiac transplant experience with cyclosporine. Transplant Proc. 2004;36:323S-30S.

98. Veinot J. Diagnostic endomyocardial biopsy pathology-general biopsy considerations, and its use for myocarditis and cardiomyopathy: a review. Can J Cardiol. 2002;18:55-65.

99. Stewart S, Winters GL, Fishbein MC, et al. Revision of the 1990 working formulation for the standardization of nomeclature in the diagnosis of heart rejection. J Heart Lung Transplant. 2005;24:1710-20.

100. Fishbein MC, Bell G, Lones MA, et al. Grade 2 cellular heart rejection: does it exist? J Heart Lung Transplant. 1994;13:1051-7.

101. Brunner-La Rocca HP, Sutsch G, Schneider J, et al. Natural course of moderate cardiac allograft rejection (International Society for Heart Transplantation grade 2) early and late after transplantation. Circulation. 1996;94:1334-8.

102. Fishbein MC, Kobashigawa J. Biopsy-negative cardiac transplant rejection: etiology, diagnosis, and therapy. Curr Opin Cardiol. 2004;19:166-9.

103. Hausen B, Rohde R, Demertizis S, et al. Strategies for routine biopsies in heart transplantation based on 8-year results with more than 13,000 biopsies. Eur J Cardiothorac Surg. 1995;9:592-8.

104. White JA, Guiraudon C, Pflugfelder PW, et al. Routine surveillance myocardial biopsies are unneccesary beyond one year after heart transplantation. J Heart Lung Transplant. 1995;14:1052-6.

105. Deng MC, Eisen HJ, Mehra MR, et al. Noninvasive discrimination of rejection in cardiac allograft recipients using gene expression profiling. Am Journal of Transplantation. 2006;6:150-60.

106. Butler CR, Thompson R, Haykowsky M, et al. Cardiovascular magnetic resonance in the diagnosis of acute heart transplant rejection: a review. Journal of Cardiovascular Magnetic Resonance. 2009;11:7.

107. Wu YL, Ye Q, Sato K, et al. Noninvasive evaluation of cardiac allograft rejection by cellular and functional cardiac magnetic resonance. JACC Cardiovasc Imaging. 2009;2:731-41.

108. Roshanali F, Mandegar MH, Bagheri J, et al. Echo rejection score: new echocardiographic approach to diagnosis of heart transplant rejection. Eur J Cardiothorac Surg. 2010;38:176-80.

109. Starling RC, Pham M, Valantine H, et al. Molecular testing in the management of cardiac transplant recipients: initial clinical experience. J Heart Lung Transplant. 2006;25:1389-95.

110. Pham MX, Teuteberg JJ, Kfoury AG, et al. Gene-expression profiling for rejection surveillance after cardiac transplantation. NEJM. 2010;362:1890-900.

SECTION 3

Diagnosis

Swan-Ganz Catheters: Clinical Applications

Dipti Gupta, Wassef Karrowni, Kanu Chatterjee

Chapter Outline

INTRODUCTION

This was demonstrated, over eighty years ago, that pulmonary artery (PA) catheterization is feasible and may be useful in understanding cardiac hemodynamics in physiologic and pathologic conditions. However, before the introduction of the balloon flotation catheters (Swan-Ganz catheters),[1] PA catheterization outside the cardiac catheterization laboratory for bedside hemodynamic monitoring was not possible. With the availability of Swan-Ganz catheters, PA catheterization can be performed even in critically ill cardiac patients. In this chapter, indications and complications of PA catheterization with the use of balloon flotation catheters for hemodynamic monitoring have been discussed.

HISTORICAL PERSPECTIVE AND EVOLUTION OF CATHETER DESIGNS

In 1929, Dr. Warner Forsmann demonstrated that right heart catheterization in humans can be performed.[2] Interestingly, he catheterized himself and introduced the catheter to his right atrium. Drs. Andre Cournand and Dickinson Richards developed catheters that could be advanced into the pulmonary arteries, and they were able to study the pathophysiology of congenital and acquired heart diseases.[3] In 1956, Drs. Forsmann, Cournand and Richards were awarded the Nobel Prize in medicine (Fig. 1). Miniature diagnostic catheters were introduced in 1964.[4] Self-guiding and flow-directed right-heart catheters were developed to measure right heart pressures.[5,6] However, balloon flotation flow-directed catheters that can be placed at the bedside without fluoroscopy were developed and introduced in clinical practice by Drs. Jeremy Swan and William Ganz in 1970 (Fig. 2). The balloon flotation catheters were further developed to measure cardiac output by thermodilution technique.[7] The pacing electrodes were also incorporated for right atrial (RA) and right ventricular (RV) pacing.[8] The multipurpose catheters

CARDIAC CATHETERIZATION

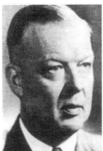 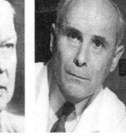 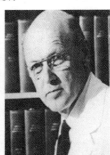

Werner Forsmann
1929

Andre Cournand and Dickinson Richards
1941

FIGURE 1: Drs. Forsmann, Cournand and Richards who developed pulmonary artery catheters and were awarded the Nobel Prize in medicine for their discoveries

that are often used in clinical practice are illustrated in Figure 3.

PLACEMENT OF BALLOON FLOTATION CATHETERS

In most instances the balloon flotation catheters can be placed at the bedside without the use of fluoroscopy. In patients with markedly dilated right atrium and right ventricle or with severe pulmonary hypertension, it is preferable to use fluoroscopy, which allows rapid placement of the catheters. Presently in most institutions, portable fluoroscopy units are available and are frequently used for placement of balloon flotation catheters.

Venous access is obtained by using one of multiple venous sites, the choice of which is determined by the preferences of the operator as well as clinical circumstances. The internal jugular or subclavian veins are the preferred route of entry due to proximity to the right heart. However, since direct pressure

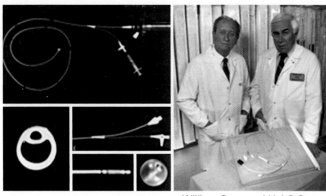

William Ganz and H.J.C Swan

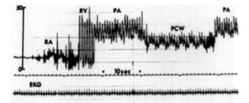

FIGURE 2: Drs. William Ganz and Jeremy Swan who developed balloon flotation catheter that can be used without fluoroscopy. The double-lumen catheter that was first introduced is also illustrated. Its placement with monitoring of hemodynamics is also illustrated. (Abbreviations: RA: Right atrial pressure; RV: Right ventricular pressure; PA: Pulmonary artery pressure; PCW: Pulmonary capillary wedge pressure)

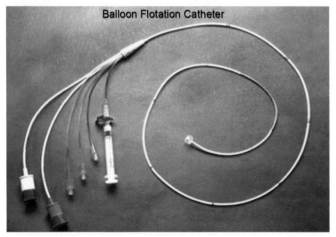

FIGURE 3: The multipurpose thermodilution triple-lumen catheters with pacing electrodes are illustrated

cannot be applied over the subclavian vein, this route should be avoided if the patient has a coagulopathy or is receiving anticoagulation therapy. The femoral vein is usually used during diagnostic catheterizations in the cardiac catheterization laboratories. For prolonged hemodynamic monitoring, the femoral vein approach should be avoided because there is a higher risk of infection. For hemodynamic monitoring for longer periods, internal jugular, subclavian or anticubital veins should be used.

Strict sterile conditions should be observed during insertion of the balloon flotation catheters, and the appropriate preparation of the skin is extremely important to minimize the risk of infection.

The catheter system must be appropriately zeroed to ambient air pressure. The catheter should be referenced, which is done by placing the air-fluid interface of the catheter (or the transducer) at a specific point to negate the effects of the length of the tubing and the fluid column.[9] The catheter is always advanced with the balloon inflated and withdrawn with the balloon deflated. The placement of the catheter is schematically illustrated in Figures 4A to D. After the catheter is in the right atrium and recognized by the RA pressure waveform, the catheter is advanced to the right ventricle. With the balloon inflated, the catheter is then advanced to the PA across the pulmonary valve. The catheter usually floats to the smaller PA branches and pulmonary capillary wedge pressure (PCWP) (PA occlusion pressure) is recognized. After deflation of the balloon, the PA pressure waveform is again recognized.

The PCWP (PA occlusion) is frequently used for indirect assessment of pulmonary venous and left atrial pressure. For the accurate measurement of PCWP, a continuous fluid column needs to be present between the distal tip of the catheter and the left atrium. The continuous fluid column is present when the pulmonary capillary pressure is higher than the surrounding alveolar pressure. If the alveolar pressure is much higher than the pulmonary capillary pressure, the capillaries collapse and a continuous fluid column between the distal tip of the catheter and the left atrium is no longer present. The measured PCWP in these locations does not reflect left atrial pressure. When there is partial obstruction of the capillaries due to increased alveolar pressure, an accurate assessment of left atrial pressure by measuring PCWP is also not possible.

Based on the relationship between pulmonary capillary blood flow, pulmonary capillary pressure and alveolar pressure, the lungs are divided into three physiologic zones.[10] Zone (1) is above the level of the left atrium where the alveolar pressure is much higher than the capillary pressure and there is compression of the capillaries. Zone (3) is located in the most dependent portion of the lung, below the level of the left atrium. In this zone, the pulmonary capillary pressure is higher than the alveolar pressure and there is a continuous fluid column between the distal tip of the catheter and the left atrium. If the catheter tip is placed in this zone, the measured PCWP reflects left atrial pressure. Whether the catheter tip is placed in Zone (3) or not can be verified by obtaining a lateral chest radiograph.

NORMAL PRESSURES AND WAVEFORMS

The normal range of RA pressure is 0–7 mm Hg, and of RV systolic pressure is 15–25 mm Hg. The mean pulmonary artery pressure (MPAP) is less than 18 mm Hg and mean PCWP is less than 15 mm Hg. The normal RV end-diastolic pressure ranges 0–8 mm Hg.

The RA pressure waveforms are characterized by two positive waves: (a) during RA systole and (b) at the end of RV rapid filling phase. There are two negative waves: (x) and (y) descents. The (x) descent is related to atrial relaxation, and (y) descent due to rapid ventricular filling. The RV pressure waveform is characterized by a sharp upstroke and a sharp down stroke during systole. During diastole, a rapid filling wave, diastasis, and atrial filling waves are recognized. The normal PA pressure waveform is characterized by a sharp upstroke and,

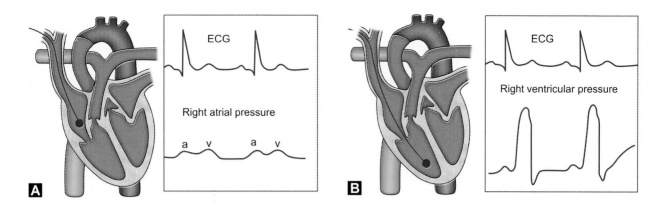

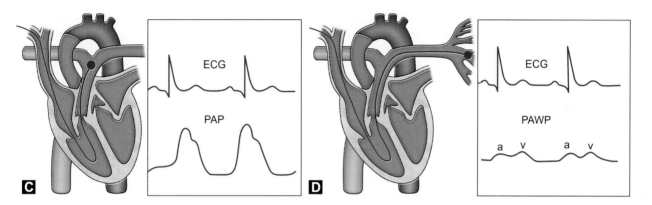

FIGURES 4A TO D: The schematic illustration of insertion of the balloon flotation catheter and the right atrial, right ventricular, pulmonary artery and pulmonary capillary wedge pressure waveforms are illustrated. The catheter is inserted into the right atrium (Panel A). In the right atrial pressure waveform there are two positive waveforms: "a" and "v." Then, the catheter is advanced to the right ventricle (Panel B). In the right ventricular pressure waveform, a rapid upstroke in systole is followed by the end-systolic dip. After the rapid filling phase, there is the phase of diastasis and atrial filling phase. Then, the catheter is advanced to the pulmonary artery (Panel C). The pulmonary artery pressure waveform is characterized by a rapid upstroke at the beginning of the ejection phase and the dicrotic notch and the dicrotic wave during the down stroke. The catheter is then advanced to a distal pulmonary artery branch to record the pulmonary capillary wedge pressure (Panel D). The pulmonary capillary wedge pressure waveform is similar to that of right atrial pressure waveform

during down stroke, by the dicrotic notch and the dicrotic wave. The PCWP waveforms are similar to those of RA pressure waveforms. The pressures, however, are higher than RA pressures.

During bedside hemodynamic monitoring, usually RA, PA and PCWPs and cardiac output are monitored. The RA pressure reflects RV diastolic pressure in absence of tricuspid valve obstruction. The RA pressure has a modest correlation with the PCWP in the absence of cardiopulmonary disease.[11] This correlation is further compromised in the presence of left ventricular dysfunction, valvular heart disease, coronary artery disease and pulmonary hypertension.[12,13]

The PCWP is frequently used to represent left ventricular preload. Left ventricular preload, however, is left ventricular end-diastolic volume. To assess left ventricular volume, it is preferable to perform transthoracic echocardiogram or other imaging techniques such as computerized cardiac tomography or cardiac magnetic resonance imaging.

Mean RA and mean PCWPs are used as right and left ventricular filling pressures respectively. It should be appreciated

that the true ventricular filling pressures are transmural pressures.[14-16] The transmural pressure is the difference between ventricular distending pressure (diastolic pressure) and the pressures opposing filling (pericardial and mediastinal pressures). Normally the intrapericardial pressure is 0 and the mediastinal pressure is from –1 mm Hg to –3 mm Hg. Thus, in normal conditions, RA and PCWPs can be used to represent right and left ventricular filling pressures. However, when intrapericardial pressure is increased as in cardiac tamponade, RA and PCWPs cannot be used as right and left ventricular filling pressures. It should be appreciated that there is a close correlation between RA and pericardial pressures. The RA pressures are 2–5 mm Hg higher than the pericardial pressures. Thus, it is possible to use RA pressure for approximate estimation of pericardial pressure.

Normally there is a good correlation between PA end-diastolic and mean PCWPs.[17-19] Usually, the difference between PA end-diastolic and mean PCWP does not exceed 5 mm Hg. A greater difference indicates increased pulmonary vascular resistance (PVR).[20]

The PCWP is similar to mean left ventricular diastolic pressure in absence of mitral valve obstruction. However, left ventricular end-diastolic pressure is usually higher than the mean PCWP. In mitral stenosis, LA and PCWPs are higher than left ventricular diastolic pressure and thus, in these patients, PCWP cannot be used to represent left ventricular filling pressure.

The accurate determination of RA or PCWPs is difficult in ventilated patients, in patients with pulmonary diseases and in patients with sleep disordered breathing. There may be a wide swing in pressures during respiratory phases. It has been suggested that the pressure measurements should be done at end expiration. For practical purposes, one can use the mean of (mean wedge pressure) to approximate the left ventricular filling pressure.

In the presence of significant tricuspid regurgitation, the cardiac output measurements with the indicator dilution technique (whether with the thermodilution or by the dye dilution) can be erroneous. In these patients the cardiac output measurements may be more accurate with the use of Fick principle. However, it is difficult to use the Fick method during hemodynamic monitoring because frequent measurement of oxygen consumption is not yet possible. It is, however, reasonable to determine changes in PA (mixed venous) oxygen saturation to assess the trend in changes in cardiac output. An increase in the PA oxygen saturation suggests an increase in cardiac output and a decrease in oxygen saturation indicates a decrease in cardiac output.

The various hemodynamic indices can be measured to establish the diagnosis of the pathologic conditions.

The hemodynamic differential diagnosis of some of the commonly encountered clinical conditions with pre-shock or shock syndromes in the intensive care units are summarized in Table 1. In cardiogenic shock, whether complicating acute coronary syndromes or chronic systolic heart failure, PCWP is much higher than the RA pressure and the cardiac output and stroke volume are reduced. In cardiogenic shock complicating RV myocardial infarction, however, RA pressure is disproportionately higher than the PCWP. In these patients, PA pressure is normal. In cardiogenic shock resulting from severe chronic RV failure such as in patients with idiopathic pulmonary arterial hypertension, PA pressure and PVR are elevated.

In hypovolemic shock, both RA pressure and PCWP are low. The characteristic hemodynamic features of septic shock are abnormally low systemic vascular resistance (usually < 700 dynes/sec/cm-5) and high cardiac output and decreased mean arterial pressure. The RA pressure and PCWP are normal or lower than normal.

In septic shock, vascular paralysis and reduction in systemic vascular resistance is the primary pathologic mechanism. The increase in cardiac output results from unloading of the left ventricle. The syndrome of "pseudosepsis" is encountered in patients with chronic advanced systolic heart failure treated with vasodilators and angiotensin inhibitors. The hemodynamic features are relatively low systemic vascular resistance, normal cardiac output, and elevated PCWP and RA pressure. Frequently there is renal failure as well. In these patients temporary discontinuation of vasodilator therapy is required.

Cardiac tamponade is also associated with cardiogenic shock. The hemodynamic features are hypotension, low cardiac output, and elevated RA and PCWPs. The mean RA pressure and PCWP are also equal (equalization of diastolic pressures). There is significant pulsus paradoxus. It should be emphasized that the diagnosis of cardiac tamponade should not be made based on hemodynamic abnormalities. Transthoracic echocardiography is the investigation of choice for the diagnosis of cardiac tamponade. The hemodynamic abnormalities of adult respiratory distress syndrome (ARDS) are similar to those of septic shock. The systemic vascular resistance and mean arterial pressure are less than normal and RA pressure and PCWP are normal or less than normal. Cardiac output is usually normal but may be reduced.

ABNORMAL PRESSURES AND WAVEFORMS

A prominent (a) wave in RA pressure tracing indicates abnormally elevated RA pressure due to increased resistance to RA emptying during atrial systole. The increased resistance may be at the level of the tricuspid valve or distal to the tricuspid valve. The tricuspid valve obstruction is characterized by increased pressure gradient across the tricuspid valve. The more severe the tricuspid valve obstruction is, the higher is the pressure gradient. In tricuspid valve obstruction the (y) descent

TABLE 1

The hemodynamic features of a few clinical conditions that can be associated with shock are summarized

	CO L/minute	MAP mm Hg	PCWP mm Hg	SVR Dynes/s/cm-5	PVR Dynes/s/cm-5	RAP mm Hg
Cardiogenic shock	Low	Low	High	High or normal	Normal or high	Normal
Right ventricular infarction	Low	Low	Normal	High	Normal	High
Hypovolemic shock	Low	Low	Low	Normal	Normal	Low
Septic shock	High	Low	Low	Low	Low	low
Pseudosepsis	Normal	Low	High	Low	High	High
Cardiac tamponade	Low	Low	High	Normal	Normal	High
ARDS	Normal or low	Normal or low	Normal or high	Normal or low	Normal or low	Normal or high

(Abbreviations: CO: Cardiac output; PCWP: Pulmonary capillary wedge pressure; RAP: Right atrial pressure; SVR: Systemic vascular resistance; PVR: Pulmonary vascular resistance; ARDS: Adult respiratory disease syndrome; MAP: Mean arterial pressure)

is slower than normal. In adults, increased resistance to RA emptying is more often due to RV failure resulting from pressure overload or volume overload.

Another cause of a prominent (a) wave is a cannon wave. It results from atrial contraction when the tricuspid valve is closed. Cannon (a) waves may occur regularly or irregularly in abnormalities of atrioventricular conduction, ventricular tachycardia, atrioventricular nodal tachyarrhythmias and ventricular pacing.

The most common cause of an absent (a) wave is atrial fibrillation. An infrequent cause is (silent giant right atrium). A prominent (v) wave in the RA pressure waveform usually indicates tricuspid valve regurgitation. In severe tricuspid regurgitation, RA pressure waveform may appear like that of RV pressure waveform (Fig. 5). It is characterized by a prominent (v) wave followed by a sharp (y) descent. The steep "y" descent is also observed in constrictive pericarditis. A "dip and plateau" filling pattern is observed in constrictive pericarditis and in restrictive cardiomyopathy.

CLINICAL APPLICATIONS

CARDIAC CATHETERIZATION LABORATORY

The balloon flotation catheters are most frequently used in the cardiac catheterization laboratory. The RA, RV, PA and PCWPs are determined routinely. Cardiac output and oxygen saturations in the different cardiac chambers are determined to assess presence of intracardiac and intrapulmonary shunts. For example, left to right shunt due to interventricular septal rupture complicating acute coronary syndromes can be diagnosed (Fig. 6). The oxygen saturation is higher in the PA than in the right atrium and the right ventricle. Severe acute or subacute mitral regurgitation can be diagnosed by analysis of PA and

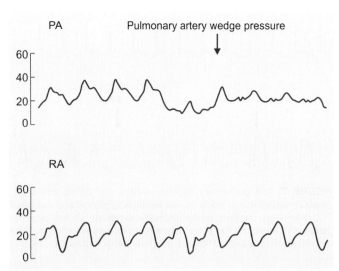

FIGURE 5: The right atrial pressure waveforms in severe tricuspid regurgitation are illustrated. There is a prominent "v" wave followed by a sharp "y" descent. The mean right atrial pressure and pulmonary capillary wedge pressure are also similar, illustrating equalization of diastolic pressures. (Abbreviations: PA: Pulmonary artery; RA: Right atrial)

PCWP waveforms (Fig. 7). The PCWP waveform reveals a large tall peaked (v) wave. In the PA pressure waveform, there is a reflected (v) wave which occurs before the dicrotic notch.

Cardiac output is determined by thermodilution technique with the use of multipurpose balloon flotation catheters. Systemic and PVRs are calculated. The shunt calculations are also made whenever is indicated. In most cardiac catheterization laboratories and in the intensive care units, automated computerized systems are available to measure the hemodynamic indices.

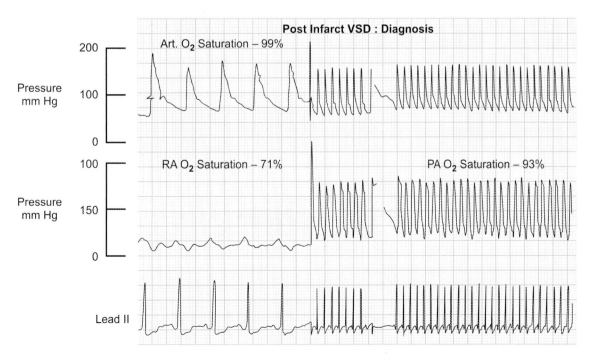

FIGURE 6: Diagnosis of severe left to right shunt due to ventricular septal rupture is illustrated. Pulmonary artery oxygen saturation is much higher than that in the right atrium. (Abbreviations: VSD: Ventricular septal defect; RA: Right atrial; PA: Pulmonary artery)

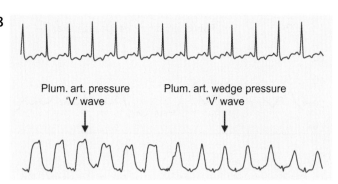

FIGURE 7: The pulmonary capillary wedge and pulmonary artery pressure waveforms in acute severe mitral regurgitation are illustrated. The pulmonary capillary wedge pressure waveform shows large tall peaked "v" waves. In the pulmonary artery pressure waveforms, there are reflected "v" waves which occur before the dicrotic notch

ACUTE CORONARY SYNDROMES

The treatment of ST-segment and non-ST segment elevation myocardial infarction consists of myocardial reperfusion therapy by either percutaneous coronary interventions or thrombolysis. Routine hemodynamic monitoring is not indicated in patients with acute coronary syndromes except in patients with cardiogenic shock.

Before the advent of echocardiography, determination of hemodynamics was employed for the diagnosis of complications of acute myocardial infarction such as severe mitral regurgitation and ventricular septal rupture. Severe mitral regurgitation is characterized by a large peaked "v" wave in the pulmonary capillary wedge pressure tracing. There is also a reflected "v" wave in the pulmonary artery pressure tracing.[7] In patients with ventricular septal rupture, there is a step up in oxygen saturation in the left ventricle and the oxygen saturation in the pulmonary artery is higher (Fig. 6). Severe right ventricular myocardial infarction can also be diagnosed by determination of hemodynamics (Fig. 8). Right atrial and right ventricular diastolic pressures are elevated. Mean right atrial and pulmonary capillary wedge pressures are equal (equalization of the diastolic pressures). The pulmonary artery pressure waveform is distorted.

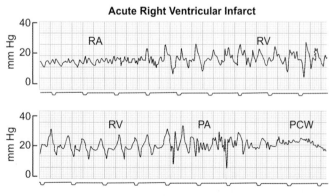

Acute Right Ventricular Infarct

FIGURE 8: The hemodynamic features of acute right ventricular myocardial infarction. Right atrial (RA) and right ventricular (RV) end-diastolic pressures are elevated. The mean RA and pulmonary capillary wedge pressure (PCWP) are equal. There is also distortion of the pulmonary (PA) pressure waveform

TABLE 2

Pulmonary artery catheters: Hemodynamic subsets in acute myocardial infarction

Subset	Signs	Cardiac index (L/min/m²)	PAWP (mm Hg)
I	PC– HYP–	> 2.2	< 18
II	PC + HYP –	> 2.2	> 18
III	PC – HYP +	< 2.2	< 18
IV	PC + HYP +	< 2.2	> 18

(Abbreviations: PC: Pulmonary congestion; HYP: Hypoperfusion; PAWP: Pulmonary artery wedge pressure)

Before the introduction of current therapies, hemodynamic measurements were made to determine the hemodynamic subsets, and therapies were recommended based on these hemodynamic subsets.[21-23] Based on cardiac output and PCWP, four hemodynamic subsets were recognized (Table 2).

In the hemodynamic subset I, the cardiac index was greater than 2.2 L/min/m² with the PCWP less than 18 mm Hg. In these patients there were also no clinical signs of pulmonary congestion or hypoperfusion. In the subset II, the cardiac index was more than 2.2 L/min/m² and the PCWP was greater than 18 mm Hg. Clinically, these patients did not have evidence of hypoperfusion but had evidence of pulmonary congestion. In the patients in subset III, the cardiac index was less than 2.2 L/min/m² and also the PCWP less than 18 mm Hg (hypovolemic shock). Clinically, the patients in this subset had evidence of hypoperfusion but no evidence of pulmonary congestion. In the hemodynamic subset IV, the cardiac index was less than 2.2 L/min/m² and the PCWP greater than 18 mm Hg (cardiogenic shock). Clinically, in these patients there was evidence of hypoperfusion and pulmonary congestion.

Suggested therapies according to the hemodynamic subsets are summarized in Table 3.

In patients in subset I, no specific therapy was recommended. In subset II, diuretics were recommended. Diuretics are necessary to relieve pulmonary congestion following reperfusion therapy in patients with acute coronary syndromes. In subset III, fluid replacement treatments were recommended. Hypovolemic shock is an uncommon complication of acute myocardial infarction. Following reperfusion therapy by percutaneous coronary intervention, hypovolemic shock is

TABLE 3

Pulmonary artery catheters: Acute myocardial infarction. Suggested therapy according to hemodynamic subsets

Subset	Therapy
I	None
II	Volume expansion
III	Diuretics, vasodilators
IV	Vasodilators, IABP, vasopressors, inotropes

(Abbreviation: IABP: Intra-aortic balloon pump)

occasionally encountered due to excessive blood loss and in these patients fluid replacement treatments are necessary. In patients in subset IV, hemodynamic monitoring is useful after reperfusion treatments and recommended for management of cardiogenic shock complicating acute coronary syndromes.

The issue, however, is whether routine hemodynamic monitoring with the use of balloon flotation catheters is required for management of patients with acute coronary syndromes. That routine hemodynamic monitoring may be associated with increased mortality and morbidity has been reported. In 1987, Gore et al. reported that routine hemodynamic monitoring in patients with acute myocardial infarction was associated with higher in-hospital mortality even in the presence of congestive heart failure, hypotension, or both.[24] In patients with congestive heart failure, the mortality was 44.8% of those who had hemodynamic monitoring and 25.3% who did not. In patients with hypotension, it was 48.3% of those who had hemodynamic monitoring and 32.2% who did not. However, in patients with cardiogenic shock, it was 74.4% of those who had hemodynamic monitoring and 79.1% who did not. Thus, in patients with cardiogenic shock, the use of balloon flotation catheters was not associated with increased in-hospital mortality. In Gusto IIb and III randomized clinical trials, the hazard ratio for the 30-day mortality in patients without cardiogenic shock was 4.80 and in patients with cardiogenic shock it was 0.99.[25] Thus, PA catheterization is not recommended in patients with acute coronary syndromes without cardiogenic shock.

These studies suggest that routine PA catheterization is not indicated in the absence of cardiogenic shock. In patients with cardiogenic shock, however, either due to left ventricular or RV myocardial infarction hemodynamic monitoring is useful and recommended for appropriate management and assessment of response to therapy.

In patients with ventricular septal rupture or severe mitral regurgitation due to papillary muscle dysfunction, hemodynamic monitoring is useful to assess response to therapy. For example, in patients with severe mitral regurgitation, response to vasodilator therapy can be determined by hemodynamic monitoring (Fig. 9).[25] It should be emphasized, however, that for the diagnosis of the mechanical complications of acute coronary syndromes, determinations of hemodynamics are not indicated and transthoracic echocardiography should be performed for the diagnosis.

NON-ACUTE CORONARY SYNDROME

The balloon flotation catheter has been used in the high-risk patients in the medical and surgical intensive care units for the management of volume status, hypotension and shock. The PA catheterization has also been used to distinguish between hemodynamic and permeability pulmonary edema. The PA catheterization has been used in high-risk surgical patients for optimization of oxygen delivery by increasing cardiac output by pharmacologic agents and by maintaining adequate volume status with fluid therapy.[26] However, randomized clinical trials reported lack of any benefit with maximizing oxygen consumption by hemodynamic monitoring.[27]

In one randomized trial in intensive care units, 579 patients received PA catheterization and 522 patients did not. The hospital mortality was 68% in patients who received PA catheterization and 66% in those who did not receive catheterization.[28]

In another randomized trial in high-risk surgical patients, 997 patients received PA catheterization and 997 patients did not.[29] The hospital mortality was 7.8% in patients receiving PA catheterization and 7.7% who did not receive catheterization. The incidence of pulmonary embolism was 8% in patients who had PA catheterization and 0% in those not receiving catheterization. The results of these studies suggest that routine PA catheterization do not provide any survival benefit and can be associated with increased morbidity.

The balloon flotation catheter has been used for the management of patients with ARDS. It has been suggested that

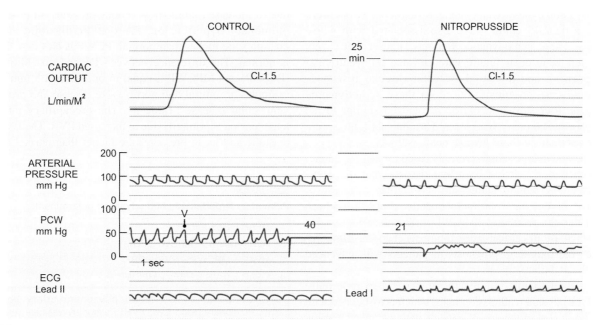

FIGURE 9: The hemodynamic response to vasodilator sodium nitroprusside in a patient with severe mitral regurgitation complicating acute myocardial infarction is illustrated. With nitroprusside, there was a marked decrease in the amplitude of the "v" wave along with an increase in cardiac output. (Abbreviations: PCW: Pulmonary capillary wedge; ECG: Electrocardiography)

monitoring of RA pressure and PCWP and cardiac output will facilitate maintenance of the volume status and regulation of vasopressors and inotropic agents. Indeed, some earlier randomized clinical trials have reported survival benefit of patients who received hemodynamic monitoring.[30]

However, in a large National Heart, Lung, and Blood Institute sponsored randomized trial, there was no benefit of PA catheterization. In this trial, 513 patients received PA catheterization and 488 patients received central venous monitoring. There were 37% of patients with shock in the PA catheterization group and 32% in the central venous monitoring group. The percentage of patients who received vasopressors was 36 in the PA group and 32 in the central venous catheter group. The 60-day mortality in patients receiving PA catheterization was 27.4% and 26.3% in patients receiving central venous monitoring. The ventilator-free and intensive care-free days were 13.2 and 12.0 days in patients who received PA catheterization respectively. In patients who received central venous catheterization, the ventilator-free and intensive care-free days were 13.5 and 12.5 days respectively. The complications rate, however, was higher in patients receiving PA catheterization (0.08%) than in patients receiving central venous catheterization (0.06%).

In this study it was concluded that "pulmonary artery catheterization (PAC) guided therapy did not improve survival or organ perfusion and complications were higher than central venous catheterization (CVC) guided therapy". Thus, there is no indication for routine use of PA catheters for hemodynamic monitoring during management of patients with acute respiratory distress syndrome.

CHRONIC HEART FAILURE

In patients with severe chronic systolic heart failure, hemodynamic subsets have been recognized not only to formulate therapy but also to assess prognosis. In patients with cardiac index of less than 2.2 L/min/m^2 and PCWP greater than 25 mm Hg, the prognosis was worse.[31,32] Systemic vascular resistance more than 1,800 dynes/sec/cm-5 and left ventricular stroke work index less than 45 gm/m^2 were also associated with worse prognosis. These hemodynamic findings suggest that severe chronic left ventricular failure with elevated left ventricular filling pressure and increased systemic vascular resistance indicate adverse prognosis. Based on these hemodynamic indices, the four subsets could be recognized similar to the subsets of acute coronary syndromes. The clinical findings were also incorporated in these hemodynamic subsets.

The hemodynamic subsets were also used for hemodynamic-tailored therapy.[33,34] It has been hypothesized that the determination of the hemodynamic subsets facilitates the use of aggressive diuretic, inotropic and vasoactive drugs. It has been reported that the reduction of PCWP to less than 18 mm Hg and the increase in cardiac index to greater than 2.2 L/min/m^2 improves the long-term prognosis of patients with advanced systolic heart failure.

The hemodynamic-tailored therapy was also reportedly reduced the hospital readmission rates, which is associated with a decrease in cost of therapy of patients with advanced chronic heart failure. The hemodynamic subsets were widely accepted by the heart failure specialists for the management of these patients. The PAC was regarded necessary for appropriate management of these patients. It should be appreciated that these studies were not randomized and were retrospective.

To assess the necessity and effectiveness of bedside hemodynamic monitoring by PAC with the use of balloon flotation catheters, a prospective randomized trial was performed.[35] The primary objective of this study was to determine whether hemodynamic monitoring is helpful for the management of patients with advanced systolic heart failure. Hemodynamic monitoring was compared to clinical assessment. The differences in mortality and number of days in hospital were compared. There was no difference in total and cardiovascular mortality and in the length of hospital stay between the patients who received PAC and patients managed by clinical assessment alone. The results of this study demonstrate that routine PA catheterization is not helpful in the management of patients with chronic advanced systolic heart failure.

It is apparent that routine PAC with the use of balloon flotation catheters is not helpful for the management of patients with acute coronary syndromes, high-risk surgical patients, patients with acute respiratory distress syndrome and patients with severe chronic heart failure (Fig. 10).[36] However, in individual critically ill patients, PAC is still necessary for appropriate management.

PULMONARY HYPERTENSION

The PAC is necessary to determine the cause of pulmonary arterial hypertension.[37] Bedside hemodynamic monitoring is also employed to assess response to therapy. Pulmonary hypertension is defined when the MPAP is greater than 25 mm Hg at rest or greater than 30 mm Hg with exercise.

PA pressure is the product of pulmonary blood flow (PBF) and PVR. In Table 4, the hemodynamic relationship between MPAP, PVR, PBF and mean pulmonary capillary wedge pressure (MPCWP) is illustrated.

The PA hypertension can be postcapillary, which is primarily due to increased pulmonary venous pressure. In postcapillary pulmonary hypertension, PA systolic/diastolic and mean pressures are higher than normal. PCWP is elevated. The PVR is normal. The difference between PA end diastolic pressure (PAEDP) and MPCWP is equal to or less than 5 mm Hg. The examples are mitral and aortic valve disease and primary left ventricular disease (Table 5). The precapillary pulmonary hypertension is primarily due to increased PVR. The PA systolic, diastolic and mean pressures are higher than normal and PVR

TABLE 4

Pulmonary hypertension hemodynamic determinants

1. MPAP = PBF × PVR
2. PVR = (MPAP − MPCWP)/PBF
3. MPAP = MPCWP = PVR × PBF
4. MPAP = (PVR × PBF) + MPCWP

(Abbreviations: MPAP: Mean pulmonary artery pressure; PBF: Pulmonary blood flow; PVR: Pulmonary vascular resistance; MPCWP: Mean pulmonarry capillary wedge pressure)

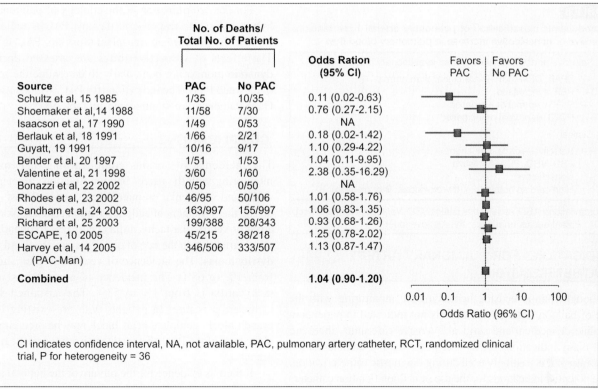

Source	No. of Deaths/ Total No. of Patients		Odds Ration (95% CI)
	PAC	No PAC	
Schultz et al, 15 1985	1/35	10/35	0.11 (0.02-0.63)
Shoemaker et al,14 1988	11/58	7/30	0.76 (0.27-2.15)
Isaacson et al, 17 1990	1/49	0/53	NA
Berlauk et al, 18 1991	1/66	2/21	0.18 (0.02-1.42)
Guyatt, 19 1991	10/16	9/17	1.10 (0.29-4.22)
Bender et al, 20 1997	1/51	1/53	1.04 (0.11-9.95)
Valentine et al, 21 1998	3/60	1/60	2.38 (0.35-16.29)
Bonazzi et al, 22 2002	0/50	0/50	NA
Rhodes et al, 23 2002	46/95	50/106	1.01 (0.58-1.76)
Sandham et al, 24 2003	163/997	155/997	1.06 (0.83-1.35)
Richard et al, 25 2003	199/388	208/343	0.93 (0.68-1.26)
ESCAPE, 10 2005	45/215	38/218	1.25 (0.78-2.02)
Harvey et al, 14 2005 (PAC-Man)	346/506	333/507	1.13 (0.87-1.47)
Combined			**1.04 (0.90-1.20)**

CI indicates confidence interval, NA, not available, PAC, pulmonary artery catheter, RCT, randomized clinical trial, P for heterogeneity = 36

FIGURE 10: The results of a meta-analysis for the use of pulmonary artery catheters (PAC) in intensive care units. There was no benefit from the routine use of pulmonary artery catheters. (*Source:* Reproduced with permission from reference 36)

is increased. The PAEDP is significantly higher than MPCWP. The examples are "idiopathic pulmonary hypertension", collagen vascular disease, and congenital heart diseases (Table 6). The mixed type of PA hypertension is defined when pulmonary arterial hypertension results from both increased pulmonary venous pressure and PVR. The systolic, diastolic and MPAPs are higher than normal. Both MPCWP and PVR are elevated. The PAEDP is higher than the MPCWP. The examples are mitral and aortic valve diseases and chronic primary left ventricular myocardial disease (Table 7).

A selective (left to right shunt) or non-selective (high-cardiac output) increase in PBF may be associated with pulmonary hypertension (Tables 7 and 8). The PA systolic, diastolic and mean pressures are higher than normal. The MPCWP is normal or increased .The PAEDP is equal to or higher than MPCWP. The PVR is normal or decreased.

TABLE 5

Hemodynamic classification of pulmonary arterial hypertension (postcapillary)

Postcapillary pulmonary hypertension
- SPAP, DPAP, MPAP are higher than normal
- PCWP is normal
- PVR is normal
- PAEDP is ≤ 5 mm Hg of MPCWP

Clinical
- Left ventricular systolic or diastolic failure
- Aortic and mitral valve disease
- Pulmonary veno occlusive disease (congenital or acquired)

(Abbreviation: DPAP: Diastolic pulmonary artery pressure)

TABLE 6

Hemodynamic classification of pulmonary arterial hypertension (precapillary)

Precapillary pulmonary hypertension
- SPAP, DPAP, MPAP are higher than normal
- MPCWP is normal
- PVR is elevated
- PAEDP is higher than MPCWP

Clinical
- Primary pulmonary hypertension (PPH)
- PH associated with collagen vascular disease
- Eisemenger syndrome, porto-pulmonary hypertension
- HIV, high altitude PH, thromboembolic PH, peripheral pulmonary arterial branch stenosis

TABLE 7

Hemodynamic classification of pulmonary arterial hypertension (mixed)

Mixed
- SPAP, DPAP, MPAP are higher than normal
- MPCWP is elevated
- PAEDP is modestly higher than MPCWP
- PVR is modestly elevated

Clinical
- Chronic LV systolic and diastolic failure
- Chronic aortic and mitral valve diseases

It is apparent that the PAC is necessary for the diagnosis of the various types of PA hypertension. In addition, determination of hemodynamics is useful to decide what therapy should be employed and also to assess response to therapy.

CHAPTER 27

Swan-Ganz Catheters: Clinical Applications

TABLE 8

Hemodynamic classification of pulmonary arterial hypertension: Selective or nonselective increase in pulmonary blood flow

- Selective or nonselective increase in pulmonary blood flow
  - SPAP, DPAP, MPAP are higher than normal
  - PBF is increased
  - PVR is normal or increased
  - PCWP is normal or increased
- Clinical
  - Selective—left to right shunt
    ASD, VSD, PDA, AV fistula
  - Nonselective
    High cardiac output (e.g. thyrotoxicosis, liver disease)

(Abbreviations: ASD: Atrial septal defect; VSD: Ventricular septal defect; PDA: Patent ductus arteriosus; AV: Ateriovenous)

INDICATIONS FOR PULMONARY ARTERY CATHETERIZATION

Although routine bedside hemodynamic monitoring with the use of balloon flotation catheters is not indicated in patients in cardiac or medical and surgical intensive care units, there are still many indications for its use. In the cardiac catheterization laboratory, it is routinely used during diagnostic catheterization. The potential indications for the use of balloon flotation catheters are summarized in Table 9.

In patients with cardiogenic shock complicating acute coronary syndromes, PAC is indicated. In patients with cardiogenic shock due to chronic severe systolic heart failure, hemodynamic monitoring is frequently required to determine appropriate therapeutic approach. In patients with discordant right and left ventricular failure, measurement of hemodynamics is extremely useful to determine the relative contributions of right and left ventricular function to the hemodynamic abnormalities. Hemodynamic monitoring is also recommended in patients requiring aggressive inotropic and vasoactive drug therapy.

For the differential diagnosis of sepsis and "pseudosepsis" determination of hemodynamics are essential.

Hemodynamic monitoring is useful in some patients with potentially reversible systolic heart failure such as with fulminant myocarditis or peripartum cardiomyopathy.

TABLE 9

The indications for the use of the Swan-Ganz catheters

- Routine application is not indicated even in high-risk cardiac or noncardiac patients
- In patients with cardiogenic shock complicating acute coronary syndromes during supportive therapy
- In patients with cardiogenic shock due to severe chronic systolic heart failure
- In patients with discordant right and left ventricular function
- In patients with severe chronic systolic or diastolic heart failure requiring inotropic, vasoactive drugs
- For the differential diagnosis of sepsis and "pseudosepsis"
- In some patients with potentially reversible systolic heart failure such as fulminant myocarditis and peripartum cardiomyopathy
- For determination of the etiology of pulmonary artery hypertension and response to therapy
- For the cardiac transplantation work up

For the determination of the etiology of pulmonary arterial hypertension and response to therapy, PAC is indicated.

For the pre-cardiac transplant work-up, PAC is necessary. The effects of vasoactive drugs are assessed during hemodynamic monitoring particularly to determine the reversibility of elevated PVR. The indications for PAC with the use of Swan-Ganz catheters are summarized in Table 9).[38]

COMPLICATIONS

The incidence of serious complications of hemodynamic monitoring with the use of balloon flotation catheters is low.[37] Atrial and ventricular premature beats occur almost universally during the placement of balloon flotation catheter. Non-sustained atrial or ventricular tachycardia occurs less frequently. There is wide variability in the rate of occurrence of atrial and ventricular dysrhythmias. The incidence of ventricular premature beats is from 1% to 68%. The incidence of nonsustained ventricular tachycardia is from 1% to 53%. The sustained ventricular tachycardia is rare. In patients with pre-existing left bundle branch block, complete heart block may be precipitated during placement of the PA catheters due to irritation of the right bundle branch.

If there is evidence for the rupture of the balloon at the distal tip of the catheter, it should be replaced.

It is difficult to estimate the incidence of thromboembolic complications during hemodynamic monitoring. However, the longer the duration of monitoring, the higher is the incidence of thromboembolism. The incidence of pulmonary infarction is approximately 7%. It results from embolization of thrombi formed around the catheter.

The PA perforation is a rare but almost always a fatal complication of PAC with the use of balloon flotation catheters. The incidence is about 0.2%. Sudden hemoptysis of bright red blood is indication of PA perforation. Emergency surgery may be required to prevent the fatal outcome.

Endocardial lesions, including subendocardial hemorrhage, formation of sterile thrombus and infective endocarditis, are infrequent complications of PAC.

The incidence of sepsis is about 4%, and it is more frequent when prolonged hemodynamic monitoring is required. To reduce the risk of sepsis, the insertion of the catheter via femoral vein should be avoided.

The rare complications are Bernard-Horner syndrome, pneumoperitoneum, fracture of the catheter and inadvertent insertion to the carotid artery. Knotting of the balloon flotation catheter around the cardiac structures is infrequently encountered.

CONCLUSION

The feasibility of PAC was demonstrated almost a century ago. With the introduction of balloon flotation (Swan-Ganz) catheters, it has been used indiscriminately in cardiac, medical and surgical intensive care units which were associated with undesirable complications including death. Following a number of randomized clinical trials, the appropriate indications for PAC have been reasonably established. However, there are a number of indications for PAC in critically ill patients.

GUIDELINES
SUMMARY OF GUIDELINES RECOMMENDATIONS (MODIFIED)

(Source: Mueller H, Chatterjee K, Davis KB, et al. Present use of bedside right heart catheterization in patients with cardiac disease. J Am Coll Cardiol. 1998;32:840-64)

GRADING OF RECOMMENDATIONS

1. Conditions in which there is general agreement that right heart catheterization is indicated.
2. Conditions in which reasonable differences of opinion exist regarding right heart catheterization.
3. Conditions in which right heart catheterization is not warranted.
4. Conditions in which a relative contraindication to right heart catheterization exists.
5. Conditions in which an absolute contraindication to right heart catheterization exists.

RECOMMENDATIONS: HEART FAILURE

Conditions in which right heart catheterization is warranted:
1. For differentiation between hemodynamic and permeability pulmonary edema, and when a trial of diuretic and/or vasodilator therapy has failed to distinguish or associated with high risk.
2. For differentiation between cardiogenic and noncardiogenic shock and for guidance of pharmacologic and/or mechanical support.
3. For guidance of therapy in patients with concomitant manifestations of "forward" and "backward" heart failure.
4. For guidance of perioperative management in selected patients with decompensated heart failure undergoing intermediate or high-risk non-cardiac surgery.
5. For pre-heart transplant work up.

Conditions in which a relative contraindication to right heart catheterization exists:
1. Coagulopathy or anticoagulation therapy that can not be temporarily discontinued.
2. Recent implantation of permanent pacemaker or cardioverter-defibrillator.
3. Left bundle branch block.
4. Bioprosthetic tricuspid or pulmonic valve.

Conditions in which an absolute contraindication to right heart catheterization exists:
1. Right-sided endocarditis.
2. Mechanical tricuspid or pulmonic valve prosthesis.
3. Presence of thrombus or tumor in right heart chambers.
4. Terminal illness for which aggressive management is considered futile.

RECOMMENDATIONS: ACUTE CORONARY SYNDROME.

Conditions in which there is general agreement that right heart catheterization is warranted:
1. Differentiation between cardiogenic and hypovolemic shock.
2. Guidance of therapy of patients with cardiogenic shock with pharmacologic and/or mechanical support with or without reperfusion therapy.
3. During short-term treatments of complications such as mitral regurgitation and ventricular septal rupture.
4. During management of patients with right ventricular myocardial infarction with hypotension.
5. For guidance of therapy of patients with refractory pulmonary edema.

Conditions in which right heart catheterization is not warranted:
1. For guidance of management of patients with postinfarction angina.
2. For guidance of therapy of pulmonary edema responding to standard therapy.

Conditions in which an absolute contraindication to right heart catheterization exist:
1. Same as in heart failure.

RECOMMENDATIONS: PERIOPERATIVE USE IN CARDIAC SURGERY.

Conditions in which there is general agreement that right heart catheterization is warranted:
1. For the diagnosis of the causes of low cardiac output.
2. For differentiation of right and left ventricular dysfunction.
3. For guidance of management of patients with low cardiac output syndromes.

Conditions in which right heart catheterization is not warranted:
1. For routine management of uncomplicated cardiac surgical patients.
2. For assessment of prognosis of cardiac surgery.

Conditions in which an absolute contraindication to right heart catheterization exists:
Same as in "heart failure".

RECOMMENDATIONS: PULMONARY ARTERIAL HYPERTENSION.

Conditions in which there is general agreement that right heart catheterization is warranted:
1. For the differential diagnosis of "postcapillary," "precapillary" and "mixed" pulmonary hypertension.
2. For the diagnosis of severity of precapillary pulmonary arterial hypertension and the prognosis.
3. For the assessment of therapy in patients with precapillary pulmonary arterial hypertension.

Conditions in which right heart catheterization is not warranted:
None

Conditions in which a relative or absolute contraindication to right heart catheterization exists:
Same as in "heart failure".

REFERENCES

1. Swan HJC, Ganz W, Forrester J, et al. Catheterization of the heart in man with the use of a flow-directed balloon-tipped catheter. N Engl J Med. 1970;283:447-51.
2. Forssmann W. Die Sondierung des rechten Herzens. Klinische Wochenschrift. 1929;8:2085-87.
3. Cournand A. Cardiac catheterization; development of the technique, its contributions to experimental medicine, and its initial application in man. Acta Med Scand. 1975;579:1-32.
4. Bradley RD. Diagnostic right-heart catheterization with miniature catheters in severely ill patients. Lancet. 1964;2:941-2.
5. Fife WP, Lee BS. Construction and use of self guiding right heart and pulmonary artery catheter. J Appl Physiol. 1965;20:148-9.
6. Scheinman MM, Abbott JA, Rapaport E. Clinical use of a flow-directed right heart catheter. Arch Intern Med. 1969;124:19-24.
7. Forrester JS, Ganz W, Diamond G, et al. Thermodilution cardiac output determination with a single flow directed catheter for cardiac monitoring. Am Heart J. 1972;83:306-11.
8. Chatterjee K, Swan HJC, Ganz W, et al. Use of a balloon-tipped flotation electrode catheter for cardiac monitoring. Am J Cardiol. 1975;36:56-61.
9. Summerhill EM, Baram M. Principles of pulmonary artery catheterization in the critically ill. Lung. 2005;183:209-19.
10. West JB, Dollery CT, Naimark A. Distribution of blood flow in isolated lung: relation to vascular and alveolar pressures. J Appl Physiol. 1964;19:713-24.
11. Mangano DT. Monitoring pulmonary arterial pressure in coronary artery disease. Anesthesiology. 1980;53:364-70.
12. Sarin CL, Yalav E, Clement AJ, et al. The necessity for measurement of left atrial pressure after cardiac surgery. Thorax. 1970;25:185-9.
13. Bell H, Stubbs D, Pugh D. Reliability of central venous pressure as an indication of left atrial pressure: a study in patients with mitral valve disease. Chest. 1971;59:169-73.
14. O'Quin R, Marini JJ. Pulmonary artery occlusion pressure; clinical physiology, measurement and interpretation. Am Rev Respir Dis. 1983;128:319-26.
15. Putterman C. The Swan-Ganz catheter: a decade of hemodynamic monitoring. J Crit Care. 1989;4:127-46.
16. Sharkey SW. Beyond the wedge; clinical physiology and the Swan-Ganz catheter. Am J Med. 1987;83:111-22.
17. Falicov RE, Resnekov L. Relationship of the pulmonary artery end-diastolic pressure to the left ventricular end-diastolic and mean filling pressures in patients with and without left ventricular dysfunction. Circulation. 1970;42:65-73.
18. Rahimtoola SH, Loeb HS, Ehsani A, et al. Relationship of pulmonary artery to left ventricular diastolic pressures in acute myocardial infarction. Circulation. 1972;46:283-90.
19. Scheinman M, Evans GT, Weiss A, et al. Relationship between pulmonary artery end-diastolic pressure and left ventricular filling pressure in patients in shock. Circulation. 1973;47:317-24.
20. Wilson RF, Beckman SB, Tyburski JG, et al. Pulmonary artery diastolic and wedge pressure relationships in critically ill and injured patients. Arch Surg. 1988;123:933-6.
21. Forrester JS, Diamond G, Chatterjee K, et al. Medical therapy of acute myocardial infarction by application of hemodynamic subsets (Part I). N Engl J Med. 1976;295:1356-62.
22. Forrester JS, Diamond G, Chatterjee K, et al. Medical therapy of acute myocardial infarction by application of hemodynamic subsets (Part II). N Engl J Med 1976;295:1404-13.
23. Gore JM, Goldberg RJ, Spodick DH, et al. A community-wide assessment of the use of pulmonary artery catheters in patients with acute myocardial infarction. Chest. 1987;92:721-7.
24. Cohen MG, Kelly RV, Kong DF, et al. Pulmonary artery catheterization in acute coronary syndromes; insights from the GUSTO IIb and GUSTO III trials. Am J Med. 2005;118:482-8.
25. Chatterjee K, Parmley WW, Swan HJC, et al. Beneficial effects of vasodilator agents in severe mitral regurgitation due to dysfunction of subvalvar apparatus. Circulation 1973;48:684-90.
26. Shoemaker WC, Appel PL, Kram HB, et al. Prospective trial of supranormal values of survivors as therapeutic goals in high-risk surgical patients. Chest. 1988;94:1176-86.
27. Hays MA, Timmins AC, Yau EH, et al. Elevation of systemic oxygen delivery in the treatment of critically ill patients. N Engl J Med. 1994;330:1717-22.
28. Harvey S, Harrison DA, Singer M, et al. Assessment of the clinical effectiveness of pulmonary artery catheters in management of patients in intensive care (PAC-Man): a randomized controlled trial. Lancet. 2005;366:472-7.
29. Sandham JD, Hull RD, Brant RF, et al. A randomized, controlled trial of the use of pulmonary-artery catheters in high-risk surgical patients. N Engl J Med. 2003;348:5-14.
30. Richard C, Warszawski J, Anguel N, et al. Early use of the pulmonary artery catheter and outcome in patients with shock and acute respiratory distress syndrome: a randomized controlled trial. JAMA. 2003;290:2713-20.
31. Franciosa JA, Wilen M, Ziesche S, et al. Survival in men with severe chronic heart left ventricular failure due to either coronary heart disease or idiopathic dilated cardiomyopathy. Am J Cardiol. 1983;51:831-6.

32. Unverferth DV, Magorien RD, Moeschberger ML, et al. Factors influencing the one-year mortality of dilated cardiomyopathy. Am J Cardiol. 1984;54:147-52.

33. Stevenson LW, Tillisch JH. Maintenance of cardiac output with normal filling pressures in patients with dilated heart failure. Circulation. 1986;74:1303-8.

34. Steimle AE, Stevenson LW, Chelimsky-Fallick C, et al. Sustained hemodynamic efficacy of therapy tailored to reduce filling pressures in survivors with advanced heart failure. Circulation. 1997;96:1165-72.

35. The ESCAPE Investigators and ESCAPE and Study Coordinators. Evaluation study of congestive heart failure and pulmonary artery catheterization effectiveness: the ESCAPE trial. JAMA. 2005;294:1625-33.

36. Shah MR, Hasselblad V, Stevenson LW, et al. Impact of the pulmonary artery catheterization in critically patients: meta-analysis of randomized clinical trials. JAMA. 2005;294:1664-70.

37. Chatterjee K. Bedside hemodynamic monitoring. In: Parmley WW, Chatterjee K (Eds). Cardiology. Philadelphia, PA: JB Lippincott Publishing Co; 1988. pp. 1-19.

38. Chatterjee K, DeMarco T, Alpert JS. Pulmonary hypertension, hemo-dynamic diagnosis and management. Arch Inter Med. 2002;162:e187-90.

Coronary Angiography and Catheter-based Coronary Intervention

Elaine M Demetroulis, Mohan Brar

Chapter Outline

INTRODUCTION

The first attempt to image the coronary arteries began in the late 1940s. In 1953, Seldinger first introduced a method of percutaneous arterial catheterization to study the coronary arteries.[1] However, this percutaneous approach was not initially widely adopted.In the late 1950s, Sones developed a safe and reliable method of selective coronary angiography using a brachial artery cut down approach to arterial access.[2] In the late 1960s, Amplatz et al.[3] and Judkins[4] developed modifications of catheters for selective coronary angiography while also employing the percutaneous method previously introduced by Seldinger. This combination and modification of previous approaches ushered in the beginning of the modern era of coronary angiography as we recognize it today.

Coronary angiography has subsequently become one of the most widely used invasive procedures in cardiovascular medicine and remains the gold standard for identifying the presence or absence of atherosclerotic coronary artery disease (CAD). It provides not only the most reliable anatomic information but also along with adjunctive invasive modalities; it can now provide the clinician with a more precise characterization of the extent of atherosclerotic disease burden. This greatly assists the practitioner in selection of the most appropriate form of therapy for a given patient. More than two million patients will undergo coronary angiography in the United States this year alone.

The methods used to perform coronary angiography have continued to improve substantially over time. Smaller (5–6 French) high-flow injection catheters have replaced larger (8 French) thick-walled catheters. The smaller sheath sizes and the introduction and development of radial artery access for coronary catheterization have allowed same-day outpatient coronary angiography, early ambulation and discharge. Complication rates associated with coronary angiography have decreased secondary to a better understanding of the periprocedural management of patients undergoing cardiac catheterization.

This chapter discusses the indications for and techniques of coronary angiography, normal coronary anatomy, some pathological coronary variants, various pitfalls to avoid in the safe and successful performance of this procedure, and a brief introductory discussion of coronary intervention.

INDICATIONS FOR CORONARY ANGIOGRAPHY

The American College of Cardiology/American Heart Association (ACC/AHA) Task Force has established indications for coronary angiography in patients with known or suspected CAD (Table 1).[5]

Despite the recent advances in noninvasive imaging of the coronary arteries, coronary angiography remains the gold standard for the delineation of coronary arterial anatomy. Patients who have a clear indication for coronary angiography include: individuals with known or suspected CAD who have severe stable angina [Canadian Cardiovascular Society (CCS) class III or IV], individuals with less severe symptoms but an abnormal noninvasive test, or asymptomatic individuals who demonstrate "high-risk" criteria on noninvasive testing. Patients resuscitated from sudden cardiac death (SCD)—particularly those with residual ventricular arrhythmias—are also candidates for coronary angiography, given the favorable outcomes associated with revascularization in this patient population. In the absence of symptoms or signs of ischemia, the presence of coronary calcification on fluoroscopy or a high calcium score by ultrafast computed tomographic (CT) scanning alone are not indications for coronary angiography.

Patients with ST segment elevation myocardial infarction (STEMI) should undergo emergent coronary angiography with intent of primary coronary intervention. Diagnostic coronary angiography should also be undertaken in patients presenting in cardiogenic shock, who are candidates for revascularization in the setting of STEMI. Additionally, patients with non-ST segment elevation myocardial infarction (NSTEMI) or unstable angina benefit from early invasive treatment with urgent coronary angiography and coronary revascularization. Coronary

TABLE 1

Indications for coronary angiography

ACC/AHA guideline summary: Coronary angiography for risk stratification in patients with chronic stable angina
Class I: There is evidence and/or general agreement that coronary angiography should be performed to risk stratify patients with chronic stable angina in the following settings: • Disabling anginal symptoms [Canadian Cardiovascular Society (CCS) classes III and IV] despite medical therapy • High-risk criteria on noninvasive testing independent of the severity of angina • Survivors of sudden cardiac death or serious ventricular arrhythmia • Symptoms and signs of heart failure • Clinical features suggest that the patient has a high likelihood of severe coronary artery disease
Class IIa: The evidence or opinion is in favor of performing coronary angiography to risk stratify patients with chronic stable angina in the following settings: • Left ventricular ejection fraction less than 45%, CCS class I or II angina and evidence, on noninvasive testing, of ischemia that does not meet high-risk criteria • Noninvasive testing does not reveal adequate prognostic information
Class IIb: The evidence or opinion is less well established for performing coronary angiography to risk stratify patients with chronic stable angina in the following settings: • Left ventricular ejection fraction greater than 45%, CCS class I or II angina and evidence, on noninvasive testing, of ischemia that does not meet high-risk criteria • CCS class III or IV angina that improves to class I or II with medical therapy • CCS class I or II angina but unacceptable side effects to adequate medical therapy
Class III: There is evidence and/or general agreement that coronary angiography should not be performed to risk stratify patients with chronic stable angina in the following settings: • CCS class I or II angina that responds to medical therapy and, on noninvasive testing, shows no evidence of ischemia • Patient preference to avoid revascularization
(*Source:* Gibbons RJ, Abrams J, Chatterjee K, et al. ACC/AHA 2002 guidelines update for the management of patients with chronic stable angina—summary article: a report of the American College of Cardiology/American Heart Association Task Force on Practice Guidelines (Committee on the Management of Patients with Chronic Stable Angina). Circulation. 2003;107:149.)

angiography should also be considered in patients with myocardial infarction (MI) complicated by congestive heart failure (CHF), hemodynamic instability, frequent complex arrhythmias, cardiac arrest or severe mitral regurgitation. Patients with angina or provocable ischemia after MI should also undergo coronary angiography, as revascularization may reduce the risk of reinfarction in these patients. Furthermore, there is evidence to support an early invasive strategy in patients with repeated presentations for acute coronary syndrome despite therapy and without evidence for ongoing ischemia or high risk, especially if these patients have not had a previous coronary angiogram. However, coronary angiography is not recommended for the subset of patients who present with chest discomfort suggestive of unstable angina, but no objective signs of ischemia and with normal coronary angiogram during the past 5 years.[5] Patients with chest pain of unclear etiology, particularly those with high-risk criteria on noninvasive cardiac testing, may benefit from coronary angiography to evaluate for the presence of significant CAD.[5] Patients who have undergone prior revascularization, especially recently, should undergo coronary angiography if there is recurrent angina or the suspicion of abrupt vessel closure.

Coronary angiography should be performed in patients before noncardiac surgery who demonstrate high-risk criteria on noninvasive testing, have angina unresponsive to medical therapy, develop unstable angina, or have equivocal noninvasive test results and are scheduled to undergo high-risk surgery. It is also recommended for patients prior to surgery for valvular heart disease or congenital heart disease—particularly those with cardiac risk factors—and in patients with infective endocarditis with evidence of coronary embolization.[5]

Finally, surveillance coronary angiography should be performed in patients after cardiac transplantation. These angiograms should be performed at specified intervals even in the absence of clinical symptoms, secondary to the often asymptomatic nature of allograft atherosclerosis. Coronary angiography is also an important assessment in potential donors for cardiac transplantation whose age or cardiac risk profile increases the likelihood of CAD.

CONTRAINDICATIONS FOR CORONARY ANGIOGRAPHY

With the exception of patient refusal, there are no absolute contraindications to coronary angiography. Significant relative contraindications include: ongoing stroke or cerebrovascular accident (CVA) within a month, recent head trauma, significant active bleeding, anemia with hemoglobin less than 8 mg/dl, uncontrolled systemic hypertension, digitalis toxicity, previous contrast reaction without pretreatment with corticosteroids, severe electrolyte imbalance, unexplained fever and untreated infection. Other disease states that are relative contraindications to coronary angiography include: acute renal failure, decompensated CHF, severe intrinsic or iatrogenic coagulopathy [International Normalized Ratio (INR greater than 2.0)]—unless transradial approach is performed, and active endocarditis. Given that the majority of these conditions are self-limited, deferral of coronary angiography until important comorbidities have been stabilized is generally preferred, unless there is evidence of ongoing myocardial necrosis. It is well recognized that coronary angiography performed under emergency conditions is associated with a higher risk of procedural complications. The risks and benefits of the procedure and alternative evaluation techniques—if potentially indicated—should always be carefully reviewed with the patient and family in all circumstances prior to coronary angiography, but especially in the presence of relative contraindications (Table 2).

PATIENT PREPARATION

The procedure should be explained to the patient in simple terms and informed consent to perform the procedure is then obtained. The operator should clearly explain the potential risks and benefits for cardiac catheterization to the patient and family. Patient information should be tailored to the specific individual and the associated clinical question to be addressed. Patients with diabetes mellitus, renal insufficiency or previous reported hypersensitivity to iodinated contrast media constitute groups

TABLE 2

Contraindications to cardiac catheterization

Absolute contraindications
- Inadequate equipment or catheterization facility
- Patient refusal

Relative contraindications
- Acute gastrointestinal bleeding or anemia
- Anticoagulation (or known uncontrolled bleeding diathesis)
- Electrolyte imbalance
- Infection or fever
- Medication intoxication (e.g. digitalis, phenothiazine)
- Pregnancy
- Recent cerebral vascular accident (> 1 mo)
- Renal failure
- Uncontrolled congestive heart failure, high blood pressure, arrhythmias
- Uncooperative patient

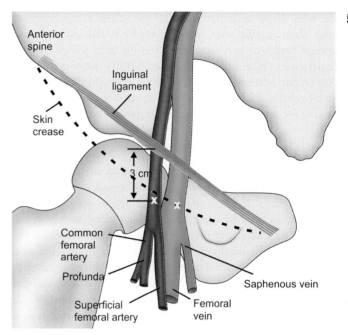

FIGURE 1: Femoral artery access site. Anatomy relevant to percutaneous catheterization of the femoral artery (FA) and vein. The right FA vein passes underneath the inguinal ligament, which connects the anterior-superior iliac spine and pubic tubercle. The arterial skin nick (indicated by X) should be placed approximately 1-1/2–2 fingerbreadths (3 cm) below the inguinal ligament and directly over the FA pulsation. (*Source:* Baim DS, Grossman W. Percutaneous approach including transseptal and apical puncture. In: Baim DS, Grossman W (Eds). Grossman's Cardiac Catheterization, Angiography, and Intervention, 6th edition. Baltimore: Lippincott, Williams and Wilkins; 2000.)

who need special consideration. For diabetic patients, insulin dosing should be adjusted to minimize the risk of periprocedural hypoglycemia. Patients with renal insufficiency should have interventions for renal function preservation following contrast administration. These should include: volume repletion with intravenous (IV) fluids before contrast administration, consideration of N-acetylcysteine administration and consideration of biplane angiography if available. At our institution, all patients with renal insufficiency receive N-acetylcysteine prior to coming to catheterization laboratory. IV fluid administration is also given to patients with renal insufficiency who are not volume overloaded before their procedure. When available, biplane angiography is performed in a select subset of patients at very high risk of clinically significant contrast nephropathy. Patients with known hypersensitivity to iodinated contrast should be premedicated using established protocols—usually including steroid and antihistamine medications—to reduce the risk of a reaction with contrast administration.

Once the patient arrives in the catheterization laboratory, the designated access site is prepped and the patient is given IV sedative medications to keep them comfortable through the procedure.

SITES AND TECHNIQUES OF VASCULAR ACCESS

The site of vascular access is determined by the anticipated pathologic and anatomic findings relevant to the patient. Documentation of any difficulties encountered during a previous procedure, especially of vascular access, should be reviewed. Prior to the procedure, assessment of all peripheral pulses is mandatory. If a transradial approach is being considered, an Allen's test should also be performed to confirm candidacy for this approach.

FEMORAL ARTERY APPROACH

Percutaneous femoral arterial catheterization remains the most widely used vascular access site for coronary angiography in the United States, although the use of radial arterial access is steadily increasing. In patients with claudication, chronic lower extremity arterial insufficiency, diminished or absent pulses, or bruits over the iliofemoral area, alternate entry sites should be considered. In order to reduce access site complications,

obtaining access to the common femoral artery below the inguinal ligament is strongly recommended. The common femoral artery passes underneath the inguinal ligament, which connects the anterior-superior iliac spine and pubic tubercle. Palpation of the femoral pulse and the previously mentioned anatomical landmarks is the first step in obtaining arterial access. Before the puncture, fluoroscopy of the tip of a metal clamp placed near the medial edge of the middle of the head of the femur is often performed. This step is done to enhance the likelihood of puncturing the common femoral artery, while remaining below the inguinal ligament. This location in the middle of the femoral head is typically the location of the common femoral artery in most patients, although there is certainly anatomic variation (Fig. 1). Adequate local anesthesia should be administered. A skin nick is then placed approximately 1-1/2–2 fingerbreadths (3 cm) below the inguinal ligament and directly over the femoral artery pulsation. Palpation identifies the middle of the artery and the needle is advanced at a 30–45° angle to the vessel, preferably puncturing only the front wall. Once brisk arterial flow through the needle is established, the guidewire is advanced through the needle to the descending aorta. The guidewire should pass freely without any resistance. If any resistance to passage of the wire is encountered, the operator should stop immediately and use fluoroscopy to visualize advancement of the wire. If the wire has not yet exited the needle tip, the wire should be removed to confirm pulsatile flow through the needle before attempting to readvance the wire, as there is concern of subintimal or extravascular passage of the wire. If pulsatile flow through the needle is not apparent after removing the wire, then the needle is repositioned until arterial backflow is reestablished and the wire passes without resistance. Once the wire is successfully placed into the descending aorta to the level of the diaphragm, the needle is then exchanged for a valved sheath, which is usually 4–6 French in size for femoral access diagnostic procedures.

TRANSRADIAL APPROACH

The radial artery approach has several distinct advantages[6,7] and is becoming more commonly used for coronary angiography. The superficial location of the radial artery makes it easily accessible in most patients. There is dual blood supply to the hand via the radial and the ulnar arteries which decreases the potential of any meaningful clinical sequelae in the case of a procedural related radial artery occlusion. Patient comfort is enhanced as there is no need for flat bedrest after a transradial procedure. Also, radial artery access provides the most secure hemostasis in the fully anticoagulated patient. Patients with a palpable radial pulse and a normal Allen's test are generally candidates for the transradial approach, although there are some contraindications including: abnormal Allen's test, known upper extremity vascular disease including Reynaud's Disease, need for intra-aortic balloon pump or other left ventricular (LV) assist devices, patient refusal, planned or existing dialysis AV fistula or planned use of radial artery for bypass conduit. In appropriately selected patients, the ideal point to access the radial artery is just proximal to the styloid process of the radius. This is usually about 2–3 cm above the flexor crease (Fig. 2). A small amount of local anesthesia is given to the area. The radial artery can be accessed with two different techniques. In the first, the radial pulse is palpated at the site indicated previously. Then, a short (2.5 cm) 21-gauge needle is advanced into the radial artery at a 30–40°angle. Once pulsatile flow is obtained, a 0.021 inch diameter guidewire is advanced in the radial artery. A hydrophilic coated sheath (typically 5 French) is advanced into the radial artery—no skin nick is usually needed. As soon as the sheath is placed, intra-arterial administration of spasmolytic cocktail is given to prevent radial artery spasm. This spasmolytic cocktail typically contains a calcium channel blocker and nitroglycerin. Heparin is also always given during transradial catheterization as this is known to decrease the chance of procedural related radial artery occlusion. Although usually

asymptomatic and without clinical sequelae in appropriately selected patients, radial artery occlusion may preclude access for future procedures.

The second technique for obtaining radial arterial access involves the use of an IV catheter to puncture the radial artery instead of a bare needle. Once a backflow of blood is noted in the hub of the IV catheter, the catheter is advanced to also puncture the posterior wall of the vessel. The needle is then removed and the plastic cannula is slowly withdrawn until pulsatile flow is obtained. Then a guidewire (0.021–0.025 inch) is advanced into the radial artery and the IV catheter is then exchanged for the sheath and spasmolytic cocktail and heparin are given.

Both of these techniques are accepted methods of obtaining radial artery access for performing coronary angiography. An important difference to note between femoral and radial access is that the radial artery is much more prone to spasm which can affect the successful performance of the procedure. It is vital to give spasmolytic medications (usually consisting of a calcium channel blocker and nitroglycerin) into the sheath on initial insertion as well as with any necessary catheter exchange, as prevention of spasm is usually more effective than attempting to treat it once it occurs. Young or female patients (those with smaller radial arteries) are more likely to have spasm of the radial artery. In addition to spasmolytic medications, adequate patient sedation helps in reducing radial artery spasm.

BRACHIAL ARTERY APPROACH

With the recent development and increase in the use of transradial catheterization, the brachial approach for catheterization has become less commonly used. There are more access site complications (bleeding, pseudoaneurysm, etc.) with brachial access compared to radial access. Accessing the brachial artery removes the advantage of dual blood supply to the hand that exists with radial access. However, when needed, the brachial approach is still a viable option for coronary angiography. For example, if femoral access is technically not possible and larger sheaths than can be accommodated by the radial artery are needed, brachial access may be indicated. In the past, brachial arterial access for coronary angiography was performed primarily with a cutdown approach. However, this technique has largely fallen out of favor in the performance of coronary angiography. Currently, when brachial access is used for coronary angiography, access is gained percutaneously, often with a 21G needle and 0.021 inch guidewire. The brachial artery is typically accessed 2–3 cm above the antecubital fossa, where the vessel is still relatively superficial. Accessing the vessel more proximal than this typically increases the risk of access difficulty and complications as the vessel is generally deeper in this area. There can be spasm of the brachial artery, but this is much less common than is observed with the radial artery. If encountered, it can be treated with spasmolytic medications including calcium channel blockers and/or nitrates.

CATHETERS FOR CORONARY ANGIOGRAPHY

Numerous shapes and sizes of catheters are available to the angiographer. Routinely used catheters that are preshaped for normal anatomy are available for both the radial and the femoral

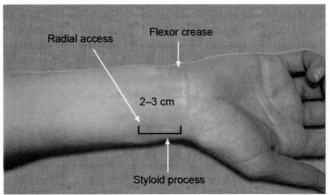

FIGURE 2: Ideal radial artery access site: just proximal to the styloid process (usually 2–3 cm from the flexor crease)

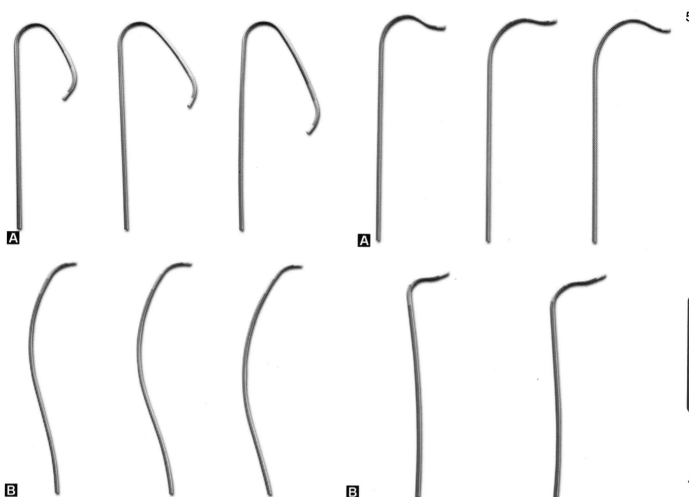

FIGURES 3A AND B: (A) Judkins left 4,5,6 catheters (left to right); (B) Judkins right 3.5,4,5 catheters (left to right). (*Source:* Boston Scientific.)

FIGURES 4A AND B: (A) Amplatz left 1,2,3 catheters (left to right); (B) Amplatz right 1,2 catheters (left to right). (*Source:* Boston Scientific.)

approaches. There is an additional array of shapes and sizes to aid the operator with the various coronary artery anatomical variations that are encountered (Figs 3 and 4). Regardless of access site, all catheters should be advanced into the ascending aorta over a wire. The wire is then removed; the catheter is aspirated and then flushed with heparinized saline and connected to either a coronary manifold or power injector system. There are many different types of catheters that are used to perform coronary and bypass graft angiography. We have described and illustrated some of the most commonly used catheters; however, there are certainly many other less commonly used catheters that have not be discussed here.

JUDKINS-TYPE CORONARY CATHETERS

The Judkins catheters have unique preshaped curves and end-hole tips. The Judkins left coronary catheter has a double curve. The length of the segment between the primary and the secondary curve determines the size of the catheter (i.e. 3.5, 4.0, 5.0 or 6.0 cm) (Figs 3A and B). The proper size of the left Judkins catheter is selected depending on the length and width of the ascending aorta. The ingenious design of the left Judkins catheter permits cannulation of the left coronary artery most

often without any major catheter manipulation except the slow advancement of the catheter under fluoroscopic guidance. With advancement, the catheter tip usually follows the ascending aortic border and falls into the left main coronary ostium. A Judkins left 4.0 catheter is generally appropriate for most adult patients with a presumed normal sized ascending aorta. When catheter size is appropriate, the catheter tip is aligned with the long axis of the left main coronary trunk in a coaxial fashion. At times, it may be necessary to upsize or downsize the catheter in order to obtain a coaxial position. This will allow the best opacification of the vessels and lessen the chance of a complication from injecting through a malpositioned catheter. If the catheter tip is pointed too superior, then a larger size catheter should be chosen. On the contrary, if the catheter tip is pointing below the level of the left main, then a shorter catheter may be needed. The Judkins left catheter is not only best suited for use from the femoral or left upper extremity approach but can also be helpful from the right upper extremity approach in selected cases.

The Judkins right coronary catheter is commonly used to cannulate the right coronary artery (RCA). It is sized by the length of the secondary curve (3.5, 4.0 and 5.0 cm sizes).

The 4.0 cm catheter is adequate for most cases and rarely is another size required—unlike with the Judkins left catheter. Also unlike the Judkins left catheter, the Judkins right catheter requires manipulation beyond just advancement in order to engage the coronary vessel. This catheter is advanced into the ascending aorta [usually in the left anterior oblique (LAO) projection] down to the level of the aortic valve. The catheter is then slightly withdrawn and torqued in a clockwise fashion to gently rotate the catheter into the right coronary sinus toward the right coronary ostium. A common error in attempting RCA cannulation is excessive rotation of the catheter. This results in an abrupt jumping of the catheter and often a very deep cannulation of the vessel. When this occurs, there is often pressure damping requiring additional manipulation of the catheter before safe performance of angiograms can be accomplished. Coronary spasm or even dissection can also result from this suboptimal method of cannulation. The Judkins right catheter is suited for use from the femoral approach as well as either upper extremity approach.

AMPLATZ-TYPE CATHETERS

The left Amplatz-type catheter is a preshaped half circle with the tip extending perpendicular to the curve. Amplatz catheter sizes (left 1, 2 and 3 and right 1 and 2) indicate the diameter of the tip's curve (Figs 4A and B). In the LAO projection, the Amplatz left catheter is advanced into the left coronary sinus. Further advancement of the catheter causes the tip to move upward and toward the left main ostium. Engagement of the left main ostium often requires additional rotational maneuvering of the catheter. After completion of the angiograms, it is most often necessary to advance the Amplatz left catheter slightly in order to safely disengage the catheter tip from the left main ostium. If the catheter is initially withdrawn instead of initially being slightly advanced, the tip often moves downward and deeper into the left main, potentially causing trauma to the vessel. An Amplatz left catheter is generally more challenging to manipulate compared to a Judkins left catheter and as a result its usage is less common. Unlike the Judkins left catheter, the Amplatz left catheter can also be used to cannulate the RCA, especially in the case of a high and/or anterior takeoff of the RCA.

The Amplatz right catheter has a much smaller but similar hook-shaped curve with a slightly downgoing tip. This catheter is advanced into the right coronary cusp. Then, like with a Judkins right catheter, it is advanced further to the level of the aortic valve, then slowly withdrawn and rotated in a clockwise direction to cannulate the RCA. Unlike the Amplatz left catheter, this catheter may be safely pulled or rotated out of the coronary artery upon completion of the angiograms.

MULTIPURPOSE CATHETER

This catheter is a gently curved catheter with an end hole and two side holes which are positioned close to the tapered tip. The multipurpose catheter can be used for both left and right coronary cannulation and theoretically for left ventriculography, although performance of left ventriculography is most safely and effectively performed with a pigtail catheter. This catheter is used much less frequently since the development of the many preshaped catheters that are generally easier to manipulate.

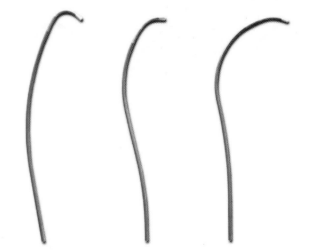

FIGURE 5: IMA, right and left bypass catheters. (*Source:* Boston Scientific.)

CATHETERS FOR BYPASS GRAFTS

Many of the bypass grafts that originate from the aorta (vein, radial or other arterial conduit) can be engaged with either a Judkins right catheter or an Amplatz right catheter. There are also dedicated bypass graft catheters that sometimes need to be used when one is unable to cannulate grafts with the Judkins or Amplatz shapes (Fig. 5). The right coronary bypass catheter is somewhat similar to a right Judkins catheter but has a wider, more open primary curve. This allows more reach that is typically needed for cannulation of the cranially and more rightward location of the bypass grafts to the right coronary and its branches. The left bypass graft catheter is also somewhat similar to the Judkins right catheter, but has a smaller secondary curve. This allows easier cannulation of grafts to the left coronary system, which usually are placed higher and more anterior than grafts to the right coronary system. The internal mammary artery (IMA) catheter has a hook-shaped tip that facilitates the engagement of pedicled IMA grafts. Cannulation of the IMA grafts first requires engagement of the brachio-cephalic artery (in the case of a right internal mammary graft) or the left subclavian artery (in the case of a left internal mammary graft).Once this has been accomplished, the IMA catheter is used to engage the IMA. The technique for IMA graft cannulation has been discussed later in more detail.

TRANSRADIAL SPECIFIC CATHETERS

With the increasing use of radial arterial access for coronary angiography, diagnostic coronary catheters with unique shapes have been and continue to be developed for transradial use (Fig. 6). Although there are different shapes, all of the catheters developed for use from the transradial approach are intended to be used to perform a complete coronary angiogram with one catheter. Many of the catheters have a hydrophilic coating to help minimize radial artery spasm. Some of the most commonly used catheters are shown (Fig. 6) and include the Tiger and Jacky shapes. More transradial specific catheter shapes currently exist (Barbeau is another) and as transradial catheterization continues to increase in use, likely more new diagnostic and guide catheter shapes will be developed. Generally, transradial operators begin with one of the more common radial specific

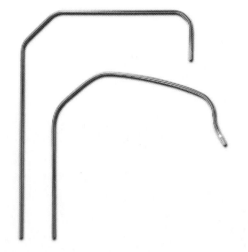

FIGURE 6: Tiger and Jacky catheters (left to right).
(*Source:* Terumo)

The major epicardial vessels and their second- and third-order branches can be visualized using coronary angiography. The network of smaller intramyocardial branches is generally not seen secondary to their size, cardiac motion and limitations in resolution of angiographic systems. These fourth-order and higher "resistance" vessels play a major role in autoregulation of coronary blood flow. Although we cannot visualize these vessels with angiography, they may limit myocardial perfusion during stress and can contribute to ischemia in patients with LV hypertrophy or systemic hypertension. Coronary perfusion in these smaller branch vessels can be quantitatively assessed using the myocardial blush score which has important prognostic significance in patients with STEMI and those undergoing percutaneous coronary intervention (PCI).[8]

The Coronary Artery Surgery Study (CASS) investigators established the nomenclature most commonly used to describe the coronary anatomy, defining 27 segments in three major coronary arteries (Table 3, Fig. 7). The Bypass Angioplasty Revascularization Investigators (BARI) modified these criteria with the addition of two segments for the ramus intermedius and addition of the third diagonal branch. In this system, the major coronary arteries include: the left main coronary artery (LMCA), the left anterior descending artery (LADA), left circumflex artery (LCX) and RCA. These are described as being a part of a right-dominant, co-dominant or left-dominant circulation. Dominance is determined by which coronary vessel

catheters and are usually able to complete the diagnostic angiogram with one catheter. However, even if they are unable to complete all of the needed angiograms with one catheter, manipulation of that catheter usually helps to at least identify the origin of the vessel that cannot be selectively engaged, which facilitates the choice of an alternative catheter that will then likely engage the vessel. Sometimes this is another radial specific catheter, but at other times a catheter that is more typically used with femoral access procedures may be more appropriate.

CHAPTER 28 — Coronary Angiography and Catheter-based Coronary Intervention

TABLE 3

Classification system for coronary segments

Number	Map location	Number	Map location	Number	Map location
Right coronary artery		Left main coronary artery		Left circumflex artery	
1	Proximal RCA	11	Left main coronary artery	18	Proximal LCX artery
2	Mid RCA	Left anterior descending artery			19	Distal LCX artery
3	Distal RCA	12	Proximal LADA	20	1st obtuse marginal
4	Right posterior descending branch	13	Mid LADA	21	2nd obtuse marginal
5	Right posterior atrioventricular	14	Distal LADA	22	Third obtuse marginal
6	First right posterolateral	15	1st diagonal	23	LCX atrioventricular groove
7	Second right posterolateral	16	2nd diagonal	24	1st left posterolateral branch
8	Third right posterolateral	17	LADA septal perforator	25	2nd left posterolateral branch
9	Posterior descending septals	29	3rd diagonal	26	3rd left posterolateral branch
10	Acute marginal segment	27	Left posterior descending branch		
		28	Ramus intermedium branch		

(Abbreviations: LADA: Left anterior descending artery; LCX: Left circumflex artery; RCA: Right coronary artery). (*Source:* CASS Principal Investigators and their Associates: Coronary Artery Surgery Study (CASS): A randomized trial of coronary artery surgery: Survival data. Circulation. 1983.68:939)

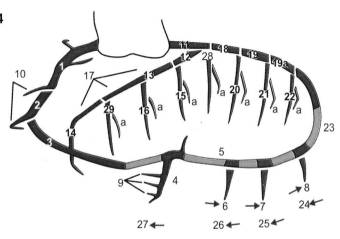

FIGURE 7: The coronary artery map used by the BARI investigators. The map is derived from that used in CASS with the addition of branch segments for the diagonal, marginal and ramus vessels

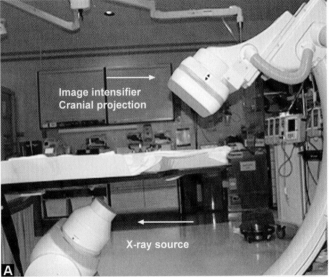

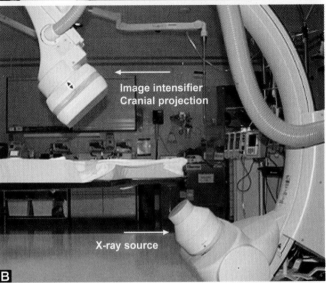

FIGURES 8A AND B: Geometry of angulated views. Head of the patient would be placed to the right (in these pictures). Cranial projection (A) and caudal projection (B)

gives rise to the posterior descending artery (PDA)—the RCA in right dominant circulation, and the lcx in a left dominant circulation. Obstructive CAD is defined as a more than 50% diameter stenosis in one or more of these vessels, although it is clear that stenoses of less than 50% do have prognostic implications because these lesions are most susceptible to plaque rupture and resulting acute MI. Subcritical stenoses of less than 50% are best characterized as nonobstructive CAD. Obstructive CAD is further classified as one, two or three-vessel disease.

In CASS, the major determinants of 6-year outcome included the number of diseased vessels, the number of diseased proximal segments and the global LV function. These three factors accounted for 80% of the prognostic information from the CASS study.

ANGIOGRAPHIC PROJECTIONS

The major coronary arteries traverse the interventricular and atrioventricular (AV) grooves, aligned with the long and short axes of the heart, respectively. Since the heart is oriented obliquely in the thoracic cavity, the coronary circulation is generally visualized in the right anterior oblique (RAO) and LAO projections to furnish true posteroanterior and lateral views of the heart. However, without sagittal angulations, these views are limited by vessel foreshortening and superimposition of branches. Simultaneous rotation of the X-ray beam in the sagittal plane provides a better view of the major coronary arteries and their branches. A simple nomenclature has evolved for the description of these sagittal views, which characterizes the relationship between the image intensifier and the patient. Assuming that the X-ray tube is under the table and the image intensifier is over the table, the projection is referred to as the "cranial" view if the image intensifier is tilted toward the head of the patient (Figs 8A and B). The projection is referred to as the "caudal" view if the image intensifier is tilted down toward the feet of the patient. It is difficult to predict which angulated views will be most useful for any particular patient because the "optimal" angiographic projection depends largely on body habitus, variation in the coronary anatomy, location of the lesion and position of the heart within the chest. It is recommended

that the coronary arteries be visualized in both the LAO and RAO projections using both cranial and caudal angulation with all segments of the vessels visualized in at least two preferably orthogonal views.

NORMAL CORONARY ANATOMY

LEFT MAIN CORONARY ARTERY

The left main coronary artery (LMCA) arises from the superior portion of the left aortic sinus, just below the sinotubular ridge of the aorta, which defines the border separating the left sinus of Valsalva from the smooth (tubular) portion of the aorta. The LMCA ranges 3–6 mm in diameter and may be up to 10–15 mm in length. The LMCA courses behind the right ventricular outflow tract and usually bifurcates into the LAD artery and LCX artery. In some patients, the LMCA trifurcates into the LAD, LCX and Ramus intermedius. When present, the ramus intermedius arises from the LMCA, between the LAD and LCX arteries and is somewhat analogous to either a diagonal branch

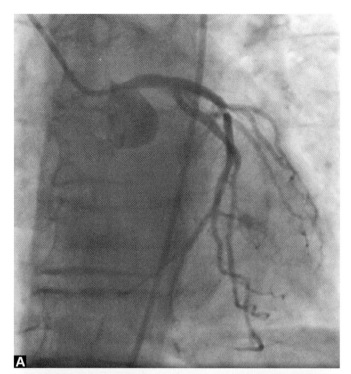

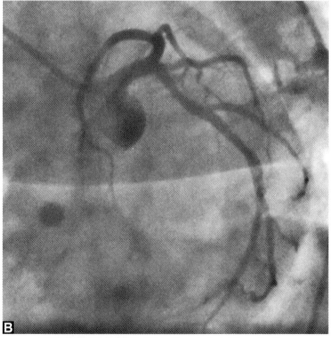

FIGURES 9A AND B: (A) Left main in LAO projection;
(B) Left main in LAO caudal projection

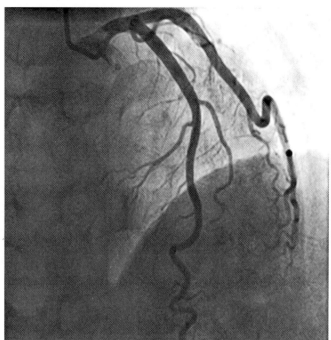

FIGURE 10: Anteroposterior cranial projection of
left anterior descending

be viewed in several projections to exclude LMCA stenosis (Figs 9A and B).

LEFT ANTERIOR DESCENDING ARTERY

The LAD courses along the epicardial surface of the anterior interventricular groove toward the cardiac apex. In the RAO projection, it extends along the anterior aspect of the heart; in the LAO projection, it passes down the cardiac midline, between the right and left ventricles (Fig. 10).

Generally the best angiographic projections for viewing the entire course of the LAD are the cranially angulated AP, LAO and RAO views. The LAO cranial view displays the mid-portion of the LAD and separates the diagonal and septal branches. The proximal LAD is often somewhat foreshortened in the LAO cranial view. The AP cranial view displays the proximal, middle and distal segment of the LAD and also allows separation of the diagonal branches superiorly and the septal branches inferiorly. In some patients, a RAO cranial angulation is needed in addition to the AP cranial to further separate the origins of the branches. The LAO caudal view displays the origin of the LAD in a horizontally oriented heart and the AP or shallow RAO with deep caudal angulation visualizes the proximal LAD as it arises from the LMCA, as well as the origins of diagonal branches with proximal origins off of the LAD. A flat RAO is not often a standard view taken of the LAD, but can be very useful for visualizing the mid to distal LAD and its apical termination when additional views of this segment of the vessel are required.

The major branches of the LAD are the septal and diagonal branches. The septal branches arise from the LAD at approximately 90° angles and pass into the interventricular septum, varying in size, number and distribution. In some cases there is a large first septal branch that is vertically oriented and divides into a number of secondary branches that spread

or an obtuse marginal branch in the territory it serves, depending on its anterior or posterior course along the lateral aspect of the left ventricle. The ramus is often best visualized in the same views as used for proximally oriented diagonal or marginal branches, namely: AP, LAO and/or RAO with steep caudal angulation to see the origin, with progressively less caudal angulation needed to visualize the mid and distal vessel. Rarely, the LMCA is absent, and there are separate ostia of the LAD and lcx arteries. The ostium of the LMCA is often best visualized in a shallow LAO projection (20–30°) sometimes with slight (0–20°) caudal angulation. The distal LMCA is often best seen in the RAO or LAO caudal views. The LMCA should always

throughout the septum. In other cases, a more horizontally oriented, large first septal branch is present that passes parallel to the LAD itself within the myocardium. In still other cases, a number of septal arteries are roughly comparable in size. These septal branches interconnect with similar septal branches passing upward from the posterior descending branch of the RCA to produce a network of potential collateral channels. The interventricular septum is the most densely vascularized area of the heart.

The diagonal branches of the LAD extend to the anterolateral aspect of the heart. Although virtually all patients have a single LAD in the anterior interventricular groove, there is wide variability in the number and size of diagonal branches. Most patients (90%) have one to three diagonal branches. Acquired atherosclerotic occlusion of the diagonal branches should be suspected if no diagonal branches are seen, particularly if there are unexplained wall motion abnormalities of the anterolateral left ventricle. Visualization of the origins of the diagonal branches often requires steep LAO (40–45°) and cranial (30–40°) angulated views, but can often be seen in the AP or RAO cranial views as well. The origins of diagonal branches with a rather proximal takeoff are often best visualized in LAO, AP or RAO projections, but with steep caudal angulation (35–45°).

In most patients, the LAD courses around the LV apex and terminates along the diaphragmatic aspect of the left ventricle. In the remaining patients, the LAD fails to reach the diaphragmatic aspect of the left ventricle, terminating instead either at or before the cardiac apex. In this circumstance, the PDA of the RCA or LCX is larger and longer than usual and supplies the apical portion of the ventricle.

In patients with no LMCA (i.e. separate ostia for the LAD and LCX), the LAD generally has a more anterior origin than the LCX. The LAD can be engaged with the Judkins left catheter in this setting with a slight counterclockwise rotation on withdrawal of the catheter and then gentle clockwise rotation on readvancement. This maneuver generally rotates the secondary bend of the catheter to a posterior position in the aorta and turns the primary bend and tip of the catheter to an anterior position. The opposite maneuver may be used to engage the LCX selectively in the setting of separate LAD and LCX ostia. Sometimes a single Judkins left catheter can be used to engage both of these vessels individually, but at other times, two different catheters are required. In this case, the larger sized Judkins left catheter will usually selectively engage the downward coursing LCX, and the shorter Judkins left catheter is used to engage the more anteriorly and superiorly located LAD.

LEFT CIRCUMFLEX ARTERY

The LCX artery originates from the LMCA and courses within the posterior (left) AV groove toward the inferior interventricular groove (Fig. 11). The LCX artery is the dominant vessel in approximately 15% of patients, supplying the left PDA from the distal continuation of the LCX. In right dominant systems, the distal LCX varies in size and length, depending on the number of posterolateral branches supplied by the distal RCA. The LCX usually gives off one to three large obtuse marginal branches as it passes down the AV groove. These are the

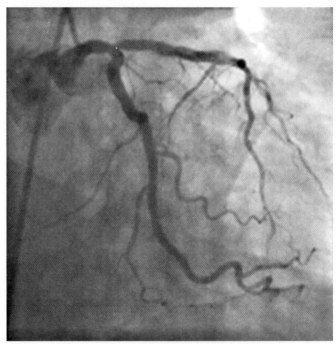

FIGURE 11: Left circumflex in RAO caudal view

principal branches of the LCX that supply the lateral free wall of the left ventricle. Beyond the origins of the obtuse marginal branches, the distal LCX tends to be small in most patients with a right dominant system.

The RAO caudal and LAO caudal projections are best for visualizing the proximal and middle LCX and obtuse marginal branches. The AP (or shallow RAO/LAO) caudal projections also show the origins of the obtuse marginal branches. More severe rightward angulation often superimposes the origins of the obtuse marginal branches on the LCX. If the LCA is dominant, the optimal projection for the left PDA is the LAO cranial view. The LCX artery also gives rise to one or two left atrial circumflex branches. These branches supply the lateral and posterior aspects of the left atrium.

RIGHT CORONARY ARTERY

The RCA originates from the right aortic sinus somewhat inferior to the origin of the LCA (Fig. 12). It passes along the right AV groove toward the crux—a point on the diaphragmatic surface of the heart where the anterior AV groove, the posterior AV groove and the inferior interventricular groove coalesce. The first branch of the RCA is generally the conus artery, which arises at the right coronary ostium or within the first few millimeters of the RCA in about 50% of patients. In the remaining patients, the conus artery arises from a separate ostium in the right aortic sinus just above the right coronary ostium. The second branch of the RCA is usually the sinoatrial node artery. It has been found that this vessel arises from the RCA in just under 60% of patients, from the lcx artery in just under 40% and from both arteries in the remaining cases. The midportion of the RCA usually gives rise to one or several medium-sized acute marginal branches. These branches supply the anterior wall of the right ventricle and may provide collateral circulation in patients with LAD occlusion. The RCA terminates

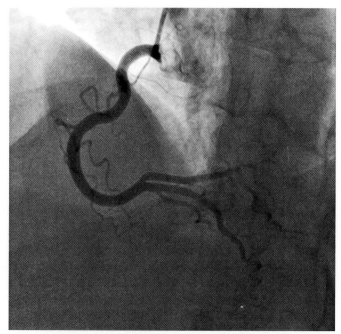

FIGURE 12: Right coronary artery in LAO cranial projection displaying the bifurcation

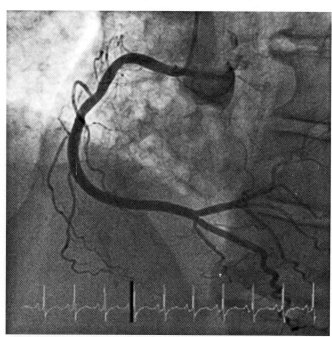

FIGURE 13: Right dominant circulation, PDA is seen coming of the RCA

in an RPDA (in right dominant circulation) and one or more right posterolateral branches.

Because the RCA traverses both the AV and the interventricular grooves, multiple angiographic projections are needed to visualize each segment of the RCA. The ostium of the RCA is best evaluated in the LAO views, with or without cranial or caudal angulation. The left lateral view is also useful for visualizing the ostium of the RCA in difficult cases. The ostium is identified by the reflux of contrast material from the RCA that also delineates the aortic root with swirling of contrast in the region of the ostium. The proximal RCA is generally evaluated in the flat LAO or LAO cranial projections but is markedly foreshortened in the RAO projections. The mid-portion of the RCA is best seen in the flat LAO, LAO cranial and flat RAO projections. The origin of the PDA and the posterolateral branches are best evaluated in the LAO cranial or AP cranial views, whereas the mid-portion of the PDA can be shown in the AP cranial or RAO projection.

RIGHT DOMINANT CORONARY CIRCULATION

The RCA is dominant in about 82–84% of patients, supplying the PDA and at least one posterolateral branch (Fig. 13). The PDA courses in the inferior interventricular groove and gives rise to a number of small inferior septal branches. These septal branches extend upward to supply the lower portion of the interventricular septum and interdigitate with superior septal branches extending down from the LAD artery. After giving rise to the PDA, the dominant RCA continues beyond the crux cordis (the junction of the AV and interventricular grooves) as the right posterior AV branch along the distal portion of the posterior (left) AV groove. This vessel then terminates in one or several posterolateral branches that supply the diaphragmatic surface of the left ventricle. There are significant anatomical variations in the origin of the PDA in a right dominant system. These variations include partial supply of the PDA territory by

acute marginal branches, double PDA and early origin of the PDA proximal to the crux. In patients with right dominance, the LCX continues in the AV groove, but generally becomes rather small after it gives off a variable number of obtuse marginal and perhaps a posterolateral branch.

LEFT DOMINANT CORONARY CIRCULATION

The LCX is dominant in about 12 to 14% of patients. In these patients, the LCX artery continues in the AV groove giving off both obtuse marginal as well as posterolateral branches through its course. The LCX then extends into the posterior interventricular groove and terminates as the left PDA. In these cases, the RCA is very small, terminates well before reaching the crux and does not supply any blood to the LV myocardium (Figs 14A and B).

CO-DOMINANT OR BALANCED CORONARY CIRCULATION

The remaining approximately 4% of patients have a co-dominant or balanced circulation. This is characterized by an RCA that gives rise to the PDA, but not to any posterolateral branches. In a balanced circulation, the LCX artery does not give rise to the PDA, but does provide essentially all of the posterolateral branches.

CORONARY COLLATERAL CIRCULATION

Networks of small anastomotic branches interconnect the major coronary arteries and serve as precursors for the collateral circulation that maintains myocardial perfusion in the presence of severe proximal atherosclerotic narrowings.[9] Collateral channels may not be seen in patients with normal or mildly diseased coronary arteries because of their small (< 200 mm) caliber. But, as CAD progresses and becomes more severe (> 90% stenosis), a pressure gradient is generated between the

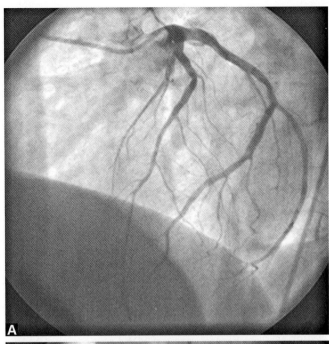

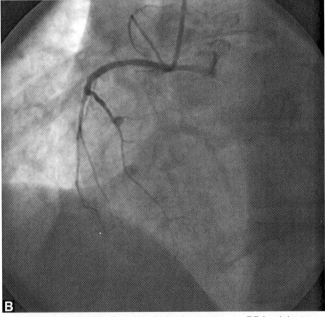

FIGURES 14A AND B: (A) Left dominant system. PDA originates from LCX; (B) RCA as non-dominant vessel in same patient

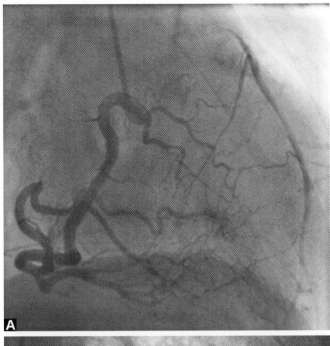

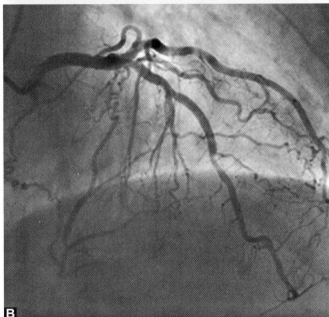

FIGURES 15A AND B: (A) LAD filling via collaterals from RCA; (B) RCA filling via collaterals from LAD

anastomotic channels and the distal vessel that is hypoperfused.[10] The trans-stenosis pressure gradient facilitates blood flow through the anastomotic channels, which progressively dilate and eventually become visible with angiography as collateral vessels (Figs 15A and B).

The visible collateral channels arise either from the contralateral coronary artery, or from the ipsilateral coronary artery through intracoronary collateral channels, or through "bridging" channels that have a serpiginous course from the proximal coronary artery to the coronary artery distal to the occlusion. These collaterals may provide up to 50% of anterograde coronary flow in chronic total occlusions. This in turn may allow the development of a "protected" region of myocardial perfusion that does not develop ischemia during times of increased myocardial oxygen demands. Recruitment

of collateral channels typically occurs over time with the gradual progression of atherosclerotic disease, but may also occur relatively quickly in patients who develop an acute STEMI caused by a sudden thrombotic occlusion. Other factors that affect collateral development are: patency of the arteries supplying the collateral, and the size and vascular resistance of the segment distal to the stenosis.

CONGENITAL ANOMALIES OF THE CORONARY CIRCULATION

Coronary anomalies may occur in 1–5% of patients undergoing coronary angiography, depending on the threshold for defining an anatomical variant (Table 4).[11,12]

The major reason for appropriately identifying and classifying coronary anomalies is to determine their propensity to

TABLE 4

Incidence of coronary anomalies among 1950 angiograms

Variable	Number	Percent
Coronary anomalies	110	5.64
Split RCA	24	1.23
Ectopic RCA (right cusp)	22	1.13
Ectopic RCA (left cusp)	18	0.92
Fistulas	17	0.87
Absent left main coronary artery	13	0.67
LCX artery arising from right cusp	13	0.67
LCA arising from right cusp	3	0.15
Low origin of RCA	2	0.1
Other anomalies	3	0.15

(*Source:* Angelini P (Ed). Coronary Artery Anomalies: A Comprehensive Approach. Philadelphia: Lippincott Williams and Wilkins; 1999. p. 42.)

develop fixed or dynamic myocardial ischemia and SCD, particularly in young and otherwise healthy individuals.[13] Documentation of precise ischemia risk for some of these anomalies using conventional exercise stress testing or intravascular Doppler flow studies is poorly predictive and may fail to detect significant anatomic abnormalities.[12,14,15] Accordingly, coronary artery anomalies are divided into those that cause and those that do not cause myocardial ischemia (Table 5).[12]

ANOMALOUS PULMONARY ORIGIN OF THE CORONARY ARTERIES

This syndrome is characterized by the origin of the coronary artery arising from the pulmonary artery. The most common variant is an anomalous origin of the LCA from the pulmonary artery (ALCAPA). Single vessel origins of the RCA, LCX coronary artery or LAD artery from the pulmonary artery have also been reported however.[15] Untreated and in the absence of an adequate collateral network, most infants (95%) with anomalous pulmonary origin of the coronary arteries (APOCA) die within the first year. In the presence of an extensive collateral network, patients may survive into adulthood. Aortography typically shows a large RCA with absence of a left coronary ostium in the left aortic sinus. During the late phase of the aortogram, patulous LAD and LCX branches fill by means of

TABLE 5

Ischemia occurring in coronary anomalies

Type of ischemia	Coronary anomaly
No ischemia	Majority of anomalies (split RCA, ectopic RCA from right cusp, ectopic RCA from left cusp)
Episodic ischemia	Anomalous origin of a coronary artery from the opposite sinus (ACAOS); coronary artery fistulas; myocardial bridge
Obligatory ischemia	Anomalous left coronary artery from the pulmonary artery (ALCAPA); coronary ostial atresia or severe stenosis

(Abbreviations: RCA: Right coronary artery; ACAOS: Anomalous origin of a coronary artery from the opposite sinus; ALCAPA: Anomalous left coronary artery from the pulmonary artery). (*Source:* Angelini P (Ed). Coronary Artery Anomalies: A Comprehensive Approach. Philadelphia; Lippincott Williams and Wilkins: 1999. p. 42)

collateral circulation from RCA branches. Still later in the filming sequence, retrograde flow from the LAD and lcx arteries opacifies the LMCA and its origin from the main pulmonary artery.[15] Once detected, coronary artery bypass surgery is recommended because of the high incidence of sudden death, cardiomyopathy and arrhythmias associated with APOCA.

ANOMALOUS CORONARY ARTERY FROM THE OPPOSITE SINUS

Origin of the LCA from the proximal RCA or the right aortic sinus with subsequent passage between the aorta and the right ventricular outflow tract has been associated with sudden death during or shortly after exercise in young persons (Figs 16A and B).[15,16] The increased risk of sudden death may be due to

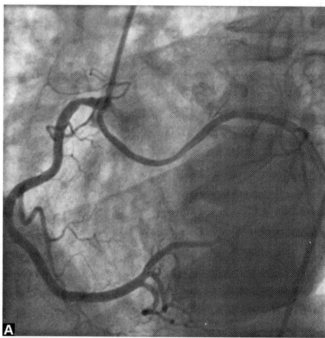

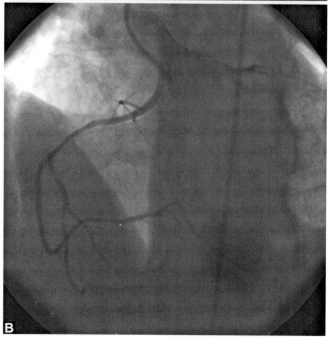

FIGURES 16A AND B: (A) Anomalous circumflex from right cusp; (B) Anomalous origin of RCA from left cusp

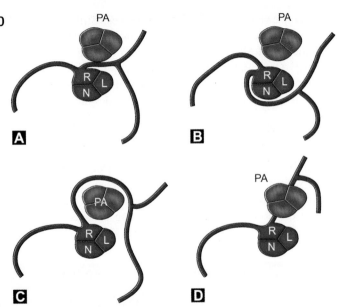

FIGURES 17A TO D: Four possible pathways of the anomalous left coronary artery arising from the right coronary sinus (R): (A) interarterial, between the aorta and the pulmonary artery (PA); (B) retroaortic; (C) prepulmonic; (D) septal, beneath the right ventricular outflow tract

a slit-like ostium, a bend with acute takeoff angles of the aberrant coronary arteries, or arterial compression between the pulmonary trunk and aorta when there is increased blood flow through these vessels with exercise and stress. Origin of the RCA from the LCA or left aortic sinus with passage between the aorta and the right ventricular outflow tract is also associated with myocardial ischemia and sudden death.[16,17] In rare cases of anomalous origin of the LCA from the right sinus, myocardial ischemia may occur even if the LCA passes anterior to the right ventricular outflow tract or posterior to the aorta (i.e. not through a tunnel between the two great vessels). Although coronary bypass surgery has been the traditional revascularization approach in patients with anomalous coronary artery from the opposite sinus(ACAOS), coronary stenting has also been reported with acceptable medium-term success.[18]

The course of the anomalous coronary arteries can be assessed by angiography. Usually the RAO view is most helpful. The four common courses for the anomalous LCA arising from the right sinus of Valsalva include a septal, anterior, interarterial or posterior course (Figs 17A to D).[19] The posterior course of the anomalous LCA arising from the right sinus of Valsalva is similar to the course of the anomalous LCX artery arising from the right sinus of Valsalva, whereas the common interarterial course of the anomalous RCA from the left sinus of Valsalva is similar to the interarterial course of the anomalous LCA arising from the right sinus of Valsalva.

Although angiography is useful for establishing the presence of anomalous coronary arteries, CT angiography is a very important adjunctive diagnostic tool for establishing the course of the vessels and relationship to the great vessels.[19,20] If a coronary anomaly is identified during coronary angiography, it may in fact be most prudent to obtain a coronary CT angiogram to best delineate the course of the coronary arteries and their relationship to the great vessels.

CORONARY ARTERY FISTULAE

A coronary artery fistula is defined as an abnormal communication between a coronary artery and a cardiac chamber or major vessel, such as the vena cava, right or left ventricle, pulmonary vein or pulmonary artery.[21,22] Congenital fistulae arise from the RCA or its branches in about one-half of the cases, and drainage generally occurs into the right ventricle, right atrium or pulmonary arteries. Coronary artery fistulas terminating in the left ventricle are uncommon (3%).[21] Coronary angiography is the best method for demonstrating these fistulae. Acquired coronary fistulae may develop in heart transplant patients who have had multiple endomyocardial biopsies of the right ventricular septum. Over time, coronary fistulae may develop from the septal arteries to the right ventricle. These coronary fistulae are usually small and not clinically significant, but are not unusual to observe with routine coronary angiography in this subset of patients.

The clinical presentation associated with a coronary artery fistula is dependent on the type of fistula, shunt volume, site of the shunt and presence of other cardiac comorbidities. Dyspnea on exertion, fatigue, CHF, pulmonary hypertension, bacterial endocarditis and arrhythmias are common presentations in symptomatic patients. Myocardial ischemia may also occur, but the mechanism remains speculative.[21] More than half of these patients are asymptomatic and the fistula is incidentally detected while performing angiography for unrelated reasons. Symptomatic patients or those with severe shunts may be treated with surgical closure, although some reports of percutaneous closure with coil embolization have had promising results.

CONGENITAL CORONARY STENOSIS OR ATRESIA

Congenital stenosis or atresia of a coronary artery can occur as an isolated lesion or in association with other congenital diseases, such as calcific coronary sclerosis, supravalvular aortic stenosis, homocystinuria, Friedreich's ataxia, Hurler syndrome, progeria and Rubella syndrome. In these cases, the atretic vessel usually fills by means of collateral circulation from the contralateral side.

MYOCARDIAL BRIDGING

The three major coronary arteries generally course along the epicardial surface of the heart. On occasion, short segments of a coronary artery may descend into the myocardium for a variable distance. This abnormality, termed myocardial bridging, occurs in 5–12% of patients and is usually confined to the LAD (Figs 18A and B).[23] Because a "bridge" of myocardial fibers passes over the involved segment of the LAD, each systolic contraction of these fibers can cause narrowing of the artery. Myocardial bridging has a characteristic appearance on angiography with the bridged segment of normal caliber during diastole but abruptly narrowed with each systole. Although bridging is not thought to have any hemodynamic significance in most cases, myocardial bridging has been associated with angina, arrhythmia, depressed LV function, myocardial stunning, early death after cardiac transplantation and sudden death.[23,24]

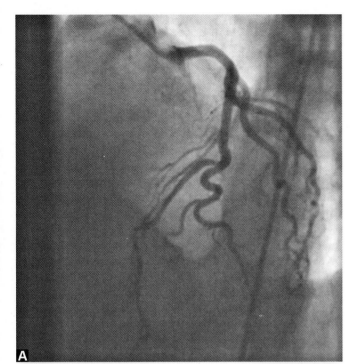

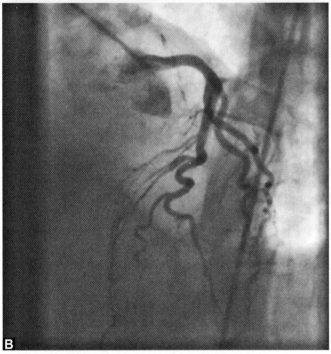

FIGURES 18A AND B: Myocardial bridge in the mid LAD in diastole (A) and systole (B)

GENERAL PRINCIPLES FOR CORONARY AND/OR GRAFT CANNULATION

Coronary cannulation is typically performed using an approximate 30° LAO projection. Pressure is constantly transduced from the tip of the catheter throughout the procedure to monitor for pressure damping or ventricularization. Either of these phenomena may indicate a severe stenosis with wedging of the catheter into the stenosis, or that the catheter tip is positioned against the coronary vessel wall. Injection of contrast when there is damping or ventricularization of the pressure waveform should be avoided as the incidence of coronary

dissection or ventricular arrhythmia is clearly increased in this situation. When pressure damping is present, care should be taken to adjust the position of the catheter until it is resolved before performing contrast injections. In the case of the RCA, dampening could also signify selective engagement of the conus branch. Whenever pressure waveform damping is present, the catheter should be repositioned until a normal waveform appears or nonselective injections performed to assess the possibility of an ostial stenosis or other anatomical reason for the pressure damping. Subsequently, a smaller French or different shape catheter may be considered to safely perform the angiogram. The basic principles regarding pressure waveform ventricularization or damping briefly described above apply to the cannulation and angiography of all coronary vessels and bypass grafts.

LEFT MAIN CORONARY ARTERY CANNULATION

As previously noted, the Judkins left 4.0 coronary catheter is used most often to engage the LMCA in femoral access procedures, with a gentle advancement under fluoroscopic guidance. However, if the Judkins left catheter begins to turn out of profile (so that one or both curves of the catheter are no longer visualized en face), it can be rotated clockwise very slightly and advanced slowly to enter the left sinus of Valsalva, permitting the catheter tip to engage the ostium of the LMCA. If the ascending aorta is dilated, advancement of the Judkins left 4.0 coronary catheter may result in the formation of an acute secondary angle of the catheter, pointing the tip of the catheter upward, away from the left coronary ostium. Further advancement of the Judkins left catheter in this position should be avoided because the catheter will then prolapse on itself and become folded in the ascending aortic arch. In the event this does occur, a guidewire should be temporarily reinserted into the catheter to straighten the secondary bend and permit the catheter to be advanced to the left sinus of Valsalva. If the ascending aorta is significantly dilated, the Judkins left 4.0 catheter should be exchanged for a larger size (e.g. Judkins left 4.5, 5.0 or 6.0). If the tip of the Judkins left catheter advances beyond the ostium of the LMCA without engagement, the primary bend of the catheter can sometimes be reshaped within the patient's body by further careful advancement to the aortic valve to gently bend the catheter tip. Then, the catheter is withdrawn to the level of the LMCA. This maneuver, along with gentle clockwise or counterclockwise rotation, frequently permits selective engagement of the LMCA when the initial attempt has failed. If the LMCA is still not cannulated and the catheter tip remains below the origin of the LMCA, a shorter Judkins left catheter can be used to allow coaxial engagement of the LMCA.

Use of an Amplatz left catheter to cannulate the LMCA generally requires more catheter manipulation than with the Judkins left catheter. When using an Amplatz left catheter, the broad secondary curve of the catheter is positioned so that it rests on the right aortic cusp with its tip pointing toward the left aortic cusp. Alternating advancement and withdrawal of the catheter with slight clockwise rotation allows the catheter tip to advance slowly and superiorly along the left sinus of Valsalva to enter the left coronary ostium. When the tip enters the ostium, the position of the catheter can usually be stabilized with slight withdrawal of the catheter. After the left coronary ostium has been cannulated, the pressure at the tip of the catheter should be checked immediately to ensure that there is no damping or ventricularization of the pressure contour. If the pressure measured at the catheter tip is normal, left coronary angiography is then performed using standard techniques. To remove the Amplatz left catheter from the coronary artery, the catheter should be advanced slightly to disengage the catheter tip superiorly from the coronary ostium. Simply withdrawing the Amplatz left catheter often results in deep seating of the catheter tip within the coronary artery—which should be avoided, as that could potentially result in catheter-induced arterial dissection.

RIGHT CORONARY ARTERY CANNULATION

As with the LMCA, cannulation of the RCA is also generally performed in the LAO view but requires different maneuvers than those for cannulation of the LMCA. Whereas the Judkins left catheter naturally seeks the ostium of the LMCA, the Judkins right or Amplatz right catheters that are typically used to engage the RCA must be rotated to engage the vessel. This is usually accomplished by first advancing the catheter into the right coronary sinus to the level of the aortic valve. The catheter is then slowly withdrawn slightly and rotated clockwise to turn the tip of the catheter toward the RCA ostium. The catheter is gently rotated until a further rightward and sometimes a slight downward movement of the catheter tip is noted. This typically signifies entry of the catheter into the right coronary ostium. If the ostium of the RCA is not easily located, the most common reason is that the ostium has a more superior and leftward origin than anticipated. Nonselective contrast injections in the right sinus of Valsalva may reveal the site of the origin of the RCA and allow successful cannulation, or selection of a different catheter (sometimes as Amplatz left catheter is helpful in this case) to accomplish this. An Amplatz left catheter can also be used to cannulate the RCA when it is in a more conventional location as well. Positioning an Amplatz left catheter in the ostium of the RCA requires a technique similar to that used with the Judkins right catheter. However, the Amplatz left catheter often engages the RCA rather deeply, increasing the risk of catheter induced dissection. So, the use of an Amplatz left catheter to engage the RCA is usually reserved for cases where the RCA ostium is not in the usual location. As in removing this catheter from the left coronary artery, removal of the Amplatz left catheter from the RCA can be achieved by slight clockwise or counterclockwise rotation and gentle advancement to disengage the catheter tip from the ostium. Initial withdrawal of the Amplatz left catheter usually leads to deep seating of the catheter into the coronary vessel and should be avoided.

An abnormal pressure tracing showing damping or ventricularization may suggest the presence of an ostial stenosis or spasm, selective engagement of the conus branch, or deep intubation of the RCA. If an abnormal pressure tracing has been encountered, injections should not be performed until this situation is rectified. In the case of pressure damping in the RCA specifically, the catheter tip should initially be gently rotated counterclockwise and sometimes withdrawn slightly in an effort to free the tip of the catheter from the vessel wall. If persistent damping occurs, the catheter should be withdrawn until it is disengaged and the pressure waveform normalizes. Attempts to re-engage the vessel can be made, but if dampening with engagement persists, a nonselective cusp injection should be performed to help assess the etiology of the damping. Sometimes this will reveal the reason and appropriate changes can be made to safely perform the angiogram including different positioning of the catheter, use of a different shaped catheter or use of a smaller French size catheter. If selective engagement of the conus branch is determined to be the etiology of the pressure damping, sometimes the catheter can be further rotated in a clockwise manner to free the catheter from the conus and engage the RCA. However, if this is not successful, the catheter should be disengaged and further attempts to successfully engage the RCA be made. If the pressure tracing is normal on initial entry into the RCA, the vessel should be imaged in at least two, preferably three projections. The initial injection should be gentle because of the possibility that forceful injection through a catheter whose tip is immediately adjacent to the vessel wall may also lead to dissection of the coronary artery, particularly when the catheter engagement is not coaxial. Coronary spasm of the proximal or ostial RCA may also occur as a result of catheter intubation. When an ostial stenosis of the RCA is seen, intracoronary nitroglycerin or calcium channel antagonists should be administered to eliminate the possibility of catheter-induced spasm as a cause of the coronary artery narrowing.

CORONARY BYPASS GRAFT CANNULATION

Selective cannulation of bypass grafts is generally more challenging than cannulation of the native coronary arteries because the locations of graft origins are more variable, even when surgical clips or graft markers are present to assist with graft location. Knowledge of the number, course and type of bypass grafts obtained from the operative report is invaluable for the identification of the bypass grafts during coronary bypass graft angiography.

SAPHENOUS VEIN GRAFTS

Saphenous vein grafts (SVGs) from the aorta to the distal RCA or PDA generally originate from the right anterolateral aspect of the aorta approximately 5 cm superior to the sinotubular ridge. SVGs to the LAD artery (or diagonal branches) originate from the anterior portion of the aorta about 7 cm superior to the sinotubular ridge. SVGs to the obtuse marginal branches arise from the left anterolateral aspect of the aorta approximately 9–10 cm superior to the sinotubular ridge. In most patients, all SVGs can be engaged with a single catheter, such as a Judkins right 4.0 or a modified Amplatz right 1. Other catheters useful for engaging SVGs include the right and left bypass graft catheters (Fig. 5). Amplatz left catheters can occasionally be useful for superiorly oriented SVGs. A multipurpose catheter may very occasionally be useful for the cannulation of an SVG to the RCA or one of its branches that has a particularly downgoing origin and was not able to be successfully cannulated with one of the aforementioned catheters.

Viewed in the LAO projection, the Judkins or Amplatz right catheters rotate anteriorly from the leftward position as the catheter is rotated in a clockwise direction. Steady advancement and withdrawal of the catheter tip in the ascending aorta (approximately 5–10 cm above the sinotubular ridge) with varying degrees of rotation usually results in cannulation of an SVG. A well-circumscribed "stump" is almost always present if the SVG is occluded at the origin. Each patent SVG or "stump" (occluded SVG) should be viewed in nearly orthogonal views. The relation between the origin of the SVGs and the surgical clips or graft markers may help to confirm whether all targeted SVGs have been visualized. However, knowing which grafts are present (by review of operative report and/or previous angiogram when available) is a much more reliable method. Additionally, if this previous data is not present, being sure that all vascular territories have been accounted for on the current study is another important element in helping to confirm that all grafts have been visualized. If a patent SVG or a stump cannot be located, it may be necessary to perform an ascending aortogram in an attempt to visualize all SVGs and their course to the coronary arteries. If a graft is noted to be patent on the aortogram, then further attempts to selectively cannulate the graft should be performed, perhaps with a different catheter if needed.

The goal of SVG angiography is to image and assess the origin of the SVG, its entire course (body of the graft) and the distal insertion site at the anastomosis between the bypass graft and the native coronary vessel. The origin of the SVG is best evaluated by achieving a coaxial engagement of the catheter tip with the origin of the SVG. The mid-portion (body) of the SVG should be evaluated with complete contrast filling of the SVG, as inadequate opacification may produce an angiogram suggestive of obstructive defects. SVGs, as all veins, have valves which should not be interpreted as being pathologic narrowings. It is critical to assess the SVG insertion or anastomotic site in full profile without overlap of the distal SVG or the native vessel. This can sometimes be challenging, but is a very important aspect of performing a diagnostically adequate angiogram. Angiographic assessment of the native vessels beyond SVG anastomotic sites generally requires views that are conventionally used for the native vessels themselves. Sequential grafts are those that supply two different epicardial branches in a side-to-side fashion (for the more proximal epicardial artery) and terminating in an end-to-side anastomosis (for the more distal epicardial artery). A "Y" graft is one in which there is a proximal anastomosis in an end-to-side fashion to another saphenous vein or arterial graft with two distal end-to-side anastomoses to the two epicardial vessels from these two grafts. Visualization of all segments and anastamoses of each of these types of grafts is imperative and may take several different projections of each graft to accomplish.

INTERNAL MAMMARY ARTERY GRAFTS

The left IMA usually arises inferiorly from the left subclavian artery at a variable distance from the origin of the subclavian. The origin of the IMA is however typically located near, but inferior to the origin of the thyrocervical trunk. Cannulation of the left IMA is usually performed with an IMA catheter (Fig. 5). Usually in the LAO projection, the catheter is advanced over a wire into the aortic arch to an area near the junction of the ascending aorta and the transverse portion of the aortic arch. The catheter is then slowly withdrawn and rotated counterclockwise to turn the tip in a cranial direction, allowing entry into the left subclavian artery. Once the left subclavian artery is engaged, a guidewire is advanced into the left subclavian artery under fluoroscopic guidance. The catheter is then advanced into the subclavian artery over the wire to a point distal to the expected origin of the left IMA. IMA cannulation is performed typically in the AP projection by withdrawing and slightly rotating the catheter counterclockwise to bring the tip anteriorly. Successful cannulation of the IMA is usually noted with a slight drop of the catheter tip in a downward and slightly anterior direction.

The right IMA is also typically cannulated with the IMA catheter. The brachiocephalic artery is entered in the LAO projection in a manner similar to how the left subclavian is entered in the case of a left IMA. However, the brachiocephalic artery tends to be more tortuous than the left subclavian. Additionally, the right common carotid artery origin is off the brachiocephalic artery, so care should be taken to avoid inadvertently advancing the guidewire into the right common carotid artery. When the guidewire is successfully positioned in the distal right subclavian artery, the IMA catheter is advanced over the wire to a point distal to the expected origin of the right IMA. The catheter is then gently withdrawn and rotated to cannulate the right IMA, similar to the method used with the left IMA.

Unlike SVGs, the IMA itself is generally less affected by atherosclerotic disease. As with all graft studies, angiograms of the IMA graft should assess all portions of the graft completely—the origin, the body and the anastomosis. This can generally be accomplished with a flat LAO, flat RAO and one cranially angulated view, typically an AP cranial view. It is important to keep in mind that visualization of the native vessel after the graft insertion site is also of importance. So, using views that one would typically use for native coronary angiography of that vessel is often a good starting point in performing coronary graft angiography. Although the LAO cranial view may be limited in its ability to demonstrate the anastomosis of the LIMA and the LAD because of vessel overlap, it may be a very good view to visualize the body of the graft and the native LAD and diagonal branches. An additional view that is sometimes helpful is assessing a "difficult to see" LIMA to LAD anastomosis is a left lateral projection, with the patient's arms placed above his or her head. In cases where there is a potential need for a repeat sternotomy (e.g. the patient had a previous bypass surgery and now needs a valve surgery), it is helpful to also obtain an AP angiogram of the IMA grafts so that their location with respect to the sternum is known to limit the chance of damage to the graft during the next sternotomy. The risk of catheter-induced dissection of the origin of the IMA can be reduced by careful manipulation of the catheter tip and avoidance of forceful advancement of the catheter in the subclavian artery without the protection of the guidewire. If the IMA cannot be selectively engaged because of tortuosity of the subclavian artery, nonselective angiography is sometimes adequate and can be enhanced by placing a blood pressure cuff on the ipsilateral arm and inflating it to a pressure

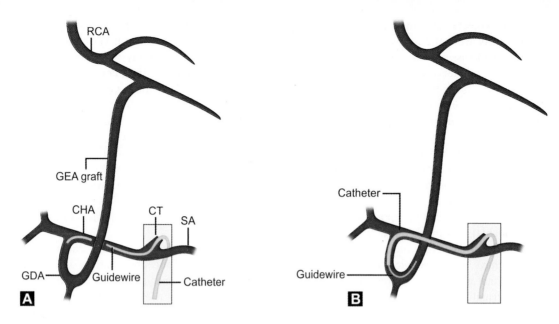

FIGURES 19A AND B: Catheterization of the right gastroepiploic artery (GEA) graft. The celiac trunk (CT) is selectively engaged with a cobra catheter, and a guidewire is gently advanced to the gastroduodenal artery (GDA) and the GEA. The catheter is advanced over the guidewire for selective arteriography of the GEA graft. (Abbreviations: CHA: Common hepatic artery; RCA: Right coronary artery; SA: Splenic artery). (*Source:* Bonow RO. Braunwald's Heart Disease—A Textbook of Cardiovascular Medicine, 9th edition.)

above systolic arterial pressure before the nonselective injection is performed. Alternatively, if nonselective angiography does not result in an adequate angiogram, the ipsilateral radial or brachial artery may need to be accessed to facilitate selective IMA engagement. IMA spasm is not uncommon and should be treated with intra-arterial nitrates or calcium channel blockers. Before performing IMA injections, the patient should be warned that they may feel chest warmth or discomfort with contrast injection due to injection into small IMA branches supplying the chest wall.

GASTROEPIPLOIC ARTERY

The right gastroepiploic artery (GEA) is the largest terminal artery of the gastroduodenal artery and was briefly used as an alternative in situ arterial conduit to the PDA in patients undergoing CABG. Use of this arterial conduit has largely been abandoned, but there is an occasional patient who may still have this type of graft so it will be briefly discussed here. The gastroduodenal artery arises from the common hepatic artery in 75% of cases, but it may also arise from the right or left hepatic artery or the celiac trunk. Catheterization of the right GEA is carried out by first entering the common hepatic artery, usually with a cobra catheter (Figs 19A and B). A torquable, hydrophilic-coated guidewire is then advanced to the gastroduodenal artery and then to the right GEA. The cobra catheter is then exchanged for a multipurpose or Judkins right coronary catheter, which then permits selective angiography of the right GEA.

STANDARDIZED PROJECTION ACQUISITION

General recommendations can be made for a sequence of angiographic image acquisition that is applicable to most patients. However, tailored views are often needed to accommodate individual variations in anatomy. As a general rule, each coronary artery should be visualized with number of (at least two) different projections that minimize vessel foreshortening and overlap. An LAO view (sometimes with shallow caudal angulation) is often performed first to evaluate the possibility of ostial LMCA disease. Other important views include the LAO cranial view to evaluate the middle and distal LAD. The LAO cranial view should have sufficient leftward positioning of the image intensifier to allow separation of the LAD, diagonal and septal branches, and enough cranial angulation to minimize foreshortening of the LAD. An LAO caudal view should be performed to clearly evaluate the distal LMCA and ostia of the LAD and LCX. The RAO caudal view best assesses the LCX and marginal branches. The distal LMCA and ostial LAD are often also well visualized in this view. A shallow RAO or AP cranial view should be obtained to evaluate the mid and distal portions of the LAD. A general sequence of views to obtain for the left coronary system may be: flat LAO, RAO caudal, AP (or slight RAO) cranial, LAO cranial and LAO caudal. The RCA should be visualized in at least two views, possibly three. A flat LAO view is useful to visualize the ostium and mid-portion of the RCA with separation of the RCA and its right ventricular branches. An LAO cranial view usually demonstrates most of the course of the RCA, but specifically visualizes the distal bifurcation of a dominant RCA into the PDA and posterolateral branches. Occasionally, a more AP cranial view is needed to assess the distal bifurcation. A flat RAO view demonstrates the mid-RCA and proximal, middle and distal termination of the PDA. A general sequence for RCA angiography may include: flat LAO, LAO cranial and then flat RAO. It cannot be overstated, that with all angiographic studies, individual

TABLE 6
Angiographic views

Vessel segment	Angiographic view	Comments
Left main	• AP projection with slight caudal angulation • LAO caudal view • RAO caudal	• Left main should be visualized in multiple projections • LAO cranial and RAO cranial views are sometimes helpful in visualization of body and distal left main
Left anterior descending	• LAO cranial • AP cranial • RAO cranial	• RAO cranial views display proximal, mid and distal segments. It also separates diagonal branches superiorly and septal inferiorly • LAO caudal for origin of lad • AP cranial views to see the proximal and mid segments • AP cranial for also the ostium of lad • Lateral projections for mid LAD and also for bifurcating disease of lad and diagonal branch
Left circumflex	• RAO caudal • AP caudal • LAO caudal (spider view)	• RAO and LAO caudal views are best to visualize proximal and mid segments along with the marginals • For left dominant system LAO cranial for left PDA branch
Right coronary artery	• LAO • LAO or AP cranial • RAO	• Ostium is best seen in LAO or LAO with caudal angulation • RAO is good view for mid segment of RCA • Distal bifurcation is best visualized with LAO cranial projection • RAO is helpful for coaxial cannulation • Left lateral is sometimes helpful for mid segment

variations may be necessary to view all of the needed segments of the coronary arteries in a given patient. It is incumbent upon the angiographer to ensure that a complete study is performed (Table 6).

THE FLUOROSCOPIC IMAGING SYSTEM

The basic principle of radiographic coronary imaging is that radiation produced by the X-ray tube is attenuated as it passes through the body. This attenuation of the X-ray is detected by the image intensifier (Fig. 20). Iodinated contrast medium is injected into the coronary arteries which enhances the absorption of the X-rays and produces a sharp contrast with the surrounding cardiac tissues. The X-ray shadow is then converted into a visible light image by the image intensifier and displayed on fluoroscopic monitors. Previously, these images were then stored on 35 mm cinefilm. However, storage of images digitally has now replaced 35 mm cinefilm for coronary angiography because of its versatility with respect to image transfer, low-cost acquisition and storage, and capability for image enhancement after image acquisition. More recently, direct digital imaging systems have eliminated the need for analog to digital converters which were previously required with conventional image intensifiers. This has all been accomplished without compromise of the image integrity[25] and has resulted in significantly reduced radiation exposure while enhancing image quality.

Passage of catheters and acquisition of angiographic images requires a high-resolution image-intensifier system with digital cineangiographic capabilities. The components are mounted on a U or C arm (which acts as a support) with the X-ray tube beneath the patient and the image intensifier above. Rotation of the arm allows viewing over a wide range of angles and positions. Some laboratories have two support systems perpendicular to one another (biplane) and use a double monitoring system, providing simultaneous angiography from two different angles (Fig. 18 Biplane). This is particularly helpful in patients with renal insufficiency as less contrast will generally be delivered for a complete study when two images are obtained with each contrast injection.

The operators stand on the patient's right side facing the fluoroscopic and hemodynamic monitors. The image intensifier is positioned over the patient's left shoulder to produce an LAO cranially angulated view of the heart. The image intensifier can be rotated to other positions e.g. caudal or RAO as well to visualize the cardiac structures from any angle. During catheterization, it is necessary to monitor and record electrocardiographic and hemodynamic data—particularly pressure waveforms.

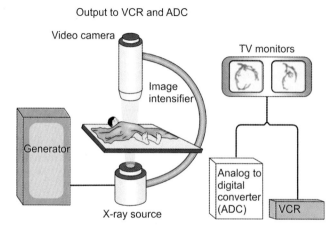

FIGURE 20: Cineangiographic equipment. The major components include: a generator, X-ray tube, image intensifier attached to a positioner such as a C-arm, optical system, video camera, videocassette recorder (VCR), analog to digital converter (ADC) and television monitors

CHARACTERISTICS OF CONTRAST MEDIA

All types of contrast media contain three iodine molecules attached to a fully substituted benzene ring. The fourth position in the standard ionic agent is taken up by sodium or methylglucamine as a cation; the remaining two positions of the benzene ring have side chains of diatrizoate, metrizoate, or iothalamate. All contrast media is excreted predominantly (99%) by glomerular filtration with about 1% excreted by the biliary system. The normal half-time of excretion is 20 minutes. The vasodilator effect and transient decrease in systemic vascular resistance are directly related to the degree of osmolality of the contrast medium used. Transient hypervolemia and depressed contractility are related to both osmolality and ionic charge and in part responsible for the elevation of left atrial and LV end-diastolic pressure after contrast injection. To reduce the osmotic effects of contrast medium, the number of dissolved particles must be decreased or the molal concentration of iodine per particle must be increased. New-generation, nonionic, monomeric and ionic dimeric contrast agents have approximately the same viscosity and iodine concentration but have only one-half or less of the osmolality of the ionic agents.[26] The advantages of the nonionic, low-osmolar agents include less hemodynamic loading, patient discomfort, binding of ionic calcium, depression of myocardial function and blood pressure, and possibly fewer anaphylactoid reactions.[27,28] Currently, nonionic, low-osmolar agents are preferred in all patients, but especially in adults with poor LV function; patients with renal disease, especially those with diabetes; and patients with a history of serious reaction to contrast media or with multiple allergies. Table 7 provides a summary of commonly used contrast agents for coronary and LV angiographic studies.

CONTRAST MEDIA REACTIONS

There are three types of contrast allergies: (1) minor cutaneous and mucosal manifestations; (2) smooth muscle and minor anaphylactoid responses and (3) major cardiovascular and anaphylactoid responses. Major reactions involving laryngeal or pulmonary edema often are accompanied by minor or less severe reactions. Nonionic contrast media has replaced ionic contrast media for most patients to minimize the chance of allergic or other adverse contrast reactions.[29,30] Patients reporting allergic reactions to contrast media should be premedicated typically with a steroid and diphenhydramine before the procedure. The premedication protocol for different laboratories may vary slightly, but common dosages include 60 mg prednisone the night before and 60 mg of prednisone the morning of the catheterization. Additionally, diphenhydramine 50 mg should be given on call to the catheterization lab. Premedication may not prevent the occurrence of adverse reactions completely. Additional routine treatment of patients with prior allergic reactions with an H_2 blocker (e.g. cimetidine) does not appear to have any additional benefit, so this practice has fallen out of favor. Patients with known prior anaphylactoid reactions to contrast dye should be pretreated with steroids and an H_1 blocker (e.g. diphenhydramine). Table 8 lists the adverse reactions associated with radiocontrast materials.

CONTRAST-INDUCED RENAL FAILURE

Patients with diabetes, renal insufficiency or volume depletion from any cause are at risk for contrast-induced nephropathy (CIN).[29,30] Advanced preparations to limit the chance of CIN include volume repletion (IV fluid administration, holding diuretics) and maintenance of large-volume urine flow (> 200 ml/h). Patients at risk for CIN should be volume replete before contrast is administered. Following the contrast study, IV fluids should be liberally continued unless intravascular volume overload is a problem. A decreased urine output after the procedure that is unresponsive to increased IV fluids and/or diuretics indicates that significant renal injury is probable. Consultation with a nephrologist is often helpful in these cases. All types of contrast agents (ionic, nonionic or low-osmolar) are associated with a similar incidence of CIN.

ACCESS SITE HEMOSTASIS

After the catheterization procedure has been completed and the catheters removed, the sheath is flushed. If heparin has been given, an activated clotting time (ACT) is obtained for femoral or brachial access procedures. The sheath is removed when the ACT is below a level specified by each institutional protocol—typically below 150–180 seconds. To remove the femoral arterial sheath, gentle pressure is applied proximal to the puncture site while the sheath is removed, taking care not to crush the sheath and/or strip clot into the distal artery. Once the sheath is removed, firm downward pressure is then applied just proximal

TABLE 7

Commonly used iodinated contrast agents in cardiac angiography

Product category	Proprietary name	Genetic constituent	Ratio of iodine to osmotically active particles	Calcium chelation	Anticoagulation effect	Osmolality
High-osmolar, ionic	Renografin-76	Diatrizoate and citrate	1.5	(+)	(+++)	1940
High-osmolar, ionic	Hypaque-76	Diatrizoate only	1.5	(−)	(+++)	1690
Low-osmolar, ionic	Hexabrix	Ioxaglate	3.0	(−)	(+++)	600
Low-osmolar, nonionic	Isovue	Iopamidol	3.0	(−)	(+)	790
Low-osmolar, nonionic	Omnipaque	Iohexol	3.0	(−)	(+)	844
Low-osmolar, nonionic	Optiray	Ioversol	3.0	(−)	(+)	702
Low-osmolar, nonionic	Visipaque	Iodinaol	3.0	(−)	(+)	290

(+), present; (+++), strongly present; (−), absent
(*Source:* Modified from Peterson KL, Nicod P. Cardiac Catheterization: Methods, Diagnosis, and Therapy. Philadelphia: Saunders; 1997.)

TABLE 8

Reactions associated with contrast media

Allergic (anaphylactoid) reactions
Grade I: Single episode of emesis, nausea, sneezing or vertigo
Grade II: Hives; multiple episodes of emesis, fevers or chills
Grade III: Clinical shock, bronchospasm, laryngospasm or edema, loss of consciousness, hypotension, hypertension, cardiac arrhythmia, angioedema or pulmonary edema
Cardiovascular toxicity
Electrophysiologic
Bradycardia (asystole, heart block)
Tachycardia (sinus, ventricular)
Ventricular fibrillation
Hemodynamic
Hypotension (cardiac depression, vasodilation)
Heart failure (cardiac depression, increased intravascular volume)
Nephrotoxicity
Discomfort
Nausea, vomiting
Heat and flushing
Hyperthyroidism

TABLE 9

Advantages or disadvantages of vascular closure devices

Device	Mechanism	Advantages and limitations
• Angioseal	• Collagen seal	• Secure hemostasis • Anchor may catch on side branch
• Duett	• Collagen-thrombin	• Stronger collagen-thrombin seal • Intra-arterial injection of collagen-thrombin
• Perclose	• Sutures	• Secure hemostasis of suture • Device failure may require surgical repair
• Vasoseal	• Collagen plug	• No intra-arterial components • Positioning wire may catch on side branch
• Starclose	• Nitinol Clip	• No intra-arterial material • Secure hemostasis of clip

(*Source:* Adapted and modified from Hurst's The Heart, 12 edition.)

to the arteriotomy for 15–30 minutes, with gradual reduction in pressure after the initial 10–15 minutes. After manual hemostasis is achieved, a small adhesive bandage is used to cover the wound. Large pressure dressings tend to obscure the puncture site (thus limiting ongoing site assessment) and are generally ineffective to prevent rebleeding so are best avoided in most cases. Depending on the sheath size, bedrest is required for typically 4–6 hours after sheath removal. Additional methods to secure postprocedure arterial hemostasis include external hemostasis pads, mechanical pressure clamps and vascular closure devices. A variety of vascular closure devices are currently available.[31-33] These devices do reduce the time to obtain hemostasis and allow earlier ambulation. They may be particularly helpful in anticoagulated patients, patients with back pain or an inability to lie flat. The advantages and disadvantages of closure devices are summarized in Table 9. All vascular closure devices should be used with caution in patients with peripheral arterial disease.

The brachial sheath is removed in relatively the same manner as a femoral sheath. There are however no mechanical pressure clamp devices or closure devices for use with brachial access. These lines are typically all manually pulled. After hemostasis is obtained, it is recommended that the arm be kept straight for several hours. Often an arm board is placed to help the patient refrain from bending or otherwise using the procedural arm during this time. With transradial catheterization, sheath removal is always done at the end of the procedure, regardless of anticoagulation status. There are various devices used to apply pressure on the radial artery site, but the most effective devices are able to isolate the pressure to the radial artery while not compromising flow in the ulnar artery. One commonly used device is a bracelet which has a small inflatable pillow on the inner portion of the bracelet which is placed over the radial artery. The bracelet is placed around the wrist just proximal to the puncture site. Once the bracelet is secured in place, the sheath

is gently withdrawn and the "pillow" (on the underside of the bracelet). Positioned over the radial artery is simultaneously inflated with air to obtain hemostasis. The air is gently released until there is slight bleeding from the site and then a small amount of air is reinjected into the "pillow" of the hemostatic device with the goal of providing hemostasis of the vessel but continued patency of the artery as determined by presence of the radial pulse distal to the device, but no visible bleeding. Deflation of air from the device and subsequent removal of the bracelet are usually accomplished within 1–2 hours after a diagnostic procedure.

COMPLICATIONS OF CARDIAC CATHETERIZATION

The cumulative incidence of the major risks of stroke, death and MI is approximately 0.1%. The minor risks of vascular injury, allergic reaction, bleeding, hematoma and infection range from 0.04% to 5% (Table 10). For diagnostic catheterization,

TABLE 10

Complications and risk for cardiac catheterization [SCAI Registry (%)]

Mortality	0.11
Myocardial infarction	0.05
Cerebrovascular accident	0.07
Arrhythmias	0.38
Vascular complications	0.43
Contrast reaction	0.37
Hemodynamic complications	0.26
Perforation of heart chamber	0.03
Other complications	0.28
Total of major complications	1.70

(*Source:* Adapted from Scanlon P, Faxon D, Audet A, et al. ACC/AHA guidelines for coronary angiography. J Am Coll Cardiol.1999;33:1756.)

TABLE 11

Patients at increased risk for complications after coronary angiography

Increased General Medical Risk
• Age greater than 70 years
• Complex congenital heart disease
• Morbid obesity
• General debility or cachexia
• Uncontrolled glucose levels
• Arterial oxygen desaturation
• Severe chronic obstructive lung disease
• Renal insufficiency with creatinine greater than 1.5 mg/dl
• Increased Cardiac Risk
• Three-vessel coronary artery disease
• Left main coronary artery disease
• Functional NYHA class IV (CHF)
• Significant mitral or aortic valve disease or mechanical valve prosthesis
• Ejection fraction less than 35%
• High-risk exercise treadmill testing (hypotension or severe ischemia)
• Pulmonary hypertension
• Pulmonary artery wedge pressure greater than 25 mm Hg
• Increased Vascular Risk
• Anticoagulation or bleeding diathesis
• Uncontrolled systemic hypertension
• Severe peripheral vascular disease
• Recent stroke

(*Source:* Scanlon P, Faxon D, Audet A, et al. ACC/AHA guidelines for coronary angiography. J Am Coll Cardiol.1999;33:1756.)

analysis of the complications in more than 200,000 patients indicates the incidence of risks as follows: death less than 0.2%; MI less than 0.05%, stroke less than 0.07%, serious ventricular arrhythmia less than 0.5% and major vascular complications (thrombosis, bleeding requiring transfusion or pseudoaneurysm) less than 1%.[34-38] Vascular complications are more frequent when the femoral or brachial approaches are used as compared to the transradial approach. The incidence of death during coronary angiography is higher in the presence of LMCA disease (0.55%), with LVEF less than 30% (0.30%) and with New York Heart Association functional Class IV disease (0.29%). Patients at increased risk for complications of cardiac catheterization are shown in Table 11.

ACCESS SITE COMPLICATIONS

The most common complication noted with femoral access catheterization is hemorrhage and local hematoma formation. These complications occur more frequently with increasing size of the access sheath, concomitant venous access, increased amounts of anticoagulation, female patients, obesity and also low body weight. Other possible access site complications (in order of decreasing frequency) include retroperitoneal hematoma, pseudoaneurysm, arteriovenous (AV) fistula and arterial thrombosis.[37] The frequency of access site complications is increased in obese patients, during high-risk procedures, in critically ill elderly patients with extensive atheromatous disease, in patients receiving anticoagulation therapies and with concomitant interventional procedures. A retroperitoneal

hematoma should be suspected in patients with hypotension, tachycardia, pallor, a falling hematocrit postcatheterization, lower abdominal or back pain, or neurologic changes in the procedural extremity. This complication is associated with high femoral arterial puncture and full anticoagulation.[34] Retroperitoneal hemorrhage can cause significant morbidity and even mortality, especially if not promptly recognized. Pseudoaneurysm is a complication more often associated with low femoral arterial puncture, usually below the head of the femur. This complication should be suspected in a patient with swelling at the access site and especially if there is a bruit present. The risk of pseudoaneurysm formation is higher with concomitant anticoagulation. Pseudoaneurysm can most often easily be identified with ultrasound imaging. Manual compression of the expansile growing mass guided by Doppler ultrasound with or without thrombin or collagen injection is an acceptable therapy for femoral pseudoaneurysm.[35,37] The more common treatment currently in use is ultrasound guided thrombin injection of the pseudoaneurysm. Larger pseudoaneurysms, or those not favorable for thrombin injection based on anatomic issues, may require surgical treatment.

OTHER COMPLICATIONS

Embolic stroke is a rare complication of diagnostic coronary angiography but, when it occurs, it can be devastating. Embolic stroke more commonly occurs in patients with significant aortic atheroma. Careful attention to aspiration and flushing of catheters is imperative in all procedures. Giving heparin for longer duration procedures (such as bypass graft procedures, aortic valve assessment) or in patients at higher risk for stroke should be considered. Catheter induced coronary artery dissection is an infrequent but important complication to be aware of. When it occurs, urgent or even emergent therapy may be needed in the form of PCI or sometimes even bypass surgery in the case of a left main dissection or inability to successfully percutaneously treat a catheter induced RCA dissection. This complication can often be avoided with proper coaxial positioning of catheters, avoiding abrupt or deep engagement of vessels, refraining from injecting when a dampened waveform is present and generally not injecting with excessive force. However, there are certainly times where, despite using appropriate technique and caution, this complication can still occur, especially in vessels with atherosclerotic disease. Air embolus is a rare (0.1%) complication during diagnostic coronary angiography and is generally preventable with meticulous attention to elimination of air within the manifold system. If an air embolus does occur, 100% oxygen should be administered, which theoretically allows resorption of smaller amounts of air within 2–4 minutes. Prompt and aggressive supportive care is sometimes necessary depending on the size and the location of the air embolus. Distal cholesterol embolization is also relatively uncommon, but is more common during procedures in patients with significant peripheral arterial disease. Nerve pain after diagnostic catheterization is infrequent, but can occur as a result of local anesthesia given during the procedure as well as the location of the sheath near a superficial nerve causing local irritation of the nerve. This condition generally resolves spontaneously over time. Although lactic acidosis may develop after coronary angiography in diabetic patients taking metformin, this complication is very rare and has been essentially eliminated with the practice of metformin discontinuation immediately before coronary angiography and not restarting the medication until renal function has been documented to be in the normal range postprocedure. With the expanded use of complex PCI, patients may now return for multiple procedures over their lifetime which can subject them to the risk of cumulative radiation injury.[39,40] An average PCI procedure imparts 150 times the radiation exposure received with a single chest X-ray and 6 times the annual radiation received by background environmental radiation.[39,40] Skin related radiation injury is more often related to a single long exposure with limited movement of the X-ray tube during the procedure. Reports of radiodermatitis related to prolonged X-ray exposure have led to the recommendation that patients who receive fluoroscopy for more than 60 minutes be counseled about the delayed effects of radiation injury to the skin, although proportionately significantly more radiation is received with digital cineangiography than with fluoroscopy alone. Radiation-induced skin lesions are generally identified by their location in the region of the body that was imaged and are manifest by an acute erythema, delayed pigmented telangiectasia and indurated or ulcerated plaques. The risk of causing radiation induced skin injury can be minimized with meticulous attention to limiting the amount of fluoroscopy and digital cineangiographic exposure during the case. In very complex procedures where increased amounts of X-ray exposure are difficult to control, care should be taken to use multiple different angles to reduce the exposure of one certain area of the body to the X-ray.

LESION QUANTIFICATION

QUANTITATIVE ANGIOGRAPHY

Although visual estimations of coronary stenosis severity are used by virtually all clinicians to guide clinical practice, "eyeball" estimates of percent diameter stenosis are limited by substantial observer variability and bias. However, more reliable and objective quantitative coronary measurements have had limited clinical use in the assessment of intermediate coronary lesions (40–70%), having been largely supplanted by physiological measures of stenosis significance, most often fractional flow reserve (FFR). Quantitative coronary angiography was initially performed by Greg Brown and his colleagues at the University of Washington nearly 30 years ago. Using hand-drawn arterial contours, reference vessel and minimal lumen diameters were measured and were used to evaluate the effect of pharmacological intervention for a number of angiographic plaque regression studies. These initial quantitative angiographic methods were time consuming and cumbersome and have now been largely replaced with computer-assisted methods for automated arterial contour detection. Quantitative angiographic analysis is divided into several distinct processes, including film digitization (when needed), image calibration and arterial contour detection.[25] The contrast-filled diagnostic or guiding catheter can be used as a scaling device for determining absolute vessel dimensions, yielding a calibration factor in millimeters per pixel. Catheter and arterial contours are obtained by drawing

a center line through the segment of interest. Linear density profiles are then constructed by the computer perpendicular to the center line, and a weighted average of the first and second derivative function is used to define the catheter or arterial edges. Individual edge points are then connected using an automated algorithm, and outliers are discarded and the edges are smoothed. The automated algorithm is then applied to a selected arterial segment, and absolute coronary dimensions and percent diameter stenosis are obtained.

LESION COMPLEXITY

Heterogeneity of the composition, distribution and location of atherosclerotic plaque within the native coronary artery results in unique patterns of stenosis morphology in patients with CAD. These patterns have been used to identify risk factors for procedural outcome and complications after PCI and to assess the risk for recurrent events in patients who present with an acute coronary syndrome.[41] Criteria established by a joint ACC/AHA task force suggested that procedure success and complication rates were related to a number of different lesion characteristics (Table 12). Over the decade following the publication of these criteria, the most complex lesion morphologies (i.e. "type C" lesions) remain associated with reduced procedural success in patients with ischemic CAD. This is despite substantial improvements in the techniques used for coronary intervention over this same time period.

TABLE 12

Characteristics of type A, B and C coronary lesions

Type A lesions (high success, > 85%; low risk)	
Discrete (< 10 mm)	Little or no calcium
Concentric	Less than totally occlusive
Readily accessible	Not ostial in locations
Non-angulated segment, < 45°	No major side branch involvement
Smooth contour	Absence of thrombus

Type B lesions (moderate success, 60–85%; moderate risk)	
Tubular (10–20 mm length)	Moderate to heavy calcification
Eccentric	Total occlusions < 3 months old
Moderate tortuosity of proximal segment	Ostial in location
Moderately angulated segment, $\geq 45°, < 90°$	Bifurcation lesion requiring double guidewire
Irregular contour	Some thrombus present

Type C lesions (low success, < 60%; high risk)	
Diffuse (> 2 cm length)	Total occlusion > 3 months old
Excessive tortuosity of proximal segment	Inability to protect major side branches
Extremely angulated segments, $\geq 90°$	Degenerated vein grafts with friable lesions

(*Source:* Ryan TJ, Bauman WB, Kennedy JW, et al. Guidelines for percutaneous coronary angioplasty. A report of the American Heart Association/American College of Cardiology Task Force on Assessment of Diagnostic and Therapeutic Cardiovascular Procedures (Subcommittee on Percutaneous Transluminal Coronary Angioplasty). Circulation.1993;88:2987.)

The predictive value of two other risk scores has been compared to the ACC/AHA lesion complexity score.[42,43] The Society for Cardiac Angiography and Interventions (SCAI) risk score used an ordinal ranking of two composite criteria (vessel patency and complex morphology) to classify lesions into four groups: (1) non-type C–patent; (2) type C–patent; (3) non-type C–occluded and (4) Type C–occluded.[42] For correctly classifying lesion success, the ACC/AHA classification had a C-statistic of 0.69; the modified ACC/AHA system had a C-statistic of 0.71; and the SCAI classification had a C-statistic of 0.75. The Mayo Clinic Risk Score added the integer scores for the presence of eight morphological variables and provided a better risk stratification than the ACC/AHA lesion classification for the predicting of cardiovascular complications, whereas the ACC/AHA lesion classification was a better system for identifying angiographic success of PCI.[43]

LESION LENGTH

Lesion length may be measured using a number of methods, including measurement of the "shoulder-to-shoulder" extent of atherosclerosis narrowed by more than 20%, quantifying the lesion length more than 50% narrowed, and estimating the distance between the proximal and the distal angiographically "normal" segment. The last method is used most commonly in clinical practice and provides a longer length than more quantitative methods. Diffuse (> 20 mm) lesions are associated with reduced procedural success with drug-eluting stents, primarily related to large degrees of late lumen loss and more extensive underlying atherosclerosis.[44]

OSTIAL LESIONS

Ostial lesions are defined as those arising within 3 mm of the origin of a vessel or branch and can be further characterized into aorto-ostial and non-aorto-ostial. Aorto-ostial lesions are often fibrocalcific and rigid, sometimes requiring additional ablative devices—such as rotational atherectomy (RA) in the presence of extensive calcification—in order to obtain adequate stent expansion. Positioning of the proximal portion of the stent in the aorto-ostial location so that no more than 1 mm of stent extends into the aorta requires meticulous care. Ostial stenoses that do not involve the aorta may also be more elastic and fibrotic than non-ostial lesions but also require the additional principles for treatment as bifurcation lesions.

BIFURCATION LESIONS

The optimal strategic approach for bifurcation lesions remains controversial. The risk for side branch occlusion during PCI relates to the relative size of the parent and branch vessel, the location of the disease in the parent vessel and the stenosis severity in the origin of the side branch. In general, placement of one stent in the larger vessel (usually the parent) is preferable to stent placement in both the parent vessel and the side branch.

ANGULATED LESIONS

Vessel angulations should be measured in the projection with the least amount of foreshortening at the site of maximum stenosis. Balloon angioplasty of angulated lesions increases the risk for dissections, although with the advent of coronary stenting, this is now most often readily treated. If a stent is placed in a highly angulated lesion, there is subsequent straightening of the vessel that may predispose to late stent strut fracture, although this is a largely theoretic risk.

DEGENERATED SAPHENOUS VEIN GRAFTS

A serial angiographic study in patients undergoing coronary bypass surgery showed that 25% of SVGs occlude within the first year after coronary bypass surgery.[45] Drug-eluting stents may reduce the restenosis rate and resulting need for PCI, in SVGs[46] but only embolic protection devices (EPD) have reduced procedural complications during SVG PCI. A study that evaluated the extent of graft degeneration and estimated volume of plaque in the target lesion found that the independent correlates of increased 30-day major adverse cardiac event rates were more extensive vein graft degeneration ($p = 0.0001$) and bulkier lesions (larger estimated plaque volume, $p = 0.0005$).[47]

LESION CALCIFICATION

Coronary artery calcium is an important marker for coronary atherosclerosis. Conventional angiography is moderately sensitive for the detection of extensive lesion calcification, but is less sensitive for detecting the presence of milder degrees of lesion calcification. Severely calcified lesions tend to be more rigid and difficult to dilate with a balloon than noncalcified lesions. In heavily calcified lesions, RA may be useful before stenting to ensure both stent delivery and more importantly, complete stent expansion.

THROMBUS

Conventional angiography is a relatively insensitive method for detecting coronary thrombus. However, its presence is associated with a higher risk of procedural complications, primarily relating to embolization of thrombotic debris into the distal circulation. Large intracoronary thrombi are most often noted as intraluminal filling defects during angiography in STEMI and may be treated with a combination of pharmacological agents (e.g. glycoprotein IIb/IIIa inhibitors) and mechanical devices (e.g. rheolytic thrombectomy, manual aspiration catheters).

TOTAL OCCLUSION

Total coronary vessel occlusion is identified as an abrupt termination of an epicardial vessel. Anterograde and retrograde collaterals may be present and are helpful in quantifying the length of the totally occluded segment. The success rate of passage of a coronary guidewire across the occlusion depends on the occlusion duration and on certain lesion morphological features. The following are lesion features that decrease the chance of procedural success: the presence of bridging collaterals, occlusion length greater than 15 mm, branches that originate at or near the occlusion point and the absence of an angiographic "beak" at the occlusion site. Newer guidewires and improved operator experience have improved procedural success rates, although the presence of a total l occlusion remains one of the major reasons for referring patients for coronary bypass surgery.

TABLE 13

Thrombolysis in myocardial infarction (TIMI) flow

Grade 3 (complete reperfusion)	Anterograde flow into the terminal coronary artery segment through a stenosis is as prompt as anterograde flow into a comparable segment proximal to the stenosis. Contrast material clears as rapidly from the distal segment as from an uninvolved, more proximal segment
Grade 2 (partial reperfusion)	Contrast material flows through the stenosis to opacify the terminal artery segment. However, contrast material enters the terminal segment perceptibly more slowly than more proximal segments
	Alternatively, contrast material clears from a segment distal to a stenosis noticeably more slowly than from a comparable segment not preceded by a significant stenosis
Grade 1 (penetration with minimal artery perfusion)	A small amount of contrast material flows through the stenosis but fails to opacify fully the epicardial vessel
Grade 0 (no perfusion)	No contrast flow through the stenosis

(*Source:* Modified from Sheehan F, Braunwald E, Canner P, et al. The effect of IV thrombolytic therapy on LV function: a report on the tissue-type plasminogen activator and streptokinase from the thrombolysis in myocardial infarction (TIMI) phase 1 trial. Circulation.1989;72:817.)

CORONARY PERFUSION

Perfusion distal to a coronary stenosis can occur anterograde by means of the native vessel, retrograde through collaterals, or through a coronary bypass graft. The rate of anterograde coronary flow is influenced by both the severity and complexity of the stenosis and the status of the microvasculature. The Thrombolysis in Myocardial Infarction (TIMI) study group established criteria to assess the degree of anterograde coronary perfusion in patients with acute MI and found that complete restoration of anterograde perfusion to TIMI 3 flow was associated with the lowest mortality rate (Table 13).

PHYSIOLOGIC ASSESSMENT OF ANGIOGRAPHICALLY INDETERMINATE CORONARY LESIONS

FRACTIONAL FLOW RESERVE

Coronary artery physiologic data can be used to facilitate clinical decisions regarding revascularization in the catheterization laboratory. Angiography alone cannot always determine the clinical or physiologic importance of a coronary stenosis that narrows the vessel by between 40% and 70% of its normal diameter.[48,49] In order to overcome this limitation, physiologic testing is often performed before making a recommendation for revascularization. Guidewires with a pressures sensor have been developed that can safely be used[50] to permit pressure measurement distal to a coronary stenosis. Some of these guidewires can measure both pressure and flow velocity. Translesional pressure at maximal hyperemia is measured. Maximal hyperemia is induced by IV (140 mcg/kg/min) or intracoronary (30–60 mcg bolus) adenosine. FFR is the ratio of the pressure distal to a coronary stenosis and pressure proximal to the stenosis. It is a pressure-derived estimate of the percent of normal coronary blood flow that would be available to the myocardium. A normal value is 1, while values less than 0.80 are associated with provocable ischemia on myocardial perfusion imaging.

CLINICAL USE OF TRANSLESIONAL PHYSIOLOGIC MEASUREMENTS

Intermediate coronary stenosis, defined as a 40–70% diameter narrowing, is encountered in almost 50% of patients undergoing coronary angiography. FFR measurements parallel noninvasive stress testing results and can identify hemodynamically significant lesions, thereby assisting in immediate decision-making regarding revascularization at the time the diagnostic angiogram. A high degree of correlation between the noninvasive stress testing and the FFR measurement has been found in analyses of patients with stable angina[51-53] non-ST elevation acute coronary syndrome[54] and chest pain of uncertain origin.[55]The FFR is useful for critical decision-making regarding stenting in patients with single or multivessel disease.[56-58] In patients with intermediate lesions, translesional hemodynamic data can be easily acquired. If the FFR is normal, intervention can be safely deferred.[57,59-61]Patients with CAD often have multiple sequential stenoses. It is important to objectively select the most appropriate of several stenoses to be treated. Coronary artery pressure measurements for calculation of FFR of each stenosis can be made by a pull-back pressure recording at maximal hyperemia.[62] In vessels with diffuse disease and long lesions (not uncommon in diabetic patients) FFR measurements can be useful in decision-making regarding the optimal location for PCI within a given artery, or perhaps to recommend CABG as an alternative to PCI. The practice of attempting complete or near complete revascularization in the catheterization laboratory for patients with symptomatic CAD has become more frequent. However, this approach has not been shown to be associated with better outcomes. Attempts to identify which arteries need to be revascularized have been made using both invasive and noninvasive techniques to assess for myocardial ischemia. Noninvasive assessment of myocardial ischemia with myocardial perfusion imaging may not accurately identify the severity of any given lesion in the setting of multivessel disease. However, FFR measurements can identify the clinical severity of individual lesions in patients with multivessel disease[53] thus helping to direct the most appropriate revascularization strategy.[58] The clinical significance of an ostial stenosis can also be further evaluated with FFR, which may be especially beneficial in patients with ostial left main disease.[63,64] Assessment of the physiologic significance of individual coronary stenosis is not only an economically viable strategy, but it also favorably modifies outcomes for patients.[54,59,65]

Historically, improvement in physiology after balloon angioplasty has been poorly correlated to both angiographic results and clinical outcomes because of the inherent limitations of the angiogram. Stenting has replaced balloon angioplasty as the mainstay for the percutaneous treatment of CAD. Unlike with percutaneous transluminal coronary angioplasty (PTCA), coronary pressure measurements after stenting can be used to predict adverse cardiac events.[66]

NON-ATHEROSCLEROTIC CORONARY ARTERY DISEASE AND TRANSPLANT VASCULOPATHY

CORONARY ARTERY SPASM

Coronary artery spasm is defined as a dynamic and reversible stenosis of an epicardial coronary artery caused by focal constriction of the smooth muscle cells within the arterial wall. Initially described by Prinzmetal and his colleagues ("Prinzmetal" or "variant" angina) in 1959, this form of angina was not provoked by the usual factors such as exercise, emotional upset, cold or ingestion of a meal. Coronary artery spasm is more commonly invoked by cigarette smoking, cocaine use, alcohol, intracoronary radiation and administration of catecholamines during general anesthesia. It is characterized by chest discomfort associated with ST elevations on ECG. Although the ST segment elevation is often striking with coronary spasm, the ST elevations rapidly revert to normal when the pain disappears spontaneously or is terminated by the administration of nitroglycerin. Coronary artery spasm may be accompanied by AV block, ventricular ectopy, ventricular tachycardia or ventricular fibrillation. MI and death are rare manifestations of coronary artery spasm. Coronary artery spasm can also be superimposed on an intramyocardial bridge.[24]

Coronary angiography is useful in patients with suspected coronary artery spasm to exclude the presence of concomitant atherosclerotic CAD and to document an episode of coronary artery spasm using provocative IV medications. Three provocative tests can be performed to detect the presence of coronary artery spasm. IV ergonovine maleate can elicit two types of responses. A diffuse coronary vasoconstriction that occurs in all the epicardial arteries is a physiological response to ergonovine and is not diagnostic of coronary artery spasm. The second response to ergonovine is a focal, occlusive spasm of the epicardial artery that is associated with chest pain and ST segment elevation on ECG. This is diagnostic of coronary spasm. Nitroglycerin should be administered directly into the coronary artery to relieve the coronary spasm. A second provocative test is the use of IV acetylcholine. Although it is more sensitive than ergonovine, it may be less specific because of the positive response in patients with atherosclerotic CAD. The final provocative test is hyperventilation during coronary angiography, which is less sensitive but highly specific for the presence of coronary artery spasm.

In the absence of a positive stimulation test, the diagnosis of coronary artery spasm must rely instead on clinical features and response to treatment with nitrates and calcium channel blockers. Sole therapy with beta blockers should be avoided because it can increase the occurrence and severity of coronary artery spasm.

SPONTANEOUS CORONARY ARTERY DISSECTION

Spontaneous coronary artery dissection is a rare cause of acute MI that is more common in younger patients and in women.[67]

SCD is often the first manifestation[68] and the majority of cases have been diagnosed at autopsy.[68] However, the entire spectrum of acute coronary syndromes may be seen.[68]The etiology of spontaneous coronary dissection is not known. Most patients presenting with this entity do not have risk factors for atherosclerotic CAD. Histologically, an inflammatory reaction in the adventitia has been described, suggestive of periarteritis. However, this inflammatory response may be reactive rather than causative.[68]In women, the risk of spontaneous coronary dissection appears to be increased during the peripartum period.[68-70,] It has been suggested that the association between coronary dissection and pregnancy may be a consequence of increased hemodynamic stress or of hormonal effects on the arterial wall.[68]

VASCULITIS

Kawasaki disease (KD) is a vasculitis of infancy and early childhood. The typical presentation is an acute febrile illness in children under the age of five; the incidence is higher in Asian and Asian-American populations than in other groups. The etiology of KD is unknown, although an inflammatory response precipitated by an infectious agent is suggested by some epidemiologic data. The most important complication of KD is coronary vasculitis, leading to coronary aneurysm formation in 20–25% of untreated patients during the acute stage of the disease. Nearly half of acute aneurysms regress, but approximately 20% lead to the development of coronary stenosis in the long term. Patients can present with MI or SCD.

While patients with known KD are followed for the development of coronary artery stenoses, some patients who were not previously diagnosed are recognized only after presenting with sequelae of CAD, including MI, heart failure and SCD.[71,72] Thus, young patients with MI should be asked about a possible childhood history of KD.

TRANSPLANT VASCULOPATHY

The incidence of angiographic allograft coronary vasculopathy is approximately 7% at 1 year. Long-term incidence of allograft coronary vasculopathy is about 32% at 5 years and 53% at 10 years.[73] Risk is slightly greater in patients transplanted because of ischemic heart disease compared to those with nonischemic heart disease.[73] Additional risk factors for transplant vasculopathy are: donor age (curvilinear), recipient age (inverse), gender (male donor), donor hypertension and number of HLA-DR mismatches. Higher transplant center volume was unexpectedly found to be associated with increased risk of vasculopathy. This may be due to higher volume centers either accepting more diverse donors or more aggressive screening for vasculopathy over time.

The diagnosis of transplant vasculopathy is often difficult to establish based upon clinical evaluation alone. Cardiac transplant recipients have both afferently and efferently denervated hearts. Although there is evidence for some reinnervation in select patients by 5 years after transplantation, the degree of reinnervation is generally incomplete.[74,75] As a result, patients with transplant vasculopathy seldom experience the classic symptom of angina pectoris. Silent MI, sudden death and progressive heart failure are common presentations of transplant vasculopathy. Symptoms associated with exertion such as dyspnea, diaphoresis, gastrointestinal distress, presyncope or syncope, are often infrequent, atypical and may be misleading.[76]Thus, to improve long-term outcomes, early diagnosis is essential. Serial screening studies are the preferred approach for detection of vasculopathy in this population.

Prospective coronary angiography is used to establish the diagnosis of transplant coronary vasculopathy. At some centers, coronary angiography is performed prior to discharge after transplantation (as a baseline) and at most centers it is performed annually starting at 1 year postoperatively. Coronary angiography yields important prognostic information, as the absence of angiographic coronary disease was a significant predictor of survival without adverse cardiac events.[77]

Although coronary angiography is the gold standard for the diagnosis of nontransplant atherosclerosis, it is less sensitive in detecting transplant vasculopathy. This is due to the often diffuse and concentric nature of this form of coronary disease. As a result, many patients who develop clinical events that are presumably due to transplant vasculopathy do not have angiographically significant disease.[78,79]

Due to these limitations, adjuncts to angiography have been sought that might improve the detection of early transplant vasculopathy. These include the TIMI frame count, Doppler measurement of coronary flow reserve and, in some centers, intravascular ultrasound imaging.

POTENTIAL ERRORS IN INTERPRETATION OF THE CORONARY ANGIOGRAM

Errors in image acquisition and interpretation of the coronary angiogram can have a profound impact on management strategies in patients with ischemic CAD, particularly when there is disagreement between angiographic, physiological and clinical findings. Attention to factors that affect angiographic image quality at the time of image acquisition will improve the ultimate course selected for patients who undergo angiography.

INADEQUATE VESSEL OPACIFICATION

Inadequate filling of the coronary artery with contrast medium results in incomplete vessel opacification or "streaming" of contrast. When this occurs, there may be an overestimation of the severity of a stenosis within the vessel. Some common causes of inadequate vessel opacification include: suboptimal position of the diagnostic catheter (i.e. not coaxial with the coronary ostium), inadequate force of contrast injection and competition from increased native coronary blood flow in cases of very large coronary vessels or high cardiac output states. Inadequate filling of the coronary vessels with contrast can often be overcome by various techniques (depending on the cause of the underfilling) including: coaxial catheter engagement (this may involve changing the catheter), a more forceful contrast agent injection (as long as catheter tip position and pressure recording confirm the safety of such a maneuver), upsizing catheter diameter or use of a guide catheter for diagnostic angiograms. In cases of absent or very short left main, selective injection of contrast medium into the LCX artery (or LAD) may give the impression of severe disease of even total occlusion of the LAD (or LCX).

This situation must be recognized and care taken to repeat the angiograms with adequate filling of both vessels.

CATHETER INDUCED SPASM

Catheter induced spasm is a relatively common occurrence during coronary angiography and important to recognize. It is more common with engagement of the RCA but can certainly also occur in the left main as well as in bypass grafts—especially free radial artery and IMA bypass grafts. Catheter induced spasm is characterized by a focal stenosis which is typically seen at or near the tip of the catheter. This often results in dampening of the pressure waveform and the need to adjust the catheter until the waveform normalizes before injecting. Often, even after adjusting the catheter until the waveform has normalized, there will appear to be a stenosis in the vessel. It is very important to give intracoronary nitroglycerin and repeat the angiogram to confirm that there is not an atherosclerotic stenosis at that site, but rather that there was coronary spasm that has been relieved with nitrates. Other maneuvers to consider in this assessment are performing a nonselective injection to assess the ostium or using a smaller French size catheter. Failure to recognize catheter induced spasm could result in the erroneous interpretation of an obstructive atherosclerotic stenosis and a subsequent unnecessary recommendation for revascularization.

INCOMPLETE STUDY

A study is considered incomplete when an inadequate number of angiographic images are taken. There is no standard number of views that should be taken, but it is critical to completely define the coronary anatomy and account for all vascular territories. This can certainly be more challenging in cases of chronically occluded vessels, after bypass surgery, or with coronary anomalies. When previous angiograms are available for review, they should be reviewed before the current procedure to ensure that all necessary angiograms have been obtained. If no previous angiogram is available and not all vascular territories are accounted for then further investigation is warranted. In procedures performed after a bypass surgery when bypass grafts are not initially able to be selectively engaged and there is no filling seen (either antegrade or by collaterals) of the vessel that was reported to be bypassed, performance of an ascending aortogram to confirm the number of grafts patent from the aorta is indicated. If additional grafts are then visualized, further attempts to selectively cannulate the grafts can be made. In cases where patients have not had previous bypass surgery but not all vascular territories are accounted for in the obtained angiograms, coronary anomaly should be suspected and investigated as described below.

CORONARY ANOMALIES

Coronary anomalies are rare but important to recognize. When unrecognized, the erroneous conclusion that a coronary vessel occlusion is present can occur. For example, if there is no LCX apparent with initial injection of the left main and there is no collateral filling of the vessel, a nonselective injection of the left coronary cusp can be performed to exclude separate LAD and LCX ostia. If there are separate ostia, then these vessels can be selectively engaged and a complete angiogram obtained. If this is not the case, than suspicion of an anomalous LCX off the proximal RCA or right coronary cusp can be suspected and investigated accordingly. Additionally, if on attempted engagement of the RCA, there is no apparent ostium in the right coronary cusp on nonselective injection, suspicion of an anomalous RCA (often with a high and leftward takeoff from the aorta) should be raised. Switching catheters and interrogating the aorta in the suspected area often results in successful cannulation of the RCA. If cannulation is still not successful, then aortography can be performed to further evaluate the RCA origin. These are some of the most commonly seen coronary anomalies with a few ideas on how to avoid performing an incomplete angiogram when they are present. Certainly there are many other anomalous coronary artery possibilities that may occur which all cannot be described here. The important concept to take away is to be aware of the possibility of coronary anomaly when all vascular territories are not accounted for while performing a coronary angiogram and be vigilant in making a full assessment. This may include recommending coronary CT angiography in some cases.

TOTAL OCCLUSION OF A CORONARY ARTERY

Total occlusion of a coronary vessel can sometimes be difficult to identify, particularly when there is a "flush" occlusion at the origin making identification of the origin very difficult. This can be especially challenging in the case of a flush occlusion of the RCA. It is important for the angiographer to make sure that all vascular territories are accounted for in the angiograms that have been obtained. If there seems to be a portion of the myocardium that does not have a clearly visible epicardial vascular supply, careful attention should be directed to the possibility of faint collateral filling of an occluded vessel in that area.

ECCENTRIC STENOSES

Coronary atherosclerosis is a ubiquitous process that leads to asymmetrical plaque distribution within the coronary artery. Although most segments of the artery wall are involved in the atherosclerotic process, eccentric lesions may appear non-obstructive in one angiographic view, while quite severe in another. This phenomenon reinforces the importance of obtaining multiple (at least two orthogonal) views of each coronary artery. If there is still question about the severity of an eccentric stenosis, then further evaluation [noninvasive physiologic assessment, pressure wire assessment or intra-vascular ultrasound (IVUS)] can be recommended and completed.

SUPERIMPOSITION OF VESSELS

Superimposition of the left and the right coronary arteries with their respective branches can result in failure to detect significant stenoses or even total occlusions. Overlap of vessels can occur in any area during a coronary angiogram, but it is especially important to adequately evaluate the distal left main, LAD ostium, LCX ostium and ramus intermedius origin (when present) without superimposition of branches. Other areas that may be more difficult to image can include the LAD and parallel diagonal branches, the origins of obtuse marginal branches of the LCX, and the distal bifurcation of the RCA into the RPDA and RPLA. It is important to obtain sufficient angulations to clearly visualize these areas. Typical views used for visualization of these various areas were discussed earlier, but in some cases there will need to be further adjustments made based on individual anatomical considerations.

MICROCHANNEL RECANALIZATION

It is sometimes difficult to differentiate very severe (> 90%) coronary stenoses (with an anterograde lumen) from total coronary occlusions (with no anterograde lumen) that have been recanalized with microchannels and bridging collaterals. Pathological studies suggest that approximately one-third of totally occluded coronary arteries ultimately recanalize, resulting in the development of multiple tortuous channels that are quite small and close to one another, creating the impression on angiography of a single, slightly irregular channel. As angiography lacks sufficient spatial resolution to demonstrate this degree of detail in most patients with recanalized total occlusions, wire crossing may not be possible in some cases unless advanced wire techniques are used.

PERCUTANEOUS CORONARY INTERVENTION

The term "angina pectoris" was introduced by Heberden in 1772 to describe a syndrome characterized by a sensation of "strangling and anxiety" in the chest. This was attributed to myocardial ischemia arising from increased myocardial oxygen consumption due to obstructive CAD. Treatment of this syndrome was initially done with coronary artery bypass surgery, first introduced in 1968. In 1977, the first PTCA was performed by Andreas Gruentzig.

The early percutaneous revascularization procedures used cumbersome equipment, which limited the success and use of these procedures. Guide catheters were large and could easily traumatize the vessel. There were no guidewires, and balloon catheters were large with low burst pressures. As a result, the procedure was limited to patients with refractory angina, good LV function, and a discrete, proximal and non-calcific lesion in a single major coronary artery. Additional requirements were that there were no involvement of major side branches or significant angulations at the lesion site. Due to these limitations, percutaneous treatment was considered feasible in only 10% of all patients needing revascularization.

The next several decades saw significant advancements and refinement of guide catheters and guidewire technology. Balloon catheters were also improved, with slimmer crossing profiles and increased tolerance to high inflation pressures. Coronary stents were developed which greatly improved the overall success of percutaneous coronary interventions (PCIs) and significantly reduced the risk of abrupt vessel closure after angioplasty. As equipment improved, experience increased and adjunctive pharmacological therapies were better understood, more complex lesions were treated in both elective and acute situations. Although femoral access has been and currently continues to be the favored approach by most for the performance of PCI, the radial artery is an increasingly attractive alternative access site. The radial artery access site is becoming more practical as the development of coronary interventional equipment (specifically radial specific guide shapes, lower profiles of balloons and stents) allows many PCI procedures to be able to be successfully completed with either 5 or 6 French systems.

Today, PCI encompasses a broad array of procedures including angioplasty, stenting and various "niche" devices which all together allow the performance of safe and effective percutaneous revascularization in many different clinical situations (Table 14).

PHARMACOTHERAPY FOR PCI

Treatment with antiplatelet and anticoagulant medications is a requirement for the safe and successful performance of any PCI. Some of the most commonly used medications during PCI are described below.

ANTIPLATELET THERAPY

Aspirin

Aspirin irreversibly inhibits cyclooxygenase and thus blocks the synthesis of thromboxane A_2, a vasoconstricting agent that promotes platelet aggregation. Aspirin substantially reduces periprocedural MI caused by thrombotic occlusions compared with placebo and has been established as a standard for all patients undergoing PCI. The inhibitory effect of aspirin occurs within 60 minutes, and its effect on platelets lasts for up to 7 days after discontinuation. Although the minimum effective aspirin dosage in the setting of PCI remains uncertain, patients taking daily aspirin should receive 75–325 mg aspirin before PCI. Patients not already taking daily long-term aspirin therapy should be given 300–325 mg of aspirin at least 2 hours and preferably 24 hours before PCI is performed.

Thienopyridines

Dual antiplatelet therapy with aspirin and a thienopyridine is required in any PCI that includes stenting. The indicated duration of dual antiplatelet therapy specifically related to stenting varies, depending on if bare metal or drug-eluting stents are used. Dual antiplatelet therapy is needed for at least 1 month with bare metal stent placement and for at least 1 year if a drug-eluting stent is placed. The initial thienopyridine developed and used was ticlopidine. It has been largely replaced by newer generations of thienopyridines that are described below as these newer medications have more favorable side effect profiles.

Clopidogrel inhibits platelet activation by irreversibly blocking the ADP (P_2Y_{12}) receptor. It has better tolerability, fewer side effects, and is at least as effective as ticlopidine. Along with aspirin, clopidogrel is routinely administered prior to stent implantation. Recent evidence also supports its use in non-stent PCI.[80,81] An initial clopidogrel dose of 600 mg is needed to produce potent inhibition of ADP-induced platelet aggregation within 2 hours.[82-84] A 300 mg loading dose can be used when longer pretreatment is possible and has been shown to produce maximal platelet inhibition within 24 hours with substantial inhibition at 15 hours.[85] Following PCI, long-term

(1 year) clopidogrel use is associated with a 27% relative reduction in adverse ischemic events ($p = 0.02$) compared to 4 weeks of therapy.[86] These findings extended and amplified the similar findings of the PCI-CURE (Clopidogrel in Unstable Angina to Prevent Recurrent Ischemic Events) trial.[81] Major bleeding was not significantly increased at 1 year, and clopidogrel therapy for 1 year was found to be cost-effective. Recent reports suggest that inadequate inhibition of platelet aggregation may occur in patients with higher body mass index and that insensitivity to clopidogrel is more common than previously thought. Both factors may contribute to periprocedural ischemic complications and stent thrombosis. Depending on the definition used, 10–15% of patients undergoing PCI are resistant to aspirin, and 25% are resistant to clopidogrel. In addition, about half of aspirin-resistant patients have a lower response to clopidogrel, placing them at higher risk of periprocedural myonecrosis and stent thrombosis.[87-89] However, reliable, standardized, bedside measures of resistance to dual antiplatelet therapy are not currently available.

Prasugrel is a more potent P_2Y_{12} ADP receptor inhibitor that has a more rapid onset of action and higher levels of platelet inhibition than higher dose clopidogrel.[90] In a study of 13,608 patients with moderate- to high-risk acute coronary syndromes undergoing scheduled PCI and randomly assigned to receive prasugrel (60 mg loading dose and 10 mg daily maintenance dose) or clopidogrel (300 mg loading dose and 75 mg daily maintenance dose) for 6–15 months, the primary efficacy endpoint, a composite of death from cardiovascular causes, nonfatal MI, or nonfatal stroke, occurred in 12.1% of patients receiving clopidogrel and 9.9% of patients receiving prasugrel ($P < 0.001$).[91] There were also significant reductions in the prasugrel group in the rates of MI (9.7% for clopidogrel vs 7.4% for prasugrel; $P < 0.001$), urgent target vessel revascularization (3.7% vs 2.5%; $P < 0.001$) and stent thrombosis (2.4% vs 1.1%; $P < 0.001$).[91] However, major bleeding was observed in 2.4% of patients receiving prasugrel and in 1.8% of patients receiving clopidogrel ($P = 0.03$), with more frequent rates of life-threatening bleeding in the prasugrel group (1.4% vs 0.9% with clopidogrel; $P = 0.01$), including fatal bleeding (0.4% vs 0.1% respectively; $P = 0.002$). Among persons treated with clopidogrel, carriers of reduced-function CYP_2C_{19} alleles had significantly lower levels of active metabolite, diminished platelet inhibition and higher rates of adverse cardiovascular events.[92] However, a similar relationship was not found in patients treated with prasugrel. Further research will be necessary to determine if measurement of point-of-care platelet assays of genetic polymorphisms can help in allocating therapy. In patients with an acute coronary syndrome undergoing PCI who are at low bleeding risk and have not had a previous stroke, prasugrel 60 mg loading dose should be given as soon as possible after definition of the coronary anatomy and continued for the appropriate course after stent placement, depending on the type of stent used.

Ticagrelor is a reversible oral P_2Y_{12} receptor antagonist which provides faster, greater and more consistent ADP-receptor inhibition than clopidogrel.[93] In a multicenter, double-blind trial of 18,624 patients presenting with an acute coronary syndrome with or without ST segment elevation, random assignment was made to treatment with ticagrelor (180 mg loading dose, 90 mg

TABLE 14

Indications for PCI

Common indications for percutaneous coronary interventions according to patient presentation:[1,2]

Patients with asymptomatic ischemia or CCS class I or II angina

Class IIa

PCI is reasonable in patients with 1 or more significant lesions in 1 or 2 coronary arteries suitable for PCI. The vessels intended to be treated must subtend a moderate to large area of viable myocardium or be associated with a moderate to severe degree of ischemia on noninvasive testing. It is also indicated in patients with recurrent stenosis after PCI with large area of viable myocardium. PCI can also be offered to patients with significant left main disease (> 50%), who are not eligible for CABG

Class IIb

(1) The effectiveness of PCI for patients with asymptomatic ischemia or CCS class I or II angina who have 2- or 3-vessel disease with significant proximal LAD CAD who are otherwise eligible for CABG with 1 arterial conduit and who have treated diabetes or abnormal LV function is not well established. However it can be considered in patients with non-proximal LAD disease in a vessel that serves a moderate area of viable myocardium with demonstrable ischemia on testing

Class III

PCI is generally not recommended in patients with asymptomatic ischemia or CCS class I or II angina who do not meet the criteria as listed under the class II recommendations or who have 1 or more of the following:

1. Only a small area of viable myocardium at risk
2. No objective evidence of ischemia
3. Lesions that have a low likelihood of successful dilatation
4. Mild symptoms those are unlikely to be due to myocardial ischemia
5. Factors associated with increased risk of morbidity or mortality
6. Left main disease and eligibility for CABG
7. Insignificant disease (< 50% coronary stenosis)

Patients with CCS class III angina

Class IIa

1. It is reasonable that PCI be performed in patients with CCS class III angina and single-vessel or multivessel CAD who are undergoing medical therapy and who have 1 or more significant lesions in 1 or more coronary arteries suitable for PCI with a high likelihood of success and low risk of morbidity or mortality
2. It is reasonable that PCI be performed in patients with CCS class III angina with single-vessel or multivessel CAD who are undergoing medical therapy with focal saphenous vein graft lesions or multiple stenoses who are poor candidates for reoperative surgery
3. Use of PCI is reasonable in patients with CCS class III angina with significant left main CAD (> 50% diameter stenosis) who are candidates for revascularization but are not eligible for CABG

Class IIb

1. PCI may be considered in patients with CCS class III angina with single-vessel or multivessel CAD who are undergoing medical therapy and who have 1 or more lesions to be dilated with a reduced likelihood of success
2. PCI may be considered in patients with CCS class III angina and no evidence of ischemia on noninvasive testing or who are undergoing medical therapy and have 2- or 3-vessel CAD with significant proximal LAD CAD and treated diabetes or abnormal LV function

Class III

PCI is not recommended for patients with CCS class III angina with single-vessel or multivessel CAD, no evidence of myocardial injury or ischemia on objective testing, and no trial of medical therapy, or who have 1 of the following:

1. Only a small area of myocardium at risk
2. All lesions or the culprit lesion to be dilated with morphology that conveys a low likelihood of success
3. A high risk of procedure-related morbidity or mortality
4. Insignificant disease (< 50% coronary stenosis)
5. Significant left main CAD and candidacy for CABG

Patients with UA or NSTEMI

Class I

An early invasive PCI strategy is indicated for patients with UA or NSTEMI who have no serious comorbidity and coronary lesions amenable to PCI. Patients must have any of the following high-risk features:

1. Recurrent ischemia despite intensive anti-ischemic therapy
2. Elevated troponin level
3. New ST segment depression
4. HF symptoms or new or worsening mitral regurgitation
5. Depressed LV systolic function
6. Hemodynamic instability
7. Sustained ventricular tachycardia
8. PCI within 6 months
9. Prior CABG

Class IIa

1. It is reasonable that PCI be performed in patients with UA or NSTEMI and single-vessel or multivessel CAD who are undergoing medical therapy with focal saphenous vein graft lesions or multiple stenoses who are poor candidates for reoperative surgery
2. In the absence of high-risk features associated with UA or NSTEMI, it is reasonable to perform PCI in patients with amenable lesions and no contraindication for PCI with either an early invasive or early conservative strategy
3. Use of PCI is reasonable in patients with UA or NSTEMI with significant left main CAD (> 50% diameter stenosis) who are candidates for revascularization but are not eligible for CABG

Contd...

Class IIb

1. In the absence of high-risk features associated with UA or NSTEMI, PCI may be considered in patients with single-vessel or multivessel CAD who are undergoing medical therapy and who have 1 or more lesions to be dilated with reduced likelihood of success
2. PCI may be considered in patients with UA or NSTEMI who are undergoing medical therapy who have 2- or 3-vessel disease, significant proximal LAD CAD, and treated diabetes or abnormal LV function

Class III

In the absence of high-risk features associated with UA or NSTEMI, PCI is not recommended for patients with UA or NSTEMI who have single-vessel or multivessel CAD and no trial of medical therapy, or who have 1 or more of the following:

1. Only a small area of myocardium at risk
2. All lesions or the culprit lesion to be dilated with morphology that conveys a low likelihood of success
3. A high risk of procedure-related morbidity or mortality
4. Insignificant disease (< 50% coronary stenosis)
5. Significant left main CAD and candidacy for CABG

STEMI

Class I

General considerations:

1. If immediately available, primary PCI should be performed in patients with STEMI who can undergo PCI of the infarct artery within 12 hours of symptom onset, if performed in a timely fashion (balloon inflation goal within 90 minutes of presentation)

Specific considerations:

2. Primary PCI should be performed for patients less than 75 years old with ST elevation or presumably new left bundle-branch block who develop shock within 36 hours of MI and are suitable for revascularization that can be performed within 18 hours of shock, unless further support is futile because of the patient's wishes or contraindications/unsuitability for further invasive care
3. Primary PCI should be performed in patients with severe congestive heart failure and/or pulmonary edema (Killip class 3) and onset of symptoms within 12 hours

Class IIa

1. Primary PCI is reasonable for selected patients 75 years or older with ST elevation or left bundle-branch block or who develop shock within 36 hours of MI and are suitable for revascularization that can be performed within 18 hours of shock. Patients with good prior functional status who are suitable for revascularization and agree to invasive care may be selected for such an invasive strategy
2. It is reasonable to perform primary PCI for patients with onset of symptoms within the prior 12–24 hours and 1 or more of the following:
    A. Severe congestive heart failure
    B. Hemodynamic or electrical instability
    C. Evidence of persistent ischemia

Class III

1. Elective PCI should not be performed in a noninfarct related artery at the time of primary PCI of the infarct related artery in patients without hemodynamic compromise
2. Primary PCI should not be performed in asymptomatic patients more than 12 hours after onset of STEMI who are hemodynamically and electrically stable

PCI after successful fibrinolysis or for patients not undergoing primary reperfusion

Class I

1. In patients whose anatomy is suitable, PCI should be performed when there is objective evidence of recurrent MI
2. In patients whose anatomy is suitable, PCI should be performed for moderate or severe spontaneous or provocable myocardial ischemia during recovery from STEMI
3. In patients whose anatomy is suitable, PCI should be performed for cardiogenic shock or hemodynamic instability

Class IIa

1. It is reasonable to perform routine PCI in patients with LV ejection fraction less than or equal to 40%, HF, or serious ventricular arrhythmias
2. It is reasonable to perform PCI when there is documented clinical heart failure during the acute episode, even though subsequent evaluation shows preserved LV function

Class IIb

PCI might be considered as part of an invasive strategy after fibrinolytic therapy

Percutaneous intervention in patients with prior coronary bypass surgery

Class I

1. When technically feasible, PCI should be performed in patients with early ischemia (usually within 30 days) after CABG
2. It is recommended that embolic protection devices (EPD) be used when technically feasible in patients undergoing PCI to saphenous vein grafts

Class IIa

1. PCI is reasonable in patients with ischemia that occurs 1–3 years after CABG and who have preserved LV function with discrete lesions in graft conduits
2. PCI is reasonable in patients with disabling angina secondary to new disease in a native coronary circulation after CABG
3. PCI is reasonable in patients with diseased vein grafts more than 3 years after CABG
4. PCI is reasonable when technically feasible in patients with a patent left internal mammary artery graft who have clinically significant obstructions in other vessels

Class III

1. PCI is not recommended in patients with prior CABG for chronic total vein graft occlusions
2. PCI is not recommended in patients who have multiple target lesions with prior CABG and who have multivessel disease, failure of multiple SVGs and impaired LV function unless repeat CABG poses excessive risk due to severe comorbid conditions

(*Source:* Modified from: King SB, Smith SC, Hirshfeld JW, et al. 2007 focused update of the ACC/AHA/SCAI 2005 guideline update for percutaneous coronary intervention. Circulation. 2008;117:261; and Modified from: Kushner FG, Hand M, Smith SC, et al. 2009 focused updates: ACC/AHA guidelines for the management of patients with ST-elevation myocardial infarction. Circulation. 2009;120:2271.)

twice daily thereafter) or clopidogrel (300–600 mg loading dose, 75 mg daily thereafter) for 12 months. The primary endpoint, a composite of death from vascular causes, MI or stroke at 12 months, occurred in 9.8% of patients receiving ticagrelor and 11.7% of those receiving clopidogrel (hazard ratio, 0.84; $P < 0.001$).[94] There was also a significant reduction in MI alone (5.8% in the ticagrelor group vs 6.9% in the clopidogrel group; $P = 0.005$) and death from vascular causes (4.0% vs 5.1%; $P = 0.001$) [No significant difference in the overall rates of major bleeding was found between the ticagrelor and clopidogrel groups (11.6% and 11.2% respectively; $P = 0.43$), but ticagrelor was associated with a higher rate of major bleeding not related to CABG (4.5% vs 3.8%, $P = 0.03$)[94]].

Current evidence suggests that in the absence of risk factors for bleeding, dual antiplatelet therapy should be continued for at least 1 month after BMS placement and for 1 year after drug-eluting stents (DES) placement. Prolonged thienopyridine therapy not only reduces late stent thrombosis but also reduces the risk of MI by potentially reducing embolus of thrombi that complicate plaques remote from the initial intervention. Indefinite aspirin and clopidogrel therapy is recommended in patients previously receiving brachytherapy and in those patients in whom stent thrombosis may be catastrophic, such as patients with unprotected left main artery stenting, or those with stenting of the "last remaining vessel". Finally, the heightened risk of stent thrombosis associated with premature discontinuation of dual antiplatelet therapy, especially in the setting of preparation for noncardiac surgery, deserves special consideration when choosing the stent type to implant at the time of PCI.

IIb/IIIa Platelet Receptor Inhibitors

Thrombin and collagen are potent platelet agonists that can cause ADP and serotonin release and activate glycoprotein (GP) IIb/IIIa fibrinogen receptors on the platelet surface. Functionally, active GP IIb/IIIa serves in the "final common pathway" of platelet aggregation by binding fibrinogen and other adhesive proteins that bridge adjacent platelets. There are currently three GP IIb/IIIa inhibitors approved for clinical use. Studies supporting the use of these agents during PCI were performed before the widespread use of dual antiplatelet therapy; henceforth, the routine use of these agents in current practice of interventional cardiology continues to be reevaluated.

The first such agent approved by the FDA was abciximab (reopro, Centocor, Malvern, PA), a monoclonal antibody. Abciximab was shown to reduce ischemic complications and late clinical events in high-risk angioplasty.[95] The other IIb/IIIa receptor inhibitors approved by the FDA include: eptifibitide (Integrilin, COR Therapeutics, San Francisco, CA) a peptide and tirofiban (Aggrastat, Merck, White House Station, NJ) a small nonpeptide molecule. These are both competitive inhibitors. Each of these agents reduces a composite end point of death or nonfatal MI in the setting of coronary intervention and in acute coronary syndromes.[96] Furthermore, in the EPIC trial, a subgroup of 555 patients with acute coronary syndromes treated with bolus abciximab and infusion had a significant reduction in mortality at 3 years.[97] A meta-analysis of 19 randomized trials of IIb/IIIa agents (20,137 patients) during PCI reported a significant and sustained decrease (20–30%) in the

risk of death.[98] The GP IIb/IIa inhibitors have demonstrated benefit in improving clinical outcomes within the first 30 days after PCI, primarily by reducing ischemic complications, including periprocedural MI and recurrent ischemia. They are particularly useful in patients with troponin-positive acute coronary syndromes[99] but have no consistent effect on reducing late restenosis. Although GP IIb/IIIa inhibitors differ in their structure, reversibility and duration, there is no difference between their clinical effects in patients undergoing primary PCI.[100,101] Bleeding is the major risk of GP IIb/IIIa inhibitors and a downward adjustment of the unfractionated heparin dose has been recommended. GP IIb/IIIa inhibitors are recommended in patients with NSTEMI and unstable angina who are not pretreated with clopidogrel and it is reasonable to administer them to patients who have a troponin-positive acute coronary syndrome who have also been pretreated with clopidogrel. Although GP IIb/IIIa inhibitors are recommended in selected patients at the time of PCI, the value of GP IIb/IIIa inhibitors as part of a routine preparatory strategy in patients with STEMI before their transport to the catheterization laboratory is not routinely recommended on the basis of the results of three studies that failed to show benefit of GP IIb/IIIa inhibitors in patients who were pretreated with oral dual antiplatelet therapy.[102-104]

The decision to use a IIb/IIIa platelet receptor in the era of high-dose clopidogrel pretreatment is complex and requires an assessment of the patient's risk of bleeding and ischemic complications with or without these agents. The patient who cannot receive the acute benefit of clopidogrel therapy due to allergy or intolerance should receive a IIb/IIIa receptor, a class I indication in the ACC Guideline statement. Based upon current evidence, it appears that IIb/IIIa receptor inhibitors are more effective in patients with refractory unstable angina, complex anatomy, slow flow on angiogram and troponin positive acute coronary syndromes.[105]

PARENTERAL ANTICOAGULANT THERAPY

Intravenous anticoagulation is always given during PCI to prevent thrombosis during the procedure. This practice was historically initiated because of the central role of thrombin in arterial thrombosis. Anticoagulation is used in conjunction with antiplatelet therapy for PCI. There are a few options of different agents to use for anticoagulation during PCI.

HEPARIN

For PCI, heparin monitoring is usually performed via the ACT, since the partial thromboplastin time (PTT) becomes prolonged at the heparin concentrations used in these procedures.[106] Initial studies of PCI indicated that unfractionated heparin should be administered to achieve an ACT of 250–350 seconds in patients undergoing PCI.[107] Similarly, the most recent American College of Cardiology/American Heart Association/Society for Cardiovascular Angiography and Intervention guideline update for PCI also recommends that intravenous, unfractionated heparin (UFH) should be given using a weight-adjusted bolus of 70–100 IU/kg to achieve an ACT between 250 and 350 seconds, in patients who do not receive a GP IIb/IIIa inhibitor.

Further heparin boluses are given if the goal ACT is not achieved. However, when a GP IIb/IIIa inhibitor is used, the heparin bolus should be reduced to 50–70 units/kg. In such patients, an ACT of 200–250 seconds appears to be safe and effective and is the current practice during PCI.[41]

Careful monitoring of the ACT is important because some patients have persistent thrombin activity despite heparin therapy, as documented by an elevation in fibrinopeptide A (FPA), a marker of thrombin activity. Increased FPA levels have been noted in patients with intracoronary thrombus, abrupt closure, postprocedural non-ST segment elevation MI and clinically unsuccessful procedures.[108]

Postprocedural heparin is not recommended in patients with an uncomplicated procedure. There is no evidence that prolonged use of postprocedural heparin or low-molecular weight heparin prevents stent thrombosis or restenosis, and postprocedural heparin is associated with increased bleeding and vascular complications.

ENOXAPARIN

Although seemingly safe and as effective as unfractionated heparin,[109,110] the clinical role of low molecular weight heparin remains uncertain as a routine strategy for PCI. It seems reasonable to continue enoxaparin rather than switching to unfractionated heparin once it has been initiated, but it must be re-dosed at the time of the PCI in most cases. It is important to note that ACT cannot be used to monitor anticoagulation status with enoxaparin use, as the ACT is not an accurate reflection of the anticoagulation status with use of this medication.

BIVALIRUDIN

Bivalirudin is a specific direct thrombin inhibitor. The REPLACE-2, ISAR-REACT-3 and ACUITY trials evaluated the efficacy and safety of bivalirudinas an alternative to unfractionated heparin with or without GP IIb/IIIa inhibitors in patients across a broad spectrum of illness severity. Most patients in the study were given a loading dose of clopidogrel (either 300 or 600 mg) at least 2 hours before the procedure. These trials showed that bivalirudin is statistically non-inferior to unfractionated heparin for the prevention of ischemic complications in patients undergoing PCI with stenting. Importantly, the overall rates of protocol-defined major bleeding were significantly lower with bivalirudin in all patients. In patients with renal insufficiency, specifically bivalirudin, was found to have a lower rate of both ischemic and bleeding complications.[111] Additionally, bivalirudin is one of the alternatives in patients with known or suspected heparin-induced thrombocytopenia who require PCI. One potential disadvantage of bivalirudin is its increased cost compared to unfractionated heparin. Although, reduction of bleeding complications may certainly balance out this initial increased cost. One last thing to keep in mind about bivalirudin is that there is no reversing agent for its anticoagulant effect. This is in contrast to unfractionated heparin as its effect can be reversed with administration of protamine. It should be noted, however, that this would only be required in the extremely rare case of a PCI with a complication that requires reversal of anticoagulation.

Appropriate selection and use of equipment is critical in the safe and successful performance of coronary intervention. Needless to say, performance of coronary intervention entails a thorough understanding of coronary anatomy and lesion characterization. The first step to performing a successful coronary intervention is performing an adequate diagnostic coronary angiogram to best define the area to be treated. Once this has been completed, a plan for intervention can be formulated and consideration can be given to equipment selection.

GUIDE CATHETERS

An optimal guide provides a stable platform for the operator to deliver devices to the diseased segment of the coronary artery. The guide catheter is primarily selected according to the size of the ascending aorta and the coronary vessel to be cannulated. Additional factors in guide selection may be anatomically based as extremely tortuous and/or calcified vessels may require a more supportive guide catheter to best ensure a successful intervention. The guide size (French) selection may also be influenced by the intended treatment of the chosen lesion. For example, interventions requiring athrectomy or simultaneous balloon or stent inflations will require a larger lumen guide catheter. Compared to diagnostic catheters, guides have a stiffer shaft because of reinforced construction and also have a larger internal diameter for a given French size. Guide catheters that are coaxially engaged provide the best support and best minimize the risk of guide catheter trauma to the vessel.

Passive guide support is provided by the inherent design and shape of the guide as well as the stiffness from the manufactured material. Active support is typically achieved by either guide manipulation into a configuration conforming to the aortic wall, or by sub-selective intubation with deep engagement in to the coronary vessel.[34] Sometimes this is necessary, but these types of aggressive guide manipulations do increase the risk of trauma to the vessel. It cannot be overstated that coaxial guide alignment with the coronary ostium is more important than the active or passive support. This coaxial alignment allows the operator the best support both to deliver equipment, as well as to allow for optimal contrast opacification to aid in proper positioning of equipment in the vessel.

The most commonly used guides are Judkins, Amplatz and Extra back up type guides. Others that have a niche in various clinical situations include IMA guide for IMA interventions and left and right bypass graft guide catheters. Additionally, there are transradial specific guide catheter shapes that are available for procedures performed from radial artery access. Standard safety measures for guide manipulations include and are listed in Table 15.

GUIDEWIRE

The wire manipulation is one of the most important aspects of PCI. Proper intraluminal advancement of the guidewire through the lesion and into the distal vessel is necessary for the safe delivery of various diagnostic and therapeutic devices while

TABLE 15

Standard safety measures for guide manipulations

- Vigorous aspiration of guide after it is inserted into the ascending aorta
- Generous bleed back and introduction of devices into the Y adaptor on the flush
- Flush frequently to avoid blood stagnation and thrombus formation
- Constantly watch the tip of guide while advancing or retrieving devices
- Pressure monitoring for dampening to avoid trauma to the vessel by inadvertent deep engagement

maintaining secure access to vessel lumen. The ability to negotiate the coronary arterial tree and to deliver the various devices to the diseased site to be treated depends somewhat on individual anatomy and makes guidewire selection variable. Important considerations in appropriate guidewire selection include: torque response, tip flexibility, pushability, stiffness and support for the delivery of devices. Angiographic characteristics of the lesion to be treated should also be considered in the selection of a coronary guidewire for PCI, as individual anatomical variations and lesion characteristics may make a certain wire more appropriate for the given PCI. Some "niche" devices, such as the athrectomy device, have dedicated wires that must be used with that specific device. Based on these requirements, the lesion and vessel characteristics noted above and, from experience in daily clinical practice, various guidewires are chosen for use by the operator.

BALLOONS

General Use Balloons

Balloons for use in PCI are delivered to the lesion over a coronary guidewire and inflated with a device that measures the inflation pressure. There are different types of balloons with the most widely used balloons falling into two basic categories: compliant and non-compliant. Compliant balloons are generally more flexible and therefore more deliverable. When inflated, they do increase in size more significantly with increased pressures. A non-compliant balloon differs in that is somewhat less flexible and less deliverable, but it is able to be inflated to higher pressures with less growth of the balloon diameter. Generally, compliant balloons are used for initial dilation of a lesion before stenting (when needed), but non-compliant balloons may be used for initial lesion dilation if there is concern that a lesion may be difficult to dilate (significant calcification in the lesion). Non-compliant balloons are generally used for further dilating stents after they have been placed, or for dilation of lesions that are more difficult to dilate as noted above.

OTHER SPECIALIZED INTRACORONARY BALLOONS

Cutting Balloon

A cutting balloon is a specialized angioplasty balloon that has several longitudinal atherotomes along its length. With balloon inflation, the atherotomes score the plaque to allow successful dilation of the lesion. They are generally a more difficult device to deliver, as they are stiffer than conventional balloons and are

currently relegated to a niche indication use. Cutting balloons can be useful in the treatment of lesions that have not dilated with conventional balloons. These are often in-stent restenosis lesions or lesions in ostial locations.

Perfusion Balloon Catheter

The perfusion balloon catheter has small holes in the shaft both proximal and distal to the balloon itself. This allows continued distal perfusion of the artery while the balloon is inflated. Perfusion balloons were initially used in patients who were unable to tolerate the prolonged balloon inflations that were sometimes used during angioplasty when it was the only available coronary intervention. However, in modern day practice, the widespread use of stenting has allowed the practice of prolonged balloon inflations to be very limited today. Perfusion balloons do still have a niche application of being used to help stabilize patients with coronary perforation. This balloon can be inflated at the site of the perforation to help seal it, but still allow perfusion distal to the perforation site via the distal lumen of the balloon catheter.

PERCUTANEOUS TRANSLUMINAL CORONARY ANGIOPLASTY

Percutaneous transluminal coronary angioplasty (PTCA) expands the coronary lumen by stretching and tearing the atherosclerotic plaque and vessel wall and, to a lesser extent, by redistributing atherosclerotic plaque along its longitudinal axis. Elastic recoil of the stretched vessel wall generally leaves a 30–35% residual diameter stenosis, and the vessel expansion can result in propagating coronary dissections, leading to abrupt vessel closure in 5–8% of patients.

PTCA was the first and only initial technique of PCI and was indeed a great accomplishment. Due to significant technological advances (stent development primarily) and the increased rates of abrupt vessel closure and restenosis with PTCA alone compared to stenting that has been demonstrated, "stand alone" PTCA has a limited role in PCI today. However, the basis of this technique remains the mainstay of PCI today, as the deployment of all stents is accomplished through the inflation of a balloon.

Some situations where angioplasty alone still does have a role in current PCI are: the "bailout" treatment of the origins of branch vessels that are covered by a stent in the parent vessel, focal in-stent restenosis lesions and the treatment of vessels that are of too small caliber to stent.

CORONARY STENTS

PTCA was associated with two major limitations: acute (during the procedure) or subacute (after the procedure and within 30 days) vessel closure and late (4–8 months postprocedure) restenosis. The development and use of intracoronary stents and the enhanced use of various antithrombotic therapies have resulted in significant reductions in both of these complications.[112-115]

Due to these advantages, stenting is now performed in the majority of PCIs. Despite substantial improvements in early and late outcomes with bare metal stenting compared to PTCA, restenosis of these stents can occur in the months to years after bare metal stenting. Further improvements in stent designs and more importantly, the development of drug-eluting stents, have further reduced restenosis rates. These advances in stenting technology are responsible for a further increase in stent utilization in PCI, relegating non-stenting PCI techniques to niche applications.

Intracoronary stents are increasingly used in patients with a previous MI, older patients and in those who have more extensive and more complex coronary lesions. Despite these more challenging subsets of patients, the overall success rate of PCI has actually increased. Despite this, the rates of emergent CABG, in-hospital ST segment elevation MI (STEMI) and mortality associated with PCI have all fallen.[116]

TYPES OF STENTS

There are many different types of intracoronary stents. They can generally be considered according to metal composition, open versus closed cell design, and whether or not they are capable of eluting drugs for local delivery.

Currently available intracoronary stents are generally composed of either stainless steel or a cobalt-chromium alloy. In general, cobalt-chromium stents tend to be more flexible, while the stainless steel designs may offer greater radial strength for bulky lesions or those involving the more fibro-muscular aorto-ostial locations. In general, modern stent designs make either of these stent types acceptable for use in virtually all cases.

Historically, the initial coil design of intracoronary stents was associated with poor radial strength and increased restenosis. Given these limitations, this design was abandoned. Currently available stents have a tubular configuration with either a closed or open cell design. Closed cell designs (in which each ring is interconnected) are slightly less flexible than open cell, but may provide more support. Today, most commercially available stents employ an open cell design. Additionally, thinner struts appear to reduce vessel injury. Given this, most stents have been designed with reduced strut thickness.

A more detailed discussion of the clinical use of bare metal and drug-eluting stents will follow further below.

STENT DEPLOYMENT

Today, intracoronary stents come premounted on a compliant balloon are delivered through a coronary guide catheter over a guidewire to the lesion and deployed by inflation of the balloon. Optimal stenting is performed in a way that reduces the minimal residual luminal stenosis to as small as possible. Attainment of a large luminal diameter minimizes the risk of both stent thrombosis and restenosis.[114,116] Suboptimal luminal dilation with stent deployment is generally due to inadequate balloon expansion and elastic recoil of the vessel. Both of these issues are related in part to plaque characteristics (lesion is resistant to dilation), as well as stent design.[117] Suboptimal stent dilation is associated with increases in the periprocedural incidence of non-ST elevation MI, overall 30 day mortality and clinical restenosis. Clinical restenosis specifically was associated with a smaller final lumen diameter and the use of multiple stents in a given procedure.[118]

Given the current availability of low profile stent delivery systems, many stenting procedures are completed with a direct stenting technique where the first intervention to the lesion is the placement of the stent. A number of randomized clinical trials have compared direct stenting to stenting after balloon dilation.[119-122] The major outcomes were similar, including procedural success. Based on these studies, the settings in which direct stenting can be considered include: vessel greater than or equal to 2.5 mm in diameter, absence of severe coronary calcification, absence of significant angulation (bend > 45°) and absence of occlusions and bifurcations lesions.

This being said, a lesion should always be dilated with a balloon before stent deployment is attempted if there is any concern that the lesion may not dilate optimally with initial stent deployment. Significant lesion calcification and the fibrotic, sometimes resistant plaque in cases of restenosis are situations where lesion predilation should be strongly considered. Balloon dilation of a lesion before stent deployment is virtually always done in situations where the vessel distal to the lesion is not initially visualized (during MI or with chronic vessel occlusion PCI). If a lesion is significantly calcified and not able to be dilated with a conventional balloon, cutting balloon angioplasty or RA can be considered so that the lesion can be dilated and optimal stent deployment can be achieved.

In addition to angiography, other modalities can be used to assess optimal stent deployment. The IVUS can be used to assess whether or not a stent has been optimally deployed and, if not, the stent can be further dilated to accomplish this.[123] Additionally, FFR measurement can be performed after stent deployment to assess the effectiveness of the stent placement. The prognostic information of the FFR has been demonstrated in several studies.[66,124] At a normal FFR, (> 0.95) adverse events are known to be significantly reduced.

ADJUNCTIVE CORONARY INTERVENTIONAL DEVICES

THROMBECTOMY

Visualization of thrombus by angiography is associated with increased risk of distal embolization and the no reflow phenomenon. The angiojet rheolytic thrombectomy catheter (Possis Medical, Inc., Minneapolis, MN) was introduced as a dedicated device for thrombus removal through the dissolution and aspiration of the thrombus. High-speed saline jets within the tip of the catheter create intense local suction by the Venturi effect. This results in pulling surrounding blood, thrombus and saline into the lumen of the catheter opening, propelling the debris proximally through the catheter lumen. Rheolytic thrombectomy was superior to a prolonged intraluminal urokinase infusion in patients with large thrombus burden, but its routine use in patients with STEMI was not associated with improvement in infarct size by single-photon emission computed tomography (SPECT) imaging and may have caused more complications.[125] Rheolytic thrombectomy is still useful and likely beneficial in clinical practice, however, with careful limited selection of some patients with a large angiographic thrombus burden in a native vessel or SVG. Bradyarrhythmias are common and prophylactic placement of a temporary pacemaker is recommended.

Newer lower profile manual aspiration catheters have been developed as an alternative to rheolytic thrombectomy in patients with thrombus-containing lesions. In a multicenter study of 1,071 patients with STEMI who were randomly assigned to the thrombus-aspiration group or the conventional-PCI group, a myocardial blush grade of 0 or 1 occurred in 17.1% of the patients in the thrombus-aspiration group and in 26.3% of those in the conventional-PCI group (P < 0.001).[125] At 30 days, the rate of death in patients with a myocardial blush grade of 0 or 1, 2 and 3 was 5.2%, 2.9% and 1.0% respectively (P = 0.003), and the rate of adverse events was 14.1%, 8.8% and 4.2% respectively (P < 0.001).[126] Meta-analysis of the data suggests that simple manual thrombus aspiration before PCI reduces mortality in patients with STEMI undergoing primary PCI.[127] Bradyarrhythmias are common, and prophylactic placement of a temporary pacemaker is recommended.

ROTATIONAL CORONARY ATHERECTOMY

Atherectomy refers to removal of the obstructing atherosclerotic plaque. It diminishes plaque volume by abrasion, as opposed to fracturing plaque radially.[128] The physical principal governing RA is known as differential cutting. Differential cutting results in the destruction of inelastic material, such as atherosclerotic, calcified and fibrotic plaques, while sparing normal elastic tissue. It favorably modifies vessel wall compliance and is particularly useful in treatment of calcified lesions.[128,130] The RA system consists of four main components (Boston Scientific, Natick, MA): guidewire, advancer, diamond coated burr catheter and control console system. Burrs are available from 1.25 mm to 2.5 mm in diameter. Selection of burr size should not exceed a burr or artery diameter ratio of 0.70.[129-131] Aggressive advancement of the burr should also be avoided because of higher rates of complication including dissection, slow or no reflow and perforation. Most RA is currently performed as an adjunct to either angioplasty or stenting in order to either debulk or modify plaque, usually in order to facilitate delivery and appropriate expansion of stents within the lesion. However, it should be noted that RA did not lower rates of restenosis in randomized trials.[132-134]

Contraindications to RA include: patients with occlusions in which a guidewire cannot cross the lesion, the presence of thrombus, or extensive vessel dissection. Extreme caution must also be given to patients with lesion lengths greater than 25 mm, angina at rest, poor distal run off and severe LV dysfunction (LVEF < 30%) as these patients are at increased risk for ischemic complications.[135] Patients generally should receive a prophylactic temporary pacemaker due to increased risk of bradycardia and heart block associated with this procedure.

DIRECTIONAL CORONARY ATHERECTOMY

Directional coronary atherectomy (DCA) uses a rotating cup shaped blade within a windowed cylinder to directionally excise atheroma. By physically removing plaque from coronary lumen, it was hoped that it would achieve larger coronary lumen diameters and result in lower restenosis rates. Clinical trials have showed that effective use of DCA produced only a modest reduction in restenosis compared to balloon angioplasty alone. In current practice DCA is used in less than 1% of patients.

Occasionally DCA may be useful when pathological sample of atheroma is of interest.[135] It could also be used to treat noncalcified bifurcation lesion involving a large branch or in the ostium of LAD artery. However, this modality has largely fallen out of favor and is used only very infrequently.

EMBOLIC PROTECTION DEVICES FOR VENOUS BYPASS GRAFT PCI

Sabor et al. drew attention to the importance of microembolization during PCI when they studied 32 patients who died within 3 weeks, noting that more than 80% had histologic evidence of microembolization.[137] Subsequently, there has been increasing awareness of the importance of embolization in atherosclerotic vascular disease, particularly during PCI in patients with acute coronary syndrome and SVG lesions.[138] A variety of occlusion—aspiration and filter-based strategies—have evolved for embolic protection during SVG interventions. The advent of EPD has reduced the risk of postprocedural adverse events after SVG PCI. Embolic protection for SVG PCI now constitutes a class I indication in the PCI guidelines.

Despite their potential benefit in preventing thromboembolization in patients with STEMI, none of the EPD has reduced MI size with primary intervention, possibly relating to the high profile of the devices. There has been limited application of embolic protection in native vessel PCI.

The EPD fall into three broad categories: distal occlusion devices, distal embolic filters and proximal occlusion devices.

DISTAL EMBOLIC FILTERS

Distal filters devices are advanced across the target lesion over a standard coronary wire in their smaller collapsed state and a retaining sheath is withdrawn, allowing the filter to open and to expand against the vessel wall. The filter then remains in place to catch any embolic material larger than the filter pore size (usually 120–150 micron pores) that is liberated during intervention. At the end of the intervention, the filter is collapsed by use of a special retrieval sheath and the filter containing the captured embolic material is removed from the body. This type of device has the advantages of maintaining anterograde flow during the procedure and allowing intermittent injection of contrast material to visualize underlying anatomy during stent deployment. However, it has the potential disadvantage of allowing the component of debris with a diameter less than the filter pore size to pass through. Newer filter devices with reduced crossing profiles and more efficient capture of embolic debris continue to be developed.

DISTAL OCCLUSION DEVICES

The GuardWire (Medtronic Vascular, Santa Rosa, CA) is a low-pressure balloon mounted on a hollow guidewire shaft. The device is passed across the target lesion and the balloon is gently inflated to occlude flow. The PCI is then performed and the debris liberated by intervention remains trapped in the stagnant column of blood. This debris is then aspirated with a specially designed catheter before the occlusion balloon is deflated to restore anterograde flow. Compared with SVG intervention without a distal occlusion device, the use of the guardwire reduced 30-day major adverse clinical events and no-reflow.[139] The major disadvantage of this device is that blood flow is stopped during SVG intervention while the balloon is inflated, creating an obligatory period of ischemia.

PROXIMAL OCCLUSION DEVICES

The third type of EPD occludes flow into the vessel with a balloon in the proximal part of the graft. Two proximal occlusion devices are currently in use: (1) the Proxies catheter (St. Jude Medical) and (2) the Kerberos embolic protection system (Kerberos, Sunnyvale, CA). With such inflow occlusion, retrograde flow generated by distal collaterals or infusion through a "rinsing" catheter can propel any liberated debris back into the lumen of the guiding catheter. These approaches have the potential advantage of providing embolic protection even before the first wire crosses the target lesion.[140]

CLINICAL OUTCOMES

The PCI refers to both nonstenting procedures and stent intervention. We will now discuss the evolution of PCI over the years with the focus of the discussion on clinical outcomes related to the use of bare metal and drug-eluting stents.

Progressive improvements in technology and innovations in delivery systems have led to catheter based therapy as a safe and viable alternative to coronary artery bypass graft surgery (CABG) for revascularization. The Angioplasty Compared to Medical Therapy Evaluation (ACME) trial, involving 212 patients with single-vessel disease and abnormal stress tests, revealed greater freedom from angina in the angioplasty group at 6 months (64% vs 46%) as well as better treadmill performance. There was no difference in death or MI.[141] Angina relief and treadmill performance were significantly better in the PTCA patients, but complications also were more frequent as demonstrated by RITA-2.[142] Meta-analyses of eight randomized published trials comparing PTCA and CABG reported no difference in mortality or MI at 1 year after angioplasty or CABG, but 18% of the angioplasty patients had required bypass surgery and 20% had an additional angioplasty, a significantly higher rate of repeat revascularization than in the surgery group.[143,144]

However, catheter based therapies were associated with angiographic restenosis rate of almost 40% at 6 months after PTCA alone. More than half of these patients had recurrent ischemic symptoms, most often progressive effort angina. Thus, 20–30% of patients required clinically driven repeat target lesion revascularization within the first year after PTCA. After this period, restenosis is uncommon as recurrent ischemia after 1 year is most often due to a new or progressive lesion.[145-146]

In current day practice, stand-alone balloon angioplasty is rarely used other than for very small (< 2.25 mm) vessels, or in the "bailout" of branch vessels that are jailed by a parent vessel stent. However, balloon angioplasty remains integral to PCI for predilation of lesions before stent placement, deployment of coronary stents and further expansion of stents after deployment. It also continues to have a role in treatment of some in-stent restenosis.

The introduction of bare metal stents (BMS) produced a significant improvement in the durability of balloon angioplasty.

Bare metal stenting produced better short-term results with less residual stenosis, elimination of dissection and lower rates of in-hospital CABG and MI. Additionally, the rate of angiographic restenosis fell to 20–30% and the rate of target lesion revascularization fell to 10–15%.[115,117,147,148] As with PTCA, clinical restenosis—when it occurs—typically happens within the first year. After this time, recurrent ischemia is much more likely to be due to new or progressive disease rather than restenosis.[148]

Although BMS clearly improved clinical outcomes and restenosis rates as compared to PTCA, there was still a significant amount of clinical restenosis of BMS. The DES were then developed in an effort to further reduce both the rate of restenosis and the need for target lesion revascularization. Late lumen loss and restenosis after nonstent interventions are caused by a combination of acute recoil, negative remodeling of the treated segment and local neointimal hyperplasia. In contrast, late lumen loss after stenting is due primarily to in-stent neointimal hyperplasia. The restenosis benefit of DES compared to BMS results from inhibition of in-stent neointimal hyperplasia.[149] A DES consists of a standard metallic stent platform, a polymer coating and an anti-restenotic drug (sirolimus, everolimus, paclitaxel, etc.). That reduces the local proliferative healing response to stent placement. The drug is mixed within the polymer that coats the stent and is released over a designated period of time which can vary from as short as days to as long as 1 year after implantation of the stent. Drug-eluting stents have indeed yielded a marked reduction in the incidence of restenosis and target lesion revascularization when compared to BMS.[150] "Real world" experience also shows a marked reduction in repeat revascularization, although restenosis rates were somewhat higher in more complex anatomical lesion subsets such as small vessels, long lesions and bifurcations.[151]

Based upon the marked reductions in restenosis and target lesion revascularization, DES have been used in most PCIs in the United States (71% in a report of usage in 2004 and 94% in a report of usage in 2005).[152,153] Although all currently approved DES have the same general components, they differ with respect to the stent platform, polymer and antirestenotic drug type. Thus, differences may be observed with respect to deliverability (ease of placement), efficacy (prevention of restenosis) and safety (rates of stent thrombosis and MI).

The first two DES to be approved in the United States were the sirolimus-eluting stent (SES) in 2003 and paclitaxel-eluting stent (PES) in 2004. They are now often referred to as "first generation" DES. In 2008, the zotarolimus-eluting stent and the everolimus-eluting stent were approved for use and they are referred to as "second generation" DES. The newer DES have a stent platform of a cobalt-chromium alloy and are thinner and more flexible than the first generation DES. Second generation DES are potentially more biocompatible than first generation DES, as they may generate less inflammatory response and have more rapid vessel endothelialization.[154]

DES VERSUS BMS

The United States Food and Drug Administration initially approved both SES and PES for patients who have newly diagnosed, previously untreated, single native coronary lesions that were less than 28–30 mm in length in a vessel with a diameter between 2.5 mm and 3.75 mm. Use of DES in patients with these characteristics was considered "on-label". Off-label use was defined as patients with complex anatomy (e.g. multi-lesion PCI, vessels outside the 2.5–3.75 mm range, lesions longer than 30 mm, ostial lesions, restenotic lesions, lesions of the left main, total occlusions and bifurcation lesions) and those with SVG lesions.

Multiple individual randomized trials and two large PCI registry data bases provide strong evidence of benefit (reduction in target lesion revascularization) with the use of DES compared to BMS. Benefit was noted both with "on label" and "off label" use of DES. A 2007 meta-analysis included 38 randomized trials involving over 18,000 patients with on-label indications.[149] The three largest were SIRIUS, TAXUS IV and TAXUS V, and the duration of follow-up was 1–4 years. The principal finding was that there was a significant reduction in target lesion revascularization with both SES and PES compared to BMS (odds ratios 0.30 and 0.42, 95% CI 0.24–0.37 and 0.33–0.53 respectively). There was no difference in overall mortality among the three groups (hazard ratio 1.00 for SES and 1.03 for PES compared to BMS). The greatest benefit was found in the subsets of patients who are at the highest risk for restenosis (diabetics, vessel diameter < 3 mm and lesion length > 20 mm).[154-157]

In reports from different large registries in the United States, the proportion of DES procedures performed with off-label use has been steadily increasing.[158] This is mainly due to lower rate of target vessel revascularization.[156]

For patients with off-label indications for DES, a thorough attempt to weigh the relative risks and benefits of restenosis protection, late stent thrombosis and prolonged dual antiplatelet therapy must be made. Alternative therapies including medical management, bare metal stenting, or CABG must be considered in these decisions and individualized to each patient.

Regarding efficacy of individual drug eluting stents, lower rates of clinical restenosis have been noted with SES compared to PES.[159,160]

Data from randomized trials directly comparing sirolimus and paclitaxel stents have generally shown significantly lower rates of angiographic restenosis and less late lumen loss with the sirolimus stent. However, differences in target lesion revascularization have been variable and often not statistically significant. Importantly, there was no significant difference in the composite end point of death or MI.[161] In the diabetic population, the benefit of SES over PES is less clear. This being said, the data must be interpreted with caution given the known limitations of meta-analyses. In contrast to the evidence from randomized trials, two large registries (T-SEARCH and STENT) found no significant difference between PES and SES in the rates of target vessel revascularization.[162,163]

There is, however, growing evidence to support the superiority of the sirolimus stent compared to the paclitaxel stent for reducing angiographic late lumen loss and angiographic restenosis. The advantage of the sirolimus stent also extends to lower rates of target vessel revascularization in complex lesion subsets. Utilization of the paclitaxel stent, however, is acceptable given that the outcomes are superior to BMS and several studies have observed similar outcomes in unselected patients treated with either sirolimus or paclitaxel stents at the discretion of the operator.[164]

Although restenosis rates have been significantly reduced with DES, it still does occur. The DES restenosis is often felt to be a consequence of balloon barotrauma to the artery in areas not covered by the stent, gaps in stent coverage, inadequate stent expansion, or the inability of the drug to limit neointimal hyperplasia.[165-168] In the SIRIUS trial, restenosis in the target lesion vessel segment (includes the stent and area 5 mm proximal and distal to the stent) occurred more frequently than restenosis within the stent among patients receiving a SES (8.9% vs 3.2%).[169] This further reinforces the importance of optimal stenting techniques to take advantage of the decreased restenosis benefit of DES demonstrated in the clinical trials. Diabetes, ostial lesions, stented length of greater than 36 mm, reference vessel diameter less than 2.17 and treatment of in-stent restenosis have been identified to be predictors of restenosis.[170]

It is important to understand the long-term safety of DES in comparison to BMS. Clinical events including development of late stent thrombosis, mortality, MI, impairment of coronary collateral function and hypersensitivity reactions must be considered. Available data demonstrates similar risks of death and MI after DES or BMS when used for either on-label or broader "real world" experience. Nevertheless, it is possible that there is a small but increased risk for very late stent thrombosis after DES (compared to BMS) that appears to be counter-balanced by a reduction in the risks associated with restenosis and repeat revascularization.[171,172] Large observational studies have found no difference in combined endpoints of death, MI or individual endpoint of mortality during mean follow-up of about 3 years.[173-175] More importantly, in a retrospective cohort of 76,525 Medicare (United States) beneficiaries, receipt of a DES was associated with a significantly lower adjusted mortality compared with either historical (hazard ratio 0.79, 95% CI 0.77–0.81) or contemporary controls (hazard ratio 0.83, 95% CI 0.82–0.86).[176]

The decision to use either a BMS or DES needs to balance the relative advantages and disadvantages of each type of stent. Restenosis and stent thrombosis are the two most important factors to consider. As noted above, DES are associated with less restenosis and lower rates of target lesion revascularization, but a greater risk of late or very late stent thrombosis, particularly after clopidogrel is discontinued. Circumstances in which implantation of a BMS is most appropriate are listed in Table 16.

In view of the potentially life-threatening consequences of stent thrombosis, the interventional cardiologist must evaluate the patient's ability to comply with a recommendation for continuous, long-term (at least 1 year) dual antiplatelet therapy

TABLE 16

Bare metal stent implantation recommended (when stenting indicated)

- When compliance of dual antiplatelet therapy is a question
- Patients with high risk of bleeding
- Patients who need long-term anticoagulation with Coumadin
- Use of larger stent size > 3.5, especially with shorter lesion length
- Patients who are preoperative for noncardiac surgery

as well as their potential for having to discontinue dual antiplatelet therapy for other reasons, prior to deciding to place a DES. The DES is perhaps preferred over BMS for patients with complex anatomy (e.g. multilesion PCI, small vessels, lesions longer than 30 mm, ostial lesions, restenotic lesions, lesions of the left main, total occlusions and bifurcation lesions). For patients with SVG stenosis, the current evidence appears to favor DES over BMS.[177]

PROCEDURAL SUCCESS AND COMPLICATIONS RELATED TO CORONARY INTERVENTION

Procedural success after PCI is measured both in terms of the angiographic success in treating the diseased vessel as well as in the complication rates related to the performance of the procedure. Complications during coronary interventions can be considered as those that are common to the complications that occur with diagnostic coronary angiography (as discussed previously), or those that occur specifically as a result of the coronary intervention. This section will focus primarily on those complications that are specifically related to the performance of PCI. Anatomic (or angiographic) success after PCI is defined as the attainment of a residual diameter stenosis of less than 50% after PTCA or less than 20% after stenting.[178] A number of clinical, angiographic and technical variables predict the risk of procedural failure and complications in patients undergoing PCI. Major complications include death, MI or stroke; minor complications include transient ischemic attacks, vascular access site complications, CIN and a host of angiographic complications (Table 17).[178]

COMPLICATIONS SPECIFIC TO PCI

Some of the most common mechanical complications of coronary intervention include: acute or threatened vessel closure,

---

TABLE 17

Variables associated with early failure and complications after percutaneous coronary intervention

Clinical variables
- Women
- Advanced age
- Diabetes mellitus
- Unstable or Canadian Cardiovascular Society (CCS) Class IV angina
- Congestive heart failure
- Cardiogenic shock
- Renal insufficiency
- Preprocedural instability requiring intra-aortic balloon pump support
- Preprocedural elevation of C-reactive protein
- Multivessel coronary artery disease

Anatomic variables
- Multivessel CAD
- Left main disease
- Thrombus
- SVG intervention
- ACC/AHA type B2 and C lesion morphology
- Chronic total coronary occlusion
- Large area of myocardium at risk
- PCI of vessel supplying collaterals to a large artery

Procedural factors
- A higher final percentage diameter stenosis
- Smaller minimal lumen diameter
- Presence of a residual dissection or trans-stenotic pressure gradient

---

coronary perforation and no-reflow. These events can cause prolonged ischemia, hemodynamic collapse and death. Prompt recognition and treatment of these complications can significantly reduce adverse patient outcomes.

THREATENED OR ACUTE CLOSURE

Threatened closure is defined as a more then 50% narrowing of an artery during a coronary intervention procedure with evidence of active ischemia. Major causes of acute or threatened closure include: coronary dissection, coronary spasm, distal embolization and thrombus formation with coronary dissection being the most common of these.

Excessive iatrogenic plaque fracturing from balloon inflation or device manipulation with subsequent separation of the layers of the vessel wall can lead to threatened or abrupt vessel closure. The National Heart Lung and Blood Institute (NHLBI) classification of coronary dissection is shown in Table 18.[179]

Other things to consider when there is concern for a coronary dissection during PCI include: streaming of contrast related to inadequate contrast injection, vessel straightening artifact (often related to the coronary guidewire) or overlap of branches (often very small branches) in the area of concern. Some maneuvers that can be completed in this assessment are: giving intracoronary nitroglycerin, obtaining angiograms with multiple different angles to best eliminate vessel overlap, withdrawing the guidewire so that the floppy portion of the wire is across the area of concern and repeating the angiogram. Generally, dissections of Grade C or worse are readily identified with angiography. However, sometimes dissections of Type A or B are more difficult to confirm. It is important for the operator to carefully assess all of these possibilities with angiography and if there is still a question, IVUS can be used to further clarify.

The major predictors of outcome related to coronary dissection include: the length of compromised vessel, the extent of the area of myocardium jeopardized and the integrity of antegrade flow. Minor dissections which are non-flow limiting are usually well tolerated and generally do not always require further treatment, but this decision also depends on the extent of myocardium at risk and other clinical considerations. However, any flow limiting dissection should be stented whenever possible in order to prevent abrupt vessel closure.

Most cases of abrupt vessel closure occur within minutes of the final balloon inflation, but subacute vessel closure after PCI can occur up to hours later in 0.5–1.0% of cases, typically as the antithrombotic therapy used during the procedure wears off.[180,181] Stents can reverse abrupt closure in more than 90% of cases overall and certainly in an even higher percentage of

---

TABLE 18

National Heart Lung and Blood Institute (NHLBI) classification of coronary dissection

- Type A: Luminal haziness
- Type B: Linear dissection
- Type C: Extraluminal contrast staining
- Type D: Spiral dissection
- Type E: Dissection with reduced flow
- Type F: Dissection with total occlusion

TABLE 19

Risk factors for coronary perforation during PCI

Over sizing of the angioplasty balloon (balloon to artery ratio > 1.2)
• High pressure balloon inflations outside stented segments
• Stenting of small or tapering vessel
• Stenting of lesions that are re-crossed after dissection or abrupt closure
• Treatment of chronic total occlusions
• Atherectomy device use—especially in angulated lesions

cases when the closure is related to a previously untreated dissection.

PERFORATION

Perforation or frank rupture of coronary arteries resulting from the guidewire, atherectomy devices, or balloons occurs in 0.2–0.6% of patients undergoing PTCA, with guidewire coronary artery perforation being the most common.[182,183] The incidence is higher with the use of atherectomy devices to ablate tissue for certain complex lesions.[182,183] The use of newer devices and more aggressive attempts to cross chronic total occlusions (with the use of stiffer coronary guidewires) harbor an increased risk for coronary artery perforation during PCI. The consequences of coronary perforation in the setting of the anticoagulation needed during PCI can cause significant morbidity and mortality (Table 19).

Coronary artery perforation in the stent era (at the site of the lesion) is a rare but potentially catastrophic complication. It may occur during stent deployment—particularly if the stent is oversized—if the lesion is very resistant to dilation (calcified lesions) and if extremely high deployment pressures are used. The degree of perforation varies from barely perceptible to severe. There is a classification scheme based upon angiographic appearance of the perforation.

• Class I: Intramural crater without extravasation
• Class II: Pericardial or myocardial blushing (staining)
• Class III: Perforation greater than or equal to 1 mm in diameter with visible contrast extravasation.

The incidence of complications varies with the severity of the perforation. For classes I, II and III perforations, the respective values were 0%, 14% and 50% for MI and 8%, 13% and 63% for cardiac tamponade. Emergency cardiac surgery with or without coronary bypass may be required.[182] The indications for emergency surgery are continued bleeding and/or hemodynamic compromise unrelieved by pericardiocentesis.

Serious perforations require immediate treatment in the cath lab, even if definitive surgical intervention is later needed. Rapid filling of the pericardial space secondary to coronary perforation in the setting of anticoagulation may very quickly lead to cardiac tamponade. Prompt recognition and treatment of tamponade with immediate pericardiocentesis is necessary to prevent a potentially catastrophic event.

When coronary perforation occurs, prompt recognition of the perforation is imperative to its successful treatment. An initial strategy is to inflate a balloon at the site of the perforation. Occasionally, this can seal the perforation, but, if not, further bleeding into the pericardium can be temporarily halted to provide some time (before development of pericardial tamponade) for other maneuvers. Next, reversal of anticoagulation should be considered when possible. Protamine is specific antagonist of heparin and should be administered promptly. It should be recognized that there is no similar reversal agent for bivalirudin. The infusion should be discontinued and the anticoagulant effect will wear off, but this may take up to 2 hours. If the perforation is not sealed with simple balloon inflation and reversal of anticoagulation, the placement of a covered stent should be considered.

Significant distal perforations of small branches by guidewires should be initially managed with balloon inflation as far distal in the vessel as is possible, reversal of anticoagulation and pericardiocentesis if needed. If the perforation persists despite this, coil embolization of the distal vessel may be considered. It should be recognized that this maneuver will likely be successful in stopping the bleeding, but will result in total occlusion of that arterial segment.

NO-REFLOW

No-reflow is defined as stagnant column of contrast agent in the vessel being treated without an identifiable mechanical obstruction. The cause is mainly embolization of atheromatous material and is aggravated by microembolization of platelet rich thrombi that release vasoactive agents leading to intense arteriolar spasm.[184] The incidence is about 2% with plain balloon angioplasty, 7% with use of RA and almost 40% for interventions involving degenerated SVGs. When no-reflow is suspected, it is important to ensure that there is not a mechanical obstruction that is causing the poor flow (dissection, incomplete treatment of the lesion, etc.). If no mechanical obstruction is identified, then no-reflow is the likely problem. Management includes intracoronary administration of various medications which may include: nitroglycerin, nipride, verapamil or adenosine. Use of EPD for interventions involving SVGs should always be considered to help reduce the severity of no reflow in these procedures.

ACUTE THROMBOTIC CLOSURE

Intracoronary thrombus is recognized angiographically as a progressively enlarging intraluminal lucency surrounded by contrast agent. Uncontrolled platelet aggregation along with superimposed spasm both play major roles in the formation of thrombus. An initial assessment to make when thrombus forms during PCI is to confirm that anticoagulation therapy is adequate and promptly correct it if needed. Generally, the risk for acute intraluminal thrombus formation during PCI is relatively low in stable angina patients. However, in patients presenting with acute coronary syndrome, lesions with visible thrombus before treatment begins, long and diffuse disease segments, or in degenerated vein grafts, the risk of thrombotic occlusion is high.[185] After stenting, acute closure due to subacute thrombosis may happen if there is incomplete apposition of stent struts with vessel wall or unrecognized obstruction proximal or distal to stent. This can generally be avoided with high pressure deployment of appropriately sized stents and adequate treatment of the entire diseased segment (Table 20).

SECTION 3

Diagnosis

TABLE 20

Variables associated with stent thrombosis

Anatomic variables
- Long lesions
- Smaller vessels
- Multivessel disease
- Acute myocardial infarction
- Bifurcation lesions

Procedural factors
- Stent underexpansion
- Incomplete wall apposition
- Residual inflow and outflow disease
- Margin dissections
- Crush technique
- Overlapping stent
- Polymer materials

REFERENCES

1. Seldinger SI. Catheter replacement of the needle in percutaneous arteriography: a new technique. ActaRadiol. 1953;39:368-76.
2. Sones FM, Shriey EK. Cine coronary arteriography. Mod Concepts Cardiovasc Dis. 1962;31:735-8.
3. Amplatz K, Formanek G, Stranger P, et al. Mechanics of selective coronary artery catheterization via femoral approach. Radiology. 1967;89:1040-7.
4. Judkins MP. Selective coronary arteriography: IA percutaneous transfemoral technique. Radiology.1967;89:815-24.
5. Gibbons RJ, Abrams J, Chatterjee K, et al. ACC/AHA 2002 guideline update for the management of patients with chronic stable angina—summary article: a report of the American College of Cardiology/ American Heart Association Task Force on Practice Guidelines (Committee on the Management of Patients with Chronic Stable Angina). Circulation. 2003;107:149-58.
6. Campeau L. Percutaneous radial artery approach for coronary angiography. Cathet Cardiovasc Diagn. 1989;16:3-7.
7. Kiemeneij F, Laarman GJ, Odekerken D, et al. A randomized comparison of percutaneous transluminal coronary angioplasty by the radial, brachial and femoral approaches: the access study. J Am Coll Cardiol. 1997;29:1269-75.
8. Gibson CM, Morrow DA, Murphy SA, et al. A randomized trial to evaluate the relative protection against post-percutaneous coronary intervention microvascular dysfunction, ischemia, and inflammation among antiplatelet and antithrombotic agents: the PROTECT-TIMI-30 trial. J Am Coll Cardiol. 2006;47:2364-73.
9. Koerselman J, Grobbee DE. Coronary collaterals: an important and underexposed aspect of coronary artery disease. Circulation. 2003;107:2507-11.
10. Werner GS, Ferrari M, Heinke S, et al. Angiographic assessment of collateral connections in comparison with invasively determined collateral function in chronic coronary occlusions. Circulation. 2003;107:1972-7.
11. Angelini P. Coronary artery anomalies—current clinical issues: definitions, classification, incidence, clinical relevance, and treatment guidelines. Tex Heart Inst J. 2002;29:271-8.
12. Angelini P, Velasco JA, Flamm S. Coronary anomalies: incidence, pathophysiology, and clinical relevance. Circulation. 2002;105:2449-54.
13. Eckart RE, Jones SO, Shry EA, et al. Sudden death associated with anomalous coronary origin and obstructive coronary disease in the young. Cardiol Rev. 2006;14:161-3.
14. Basso C, Marron BJ, Corrado D, et al. Clinical profiles of congenital coronary artery anomalies with origin from the wrong aortic sinus leading to sudden death in young competitive athletes. J Am Coll Cardiol. 2000;35:1493-501.
15. Von Kodolitsch Y, Franzen O, Lund GK, et al. Coronary artery anomalies. Part II: recent insights from clinical investigations. Z Kardiol. 2005;94:1-13.
16. Porto I, MacDonald ST, Selvanayagam JB, et al. Intravascular ultrasound to guide stenting of an anomalous right coronary artery coursing between the aorta and pulmonary artery. J Invasive Cardiol. 2005;17:E33-6.
17. Garcia-Rinaldi R. Right coronary arteries that course between aorta and pulmonary artery. Ann Thorac Surg. 2002;74:973-4.
18. Doorey AJ, Pasquale MJ, Lally JF, et al. Six month success of intracoronary stenting for anomalous coronary arteries associated with myocardial ischemia. Am J Cardiology. 2000;86:580-2.
19. Kim SY, Seo JB, Do KH, et al. Coronary artery anomalies: classification and ECG-gated multi-detector row CT findings with angiographic correlation. Radiographics. 2006;26:317-33.
20. Sevrukov A, Aker N, Sullivan C, et al. Identifying the course of an anomalous left coronary artery using contrast enhanced electron beam tomography and 3D reconstruction. Catheter Cardiovasc Interv. 2002;57:532-6.
21. Luo L, Kebede S, Wu S, et al. Coronary artery fistulae. Am J Med Sci. 2006;332:79-84.
22. Cebi N, Schulze-Waltrup N, FromkeJ, et al. Congenital coronary artery fistulas in adults: concomitant pathologies and treatment. Int J Cardiovasc Imaging. 2008;24:349-55.
23. Alegria JR, Herrmann J, Holmes DR, et al. Myocardial bridging. Eur Heart J. 2005;26:1159-68.
24. Rozenberg V, Nepomnyashchikh L. Pathomorphology of myocardial bridges and their role in the pathogenesis of coronary disease. Bull Exp Biol Med. 2002;134:593-6.
25. Van Herck PL, Gavit L, Gorissen P, et al. Quantitative coronary arteriography on digital flat-panel system. Catheter Cardiovasc Interv. 2004;63:192-200.
26. Kern MJ. Selection of radiocontrast media in cardiac catheterization: comparative physiology and clinical effects of nonionic and ionic dimeric formulations. Am Heart J. 1991;122:195-201.
27. Hirshfield JW. Cardiovascular effects of contrast agents. Am J Cardiol. 1990;66:9F-17F.
28. McClennan BL. Ionic and nonionic iodinated contrast media: evolution and strategies for use. AJR Am J Roentgenol. 1990;155:225-33.
29. Tepel M, va der Geit M, Schwarzfeld C, et al. Prevention of radiographic-contrast-agent-induced reductions in renal function by acetylcysteine. N Engl J Med. 2000;343:180-4.
30. Chu VL, Cheng JW. Fenoldopam in the prevention of contrast media-induced acute renal failure. Ann Pharmacother. 2001;35:1278-82.
31. Silber S. Rapid hemostasis of arterial puncture sites with collagen in patients undergoing diagnostic and interventional cardiac catheterization. Clin Cardiol.1997;20:981-2.
32. Chamberlin JA, Lardi AB, McKeever LS, et al. Use of vascular sealing devices (Vasoseal and Perclose) versus assisted manual compression (Femostop) in transcatheter coronary interventions requiring abciximab (ReoPro). Catheter Cardiovasc Interv. 1999;47:143-7.
33. Sanborn TA, Gibbs HH, Brinker JA, et al. A multicenter randomized trial comparing a percutaneous collagen hemostasis device with conventional manual compression after diagnostic angiography and angioplasty. J Am Coll Cardiol.1993;22:1273-9.
34. Krone RJ, Johnson L, Noto T. Five year trends in cardiac catheterization: a report from the Registry of the Society for Cardiac Angiography and Interventions. Cathet Cardiovasc Diagn. 1996;39:31-5.
35. Trerotola SO, Kuhlman JE, Fishman EK. Bleeding complications of femoral catheterization: CT evaluation. Radiology.1990;174:37-40.
36. Lazar JM, Uretsky BF, Denys BG, et al. Predisposing risk factors and natural history of acute neurologic complications of left-sided cardiac catheterization. Am J Cardiol.1995;75:1056-60.
37. Douglas JS, King SB. Complications of coronary arteriography: management during and following the procedure. In: King SB,

Douglas JS (Eds). Coronary Arteriography. New York: McGraw-Hill; 1984. pp. 302-13.

38. Jolly SS, Amlani S, Hamon M, et al. Radial versus femoral access for coronary angiography or intervention and the impact on major bleeding and ischemic events: a systematic review and meta-analysis of randomized trials. Am Heart J. 2009;157:132-40.

39. Efstathopoulos EP, Karvouni E, Kottou S, et al. Patient dosimetry during coronary interventions: a comprehensive analysis. Am Heart J. 2004;147:468-75.

40. Johnson LW, Moore RJ, Balter S. Review of radiation safety in the cardiac catheterization laboratory. Cathet Cardiovasc Diagn. 1992;25:186-94.

41. Smith S, Feldman TE, Hirshfeld JW, et al. ACC/AHA/SCAI 2005 guideline update for percutaneous coronary intervention: a report of the American College of Cardiology/American Heart Association Task Force on Practice Guidelines (ACC/AHA/SCAI Writing Committee to Update the 2001 Guidelines for Percutaneous Coronary Intervention). J Am Coll Cardiol. 2006;47:e1-121.

42. Krone RJ, Shaw RE, Klein LW, et al. Evaluation of the ACC/AHA/SCAI lesion classification system in the current "stent era" of coronary interventions (from the ACC–National Cardiovascular Data Registry). Am J Cardiol. 2003;92:389-94.

43. Singh M, Rihal CS, Lennon RJ, et al. Comparison of Mayo Clinic risk score and ACC/AHA lesion classification in the prediction of adverse cardiovascular outcome following percutaneous coronary interventions. J Am Coll Cardiol. 2004;44:357-61.

44. Popma J, Leon M, Moses J, et al. Quantitative assessment of angiographic restenosis after sirolimus-eluting stent implantation in native coronary arteries. Circulation. 2004;110:3773-80.

45. Alexander JH, Hafley G, Harrington RA, et al. Efficacy and safety of edifoligide, an E2F transcription factor decoy, for prevention of vein graft failure following coronary artery bypass graft surgery: PREVENT IV: a randomized controlled trial. JAMA. 2005;294:2446-54.

46. Hoye A, Lemos PA. Effectiveness of sirolimus eluting stent in the treatment of saphenous vein graft disease. J Invasive Cardiol. 2004; 16:230-3.

47. Giugliano GR, Kuntz Re, Popma JJ, et al. Determinants of 30 day adverse events following saphenous vein graft intervention with and without a distal occlusion embolic protection device. Am J Cardiol. 2005;95:173-7.

48. White CW, Wright CB, Doty DB, et al. Does visual interpretation of the coronary arteriogram predict the physiologic importance of a coronary stenosis? N Engl J Med. 1984;310:819-24.

49. Kern MJ, Samady H. Current concepts of integrated coronary physiology in the catheterization laboratory. J Am Coll Cardiol. 2010;55:173-85.

50. Qian J, Ge J, Baumgart D, et al. Safety of intracoronary Doppler flow measurement. J Am Heart. 2000;140:502-10.

51. Miller DD, Donohue TJ, Younis LT, et al. Correlation of pharmacological 99mTc-sestamibi myocardial perfusion imaging with poststenotic coronary flow reserve in patients with angiographically intermediate coronary artery stenoses. Circulation. 1994;89:2150-60.

52. Joye JD, Schulman DS, Lasorda D, et al. Intracoronary Doppler guide wire versus stress single-photon emission computed tomographic thallium-201 imaging in assessment of intermediate coronary stenoses. J Am Coll Cardiol. 1994;24:940-7.

53. Chamuleau SA, Tio RA, de Cock CC, et al. Prognostic value of coronary blood flow velocity and myocardial perfusion in intermediate coronary narrowings and multivessel disease. J Am Coll Cardiol. 2002;39:852-8.

54. Leesar MA, Abdul-Baki T, Akkus NI, et al. Use of fractional flow reserve versus stress perfusion scintigraphy after unstable angina. Effect on duration of hospitalization, cost, procedural characteristics and clinical outcome. J Am Coll Cardiol. 2003;41:1115-21.

55. Pijls NH, De Bruyne B, Peels K, et al. Measurement of fractional flow reserve to assess the functional severity of coronary-artery stenoses. N Engl J Med. 1996;334:1703-8.

56. Chamuleau SA, Meuwissen M, Koch KT, et al. Usefulness of fractional flow reserve for risk stratification of patients with multivessel coronary artery disease and an intermediate stenosis. Am J Cardiol. 2002;89:377-80.

57. Tobis J, Azarbal B, Slavin L. Assessment of intermediate severity coronary lesions in the catheterization laboratory. J Am Coll Cardiol. 2007;49:839-48.

58. Tonino PA, De Bruyne B, Pijls NH, et al. Fractional flow reserve versus angiography for guiding percutaneous coronary intervention. N Engl J Med. 2009;360:213-24.

59. Bech GJ, De Bruyne B, Bonnier HJ, et al. Long-term follow-up after deferral of percutaneous transluminal coronary angioplasty of intermediate stenosis on the basis of coronary pressure measurement. J Am Coll Cardiol. 1998;31:841-7.

60. Bech GJ, De Bruyne B, Pijls NH, et al. Fractional flow reserve to determine the appropriateness of angioplasty in moderate coronary stenosis: a randomized trial. Circulation. 2001;103:2928-34.

61. Pijls NH, van Schaardenburgh P, Manoharan G, et al. Percutaneous coronary intervention of functionally nonsignificant stenosis: 5-year follow-up of the DEFER Study. J Am Coll Cardiol. 2007;49:2105-11.

62. Pijls NH, De Bruyne B, Bech GJ, et al. Coronary pressure measurement to assess the hemodynamic significance of serial stenoses within one coronary artery: validation in humans. Circulation. 2000;102:2371-7.

63. Bech GJ, Droste H, Pijls NH, et al. Value of fractional flow reserve in making decisions about bypass surgery for equivocal left main coronary artery disease. Heart. 2001;86:547-52.

64. Courtis J, Rodés-Cabau J, Larose E, et al. Usefulness of coronary fractional flow reserve measurements in guiding clinical decisions in intermediate or equivocal left main coronary stenoses. Am J Cardiol. 2009;103:943-9.

65. Fearon WF, Yeung AC, Lee DP, et al. Cost-effectiveness of measuring fractional flow reserve to guide coronary interventions. Am Heart J. 2003;145:882-7.

66. Pijls NH, Klauss V, Siebert U, et al. Coronary pressure measurement after stenting predicts adverse events at follow-up: a multicenter registry. Circulation. 2002;105:2950-4.

67. A Leone F, Macchiusi A, Ricci R, et al. Acute myocardial infarction from spontaneous coronary artery dissection a case report and review of the literature. Cardiol Rev. 2004;12:3-9.

68. Basso C, Morgagni GL, Thiene G. Spontaneous coronary artery dissection: a neglected cause of acute myocardial ischaemia and sudden death. Heart. 1996;75:451-4.

69. DeMaio SJ, Kinsella SH, Silverman ME. Clinical course and long-term prognosis of spontaneous coronary artery dissection. Am J Cardiol. 1989;64:471-4.

70. Jorgensen MB, Aharonian V, Mansukhani P, et al. Spontaneous coronary dissection: a cluster of cases with this rare finding. Am Heart J. 1994;127:1382-7.

71. Kato H, Inoue O, Kawasaki T, et al. Adult coronary artery disease probably due to childhood Kawasaki disease. Lancet. 1992; 340:1127-9.

72. Burns JC, Shike H, Gordon JB, et al. Sequelae of Kawasaki disease in adolescents and young adults. J Am Coll Cardiol. 1996;28:253-7.

73. Taylor DO, Edwards LB, Boucek MM, et al. Registry of the International Society for Heart and Lung Transplantation: twenty-fourth official adult heart transplant report-2007. J Heart Lung Transplant. 2007;26:769-81.

74. Gao SZ, Alderman EL, Schroeder JS, et al. Accelerated coronary vascular disease in the heart transplant patient: coronary arteriographic findings. J Am Coll Cardiol. 1988;12:334-40.

75. Wellnhofer E, Stypmann J, Bara CL, et al. Angiographic assessment of cardiac allograft vasculopathy: results of a Consensus Conference

of the Task Force for Thoracic Organ Transplantation of the German Cardiac Society. Transpl Int. 2010;23:1094-104.

76. Gao SZ, Alderman EL, Schroeder JS, et al. Progressive coronary luminal narrowing after cardiac transplantation. Circulation. 1990;82:IV269-75.

77. St Goar FG, Pinto FJ, Alderman EL, et al. Detection of coronary atherosclerosis in young adult hearts using intravascular ultrasound. Circulation. 1992;86:756-63.

78. Fang JC, Kinlay S, Wexberg P, et al. Use of the thrombolysis in myocardial infarction frame count for the quantitative assessment of transplant-associated arteriosclerosis. Am J Cardiol. 2000;86:890-2.

79. Baris N, Sipahi I, Kapadia SR, et al. Coronary angiography for follow-up of heart transplant recipients: insights from TIMI frame count and TIMI myocardial perfusion grade. J Heart Lung Transplant. 2007;26:593-7.

80. Mehta S, Yusuf S, Peters R, et al. Effects of pretreatment with clopidogrel and aspirin followed by long-term therapy in patients undergoing percutaneous coronary intervention: the PCI-CURE study. Lancet. 2001;358:527-33.

81. Berger PB, Steinubl S. Clinical implications of percutaneous coronary intervention-clopidogrel in unstable angina to prevent recurrent events (PCI-CURE) study—a U.S. perspective. Circulation. 2002;106:2284-7.

82. Pache J, Kastrati A, Mehilli J, et al. Clopidogrel therapy in patients undergoing coronary stenting: value of a high-loading dose regimen. Catheter Cardiovasc Interv. 2002;55:436-41.

83. Kandzari DE, Berger PB, Kastrati A, et al. Influence of treatment duration with a 600 mg dose of clopidogrel before percutaneous coronary revascularization. J Am Coll Cardiol. 2004;44:2133-6.

84. Cuisset T, Frere C, Quilici J, et al. Benefit of a 600 mg loading dose of clopidogrel on platelet reactivity and clinical outcomes in patients with non-ST-segment elevation acute coronary syndrome undergoing coronary stenting. J Am Coll Cardiol. 2006;48:1339-45.

85. Steinhubl S, Berger PB, Brennan DM, et al. Optimal timing for the initiation of pretreatment with 300 mg clopidogrel before percutaneous coronary intervention. J Am Coll Cardiol. 2006;47:939-43.

86. Steinhubl SR, Berger PB, Mann JT, et al. Early and sustained dual oral antiplatelet therapy following percutaneous coronary interventional: a randomized controlled trial. JAMA. 2002;288:2411-20.

87. Lev EI, Patel RT, Maresh KJ, et al. Aspirin and clopidogrel drug response in patients undergoing percutaneous coronary intervention: the role of dual drug resistance. J Am Coll Cardiol. 2006;47:27-33.

88. Hochholzer W, Trenk D, Bestehorn H, et al. Impact of the degree of peri-interventional platelet inhibition after loading with clopidogrel on early clinical outcome of elective coronary stent placement. J Am Coll Cardiol. 2006;48:1742-50.

89. Wenaweser P, Dorffler-Melly J, Imboden K, et al. Stent thrombosis is associated with an impaired response to antiplatelet therapy. J Am Coll Cardiol. 2005;45:1748-52.

90. Wiviott SD, Trenk D, Frelinger AL, et al. Prasugrel compared with high loading- and maintenance-dose clopidogrel in patients with planned percutaneous coronary intervention: the Prasugrel in Comparison to Clopidogrel for Inhibition of Platelet Activation and Aggregation-Thrombolysis in Myocardial Infarction 44 Trial. Circulation. 2007;116:2923-32.

91. Wiviott SD, Braunwald E, McCabe CH, et al. Prasugrel versus clopidogrel in patients with acute coronary syndromes. N Engl J Med. 2007;357:2001-15.

92. Mega JL, Close SL, Wiviott SD, et al. Cytochrome P450 genetic polymorphisms and the response to prasugrel: relationship to pharmacokinetic, pharmacodynamic, and clinical outcomes. Circulation. 2009;119:2553-60.

93. James S, Akerblom A, Cannon CP, et al. Comparison of ticagrelor, the first reversible oral P2Y12 receptor antagonist, with clopidogrel in patients with acute coronary syndromes: rationale, design, and

94. Wallentin L, Becker RC, Budaj A, et al. Ticagrelor versus clopidogrel in patients with acute coronary syndromes. N Engl J Med. 2009;361:1045-57.

95. The EPIC Investigators. Use of a monoclonal antibody directed against the platelet glycoprotein IIb/IIIa receptor in high-risk coronary angioplasty. N Engl J Med. 1994;330:956-61.

96. PRICE Investigators. Comparative 30-day economic and clinical outcomes of platelet glycoprotein IIb/IIIa inhibitor use during elective percutaneous coronary intervention: Prairie ReoPro versus Integrilin Cost Evaluation (PRICE) Trial. Am Heart J. 2001;141:402-9.

97. Topol EJ, Ferguson JJ, Weisman HF, et al. Long-term protection from myocardial ischemic events after brief integrin beta3 blockade with percutaneous coronary intervention. JAMA.1997;278:479-84.

98. Karvouni E, Katritsis DG, Ioannidis JP. Intravenous glycoprotein IIb/IIIa receptor antagonists reduce mortality after percutaneous coronary interventions. J Am Coll Cardiol. 2003;41:26-32.

99. Kastrati A, Mehilli J, Neumann FJ, et al. Abciximab in patients with acute coronary syndromes undergoing percutaneous coronary intervention after clopidogrel pretreatment: the ISAR-REACT 2 randomized trial. JAMA. 2006;295:1531-8.

100. Gurm HS, Tamhane U, Meier P, et al. A comparison of abciximab and small-molecule glycoprotein IIb/IIIa inhibitors in patients undergoing primary percutaneous coronary intervention: a meta-analysis of contemporary randomized controlled trials. Circ Cardiovasc Interv. 2009;2:230-6.

101. De Luca G, Ucci G, Cassetti E, et al. Benefits from small molecule administration as compared with abciximab among patients with ST-segment elevation myocardial infarction treated with primary angioplasty: a meta-analysis. J Am Coll Cardiol. 2009;3:1668-73.

102. Van't Hof AW, Ten Berg J, Heestermans T, et al. Prehospital initiation of tirofiban in patients with ST-elevation myocardial infarction undergoing primary angioplasty (On-TIME 2): amulticentre, double-blind, randomised controlled trial. Lancet. 2008;372:537-46.

103. Mehilli J, Kastrati A, Schulz S, et al. Abciximab in patients with acute ST-segment-elevation myocardial infarction undergoing primary percutaneous coronary intervention after clopidogrel loading: a randomized double-blind trial. Circulation. 2009;119:1933-40.

104. Stone GW, Witzenbichler B, Guagliumi G, et al. Bivalirudin during primary PCI in acute myocardial infarction. N Engl J Med. 2008;358:2218-30.

105. Puma JA, Banko LT, Pieper KS, et al. Clinical characteristics predict benefits from eptifibatide therapy during coronary stenting: insights from the Enhanced Suppression of the Platelet IIb/IIIa Receptor with Integrilin Therapy (ESPRIT) Trial. J Am Coll Cardiol. 2006;47:715-8.

106. Hirsh J, Warkentin TE, Raschke R, et al. Heparin and low-molecular-weight heparin: mechanisms of action, pharmacokinetics, dosing considerations, monitoring, efficacy and safety. Chest. 1998;114: 489S-510S.

107. Chew DP, Bhatt DL, Lincoff AM, et al. Defining the optimal activated clotting time during percutaneous coronary intervention: aggregate results from 6 randomized, controlled trials. Circulation. 2001;103: 961-6.

108. Oltrona L, Eisenberg PR, Lasala JM, et al. Association of heparin-resistant thrombin activity with acute ischemic complications of coronary interventions. Circulation. 1996;94:2064-71.

109. Ferguson JJ, Califf RM, Antman EM, et al. Enoxaparin vs unfractionated heparin in high-risk patients with non-ST-segment elevation acute coronary syndromes managed with an intended early invasive strategy: primary results of the SYNERGY randomized trial. JAMA. 2004;292:45-54.

110. Bhatt DL, Lee BI, Casterella PJ, et al. Safety of concomitant therapy with eptifibatide and enoxaparin in patients undergoing percutaneous coronary intervention: results of the Coronary Revascularization using

Integrilin and Single bolus Enoxaparin Study. J Am Coll Cardiol. 2003;41:20-5.

111. Chew DP, Bhatt DL, Kimball W, et al. Bivalirudin provides increasing benefit with decreasing renal function: a meta-analysis of randomized trials. Am J Cardiol. 2003;92:919-23.

112. Dotter CT, Judkins MP. Transluminal treatment of arteriosclerotic obstruction. Description of new technique. Circulation. 1964;30:654-70.

113. Sutton JM, Ellis SG, Roubin GS, et al. Major clinical events after coronary stenting. The multicenter registry of acute and elective Gianturco-Roubin stent placement. The Gianturco-Roubin Intracoronary Stent Investigator Group. Circulation. 1994;89:1126-37.

114. George BS, Voorhees WD, Roubin GS. Multicenter investigation of coronary stenting to treat acute or threatened closure after percutaneous transluminal coronary angioplasty: clinical and angiographic outcomes. J Am Coll Cardiol. 1993;22:135-43.

115. Fischman DL, Leon MB, Baim DS, et al. A randomized comparison of coronary-stent placement and balloon angioplasty in the treatment of coronary artery disease. Stent Restenosis Study Investigators. N Engl J Med. 1994;331:496-501.

116. Anderson HV, Shaw RE, Brindis RG, et al. A contemporary overview of percutaneous coronary interventions. The American College of Cardiology-National Cardiovascular Data Registry (ACC-NCDR). J Am Coll Cardiol. 2002;39:1096-103.

117. Serruys PW, de Jaegere P, Kiemeneij OF, et al. A comparison of balloon-expandable-stent implantation with balloon angioplasty in patients with coronary artery disease. Benestent Study Group. N Engl J Med. 1994;331:489-95.

118. Bermejo J, Botas J, García E, et al. Mechanisms of residual lumen stenosis after high-pressure stent implantation: a quantitative coronary angiography and intravascular ultrasound study. Circulation. 1998;98:112-8.

119. Cutlip DE, Leon MB, Ho KK, et al. Acute and nine-month clinical outcomes after "suboptimal" coronary stenting: results from the STent Anti-thrombotic Regimen Study (STARS) registry. J Am Coll Cardiol. 1999;34:698-706.

120. Briguori C, Sheiban I, De Gregorio J, et al. Direct coronary stenting without predilation. J Am Coll Cardiol. 1999;34:1910-5.

121. Wilson SH, Berger PB, Mathew V, et al. Immediate and late outcomes after direct stent implantation without balloon predilation. J Am Coll Cardiol. 2000;35:937-43.

122. Carrié D, Khalifé K, Citron B, et al. Comparison of direct coronary stenting with and without balloon predilatation in patients with stable angina pectoris. BET (Benefit Evaluation of Direct Coronary Stenting) Study Group. Am J Cardiol. 2001;87:693-8.

123. Nakamura S, Colombo A, Gaglione A, et al. Intracoronary ultrasound observations during stent implantation. Circulation. 1994;89:2026-34.

124. Fearon WF, Luna J, Samady H, et al. Fractional flow reserve compared with intravascular ultrasound guidance for optimizing stent deployment. Circulation. 2001;104:1917-22.

125. Ali A, Cox D, Dib N, et al. Rheolytic thrombectomy with percutaneous coronary intervention for infarct size reduction in acute myocardial infarction: 30-day results from a multicenter randomized study. J Am Coll Cardiol. 2006;48:244-52.

126. Svilaas T, Vlaar PJ, van der HorstI C, et al. Thrombus aspiration during primary percutaneous coronary intervention.N Engl J Med. 2008;358:557-67.

127. Bavry AA, Kumbhani DJ, Bhatt DL. Role of adjunctive thrombectomy and embolic protection devices in acute myocardial infarction: a comprehensive meta-analysis of randomized trials. Eur Heart J. 2008;29:2989-3001.

128. O'Neill WW. Mechanical rotational atherectomy. J Am Coll Cardiol. 1992;69:12F-8F.

129. Ellis SG, Popma JJ, Buchbinder M, et al. Relation of clinical presentation, stenosis morphology, and operator technique to procedural results of rotational atherectomy. Circulation. 1994;89:882-902.

130. Teirstein PS, Warth DC, Haq N, et al. High speed rotational coronary atherectomy for patients with diffuse coronary artery disease. J Am Coll cardiol. 1991;18:1694-701.

131. Whitlow PL, Bass TA, Kipperman RM, et al. Results of the study to determine rotablator and transluminal angioplasty strategy (STRATAS). Am J Cardiol. 2001;87:699-705.

132. Safian RD, Feldman T, Muller DW, et al. Coronary angioplasty and Rotablator atherectomy trial (CARAT): immediate and late results of a prospective multicenter randomized trial. Catheter Cardiovasc Interv. 2001;53:213-20.

133. Dill T, Dietz U, Hamm CW, et al. A randomized comparison of balloon angioplasty versus rotational atherectomy in complex coronary lesions. Eur Heart J. 2000;21:1759-66.

134. Mauri L, Reisman M, Buchbinder M, et al. Comaparision of rotational atherectomy with conventional balloon angioplasty in prevention of restenosis of small coronary arteries. Am Heart J. 2003;145:847-54.

135. Sharma SK, Dangas G, Mehran R, et al. Risk factors for the development of slow flow during rotational coronary atherectomy. Am J Cardiol. 1997;80:219-22.

136. Virmani R, Liistro F, Stankovic G, et al. Mechanism of Late in-stent restenosis after implantation of paclitaxel derivative eluting polymer stent system in humans. Circulation. 2002;106:2649-51.

137. Saber RS, Edwards WD, Bailey KR, et al. Coronary embolization after balloon angioplasty or thrombolytic therapy: an autopsy study of 32 cases. J Am Coll Cardiol. 1993;22:1283-8.

138. Topol EJ, Yadav JS. Recognition of the importance of embolization in atherosclerotic vascular disease. Circulation. 2000;101:570-80.

139. Baim DS, Wahr D, George B, et al. randomized trial of a distal embolic protection device during percutaneous intervention of saphenous vein aorto-coronary bypass graft. Circulation. 2002;105:1285-90.

140. Mourish G, Soulez A, Roger C, et al. Proximal trial presentation. Transcatheter Therapeutics. Washington DC; 2005.

141. Parisi AF, Folland ED, Hartigan P. A comparison of angioplasty with medical therapy in the treatment of single-vessel coronary artery disease. N Engl J Med.1992;326:10-6.

142. Boden WE, O'Rourke RA, Crawford MH, et al. Outcomes in patients with acute non-Q-wave myocardial infarction randomly assigned to an invasive as compared with a conservative management strategy. N Engl J Med. 1998;338:1785-92.

143. Pocock SJ, Henderson RA, Rickards AF, et al. Meta-analysis of randomized trials comparing coronary angioplasty with bypass surgery. Lancet. 1995;346:1184-9.

144. Sim I, Gupta M, McDonald K, et al. A meta-analysis of randomized trials comparing coronary artery bypass grafting with percutaneous transluminal coronary angioplasty in multivessel coronary artery disease. Am J Cardiol. 1995;76:1025-9.

145. Ormiston JA, Stewart FM, Roche AH, et al. Late regression of the dilated site after coronary angioplasty: a 5-year quantitative angiographic study. Circulation. 1997;96:468-74.

146. Guiteras-Val P, Varas-Lorenzo C, Garcia-Picart J, et al. Clinical and sequential angiographic follow-up six months and 10 years after successful percutaneous transluminal coronary angioplasty. Am J Cardiol. 1999;83:868-74.

147. Cannan CR, Yeh W, Kelsey SF, et al. Incidence and predictors of target vessel revascularization following percutaneous transluminal coronary angioplasty: a report from the National Heart, Lung and Blood Institute Percutaneous Transluminal Coronary Angioplasty Registry. Am J Cardiol. 1999;84:170.

148. Cutlip DE, Chauhan MS, Baim DS, et al. Clinical restenosis after coronary stenting: perspectives from multicenter clinical trials. J Am Coll Cardiol. 2002;40:2082-9.

149. Costa MA, Simon DI. Molecular basis of restenosis and drug-eluting stents. Circulation. 2005;111:2257-73.

150. Stettler C, Wandel S, Allemann S, et al. Outcomes associated with drug-eluting and bare-metal stents: a collaborative network meta-analysis. Lancet. 2007;370:937-48.

151. Schofer J, Schlüter M, Gershlick AH, et al. Sirolimus-eluting stents for treatment of patients with long atherosclerotic lesions in small coronary arteries: double-blind, randomized controlled trial (E-SIRIUS). Lancet. 2003;362:1093-9.

152. Cohen HA, Williams DO, Holmes DR, et al. Use of drug-eluting stents in contemporary interventions: a comparison to bare metal stent use in the National Heart, Lung and Blood Institute Dynamic Registry (abstract). J Am Coll Cardiol. 2005;45:63A.

153. Williams DO, Abbott JD, Kip KE, DEScover Investigators. Outcomes of 6906 patients undergoing percutaneous coronary intervention in the era of drug-eluting stents: report of the DEScover Registry. Circulation. 2006;114:2154-62.

154. Kedhi E, Joesoef KS, McFadden E, et al. Second-generation everolimus-eluting and paclitaxel-eluting stents in real-life practice (COMPARE): a randomised trial. Lancet. 2010;375:201-9.

155. Tu JV, Bowen J, Chiu M, et al. Effectiveness and safety of drug-eluting stents in Ontario. N Engl J Med. 2007;357:1393-402.

156. Abbott JD, Voss MR, Nakamura M, et al. Unrestricted use of drug-eluting stents compared with bare-metal stents in routine clinical practice: findings from the National Heart, Lung and Blood Institute Dynamic Registry. J Am Coll Cardiol. 2007;50:2029-36.

157. Marroquin OC, Selzer F, Mulukutla SR, et al. A comparison of bare-metal and drug-eluting stents for off-label indications. N Engl J Med. 2008;358:342-52.

158. Win HK, Caldera AE, Maresh K, et al. Clinical outcomes and stent thrombosis following off-label use of drug-eluting stents. JAMA. 2007;297:2001-9.

159. Serruys PW, Ruygrok P, Neuzner J, et al. A randomised comparison of an everolimus-eluting coronary stent with a paclitaxel-eluting coronary stent: the SPIRIT II trial. Euro Intervention. 2006;2:286-94.

160. Park KW, Yoon JH, Kim JS, et al. Efficacy of Xience/promus versus Cypher in rEducing Late Loss after stENTing (EXCELLENT) trial: study design and rationale of a Korean multicenter prospective randomized trial. Am Heart J. 2009;157:811-7.

161. Schömig A, Dibra A, Windecker S, et al. A meta-analysis of 16 randomized trials of sirolimus-eluting stents versus paclitaxel-eluting stents in patients with coronary artery disease. J Am Coll Cardiol. 2007;50:1373-80.

162. Simonton CA, Brodie B, Cheek B, et al. Comparative clinical outcomes of paclitaxel- and sirolimus-eluting stents: results from a large prospective multicenter registry—STENT Group. J Am Coll Cardiol. 2007;50:1214-22.

163. Ong AT, Serruys PW, Aoki J, et al. The unrestricted use of paclitaxel-versus sirolimus-eluting stents for coronary artery disease in an unselected population: one-year results of the Taxus-Stent Evaluated at Rotterdam Cardiology Hospital (T-SEARCH) registry. J Am Coll Cardiol. 2005;45:1135-41.

164. Eisenstein EL, Leon MB, Kandzari DE, et al. Long-term clinical and economic analysis of the Endeavor zotarolimus-eluting stent versus the cypher sirolimus-eluting stent: 3-year results from the ENDEAVOR III trial (Randomized Controlled Trial of the Medtronic Endeavor Drug [ABT-578] Eluting Coronary Stent System Versus the Cypher Sirolimus-Eluting Coronary Stent System in De Novo Native Coronary Artery Lesions). JACC Cardiovasc Interv. 2009;2:1199.

165. Carrozza JP. Sirolimus-eluting stents: does a great stent still need a good interventionalist? J Am Coll Cardiol. 2004;43:1116-7.

166. Lemos PA, Saia F, Ligthart JM, et al. Coronary restenosis after sirolimus-eluting stent implantation: morphological description and mechanistic analysis from a consecutive series of cases. Circulation. 2003;108:257-60.

167. Fujii K, Mintz GS, Kobayashi Y, et al. Contribution of stent under-expansion to recurrence after sirolimus-eluting stent implantation for in-stent restenosis. Circulation. 2004;109:1085-8.

168. Takebayashi H, Kobayashi Y, Mintz GS, et al. Intravascular ultrasound assessment of lesions with target vessel failure after sirolimus-eluting stent implantation. Am J Cardiol. 2005;95:498-502.

169. Moses JW, Leon MB, Popma JJ, et al. Sirolimus-eluting stents versus standard stents in patients with stenosis in a native coronary artery. N Engl J Med. 2003;349:1315-23.

170. Lemos PA, Hoye A, Goedhart D, et al. Clinical, angiographic, and procedural predictors of angiographic restenosis after sirolimus-eluting stent implantation in complex patients: an evaluation from the Rapamycin-Eluting Stent Evaluated At Rotterdam Cardiology Hospital (RESEARCH) study. Circulation. 2004;109:1366-70.

171. Stone GW, Ellis SG, Colombo A, et al. Offsetting impact of thrombosis and restenosis on the occurrence of death and myocardial infarction after paclitaxel-eluting and bare metal stent implantation. Circulation. 2007;115:2842-7.

172. Garg P, Cohen DJ, Gaziano T, et al. Balancing the risks of restenosis and stent thrombosis in bare-metal versus drug-eluting stents: results of a decision analytic model. J Am Coll Cardiol. 2008;51:1844-53.

173. Ko DT, Chiu M, Guo H, et al. Safety and effectiveness of drug-eluting and bare-metal stents for patients with off- and on-label indications. J Am Coll Cardiol. 2009;53:1773-82.

174. Mauri L, Silbaugh TS, Wolf RE, et al. Long-term clinical outcomes after drug-eluting and bare-metal stenting in Massachusetts. Circulation. 2008;118:1817-27.

175. Hannan EL, Racz M, Holmes DR, et al. Comparison of coronary artery stenting outcomes in the eras before and after the introduction of drug-eluting stents. Circulation. 2008;117:2071-8.

176. Groeneveld PW, Matta MA, Greenhut AP, et al. Drug-eluting compared with bare-metal coronary stents among elderly patients. J Am Coll Cardiol. 2008;51:2017-24.

177. Brilakis ES, Lichtenwalter C, Banerjee S, et al. Continued benefit from paclitaxel-eluting compared with bare-metal stent implantation in saphenous vein graft lesions during long-term follow-up of the SOS (Stenting of Saphenous Vein Grafts) trial. JACC Cardiovasc Interv. 2011;4:176-82.

178. Smith SC, Feldman TE, Hirshfeld JW, et al. ACC/AHA/SCAI 2005 Guideline Update for Percutaneous Coronary Intervention—summary article: a report of the American College of Cardiology/American Heart Association Task Force on Practice Guidelines (ACC/AHA/SCAI Writing Committee to Update the 2001 Guidelines for Percutaneous Coronary Intervention). Circulation. 2006;113:156.

179. Maynard C, Chapko C, et al. Percutaneous transluminal angioplasty: report of complications from National Heart, Lung, and Blood Institute PTCA registry. Circulation. 1983;67:723-30.

180. Black AJR, Namay DL, Niederman AL, et al. Tear of dissection after coronary angioplasty: morphologic correlates of an ischemic complication. Circulation. 1989;79:1035-42.

181. Ellis SG, Roubin GS, King SB, et al. Angiographic and clinical predictors of acute closure after native vessel coronary angioplasty. Circulation. 1988;77:372-9.

182. Gruberg L, Pinnow E, Flood R, et al. Incidence, management, and outcome of coronary artery perforation during percutaneous coronary intervention. Am J Cardiol. 2000;86:680-2.

183. Ellis SG, Ajluni S, Arnold AZ, et al. Increased coronary perforation in the new device era. Incidence, classification, management, and outcome. Circulation. 1994;90:2725-30.

184. Kaplan BM, Benzuly KH, Kinn JW, et al. Treatment of no-reflow in degenerated SVG interventions: comparison of intracoronary verapamil and nitroglycerine. Cathet Cardiovasc Diagn. 1996;39:113-8.

185. Bergelson BA, Fishman RF, Tomasso CL, et al. Abrupt vessel closure: changing importance, management and consequences. Am heart J. 1997;134:362-81.

CHAPTER 28

Coronary Angiography and Catheter-based Coronary Intervention

ELECTROPHYSIOLOGY

Arrhythmia Mechanisms

Mark Anderson

Chapter Outline

- Arrhythmia Initiation
  - Molecular and Cellular Mechanisms
  - Action Potentials Require Orchestrated Ion Channel Opening and Inactivation
  - Action Potential Physiology is a Consequence of Ion Channel and Cellular Properties
  - Action Potentials are Designed for Automaticity and to Initiate Contraction

- Action Potential Physiology is Reflected by the Surface Electrocardiogram
- Afterdepolarizations and Triggered Arrhythmias
- Proarrhythmic Substrates
- Proarrhythmic Triggers and Substrates are Promoted in Failing Hearts

INTRODUCTION

Arrhythmias require initiating conditions and a hospitable substrate for perpetuation. Triggers and substrates are often considered as unrelated or independent events. However, new findings suggest that triggers and substrates may be connected, particularly in structural heart disease, by hyperactivity of signaling molecules, intracellular Ca^{2+} and reactive oxygen species (ROS).[1] There is now a body of evidence to support a view that the increased ROS and disturbed intracellular Ca^{2+} homeostasis that mark structural heart disease contribute to arrhythmia initiation, while actively promoting a proarrhythmic substrate. Ion channels are the fundamental effectors that determine membrane currents and arrhythmias, but ion channels are regulated by multiple factors in myocardium, including intracellular Ca^{2+}, phosphorylation and ROS. These same factors participate in responses to common forms of myocardial injury, including ischemia and infarction, which lead to proarrhythmic adaptations in myocardium. This chapter will briefly review ion channel biology, genetic diseases of ion channels, and cellular and tissue arrhythmia mechanisms in an effort to present a broad, but comprehensible, approach to understanding arrhythmia mechanisms.

At a basic level, much of our understanding is due to studies in reduced systems (e.g. isolated heart muscle cells or non-cardiac cells heterologously expressing ion channel proteins) and animal models. However, many key arrhythmia mechanisms, including afterdepolarizations[2,3] and reentry[4] have been identified in patients. In fact, clinical studies and therapies, particularly ablation of focal and reentrant arrhythmias have provided strong evidence for fundamental concepts first formulated from analysis of animal studies. However, not all basic knowledge supporting discussion in this chapter has been translated to and validated in patients.

ARRHYTHMIA INITIATION

MOLECULAR AND CELLULAR MECHANISMS

Ion channels and exchangers are the fundamental units directing physiological and pathological membrane excitability and conduction.

Equation 1:

$$E = \frac{RT}{zF} \ln \frac{[\text{ion outside cell}]}{[\text{ion inside cell}]} = 2.303 \frac{RT}{zF} \log_{10} \frac{[\text{ion outside cell}]}{[\text{ion inside cell}]}$$

Nernst Equation E-equilibrium potential or Nernst potential is the cell membrane potential that is necessary to oppose the diffusion of an ion across the cell membrane as motivated by the concentration gradient of each ion (R—universal gas constant; T—temperature in degrees Kelvin; z—valence: F—Faraday's constant). At 25°C, $RT/F = 25.693$ mV.

Selective membrane permeability coupled with active pumps (ATPases) allow for an electrochemical gradient across cell membranes. The Nernst equation[5] is a powerful, but simplified (i.e. relies exclusively on two ions), description of a half cell that predicts how ionic gradients determine cell membrane potential. The maintenance of Na^+ and K^+ gradients under conditions of selective membrane permeability requires a Na^+ and K^+ 'pump'—the Na^+/K^+ ATPase. The Na^+/K^+ pump transports extracellular Na^+ $[Na^+]_o$ and intracellular K^+ $[K^+]_i$ against their concentration gradients, a process that requires energy input from ATP hydrolysis. The Na^+/K^+ ATPase is required to maintain physiological $[Na^+]_o$ (~ 145 mM), $[K^+]_o$ (~ 4 mM) and $[Na^+]_i$ (~ 10 mM), $[K^+]_i$ (~ 140 mM) in the face of the tendency of these gradients to dissipate with repetitive opening of Na^+ and K^+ channel proteins. Under resting conditions myocardial cell membrane potentials approximate

566 the equilibrium potential for K⁺, ~ –90 mV, where the cytosolic side of the membrane is negative and the extracellular side of the membrane is positive, because the cell membrane permeability is greatest for K⁺ under resting conditions. The resting membrane permeability to K⁺ occurs because a particular ion channel, the inward rectifier, opens at the negative potentials present in resting membranes.

Equation 2:

$$E_{eq,K^+} = \frac{RT}{zF} \ln \frac{[K^+]_o}{[K^+]_i},$$

Nernst Equation for K⁺.

The resting membrane potential is highly dependent upon $[K^+]_o$ and the resting membrane potential determines membrane excitability in part because voltage-gated Na⁺ channels (mostly $Na_V1.5$) begin to inactivate at membrane potentials more positive than –100 mV. At 37 °C (~ 310 °K) the equilibrium potential for K⁺ (Eeq, K⁺) is –91 mV for $[K^+]_o$ = 4.5 mM and $[K^+]_i$ = 140 mM. If the $[K^+]_o$ is reduced to 2.5 mM the Eeq, K⁺ is –107.5 mV (and more $Na_V1.5$ channels are available to activate), and if the $[K^+]_o$ = 6.5 mM, the Eeq, K⁺ is –82 mV (with reduced $Na_V1.5$ channel availability). Thus, the Nernst equation provides quantitative insight into the importance of K⁺ homeostasis for normal cardiac electrophysiology.

Ion channels are protein complexes embedded in cell membranes (Figs 1A to D). All ion channels consist of a pore forming α subunit (Figs 1A to C). Some α subunits (e.g. K⁺ channels) aggregate with identical or similar α subunits to form a cell membrane spanning pore. This pore is the conductance pathway that allows individual ions to cross lipid bilayer membranes with high throughput. Ion channels are configured for relative ion selectivity. The specific amino acids lining the pore create a 'filter' that selects ionic species for conductance

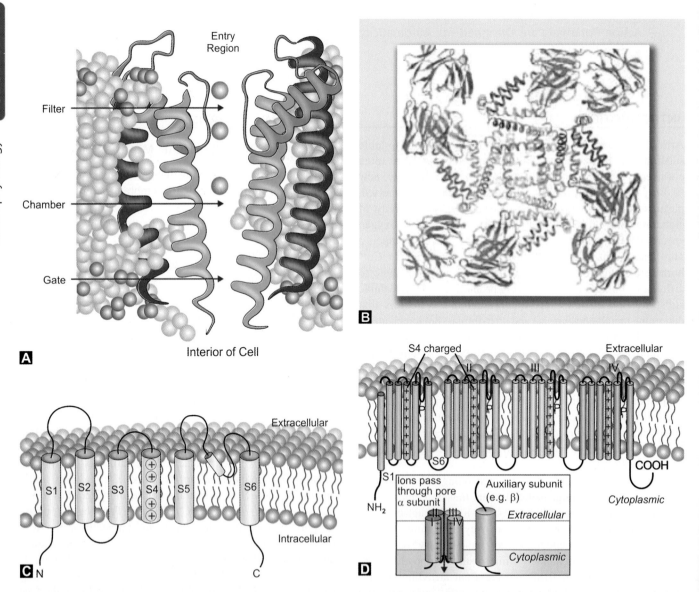

FIGURES 1A TO D: Ion channels are proteins that form a conductance pore through bilayer lipid cell membranes. (A) A ribbon diagram representation of the pore forming α subunit for a bacterial voltage-gated K⁺ channel viewed from the side. (B) Ribbon diagram of a voltage-gated K⁺ channel viewed from above. This view shows the fourfold symmetry of α subunit proteins that assemble to form a conductance pore for K⁺ (center). (C) Schematic representation of a voltage-gated K⁺ channel α subunit showing the voltage sensor (S4) and the pore (P) loop between S5 and S6. (D) A schematic representation of a voltage-gated Na⁺ or Ca^{2+} channel that is similar to four concatenated K⁺ channel α subunits

based on ionic size and charge. In solution ions are effectively larger due to a sphere of hydration that is a result of charge-associated water molecules. The selectivity filter in ion channels may remove water (dehydrate) from permeant ions as a requirement for passage through the conductance pore. Other α subunits are formed from a single large protein (e.g. Na^+ and Ca^{2+} channels). Ion channels open and close in response to a blend of various stimuli. In contracting atrial and ventricular myocardium and in specialized pacemaking [sinoatrial node (SAN)] and conduction tissue (atrioventricular node and His-Purkinje system) the most important and best understood ion channels are primarily opened by changes in membrane potential. These so-called 'voltage-gated ion channels' all contain a cell membrane spanning domain enriched in charged amino acids that act as a membrane voltage sensor (Figs 1C and D). The voltage sensor moves in response to changes in the membrane potential, and these movements are allosterically coupled to the pore domain. Voltage-gated ion channels open and close in response to a change in membrane potential, but also inactivate. Inactivation appears to be the result of various protein conformations that hinder the availability of the pore domain to open in response to a voltage stimulus, before the ion channel is 'reset' by recovering from the state of inactivation. Importantly, voltage-gated ion channels respond to additional factors, including amino acid phosphorylation and oxidation, which influence the probability of ion channels to open (Fig. 2A).

The voltage dependence of ionic current carried by voltage-dependent ion channels and exchangers is often presented as a current-voltage (I-V) relationship (Figs 2B and C). The I-V relationship is obtained in voltage-clamped cells or tissue, typically under conditions designed to isolate individual currents (e.g. by controlling the ionic constituents in the intracellular and extracellular solutions, addition of antagonist drugs or pore blocking ions, or by heterologous expression of individual ionic channels in non-excitable cells by gene transfection). The I-V relationships can reveal important ion channel behaviors such as the voltage dependence of activation and inactivation, ion selectivity, rectification and conductance. Voltage-gated ion channels activate and inactivate over a range of membrane potentials. In some cases, the voltage-range of activation and inactivation permits a 'window current' where ion channels can reactivate (Fig. 2D). An important window for voltage-gated Ca^{2+} channel (Ca_V1) currents (I_{Ca}) occurs during the membrane potentials present during the AP plateau. Excessive Ca_V1 window currents are a cause of triggered arrhythmias. Many ion channels (e.g. Na_V, K_V and Ca_V) have a very high selectivity for their namesake ions under physiological conditions. For example, K^+ channels are greater than 1,000 times more likely to conduct K^+ compared to Na^+. A simple, Ohmic, I-V relationship is linear with the line crossing through the zero point (Fig. 2B). However, the I-V relationship of most ion channels in heart is complex, and curvilinear (Fig. 2C). The point of current reversal, or equilibrium potential (mV), can be calculated by the Nernst equation: ~ +60 for Na^+, ~ –98 for K^+ and ~ +130 for Ca^{2+} under physiological conditions. The I-V relationship is influenced by the electrochemical gradient, which determines where a current transitions from inward to outward (as referenced to the cell membrane and cytoplasm). Convention

holds that inward currents are negative and outward currents are positive. The I-V relationship is also affected by a property of some ion channels called rectification. Rectification is the tendency of a current to conduct preferentially inwardly or outwardly. A prominent example is the inwardly rectifying K^+ current (I_{K1}) that is crucial for determining resting membrane potential in myocardium. I_{K1} exhibits a pronounced inward rectification that is most evident at very negative membrane potentials. However, the physiologically relevant outward current is relatively small and is present near the resting membrane potential (Fig. 2E). Ion channel current is determined by gating properties, including opening probability, conductance, rectification, the electrochemical gradient of a particular ion and ion selectivity. Some ion channels may assume more than a single conductance (i.e. a subconductance state). The Ca^{2+}-gated ryanodine receptor Ca^{2+} channel has multiple subconductance states. Ion channel activity is also regulated by ions (e.g. Ca^{2+} and H^+), oxidation and phosphorylation.

Ion channel α subunits do not exist or operate in isolation. Accessory subunit proteins, often labeled as β, δ and γ, comprise the ion channel macromolecular complex. These accessory subunits may serve as chaperones to increase expression of α subunit proteins on the cell membrane. Accessory subunits are also targets for regulatory proteins, such as kinases and phosphatases, and may influence the probability of α subunits to open in response to a voltage stimulus. Ion channel macromolecular complexes require precise localization in the cellular ultrastructure to function properly. For example, voltage-gated Ca^{2+} channels, Ca_V1, are enriched in T-tubular membranes across from intracellular Ca^{2+} channels called ryanodine receptors (RyR2) that control Ca^{2+} release from the sarcoplasmic reticulum (SR) (Fig. 3).[6,7] Distortion of the relationship of Ca_V1 and RyR channels occurs in heart failure and contributes to loss of normal intracellular Ca^{2+} homeostasis, mechanical dysfunction and promotes arrhythmia-initiating afterdepolarizations.[8] Cytoskeletal proteins also contribute to ion channel disposition and localization, and cytoskeletal diseases, such as the ankyrin syndromes,[9,10] cause arrhythmias and other pathological phenotypes in excitable cells in brain and pancreas.

The current view of ion channel structure and function arose using three fundamental investigational approaches. The first was a combination of voltage clamp and mathematical modeling. Voltage clamp uses an operational amplifier with feedback control to 'clamp' a cell membrane at a command potential. By controlling cell membrane potential and the concentration of ions in the cell interior and exterior, it was possible to study individual macroscopic currents that arose from all the ion channels of a particular type operating together on the cell membrane. Originally, voltage clamp studies were focused on very large excitable cells, such as the squid giant axon, which were amenable to early techniques such as Vaseline gap and intracellular electrodes. Hodgkin and Huxley used data obtained in squid axon to develop a model of ion channel physiology that postulated 'gates' for activation and inactivation.[11] Their studies provided a conceptual and quantitative framework for understanding ion channels that has endured, albeit with modifications, into the modern era. In 1981, Hammell et al. published the first description of voltage clamp studies using the patch clamp technique (Figs 4A to D).[12] Cardiac myocytes

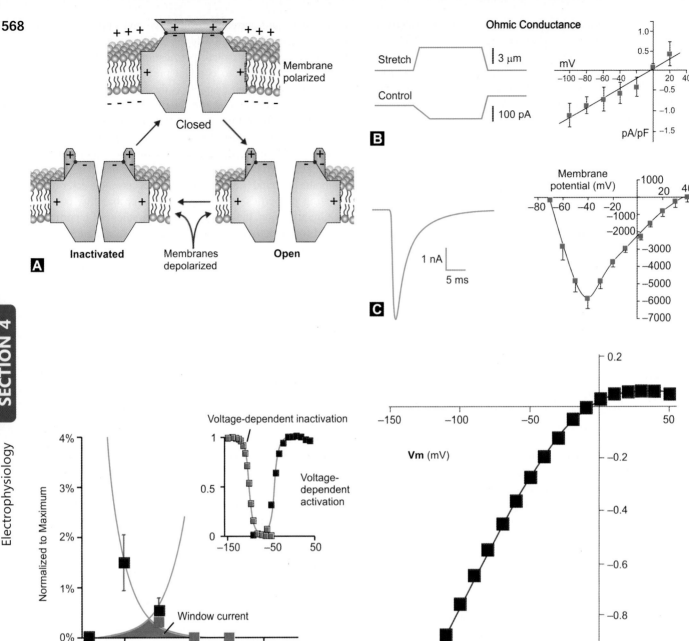

FIGURES 2A TO E: Ion channel gating is the process that determines the probability of an α subunit being available to conduct ionic current. (A) A schematic representation of basic gating states: open; closed and inactivated for a voltage-gated ion channel. (B) Examples of a non-rectifying, stretch-activated ionic current (left). The current, normalized to membrane surface area, (pA/pF)-voltage (mV) relationship for this current shows an Ohmic conductance that is linear and passes through zero. (C) The left panel shows an example of a voltage-gated Na^+ current that activates rapidly (inward deflection) and then rapidly inactivates (resolution of the inward current back to baseline within a few milliseconds). The right panel shows the parabolic current-voltage relationship that is characteristic of voltage-gated Na^+ current in myocardium. (D) An example of a 'window current' for voltage-gated Na^+ channels. The shaded overlap between the voltage-dependent loss of Na^+ channel availability to open (inactivation, pink boxes) and voltage-dependent Na^+ channel activation (purple boxes) is the window current. (E) An example of a current-voltage relationship for an inwardly rectifying K^+ channel current (I_{K1})

were the subject of one of the first studies using patch clamp that described currents flowing through individual ion channels.[13] Patch clamp allowed for high resistance, giga-Ohm, seals between a glass microelectrode and the cell membrane. This high resistance seal allowed resolution of the extremely small currents associated with individual ion channels (in the pico-Ampere range for Ca_V). Patch clamp used in the whole

cell mode allowed investigators to measure macroscopic currents in single cells grown in culture or isolated from tissue, and to control intracellular contents by dialysis of an investigator-selected solution. Modern molecular biology techniques of gene cloning and expression were developed after voltage clamp.[14] Expression of wild type and mutant ion channels studied in non-native and native cells allowed investigators to determine the

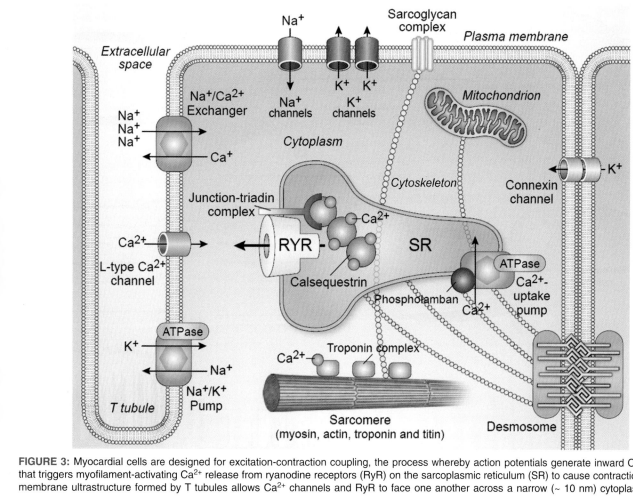

FIGURE 3: Myocardial cells are designed for excitation-contraction coupling, the process whereby action potentials generate inward Ca^{2+} current that triggers myofilament-activating Ca^{2+} release from ryanodine receptors (RyR) on the sarcoplasmic reticulum (SR) to cause contraction. The cell membrane ultrastructure formed by T tubules allows Ca^{2+} channels and RyR to face one another across a narrow (~ 10 nm) cytoplasmic space

biophysical purpose of various ion channel domains such as the voltage sensor.[15] These 'structure-function' studies provided highly detailed information that led to more complete understanding of ion channel molecular physiology in health and disease. Because ion channel proteins are expressed in cells at relatively low copy number, have prominent lipophilic regions (that allow for membrane insertion) and are large, they are difficult to crystallize. However, the MacKinnon laboratory overcame many of these obstacles by over-expressing bacterial K^+ channels,[16,17] which have served as a structural model for many of the voltage-gated cation channels present in heart. The combination of voltage clamp, molecular biology and high resolution structural information form the modern tool kit for understanding cardiac ion channels.

Ion channels are not the only source of ionic membrane currents. In myocardium, the Na^+/Ca^{2+} exchanger is the predominant mechanism for removing Ca^{2+} from the cytoplasm to the extracellular space. The Na^+/Ca^{2+} exchanger transfers a Ca^{2+} for $3Na^+$ (forward exchange mode). Because there is a single net positive charge moved to exchange a Ca^{2+} ion from the cytoplasm to the extracellular space, the Na^+/Ca^{2+} exchanger produces a small inward Na^+ current in forward mode. Although the Na^+/Ca^{2+} exchanger does not directly require ATP, the Na^+ gradient necessary for forward mode exchange depends upon the ATP-requiring Na^+/K^+ ATPase. The Na^+/K^+ ATPase and a sarcolemmal Ca^{2+} ATPase produce small, but measurable

currents. The Na^+/Ca^{2+} exchanger current, although small in magnitude compared to Na_V or Ca_V channel currents, contributes to AP duration. It is essential for the direct myocardial inotropic actions of digitalis glycosides, which inhibit the Na^+/K^+ ATPase leading to accumulation of $[Na^+]_i$ and consequent increase in $[Ca^{2+}]_i$, because the gradient for Ca^{2+} extrusion by Na^+/Ca^{2+} exchanger is less favorable than when $[Na^+]_i$ is lower. The Na^+/Ca^{2+} exchanger is a source of inward currents for arrhythmia triggering afterdepolarizations, as will be discussed below.

ACTION POTENTIALS REQUIRE ORCHESTRATED ION CHANNEL OPENING AND INACTIVATION

Action potentials are the fundamental unit of membrane excitability (Fig. 5). In most myocardial cells action potentials are initiated by opening of voltage-gated Na^+ channels, $Na_V1.5$. The inward $Na_V1.5$ current (I_{Na}) depolarizes atrial and ventricular myocytes in a few milliseconds. The brevity of I_{Na} is due to the rapidity of the inactivation process, which competes with activation to modulate the peak current. The membrane potential depolarizes (becomes more positive) from the negative resting potential (~ –80 mV) to approach the reversal potential for Na^+, estimated by the Nernst equation (~ +50 mV). Specialized myocytes that are dedicated more to automaticity (i.e. SAN) and conduction (i.e. the atrioventricular node) than contraction rely on I_{Ca} for their (phase 0) action potential

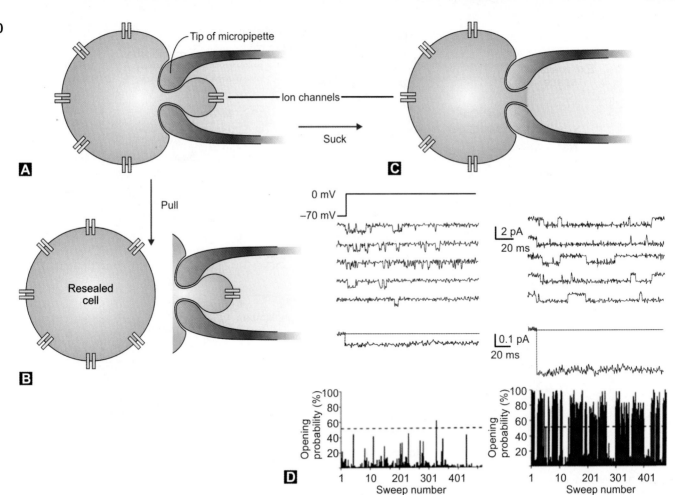

FIGURES 4A TO D: Patch clamp is a flexible approach to voltage clamp single cells or cell membrane patches. The high resistance seals (giga Ohm) between the glass micro-pipette and the cell membrane allow for resolution of very small (pA) currents. (A) On cell configuration for recording a subset of ion channels on a cell membrane. (B) Excised membrane patch for recording a subset of ion channels on a cell membrane under conditions where the cytoplasmic constituents can be easily manipulated. (C) Whole cell mode configuration for recording all the ion channels on a cell membrane and where the pipette solution can be dialyzed into the cell. (D) Examples of single Ca^{2+} channel recordings ($Ca_V1.2$) using excised cell membrane patches (as in panel B) at baseline (left panels) and after application of calmodulin kinase II to the cytoplasmic face of the membrane. The top panels show ionic currents from single $Ca_V1.2$ channels in response to a voltage clamp command from –70 to 0 mV. The downward deflections indicate channel openings. The middle tracing is an ensemble current averaged from multiple 'sweeps', as shown in the top five tracings. The bottom panels show a diary plot that indicates the opening probability of the single channel in the recording for each sweep. Panel D is adapted from Dzhura et al. 2000

upstroke. Membrane depolarization activates a combination of voltage-gated ion channels, but the most prominent are depolarizing inward $Ca_V1.2/1.3$ currents (I_{Ca}) and several distinct, but structurally related repolarizing inward K^+ channel ($K_V x$) currents (I_K). The interplay between I_{Ca} and I_K largely determines the duration of the myocardial action potentials, which last hundreds of milliseconds. Atrial and ventricular myocardial action potentials have different shapes and electrophysiological properties. In fact, there are important heterogeneities in action potential configuration within the atrium and ventricle. The ventricular endocardium, mid-myocardium and epicardium show prominent differences in action potential configuration, due to variability in expression of repolarizing K^+ currents (Fig. 6). While the physiological benefit of action potential heterogeneity is unknown, the heterogeneities are affected by K^+ channel antagonist drugs and by electrical remodeling during heart failure, where expression of various repolarizing K^+ channels is reduced.[18] In addition to

voltage-gated ion channels and exchangers, there is an increasing recognition that other non-voltage-gated ion channels contribute to action potential configuration. A more complete discussion of these channels is reviewed elsewhere.[19,20]

ACTION POTENTIAL PHYSIOLOGY IS A CONSEQUENCE OF ION CHANNEL AND CELLULAR PROPERTIES

Myocardial action potentials are distinguished from action potentials in other excitable tissues by their extreme length, lasting up to hundreds of milliseconds. In contrast, action potentials in most neurons last only a few milliseconds. Cardiac action potentials are often described in phases (Fig. 5). Phase 0 marks the abrupt depolarization from the resting potential and is attributable to $Na_V1.5$ current in most myocardial cells. Cardiac action potentials are long because of their plateau. The action potential plateau occurs because of a fine balance, mostly

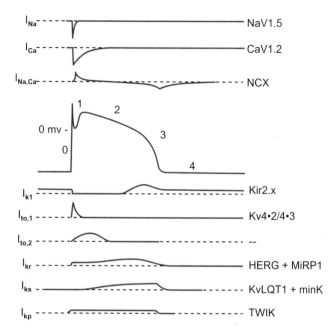

FIGURE 5: The action potential duration and configuration is shaped by the interplay between inward and outward-going ionic currents. The top two tracings represent $Na_V1.5$ and $Ca_V1.2$ inward currents that initiate and sustain action potential depolarization. The third tracing from the top is the Na^+/Ca^{2+} exchanger (NCX) that can produce inward (forward mode) and outward (reverse mode) currents at various action potential phases. The ventricular action potential is labeled by phase (0–4). The lower six tracings represent some of the K^+ currents that contribute to action potential repolarization

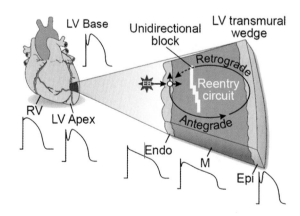

FIGURE 6: Ventricular action potentials are heterogenous and vary between base and apex and across the myocardium from endocardium to epicardium. M cells in the mid-myocardium have characteristically long action potentials with a reduced phase 1. Structural defects, such as scar tissue, can serve as a structural barrier that supports a reentry circuit for arrhythmias. Exaggeration of action potential heterogeneities, by genetic disease or acquired disease, can also support a reentry circuit, even in the absence of scar

between depolarizing inward Ca_V current, a small persistent (slowly inactivating) component of $Na_V1.5$ current, and activation of repolarizing K^+ currents. The initial plateau is referred to as phase 2, while the later plateau is referred to as phase 3. In electrically healthy myocardium phase 3 is the period of repolarization to resting membrane potential (phase 4). Phase 3 occurs as inward currents inactivate and repolarizing currents

become preeminent. Phase 1 occurs immediately after peak **571** membrane potential depolarization (i.e. the end of phase 0) and where prominent (e.g. ventricular epicardium) is marked by a 'notch' that is due to a combination of K_V channel currents that support a transient inward current (I_{to}) and a more rapid repolarizing K^+ current (the ultrarapid transient outward current, I_{Kur}). The initial component of the action potential plateau (phase 2) is marked by high membrane resistance (R), so small increases in net inward current lead to prominent positive increases in membrane voltage, according to Ohm's law (V = I × R). In automatic cells phase 4 is not stable, but instead consists of an increasing positive membrane potential in late diastole that leads to activation of Ca_V channel currents to initiate phase 1 AP depolarization. Thus, a rich diversity of ion channels contributes to various AP configurations. These AP configurations are matched to the purpose of particular myocardial cells (e.g. pacing or contraction), but in disease AP parameters are directly relevant to arrhythmia initiation and perpetuation.

Action potentials can be repetitively initiated in atrial and ventricular myocardium within the time constraints of the tissue refractory period (Figs 7A and B). The refractory period is determined in large part by the duration of the cardiac action potential. Action potentials are initiated by positive (inward) current sufficient to depolarize the membrane potential to the threshold for activation of $Na_V1.5$ in contracting myocardium or Ca_V1 in specialized conduction tissue. During phase 2 of the action potential plateau myocardial cells are absolutely refractory, meaning that no amount of inward current is adequate to elicit an action potential. Later in the course of action potential repolarization (phase 3) an action potential can be stimulated, but only by a larger inward current than would be necessary after completion of action potential repolarization. Tissue where an action potential can only be stimulated by a supranormal current is said to be relatively refractory. Under physiological conditions action potentials shorten in response to shorter stimulation intervals (i.e. faster rates), due to a process called restitution (Fig. 7C). Action potential restitution occurs, in part, because rapid simulation enhances net outward repolarizing current. Action potential restitution is impaired in genetic long QT syndromes (LQTS), where repolarizing currents are defective, or in common forms of heart failure where reduction in repolarizing currents is a signature event in the proarrhythmic electrical remodeling process. Tissue refractoriness can persist after action potential repolarization under conditions of reduced availability of inward currents responsible for phase 0 depolarization (i.e. $Na_V1.5$ in contracting myocardium and $Ca_V1.2$ and $Ca_V1.3$ in specialized conduction tissue). Various factors contribute to availability of these channels to open, including cell membrane potential (e.g. fewer Na_V and Ca_V channels are available to open at depolarized potentials because membrane depolarization favors inactivation), oxidation, pH, $[Ca^{2+}]_i$, ischemia and autonomic tone. Thus, cell membrane excitability depends on multiple input variables that ultimately converge on ion channels and APs.

The rate that APs are conducted across myocardium (i.e. the conduction velocity) is determined by two principle factors. The first are determined by inputs that affect phase 0: availability of Na_V currents in contracting myocardium and Ca_V currents in specialized conducting and automatic tissue. The second is the

CHAPTER 29

Arrhythmia Mechanisms

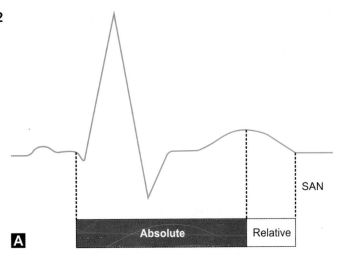

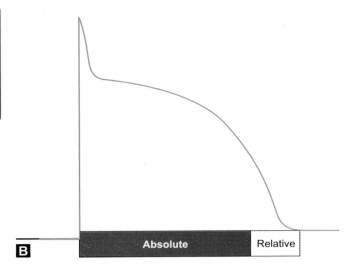

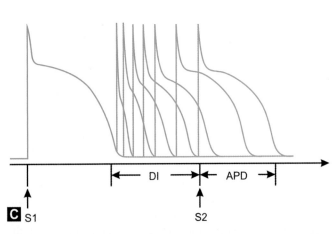

FIGURES 7A TO C: Tissue refractoriness to excitation is determined by action potential repolarization and reflected in the surface ECG. (A) A schematic ECG tracing. (B) The surface ECG is a reflection of many action potentials. Myocardial tissue is absolutely refractory to repeat stimulation (dark bars) until late in repolarization. Tissue is potentially excitable prior to completion of repolarization, but initiation of excitation requires a supranormal depolarizing current, a state of relative refractoriness (light bars). (C) Action potential restitution is revealed by a premature stimulus (S2) deployed over a range of coupling intervals

efficacy of electrical coupling between myocardial cells. Myocardial cells are electrically coupled by connexin hemi-channels that cooperate to form a conductance pore between adjacent cells. The predominant connexin (Cx) type is specific to atrium, ventricle and specialized conduction tissue. Cx 40 and 43 are the major forms in atrium, Cx 43 is the major form in ventricle and Cx 45 is the major form in sinus node, AV node and His-Purkinje cells. Longitudinal intercellular coupling is favored in ventricular myocardium, based on the greater density of Cx 43, compared to side-to-side connections. Conduction velocity is more rapid in the longitudinal direction, due to the greater density of Cx 43 and because $Na_V 1.5$ is enriched at the longitudinal junctions, analogous to Nodes of Ranvier in neurons.[21] Like voltage-gated ion channels, Cxs are part of a substantial macromolecular complex that influences intercellular conduction. Altered Cx behavior, localization and expression[22] contributes to conduction velocity dispersion and slowing that are critical components of the proarrhythmic substrate in rare genetic diseases and common forms of structural heart disease.

ACTION POTENTIALS ARE DESIGNED FOR AUTOMATICITY AND TO INITIATE CONTRACTION

Myocardial action potentials are committed to the major tasks of myocardium: rhythmic, repetitive beating and mechanical work that propels blood through the circulatory system. Sinoatrial node (SAN) action potentials have a specialized, late diastolic component or phase 4 where membrane depolarization leads to activation of Ca_V channel currents to drive phase 0 depolarization. The slope of phase 4 is the membrane potential mechanism for increasing (steeper slope) or decreasing (shallower slope) heart rate (Fig. 8). In healthy hearts, the activity of phase 4 is largely confined to the SAN, where the steady increase in net inward current during late diastolic depolarization is augmented by β adrenergic receptor stimulation

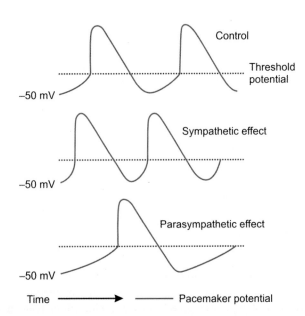

FIGURE 8: The cell membrane potential for determining heart rate in sinoatrial nodal cells is set by the steepness of phase 4 (pacemaker) potential. Steeper phase 4 allows the membrane potential to reach the threshold for action potential initiation more rapidly than shallow phase 4 depolarization

and reduced by muscarinic receptor stimulation. Multiple currents likely contribute to physiological phase 4 depolarization in SAN, but recent evidence suggests that two currents play a critical role in physiological pacing. The classical 'pacemaker' current is a Na^+/K^+ selective cation current carried by an *HCN4* gene encoded channel. The *HCN4* current, also called the funny current (I_f) is enhanced by cyclic AMP, which confers increased activity (and steeper phase 4) with α adrenergic receptor agonist stimulation.[23,24] More recent understanding of physiological automaticity in SAN cells suggests that SR Ca^{2+} release enhances inward Na^+/Ca^{2+} exchanger current. The relationship between spontaneous SAN cell SR Ca^{2+} release and inward Na^+/Ca^{2+} exchanger current that contributes to phase 4 depolarization has been called a 'Ca^{2+} clock mechanism' of pacing.[25] The Ca^{2+} clock is responsive to α adrenergic receptor agonist stimulation because cellular Ca^{2+} entry by Ca_V1 currents and SR Ca^{2+} release are both increased by catecholamines. The Ca^{2+} clock concept has important and interesting implications, because it identifies proteins and subcellular systems designed for excitation-contraction coupling in mechanically purposed atrial and ventricular myocardium as serving a dual purpose as a mechanism for automaticity—excitation-excitation coupling. While the Ca^{2+} clock appears to contribute to the normal physiology of SAN cells, SR Ca^{2+} leak and increased inward Na^+/Ca^{2+} exchanger current is known to induce DADs and trigger arrhythmias in atrial and ventricular myocardium under conditions of pathological stress. Thus, physiological automaticity resembles pathological triggering, suggesting that so-called 'triggered' arrhythmias are a natural consequence of excitation-contraction coupling. In my opinion, the similarities between automaticity and triggering suggest that bright line distinctions between these concepts are no longer warranted or appropriate.

The AP plateau is unique to cardiac muscle because cardiac muscle relies on a specific mode of excitation-contraction coupling called Ca^{2+}-induced Ca^{2+} release (CICR, Fig. 3).[26] The AP plateau is the membrane potential substrate for grading Ca^{2+} entry by voltage-gated Ca^{2+} channels. CICR is initiated by a Ca^{2+} current trigger, mostly through $Ca_V1.2$ in ventricular myocardium, and $Ca_V1.2$ and $Ca_V1.3$ in atrial myocardium. Ca_V channels are arrayed in close juxtaposition to RyRs and the Ca_V current triggers RyR opening. Ryanodine receptor (RyR) opening results in a release of myofilament-activating Ca^{2+} from the SR lumen into the cytoplasm in the vicinity of myofilaments. Ca^{2+} triggers myofilament crossbridge formation that causes myocardial contraction. Systole requires energy, in part, due to the ATP cost of sequestering Ca^{2+} into the SR. Like systole, diastole is an energy requiring process that is initiated when the SR bound Ca^{2+} ATPase pumps (SERCa 2a: sarcoplasmic endoplasmic reticulum Ca^{2+} ATPase type 2a) sequester Ca^{2+} from the cytoplasm into the SR lumen, allowing release of myofilament crossbridge formation and myocardial relaxation. SR Ca^{2+} release occurs in a highly structured subcellular domain, resulting in very high local $[Ca^{2+}]_i$. SR Ca^{2+} affects myocardial ion channels, particularly Ca_V1 and the Na^+/Ca^{2+} exchanger. The actions at Ca_V1 currents are complex, and include conflicting processes called facilitation (peak current is increased and inactivation is

reduced) and Ca^{2+} dependent inactivation (peak current is reduced and inactivation is increased). These processes are labile and may have marked influence on the shape, duration and stability of the AP plateau. In our opinion, the best available evidence suggests that Ca_V1 channel current facilitation is due to phosphorylation of a specific residue on the Ca_V1 β subunit by the multifunctional Ca^{2+} and calmodulin-dependent protein kinase II (CaMKII).[27] Ca_V1 channels current facilitation occurs because Ca_V1 channels enter a highly active gating mode after CaMKII phosphorylation where the probability of channel opening rises significantly above baseline.[28] CaMKII actions on Ca_V1 channels cause proarrhythmic afterdepolarizations and arrhythmias.[29-31]

ACTION POTENTIAL PHYSIOLOGY IS REFLECTED BY THE SURFACE ELECTROCARDIOGRAM

The electrocardiogram (ECG) is one of the most commonly ordered medical tests in most hospitals. The ECG is a surface report on myocardial electrical activity. Although multiple factors influence ECG parameters, the basic intervals (PR, QRS, QT) reflect ion channel-directed AP parameters (Figs 7A to C). The PR interval is the duration required for an electrical impulse to conduct from the point of 'break out' near the SAN, through atrial myocardium and AVN to the ventricle. In healthy myocardium, this interval will be dominated by the slowest conducting segment, which is in the AVN. In diseased myocardium, impaired atrial and His-Purkinje conduction may contribute to PR prolongation. The QRS interval reflects the speed of conduction and depolarization through the right and left ventricles. The QRS interval can be prolonged by Na_V or Cx gene defects or antagonist drugs, injury or disease in the His-Purkinje system or myocardial injury, including myocardial ischemia, infarction and scar. The QT interval corresponds to ventricular repolarization. Ventricular repolarization is complex, due to the physiological variation in repolarizing ionic currents in endocardium, mid-myocardium and epicardium, as well as between the ventricular apex and base. QT interval prolongation can occur in long QT syndromes that are due to intrinsic defects in repolarizing ionic currents or their cellular localization (LQTS). Ion channel antagonist drugs are the most common reason for QT interval prolongation. Importantly, a wide variety of drugs are antagonists of the hERG (human ether-a-go-go related gene)[32,33] or *KCNH2* encoded $K_V11.1$ K^+ channel α subunit protein that conducts the rapid delayed rectifier current (I_{Kr}).[34] Rectifier current antagonist properties are a major obstacle for drug development because of the link between QT prolongation, Torsade de Pointes ventricular arrhythmia and sudden death.[35] Diseases of ion channel encoding genes that alter membrane repolarization (Table 1) can result in AP and QT interval lengthening (Long QT syndromes) or AP and QT interval shortening (Short QT syndromes).[36] Failing myocardium from a variety of causes (e.g. myocardial infarction, valvular disease, genetic disease) undergoes a proarrhythmic electrical remodeling process where repolarizing K^+ currents are reduced resulting in AP and QT interval prolongation.[18] Understanding basic electrophysiological principles constitutes the foundation for understanding arrhythmia mechanisms and for interpreting ECGs.

TABLE 1

A compilation of genetic arrhythmia syndromes due to mutation in ion channel proteins

	Rhythm	Inheritance	Locus	Ion channel	Gene
Long QT syndrome (RW)	TdP	AD			
LQT1			11p15	I_{Ks}	KCNQ1, KvLQT1
LQT2			7q35	I_{Kr}	KCNH2, HERG
LQT3			3p21	I_{Na}	SCN5A, Na$_v$1.5
LQT4			4q25		ANKB, ANK2
LQT5			21q22	I_{Ks}	KCNE1, minK
LQT6			21q22	I_{Kr}	KCNE2, MiRP1
LQT7 (Andersen-Tawil syndrome)			17q23	I_{K1}	KCNJ2, Kir 2.1
LQT8 (Timothy syndrome)			6q8A	I_{Ca}	CACNA1C, Ca$_v$1.2
LQT9			3p25	I_{Na}	CAV3, caveolin-3
LQT10			11q23.3	I_{Na}	SCN4B, Na$_v$b4
Long QT syndrome (JLN)	TdP	AR	11p15	I_{Ks}	KCNQ1, KvLQT1
			21q22	I_{Ks}	KCNE1, minK
Brugada syndrome					
BrS1	PVT	AD	3p21	I_{Na}	SCN5A, Na$_v$1.5
BrS2	PVT	AD	3p24	I_{Na}	GPD1L
BrS3	PVT	AD	12p13.3	I_{Ca}	CACNA1C, Ca$_v$1.2
BrS4	PVT	AD	10p12.33	I_{Ca}	CACNB2b, Ca$_v\beta_{2b}$
Short QT syndrome					
SQT1	VT/VF	AD	7q35	I_{Kr}	KCNH2, HERG
SQT2			11p15	I_{Ks}	KCNQ1, KvLQT1
SQT3		AD	17q23.1–24.2	I_{K1}	KCNJ2, Kir2.1
SQT4			12p13.3	I_{Ca}	CACNA1C, Ca$_v$1.2
SQT5		AD	10p12.33	I_{Ca}	CACNB2b, Ca$_v\beta_{2b}$
Catecholaminergic VT					
CPVT1	VT	AD	1q42–43		RyR2
CPVT2	VT	AR	1p13–21		CASQ2

(Abbreviations: AD: Autosomal dominant; AR: Autosomal recessive; JLN: Jervell and Lange-Nielsen; RW: Romano-Ward; TdP: Torsade de pointes; VF: Ventricular fibrillation; VT: Ventricular tachycardia; PVT: Polymorphic VT; I_{Ks}: Slowly activating delayed rectifier current; I_{Kr}: Rapidly activating delayed rectifier current; I_{Na}: Na$^+$ channel current; I_{K1}: Inward rectifier current; I_{Ca}: Ca^{2+} channel current; GPDIL: Glycerol-3-phosphate dehydrogenase 1-like gene; RyR2: Ryanodine receptor 2 gene; CASQ2: Calsequestrin 2 gene. (*Source:* Antzelevitch 2007)

AFTERDEPOLARIZATIONS AND TRIGGERED ARRHYTHMIAS

Afterdepolarizations are arrhythmia-initiating oscillations in cell membrane potential. Early afterdepolarizations (EADs) occur during the plateau phases (2 and 3) of AP repolarization. Delayed afterdepolarizations (DADs) occur after AP repolarization, during phase 4 (Figs 9A and B). EADs and DADs can trigger an arrhythmia by propagating to adjacent tissue under favorable source-sink conditions. In theory, EAD and DADs can emerge from an essentially limitless set of conditions, sharing a common requirement that net inward current is enhanced to initiate a depolarizing oscillation in membrane potential. EADs and DADs of sufficient magnitude depolarize the cell membrane to reach the threshold for activation of Na$_V$ and/or Ca$_V$ channel currents to initiate AP phase 0. EADs and DADs that occur at the same time in a sufficient number of cells can lead to a premature AP. One or more premature APs can trigger an arrhythmia by engaging a proarrhythmic substrate supporting reentry. Although there are many potential scenarios for increasing net inward current to initiate EADs or DADs, there is an emerging body of experimental evidence that a common pathway for promoting EADs is reactivation of Ca$_V$ channel currents, while a common pathway favoring DADs is loss of synchronous SR Ca^{2+} release leading to inward Na$^+$/Ca^{2+} exchanger current. Thus, both EADs and DADs can be thought to arise as a consequence of corruption of key components of CICR.

EADs and DADs are hypothesized to initiate life-threatening arrhythmias in long QT syndromes, catecholaminergic polymorphic VT, atrial fibrillation, and ventricular arrhythmias in heart failure. Long QT syndromes are mostly the result of dominant or dominant negative mutations that cause a defect in depolarization that results in AP prolongation (Table 1),

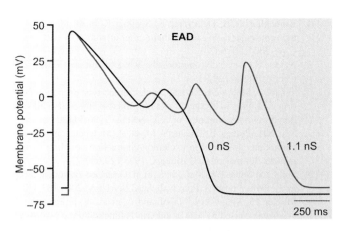

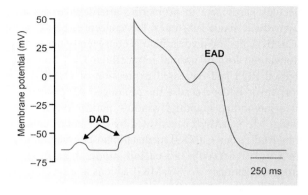

FIGURES 9A AND B: Afterdepolarizations are arrhythmia-triggering oscillations in cell membrane potential. (A) Early afterdepolarizations (EADs) occur during action potential repolarization. (B) Delayed afterdepolarizations (DADs) occur after action potential repolarization

secondary increases in Ca_V1 current and afterdepolarizations. CaMKII is activated in atrial fibrillation[37,38] and during AP prolongation,[39] due to enhanced Ca^{2+} entry, and is thought to promote arrhythmias by enhancing Ca_V1 current facilitation,[29] the non-inactivating component of $Na_V1.5$[40] and SR Ca^{2+} leak[41] in animal and cellular models. CaMKII inhibition can suppress afterdepolarizations[29,30,39] and arrhythmias[31] without AP or QT interval shortening, suggesting that CaMKII contributes to a critical proarrhythmic connection between AP prolongation and afterdepolarizations. EADs and DADs are also implicated in arrhythmogenesis in heart failure, due to a proarrhythmic electrical remodeling process where K^+ current expression is reduced—leading to AP prolongation and increased activity and expression of CaMKII in failing myocardium.[42] CaMKII activity and/or expression are increased in failing myocardium from animal models and from patients.[43] Thus, emerging concepts suggest that afterdepolarizations and excessive CaMKII activity constitute a unified mechanism for arrhythmia triggering in genetic and structural forms of heart disease.[1,44,45] CaMKII may contribute to other competing concepts favoring afterdepolarizations, including RyR2 Ca^{2+} leak due to ROS[46] and hyperphosphorylation by protein kinase A.[47]

PROARRHYTHMIC SUBSTRATES

Cardiac arrhythmias are often initiated by afterdepolarizations, but sustained by a mechanism called reentry (Fig. 10). Reentry can occur over a large tissue domain (e.g. typical atrial flutter, bundle branch reentry ventricular tachycardia, the atrioventricular reciprocating tachycardia), or in a small volume of tissue (e.g. atrioventricular nodal tachycardia, fasicular ventricular tachycardia). Processes that lead to myocardial scar formation, such as myocardial infarction, can favor reentry by producing regions of slowed conduction.[4] Reentry can be supported by an anatomically defined pathway involving scar, specialized conduction tissue, or both. However, functional reentry can occur in structurally normal tissue due to exaggerated electrical inhomogeneities of activation[48,49] or repolarization. Physiological electrical heterogeneity is exaggerated by proarrhythmic drugs, and in animal models of myocardial hypertrophy.[50] Enhanced dispersion of repolarization is thought to support a voltage gradient that constitutes a functional

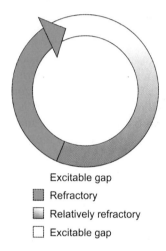

FIGURE 10: A simplified reentrant circuit with core components indicated by color coding

reentrant circuit. Reduced I_{Na}, as occurs in the Brugada Syndrome, can also induce a functional reentrant circuit by unmasking enhanced transient outward K^+ current in AP phase 1.[51] In cases of structural heart disease where scar and fibrosis contribute to anatomical reentrant pathways, the exaggeration of heterogeneity of repolarization may also contribute to creation of a sustainable arrhythmia circuit. It is likely that failing human hearts exhibit focal and reentrant arrhythmias,[52,53] with the caveat that an apparent arrhythmia focus could be a 'microreentrant' circuit. Programmed electrical stimulation (discussed in another chapter) can be used to distinguish between reentry and focal arrhythmia mechanisms.

PROARRHYTHMIC TRIGGERS AND SUBSTRATES ARE PROMOTED IN FAILING HEARTS

Although afterdepolarizations and reentry are distinct entities, there is a growing appreciation that common biological factors can promote development of proarrhythmic triggers and substrates in heart failure. CaMKII has emerged as a signal that drives structural and electrical components of myocardial injury, providing a molecular rationale to explain why failing hearts are prone to arrhythmias. While it is likely that many signaling molecules participate in promoting afterdepolarizations and proarrhythmic tissue substrates, this concept is best developed for CaMKII. Failing myocardium is consistently marked by AP prolongation, loss of normal intracellular Ca^{2+} homeostasis, increased ROS and increased expression of CaMKII. These factors favor EADs because the prolonged AP plateau occurs over a membrane potential window permissive for $Ca_V1.2$ opening.[54,55,56] CaMKII is activated by Ca^{2+} bound calmodulin and by ROS,[57] and CaMKII mediated phosphorylation leads to high $Ca_V1.2$ activity (so-called mode 2 gating)[28] and afterdepolarizations.[29,31,58] CaMKII actions at a specific site on a $Ca_V1.2$ β subunit (Thr 498)[27] lead to increased cellular Ca^{2+} entry and increased SR Ca^{2+} filling.[29] CaMKII also phosphorylates RyR2 (at Ser 2814)[59] leading to increased RyR2 opening, SR Ca^{2+} leak and afterdepolarizations that promote ventricular arrhythmia in failing hearts.[41] A similar mechanism may also favor atrial fibrillation.[38] RyR2 Ca^{2+} leak can trigger inward Na^+/Ca^{2+} exchanger current[60] that promotes DADs and phase 3 EADs. CaMKII activity at key Ca^{2+} homeostatic proteins ($Ca_V1.2$ and RyR2) promotes loss of normal intracellular Ca^{2+} homeostasis, which may reduce the efficacy of CICR resulting in reduced mechanical performance.[61]

After myocardial infarction the borderzone tissue between non-living scar and normal myocytes serves as a substrate for reentry. Surviving borderzone tissue undergoes electrical remodeling marked by reduced $Na_V1.5$ expression that is due, at least in part, to reduction in ion channel-targeting ankyrin G expression.[21] Loss of $Na_V1.5$ current contributes to conduction slowing. In addition, borderzone tissue is enriched in ROS and ROS activated CaMKII is increased in the MI borderzone,[62] where it may contribute to conduction slowing by effects, at least in part, on Na_V channels.[63] CaMKII activation contributes to scar formation by increasing myocardial death in response to ischemic injury.[64] The pro-survival effects of CaMKII inhibition are likely multifactorial, and have been mapped to $Ca_V1.2$,[29,65] SR Ca^{2+},[64] and mitochondria.[65,66] CaMKII activation after MI results in activation of inflammatory signaling by increased nuclear factor for κB (NF-κB) transcription.[67] Thus, understanding CaMKII signaling provides insight into how a properly positioned nodal signal can produce the twin phenotypes of heart failure and arrhythmias. CaMKII resides at an intersection of the β adrenergic receptor and angiotensin II signaling pathways,[57] both of which are extensively therapeutically validated to improve heart failure symptoms and reduce sudden death after MI. Improved understanding of cellular signaling important for arrhythmias has the potential to lead to more effective and novel non-invasive antiarrhythmic treatments.

REFERENCES

1. Tomaselli GF, Barth AS. Sudden cardio arrest: oxidative stress irritates the heart. Nat Med. 2010;16:648-9.
2. Kurita T, Ohe T, Shimizu W, et al. Early afterdepolarizationlike activity in patients with class IA induced long QT syndrome and torsades de pointes. Pacing and Clinical Electrophysiology. 1997;20:695-705.
3. Shimizu W, Ohe T, Kurita T, et al. Effects of verapamil and propranalol on early afterdepolarizations and ventricular arrhythmias induced by epinephrine in congenital long QT syndrome. J Am Coll Cardiol. 1995;26:1299-309.
4. Brunckhorst CB, Delacretaz E, Soejima K, et al. Identification of the ventricular tachycardia isthmus after infarction by pace mapping. Circ. 2004;110:652-9.
5. Nernst R. Die elektromotorische wirksamkeit der ionen. Z Phys Chem. 1889;4:129-81.
6. Tanabe T, Mikami A, Numa S, et al. Cardiac-type excitation-contraction coupling in dysgenic skeletal muscle injected with cardiac dihydropyridine receptor cDNA. Nature. 1990;344:451-3.
7. Sun XH, Protasi F, Takahashi M, et al. Molecular architecture of membranes involved in excitation-contraction coupling of cardiac muscle. Journal of Cell Biology. 1995;129:659-71.
8. Song LS, Sobie EA, McCulle S, et al. Orphaned ryanodine receptors in the failing heart 3. Proc Natl Acad Sci USA. 2006;103:4305-10.
9. Mohler PJ, Splawski I, Napolitano C, et al. A cardiac arrhythmia syndrome caused by loss of ankyrin-B function. Proc Natl Acad Sci USA. 2004;101:9137-42.
10. Mohler PJ, Schott JJ, Gramolini AO, et al. Ankyrin-B mutation causes type 4 long-QT cardiac arrhythmia and sudden cardiac death [comment]. Nature. 2003;421:634-9.
11. Hodgkin AL, Huxley AF. A quantitative description of membrane current and its application to conduction and excitation in nerve. Journal of Physiology. 1952;117:500-44.
12. Hamill OP, Marty A, Neher E, et al. Improved patch-clamp techniques for high-resolution current recording from cells and cell-free membrane patches. Pflugers Arch. 1981;391:85-100.
13. Colquhoun D, Neher E, Reuter H, et al. Inward current channels activated by intracellular Ca in cultured cardiac cells. Nature. 1981;294:752-4.
14. Papazian DM, Schwarz TL, Tempel BL, et al. Cloning of genomic and complementary DNA from Shaker: a putative potassium channel gene from Drosophila. Science. 1987;237:749-53.
15. Timpe LC, Schwarz TL, Tempel BL, et al. Expression of functional potassium channels from Shaker cDNA in Xenopus oocytes. Nature. 1988;331:143-5.
16. Doyle DA, Morais CJ, Pfuetzner RA, et al. The structure of the potassium channel: molecular basis of K^+ conduction and selectivity. Science. 1998;280:69-77.
17. MacKinnon R, Cohen SL, Kuo A, et al. Structural conservation in prokaryotic and eukaryotic potassium channels. Science. 1998;280:106-9.
18. Tomaselli GF, Zipes DP. What causes sudden death in heart failure? Circ Res. 2004;95:754-63.
19. Grant AO. Cardiac ion channels. Circ Arrhythm Electrophysiol. 2009;2:185-94.
20. Roden DM, Balser JR, George AL Jr., et al. Cardiac ion channels. Annu Rev Physiol. 2002;64:431-75.
21. Lowe JS, Palygin O, Bhasin N, et al. Voltage-gated Na_V channel targeting in the heart requires an ankyrin-G dependent cellular pathway 1. J Cell Biol. 2008;180:173-86.
22. Hesketh GG, Shah MH, Halperin VL, et al. Ultrastructure and regulation of lateralized connexin43 in the failing heart. Circ Res. 2010;106:1153-63.
23. Ludwig A, Zong X, Stieber J, et al. Two pacemaker channels from human heart with profoundly different activation kinetics. EMBO J. 1999;18:2323-9.
24. Seifert R, Scholten A, Gauss R, et al. Molecular characterization of a slowly gating human hyperpolarization-activated channel predominantly expressed in thalamus, heart, and testis. Proc Natl Acad Sci USA. 1999;96:9391-6.
25. Maltsev VA, Vinogradova TM, Lakatta EG. The emergence of a general theory of the initiation and strength of the heartbeat 1. J Pharmacol Sci. 2006;100:338-69.
26. Fabiato A, Fabiato F. Contractions induced by a calcium-triggered release of calcium from the sarcoplasmic reticulum of single skinned cardiac cells. J Physiol. 1975;249:469-95.
27. Grueter CE, Abiria SA, Dzhura I, et al. L-Type Ca(2+) channel facilitation mediated by phosphorylation of the beta subunit by CaMKII 1. Mol Cell. 2006;23:641-50.

28. Dzhura I, Wu Y, Colbran RJ, et al. Calmodulin kinase determines calcium-dependent facilitation of L-type calcium channels. Nat Cell Biol. 2000;2:173-7.

29. Koval OM, Guan X, Wu Y, et al. Ca$_V$1.2 beta-subunit coordinates CaMKII-triggered cardiomyocyte death and afterdepolarizations. Proc Natl Acad Sci USA. 2010;107:4996-5000.

30. Wu Y, MacMillan LB, McNeill RB, et al. CaM kinase augments cardiac L-type Ca2+ current: a cellular mechanism for long Q-T arrhythmias. American Journal of Physiology. 1999;276:H2168-H2178.

31. Wu Y, Temple J, Zhang R, et al. Calmodulin kinase II and arrhythmias in a mouse model of cardiac hypertrophy. Circ. 2002;106:1288-93.

32. Warmke JW, Ganetzky B. A family of potassium channel genes related to eag in Drosophila and mammals. Proc Natl Acad Sci USA. 1994;91:3438-42.

33. Trudeau MC, Warmke JW, Ganetzky B, et al. HERG, a human inward rectifier in the voltage-gated potassium channel family. Science. 1995;269:92-5.

34. Sanguinetti MC, Jiang C, Curran ME, et al. A mechanistic link between an inherited and an acquired cardiac arrhythmia: HERG encodes the IKr potassium channel. Cell. 1995;81:299-307.

35. Anderson ME, Al Khatib SM, Roden DM, et al. Cardiac repolarization: current knowledge, critical gaps, and new approaches to drug development and patient management. Am Heart J. 2002;144:769-81.

36. Morita H, Wu J, Zipes DP. The QT syndromes: long and short. Lancet. 2008;372:750-63.

37. Tessier S, Karczewski P, Krause EG, et al. Regulation of the transient outward K(+) current by Ca(2+)/calmodulin-dependent protein kinases II in human atrial myocytes. Circulation Research. 1999;85:810-9.

38. Chelu MG, Sarma S, Sood S, et al. Calmodulin kinase II-mediated sarcoplasmic reticulum Ca2+ leak promotes atrial fibrillation in mice. J Clin Invest. 2009;119:1940-51.

39. Anderson ME, Braun AP, Wu Y, et al. KN-93, an inhibitor of multifunctional Ca++/calmodulin-dependent protein kinase, decreases early afterdepolarizations in rabbit heart. J Pharm Exp Ther. 1998;287:996-1006.

40. Wagner S, Dybkova N, Rasenack EC, et al. Ca2+/calmodulin-dependent protein kinase II regulates cardiac Na+ channels. J Clin Invest. 2006;116:3127-38.

41. Ai X, Curran JW, Shannon TR, et al. Ca^{2+}/calmodulin-dependent protein kinase modulates cardiac ryanodine receptor phosphorylation and sarcoplasmic reticulum Ca^{2+} leak in heart failure. Circ Res. 2005;97:1314-22.

42. Sag CM, Wadsack DP, Khabbazzadeh S, et al. Calcium/calmodulin-dependent protein kinase II contributes to cardiac arrhythmogenesis in heart failure. Circ Heart Fail. 2009;2:664-75.

43. Zhang T, Brown JH. Role of Ca^{2+}/calmodulin-dependent protein kinase II in cardiac hypertrophy and heart failure. Cardiovasc Res 2004;63:476-86.

44. Anderson ME. CaMKII and a failing strategy for growth in heart. J Clin Invest. 2009;119:1082-5.

45. Qi X, Yeh YH, Chartier D, et al. The calcium/calmodulin/kinase system and arrhythmogenic afterdepolarizations in bradycardia-related acquired long-QT syndrome. Circ Arrhythm Electrophysiol. 2009;2:295-304.

46. Belevych AE, Terentyev D, Viatchenko-Karpinski S, et al. Redox modification of ryanodine receptors underlies calcium alternans in a canine model of sudden cardiac death. Cardiovasc Res. 2009;84:387-95.

47. Marx SO, Reiken S, Hisamatsu Y, et al. PKA phosphorylation dissociates FKBP12.6 from the calcium release channel (ryanodine receptor): defective regulation in failing hearts [In Process Citation]. Cell. 2000;101:365-76.

48. Ziv O, Morales E, Song YK, et al. Origin of complex behaviour of spatially discordant alternans in a transgenic rabbit model of type 2 long QT syndrome. J Physiol. 2009;587:4661-80.

49. Antzelevitch C. Role of spatial dispersion of repolarization in inherited and acquired sudden cardiac death syndromes. Am J Physiol Heart Circ Physiol. 2007;293:H2024-H38.

50. Volders PG, Sipido KR, Vos MA, et al. Cellular basis of biventricular hypertrophy and arrhythmogenesis in dogs with chronic complete atrioventricular block and acquired torsade de pointes. Circ. 1998;98:1136-47.

51. Yan GX, Antzelevitch C. Cellular basis for the Brugada syndrome and other mechanisms of arrhythmogenesis associated with ST-segment elevation. Circ. 1999;100:1660-6.

52. Pogwizd SM, McKenzie JP, Cain ME. Mechanisms underlying spontaneous and induced ventricular arrhythmias in patients with idiopathic dilated cardiomyopathy. Circ. 1998;98:2404-14.

53. Pogwizd SM, Chung MK, Cain ME. Termination of ventricular tachycardia in the human heart. Insights from three-dimensional mapping of nonsustained and sustained ventricular tachycardias. Circ. 1997;95:2528-40.

54. Antoons G, Volders PG, Stankovicova T, et al. Window Ca^{2+} current and its modulation by Ca^{2+} release in hypertrophied cardiac myocytes from dogs with chronic atrioventricular block 8. J Physiol. 2007;579:147-60.

55. January CT, Riddle JM, Salata JJ. A model for early after-depolarizations: induction with the Ca^{2+} channel agonist Bay K 8644. Circulation Research. 1988;62:563-71.

56. Wu Y, Kimbrough JT, Colbran RJ, et al. Calmodulin kinase is functionally targeted to the action potential plateau for regulation of L-type Ca^{2+} current in rabbit cardiomyocytes. J Physiol. 2004;554:145-55.

57. Erickson JR, Joiner ML, Guan X, et al. A dynamic pathway for calcium-independent activation of CaMKII by methionine oxidation. Cell. 2008;133:462-74.

58. Xie LH, Chen F, Karagueuzian HS, et al. Oxidative-stress-induced afterdepolarizations and calmodulin kinase II signaling. Circ Res. 2009;104:79-86.

59. Wehrens XH, Lehnart SE, Reiken SR, et al. Ca^{2+}/calmodulin-dependent protein kinase II phosphorylation regulates the cardiac ryanodine receptor. Circ Res. 2004;94:e61-e70.

60. Wu Y, Roden DM, Anderson ME. Calmodulin kinase inhibition prevents development of the arrhythmogenic transient inward current. Circulation Research. 1999;84:906-12.

61. Couchonnal LF, Anderson ME. The role of calmodulin kinase II in myocardial physiology and disease. Physiology (Bethesda). 2008;23:151-9.

62. Christensen MD, Dun W, Boyden PA, et al. Oxidized calmodulin kinase II regulates conduction following myocardial infarction: a computational analysis. PLoS Comput Biol. 2009;5:e1000583.

63. Hund TJ, Decker KF, Kanter E, et al. Role of activated CaMKII in abnormal calcium homeostasis and I(Na) remodeling after myocardial infarction: insights from mathematical modeling. J Mol Cell Cardiol. 2008;45:420-8.

64. Yang Y, Zhu WZ, Joiner ML, et al. Calmodulin kinase II inhibition protects against myocardial cell apoptosis in vivo 3. Am J Physiol Heart Circ Physiol. 2006;291:H3065-H75.

65. Chen X, Zhang X, Kubo H, et al. Ca^{2+} influx-induced sarcoplasmic reticulum Ca^{2+} overload causes mitochondrial-dependent apoptosis in ventricular myocytes 1. Circ Res. 2005;97:1009-17.

66. Timmins JM, Ozcan L, Seimon TA, et al. Calcium/calmodulin-dependent protein kinase II links ER stress with Fas and mito-chondrial apoptosis pathways. J Clin Invest. 2009;119:2925-41.

67. Singh MV, Kapoun A, Higgins L, et al. Ca^{2+}/calmodulin-dependent kinase II triggers cell membrane injury by inducing complement factor B gene expression in the mouse heart. J Clin Invest. 2009;119:986-96.

Antiarrhythmic Drugs

Rakesh Gopinathannair, Brian Olshansky

Chapter Outline

INTRODUCTION

Antiarrhythmic drugs (AADs) were developed to suppress cardiac arrhythmias, and therefore improve survival, symptoms and morbidity. Much of the original data were based on studies performed on cellular preparations and in vivo animal models. Despite a surfeit of supporting data demonstrating that AADs can have potent impact on various cardiac ion channels and receptors to affect arrhythmias, the lofty goal of improving survival and outcomes in patients with cardiovascular disease and arrhythmias have been less than anticipated based on results from large long-term randomized controlled clinical trials.

The AAD therapy has undergone constant evolution as new therapies have emerged and the risk benefit profile of these drugs on major clinical endpoints is better understood. The AAD therapy continues to have a critical role in the management of patients with cardiac arrhythmias, but its place is now better appreciated and understood in light of other advancements including radiofrequency catheter ablation and implantable devices. The role has transformed, as it is now realized that AADs are often not perfectly effective under all circumstances and there is risk for proarrhythmia. Many older AADs, considered the staple of arrhythmia management for years, have begun to disappear with the emergence of several purportedly safer and potentially more effective therapies.

The history of AAD therapy can be best described as a somewhat sobering transition from "panacea" to "Pandora's box". Currently, AADs, for the most part, are used as an adjunct to therapies that target and cure the rhythm like catheter ablation or those directed against the underlying structural heart disease. This role reversal has resulted from superior efficacy of newer therapies, as well as concerns over the safety and effectiveness of AADs.

Perhaps the biggest concern, notwithstanding mediocre efficacy, is the proarrhythmic, as well as systemic, side effects of AADs. Proarrhythmia may have contributed to the lack of benefit from AADs on hard clinical endpoints. The AADs are among the most complex to prescribe and monitor. Now, with a better understanding of the risks and benefits, AADs are used in a much more regulated and rigorous fashion. Several drugs disappearing from the scenery include quinidine, procainamide, phenytoin, tocainide and bretylium. Others (mexiletine and disopyramide) are used infrequently. Now, there is a better understanding of the proarrhythmic and toxic effects of these AADs. Even though guidelines are developed for their use, AADs is still often used indiscriminately without careful observation for adverse effects. AADs are available, being used and being developed. Proper and effective AAD therapy continues to play an important role to treat symptomatic and potentially life-threatening arrhythmias. The drugs are used to treat a wide variety of sustained and nonsustained atrial and ventricular tachyarrhythmias, as well as atrial and ventricular ectopy. As these drugs play an important role to treat a wide variety of arrhythmias, clinicians who use these drugs must be familiar with their indications, pharmacology, mechanisms of action, dosing, adverse effects, proarrhythmic effects and interactions with other drugs.

This chapter describes the classification schema, as well as clinical pharmacology, adverse effects and interactions of individual drugs. We will also focus on the clinical applicability of the individual agents based on available clinical data. A small section at the end of the chapter focuses on emerging and investigational AADs.

ARRHYTHMIA MECHANISMS AND ANTIARRHYTHMIC DRUGS

Cardiac tachyarrhythmias are due to several well understood mechanisms including various forms of reentry, triggered activity and automaticity. The AADs can affect cardiac ionic channels and receptors to affect properties that alter the chance of initiation, perpetuation and termination of tachyarrhythmias. The AADs can affect cardiac excitability, conduction and refractoriness. The AADs, depending on the type, can block the sodium channel and, therefore, slow down conduction in the myocardium by reducing the electrical gradient of cellular activation (Vmax, rate of rise of phase 0 of the action potential) to reduce the presence of reentrant ventricular and supraventricular arrhythmias. The AADs can also suppress spontaneous depolarization of cells leading to decreased automaticity. Many of the AADs are specific for certain cardiac tissue such as atrial, AV nodal or ventricular myocardium. Some AADs affect myocardial repolarization by affecting several potassium channels. Other AADs block calcium channels to affect other forms of reentry triggered activity, as well as automaticity dependent on the tissue and the mechanism of the arrhythmia. Some newer AADs also can affect cell-to-cell communications or work by other novel mechanisms.

INDICATIONS FOR ANTIARRHYTHMIC DRUG THERAPY

The AADs are now mainly used to treat atrial tachyarrhythmias, particularly atrial fibrillation (AF).[1] While mortality outcome with regard to rhythm control with an AAD is not superior to rate control,[2] symptom reduction and improvement in quality of life can be superior in select patients who have AF and atrial flutter. The AADs are used to treat other supraventricular tachyarrhythmias including AV node reentry, sinoatrial reentry, AV reentry tachycardia and atrial tachycardias. Occasionally, AADs are used to suppress ventricular and atrial ectopy including nonsustained and even sustained ventricular tachycardia (VT) but their use is balanced by potential adverse effects. The AADs can be used as primary therapy for patients with idiopathic VT but for patients with underlying structural heart disease and VT, AADs are not generally recommended as primary therapy unless there are specific reasons to do so in lieu of ablation therapy and/or implantable devices. The reason for this is that the proarrhythmic effects of the drugs can exceed the benefits.

PROARRHYTHMIA

The AADs suppress, and otherwise treat, arrhythmias but they can also create new ones. In some instances, this is simply an increase in the amount of atrial or ventricular ectopy but in the

worst case scenario, it can lead to ventricular fibrillation and sudden cardiac death. The proarrhythmic effects of the AADs are drug and patient specific but include the following potentially important problems:

- Sinus bradycardia
- Atrioventricular block
- Increased ventricular or atrial ectopy
- VT (monomorphic and polymorphic), including torsades de pointes related to QT interval prolongation (Fig. 1)
- Ventricular fibrillation
- Slowing of atrial tachyarrhythmias allowing one-to-one AV conduction when this was not present before the drug.

In some instances, based on the drug and the patient, a proarrhythmic response can be identified or predicted. For some drugs, starting the drug in the hospital to observe for developing proarrhythmia or the presence of QT interval prolongation that could predict proarrhythmia is effective. In other instances, this is not helpful, and only long-term monitoring can determine proarrhythmia. In some instances, it is difficult to determine if a cardiac arrest on a drug is due to drug proarrhythmia or due to lack of efficacy.

CLASSIFICATION SCHEME

The Vaughan-Williams classification, the most commonly used and by far the most clinically relevant, classifies the drugs based on their most prominent electrophysiological action[3] (Table 1). The more complex "Sicilian Gambit" scheme classifies AADs based on their cellular mechanism of action and is mostly utilized for research purposes and drug development[4] (Fig. 2). While the Sicilian Gambit held up hope for defining the potential mechanisms of AADs better, its role has all but disappeared. There are problems with both classifications. In fact, our understanding of the mechanisms of action of AADs is at best questionable, as much of the data are from animal models and isolated muscle preparations rather than from clinical assessment. Drugs can have a multiplicity of effects by themselves and by their active metabolites that do not fit neatly into one specific classification scheme.

VAUGHAN-WILLIAMS CLASSIFICATION

Class I: Sodium channel blockers:

Class IA, e.g. quinidine, procainamide, disopyramide

Class IB, e.g. lidocaine, mexiletine, phenytoin

Class IC, e.g. flecainide, propafenone

Class II: Sympathetic antagonists—beta-blockers

Class III: Prolong repolarization, e.g. sotalol, amiodarone, dofetilide, ibutilide, dronedarone, azimilide

Class IV: Calcium channel antagonists

The dosing, common uses and adverse effects of the orally available AADs are shown in Table 2. Table 3 describes the major drug interactions of AADs.

CLASS I ANTIARRHYTHMIC DRUGS: SODIUM CHANNEL BLOCKERS

The class I antiarrhythmic drugs primarily act by slowing conductance of sodium (Na⁺) across the cell membrane. These

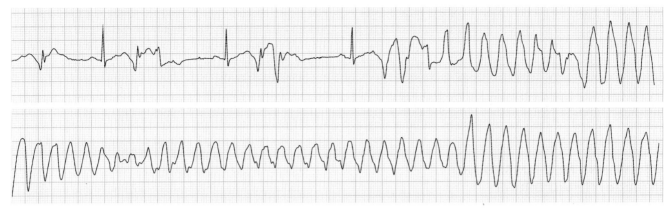

FIGURE 1: An example of sotalol-induced QTc prolongation resulting in torsades de pointes. This patient had a recent increase in his diuretic dosage and was hypokalemic at the time of presentation

TABLE 1

The Vaughan-Williams classification of antiarrhythmic drugs

Class	Drug	Ion channel effect	Electrophysiological effect
I		Block inward Na+ channel and outward K+ channels	
IA	Quinidine Procainamide Disopyramide		Slow conduction velocity (predominant effect) and increase refractoriness
IB	Lidocaine Mexiletine		Shorten APD, especially in depolarized cells
IC	Flecainide Propafenone		Marked conduction slowing (minimal effect on refractoriness)
II	Beta-blockers	Beta-adrenoceptor blockade	Sympatholytic effect
III	Sotalol	Block Ikr and beta-receptors	Prolong refractoriness and APD
	Amiodarone	Blocks multiple potassium channels, Na+ channels, Ca++ channels, beta-receptors	Prolong refractoriness and APD
	Dronedarone	Blocks multiple potassium channels, Na+ channels, Ca++ channels, beta-receptors	Prolong refractoriness and APD
	Ibutilide	Blocks Ikr and late Na+ current	Prolong refractoriness and APD
	Dofetilide	Blocks Ikr	Prolong refractoriness and APD
	Azimilide	Blocks Ikr and Iks	Prolong refractoriness and APD
IV	Calcium channel blockers	Blocks Ca++ channels	Negative chronotropic and inotropic effects

(Abbreviations: APD: Action potential duration; IKr: Rapid rectifier current; IKs: Delayed rectifier current)

drugs, therefore, interfere with the depolarization phase of the cardiac action potential ("phase 0") and also decrease responsiveness to excitation (reduction in $\dot{V}_{max}$). The magnitude of Na+ channel blockade is determined by specific cardiac tissue, specific drug properties, heart rate, autonomic (parasympathetic and sympathetic) activation, ischemic state and the state of depolarization, among others.

Based on the mechanisms by which these drugs act to block the sodium channel, as well as their effects on other channels, can alter refractoriness. Class I drugs are further classified into IA (quinidine, procainamide and disopyramide), IB (mexiletine, lidocaine), and IC (flecainide, propafenone).[5] Depending on the type, class I drugs can block sodium channels (class IC drugs) or alter the ability of the sodium channel to conduct; the effect on the channel can be short or prolonged.

Sodium channels normally transition through three distinct conformational states during the action potential: (1) open, (2) closed and (3) inactivated.[6] Only open channels conduct sodium current. Sodium channel blockers interact with open, as well as inactivated channel states, but not usually with closed channels. Thus, sodium channel blockade depends on the conformational state of the channel and blockade is phasic. The extent of sodium channel block can be increased by reducing the recovery rate of the sodium channel. This can happen in disease states, such as ischemia, or can be the property of a particular drug. For example, the class IC drugs, which unbind "very slowly" from sodium channels, are the most potent sodium channel blockers. Class I AADs exhibit use dependence. Tachycardia increases the number of sodium channels in the open and inactivated states. Since sodium channel blockers have greater affinity for the open and inactivated channels, when compared to closed

Drug	Channels: NA Fast	Channels: NA Med.	Channels: NA Show	Channels: Ca	Channels: K	Channels: I_f	Receptors: α	Receptors: β	Receptors: M_2	Receptors: P	Pumps: Na-K ATPase	Clinical effects: Left ventricular function	Clinical effects: Sinus rate	Clinical effects: Extra-cardiac	ECG effects: PR interval	ECG effects: QRS width	ECG effects: JT interval
Lidocaine	○											→	→	◉			↓
Mexiletine	○											→	→	◉			↓
Tocainide	○											→	→	●			↓
Moricizine	✦											↓	→	○		↑	
Procainamide		✧			◉							↓	→	●	↑	↑	↑
Disopyramide		✧			◉				○			↓	→	◉	↑↓	↑	↑
Quinidine		✧			◉		○		○			→	↑	◉	↑↓	↑	↑
Propafenone		✧						◉				↓	↓	○	↑	↑	
Flecainide			✧		○							↓	→	○	↑	↑	
Encainide			✧									↓	→	○	↑	↑	
Bepridil	○			●	◉							?	↓	○			↑
Verapamil	○			●			◉					↓	↓	○	↑		
Diltiazem				◉								↓	↓	○	↑		
Bretylium					●		■	■				→	↓	○			↑
Sotalol					●			●				↓	↓	○	↑		↑
Amiodarone	○			○	●		◉	◉				→	↓	●	↑		↑
Alinidine					◉	●						?	↓	●			
Nadolol								●				↓	↓	○	↑		
Propranolol	○							●				↓	↓	○	↑		
Atropine												→	↑	◉	↓		
Adenosine										□		?	↓	○	↑		
Digoxin									□		●	↑	↓	●	↑		↓

Relative potency of block: ○ Low; ● High; □ Agonist; ✦ Inactivated state blocker; ◉ Moderate; ✧ Activated state blocker; ■ Agonist/Antagonist

FIGURE 2: The Sicilian Gambit scheme for classifying antiarrhythmic drugs. [*Source:* Task Force of the Working Group on Arrhythmias of the European Society of Cardiology. Circulation. 1991;84:1831-51 (Reference 4)]

channels, the extent of sodium channel blockade and consequently, conduction slowing, is greater during faster heart rates. This phenomenon is called use dependence.

Class IA drugs (quinidine, procainamide, disopyramide) slow conduction in atrial and ventricular myocardium and have a moderate effect on slowing myocardial conduction by moderate effect on phase 0 ($\dot{V}_{max}$) but they also have other effects. These drugs prolong repolarization by their effects on potassium channels. Disopyramide, in particular, can have an anticholinergic effect. Additionally, these drugs have vasodilatory (intravenous procainamide and quinidine), negative inotropic (disopyramide) and vagolytic (quinidine and disopyramide effects).

Quinidine, disopyramide and procainamide have active metabolites (3-hydroxyquinidine, mono-N-dealkylated disopyramide and N-acetylprocainamide respectively). These drug and metabolites can be toxic by several mechanisms. In particular, they are known to prolong action potential duration in the ventricle causing QT prolongation and torsades de pointes. These drugs can have multiple adverse side effects including negative inotropic effects (disopyramide), anticholinergic effects (disopyramide), hypotensive effects (intravenous procainamide and quinidine), autoimmune effects (procainamide in particular), agranulocytosis (disopyramide and procainamide), thrombocytopenia (quinidine) and neurological side effects with nightmares (procainamide).

Due to a wide range of side effects that cause serious problems and require termination of the drug, these drugs are used rarely as the toxicity limits their utility. Furthermore, they are not necessarily the most effective AADs to suppress atrial or ventricular arrhythmias. Due to their toxicity, they have not been well tested in controlled clinical trials, but meta-analyses[7] and other observational data would suggest that their use is limited for both atrial and ventricular arrhythmias and, therefore, these drugs have become phased out for routine use in patients. Nevertheless, there may still be a role for the use of disopyramide in particular to treat some forms of AF, particularly those suspected to be due to vagal activation.

Class IA Antiarrhythmic Drugs

Quinidine: Quinidine not only blocks the rapid sodium current but also affects rapid (IKr) and slow (IKs) components of the delayed-rectifier potassium current, the inward-rectifier potassium current (IKI), the ATP-sensitive potassium channel (IKATP) and transient outward current (Ito). With regard to Ito, the effect is different from the other class IA AADs.

Dosing, uses and side effects of orally available antiarrhythmic drugs

Class	Drug	Maintenance oral dosing	Side effects	Uses
IA	Quinidine	300–600 mg every 6 hours	• Nausea, vomiting, diarrhea, anorexia, abdominal pain • Tinnitus, hearing loss, visual disturbance, confusion (cinchonism) • Thrombocytopenia, hemolytic anemia, anaphylaxis • Hypotension, QRS prolongation, syncope, torsades de pointes, QT prolongation	• PVCs • Sustained VT and VF • Short QT syndrome • Brugada syndrome • AF • Atrial flutter
	Procainamide	250–1,000 mg every 4–6 hours (no longer available)	• Rash, myalgia, vasculitis, Raynaud • Fever, agranulocytosis • Hypotension, bradycardia, QT prolongation, torsades de pointes • Drug-induced lupus	• Sustained VT • Unmasking Brugada syndrome • AF in WPW
	Disopyramide	100–200 mg every 6 hours	• Urinary retention, constipation, glaucoma, xerostomia • QT prolongation, torsades de pointes • Reduced ventricular contractility	• PVCs • VT • Hypertrophic CMP • AF
IB	Mexiletine	200–300 mg every 8 hours	• Tremor, dysarthria, dizziness, diplopia, nystagmus, anxiety • Nausea, vomiting, dyspepsia • Hypotension, bradycardia	• VT and VF • Reduction of ICD shocks
IC	Flecainide	100–200 mg two times daily	• Negative inotropy, AV block, bradycardia • Decreases pacing threshold • Confusion, irritability	• Paroxysmal AF • SVTs • VT • PVCs unmasking Brugada syndrome
	Propafenone	150–300 mg every 8 hours	• Dizziness, blurred vision • Bronchospasm • AV block, bradycardia, heart failure exacerbation • Decreases pacing threshold	• Paroxysmal AF • SVTs • VT • PVCs
II	Beta-blocker	Beta-blocker specific	• Hypotension, bradycardia, heart block, heart failure exacerbation • Bronchospasm • Depression • Impairment of sexual function	• Atrial arrhythmias • Rate control in AF • SVTs • PVCs • VT • VF
III	Amiodarone	1,200–1,800 mg daily for the first 7–10 days, then taper gradually to 200–400 mg daily	• Pulmonary fibrosis • Abnormal liver function tests • Hyperthyroidism or hypothyroidism • Bradycardia, heart failure exacerbation • Tremor, paresthesia • Photosensitivity • Corneal deposits	• VT • VF • Reduction of ICD shocks • AF • Atrial flutter • AF in WPW • Other SVTs
	Sotalol	80–160 mg every 12 hours	• Bradycardia, torsades de pointes	• Sustained VT/VF • VT in ARVD • Reduction of ICD shocks • AF • Atrial flutter
	Dofetilide	250–500 mcg twice daily	• Torsade de pointes	• AF
	Dronedarone	400 mg twice daily	• Gastrointestinal side effects	• To reduce the risk of cardiovascular hospitalization in patients with non-permanent AF and associated cardiac risk factors • Rhythm control in AF
IV	Calcium channel blocker (Verapamil)	80–160 mg every 8 hours	• Hypotension, bradycardia, AV block	• Idiopathic VT • PVCs • Rate control in AF • SVTs

(Abbreviations: AF: Atrial fibrillation; CMP: Cardiomyopathy; ICD: Implantable cardioverter defibrillator; PVCs: Premature ventricular contractions; SVTs: Supraventricular tachycardias; VF: Ventricular fibrillation; VT: Ventricular tachycardia; WPW: Wolff-Parkinson-White syndrome)

TABLE 3

Major drug interactions of antiarrhythmic drugs

Drug	Interacting drug	Interaction
Quinidine	Phenytoin	↓ Quinidine levels
	Phenobarbital	↓ Quinidine levels
	Rifampin	↓ Quinidine levels
	Ketoconazole	↑ Quinidine levels
	Verapamil	↑ Quinidine levels
	Propafenone	↑ Propafenone level
	Beta-blockers	↑ Beta-blockade
	Digoxin	↑ Digoxin concentration
Mexiletine	Phenytoin	↓ Mexiletine levels
	Phenobarbital	↓ Mexiletine levels
	Rifampin	↓ Mexiletine levels
	Ketoconazole	↑ Mexiletine levels
	Isoniazid	↑ Mexiletine levels
	Theophylline	↑ Theophylline levels
Flecainide	Digoxin	↑ Digoxin levels
	Amiodarone	↑ Flecainide levels
	Quinidine	↑ Flecainide levels
Propafenone	Digoxin	↑ Digoxin levels
	Warfarin	↓ Warfarin clearance
	Cyclosporine	↑ Cyclosporine levels
	Quinidine	↑ Propafenone levels
Amiodarone	Digoxin	↑ Digoxin effect
	Warfarin	↑ Warfarin effect
	QT prolonging drugs	↑ Risk of torsades de pointes
	Beta-blockers	Bradycardia and AV block
	Diltiazem and Verapamil	Hypotension and Bradycardia ↑ cyclosporine concentration
	Anesthetic drugs	
	Cyclosporine	
Sotalol	QT prolonging drugs	↑ Risk of torsades de pointes
Dofetilide	QT prolonging drugs	
Dronedarone		
Beta-blockers	Quinidine	↑ Beta-blockade
	Amiodarone, Digoxin,	Bradycardia
	Diltiazem, Verapamil	
Calcium channel blockers (Verapamil)	Digoxin	↑ Digoxin levels

The Ito blockade is purported to reduce the disparity of repolarization in the right ventricular outflow tract and thereby attenuate anterior precordial ST-segment elevation in the Brugada syndrome. Quinidine has been shown to reduce inducibility of ventricular arrhythmias, as well as suppress electrical storm in small studies of Brugada syndrome patients.[8,9] Thus, quinidine has been proposed as an adjunct, but not an alternative, to implantable cardioverter defibrillator (ICD) therapy in high-risk patients with Brugada syndrome.[10] Otherwise, quinidine is rarely used due to its proarrhythmic effects and its adverse effects.

Diarrhea is common; thrombocytopenia can occur or tinnitus is possible. Quinidine can cause idiosyncratic QT prolongation and torsades de pointes. There is a potential interaction between digoxin and quinidine such that quinidine will increase and even double the digoxin levels. The dose of quinidine is generally 200–400 mg every six hours but can be used in a long-acting preparation that is difficult to obtain.

Procainamide: Similar to quinidine, the adverse effects, as well as the proarrhythmic effects, outweigh the potential benefits in many cases and therefore, this drug is rarely used. It is hardly available other than in the intravenous form. Nausea, lupus-like syndrome (positive antinuclear antibodies with antihistone antibodies) and agranulocytosis, along with proarrhythmia, are some of the reasons for not using this drug. Intravenous procainamide is very useful in the acute management of supraventricular tachycardias, in particular, rapidly conducted AF and atrial flutter in patients with Wolff-Parkinson-White syndrome. Procainamide can help to facilitate pace termination of atrial arrhythmias.[11] Procainamide can cause torsades de pointes mainly due to its active class III metabolite, N-acetylprocainamide.[12]

Disopyramide: Disopyramide is still available but used rarely. The primary use of disopyramide is in patients with hypertrophic cardiomyopathy and left ventricular outflow tract obstruction, and to treat AF. A multi-center study showed that disopyramide can be an effective therapy in symptomatic hypertrophic obstructive cardiomyopathy, with 66% of patients remaining asymptomatic at 3 years with a 50% reduction in outflow gradient. Although disopyramide did not show any mortality benefit in hypertrophic cardiomyopathy, it should nevertheless be considered before invasive options such as surgical myectomy.[13]

Long-term use of disopyramide, however, is limited due to its severe anticholinergic effects, including constipation and dry mouth, as well as urinary retention (as it is about 10% as potent as atropine) and cannot be used in patients with a history of ventricular dysfunction, congestive heart failure or for men with enlarged prostate. Disopyramide is usually used in a long-acting preparation. The dosing is between 400 mg and 600 mg a day in divided doses. Disopyramide can have a marked negative inotropic effect in patients with heart failure and is contraindicated under such circumstances. It can lengthen QT interval and cause torsades de pointes.

Class IB Antiarrhythmic Drugs

Lidocaine and mexiletine are the only currently available and utilized class IB drugs. As a group, class IB drugs block sodium channels in both activated and inactivated states, but do not delay channel recovery. They affect conduction in ventricular myocardium and have little, if any, effect on atrial myocardium or on AV conduction. This results in shortening of action potential duration and refractoriness. Lidocaine may affect ischemic myocardium preferentially. Their efficacy is increased at high heart rates and also in depolarized tissues, which makes them effective in treatment of ventricular arrhythmias in the ischemic myocardium.

Lidocaine: Lidocaine is useful to treat patients who have had recurrent VT or ventricular fibrillation.[14] It does not appear to be effective or beneficial as a prophylactic drug for patients who have had myocardial infarction.[15-17] It has negligible effects on atrial electrophysiology. Lidocaine can suppress conduction, preferentially in ischemic myocardium and does not prolong the QT interval. The purported effect is to prevent reentrant arrhythmias, but it can also suppress automatic and escape rhythms.

Lidocaine dosing can be complex. It undergoes extensive first-pass metabolism in the liver and so can only be administered parenterally. Given rapid initial distribution (half-life of 8 minutes), lidocaine should be administered with multiple loading doses, followed by a maintenance infusion to maintain levels in therapeutic range. The drug has two active metabolites, monoethylglycinexylidide and glycinexylidide. Up to 70% of the drug is protein bound and this number increases in the acute phase of a myocardial infarction when alpha-1-acid glycoprotein increases (as such, over long time periods, lidocaine levels can increase despite a relatively short half-life). In congestive heart failure, where the volume of distribution is reduced, lidocaine achieves higher than normal initial concentration and so the initial dose should be reduced to avoid toxicity. Lidocaine is actively bound to alpha-1-acid glycoprotein, whose levels are increased in heart failure, and perhaps after myocardial infarction thereby decreasing drug availability.

Lidocaine has an elimination half-life of about 2 hours and steady state is reached in 4–5 half lives. Steady state concentration for lidocaine is determined by liver blood flow[18] and is reduced in both heart failure and liver disease. Thus, maintenance dosage of lidocaine should be reduced in both conditions. Renal dysfunction has no impact on lidocaine metabolism.

Lidocaine is most commonly used for acute suppression of potentially life-threatening ventricular arrhythmias (although little data support its role as a drug that improves survival). Lidocaine administration in this setting is based more on anecdotal experience than real data. Lidocaine is frequently ineffective, has a narrow therapeutic range and is frequently associated with neurological toxicity. There are no randomized controlled trials demonstrating benefits of lidocaine. Lidocaine has little effect on atrial tissue and has no value in treating supraventricular tachycardias. The effect of lidocaine in treating arrhythmias in Wolff-Parkinson-White syndrome is controversial[19] and other drugs, including procainamide, ibutilide or amiodarone, are preferred.

Lidocaine is usually administered as a loading dose followed by a maintenance infusion. A commonly used loading regimen is one suggested by Wyman et al., where an initial bolus of 75 mg is given, followed by 50 mg given every 5 minutes repeated three times, for a total loading dose of 225 mg.[20] This regimen usually achieves and maintains plasma concentrations in the therapeutic range of 1.5–5 mcg/ml. This is followed by a maintenance infusion at 1–4 mg/min. It should be noted that wide inter-individual variability in peak plasma concentration exists and, therefore, patients should be closely monitored for evidence of toxicity during loading. Lidocaine has little therapeutic effect at plasma concentrations below 1.5 mcg/ml, and the risk of toxicity increases above 5 mcg/ml.

Symptoms of central nervous system are the most frequent side effects associated with lidocaine administration. Symptoms include paresthesias, perioral numbness, drowsiness, diplopia, dysarthria, confusion and hallucinations. Nystagmus can be an early sign of neurological toxicity. Toxic levels can result in seizures and coma. In patients with known infranodal conduction abnormalities, lidocaine may worsen conduction and should be administered cautiously. Metoprolol, propranolol and cimetidine can reduce hepatic blood flow, decrease lidocaine clearance and can potentially result in lidocaine toxicity when administered concomitantly.[21,22]

Mexiletine: Mexiletine is an orally active congener of lidocaine. Mexiletine, like lidocaine, does not suppress AV conduction and has little effect on hemodynamics and ventricular function.[23] Like lidocaine, mexiletine has little effect on atrial electrophysiology. Mexiletine is almost completely absorbed orally, is primarily metabolized (90%) in the liver by the CYP2D6 system to inactive metabolites and is excreted in urine. Mexiletine has a plasma half-life of 9–12 hours. Intravenous mexiletine is not available in the United States.

Mexiletine is primarily used to suppress ventricular arrhythmias and ICD shocks in patients with structural heart disease, either as monotherapy or in combination with another AAD, such as amiodarone or, in years past, quinidine. Effectiveness of mexiletine in this setting varies widely and ranges from 6% to 60%, with majority of studies suggesting a success rate around 20%[24] depending on the condition and the type of ventricular arrhythmia being suppressed. It alone does not improve survival in a controlled trial of high-risk patients.[25] Mexiletine does not prolong and may even shorten the QT interval and can therefore be useful to suppress arrhythmias for patients with the congenital long QT syndrome type III and those with history of drug-induced torsades de pointes.[26]

Mexiletine is usually initiated at a dose of 150 mg every 8 hours. The dose can be increased at 2–3 day intervals until arrhythmia suppression or intolerable side effects develop. Suggested maximum maintenance dose is 300 mg every 6–8 hours. Patients with renal failure should be initiated at a lower dose. Dosage adjustment is also advised in patients with hepatic failure and congestive heart failure, as they impair liver blood flow and prolong elimination half-life of mexiletine.

The most common adverse events with mexiletine are gastrointestinal and neurologic. Tremor, nausea and vomiting are common; dizziness, confusion, blurred vision and ataxia are also seen. Mexiletine-induced tremor may respond to beta-blockers. Thrombocytopenia occurs infrequently.[27] Neurologic side effects are dose-dependent. Severe bradycardia and abnormal sinus node recovery times, with mexiletine have been reported in patients with otherwise or symptomatic sinus node dysfunction.

The major drug interactions of mexiletine are listed in Table 3. Inducers and inhibitors of the CYP2D6 system can influence mexiletine metabolism and can affect effectiveness and/or toxicity. Mexiletine decreases theophylline clearance and increases plasma theophylline concentrations.[28] Digoxin and warfarin levels are unaffected by mexiletine.

Class IC Antiarrhythmic Drugs

The currently available class IC drugs, flecainide and propafenone, are potent sodium channel blockers and cause marked conduction slowing in cardiac tissues without exerting any effects on refractoriness. Their sodium channel blocking effects are exaggerated at high heart rates (use dependency) and in depolarized tissues. At therapeutic doses, class IC drugs prolong the PR and QRS intervals without having significant effects on the QTc interval. Class IC drugs also exert negative inotropic effects and can worsen heart failure in patients with left ventricular dysfunction. The use of these drugs is not recommended in patients who have ventricular dysfunction, who have marked left ventricular hypertrophy or who have ischemic heart disease.[29]

Flecainide: Oral flecainide is 90–95% bioavailable and is predominantly metabolized in the liver by CYP2D6 to inactive metabolites. Flecainide is also eliminated to some extent by the kidneys and because of this, genetic variations in CYP2D6 does not seem to significantly affect pharmacological actions of flecainide. Flecainide is eliminated slowly with a half-life of 16–20 hours.

Flecainide is highly effective in suppressing a variety of ventricular and supraventricular tachycardias.[30] It is one of the most potent drugs to suppress ventricular ectopy.[29] At the present time, flecainide is commonly used for restoration and maintenance of sinus rhythm in patients with paroxysmal AF and no structural heart disease. It can be used for maintenance therapy or as a "pill-in-the-pocket" drug for AF termination.[31,32] Flecainide is also effective for suppression of idiopathic ventricular arrhythmias of right and left ventricular outflow tract origin,[33] as well as to treat supraventricular tachycardias in patients with Wolff-Parkinson-White syndrome.

Recently, flecainide has been found to be effective in suppression of catecholaminergic polymorphic VT, which is an inherited, potentially lethal arrhythmic syndrome resulting from mutations in the ryanodine and calsequestrin receptors, causing abnormal calcium handling. Flecainide was found to completely suppress adrenergically mediated polymorphic VT in a mouse model of catecholaminergic polymorphic VT, as well as in two patients with drug-refractory catecholaminergic polymorphic VT. Flecainide was shown in the mouse model to have direct inhibitory effect on the defective ryanodine receptor-mediated calcium release.[34] Flecainide may also be beneficial for patients with long QT interval syndrome type III with a specific SCN5A (D1790G) mutation.[35]

Based on results of the Cardiac Arrhythmia Suppression Trial I (CAST I), although flecainide suppressed premature ventricular contractions (PVCs) in post-myocardial infarction patients, it increased mortality compared with placebo. The same was true of another now obsolete class IC AAD—encainide.[29] Additionally, moricizine, another class I AAD, was shown to have an early proarrhythmic effect during the loading phase in the CAST II trial, even though it did not have any long-term adverse effects compared with placebo.[36] Based on these and other similar data, class IC drugs are contraindicated in patients with advanced structural heart disease and those at risk to develop myocardial ischemia.

Oral flecainide is usually initiated at a dose of 50–100 mg twice daily and can be titrated to a maximum recommended dose of 300 mg daily. At efficacious doses, QRS widening of up to 25% is seen and this is usually evaluated by exercise treadmill testing at high heart rates.[37] A one-time dose of 300 mg or 600 mg flecainide is used when employed as a "pill-in-the-pocket" dosing.[38] To reduce the incidence of adverse effects, flecainide therapy should start with a low dosage that

is maintained until steady state has been reached (at least 4 days) and altered relative to clinical response. Flecainide levels can be measured. There is little issue with regard to active metabolites. Caution should be exercised with initial dosing and up titration in patients with hepatic and renal dysfunction. Major drug interactions with flecainide are shown in Table 3.

Most common adverse effects of flecainide are dose-dependent and include headache, ataxia, and blurred vision. Flecainide can cause AF to convert to atrial flutter and, in the absence of AV blocking drugs, can result in rapid 1:1 AV conduction (often with aberrant conduction). In patients with depressed ventricular function, negative inotropic effects can precipitate heart failure.[39] In patients with pacemakers and ICDs, flecainide should be used with caution as it can significantly increase pacing and defibrillation thresholds.[40,41] There is a risk of incessant monomorphic VT in patients who have VT, but this is now uncommon as the drug is rarely, if ever, used under these circumstances. Flecainide is also contraindicated in patients with suspected sodium channelopathies, like Brugada syndrome, as it can worsen this condition (indeed, it has been used to bring out the classic ECG abnormality). Additionally, caution is needed for patients with advanced His-Purkinje conduction system disease as infra-Hisian block can ensue. Caution about using this drug in patients with substantial left ventricular hypertrophy is recommended in the current ACC/AHA/HRS AF guidelines.[31]

Propafenone: Propafenone, in addition to being a potent sodium channel blocker, has beta-adrenergic blocking (about one-thirtieth of the potency of propranolol) and calcium-channel blocking properties. The drug is structurally similar to propranolol and can have significant beta-blocking properties in patients who are slow metabolizers of propafenone.[42]

Propafenone is metabolized through the hepatic CYP2D6 pathway into 5-hydroxy propafenone and this process is largely genetically determined. Approximately 7% of the US population is deficient in CYP2D6, resulting in very slow conversion of propafenone to the active metabolites, 5-hydroxypropafenone and N-depropylpropafenone. The consequent accumulation of high concentrations of propafenone leads to significant beta-adrenoceptor antagonism in poor metabolizers.[43,44] The genetic phenotype, while determining the degree of beta-blockade, does not seem to significantly affect the antiarrhythmic effects of propafenone in most patients.

Propafenone is used to help in maintaining sinus rhythm in patients with paroxysmal or persistent AF who have no associated structural heart disease. It is usually administered in doses ranging from 150 mg to 300 mg every 8–12 hours (a long-acting preparation is available). Peak plasma concentrations are achieved in 1–3 hours following an oral dose. Propafenone increases the PR and QRS intervals on the surface electrocardiogram, but it does not prolong the QT interval. Propafenone can result in acceleration of the ventricular rate in AF if it is converted to a slow atrial flutter. Therefore, administration of an AV nodal blocking drug along with propafenone is recommended. Like flecainide, propafenone is contraindicated in patients with prior myocardial infarction, known ischemic heart disease, severe ventricular hypertrophy and history of sustained VT or severe structural heart disease.[31]

The most common side effects of propafenone are nausea, dizziness and metallic taste. Neurological side effects, like paresthesias and blurred vision, are dose-dependent and are more common in poor metabolizers. Enhanced beta-blockade resulting from poor metabolism can result in bronchospasm and asthma exacerbations. Sustained VT, as a proarrhythmic effect of sodium channel blockade, has been reported and tends to occur in patients with history of VT and underlying structural heart disease.

Propafenone decreases warfarin clearance by inhibition of CYP2C9, resulting in an increased anticoagulant effect. Propafenone markedly increases digoxin levels by decreasing non-renal clearance of digoxin. Quinidine, cimetidine and antidepressants, like fluoxetine and paroxetine, can all inhibit CYP2D6; thereby increasing propafenone levels. Levels of metoprolol[45] and propranolol, which are also metabolized by CYP2D6, are increased in the presence of propafenone.

CLASS II ANTIARRHYTHMIC DRUGS: BETA-ADRENOCEPTOR BLOCKERS

Beta-adrenergic blocking drugs are one of the most efficacious drugs used in clinical cardiology for a variety of purposes, including treatment of congestive heart failure and myocardial ischemia. Beta-blockers also have AAD properties and can reduce the risk of sudden cardiac death by a number of mechanisms, can reduce ventricular tachyarrhythmias in select patients, can inhibit AF, can prevent paroxysmal supraventricular tachyarrhythmias of various types and can have additive effects to other AADs. Additionally, beta-blockers can slow AV nodal conduction in patients with rapid atrial tachyarrhythmias including AF and atrial flutter.[46]

Specifically, beta-blockers can prevent catecholamine induced or modulated arrhythmias[47] that occur in catecholaminergic polymorphic VT, idiopathic exercise-induced VT, right ventricular outflow tract tachycardia and ventricular tachyarrhythmias due to the long QT interval syndrome; in particular, those patients with long QT interval syndrome type 1.[26]

Beta-blockers work by a variety of mechanisms. They can suppress automaticity and the triggers for atrial tachycardias, AF and ventricular fibrillation. They can also interfere with the reentry circuit in patients with AV node reentry and with AV reentry tachycardia (by facilitating blockade in the AV node).[48] Beta-blockers may facilitate the effects of class I AADs since their efficacy may be blunted under conditions of catecholamine excess. Additionally, recent data suggest that the combination of amiodarone and beta-blockers is most effective at preventing potentially life-threatening arrhythmias in an ICD population.[49] The mechanism by which this occurs is not completely known.

While a variety of beta-blockers are available for use, when it comes to arrhythmia management, it is important to have drug levels that persist throughout the day. Several beta-blockers do not do this when given on once-a-day basis; for example, atenolol. Specific beta-blockers may be effective for other reasons, including treatment of congestive heart failure and hypertension. When it comes to treating arrhythmias, although it is important to use a beta-blocker such that levels persist throughout the day. Sotalol is a beta-blocker, but it is actually a stereoisomer including d-sotalol and l-sotalol. While d-sotalol is a class III AAD; l-sotalol is a beta-blocker. When using sotalol at lower doses, the greatest effect is from the l-stereoisomer.

Some beta-blockers may have additional central nervous system effects and this effect may depend upon lipid solubility. Water-soluble and renally excreted beta-blockers, such as atenolol, rarely cross the blood-brain barrier, whereas lipid soluble beta-blockers, such as propranolol, cross the blood-brain barrier easily. It is likely that some of the benefits of beta-blockers are through central effects that are not well understood. Additionally, there are data to suggest that carvedilol may be more than just a beta-blocker as it can inhibit the rapid activating delayed-rectifier current, the L-type calcium current and the Ito, as well as the delayed-rectifier current (IKs).[50]

Beta-blockers can terminate specific acute arrhythmias, such as AF with rapid ventricular response rates that may occur in the period early after cardiac and non-cardiac surgery. In this particular case, as in other cases whereby AF is catecholamine mediated, beta-blockers can be modestly effective.[51] Additionally, AF can be treated by a beta-blocker in the setting of thyrotoxicosis.

CLASS III ANTIARRHYTHMIC DRUGS: DRUGS THAT PROLONG REPOLARIZATION

All clinically available class III drugs block the rapid component of the delayed-rectifier potassium channel (Ikr), resulting in an increase in action potential duration and refractoriness in various cardiac tissues, the hallmark of a class III AAD. With class III AADs, reverse use dependence can also occur. In this situation, the AAD effect is most pronounced during slow heart rates. The class III AADs (d-sotalol and N-acetylprocainamide—a metabolite of procainamide, but not amiodarone) demonstrate reverse use dependence. Quinidine can show reverse use dependence for the potassium channel, but use dependence for the sodium channel.

Sotalol

Sotalol is a class III AAD with beta-blocking properties. This combination results in sinus slowing, decrease in AV nodal conduction and increased refractoriness in atria, AV node, ventricle and accessory pathways. The dextro stereoisomer of sotalol (d-sotalol) is a pure class III AAD without beta-blocking properties.

Oral bioavailability of sotalol is close to 100%. Peak concentrations are seen in 2.5–4 hours following a dose. The drug has an elimination half-life of 12–16 hours and is excreted unchanged by the kidneys. Thus, drug accumulation results in the setting of renal insufficiency, increasing the risk of torsades de pointes and necessitating dose adjustment.

Sotalol is currently available in the United States only in the oral form. Usual starting dose of sotalol is 80 mg twice daily with gradual increase to 240–320 mg daily, provided the QTc is within accepted limits (< 500 msec). The following dosing algorithm is proposed in patients with renal insufficiency (Table 4A). No dose adjustment is needed in patients with hepatic disease.

Patients with heart failure and severe left ventricular dysfunction will fare poorly on this drug due to the substantial

TABLE 4A

Sotalol renal dosing algorithm

Creatinine clearance (measured by Cockcroft-Gault method) ml/min	Dosing frequency
> 60	Every 12 hours
30–60	Every 24 hours
10–30	Every 36–48 hours
< 10	Individualize

beta-blocking effects. Concern has been raised for those patients with marked left ventricular hypertrophy, as such patients have a preponderance of mid-myocardial cells and therefore can be at a greater risk for developing QT interval prolongation.

The combined class III and beta-blocking properties make sotalol effective for supraventricular and ventricular arrhythmias.[52] Sotalol is most commonly used as a rhythm control drug in AF and to suppress ventricular arrhythmias in ICD patients.

The Survival With Oral d-Sotalol (SWORD) trial evaluated the effect of d-sotalol, a pure class III drug and one that is no longer available, versus placebo on mortality in patients who had a myocardial infarction and a left ventricular ejection fraction less than or equal to 40%. The SWORD trial was stopped prematurely due to increased mortality in the d-sotalol arm which was primarily due to arrhythmic death.[53] In a multicenter, double-blind study of 1,456 patients with recent myocardial infarction randomized to d-sotalol and l-sotalol 320 mg once daily versus placebo, the mortality rate at 12-month follow-up was not significantly different between the two groups (8.9% in the sotalol group vs 7.3% in the placebo group), but the reinfarction rate was 41% lower in the sotalol group (p < 0.05). This beneficial effect was attributed to the beta-blocking properties of l-sotalol.[54]

In the Electrophysiologic Study Versus Electrocardiographic Monitoring (ESVEM) trial, a randomized, NIH-sponsored multicenter trial designed to determine the best method to guide drug therapy for patients who had malignant ventricular arrhythmias, sotalol was effective in 31% of the patients, which was the best among the different AADs tested.[55] It should be noted, however, that ESVEM did not test amiodarone or ICDs. Sotalol has been shown to be effective in an ICD population where, when compared to placebo, it significantly reduced the number of both appropriate and inappropriate ICD shocks.[56]

The Sotalol Amiodarone AF Efficacy Trial (SAFE-T) was a randomized, double-blind, placebo-controlled trial that compared sotalol versus amiodarone in restoration and maintenance of sinus rhythm in patients with persistent AF. A total of 665 patients were randomized to sotalol (n = 261), amiodarone (n = 261) and placebo (n = 137), and were monitored weekly for 1–4.5 years. The primary endpoint was time to recurrence of AF. Sotalol and amiodarone were equally efficacious in converting AF to sinus rhythm (24% in sotalol group vs 27% in amiodarone group) and both were superior to placebo. The median time to AF recurrence was 487 days in the amiodarone group when compared to 74 days in the sotalol group and 6 days in the placebo group. Amiodarone was clearly superior to sotalol and placebo for maintenance of sinus rhythm.

Sotalol, however, was equally efficacious as amiodarone in maintaining sinus rhythm in the subgroup of patients with ischemic heart disease. Major adverse events were comparable among the three groups.[57]

The effects of sotalol, a class III AAD, can result in dose-dependent QTc prolongation and risk of torsades de pointes. At doses ranging from 160 mg/day to 240 mg/day, QTc prolongation of 10–40 ms was noted. Of particular concern is the situation where patients receive concomitant diuretics with frequent dose changes and inadequate potassium replacement. The overall incidence of torsades de pointes appears to be 2% and is more common in females, structural heart disease, and is exacerbated by hypokalemia and concomitant use of other AADs or QT-prolonging drugs. Careful dose titration and dose adjustment in renal insufficiency are essential to avoid risk of torsades de pointes. Typical adverse effects of beta-blockers such as bronchospasm, masking of hypoglycemia and rebound tachycardia, and hypertension on drug withdrawal may also be seen with sotalol. Concomitant use of sotalol with other QT-prolonging drugs increases the risk of torsades de pointes.

Dofetilide

Dofetilide is a potent and selective IKr blocker that prolongs action potential duration and refractoriness, more so in the atrium than in the ventricle.[58] Dofetilide does not exhibit any negative inotropic properties and has no effect on conduction velocity.

Oral bioavailability of dofetilide exceeds 90% and peak plasma concentrations are attained in 2–3 hours. The drug is partially metabolized by CYP3A4 to inactive metabolites and excreted predominantly (80%) in the urine with an elimination half-life of 8–10 hours. Drug elimination is reduced and accumulation results in renal failure, necessitating dosage adjustment and/or drug discontinuation. Medications that can induce or inhibit CYP3A4 metabolism can affect dofetilide concentrations and can potentially lead to adverse effects.[59]

Dofetilide is primarily used in the restoration and maintenance of sinus rhythm in AF, especially in patients with structural heart disease. The Danish Investigators of Arrhythmia and Mortality on Dofetilide trial (DIAMOND), which evaluated dofetilide versus placebo on all-cause mortality in 1,518 patients with symptomatic congestive heart failure and severe left ventricular dysfunction, showed no difference in all-cause mortality between the two arms. A significant decrease in the risk of heart failure hospitalization was observed in the dofetilide group. In patients with AF, dofetilide resulted in a 12% conversion rate to sinus rhythm compared to 1% in the placebo group (p < 0.05) and once sinus rhythm was restored, dofetilide was significantly more effective in maintaining sinus rhythm than placebo (HR 0.35; 95% confidence interval 0.22–0.57; P < 0.001). Twenty-five cases of torsades de pointes were reported in the dofetilide group (3.3%) as compared with none in the placebo group.[60]

The recommended dosage of dofetilide is 500 μg twice daily, but the dose varies based on renal function. Given the risk of torsades de pointes, physicians are required to receive special training prior to prescribing dofetilide. The drug has to be initiated in the hospital with continuous electrocardiographic

CHAPTER 30

Antiarrhythmic Drugs

TABLE 4B

Dofetilide renal dosing algorithm

Creatinine clearance (measured by Cockcroft-Gault method) ml/min	Dosing frequency
> 60	500 mcg twice daily
40–60	250 mcg twice daily
20–39	125 mcg twice daily
< 20	Contraindicated
Hemodialysis	Contraindicated

monitoring for either 3 days or 12 hours after conversion to sinus rhythm, whichever is greater. Creatinine clearance needs to be measured (using the Cockcroft-Gault formula) prior to initiation. A 500 mcg twice daily dosing is initiated only in patients with creatinine clearance more than 60 ml/min. The renal dosing algorithm for dofetilide is shown in Table 4B. Once initiated, if the QTc at 2–3 hours following the first dose is more than 15% from baseline or more than 500 msec (> 550 msec for bundle branch block or intraventricular conduction delay), then the dose needs to be reduced. If the QTc is more than 500 msec (> 550 msec for bundle branch block or intraventricular conduction delay) at any time during doses 2–6, dofetilide needs to be discontinued and an alternative drug sought. Despite initial enthusiasm with regard to the use of the drug,[61] its use has been tempered by strict regulations regarding its use.

The major adverse effect of dofetilide is torsades de pointes. The incidence is dose-dependent and is also influenced by structural heart disease and concomitant usage of QT-prolonging medications.[60,62] The overall incidence, during maintenance therapy on 500 μg twice daily, is around 1.7%.[63] Verapamil, trimethoprim, thiazides, azole antifungals and cimetidine should be discontinued prior to dofetilide initiation as concomitant administration results in markedly elevated plasma concentrations of dofetilide and increases risk of torsades de pointes.[59] Inducers of CYP3A4, such as phenobarbital and rifampin, can enhance dofetilide metabolism and decrease its efficacy. Dofetilide does not interact with digoxin or warfarin.

Ibutilide

Ibutilide is a methane sulfonamide analog of sotalol that is a potent blocker of IKr, resulting in prolongation of action potential duration and refractoriness. In addition, ibutilide also activates the slow inward sodium current.[64] Ibutilide is only available for intravenous use and is currently approved for rapid conversion of recent-onset AF and atrial flutter.

The Ibutilide Repeat Dose Study was a multicenter trial that randomly assigned 266 patients with AF of atrial flutter of recent-onset (3–45 days) to ibutilide or matching placebo. Ibutilide was administered as two 10-minute infusions of 1 mg, separated by 10 minutes. The overall conversion rate was 47% with ibutilide versus 2% with placebo (p < 0.0001), with the drug being more efficacious in atrial flutter than AF (63% vs 31%; p < 0.0001). The mean time to conversion was 27 minutes postinfusion. Among patients who received ibutilide, 8.3% developed torsades de pointes during infusion.[65] Ibutilide has also been shown to be efficacious in conversion of AF in patients with Wolff-Parkinson-White syndrome.

Ibutilide is given as an intravenous infusion over 10 minutes. Recommended dose is 1 mg given over 10 minutes. A second 1 mg dose, separated from the first dose by 10 minutes, can be given if the atrial arrhythmia persists. The drug has a half-life of ~ 6 hours and is primarily metabolized by the liver. No dosage adjustments are recommended for hepatic or renal dysfunction.

The major side effect of ibutilide is QTc prolongation and torsades de pointes, which developed in 8.3% of patients in the Ibutilide Repeat Dose Study.[65] Due to this, it is essential that patients receiving ibutilide have continuous electrocardiographic monitoring for 4–6 hours following treatment, with skilled personnel and resuscitation equipment available and ready. Ibutilide should be avoided in patients with baseline QTc prolongation (> 440 msec), advanced structural heart disease, and electrolyte abnormalities such as hypokalemia or hypomagnesemia, given the higher risk of torsades de pointes in these situations.

The use of ibutilide for pharmacological conversion of AF or atrial flutter was never popular given modest efficacy, high risk of polymorphic VT, and the need for close monitoring following drug administration. Several studies have shown that concurrent administration of intravenous magnesium improves efficacy of ibutilide.[66-70] A better method to improve the safety and efficacy of ibutilide was addressed in a recent randomized trial. Fragakis, et al. randomly assigned patients with recent-onset AF with rapid ventricular rate to receive ibutilide alone or a combination of ibutilide and esmolol and showed that intravenous beta-blockade resulted in a significant improvement in conversion rate (67% for the combination vs 46% for ibutilide alone) with marked reduction in immediate recurrence of AF. The combination of ibutilide plus esmolol proved to be safer also (no cases of polymorphic VT in the combination group vs 6.5% in the ibutilide group).[71] This combination of ibutilide and esmolol, along with newer drugs like vernakalant, may result in an expanded role for pharmacological agents in the restoration of sinus rhythm in AF.[72]

Amiodarone

Amiodarone, a synthesized, iodinated benzofuran derivative, structurally similar to thyroxine, was identified with initial work with the ammi visnaga plant.[73] Although classified as a class III AAD, it is a complex and unique drug with properties spanning all four Vaughan-Williams classes. The exact mechanism responsible for its antiarrhythmic actions remains unclear. In animal studies, amiodarone has been shown to prolong action potential duration and refractoriness in the atria and the ventricles, the AV node, and Purkinje fibers.[74] Amiodarone also blocks inactivated sodium channels, slows phase 4 depolarization in sinus node, and delays AV nodal conduction.[75] Electrophysiological properties of amiodarone differ between intravenous and oral use. During intravenous use, amiodarone exhibits sodium and calcium channel blocking properties, has greater effect at higher heart rates and in depolarized tissue. This property makes it useful in treatment of ventricular arrhythmias in the setting of myocardial ischemia. Chronic oral therapy with amiodarone prolongs the PR and QT intervals on the surface electrocardiogram.

Amiodarone is highly lipid-soluble and has a large volume of distribution (20–200 l/kg).[76] Oral bioavailability is highly variable and it usually takes weeks before a steady state is reached, as it accumulates slowly in the adipose tissue. A dose of more than 10 g is usually needed to saturate the fat stores. Amiodarone is mostly metabolized to desethylamiodarone. Plasma half-life after intravenous administration ranges from 4.8 hours to 68.2 hours.[77] Elimination is slow and extremely variable with a half-life ranging from 13 days to 103 days. Dosage adjustment is not required in renal disease. Neither hemodialysis nor peritoneal dialysis removes amiodarone.

US Food and Drug Administration has currently approved amiodarone only for refractory, life-threatening ventricular arrhythmias, although the drug is widely used in the treatment of a variety of atrial and ventricular arrhythmias. Clinical data supporting the use of the amiodarone in ventricular arrhythmias is summarized below.

The European Myocardial Infarction Amiodarone Trial (EMIAT)[78] and Canadian Amiodarone Myocardial Infarction Arrhythmia Trial (CAMIAT)[79] were large randomized trials that evaluated the impact of amiodarone after myocardial infarction. In EMIAT, 1,486 post-myocardial infarction patients with a left ventricular ejection fraction less than 40% were randomly assigned to receive either amiodarone ($n = 743$; loading period followed by 200 mg/day), or matching placebo ($n = 743$). Presence of ventricular arrhythmia was not needed for inclusion. No difference in all-cause or cardiovascular death was seen after a median follow-up of 21 months. A 35% risk reduction ($p < 0.05$) in arrhythmic deaths was seen in the amiodarone group.[78]

In CAMIAT, 1,202 patients who were 6–45 days post-myocardial infarction and had a mean of at least 10 PVCs/hour were randomly assigned to amiodarone ($n = 606$) or placebo ($n = 596$) and followed for a mean of 1.8 years. Patients in the amiodarone group had a 48.5% reduction ($p = 0.016$) in the combined endpoint of resuscitation from ventricular fibrillation or arrhythmic death (3.3% in the amiodarone group vs 6.6% in the placebo group). There was no significant difference in all-cause mortality ($p = 0.13$) between the two groups.[79]

The EMIAT and CAMIAT showed that amiodarone given post-myocardial infarction can reduce arrhythmic death but did not improve total mortality. In a pooled post-hoc analysis of EMIAT and CAMIAT, the combination of amiodarone with a beta-blocker resulted in significant improvements in arrhythmic death or resuscitated cardiac arrest when compared to beta-blockers alone, amiodarone alone, or placebo. Non-significant reductions in total mortality were noted with the combination compared to those not receiving beta-blockers.[80]

Estudio Piloto Argentino de Muerte Sfibita y Amiodarone (EPAMSA), Grupo de Estudio de la Sobrevida en la Insuficiencia Cardiaca en Argentina (GESICA) and Congestive Heart Failure Survival Trial of Antiarrhythmic Therapy (CHF-STAT) were trials that evaluated the role of amiodarone in patients with congestive heart failure.[81-83] The EPAMSA randomized patients with a left ventricular ejection fraction less than or equal to 35% and asymptomatic ventricular arrhythmias to receive either amiodarone ($n = 66$) or no drug ($n = 61$). During a 12-month follow-up period, total mortality (10.6% vs 28.8%,

$p = 0.02$) and sudden death (7% vs 20.4%, $p = 0.04$) were reduced in patients receiving amiodarone compared to placebo.[81]

The GESICA was a multicenter, randomized trial of 516 patients in Argentina with congestive heart failure and left ventricular systolic function less than or equal to 35% (39% with ischemic cardiomyopathy), but no history of symptomatic ventricular arrhythmias. The trial showed that patients receiving amiodarone had a 28% reduced risk of death and a 31% reduced risk of heart failure hospitalizations, when compared to placebo.[82]

The CHF-STAT, on the other hand, randomized 674 patients with congestive heart failure, a left ventricular ejection fraction less than or equal to 40%, and at least 10 PVCs/hour, to amiodarone ($n = 336$) or matching placebo ($n = 338$). Over a median follow-up of 45 months, amiodarone was associated with PVC suppression and improved left ventricular function. No difference in total mortality ($p = 0.6$) or sudden death ($p = 0.43$) was found between the two groups.[83] The reason for the difference in outcomes between GESICA and EPAMSA versus CHF-STAT has been attributed to the presence of a higher percentage of patients with ischemic cardiomyopathy in CHF-STAT. Drug discontinuation rate of amiodarone in these studies ranged from 20% to 40%.

A meta-analysis of 15 randomized controlled trials ($n = 8,522$) of amiodarone versus placebo for prevention of sudden cardiac death showed that amiodarone was associated with a 29% reduced risk of sudden cardiac death (7.1% vs 9.7%; OR 0.72, $p < 0.001$) and an 18% reduced risk of cardiovascular death (14.0% vs 16.3%; OR 0.82, $p = 0.004$). No significant difference in all-cause mortality was demonstrated. Patients who received amiodarone were more likely to have thyroid problems (OR 5.68; $p < 0.0001$), pulmonary toxicity (OR 1.97; $p = 0.002$), hepatotoxicity (OR 2.1; $p = 0.015$), or bradyarrhythmias (OR 1.78; $p = 0.008$) when compared to the control group.[84] The literature thus suggests that amiodarone is beneficial in treatment of ventricular arrhythmias in patients with cardiomyopathy and congestive heart failure. These findings also suggest that amiodarone is a reasonable option, albeit with risk for long-term side effects and no all-cause mortality benefit, for prevention of sudden cardiac death in patients who are not ICD candidates.

For most patients, however, the reason to use amiodarone to treat ventricular arrhythmias in patients with implantable devices is to suppress recurrent episodes of VT and ventricular fibrillation leading to ICD shocks. It is important to recognize that amiodarone can increase the threshold of energy necessary to defibrillate the patient and can slow the VT rates.[40]

Amiodarone is by far the most effective AAD to maintain sinus rhythm in patients with AF. The Canadian Trial of AF (CTAF) was a prospective, multicenter, randomized trial that randomly assigned 403 patients with at least one episode of AF in the past 6 months to receive amiodarone or either sotalol or propafenone. After a mean follow-up of 16 months, AF recurrence was noted in 35% of patients in the amiodarone group versus 63% in the sotalol or propafenone groups ($p < 0.001$). Adverse effects resulting in drug discontinuation was higher in the amiodarone group (18% vs 11% in the sotalol/propafenone group) but was not statistically significant ($p = 0.06$).[85]

The SAFE-T trial, which compared amiodarone against sotalol in the restoration and maintenance of sinus rhythm in patients with persistent AF, showed that amiodarone was equally efficacious as sotalol in restoring sinus rhythm but was vastly superior to sotalol in maintaining sinus rhythm. Major adverse events in the amiodarone group were comparable to placebo.[57] The relative safety of amiodarone when used in treatment of AF was illustrated in a Cochrane database review of 45 randomized controlled studies ($n = 12,559$) that evaluated the different AADs used for maintenance of sinus rhythm in AF. The effect on these drugs on mortality, thromboembolic events, and proarrhythmia were noted. The study found that class IA, class IC and class III drugs showed a significant reduction in AF recurrence (odds ratio 0.19–0.60, number needed to treat: 2–9) compared to placebo, but none improved mortality. Class IA drugs were associated with increased mortality and all drugs, except propafenone and amiodarone, increased the risk of proarrhythmia.[7]

Given huge volume of distribution, a loading dose regimen is essential to ensure onset of therapeutic action within a reasonable time frame. Loading can be done using intravenous or oral dosing. For outpatient initiation, we routinely employ a loading regimen (400 mg three to four times a day) that ensures a 10–15 g load within 7–10 days after initiation. Once the 10 g load is complete, the patient is switched to a maintenance dose of 200–400 mg a day. The loading dose is generally higher in those patients who have ventricular tachyarrhythmias and the long-term maintenance dose is higher as well. For patients with AF or other atrial arrhythmias, the maintenance dose can be as low as 100–200 mg a day with a load less than 10 g orally.

The manufacturer recommended and routinely used intravenous infusion regimen follows three phases over 24 hours: 150 mg over 10 minutes (with an additional bolus dose of 150 mg for patients with recurrent VT), followed by 1 mg/min over the next 6 hours, followed by 0.5 mg/min over next 18 hours. Infusion should preferably be through a central line to avoid risk of phlebitis. Intravenous amiodarone can result in hypotension and negative inotropy.

Amiodarone is well-tolerated in the long-term if close attention is paid to screen for and recognize adverse events.[86] Side effects are common and can range from 15% in the first year to 50% with long-term use. The majority of the side effects are extracardiac, with the most serious one being interstitial pneumonitis leading to pulmonary fibrosis.[87] This can be difficult to predict and challenging to diagnose.[87,88]

Amiodarone frequently affects thyroid function, but it can also cause hypersensitivity to the sun, cause skin color changes, have neurological effects (weakness, difficulty in walking especially in the elderly), effects on hepatic function and potentially optic neuritis. Corneal microdeposits are common but of little importance. Amiodarone can also cause sinus bradycardia and AV block.[86]

Amiodarone can increase serum levels of digoxin, quinidine, procainamide, flecainide, cyclosporine and warfarin. Although amiodarone can prolong QTc interval, risk of torsades de pointes is extremely rare, perhaps secondary to its multichannel blocking properties or to the uniformity by which it prolongs repolarization.

A comprehensive list of adverse reactions to amiodarone and their management is shown in Table 5. Fortunately, the majority of the adverse reactions can be easily managed and do not necessitate discontinuation of the drug. Adverse reactions to amiodarone depend, in part, on the dose and the duration of therapy. If long-term administration is considered, the lowest effective dose should be selected to minimize toxicity. Even then, regular and careful monitoring is essential to ensure patient safety. All patients at initiation of therapy should have a 12-lead electrocardiogram, chest X-ray, pulmonary function test (including DLCO), and laboratory evaluation for electrolytes and renal function, liver function, and thyroid function. An ophthalmological evaluation is recommended at baseline if there is visual impairment, and a follow-up evaluation should be done for new eye-related symptoms. Liver function and thyroid function tests are assessed every 6 months. An electrocardiogram and a chest X-ray should be repeated yearly. Follow-up pulmonary function tests should be done for new or unexplained dyspnea or if there are abnormalities in the chest X-ray compared to baseline.[86]

Amiodarone interferes with the clearance of many drugs, especially those that are highly protein bound. The major drug interactions of amiodarone are listed in Table 3. Of particular importance is the inhibition of warfarin and digoxin clearance by amiodarone, resulting in higher plasma levels of these drugs and necessitating dosage reduction or discontinuation. Warfarin dose should be reduced to half and digoxin should be discontinued if that particular patient is started on amiodarone.

Dronedarone

Dronedarone is structurally similar to amiodarone but lacks the iodine moiety. It has multichannel blocking properties similar to amiodarone but it is not as potent. Dronedarone was initially developed with the aim to reducing or eliminating amiodarone-induced toxicity while maintaining efficacy. For clinical purposes, dronedarone is classified as a Vaughan-Williams Class III AAD. Electrophysiological properties of dronedarone include inhibitory effects on the rapid delayed-rectifier, slow delayed-rectifier, acetylcholine-activated, and inward-rectifier potassium channels, inward sodium current, T-type and L-type calcium channels, and alpha-adrenoceptors and beta-adrenoceptors.[89,90] Dronedarone slows down sinus rate by suppression of sinus node automaticity and by changing the slope of phase 4 depolarization in the sinus node.[91] The drug also slows AV conduction, increase SAV nodal and ventricular effective refractory period, and has been shown to reduce VT and PVCs in ischemic animal models.[89,92]

Dronedarone has negligible proarrhythmic effect but has been shown to increase mortality in patients with acute heart failure.[93] Dronedarone is devoid of the many adverse effects and drug interactions associated with amiodarone. Pulmonary toxicity has not been reported with dronedarone. When compared to placebo, there was no significant difference in hyperthyroidism, hypothyroidism, neurological abnormalities, gastrointestinal and hepatic abnormalities with dronedarone. Similar to amiodarone, dronedarone causes mild increases in serum creatinine by inhibiting cation transport in the renal tubules. Glomerular filtration rate, however, is not affected.[94]

TABLE 5

Incidence, diagnosis, and management of major adverse reactions to amiodarone

Reaction	Incidence (%)	Diagnosis	Management
Pulmonary	2	Couth and/or dyspnea, especially with local or diffuse opacities on high-resolution CT scan and decrease in DLCO from baseline	Usually discontinue drug; corticosteroids may be considered in more severe cases; occasionally, can continue drug if levels high and abnormalities resolve; rarely, continue amiodarone with corticosteroid if no other option
Gastrointestinal tract	30 15–30 <3	Nausea, anorexia and constipation AST or ALT level greater than 2 times normal Hepatitis and cirrhosis	Symptoms may decrease with decrease in dose If hepatitis considered, exclude other causes Consider discontinuation, biopsy or both to determine whether cirrhosis is present
Thyroid	4–22 2–12	Hypothyroidism Hyperthyroidism	L-Thyroxine Corticosteroids, propylthiouracil or methimazole; may need thyroidectomy
Skin	<10 25–75	Blue discoloration Photosensitivity	Reassurance; decrease in dose Avoidance of prolonged sun exposure; sunblock; decrease in dose
Central nervous system	3–30	Ataxia, paresthesias, peripheral polyneuropathy, sleep disturbance, impaired memory and tremor	Often dose dependent, and may improve or resolve with dose adjustment
Ocular	<5 ≤1 >90	Halo vision, especially at night Optic neuropathy Photophobia, visual blurring and microdeposits	Corneal deposits the norm; if optic neuropathy occurs, discontinue Discontinue drug and consult an ophthalmologist
Heart	5 <1	Bradycardia and AV block Proarrhythmia	May need permanent cardiac pacing May need to discontinue the drug
Genitourinary	<1	Epididymitis and erectile dysfunction	Pain may resolve spontaneously

(Abbreviations: ALT: Alanine aminotransferase; AST: Aspartate aminotransferase; DLCO: Diffusion capacity of carbone monoxide). [*Source:* Goldschlager N, Epstein AE, Naccarelli GV, et al. A practical guide for clinicians who treat patients with amiodarone: 2007. Heart Rhythm. 2007;4:1250-9 (Reference 86)]

CHAPTER 30

Antiarrhythmic Drugs

Dronedarone is metabolized by the hepatic CYP3A4 system and in turn is also a moderate inhibitor of the CYP3A4 system and weak CYP2D6 and P-glycoprotein inhibitor. These properties result in increased effects of drugs like cyclosporine, digoxin and some statins when coadministered with dronedarone.[94] Unlike amiodarone, dronedarone does not have any drug interactions with warfarin.

A synopsis of the randomized clinical trials that evaluated the impact of dronedarone in AF and heart failure are shown in Table 6 and have been summarized in detail.[95] The European Trial in AF or Flutter Patients Receiving Dronedarone for the Maintenance of Sinus Rhythm (EURIDIS) and the American-Australian-African Trial with Dronedarone in AF or Flutter Patients for the Maintenance of Sinus Rhythm (ADONIS) compared dronedarone to placebo in maintaining sinus rhythm after conversion from atrial flutter or AF. The EURIDIS showed that at the end of 1 year of follow-up, 67% of patients on dronedarone had a recurrence of AF compared to 78% in the placebo group. In the ADONIS trial, 61% in the dronedarone group had recurrent AF compared to 73% in the placebo. Although significantly different from placebo, the high recurrence rate of AF with dronedarone cast doubts on its efficacy to maintain sinus rhythm.[96]

The DIONYSOS trial[97] [Randomized, Double-Blind TrIal to Evaluate the Efficacy and Safety of DrOnedarone (400 mg bid) Vs AmiodaroNe (600 mg qd for 28 daYS, then 200 mg qd Thereafter) for at least 6 months for the Maintenance of Sinus Rhythm in Patients with AF] directly compared dronedarone (400 mg twice daily) to amiodarone (600 mg every day for 28 days, then 200 mg every day thereafter) in restoration and maintenance of sinus rhythm in patients with AF. During a mean follow-up of 7 months, 64% of patients in the dronedarone arm had AF recurrence when compared to 42% in the amiodarone arm. Adverse event rates were high, but comparable between both drugs (39% with dronedarone vs 45% with amiodarone; HR 0.80, $p = 0.13$). There were fewer thyroid, neurological, skin, and eye-related adverse events with dronedarone except gastrointestinal side effects, which were higher in the dronedarone group. In summary, dronedarone was inferior to amiodarone in efficacy, but was more favorable than amiodarone in terms of safety.[97]

The Efficacy and Safety of Dronedarone for the Control of Ventricular Rate during AF (ERATO) study found dronedarone to be effective for ventricular rate control in patients with AF, both at rest and with exercise.[98]

The ATHENA (A Placebo-Controlled, Double-Blind, Parallel Arm Trial to Assess the Efficacy of Dronedarone 400 mg bid for the Prevention of Cardiovascular Hospitalization or Death from Any Cause in Patients with Atrial Fibrillation/Atrial Flutter) trial evaluated the effect of dronedarone in reducing a

TABLE 6

Summary of randomized clinical trials that assessed the efficacy and safety of dronedarone in patients with atrial fibrillation and heart failure

Clinical trial	Patient profile	Number of patients	Intervention	Primary end point	Follow-up (months)	Results/Conclusions
DAFNE	Persistent AF post-cardio-version	199	Dronedarone (400–800 mg twice daily) versus placebo	Time to first recurrence of AF	6	Use of dronedarone was associated with a longer median time to AF recurrence (60 days vs 5.3 days for dronedarone and placebo respectively, $p = 0.026$; 55% relative risk reduction, $p = 0.001$); likewise, patients receiving dronedarone, 400 mg orally twice daily, were more likely to maintain sinus rhythm compared with patients receiving placebo
EURIDIS and ADONIS	Paroxysmal AF	1,237	Dronedarone 400 mg twice daily versus placebo	Time to first recurrence of AF	12	Dronedarone significantly lengthened the time to AF recurrence [41 days vs 96 days (EURIDIS) and 59 days vs 158 days (ADONIS) for dronedarone and placebo respectively], as well as symptoms associated with atrial fibrillation, compared with placebo. Ventricular rates during AF recurrence were significantly lower with dronedarone
DIONYSOS	Persistent AF for > 3 days	504	Dronedarone (400 mg twice daily) versus amiodarone (600 mg and then 200 mg per day)	AF recurrence or drug intolerance resulting in discontinuation	7	More patients on dronedarone had AF recurrence or stopped the drug due to intolerance or lack of efficacy compared with patients receiving amiodarone (75.1% vs 58.8% for dronedarone and amiodarone respectively, HR 1.59).
ERATO	Permanent AF with ventricular rates > 80 bpm on rate-controlling agents	630	Dronedarone 400 mg twice daily versus placebo	Mean ventricular rate at 2 weeks	1	Dronedarone use was associated with decrease in ventricular rate, both at rest (12.3 bpm with dronedarone vs 0.2 bpm with placebo) and with exercise (25.6 bpm with dronedarone vs 2.2 bpm with placebo)
ATHENA	Paroxysmal or persistent AF or atrial flutter with one or more associated risk factors	4,628	Dronedarone (400 mg twice daily) versus placebo	Composite of all-cause mortality and cardiovascular hospitalization	21±5	The use of dronedarone was associated with decreased cardiovascular deaths and arrhythmic deaths compared with placebo (31.9% in dronedarone arm vs 39.8% in placebo arm, HR 0.76). There was also a decrease in hospitalizations for AF and acute coronary syndrome in patients receiving dronedarone compared with placebo
ANDROMEDA	Congestive heart failure (NYHA Class III–IV); left ventricular ejection fraction < 35%	617	Dronedarone (400 mg twice daily) versus placebo	All-cause mortality or heart failure hospitalization	2	Trial was stopped early as dronedarone was associated with a significant increase in all-cause mortality (8.1% in the dronedarone arm vs 3.8% in placebo arm, HR 2.13)

composite endpoint of death or cardiovascular hospitalizations in AF patients.[99] A total of 4,628 patients with paroxysmal or persistent AF and presence of risk factors for stroke and/or death were randomized to dronedarone or matching placebo and were followed for a median period of 21 ± 5 months. The study found that patients randomized to dronedarone had fewer cardiovascular deaths (HR = 0.71; 95% CI, 0.51–0.98; $P = 0.03$), as well as arrhythmic deaths (HR = 0.55; 95% CI, 0.34–0.88; $P = 0.01$), when compared to placebo. There were also fewer cardiovascular hospitalizations in the dronedarone arm. A post-hoc analysis of ATHENA showed that there were fewer strokes or transient ischemic attacks in the dronedarone group.[100] The ATHENA was the first trial to show mortality benefit with an AAD and was largely responsible for approval of dronedarone in the United States.

The Antiarrhythmic Trial with Dronedarone in Moderate to Severe Congestive Heart Failure Evaluating Morbidity Decrease (ANDROMEDA) compared dronedarone with placebo in patients with AF hospitalized with new or worsening heart failure and a left ventricular ejection fraction less than 35%.[93] The study had to be terminated prematurely after a median follow-up of 2 months, as mortality was significantly increased in the dronedarone arm (8.1% vs 3.8% in the placebo arm). The increased mortality was predominantly attributed to deaths from worsening heart failure and treatment with dronedarone was the most powerful predictor of death. This study resulted in a black box warning for dronedarone that warns against its use in patients with New York Heart Association (NYHA) class IV heart failure or NYHA class II and III heart failure with recent decompensation requiring hospitalization or referral to a heart failure clinic.[94] Recent post-marketing data released by the manufacturer reports several cases of hepatocellular injury and at least two cases of acute hepatic failure requiring liver transplantation, which occurred at 4.5 months and 6 months following drug initiation. This has prompted a manufacturer recommendation to consider serial liver enzyme monitoring at least for the first 6 months while being on dronedarone.[101] PALLAS included patients at least 65 years old with at least 6-month history of permanent atrial fibrillation and risk factors for major vascular events. Patients received dronedarone or placebo. Of 3236 enrolled, the co-primary outcome of stroke, myocardial infarction, systemic embolism, or death from cardiovascular causes was higher with drenedarone (HR: 2.29; 95% confidence interval 1.34-3.94; P = 0.002). The death rate was higher with dronedarone (HR, 3.11; 95% confidence interval, 1.00-4.49; P = 0.046), including death from arrhythmia (HR, 3.26; 95% confidence interval 1.06-10.00; P = 0.03). There were more strokes (HR, 2.32; 95% confidence interval 1.11-4.88; P = 0.02) and more heart failure hospitalizations (HR, 1.81; 95% confidence interval 1.10 to 2.99; P = 0.02) with drenedarone.[101a]

Dronedarone, although not a very effective rhythm control drug by itself, remains the first AAD to show a reduction in cardiovascular mortality in AF patients with risk factors for stroke and/or death. Although mortality reduction is a significant finding, its clinical utility is unclear, as the primary goal in AF management is symptom reduction and improving quality of life. The favorable safety profile, as well as the fact that a loading dose is not needed, makes dronedarone an ideal drug to start as an outpatient. The fact that it improves mortality and reduces cardiovascular hospitalizations in patients with AF makes it attractive from a health care expenditure standpoint. On the other hand, it is our opinion that use of dronedarone should be avoided in patients with congestive heart failure and severe left ventricular dysfunction or for those patients with permanent AF. The 2011 ACCF/AHA/HRS focused update of the 2006 AF guidelines now include dronedarone.[31] It is fair to say that dronedarone has definitely expanded the horizon in terms of management options for AF.

Azimilide

Azimilide dihydrochloride is a class III AAD that blocks both the rapid (IKr) and the slow (IKs) delayed-rectifier potassium channels.[102] It is different from the other class III drugs that only block IKr. Azimilide prolongs the action potential duration and refractoriness in atrial and ventricular myocardium and has been shown to cause dose-dependent QTc prolongation.[102] Unlike other class III drugs, azimilide does not exhibit reverse use-dependence, which is thought to be secondary to IKs blockade.

The AzimiLide post-Infarct surVival Evaluation (ALIVE) trial assessed the effect of azimilide on survival in patients who were 6–21 days post-myocardial infarction and had a left ventricular ejection fraction ranging from 15% to 35%. No survival advantage was seen with azimilide but the drug caused no excessive harm.[103] Azimilide is not approved for clinical use in the United States but is available in Europe, where it has been primarily used for suppressing ventricular arrhythmias in ICD patients.

The SHock Inhibition Evaluation with azimiLiDe (SHIELD) trial was a randomized, double-blind, placebo controlled, international trial of 633 patients that evaluated the effect of azimilide, either 75 mg (n = 220) or 125 mg (n = 199) daily, versus placebo (n = 214) on all-cause shocks plus symptomatic tachycardias terminated by antitachycardia pacing and appropriate ICD therapies.[104] All patients enrolled in the trial had an ICD implanted and had either a documented episode of cardiac arrest or spontaneous sustained VT with left ventricular ejection fraction less than or equal to 0.40 during 42 days prior to the first ICD implantation or an ICD shock for spontaneous VT or ventricular fibrillation within the previous 180 days. Over a median follow-up of 367 days, there was a significant 57% reduction in all-cause shocks plus antitachycardia pacing (ATP) therapies in the azimilide 75 mg per day group compared to placebo (HR = 0.43; CI 0.26–0.69, P = 0.0006). A 47% reduction was seen in the azimilide 125 mg per day group (HR = 0.53; CI 0.34–0.83, P = 0.0053). Both doses of azimilide decreased all-cause shocks but this was not statistically significant. When compared to placebo, azimilide 75 mg and 125 mg per day reduced appropriate ICD shocks and ATP by 48% (p = 0.017) and 62% (p = 0.0004) respectively. High (35–40%) but comparable rates of drug discontinuation was seen in both azimilide and placebo groups. Four patients in the azimilide group and one in the placebo group had torsades de pointes. Thus, it appears that azimilide has beneficial effects in prevention of ventricular arrhythmias in ICD patients.

On the other hand, azimilide was disappointing as a rhythm control drug for restoration and maintenance of sinus rhythm in AF. The North American Azimilide Cardioversion Maintenance Trial (ACOMET II) study compared azimilide (125 mg daily) with sotalol (160 mg twice daily) or placebo for maintaining sinus rhythm in 658 patients with persistent AF undergoing electrical cardioversion.[105] The primary endpoint was recurrence of AF. Azimilide was found to be superior to placebo, but was significantly inferior to sotalol in maintaining sinus rhythm.

The Azimilide Supraventricular Tachyarrhythmia Reduction (A-STAR) trial evaluated the effect of azimilide in maintaining sinus rhythm in patients with structural heart disease.[106] The trial randomized 220 patients to azimilide (125 mg daily) versus matching placebo, and patients were followed for time to first symptomatic AF recurrence. There was no significant difference between the azimilide and the placebo groups with respect to the primary endpoint. In terms of adverse effects, neutropenia was seen in 1% of patients who were on azimilide. A dose-dependent increase in torsades de pointes was noted with the incidence rates ranging from 0.3% for the 75 mg dose to 1.2% for the 100 mg dose.[107] Thus, in terms of AF rhythm control, the risk-benefit ratio was definitely not in favor of azimilide, and it is doubtful that this drug will be available for use in AF.

CLASS IV ANTIARRHYTHMIC DRUGS: CALCIUM CHANNEL ANTAGONISTS

Verapamil blocks the L-type calcium channel and can be used to slow AV nodal conduction to control the ventricular response rate atrial flutter and AF, but it could also be used to prevent recurrence of AV nodal reentry and AV reentry supraventricular tachycardia. Furthermore, verapamil can prevent triggered activity and inhibit idiopathic right ventricular outflow tract tachycardias by this mechanism. Additionally, verapamil can affect reentrant mechanisms responsible for idiopathic left VT. The dose of verapamil is 120–480 mg a day in single or divided doses. Diltiazem, another calcium channel blocker that can be used to control the ventricular response rate in AF, is available in both intravenous and oral formulations.

MISCELLANEOUS DRUGS

ADENOSINE

Adenosine is an ultrashort acting purinergic agonist; it is vagotonic. It binds to the adenosine A1 receptor. Adenosine activates the $IK_{ACH,ADO}$ channels present in the atrium, sinus node and the AV node. This results in increased outward potassium current which leads to shortening of atrial action potential and membrane hyperpolarization and transient AV nodal block and sinus node depression.[108] These IK_{ADO} channels are not present in the ventricular myocytes and, therefore adenosine has not much of an effect in the ventricular myocardium. Indirectly, adenosine has an antiadrenergic action due to a decrease in cyclic AMP. This property might be responsible for its suppressive effect on outflow tract ventricular arrhythmias as well as a subgroup of focal atrial tachycardias, which probably are delayed after depolarization-mediated triggered rhythms resulting from catecholamine-mediated calcium overload.

Adenosine has a rapid onset of action and intravenous administration of 6–12 mg adenosine results in sinus node slowing and transient AV block. This property is most often used to terminate AV node dependent paroxysmal AV nodal reentry and orthodromic AV reentry supraventricular tachycardias. Adenosine can stop idiopathic VTs, especially those that originate from the right ventricular outflow tract.[109] It can also terminate some atrial tachycardias.[110] Adenosine is commonly used during an electrophysiology study to determine the presence of a concealed accessory pathway. The vasodilatory properties of adenosine make it useful as a chemical alternative to exercise in the diagnosis of myocardial ischemia.

Adverse effects with adenosine typically include dyspnea, chest tightness, flushing and exacerbation of bronchospasm. These are typically short-lasting and resolve quickly. Adenosine should be used with caution in patients with severe reactive airway disease. Use of adenosine can result in AF in 10–15% of patients due to shortening of atrial refractory periods. Transplanted hearts are exquisitely sensitive to adenosine and significant dose reduction is required.[111] Methylxanthines, such as caffeine and theophylline, block adenosine receptors and counteract the effects of adenosine. Dipyridamole reduces the reuptake of adenosine, thereby prolonging the effect of adenosine. Due to this, those who are on oral dipyridamole undergoing a stress test should receive intravenous dipyridamole and not adenosine.

NEWER DRUGS

TEDISAMIL

Tedisamil is a class III AAD that blocks multiple potassium channels, including IKr, IKs, IKur, Ito and IKATP.[112] Tedisamil

prolong atrial and ventricular action potentials, but its effects are more pronounced in the atrial tissue. It also suppresses sinus node function and has antianginal properties.[107] Tedisamil has a half-life of 8–13 hours, is not metabolized, and is renally excreted.

A randomized, placebo-controlled dose-response study ($n = 175$) showed that tedisamil at doses of 0.4 mg/kg and 0.6 mg/kg was superior to placebo in converting new-onset AF to sinus rhythm. Efficacy was modest with a 41% conversion rate for 0.4 mg/kg and 51% conversion rate for the 0.6 mg/kg tedisamil group. There were two cases of ventricular arrhythmias (one case of torsades de pointes and one case of monomorphic VT) in the tedisamil group.[112] Clearly, more studies are needed to evaluate the safety and efficacy of tedisamil in AF.

VERNAKALANT

Vernakalant is the first in a class of AADs that are "atrial-selective". Atrial-selective drugs are being developed to target the ion channels or currents that are present in the atria and not in the ventricles. These include the ultra rapid potassium current IKur and the acetylcholine-mediated potassium channel IK_{ACH}. The goal for developing these drugs is to restore and maintain sinus rhythm in AF while avoiding the adverse ventricular events such as QTc prolongation and torsades de pointes.[113]

Vernakalant acts selectively in the atrium, targeting the following ion channels: IKur, IK_{ACH}, Ito and late INA.[114] The efficacy and safety of intravenous vernakalant (administered as a 10-minute intravenous infusion at a dose of 3 mg/kg; if AF had not been terminated within 15 minutes, a second 10-minute infusion be followed at a dose of 2 mg/kg) for the treatment of AF was assessed in the randomized, placebo-controlled, double-blind Atrial Arrhythmia Conversion Trials (ACT) I–III.[115-117] The ACT I and ACT III trials investigated vernakalant in the treatment of patients with sustained AF (duration > 3 hours, but not more than 45 days). A total of 336 patients were enrolled in ACT I and 276 patients in ACT III. The primary endpoint was conversion to sinus rhythm for at least 1 minute within 90 minutes of drug infusion. In both these trials, vernakalant was significantly better than placebo in converting AF to sinus rhythm.

In ACT I, sinus rhythm was achieved in 62% of patients receiving vernakalant compared with 4.9% of patients receiving placebo for AF of 3–48 hour duration.[115] In ACT III, 51.2% of patients receiving vernakalant converted to sinus rhythm compared with 3.6% of patients receiving placebo for AF of 3 hours to 7 days.[117] The median time to conversion was 10 minutes from the start of infusion and sinus rhythm was maintained for more than 24 hours in 97% of patients. Data from the ACT II trial, which investigated the efficacy of intravenous vernakalant in 150 patients with sustained AF (3–72 hours duration) that occurred between 24 hours and 7 days after coronary artery bypass graft and/or valvular surgery, showed a 47% conversion rate compared to 14% for placebo.[116]

In the AVRO (A Phase III Superiority Study of Vernakalant versus Amiodarone in Subjects With Recent Onset Atrial Fibrillation) trial, 254 patients with recent-onset AF (3–48 hours duration) were randomized to receive either intravenous vernakalant or intravenous amiodarone. Treatment with vernakalant converted 51.7% of patients to sinus rhythm at

90 minutes compared with 5.2% of patients treated with amiodarone. Both drugs were well tolerated.[118]

Vernakalant does not appear to be effective in AF of longer duration (> 7 days) or in atrial flutter.[117] Preliminary studies have shown that oral vernakalant (5 mg/kg) is rapidly absorbed and well-tolerated. Studies are ongoing to determine efficacy and safety of the oral formulation. Vernakalant appears to have a good safety profile but concerns still exist. Most common side effects are nausea, dysgeusia, paresthesias and hypotension.[117] No episodes of drug-induced torsades de pointes were reported in the ACT trials.

Currently, vernakalant is approved in Europe for rapid conversion of recent-onset AF ($\leq$ 7 days duration for non-surgery patients, and less than or equal to 3 days duration for post-cardiac surgery patients) to sinus rhythm in adults. The atrial selectivity, modest efficacy rate and excellent safety profile makes vernakalant an important addition to the armamentarium for pharmacological conversion of AF.

IVABRADINE

High resting sinus heart rates have been independently associated with mortality and adverse cardiovascular outcomes.[119,120] Ivabradine is a selective cardiac pacemaker (I_f) current blocker that slows sinus rates.[121] When compared to placebo in the BEAUTIFUL (morBidity mortality EvAlUaTion of the I_f inhibitor ivabradine in patients with coronary disease and left ventricULar dysfunction) trial, ivabradine did not improve the composite outcome of cardiovascular death, hospitalizations for heart failure and/or acute myocardial infarction in patients with coronary artery and left ventricular dysfunction.[122] However, it did reduce fatal- and non-fatal myocardial infarction and coronary revascularization[122] and so may be useful as an antianginal drug, especially in combination with a beta-blocker.[123] Recent data would suggest that slowing heart rate may, in fact, improve outcomes in select patients with congestive heart failure[124] and with inappropriate sinus tachycardia.[125] Usual dosing range is 5–7.5 mg twice daily.

RANOLAZINE

Ranolazine is an antianginal drug that also can affect the late and the peak inward sodium current, the late calcium current and the IKr and IKs currents, as well as the sodium/calcium exchanger.[126] In the Efficiency with Ranolazine for Less Ischemia in Non-ST elevation acute coronary syndromes (MERLIN)-TIMI 36 trial, ranolazine significantly lowered nonsustained VT and supraventricular tachyarrhythmias in patients with non-ST elevation myocardial infarction when compared to placebo.[127] Recent data from a canine model suggests that ranolazine, in combination with dronedarone, may be a potent combination to reduce AF.[128]

EMERGING ANTIARRHYTHMIC DRUGS

Various novel AADs are presently being tested but they are nowhere near being considered valuable and/or valid therapies for arrhythmia suppression. Research continues with nifekalant, an IKr blocker for ventricular arrhythmias, celivarone, an amiodarone analogue, several IKur (and multichannel) blockers (AVE0118, AZD7009, NIP-141/142), sodium current blockers

(pilsicainide and ranolazine), other amiodarone analogues (celivarone, ATI-2042 and PM101), selective IKs blockers (HMR1556) and Kv1.5 blockers (XEN-D0101).[129] Additionally, drugs are being tested that work by novel mechanisms including those that inhibit the atrial acetylcholine regulated potassium current, IK_{ACH} (tertiapin-Q), those that target abnormal calcium handling via the ryanodine receptor RyR2 (calstabin-2), those that act as sodium/calcium exchange inhibitors (KB-R7943), those that block the stretch activated channels, those that are gap junction modifiers (rotigaptide, GAP-134), those that antagonize the serotonin 5-hydroxytryptamine receptors (RS-100-302) and those that are long-acting adenosine A1 receptors (tecadenoson and selodenoson).[129] Likely, new drugs will be developed that will focus on other approaches rather than simply blocking specific cardiac channels.

ANTIARRHYTHMIC DRUG SELECTION IN ATRIAL FIBRILLATION

The 2011 ACC/AHA/ESC Guidelines for Management of AF provides recommendations regarding AAD selection if rhythm control is planned for AF (Flow chart 1).[31] The recommendations are primarily based on AAD safety than on drug efficacy. For patients with no evidence of structural heart disease or have hypertension without substantial left ventricular hypertrophy, flecainide, propafenone, sotalol or dronedarone is first-line therapy, followed by amiodarone, dofetilide, or catheter ablation. For patients with hypertension and substantial left ventricular hypertrophy, amiodarone is the first choice drug, with catheter ablation as the second-line choice. In patients with coronary artery disease, dofetilide or sotalol is first-line, followed by amiodarone or catheter ablation. For heart failure patients, amiodarone or dofetilide is first-line therapy, followed by catheter ablation. Most recently, dronedarone has been included in the guidelines and has a role in the treatment of AF as stated in the package insert as "an AAD indicated to reduce the risk of cardiovascular hospitalization in patients with paroxysmal or persistent AF or atrial flutter, with a recent episode of AF or atrial flutter and associated cardiovascular risk factors (i.e. age > 70, hypertension, diabetes, prior cerebrovascular accident, left atrial diameter $\geq$ 50 mm or left ventricular ejection fraction < 40%), who are in sinus rhythm or who will be cardioverted".[94]

OUT-PATIENT VERSUS IN-HOSPITAL INITIATION FOR ANTIARRHYTHMIC DRUG THERAPY

The location of initiation of an AAD depends on the severity of the arrhythmia and the risk of starting the AAD. It is recommended that all class IA AADs be initiated in the hospital due to risk of torsades de pointes, which at times can be idiosyncratic and non-dose dependent. Class IB AADs, specifically mexiletine, can be started and titrated as an outpatient because the risk of proarrhythmia is small but, in most cases, this drug is started in the hospital due to the fact that most patients whom this drug is initiated have unstable ventricular arrhythmias. Class IC AADs can generally be started outside the hospital for AF as the early risk of proarrhythmia is low as long as the patient has no underlying structural heart disease and no evidence for cardiac ischemia. There is a small risk of rapid rates in AF with one-to-one conduction and atrial

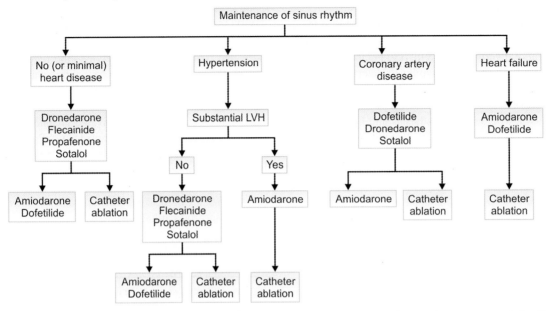

[*Source:* Modified from Wann LS, Curtis AB, January CT, et al. 2011 ACCF/AHA/HRS focused update on the management of patients with atrial fibrillation (updating the 2006 guideline): a report of the American College of Cardiology Foundation/American Heart Association Task Force on Practice Guidelines. Circulation. 2011;123:104-23 (Reference 31)]

flutter but, with proper AV nodal blocking drugs, this risk can be offset. Amiodarone can be started as an outpatient for patients who have AF and atrial flutter as the proarrhythmic risk is low. On the other hand, most patients with VT are considered unstable and, therefore, the initiation of amiodarone normally begins in the hospital. A patient may not be fully loaded with amiodarone, but nevertheless the drug should be started in the hospital. Sotalol and dofetilide should be initiated in the hospital due to the risk of developing QT prolongation and torsades de pointes. Dofetilide must be started in the hospital based on strict guidelines about how the drug should be initiated and titrated. Dronedarone is generally not proarrhythmic and can be started outside the hospital.

ANTIARRHYTHMIC DRUGS IN PREGNANCY AND LACTATION

An overview of the effect of various AADs in pregnancy and lactation is presented in Table 7. Sotalol is the only pregnancy category B drug [either animal-reproduction studies have not demonstrated a fetal risk but there are no controlled studies in pregnant women, or animal-reproduction studies have shown an adverse effect (other than a decrease in fertility) that was not confirmed in controlled studies in women in the first trimester (and there is no evidence of a risk in later trimesters)], while amiodarone is classified as pregnancy category D drug [there is positive evidence of human fetal risk, but the benefits from use in pregnant women may be acceptable despite the risk (e.g. if the drug is needed in a life-threatening situation or for a serious disease for which safer drugs cannot be used or are ineffective)]. Dronedarone is a pregnancy category X drug (studies in animals or human beings have demonstrated fetal abnormalities, or there is evidence of fetal risk based on human experience or both, and the risk of the use of the drug in pregnant women clearly outweighs any possible benefit. The drug is

TABLE 7

Antiarrhythmic drugs in pregnancy and lactation

Drug	Pregnancy	Lactation
Quinidine	C	Excreted
Procainamide	C	Excreted
Disopyramide	C	Excreted
Mexiletine	C	Excreted
Flecainide	C	Excreted
Propafenone	C	?
Sotalol	B	Excreted
Dofetilide	C	?
Dronedarone	X	?
Amiodarone	D	Excreted

contraindicated in women who are or may become pregnant) and so is contraindicated in women who are or may become pregnant. The rest of the AADs are considered pregnancy category C drug [either studies in animals have revealed adverse effects on the fetus (teratogenic or embryocidal or other) and there are no controlled studies in women, or studies in women and animals are not available. Drugs should be given only if the potential benefit justifies the potential risk to the fetus]. The use of beta-blockers during pregnancy is relatively safe. The only exception is atenolol, which is a pregnancy category D drug.

COMPARING ANTIARRHYTHMIC DRUGS TO IMPLANTABLE CARDIOVERTER DEFIBRILLATORS IN PATIENTS AT RISK OF ARRHYTHMIC DEATH

Several large, randomized, prospective, multicenter, controlled clinical trials compared ICDs versus AADs.[130,131] The Antiarrhythmics Versus Implantable Defibrillators (AVID) trial randomized patients resuscitated from a cardiac arrest to an ICD, empiric amiodarone (mean dose of 300 mg; 90% of patients) or sotalol (mean dose 250 mg) guided by electrophysiology study or Holter monitoring. The group runnings ICDs had a significant 39% (one year), 27% (two year) and 31% (three year) mortality reduction when compared to AADs. Only those patients with left ventricular ejection fraction between 20% and 34% showed a survival benefit with ICD (83%) when compared to amiodarone (72%).[130] The multicenter, prospective Sudden Cardiac Death Heart Failure Trial (SCD-HeFT) randomly assigned 2,521 medically managed ischemic and non-ischemic cardiomyopathy patients with a left ventricular ejection fraction less than or equal to 35%, and NYHA functional class II–III heart failure to an ICD, amiodarone and placebo. Patients were followed for a median of 46 months. The primary endpoint was total mortality. The study showed that the ICD resulted in a 7.2% absolute and a 22% relative reduction in mortality, when compared to placebo and amiodarone. Amiodarone was no better than placebo in improving mortality. Patients with NYHA class III heart failure symptoms fared worse with amiodarone when compared to placebo (HR1.44, confidence interval 1.05–1.97, $P = 0.01$).[131]

In summary, ICDs are superior to AADs for both primary and secondary prevention of mortality, presumably due to sudden cardiac death. The AADs should be reserved only for patients who are not candidates for an ICD, who refuse ICD therapy, and for select patients with genetic disorders that respond well to a specific AAD.

ANTIARRHYTHMIC DRUG-DEVICE INTERACTIONS

The ICD has emerged as the primary therapeutic modality for prevention of sudden cardiac death. Concomitant AAD therapy may be required in select ICD patients to suppress recurrent atrial and ventricular arrhythmias and to reduce the incidence and frequency of both appropriate and inappropriate shocks.[40] When used in this setting, AADs can affect device functioning in several ways:

- AADs can increase defibrillation and pacing thresholds
- AADs can slow VT rate to below the programmed ICD detection rate
- AADs can cause sinus and AV node dysfunction, resulting in bradycardia and AV block
- AADs can be proarrhythmic

It is important to be aware of these potential interactions when selecting an appropriate AAD and also during device programming. Amiodarone and sotalol are the two most common AADs used in an ICD population. Table 8 lists the effect of various AADs on pacing and defibrillation thresholds. Class I AADs and amiodarone have been shown to raise the defibrillation threshold, whereas class III drugs such as sotalol and dofetilide tend to decrease the energy needed to defibrillate.[40] The results of the prospective, randomized, Optimal Pharmacologic Therapy in Cardioverter Defibrillator Patients (OPTIC) trial casts doubts regarding the clinical significance of these above-mentioned effects in the current era of high energy ICD devices. The OPTIC trial compared the effects of beta-blockers, beta-blocker plus amiodarone and sotalol on defibrillation energy requirements in 94 patients. The study

TABLE 8

Effect of antiarrhythmic drugs on defibrillation and pacing thresholds

Drug	Pacing threshold	Defibrillation threshold
Quinidine	Increase	Increase
Procainamide	Increase	No change/increase
Lidocaine	No change	Increase
Flecainide	Increase	Increase
Beta-blockers	Increase	Decreases
Digoxin	Decrease	Decrease/no change
Ibutilide	Not known	Decrease
Sotalol	No effect	Decrease
Amiodarone	No effect	Increase
Dofetilide	No change	Decrease
Verapamil	Increase	Not known

showed that changes in defibrillation threshold with amiodarone and sotalol are at best modest and argues against repeat defibrillation threshold testing after initiating therapy with either drug.[132] The study also showed that amiodarone plus a beta-blocker was most effective in preventing ICD shocks at 1 year and was more effective than sotalol (10.3% vs 24.3% for sotalol; HR, 0.43; $P = 0.02$).[49]

CONCLUSION

Antiarrhythmic drug therapy continues to play a critical role in the management of atrial and ventricular arrhythmias. The role of AADs has evolved in the face of advances in curative therapy for specific arrhythmias, as well as for underlying diseases. It is fair to say that the history of AAD therapy has come full circle: from the days of the CAST and SWORD trials showing increased mortality to demonstration of mortality benefit with dronedarone in the recent ATHENA trial. Irrespective of effects on survival, AADs are an integral part of the pharmacological armamentarium to combat AF, to treat ventricular arrhythmias in the structurally normal heart and in those with channelopathies, to suppress sustained ventricular arrhythmias in patients with structural heart disease who either have an ICD or are not candidates for one. The field of AAD therapy continues to evolve as newer drugs that target novel mechanisms are being actively developed and, with currently available drugs finding new indications for their use.

REFERENCES

1. Gopinathannair R, Sullivan RM, Olshansky B. Update on medical management of atrial fibrillation in the modern era. Heart Rhythm. 2009;6:S17-22.
2. Wyse DG, Waldo AL, DiMarco JP, et al. A comparison of rate control and rhythm control in patients with atrial fibrillation. N Engl J Med. 2002;347:1825-33.
3. Vaughan Williams EM. A classification of antiarrhythmic actions reassessed after a decade of new drugs. J Clin Pharmacol. 1984;24: 129-47.
4. The Sicilian gambit. A new approach to the classification of antiarrhythmic drugs based on their actions on arrhythmogenic mechanisms. Task Force of the Working Group on Arrhythmias of the European Society of Cardiology. Circulation. 1991;84:1831-51.
5. Harrison DC. Antiarrhythmic drug classification: new science and practical applications. Am J Cardiol. 1985;56:185-7.

6. Hodgkin AL, Huxley AF. A quantitative description of membrane current and its application to conduction and excitation in nerve. J Physiol. 1952;117:500-44.

7. Lafuente-Lafuente C, Mouly S, Longas-Tejero MA, et al. Antiarrhythmic drugs for maintaining sinus rhythm after cardioversion of atrial fibrillation: a systematic review of randomized controlled trials. Arch Intern Med. 2006;166:719-28.

8. Belhassen B, Glick A, Viskin S. Efficacy of quinidine in high-risk patients with Brugada syndrome. Circulation. 2004;110:1731-7.

9. Mok NS, Chan NY, Chiu AC. Successful use of quinidine in treatment of electrical storm in Brugada syndrome. Pacing Clin Electrophysiol. 2004;27:821-3.

10. Mizusawa Y, Sakurada H, Nishizaki M, et al. Effects of low-dose quinidine on ventricular tachyarrhythmias in patients with Brugada syndrome: low-dose quinidine therapy as an adjunctive treatment. J Cardiovasc Pharmacol. 2006;47:359-64.

11. Olshansky B, Okumura K, Hess PG, et al. Use of procainamide with rapid atrial pacing for successful conversion of atrial flutter to sinus rhythm. J Am Coll Cardiol. 1988;11:359-64.

12. Olshansky B, Martins J, Hunt S. N-acetyl procainamide causing torsades de pointes. Am J Cardiol. 1982;50:1439-41.

13. Sherrid MV, Barac I, McKenna WJ, et al. Multicenter study of the efficacy and safety of disopyramide in obstructive hypertrophic cardiomyopathy. J Am Coll Cardiol. 2005;45:1251-8.

14. Lie KI, Wellens HJ, van Capelle FJ, et al. Lidocaine in the prevention of primary ventricular fibrillation. A double-blind, randomized study of 212 consecutive patients. N Engl J Med. 1974;291:1324-6.

15. Alexander JH, Granger CB, Sadowski Z, et al. Prophylactic lidocaine use in acute myocardial infarction: incidence and outcomes from two international trials. The GUSTO-I and GUSTO-IIb Investigators. Am Heart J. 1999;137:799-805.

16. Singh BN. Routine prophylactic lidocaine administration in acute myocardial infarction. An idea whose time is all but gone? Circulation. 1992;86:1033-5.

17. Hine LK, Laird N, Hewitt P, et al. Meta-analytic evidence against prophylactic use of lidocaine in acute myocardial infarction. Arch Intern Med. 1989;149:2694-8.

18. Stenson RE, Constantino RT, Harrison DC. Interrelationships of hepatic blood flow, cardiac output, and blood levels of lidocaine in man. Circulation. 1971;43:205-11.

19. Josephson ME, Kastor JA, Kitchen JG 3rd. Lidocaine in Wolff-Parkinson-White syndrome with atrial fibrillation. Ann Intern Med. 1976;84:44-5.

20. Wyman MG, Slaughter RL, Farolino DA, et al. Multiple bolus technique for lidocaine administration in acute ischemic heart disease. II. Treatment of refractory ventricular arrhythmias and the pharmacokinetic significance of severe left ventricular failure. J Am Coll Cardiol. 1983;2:764-9.

21. Ochs HR, Carstens G, Greenblatt DJ. Reduction in lidocaine clearance during continuous infusion and by coadministration of propranolol. N Engl J Med. 1980;303:373-7.

22. Feely J, Wilkinson GR, McAllister CB, et al. Increased toxicity and reduced clearance of lidocaine by cimetidine. Ann Intern Med. 1982;96:592-4.

23. Stein J, Podrid P, Lown B. Effects of oral mexiletine on left and right ventricular function. Am J Cardiol. 1984;54:575-8.

24. Campbell RW. Mexiletine. N Engl J Med. 1987;316:29-34.

25. International mexiletine and placebo antiarrhythmic coronary trial: I. Report on arrhythmia and other findings. Impact Research Group. J Am Coll Cardiol. 1984;4:1148-63.

26. Shimizu W, Aiba T, Antzelevitch C. Specific therapy based on the genotype and cellular mechanism in inherited cardiac arrhythmias. Long QT syndrome and Brugada syndrome. Curr Pharm Des. 2005;11:1561-72.

27. Fasola GP, D'Osualdo F, de Pangher V, et al. Thrombocytopenia and mexiletine. Ann Intern Med. 1984;100:162.

28. Bigger JT Jr. The interaction of mexiletine with other cardiovascular drugs. Am Heart J. 1984;107:1079-85.

29. Preliminary report: effect of encainide and flecainide on mortality in a randomized trial of arrhythmia suppression after myocardial infarction. The Cardiac Arrhythmia Suppression Trial (CAST) Investigators. N Engl J Med. 1989;321:406-12.

30. Roden DM, Woosley RL. Drug therapy. Flecainide. N Engl J Med. 1986;315:36-41.

31. Wann LS, Curtis AB, January CT, et al. 2011 ACCF/AHA/HRS focused update on the management of patients with atrial fibrillation (updating the 2006 guideline): a report of the American College of Cardiology Foundation/American Heart Association Task Force on Practice Guidelines. Circulation. 2011;123:104-23.

32. Konety SH, Olshansky B. The "pill-in-the-pocket" approach to atrial fibrillation. N Engl J Med. 2005;352:1150-1.

33. Buxton AE, Waxman HL, Marchlinski FE, et al. Right ventricular tachycardia: clinical and electrophysiologic characteristics. Circulation. 1983;68:917-27.

34. Watanabe H, Chopra N, Laver D, et al. Flecainide prevents catecholaminergic polymorphic ventricular tachycardia in mice and humans. Nat Med. 2009;15:380-3.

35. Benhorin J, Taub R, Goldmit M, et al. Effects of flecainide in patients with new SCN5A mutation: mutation-specific therapy for long-QT syndrome? Circulation. 2000;101:1698-706.

36. Effect of the antiarrhythmic agent moricizine on survival after myocardial infarction. The Cardiac Arrhythmia Suppression Trial II Investigators. N Engl J Med. 1992;327:227-33.

37. Vik-Mo H, Ohm OJ, Lund-Johansen P. Electrophysiologic effects of flecainide acetate in patients with sinus nodal dysfunction. Am J Cardiol. 1982;50:1090-4.

38. Alboni P, Botto GL, Baldi N, et al. Outpatient treatment of recent-onset atrial fibrillation with the "pill-in-the-pocket" approach. N Engl J Med. 2004;351:2384-91.

39. Muhiddin KA, Turner P, Blackett A. Effect of flecainide on cardiac output. Clin Pharmacol Ther. 1985;37:260-3.

40. Rajawat YS, Dias D, Gerstenfeld EP, et al. Interactions of anti-arrhythmic drugs and implantable devices in controlling ventricular tachycardia and fibrillation. Curr Cardiol Rep. 2002;4:434-40.

41. Hellestrand KJ, Burnett PJ, Milne JR, et al. Effect of the antiarrhythmic agent flecainide acetate on acute and chronic pacing thresholds. Pacing Clin Electrophysiol. 1983;6:892-9.

42. McLeod AA, Stiles GL, Shand DG. Demonstration of beta adreno-ceptor blockade by propafenone hydrochloride: clinical pharmacologic, radioligand binding and adenylate cyclase activation studies. J Pharmacol Exp Ther. 1984;228:461-6.

43. Siddoway LA, Thompson KA, McAllister CB, et al. Polymorphism of propafenone metabolism and disposition in man: clinical and pharmacokinetic consequences. Circulation. 1987;75:785-91.

44. Lee JT, Kroemer HK, Silberstein DJ, et al. The role of genetically determined polymorphic drug metabolism in the beta-blockade produced by propafenone. N Engl J Med. 1990;322:1764-8.

45. Wagner F, Kalusche D, Trenk D, et al. Drug interaction between propafenone and metoprolol. Br J Clin Pharmacol. 1987;24:213-20.

46. Olshansky B, Rosenfeld LE, Warner AL, et al. The Atrial Fibrillation Follow-up Investigation of Rhythm Management (AFFIRM) study: approaches to control rate in atrial fibrillation. J Am Coll Cardiol. 2004;43:1201-8.

47. Olshansky B, Martins JB. Usefulness of isoproterenol facilitation of ventricular tachycardia induction during extrastimulus testing in predicting effective chronic therapy with beta-adrenergic blockade. Am J Cardiol. 1987;59:573-7.

48. Zicha S, Tsuji Y, Shiroshita-Takeshita A, et al. Beta-blockers as antiarrhythmic agents. Handb Exp Pharmacol. 2006;171:235-66.

49. Connolly SJ, Dorian P, Roberts RS, et al. Comparison of beta-blockers, amiodarone plus beta-blockers, or sotalol for prevention of shocks from implantable cardioverter defibrillators: the OPTIC Study: a randomized trial. JAMA. 2006;295:165-71.

50. Cheng J, Niwa R, Kamiya K, et al. Carvedilol blocks the repolarizing K+ currents and the L-type Ca2+ current in rabbit ventricular myocytes. Eur J Pharmacol. 1999;376:189-201.

51. Olshansky B. Management of atrial fibrillation after coronary artery bypass graft. Am J Cardiol. 1996;78:27-34.

52. Hohnloser SH, Woosley RL. Sotalol. N Engl J Med. 1994;331:31-8.

53. Waldo AL, Camm AJ, deRuyter H, et al. Effect of d-sotalol on mortality in patients with left ventricular dysfunction after recent and remote myocardial infarction. The SWORD Investigators. Survival With Oral d-Sotalol. Lancet. 1996;348:7-12.

54. Julian DG, Prescott RJ, Jackson FS, Szekely P. Controlled trial of sotalol for one year after myocardial infarction. Lancet. 1982;1:1142-7.

55. Mason JW. A comparison of seven antiarrhythmic drugs in patients with ventricular tachyarrhythmias. Electrophysiologic Study versus Electrocardiographic Monitoring Investigators. N Engl J Med. 1993;329:452-8.

56. Pacifico A, Hohnloser SH, Williams JH, et al. Prevention of implantable-defibrillator shocks by treatment with sotalol. d,l-Sotalol Implantable Cardioverter-Defibrillator Study Group. New Engl J Med. 1999;340:1855-62.

57. Singh BN, Singh SN, Reda DJ, et al. Amiodarone versus sotalol for atrial fibrillation. N Engl J Med. 2005;352:1861-72.

58. Baskin EP, Lynch JJ Jr. Differential atrial versus ventricular activities of class III potassium channel blockers. J Pharmacol Exp Ther. 1998;285:135-42.

59. Abel S, Nichols DJ, Brearley CJ, et al. Effect of cimetidine and ranitidine on pharmacokinetics and pharmacodynamics of a single dose of dofetilide. Br J Clin Pharmacol. 2000;49:64-71.

60. Torp-Pedersen C, Møller M, Bloch-Thomsen PE, et al. Dofetilide in patients with congestive heart failure and left ventricular dysfunction. Danish Investigations of Arrhythmia and Mortality on Dofetilide Study Group. N Engl J Med. 1999;341:857-65.

61. Olshansky B. Dofetilide versus quinidine for atrial flutter: viva la difference!? J Cardiovasc Electrophysiol. 1996;7:828-32.

62. Yap YG, Camm AJ. Drug induced QT prolongation and torsades de pointes. Heart. 2003;89:1363-72.

63. Elming H, Brendorp B, Pedersen OD, et al. Dofetilide: a new drug to control cardiac arrhythmia. Expert Opin Pharmacother. 2003;4:973-85.

64. Murray KT. Ibutilide. Circulation. 1998;97:493-7.

65. Stambler BS, Wood MA, Ellenbogen KA, et al. Efficacy and safety of repeated intravenous doses of ibutilide for rapid conversion of atrial flutter or fibrillation. Ibutilide Repeat Dose Study Investigators. Circulation. 1996;94:1613-21.

66. Tercius AJ, Kluger J, Coleman CI, et al. Intravenous magnesium sulfate enhances the ability of intravenous ibutilide to successfully convert atrial fibrillation or flutter. Pacing Clin Electrophysiol. 2007;30:1331-5.

67. Patsilinakos S, Christou A, Kafkas N, et al. Effect of high doses of magnesium on converting ibutilide to a safe and more effective agent. Am J Cardiol. 2010;106:673-6.

68. Coleman CI, Sood N, Chawla D, et al. Intravenous magnesium sulfate enhances the ability of dofetilide to successfully cardiovert atrial fibrillation or flutter: results of the Dofetilide and Intravenous Magnesium Evaluation. Europace. 2009;11:892-5.

69. Steinwender C, Honig S, Kypta A, et al. Pre-injection of magnesium sulfate enhances the efficacy of ibutilide for the conversion of typical but not of atypical persistent atrial flutter. Int J Cardiol. 2010;141:260-5.

70. Coleman CI, Kalus JS, Caron MF, et al. Model of effect of magnesium prophylaxis on frequency of torsades de pointes in ibutilide-treated patients. Am J Health Syst Pharm. 2004;61:685-8.

71. Fragakis N, Bikias A, Delithanasis I, et al. Acute beta-adrenoceptor blockade improves efficacy of ibutilide in conversion of atrial fibrillation with a rapid ventricular rate. Europace. 2009;11:70-4.

72. Gopinathannair R, Olshansky B. Ibutilide revisited: stronger and safer than ever. Europace. 2009;11:9-10.

73. Anrep GV, Barsoum GS, Kenawy MR, et al. Ammi visnaga in the treatment of the anginal syndrome. Br Heart J. 1946;8:171-7.

74. Mason JW. Amiodarone. N Engl J Med. 1987;316:455-66.

75. Mason JW, Hondeghem LM, Katzung BG. Amiodarone blocks inactivated cardiac sodium channels. Pflugers Arch. 1983;396:79-81.

76. Holt DW, Tucker GT, Jackson PR, et al. Amiodarone pharmacokinetics. Br J Clin Pract Suppl. 1986;44:109-14.

77. Plomp TA, van Rossum JM, Robles de Medina EO, et al. Pharmacokinetics and body distribution of amiodarone in man. Arzneimittelforschung. 1984;34:513-20.

78. Julian DG, Camm AJ, Frangin G, et al. Randomised trial of effect of amiodarone on mortality in patients with left-ventricular dysfunction after recent myocardial infarction: EMIAT. European Myocardial Infarct Amiodarone Trial Investigators. Lancet. 1997;349:667-74.

79. Cairns JA, Connolly SJ, Roberts R, et al. Randomised trial of outcome after myocardial infarction in patients with frequent or repetitive ventricular premature depolarisations: CAMIAT. Canadian Amiodarone Myocardial Infarction Arrhythmia Trial Investigators. Lancet. 1997;349:675-82.

80. Boutitie F, Boissel JP, Connolly SJ, et al. Amiodarone interaction with beta-blockers: analysis of the merged EMIAT (European Myocardial Infarct Amiodarone Trial) and CAMIAT (Canadian Amiodarone Myocardial Infarction Trial) databases. The EMIAT and CAMIAT Investigators. Circulation. 1999;99:2268-75.

81. Garguichevich JJ, Ramos JL, Gambarte A, et al. Effect of amiodarone therapy on mortality in patients with left ventricular dysfunction and asymptomatic complex ventricular arrhythmias: Argentine Pilot Study of Sudden Death and Amiodarone (EPAMSA). Am Heart J. 1995;130:494-500.

82. Doval HC, Nul DR, Grancelli HO, et al. Randomised trial of low-dose amiodarone in severe congestive heart failure. Grupo de Estudio de la Sobrevida en la Insuficiencia Cardiaca en Argentina (GESICA). Lancet. 1994;344:493-8.

83. Singh SN, Fletcher RD, Fisher SG, et al. Amiodarone in patients with congestive heart failure and asymptomatic ventricular arrhythmia. Survival Trial of Antiarrhythmic Therapy in Congestive Heart Failure. N Engl J Med. 1995;333:77-82.

84. Piccini JP, Berger JS, O'Connor CM. Amiodarone for the prevention of sudden cardiac death: a meta-analysis of randomized controlled trials. Eur Heart J. 2009;30:1245-53.

85. Roy D, Talajic M, Dorian P, et al. Amiodarone to prevent recurrence of atrial fibrillation. Canadian Trial of Atrial Fibrillation Investigators. N Engl J Med. 2000;342:913-20.

86. Goldschlager N, Epstein AE, Naccarelli GV, et al. A practical guide for clinicians who treat patients with amiodarone: 2007. Heart Rhythm. 2007;4:1250-9.

87. Olshansky B, Sami M, Rubin A, et al. Use of amiodarone for atrial fibrillation in patients with preexisting pulmonary disease in the AFFIRM study. Am J Cardiol. 2005;95:404-5.

88. Olshansky B. Images in clinical medicine. Amiodarone-induced pulmonary toxicity. N Engl J Med. 1997;337:1814.

89. Manning AS, Bruyninckx C, Ramboux J, et al. SR 33589, a new amiodarone-like agent: effect on ischemia- and reperfusion-induced arrhythmias in anesthetized rats. J Cardiovasc Pharmacol. 1995;26:453-61.

90. Djandjighian L, Planchenault J, Finance O, et al. Hemodynamic and antiadrenergic effects of dronedarone and amiodarone in animals with a healed myocardial infarction. J Cardiovasc Pharmacol. 2000;36:376-83.

91. Sun W, Sarma JS, Singh BN. Electrophysiological effects of dronedarone (SR33589), a noniodinated benzofuran derivative, in the rabbit heart: comparison with amiodarone. Circulation. 1999;100:2276-81.

92. Finance O, Manning A, Chatelain P. Effects of a new amiodarone-like agent, SR 33589, in comparison to amiodarone, D,L-sotalol, and lignocaine, on ischemia-induced ventricular arrhythmias in anesthetized pigs. J Cardiovasc Pharmacol. 1995;26:570-6.

93. Kober L, Torp-Pedersen C, McMurray JJ, et al. Increased mortality after dronedarone therapy for severe heart failure. N Engl J Med. 2008;358:2678-87.

94. Dronedarone prescribing information. [online] MULTAQ website. Available from http://www.multaq.com/docs/consumer_pdf/pi.aspx [Accessed February 2011]

95. Sullivan RM, Olshansky B. Dronedarone: evidence supporting its therapeutic use in the treatment of atrial fibrillation. Core Evid. 2010;5:49-59.

96. Singh BN, Connolly SJ, Crijns HJ, et al. Dronedarone for maintenance of sinus rhythm in atrial fibrillation or flutter. N Engl J Med. 2007;357:987-99.

97. Le Heuzey JY, De Ferrari GM, Radzik D, et al. A short-term, randomized, double-blind, parallel-group study to evaluate the efficacy and safety of dronedarone versus amiodarone in patients with persistent atrial fibrillation: the DIONYSOS study. J Cardiovasc Electrophysiol. 2010;21:597-605.

98. Davy JM, Herold M, Hoglund C, et al. Dronedarone for the control of ventricular rate in permanent atrial fibrillation: the Efficacy and safety of dRonedArone for the cOntrol of ventricular rate during atrial fibrillation (ERATO) study. Am Heart J. 2008;156:527,e1-9.

99. Hohnloser SH, Crijns HJ, van Eickels M, et al. Effect of dronedarone on cardiovascular events in atrial fibrillation. N Engl J Med. 2009;360:668-78.

100. Connolly SJ, Crijns HJ, Torp-Pedersen C, et al. Analysis of stroke in ATHENA: a placebo-controlled, double-blind, parallel-arm trial to assess the efficacy of dronedarone 400 mg BID for the prevention of cardiovascular hospitalization or death from any cause in patients with atrial fibrillation/atrial flutter. Circulation. 2009;120:1174-80.

101. Sanofi Aventis. Important Drug Warning on Multaq: Letter to Healthcare Provider - Jan 14, 2011

101a. Connolly SJ, CammAJ, Halperin JL, et al. Dronedarone in high risk permanent atrial fibrillation. The New England Journal of Medicine. 2011;365:2258-76.

102. Lombardi F, Terranova P. Pharmacological treatment of atrial fibrillation: mechanisms of action and efficacy of class III drugs. Curr Med Chem. 2006;13:1635-53.

103. Camm AJ, Pratt CM, Schwartz PJ, et al. Mortality in patients after a recent myocardial infarction: a randomized, placebo-controlled trial of azimilide using heart rate variability for risk stratification. Circulation. 2004;109:990-6.

104. Dorian P, Borggrefe M, Al-Khalidi HR, et al. Placebo-controlled, randomized clinical trial of azimilide for prevention of ventricular tachyarrhythmias in patients with an implantable cardioverter defibrillator. Circulation. 2004;110:3646-54.

105. Lombardi F, Borggrefe M, Ruzyllo W, et al. Azimilide vs. placebo and sotalol for persistent atrial fibrillation: the A-COMET-II (Azimilide-CardiOversion MaintEnance Trial-II) trial. Eur Heart J. 2006;27:2224-31.

106. Kerr CR, Connolly SJ, Kowey P, et al. Efficacy of azimilide for the maintenance of sinus rhythm in patients with paroxysmal atrial fibrillation in the presence and absence of structural heart disease. Am J Cardiol. 2006;98:215-8.

107. Conway E, Musco S, Kowey PR. New horizons in antiarrhythmic therapy: will novel agents overcome current deficits? Am J Cardiol. 2008;102:12H-9H.

108. Lerman BB, Belardinelli L. Cardiac electrophysiology of adenosine. Basic and clinical concepts. Circulation. 1991;83:1499-509.

109. Wilber DJ, Baerman J, Olshansky B, et al. Adenosine-sensitive ventricular tachycardia. Clinical characteristics and response to catheter ablation. Circulation. 1993;87:126-34.

110. Kall JG, Kopp D, Olshansky B, et al. Adenosine-sensitive atrial tachycardia. Pacing Clin Electrophysiol. 1995;18:300-6.

111. Ellenbogen KA, Thames MD, DiMarco JP, et al. Electrophysiological effects of adenosine in the transplanted human heart. Evidence of supersensitivity. Circulation. 1990;81:821-8.

112. Hohnloser SH, Dorian P, Straub M, et al. Safety and efficacy of intravenously administered tedisamil for rapid conversion of recent-onset atrial fibrillation or atrial flutter. J Am Coll Cardiol. 2004;44:99-104.

113. Wijffels MC, Crijns HJ. Recent advances in drug therapy for atrial fibrillation. J Cardiovasc Electrophysiol. 2003;14:S40-7.

114. Naccarelli GV, Wolbrette DL, Samii S, et al. Vernakalant—a promising therapy for conversion of recent-onset atrial fibrillation. Expert Opin Investig Drugs. 2008;17:805-10.

115. Roy D, Pratt CM, Torp-Pedersen C, et al. Vernakalant hydrochloride for rapid conversion of atrial fibrillation: a phase 3, randomized, placebo-controlled trial. Circulation. 2008;117:1518-25.

116. Kowey PR, Dorian P, Mitchell LB, et al. Vernakalant hydrochloride for the rapid conversion of atrial fibrillation after cardiac surgery: a randomized, double-blind, placebo-controlled trial. Circ Arrhythm Electrophysiol. 2009;2:652-9.

117. Pratt CM, Roy D, Torp-Pedersen C, et al. Usefulness of vernakalant hydrochloride injection for rapid conversion of atrial fibrillation. Am J Cardiol. 2010;106:1277-83.

118. Camm AJ, Capucci A, Hohnloser SH, et al. A randomized active-controlled study comparing the efficacy and safety of vernakalant to amiodarone in recent-onset atrial fibrillation. J Am Coll Cardiol. 2011;57:313-21.

119. Fox K, Borer JS, Camm AJ, et al. Resting heart rate in cardiovascular disease. J Am Coll Cardiol. 2007;50:823-30.

120. Gopinathannair R, Sullivan RM, Olshansky B. Slower heart rates for healthy hearts: time to redefine tachycardia? Circ Arrhythm Electrophysiol. 2008;1:321-3.

121. DiFrancesco D, Camm JA. Heart rate lowering by specific and selective I(f) current inhibition with ivabradine: a new therapeutic perspective in cardiovascular disease. Drugs. 2004;64:1757-65.

122. Fox K, Ford I, Steg PG, et al. Ivabradine for patients with stable coronary artery disease and left-ventricular systolic dysfunction (BEAUTIFUL): a randomised, double-blind, placebo-controlled trial. Lancet. 2008;372:807-16.

123. Tardif JC, Ponikowski P, Kahan T. Efficacy of the I(f) current inhibitor ivabradine in patients with chronic stable angina receiving beta-blocker therapy: a 4-month, randomized, placebo-controlled trial. Eur Heart J. 2009;30:540-8.

124. Swedberg K, Komajda M, Bohm M, et al. Ivabradine and outcomes in chronic heart failure (SHIFT): a randomised placebo-controlled study. Lancet. 2010;376:875-85.

125. Calo L, Rebecchi M, Sette A, et al. Efficacy of ivabradine administration in patients affected by inappropriate sinus tachycardia. Heart Rhythm. 2010;7:1318-23.

126. Antzelevitch C, Belardinelli L, Zygmunt AC, et al. Electrophysiological effects of ranolazine, a novel antianginal agent with antiarrhythmic properties. Circulation. 2004;110:904-10.

127. Scirica BM, Morrow DA, Hod H, et al. Effect of ranolazine, an antianginal agent with novel electrophysiological properties, on the incidence of arrhythmias in patients with non ST-segment elevation acute coronary syndrome: results from the Metabolic Efficiency With Ranolazine for Less Ischemia in Non ST-Elevation Acute Coronary Syndrome Thrombolysis in Myocardial Infarction 36 (MERLIN-TIMI 36) randomized controlled trial. Circulation. 2007;116:1647-52.

128. Burashnikov A, Sicouri S, Di Diego JM, Belardinelli L, Antzelevitch C. Synergistic effect of the combination of ranolazine and dronedarone to suppress atrial fibrillation. J Am Coll Cardiol. 2010;56:1216-24.

129. Savelievap I, Camm J. Anti-arrhythmic drug therapy for atrial fibrillation: current anti-arrhythmic drugs, investigational agents, and innovative approaches. Europace. 2008;10:647-65.

130. A comparison of antiarrhythmic-drug therapy with implantable defibrillators in patients resuscitated from near-fatal ventricular arrhythmias. The Antiarrhythmics versus Implantable Defibrillators (AVID) Investigators. N Engl J Med. 1997;337:1576-83.

131. Bardy GH, Lee KL, Mark DB, et al. Amiodarone or an implantable cardioverter-defibrillator for congestive heart failure. N Engl J Med. 2005;352:225-37.

132. Hohnloser SH, Dorian P, Roberts R, et al. Effect of amiodarone and sotalol on ventricular defibrillation threshold: the optimal pharmacological therapy in cardioverter defibrillator patients (OPTIC) trial. Circulation. 2006;114:104-9.

SECTION 4

Electrophysiology

Chapter 31

Electrophysiology Studies

Indrajit Choudhuri, Masood Akhtar

Chapter Outline

INTRODUCTION

Clinical cardiac electrophysiology (EP) is a relatively new and continually evolving investigative field. Its modern underpinnings date back to the first description of the cardiac Purkinje fibers in 1839 by Czech neuroscientist Jan Evangelista Purkynê,[1] and description of the atrioventricular (AV) bundle by Wilhelm His Jr.[2] and accessory "AV bundles" by Albert Kent in 1893.[3] Such anatomic discoveries of the cardiac conduction system were the first murmurings of what would spawn an entirely independent arena of cardiac investigation that continued in this vein into the early 20th century with description of the AV node by Sunao Tawara[4] in 1906 and, finally, the sinoatrial node[5] in 1907 by Arthur Keith and his student Martin Flack. Einthoven's 1908 description of the modern electrocardiograph[6] heralded a new phase of cardiac electrophysiologic discovery, permitting arrhythmia description and electrocardiogram (ECG) correlation with clinical presentation. During his Nobel speech, Einthoven foretold that "a new chapter has been opened in the study of heart diseases ...." This was the primary mode of "electrophysiology study" during the first half of the 20th century, during which time the first case of idiopathic ventricular fibrillation (VF) was described, in 1929,[7] and the first long QT case reports were described by Jervell and Lange-Nielsen.[8]

Percutaneous and open-chest techniques for arrhythmia mapping were first described in the 1950s, but it was not until the late 1960s and 1970s that a reproducible technique for recording the His bundle potential[9] was demonstrated and utilized. Its role, as well as that of programed electrical stimulation, for identification of site of origin and arrhythmia mechanism established the invasive cardiac EP study as a

mainstay in diagnostic cardiology, expanding the frontiers of cardiac EP and cardiovascular disease. This breakthrough was accompanied by an increase in open-chest surgical therapy and ablation, providing further insight into the mechanisms of arrhythmias. However, demonstration of a closed-chest catheter technique for destruction of cardiac tissue[10] truly revolutionized the field. It provided a percutaneous option for patients to undergo diagnosis and treatment in the same setting.

Since those early and formative years, the comprehensive EP study has gradually evolved from a prolonged undertaking to a streamlined diagnostic process that attempts to identify clinically relevant mechanisms of arrhythmogenesis, and correlate these with symptomatology to guide therapy. This chapter focuses on fundamental aspects of the contemporary intracardiac EP study and should serve as a foundation for all cardiovascular disease practitioners seeking further insight into the electrophysiologic mechanisms of the human heart.

CARDIAC ELECTROPHYSIOLOGY STUDY: PHILOSOPHY, REQUIREMENTS AND BASIC TECHNIQUES

The contemporary EP study has been condensed, abbreviated and streamlined to capitalize on the basic science, and clinical foundations established since the 1800s to efficiently evaluate tendency toward arrhythmia and its underlying mechanisms. The EP studies are performed to investigate clinically documented rhythm disturbances or evaluate symptoms compatible with arrhythmic etiology, such as palpitations or syncope, for risk stratification of sudden death and evaluation of pharmacologic therapy.[11] Alternatively, not all arrhythmias and arrhythmic mechanisms may be evaluated by or necessitate study. For instance, an EP study is not generally indicated for evaluation of symptomatic bradycardia. Whether the mechanism is sinus node dysfunction or conduction disease in the AV node, His bundle or Purkinje system, permanent pacing is usually required, and demonstrating mechanism may be of more "academic" concern. In specific situations, however, demonstration of the level and mechanism of conduction block may be instrumental in guiding therapy, such as in apparent conduction block attributable to junctional extrasystoles in which beat suppression is required, whether medical or ablative, rather than pacing. Indications for EP study are shown in Tables 1 to 13.[12]

TABLE 1

Indications for electrophysiology study to evaluate sinus node function

Class I
- Symptomatic patients in whom sinus node dysfunction is suspected as the cause of symptoms, but a causal relation between an arrhythmia and the symptoms has not been established after appropriate evaluation

Class II
- Patients with documented sinus node dysfunction in whom evaluation of AV or VA conduction or susceptibility to arrhythmias may aid in selection of the most appropriate pacing modality
- Patients with electrocardiographically documented sinus bradyarrhythmias to determine if abnormalities are due to intrinsic disease, autonomic nervous system dysfunction or the effects of drugs so as to help select therapeutic options
- Symptomatic patients with known sinus bradyarrhythmias to evaluate potential for other arrhythmias as the cause of symptoms

Class III
- Symptomatic patients in whom an association between symptoms and a documented bradyarrhythmia has been established and choice of therapy would not be affected by results of an electrophysiology study
- Asymptomatic patients with sinus bradyarrhythmias or sinus pauses observed only during sleep, including sleep apnea

Abbreviations: AV: Atrioventricular; VA: Ventriculoatrial

TABLE 2

Electrophysiology study indications for acquired AV block

Class I
- Symptomatic patients in whom His-Purkinje block, suspected as a cause of symptoms, has not been established
- Patients with second-degree or third-degree AV block treated with a pacemaker who remain symptomatic and in whom another arrhythmia is suspected as a cause of symptoms

Class II
- Patients with second-degree or third-degree AV block in whom knowledge of the site of block or its mechanism or response to pharmacological or other temporary intervention may help to direct therapy or assess prognosis
- Patients with premature, concealed junctional depolarizations suspected as a cause of second-degree or third-degree AV block pattern (i.e. pseudo-AV block)

Class III
- Symptomatic patients in whom the symptoms and presence of AV block are correlated by ECG findings
- Asymptomatic patients with transient AV block associated with sinus slowing (e.g. nocturnal type I second-degree AV block)

Abbreviations: AV: Atrioventricular; ECG: Electrocardiogram

The cardiac EP study itself is a systematic evaluation of clinically relevant aspects of myocardial electrical stimulation and propagation and arrhythmic potential. It is conducted in a diagnostic cardiac EP or angiography suite, with minimum

TABLE 3

Electrophysiology study indications for chronic intraventricular conduction delay

Class I
- Symptomatic patients in whom the cause of symptoms is not known

Class II
- Asymptomatic patients with bundle branch block in whom pharmacological therapy that could increase conduction delay or produce heart block is contemplated

Class III
- Asymptomatic patients with intraventricular conduction delay
- Symptomatic patients whose symptoms can be correlated with or excluded by ECG events

Abbreviations: ECG: Electrocardiogram

TABLE 4

Electrophysiology study indications for narrow QRS complex tachycardias

Class I
- Patients with frequent or poorly tolerated episodes of tachycardia that do not adequately respond to drug therapy and for whom information about site of origin, mechanism and electrophysiological properties of the pathways of the tachycardia is essential for choosing appropriate therapy (drugs, catheter ablation, pacing or surgery)
- Patients who prefer ablative therapy to pharmacological treatment

Class II
- Patients with frequent episodes of tachycardia requiring drug treatment for whom there is concern about proarrhythmia or the effects of the antiarrhythmic drug on sinus node or AV conduction

Class III
- Patients with tachycardias easily controlled by vagal maneuvers and/or well-tolerated drug therapy who are not candidates for nonpharmacological therapy

Abbreviations: AV: Atrioventricular

TABLE 5

Electrophysiology study indications for wide QRS complex tachycardias

Class I
- Patients with wide QRS complex tachycardia in whom correct diagnosis is unclear after analysis of available ECG tracings, and for whom knowledge of the correct diagnosis is necessary for patient care

Class II
- None

Class III
- Patients with ventricular or supraventricular tachycardia with aberrant conduction or preexcitation syndromes diagnosed with certainty by ECG criteria, and for whom invasive electrophysiological data would not influence therapy. However, data obtained at baseline EP study in these patients might be appropriate as a guide for subsequent therapy

Abbreviations: ECG: Electrocardiogram; EP: Electrophysiology

TABLE 6

Electrophysiology study indications for prolonged QT intervals

Class I
- None

Class II
- Identification of a proarrhythmic effect of a drug in patients experiencing sustained ventricular tachycardia or cardiac arrest while receiving the drug
- Patients who have equivocal abnormalities of QT interval duration or TU wave configuration, with syncope or symptomatic arrhythmias, in whom catecholamine effects may unmask a distinct QT abnormality

Class III
- Patients with clinically manifest congenital QT prolongation, with or without symptomatic arrhythmias
- Patients with acquired prolonged QT syndrome with symptoms closely related to an identifiable cause or mechanism

TABLE 7

Electrophysiology study indications for Wolff-Parkinson-White syndrome

Class I
- Patients being evaluated for catheter ablation or surgical ablation of an accessory pathway
- Patients with ventricular preexcitation who have survived cardiac arrest, or who have unexplained syncope
- Symptomatic patients in whom determination of the mechanism of arrhythmia, or knowledge of the electrophysiological properties of the accessory pathway and normal conduction system would help in determining appropriate therapy

Class II
- Asymptomatic patients with a family history of sudden cardiac death or with ventricular preexcitation, but no spontaneous arrhythmia, who engage in high-risk occupations or activities, and in whom knowledge of the electrophysiological properties of the accessory pathway or inducible tachycardia may help to determine recommendations for further activities or therapy
- Patients with ventricular preexcitation who are undergoing cardiac surgery for other reasons

Class III
- Asymptomatic patients with ventricular preexcitation, except those in Class II above

TABLE 8

Electrophysiology study indications for premature ventricular complexes, couplets and nonsustained ventricular tachycardia

Class I
- None

Class II
- Patients with other risk factors for future arrhythmic events, such as a low ejection fraction, positive signal-averaged ECG, and non-sustained VT on ambulatory ECG recordings in whom electrophysiology studies will be used for further risk assessment and for guiding therapy in patients with inducible VT
- Patients with highly symptomatic, uniform morphology premature ventricular complexes, couplets and nonsustained VT, who are considered as potential candidates for catheter ablation

Class III
- Asymptomatic or mildly symptomatic patients with premature ventricular complexes, couplets and nonsustained VT without other risk factors for sustained arrhythmias

Abbreviations: ECG: Electrocardiogram; VT: Ventricular tachycardia

TABLE 9

Electrophysiology study indications for unexplained syncope

Class I
- Patients with suspected structural heart disease and syncope that remains unexplained after appropriate evaluation

Class II
- Patients with recurrent unexplained syncope without structural heart disease and a negative head-up tilt test

Class III
- Patients with a known cause of syncope for whom treatment will not be guided by electrophysiological testing

TABLE 10

Electrophysiology study indications for survivors of cardiac arrest

Class I
- Patients surviving cardiac arrest without evidence of an acute Q-wave MI
- Patients surviving cardiac arrest occurring more than 48 hours after the acute phase of MI in the absence of a recurrent ischemic event

Class II
- Patients surviving cardiac arrest caused by bradyarrhythmia
- Patients surviving cardiac arrest thought to be associated with a congenital repolarization abnormality (long-QT syndrome) in whom the results of noninvasive diagnostic testing are equivocal

Class III
- Patients surviving a cardiac arrest that occurred during the acute phase (< 48 hours) of MI
- Patients with cardiac arrest resulting from clearly definable specific causes such as reversible ischemia, severe valvular aortic stenosis or noninvasively defined congenital or acquired long-QT syndrome

Abbreviation: MI: Myocardial infarction

TABLE 11

Electrophysiology study indications for unexplained palpitations

Class I
- Patients with palpitations who have a pulse rate documented by medical personnel as inappropriately rapid and in whom ECG recordings fail to document the cause of the palpitations
- Patients with palpitations preceding a syncopal episode

Class II
- Patients with clinically significant palpitations suspected to be of cardiac origin in whom symptoms are sporadic and cannot be documented. Studies are performed to determine the mechanisms of arrhythmias, direct or provide therapy, or assess prognosis

Class III
- Patients with palpitations documented to be due to extracardiac causes (e.g. hyperthyroidism)

Abbreviation: ECG: Electrocardiogram

requirements of single-plane fluoroscopy and patient table/gantry; electrocardiac stimulator, signal filtering and recording system; and diagnostic electrode catheters through which cardiac stimulation and intracardiac signals/impulses may be sensed and delivered. Patients are generally studied in the postabsorptive state so as to minimize risk of aspiration while sedated or during arrhythmia induction that, at times, may provoke hemodynamic instability necessitating rapid arrhythmia termination including external cardioversion/defibrillation. Patients undergo sterile

TABLE 12

Electrophysiology study indications for guiding drug therapy

Class I
- Patients with sustained ventricular tachycardia or cardiac arrest, especially those with prior MI
- Patients with AVNRT, AV reentrant tachycardia using an accessory pathway, or atrial fibrillation associated with an accessory pathway, for whom chronic drug therapy is planned

Class II
- Patients with sinus node reentrant tachycardia, atrial tachycardia, atrial fibrillation or atrial flutter without ventricular preexcitation syndrome, for whom chronic drug therapy is planned
- Patients with arrhythmias not inducible during control EPS, for whom drug therapy is planned

Class III
- Patients with isolated atrial or ventricular premature complexes
- Patients with ventricular fibrillation with a clearly identified reversible cause

Abbreviations: AVNRT: Atrioventricular nodal reentrant tachycardia; EPS: Electrophysiology study; MI: Myocardial infarction

TABLE 13

Electrophysiology study indications for candidates and recipients of implantable electrical devices

Class I
- Patients with tachyarrhythmias, before and during implantation, and final (predischarge) programing of an electrical device to confirm its ability to perform as anticipated
- Patients with an implanted electrical antitachyarrhythmia device in whom changes in status or therapy may have influenced the continued safety and efficacy of the device
- Patients who have a pacemaker to treat a bradyarrhythmia and receive a cardioverter-defibrillator, to test for device interactions

Class II
- Patients with previously documented indications for pacemaker implantation to test for the most appropriate long-term pacing mode and sites to optimize symptomatic improvement and hemodynamics

Class III
- Patients who are not candidates for device therapy

A complete study evaluates sinus node automaticity and impulse propagation, atrial myocardial conduction properties, anterograde and retrograde conduction patterns, ventricular myocardial conduction properties and associated arrhythmic tendency, both spontaneous and stimulated.[13] Not all assessments may be possible in every patient. Pharmacologic agents also are administered to modify intrinsic automaticity and conduction properties to expose occult arrhythmic potential.

CARDIAC ACCESS AND CATHETERIZATION

The recording of local activation signals during EP study is obtained through stationary electrode catheters (Fig. 1), usually varying in size from 4 to 8 French. Standard diagnostic multipolar electrode catheters are introduced percutaneously through peripheral veins, such as the antecubital, femoral, subclavian or internal jugular veins, and then guided fluoroscopically to their intended intracardiac position. For safety and convenience, sites accessible transvenously via right cardiac chambers are chosen, usually the high-lateral right atrium or right atrial appendage, approximating the site of sinus endocardial breakthrough; His bundle region, approximating the site of atrioventricular nodal (AVN) conduction; within the coronary sinus (CS) that is posteriorly located, approximating a septal-lateral axis of activation of both the left atrium and ventricle; and the right ventricle (RV) (Fig. 2). This "standard" catheter positioning approximates the normal conduction system axis, creating a skeleton of recording sites that define the sequence and timing of activation from all four cardiac chambers. Other recording sites, such as the right bundle-branch

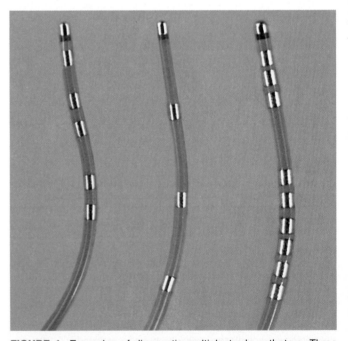

FIGURE 1: Examples of diagnostic multielectrode catheters. Three diagnostic catheters with different interelectrode spacing and electrode distribution are shown. Closer-spaced electrodes permit detection of high-frequency signals such as His or accessory pathway potentials, with high degree of localization though at the expense of signal amplitude, whereas wider-spaced electrodes yield larger-amplitude signals, at the expense of localization accuracy

skin preparation using iodine and other alcohol-based and nonalcohol-based scrubs, followed by draping to prevent cross-contamination from nonsterilized areas and to maintain patient dignity while permitting access to anticipated sites of vascular entry. Local anesthesia, as well as mild conscious sedation, is warranted to facilitate painless percutaneous vascular access, particularly in apprehensive patients. After diagnostic catheters are introduced, sedation may be lightened so as not to hinder arrhythmia induction, as some sedative drugs may alter properties of the cardiac conduction system. The awake patient should be continuously reassured to promote relaxation and to prevent sudden movements that may result in catheter dislodgement and vascular injury, not to mention intracardiac trauma. Antiarrhythmic drugs are usually withheld prior to the study, although in select cases, they may be continued if clinical events occurred on specific agents or in an effort to promote tolerability of arrhythmias that may otherwise provoke severe symptoms or hemodynamic collapse.

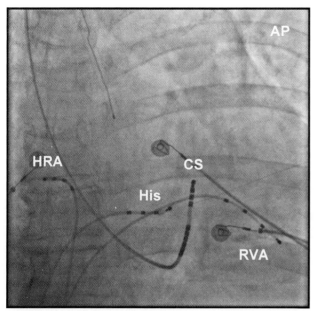

FIGURE 2: Anteroposterior (AP) fluoroscopic projection of "standard" intracardiac catheter locations. The high right atrial (HRA) catheter is positioned laterally in the right atrial appendage. The His catheter is positioned across the atrioventricular junction at the mid-to-superior septal aspect of the tricuspid valve. The right ventricular catheter is seated in the apex (RVA). The coronary sinus (CS) catheter is positioned with the proximal electrode approximately 1 cm from the CS ostium. (*Source:* Reproduced from Choudhuri et al. Principles and techniques of cardiac catheter mapping. In: Camm AJ, Saksena S (Eds). Electrophysiologic Disorders of the Heart, 2nd edition. St. Louis: Churchill-Livingstone (Elsevier) Inc; 2010. With permission from Elsevier.)

region just across the tricuspid valve and right ventricular septum or outflow tract, and even the pulmonary veins, may be sampled using traditional and specially designed catheters to further augment and enhance the diagnostic framework based on the suspected arrhythmia.

Transseptal catheterization (see below) via the right atrium to access left atrium is invaluable, particularly to approach pulmonary veins in atrial fibrillation (AF) ablation and for ventricular tachycardia (VT) ablation in patients with mechanical aortic valve in whom the left ventricle (LV) would be otherwise inaccessible through the aortic retrograde approach. Continuous heparinization is desirable for left-heart catheterization to avoid thromboembolic complications. Catheterization into the pericardial space using a subxiphoid or subcostal approach permits access for mapping and ablation of arrhythmias of epicardial origin.

SIGNALS AND FILTERING

Once intracardiac diagnostic catheters are appropriately positioned and connectivity established, the recorded signals, intracardiac electrograms (EGMs), are displayed simultaneously on a multichannel digital recording system along with several unfiltered surface ECG leads. Signal filtering between 30–40 Hz and 500 Hz is best suited for sharp intracardiac signals such as those from the His bundle and accessory pathways (Figs 3A to F). A high-pass filter setting of more than 50–100 Hz reduces undesirable low-frequency signals. In addition, 60-cycle interference and its harmonics can be eliminated with

a notch filter tuned to 60 Hz,[11] although potentially at the expense of other low-amplitude physiologic signals in that frequency range.

FUNDAMENTALS OF THE CARDIAC ELECTROPHYSIOLOGY STUDY

Identifying pathology during the cardiac EP study requires a keen awareness of normal electrophysiologic characteristics, an understanding of the principles guiding intracardiac EGM interpretation and knowledge of expected responses to programed stimulation.[14] Further, these assessments must be universally understood and communicable to other practitioners at various levels of training and expertise including electrophysiologists, cardiologists, physician extenders, lab technicians, nurses and even health care providers not directly practicing in the field of cardiovascular diseases.

CONVENTIONS

Several conventions are used to describe electrical events in a standardized manner, which are briefly described in this chapter. The most fundamental of these is that of timing and intervals. Measurements of most EP intervals are made in milliseconds, similar to usual intervals on the standard ECG. However, rates of atrial and ventricular events are determined in beats per minute and are converted to milliseconds by dividing the rate into 60,000 (the number of milliseconds per minute), yielding the rate of that particular event (e.g. heart rate) in milliseconds (per beat or occurrence). Hence sinus rhythm, usually 60–100 beats per minute, corresponds to cycle length 1,000–600 ms, respectively.

Diagnostic EP catheters have multiple electrodes, which create various recording unipoles and bipoles. By convention, the distal or tip electrode is designated electrode "1" and more proximal electrodes are numbered sequentially with increasing distance from the tip electrode. Further, whereas intracardiac EGMs are typically bipolar signals—and hence require two electrodes (usually adjacent) to generate the signal—a quadripolar catheter can generate up to three bipolar EGMs ("1–2", "2–3", "3–4"), and a decapolar catheter can display up to nine bipoles from adjacent electrodes. Other pairs can be configured as well. Often, all bipoles are not displayed; it depends on the clinical utility, particular catheter and/or its location and mapping resolution required.

NORMAL CARDIAC ELECTROPHYSIOLOGY

Normal Propagation Patterns

An awareness of two principles aids in proper interpretation of intracardiac EGMs. The first is that propagation within myocardium is generally radial, although with some directionality, due to anisotropic conduction and presence of structural barriers. This pattern of propagation during a stable rhythm results in activation at various myocardial areas simultaneously. Consider an atrial tachycardia arising from the low crista terminalis (Fig. 4A). Repetitive depolarization at this site is itself not detected, as this location is not standard for

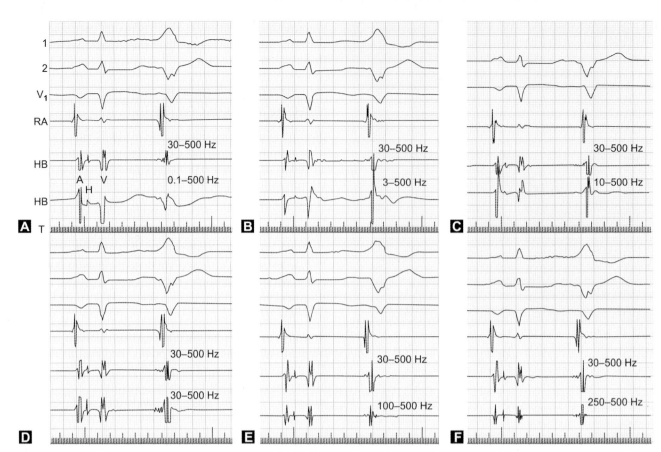

FIGURES 3A TO F: Effects of various filtering frequencies on the morphologic appearance of intracardiac electrograms. The tracings from top to bottom are electrocardiographic leads 1, 2, V1, right atrial (RA), two His bundle (HB) electrograms and timeline (T). In each Panel, the first beat is of sinus origin and is followed by a spontaneous ventricular premature beat. The top HB, RA and right ventricle are filtered at 30–500 Hz (i.e. the usual filtering frequencies). The bottom HB tracing shows the effect of various filtering frequencies on the appearance. The low-frequency signals are mostly eliminated at high-band-pass filter frequency settings above 10 Hz (Panel C). The low-band-pass filter settings above 500 Hz generally do not have a significant effect on the intracardiac electrogram appearance. It should be pointed out that the high-band-pass setting reduces the overall magnitude of the electrogram, necessitating an increase in amplification. It should also be noted that, at all frequencies depicted, the HB deflection can be clearly identified. (*Source:* Akhtar M. Invasive cardiac electrophysiologic studies: An introduction. In: Parmley WW, Chatterjee K (Eds). Cardiology: Physiology Pharmacology Diagnosis. Philadelphia: Lippincott; 1991. With permission from Lippincott Williams and Wilkins)

diagnostic catheters. Only after radial propagation through the right atrium, away from the tachycardia origin, and arrival at sites where catheters are located, e.g. the high right atrium (HRA) and His, are EGMs first recorded. In this case conduction times to these locations are fairly similar, resulting in near-simultaneous activation at both sites. The EGMs should neither be interpreted as representing a tachycardia arising simultaneously from those sites nor rapidly propagating from one site to the other so as to "appear" near-simultaneous, but rather more accurately explained by radial spread of a wave of activation arising from a location that has relatively similar conduction times to those catheter locations. This principle is inherently not specific, and other endocardial sites may also be equidistant from the HRA and His catheters (Fig. 4B). Hence, radial spread permits tachycardias arising from various intracardiac sites to produce similar EGM patterns (Fig. 4C). Definitive identification of involved sites requires more detailed cardiac mapping.

With respect to the AV conduction system, such tissues, in fact, should be considered to exhibit at least bidirectional propagation unless absence of this capability is demonstrated, even if unidirectional propagation predominates. For instance, in sinus rhythm or when pacing the atrium, it is expected that the impulse will conduct to the ventricles in an otherwise healthy heart. However, it should not be discounted that retrograde, i.e. ventriculoatrial (VA), conduction may also be responsible for cardiac rhythm events. Consider the situation of aberrant conduction induced by cycle length variation. Often one finds aberrancy, i.e. "bundle branch block," persists for several beats. This phenomenon develops due to anterograde conduction of a supraventricular impulse solely along the unblocked bundle and then spread of activation across the interventricular septum to invade and travel retrogradely along the previously blocked bundle, rendering it refractory to anterograde conduction by the next arriving supraventricular impulse and thereby maintaining aberrancy (Figs 5A to C).

In addition to these technical and physiologic aspects, it should be recognized that microscopic, molecular and cellular properties underlying myocardial membrane ion channel function, excitation-contraction, cellular automaticity, conduction velocity and tissue refractoriness to name a few, directly impact EGMs observed during EP study. These aspects are critical to a fundamental foundation on which to develop

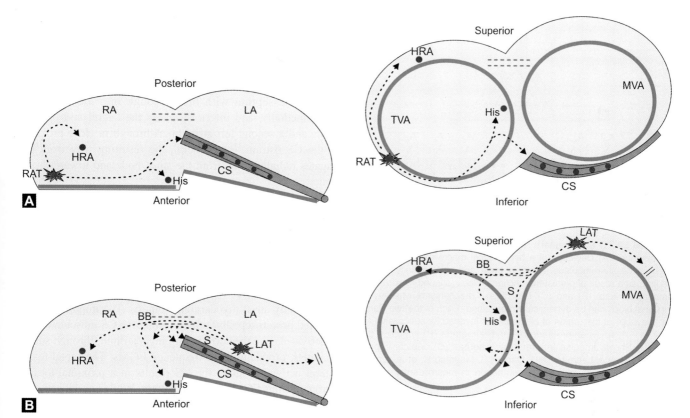

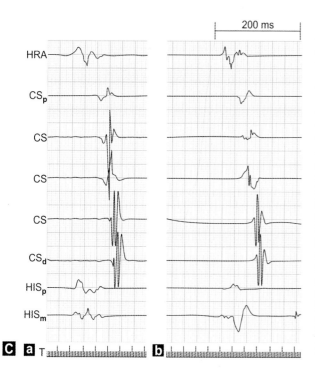

FIGURES 4A TO C: Radial propagation from two different focal tachycardia origins resulting in similar electrogram (EGM) activation sequences. (A) Cranial (upper) and left anterior oblique caudal (lower) schematic depictions of the atria with focal tachycardia site of origin in the low crista terminalis and (B) anterior left atrium (LA) above the mitral valve annulus (MVA). (A) Low crista terminalis (CT) tachycardia focus: wavefronts propagate superiorly along the CT into the right atrial (RA) appendage as well as simultaneously along the floor of the RA and then anteriorly and superiorly to arrive at the His region. Local conduction properties and similarity in distance between the tachycardia focus and the high right atrium (HRA) and His results in similar activation times to these two sites. The wavefront traveling along the RA floor also penetrates the septum posteriorly and activates the coronary sinus (CS) from proximal to distal. (B) Anterior LA tachycardia focus: wavefronts are shown to propagate along Bachmann's bundle (BB) and the interatrial septum (S). The rapidly conducted BB wavefront then propagates radially within the RA to arrive at the HRA and His electrodes with relatively similar activation times. Conduction block to the lateral LA (from scar or ablation) prevents a wavefront from activating the CS electrodes from distal to proximal. The S-wavefront travels inferiorly along the interatrial septum and then activates the CS from proximal to distal, possibly through direct penetration or after crossing the septum and entering the RA. The more rapid conduction across BB may explain earlier activation at the HRA and His as compared to the CS. (C) EGM patterns from a (left) and b (right). Surface ECG leads and intracardiac EGM channels are shown with timeline (T). In both tachycardias, activation is earliest at HRA and His, followed by proximal to distal activation in the coronary sinus. Red—arrhythmia focus; lime green—valve annuli; teal—coronary sinus; violet dashed lines—Bachmann's bundle; dotted lines with arrowhead—activation wavefronts. HRA, His and CS electrodes are shown. Gray signifies "behind" other structures. TVA: Tricuspid valve annulus

an understanding of cardiac EP in all its manifestations. As an initial consideration of the final consequence of these processes, we will introduce here normal conduction patterns, and a perspective on the most normal of electrophysiologic manifestations—sinus rhythm.

Sinus Rhythm and Normal Atrioventricular Conduction Parameters

An almost tacit assumption in the interpretation of intracardiac EGMs and, more importantly, in the understanding of cardiology

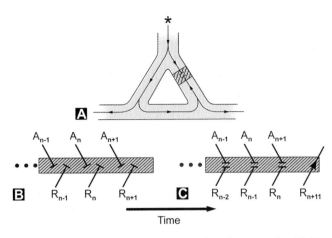

FIGURES 5A TO C: Schematic representation of a generalized linking phenomenon. (A) Depiction of a hypothetical macroreentry circuit into which successive impulses (asterisk) enter and preferentially traverse one limb as a result of persistent functional block (shaded region) in the contralateral limb. (B) and (C) Two distinct mechanisms whereby the functional block can be dynamically maintained. Each of the two Panels is a "blow-up" of the region of block as it is invaded by successive (i.e. n − 2, n − 1, n, ...) anterograde (A) and retrograde (R) impulses over time. (B) Shows impulse interference, whereas (C) depicts impulse collision. (*Source:* Lehmann MH, Denker S, Mahmud R, et al. Linking: a dynamic electrophysiologic phenomenon in macroreentry circuits. Circulation. 1985;71:254-65)

as well as EP is the recognition of sinus rhythm. It remains the most important and common cardiac rhythm, yet its study and comprehension are typically limited to the identification of regular cardiac activity with ECG demonstration of a P-wave preceding a QRS complex. Understanding sinus rhythm through intracardiac EGMs conveys a wealth of fundamental EP, and cardiovascular physiology that is critical to understanding normal phenomena and pathology. It is also important to recognize that the depiction of sinus rhythm through intracardiac EGMs, and all rhythms for that matter, is in large part dependent upon the established construct that anticipates catheters positioned in standard locations, such as HRA, CS, His bundle region and RV, as described above.

Sinus rhythm originates from the sinoatrial node, located epicardially at the junction of the right atrium with the anterolateral aspect of the superior vena cava. Its important property of automaticity generates an electrical depolarization in a regular manner that is the sinus rhythm. Depolarizations occur usually every 1,000–600 ms, termed the sinus cycle length, corresponding to a heart rate of 60–100 bpm. Once the sinus node depolarizes, resulting phenomena, including propagation to and within the atrium, atrial contraction, conduction along the normal AV pathway and activation of the ventricles, are all secondary and need not necessarily occur while in sinus rhythm. However, these secondary phenomena signify that sinus rhythm is associated with the other normal electromechanical cardiac events necessary for maintenance of circulation.

After exiting the sinoatrial node, the sinus impulse propagates both epicardially and endocardially. The endocardial breakthrough is in the posterior lateral right atrium, typically somewhat below but still in close proximity to the actual sinus node. Hence, a catheter in this region will be the first to detect

an EGM during sinus rhythm. By the time endocardial breakthrough has occurred, the impulse has also stimulated enough atrial myocardium to initiate inscription of the ECG P-wave. The impulse spreads rapidly due to presence of sodium channels, with some degree of preferential conduction anteriorly toward the septum with breakthrough into the left atrium anteromedially, and inferiorly along the lateral and posterior walls and a second left atrial breakthrough in close proximity to the CS ostium.[15] In general, the resulting wavefront propagates radially away from the sinus node and toward the AV node.

The proximal electrodes of a correctly positioned His catheter lie intra-atrially, mid to anteriorly, and are the poles that typically identify the next atrial deflection of sinus rhythm as the impulse propagates toward the AV node. The time interval between the onset of the P-wave and the arrival of the atrial impulse at the His bundle catheter is a measure of intra-atrial conduction time (IACT) and typically is less than 30 ms in adults with healthy atrial myocardium (Fig. 6). The impulse also has traveled posteroseptally into and along the CS musculature that is activated, like the surrounding myocardium, through sodium channels, producing high-frequency EGMs. The septal-to-left-lateral activation along the CS results in a proximal-to-distal coronary sinus EGM activation pattern. While biatrial activation is occurring, the impulse also encounters the AVN region, where absence of sodium channels rendering conduction dependent primarily upon slow calcium channels, as well as other anatomic, histologic and electrical phenomena results in slow conduction within the AV node. The resultant low-amplitude and slowly propagating electrical wavefronts do not generate a discernable wave or deflection on surface ECG or intracardiac electrodes using standard catheters and filtering. The delay permits completion of passive ventricular filling, allowing the eventual atrial contraction to prime the ventricles, thereby augmenting stroke volume. After the impulse leaves the AV node, it encounters the His bundle where cell membranes do once again incorporate sodium channels, and rapid conduction resumes, generating a high-frequency deflection. The location of the His bundle, anatomically within several millimeters to 1 cm anterior and superior to the AV node, provides a surrogate marker to measure AVN conduction time, which is measured between the atrial EGM on the bipole identifying the largest His EGM and the first rapid deflection of the His EGM (A-H interval), and is typically less than 125 ms (Fig. 6). Propagation along the His-Purkinje system (HPS) results in myocardial breakout at various points along the LV septum and soon after at the mid-to-distal RV septum. Standard catheter positioning does not typically employ LV catheters but does incorporate an RV catheter, usually at the apex, and it is this catheter that displays the first ventricular EGM. The time for normal HPS activation to reach the ventricles, measured from the His bundle recording to the earliest ventricular activation (H-V interval), whether on surface ECG or intracardiac EGMs, is 35–55 ms (Fig. 6). The IACT, A-H and H-V intervals together comprise the ECG P-R interval.

Simultaneously or very soon after RV activation, RV septal activation is detected as ventricular EGMs on the His bundle electrodes across the tricuspid valve and along the basal ventricular septum, resulting from both transseptal impulse

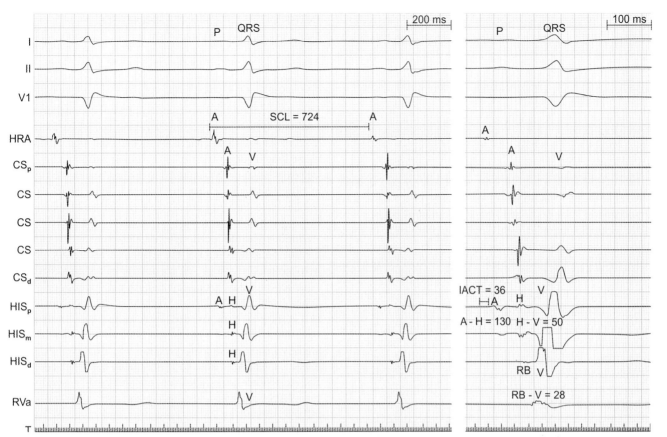

FIGURE 6: Baseline conduction parameters. Surface electrocardiographic (ECG) leads and intracardiac channels are shown during sinus rhythm at 100 mm/s (left) and 200 mm/s (right) sweep. Atrial electrograms (AEGMs) span the duration of the P-wave while ventricular electrograms (VEGMs) are aligned with and span the QRS duration. Sinus cycle length is measured from onset of AEGM on the HRA channel to the onset of the next HRA EGM (calipers, left Panel). The His bundle EGM (H) is the largest high-frequency signal between the AEGM and ventricular electrogram (VEGM) on the His recording channels. Intra-atrial conduction time (IACT) estimates the conduction time from the sinus to the atrioventricular (AV) node and is measured from onset of the P-wave to onset of the AEGM on the His catheter (calipers, right Panel). A-H interval, analogous to AV nodal conduction, is measured from onset of AEGM on His catheter to first high-frequency component of the His bundle deflection. The H-V interval assesses His-Purkinje conduction and is measured from the first high-frequency deflection of the His EGM to the onset of the ventricular depolarization whether VEGM or surface QRS. Right Panel: A low-amplitude high-frequency EGM is seen on the distal His channel just preceding the VEGM. There is no discernable AEGM on this channel, signifying the electrode is far enough distal across the tricuspid valve so as not to be able to detect atrial activity. This EGM is generated by the right bundle branch. The RB–V interval is typically less than 30 ms. (Abbreviations: CS: Coronary sinus; HRA: High right atrium; RB: Right bundle; SCL: Sinus cycle length)

spread and radial propagation of the impulse from the RV septal breakout site (Figs 6 and 7).[16] The CS catheter also detects ventricular signals; however, these are not the signals of earliest LV activation. Rather, the latest area to be activated in the LV is the base, and it is this basal posterior LV activation that is detected on the CS catheter. Unlike the ventricular EGMs seen on the RV and His catheter, the CS ventricular EGMs are of lower amplitude and lower frequency because the CS electrodes are not in contact with LV myocardium and may even reside more than 10 mm away, due to the location of the CS catheter within the coronary sinus and anatomic variations in the relationship between the coronary sinus and the mitral valve annulus.[17]

PROGRAMMED ELECTRICAL STIMULATION AND ASSOCIATED ELECTROPHYSIOLOGY

Two distinct patterns of pacing are applied during an EP study: (1) continuous pacing and (2) interrupted pacing. These techniques permit comprehensive assessment of all relevant

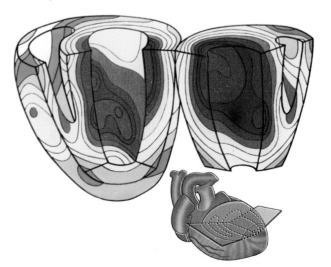

FIGURE 7: Three-dimensional isochronic representation of activation of the heart. Inset shows section levels. (*Source:* Durrer et al. Total excitation of the isolated human heart. Circulation. 1970;41: 899-912. Wolters Kluwer Health, with permission)

aspects of myocardial conduction and clinical arrhythmia tendency. If arrhythmia is induced, variations of these techniques may be employed during tachycardia to diagnose underlying mechanism(s).

CONTINUOUS PACING

Continuous pacing, in which each stimulus is referred to as "S1," is performed at fixed cycle lengths or with gradual decrementation in cycle length (i.e. gradual increase in heart rate). Continuous fixed-cycle-length pacing is used for study of sinus node function and integrity of subsidiary pacemakers, arrhythmia induction and overdrive pacing of a tachycardia ("entrainment," not discussed here). Continuous pacing with gradual decrementation in cycle length is performed to evaluate myocardial stimulation limits, and usually delivered until the occurrence of a desired event such as induction of tachycardia, conduction block (Fig. 8) or failure to achieve 1:1 myocardial capture. As such, this technique provides an overall measure of ability of a particular tissue, chamber or region to respond to sequential stimuli; is a measure of absolute limits of myocardial responsiveness; and may provide insight into tachycardia mechanism.

With fixed-cycle-length pacing at cycle lengths that are not excessively short, but shorter than sinus so as to avoid competition and interference, healthy atrial and ventricular tissue will respond in a 1:1 manner with minimal conduction delay (latency) between the stimulus artifact and the onset of the associated EGM and P-wave or QRS down to cycle lengths shorter than 250 ms.[14] As cycle length is decremented, a point is reached beyond which latency increases. This observation suggests the pacing cycle length is encroaching on the ability of local tissue capture and propagation to the surrounding myocardium in a 1:1 manner, and further pacing acceleration can result in failure of capture or breakup and fractionation of the propagating wavefront, provoking fibrillation, whether atrial or ventricular. The observation of increased latency should signal the operator to discontinue the pacing drive as induction of fibrillation may, at the least, prevent complete electrophysiologic evaluation in the case of AF, unless fibrillation is the desired result, and may require emergent electrical conversion if VF is induced.

INTERMITTENT OR INTERRUPTED PACING WITH EXTRASTIMULI

The second pacing format is intermittent pacing with delivery of premature (or extra) stimuli. This pacing format is advantageous for studying myocardial and conduction system refractory periods and for creation of local conduction block to facilitate induction of reentrant arrhythmias. With this approach, a series of six to ten paced beats are delivered at a constant cycle length (drive train of S1s) and are followed by at least one extrastimulus (S2) coupled to the last beat of the basic drive at a cycle length shorter than the S1 drive cycle. The S2 is initiated late during electrical diastole and the coupling interval is progressively decreased with successive drives, thereby "scanning diastole" until myocardial capture and/or conduction cannot be achieved, i.e. the effective refractory period of myocardial (Fig. 9) or AV conduction (Figs 10A to C)[11,18] or conduction delay promotes arrhythmia induction (Fig. 11). When latency or frank tissue refractoriness is encountered, the refractory period of downstream tissues may not be determinable. In such cases, the S2 coupling interval may be slightly increased so as to permit myocardial capture or avoid latency, then additional extrastimuli may be introduced (S3, S4, S5, etc.). Since antegrade AVN conduction is generally poorer than HPS conduction, evaluating the refractory period of the HPS is limited by AVN conduction and may not always be determinable. Various agents can be administered to shorten refractoriness and improve conduction, thereby permitting evaluation of HPS conduction if AVN conduction improves adequately. Refractory periods of myocardial tissue are dependent upon and vary directly with drive cycle length. Therefore multiple drive cycles are used to assess dynamicity of refractoriness. Whereas a 600 ms cycle length drive may yield a tissue-effective refractory period of 300 ms, a 400 ms cycle length drive would be expected to shorten tissue refractoriness.[19]

SIGNIFICANCE OF "SHORT-LONG-SHORT" PACING CYCLES

At times, the aforementioned pacing maneuvers are unsuccessful in inducing a suspected arrhythmia. For documented or

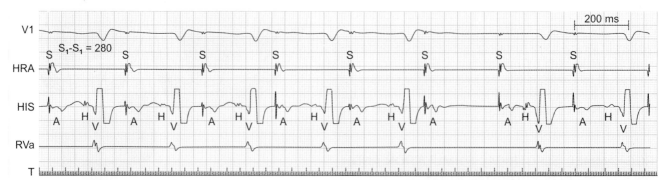

FIGURE 8: Demonstration of atrioventricular (AV) conduction block. Surface lead (V_1), intracardiac channels (HRA, His, RVa), and timeline (T) are shown. Continuous atrial pacing at 280 ms (S_1–S_1) results in conduction to the ventricle with progressive prolongation in A–H interval until conduction block. Notice that each pacing stimulus is associated with an atrial electrogram (A) and the A–H interval prolongs with each successive paced stimulus until no H is seen after the sixth paced A. Conducted beats are associated with a fixed H–V interval, confirming conduction delay above the His, i.e. in the AV node. With continued pacing, a new Wenckebach cycle ensues

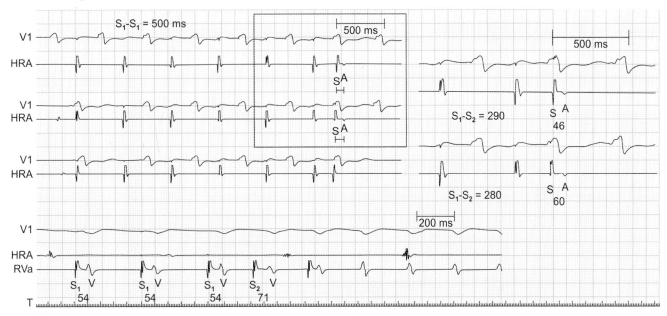

FIGURE 9: Latency and atrial effective refractory period. Surface lead (V1) and intracardiac channel (HRA) are shown with three successive atrial pacing drives at 500-ms cycle length (S_1–S_1) and progressively abbreviated extrastimuli (S_2) (upper left Panel). In the first drive, atrial extrastimulation coupled at 290 ms results in a stim-A (latency) time of 46 ms (inset; expanded view to the right). In the second drive, the extrastimulation at 280 ms is associated with increased latency (60 ms) (inset; expanded view to the right). In the third drive, further decrementation in the extrastimulus coupling interval to 270 ms results in loss of atrial capture with no atrial electrogram associated with the extrastimulus, thereby establishing the atrial effective refractory period as 600:270 ms. Surface lead (V1) and intracardiac channels (HRA, RVa) are shown (lower Panel). Ventricular pacing at 350 ms (S_1–S_1) is associated with a S_1–V time (latency) of 54 ms. The first ventricular extrastimulus is associated with increased latency, S_2–V time of 71 ms

suspected arrhythmias that rely on conduction delay for arrhythmia initiation (i.e. reentrant arrhythmias), "short-long-short" pacing—a variation on the extrastimulus technique—may prove useful in promoting conduction delay that initiates tachyarrhythmias when other maneuvers do not. This is applicable to all forms of reentrant tachyarrhythmias, whether in the atrium, ventricle or involving the HPS. A drive of six to eight beats is delivered at a specific cycle length, followed by the last beat of the drive coupled at a cycle length greater than that of the preceding beats in the drive. This long-coupled beat has the effect of shortening myocardial refractoriness (Figs 12A to F).[19,20] This allows an extrastimulus to be coupled at shorter cycle lengths ("short-long-short") than with fixed-cycle-length pacing, which may then create adequate myocardial propagation slowing to support reentry. This pacing technique has a divergent effect in the HPS, that is, HPS refractoriness increases with "short-long-short" sequences, which may directly enhance conduction delay and promote reentry within the HPS (Figs 13A to F).

For induction of reentrant supraventricular tachycardias (SVTs), single, double or more extrastimuli may be delivered (Fig. 14). For induction of VT, up to three ventricular extrastimuli are typically employed. The sensitivity of pacing protocols seems to be directly related to the number of extrastimuli utilized.[16] However, this occurs at the expense of specificity as polymorphic VT/VF can be induced at very short coupling intervals by using multiple ventricular extrastimuli in patients otherwise without arrhythmic risk. Regardless of pacing protocol, induction of sustained monomorphic VT constitutes a specific response and is seldom induced in patients who are not clinically prone to such arrhythmias. In contrast, the induction of polymorphic VT/VF with three extrastimuli at short coupling intervals can be nonspecific.[11]

Relation of Pacing Technique to Anticipated Arrhythmia Mechanism and Inducibility

Reentrant arrhythmias lend themselves best to study because the reentrant nature of arrhythmias creates a reproducible and regular activation sequence that can be evaluated when the arrhythmia is sustained. Tissue refractoriness and conduction slowing are necessary factors in the initiation and maintenance of reentrant arrhythmias, which can be achieved readily through continuous pacing with progressive cycle length decrementation and premature extrastimulation, with or without pharmacologic facilitation.

Unifocal triggered rhythms also can be evaluated by EP study. However, their tendency toward arrhythmia induction can be more challenging, being somewhat more sensitive to hormonal changes and limited by sedation and attendant varying catecholamine levels. Rapid, long pacing drives, through promotion of myocyte calcium overload and associated delayed afterdepolarizations, may permit induction of arrhythmias known to occur related to this mechanism, such as focal atrial tachycardias and certain idiopathic VT. Further, catecholamine administration (e.g. isoproterenol) enhancing cAMP-mediated adrenergic stimulation and associated diastolic calcium overload may facilitate induction with or without pacing. Interestingly, often it is not a specific level of catecholamine but rather the flux in serum concentration that permits induction (e.g. wash-in or wash-out phases).

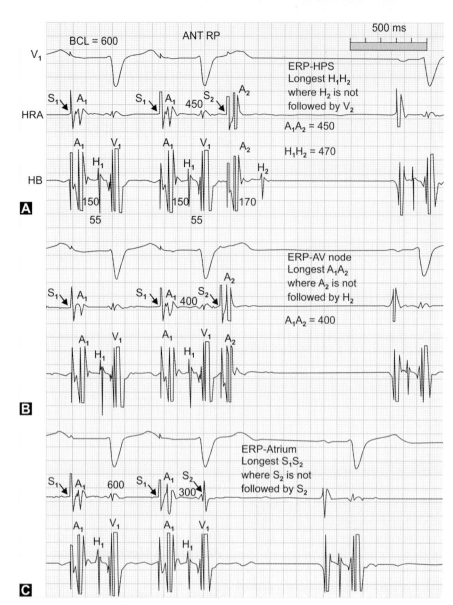

FIGURES 10A TO C: Determination of cardiac refractory periods during atrial pacing. During a basic cycle-length pacing at 600 ms (S_1S_1 or A_1A_1), atrial premature stimulation (S_2 or A_2) at progressively shorter coupling intervals (S_1S_2 or A_1A_2) is depicted. The definition of the effective refractory period (ERP) of the His-Purkinje system (HPS), atrioventricular (AV) node, and atrium are labeled. ANT RP: Antegrade refractory period. (*Source:* Reproduced from Akhtar M. Invasive cardiac electrophysiologic studies: an introduction. In: Parmley WW, Chatterjee K (Eds). Cardiology: Physiology, Pharmacology, Diagnosis. Philadelphia: Lippincott; 1991. With permission from Lippincott Williams and Wilkins)

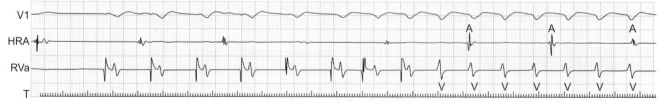

FIGURE 11: Ventricular tachycardia (VT) induction with extrastimuli. Surface lead (V1) and intracardiac channels (HRA, RVa) are shown. A six-beat ventricular drive at 350 ms is followed by two premature extrastimuli, inducing a wide complex tachycardia (V) with left bundle branch block morphology at 230 ms and atrioventricular dissociation, i.e. VT. A, atrial electrogram

CLINICAL APPLICATION OF "ROUTINE" ELECTROPHYSIOLOGY STUDY AND ANTICIPATED RESPONSES TO PROGRAMMED STIMULATION

While few would consider the findings of even a normal comprehensive EP study "routine," it is important to utilize a

systematic approach that permits complete evaluation of the myocardium and conduction system, including sinus node automaticity and impulse propagation, atrial myocardial conduction properties, anterograde and retrograde AV conduction patterns, ventricular myocardial conduction properties and associated arrhythmic tendency including

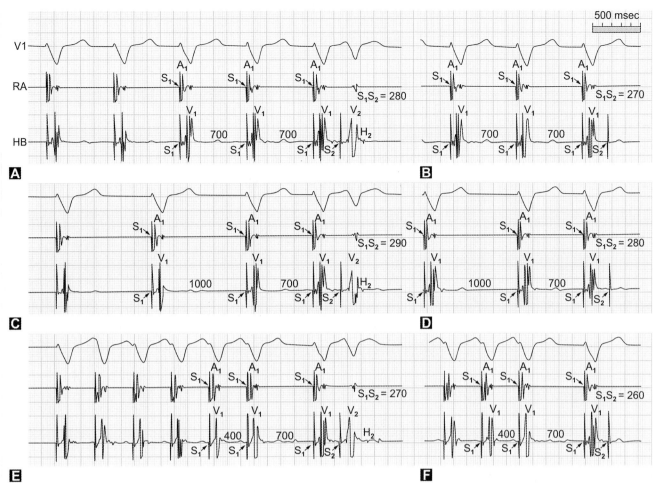

FIGURES 12A TO F: Effect of abrupt cycle length change on refractoriness of the ventricular muscle. The effective refractory period (ERP) of the ventricular muscle during constant cycle length (method I) is 270 ms (A and B). A change of $CL_p \rightarrow CL_R$ from 1,000 $\rightarrow$ 700 ms (method IIA, C and D) lengthens ERP of the ventricular muscle to 280 ms, whereas a change of $CL_P \rightarrow CL_R$ from 400 $\rightarrow$ 700 ms (method IIB, E and F) shortens the ERP of the ventricular muscle to 260 ms. Note that for the same CL_R, ERP of the ventricular muscle varies directly with CL_p. (*Source:* Modified from Denker S, Lehmann MH, Mahmud R, et al. Divergence between refractoriness of His-Purkinje system and ventricular muscle with abrupt changes in cycle length. Circulation. 1983;68;1212-21)

attempts at arrhythmia induction in the baseline state and during pharmacologic facilitation. The comprehensive EP study is performed in the following stages:

- Atrial continuous pacing with and without cycle length decrementation
- Atrial premature stimulation with extrastimuli
- Ventricular continuous pacing with and without cycle length decrementation
- Ventricular premature stimulation with extrastimuli
- Short bursts of rapid atrial or ventricular pacing[14]

While not all aspects may be assessed in each patient and the order may vary according to patients' needs and tolerances, this framework provides a method to perform a comprehensive electrophysiologic evaluation of intrinsic conduction properties and arrhythmogenic tendency. Burst pacing is rarely employed for the study of normal cardiac EP and is generally used in arrhythmia induction or termination and will not be elaborated upon here.[14]

Baseline Observations

Irrespective of the presenting rhythm or potential rhythm of interest, the surface ECG provides valuable information against which the intracardiac patterns of activation can be compared. It is negligent to disregard the baseline surface ECG, and basic observations of P-R, R-P, QRS and QT intervals should be made at the initiation of and throughout every study. Once baseline observations have been made, including intrinsic cycle length, activation sequence and parameters of AV conduction (Fig. 6), the active study can be performed with particular attention to appropriate stimulation protocols, myocardial capture and conduction, and activation of other chambers in response to each stimulus and nonstimulated responses. The large majority of patients, undergoing diagnostic EP study, are present in sinus rhythm; hence, the study usually starts with atrial stimulation. Alternately, as induction of AF presents a barrier to study completion, it may be pragmatic to perform atrial stimulation last in patients with a history of AF or sick sinus.

Atrial Stimulation for Evaluation of Sinus Node Function; and Atrial and Atrioventricular Nodal Conduction Properties

The assessment of sinus node automaticity should be included in all comprehensive EP studies, but particularly in patients

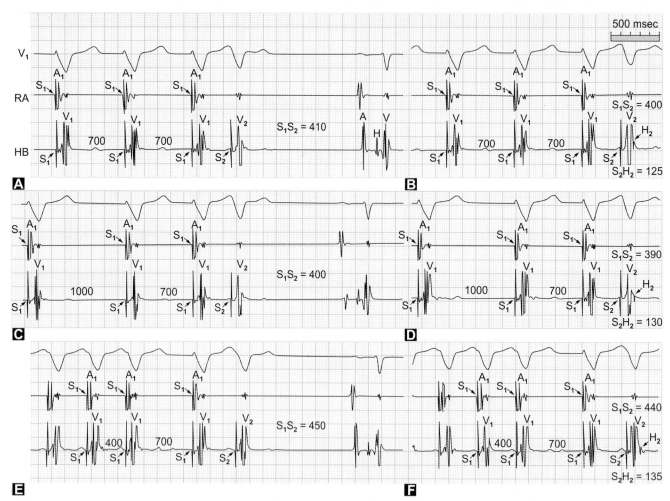

FIGURES 13A TO F: Effect of abrupt cycle length change on refractoriness of the His-Purkinje system (HPS). The tracings show the retrograde relative refractory period (RRP) of the HPS during methods I, IIA and IIB. With method I (A and B), H_2 emergence from the local ventricular electrogram is noted at an S_1S_2, interval of 400 ms. A change of $CL_p \rightarrow CL_R$ from 1,000 → 700 ms (method IIA, C and D) shortens the RRP of the HPS to 390 ms, whereas a change of $CL_p \rightarrow CL_R$ from 400 → 700 ms (method IIB, E and F) lengthens the RRP of the HPS to 440 ms. Note that for the same CL_R, the RRP of the HPS is 50 ms longer during method IIB compared with method IIA, but remarkably CL_p is 600 ms shorter during method IIB compared with method IIA. (Abbreviations: V_1: Surface electrocardiographic lead; RA: Right atrial electrogram; HB: His bundle electrogram. All measurements are in milliseconds). (*Source:* Modified from Denker S, Lehmann MH, Mahmud R, et al. Divergence between refractoriness of His-Purkinje system and ventricular muscle with abrupt changes in cycle length. Circulation. 1983;68;1212-21)

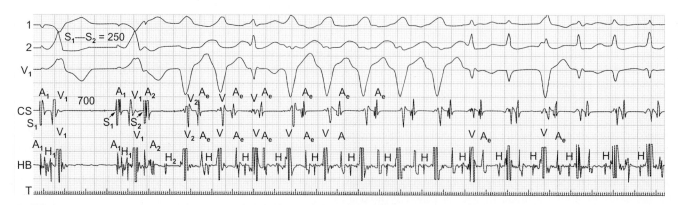

FIGURE 14: Induction of supraventricular tachycardia (SVT) in Wolff-Parkinson-White syndrome. The tracings are labeled. Atrial pacing from coronary sinus (CS) is done at a 700-ms basic cycle. During the basic drive pacing, left free-wall accessory pathway conduction to the ventricle produces ventricular preexcitation. A single premature beat (S_2) blocks in the accessory pathway and conducts over the normal pathway with a left bundle branch block morphology, and the SVT is initiated. Note the intermittent normalization of the QRS complex during this SVT. (*Source:* Modified from Jazayeri MR, Caceres J, Tchou P, et al. Electrophysiologic characteristics of sudden QRS axis deviation during orthodromic tachycardia. J Clin Invest. 1989;83:952-9. With permission from American Society for Clinical Investigation)

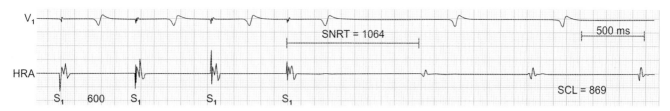

FIGURE 15: Measurement of sinus node recovery time (SNRT). A train of S_1's at 600 ms is delivered over 30 seconds to achieve sinus suppression. With discontinuation of pacing, the time for first sinus return cycle is 1,064 ms, which is within normal limits. Correcting for the predominant sinus cycle length (SCL), 869 ms, yields a corrected SNRT of 195 ms, also within normal limits

presenting with dizziness, dyspnea on exertion, presyncope, syncope or other manifestations of sinus node dysfunction in whom diagnosis cannot be made noninvasively.[14] Right atrial pacing for 30 sec to 1 min at a fixed cycle length shorter than sinus causes sinus suppression. Abrupt discontinuation of pacing permits determination of the time for the first automatic intrinsic/escape sinus beat to return, this interval is termed the sinus node recovery time (SNRT). The SNRT is evaluated at various drive cycles ranging between the sinus cycle length and usually 400 ms. Sinus node recovery times less than 1,525 ms are generally considered normal. By deducting the predominant sinus cycle length from this interval, one can obtain the so-called corrected SNRT (Fig. 15). In one series[21] the value for corrected SNRT was less than 525 ms in normal individuals but exceeded this in patients with overt sinus node dysfunction.

In the vast majority of patients with true sinus node disease, sinoatrial conduction abnormalities are the predominant reason for sinus node dysfunction. Sinoatrial conduction time (SACT) in the absence of obvious sinus node disease is less than 100 ms. The SACT is evaluated in similar fashion to the SNRT by atrial pacing, in this case, just faster than sinus, hence avoiding significant sinus node suppression. The return cycle then represents the time for the last paced beat to enter the sinus node, reset it and propagate back to the pacing catheter. Again, deducting the predominant sinus cycle from the return cycle should approximate the propagation time to and from the sinus node, and the SACT is thus one-half of this value. SACTs in excess of 125 ms[14] are felt to represent important sinoatrial conduction disease. This interval is most accurate when the HRA catheter is positioned in close proximity to the sinus node, in the posterolateral aspect of the right atrium, and not in the right atrial appendage, which may be associated with prolonged conduction intervals between it and the sinus node.

The sensitivity of SNRT for the detection of sinus node dysfunction is 54%, whereas that of SACT is 51%, with a combined sensitivity of approximately 64%. Poor sensitivity of such testing relates in part to the possibility that in previous studies, documented episodes of sinus bradycardia or sinus arrest due to neurocardiogenic mechanisms may not have been excluded.[22] The specificity of both tests combined is approximately 88%. In patients with bradycardia/tachycardia syndrome, EP testing may also be necessary for the proper diagnosis and therapy of the concomitant tachyarrhythmia or bradyarrhythmia, as AV conduction is frequently abnormal in patients with sinus node dysfunction.[14]

After evaluation of sinus node automaticity, AV conduction capabilities are assessed in patients presenting in sinus rhythm. With successively faster pacing or shorter cycle length, AVN conduction time as measured by the A-H interval initially accommodates to the pacing drive, then prolongs until a pacing cycle length at which the Wenckebach pattern of conduction block is observed (Fig. 8). In most, this AV block cycle length is reached between 600 ms and 300 ms, although in some patients with "enhanced AVN conduction" 1:1 conduction may be maintained at cycle lengths less than 300 ms, often with electrocardiographically abbreviated P-R intervals. The clinical significance of this is unclear but has been seen in patients with rapid ventricular response in AF and atrial flutter. At the other extreme, observing a pattern of Wenckebach at cycle lengths greater than 600 ms is unusual but may be seen in healthy young adults with elevated vagal tone and should not be considered abnormal unless it is not reversible by vagolytic or sympathomimetic agents or occurs during exercise.[14]

Next, atrial premature extrastimuli are introduced for evaluation of atrial myocardial refractoriness and effective refractory period of the AV node. As mentioned previously, a fixed drive cycle coupled with a single premature extrastimulus is repeatedly delivered to scan diastole until absence of a particular event, whether that be conduction to the ventricles, arrival at the His, or myocardial capture, thereby establishing effective refractory periods at that cycle length (Figs 10A to C). If the atrial effective refractory period is reached before demonstrating AV nodal refractoriness, then prolongation of the extrastimulus coupling interval and introduction of additional extrastimuli may permit such demonstration (Figs 16A and B).

In addition, with atrial extrastimulus testing, "dual AVN physiology" may be observed. With gradual decrementation in the extrastimulus coupling interval, there is an abrupt prolongation in the H1-H2 interval, signifying conduction block in the AVN "fast" pathway but resulting in the atrial paced impulse arriving at the AV node by an alternate pathway that is associated with longer H1-H2 intervals ("slow-pathway"). Dual AVN pathways are felt to underlie the mechanism of AVN reentry tachycardia, and both continuous atrial pacing and atrial premature extrastimuli will often induce AVN reentry (Figs 17A and B), although other SVTs may be initiated by this mechanism as well.

Evaluation of Atrioventricular Conduction Disease

In appropriate patients, EP study is warranted to evaluate the site and mechanism of AV block. A discernible His bundle

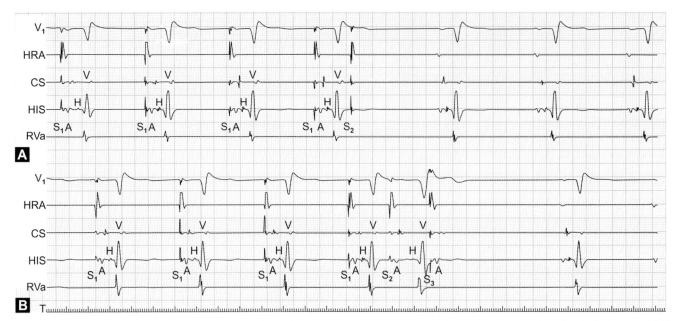

FIGURES 16A AND B: Atrial effective refractory period (AERP) and atrioventricular nodal effective refractory period (AVNERP). Surface lead (V_1) and intracardiac channels (HRA, CS, HIS, RVa) are shown. (A) Atrial pacing results in 1:1 atrial capture and conduction through AVN to the ventricle during the basic drive (S_1). The single premature atrial extrastimulus (S_2) fails to capture the atrial myocardium (AERP)—observe no atrial electrogram follows the S_2, unlike the S_1's—so no impulse propagates through the AVN to activate the ventricle. Sinus rhythm ensues in the absence of atrial pacing. (B) Having reached AERP, the S_2 coupling is increased by 30 ms to permit atrial capture and evaluation of AVN refractoriness. In this case the S_2 captures atrial myocardium as evidenced by presence of an A electrogram and conducts through the AVN to the ventricle, and an S_3 that also captures the atrium fails to conduct to the ventricles and blocks above the His bundle as no His deflection is seen, i.e. in the AVN. In this case, the AVNERP was established at 600:300:360 ms

recording enables one to determine the exact site of AV conduction abnormality, i.e. proximal, within or distal to the His bundle region. This, in combination with surface ECG morphology of conducted beats, enables one to identify precisely the location of conduction abnormality. The finding of a prolonged H-V interval, greater than 60 ms, is evidence of HPS conduction disease (Figs 18A and B). If 1:1 AV conduction is present in patients suspected of intermittent AV block, atrial pacing with cycle length decrementation should be performed to evaluate reproducibility of AV block. AV block in the HPS is abnormal during continuous atrial pacing (Fig. 19) but may be a physiologic response during atrial extrastimulation or with sudden rate change related to asynchronous initiation of atrial pacing.[14]

In asymptomatic patients with first-degree AV block (prolonged P-R interval), electrophysiologic assessment is unnecessary regardless of the QRS morphology of the conducted beats, although in asymptomatic individuals with second-degree AV block electrophysiologic assessment is used to identify site of block (Figs 20A to C). Patients with intra-Hisian or infra-Hisian block tend to have a more unpredictable course, and permanent pacing is desirable.[23] Even though intranodal block usually presents as Wenckebach's phenomenon or Mobitz type I, it is not uncommon to see Wenckebach within the His or in the HPS distal to the His bundle. There is no difference in prognosis regardless of how the intra-Hisian or infra-Hisian second-degree block manifests itself, i.e. type I versus type II. In symptomatic patients with second-degree AV block, the role of EP study is limited because permanent pacing is the appropriate intervention. On

the other hand, if the patient's symptoms cannot be explained on the basis of AV block and may be related to another arrhythmia such as VT, EP study should be considered. In patients with third-degree or complete AV block, EP studies are seldom required; permanent pacing is the obvious option in symptomatic patients.[11]

Ventricular Stimulation and Assessment of Ventriculoatrial Conduction, Wide QRS Tachycardia and Sudden Death Risk

As a construct, the AV conduction system can be considered as a pair of cables, the left and right bundle branches, joined proximally at the AV junction; all capable of bidirectional conduction. Similar to anterograde conduction, retrograde AV conduction can be assessed with gradual decrementation in a continuous ventricular drive (Fig. 21). The importance of the specific cycle length at which retrograde conduction block occurs is particularly relevant in determining arrhythmia mechanisms. For example, in a patient with narrow complex tachycardia with 1:1 conduction to the ventricle of unknown mechanism at a heart rate of 190 bpm (~320 ms), identifying retrograde AV conduction block at 450 ms (~135 bpm) would suggest that the tachycardia cannot be one in which the ventricles would be required to conduct to the atrium to maintain the tachycardia. Instead, the tachycardia mechanism is more likely entirely independent of VA conduction, i.e. atrial tachycardia.

The specific pattern of VA conduction should be closely observed. Whereas retrograde conduction over the normal

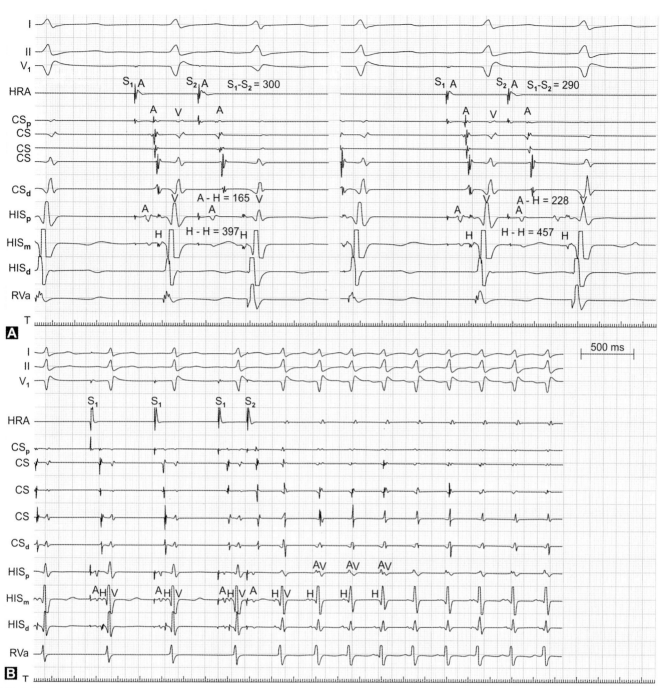

FIGURES 17A AND B: Dual atrioventricular node (AVN) physiology and induction of AVNRT. (A) On left side: the last paced beat of a 600-ms basic drive (S_1) is shown, with a single atrial extrastimulus coupled at 300 ms (S_2) that conducts through the AVN to the ventricles with A-H 165 ms and H-H 397 ms. On right side: with the same basic drive, the atrial extrastimulus coupling interval is decremented by 10 ms to 290 ms, resulting in conduction through the AVN to the ventricle with marked conduction delay in excess of 50 ms (A-H 228 ms, H-H 457 ms) compared to the previous drive, compatible with "jump" to a slow AVN pathway. (B) Induction of common AVN reentry tachycardia (AVNRT). Atrial pacing at 600 ms (in a different patient) is followed by a single extrastimulus coupled at 360 ms (S_2) that is associated with A-H delay and initiation of a tachycardia with narrow QRS identical to sinus, and electrogram (EGM) pattern with nearly simultaneous atrial and ventricular activation preceded by a His deflection. A narrow QRS tachycardia preceded by His EGM must be, in general, supraventricular as each impulse activates the His before activating the ventricles and hence must be arising above the His, i.e. atrium or AVN. In AVNRT, an atrial premature complex or premature extrastimulus provokes AVN fast pathway block and results in conduction over a slow AVN pathway manifested by a prolonged P-R and A-H. After conducting over the slow AVN pathway, the wavefront reaches a lower turnaround/branch point and propagates along the AVN "fast pathway" retrogradely to the atria while continuing along the His-Purkinje system (HPS) toward the ventricles. This results in nearly simultaneous atrial and ventricular activation, and the distinctive pattern of complete alignment of all atrial and ventricular EGM and superimposed P's and QRS's

pathway would be expected to activate the atria earliest at the His catheter, which is in closest proximity to the AV node (Fig. 22A), retrograde AV conduction over other pathways would result in altered activation sequences (aside from path-

ways very close to the AV node such as anteroseptal accessory pathways). For instance, retrograde activation that is earliest in the proximal CS is suggestive of a posteriorly located midline pathway (Fig. 22B), such as an AVN slow pathway or a

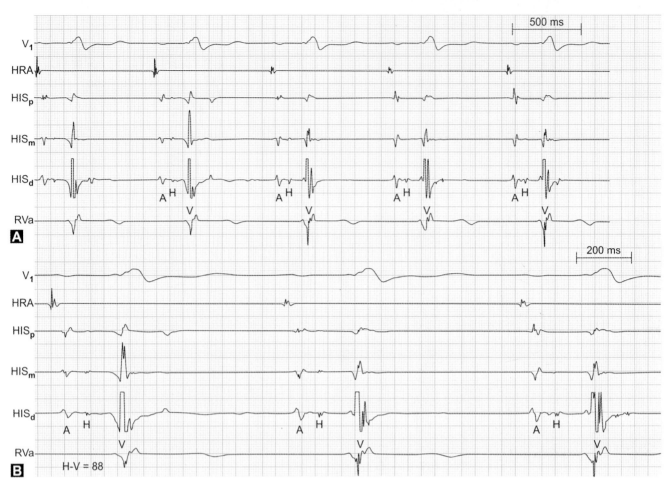

FIGURES 18A AND B: His-Purkinje disease. Sinus rhythm is shown in a patient with recurrent syncope and right bundle branch block at 50 mm/s (A) and 100 mm/s (B) sweep. The A-H interval is 138 ms and H-V interval is 88 ms at baseline heart rate of 69 bpm

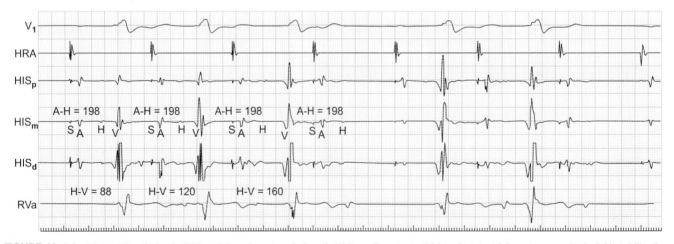

FIGURE 19: Infra-Hisian Wenckebach. With atrial pacing at cycle length 700 ms (heart rate 86 bpm), 1:1 atrial capture results in A-H stabilization at 198 ms and progressive prolongation in the H-V until the fourth paced complex fails to conduct beyond the His to reach the ventricles. The prolonged but stable A-H interval of 198 ms signifies atrioventricular conduction disease, but the Wenckebach pattern of conduction and block below the His implies significant distal conduction system disease as well

posteroseptal accessory pathway; retrograde activation earliest at the distal CS would suggest presence of a left free-wall accessory pathway or left-sided AVN;[24] and retrograde activation that is earliest at the HRA would suggest presence of a right free-wall accessory pathway.

Retrograde conduction refractory periods of HPS, AV node and accessory pathways may be determined through the use of ventricular premature extrastimuli. It is once again identified as the longest ventricular S1-S2 that fails to conduct beyond His or to the atria and is analogous to the anterograde refractory

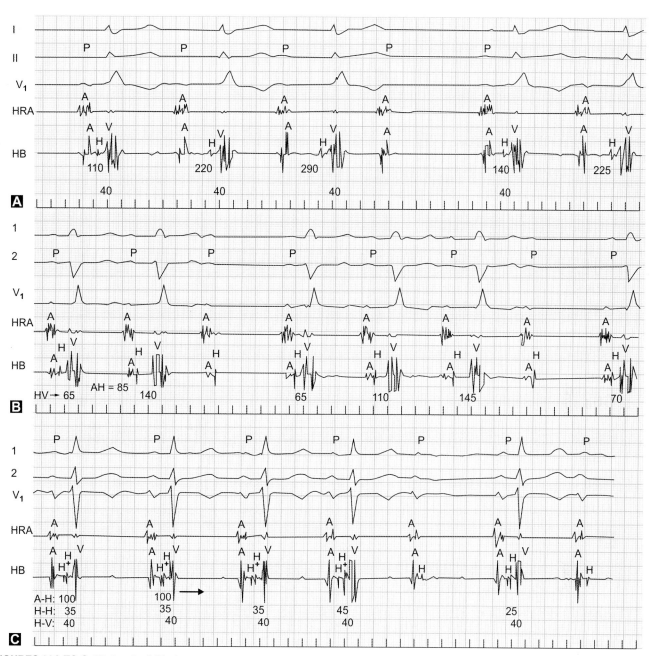

FIGURES 20A TO C: His bundle (HB) electrograms in atrioventricular (AV) block. The tracings are from three different patients with second-degree AV block. In Figures A and B, the conducted QRS complexes are wide and associated with bundle branch block. (A) The block is within the AV node (i.e. the A-wave on the HB is not followed by an HB deflection). (B) It can be appreciated that the block is distal to the HB even though the surface electrocardiogram (ECG) demonstrates a Wenckebach phenomenon. The latter can obviously occur in the His-Purkinje system as well, as depicted in this figure. (C) The site of the block is within the HB. This is suggested by split HB potentials (labeled H and H⁺), and the block is distal to the H but proximal to the H⁺. Intra-His block is difficult to diagnose from the surface ECG but can be suspected when a Mobitz type II occurs in association with a normal P-R interval and a narrow QRS complex. (*Source:* Modified from Akhtar M. Invasive cardiac electrophysiologic studies: an introduction. In: Parmley WW, Chatterjee K (Eds). Cardiology: Physiology, Pharmacology, Diagnosis. Philadelphia: Lippincott; 1991. With permission from Lippincott, Williams and Wilkins)

periods. Ventricular extrastimuli are also of use in assessing ventricular refractoriness and for arrhythmia induction, whether supraventricular or ventricular. Multiple extrastimuli are important for induction protocols when assessing tendency toward arrhythmia, particularly wide QRS tachycardia, which may occur due to a variety of electrophysiologic mechanisms, both from supraventricular and ventricular origins (Figs 23A to D).[25] The underlying nature of the wide QRS tachycardia is critical for both prognosis and therapy, and EP studies have

proven invaluable for distinguishing the various etiologies. With few exceptions, when the nature of the arrhythmic problem is not known and the direction of therapy is not clear, patients with wide QRS tachycardia should undergo EP study. This is particularly true in situations where nonpharmacologic therapy is the desired goal.[11]

In patients with features suggesting high risk of sudden death, such as structural heart disease and LV dysfunction as well as evidence of ventricular ectopy or arrhythmia in this

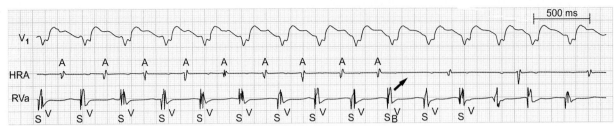

FIGURE 21: Retrograde conduction block. Continuous ventricular pacing (S) with gradual decrementation in cycle length results in 1:1 ventricular capture (V) and conduction to the atria (A) with progressive prolongation in V-A time until the 10th paced complex (S$_B$V) fails to conduct to the atrium and a 2:1 retrograde conduction pattern is established

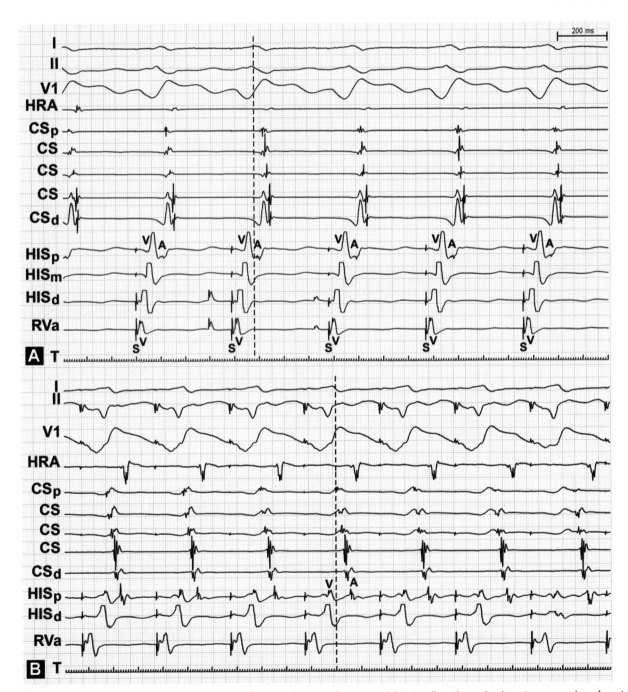

FIGURES 22A AND B: Retrograde conduction patterns. Surface electrocardiogram and intracardiac channels show two examples of ventricular pacing resulting in 1:1 myocardial capture and conduction to the atria over different pathways. (A) Retrograde atrial activation is earliest at the proximal His (A) followed by coronary sinus (CS) activation from proximal to distal, suggesting retrograde conduction over an anteriorly located pathway, i.e. the atrioventricular node (AVN) fast pathway. (B) Retrograde atrial activation is earliest in the proximal CS and later in the His (A), suggesting retrograde conduction over a posteriorly located pathway, i.e. AVN slow pathway or posteroseptal accessory pathway. Dashed lines identify earliest atrial activation. (Abbreviations: V: Ventricular electrogram; S: Stimulus artifact)

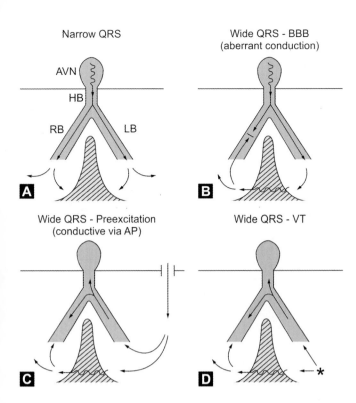

FIGURES 23A TO D: Wide QRS tachycardia mechanisms. Routes of impulse propagation during a wide QRS tachycardia in various settings are depicted. It should be noted that only in A and B, His bundle activation expected to precede ventricular activation. This helps the delineation from other causes of wide QRS tachycardia, shown in C and D. (Abbreviations: AP: Accessory pathway; BBB: Bundle branch block; VT: Ventricular tachycardia). (*Source:* Modified with permission from Akhtar M. Techniques of electrophysiologic evaluation. In: Fuster V, O'Rourke RA, Walsh RA, Poole-Wilson P (Eds). Hurst's The Heart, 12th edition. New York: The McGraw-Hill Companies, Inc.; 2007. With permission from The McGraw-Hill Companies, Inc.)

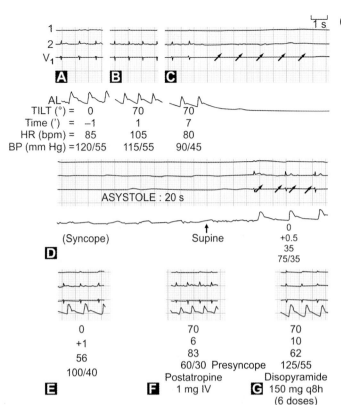

FIGURES 24A TO G: Asystole in neurocardiogenic syncope. Note the normal heart rate (HR) and blood pressure (BP) in supine position. At the beginning of head-up tilt at 70 degrees (B), some degree of tachycardia is noted. Seven minutes after the onset of tilt (C), an episode of atrioventricular block occurs and is followed by sinus arrest and a total asystole of 20 seconds. Syncopal episodes follow. Presyncope is still present when asystole is prevented by atropine (F). Findings in C might tempt one to prescribe permanent pacing, an inappropriate choice of therapy. In this patient with neurocardiogenic syncope, disopyramide (G) prevented hypotension and syncope without the need for a permanent pacemaker. (*Source:* Modified from Sra JS, Jazayeri MR, Avitall B, et al. Comparison of cardiac pacing with drug therapy in the treatment of neurocardiogenic (vasovagal) syncope with bradycardia or asystole. N Engl J Med. 1993;328:1085-90. With permission from Massachusetts Medical Society)

setting, utilization of multiple extrastimuli (maximum 3), including short-long-short sequences, from multiple ventricular sites in the baseline state and under pharmacologic stress or stimulation is necessary. The induction of monomorphic VT is a specific response reflecting tendency of the myocardial substrate to support this type of arrhythmia and clinically appropriate therapy should be rendered accordingly. Alternately, the induction of polymorphic VT can be a nonspecific response in patients without structural heart disease, when triple extrastimuli at short coupling intervals are utilized; hence, the delivery of additional ventricular extrastimuli should be weighed carefully against the risk of a nonspecific finding.[11]

Role of Electrophysiology Study in Evaluation of Unexplained Syncope

While neurocardiogenic mechanisms constitute the most common causes of syncope in patients with ostensibly normal hearts and should be evaluated through tilt testing (Figs 24A to G),[22,23,25,26] EP study is integral in evaluating patients with syncope that remains unexplained, particularly those with heart disease.[27] During such studies, all arrhythmic possibilities, such as sinus node dysfunction, AV conduction abnormalities, SVT and VT, should be excluded. Patients with underlying structural heart disease, such as old myocardial infarction, primary myocardial disease or poor LV function, generally have underlying VT to explain syncope (Figs 25A and B). When arrhythmias occur in patients without overt structural heart disease, sinus node dysfunction, AV block (particularly intra-Hisian block) or SVT may be more likely. Less frequently, VT can occur in the absence of an overt structural heart disease.[11]

SURVIVORS OF SUDDEN CARDIAC ARREST

In many patients with documented episodes of cardiac arrest from the onset, VF can be documented as the initial cause. Patients dying suddenly often have underlying structural heart disease (usually coronary artery disease or primary myocardial disease) and are prone to VT/VF due to electrical instability. It seems prudent to investigate both the nature and extent of organic heart disease and also to assess vulnerability to recurrent VT/VF. At present, EP study is considered a routine part of the overall patient assessment in this group of individuals.[11,28,29]

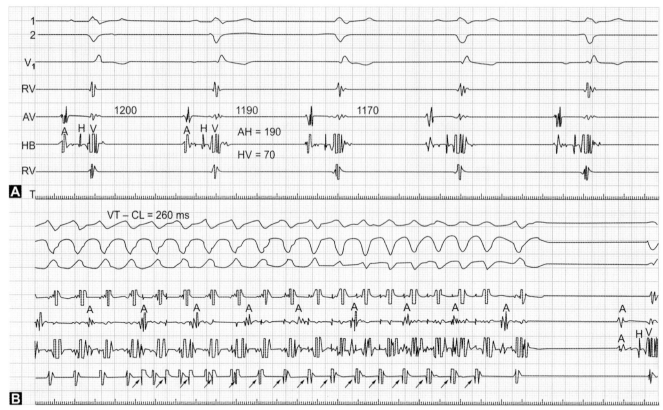

FIGURES 25A AND B: Arrhythmic causes of syncope. (A) Sinus rhythm in a patient with unexplained syncope. Sinus bradycardia, bifascicular block, and a long P-R interval from surface electrocardiogram suggest possible conduction system disease etiology. (B) In this patient, however, ventricular tachycardia was inducible with ventricular extrastimulation and was the actual cause of syncope. Control of ventricular tachycardia (VT) without a pacemaker was sufficient to prevent syncope in this patient. Termination of tachycardia and restoration of sinus rhythm are shown in Figure B. (Abbreviation: CL: Cycle length). (*Source:* Modified from Akhtar M. Techniques of electrophysiologic evaluation. In: Fuster V, O'Rourke RA, Walsh RA, Poole-Wilson P (Eds). Hurst's The Heart, 12th edition. New York: The McGraw-Hill Companies Inc.; 2007. With permission from The McGraw-Hill Companies Inc.)

In survivors of VT/VF, EP study is desirable for a variety of reasons:

- In our experience, almost 40% of patients with monomorphic VT in association with idiopathic dilated cardiomyopathy and valvular heart disease have bundle branch reentry (BBR) as the underlying mechanism (Fig. 26). We feel this arrhythmia is preferably managed with bundle branch ablation, which is curative, rather than with an implantable cardioverter-defibrillator (ICD) alone.
- Several VT morphologies or other arrhythmias may be identified in addition to the presenting/clinical VT. Lack of awareness of such arrhythmias may complicate patient management. For example, rapid SVT may require separate attention to prevent unnecessary ICD shocks, either through antiarrhythmic therapy or by ablation. The coexistence of sick sinus or conduction system disease may be aggravated by antiarrhythmic therapy and necessitate pacing. Identification preoperatively could contribute to appropriate device selection.
- Rarely, supraventricular arrhythmia may trigger VT/VF. This may happen in patients with severe coronary artery disease, congestive heart failure or Wolff-Parkinson-White syndrome to name a few scenarios. Elimination of the underlying triggers should be the primary therapeutic approach with the need for an ICD, a secondary concern.

Cardioactive Agents

The invasive EP study often incorporates a phase in which observation and programed stimulation is conducted under pharmacologic influence in an attempt to facilitate arrhythmia induction. Two agents are commonly employed, isoproterenol and procainamide.

Isoproterenol is a sympathomimetic amine with primary activity on beta-adrenergic receptors type 1 and type 2. Its overall effects are to increase inotropic and chronotropic response as well as improve conduction system and myocardial propagation. Usually a dose of 1–3 mcg/min is adequate to achieve at least a 20–25% increase in sinus rate in normal patients. Its role during EP study is primarily threefold:

1. Evaluation of chronotropic response;
2. Assessment of AV conduction; and
3. Facilitation of arrhythmia induction.

In patients being evaluated for sinus node dysfunction, in addition to SNRT and SACT evaluation, a blunted response to catecholamine stimulation correlates with impaired chronotropic response during exercise testing in patients with sinus node dysfunction. As mentioned previously, AV conduction with Wenckebach at cycle lengths greater than 600 ms should be considered unusual, but may be seen in patients with high vagal tone. However, this finding should not be considered abnormal in isolation, and only if a lack of

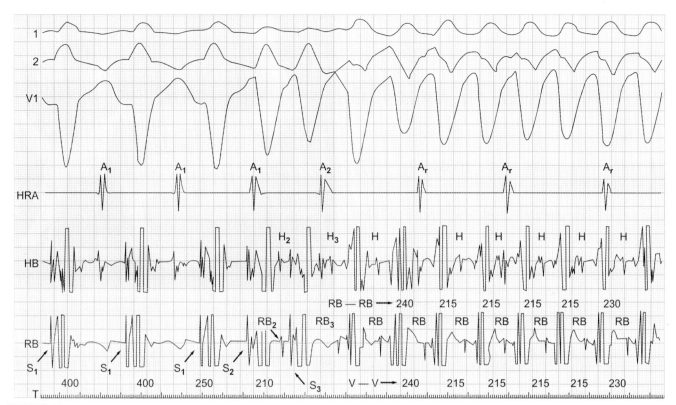

FIGURE 26: Induction of sustained ventricular tachycardia due to bundle branch reentry (BBR). The surface electrocardiogram and intracardiac tracings are labeled. Basic cycle length (S_1S_1) is 400 ms during ventricular pacing. Sustained BBR is induced with two extrastimuli (S_2S_3). Note that the His bundle and right bundle (RB) deflections precede the QRS, suggesting supraventricular tachycardia with aberrant conduction. However, there is 2:1 ventriculoatrial (VA) block, indicating the ventricular nature of this tachycardia. Without His bundle/right bundle (HB/RB) recordings, the diagnosis can be difficult and, consequently, the likelihood of inappropriate therapy will be high. RB-RB and V-V (ventricular) intervals are labeled. (*Source:* Modified from Caceres J, Jazayeri M, McKinnie J, et al. Sustained bundle branch reentry as a mechanism of clinical tachycardia. Circulation. 1989;79:256-70. With permission from Wolters Kluwer Health)

improvement with adrenergic stimulation is demonstrated should pathology be suspected. Isoproterenol infusion aids such evaluation in that it can improve both AVN and HPS conduction. In addition to assessment of sinus node automaticity and AV conduction, isoproterenol facilitates arrhythmia induction and sustainability both through modulation of AVN and accessory pathway conduction; and by provoking myocardial refractory period shortening that permits shorter coupling during atrial and ventricular premature extrastimulation to enhance tissue conduction delay, thereby promoting reentry. A pronounced benefit of isoproterenol is seen in patients with structurally normal hearts and idiopathic VT, in whom rapid atrial pacing and isoproterenol facilitates induction of triggered activity.[30] Finally, isoproterenol can reverse antiarrhythmic effects, primarily through its actions on ion channels. Therefore, efficacy of antiarrhythmic therapy is also an important contribution of isoproterenol to the EP study.

Procainamide is a class IA antiarrhythmic drug with primary effects in blocking sodium channels. It increases tissue refractoriness and slows conduction in the atria, HPS and ventricles, with variable effects on the AV node.[31,32] Its primary role in the clinical EP study is to assess propensity toward AV conduction block and VT induction. In patients with normal HPS conduction, procainamide may introduce mild conduction delay. However, in patients with moderate conduction disease,

manifested by H-V intervals greater than 65 ms, a dose of 10 mg/kg can unmask a profound tendency toward conduction block. If the H-V prolongs beyond 100 ms, this is an indication for permanent pacing. As stated, conduction slowing is an anticipated effect of procainamide therapy and hence is the primary mechanism of its antiarrhythmic qualities in acute VT suppression. However, conduction slowing can also promote reentry, particularly in patients with structural heart disease. Hence, it is employed during EP study to evaluate VT inducibility but also explains why class I antiarrhythmics are contraindicated for long-term maintenance therapy in patients with structural heart disease.

CARDIAC ELECTROPHYSIOLOGY STUDY FOR EVALUATION OF DRUG THERAPY

In patients with relatively benign cardiac arrhythmias, EP testing to assess efficacy of pharmacologic therapy is unnecessary in most situations, and clinical course can be observed to determine whether control has been achieved. Also, in patients with ICDs, antiarrhythmic therapy can be assessed clinically as the device will record and treat events according to its specific programing. However, for patients with potentially life-threatening tachycardias like VT or with severe manifestations of cardiac arrhythmias, such as syncope or presyncope, in whom device therapy is not present, it is desirable to assess efficacy of pharmacologic intervention. A technique of drug testing has been developed whereby the elimination of inducibility of a given tachycardia is assessed following a drug administration. If drug therapy eliminates induction, addition of isoproterenol may demonstrate reversal of therapeutic drug effect.[33] This is helpful in considering additional or alternative therapy. Failure of serial drug testing is associated with a significant recurrence rate and is a strong indication for nonpharmacologic intervention.[11]

ELECTROPHYSIOLOGY STUDY TO GUIDE ABLATIVE THERAPY

ROLE OF THREE-DIMENSIONAL MAPPING SYSTEMS

Treatment of cardiac arrhythmias is dictated by various factors impacting risk related to therapy including potential adverse effects, tolerance of the patient to specific treatment and anticipated likelihood of long-term success. One modality employed for arrhythmia diagnosis and treatment is catheter ablation, through which sites involved in arrhythmia genesis and maintenance are mapped and targeted for local tissue destruction via a percutaneous catheter-based procedure. Identification of specific location(s) that initiate or maintain arrhythmia is challenging for a variety of reasons, but particularly so due to difficulty in returning the catheter to a particular location with any measure of precision and accuracy, given the various cardiac and respiratory motions that impact how catheters and the heart interface, as well as the ambiguity of depth perception on two-dimensional (2D) fluoroscopy.

Three-dimensional (3D) electroanatomic mapping systems are an integral tool in interventional EP as they provide a manner to visualize inside of the heart and reliably guide catheters to specific locations that would otherwise prove challenging with 2D fluoroscopy alone.[34,35] These systems have two important capabilities: (1) creating and visualizing endocardial geometry as a 3D model and (2) superimposing timing and voltage information to create "maps" that visually indicate whether a particular region is activated earlier or later than others, and if a particular region is healthy or scarred according to the amplitude of the local EGM (Supplemental Video 1). These color-coded maps are displayed with a virtual rendition of the mapping catheter, so as to convey visually the relationship of the catheter to the surrounding myocardial chamber—a relationship that is often ambiguous on fluoroscopy. These systems are able to achieve a fairly high level of precision and can annotate catheter tip locations in the 3D model to provide targets for navigation and provide a "history" of previous sites mapped. However, as the true 3D anatomical position of the virtual catheter is not known to the system—only the relative position of the catheter within the mapping system's 3D coordinate space is known—accuracy is compromised. To address this, these systems can import an actual 3D anatomic volume, such as a computed tomography (CT) scan or magnetic resonance image (MRI), of a particular cardiac chamber to define the anatomic coordinate system.[36] The anatomic volume can be aligned and rotated to best approximate the orientation of 3D map, which is then superimposed (Fig. 27). This process of "registering" the volume and map permits better anatomical

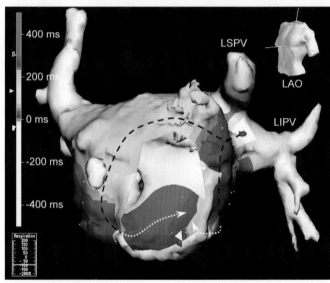

FIGURE 27: Left atrial (LA) computed tomography (CT) with 3D electroanatomic map (LAO projection). Electroanatomic mapping data is superimposed on a 3D LA geometry and then registered with a CT of the LA and pulmonary veins (PVs) to convey activation timing. Activation with respect to a timing reference is depicted according to the color scale (left). The mitral valve annulus is demarcated by a green perimeter. Earliest activation, displayed in white, is seen arising from between the left superior and inferior PVs, and then propagates (red to orange to yellow, etc. according to color scale) counterclockwise and clockwise around the mitral valve annulus (black dashed lines). The two wavefronts pass posteriorly (white dashed arrow) and meet (seen by looking through the mitral valve annulus into the LA) where crowding of isochrones suggests conduction block, in this case, between the mitral valve annulus and the inferior aspect of the inferior pulmonary vein, i.e. across the posterior mitral isthmus

localization by comparing the created 3D map to the known anatomy to verify that all areas have been accounted for and to identify true location of the catheter and its relationship to sometimes highly important and sensitive structures, such as pulmonary veins for AF ablation.[37] Whether a mapping system is used with or without a 3D volume, the images are displayed on a separate view from live fluoroscopy, requiring the operator to incorporate information from both image sources and perform a mental real-time registration of these images. The latest commercial fluoroscopy systems have the capability to register a 3D volume directly with live fluoroscopy so true catheter location can be visualized within a registered anatomic model[38] (Fig. 28). The registered volumetric and fluoroscopic image can then be compared to the image of the 3D map, which may also be registered to the 3D volume. In an effort to achieve both accuracy and precision, this method still requires operator to assimilate information from multiple image sources. The systems that register various imaging modalities with live fluoroscopy must also overcome the challenges posed by cardiac and respiratory motion evident on live fluoroscopy but not accounted for by the static anatomic and virtual models. Techniques to compensate for this motion, cardiac and respiratory "gating,"[39] permit a method of continuous and real-time registration between the live fluoroscopy and the 3D model. Incorporating voltage and timing maps directly into the CT or MRI volumes that are registered to fluoroscopy would provide a means to

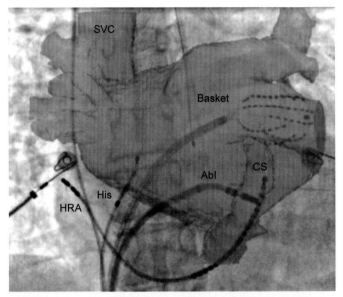

FIGURE 28: Live fluoroscopy with overlay of registered left atrial (LA) computed tomography (CT). An anteroposterior projection of live fluoroscopy shows multiple catheters including a multielectrode basket catheter and ablation catheter positioned through transseptal sheaths into the LA. The LA CT reconstruction is registered with fluoroscopy to demonstrate specific anatomy and catheter locations. The basket catheter is positioned in the left inferior pulmonary vein and the ablation catheter is positioned at the mitral valve annulus and, hence, appears in close proximity to the duodecapolar catheter within the coronary sinus (CS). The CT is depicted in posteroanterior projection in order for anatomical alignment between the two modalities. (Abbreviations: Abl: Ablation catheter; HRA: High right atrium; SVC: Superior vena cava)

unite all these imaging modalities and technologies into a single system.

COMPLICATIONS

The contemporary EP study is safe when performed in appropriate facilities by trained physicians and personnel. Although patient factors, such as age, anatomy and associated comorbidities, must be considered in individualizing procedural risk, the major complication rate is approximately 1% and for death is 1:1,000. The complications are the same as those anticipated with other forms of cardiac catheterization as well some more particular to the EP study. These include inadequate hemostasis with or without vascular injury including local bleeding from access sites with adjacent extension, hematoma, AV fistula, pseudoaneurysm and major vessel perforation; vascular and intracardiac thrombosis with or without pulmonary or systemic embolism including stroke; cardiac injury including myocardial infarction, coronary artery and CS dissection, and myocardial perforation and associated pericardial effusion with or without cardiac tamponade; tachyarrhythmias and bradyarrhythmias and injury to the conduction system rarely necessitating permanent pacing; esophageal injury and pulmonary vein stenosis in left atrial ablation; skin injuries associated with direct cardioversion and radiation/fluoroscopy exposure; phrenic nerve injury and paralysis; decompensated heart failure; infection; and allergic reactions primarily to administered agents such as iodine, anesthetics, antibiotics, blood products and protamine.

CONCLUSION

It remains a truism that the past offers insight into the present and future. The historical discoveries that have coalesced into the field of clinical cardiac EP are truly awesome and compel one to take pause and reflect on the origins of this burgeoning field. Cardiologists of the 21st century must still see in the electrocardiogram all the electrical processes and associated physical manifestations underlying cardiac EP described over the past 100 years to fully appreciate normal processes and cardiovascular pathology. These fundamental principles, outlined here, form a clinical foundation for every student of the medical arts who is interested and invested in cardiovascular diseases to begin to comprehend the most fundamental of physiologic questions, "Why does the heart beat?"

ACKNOWLEDGMENTS

The authors gratefully acknowledge the assistance of Brian Miller and Brian Schurrer in the preparation of illustrations and Barbara Danek, Joe Grundle and Katie Klein in editing the manuscript.

VIDEO LEGEND

Electroanatomic mapping of VT substrate. Point-by-point mapping of the left ventricle was performed in sinus rhythm to create a "scar map." Tissue zones are depicted through the color scheme: red—dense scar; purple—healthy myocardium; colored "infarct border zone" separates red and purple regions. The specific color scheme is determined by the voltage window shown at right. In this case dense scar is defined as tissue producing EGM amplitudes less than 0.52 mV and healthy myocardium is defined as tissue producing EGM amplitude more than 1.50 mV. EGM amplitudes between 0.52 mV and 1.50 mV then define the border zone. The left ventricle is shown in anteroposterior view with apex to the right and base to the left. The geometry is rotated to demonstrate the distribution of healthy tissue, seen involving most of the LV, and scar involving the basal septum and small portions of the lateral wall and apex. After one revolution, the LV geometry is tilted upward to show the inferior wall. The blue sphere locates the presumed VT exit site and the red spheres annotate ablation lesions that connect the exit site with the mitral valve annulus to prevent reentry. (Abbreviations: EGM: Electrogram; LV: Left ventricle; VT: Ventricular tachycardia)

REFERENCES

1. John HJ. Jan Evangelista Purkyně: Czech Scientist and Patriot, 1787-1869. Philadelphia: American Philosophical Society; 1959.
2. His W Jr. Die Thätigkeit des embryonalen Herzens und deren Bedeutung für die Lehre von der Herzbewegung beim Erwachsenen. Arb Med Klinik Leipzig. 1893;1:14-50.
3. Kent AF. Researches on the structure and function of the mammalian heart. J Physiol. 1893;14:i2-254.
4. Tawara S. Eine anatomisch-histologische studie über das atrio-ventrikular bündel und die Purkinjeschen fäden. Das Reizleitungssystem des Säugetierherzens. Jena, Germany: Verlag von Gustav Fischer; 1906. p. 200.

5. Keith A, Flack M. The form and nature of the muscular connections between the primary divisions of the vertebrate heart. J Anat Physiol. 1907;41:172-89.

6. Einthoven W. Weiteres über das elektrokardiogram. Pflüger Arch ges Physiol. 1908;122:517-48.

7. Dock W. Transitory ventricular fibrillation as a cause of syncope and its prevention by quinidine sulfate. Am Heart J. 1929;4:709-14.

8. Jervell A, Lange-Nielsen F. Congenital deaf-mutism, functional heart disease with prolongation of the Q-T interval and sudden death. Am Heart J. 1957;54:59-68.

9. Scherlag BJ, Lau SH, Helfant RH, et al. Catheter technique for recording His bundle activity in man. Circulation. 1969;39:13-8.

10. Scheinman MM, Morady F, Hess DS, et al. Catheter-induced ablation of the atrioventricular junction to control refractory supraventricular arrhythmias. JAMA. 1982;248:851-5.

11. Akhtar M. Techniques of electrophysiologic evaluation. In: Fuster V, O'Rourke R, Walsh R, Poole-Wilson P (Eds). Hurst's The Heart, 12th edition. New York: The McGraw-Hill Companies; 2008. pp. 1064-76.

12. Guidelines for Clinical Intracardiac Electrophysiological and Catheter Ablation Procedures. A report of the American College of Cardiology/American Heart Association Task Force on practice guidelines. (Committee on Clinical Intracardiac Electrophysiologic and Catheter Ablation Procedures), Developed in collaboration with the North American Society of Pacing and Electrophysiology. Circulation. 1995;92:673-91.

13. Buxton AE, Calkins H, Callans DJ, et al. ACC/AHA/HRS 2006 key data elements and definitions for electrophysiological studies and procedures: a report of the American College of Cardiology/American Heart Association Task Force on Clinical Data Standards (ACC/AHA/HRS Writing Committee to Develop Data Standards on Electrophysiology). J Am Coll Cardiol. 2006;48:2360-96.

14. Akhtar M, Mahmud R, Tchou P, et al. Normal electrophysiologic responses of the human heart. Cardiol Clin. 1986;4(3):365-86.

15. Lemery R, Birnie D, Tang AS, et al. Normal atrial activation and voltage during sinus rhythm in the human heart: an endocardial and epicardial mapping study in patients with a history of atrial fibrillation. J Cardiovasc Electrophysiol. 2007;18:402-8.

16. Durrer D, van Dam RT, Freud GE, et al. Total excitation of the isolated human heart. Circulation 1970;41:899-912.

17. Becker AE. Left atrial isthmus: anatomic aspects relevant for linear catheter ablation procedures in human. J Cardiovasc Electrophysiol. 2004;15:809-12.

18. Josephson ME. Clinical Cardiac Electrophysiology: Techniques and Interpretations, 4th edition. Philadelphia: Lippincott Williams and Wilkins; 2008. pp. 39-47.

19. Denker S, Lehmann MH, Mahmud R, et al. Divergence between refractoriness of His-Purkinje system and ventricular muscle with abrupt changes in cycle length. Circulation. 1983;68:1212-21.

20. Denes P. The effect of cycle length on the atrial refractory period. Pacing Clin Electrophysiol. 1984;7:1108-14.

21. Narula OS, Scherlag BJ, Samet P, et al. Atrioventricular block. Localization and classification by His bundle recordings. Am J Med. 1971;50:146-65.

22. Sra JS, Jazayeri MR, Avitall B, et al. Comparison of cardiac pacing with drug therapy in the treatment of neurocardiogenic (vasovagal) syncope with bradycardia or asystole. N Engl J Med. 1993;328:1085-90.

23. Dhingra RC, Wyndham C, Bauernfeind R, et al. Significance of block distal to the His bundle induced by atrial pacing in patients with chronic bifascicular block. Circulation. 1979;60:1455-64.

24. Nakagawa H, Jackman WM. Catheter ablation of paroxysmal supraventricular tachycardia. Circulation. 2007;116:2465-78.

25. Akhtar M, Jazayeri M, Avitall B, et al. Electrophysiologic spectrum of wide QRS complex tachycardia. In: Zipes DP, Jalife J (Eds). Cardiac Electrophysiology: From Cell to Bedside. Orlando: WB Saunders; 1990. p. 635.

26. Sra JS, Anderson AJ, Sheikh SH, et al. Unexplained syncope evaluated by electrophysiologic studies and head-up tilt testing. Ann Intern Med. 1991;114:1013-9.

27. Strickberger SA, Benson DW, Biaggioni I, et al. AHA/ACCF scientific statement on the evaluation of syncope: from the American Heart Association Councils on Clinical Cardiology, Cardiovascular Nursing, Cardiovascular Disease in the Young, and Stroke, and the Quality of Care and Outcomes Research Interdisciplinary Working Group; and the American College of Cardiology Foundation: in collaboration with the Heart Rhythm Society: endorsed by the American Autonomic Society. Circulation. 2006;113:316-27.

28. Akhtar M, Garan H, Lehmann MH, et al. Sudden cardiac death: management of high-risk patients. Ann Intern Med. 1991;114:499-512.

29. Morady F, Scheinman MM, Hess DS, et al. Electrophysiologic testing in the management of survivors of out-of-hospital cardiac arrest. Am J Cardiol. 1983;51:85-9.

30. Lerman BB, Stein K, Engelstein ED, et al. Mechanism of repetitive monomorphic ventricular tachycardia. Circulation. 1995;92:421-9.

31. Pronestyl injection package insert (Princeton Pharmaceutical—US), Rev 8/91, Rec 2/93.

32. Coyle JD, Lima JJ. Procainamide. In: Evans WE, Schentag JJ, Jusko WJ (Eds). Applied Pharmacokinetics: Principles of Therapeutic Drug Monitoring, 3rd edition. Vancouver: Applied Therapeutics; 1992. pp. 1-33.

33. Jazayeri MR, Van Wyhe G, Avitall B, et al. Isoproterenol reversal of antiarrhythmic effects in patients with inducible sustained ventricular tachyarrhythmias. J Am Coll Cardiol. 1989;14:705-11.

34. Gepstein L, Hayam G, Ben-Haim SA. A novel method for nonfluoroscopic catheter-based electroanatomical mapping of the heart. Circulation. 1997;95:1611-22.

35. Sra J, Thomas JM. New techniques for mapping cardiac arrhythmias. Indian Heart J. 2001;53:423-44.

36. Dong J, Calkins H, Solomon SB, et al. Integrated electroanatomic mapping with three-dimensional computed tomographic images for real-time guided ablations. Circulation. 2006;113:186-94.

37. Sra J. Cardiac image registration. J Atr Fibrillation. 2008;1:145-60.

38. Sra J, Krum D, Malloy A, et al. Registration of three-dimensional left atrial computed tomographic images with projection images obtained using fluoroscopy. Circulation. 2005;112:3763-8.

39. Sra J, Ratnakumar S. Cardiac image registration of the left atrium and pulmonary veins. Heart Rhythm. 2008;5:609-17.

SECTION 4

Electrophysiology

Syncope

Vijay Ramu, Fred Kusumoto, Nora Goldschlager

Chapter Outline

INTRODUCTION

Syncope is a sudden and transient loss of consciousness associated with loss of postural tone, followed by complete and spontaneous recovery. The term "syncope" originates from the Greek word "Synkoptein" which means—cutting short (koptein-"to cut"). In the first six centuries, many Greek philosophers and physicians speculated on the causes of syncope. Claudius Galen, a famous Greek physician, suggested that syncope was a problem of both the stomach and the heart.[1] The mechanism for transient loss of consciousness associated with syncope is cerebral hypoperfusion with reduced blood flow to the reticular activating system. A common phrase used in clinical medicine is presyncope which is considered to represent a warning or prodrome for frank syncope. In the case of presyncope, symptoms, such as dizziness and graying out, are not followed by frank loss of consciousness. Many physicians evaluate and treat presyncope in a similar manner to syncope; although a reasonable approach, there is no strong clinical data to support similar etiologies and outcomes.

It is important to acknowledge that the definition of syncope (and thus etiologic classification) varies even among experts. Using a more general definition of transient loss of consciousness, some experts include neurologic (e.g. seizure and concussion), metabolic (e.g. hypoxia) and psychiatric conditions as forms of syncope, while others who emphasize cerebral hypoperfusion consider syncope as one of the several causes of transient loss of consciousness and classify some

neurologic, metabolic and psychiatric mechanisms as separate entities (Flow chart 1).[2,3] Using this more restrictive definition of syncope, the three most important causes of transient loss of consciousness are: (1) syncope; (2) seizure and (3) psychogenic blackouts. Other rare causes include metabolic disorders, such as hypoglycemia or hypoxia, intoxication, and psychiatric problems such as cataplexy or pseudosyncope. Determining the correct cause of syncope is the key to approaching therapy, if the initial working clinical diagnosis is erroneous, subsequent investigations and even the final diagnosis and treatment may also be incorrect.[4] Regardless of definition, syncope may represent a harbinger for sudden death, and often the diagnostic evaluation focuses on identifying or ruling out potential life-threatening causes of syncope such as ventricular arrhythmias or aortic stenosis. For this reason, the diagnostic workup for the patient with syncope revolves around two different but related issues: (1) identification of the specific mechanism for syncope and (2) risk stratification to estimate short-term and long-term risk of adverse outcomes. It is important for the clinician to remember that the diagnostic workup of syncope requires a patient-specific approach and diagnostic tests must carefully be chosen. Several medical societies including the European Society of Cardiology (ESC) and the American Heart Association/American College of Cardiology Foundation (AHA/ACCF) have provided comprehensive guidelines or scientific statements for the diagnosis and management of syncope, although some aspects are not without controversy.[2-5]

FLOW CHART 1: Classification of mechanistic causes for transient loss of consciousness and syncope

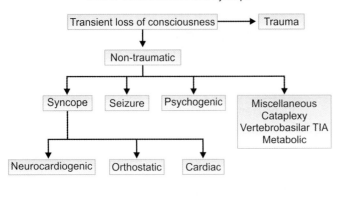

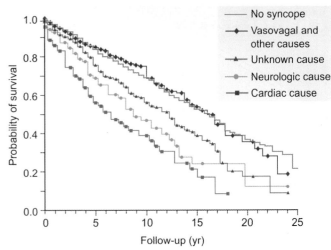

FIGURE 1: Survival curves from Framingham data for patients with different types of syncope. (*Source:* Soteriades ES, Evans JC, Larson MG, et al. Incidence and prognosis of syncope. N Engl J Med. 2002;347: 878-85)

EPIDEMIOLOGY

INCIDENCE AND PREVALENCE OF SYNCOPE

Several studies have attempted to evaluate the incidence and prevalence of syncope. Obtaining accurate figures is difficult, since it has been estimated that only 25–50% of syncopal episodes are reported to medical professionals and only 2–5% of episodes are evaluated in emergency department settings.[2] In the most recent report from the Framingham study, the incidence of a first report of syncope was 6.2/1000 person-years follow-up and a ten-year cumulative incidence of 6%.[6] In addition, a sharp increase in the incidence of syncope after age 70 years, particularly in the presence of cardiovascular disease, was reported. Several studies suggest that syncope is quite common in younger populations.[7-9] For example, in a cohort of 62 medical students, 32% reported a prior episode of syncope, with a higher rate in women than in men (42% and 31% respectively).[9] Collectively, the data suggest a bimodal distribution of a first episode of syncope, with a first peak between the first and the second decade (with a female predominance) and another peak that begins after the age of 60 years and is gender-independent.[2] To summarize, up to approximately 30–40% of people will have an episode of syncope during their lifetime, and of these 30–40% will have a recurrent episode within three years.[1-9]

Although syncope may be the first symptom for a patient at high risk for sudden death and adverse clinical outcomes, examination of cohort studies suggests that the mortality rate ranges from 1–2% at 30 days to 7–8% at one year.[6,10] Examination of large hospital databases suggests that in-hospital mortality for syncope is also low (0.28%) with almost all deaths occurring in patients over 60 years of age.[8] However, in the Framingham report, patients who were thought to have a cardiac cause of syncope had a six month mortality rate of 10%.[6] The additional risk conferred simply by the presence of syncope is controversial and has varied from no additional risk to a 30% increase in risk in cohort studies using matched controls.[6,11] For example, Kapoor and his colleagues found that mortality was the same in patients with or without syncope and was instead dependent on the presence and type of underlying cardiac disease and other comorbidities.[11] In contrast, in a population based study from the Framingham data, syncope was associated with a 30% increase in mortality compared to patients without syncope (Fig. 1).[6]

ECONOMIC BURDEN OF SYNCOPE

It has been estimated that syncope accounts for 1–3% of emergency department evaluations and 1–6% of hospital admissions.[12,13] Several studies have estimated that the annual cost of management and treatment of patients with syncope ranges 1.7–2.4 billion dollars in the United States.[8,14] The cost for the management of patients with syncope varies widely, dependent on the diagnostic tests ordered and whether or not an implantable cardiac rhythm device (pacemaker or ICD) is used.[8] In addition to the cost of diagnostic evaluation and specific therapies, syncope can be associated with injuries and significant psychological disability that can increase cost and have a significant impact on quality-of-life.[15-17] Major injuries, such as fractures and motor vehicle accidents were reported in about 6% of patients.[15] Minor injuries including bruises and lacerations were reported in 27–29% of patients with syncope.[15] Elderly patients have a higher incidence of injuries when compared to younger patients, with a dramatic increase after age of 70 years, the incidence almost doubles between the sixth and the seventh decades of life.[15-17] Syncope is associated with a significant reduction in quality-of-life indices, particularly in the presence of recurrent episodes, associated comorbidities and in women.[15-17]

CAUSES AND CLASSIFICATION OF SYNCOPE

As discussed earlier, syncope is but one cause of transient loss of consciousness. Syncope can further be classified into three general causes: (1) reflex or neurally mediated syncope; (2) syncope due to orthostatic hypotension and (3) cardiac syncope (Flow chart 1).

Reflex or neurally mediated syncope is the most common cause of syncope. One form, often called vasovagal syncope or the "common faint", is the single most common cause of syncope. The pathophysiological basis for vasovagal syncope was described by Sir Thomas Lewis in the early 1900s and importantly noted that although the bradycardia component could be reversed by atropine, hypotension and altered state of consciousness persisted. Although vasovagal syncope is the most common cause of syncope in younger patients, accounting for up to 50% of cases, it is important to recognize that even in patients more than 65 years old vasovagal syncope accounts for approximately 30% of cases. In all forms of reflex syncope, triggering of the afferent limb of a reflex arc leads to hypotension due to vasodilation (vasodepressor effect) and decreased heart rate (vagal effect). In vasovagal syncope the afferent limb can be triggered by a variety of conditions such as heat, hypovolemia, pain, or fear and anxiety while in conditions often called—situational syncope, triggering occurs from specific actions such as micturition, cough or swallow. Finally, particularly in older patients, the afferent limb can be triggered by carotid sinus stimulation.

A second cause of syncope is orthostatic hypotension. Normally with standing, accumulation of fluid in the legs results in the initiation of a complex neurologic reflex response that maintains systemic blood pressure. In orthostatic hypotension this response is insufficient, leading to a decrease in systemic blood pressure. An abnormal response is usually defined as a 20–30 mm Hg drop in systolic blood pressure on standing. Reduction in blood pressure and the increase in heart rate (which may be attenuated in older patients and in those with diabetes) are usually observed immediately after standing but can be delayed for a short period of time and thus blood pressure measurements should continue for several minutes after standing. Orthostatic hypotension can be due to a primary abnormality of the autonomic nervous system (either isolated or affecting multiple systems) or secondary (e.g. diabetes, Parkinson's disease and uremia). Diabetes is the most common cause of autonomic neuropathy in the United States and can be associated with relatively high mortality rates (25–50% mortality at 5–8 years).[18] Another form of autonomic dysfunction that can be associated with syncope is the postural orthostatic tachycardia syndrome (POTS); up to 20–30% of patients with POTS will report a prior history of syncope or presyncope.[19] Investigators believe that in POTS, hypotension on standing does not occur but maintenance of upright blood pressure requires an abnormal increase in heart rate, leading to sustained sinus tachycardia (usually > 110 bpm). Although patients with POTS and orthostatic hypotension can present with symptoms of syncope they more commonly complain of symptoms such as fatigue, palpitations, rapid and pounding heart rates, and dizziness.

The third cause of syncope is a cardiac abnormality. Etiologies of cardiac syncope can broadly be divided into abnormal heart rhythms and obstruction to flow. Both rapid heart rates and slow heart rates can cause cerebral hypoperfusion and syncope. Obstruction to blood flow can be due aortic stenosis, pulmonary valve stenosis or dynamic left ventricular outflow tract obstruction in some patients with hypertrophic cardiomyopathy (HCM). Patients with anomalous coronary arteries can sometimes present with exertional syncope, particularly in those whose right coronary artery originates from the left system with the right coronary artery passing between the aorta and pulmonary artery.[20] Large population studies have shown that of the multiple causes of syncope, a cardiac etiology carries the worst prognosis (Fig. 1).[6]

The evaluation of syncope is often challenging and in up to 40% of cases no specific cause can be identified; this is specially true in older patients.[2,3,6] The history and physical examination play an essential role in evaluating patients with syncope. Several studies have attempted to evaluate the diagnostic yield of different tests in clinical practice.[2,3,21] It is important to acknowledge that the highest diagnostic yield of any test in unselected populations of patients with syncope is at best probably 25–30% with no test providing a "gold standard", underscoring the importance of careful initial evaluation by the history and the physical examination and choosing subsequent tests based on this initial assessment.[2–4]

HISTORY AND PHYSICAL EXAMINATION

The history and physical examination play an important role in establishing cause of transient loss of consciousness and, in particular, for differentiating between syncope and seizure as this distinction can be difficult (Flow chart 1). For example, up to 40% of patients with syncope will have generalized seizure-like activity and myoclonic jerking due to cerebral hypoperfusion.[22] Symptoms, such as prolonged confusion after the episode (postictal state) and tongue biting, are suggestive of seizure.[23,24] An altered sense of smell, taste or an aura such as a sense of déjà vu prior to the event are suggestive of a temporal lobe seizure.[24] Focal neurologic signs and symptoms during or after the event (Todd's palsy), also make seizure more likely than syncope. Urinary incontinence, although more commonly observed with seizures, does not completely rule out syncope. In syncopal patients, recovery is complete and often, but not always, rapid, as contrasted with seizures in which recovery is slow due to the postictal state and associated confusion. Petit mal or absence seizures are occasionally misdiagnosed as syncope. A key feature that favors the diagnosis of absence seizures is preserved postural tone despite unresponsiveness. Temporal lobe seizures can have a long duration with varied levels of consciousness. Several investigators have evaluated specific characteristics of the history for differentiating among the various causes of syncope and between syncope and seizure.[24,25] In a cohort of 539 patients a simple point score system correctly differentiated seizure from syncope in 94% of patients with a sensitivity of 94% and a specificity of 94%.[24] Tongue biting, postictal confusion, head turning to one side and prodromal déjà vu or jamais vu were more suggestive of seizures while presyncope, diaphoresis prior to the episode, or loss of consciousness associated with standing made seizure less likely.

Once the clinician has decided that an episode of transient loss of consciousness is most likely due to syncope, the history and physical examination can provide further clues as to its specific cause.[26,27] Pertinent questions should include a history prior of cardiac disease and diagnosis, if known; family history of arrhythmias, syncope and sudden death; knowledge of an abnormal electrocardiogram; medications; positional changes that occurred prior to the syncopal spell (including head-turning); prodromal symptoms; and history of prior syncopal events. Features of the clinical history that are more commonly associated with significant arrhythmias such as ventricular tachycardia or bradycardia due to advanced or complete heart block include male sex, age older than 50 years, fewer than three episodes of syncope and duration of warning prior to syncope of less than 6 seconds.[26–28] Conversely, symptoms, such as blurred vision, nausea, vomiting, warmth, diaphoresis and prolonged fatigue after syncope, have been associated with neurally mediated syncope rather than ventricular tachycardia or complete heart block. In a cohort of 341 patients, the presence of suspected cardiac disease was the strongest predictor of cardiac cause of syncope and absence of cardiac disease had a negative predictive value for a cardiac cause of 97%.[26] However, a more recent study found that the value of clinical history for distinguishing between cardiac and neurally mediated syncope was significantly reduced in older patients.[21] Finally, syncope associated with exertion has traditionally been identified as "high-risk" due to its association with valvular aortic stenosis, HCM, congenital coronary anomalies and channelopathies such as Long QT syndrome, but no large studies have been performed in these groups.[29] Using a similar approach for distinguishing between syncope and seizure, Sheldon and his coworkers identified several historical features that can help to differentiate between vasovagal syncope and cardiac causes of syncope (Fig. 2).[30,31] Symptoms such as lightheadedness associated with pain or medical settings or with prolonged sitting or standing, and a sensation of warmth or sweatiness prior to the episode made vasovagal syncope more likely. Conversely, a history of diabetes, prior arrhythmia, no recollection of the episode and palpitations preceding syncope more likely made a cardiac cause. Similarly a first event over 35 years of age or bystanders describing the patient "turning blue" were also associated with a cardiac cause of syncope.

The physical examination has a central role in evaluation of syncope. A complete cardiac examination should be performed to assess the presence of structural cardiac disease. Orthostatic vital signs are an essential part of the physical examination in a patient. A drop of systolic blood pressure exceeding 20 mm Hg or a decrease in diastolic blood pressure of more than 10 mm Hg is considered to be diagnostic for orthostatic hypotension. The POTS is defined as an increase in heart rate more than 25–30 beats per minute within 5 minutes of standing with symptoms. Cardiac auscultatory findings, such as murmurs or gallops, are important for identifying the presence and severity of structural cardiac disease such as aortic stenosis and HCM. On palpation, findings, such as a left ventricular heave or a sustained left ventricular impulse, can alert the clinician to the presence of structural heart disease, such as left ventricular hypertrophy or ventricular dilation, due to cardiomyopathy or past myocardial infarction that will make more likely a cardiac cause of syncope.

Finally, performing carotid sinus massage (CSM) is important in patients with syncope over 40 years of age.[2] Neurologic complications during CSM occur rarely (0.17–0.45% of patients) and it is important to confirm the absence of carotid bruits or neurologic symptoms suggestive of a stroke or transient ischemic attack and before performing the maneuver.[2] Continuous electrocardiographic monitoring is essential and continuous blood pressure monitoring is highly desirable. To perform CSM, firm continuous pressure for 5–10 seconds should be applied to the right carotid artery at the level of the cricoid cartilage and after several minutes the same maneuver should be repeated on the left side. Ideally, CSM should be performed in both the supine and upright positions since an abnormal vasodepressor response may be detected only when the patient is upright. An abnormal response (carotid sinus hypersensitivity) is usually defined as ventricular asystole more than 3 seconds (due either to sinus pause or AV block) or a fall in systemic blood pressure more than 50 mm Hg (Fig. 2). Formal CSM is often included as a part of the tilt table test in some institutions. It is important to remember that the history and physical examination play a critical role for risk stratification of the patient with syncope.[2,3] As outlined previously, patients with a cardiac cause of syncope have a far worse short-term and long-term prognosis compared to syncope due to other causes. For this reason, the history and physical examination help the clinician decide whether structural cardiac disease is present and provide an initial estimate for the likelihood of a cardiac cause for syncope.

BLOOD TESTS

Routine blood tests including electrolytes, tests for anemia (hematocrit or hemoglobin) and glucose, although commonly performed, generally have a low diagnostic yield in evaluation of syncope.[2,3] The exception may be the presence of anemia; anemia has been incorporated into several prognostic algorithms used for risk stratification of patients with syncope.[32,33] Frequently, patients with syncope are evaluated for myocardial infarction, even in the absence of an infarction pattern on the electrocardiogram. Despite this approach, the yield of diagnostic evaluation for myocardial infarction for patients with syncope is less than 1%.[34] In a small study investigators found that higher brain natriuretic peptide (BNP) levels could be used to identify patients with syncope due to cardiac causes or worse outcomes, and a recently published risk stratification schema for patients with syncope used a BNP more than 300 pg/ml as one criteria for identifying high-risk patients.[33,35] It is important to note that the most recent guidelines do not specifically recommend any blood tests for the evaluation of syncope.[2,3]

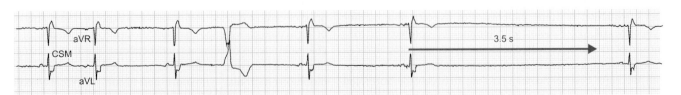

FIGURE 2: Simultaneously recorded leads aVR and aVF rhythm strips obtained during carotid sinus massage (CSM). Initially sinus slowing is observed and ultimately a 3.5 second sinus pause is noted. A pause with ventricular asystole more than 3 seconds, due either to sinus pause/arrest or AV block, defines carotid sinus hypersensitivity

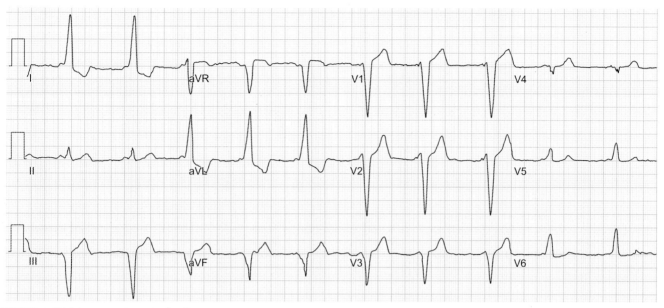

FIGURE 3: ECG from a patient with Wolff Parkinson White syndrome due to the presence of a right freewall accessory pathway. Pre-excitation of the right ventricle leads to a short PR interval and a QRS complex with a left bundle branch block morphology and a negative delta wave in aVR [*Source:* Kusumoto FM. ECG Interpretation. Pathophysiology to Clinical Application. New York: Blackwell-Springer; 2009 (with permission)]

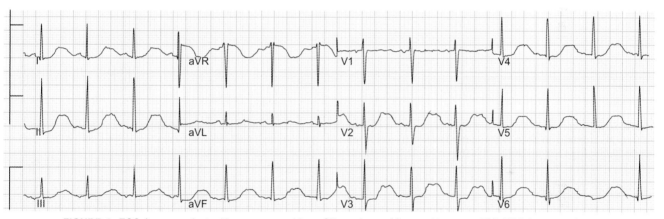

FIGURE 4: ECG from a patient with syncope and long QT syndrome (*Source:* Kusumoto FM. ECG Interpretation. Pathophysiology to Clinical Application. New York: Blackwell-Springer; 2009)

ELECTROCARDIOGRAM

A 12 lead ECG is a basic part of the workup in all patients with syncope.[2,3] Although the diagnostic yield of a baseline ECG is low (5–10%), it is an inexpensive and widely available test that can be used to quickly risk stratify patients, particularly if it is abnormal.[2,3,29] Baseline sinus bradycardia, atrioventricular block and intraventricular conduction block (left or right bundle branch block) suggest the possibility of bradycardia as a cause for syncope. Presence of Q waves that suggest the possibility of a prior myocardial infarction or other findings such as left ventricular hypertrophy make structural heart disease, and thus a cardiac cause of syncope, more likely. The presence of premature ventricular depolarizations may have some prognostic information in patients with syncope. In an older study of 235 patients with syncope, the presence of frequent or paired premature ventricular contractions was associated with higher mortality and risk of sudden death.[36]

Finally, there are some ECG patterns that can be used to identify potential causes for syncope: Wolff Parkinson White Syndrome, Long QT Syndrome, Brugada syndrome, arrhythmogenic right ventricular cardiomyopathy and HCM (Figs 3 to 7A and B).

ECHOCARDIOGRAPHY

Both the AHA/ACCF and ESC guidelines state that the echocardiogram plays a central role in syncopal patients with suspected cardiac disease.[2,3] In a review of over 2,000 elderly patients admitted for syncope at a single center, echocardiograms were obtained in 40% of patients and abnormalities were identified in almost 70%.[21] However, results from the echocardiogram affected management in less than 5% of the cases.[21] Echocardiography has a low diagnostic yield in patients with a normal physical examination and normal ECG and need not necessarily be obtained in all patients with syncope. A structural abnormality noted during echocardiography does not per se establish a diagnostic cause for syncope. However, the presence of severe aortic stenosis or rarer conditions, such as atrial myxoma, is usually diagnostic of etiology (Figs 8A and B).

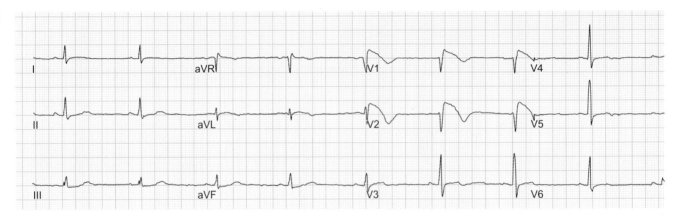

FIGURE 5: ECG from a patient with Brugada syndrome showing the characteristic Type I right bundle branch block pattern and downsloping ST segment elevation in V_1 and V_2. Type I Brugada syndrome is more specific than the "saddle back" ST segment contour in the Type II pattern. ECG patterns in Brugada syndrome can be quite variable, even over short periods of time; questionable diagnoses can be clarified during the intravenous infusion of a sodium-channel blocking drug (*Source:* Kusumoto FM. ECG Interpretation. Pathophysiology to Clinical Application. New York: Blackwell-Springer; 2009)

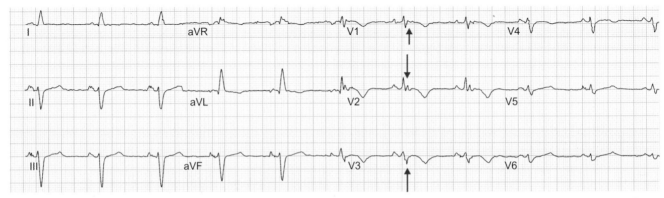

FIGURE 6: ECG from a patient with arrhythmogenic right ventricular cardiomyopathy. There are prominent anterior forces and precordial T wave inversion is present in addition to the highly specific epsilon waves (arrows) that represent delayed conduction in the right ventricle. (*Source:* Kusumoto FM. ECG Interpretation. Pathophysiology to Clinical Application. New York: Blackwell-Springer; 2009)

EXERCISE TESTING

Exercise testing has a low diagnostic yield in the evaluation of syncope (< 5%).[29] However, it may particularly be useful in those patients with exertional syncope. Published guidelines are not uniform in their recommendations; however, the AHA/ACCF scientific statement (but not the ESC guidelines) suggest that exercise testing should be more widely applied to any patient with unexplained syncope, particularly those with coronary artery disease or those at risk for coronary artery disease.

Perhaps even more useful than the identification of ischemia in the patient with syncope is the evaluation of hemodynamic and heart rhythm responses to exercise testing. Development of atrioventricular block with exercise is always abnormal and suggests bradycardia as the mechanism for symptoms. An abnormal decrease in blood pressure during or after exercise may be an important clue for the mechanism of exertional syncope in a patient with HCM.

CONTINUOUS ECG MONITORING

External Devices (24 Hours Ambulatory ECG Recorders, Event Recorders)

Since intermittent bradycardia or tachycardia are the most common cardiac etiologies for syncope, an ECG obtained when the patient is having symptoms is critical for determining whether an arrhythmia is the cause of symptoms. Although asymptomatic arrhythmias can be helpful in suggesting a possible mechanism in some settings, the diagnostic yield of short periods of rhythm monitoring, whether telemetry monitoring during a hospital admission or traditional 24–48 hours ambulatory ECG (Holter) monitoring, is very low.[29] Since most episodes of syncope are usually separated by long periods of time the yield of monitoring less than 48 hours is at best 1–2%.[29]

External recorders that have a loop memory that continuously acquires and deletes ECG information can provide longer periods of rhythm monitoring but studies have provided conflicting reports on the utility of these devices due to the sporadic nature of syncope events. An external event recorder is an attractive diagnostic test for patients with near syncope that occurs frequently (e.g. weekly) (Fig. 9). Event monitors that do not provide continuous ECG monitoring and instead are applied by the patient to the chest when symptoms occur may be useful in the patient with palpitations or dizziness, but are of little use in the diagnostic evaluation of syncope due to patient incapacitation during the episodes.

Implantable Loop Recorders

More recently implantable loop recorders (ILRs) that are placed subcutaneously in the left upper chest and that have larger

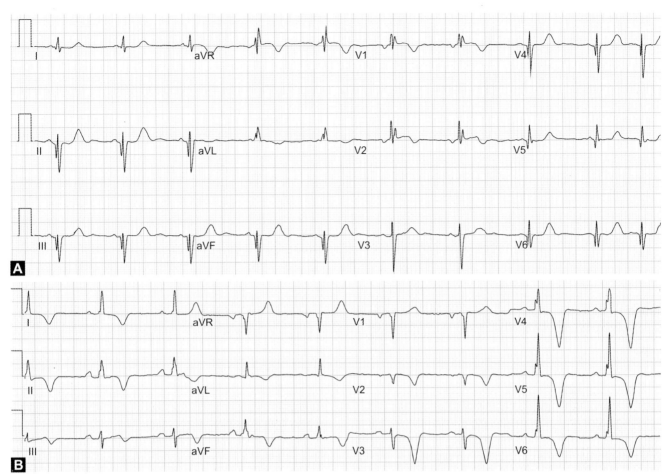

FIGURES 7A AND B: (A) ECGs from two patients with hypertrophic cardiomyopathy. Hypertrophy predominantly affecting the septum, leading to a larger than expected R wave in V1 and "pseudo Q waves in the inferolateral leads. (B) Hypertrophy affecting the cardiac apex, leading to deep lateral T wave inversions (*Source:* Kusumoto FM. ECG Interpretation. Pathophysiology to Clinical Application. New york: Blackwell-Springer; 2009)

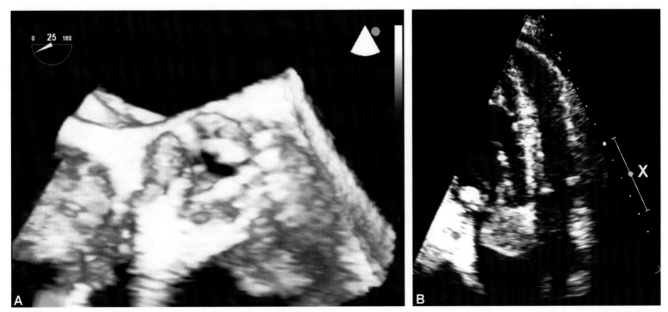

FIGURES 8A AND B: (A) Diagnostic echocardiographic images in patients that presented with syncope. Three-dimensional transesophageal echocardiographic image of a patient with severe aortic stenosis. (B) Four chamber transthoracic echocardiographic image of a sessile left atrial myxoma attached to the interatrial septum (*Source:* Emery Kapples, Jeannine Hiers and Carolyn Landolfo)

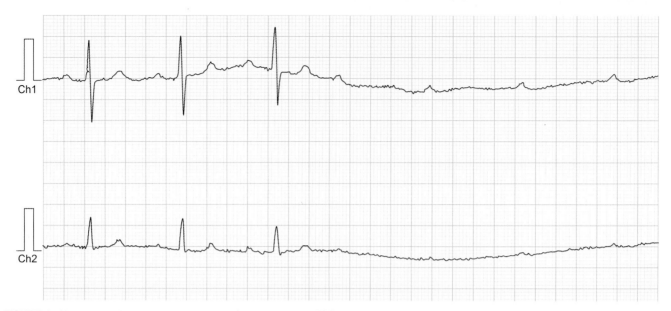

FIGURE 9: Simultaneously recorded rhythm strips from an external ECG event monitor with looping memory documenting intermittent high grade AV block associated with symptoms. The patient had a prior positive tilt table test for a diagnosis of vasovagal syncope, but due to continued symptoms despite medical treatment underwent further diagnostic testing for arrhythmias. A permanent pacemaker was placed with resolution of symptoms

memories and the ability to continuously monitor the ECG for more than 1 year have been developed by several manufacturers. These small devices have a battery life that lasts for 18–24 months. Some clinicians use a program system analyzer to optimize placement of the device to obtain good cardiac signals. The two electrodes used for recording cardiac electrical activity are usually placed on either end of a rectangular shaped device.

Once implanted the ILR will record tachycardia or bradycardia using rate parameters defined and programmed by the clinician. The ILR can also be manually activated with a hand-held activator by a bystander or by the patient after the episode. The ILR is usually programmed to save data for a prespecifed time (e.g. 5 minutes) prior to manual activation. Several studies have documented the usefulness of the ILR for evaluating patients with syncope.[2,37–39] In the largest study to date, of 392 patients with syncope who underwent placement of an ILR, 103 (26%) had recurrent syncope and of these, 53 received specific therapy based on the findings recorded on the ILR (usually bradycardia requiring implantation of a permanent pacemaker).[39] Patients that received specific therapy based on the ILR results had a significant reduction in the incidence of recurrent syncope (10% vs 41%).[39] Importantly, approximately 30–40% of patients will have a recurrent episode of syncope not associated with an arrhythmia, and while this finding does not allow definitive therapy it does essentially rule out arrhythmia as a cause for the patient's symptoms and can be reassuring to the patient.[40]

Current guidelines recommend an ILR for patients with recurrent but infrequent episodes of syncope in whom there is a high index of suspicion for an arrhythmogenic cause after a negative initial workup.[2,3] The ILR has gradually supplanted invasive electrophysiology studies and tilt table testing as the diagnostic test of choice for patients with syncope. The ILR is ideal for obtaining a heart rhythm correlation for a patient with intermittent symptoms. As discussed above, the most common

abnormal finding recorded by the ILR is transient bradycardia, although supraventricular and ventricular tachycardias (Fig. 10) can sometimes be observed. In addition, identifying normal heart rates during an episode of syncope is extremely useful as this finding essentially rules out a primary arrhythmia mechanism for syncope.

SIGNAL AVERAGED ECG

In some patients with structural heart disease (cardiomyopathy or prior myocardial infarction), low amplitude signals in the terminal portion of the QRS complexes can sometimes be observed using special recording techniques that obtain a number of QRS complexes (allowing random noise to cancel out) and use special filtering algorithms. Late potentials are thought to arise from delayed depolarization of the abnormal myocardium and thus reflect nonhomogeneous depolarization. The signal averaged ECG (SAECG) may be useful in rare circumstances, for example in some cases the SAECG can help to identify patients with arrhythmogenic right ventricular cardiomyopathy.[41] In these patients, fatty infiltration of the right ventricle leads to an abnormal SAECG recording that appears to correlate with myocardial fibrosis obtained by biopsy. Other preliminary data suggest that the SAECG may also be useful in identifying patients with Brugada syndrome who are at higher risk for ventricular arrhythmias.[42] In general, however, the SAECG provides little additional diagnostic information and is not routinely used.

UPRIGHT TILT TABLE TESTING

Upright tilt table testing is commonly obtained in the diagnostic workup of syncope.[2,43] The physiology of standing is complex, but when the patient is moved from the supine to the upright position, approximately 300–600 ml of blood pools in the lower extremities and lower portion of the abdomen, which in turn

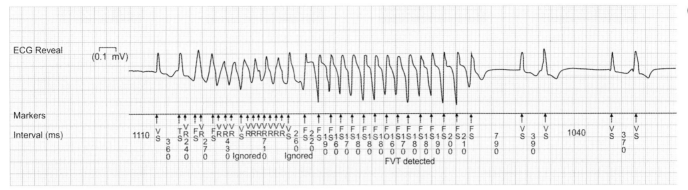

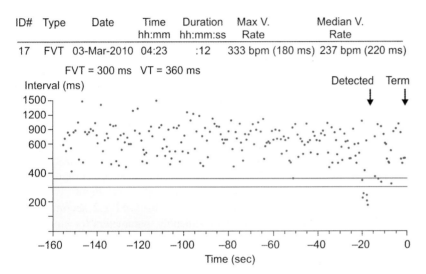

ID#	Type	Date	Time hh:mm	Duration hh:mm:ss	Max V. Rate	Median V. Rate
17	FVT	03-Mar-2010	04:23	:12	333 bpm (180 ms)	237 bpm (220 ms)

FVT = 300 ms   VT = 360 ms

FIGURE 10: Tracings from an ILR showing nonsustained polymorphic ventricular tachycardia that was recorded during sleep (04:23). The device was set to automatically capture rapid heart rates (FVT: Fast ventricular tachycardia, in this case defined as a rhythm with a cycle length < 300 ms). Actual electrograms (Top) and histograms (Bottom) from the event can be obtained. The histogram shows sudden onset of rapid ventricular activity (FS: fibrillation sense) separated by short cycle lengths. The rhythm spontaneously terminates with normal ventricular signal and bigeminy (VS: ventricular sense). Although this abnormal rhythm was not recorded during symptoms results from the ILR suggest ventricular arrhythmias as the cause for the patient's symptoms

leads to a 25–50% decrease in intravascular volume.[43] In response to the decrease in stroke volume a complex interplay of various cardioregulatory systems normally results in maintenance of blood pressure despite the redistribution of blood.

Upright tilt table testing was first applied in clinical medicine 25 years ago as a method for evaluating a patient's hemodynamic response to orthostatic stress and identifying patients likely to develop vasovagal syncope.[44] Several protocols have been developed and there is no uniformity of approach, but generally the patient is positioned on a table at an angle of 60–70 degrees for 30–45 minutes, with only foot support. Some protocols use isoproterenol infusion or nitroglycerin to increase the likelihood of eliciting a vasovagal response. The tilt table test is used to quantify orthostatic hypotension and to attempt to induce a vasovagal response. In those patients who have a vasovagal response, hemodynamic monitoring during the test can quantify the relative and absolute changes in blood pressure and heart rate. Several different hemodynamic responses to tilt table testing can be observed in (Fig. 11):

1. The *normal response* consists of an increase in heart rate of approximately 10–15 beats per minute, an elevation of diastolic blood pressure of about 10 mm Hg and little change in systolic blood pressure.

2. *Orthostatic/POTS response*: Orthostatic hypotension is defined as a reduction in systolic blood pressure of at least 20 mm Hg or a reduction in diastolic blood pressure of at least 10 mm Hg. The POTS pattern consists of a sustained increase in heart rate of at least 30 beats/min or a sustained pulse rate of 120 beats per minute with no profound hypotension. Both of these responses are usually observed within the first 5–15 minutes of tilting; however, in older patients the orthostatic response may be delayed.[45]

3. *Neurocardiogenic response*: Initially, blood pressure and heart rate remain stable. However, after 10–20 minutes a sudden decrease in blood pressure and heart rate will be observed. Some investigators further divide this response into primary vagal, primary vasodepressor or a mixed response, depending on the relative magnitude of blood pressure and heart rate changes.

4. Some investigators also classify as a response of *psychogenic reaction* in which patients develop symptoms with no changes in heart rate or blood pressure.

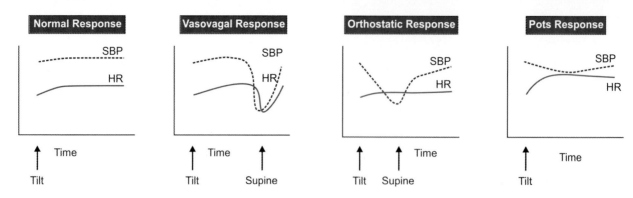

FIGURE 11: Tilt table hemodynamic responses in different conditions. Normally in tilt table testing, with the upright position normal baroceptor function maintains a relatively constant heart rate (HR) and systolic blood pressure (SBP). In the vasovagal response after a relatively long period of time a drop in SBP rapidly followed by a drop in HR is observed. In the orthostatic response, with standing an almost immediate but gradual drop in SBP is observed and HR remains unchanged. In the postural orthostatic tachycardia syndrome (POTS) response SBP is maintained by a significant increase in HR

In patients referred for evaluation for syncope, the most commonly observed abnormal finding during tilt table testing is a mixed form of the neurocardiogenic response (35–45%) in all age groups. The second most common response is age dependent: a bradycardia response observed in patients less than 35 years of age and a pure vasodepressor response in older patients.[46]

Although tilt table testing has been useful as an experimental test for providing physiologic data in patients with vasovagal syncope and orthostatic hypotension and is widely performed, its clinical application has not been well defined. First, it is important to note that the tilt table test has poor reproducibility. When patients with a positive tilt table test are subsequently reevaluated, approximately 50% will have a negative test regardless of whether they were treated or not.[47,48] Second, several studies have found that the likelihood of recurrent episodes of syncope was similar in patients with a positive response and a negative response. Third, abnormalities identified by tilt table testing do not predict the likelihood of bradycardia events that are documented by stored ILR data.[49] Despite these shortcomings tilt table testing may be useful for evaluating some patients with syncope, particularly those with orthostatic hypotension. The ESC has developed detailed guidelines for the methodology, indications and diagnostic criteria for tilt table testing.[2] In general, tilt table testing is recommended when it is important to identify whether the patient is susceptible to vasovagal syncope (e.g. a patient with a structurally normal heart that has a single episode of syncope associated with significant injury) or to help differentiate between reflex syncope from orthostatic hypotension. The tilt table test has been shown to have little use for guiding therapy or as a follow-up tool.[50]

ELECTROPHYSIOLOGY STUDY

The electrophysiology study (EPS) is an invasive test that may be useful for workup of syncope in selected patients.[29] In EPS, using specialized electrode catheters placed in the heart, the clinician can define cardiac electrophysiologic properties, such as sinus node and AV node function, and evaluate the mechanism for any inducible ventricular tachycardia or supraventricular tachycardia under controlled conditions.

Bradycardia can be due to siunus node dysfunction and/or atrioventricular conduction abnormalities. There are several parameters used in EPS for evaluation of the sinus node. The most commonly used parameter is the sinus node recovery time (SNRT). To measure the SNRT, atrial pacing is performed for 30 seconds and the sinus node response on cessation of pacing is evaluated. An abnormal SNRT is shown in Figure 12. In this case, sinus node activation is observed 2.2 seconds after cessation of pacing. Unfortunately, parameters for sinus node dysfunction have highly variable sensitivity (25–70%) and specificity (45–100%) for the clinical diagnosis. The EPS is more useful for evaluation of atrioventricular function and can be used to determine the site of AV conduction block (Fig. 13). Atrioventricular block that develops at or below the level of the His bundle (infra-Hisian block) portends a poor prognosis since intrinsic pacemaker activity of ventricular tissue is not only slow and unresponsive to autonomic influences, but is also notoriously unreliable, even in the short term. A baseline His-to-ventricular (HV) interval more than 100 ms or prolongation of the HV interval to more than 100 ms with procainamide stress has also been shown to be useful for identifying patients at high risk for the development of syncope due to bradycardia. It is important to acknowledge that EPS is useful for defining the site of block in the presence of fixed block but is not useful for evaluating the patient that develops intermittent atrioventricular block at the level of the AV node.

Tachycardia accounts for approximately 15–25% of patients with syncope.[51,52] The EPS may be useful for identifying supraventricular tachycardia but usually this diagnosis is made with continuous ECG monitoring since any arrhythmia induced at EPS may not represent a clinically relevant arrhythmia or the mechanism for syncope. Traditionally, the utility of EPS in the patient with syncope has focused on induction of ventricular tachycardia. In patients with myocardial scars (due to past myocardial infarction or any process that produces myocardial fibrosis) and ventricular tachycardia due to reentry utilizing slowly conducting channels within the scar, programmed stimulation of the ventricle during EPS can be used to assess risk for future ventricular arrhythmias. Although protocols vary among institutions, generally pacing is performed from two sites in the right ventricle delivering one, two or three extrastimuli

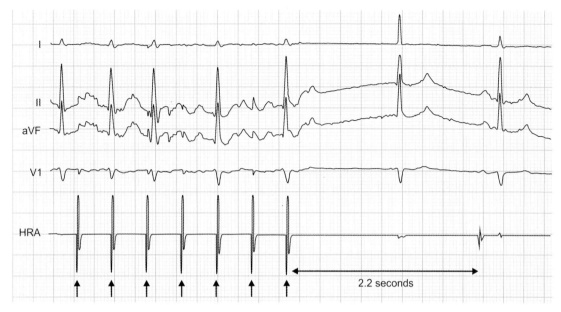

FIGURE 12: Abnormal sinus node recovery time (SNRT). The atria are paced (arrows) at 150 bpm for 30 seconds. Notice the patient has AV block during atrial pacing (this would be expected due to normal decremental conduction properties of the AV node). With cessation of pacing a junctional beat occurs but it takes 2.2 seconds for sinus node activity to return. (*Source:* Kusumoto FM, Goldschlager N. Cardiac Pacing for the Clinician, 2nd edition. New York: Springer; 2008. pp. 647-94)

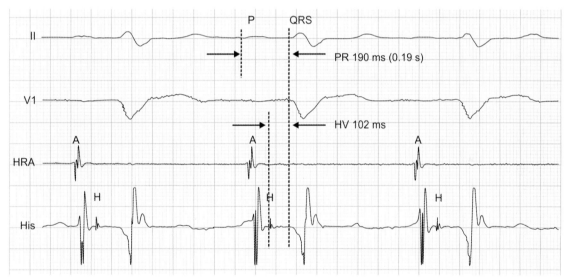

FIGURE 13: Electrograms demonstrating significant prolongation of the HV interval (102 ms) in the setting of a PR interval at the upper limit of normal (190 ms) that suggests infra-Hisian disease. (Abbreviations: H: His bundle electrogram; A: Atrial electrogram). (*Source:* Kusumoto FM. Understanding Intracardiac EGMs and ECGs, 1st edition. Hoboken New Jerse: Wiley-Blackwell; 2010)

after a basic pacing train of eight beats that ensures uniform capture of ventricular tissue. Data from older studies suggest that EPS can be useful for evaluating risk of sudden death in patients with syncope and a prior myocardial infarction.[53,54]

A decade ago, EPS and ventricular stimulation protocols for induction of ventricular tachycardia played a central role in the diagnostic evaluation of syncope in patients with structural heart disease. Since then several important trends have relegated EPS to only occasional use in certain patient groups with syncope. First, several landmark studies have shown that many patients with structural heart disease will receive a mortality benefit from an empiric implantable cardiac defibrillator (ICD) irrespective of the presence or absence of syncope. For example, many patients with an ejection fraction less than 30% due to prior myocardial infarction or an ejection fraction less than 35% in the presence of heart failure symptoms are candidates for ICD placement whether or not they have syncope.[55,56] Second, the ILR appears to be an excellent option for many patients with structural heart disease and syncope who are not candidates for empiric ICD implantation based on ejection fraction and heart failure symptoms alone.[51,52,57] Currently, EPS is reasonable for evaluating patients with syncope and coronary artery disease with prior myocardial infarction that do not meet criteria for an ICD implant or those patients that meet criteria for ICD implant, but where further risk stratification information might change a clinical decision (usually whether or not to implant an ICD). The EPS is also reasonable for the patient with syncope and evidence for abnormal atrioventricular conduction where defining the site of block will impact clinical decision-making. For example, if infra-Hisian block was found at EPS a permanent pacemaker would be implanted.

CARDIAC CATHETERIZATION

Cardiac catheterization is generally not indicated for the workup of syncope unless accompanied by symptoms suggestive of significant coronary artery disease.

NEUROLOGIC TESTS

Computed tomography (CT) scans, electroencephalography (EEG) and carotid duplex scans are often obtained for the evaluation of patients with transient loss of consciousness. Multiple studies have shown that the diagnostic yield of these tests is extremely low (1–3%) in unselected patient populations.[2,3,29] It is recommended that these tests should be ordered only if indicated by clinical findings that specifically suggest a neurologic process.

APPROACH TO THE EVALUATION OF SYNCOPE

As outlined in the preceding sections, there are many tests available for the assessment of syncope and indiscriminate use of diagnostic tests can lead to an expensive evaluation that provides little insight into the management of the patient. Although it is difficult to provide a "one size fits all" algorithm for managing patients with syncope some general guidelines are useful. Recently published guidelines emphasize the importance of the history and a comprehensive physical examination in the initial evaluation of syncope and also recommend a baseline ECG. Since future risk is largely dependent on whether the patient has a cardiac cause of syncope and whether the patient has structural heart disease most diagnostic and risk-stratification algorithms use this issue as the first decision point (Flow chart 2).

Patients with no history, physical examination or ECG findings suggestive of cardiac disease have a fairly low likelihood of a significant cardiac cause for syncope. If the history is suggestive of vasovagal syncope no further evaluation will be required in many patients. Similarly if the patient presents to the emergency department with symptoms that correlate with an arrhythmia then specific treatment can be initiated. However, even after a comprehensive initial evaluation, the clinician may be unsure of the mechanism of syncope. If the clinician is confident that the patient has no cardiac disease, but is uncertain of whether an arrhythmia is present extended ECG monitoring will be useful. Particularly, in patients with syncope associated with injury, an external event recorder or an ILR may be appropriate depending on the frequency of symptoms. If the patient does not have structural heart disease and the clinician is unsure of the patient's hemodynamic response to orthostatic stress, tilt table testing may be a reasonable next test. Tilt table testing may be helpful particularly for identifying patients with orthostatic hypotension or POTS.

When the clinician is uncertain as to whether structural heart disease is present an echocardiogram can be extremely useful for obtaining information on cardiac anatomy and function. An exercise test may be useful in selected patients with exertional syncope. Cardiac tests, such as 24-hour ambulatory ECG monitoring (duration of evaluation is too short), cardiac enzymes, electrophysiologic tests and cardiac catheterization, and neurologic tests, such as carotid ultrasound, CT scan and EEG, have very little utility.

In the patient with structural heart disease identified by history, physical examination and ECG the appropriate workup will depend on the type of disease present (Flow chart 3). Issues with specific cardiac conditions are described in the following section, but several general comments can be made. Patients with structural heart disease can often have vasovagal syncope but the physician should have a low threshold for further cardiac evaluation. Patients at high risk for ventricular arrhythmias (prior myocardial infarction and EF < 30%, EF < 30–35% with Class II or III heart failure symptoms) can be referred directly for an ICD. For patients with syncope who have coronary artery disease and prior myocardial infarction associated with wall

FLOW CHART 2: Diagnostic evaluation of a patient with syncope

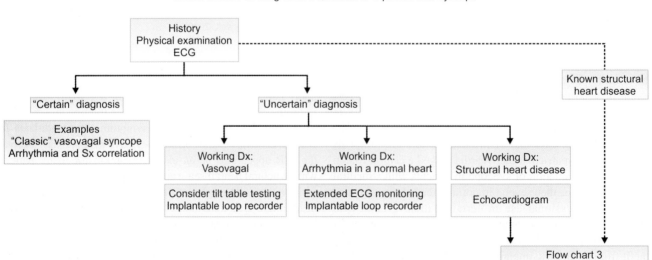

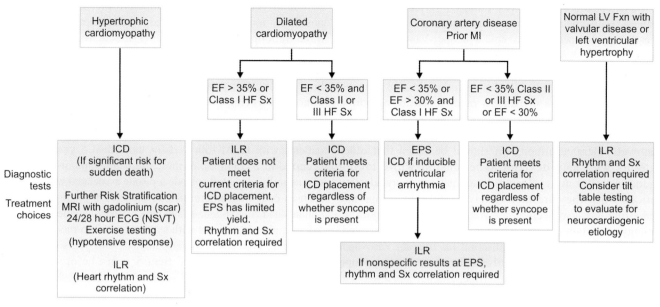

(Abbreviations: ICD: Implantable cardiac defibrillator; ILR: Implantable loop recorder; EF: Ejection fraction)

motion abnormalities, EPS may be useful for determining whether ventricular arrhythmias can be induced with premature ventricular stimulation. The EPS may also be useful for patients with atrioventricular conduction disease identified on ECG to assess the site of block and therefore prognosis and management strategies. Often, an ILR to evaluate the cardiac rhythm during a subsequent episode of syncope will be the most useful diagnostic test for determining the cause of syncope.

SPECIFIC PATIENT GROUPS

VASOVAGAL (NEUROCARDIOGENIC) SYNCOPE

In vasovagal syncope there are widely spaced episodes of a temporary loss of consciousness associated with a fall in arterial blood pressure followed by an almost instantaneous profound slowing of the heart rate. Neurocardiogenic fainting usually occurs in a standing position and is triggered by stressful conditions or pain. The onset may be abrupt or associated with warning symptoms such as fatigue, weakness, nausea, sweating, pallor, visual disturbances, abdominal discomfort, headache, pins-and-needles sensations and feelings of depersonalization, lightheadedness or vertigo. Vasovagal syncope is the most common etiology of syncope regardless of the population studied. The diagnosis of vasovagal syncope is generally made by the history and physical examination although tilt table testing may be necessary in some cases to provide confirmatory evidence in some patients; this may especially be the case in patients who are amnesic for the syncopal spell and who cannot therefore provide a sufficiently detailed history.

Treatment of vasovagal syncope, particularly in patients with frequent symptoms, can be challenging due to the sporadic nature of symptoms and the absence of therapeutic options that have been validated by large clinical trials. As emphasized by the 2009 European Society Guidelines, explanation of the diagnosis and counseling and reassurance of the patient remain the cornerstone of treatment for patients

with neurally mediated syncope.[2] About one-third of patients will have recurrent symptoms but many patients will have only a single event. Recurrent episodes of vasovagal syncope are more likely in women and in patients with more than 3 prior episodes.[58]

Physical counter pressure maneuvers have emerged as a first line therapy in management of neurally mediated syncope.[2,59] These maneuvers include leg crossing, hand gripping and arm or buttock muscle tensing in an effort to raise the blood pressure during the impending phase. A recent multicenter trial found that training in counter pressure maneuvers was associated with a 40% decrease in the likelihood of recurrent syncope. Similarly, "tilt training" or "standing training" is a management option in a patient who is educated and highly motivated.[60] Patients are asked to stand approximately 10–15 cm from a wall (to reduce the likelihood of significant injury in case of a fall) for gradually longer periods, usually 3–5 minutes twice daily initially, increasing to 30 minutes twice daily over time. This form of training improves tolerance to standing although long-term compliance with the training regimen can sometimes be a limiting factor in successful treatment.

Many drugs including beta blockers, selective serotonin receptor inhibitors (SSRI), disopyramide, theophylline, scopolamine, ephedrine, midodrine, clonidine and other medications have been tried in treatment of this condition.[47,61–64] Although small studies and trials have been published that suggest benefit from therapy, the intermittent and inconsistent occurrence of symptoms make evaluation of treatment extremely difficult. In addition, the pathophysiology-triggers, relative degrees/importance of bradycardia and hypotension are probably extremely heterogeneous and thus it is not surprising that individual responses vary markedly. Beta blockade, although traditionally popular, has recently been shown in a randomized multicenter trial to have no clinical benefit.[61] In the prevention of syncope trial (POST), 208 patients with vasovagal syncope were randomized to metoprolol or placebo, and after one year follow-up there were no differences in symptoms or quality-of-life detected between the two groups.[61] At least in part due to these results, beta blockade is no longer considered a front-line therapy for neurocardiogenic syncope. Vasoconstrictors, such as the alpha-agonist midodrine, have been used for treatment of neurocardiogenic syncope in an effort to treat the hypotension associated with the episodes. In one placebo controlled study, 80% of patients randomized to midodrine did not have recurrent symptoms at one year follow-up compared to 13% in the placebo group.[62] In general, midodrine was well tolerated although it should be noted that older patients who may develop hypertension while taking midodrine were not evaluated. Since patients may identify periods when they are more likely to develop symptoms, midodrine has also been administered as a "pill in pocket" strategy in certain patients who are educated and motivated. Not all studies using vasoconstriction for treating vasovagal syncope have been successful. In the vasovagal syncope international study (VASIS), etilefrine, another alpha agonist, was studied in patients with vasovagal syncope.[47] One hundred twenty six patients were randomized to oral etilefrine or placebo and after one year follow-up syncope occurred in 22–24% of patients, without a difference between the two treatment arms and no change in the time to first occurrence of syncope.

Almost two decades ago, permanent cardiac pacing was proposed as a potential treatment option for patients with neurally mediated syncope associated with significant bradycardia.[65,66] Initial nonrandomized trials suggested an important effect of pacing for reducing episodes of syncope.[65,66] Subsequent placebo controlled studies, however, suggested that there was a significant placebo effect associated with pacing therapy and that therefore pacing therapy per se could not be shown to have a beneficial effect.[67,68] The most recent study, the International Study of Syncope of Uncertain Etiology (ISSUE)-2 evaluated whether significant bradycardia identified by ILRs could be used to better identify patients that could benefit from pacing therapy.[69] Interestingly, 53 patients that received pacemakers due to bradycardia identified by ILR reported a statistically significant 41% decrease in recurrent syncope compared to those patients that did not receive an ILR (and consequently did not receive a permanent pacemaker). A large randomized trial (ISSUE-3) has been initiated to validate this diagnostic and therapeutic strategy. At this time, pacing therapy plays a small role in management and only in selected patients with neurocardiogenic syncope who have frequent recurrent symptoms primarily associated with bradycardia or asystolic pauses in rhythm.

HYPERTROPHIC CARDIOMYOPATHY

Hypertrophic cardiomyopathy (HCM) is a diverse genetic disorder that often affects proteins in the sarcomere and that is associated with left ventricular hypertrophy. In a small percentage of patients the interventricular septum is preferentially affected and during systole a dynamic gradient in the left ventricular outflow tract can be observed (hypertrophic obstructive cardiomyopathy or HOCM). Several cohort studies have found that the occurrence of syncope is a major risk factor

for sudden death with a 1.7–5-fold increase in risk.[70–72] Although ventricular arrhythmias are the most concerning possibility for the cause of syncope in these patients, they can have syncope from many other mechanisms, including supraventricular arrhythmias (particularly atrial fibrillation with loss of atrial contraction and rapid ventricular rates), bradycardia, left ventricular outflow tract obstruction and abnormal reflex peripheral blood pressure responses (hypotension) due to stimulation of pressure receptors in the body of the left ventricle. In the largest study to date, in 1,511 patients with HCM followed for more than 5 years, syncope occurred in 205 (14%), of these, 52 had symptoms suggestive of a neurally mediated episode (episode associated with a trigger such as coughing, micturition or change in position) and 153 patients had "unexplained" syncope.[73] Risk of sudden death was 5-fold higher in patients with syncope within 6 months of their evaluation; conversely, older patients (> 40 years old) and an episode of syncope more than 5 years before the initial evaluation were not found to be at increased risk of sudden cardiac death.

Collectively, the data from published studies suggest that while syncope is an important symptom that may herald an increased risk of sudden death, it requires thoughtful clinical evaluation of the patient. Family history of sudden cardiac death (first degree relative with sudden death before age 50), documented nonsustained ventricular tachycardia and degree of left ventricular hypertrophy (> 3 cm) have been identified as risk factors for sudden death. Emerging risk factors include a hypotensive response after exercise and late gadolinium enhancement on magnetic resonance imaging. Although some have advocated ICD placement in HCM patients with multiple risk factors, one cohort study found similar rates of appropriate ICD therapy in patients with 1, 2 or 3 risk factors.[72] For patients who do not receive an ICD, an ILR may be a reasonable diagnostic option.[53,71,74]

NONISCHEMIC CARDIOMYOPATHY

For many years the presence of syncope in a patient with nonischemic cardiomyopathy has been considered an ominous sign, associated with increased risk of sudden cardiac death due to ventricular arrhythmias.[75,76] In the largest cohort to date, 26% of 108 patients with nonischemic cardiomyopathy and syncope had significant ventricular arrhythmias during follow-up, a rate that was not statistically different from a comparison group of patients that presented with sustained ventricular arrhythmias.[76] Post-hoc analysis from two of the large ICD trials suggests that syncope in patients with nonischemic cardiomyopathy can have multiple mechanisms other than ventricular arrhythmias. In the defibrillators in non-ischemic cardiomyopathy treatment evaluation (DEFINITE) Trial, 458 patients with nonischemic cardiomyopathy were randomized to receive standard medical therapy or standard medical therapy and an ICD.[77] After randomization, there was no significant difference for the development of syncope between the two groups (standard therapy: 34% vs standard therapy + ICD: 39%). Of the patients in the ICD arm that had syncope, two-thirds were not associated with delivery of ICD therapy, suggesting a mechanism other than ventricular arrhythmias for the symptoms. The sudden cardiac death heart failure trial (SCD-HeFT) randomized patients with heart failure symptoms and reduced ejection fraction less than 35% (approximately 50% were nonischemic) to placebo, ICD or amiodarone.[78] Regardless of the treatment arm, syncope occurred in approximately 14% of patients after randomization. Although syncope was associated with appropriate ICD therapy in patients randomized to the ICD arm, total mortality was increased by 40% equally in all three arms. Ventricular arrhythmias were thought to be the presumptive cause of syncope in less than 15% of cases. Syncope may be an important symptom for increased risk of sudden death in patients with nonischemic cardiomyopathy but may be due to mechanisms other than ventricular arrhythmias and may identify a group of patients at higher risk for total mortality.

CONGENITAL HEART DISEASE

Approximately one million adults in the United States have congenital heart disease. Depending on the abnormality, patients with congenital heart disease are at higher risk for different arrhythmias. For example, significant arrhythmias will develop in approximately 80% of patients with D-transposition of the great arteries (dTGA) who have undergone an atrial switch repair (Mustard or Senning) (Fig. 14).[79-85] Sinus node dysfunction (20–40%) that often requires permanent pacing is very common as are development of atrial tachycardias (4–20%).[79-81] Atrioventricular block and ventricular tachycardia (due to right ventricular dysfunction and fibrosis that develop due to long-term contraction against systemic pressures) have all been described as causes of syncope. In one long-term follow-up study, syncope developed in 6% of patients. In addition, sudden death occurred in approximately 7% of patients between 6–19 years after repair.[82] In a recently published multicenter study of a 149 patient cohort, sudden death and sustained ventricular arrhythmias occurred in approximately 9% of patients.[83] A QRS duration more than 140 ms was associated with a 14-fold increase in risk of ventricular arrhythmias. Atrial tachycardias were present in 44% of patients but was not a significant predictor for risk of ventricular arrhythmias or sudden death. Finally, in a cohort study of 37 patients with d-TGA who

received ICDs, the annual rate of appropriate shocks was 0.5% for primary prevention and 6.0% for secondary prevention.[84] Taken together the data illustrate the complexity of managing adults with repaired congenital heart disease who present with syncope.

ELDERLY PATIENTS

Syncope in the elderly patients can particularly be difficult from both a diagnostic and therapeutic viewpoint. First, there is significant overlap between syncope and "unexplained falls" and many older patients have limited recall of events surrounding the symptoms.[84] In studies that have specifically evaluated syncope in the elderly patients, in approximately 50% the mechanism cannot be determined, although neurally mediated syncope was, somewhat surprisingly, found to be the most common cause (22%).[19,21,45,46] The natural history of vasovagal syncope may be different in the elderly patients with some reports suggesting an association with malignancy and other terminal conditions.[86] Elderly patients often do not have the typical prodrome of vasovagal syncope that is commonly noted in younger patients.[19,21,46] In addition, there is more overlap between vasovagal symptoms and orthostatic hypotension and carotid hypersensitivity, both are more common in the elderly patients, with the former often iatrogenic in origin. Although a vasovagal etiology is most commonly found in the elderly patients with syncope, orthostatic hypotension (13%) and arrhythmia (12%) are also more commonly observed in the elderly patients than in younger patients.[19]

Treatment of syncope in the elderly patients can be more challenging due to the multifactorial etiology and difficulty in determining a precise cause despite multiple diagnostic tests. In particular, neurologic tests, such as CT scans and EEGs, have very low diagnostic yield (< 5%), as is true for younger patients.[19] Some treatment strategies are limited in the elderly patients, as, for example, the older patient with vasovagal syncope, in whom medications, such as midodrine and fludrocortisone, are not tolerated due to accompanying hypertension.

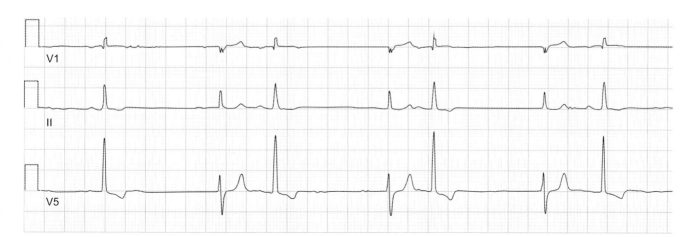

FIGURE 14: Three lead ECG rhythm strip from a syncopal patient with d-transposition of the great arteries who had undergone a Mustard procedure. Severe sinus node dysfunction is present with a slow sinus rate. In addition a prominent R wave diagnostic for right ventricular hypertrophy is observed in lead V₁. Cardiac rhythm causes for syncope in this patient include bradycardia due to sinus node dysfunction, ventricular tachycardia due to right ventricular dilation and, less likely, atrial flutter

The clinician is often faced with questions about the safety of driving in patients with syncope. In the largest study to date, 3,877 consecutive patients with syncope were identified from a large database.[87] Within this group, 381 patients (9.8%) had an episode of syncope while driving (driving group). When compared to the non-driving group, the syncope while driving group was younger, more likely to be male, and more likely to have cardiovascular disease. Syncope during driving was most commonly due to neurocardiogenic causes (37%) with no cause determined in 23% and arrhythmia in 12%. Patients in the driving group had a slightly higher prevalence of accompanying injury (driving: 29% vs non-driving: 24%) but no difference in hospitalization rates (driving: 17% vs non-driving: 15%). Recurrent syncope in the driving group occurred in 72 patients, out of which 35 of whom had recurrent syncope more than 6 months after the initial evaluation.

Driving has become almost an essential component for functioning in today's society for many people. Driver incapacitation for medical reasons (e.g. seizure or syncope) has important public safety ramifications.[88–90] Laws for mandatory physician reporting of medical conditions that can impact driving exist in some states (e.g. New Jersey, Pennsylvania), but not in other states (e.g. Florida, New Mexico). What constitutes an important reportable medical condition varies significantly, particularly in the case of syncope where etiology and prognosis vary widely. In the United Kingdom, for a noncommercial license, a simple faint with definite provocative factors does not lead to any driving restrictions, while unexplained syncope with a high risk of recurrence leads to a mandatory 6 month period during which driving is not permitted. The overall impact of mandatory physician reporting of patients with cardiac conditions probably has a negligible impact on motor vehicle accident-related mortality and morbidity in a larger population. As emphasized in a recent editorial, the risk of driving accidents related to recurrent syncope is significantly lower than the risk of severe accidents from high risk groups such as young drivers, the elderly patients, or distracted drivers.[88] The most recent published guidelines recommend a minimum of 6 months of abstinence from driving after a syncopal event, with resumption of driving permitted if no further episodes have occurred.[90]

GUIDELINES FOR EMERGENCY DEPARTMENT EVALUATION

One of the most significant sources for high cost in patients with syncope is hospital admission that ranges 26–60%.[2,3,37,91] For this reason a number of investigators have evaluated the utility of algorithms for identifying patients at higher risk for significant events and have developed syncope management units (similar to the concept of chest pain units) that allow expedited and more efficient management of patients with syncope. The components of the risk stratification rules vary and some have debated whether the rules are effective for reducing cost (Table 1).

The Osservatorio Epidemiologico sulla Sincope nel Lazio (OESIL) risk score was derived from a patient cohort of 270 patients that presented with syncope in 6 community hospitals in the Lazio region of Italy.[91,92] Multivariate analysis identified four independent predictors that predicted risk: History of cardiovascular disease, age more than 65 years, syncope without a prodrome and an abnormal ECG. The 12 month mortality increased linearly from 0% (no risk factors present) to 57% (all four risk factors present). Several subsequent studies have validated the OESIL risk score for predicting one year risk in other patient cohorts.[91–93]

The San Francisco Syncope Rule was developed to predict short-term outcomes (7 days after the index event).[32] The investigators evaluated multiple variables but simplified their rule to include five elements: (1) abnormal ECG; (2) shortness of breath; (3) hematocrit less than 30%; (4) systolic blood pressure less than 90 mm Hg and (5) a history heart failure. Often the mnemonic chess is used to more easily remember the components: C: Congestive heart failure; H: Hematocrit; E: ECG; S: Systolic blood pressure; S—shortness of breath. Similar to the OESIL risk score subsequent studies have generally validated the utility of the San Francisco Syncope Rule.[93]

In the short term prognosis of syncope (STePS) study 676 patients with syncope were evaluated at both 10 days and 1 year.[94] Severe outcomes (death, major therapeutic procedures, readmission to the hospital within 10 days) were observed in 6.1% of patients (mainly rehospitalization) at 10 day follow-up. Severe outcomes were observed mainly in patients who were admitted (14.7%) compared to those who were discharged from the emergency department (2.0%). The main mechanistic cause for severe outcomes was arrhythmia-related (25/41 patients, most often due to implantation of a permanent pacemaker), although five patients died had a variety of causes, none specifically arrhythmia related (disseminated intravascular coagulation, pulmonary edema, aortic dissection, pulmonary embolism and stroke). Predictors of short-term risk included an abnormal ECG, concomitant trauma and absence of preceding symptoms. Interestingly, factors associated with long-term adverse outcomes were different from the short-term risk predictors and included age more than 65 years and history of neoplasm, cerebrovascular disease and heart disease (structural heart disease or ventricular arrhythmias).

In the risk stratification of syncope in the emergency department (ROSE) study a cohort of 550 patients with syncope was evaluated.[33] One-month serious outcome (acute myocardial infarction, life-threatening arrhythmia, requirement for ICD or permanent pacemaker implant, hemorrhage requiring transfusion, pulmonary embolus or significant neurologic event) or all-cause death occurred in 40 (7.3%) patients in the derivation cohort. Independent predictors were B-type BNP concentration ≥ 300 pg/ml [odds ratio (OR): 7.3], positive fecal occult blood (OR: 13.2), hemoglobin ≤ 9.0 g/dL (OR: 6.7), oxygen saturation ≤ 94% (OR: 3.0) and Q-wave on the presenting ECG (OR: 2.8). One-month serious outcome or all-cause death occurred in 39 (7.1%) patients in the validation cohort. The ROSE rule (the presence of any of the independent predictors) had a sensitivity

TABLE 1

Comparison of the components and primary outcomes for four different risk stratification schemes

Algorithm	Age	Sx and Hx	PE	Components: ECG	Anemia	O₂	BNP	Endpoint
OESIL	≥ 65 y	Sudden onset CVD		Q waves, ST Δ's, LVH, BBB, Arrhythmia				1 year Mortality
SFSR*		SOB, HF Hx	SBP < 90 mm Hg	Δ's, from a prior ECG, Arrhythmia	Hct ≤ 30%			7 day Mortality and serious outcomes
STePS†	> 65 y	Trauma, Sudden onset Hx CVA or CVD, Male		Q waves LVH, LBBB, Arrhythmia				10 day and 1 year Mortality and serious outcomes
ROSE**		Chest pain		Q waves, LBBB, HR ≤ 50 bpm	Hb ≤ 9 g/dL; fecal blood	≤ 94%	> 300 pg/ml	30 day serious outcomes

(Abbreviations: OESIL: Osservatorio Epidemiologico sulla Sincope nel Lazio; SFSR: *San Francisco Syncope Rule. Serious Outcomes: Myocardial infarction, arrhythmia, pulmonary embolism, stroke, subarachnoid hemorrhage, significant hemorrhage or any condition causing or likely to cause a return ED visit and hospitalization for a related event; †STePS: Short Term Prognosis of Syncope. Serious Outcomes: Need for major therapeutic procedures and early (within 10 days) readmission to hospital; **ROSE: Risk stratification of Syncope in the Emergency Department. Serious Outcomes: Acute myocardial infarction, serious arrhythmia, hemorrhage, pulmonary embolus; Hx: History; PE: Physical examination; O₂: Oxygen saturation; BNP: Brain natriuretic peptide; Time frame: Time of endpoint evaluation; HR: Heart rate; PVC: Premature ventricular contractions; SOB: Shortness of breath; CVD: Cardiovascular disease; CVA: Cerebrovascular accident; LVH: Left ventricular hypertrophy; LBBB: Left bundle branch block)

CHAPTER 32

Syncope

and specificity of 87.2% and 65.5% respectively, and a negative predictive value of 98.5% for a serious outcome or death at one month. An elevated BNP concentration alone was a major predictor of serious cardiovascular outcomes (8 of 22 events, 36%) and all-cause deaths (8 of 9 deaths, 89%).

Another strategy for reducing the cost of syncope is streamlining the process of evaluation using syncope or transient loss of consciousness units. In the Syncope Evaluation in the Emergency Department Study (SEEDS), 103 patients were randomized to standard care or a specialized syncope unit that provided early evaluation and focused diagnostic testing.[95] Patients randomized to the syncope unit were less likely to require hospital admission (syncope unit: 43% vs standard care: 98%) and more likely to have a presumptive diagnosis (syncope unit: 67% vs standard care: 10%) on discharge from the emergency department or from the syncope unit.

Several groups have argued the obvious importance of developing a consistent method for risk stratification of patients with syncope.[2,3,37] Although the currently published rules vary some basic points can be made. First it is important to decide whether or not to assign a working diagnosis of a cardiac cause of syncope. All of the risk stratification schemes use two or more criteria for identifying a group of patients with a higher likelihood for cardiac syncope. An abnormal ECG (Q waves, bundle branch block or atrioventricular block) is a component in all of the risk stratification schemes. Criteria, such as age more than 65 (OESIL),[90] history of cardiovascular disease (OESIL)[91] or presence of congestive heart failure (San Francisco Syncope Rule)[32] and elevated BNP (ROSE)[33] are all parameters that increase the likelihood of identifying a patient with a cardiac cause for syncope. Second, criteria that evaluate for noncardiac causes of syncope focus on conditions associated with higher short-term risk such as pulmonary embolus (O₂ saturation < 90% in the San Francisco Syncope Rule or < 94% in ROSE),[32,33] significant anemia (hematocrit < 30% in the San Francisco Syncope Rule and hemoglobin < 9.0 g/dL in ROSE),[32,33] or shock from any cause (SBP < 90 mm Hg in the San Francisco Syncope Rule)[32] or gastrointestinal bleeding (fecal occult blood in ROSE).[33]

GUIDELINES/OFFICIAL RECOMMENDATIONS

There have been formal statements on syncope from two cardiology groups. The AHA/ACCF in collaboration with the Heart Rhythm Society published a scientific statement on the evaluation of syncope in 2006.[3] The writing group recommends a history, physical examination and ECG in all patients with syncope. If the cause of syncope remains unexplained (not neurally mediated or orthostatic) they recommend an echocardiogram, an exercise test and ischemia evaluation. If these tests are normal, no additional testing is required for an isolated benign event. However, if recurrent episodes of syncope or if the episode is associated with significant injury, the clinician should use tests that evaluate the cardiac rhythm during symptoms. The choice among 24–48 hour ambulatory ECG monitoring, external event recorder or an ILR will depend on the frequency of the episodes and the severity of symptoms (syncope vs presyncope). The scientific statement provides a concise practical framework on the evaluation of syncope but does not address emergency room evaluation or subsequent treatment.

More recently, the ESC has published a comprehensive guidelines document that discusses both diagnosis and management of syncope.[2] Similar to the scientific statement from the cardiology societies based in the United States, they recommend an initial evaluation that includes history, physical examination (with orthostatic blood pressure measurements) and an ECG. They emphasize that the clinician should attempt to answer three specific questions:

1. Is it a syncopal episode or not?
2. Has an etiologic diagnosis been determined?
3. Is there evidence for a high risk of a cardiovascular event or death?

If these questions cannot be answered with the initial evaluation, additional tests, such as an echocardiography and other types of cardiac imaging, exercise testing, tilt table testing, cardiac rhythm monitoring and other tests, can be chosen depending on the clinical situation. The European Guidelines do not provide a simple algorithmic approach but rather emphasize that the clinician must carefully choose tests in individual patients to risk stratify the patient and identify a specific etiology of syncope so that a diagnosis for specific treatment plan can be developed.

REFERENCES

1. Papavramidou N, Tziakas D. Galen on "syncope". Int J Cardiol. 2010;142:242-4.

2. European Heart Rhythm Association (EHRA), Heart Failure Association (HFA), Heart Rhythm Society (HRS), et al. Guidelines for the diagnosis and management of syncope (version 2009): the Task Force for the Diagnosis and Management of Syncope of the European Society of Cardiology (ESC). Eur Heart J. 2009;30:2631-71.

3. Strickberger SA, Benson DW, Biaggioni I, et al. AHA/ACCF scientific statement on the evaluation of syncope: from the American Heart Association Councils on Clinical Cardiology, Cardiovascular Nursing, Cardiovascular Disease in the Young, and Stroke, and the Quality of Care and Outcomes Research Interdisciplinary Working Group; and the American College of Cardiology Foundation In Collaboration With the Heart Rhythm Society. J Am Coll Cardiol. 2006;47:473-84.

4. Petkar S, Cooper P, Fitzpatrick AP. How to avoid a misdiagnosis in patients presenting with transient loss of consciousness. Postgrad Med J. 2006;82:630-41.

5. Benditt DG, Olshansky B, Wieling W. The ACCF/AHA scientific statement on syncope needs rethinking. J Am Coll Cardiol. Ad Hoc Syncope Consortium. 2006;48:2598-9; (author reply) Epub 2006;2599.

6. Soteriades ES, Evans JC, Larson MG, et al. Incidence and prognosis of syncope. N Engl J Med. 2002;347:878-85.

7. Dermaskin G, Lamb LE. Syncope in a population of healthy young adults; incidence, mechanisms, and significance. J Am Med Assoc. 1958;168:1200-7.

8. Alshekhlee A, Shen WK, Mackall J, et al. Incidence and mortality rates of syncope in the United States. Am J Med. 2009;122:181-8.

9. Serletis A, Rose S, Sheldon AG, et al. Vasovagal syncope in medical students and their first degree relatives. Eur Heart J. 2006;27:1965-70.

10. Quinn J, McDermott, Kramer N, et al. Death after emergency department visits for syncope: how common and can it be predicted? Ann Emerg Med. 2007;49:420-7.

11. Kapoor WN, Hanusa BH. Is syncope a risk factor for poor outcomes? Comparison of patients with and without syncope. Am J Med. 1996;100:646-55.

12. Day SC, Cook EF, Funkenstein H, et al. Evaluation and outcome of emergency room patients with transient loss of consciousness. Am J Med. 1982;73:15-23.

13. Silverstein MD, Singer DE, Mulley AG, et al. Patients with syncope admitted to medical intensive care units. JAMA. 1982;248:1185-9.

14. Sun BC, Emond JA, Camargo CA. Direct medical costs of syncope-related hospitalizations in the United States. Am J Cardiol. 2005;95:668-71.

15. van Dijk N, Sprangers MA, Boer KR, et al. Quality of life within one year following presentation after transient loss of consciousness. Am J Cardiol. 2007;100:672-6.

16. van Dijk N, Sprangers MA, Colman N, et al. Clinical factors associated with quality of life in patients with transient loss of consciousness. J Cardiovasc Electrophysiol. 2006;17:998-1003.

17. Bartoletti A, Fabiani P, Bagnoli L, et al. Physical injuries caused by a transient loss of consciousness: main clinical characteristics of patients and diagnostic contribution of carotid sinus massage. Eur Heart J. 2008;29:618-24.

18. Ewing DJ, Campbell IW, Clarke BF. The natural history of diabetic autonomic neuropathy. Q J Med. 1980;49:95-108.

19. Ojha A, McNeeley K, Heller E, et al. Orthostatic syndromes differ in syncope frequency. Am J Med. 2010;123:245-9.

20. Cheitlin MD, MacGregor J. Congenital anomalies of coronary arteries: role in the pathogenesis of sudden cardiac death. Herz. 2009;34:268-79.

21. Mendu ML, McAvay G, Lampert R, et al. Yield of diagnostic tests in evaluating syncopal episodes in older patients. Arch Intern Med. 2009;169:1299-305.

22. Grubb BP, Gerard G, Roush K, et al. Differentiation of convulsive syncope and epilepsy with head-up tilt testing. Ann Intern Med. 1991;115:871-6.

23. Sheldon R, Rose S, Ritchie D, et al. Historical criteria that identify Syncope from Seizures. J Am Coll Cardiol. 2002;40:142-8.

24. Benbadis SR, Wolgamuth BR, Goren H, et al. Value of tongue biting in the diagnosis of seizures. Arch Intern Med. 1995;155:2346-9.

25. Hoefnagels WA, Padberg GW, Overweg J, et al. Syncope or seizure? A matter of opinion. Clin Neurol Neurosurg. 1992;94:153-6.

26. Alboni P, Brignole M, Menozzi C, et al. Diagnostic value of history in patients with syncope with or without heart disease. J Am Coll Cardiol. 2001;37:1921-8.

27. Del Rosso A, Ungar A, Maggi R. Clinical predictors of cardiac syncope at initial evaluation in patients referred to general hospital EGSYS Score. Heart. 2008;94:1620-6.

28. Sheldon R, Hersi A, Ritchie D, et al. Syncope and structural heart disease: historical criteria for vasovagal syncope and ventricular tachycardia. J Cardiovasc Electrophysiol. 2010;21:1358-64.

29. Linzer M, Yang EH, Estes NA 3rd, et al. Diagnosing syncope. Part 1: value of history, physical examination, and electrocardiography. Clinical efficacy assessment project of the American College of Physicians. Ann Intern Med. 1997;126:989-96.

30. Sheldon R, Rose S, Connolly S, et al. Diagnostic criteria for vasovagal syncope based on a quantitative history. Eur Heart J. 2006;27:344-50.

31. Sheldon R, Hersi A, Ritchie D, et al. Syncope and structural heart disease: historical criteria for vasovagal syncope and ventricular tachycardia. J Cardiovasc Electrophysiol. 2010;21:1358-64.

32. Quinn JV, Stiell IG, McDermott DA, et al. Derivation of the San Francisco Syncope Rule to predict patients with short-term serious outcomes. Ann Emerg Med. 2004;43:224-32.

33. Reed MJ, Newby DE, Coull AJ, et al. The ROSE (risk stratification of syncope in the emergency department) study. J Am Coll Cardiol. 2010;55:713-21.

34. Link MS, Lauer EP, Homoud MK, et al. Low yield of rule-out myocardial infarction protocol in patients presenting with syncope. Am J Cardiol. 2001;88:706-7.

35. Reed MJ, Newby DE, Coull AJ, et al. Role of brain natriuretic peptide (BNP) in risk stratification of adult syncope. Emerg Med J. 2007;24:769-73.

36. Kapoor WN, Cha R, Peterson JR, et al. Prolonged electrocardiographic monitoring in patients with syncope: importance of frequent or repetitive ventricular ectopy. Am J Med. 1987;82:20-8.

37. Huff JS, Decker WW, Quinn JV, et al. American College of Emergency Physicians. Clinical policy: critical issues in the evaluation and management of adult patients presenting to the emergency department with syncope. Ann Emerg Med. 2007;49:431-44.

38. Krahn AD, Klein GJ, Yee R, et al. Randomized assessment of syncope trial: conventional diagnostic testing versus a prolonged monitoring strategy. Circulation. 2001;104:46-51.

39. Brignole M, Sutton R, Menozzi C, et al. International Study on Syncope of Uncertain Etiology 2 (ISSUE 2) Group. Early application of an implantable loop recorder allows effective specific therapy in patients with recurrent suspected neurally mediated syncope. Eur Heart J. 2006;27:1085-92.

40. Pierre B, Fauchier L, Breard G, et al. Implantable loop recorder for recurrent syncope: influence of cardiac conduction abnormalities showing up on resting electrocardiogram and of underlying cardiac disease on follow-up developments. Europace. 2008;10:477-81.

41. Marcus FI, Zareba W, Calkins H, et al. Arrhythmogenic right ventricular cardiomyopathy/dysplasia clinical presentation and diagnostic evaluation: results from the North American Multidisciplinary Study. Heart Rhythm. 2009;6:984-92.

42. Furushima H, Chinushi M, Hirono T, et al. Relationship between dominant prolongation of the filtered QRS duration in the right precordial leads and clinical characteristics in Brugada syndrome. J Cardiovasc Electrophysiol. 2005;16:1311-7.

43. Benditt DG, Ferguson DW, Grubb BP, et al. Tilt table testing for assessing syncope. J Am Coll Cardiol. 1996;28:263-75.

44. Kenny RA, Ingram A, Bayliss J, et al. Head-up tilt: a useful test for investigating unexplained syncope. Lancet. 1986;1:1352-5.

45. Podoleanu C, Maggi R, Brignole M, et al. Lower limb and abdominal compression bandages prevent progressive orthostatic hypotension in elderly persons: a randomized single-blind controlled study. J Am Coll Cardiol. 2006;48:1425-32.

46. Kurbaan AS, Bowker TJ, Wijesekera N, et al. Age and hemodynamic responses to tilt testing in those with syncope of unknown origin. J Am Coll Cardiol. 2003;41:1004-7.

47. Raviele A, Brignole M, Sutton R, et al. Effect of etilefrine in preventing syncopal recurrence in patients with vasovagal syncope: a double-blind, randomized, placebo-controlled trial. The Vasovagal Syncope International Study. Circulation. 1999;99:1452-7.

48. Moya A, Permanyer-Miralda G, Sagrista-Sauleda J, et al. Limitations of head-up tilt test for evaluating the efficacy of therapeutic interventions in patients with vasovagal syncope: results of a controlled study of etilefrine versus placebo. J Am Coll Cardiol. 1995;25:65-9.

49. Moya A, Brignole M, Menozzi C, et al. International Study on Syncope of Uncertain Etiology (ISSUE) Investigators. Mechanism of syncope in patients with isolated syncope and in patients with tilt-positive syncope. Circulation. 2001;104:1261-7.

50. Petkar S, Fitzpatrick A. Tilt table testing: transient loss of consciousness discriminator or epiphenomenon? Europace. 2008;10:747-50.

51. Sud S, Klein GJ, Skanes AC, et al. Predicting the cause of syncope from clinical history in patients undergoing prolonged monitoring. Heart Rhythm. 2009;6:238-43.

52. Entem FR, Enriquez SG, Cobo M, et al. Utility of implantable loop recorders for diagnosing unexplained syncope in clinical practice. Clin Cardiol. 2009;32:28-31.

53. Lacroix D, Dubuc M, Kus T, et al. Evaluation of arrhythmic causes of syncope: correlation between Holter monitoring, electrophysio-logic testing, and body surface potential mapping. Am Heart J. 1991;122:1346-54.

54. Ruskin JN. Role of invasive electrophysiological testing in the evaluation and treatment of patients at high risk for sudden cardiac death. Circulation. 1992;85:I152-9.

55. Moss AJ, Zareba W, Hall WJ, et al. Multicenter Automatic Defibrillator Implantation Trial II Investigators. Prophylactic implantation of a defibrillator in patients with myocardial infarction and reduced ejection fraction. N Engl J Med. 2002;346:877-83.

56. Maron BJ, Shen WK, Link MS, et al. Efficacy of implantable cardioverter-defibrillators for the prevention of sudden death in patients with hypertrophic cardiomyopathy. Efficacy of implantable cardioverter-defibrillators for the prevention of sudden death in patients with hypertrophic cardiomyopathy. N Engl J Med. 2000;342:365-73.

57. Menozzi C, Brignole M, Garcia-Civera R, et al. International Study on Syncope of Uncertain Etiology (ISSUE) Investigators. Mechanism of syncope in patients with heart disease and negative electrophysiologic test. Circulation. 2002;105:2741-5.

58. Aydin MA, Maas R, Mortensen K, et al. Predicting recurrence of vasovagal syncope: a simple risk score for the clinical routine. J Cardiovasc Electrophysiol. 2009;20:416-21.

59. van Dijk N, Quartieri F, Blanc JJ, et al. PC-Trial Investigators. Effectiveness of physical counterpressure maneuvers in preventing vasovagal syncope: the Physical Counterpressure Manoeuvres Trial (PC-Trial). J Am Coll Cardiol. 2006;48:1652-7.

60. Duygu H, Zoghi M, Turk U, et al. The role of tilt training in preventing recurrent syncope in patients with vasovagal syncope: a prospective and randomized study. Pacing Clin Electrophysiol. 2008;31:592-6.

61. Sheldon RS, Amuah JE, Connolly SJ, et al. Prevention of syncope trial. Effect of metoprolol on quality of life in the prevention of syncope trial. J Cardiovasc Electrophysiol. 2009;20:1083-8.

62. Perez-Lugones A, Schweikert R, Pavia S, et al. Usefulness of midodrine in patients with severely symptomatic neurocardiogenic syncope: a randomized control study. J Cardiovasc Electrophysiol. 2001;12:935-8.

63. Grubb BP, Wolfe DA, Samoil D, et al. Usefulness of fluoxetine hydrochloride for prevention of resistant upright tilt induced syncope. Pacing Clin Electrophysiol. 1993;16:458-64.

64. Takata TS, Wasmund SL, Smith ML. Serotonin reuptake inhibitor (paxil) does not prevent the vasovagal reaction associated with carotid sinus massage and/or lower body negative pressure in healthy volunteers. Circulation. 2002;106:1500-4.

65. Connolly SJ, Sheldon R, Roberts RS, et al. The North American Vasovagal Pacemaker Study (VPS). A randomized trial of permanent cardiac pacing for the prevention of vasovagal syncope. J Am Coll Cardiol. 1999;33:16-20.

66. Sutton R, Brignole M, Menozzi C, et al. Dual-chamber pacing in the treatment of neurally mediated tilt-positive cardioinhibitory syncope: pacemaker versus no therapy: a multicenter randomized study. The Vasovagal Syncope International Study (VASIS) Investigators. Circulation. 2000;102:294-9.

67. Connolly SJ, Sheldon R, Thorpe KE, et al. VPS II Investigators. Pacemaker therapy for prevention of syncope in patients with recurrent severe vasovagal syncope: Second Vasovagal Pacemaker Study (VPS II): a randomized trial. JAMA. 2003;289:2224-9.

68. Sud S, Massel D, Klein GJ, et al. The expectation effect and cardiac pacing for refractory vasovagal syncope. Am J Med. 2007;120:54-62.

69. Brignole M, Sutton R, Menozzi C, et al. International Study on Syncope of Uncertain Etiology 2 (ISSUE 2) Group. Early application of an implantable loop recorder allows effective specific therapy in patients with recurrent suspected neurally mediated syncope. Eur Heart J. 2006;27:1085-92.

70. Dimitrow PP, Chojnowska L, Rudzinski T, et al. Sudden death in hypertrophic cardiomyopathy: old risk factors re-assessed in a new model of maximalized follow-up. Eur Heart J. 2010;31:842-8.

71. Haghjoo M, Faghfurian B, Taherpour M, et al. Predictors of syncope in patients with hypertrophic cardiomyopathy. Pacing Clin Electrophysiol. 2009;32:642-7.

72. Maron BJ, Spirito P, Shen WK, et al. Implantable cardioverter-defibrillators and prevention of sudden cardiac death in hypertrophic cardiomyopathy. JAMA. 2007;298:405-12. Erratum in: JAMA. 2007;298:1516.

73. Spirito P, Autore C, Rapezzi C, et al. Syncope and risk of sudden death in hypertrophic cardiomyopathy. Circulation. 2009;119:1703-10.

74. Pezawas T, Stix G, Kastner J, et al. Implantable loop recorder in unexplained syncope: classification, mechanism, transient loss of consciousness and role of major depressive disorder in patients with and without structural heart disease. Heart. 2008;94:e17.

75. Knight BP, Goyal R, Pelosi F, et al. Outcome of patients with nonischemic dilated cardiomyopathy and unexplained syncope treated with an implantable defibrillator. J Am Coll Cardiol. 1999;33:1964-70.

76. Phang RS, Kang D, Tighiouart H, et al. High risk of ventricular arrhythmias in patients with nonischemic dilated cardiomyopathy presenting with syncope. Am J Cardiol. 2006;97:416-20.

77. Ellenbogen KA, Levine JH, Berger RD, et al. Defibrillators in Non-Ischemic Cardiomyopathy Treatment Evaluation (DEFINITE) Investigators. Are implantable cardioverter defibrillator shocks a surrogate for sudden cardiac death in patients with nonischemic cardiomyopathy? Circulation. 2006;113:776-82.

78. Olshansky B, Poole JE, Johnson G, et al. SCD-HeFT Investigators. Syncope predicts the outcome of cardiomyopathy patients: analysis of the SCD-HeFT study. J Am Coll Cardiol. 2008;51:1277-82.

79. Hayes CJ, Gersony WM. Arrhythmias after the Mustard operation for transposition of the great arteries: a long-term study. J Am Coll Cardiol. 1986;7:133-7.

80. Gillette PC, Wampler DG, Shannon C, et al. Use of cardiac pacing after the Mustard operation for transposition of the great arteries. J Am Coll Cardiol. 1986;7:138-41.

81. Gelatt M, Hamilton RM, McCrindle BW, et al. Arrhythmia and mortality after the Mustard procedure: a 30-year single-center experience. J Am Coll Cardiol. 1997;29:194-201.

82. Wilson NJ, Clarkson PM, Barratt-Boyes BG, et al. Long-term outcome after the mustard repair for simple transposition of the great arteries. 28-year follow-up. J Am Coll Cardiol. 1998;32:758-65.

83. Schwerzmann M, Salehian O, Harris L, et al. Ventricular arrhythmias and sudden death in adults after a Mustard operation for transposition of the great arteries. Eur Heart J. 2009;30:1873-9.

84. Khairy P, Harris L, Landzberg MJ, et al. Sudden death and defibrillators in transposition of the great arteries with intra-atrial baffles: a multicenter study. Circ Arrhythm Electrophysiol. 2008;1:250-7.

85. Cummings SR, Nevitt MC, Kidd S. Forgetting falls. The limited accuracy of recall of falls in the elderly. J Am Geriatr Soc. 1988;36:613-6.

86. Venkatraman V, Lee L, Nagarajan DV. Lymphoma and malignant vasovagal syndrome. Br J Haematol. 2005;130:323.

87. Sorajja D, Nesbitt GC, Hodge DO, et al. Syncope while driving: clinical characteristics, causes, and prognosis. Circulation. 2009;120:928-34.

88. Curtis AB, Epstein AE. Syncope while driving: How safe is safe? Circulation. 2009;120:921-3.

89. Simpson CS, Hoffmaster B, Mitchell LB, et al. Mandatory physician reporting of drivers with cardiac disease: Ethical and practical considerations. Can J Cardiol. 2004;20:1329-34.

90. Epstein AE, Baessler CA, Curtis AB, et al. Addendum to "personal and public safety issues related to arrhythmias that may affect consciousness: implications for regulation and physician recommendations: a medical/scientific statement from the American Heart Association and the North American Society of Pacing and Electrophysiology": public safety issues in patients with implantable defibrillators: a scientific statement from the American Heart Association and the Heart Rhythm Society. Circulation. 2007;115:1170-6.

91. Brignole M, Disertori M, Menozzi C, et al. Management of syncope referred urgently to general hospitals with and without syncope units evaluation of guidelines in syncope study group. Europace. 2003;5:293-8.

92. Colivicchi F, Ammirati F, Melina D, et al. OESIL (Osservatorio Epidemiologico sulla Sincope nel Lazio) Study Investigators Development and prospective validation of a risk stratification system for patients with syncope in the emergency department: the OESIL risk score. Eur Heart J. 2003;24:811-9.

93. Dipaola F, Costantino G, Perego F, et al. STePS investigators. San Francisco Syncope Rule, Osservatorio Epidemiologico sulla Sincope nel Lazio risk score, and clinical judgment in the assessment of short-term outcome of syncope. Am J Emerg Med. 2010;28:432-9.

94. Costantino G, Perego F, Dipaola F, et al. STePS Investigators. Short-and long-term prognosis of syncope, risk factors, and role of hospital admission: results from the STePS (Short-Term Prognosis of Syncope) study. J Am Coll Cardiol. 2008;51:276-83.

95. Shen WK, Decker WW, Smars PA, et al. Syncope Evaluation in the Emergency Department Study (SEEDS): a multidisciplinary approach to syncope management. Circulation. 2004;110:3636-45.

Atrial Fibrillation

Vasanth Vedantham, Jeffrey E Olgin

Chapter Outline

INTRODUCTION

Atrial fibrillation (AF) is the most common sustained arrhythmia in adults and is associated with substantial morbidity, mortality and cost. AF is characterized by disorganized atrial electrical activity and irregular ventricular rates. AF can result in heart failure, thromboembolism, impaired quality of life and may increase mortality. While AF is frequently associated with structural heart disease, it can occur in isolation (lone AF) or in association with non-cardiac diseases. In the coming years it is projected that AF will be seen with increasing frequency both by cardiologists and by non-specialists. The purpose of this chapter is to provide a broad overview of our current understanding of this complex arrhythmia, and to provide a framework for clinical decision making in patients with AF.

DEFINITION AND CLASSIFICATION

Atrial fibrillation (AF) is easily recognized on the surface of ECG as an irregular supraventricular rhythm (irregular QRS complexes), with a loss of clear P-waves and/or the presence of fibrillatory waves (Fig. 1). AF in response to a reversible cause (e.g. hyperthyroidism, pericarditis, hypoxia, pneumonia, surgery, pulmonary embolism) is called "secondary AF". AF can also occur in association with valve disease (typically mitral stenosis or regurgitation), in association with other structural heart disease (congestive heart failure, right ventricular dysfunction) or other known risks (e.g. hypertension, pulmonary disease, sleep apnea). AF that occurs without any overt heart disease, pulmonary disease or hypertension (HTN) is called "lone AF".

While several classification schemes have been proposed for AF, the most widely used is based on the duration of AF episodes and whether intervention is required to terminate AF.[1] AF is called "paroxysmal" when episodes terminate spontaneously in less than seven days from onset. When two or more such episodes occur, paroxysmal AF is called "recurrent". When AF lasts longer than seven days or requires pharmacological or electrical conversion, it is called "persistent". AF that is resistant to drugs or cardioversion is called "permanent". It should be noted that these definitions are not necessarily always clean; for example, some patients with persistent AF may have periods where their AF is paroxysmal. Moreover, while there is evidence that there is a progression of AF from paroxysmal to persistent to permanent, this does not occur in every patient.

EPIDEMIOLOGY

INCIDENCE AND PREVALENCE

Atrial fibrillation is the most common clinical arrhythmia, both in the population at large and in hospitalized patients. According to a large population-based study (ATRIA), the prevalence of AF in the general population is roughly 1%, translating to about 3 million patients in the United States.[2] The prevalence of AF in ATRIA also rose steeply with age, with a prevalence of 0.1% in patients less than 50 years old and 9% in patients over 80 years old. Data from ATRIA also show higher incidence of AF

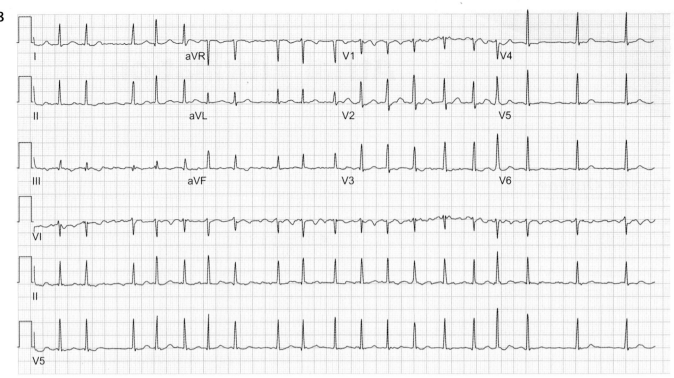

FIGURE 1: Typical ECG of atrial fibrillation showing an absence of P waves, the presence of fibrillatory waves (visible in lead V1), and a rapid, irregular ventricular response

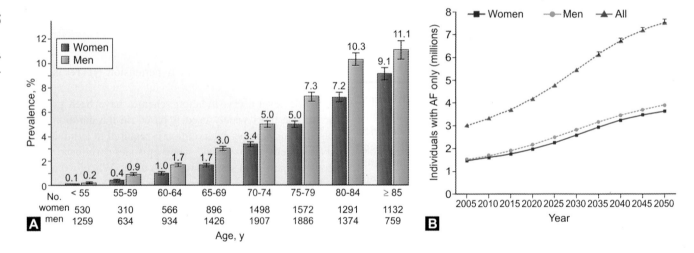

FIGURES 2A AND B: (A) Increasing prevalence of AF as a function of age in men and women in a large cross-sectional study. (B) Projected increase in the prevalence of AF to 2050. (*Source:* Reproduced with permission from reference 2 (A) and reference 5 (B)

among men than women (1.1% vs 0.9%), and among whites than blacks (2.2% vs 1.5% among patients older than 50 years). Other prospective longitudinal population-based studies[3,4] have explored the incidence of AF, and have shown a marked increase with age, from about 0.1% per year in patients between 55–60 years old to as high as 5% per year in patients older than 80 years, consistent with the studies of AF prevalence (Fig. 2A). Since the age distribution of the population in the developed world is shifting toward older ages, the overall incidence of AF is rising. Available projections based on these longitudinal studies forecast about 5 million patients in the United States with AF by 2025 (Fig. 2B).[5] In addition, since many episodes of paroxysmal AF are either asymptomatic, self-limited or occur in unmonitored patients, the true prevalence of AF is likely to be significantly higher than that of diagnosed AF.

NATURAL HISTORY

Left untreated, the rapid ventricular rates associated with AF and the loss of atrial mechanical activity can lead to cardiomyopathy and heart failure, conditions which themselves can perpetuate AF through their effects on cardiac hemodynamics. While AF is often thought of as a progressive disease, with paroxysmal AF eventually progressing to persistent and permanent AF, they are patients in whom it does not progress. Although long-term data from large studies are not available, smaller studies have shown that about 25% of patients with paroxysmal AF will progress to permanent AF within 5 years.[6]

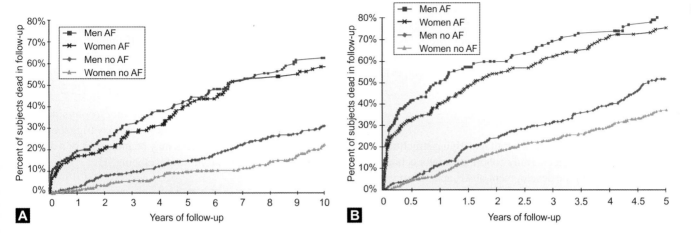

FIGURES 3A AND B: Kaplan-Meier curves for patients with AF and matched controls from the Framingham Study cohort. (A) Data for patients aged 55–74 (B) Data from patients aged 75–94. (*Source:* Modified from reference 9)

Not surprisingly, given its association with cardiovascular and systemic disease, the diagnosis of AF is associated with adverse long-term and short-term clinical outcomes. Although longitudinal studies in patients with lone AF have not revealed an adverse prognosis,[7] patients with AF in the context of cardiovascular disease had an approximate doubling of all-cause mortality in two large population-based studies, even after adjustment for the contributions of age, sex and comorbid conditions (Figs 3A and B).[8,9]

The most common serious complication of AF is thromboembolic stroke. Compared to the general population, the relative risk of stroke in patients with AF is 2.4 for women and 3.0 for men.[10] Additional factors, such as congestive heart failure, diabetes, HTN, prior stroke and age, increase the risk of stroke. The CHADS2 score is a useful risk assessment tool to calculate risk of stroke in patients with AF.[11] Compared to patients with carotid artery disease, strokes associated with AF are on average more severe (larger territory) and transient ischemic attacks are longer lasting, presumably because embolic particles are larger in AF patients.[12] As a result, long-term outcomes, both in terms of morbidity and mortality, are worse for patients who suffer strokes due to AF than for those whose strokes are due to carotid disease.[13–15] Recent epidemiological studies have also shown an increased risk of Alzheimer's disease and other forms of dementia in patients with AF, even in the absence of stroke.[16,17] This association appears to be independent of common risk factors for both conditions and confers increased mortality in the subset of AF patients who experience cognitive decline.[18] Conflicting data exists on the effect of AF on heart failure progression and mortality in heart failure patients. In the studies of left ventricular dysfunction (SOLVD) and Candesartan in heart failure—assessment of reduction in mortality (CHARM) trials, development of AF was associated with significantly worse outcomes than patients without AF.[19,20] However, no significant outcomes differences attributable to AF were observed in the vasodilator heart failure trial (V-HeFT) studies.[21]

ETIOLOGY AND PATHOGENESIS

While short episodes of AF lasting a few seconds can be induced in normal atria, longer episodes require a vulnerable atrial substrate. This vulnerable substrate can be due to atrial enlargement, atrial fibrosis or other electrophysiological abnormalities of the atrial myocardium (Table 1). For spontaneous

---

TABLE 1

Factors predisposing to atrial fibrillation

Electrophysiological abnormalities
- Enhanced automaticity (focal AF)
- Conduction abnormality (reentry)

Atrial pressure elevation
- Mitral or tricuspid valve disease
- Myocardial disease (primary or secondary, leading to systolic or diastolic dysfunction)
- Semilunar valve abnormalities (causing ventricular hypertrophy)
- Systemic or pulmonary hypertension
- Intracardiac tumors or thrombi

Atrial ischemia
- Coronary artery disease

Inflammatory or infiltrative atrial disease
- Pericarditis
- Amyloidosis
- Myocarditis
- Age-induced atrial fibrotic change

Drugs
- Alcohol
- Caffeine

Endocrine disorders
- Hyperthyroidism
- Pheochromocytoma

Changes in autonomic tone
- Increased parasympathetic activity
- Increased sympathetic activity

Primary or metastatic disease in or adjacent to the atrial wall

Postoperative
- Cardiac, pulmonary or esophageal surgery

Congenital heart disease

Neurogenic
- Subarachnoid hemorrhage
- Nonhemorrhagic, major stroke

Idiopathic (lone AF)

Familial AF

(*Source:* Reference 1)

AF to occur, there also needs to be a trigger. This is typically premature atrial depolarizations or short bursts of atrial tachycardia that interact with a vulnerable substrate to spontaneously induce AF. While the triggering activity may arise from anywhere in the atria, evidence to date suggests that majority arise from the pulmonary veins.

STRUCTURAL HEART DISEASE

AF is most frequently associated with underlying structural heart disease. In the Framingham Study cohort, the major echocardiographic predictors of the development of AF, apart from valvular disease, were LV systolic dysfunction, LV hypertrophy and atrial enlargement.[22] In addition, a variety of non-cardiac conditions can result in AF, and AF can occur in the absence of any other discernable cardiac or non-cardiac disease.

Valvular Heart Disease

Diseases of the mitral and tricuspid valves result in pressure and/or volume overload of the atria, causing marked dilation and adverse atrial remodeling, predisposing to AF. Depending on the number of valves involved and the severity of the lesions, the prevalence of AF in patients with rheumatic heart disease ranges from 16% for isolated mitral regurgitation to as high as 70% for patients with a combination of mitral stenosis, mitral regurgitation and tricuspid regurgitation.[23]

Heart Failure

Heart failure is a major cause of AF, due to the effects of chronically elevated left-sided pressures on left atrial structure and function, and the activation of neurohormonal cascades that lead to atrial remodeling. Between 10 and 50% of patients with LV dysfunction have also AF, depending on the severity of LV dysfunction and NYHA functional class.[24] Rapid rates associated with AF can also cause heart failure. In such cases, treatment of AF or rate control can result in significant improvement in heart failure symptoms and ejection fraction.[25,26]

Ischemic Heart Disease

Cardiac ischemia is a common cause of AF, likely due to a combination of elevated filling pressures in the left atrium, metabolic stress and inflammation. Approximately 5–10% of patients experiencing an acute MI will present in AF and this subset has a worse prognosis.[27,28]

Hypertrophic Cardiomyopathy

The estimated incidence of AF among patients with hypertrophic cardiomyopathy varies from around 10% to 30%.[29] Because of poor LV compliance, these patients often depend on the atrial contribution to cardiac output and require relatively longer times for ventricular filling. As a result, they tolerate AF poorly, and can exhibit marked hemodynamic deterioration and severe symptoms associated with rapid AF.

In addition to the above-mentioned lesions, adult survivors of congenital heart disease often develop AF, either alone or in combination with other atrial tachyarrhythmias. Pericardial disease can also cause AF, both due to the effects of inflammation and hemodynamic sequelae of compromised ventricular filling. Related to this, patients undergoing cardiac surgery have an incidence of mostly self-limited postoperative AF as high as 30–40%.[30,31]

ELECTROPHYSIOLOGICAL ABNORMALITIES

AF is associated with several other electrophysiological disorders of the heart, which in some cases may trigger episodes of AF directly and in other cases may be indicators of a diseased atrial substrate that is prone to developing AF.

Atrial Tachycardia and Pulmonary Venous Activity

The pulmonary venous myocardium has been identified as a major source of AF triggers, through a combination of abnormal automaticity, triggered activity and the proximity of autonomic ganglia.[32,33] Other thoracic venous structures (superior vena cava and coronary sinus) and embryological venous remnants (vein and ligament of Marshall) may also trigger AF.[34] The precise mechanisms that regulate electrical activity of the pulmonary venous myocardium are unknown. Intensive research is ongoing into the anatomy, embryology and electrophysiological properties of the myocardial cells within the pulmonary veins.[35]

Supraventricular Tachycardia

AV node reentry tachycardia and AV reentry tachycardia utilizing an accessory pathway can trigger AF. In such cases, elimination of the SVT with catheter ablation or treatment with medications may eliminate the trigger for AF.[36,37] Other reentrant arrhythmias, such as atrial flutter, can similarly degenerate into AF, and catheter ablation of the predisposing arrhythmia may reduce AF frequency. An increased incidence of AF has been documented in patients with ventricular preexcitation due to an accessory pathway, even in the absence of spontaneous or inducible tachycardia.[38,39]

Conduction System Disease

Sinus node dysfunction and prolongation of the PR interval are both associated with AF, presumably due to common underlying atrial pathophysiology.[40,41] Some evidence supports the idea that bradycardia in patients with sinus node dysfunction may itself predispose to AF episodes, and that atrial pacing may reduce AF burden in such patients.

Cardiac Nervous System Dysfunction

Imbalance between the sympathetic and parasympathetic arms of the cardiac autonomic nervous, in either direction, can lead to AF. Sympathetic activation can lead to enhanced activity of ectopic foci, which can trigger AF.[42] Prolonged sympathetic activation, as occurs in heart failure, can also lead to adverse structural remodeling of atrial tissue. On the other hand, enhanced vagal tone shortens the refractory period of atrial tissue, facilitating atrial reentry. The latter mechanism may account for a subset of patients with lone AF, such as highly trained athletes with high vagal tone, and those whose episodes of AF occur predominantly in sleep.[43]

Hypertension is the most common non-cardiac cause of AF, with a prevalence of 70% among AF patients enrolled in the atrial fibrillation follow-up investigation of rhythm management (AFFIRM) trial.[44] In population-based series, hypertension confers an adjusted relative risk of 1.5 for the development of AF.[45] While hypertension undoubtedly can lead to AF via an increased LV stiffness and left-sided filling pressures, the increased activation of the renin-angiotensin-aldosterone system (RAAS) may directly cause adverse electrical remodeling within the atria. Hyperthyroidism is common cause of AF. One percent of patients with new-onset AF have overt hyperthyroidism, while an additional 5–6% have subclinical hyperthyroidism.[46] In other studies, subclinical hyperthyroidism confers a relative risk of 3–5% for the development of AF.[47,48] Conversely, about 5–15% of patients with hyperthyroidism develop AF.[49] Conditions associated with systemic inflammation, metabolic stress or atrial enlargement, such as diabetes,[45] obesity,[50] postsurgical state[51] and sepsis[52] are all associated with the development of AF.

Chronic obstructive pulmonary disease (COPD) is associated with a relative risk of 1.3–1.8 for the development of AF, depending on the severity of lung disease.[53] The pathogenesis of AF in the setting of lung disease is likely to be a combination of direct effects of inflammation on the atria, metabolic stress of hypoxia and hemodynamic effects of chronically elevated right-sided pressures. Obstructive sleep apnea (OSA) is also associated with AF, and may be an under-recognized cause of the arrhythmia. The relative risk of AF in patients with OSA is as high as 2.8.[54] Treatment of OSA with continuous positive airway pressure can reduce the frequency of episodes of AF. With the increasing incidence of obesity, AF related to OSA is likely to occur with increasing frequency.

A number of substances are known causes of AF. While moderate alcohol consumption does not significantly increase the risk of AF, heavy alcohol use is strongly associated with AF.[55–57] In addition, a variety of medications can precipitate episodes of AF, including modulators nervous system function, diuretics and cardiac inotropic agents.[58] Although anecdotal evidence exists in support of caffeine as a precipitant of AF, an association between AF and caffeine consumption has not been proven in larger studies.[59]

LONE ATRIAL FIBRILLATION

About 20–30% of patients with AF have no discernable cardiac or non-cardiac cause.[60,61] Studies of tissue in patients with lone AF have identified numerous abnormalities including subclinical cardiomyopathy as well as atrial fibrosis, but it is not clear whether these are a cause or a consequence of the arrhythmia.[62] Propensity to develop AF is highly heritable, even after adjustment for other risk factors.[63,64] Genetic mapping studies in patients with familial AF have identified rare monogenic causes for AF, including mutations in cardiac ion channels and accessory proteins, gap junctions, and other genes relevant to atrial biology (Table 2).[65] However, the vast majority of lone AF appears to be non-Mendelian, implying polygenic or epigenetic etiology. Candidate gene association studies in AF have identified several alleles that confer increased risk of AF,

651

CHAPTER 33

Atrial Fibrillation

TABLE 2
Genetic causes of atrial fibrillation

Mendelian AF, Candidate gene resequencing, and rare variants	
Gene symbol/ Locus	Gene name
GJA5	Connexin 40
KCNQ1	Potassium voltage-gated channel, KQT-like subfamily, member 1
NPPA	Natriuretic peptide precursor A
LMNA	Lamin A/C
KCNA5	Potassium voltage-gated channel, shaker-related subfamily, member 5
KCNE2	Potassium voltage-gated channel, Isk-related family, member 2
KCNH2	Potassium voltage-gated channel, subfamily H, member 2
KCNJ2	Potassium inwardly rectifying channel, subfamily J, member 2
SCN5A	Sodium channel, voltage-gated, type V, alpha-subunit
Chr 5p13	Unknown
Chr 6q14-q16	Unknown
Chr 10q22-q24	Unknown
Chr 10p11-q21	Unknown
Candidate gene association studies	Gene name
ACE	Angiotensin-converting enzyme
AGT	Angiotensinogen
GJA5	Connexin 40
KCNE1	Potassium voltage-gated channel, Isk-related family, member 1
KCNH2	Potassium voltage-gated channel, subfamily H, member 2
Genome-Wide association studies	Candidate gene symbol and name
Chr 4q25	PITX2 Paired-like homeodomain 2
Chr 16q22	ZFHX3 Zinc finger homeodomain
Chr 1p21	KCNN3 Calcium-activated potassium channel
(Source: Reference 65)	

including variants in ion channels and associated proteins as well as regulators of the RAAS system (Table 2). More recent candidate gene data have uncovered genetic mosaicism in AF patients, in which atrial cardiomyocytes, but not peripheral blood lymphocytes, harbor disease-causing gap junction mutations.[66,67] Unbiased genome-wide association studies have also identified risk-conferring polymorphisms, including one at a non-coding locus on Chr 4q25, which confers a roughly fourfold lifetime relative risk for AF in carriers.[68] The polymorphism is in a non-transcribed area of the genome where it likely confers a regulatory function on nearby genes. PITX2c is located downstream of this polymorphism, and is important for establishing the identity of the pulmonary venous myocardium and in suppressing automaticity in left-sided remnants of embryonic cardiac pacemaking tissue.[69] Intensive research is ongoing to determine precisely how this allele might contribute to AF pathogenesis via an effect on PITX2C. Clinical implications of this research might include identifying novel drug targets, but such advances will require considerable progress in our understanding of the regulatory networks controlling atrial structure and function.

DIAGNOSIS

PRESENTATION

As assessed by remote monitoring, most individual episodes of AF are asymptomatic and many patients are unaware of their arrhythmia.[70] Those who are symptomatic exhibit a broad spectrum of complaints, most commonly palpitations, dyspnea and symptoms of congestive heart failure.[71] The hemodynamic consequences and symptoms associated with AF are usually related to the ventricular rate and the presence or absence of underlying heart disease such as valvular disease, LV dysfunction or active coronary disease. Patients in any of the latter categories may tolerate AF poorly. Rarely, when a rapidly conducting accessory pathway is present (WPW syndrome), AF can lead to ventricular fibrillation and sudden cardiac death.[72] In otherwise healthy patients without accessory pathways, syncope is an unusual presentation for AF. Non-cardiac symptoms associated with AF include polyuria (related to ANF release by distended atria) and thromboembolic events, most commonly acute embolic stroke.

PHYSICAL EXAMINATION

The physical examination of patients with AF is also highly variable. Patients in AF can have heart rates ranging from bradycardia to extreme tachycardia depending on the integrity of AV nodal conduction, medications, autonomic tone and the presence of accessory pathways. Due to loss of atrial mechanical function, A-waves are absent from the jugular venous pulsation and a fourth heart sound is not audible in AF. Owing to the variable ventricular filling time in AF, the intensity of heart sounds can change beat to beat. It should also be recognized that commonly used diagnostic maneuvers used to evaluate heart murmurs, such as Valsalva, handgrip and respiratory variation, are of limited utility in the patient with AF because the variable filling time will cause variation in murmur intensity independent of the effects of preload and afterload. Signs of poor perfusion or congestive heart failure can be seen when AF occurs in the setting of valvular disease, LV systolic or diastolic dysfunction, acute myocardial infarction, or when long-standing tachycardia leads to cardiomyopathy.

ELECTROCARDIOGRAM

Although the hallmarks of AF on the surface ECG are loss of P-waves and an irregular ventricular response, AF must still be distinguished from other supraventricular tachycardias associated with an irregular ventricular response, including atrial flutter with variable block and multifocal atrial tachycardia (Fig. 4). The latter is typically associated with lung disease, and is characterized by at least three distinct P-wave morphologies on the surface ECG, whereas the fibrillatory waves in AF are more rapid and variable in morphology. In certain patients, however, fibrillatory waves can be "coarse" and at first glance may be difficult to distinguish from flutter waves. Careful examination of the surface ECG in such patients usually

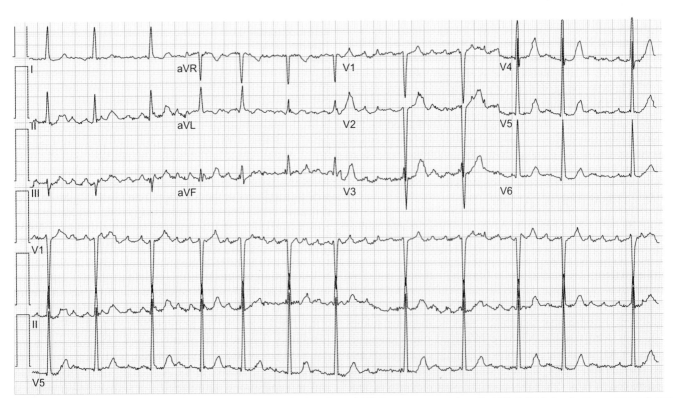

FIGURE 4: ECG shows coarse atrial fibrillation, sometimes mistaken for atrial flutter or erroneously called "fib-flutter" due to the apparent flutter waves in lead V1. However, the variable atrial cycle length and changing morphology of atrial depolarizations makes this ECG diagnostic of atrial fibrillation

unmasks subtle variation in the amplitudes and frequency of apparent flutter waves that reveal the true rhythm to be AF. In the setting of complete AV block with a junctional escape, accelerated junctional rhythms, ventricular tachycardia or ventricular pacing, the ventricular rate in AF can be regular. In such cases, it is important to focus on the nature of the atrial activity to make the diagnosis of AF. Sometimes, temporary inhibition of pacing function may be necessary to unmask AF. When QRS morphology is highly variable in AF and ventricular rate exceeds 200 beats per minute, ventricular pre-excitation or ventricular tachycardia should be suspected.

DIAGNOSTIC TESTING

All patients presenting with new-onset AF should undergo appropriate testing for a reversible cause.[1] A careful history of medication use and substance use, particularly alcohol, should be obtained. AF can often be the only presenting sign of hyperthyroidism, so all patients with new-onset AF should receive an assessment of thyroid function. Additional laboratory testing should be guided by the history and physical examination. Although AF frequently accompanies acute coronary syndromes and stable coronary artery disease, it is rarely the only sign of active ischemia. Thus, in the absence of other symptoms suggestive of active ischemic heart disease, it is not necessary for patients with AF to undergo stress testing or coronary angiography. All patients with AF should receive an echocardiogram, since the most common cause of AF is structural heart disease.

Because episodes of AF can be brief, can occur in sleep and can be asymptomatic, the clinical history is often not reflective of a patient's overall burden of AF (the fraction of time the patient is in AF).[70,73] In patients with symptoms compatible with AF, but no clear evidence at presentation, cardiac monitoring for extended periods can be helpful. Unless episodes are very frequent, Holter monitoring is often of insufficient duration to capture the episodes. Event monitors with telephonic transmission and automatic triggering algorithms for detecting and recording AF can be very useful to confirm a diagnosis, determine whether symptoms are due to AF, determine the burden of AF and determine whether symptoms are due to poorly controlled ventricular rates.[74]

MANAGEMENT

NEW-ONSET ATRIAL FIBRILLATION

Newly diagnosed AF should prompt a diagnostic work up as outlined above for a reversible cause. In general, when a reversible cause is identified, initial treatment should be directed at the underlying precipitating factor rather than the AF. Patients with new-onset AF presenting to the emergency room can in most cases be managed safely without hospital admission.[75] Hospital admission may be warranted for patients with concurrent medical conditions requiring inpatient treatment, for the elderly, and for patients with significant structural heart disease, ischemia, hemodynamic instability or preexcited AF.

Immediate reversion to sinus rhythm is warranted in patients with hemodynamic instability, active ischemia, severe heart failure symptoms, or AF with ventricular preexcitation.[1] In such cases, while it is ideal to confirm absence of an intracardiac thrombus using a transesophageal echocardiogram, this may not be possible due to the urgency of the situation. At a minimum, systemic anticoagulation should be administered prior to cardioversion unless strongly contraindicated.

When urgent cardioversion is not indicated, it is acceptable to pursue an initial rate control strategy for patients who are mildly or moderately symptomatic. This approach allows time for a diagnostic workup, treatment of a potentially reversible cause of AF, and for an assessment of thromboembolic risk. About 70% of patients with new-onset AF of less than 72 hours duration will spontaneously convert to sinus rhythm without intervention.[76] For the remainder, reversion to sinus rhythm with cardioversion, either electrical or chemical, may be reasonable if the risk of short-term AF recurrence is relatively low or unknown. This is the case in younger patients (< 65) with structurally normal hearts and in patients with reversible causes for AF once the underlying cause is addressed. Antiarrhythmic drug therapy is generally reserved for patients with recurrent AF and is not routinely administered to patients after cardioversion for new-onset AF. Appropriate thromboembolic prophylaxis is essential before and after cardioversion (discussed under heading "Prevention of Thromboembolism").

RATE CONTROL VERSUS RHYTHM CONTROL IN RECURRENT AF

In approaching the patient with recurrent paroxysmal or persistent AF, the clinician must decide whether to attempt to maintain sinus rhythm. Theoretically, maintaining sinus rhythm would prevent symptoms associated with AF, normalize heart rate, maintain AV synchrony and the atrial contribution to cardiac output, and prevent deleterious atrial remodeling. Moreover, the epidemiological data on outcomes in AF raise hope that patients in whom sinus rhythm can be maintained might have improved quality of life and reduced mortality. On the other hand, the pharmacological tools available to maintain sinus rhythm are limited, and the attempt to maintain AF may be associated with side effects of these medications.

Two large clinical trials, AFFIRM and rate control versus electrical cardioversion (RACE), along with several smaller trials, have tested prospectively whether attempting to maintain sinus rhythm using antiarrhythmic drugs in patients with AF results is better clinical outcomes than simply controlling the ventricular rate in AF.[77,78] Two critical findings emerged from these studies: first, that there was no clear mortality benefit, cardiovascular benefit or clinically significant functional improvement associated with pursuing a rhythm control strategy in the patients enrolled in these studies; and second, that the incidence of thromboembolic events was similar regardless of the strategy chosen (Figs 5A and B). The latter finding likely reflected the relatively poor efficacy of rhythm control in these patients: although 63% remained free of symptomatic AF in AFFIRM at 5 years after randomization, many of these patients had subclinical episodes of AF that contribute to thrombo-embolic risk.

It is important to recognize that the failure to demonstrate benefit to rhythm control is not due to a clinical equivalence

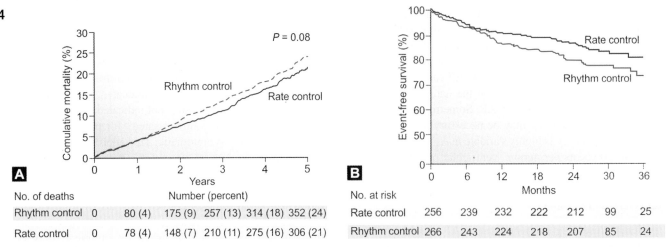

FIGURES 5A AND B: Comparison of outcomes in patients with AF pursuing a rhythm control and rate control strategy in two large clinical trials: (A) Data from AFFIRM shows no statistically significant difference in overall mortality, although there is a trend toward increased mortality with rhythm control. (*Source:* Wyse DG, Waldo AL, DiMarco JP, et al. A comparison of rate control and rhythm control in patients with atrial fibrillation. N Engl J Med. 2002;347:1825-33, with permission). (B) Similar findings were seen in the RACE trial for a composite endpoint including mortality and other adverse events. (*Source:* Van Gelder IC, Hagens VE, Bosker HA, et al. A comparison of rate control and rhythm control in patients with recurrent persistent atrial fibrillation. N Engl J Med. 2002;347:1834-40, with permission)

between sinus rhythm and rate-controlled AF. Rather, patients in the rhythm control arms of these trials had antiarrhythmic drug-related side effects and an overall increase in non-cardiovascular death,[79] along with frequent recurrences of AF despite the attempt at rhythm control. Indeed, analysis of mortality data from AFFIRM and RACE has shown that patients who were in sinus rhythm throughout the study, regardless of treatment arm chosen, had a hazard ratio for mortality of 0.53 compared to those in AF.[79,80] However, it is unclear whether the improved mortality was due to the fact that they were in sinus rhythm or whether those patients in whom sinus rhythm could be maintained with available therapy had fewer co-morbidities or other factors that was associated with lower mortality risks regardless of what rhythm they were in. In these studies, any benefit was likely counterbalanced by drug toxicity and limited efficacy in the other patients, yielding a net equivalence of the two approaches. Thus, while maintaining sinus rhythm is in general a desirable outcome, the pharma-cological tools employed in these studies lacked the safety and efficacy to do so in a way that provided net benefit in an unselected patient population. It should be noted that these studies were undertaken prior to the wide availability of catheter ablation for AF, which might significantly change the efficacy of sinus rhythm maintenance and the frequency of adverse events associated with rhythm control.

At a minimum, these studies legitimized rate control as a reasonable treatment option in asymptomatic patients. Currently, there is no algorithmic or guideline-driven approach that determines in whom rhythm control should be attempted. Relevant considerations are age, comorbidities, patient preference, risk of antiarrhythmic drugs, the likelihood of maintaining sinus rhythm, and whether the patient has symptoms due to AF even with adequate rate control. Thus, in older patients with structural heart disease and/or hypertension and no symptoms, rate control may be a reasonable first strategy; while in younger patients or in patients with lone AF with symptoms, rhythm control may be a reasonable initial choice.

RESTORATION OF SINUS RHYTHM

Once a rhythm control strategy is selected, the initial step is to restore sinus rhythm. Reversion to sinus rhythm without early recurrence of AF is more likely when the duration of AF is less than one year, the left atrium is not markedly enlarged, and structural heart disease is minimal.[81] In unselected patients with AF, electrical cardioversion is associated with a 1–2% short-term risk of clinical thromboembolism in the absence of anticoagulation.[82] This risk can be reduced to an acceptable level if patients are therapeutic on warfarin for 1 month prior to the procedure, or if a transesophageal echo performed immediately prior to cardioversion reveals no intracardiac thrombus and intravenous heparin is administered prior to cardioversion.[83] It is also safe to cardiovert low-risk patients without a history of rheumatic heart disease or prior thromboembolism when the duration of the AF episode is less than 48 hours without a TEE. In these cases, intravenous heparin or equivalent should be administered before cardioversion.[84] After cardioversion, either electrical or chemical, a period of atrial stunning ensues, in which atrial function is reduced and the potential for thrombus formation remains high.[85] For that reason, patients should be therapeutically anticoagulated from the time of cardioversion for at least 1 month. After that, thromboembolic risk should be reassessed and addressed as indicated.

Electrical cardioversion is highly effective for restoration of sinus rhythm in patients with paroxysmal AF. Seventy to ninety percent of patients can be converted to SR using biphasic shocks.[86] Chemical cardioversion is also effective for reversion to sinus rhythm, but in general it is not as effective as electrical cardioversion. Class III agents, such as amiodarone, ibutilide and dofetilide, are the most effective drugs for cardioversion of long-standing AF, while class 1C agents flecainide and propafenone are also effective when the duration of AF is less than 7 days.[1] When using ibutilide or dofetilide, special attention should be paid to electrolytes and QT interval, as these medications confer a significant short-term risk of torsades-de-pointes. Facilitated electrical cardioversion, in which patients are loaded on an antiarrhythmic drug prior to cardioversion, can improve the success rate for patients who fail conventional electrical cardioversion.[87]

MAINTENANCE OF SINUS RHYTHM—PHARMACOLOGICAL APPROACHES

In general, once a decision to attempt rhythm control has been made, the choice of anti-arrhythmic drugs is primarily dictated by risks and side-effect potential, which are largely determined by the presence or absence of structural heart disease. Flow chart 1 shows a scheme recommended in the 2006 ACC/AHA/ESC Guidelines for management of AF. This section presents an overview of the Class 1 and Class 3 medications used to maintain sinus rhythm and the evidence supporting their use in specific populations.

Class 1: Antiarrhythmic Drugs

The class 1C medications flecainide and propafenone are effective for maintaining sinus rhythm in patients with paroxysmal AF and are widely used as first-line therapy in selected patients.[88–90] While these medications can be taken on a standing basis for rhythm maintenance, they can also be used on an as-needed basis ("pill-in-the-pocket" approach) for patients with symptomatic paroxysmal AF.[91] The main cardiac side effects of these agents are pro-arrhythmia and increased mortality in patients with ischemic or structural heart disease,[92] brady-arrhythmias in patients with infranodal conduction system disease, and worsening heart failure in patients with LV dysfunction. 1C agents are therefore not recommended for use in patients with any structural heart lesions. Since the ventricular pro-arrhythmia is thought to occur during ischemia, even asymptomatic patients on 1C agents should be screened for ischemic heart disease while receiving drug therapy. In addition, class 1C medications can convert AF to atrial flutter that can be conducted 1:1 by the AV node, resulting in extremely rapid ventricular response.[93] Patients on 1C medications should therefore also take an AV nodal blocking agent unless AV conduction is not present or is significantly impaired. In the past, the Class 1A antiarrhythmic drugs, such as quinidine or procainamide, have been used for sinus rhythm maintenance in patients with AF. These agents are no longer widely used for treatment of AF because they are often poorly tolerated.[94]

Class 3: Antiarrhythmic Drugs

Although amiodarone is not FDA approved for the treatment of AF, it is widely used for this indication and is the most effective antiarrhythmic agent for sinus rhythm maintenance.[95] Although it has minimal proarrhythmic effects, its extra-cardiac side effect profile is significant, particularly at higher doses and with prolonged treatment.[96] In clinical trials, amiodarone was discontinued due to side effects more often than sotalol or propafenone. Nevertheless, amiodarone had significantly greater efficacy than the other drugs.[97] Despite its side effects, it is also safe to use in patients with heart failure and in patients with CAD.[98,99] For these reasons (efficacy and safety), amiodarone is frequently the drug of choice for short-term use and for patients with significant comorbidities. Nevertheless, because of extra-cardiac side effects, the 2006 ACC/AHA/ESC guidelines recommend that amiodarone be used as a second-line therapy except for patients with heart failure, moderate-to-severe systolic dysfunction, or hypertension and significant left ventricular hypertrophy. Amiodarone has an additional use in the prevention of postoperative AF after cardiac surgery, where a short perioperative course cuts the incidence of AF by about 50%.[100]

CHAPTER 33

Atrial Fibrillation

FLOW CHART 1: 2006 American College of Cardiology (ACC)/American Heart Association (AHA)/European Society of Cardiology (ESC) algorithm for antiarrhythmic drug therapy to maintain sinus rhythm in patients with recurrent paroxysmal or persistent AF. Patients should first be categorized by severity of heart disease (left to right) and treatment selection should proceed from top to bottom. Within boxes, drugs are listed alphabetically and not by order of preference

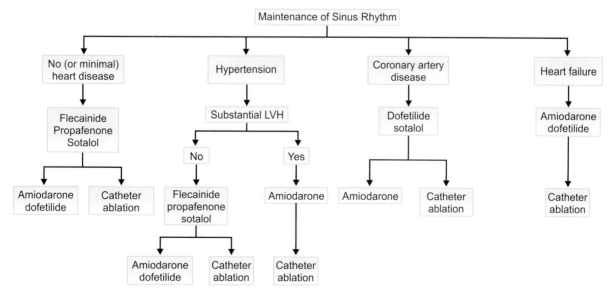

(*Source:* Reference 1)

Sotalol is roughly equal in efficacy to propafenone in randomized trials and significantly less effective that amiodarone in maintaining sinus rhythm.[97] Its effects are highly dose-dependent, with greater rhythm maintenance effects at higher doses and predominantly beta-blocking effects at lower doses.[101] The presence of beta-blocking effects can be helpful in slowing ventricular rate during recurrences of AF.[102] Side effects can include bradycardia and QT interval prolongation. For that reason, it is essential to monitor the QT interval in patients taking sotalol and to avoid use of the drug in patients at risk for QT interval prolongation or with significant impairment in drug clearance due to kidney disease. In most cases, inpatient monitoring is required for initiation of sotalol due to the risk of torsades de pointes and bradyarrhythmias.

Dofetilide is at least as effective as sotalol in maintaining sinus rhythm in patients with recurrent AF.[103] Although dofetilide prolongs the QT interval in a dose-dependent fashion and can cause torsades de pointes, an increase in mortality has not been observed in clinical trials of dofetilide use for AF.[104] This is likely because dofetilide is administered during inpatient monitoring with careful assessment of QT interval and dose adjustment or discontinuation as needed. Dofetilide is also safe and effective in patients with severe heart failure, in whom it reduces AF recurrences and heart failure hospitalizations without affecting mortality.[105] However, because of the potential for proarrhythmia with this medication, dofetilide is as considered a second-line medication except for patients with heart failure or coronary artery disease.

Dronedarone is a non-iodinated chemical derivative of amiodarone that lacks extracardiac side effects such as pulmonary, thyroid and ocular toxicity. Several large clinical trials have found that it can be effective in maintaining sinus rhythm, although less than amiodarone. However, unlike amiodarone, dronedarone appears to cause increased mortality in patients with severe heart failure.[106] In patients with normal cardiac function or mild-to-moderate heart failure, a large prospective randomized trial found a significant reduction in a composite primary outcome of hospitalization for cardiovascular causes and cardiovascular death, without a significant effect on overall mortality.[107]

Modulators of the RAAS System

Due to the role of the RAAS system in the pathogenesis of AF, the use of angiotensin receptor blockers (ARB) and angiotensin converting enzyme inhibitors has been explored in AF. A recent meta-analysis of 23 randomized trials showed a roughly 33% reduction in AF episodes associated with RAAS inhibition.[108] Particularly for patients with hypertension, left ventricular dysfunction or diabetes, but possibly even for patients without many comorbidities, RAAS inhibition can be an important adjunctive therapy for AF.

MAINTENANCE OF SINUS RHYTHM—INVASIVE APPROACHES

Nonpharmacological approaches to maintenance of sinus rhythm include catheter ablation, surgical ablation, pacing, and atrial defibrillation. The finding that physiological pacing modes in bradycardic patients with AF can prevent recurrences has led to a variety of pacing strategies to maintain sinus rhythm, including multisite pacing, alternative site pacing, and overdrive suppression of AF. With the exception of small subpopulations these strategies have not been shown to be effective.[109] Patients with AF should therefore not receive permanent pacemakers for the purpose of AF suppression, although selection of physiological pacing modes and minimization of ventricular pacing can prevent AF episodes in patients receiving pacemakers for other reasons. Thus far, the safety, efficacy and tolerability of implantable atrial defibrillators have not been demonstrated in large trials, and therefore these devices remain largely investigational.

Catheter Ablation

The development of catheter ablation for AF began with the observation that rapid firing originating in the pulmonary veins frequently triggered AF.[32] This finding led to the idea of electrically isolating the pulmonary venous myocardium from the left atrium using radiofrequency ablation.[110–112] Since the original description of this approach, intensive development and testing of different approaches and techniques has taken place (Figs 6A and B).

At present, ablation techniques for AF vary widely among practitioners and the optimal approach has yet to be defined.[113] Most commonly, contiguous or nearly contiguous lesions are created around each of the four pulmonary veins, and electrical isolation is confirmed with a combination of recording and pacing within the pulmonary veins. Many ablationists also target non-pulmonary vein AF triggers such as autonomic ganglia, the ligament and vein of Marshall, the superior vena cava,[114] the posterior left atrial wall and the left atrial appendage.[115] There has also been interest in modifying the atrial substrate using catheter ablation, particularly for patients with permanent AF. Additional ablations are sometimes performed in areas displaying complex, fractionated electrograms that may play a role in AF maintenance,[116] although the added benefit of such an approach has yet to be established in large clinical trials.[117]

Because ablation causes atrial inflammation in the short run, early recurrence of AF is common after ablation and does not necessarily indicate long-term procedural non-success.[118] For this reason, success is usually defined as symptomatic improvement with no evidence of AF after a post-procedure blanking period. When AF recurs after the blanking period, the most common reason is reconnection of pulmonary venous myocardium to the atria, which may necessitate additional ablation procedures.[119] Catheter ablation is most effective in patients with paroxysmal AF, normal atrial size and minimal structural heart disease.[120] Success rates of 70–90% at 1 year have been reported for such patients.[113] When patients with structural heart disease, heart failure and increased atrial size are included in such studies, success rate declines. Success can be achieved in some patients by adding an antiarrhythmic medication after ablation, even when the medication was not effective prior to ablation.

Although AF ablation has become safer as techniques have improved, there is potential for serious complications. In addition to the usual risks associated with invasive cardiac procedures, such as thromboembolism, cardiac perforation, and vascular complications, AF ablation also carries the risks of

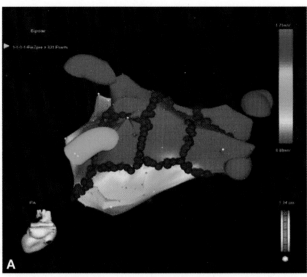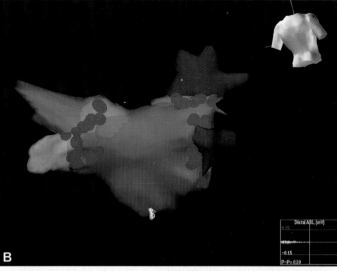

FIGURES 6A AND B: Two approaches to atrial fibrillation ablation: (A) Linear left atrial ablation. Linear lesions (red balls) are shown superimposed on a posterior-anterior view of the left atrium generated with the CARTO electroanatomical mapping system (Biosense). The following lines are represented: A wide area circumferential ablation around the left and right pulmonary veins, a line from the left inferior pulmonary vein to the mitral annulus, lines between the upper and the lower pulmonary veins, and two lines along the posterior left atrium connecting the circumferential ablations. Reproduced with permission from: Pappone C and Santinelli V. Heart Rhythm. 2006;3:1105-9. (B) Segmental pulmonary vein isolation. In this approach, lesions (red balls) are created surrounding the ostia of the four pulmonary veins in ordert to achieve electrical isolation. A PA view is shown, with lesions superimposed on a CT registered electroanatomic map created with the NavX system (St. Jude Medical). (*Source.* Dr Nitish Badhwar)

iatrogenic left atrial flutter,[121] pulmonary vein stenosis,[122] extracardiac nerve injury[113] and atrial-esophageal fistula.[123] Although these complications are uncommon, they can be devastating when they occur. These concerns, along with limited data on long-term efficacy, are reflected in the 2006 ACC/AHA/ESC guidelines, in which ablation is second-line therapy for AF. While the results of initial trials of ablation versus antiarrhythmic drug therapy for paroxysmal AF have generally favored the invasive approach,[124–126] this comparison has not yet been made in large multicenter trials, nor has the question of whether anticoagulation can be discontinued after successful AF ablation. Trials currently underway will hopefully shed additional light on these issues and help to clarify the proper place of catheter ablation in a rhythm maintenance strategy.

Surgical Procedures for AF Maintenance

Surgical procedures to maintain sinus rhythm in patients with AF predate the era of catheter ablation.[127] The Cox MAZE procedure, which may include a "cut and sew" approach or an ablation approach, involves making a patchwork of lesions in the atrium to create lines of scar. The lines of scar presumably prevent reentry circuits from sustaining and are believed to prevent vulnerable atrial substrate from maintaining AF. As with catheter ablation, many different lesion sets, ablative methods and strategies have been employed for surgical AF ablation.[128–130] Observational studies suggest that these techniques are highly effective; however, large randomized trials have not been carried out and surgical technique is highly variable, so overall efficacy of surgical management of AF is not known.[131,132] In addition, sinus node injury or exit block requiring permanent pacing can complicate the procedures, and atrial function may be permanently impaired.[133,134] Finally, as with catheter ablation, lesion sets can be proarrhythmic by creating conduction barriers and

slowing conduction velocity, thereby facilitating macro-reentrant circuits.[135] Because these procedures require open cardiac surgery with cardioplegia and cross-clamping of the aorta, they are usually performed on patients who require cardiac surgery for a structural lesion associated with AF such as mitral valve disease.

STRATEGIES FOR RATE CONTROL

The recommended target for rate control in AF is 80 bpm at rest and less than 120 bpm with moderate activity, although these numbers are not based on prospective trials.[1] Recent prospective data, in which patients randomized to a permissive rate control arm had no worse outcomes than patients in whom strict rate control was achieved have called these numbers into question.[136] Further research will be necessary to determine the optimal targets for rate control.

The mainstays for rate control in AF are beta-adrenergic blockers and the non-dihydropyridine calcium channel blockers diltiazem and verapamil. These medications slow AV nodal conduction and prolong AV nodal refractoriness, thereby reducing the frequency of fibrillatory waves that can be conducted to the ventricles. In retrospective studies of AFFIRM patients, beta-blockers alone or combined with digoxin were most effective for rate control.[137] In patients with reduced EF and symptoms of heart failure in AF, intravenous calcium channel blockers should be avoided due to the potential for causing symptomatic hypotension and in severe cases precipitating cardiogenic shock. In such patients, beta-blockers, amiodarone or digoxin are preferred. As oral therapy for ambulatory AF patients, digoxin can be a useful adjunctive agent for rate control, but is less effective as monotherapy for rate control in AF and should not be used in this way.[137] Dronederone is also an effective rate control agent and can be used for this purpose even if not effective at maintaining sinus rhythm. The side-effect profile and pharmacokinetics may make this more attractive than amiodarone for this purpose.

Not infrequently, patients with paroxysmal AF and rapid ventricular response requiring rate control medications will experience sinus pauses or symptomatic bradycardia when AF converts spontaneously to sinus rhythm. Since rate control medications are essential in these patients, permanent pacemaker implantation may become necessary to permit higher doses of nodal agents. Conversely, in patients in whom attempts at rate control have failed or are not tolerated and are not candidates for rhythm control, catheter ablation of the AV junction with pacemaker implantation is highly effective for rate control.[138,139] For patients whose symptoms are primarily due to elevated heart rates, this is a very effective therapy for symptomatic AF.

PREVENTION OF THROMBOEMBOLISM

It is imperative that all patients with AF undergo risk stratification for thromboembolic events, regardless of AF type and regardless of treatment strategy (rhythm control vs rate control).[1] Anticoagulation with warfarin lowers the risk of stroke for nearly all patients with AF;[140] however, in the lowest risk patients, the risk of major bleeding due to warfarin therapy exceeds the value of this marginal risk reduction.[141] For such patients, aspirin can be an acceptable alternative. To facilitate the categorization of AF patients by stroke risk, prediction tools have been developed based on pooled data from several large stroke prevention trials and other smaller studies.

Patients with AF due to rheumatic heart disease represent the highest risk group because of the marked atrial enlargement and consequent stasis that typically accompanies mitral stenosis. These patients should be anticoagulated with warfarin unless a strong contraindication is present. For patients with non-valvular AF, several studies have evaluated the clinical predictors for stroke. The Atrial Fibrillation Investigators (AFI), using pooled data from several trials, and the Stroke Prevention and Atrial Fibrillation (SPAF) investigators each used data from the non-treatment arms of primary prevention trials of stroke in AF patients.[142,143] Clinical factors that predicted risk of stroke were then integrated to form the CHADS2 score, and this tool was validated using results from the National Registry of Atrial Fibrillation.[11] The CHADS2 score assigns 1 point each for a history of congestive heart failure, hypertension, age greater than 74, diabetes mellitus and two points for a prior history of systemic embolic event. An overall risk score of 0 suggests low risk, 1 or 2 suggests intermediate risk and greater than 2 is considered high risk (Table 3). Based on these data, current guidelines recommend aspirin for patients with a CHADS2 score of 0 and warfarin in patients with a CHADS2 score of 2 or greater. Patients with a CHADS2 score of 1 may use aspirin or warfarin depending on comorbidities and patient preference. Currently there are no other approved pharmacological treatments to prevent strokes; however, there are several direct thrombin inhibitors and factor Xa inhibitors under various phases of study.[144] Nonpharmacological treatments to prevent strokes in AF have targeted the left atrial appendage, either by occlusion or removal. While this has traditionally been accomplished by surgery,[145] there are several transvenous devices under investigation that occlude or ligate the left atrial appendage.[146] These approaches may be useful in patients at high risk for stroke, but who are not capable of taking Coumadin or in patients who have had a stroke from AF on therapeutic doses of Coumadin. While small clinical trials have demonstrated the feasibility of percutaneous approaches,[147,148] large randomized clinical trials to test rigorously for reduction in stroke have not been carried out.

CONCLUSION

Although major advances in the understanding and treatment of AF have occurred recently—such as the understanding of the role of the pulmonary veins in AF and the development of catheter ablation for AF—we still do not have an understanding of the etiology of the underlying substrate of AF and thus no targeted treatments to prevent or reverse AF exist. Current treatment strategies are aimed at preventing stroke, and either rate control or rhythm control to prevent rapid ventricular rates and symptoms. If the latter approach is chosen, the choice of rhythm control drugs is dictated by side-effect profile and risk, rather than efficacy, since efficacies are similar for long term. Until rigorous multi-center randomized trials have been completed, ablation is reserved for symptomatic patients with paroxysmal AF who are intolerant or resistant to pharmacological rhythm control. Success rate for ablation of persistent and permanent AF is significantly lower than that for paroxysmal AF. In general, treatment options for persistent and permanent AF are limited to stroke prevention and rate control. Future research will hopefully define the substrate(s) that predispose to AF and thereby allow directed therapy to prevent or reverse AF.

TABLE 3

Event rates by stroke risk factor, baseline CHADS2 score, and anticoagulation status in 11,526 adults with atrial fibrillation and no conraindications to warfarin therapy at baseline

CHADS2 score (no. of patients)	Event rate (per 100 person-years) (95% confidence interval)		
	Taking warfarin	Not taking warfarin	Crude rate ratio (95% confidence interval)
0 (2557)	0.25 (0.11–0.55)	0.49 (0.30–0.78)	0.50 (0.2–1.28)
1 (3662)	0.72 (0.50–1.03)	1.52 (1.19–1.94)	0.47 (0.30–0.73)
2 (2955)	1.27 (0.94–1.72)	2.50 (1.98–3.15)	0.51 (0.35–0.75)
3 (1555)	2.20 (1.61–3.01)	5.27 (4.15–6.70)	0.42 (0.28–0.62)
4 (556)	2.35 (1.44–3.83)	6.02 (3.90–9.29)	0.39 (0.20–0.75)
5 or 6 (241)	4.60 (2.72–7.76)	6.88 (3.42–13.84)	0.67 (0.28–1.60)
(*Source:* Reference 148)			

2006 ACC/AHA ESC guidelines: Pharmacological management of newly discovered AF

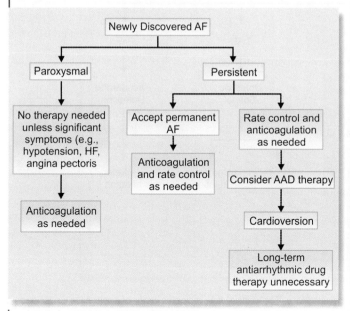

(Abbreviation: AAD: Antiarrhythmic drugs). (*Source:* Fuster V, et al. J Am Coll Cardiol. 2006;48(4):e149-e246)

2006 ACC/AHA/ESC guidelines: Pharmacological management of recurrent paroxysmal AF

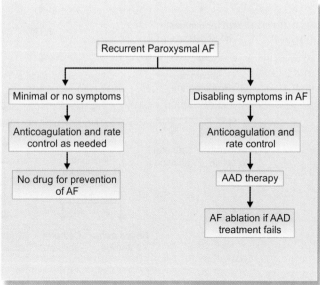

(*Source:* Fuster V, et al. J Am Coll Cardiol. 2006;48(4):e149-e246)

2006 ACC/AHA ESC guidelines: Pharmacological management of recurrent persistent or permanent AF

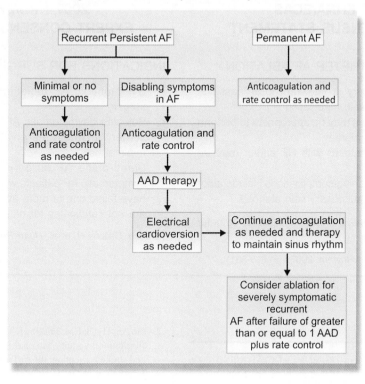

(*Source:* Fuster V, et al. J Am Coll Cardiol. 2006;48(4):e149-e246)

CHAPTER 33

Atrial Fibrillation

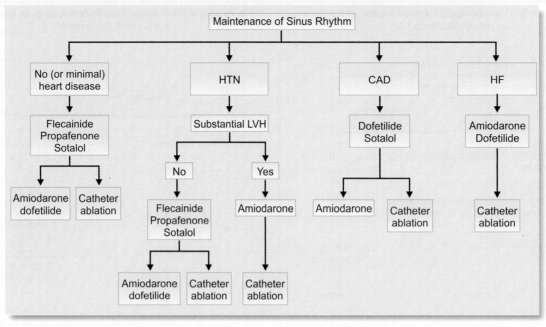

2006 ACC/AHA/ESC guidelines: Antiarrhythmic approaches to maintain sinus rhythm in patients with recurrent paroxysmal or persistent AF who require sinus rhythm*

*Within each box, drugs are listed alphabetically and not in order of suggested use. The vertical flow indicates order of preference under each condition. The seriousness of heart disease proceeds from left to right, and selection of therapy in patientw with multiple conditions depends on the most serious condition present. (Abbreviation: LVH: Left ventricular hypertrophy). (*Source:* Fuster V, et al. J Am Coll Cardiol. 2006;48(4):e149-e246).

2007 HRS/EHRA/ECAS EXPERT CONSENSUS STATEMENT

INDICATIONS FOR CATHETER AF ABLATION

- Symptomatic AF refractory or intolerant to at least one Class 1 or 3 antiarrhythmic medication
- In rare clinical situations, it may be appropriate to perform AF ablation as first-line therapy
- Selected symptomatic patients with HF and/or reduced ejection fraction
- Potential rare, life-threatening complications include atrio-esophageal fistula and pulmonary vein stenosis

[Presence of a LA thrombus is a contraindication to catheter ablation of AF]

(*Source:* Calkins H, et al. *Heart Rhythm.* 2007;4(6):816-861)

2007 HRS/EHRA/ECAS EXPERT CONSENSUS STATEMENT

INDICATIONS FOR SURGICAL ABLATION

- Symptomatic AF patients undergoing other cardiac surgery
- Selected asymptomatic AF patients undergoing cardiac surgery in whom the ablation can be performed with minimal risk
- Stand-alone AF surgery should be considered for symptomatic AF patients who prefer a surgical approach, have failed one or more attempts at catheter ablation, or are not candidates for catheter ablation

(*Source:* Calkins H, et al. *Heart Rhythm.* 2007;4(6):816-861)

REFERENCES

1. Fuster V, Rydén LE, Cannom DS, et al. ACC/AHA/ESC 2006 Guidelines for the Management of Patients with Atrial Fibrillation: a report of the American College of Cardiology/American Heart Association Task Force on Practice Guidelines and the European Society of Cardiology Committee for Practice Guidelines (Writing Committee to Revise the 2001 Guidelines for the Management of Patients With Atrial Fibrillation): developed in collaboration with the European Heart Rhythm Association and the Heart Rhythm Society. Circulation. 2006;114:e257-e354.

2. Go AS, Hylek EM, Phillips KA, et al. Prevalence of diagnosed atrial fibrillation in adults: national implications for rhythm management and stroke prevention: the AnTicoagulation and Risk Factors in Atrial Fibrillation (ATRIA) study. JAMA. 2001;285:2370-5.

3. Miyasaka Y, Barnes ME, Gersh BJ, et al. Secular trends in incidence of atrial fibrillation in Olmsted County, Minnesota, 1980 to 2000, and implications on the projections for future prevalence. Circulation. 2006;114:119-25.

4. Heeringa J, van der Kuip DAM, Hofman A, et al. Prevalence, incidence and lifetime risk of atrial fibrillation: the Rotterdam study. European Heart Journal. 2006;27:949-53.

5. Naccarelli GV, Varker H, Lin J, et al. Increasing prevalence of atrial fibrillation and flutter in the United States. Am J Cardiol. 2009;104:1534-9.

6. Kerr CR, Humphries KH, Talajic M, et al. Progression to chronic atrial fibrillation after the initial diagnosis of paroxysmal atrial fibrillation: results from the Canadian Registry of Atrial Fibrillation. Am Heart J. 2005;149:489-96.

7. Kopecky SL, Gersh BJ, McGoon MD, et al. The natural history of lone atrial fibrillation. A population-based study over three decades. N Engl J Med. 1987;317:669-74.

8. Stewart S, Hart CL, Hole DJ, et al. A population-based study of the long-term risks associated with atrial fibrillation: 20-year follow-up of the Renfrew/Paisley study. Am J Med. 2002;113:359-64.

9. Benjamin EJ, Wolf PA, D'Agostino RB, et al. Impact of atrial fibrillation on the risk of death: the Framingham heart study. Circulation. 1998;98:946-52.

10. Frost L, Engholm G, Johnsen S, et al. Incident stroke after discharge from the hospital with a diagnosis of atrial fibrillation. Am J Med. 2000;108:36-40.

11. Gage BF, Waterman AD, Shannon W, et al. Validation of clinical classification schemes for predicting stroke: results from the National Registry of Atrial Fibrillation. JAMA. 2001;285:2864-70.

12. Anderson DC, Kappelle LJ, Eliasziw M, et al. Occurrence of hemispheric and retinal ischemia in atrial fibrillation compared with carotid stenosis. Stroke. 2002;33:1963-7.

13. Lin HJ, Wolf PA, Kelly-Hayes M, et al. Stroke severity in atrial fibrillation. The Framingham Study. Stroke. 1996;27:1760-4.

14. Jorgensen HS, Nakayama H, Reith J, et al. Acute stroke with atrial fibrillation. The Copenhagen Stroke Study. Stroke. 1996;27:1765-9.

15. Lamassa M, Di Carlo A, Pracucci G, et al. Characteristics, outcome, and care of stroke associated with atrial fibrillation in Europe: data from a multicenter multinational hospital-based registry (The European Community Stroke Project). Stroke. 2001;32:392-8.

16. Ott A, Breteler MM, de Bruyne MC, et al. Atrial fibrillation and dementia in a population-based study. The Rotterdam Study. Stroke. 1997;28:316-21.

17. Kilander L, Andren B, Nyman H, et al. Atrial fibrillation is an independent determinant of low cognitive function: a cross-sectional study in elderly men. Stroke. 1998;29:1816-20.

18. Miyasaka Y, Barnes ME, Petersen RC, et al. Risk of dementia in stroke-free patients diagnosed with atrial fibrillation: data from a community-based cohort. Eur Heart J. 2007;28:1962-7.

19. Dries DL, Exner DV, Gersh BJ, et al. Atrial fibrillation is associated with an increased risk for mortality and heart failure progression in patients with asymptomatic and symptomatic left ventricular systolic dysfunction: a retrospective analysis of the SOLVD trials. Studies of left ventricular dysfunction. J Am Coll Cardiol. 1998;32:695-703.

20. Olsson LG, Swedberg K, Ducharme A, et al. Atrial fibrillation and risk of clinical events in chronic heart failure with and without left ventricular systolic dysfunction: results from the Candesartan in Heart failure-Assessment of Reduction in Mortality and morbidity (CHARM) program. J Am Coll Cardiol. 2006;47:1997-2004.

21. Carson PE, Johnson GR, Dunkman WB, et al. The influence of atrial fibrillation on prognosis in mild to moderate heart failure. The V-HeFT Studies. The V-HeFT VA Cooperative Studies Group. Circulation. 1993;87:VI102-10.

22. Vaziri SM, Larson MG, Benjamin EJ, et al. Echocardiographic predictors of nonrheumatic atrial fibrillation. The Framingham Heart Study. Circulation. 1994;89:724-30.

23. Diker E, Aydogdu S, Ozdemir M, et al. Prevalence and predictors of atrial fibrillation in rheumatic valvular heart disease. Am J Cardiol. 1996;77:96-8.

24. Maisel WH, Stevenson LW. Atrial fibrillation in heart failure: epidemiology, pathophysiology, and rationale for therapy. Am J Cardiol. 2003;91:2D-8D.

25. Kieny JR, Sacrez A, Facello A, et al. Increase in radionuclide left ventricular ejection fraction after cardioversion of chronic atrial fibrillation in idiopathic dilated cardiomyopathy. Eur Heart J. 1992;13:1290-5.

26. Redfield MM, Kay GN, Jenkins LS, et al. Tachycardia-related cardiomyopathy: a common cause of ventricular dysfunction in patients with atrial fibrillation referred for atrioventricular ablation. Mayo Clin Proc. 2000;75:790-5.

27. Crenshaw BS, Ward SR, Granger CB, et al. Atrial fibrillation in the setting of acute myocardial infarction: the GUSTO-I experience. Global utilization of streptokinase and TPA for occluded coronary arteries. J Am Coll Cardiol. 1997;30:406-13.

28. Wong CK, White HD, Wilcox RG, et al. New atrial fibrillation after acute myocardial infarction independently predicts death: the GUSTO-III experience. Am Heart J. 2000;140:878-85.

29. Robinson K, Frenneaux MP, Stockins B, et al. Atrial fibrillation in hypertrophic cardiomyopathy: a longitudinal study. J Am Coll Cardiol. 1990;15:1279-85.

30. Pires LA, Wagshal AB, Lancey R, et al. Arrhythmias and conduction disturbances after coronary artery bypass graft surgery: epidemiology, management, and prognosis. Am Heart J. 1995;129:799-808.

31. Maisel WH, Rawn JD, Stevenson WG. Atrial fibrillation after cardiac surgery. Ann Intern Med. 2001;135:1061-73.

32. Haissaguerre M, Jais P, Shah DC, et al. Spontaneous initiation of atrial fibrillation by ectopic beats originating in the pulmonary veins. N Engl J Med. 1998;339:659-66.

33. Chen SA, Hsieh MH, Tai CT, et al. Initiation of atrial fibrillation by ectopic beats originating from the pulmonary veins: electrophysiological characteristics, pharmacological responses, and effects of radiofrequency ablation. Circulation. 1999;100:1879-86.

34. Chen SA, Tai CT, Hsieh MH, et al. Radiofrequency catheter ablation of atrial fibrillation initiated by spontaneous ectopic beats. Curr Cardiol Rep. 2000;2:322-8.

35. Wit AL, Boyden PA. Triggered activity and atrial fibrillation. Heart Rhythm. 2007;4:S17-S23.

36. Sauer WH, Alonso C, Zado E, et al. Atrioventricular nodal reentrant tachycardia in patients referred for atrial fibrillation ablation: response to ablation that incorporates slow-pathway modification. Circulation. 2006;114:191-5.

37. Katritsis DG, Giazitzoglou E, Wood MA, et al. Inducible supra-ventricular tachycardias in patients referred for catheter ablation of atrial fibrillation. Europace. 2007;9:785-9.

38. Sharma AD, Klein GJ, Guiraudon GM, et al. Atrial fibrillation in patients with Wolff-Parkinson-White syndrome: incidence after surgical ablation of the accessory pathway. Circulation. 1985;72:161-9.

39. Hamada T, Hiraki T, Ikeda H, et al. Mechanisms for atrial fibrillation in patients with Wolff-Parkinson-White syndrome. J Cardiovasc Electrophysiol. 2002;13:223-9.

40. Cheng S, Keyes MJ, Larson MG, et al. Long-term outcomes in individuals with prolonged PR interval or first-degree atrioventricular block. JAMA. 2009;301:2571-7.

41. Sanders P, Morton JB, Kistler PM, et al. Electrophysiological and electroanatomic characterization of the atria in sinus node disease: evidence of diffuse atrial remodeling. Circulation. 2004;109:1514-22.

42. Coumel P. Autonomic influences in atrial tachyarrhythmias. J Cardiovasc Electrophysiol. 1996;7:999-1007.

43. Herweg B, Dalal P, Nagy B, et al. Power spectral analysis of heart period variability of preceding sinus rhythm before initiation of paroxysmal atrial fibrillation. Am J Cardiol. 1998;82:869-74.

44. Baseline characteristics of patients with atrial fibrillation: the AFFIRM study. Am Heart J. 2002;143:991-1001.

45. Benjamin EJ, Levy D, Vaziri SM, et al. Independent risk factors for atrial fibrillation in a population-based cohort. The Framingham Heart Study. JAMA. 1994;271:840-4.

46. Krahn AD, Klein GJ, Kerr CR, et al. How useful is thyroid function testing in patients with recent-onset atrial fibrillation? The Canadian Registry of Atrial Fibrillation Investigators. Arch Intern Med. 1996;156:2221-4.

47. Sawin CT, Geller A, Wolf PA, et al. Low serum thyrotropin concentrations as a risk factor for atrial fibrillation in older persons. N Engl J Med. 1994;331:1249-52.

48. Auer J, Scheibner P, Mische T, et al. Subclinical hyperthyroidism as a risk factor for atrial fibrillation. Am Heart J. 2001;142:838-42.

49. Frost L, Vestergaard P, Mosekilde L. Hyperthyroidism and risk of atrial fibrillation or flutter: a population-based study. Arch Intern Med. 2004;164:1675-8.

50. Wang TJ, Parise H, Levy D, et al. Obesity and the risk of new-onset atrial fibrillation. JAMA. 2004;292:2471-7.

51. Polanczyk CA, Goldman L, Marcantonio ER, et al. Supraventricular arrhythmia in patients having noncardiac surgery: clinical correlates and effect on length of stay. Ann Intern Med. 1998;129:279-85.

52. Salman S, Bajwa A, Gajic O, et al. Paroxysmal atrial fibrillation in critically ill patients with sepsis. J Intensive Care Med. 2008;23:178-83.

53. Buch P, Friberg J, Scharling H, et al. Reduced lung function and risk of atrial fibrillation in the Copenhagen City Heart Study. Eur Respir J. 2003;21:1012-6.

54. Gami AS, Pressman G, Caples SM, et al. Association of atrial fibrillation and obstructive sleep apnea. Circulation. 2004;110:364-7.

55. Frost L, Vestergaard P. Alcohol and risk of atrial fibrillation or flutter: a cohort study. Arch Intern Med. 2004;164:1993-8.

56. Mukamal KJ, Tolstrup JS, Friberg J, et al. Alcohol consumption and risk of atrial fibrillation in men and women: the Copenhagen City Heart Study. Circulation. 2005;112:1736-42.

57. Djousse L, Levy D, Benjamin EJ, et al. Long-term alcohol consumption and the risk of atrial fibrillation in the Framingham study. Am J Cardiol. 2004;93:710-3.

58. van der Hooft CS, Heeringa J, van Herpen G, et al. Drug-induced atrial fibrillation. J Am Coll Cardiol. 2004;44:2117-24.

59. Frost L, Vestergaard P. Caffeine and risk of atrial fibrillation or flutter: the Danish Diet, Cancer, and Health Study. Am J Clin Nutr. 2005;81:578-82.

60. Levy S, Maarek M, Coumel P, et al. Characterization of different subsets of atrial fibrillation in general practice in France: the ALFA study. The College of French Cardiologists. Circulation. 1999;99:3028-35.

61. Kannel WB, Abbott RD, Savage DD, et al. Epidemiologic features of chronic atrial fibrillation: the Framingham study. N Engl J Med. 1982;306:1018-22.

62. Frustaci A, Chimenti C, Bellocci F, et al. Histological substrate of atrial biopsies in patients with lone atrial fibrillation. Circulation. 1997;96:1180-4.

63. Fox CS, Parise H, D'Agostino RB, Sr, et al. Parental atrial fibrillation as a risk factor for atrial fibrillation in offspring. JAMA. 2004;291:2851-5.

64. Marcus GM, Smith LM, Vittinghoff E, et al. A first-degree family history in lone atrial fibrillation patients. Heart Rhythm. 2008;5:826-30.

65. Lubitz SA, Ozcan C, Magnani JW, et al. Genetics of atrial fibrillation: implications for future research directions and personalized medicine. Circ Arrhythm Electrophysiol. 2010;3:291-9.

66. Gollob MH, Jones DL, Krahn AD, et al. Somatic mutations in the connexin 40 gene (GJA5) in atrial fibrillation. N Engl J Med. 2006;354:2677-88.

67. Thibodeau IL, Xu J, Li Q, et al. Paradigm of genetic mosaicism and lone atrial fibrillation: physiological characterization of a connexin 43-deletion mutant identified from atrial tissue. Circulation. 2010;122:236-44.

68. Gudbjartsson DF, Arnar DO, Helgadottir A, et al. Variants conferring risk of atrial fibrillation on chromosome 4q25. Nature. 2007;448:353-7.

69. Mommersteeg MT, Brown NA, Prall OW, et al. Pitx2c and Nkx2-5 are required for the formation and identity of the pulmonary myocardium. Circ Res. 2007;101:902-9.

70. Israel CW, Gronefeld G, Ehrlich JR, et al. Long-term risk of recurrent atrial fibrillation as documented by an implantable monitoring device: implications for optimal patient care. J Am Coll Cardiol. 2004;43:47-52.

71. Lok NS, Lau CP. Presentation and management of patients admitted with atrial fibrillation: a review of 291 cases in a regional hospital. Int J Cardiol. 1995;48:271-8.

72. Timmermans C, Smeets JL, Rodriguez LM, et al. Aborted sudden death in the Wolff-Parkinson-White syndrome. Am J Cardiol. 1995;76:492-4.

73. Page RL, Wilkinson WE, Clair WK, et al. Asymptomatic arrhythmias in patients with symptomatic paroxysmal atrial fibrillation and paroxysmal supraventricular tachycardia. Circulation. 1994;89:224-7.

74. Kinlay S, Leitch JW, Neil A, et al. Cardiac event recorders yield more diagnoses and are more cost-effective than 48-hour Holter monitoring in patients with palpitations. A controlled clinical trial. Ann Intern Med 1996;124:16-20.

75. Michael JA, Stiell IG, Agarwal S, et al. Cardioversion of paroxysmal atrial fibrillation in the emergency department. Ann Emerg Med. 1999;33:379-87.

76. Danias PG, Caulfield TA, Weigner MJ, et al. Likelihood of spontaneous conversion of atrial fibrillation to sinus rhythm. J Am Coll Cardiol. 1998;31:588-92.

77. Wyse DG, Waldo AL, DiMarco JP, et al. A comparison of rate control and rhythm control in patients with atrial fibrillation. N Engl J Med. 2002;347:1825-33.

78. Van Gelder IC, Hagens VE, Bosker HA, et al. A comparison of rate control and rhythm control in patients with recurrent persistent atrial fibrillation. N Engl J Med. 2002;347:1834-40.

79. Corley SD, Epstein AE, DiMarco JP, et al. Relationships between sinus rhythm, treatment, and survival in the Atrial Fibrillation Follow-Up Investigation of Rhythm Management (AFFIRM) study. Circulation. 2004;109:1509-13.

80. Steinberg JS, Sadaniantz A, Kron J, et al. Analysis of cause-specific mortality in the Atrial Fibrillation Follow-up Investigation of Rhythm Management (AFFIRM) study. Circulation. 2004;109:1973-80.

81. Dittrich HC, Erickson JS, Schneiderman T, et al. Echocardiographic and clinical predictors for outcome of elective cardioversion of atrial fibrillation. Am J Cardiol. 1989;63:193-7.

82. Gentile F, Elhendy A, Khandheria BK, et al. Safety of electrical cardioversion in patients with atrial fibrillation. Mayo Clin Proc. 2002;77:897-904.

83. Klein AL, Grimm RA, Murray RD, et al. Use of transesophageal echocardiography to guide cardioversion in patients with atrial fibrillation. N Engl J Med. 2001;344:1411-20.

84. Weigner MJ, Caulfield TA, Danias PG, et al. Risk for clinical thromboembolism associated with conversion to sinus rhythm in patients with atrial fibrillation lasting less than 48 hours. Ann Intern Med. 1997;126:615-20.

85. Black IW, Fatkin D, Sagar KB, et al. Exclusion of atrial thrombus by transesophageal echocardiography does not preclude embolism after cardioversion of atrial fibrillation. A multicenter study. Circulation. 1994;89:2509-13.

86. Wozakowska-Kaplon B, Janion M, Sielski J, et al. Efficacy of biphasic shock for transthoracic cardioversion of persistent atrial fibrillation: can we predict energy requirements? Pacing Clin Electrophysiol. 2004;27:764-8.

87. Oral H, Souza JJ, Michaud GF, et al. Facilitating transthoracic cardioversion of atrial fibrillation with ibutilide pretreatment. N Engl J Med. 1999;340:1849-54.

88. Meinertz T, Lip GY, Lombardi F, et al. Efficacy and safety of propafenone sustained release in the prophylaxis of symptomatic paroxysmal atrial fibrillation (The European Rythmol/Rytmonorm Atrial Fibrillation Trial [ERAFT] study). Am J Cardiol. 2002;90:1300-6.

89. Pritchett EL, Page RL, Carlson M, et al. Efficacy and safety of sustained-release propafenone (propafenone SR) for patients with atrial fibrillation. Am J Cardiol. 2003;92:941-6.

90. Aliot E, Denjoy I. Comparison of the safety and efficacy of flecainide versus propafenone in hospital out-patients with symptomatic paroxysmal atrial fibrillation/flutter. The Flecainide AF French Study Group. Am J Cardiol. 1996;77:66A-71A.

91. Alboni P, Botto GL, Baldi N, et al. Outpatient treatment of recent-onset atrial fibrillation with the "pill-in-the-pocket" approach. N Engl J Med. 2004;351:2384-91.

92. Echt DS, Liebson PR, Mitchell LB, et al. Mortality and morbidity in patients receiving encainide, flecainide, or placebo. The cardiac arrhythmia suppression trial. N Engl J Med. 1991;324:781-8.

93. Feld GK, Chen PS, Nicod P, et al. Possible atrial proarrhythmic effects of class 1C antiarrhythmic drugs. Am J Cardiol. 1990;66:378-83.

94. Stafford RS, Robson DC, Misra B, et al. Rate control and sinus rhythm maintenance in atrial fibrillation: national trends in medication use, 1980-1996. Arch Intern Med. 1998;158:2144-8.

95. Zimetbaum P. Amiodarone for atrial fibrillation. N Engl J Med. 2007;356:935-41.

96. Goldschlager N, Epstein AE, Naccarelli GV, et al. A practical guide for clinicians who treat patients with amiodarone: 2007. Heart Rhythm. 2007;4:1250-9.

97. Roy D, Talajic M, Dorian P, et al. Amiodarone to prevent recurrence of atrial fibrillation. Canadian Trial of Atrial Fibrillation Investigators. N Engl J Med. 2000;342:913-20.

98. Effect of prophylactic amiodarone on mortality after acute myocardial infarction and in congestive heart failure: meta-analysis of individual data from 6500 patients in randomised trials. Amiodarone Trials Meta-Analysis Investigators. Lancet. 1997;350:1417-24.

99. Bardy GH, Lee KL, Mark DB, et al. Amiodarone or an implantable cardioverter-defibrillator for congestive heart failure. N Engl J Med. 2005;352:225-37.

100. Daoud EG, Strickberger SA, Man KC, et al. Preoperative amiodarone as prophylaxis against atrial fibrillation after heart surgery. N Engl J Med. 1997;337:1785-91.

101. Benditt DG, Williams JH, Jin J, et al. Maintenance of sinus rhythm with oral d,l-sotalol therapy in patients with symptomatic atrial fibrillation and/or atrial flutter. d,l-Sotalol Atrial Fibrillation/Flutter Study Group. Am J Cardiol. 1999;84:270-7.

102. Juul-Moller S, Edvardsson N, Rehnqvist-Ahlberg N. Sotalol versus quinidine for the maintenance of sinus rhythm after direct current conversion of atrial fibrillation. Circulation. 1990;82:1932-9.

103. Singh S, Zoble RG, Yellen L, et al. Efficacy and safety of oral dofetilide in converting to and maintaining sinus rhythm in patients with chronic atrial fibrillation or atrial flutter: the symptomatic atrial fibrillation investigative research on dofetilide (SAFIRE-D) study. Circulation. 2000;102:2385-90.

104. Pritchett EL, Wilkinson WE. Effect of dofetilide on survival in patients with supraventricular arrhythmias. Am Heart J. 1999;138:994-7.

105. Torp-Pedersen C, Moller M, Bloch-Thomsen PE, et al. Dofetilide in patients with congestive heart failure and left ventricular dysfunction. Danish Investigations of Arrhythmia and Mortality on Dofetilide Study Group. N Engl J Med. 1999;341:857-65.

106. Kober L, Torp-Pedersen C, McMurray JJ, et al. Increased mortality after dronedarone therapy for severe heart failure. N Engl J Med. 2008;358:2678-87.

107. Hohnloser SH, Crijns HJ, van Eickels M, et al. Effect of dronedarone on cardiovascular events in atrial fibrillation. N Engl J Med. 2009;360:668-78.

108. Schneider MP, Hua TA, Bohm M, et al. Prevention of atrial fibrillation by Renin-Angiotensin system inhibition a meta-analysis. J Am Coll Cardiol. 2010;55:2299-307.

109. Knight BP, Gersh BJ, Carlson MD, et al. Role of permanent pacing to prevent atrial fibrillation: science advisory from the American Heart Association Council on Clinical Cardiology (Subcommittee on Electrocardiography and Arrhythmias) and the Quality of Care and Outcomes Research Interdisciplinary Working Group, in collaboration with the Heart Rhythm Society. Circulation. 2005;111:240-3.

110. Oral H, Knight BP, Tada H, et al. Pulmonary vein isolation for paroxysmal and persistent atrial fibrillation. Circulation. 2002;105:1077-81.

111. Pappone C, Rosanio S, Oreto G, et al. Circumferential radiofrequency ablation of pulmonary vein ostia: a new anatomic approach for curing atrial fibrillation. Circulation. 2000;102:2619-28.

112. Haissaguerre M, Shah DC, Jais P, et al. Electrophysiological breakthroughs from the left atrium to the pulmonary veins. Circulation. 2000;102:2463-5.

113. Cappato R, Calkins H, Chen SA, et al. Updated worldwide survey on the methods, efficacy, and safety of catheter ablation for human atrial fibrillation. Circ Arrhythm Electrophysiol. 2010;3:32-8.

114. Tsai CF, Tai CT, Hsieh MH, et al. Initiation of atrial fibrillation by ectopic beats originating from the superior vena cava: electrophysiological characteristics and results of radiofrequency ablation. Circulation. 2000;102:67-74.

115. Di Biase L, Burkhardt JD, Mohanty P, et al. Left atrial appendage: an underrecognized trigger site of atrial fibrillation. Circulation. 2010;122:109-18.

116. Nademanee K, McKenzie J, Kosar E, et al. A new approach for catheter ablation of atrial fibrillation: mapping of the electrophysiologic substrate. J Am Coll Cardiol. 2004;43:2044-53.

117. Oral H, Chugh A, Yoshida K, et al. A randomized assessment of the incremental role of ablation of complex fractionated atrial electrograms after antral pulmonary vein isolation for long-lasting persistent atrial fibrillation. J Am Coll Cardiol. 2009;53:782-9.

118. Oral H, Knight BP, Ozaydin M, et al. Clinical significance of early recurrences of atrial fibrillation after pulmonary vein isolation. J Am Coll Cardiol. 2002;40:100-4.

119. Verma A, Kilicaslan F, Pisano E, et al. Response of atrial fibrillation to pulmonary vein antrum isolation is directly related to resumption and delay of pulmonary vein conduction. Circulation. 2005;112:627-35.

120. Berruezo A, Tamborero D, Mont L, et al. Pre-procedural predictors of atrial fibrillation recurrence after circumferential pulmonary vein ablation. Eur Heart J. 2007;28:836-41.

121. Oral H, Scharf C, Chugh A, et al. Catheter ablation for paroxysmal atrial fibrillation: segmental pulmonary vein ostial ablation versus left atrial ablation. Circulation. 2003;108:2355-60.

122. Saad EB, Marrouche NF, Saad CP, et al. Pulmonary vein stenosis after catheter ablation of atrial fibrillation: emergence of a new clinical syndrome. Ann Intern Med. 2003;138:634-8.

123. Pappone C, Oral H, Santinelli V, et al. Atrio-esophageal fistula as a complication of percutaneous transcatheter ablation of atrial fibrillation. Circulation. 2004;109:2724-6.

124. Pappone C, Augello G, Sala S, et al. A randomized trial of circumferential pulmonary vein ablation versus antiarrhythmic drug therapy in paroxysmal atrial fibrillation: the APAF study. J Am Coll Cardiol. 2006;48:2340-7.

125. Piccini JP, Lopes RD, Kong MH, et al. Pulmonary vein isolation for the maintenance of sinus rhythm in patients with atrial fibrillation: a meta-analysis of randomized, controlled trials. Circ Arrhythm Electrophysiol. 2009;2:626-33.

126. Wilber DJ, Pappone C, Neuzil P, et al. Comparison of antiarrhythmic drug therapy and radiofrequency catheter ablation in patients with paroxysmal atrial fibrillation: a randomized controlled trial. JAMA. 2010;303:333-40.

127. Cox JL, Boineau JP, Schuessler RB, et al. Electrophysiologic basis, surgical development, and clinical results of the maze procedure for atrial flutter and atrial fibrillation. Adv Card Surg. 1995;6:1-67.

128. Nitta T, Ishii Y, Ogasawara H, et al. Initial experience with the radial incision approach for atrial fibrillation. Ann Thorac Surg. 1999;68:805-10.

129. Defauw JJ, Guiraudon GM, van Hemel NM, et al. Surgical therapy of paroxysmal atrial fibrillation with the "corridor" operation. Ann Thorac Surg. 1992;53:564-70.

130. Mantovan R, Raviele A, Buja G, et al. Left atrial radiofrequency ablation during cardiac surgery in patients with atrial fibrillation. J Cardiovasc Electrophysiol. 2003;14:1289-95.

131. Cox JL, Boineau JP, Schuessler RB, et al. Five-year experience with the maze procedure for atrial fibrillation. Ann Thorac Surg. 1993;56:814-823.

132. Gaynor SL, Schuessler RB, Bailey MS, et al. Surgical treatment of atrial fibrillation: predictors of late recurrence. J Thorac Cardiovasc Surg. 2005;129:104-11.

133. Izumoto H, Kawazoe K, Kitahara H, et al. Operative results after the Cox/maze procedure combined with a mitral valve operation. Ann Thorac Surg. 1998;66:800-4.

134. Pasic M, Musci M, Siniawski H, et al. The Cox maze iii procedure: parallel normalization of sinus node dysfunction, improvement of atrial function, and recovery of the cardiac autonomic nervous system. J Thorac Cardiovasc Surg. 1999;118:287-95.

135. McElderry HT, McGiffin DC, Plumb VJ, et al. Proarrhythmic aspects of atrial fibrillation surgery: mechanisms of postoperative macroreentrant tachycardias. Circulation. 2008;117:155-62.

136. Van Gelder IC, Groenveld HF, Crijns HJ, et al. Lenient versus strict rate control in patients with atrial fibrillation. N Engl J Med. 2010;362:1363-73.

137. Olshansky B, Rosenfeld LE, Warner AL, et al. The Atrial Fibrillation Follow-up Investigation of Rhythm Management (AFFIRM) study: approaches to control rate in atrial fibrillation. J Am Coll Cardiol. 2004;43:1201-8.

138. Curtis AB, Kutalek SP, Prior M, et al. Prevalence and characteristics of escape rhythms after radiofrequency ablation of the atrioventricular junction: results from the registry for AV junction ablation and pacing in atrial fibrillation. Ablate and Pace Trial Investigators. Am Heart J. 2000;139:122-5.

139. Scheinman MM, Huang S. The 1998 NASPE prospective catheter ablation registry. Pacing Clin Electrophysiol. 2000;23:1020-8.

140. Stroke Prevention in Atrial Fibrillation Study. Final results. Circulation. 1991;84:527-39.

141. Hughes M, Lip GY. Risk factors for anticoagulation-related bleeding complications in patients with atrial fibrillation: a systematic review. QJM. 2007;100:599-607.

142. Risk factors for stroke and efficacy of antithrombotic therapy in atrial fibrillation. Analysis of pooled data from five randomized controlled trials. Arch Intern Med. 1994;154:1449-57.

143. Patients with nonvalvular atrial fibrillation at low risk of stroke during treatment with aspirin: stroke Prevention in Atrial Fibrillation III study. The SPAF III Writing Committee for the Stroke Prevention in Atrial Fibrillation Investigators. JAMA. 1998;279:1273-7.

144. Rother J, Crijns H. Prevention of stroke in patients with atrial fibrillation: the role of new antiarrhythmic and antithrombotic drugs. Cerebrovasc Dis. 2010;30:314-22.

145. Johnson WD, Ganjoo AK, Stone CD, et al. The left atrial appendage: our most lethal human attachment! Surgical implications. Eur J Cardiothorac Surg. 2000;17:718-22.

146. Onalan O, Crystal E. Left atrial appendage exclusion for stroke prevention in patients with nonrheumatic atrial fibrillation. Stroke. 2007;38:624-30.

147. Block PC, Burstein S, Casale PN, et al. Percutaneous left atrial appendage occlusion for patients in atrial fibrillation suboptimal for warfarin therapy: 5-year results of the PLAATO (Percutaneous Left Atrial Appendage Transcatheter Occlusion) study. JACC Cardiovasc Interv. 2009;2:594-600.

148. Go AS, Hylek EM, Chang Y, et al. Anticoagulation therapy for stroke prevention in atrial fibrillation: hsow well do randomized trials translate into clinical practice? JAMA. 2003;s290:2685-92.

Supraventricular Tachycardia

Renee M Sullivan, Wei Wei Li, Brian Olshansky

Chapter Outline

INTRODUCTION

Supraventricular tachycardia (SVT) is a heart rhythm distur-bance, initiated in the atria or ventricles, with atrial rates exceeding 100 beats per minute (bpm), that requires tissue above the His bundle in order to be perpetuated (Fig. 1). SVTs can be symptomatic or asymptomatic, slow or fast, regular or irregular, sustained or nonsustained, paroxysmal, persistent or permanent, and may be due to various mechanisms involving tissue in the atria, AV node, His Purkinje system and/or the ventricles. SVT is generally not life threatening. Occasionally, SVT impairs hemodynamics, provokes hypotension, precipitates heart failure (either acutely or as a result of long-standing tachycardia), or leads to syncope or causes debilitating symptoms including palpitations, lightheadedness, dizziness, chest discomfort, dyspnea or weakness. The treatment depends upon each patient's specific symptom complex, the hemodynamic response to the tachycardia, the relationship of the tachycardia to other comorbidities and the concerns of each patient.

Tremendous advances have occurred in the management of SVT over the past 60 years. No longer do we use deslanoside,

lantanoside, atabrine, quinidine, pressors, cholinergics or a host of other therapies[1-9] to attempt to convert episodes of SVT; we have much better therapies. No longer do we have to worry about side effects and long-term treatment of highly sympto-matic episodes of SVT as we now have ablation to cure many forms of SVT. While advances continue in the field, most of the attention on the management of SVT has shifted to atrial fibrillation (AFib), leaving few new therapies or modalities to evaluate or manage SVT in the past decade.

This chapter will address a modern approach to the overall evaluation and the management of those patients who have SVT.

CLASSIFICATION

Supraventricular tachycardias are either AV nodal dependent or AV nodal independent (Table 1). AV nodal dependent SVTs require AV nodal conduction in order to perpetuate. These SVTs generally have a regular ventricular rate. The two common forms of SVT are atrioventricular nodal reentry tachycardia (AVNRT) and atrioventricular reciprocating tachycardia

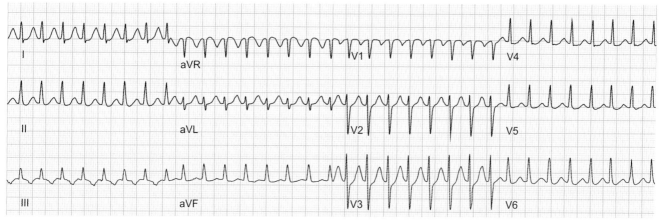

FIGURE 1: Typical regular supraventricular tachycardia. No P wave is visible. The most likely diagnosis of this particular supraventricular tachycardia is AV nodal reentry supraventricular tachycardia

Classification of supraventricular tachycardias

- AV nodal dependent
  - AV nodal reentry
  - AV reentry
    Orthodromic AV reciprocating tachycardia
    Antidromic AV reciprocating tachycardia
- AV nodal independent
  - Atrial tachycardias
    Sinoatrial reentry
    Focal (triggered, automatic, microreentry)
    Macroreentry (scar mediated, congential heart disease)
  - Junctional ectopic tachycardia
  - Atria flutter
    Right atrial flutter
      Clockwise
      Counterclockwise
    Left atrial flutter
      Mitral reentry
      Scar mediated
      Pulmonary vein
  - Atrial fibrillation

FLOW CHART 1: Supraventricular tachycardia—AVRT (Panel A), AVNRT (Panel B) and AT (Panel C)

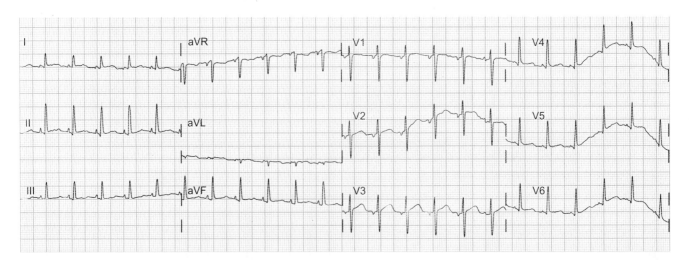

(AVRT). AV nodal independent SVTs require only atrial tissue and do not require AV nodal activation for the tachycardia to occur. They can have a regular ventricular response, as seen in sinoatrial reentry, nonparoxysmal junctional ectopic tachycardia (JET), monomorphic atrial tachycardia (AT), and atrial flutter (AFL) with a fixed or variable AV conduction ratio or an irregular ventricular response as seen with AFib (discussed in detail in another chapter), AFL with variable AV conduction and multifocal atrial tachycardia (MAT). Almost all irregular SVTs are AV nodal independent. AV nodal dependent SVTs can occasionally be irregular, especially at the initiation and termination of the tachycardia. AV nodal independent SVTs can be associated with complete AV block such that the ventricular rhythm is a junctional or ventricular escape (Flow chart 1).

ATRIAL-BASED AV NODAL INDEPENDENT SVT

Sinus Tachycardia

Sinus tachycardia is ubiquitous, occurs with sympathetic activation and may be due to specific triggers such as infection,

heart failure, pulmonary embolus or hyperthyroidism,[10] to name a few. It is not generally considered to be SVT. Sinus tachycardia tends to start with gradual acceleration and usually stops with an even more gradual deceleration. In some instances, it can be difficult to distinguish sinus tachycardia from SVT. The P wave morphology in sinus tachycardia is similar to that in sinus rhythm (Fig. 2), although due to sympathetic stimulation of the sinus node, exit from the sinus node may be more superior and thus the P wave may shift slightly in sinus tachycardia. Rates rarely exceed 200 bpm, except in children or during extreme physical activity. The P wave normally precedes the QRS complex but this depends on AV nodal conduction. Adenosine may appear to stop the tachycardia, but after slowing, the rate will increase gradually, indicative of sinus tachycardia rather than SVT.

Sinus tachycardia, considered abnormal for the physiological condition, is termed "inappropriate". If extreme sinus tachycardia is dependent upon an upright posture, and unrelated to fluid depletion or other explainable cause, it is termed Postural Orthostatic Tachycardia Syndrome (POTS).[11]

In some instances, it can be difficult to distinguish POTS from inappropriate sinus tachycardia or an AT.[12] When SVT persists without change during day or night and is independent of activity, fever or another explainable cause, it is more likely

FIGURE 2: In sinus tachycardia, the P wave is similar to that seen during sinus rhythm and the PR interval is normal. In some instances, it can be difficult to distinguish sinus tachycardia from an atrial tachycardia but there is generally more variability in the rate in patients with persistent narrow QRS tachycardia due to sinus tachycardia

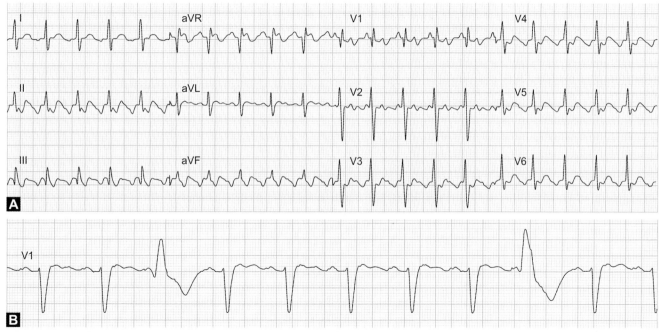

FIGURES 3A AND B: (A) In atrial flutter with a 2 to 1 conduction ratio, the ventricular rate is constant at rest and with activity. There appears to be an upright P wave in V_1 that may be suspicious for sinus tachycardia but it is clear looking at the inferior leads that this is atrial flutter with 2:1 AV conduction with a flutter wave buried in the ST segment. The fact that the rate does not change is a tipoff that this is not sinus tachycardia as well. (B) This is a constant atrial tachycardia with 2 to 1 conduction and PVCs. The fact that the rate does not change again is an indication that this is not sinus tachycardia

to be AT or AFL with a fixed AV conduction ratio (Figs 3A and B). Vagal maneuvers or adenosine may be required to secure the diagnosis.

Atrial Flutter

Atrial flutter is a macroreentrant rapid AT typically involving the right atrium.[13] It tends to coexist with AFib (although most AFib originates from the left atrium) and tends to occur in patients with structural heart disease. The atrial rate, without drug therapy, exceeds 200 bpm but can be as high as 350 bpm. In patients treated with antiarrhythmic drugs, such as amiodarone, flecainide or propafenone, and in patients with large

atria, the rates of AFL can be slower than 200 bpm. The most common form of AFL, due to counterclockwise electrical activation in the right atrium around the tricuspid ring utilizing an isthmus of tissue, the cavotricuspid isthmus, has a "saw tooth" appearance in the inferior leads with no isoelectric segment between beats (Fig. 4). Approximately 10% of typical AFL is perpetuated by clockwise activation around the tricuspid ring. Atypical forms of right AFL involve upper loop or lower loop reentry mechanisms[14,15] (Figs 5A and B). These flutters do not show the "typical" electrocardiographic appearance or rate and may require an alternative approach during ablation procedures. Left AFL not only often involves a reentry circuit around the mitral annulus but also can be due to reentry around or in

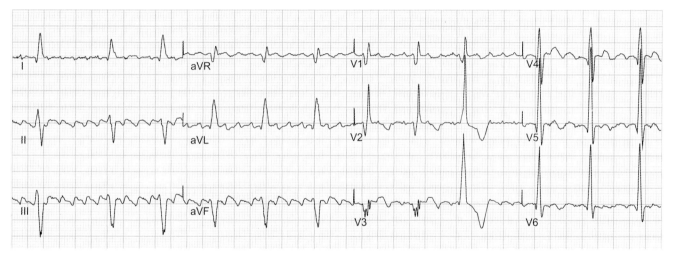

FIGURE 4: "Saw tooth" flutter waves are seen in the inferior leads in "typical" counterclockwise, isthmus dependent atrial flutter. Usually, this form of atrial flutter demonstrates upright P waves in lead V1. Here, there is variable AV conduction

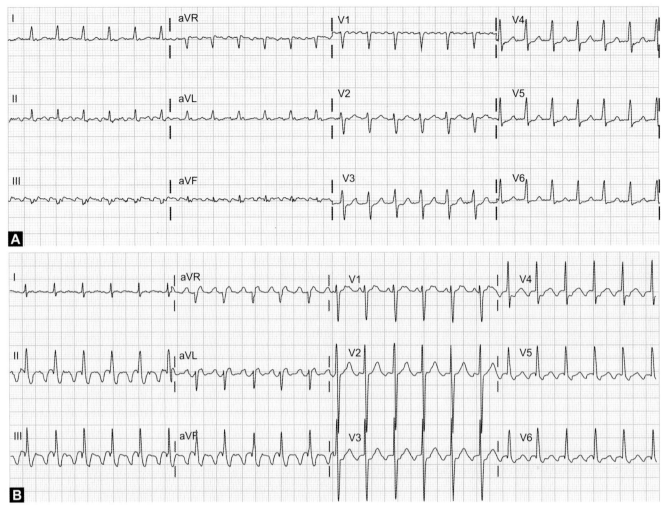

FIGURES 5A AND B: Unusual flutter waves in the inferior leads. These flutters may not be isthmus dependent. It can be difficult to distinguish from left atrial flutters and unusual right atrial reentry circuits in some instances

pulmonary veins and/or scar (Fig. 6).[16] Left AFL is often associated with, and may be present after attempts to ablate AFib,[17] requiring further ablation procedures.[18] Some AFL due to scar can be associated with congenital heart disease; these often have very unusual reentrant pathways. The distinction between AFL and AT in complex congenital heart disease (or its repair) is more dependent on the rate than the mechanism or the appearance on the surface electrocardiogram (ECG).

Atrial Tachycardia

Atrial tachycardia can originate from the left atrium, right atrium, vena cavae or pulmonary veins [Flow chart 1 (panel C)]. The tachycardia can be focal or macroreentrant involving large areas of the atria. Focal forms can be microreentrant or due to an automatic or triggered mechanism.

Monomorphic AT represents about 5–10% of all regular SVTs. The P wave precedes the QRS complex but generally has a morphology distinct from the sinus P wave. The PR interval may vary. The atrial rates are generally 120–200 bpm. The conduction can be 1:1 but AV block can be present. An "A-A-V" pattern can be seen during AT.[19] Adenosine may occasionally stop the tachycardia;[20] more commonly, only AV block occurs. Digoxin toxicity may precipitate AT with AV block.

Focal Atrial Tachycardia

Automatic AT represents less than 2–5% of SVTs. It may have a gradual onset and offset, sometimes similar to sinus tachycardia, in contrast to atrial reentrant tachycardias that start with a premature beat and have a sudden offset. As such, focal ATs may be difficult to distinguish from sinus tachycardia but tend to be faster and occur at rates inappropriate for physiological needs. Furthermore, the P wave morphology is usually distinctly different from that seen in sinus tachycardia.

Triggered ATs have a sudden onset and offset. Some ATs are catecholamine-dependent and begin with exercise. ATs can be associated with acute myocardial infarction (AMI), alcohol intoxication, exacerbation of chronic obstructive lung disease, electrolyte abnormalities, and digoxin use. Chronic, persistent, automatic AT, like other forms of persistent SVTs, can cause tachycardia-induced cardiomyopathy.

Intra-atrial Reentrant Tachycardia

Macroreentry or microreentry AT often utilizes areas of scar at incisions from prior cardiac surgery or corrected congenital heart disease (such as a Fontan procedure) and represents 5–10% of SVTs.[21-24] This type of tachycardia is distinguishable from AFL as there are discrete P waves separated by an

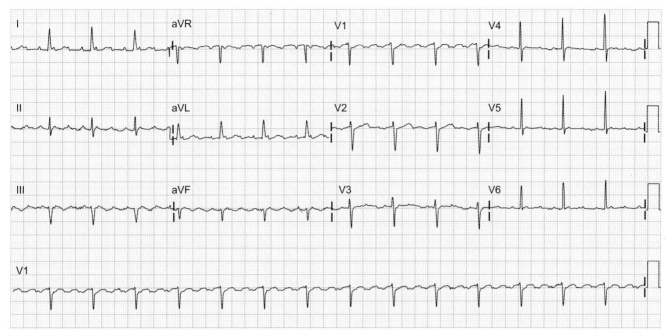

FIGURE 6: The left atrial flutter shown here has negative flutter waves in V1 and upright flutter waves in the inferior leads

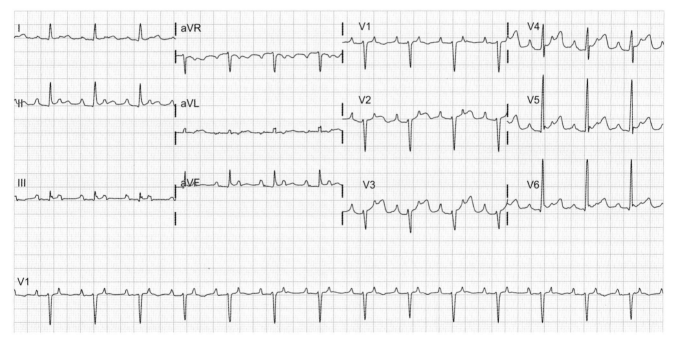

FIGURE 7: Atrial tachycardia with 2:1 AV conduction. Discrete P waves are separated by an isoelectric interval, in sharp contrast to atrial flutter in which an isoelectric interval is usual, not present. Occasionally, an atrial flutter is slow, especially if an antiarrhythmic drug is given, but generally, the rate is faster than 250 bpm. This atrial tachycardia is due to attempted ablation of atrial fibrillation in the left atrium and this is a left atrial tachycardia. The P wave morphology can help distinguish the location of atrial tachycardia origination

isoelectric baseline. Adenosine may terminate atrial reentrant SVTs in 15% of cases.

Sinoatrial Re-entry Tachycardia

Sinoatrial re-entry tachycardia (SART) is a unique, uncommon form of regular AT due to a re-entrant mechanism involving the sinoatrial node.[25] The P wave morphology is often similar to that in sinus rhythm with the exit point in the right atrium slightly below the sinus node (Figs 8A and B) but it can

masquerade as other forms of SVT.[26] This tachycardia starts and stops abruptly and tends to be slower and more irregular than other types of SVT. Patients with AVNRT may also have associated SVTs such as sinoatrial reentry.[27]

Multifocal Atrial Tachycardia

In MAT, atrial activation occurs from multiple locations leading to at least three different morphologies of P waves (Fig. 9). The atrial rate is between 110 bpm and 170 bpm. In some cases, it

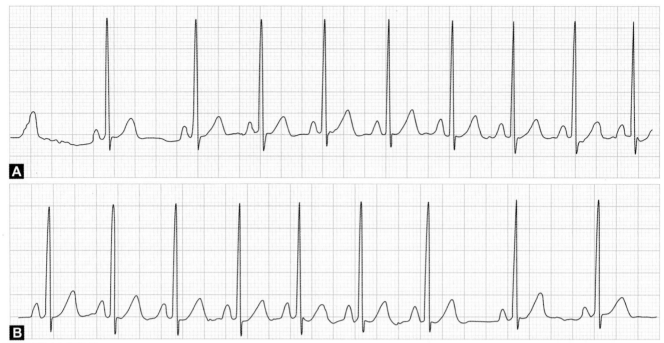

FIGURES 8A AND B: This rhythm strip demonstrates an abrupt change (speeding and slowing) in heart rate with an upright P wave in the inferior leads. The P wave morphology does not change and is similar to that in sinus rhythm. This is expected in typical sinoatrial reentrant supraventricular tachycardia

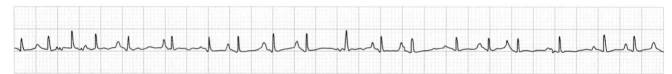

FIGURE 9: This rhythm strip shows multifocal atrial tachycardia, with at least three distinct P wave morphologies present. This type of tachycardia is often related to severe pulmonary disease and treatment of the underlying disease is the best way to eliminate the tachycardia. The prognosis is generally poor but not directly related to the atrial tachycardia itself. While there is no specific antiarrhythmic treatment for this tachycardia, amiodarone or verapamil may be effective

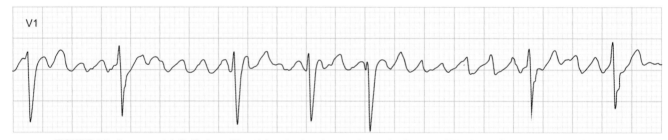

FIGURE 10: Coarse atrial fibrillation with atrial activation that continuously changes. This is not flutter or atrial tachycardia

can be difficult to distinguish from "coarse" AFib (Fig. 10). The vast majority (60–85%) of cases occurs in acutely ill, older individuals and those with severe chronic obstructive lung disease but also can occur in patients with cor pulmonale, pneumonia, sepsis, hypertensive heart disease, and systolic heart failure. Approximately up to 0.40% of hospitalized patients have this arrhythmia.[28] Exacerbating factors include theophylline toxicity, hypokalemia, hypoxia, acidosis and catecholamine infusion. The acute mortality associated with, but not directly due to, MAT is 30–60% but this reflects the underlying disease and not necessarily the arrhythmia itself. Treatment is aimed at

the underlying disease and while verapamil has been advocated, it is not particularly effective in all patients.[29]

AV NODAL DEPENDENT SVT

Atrioventricular Nodal Reentrant Tachycardia

Atrioventricular nodal reentrant tachycardia is due to the presence of two physiological and anatomical ("slow" and "fast") AV nodal pathways.[30] About 65% of all regular SVTs are due to AVNRT. Typically, activation proceeds down the "slow" perinodal pathway and returns via the retrograde "fast"

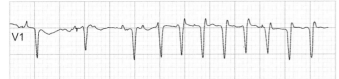

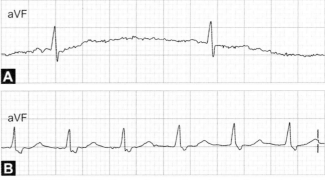

FIGURE 11: Atrioventricular nodal reentrant supraventricular tachycardia AVNRT is a narrow QRS complex tachycardia with no obvious P waves present. A pseudo R' can be observed in lead V1 as depicted here. The initiation is with a long PR interval suggesting conduction down a slow AV nodal pathway. This tachycardia can generally be terminated by carotid sinus massage, vagal maneuvers or adenosine

FIGURES 12A AND B: Comparing baseline sinus rhythm tracing to that during tachycardia shows a retrograde P wave buried at the end of the QRS complex. In this particular instance, it occurs in lead AVF rather than in V1

perinodal pathway [Flow chart 1 (Panel B)]. The rates of AVNRT are usually between 150 bpm and 200 bpm but it can be as fast as 250 bpm. Slow or fast AVNRT usually begins with a premature atrial depolarization followed by a long PR interval. There can be a pseudo R' in lead V1 (Fig. 11) and a pseudo S wave in the inferior leads, a retrograde P wave seen in other leads (Figs 12A and B) or not (Fig. 13). AVNRT can be present with a bundle branch block (Fig. 14) and this can be tachycardia dependent. The atypical form of AVNRT involves a short PR (long RP) interval with antegrade conduction down a fast

pathway and retrograde conduction via the slow pathway. A rare form of AVNRT involves slow antegrade activation and slow retrograde activation ("slow-slow" AVNRT).[31]

Atrioventricular nodal reentry tachycardia (AVNRT) can begin at any age and occurs more commonly in women than men. It is more likely to occur in the adult population even

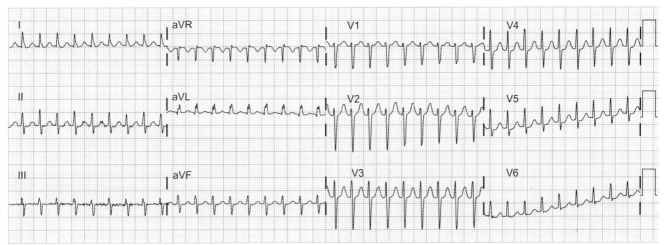

FIGURE 13: Typical AVNRT with a faster rate and no obvious P waves associated with the QRS complexes. A regular narrow QRS complex supraventricular tachycardia in which P waves are absent is most likely to be AVNRT

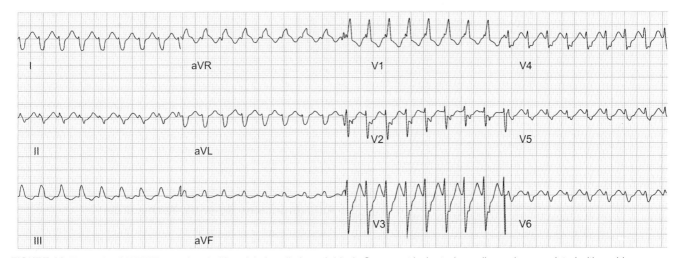

FIGURE 14: Example of AVNRT associated with a right bundle branch block. Supraventricular tachycardia can be associated with a wide or narrow QRS complex. In some cases a wide QRS complex supraventricular tachycardia is due to an underlying bundle branch block. Alternatively, there can be tachycardia dependent right bundle branch block aberration. In this case, it is possible to see a retrograde P wave in leads V2–V5

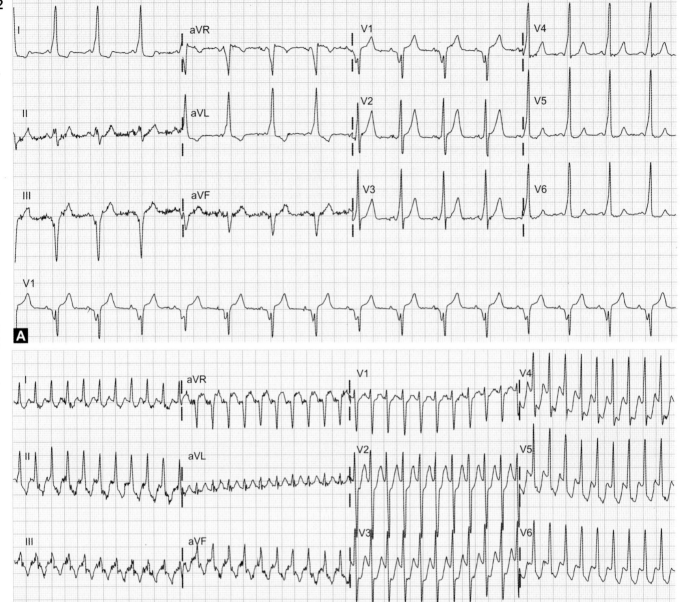

FIGURES 15A AND B: (A) This tracing shows evidence for a posteroseptal accessory pathway in sinus rhythm. There is evidence that this is Wolff-Parkinson-White syndrome with a negative delta wave in V1 and a positive delta wave in V2. The delta wave in the inferior leads, i.e. III and AVF, are negative. This delta wave vector is consistent with a posteroseptal accessory pathway (B) This tracing, seen in the same patient who had an EKG in sinus rhythm shown in 15A, shows a rapid narrow QRS complex supraventricular tachycardia with a retrograde inverted P wave present in the ST segment. The P wave is best seen in leads II, III and AVF. This is orthodromic AV reciprocating tachycardia. The supraventricular tachycardia does not demonstrate conduction down the accessory pathway. Since conduction is going down the AV node and up the accessory pathway, there is no evidence for a delta wave during tachycardia. This is typical orthodromic AV reciprocating tachycardia

though dual AV nodal pathways are common in children.[32] Likely, AV nodal pathways change over time. Although dual AV nodal pathways are common, only a small percentage of individuals with dual pathways have AVNRT as specific characteristics are required for the tachycardia to occur: the slow pathway must have a longer refractory period than the fast pathway[33] and there may be specifics about AV nodal pathway conduction and connectedness that play a role.[34,35] High catecholamine states can exacerbate AVNRT. Symptoms, such as palpitations, neck pounding, lightheadedness, weakness, anxiety, shortness of breath, chest discomfort, pulmonary congestion and syncope due to simultaneous atrial and ventricular contraction, may occur during typical forms of

AVNRT.[36,37] Although conceivable but rare, AVNRT may occur with conduction block at the lower portion of the AV node or below, demonstrating 1:1 conduction but no evidence for conduction block between the atria and the ventricles. These forms of AVNRT stop abruptly with adenosine, vagal maneuvers, and verapamil.

Atrioventricular Re-entry Tachycardia

Atrioventricular reciprocating tachycardia is a macroreentrant tachycardia involving activation of the atria and ventricles through anterograde and retrograde conducting AV pathways [the AV node and an accessory pathway[38] (Figs 15A and B)]. Typically, the antegrade conduction during AVRT is via the

AV node with retrograde conduction via an independent accessory pathway. When this occurs, it is known as "orthodromic AV reciprocating tachycardia" [Flow chart 1 (Panel A)], representing approximately 30% of all regular SVTs. It is more common in young males and tends to be faster than AVNRT. During this tachycardia, the P wave is distinctly after the QRS complex and this tachycardia is often termed "long RP tachycardia". The symptoms of neck pounding experienced by the patients with AVNRT tend not to be present for those with AVRT as atrial and ventricular activation is not simultaneous. Cannon A waves do not tend to occur in AVRT.

As AVRT can be faster than AVNRT, it is more often associated with QRS alternans[39] (Fig. 16). The accessory pathway responsible for AVRT can be "concealed", that is, not present as a "delta wave" on the ECG recording. Like AVNRT, this tachycardia stops abruptly with vagal maneuvers or adenosine due to blockage in the AV node.

Pre-excitation Syndromes

Manifest antegrade conduction through an accessory pathway can "pre-excite" the ventricles and cause a fusion complex or complete conduction via the antegrade accessory pathway. The AV connection can occur by way of the left ventricle, the right ventricle, or the septum at virtually any location between the atria and the ventricles. When this is present in sinus rhythm, the pattern on the ECG is known as the "Wolff-Parkinson-White" (WPW) pattern.[40] When this pattern is associated with palpitations, this is known as WPW syndrome.

Orthodromic atrioventricular re-entry tachycardia (AVRT) is the most common SVT that occurs with the WPW syndrome

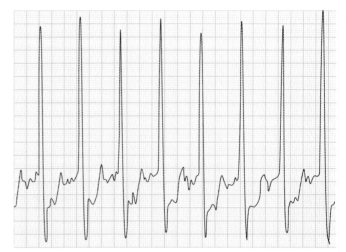

FIGURE 16: Example of a recording orthodromic AV reciprocating tachycardia in which there is a retrograde P wave and evidence for QRS alternans

and other preexcitation syndromes. In less than 10% of cases of WPW syndrome, antegrade conduction is via an accessory pathway and retrograde conduction is via the AV node ("antidromic tachycardia") (Fig. 17). In rare instances, antegrade conduction proceeds down an accessory pathway and comes up another accessory pathway (Fig. 18). In the case of AVRT, in which conduction proceeds antegrade via an accessory pathway, the QRS complex is bizarre and wide. Irregular and rapid conduction via an accessory pathway during AFib can be potentially life-threatening and is dependent upon conduction via the AV node and/or the accessory pathway (Fig. 19).

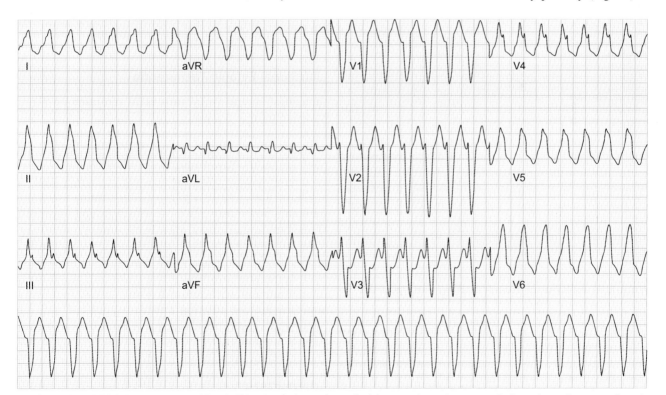

FIGURE 17: 12 lead ECG demonstrates antidromic AV reciprocating tachycardia. It is a rare form of supraventricular tachycardia present in patients with preexcitation syndromes. This wide QRS complex tachycardia can be difficult to distinguish from ventricular tachycardia. Preexcitation is likely to be seen in sinus rhythm with a similar QRS complex morphology. An electrophysiology study might be necessary to confirm that this is in fact antidromic tachycardia rather than ventricular tachycardia. During an electrophysiology study, an atrial premature can preexcite the ventricle with a similar QRS morphology when retrograde His bundle activation is refractory during antidromic AVRT. Antegrade conduction proceeds via the accessory pathway rapidly, with a short PR interval (best seen here in lead aVL). There is retrograde conduction via the AV node. This pathway is right-sided based on the QRS morphology (a negative QRS in lead V1). It was located close to the His bundle/AV node region

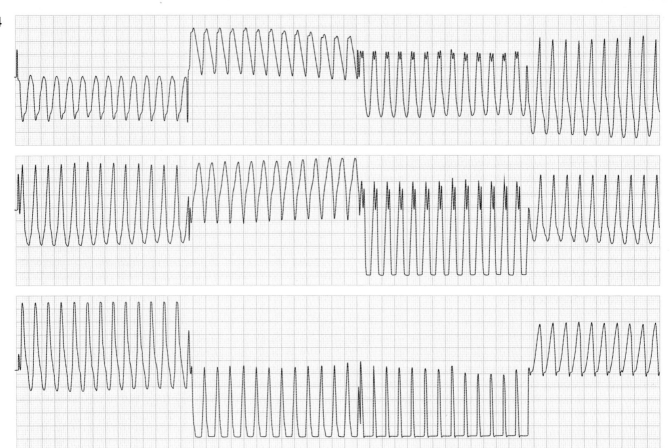

FIGURE 18: Very rapid wide QRS complex tachycardia is difficult to distinguish from ventricular tachycardia but is a form of antidromic AV reciprocating tachycardia in which antegrade conduction proceeds down an accessory pathway and goes up another accessory pathway. In this particular case, adenosine changed a slower form of antidromic tachycardia to a faster form after blocking the AV node. In this particular patient, the retrograde accessory pathway was a septal pathway and the antegrade pathway was a left-sided pathway that was anterior. The location of the antegrade conducting accessory pathway is the reason for the morphology of the QRS complex

Other "preexcitation syndromes" can be due to His-Purkinje system preexcitation, particularly of the right bundle. An atriofascicular pathway can occur that bypasses the AV node and inserts into or next to the right bundle known as a "Mahaim fiber". Such a pathway tends to have "decremental" properties in which premature beats can be associated with progressively slower conduction through the pathway.[41] These are antegrade only conducting "atriofascicular" pathways (Fig. 20). Mahaim fibers can be "innocent bystanders" whereby AVNRT proceeds down the Mahaim fiber to the ventricles or they can be the antegrade limb of a macroreentrant SVT in which the retrograde limb involves the AV node.[42]

Permanent Junctional Reciprocating Tachycardia

Permanent junctional reciprocating tachycardia (PJRT) is a persistent form of AVRT in which conduction proceeds down the AV node and up a posteroseptal, slowly conducting accessory pathway (Fig. 21). As this tachycardia is persistent and often rather slow, it may go undetected for years and lead to tachycardia-induced cardiomyopathy.[43,44] In some instances, a macroreentrant SVT involving the AV node is dependent upon slow conducting accessory tissue that is independent of the AV node and often (but not always) in a portion of the posterior right atrium.[45]

Junctional Ectopic Tachycardia

Junctional ectopic tachycardia is an automatic or triggered tachycardia that originates from tissue surrounding the AV node (Fig. 22). The rhythm tends to be persistent and nonparoxysmal and may slow but does not generally terminate with adenosine. This rhythm is more common in children but also tends to occur after cardiac surgery, during AMI, after cardioversion of AFib, with myocarditis, during exercise, and in healthy individuals and those with sinus node dysfunction. This tachycardia may also occur under situations of catecholamine excess or in digoxin toxicity. SVT with AV dissociation is most likely JET. The JET can be associated with a poor prognosis but a recent multicenter report suggests that treatment with antiarrhythmic drugs (particularly amiodarone) or ablation can be associated with good outcomes.[46] Rarely, rapid forms of JET can be seen in specific situations, such as the postoperative period, in which catecholamine stimulation is high (Fig. 23).

DIAGNOSIS

The clinical presentation can be diagnostic of SVT and it may be possible to proceed with further evaluation and therapy on this basis alone. Classic symptoms include the abrupt onset of rapid palpitations with associated dyspnea, chest discomfort,

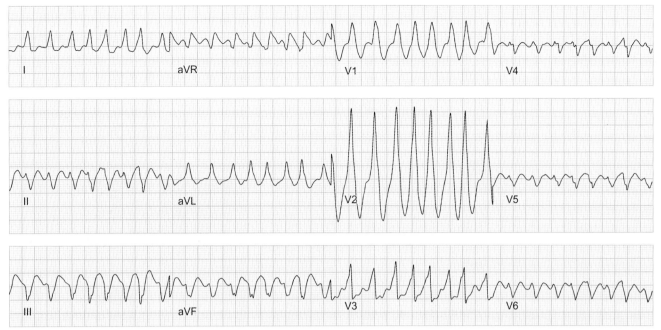

FIGURE 19: Atrial fibrillation in a patient with the Wolff-Parkinson-White. This is an irregularly irregular wide QRS complex tachycardia with occasional conducted beats via the AV node. The QRS complexes are due to ventricular activation by way of the left-sided posterior accessory pathway (as determined by the QRS morphology with a positive delta wave in V1). The best long-term treatment is ablation of the accessory pathway. Acutely, cardioversion or drug therapy (procainamide or amiodarone) are the treatments of choice. If the patient is not tolerating this tachycardia hemodynamically, it is important to proceed rapidly to electrical cardioversion. It is important to avoid digoxin, calcium channel blockers and even beta blockers acutely in patients who present with this tachycardia

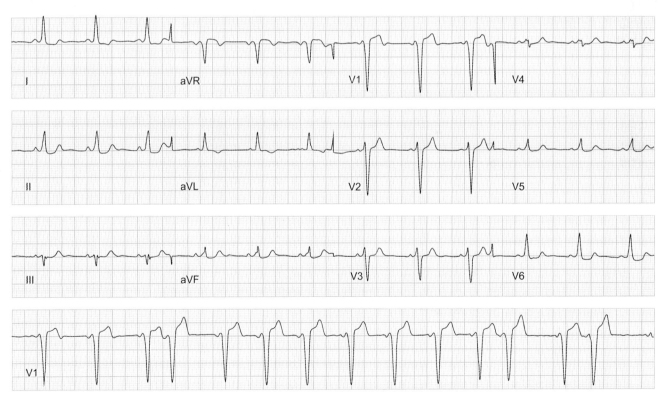

FIGURE 20: A Mahaim fiber is noted in sinus rhythm in this tracing from a 19-year-old female who has supraventricular tachycardia. There is evidence for a left bundle branch block without manifest preexcitation but with a short PR interval. There is no obvious delta wave but the QRS morphology becomes slightly wider. There may be slight accentuation of the QRS width with the premature atrial contraction as it may be fused conduction between the atriofascicular ("Mahaim") fiber, connecting the right atrium to the right bundle and normal antegrade AV nodal conduction. A Mahaim fiber may be suspected based on the clinical presentation. It is unlikely for a 19-year-old to have a left bundle branch block with a short PR interval. Patients with this abnormality can have a macroreentrant supraventricular tachycardia involving antegrade conduction down the Mahaim fiber and retrograde conduction up the AV node or they may have AV nodal reentry with "innocent bystander" Mahaim conduction. Mahaim fibers tend to conduct only in the antegrade direction. These are right-sided pathways that insert into the right bundle

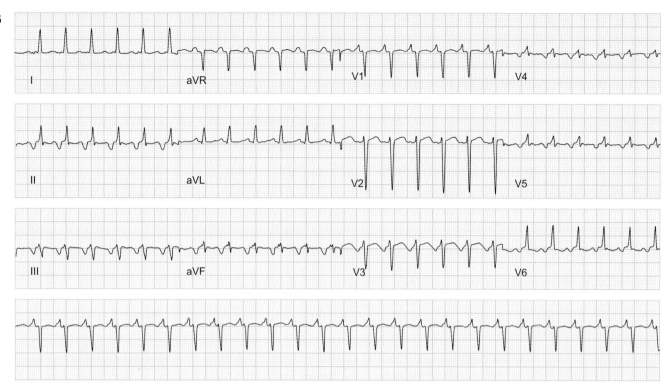

FIGURE 21: Supraventricular tachycardia is permanent junctional reciprocating tachycardia (PJRT). The P wave precedes the QRS complex and is inverted in leads II, III and AVF and upright in V1. The differential diagnosis for this tachycardia is atypical AV nodal reentry (antegrade fast pathway and retrograde slow pathway), atrial tachycardia and permanent junctional reciprocating tachycardia. This patient had permanent junctional reciprocating tachycardia with retrograde conduction by way of an accessory pathway that was conducting slowly as determined by electrophysiology testing. This patient developed heart failure and a cardiomyopathy due to persistent tachycardia. With ablation of the slow retrograde accessory pathway, the tachycardia was eliminated, thereby returning the ejection fraction to normal and resolving the heart failure

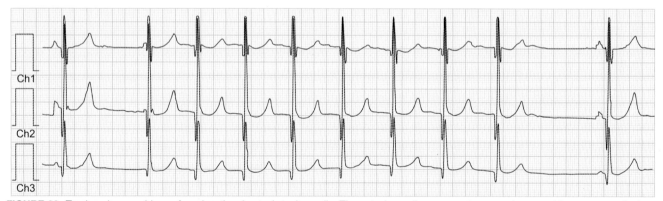

FIGURE 22: Tracing shows evidence for a junctional ectopic tachycardia. These tachycardias are most commonly present in younger patients and they originate from tissue surrounding the AV node. This tachycardia can be associated with AV dissociation. The first beat of this tachycardia occurs at the same time as a P wave demonstrating the dissociation of the A and the V during the tachycardia

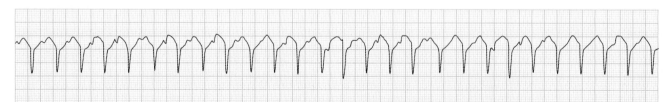

FIGURE 23: Rarely, an accelerated junctional tachycardia, faster than junctional ectopic tachycardia, can occur in older people who have high catecholamine states. In this particular case, the patient was postoperative after cardiac surgery. There is a narrow complex tachycardia with retrograde atrial activation but not in a one-to-one fashion. There is retrograde a conduction block

dizziness, and lightheadedness. These symptoms often abruptly terminate when the patient utilizes vagal maneuvers that are learned over time in an attempt to abate the symptoms.

The physical examination can aid in determining the specific type of SVT. The neck veins may show prominent pulsations with each beat, consistent with cannon A waves, common in typical AVNRT. Alternatively, patients with AFL may have flutter waves seen as pulsations in the neck at a rate faster than the pulse itself. An irregularly irregular pulse or a pulse deficit would be consistent with AFib. Additionally, important information from the physical examination includes blood pressure recordings as well as evidence for hemodynamic compromise or the presence of congestive heart failure. These findings are indicators that a more aggressive approach is necessary to control the rate and the rhythm.

Bedside maneuvers, such as carotid sinus massage or Valsalva, can terminate tachycardia abruptly. They can also uncover the presence of an AV nodal independent tachycardia such as AFL (Fig. 24). These maneuvers can also slow down the sinus rate and stop sinoatrial reentry as well. Adenosine can stop some ATs.

ELECTROCARDIOGRAPHIC RECORDINGS

Supraventricular tachycardia may be diagnosed by a single ECG lead but a multiple lead ECG recording is generally more useful to help distinguish one form of SVT from another. A 12-lead ECG during sinus rhythm can help to determine if there is preexcitation or a bundle branch block. Ambulatory event recorders, including Holter monitors or even an implantable loop recorder, may be necessary to detect intermittent episodes of SVT.

During recorded episodes, clues to the diagnosis of the presence and type of SVT can be discerned from the initiation and termination of the tachycardia (Fig. 11), the relationship between the P waves and the QRS complexes (Fig. 7), the P wave and QRS morphologies, as well as the presence of AV block and the tachycardia regularity and rate. In some cases, the type of SVT may not be clear based on available recordings even with bedside interventions (vagal maneuvers or intravenous adenosine) (Fig. 24). An invasive electrophysiology test may be needed to ascertain the SVT type and mechanism.

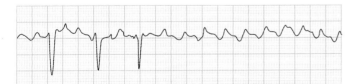

FIGURE 24: In this particular tracing, a patient who had atrial flutter was given adenosine to secure the diagnosis. There was transient AV block with a long pause and the presence of flutter waves becoming evident. Prior to the adenosine, there was 2 to 1 conduction during atrial flutter and it was difficult to make the diagnosis for certain. This tracing shows the effect of adenosine uncovering the mechanism of this particular tachycardia, typical atrial flutter. Adenosine will not stop atrial flutter but will stop AV nodal dependent supraventricular tachycardias such as AVNRT and AVRT. It can also stop sinoatrial reentry and some atrial tachycardias. Adenosine can be useful to help distinguish atrial versus AV nodal dependent supraventricular tachycardias

In typical (slow antegrade, fast retrograde) AVNRT, the P wave is nearly simultaneous with the QRS complex. Characteristically there is a small upright P wave in lead V1 just at the end of the QRS complex known as a pseudo R' (Fig. 11). At tachycardia initiation, a long PR interval may be seen indicating antegrade conduction via a slow conducting AV nodal pathway. In atypical (fast antegrade, slow retrograde) AVNRT, there is an inverted P wave in the inferior leads often just before the next QRS complex. AVNRT of this type or AVRT should be suspected if inverted P waves are present in leads II, III and aVF.

In monomorphic AT, the P wave is inconsistent with sinus tachycardia. AV block may be present but conduction tends to be at a fixed ratio (Fig. 7). Similarly, for AFL, variable conduction or 2:1 conduction may occur and one of the P waves could be buried in the ST segment (Fig. 3A). In sinus tachycardia, the P wave is before the QRS complex and is upright in the inferior leads (Fig. 2). It may be difficult to distinguish from SART as the P wave morphology can be virtually identical (Figs 8A and B). In JETs, AV dissociation may be present as the tachycardia can be independent of atrial activation. In MAT, at least three morphologies of P waves are present (Fig. 9).

Wide QRS Tachycardia—Is It SVT?

Wide QRS complex tachycardia (QRS width ≥ 120) is generally ventricular tachycardia but approximately 10% of wide QRS tachycardias are SVT (Table 2). A wide QRS complex during SVT can be due to a bundle branch block that may be present in sinus rhythm. The baseline ECG can, therefore, be of some help in diagnosing the mechanism as the morphology may be the same as in sinus rhythm but the QRS can change during SVT when there is an underlying bundle branch block[47] and the QRS morphology during ventricular tachycardia can mimic the morphology in sinus rhythm.[48]

There can be rate-dependent ("phase 3") aberration (QRS widening with a bundle branch block pattern) that is due to rate dependent block in one of the bundles due to rate related refractoriness. When this occurs, it is often present when there is an acceleration of the tachycardia or if there is irregular AV conduction such that there is long-short conduction. This is known as "Ashman's phenomenon" which tends to occur during AFib. Tachycardia-dependent aberration can be continuous or intermittent and related to refractoriness in the right or left bundle branch. A phenomenon of "concealed perpetuated aberration" is also possible in which persistent bundle branch

TABLE 2

Differential diagnosis of wide QRS tachycardia

- SVT with fixed bundle branch block
- SVT with intermittent aberration including concealed perpetuated aberration
- SVT with persistent rate dependant aberration
- SVT with passive conduction down a bypass tract
- SVT due to antidromic AV reciprocating tachycardia
- Ventricular tachycardia

block aberration can occur even though there is fluctuation in rate.

In some patients, both wide and narrow QRS SVT coexist. If the rates of the wide and narrow QRS SVT are similar, or if the rate during the wide QRS tachycardia is faster, the cause of the tachycardia remains uncertain. If the wide QRS SVT is due to bundle branch block aberration and it is slower than the narrow QRS SVT, this likely indicates the presence of AVRT with retrograde conduction via the accessory pathway on the same side as the bundle branch block. The slower rate during the wide QRS complex tachycardia is because the bundle branch block causes the contralateral ventricle to activate first and there is conduction delay through the ventricular myocardium before conduction can proceed up the retrograde pathway. A bundle branch block located on the side ipsilateral to the accessory pathway will lengthen the reentry circuit pathway (e.g. a left bundle branch block tachycardia with a left sided retrograde accessory pathway is likely to be slower than SVT with a narrow QRS complex in the same patient) and the VA interval can lengthen with the bundle branch block aberration. Occasionally, tachycardia can begin in a fascicle with a relatively narrow, yet wide, QRS complex, and with AV dissociation. This tachycardia can be confused with SVT.

In rare instances, antegrade conduction via an accessory pathway during tachycardia can present as a wide QRS complex SVT. Antidromic AVRT (conduction down an accessory pathway and up the AV node or another accessory pathway) occurs rarely. Preexcited AFib with intermittent AV conduction down an accessory pathway is also possible.

Adenosine is potentially diagnostic and can be given in a patient with a wide QRS complex tachycardia that is well tolerated.[49] If adenosine or a vagal maneuver stops a wide QRS tachycardia, it is likely SVT even though some idiopathic ventricular tachycardias may stop with adenosine or even a vagal maneuver. Despite careful analysis, and even bedside maneuvers, the diagnosis of the type of SVT may be incorrect in as many as 20% of recorded episodes.

ELECTROPHYSIOLOGY STUDIES

Invasive electrophysiology studies are used either for diagnosis of SVT in patients with classic symptoms or for determination of the mechanism of SVT for those who have recorded episodes or have a wide QRS tachycardia that may be SVT or VT. During the electrophysiology study, 2–5 intravenous catheter sheaths are placed and recording and stimulating catheter electrodes are placed in specific sites of the heart to record electrical activation and to stimulate the heart to initiate tachycardia and understand its mechanism. Catheters can also be used to locate specific tissues that are responsible for the tachycardia. SVTs with regular rate (AVNRT and AVRT), if present, are often readily inducible with delivery of premature atrial or ventricular extrastimuli. In some cases, AT and rare cases of AVNRT or AVRT, the SVTs are not inducible. Increasing the aggressiveness of the atrial and ventricular extrastimuli by pacing at faster rates and adding more extra stimuli may be useful. Sometimes, catecholamine stimulation with isoproterenol, and/or atropine may be necessary to initiate the tachyarrhythmia during extrastimulus testing. In rare instances, a beta-blocker is required to initiate SVT.

After SVT is initiated in the electrophysiology laboratory, the relationships of the atria, ventricles and His bundle during extrastimulus testing and during tachycardia can help to determine the tachycardia mechanism. Transient entrainment may help to understand the location and mechanism of the SVT.[50]

During SVT, if specifically timed ventricular extrastimuli activate the atria when the His bundle is refractory, the presence of an accessory pathway is diagnosed and the tachycardia is likely orthodromic AVRT. Similarly, if during SVT specifically timed atrial extrastimuli activate the ventricles when the His bundle is refractory, the tachycardia is like antidromic AVRT. AV relationships can also help to determine if there is an accessory pathway.

In some instances, detailed electroanatomical mapping is necessary to understand the tachycardia mechanism or the origin of the tachycardia (such as focal or reentrant AT). Similarly, simultaneous atrial record map may be helpful to understand the mechanism of the tachycardia. In some instances, it is a transseptal catheterization or even an arterial approach in needed to reach the tissue responsible for tachycardia.

TREATMENTS

The goal of treatment is to terminate tachycardia acutely, maintain normal sinus rhythm, control ventricular response rate, eliminate symptoms, normalize hemodynamics, and prevent worsening of any underlying cardiovascular conditions due to SVT.

ACUTE CARE

Acute management depends on the type and severity of symptoms related to the SVT and the type of SVT (Table 3). Acute interventions are designed to slow the ventricular rate (for AV nodal independent SVTs) and/or terminate the tachycardia. Therapies include drugs to cardiovert and prevent recurrence, drugs used to slow the AV conduction and the ventricular rate, and direct current cardioversion. Acute management requires careful electrocardiographic and hemo-dynamic monitoring. Patients remaining in SVT and having ventricular rates that cannot be controlled require hospital admission. Other indications for admission include frequent recurrences, resistance to initial drug therapy, initiation of new antiarrhythmic drugs, radiofrequency (RF) catheter ablation (elective or urgent) or adverse consequences from SVT (heart failure exacerbation, hypotension, myocardial ischemia) (Flow chart 2).

AV Nodal Dependent SVT or Regular SVT

AV Nodal dependent SVT or regular SVT for which mechanism is unknown. The first line treatment for an AV nodal dependent tachycardia is a vagal maneuver, such as carotid sinus massage, to create transient AV block and terminate the tachycardia. Patients can learn to perform vagal maneuvers and stop tachycardia on their own without the need for medical intervention.

TABLE 3 679

Pharmacologic management for supraventricular tachycardia

Drugs	Mechanisms	Dosage	Side effects	Contraindications
Adenosine	Purinergic agonist Inhibition sinus node and AV node	6 mg by rapid IV. If ineffective,12 mg and 18 mg	Nausea, light-headedness, headache, flushing, chest pain, bradycardia, brief asystole	Persantine Cardiac transplant Bronchospasm
Verapamil	Slow or block AV nodal conduction and slow sinus rate	2.5–5 mg over 1–2 min	Negative inotropic effect, hypotension, cardiogenic shock, marked bradycardia	Hypotension Systolic dysfunction Atrial fibrillation with preexcitation
Diltiazem	Slow or block AV nodal conduction and slow sinus rate	0.25 mg/kg IV bolus then 5–15 mg/hour gtt	Negative inotropic effect, hypotension, bradycardia	Hypotension Systolic dysfunction Atrial fibrillation with preexcitation
Metoprolol	Block β-sympathetic nervous system at the receptor level Inhibitory effects on sinus node, AV node and myocardial contraction	2.5–5 mg 3x at 2-min interval	Negative inotropic effect, hypotension	Hypotension Cardiogenic shock Bradycardia Decompensated heart failure Bronchospasm
Esmolol	Inhibitory effects on sinus node, AV node and myocardial contraction	IV 500 mcg/min loading dose over 1 min before each titration	Negative inotropic effect, hypotension, peripheral ischemia, confusion, bradycardia, bronchospasm	Hypotension Cardiogenic shock Bradycardia Decompensated heart failure Bronchospasm
Digoxin	Na^{+}/K^{+} ATPase inhibition Parasympathetic activation leading to sinus lowing and AV nodal inhibition	0.75–1.5 mg in divided doses over 12–24 hours	Nausea, vomiting, diarrhea, fatigue, confusion, colored vision, palpitation, arrhythmia, syncope	WPW syndrome Atrial fibrillation with preexcitation
Amiodarone	Class III AAD but with classes I, II and IV activity, block sodium, calcium and potassium channels	Oral: loading 1200–1600 mg daily, maintenance 200–400 mg daily IV: 150 mg over 10 min, then 360 mg over 6 hours, 540 mg over remaining 24 hours, then 0.5 mg/min	Thyroid abnormalities, pulmonary fibrosis, QT prolongation, liver function abnormalities	Severe sinus node dysfunction Hepatic dysfunction Pregnancy

Carotid sinus massage is an easy and effective methodology to stop AV nodal dependent SVT but should only be used in the absence of a carotid bruit and/or absence of significant carotid disease.[51] In this procedure, the head should be turned away from the side being compressed (usually the right side) and a firm compression with 2–3 fingers is applied over the bulb of the carotid. A strong arterial impulse must be felt with firm pressure and rubbing. Sometimes, carotid massage can be combined with a Valsalva maneuver and even the Trendelenburg position to facilitate conversion. The success of the carotid sinus massage depends, in part, on the technique. A Valsalva maneuver can similarly increase parasympathetic tone and therefore slow down the conduction in the antegrade slow pathway. Another vagal reflex, the "diving reflex" in which the face is placed in cold water, may be effective.[52] These maneuvers are unlikely to be effective if hypotension is present.

Adenosine (Flow chart 3) can differentiate AV nodal independent versus AV nodal dependent SVT and can be used to help to make a diagnosis (Fig. 24) but, like AVNRT, SART can respond to autonomic maneuvers and adenosine. Adenosine effectively and rapidly terminates AV nodal dependent SVTs.[53] It is generally effective even if borderline hypotension is present.

The advantage of adenosine is its rapid onset and short half-life. Adenosine must be given as a rapid intravenous bolus followed by a rapid saline infusion and should be given via a reliable, large bore IV access. The doses are between 6 mg and 12 mg, and occasionally up to 18 mg for highly resistant patients.

Adenosine must be used with caution in patients who are already taking persantine and also in patients who have cardiac transplant because asystole may occur. Furthermore, adenosine can cause long-lasting bronchoconstriction in patients with chronic obstructive lung disease or uncontrolled asthma. Caffeine and phosphodiesterase inhibitors will inhibit the effects of adenosine.[54] Some patients are reticent to have adenosine due to its short but potentially noxious side effects. Nevertheless, it is the preferred intervention to stop AVNRT and AVRT and it is effective in over 95% of individuals.[55,56]

Intravenous calcium channel antagonists, verapamil and diltiazem, can also terminate SVT.[57-59] Intravenous verapamil at doses of 5 mg, 10 mg and 15 mg can be effective; the duration of action is 5–45 minutes. Intravenous diltiazem can be used in doses of 0.15 mg/kg, 0.25 mg/kg and 0.45 mg/kg. Calcium channel blockers have negative inotropic effects and therefore can cause hypotension; use is not recommended when the patient

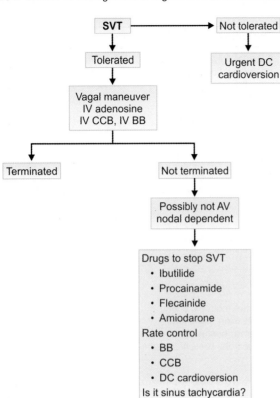

The use of digoxin for the acute management of SVT is now rare. Digoxin requires a loading dose and takes prolonged time to effect. It is less efficacious than other drugs and contraindicated in the WPW syndrome. It may be used in combination with beta-adrenergic blockers or calcium channel blockers to control recurrent episodes of SVT.

AV Nodal Independent SVT

Intravenous beta-blockers, digoxin and/or calcium channel blockers can control the ventricular rate in patients who have atrial-based, AV nodal independent SVT (AT, AFL and AFib). The one exception is SART that responds reliably to adenosine.

The preference of the drug class is related to the underlying conditions, blood pressure and ventricular function. Beta-blockers (in combination with digoxin), for example, are useful in controlling the ventricular response rate in AFL and AFib, especially in the postoperative period. Intravenous diltiazem has less negative inotropic effect than verapamil and can be used to control the ventricular rate when there is borderline low blood pressure. Diltiazem also may be useful when there is concern about bronchospasm. Digoxin may require a large loading dose and a protracted period but is more useful for patients with ventricular dysfunction or hypotension.

For patients with poorly tolerated AV nodal independent SVTs (AFL, AT and AFib), IV amiodarone is used to control the ventricular response rate.[60,61] Amiodarone has little role in the management of SVT otherwise.[62] For children, procainamide appears more effective than amiodarone for SVT.[63] Several drugs can stop AFL and AFib including intravenous procainamide and ibutilide. Acute treatments for AFL and AFib have been discussed in this chapter.

The WPW syndrome, when it is manifest as rapid AFib, should be treated with a drug that blocks the accessory pathway: either procainamide or amiodarone.[64,65] Digoxin, calcium channel blockers and beta-adrenergic blockers are strictly prohibited in these patients during acute management.[65]

Sinus tachycardia and MAT are likely due to underlying conditions. There is no specific treatment for the tachyarrhythmia and the goal is to treat the underlying conditions that are responsible for these problems.[66] When it is uncertain if a wide QRS complex tachycardia is SVT, drugs that block the AV node are not recommended.

is hypotensive or has ventricular dysfunction. It should be avoided in patients with preexcited AFib (i.e. antegrade activation via an accessory pathway). It should never be used when there is an undiagnosed wide QRS complex tachycardia as the results could be disastrous. Verapamil (and, less commonly, diltiazem) can be used when SVT is terminated with adenosine but recurs or in patients who ingest large amounts of caffeine.

Intravenous beta-adrenergic blockade (metoprolol or esmolol) may be effective in terminating SVT as well.[59] Esmolol has a short half-life of less than 10 minutes. Metoprolol has a longer half-life but is less expensive. Both of these drugs have a negative inotropic effect and may cause hypotension. Beta blockade and intravenous digoxin are third line drugs for termination of AV nodal dependent SVT.

FLOW CHART 3: Response of SVT to IV adenosine

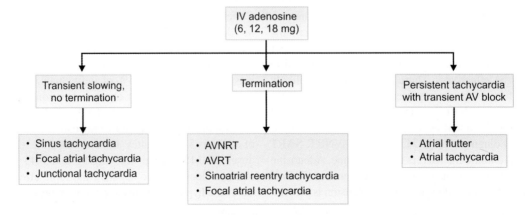

When to Use DC Cardioversion

Cardioversion is the best option for patients with an undiagnosed wide QRS complex tachycardia not tolerated hemodynamically and for any poorly tolerated (hemodynamic instability or evidence of heart failure or myocardial ischemia) SVT in which the rate cannot be controlled and the rhythm cannot be restored to sinus.

In patients who have hemodynamic collapse due to any type of SVT other than sinus tachycardia, synchronized DC cardioversion is recommended. However, it is important to ascertain that the SVT is not sinus tachycardia, as it will not respond to cardioversion.

LONG-TERM MANAGEMENT

Several issues must be considered before the long-term treatment is contemplated:

- Is it required?
- What are the implications of no treatment?
- How old is the patient? Are there comorbidities?
- Is the rhythm triggered by any acute nonarrhythmic condition such as pneumonia or pulmonary embolus?
- Is there any evidence of worsening congestive heart failure?
- How chronic is the rhythm and what is the rate of the tachycardia?
- Is there hemodynamic compromise?
- How symptomatic is the patient?
- How often does tachycardia occur?
- What are the patient's wishes regarding treatment?

The long-term management of SVT depends on multiple factors, including the symptoms related to SVT, the recurrence rates, the underlying clinical conditions and the presence of structural heart disease. For example, the treatment of a patient who has one episode of a mildly symptomatic SVT terminated by vagal maneuvers or adenosine, treatment will be different from a person with frequent recurrence. Other ensuing factors must be considered such as the necessity for medication to prevent SVT during pregnancy. In this case, more definitive treatment by an ablation would likely be the primary choice.

The choice of drug for long-term management of SVT depends on the mechanism of the SVT and the goal of treatment. For ATs, AFL and AFib a simple strategy is to control the ventricular rate instead of maintaining sinus rhythm (Fig. 25). Beta-adrenergic blockers, calcium channel blockers and digoxin, in combination, can be effective.[66,67] This approach alone may not make sense as symptoms continue. Furthermore, it can be very difficult to control the ventricular response rate for some SVTs, such as in AT and AFL. Therefore, it may be necessary to cardiovert the patient, use an antiarrhythmic drug or even

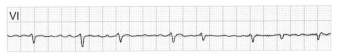

FIGURE 25: Atrial fibrillation with a controlled ventricular response rate. Normally, the ventricular response rate to atrial fibrillation is fast as long as there is an intact AV node and the patient is not taking medical therapy to slow or block conduction in the AV node

ablate the tachycardia. Antiarrhythmic drugs are often not effective for AFL and ablation may be necessary.[68,69] Occasionally, the ventricular rate cannot be controlled and maintenance of sinus rhythm is not an option; in this case, AV nodal ablation with permanent pacemaker may be required (Fig. 26).

For monomorphic AT, antiarrhythmic drugs can be given to help to maintain the sinus rhythm. The choice of antiarrhythmic drugs is similar to a methodology used for AFib, mainly based on the underlying structural heart disease. For patients without underlying structural heart disease, sotalol, propafenone and flecainide are possibilities. For patients with underlying structural heart disease, sotalol and amiodarone could be used to maintain sinus rhythm without a proarrhythmic effect.[70]

Like AFib and AFL, ATs can increase the risk of thromboembolic events.[71] Consideration must be given to the use of routine long-term anticoagulation for SVTs at risk for stroke. While guidelines address this issue for patients with AFib, they do not for ATs as data are scarce in this regard. Various antiarrhythmic drugs may suppress AFL. However, the safety and efficacy of antiarrhythmic drugs for AFL have not been well tested in the long term.[71] Furthermore, recent data suggest that ablation techniques especially for isthmus-dependent right AFL are more effective and cost-effective than drug therapy. Similarly, there are no specific guidelines with respect to anticoagulation for AFL. Recent data indicate that AFL has a similar or slightly lower risk of thromboembolic risk when compared with AFib. Therefore, AFL should be considered very much like AFib when contemplating the use of anticoagulation.

Catheter Ablation

Catheter ablation has emerged as a curative approach for the patients who have SVT.[72-75] The mechanism by which catheter ablation may work is dependent upon the type of tachycardia. Catheter ablation involves the purposeful destruction or isolation of selective tissue responsible for the tachycardia. Even extensive ablation rarely has a significant effect on cardiac function and may only require lesions that are rather small. Delivery of heat to the tissue via RF energy remains the standard approach in the ablation of most arrhythmias. Cryoablation has

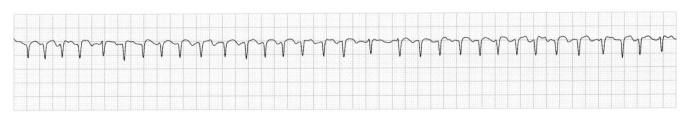

FIGURE 26: Irregularly irregular narrow QRS complex tachycardia is atrial fibrillation with a rapid ventricular response rate

been used with some success in selected patients who have arrhythmias.[76]

RF ablation can successfully cure AVNRT,[77] AVRT,[74] sinoatrial reentry,[78] WPW,[79] Mahaim tachycardias,[80] focal AT,[81,82] AFL,[83,84] and even AFib.[85] Additionally, ablation may be useful for JETs and occasionally for inappropriate sinus tachycardia.[11,86] Ablation can substantially improve the quality of life in patients with SVT.[87] Candidates for ablation include those patients who want their SVT eliminated and for whom the benefits outweigh the risks. The success rates for RF ablation vary by the rhythm disturbance and its location. RF ablation is strongly considered for those patients who have frequent, recurrent and symptomatic episodes that are either fast and/or refractory to the drugs.[88] The age distribution of RF ablation is a bell shaped curve with the average being 27 ± 17 years for accessory pathways and 44 ± 18 years for AVNRT.[75] Data suggests that there is a substantial decrease in frequency and severity of arrhythmias and decrease in self-imposed restrictions.[87] Cost-effectiveness data, based on older studies, indicates that the cost per quality adjusted life-year gained is $6,600 to $19,000.[89-91]

Generally, an electrophysiology study is performed as a diagnostic procedure with an ablation.[92] The procedure includes arrhythmia induction, mapping of the pathways or location, ablation and post-ablation attempts at arrhythmia induction. Conscious sedation is used and 3–5 transvenous catheters are placed. A transseptal approach may be needed to ablate a left-sided accessory pathway or for a left AT or AFL. In some instances, retrograde ablation approaches are performed from the aortic route.

Catheter ablation with a 4 mm tip catheter can eliminate the slow pathway in AVNRT, the accessory pathway in AVRT, and select focal ATs safely and effectively. In most cases, the lesions are focal but for AFL and specific ATs associated with complex macroreentry circuits (including patients with congenital heart disease)[93] linear lesions must be delivered to achieve the success. In rare instances, irrigated tipped catheters or an 8 mm tipped catheter is required to deliver extensive or deep lesions.[94] For younger patients and for specific tachycardias that originate from areas directly adjacent to the AV node, such as JET or in some cases, AVNRT, cryoablation may be safer and yet potentially effective.[95] However, RF generally remains the standard for ablation for most SVTs.

The success rate for ablation of AVNRT and many accessory pathway related SVTs exceeds 95%.[96] For typical AVNRT, the success rate is approximately 98% in experienced laboratories. The success rates for accessory pathway ablation may vary depending upon the location and are between 85% and 99% even for PJRT[45] and Mahaim tachycardias.[97] The recurrence rates after ablation, especially for accessory pathways, can be between 3% and 9%. The success rate for typical AFL is greater than 90% and recurrence rates are less than 10%[83,96] but AFib can follow.[98] The success rates for more unusual or AFib ablation-created AFL is less.[99] Ablation of AT has an approximately 70–90% success rate depending on the location and mechanism of the tachycardia.[100] In some instances, the tachycardias are close to the normal conduction system or in unusual locations.[101-105] The efficacy of ablation for ATs is from 80% to 98% with recurrences between 5% and 20% and

TABLE 4

Complications of catheter ablation for SVT (depends on SVT type)

Complications	Prevalence
AV block	0.67–1%
Cardiac tamponade	0.22–1.1%
Pericarditis	0.31%
Pneumothorax	0.15–0.22%
Tricuspid regurgitation	0.22%
Acute myocardial infarction	0.15%
Femoral artery pseudoaneurysm	0.15%
Death	0.1%

complications of 1.6% in one series.[106] AFib ablation is not as successful as ablation of AVNRT or AVRT and complication rates are higher.

Complications in ablation include death (0.1%)[107,108] (Table 4). There is approximately 0.4% risk of AV nodal block requiring a pacemaker with AVNRT "slow pathway" ablation. There are also risks of cardiac tamponade, pericarditis, hematoma and deep venous thrombosis. In general, the risks of the procedure are relatively low and all risks are less than 1%. Thus, ablation should be performed in patients who are highly symptomatic and with frequent recurrences, for those who have a high-risk profession, and for those with hemodynamic impairment or cardiomyopathy due to the persistent tachycardia.[92]

CONCLUSION

Supraventricular tachycardia remains a common and often symptomatic problem for many patients. A wide variety of types and clinical presentations of SVT exist. The diagnosis requires careful observation and interpretation of electrocardiographic recordings. Evaluation involves thoughtful assessment of the relationship between the tachycardia, hemodynamics and symptoms. While rarely life-threatening, treatment is often required. Remarkable advances have been made in the treatment of most forms of SVT.

REFERENCES

1. Gertler MN, Yohalem SB. The effect of atabrin on auricular fibrillation and supraventricular tachycardia in man. J Mt Sinai Hosp N Y. 1947;13:323-7.
2. Waldman S, Pelner L. The action of neostigmine in supraventricular tachycardias. Ann Intern Med. 1948;29:53-63.
3. Youmans WB, Goodman MJ, Gould J. Neosynephrine in treatment of paroxysmal supraventricular tachycardia. Am Heart J. 1949;37:359-73.
4. Elek SR, Bernstein JC, Griffith GC. Pressor drugs in the treatment of supraventricular tachycardia. Ann West Med Surg. 1952;6:497-9.
5. Furman RH, Geiger AJ. Use of cholinergic drugs in paroxysmal supraventricular tachycardia; serious untoward reactions and fatality from treatment with methacholine and neostigmine. JAMA. 1952;149:269-72.
6. Levenson RM, Thayer RH. Lanatoside C in the treatment of supraventricular tachycardia. Am Pract Dig Treat. 1952;3:635-7.
7. Levine EB, Blumfield G. Neostigmine bromide orally in prevention of paroxysmal supraventricular tachycardia. Ann West Med Surg. 1952;6:642-7.

8. Chotkowski LA, Powell CP, Rackliffe RL. Methoxamine hydrochloride in the treatment of paroxysmal supraventricular tachycardia; report of three cases. N Engl J Med. 1954;250:674-6.

9. Donegan CK, Townsend CV. Phenylephrine hydrochloride in paroxysmal supraventricular tachycardia. JAMA. 1955;157:716-8.

10. Yusuf S, Camm AJ. The sinus tachycardias. Nat Clin Pract Cardiovasc Med. 2005;2:44-52.

11. Low PA, Opfer-Gehrking TL, Textor SC, et al. Postural tachycardia syndrome (POTS). Neurology. 1995;45:S19-25.

12. Bhatt AG, Monahan KM. Nonreentrant supraventricular tachycardia misdiagnosed as inappropriate sinus tachycardia. Pacing Clin Electrophysiol. 2011;34:e70-3.

13. Olshansky B, Wilber DJ, Hariman RJ. Atrial flutter—update on the mechanism and treatment. Pacing Clin Electrophysiol. 1992;15:2308-35.

14. Garan H. Atypical atrial flutter. Heart Rhythm. 2008;5:618-21.

15. Cosio FG, Martin-Penato A, Pastor A, et al. Atypical flutter: a review. Pacing Clin Electrophysiol. 2003;26:2157-69.

16. Jais P, Hocini M, Weerasoryia R, et al. Atypical left atrial flutters. Card Electrophysiol Rev. 2002;6:371-7.

17. Cummings JE, Schweikert R, Saliba W, et al. Left atrial flutter following pulmonary vein antrum isolation with radiofrequency energy: linear lesions or repeat isolation. J Cardiovasc Electrophysiol. 2005;16:293-7.

18. Chugh A, Oral H, Good E, et al. Catheter ablation of atypical atrial flutter and atrial tachycardia within the coronary sinus after left atrial ablation for atrial fibrillation. J Am Coll Cardiol. 2005;46:83-91.

19. Knight BP, Ebinger M, Oral H, et al. Diagnostic value of tachycardia features and pacing maneuvers during paroxysmal supraventricular tachycardia. J Am Coll Cardiol. 2000;36:574-82.

20. Kall JG, Kopp D, Olshansky B, et al. Adenosine-sensitive atrial tachycardia. Pacing Clin Electrophysiol. 1995;18:300-6.

21. Nakagawa H, Shah N, Matsudaira K, et al. Characterization of reentrant circuit in macroreentrant right atrial tachycardia after surgical repair of congenital heart disease: isolated channels between scars allow "focal" ablation. Circulation. 2001;103:699-709.

22. Triedman JK, Jenkins KJ, Colan SD, et al. Intra-atrial reentrant tachycardia after palliation of congenital heart disease: characterization of multiple macroreentrant circuits using fluoroscopically based three-dimensional endocardial mapping. J Cardiovasc Electrophysiol. 1997;8:259-70.

23. Kalman JM, VanHare GF, Olgin JE, et al. Ablation of 'incisional' reentrant atrial tachycardia complicating surgery for congenital heart disease. Use of entrainment to define a critical isthmus of conduction. Circulation. 1996;93:502-12.

24. Walsh EP. Arrhythmias in patients with congenital heart disease. Card Electrophysiol Rev. 2002;6:422-30.

25. Gomes JA, Mehta D, Langan MN. Sinus node reentrant tachycardia. Pacing Clin Electrophysiol. 1995;18:1045-57.

26. Gomes JA, Hariman RJ, Kang PS, et al. Sustained symptomatic sinus node reentrant tachycardia: incidence, clinical significance, electrophysiologic observations and the effects of antiarrhythmic agents. J Am Coll Cardiol. 1985;5:45-7.

27. Paulay KL, Ruskin JN, Damato AN. Sinus and atrioventricular nodal reentrant tachycardia in the same patient. Am J Cardiol. 1975;36:810-6.

28. Scher DL, Arsura EL. Multifocal atrial tachycardia: mechanisms, clinical correlates, and treatment. Am Heart J. 1989;118:574-80.

29. Salerno DM, Anderson B, Sharkey PJ, et al. Intravenous verapamil for treatment of multifocal atrial tachycardia with and without calcium pretreatment. Ann Intern Med. 1987;107:623-8.

30. Akhtar M, Jazayeri MR, Sra J, et al. Atrioventricular nodal reentry. Clinical, electrophysiological, and therapeutic considerations. Circulation. 1993;88:282-95.

31. Heidbuchel H, Jackman WM. Characterization of subforms of AV nodal reentrant tachycardia. Europace. 2004;6:316-29.

32. Blaufox AD, Rhodes JF, Fishberger SB. Age related changes in dual AV nodal physiology. Pacing Clin Electrophysiol. 2000;23:477-80.

33. Wu D, Denes P, Dhingra R, et al. Determinants of fast- and slow-pathway conduction in patients with dual atrioventricular nodal pathways. Circ Res. 1975;36:782-90.

34. McGuire MA, Janse MJ, Ross DL. "AV nodal" reentry: Part II: AV nodal, AV junctional, or atrionodal reentry? J Cardiovasc Electrophysiol. 1993;4:573-86.

35. Janse MJ, McGuire MA, Loh P, et al. Electrophysiology of the A-V node in relation to A-V nodal reentry. Jpn Heart J. 1996;37:785-91.

36. Laurent G, Leong-Poi H, Mangat I, et al. Influence of ventriculoatrial timing on hemodynamics and symptoms during supraventricular tachycardia. J Cardiovasc Electrophysiol. 2009;20:176-81.

37. Gonzalez-Torrecilla E, Almendral J, Arenal A, et al. Combined evaluation of bedside clinical variables and the electrocardiogram for the differential diagnosis of paroxysmal atrioventricular reciprocating tachycardias in patients without pre-excitation. J Am Coll Cardiol. 2009;53:2353-8.

38. Obel OA, Camm AJ. Accessory pathway reciprocating tachycardia. Eur Heart J. 1998;19:E13-24, E50-1.

39. Morady F, DiCarlo LA, Baerman JM, et al. Determinants of QRS alternans during narrow QRS tachycardia. J Am Coll Cardiol. 1987;9:489-99.

40. Wolff L, Parkinson J, White PD. Bundle branch block with short P-R interval in healthy young people prone to paroxysmal tachycardia. Am Heart J. 1930;5:685.

41. Sternick EB, Timmermans C, Rodriguez LM, et al. Mahaim fiber: an atriofascicular or a long atrioventricular pathway? Heart Rhythm. 2004;1:724-7.

42. Gallagher JJ, Smith WM, Kasell JH, et al. Role of Mahaim fibers in cardiac arrhythmias in man. Circulation. 1981;64:176-89.

43. Dorostkar PC, Silka MJ, Morady F, et al. Clinical course of persistent junctional reciprocating tachycardia. J Am Coll Cardiol. 1999;33:366-75.

44. Nerheim P, Birger-Botkin S, Piracha L, et al. Heart failure and sudden death in patients with tachycardia-induced cardiomyopathy and recurrent tachycardia. Circulation. 2004;110:247-52.

45. Meiltz A, Weber R, Halimi F, et al. Permanent form of junctional reciprocating tachycardia in adults: peculiar features and results of radiofrequency catheter ablation. Europace. 2006;8:21-8.

46. Collins KK, Van Hare GF, Kertesz NJ, et al. Pediatric nonpostoperative junctional ectopic tachycardia medical management and interventional therapies. J Am Coll Cardiol. 2009;53:690-7.

47. Datino T, Almendral J, Gonzalez-Torrecilla E, et al. Rate-related changes in QRS morphology in patients with fixed bundle branch block: implications for differential diagnosis of wide QRS complex tachycardia. Eur Heart J. 2008;29:2351-8.

48. Olshansky B. Ventricular tachycardia masquerading as supraventricular tachycardia: a wolf in sheep's clothing. J Electrocardiol. 1988;21:377-84.

49. Marill KA, Wolfram S, Desouza IS, et al. Adenosine for wide-complex tachycardia: efficacy and safety. Crit Care Med. 2009;37:2512-8.

50. Olshansky B, Okumura K, Hess PG, et al. Demonstration of an area of slow conduction in human atrial flutter. J Am Coll Cardiol. 1990;16:1639-48.

51. Lim SH, Anantharaman V, Teo WS, et al. Comparison of treatment of supraventricular tachycardia by Valsalva maneuver and carotid sinus massage. Ann Emerg Med. 1998;31:30-5.

52. Belz MK, Stambler BS, Wood MA, et al. Effects of enhanced parasympathetic tone on atrioventricular nodal conduction during atrioventricular nodal reentrant tachycardia. Am J Cardiol. 1997;80:878-82.

53. DiMarco JP, Miles W, Akhtar M, et al. Adenosine for paroxysmal supraventricular tachycardia: dose ranging and comparison with verapamil. Assessment in placebo-controlled, multicenter trials. The

Adenosine for PSVT Study Group. Ann Intern Med. 1990;113: 104-10.

54. Cabalag MS, Taylor DM, Knott JC, et al. Recent caffeine ingestion reduces adenosine efficacy in the treatment of paroxysmal supraventricular tachycardia. Acad Emerg Med. 2010;17:44-9.

55. Cairns CB, Niemann JT. Intravenous adenosine in the emergency department management of paroxysmal supraventricular tachycardia. Ann Emerg Med. 1991;20:717-21.

56. Rankin AC, Brooks R, Ruskin JN, et al. Adenosine and the treatment of supraventricular tachycardia. Am J Med. 1992;92:655-64.

57. Sung RJ, Elser B, McAllister RG. Intravenous verapamil for termination of re-entrant supraventricular tachycardias: intracardiac studies correlated with plasma verapamil concentrations. Ann Intern Med. 1980;93:682-9.

58. Dougherty AH, Jackman WM, Naccarelli GV, et al. Acute conversion of paroxysmal supraventricular tachycardia with intravenous diltiazem. IV Diltiazem Study Group. Am J Cardiol. 1992;70: 587-92.

59. Das G, Tschida V, Gray R, et al. Efficacy of esmolol in the treatment and transfer of patients with supraventricular tachyarrhythmias to alternate oral antiarrhythmic agents. J Clin Pharmacol. 1988;28: 746-50.

60. Dilber E, Mutlu M, Dilber B, et al. Intravenous amiodarone used alone or in combination with digoxin for life-threatening supraventricular tachyarrhythmia in neonates and small infants. Pediatr Emerg Care. 2010;26:82-4.

61. Delle Karth G, Geppert A, Neunteufl T, et al. Amiodarone versus diltiazem for rate control in critically ill patients with atrial tachyarrhythmias. Crit Care Med. 2001;29:1149-53.

62. Blomstrom-Lundqvist C, Scheinman MM, Aliot EM, et al. ACC/AHA/ESC guidelines for the management of patients with supraventricular arrhythmias—executive summary: a report of the American College of Cardiology/American Heart Association Task Force on Practice Guidelines and the European Society of Cardiology Committee for Practice Guidelines (Writing Committee to Develop Guidelines for the Management of Patients With Supraventricular Arrhythmias). Circulation. 2003;108:1871-909.

63. Chang PM, Silka MJ, Moromisato DY, et al. Amiodarone versus procainamide for the acute treatment of recurrent supraventricular tachycardia in pediatric patients. Circ Arrhythm Electrophysiol. 2010;3:134-40.

64. Simonian SM, Lotfipour S, Wall C, et al. Challenging the superiority of amiodarone for rate control in Wolff-Parkinson-White and atrial fibrillation. Intern Emerg Med. 2010;5:421-6.

65. Redfearn DP, Krahn AD, Skanes AC, et al. Use of medications in Wolff-Parkinson-White syndrome. Expert Opin Pharmacother. 2005;6:955-63.

66. Kastor JA. Multifocal atrial tachycardia. N Engl J Med. 1990;322): 1713-7.

67. Arsura EL, Solar M, Lefkin AS, et al. Metoprolol in the treatment of multifocal atrial tachycardia. Crit Care Med. 1987;15:591-4.

68. Olshansky B. Dofetilide versus quinidine for atrial flutter: viva la difference!? J Cardiovasc Electrophysiol. 1996;7:828-32.

69. Natale A, Newby KH, Pisano E, et al. Prospective randomized comparison of antiarrhythmic therapy versus first-line radiofrequency ablation in patients with atrial flutter. J Am Coll Cardiol. 2000;35: 1898-904.

70. Chiang CE, Chen SA, Wu TJ, et al. Incidence, significance, and pharmacological responses of catheter-induced mechanical trauma in patients receiving radiofrequency ablation for supraventricular tachycardia. Circulation. 1994;90:1847-54.

71. Fuster V, Ryden LE, Cannom DS, et al. ACC/AHA/ESC 2006 guidelines for the management of patients with atrial fibrillation—executive summary: a report of the American College of Cardiology/American Heart Association Task Force on Practice Guidelines and the European Society of Cardiology Committee for Practice Guidelines (Writing Committee to Revise the 2001 Guidelines for the Management of Patients With Atrial Fibrillation). J Am Coll Cardiol. 2006;48:854-906.

72. Kay GN, Epstein AE, Dailey SM, et al. Role of radiofrequency ablation in the management of supraventricular arrhythmias: experience in 760 consecutive patients. J Cardiovasc Electrophysiol. 1993;4:371-89.

73. O'Hara GE, Philippon F, Champagne J, et al. Catheter ablation for cardiac arrhythmias: a 14-year experience with 5330 consecutive patients at the Quebec Heart Institute, Laval Hospital. Can J Cardiol. 2007;23:67B-70B.

74. Calkins H, Langberg J, Sousa J, et al. Radiofrequency catheter ablation of accessory atrioventricular connections in 250 patients. Abbreviated therapeutic approach to Wolff-Parkinson-White syndrome. Circulation. 1992;85:1337-46.

75. Calkins H, Yong P, Miller JM, et al. Catheter ablation of accessory pathways, atrioventricular nodal reentrant tachycardia, and the atrioventricular junction: final results of a prospective, multicenter clinical trial. The Atakr Multicenter Investigators Group. Circulation. 1999;99:262-70.

76. Friedman PL, Dubuc M, Green MS, et al. Catheter cryoablation of supraventricular tachycardia: results of the multicenter prospective "frosty" trial. Heart Rhythm. 2004;1:129-38.

77. Jackman WM, Wang XZ, Friday KJ, et al. Catheter ablation of atrioventricular junction using radiofrequency current in 17 patients. Comparison of standard and large-tip catheter electrodes. Circulation. 1991;83:1562-76.

78. Sanders WE, Sorrentino RA, Greenfield RA, et al. Catheter ablation of sinoatrial node reentrant tachycardia. J Am Coll Cardiol. 1994;23:926-34.

79. Jackman WM, Wang XZ, Friday KJ, et al. Catheter ablation of accessory atrioventricular pathways (Wolff-Parkinson-White syndrome) by radiofrequency current. N Engl J Med. 1991;324:1605-11.

80. McClelland JH, Wang X, Beckman KJ, et al. Radiofrequency catheter ablation of right atriofascicular (Mahaim) accessory pathways guided by accessory pathway activation potentials. Circulation. 1994;89: 2655-66.

81. Kay GN, Chong F, Epstein AE, et al. Radiofrequency ablation for treatment of primary atrial tachycardias. J Am Coll Cardiol. 1993;21: 901-9.

82. Steinbeck G, Hoffmann E. 'True' atrial tachycardia. Eur Heart J. 1998;19:E10-2, E48-9.

83. Feld GK, Fleck RP, Chen PS, et al. Radiofrequency catheter ablation for the treatment of human type 1 atrial flutter. Identification of a critical zone in the reentrant circuit by endocardial mapping techniques. Circulation. 1992;86:1233-40.

84. Cosio FG, Lopez-Gil M, Goicolea A, et al. Radiofrequency ablation of the inferior vena cava-tricuspid valve isthmus in common atrial flutter. Am J Cardiol. 1993;71:705-9.

85. Haissaguerre M, Jais P, Shah DC, et al. Spontaneous initiation of atrial fibrillation by ectopic beats originating in the pulmonary veins. N Engl J Med. 1998;339:659-66.

86. Shen WK. Modification and ablation for inappropriate sinus tachycardia: current status. Card Electrophysiol Rev. 2002;6:349-55.

87. Bubien RS, Knotts-Dolson SM, Plumb VJ, et al. Effect of radiofrequency catheter ablation on health-related quality of life and activities of daily living in patients with recurrent arrhythmias. Circulation. 1996;94:1585-91.

88. Goldberg AS, Bathina MN, Mickelsen S, et al. Long-term outcomes on quality-of-life and health care costs in patients with supraventricular tachycardia (radiofrequency catheter ablation versus medical therapy). Am J Cardiol. 2002;89:1120-3.

89. Bathina MN, Mickelsen S, Brooks C, et al. Radiofrequency catheter ablation versus medical therapy for initial treatment of supraventricular tachycardia and its impact on quality of life and healthcare costs. Am J Cardiol. 1998;82:589-93.

90. Ikeda T, Sugi K, Enjoji Y, et al. Cost effectiveness of radiofrequency catheter ablation versus medical treatment for paroxysmal supraventricular tachycardia in Japan. J Cardiol. 1994;24:461-8.

91. Kertes PJ, Kalman JM, Tonkin AM. Cost effectiveness of radio-frequency catheter ablation in the treatment of symptomatic supraventricular tachyarrhythmias. Aust N Z J Med. 1993;23:433-6.

92. Morady F. Radio-frequency ablation as treatment for cardiac arrhythmias. N Engl J Med. 1999;340:534-44.

93. Yap SC, Harris L, Silversides CK, et al. Outcome of intra-atrial re-entrant tachycardia catheter ablation in adults with congenital heart disease: negative impact of age and complex atrial surgery. J Am Coll Cardiol. 2010;56:1589-96.

94. Feld G, Wharton M, Plumb V, et al. Radiofrequency catheter ablation of type 1 atrial flutter using large-tip 8- or 10-mm electrode catheters and a high-output radiofrequency energy generator: results of a multicenter safety and efficacy study. J Am Coll Cardiol. 2004;43:1466-72.

95. Collins KK, Schaffer MS. Use of cryoablation for treatment of tachyarrhythmias in 2010: survey of current practices of pediatric electrophysiologists. Pacing Clin Electrophysiol. 2011;34:304-8.

96. Spector P, Reynolds MR, Calkins H, et al. Meta-analysis of ablation of atrial flutter and supraventricular tachycardia. Am J Cardiol. 2009;104:671-7.

97. Bohora S, Dora SK, Namboodiri N, et al. Electrophysiology study and radiofrequency catheter ablation of atriofascicular tracts with decremental properties (Mahaim fibre) at the tricuspid annulus. Europace. 2008;10:1428-33.

98. Chinitz JS, Gerstenfeld EP, Marchlinski FE, et al. Atrial fibrillation is common after ablation of isolated atrial flutter during long-term follow-up. Heart Rhythm. 2007;4:1029-33.

99. Satomi K, Bansch D, Tilz R, et al. Left atrial and pulmonary vein macroreentrant tachycardia associated with double conduction gaps: a novel type of man-made tachycardia after circumferential pulmonary vein isolation. Heart Rhythm. 2008;5:43-51.

100. Feld GK. Catheter ablation for the treatment of atrial tachycardia. Prog Cardiovasc Dis. 1995;37:205-24.

101. Rillig A, Meyerfeldt U, Birkemeyer R, et al. Catheter ablation within the sinus of Valsalva—a safe and effective approach for treatment of atrial and ventricular tachycardias. Heart Rhythm. 2008;5:1265-72.

102. Sacher F, Vest J, Raymond JM, et al. Incessant donor-to-recipient atrial tachycardia after bilateral lung transplantation. Heart Rhythm. 2008;5:149-51.

103. Yamada T, Huizar JF, McElderry HT, et al. Atrial tachycardia originating from the noncoronary aortic cusp and musculature connection with the atria: relevance for catheter ablation. Heart Rhythm. 2006;3:1494-6.

104. Iwai S, Badhwar N, Markowitz SM, et al. Electrophysiologic properties of para-hisian atrial tachycardia. Heart Rhythm. 2011. [Epub ahead of print]

105. Ouyang F, Ma J, Ho SY, et al. Focal atrial tachycardia originating from the non-coronary aortic sinus: electrophysiological characteristics and catheter ablation. J Am Coll Cardiol. 2006;48:122-31.

106. Tracy CM. Catheter ablation for patients with atrial tachycardia. Cardiol Clin. 1997;15:607-21.

107. Chen SA, Chiang CE, Tai CT, et al. Complications of diagnostic electrophysiologic studies and radiofrequency catheter ablation in patients with tachyarrhythmias: an eight-year survey of 3,966 consecutive procedures in a tertiary referral center. Am J Cardiol. 1996;77:41-6.

108. Scheinman MM, Huang S. The 1998 NASPE prospective catheter ablation registry. Pacing Clin Electrophysiol. 2000;23:1020-8.

Chapter 35

Clinical Spectrum of Ventricular Tachycardia

Masood Akhtar

Chapter Outline

INTRODUCTION

In this communication, it is assumed that the clinician has already made the distinction between the various causes of wide QRS tachycardias, of which ventricular tachycardia (VT) is only one, albeit the most common one.[1-4]

As the field of invasive interventional electrophysiology has grown, interest in finding the cellular/molecular basis for arrhythmias has escalated. At this time, however, we clinically deal with myriad complex VTs, often with incomplete understanding and the desire to simplify information for clinical purposes.[5-10] While ultimately VT-VF (ventricular fibrillation) may find a better classification based solely on genetic and cellular knowledge, their definition within the parameters of the current science is still evolving and mostly based on clinical presentation. For all practical purposes, generally only the clinical classifications are used to manage patients. When the word VT is mentioned, a number of natural questions cross one's mind. Is the episode brief or sustained? What are the patient's symptoms? Is there underlying heart disease? In this chapter, we have taken a clinician's approach as practiced today. It is,

however, important to realize that, increasingly, new entities are being introduced that may or may not fit into a given classification, and words, like miscellaneous, idiopathic and other descriptive terms, will continue to be used.

Table 1 is an attempt to present a simple and clinically relevant classification. The usual first encounter for an arrhythmologist to a patient with documented VT is a rhythm strip from telemetry, monitor, ambulatory recorder, during device interrogation or, occasionally, a 12-lead ECG (Fig. 1) showing a monomorphic (Panel A) or polymorphic (Panel B) VT. This is a striking feature of VT and is seldom missed by a clinician, unless, in a given lead, the polymorphic nature of the VT is not appreciable. There can be serious consequences for not knowing polymorphic versus monomorphic VT (MMVT). For example, administering an additional dose of an antiarrhythmic drug in the presence of a polymorphic variant of VT may aggravate the situation. Hence, it is prudent to emphasize at the outset that the distinction between the monomorphic and the polymorphic nature of the VT is important and can be deciphered by recording two leads perpendicular to each other.

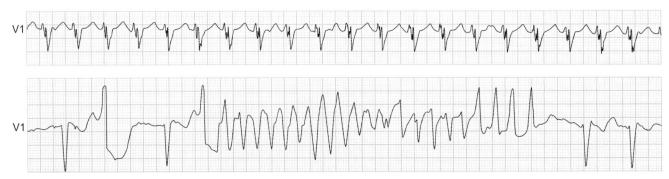

FIGURE 1: Rhythm strip (V1) shown. Note the monomorphic appearance of the VT in the top panel. P-wave is not clearly visible but its presence is suggested in some ST-T signals. The bottom tracing shows a prolongation of the QT interval, an episode of torsades de pointes, with rapid polymorphic VT of a constantly changing morphology that appears to be twisting around a central axis, which is the literal meaning of torsades de pointes (twisting of the points)

TABLE 1

Clinical spectrum of ventricular tachycardia

Monomorphic VT		Polymorphic VT		
SHD	No SHD	Long QT	Normal QT	Short QT
Myocardial Fibrosis	RV outflow	Congenital (QT-1 to QT-12)	Brugada* (Type 1-3)	Short QT (1-5)
BBR (HPS Disease)	Idiopathic LV-VT	Acquired: Drugs, electrolyte (Table 2)	Active ischemia	
ARVD (RV fatty infiltration) regional and familial forms of ARVD Naxos, Venetian	From Sinus Valsalva, Mitral, Pulmonic Cusp		Myocardial hypertrophy	
	Bidirectional		LV Noncompaction	
VT Post Surgical Scar	Iatrogenic device leads		Catecholaminergic PVT J-wave syndromes early repolarization syndromes hypothermia Idiopathic VF	

(Abbreviations: SHD: Structural heart disease; BBR: Bundle branch reentry; ARVD: Arrhythmic RV dysplasia; RV: Right ventricular; LV: Left ventricular; PVT: Polymorphic ventricular tachycardia; VF: Ventricular fibrillation.
• Regional expressions for Brugada-like syndromes:
  — Thailand – Tai Lai (death during sleep)
  — Phillipines – Bangungut (scream followed by sudden death-at night)
  — Japan – Pokkuri – (unexpected sudden death at night)

Once that distinction is settled, the usual next line of questioning regards the underlying pathology or structural heart disease (SHD) such as ischemia, myopathy, etc. When there is no SHD detected, attention is then directed to various VT syndromes. These somewhat newer entities are currently hard to classify. In the future, expressions, like channelopathies, repolarization syndromes, J-wave abnormalities or other such terminology, will be used routinely, and it seems this trend has already begun.[11,12]

MONOMORPHIC VENTRICULAR TACHYCARDIA

MYOCARDIAL VT IN ASSOCIATION WITH STRUCTURAL HEART DISEASE

Myocardial VT in Association with Fibrosis/Scar[8-10,13-15] (Table 1)

Coronary artery disease (CAD) remains the most common form of VT. Both monomorphic and polymorphic forms exist. However, the monomorphic forms [Fig. 1 (top panel)] are better understood and the underlying mechanism is easier to comprehend. Its distinction from other forms of wide QRS tachycardias has been extensively published.[1-4] The classic model used to visualize this circuit of reentry is depicted in Figure 2.[9] The fibrotic scar zone, shown as islands, the paths of impulse propagation in various directions, is indicated by arrows. On the surface ECG, QRS starts when the impulse exits from within the circuit. If one was to electrically stimulate this exit site, the surface ECG QRS would look identical to the spontaneous VT with a short stimulus artifact to QRS interval (Fig. 3). Depending upon the geometry of the scar, the impulse could go in several directions, dictated by the shape of the scar and the state of the myocardium. As an example shown in Figure 2, the impulse travels in all the directions in a three-dimensional tissue. During activation of a normal myocardium

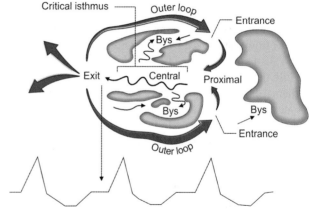

FIGURE 2: Classical model used to demonstrate reentry through the surviving muscle bands among the myocardial scar (shown as five islands). The QRS on the surface ECG starts where the impulse exits from the critical isthmus and turns around in a figure-of-eight fashion to reenter from the proximal end. Ablation at sites other than beside the central blue line is unlikely to be successful. This is why it is termed a critical area of slow conduction or as critical isthmus. (*Source:* Modified from Stevenson W, Soejima K. Catheter ablation of ventricular tachycardia. In: Zipes DP, Jalife J (Eds). Cardiac Electrophysiology: From Cell to Bedside, 4th edition. Philadelphia: WB Saunders; 2004. pp. 1087-96)

the impulse will reenter the circuit at the proximal end or some other points. Depending on its length, the location of surviving myocardial cells within the scar and the speed of conduction, the local electrical signal produced may bear a variable relation with the surface QRS. For example, the interval recorded between the electrogram and pacing artifact from the same catheter site in the critical isthmus to the next QRS will measure the same.[9] However, from the adjacent bystander, the interval from the local electrogram to next QRS will be considerably shorter compared to the pacing to the next artifact QRS interval from the same site. These maneuvers are very helpful in finding the right location for catheter ablation.

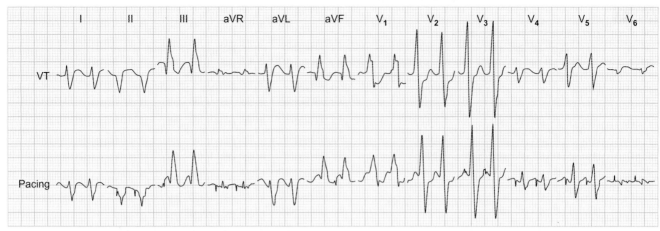

FIGURE 3: Example of spontaneous ventricular tachycardia (VT) recorded on a 12-lead ECG. The bottom shows 12-lead pace map. Note that the QRS is identical to spontaneous VT and the stimulus artifact to QRS is relatively short—best appreciated in leads II, V$_{4-6}$

It should be pointed out that the diastolic interval between the QRS complexes is increased when the reentrant impulse is travelling through the isthmus (surviving muscle band, area of slow conduction), which is critical for the VT to continue. While this electrical activity is not visible on the surface ECG, it can be recorded by placing electrode catheters along the pathway. Penetration of this pathway occurs during sinus rhythm as well, and it can be recorded both by intracardiac recording techniques as well as from the surface by proper magnification and filters (the so-called signal-averaged ECG).[16]

While the actual reentrant circuits may be more complex, the schema shown in Figure 2 gives one broad concept of how a VT can be mapped. When appropriate location of slow conduction is isolated, it leads to a successful ablation using radiofrequency or another form of energy. The baseline ECG is seldom normal in these patients, and likely to be suggestive of some cardiac pathology.

Therapy for a scar-related VT can be manifold:[17,18]

- In patients with an ejection fraction of less than 35%, implantable cardioverter defibrillator (ICD) is advised. The main reason is the prevention of sudden VT-related death from an existing or new arrhythmia (Fig. 4).[19] In many cases, particularly with slow VT ($\geq$ 280 ms), antitachycardia pacing will also terminate an organized MMVT, which is more comfortable for the patient
- With better left ventricular ejection fractions (LVEF), antiarrhythmic agents, particularly Class III drugs, such as sotalol, amiodarone and dronedarone, may be sufficient. In patients with CAD and VT, the addition of beta-blockers is beneficial because the role of ischemia in the initiation and maintenance of VT cannot be excluded with certainty at a given time. In high-risk patients post-myocardial infarction or cardiac surgery, an external defibrillator in the form of a life vest can be recommended

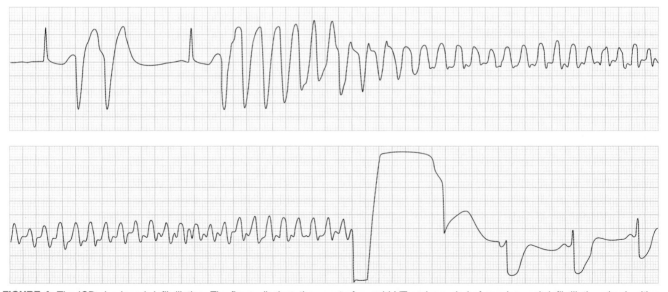

FIGURE 4: The ICD shock and defibrillation. The figure displays the onset of a rapid VT and a period of sensing and defibrillation shock with an ICD and restoration of sinus rhythm. The effect of acute injury from ICD can be appreciated in subsequent sinus complexes. This tachycardia was different than previously documented (*Source:* Tchou PJ, Kadri N, Anderson J, et al. Automatic implantable cardioverter defibrillators and survival of patients with left ventricular dysfunction and malignant ventricular arrhythmias. Ann Intern Med. 1988;109:529-34, with permission)

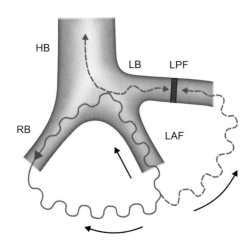

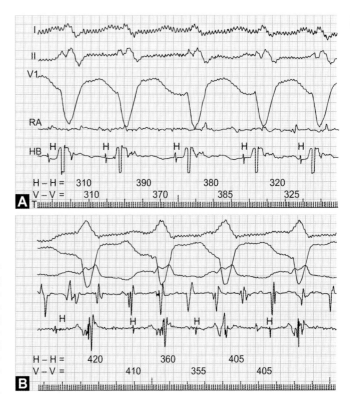

FIGURE 5: Schema demonstrates the circuit of bundle branch reentry VT. In this example, the impulse reaches the right ventricle via the right bundle (RB) and returns to the His bundle through the inferior fascicle of the left bundle (LB). While the same impulse approaches the His bundle via the superior fascicle, the two impulses will collide somewhere in that region. Activation of the His bundle will occur as a necessity since the left and right bundle are connected via the His bundle. The arrows depict the direction of impulse propagation. Tracings from top to bottom in each panel are surface ECG leads I, II and V$_1$. The intracardiac tracings are HRA (high right atrial electrogram) and HB (His bundle electrogram). Time lines at the bottom are consecutive (Abbreviations: LAF: Left anterior fascicle; LPF: Left posterior fascicle)

FIGURES 6A AND B: Bundle branch reentry with a left bundle branch block pattern (A) and right bundle branch block pattern (B) are shown. The axis is normal in A and leftward in B. The atrial rhythm is atrial fibrillation. Note that His deflection precedes the QRS and the change in the cycle length of H-H (labeled) precedes that of V-V (also labeled). In other words, the His bundle activation drives the ventricle, which is the opposite of what happens in myocardial VT, where the His bundle deflection follows the local V electrogram or is obscured by it. Nonetheless, the V-V cycle drives the H-H cycle in myocardial VT. (*Source:* Blanck Z, Jazayeri M, Akhtar M. Facilitation of sustained bundle branch reentry by atrial fibrillation. J Cardiovasc Electrophysiol. 1996;7:348-52, with permission)

- When VT is incessant, endocardial and/or epicardial mapping and catheter ablation may be necessary
- Although surgical ablation is seldom necessary, it remains an option
- In rare situations, cardiac transplantation with or without ventricular assist devices may be the only option when there are no contraindications

Monomorphic VT due to Bundle Branch Reentry[20-25]

In this form of monomorphic VT, the underlying pathological substrate is the His-Purkinje system, which has markedly prolonged conduction time. More specifically, the right and left bundle branches are used for propagation to the ventricle via one bundle, returning to the His bundle through the contralateral bundle branch. Sometimes the electrical circuit is localized to the two fascicles of the left bundle; in that case it is termed interfascicular reentry. The schema in Figure 5 depicts the reentry circuits and Figures 6A and B shows bundle branch reentry (BBR)-VT, both a left bundle branch block (LBBB) pattern (A) and a right bundle branch block (RBBB) pattern (B). While the general incidence of BBR as the mechanism of MMVT is 6%, it is much higher in patients with idiopathic dilated cardiomyopathy and aortic valve disease.[24-26] In patients with aortic valve disease, this is particularly common in the early post-surgical period.[24] This form of VT is apparently a common finding in patients with myotonic dystrophy, when VT is observed in that population.[25] The common theme among all of the above scenarios is the presence of His-Purkinje pathology manifested by nonspecific intraventricular conduction defect (IVCD), incomplete-to-complete bundle branch block on surface ECG with prolonged H-V interval on the His bundle

electrogram recording.[20] Unlike patients with myocardial disease, where the His bundle potential follows QRS, in BBR it always precedes QRS with equal to or longer H-V than sinus, and H-H cycle length changes precede V-V cycle length changes (Fig. 6).

While typically these individuals have low LVEF, BBR can recur in patients without SHD and normal LVEF[27] and in some patients with valvular disease, myocardial dystrophy and preserved left ventricular (LV) function.[24,25] Common to all of the above is the IVCD, and prolonged H-V interval and myocardial damage is not a prerequisite.

The tachycardia morphology is either an LBBB or, less frequently, an RBBB pattern (Figs 6 and 7). Since the reentrant impulse depolarizes the ventricle via the bundle branch, the surface ECG appearance of the QRS has some features common to QRS complex due to aberrant conduction, such as rapid initial inscription of the QRS, unlike the slurred beginning of QRS seen in myocardial VT or pre-excited QRS. These tachycardias are often rapid and poorly tolerated by patients with poor LV function, frequently lead to syncope and may degenerate into VF.

Bundle branch ablation is the preferred therapy in patients with good LV function (Fig. 7), while an ICD should be

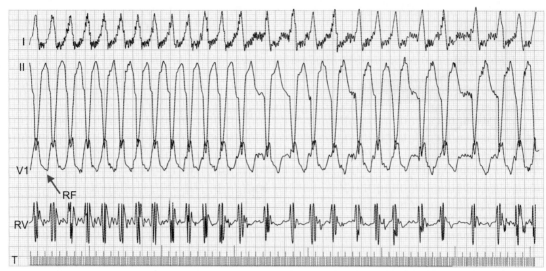

FIGURE 7: Ablation of bundle branch reentry (BBR). The first 13 complexes are due to BBR-VT. The underlying atrial rhythm is atrial fibrillation, which becomes obvious when the VT stops due to right bundle ablation. Note, there is no change in QRS configuration but now the ventricular rate is irregular due to AF

implanted in cases where the LVEF is less than 35%. Although BBR is easily pace-terminable, RBBB ablation may still be necessary in some cases to prevent frequent recurrences.

Monomorphic VT in Association with Arrhythmogenic Right Ventricular Dysplasia[28,29]

In arrhythmogenic right ventricular dysplasia (ARVD), the right ventricular (RV) muscle is replaced by fatty tissue, which in effect creates a model very similar to that shown in Figure 2. The disease may be patchy; affecting only RV apex, outflow or other parts, but may be quite extensive, replacing most RV myocardium with fatty infiltrates. At times the LV may also be affected.

For the most part, the main clinical problem these patients have is with nonsustained or sustained VT with a left bundle branch configuration with variable axis. While any axis may be noted, left bundle and left atrial (LA) morphology is very suggestive of ARVD; surface ECG also characteristically shows T-wave inversion in V_1–V_3 (Fig. 8) and may extend to V_4 or V_5. A late small deflection may be seen at the end of the QRS (epsilon wave) (Fig. 8 inset). Signal-averaged ECG is often positive. Diagnostic work should include magnetic resonance imaging (MRI), which is more sensitive than ultrasound, particularly in the early stages when the dysplasia is patchy.

Several genetic abnormalities are associated with this syndrome. In several areas of the world, such as Naxos (Greece) and the Venetian region (Italy), a large prevalence of these VTs is noted among some families.[30] The VTs generally have a monomorphic configuration, but sudden cardiac death (SCD) may occur. Sotalol and amiodarone have been used to control VT. Catheter ablation is not encouraged due to the risk of perforation. The ICD therapy is recommended for the prevention of SCD. This topic is more extensively covered elsewhere in this book.

Monomorphic VT Post Surgery for Congenital Heart Disease[31,32]

This type of tachycardia is mechanistically akin to a scar-related reentry. Since most of these incisional scars are in the right ventricle, the morphology is likely to be an LBBB configuration and a variable axis, usually right. Associated congenital heart disease (CHD), adhesions post surgery and other factors, such as development of thorax, etc., may create a somewhat atypical QRS configuration, but endocardial mapping will localize the VT in the neighborhood of the scar. Antiarrhythmic drugs and catheter ablation (while they may be sufficient to control the VT), concomitant pulmonary hypertension or pulmonic valve regurgitation would increase the risk for SCD. This scenario may require serious consideration for ICD implant; not an easy decision in this young population.

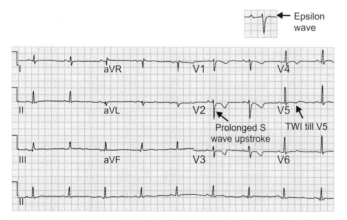

FIGURE 8: Twelve-lead ECG in arrhythmic right ventricular dysplasia (ARVD), the T-wave inversion V_{1-5} (usually up to V_3) and late wave (epsilon wave in the insert) are characteristic findings in the baseline ECG of these patients (*Source:* Nasir K, Bomma C, Tandri H, et al. Electrocardiographic features of arrhythmogenic right ventricular dysplasia/cardiomyopathy according to disease severity: a need to broaden diagnostic criteria. Circulation. 2004;110:1527-34, with permission)

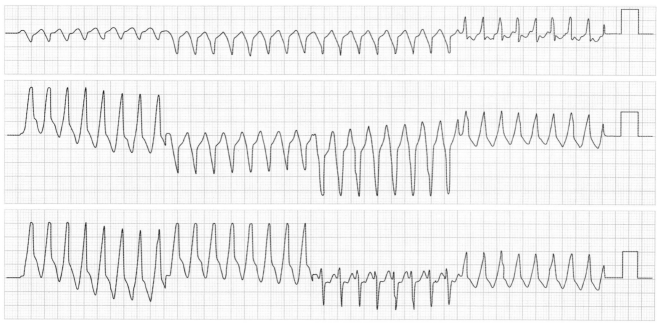

FIGURE 9: Right ventricular outflow tract (RVOT) VT. Typically, VT arises in RVOT. The orientation of the 12-lead ECG is leads I, II and III are on the left from top to bottom. The AVR, AVL, AVF are the next three leads, V_{1-3} and V_{4-6} are next. The same designation is used with all of the 12-lead ECGs unless labeled otherwise. Note left bundle branch block pattern and right axis typical of this type of VT

MONOMORPHIC VT IN ASSOCIATION WITH STRUCTURALLY NORMAL HEART

VT from Right Ventricular Outflow Tract

As the name suggests, the most common location of this VT is outflow which produces a characteristic LBBB and right atrial morphology (Fig. 9).[33,34] If the breakthrough occurs on the left side, an RBBB morphology may be seen. The baseline ECG is usually normal. The process could present in the form of isolated premature ventricular complexes, repetitive MMVT, nonsustained or sustained VT. When RV outflow VT is symptomatic, palpitation, lightheadedness and presyncope are common. Syncope may occur, but SCD is rare in these patients. The mechanism is not completely clear, but the tachycardia often is initiated by isoproterenol. Triggered delayed afterdepolarization driven by catecholamines is the prevailing view regarding the arrhythmogenic mechanism. Clinically increased sympathetic drive, such as physical exercise, often triggers the episode and, not infrequently, beta-blockers may be effective in controlling the VT. Thus, antiarrhythmic drugs, such as sotalol and amiodarone, may also be effective. Considering a good long-term outcome, catheter ablation is increasingly used as a preferred form of therapy. Even though the diagnosis is often clear from clinical data, ARVD should be excluded with MRI prior to catheter ablation.

Idiopathic Left Ventricle VT[35,36]

The electrophysiologic basis of this VT is reentry within the peripheral Purkinje system. The QRS morphology is that of right bundle and LA (Fig. 10), but other ranges of axis are occasionally observed. The baseline ECG and LVEF as a rule are normal. Intravenous verapamil will often terminate the VT but is less effective orally. Class III antiarrhythmic agents, such

as amiodarone, are effective, but, at this time, catheter ablation is the first-line treatment considering this VT is easily inducible in the laboratory.

As with RV outflow VT, the ventricle is usually normal. Sudden death is rare but the usual symptoms of arrhythmias, such as palpitations, dizziness and occasional presyncope and syncope, are noted.

Aortic Sinus of Valsalva, Pulmonic, Mitral Cusp VT

Monomorphic VT with right axis occasionally arises from structures outside the traditional ventricular myocardium.[37,38] While they mimic the outflow VT, awareness of these loci helps to improve mapping. Catheter ablation is the usual treatment. Although experience with these types of VT is limited, it is likely that the traditional antiarrhythmic drugs may be successful.

Bidirectional Tachycardia

Bidirectional tachycardia seen with digitalis toxicity is rare, but is seen in the early stages of the exercisein patients with catecholaminergic VT (discussed later). Its classic picture is that of two sets of monomorphic QRS complexes alternating in QRS morphologies. In a sense, bidirectional tachycardia has not a true polymorphic but rather a pleomorphic appearance.

Iatrogenic VT

Whenever a lead is placed in the ventricle, it is not surprising that a monomorphic VT from mechanical movement may be created that can be mistaken for a spontaneous VT, particularly with ICD leads since these patients also have clinical VT. Whenever a resistant VT is found with morphology that could be generated from the location of the catheter, nothing but catheter withdrawal and repositioning will fix this type of VT,

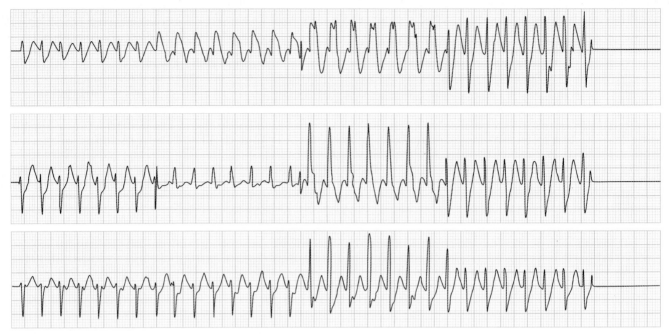

FIGURE 10: Idiopathic left ventricular VT. The typical QRS morphology is that of right bundle branch block and left-axis pattern. Note the initial part of the QRS has rapid inscription due to the fascicular origin of this VT. Contrast this with Figure 9 where the initial part of the QRS has a slow inscription

so keeping this in mind is important as part of the differential diagnosis in patients with device implant.

POLYMORPHIC VENTRICULAR TACHYCARDIA

Polymorphic ventricular tachycardia can be broadly separated into three categories: (1) PVT in association with long QT interval; (2) PVT in association with normal QT and (3) VT in association with short QT interval. Long QT itself has been traditionally divided into congenital and acquired forms.

PVT IN ASSOCIATION WITH LONG QT INTERVAL (TABLE 1)

Congenital Long QT Interval Syndrome[39-42]

At this writing, at least 12 entities (QT-1–12) have been described here briefly, as long QT syndrome is covered elsewhere in the book. Other less-understood entities will not be discussed here.

QT-1: QT-1 is the most common form [Fig. 11 (left panel)]. The recessive variety may be associated with deafness. The PVT

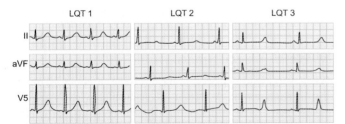

FIGURE 11: Congenital long QT (LQT). The three most common genetic varieties are shown. The corresponding chromosomes are labeled. See text for other details. (*Source:* Moss AJ, Zareba W, Benhorin J, et al. ECG T-wave patterns in genetically distinct forms of the hereditary long QT syndrome. Circulation. 1995;92:2929-34, with permission)

is typically triggered with physical activity, emotional stress, diving and swimming. Syncope, presyncope and SCD are the most serious clinical manifestations. The surface ECG shows a broad, prolonged T-wave and a long QT interval (Fig. 11). Early onset of symptoms, syncope, excessive QT prolongation is more than or equal to 550 msec in QT-1 and QT-2, and males with QT-3 are associated with a high risk of SCD (Fig. 11). Nonselective beta-blockers, such as propranolol and nadolol, are preferred, but others have been used. A dose of propranolol (5 mg/kg is usual) and avoidance of triggering events, such as adrenergic stress or diving, is highly recommended. Drugs that prolong QT (Table 2) and electrolyte imbalance, such as hypokalemia, can be lethal in this population with prolonged QT syndrome.

The gene involved in QT-1 is $KCNQ^1$ and affects K^+ current (delayed rectifier current 1Ks), which is reduced, causing the lengthening of QT [Fig. 11 (left panel)]. If a proband is found, it is likely that a high percentage of blood relatives may carry the abnormal gene. Genetic screening should be recommended. Beta-blockers are effective in controlling the symptoms. Left stellate ganglionectomy has been successful in controlling symptoms. In patients with malignant manifestation, i.e. SCD or PVT-related syncope, ICD should be seriously considered.

QT-2: QT-2 [Fig. 11 (middle panel)] is the second most common, and carried by 1Kr (delayed rectifiers), which encodes the gene KCNH2. The QT is prolonged as expected, but the T-wave is somewhat flat and less pronounced than QT-1. While adrenergic stress remains important, auditory stimuli in particular may trigger malignant arrhythmia.

QT-3: Compared to QT-1 and QT-2, QT-3 is less common but has a worse outcome. The QT-3 is prolonged [Fig. 11 (right panel)] due to increased inward Na^+ current. The Na^+ channel is encoded by the gene SCN5A and, consequently, the ECG shows a prolonged ST segment, short T-wave and a long QT

TABLE 2

Abbreviated list of drugs reported to cause prolongation of the QT interval or torsades de pointes

Antiarrhythmic:	
Class 1A	Disopyramide, procainamide, quinidine
Class III	Amiodarone, bretylium, sotalol, dofetilide, ibutilide
Antimicrobial	Erythromycin, trimethoprim-sulfamethoxazole, clarithromycin
Antifungal	Fluconazole, ketoconazole, itraconazole
Antimalarial or antiprotozoal	Chloroquine, halofantrine, mefloquine, pentamidine, quinine
Antihistamine	Astemizole, terfenadine, diphenhydramine
Gastrointestinal prokinetic	Cisapride
Psychoactive	Chloral hydrate, haloperidol, lithium, phenothiazines, pimozide, tricyclic antidepressants
Anti-human immunodeficiency virus	Efavirenz
Miscellaneous	Amantadine, indapamide, probucol, tacrolimus, vasopressin

Source: Modified from El-Sherif N, Turitto G. Torsades de pointes. In: Zipes DP, Jalife J (Eds). Cardiac Electrophysiology: From Cell to Bedside, 4th edition. Philadelphia: WB Saunders; 2004. pp. 687-98

CHAPTER 35

Clinical Spectrum of Ventricular Tachycardia

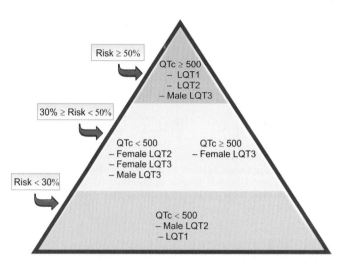

FIGURE 12: A pyramid showing risk stratification in congenital long QT (LQT) syndrome. (*Source:* Modified from Schwartz PJ, Priori SG. Long QT syndrome: genotype-phenotype correlations. In: Zipes DP, Jalife J (Eds). Cardiac Electrophysiology: From Cell to Bedside, 4th edition. Philadelphia: WB Saunders; 2004. pp. 651-9

interval. Prognosis without therapy is poor, particularly in young males (Fig. 12). Bradycardia is one of the main triggers, such that the most fatal events occur at night or during sleep. The role of beta-blockers is still controversial and, without bradycardia support (i.e. pacemaker), somewhat risky. Patients who have exhibited symptoms due to PVT, such as syncope or cardiac arrest, should have ICD implantation. The role of gene-specific drugs and other agents that shorten the QT interval, such as mexiletine, has not been systematically studied sufficiently to be utilized as the sole therapy for prevention of SCD. Risk stratification among patients with congenital long QT is shown in Figure 12.

Acquired Long QT Syndrome

Although the exact underlying etiology of acquired long QT is not understood, it is widely believed and sometimes reported that a genetic basis with low penetrance may account for some of these cases.[43,44] An external trigger, such as an antiarrhythmic drug, electrolyte imbalance, etc., is required for the clinical manifestations of this form, i.e. prolongation of QT and torsades de pointes.

There are an increasing number of pharmaceutical agents that have been documented to be the culprit (Table 2). In addition to the Class I or Class III antiarrhythmic drugs [Fig. 1 (top panel)], many other agents and situations have produced similar adverse affects. Low Mg^{++}, Ca^{++} and K^+ may trigger torsades de pointes in vulnerable populations. Some drugs, by blocking or binding with certain liver enzymes, may lower metabolism, raising the blood level of the parent compound that in turn may produce prolonged QT and torsades de pointes.

Acute treatment is usually the administration of IV Mg^{++}, which often effectively halts torsades, but recognizing and discontinuing the offending agent is usually sufficient. Isoproterenol infusion and overdrive pacing are also used to stop the torsades de pointes. Patients are advised to avoid similar agents and situations, such as over-the-counter medication, where the contents are not clearly labeled. This aspect of long QT is important to realize because the blood relatives of a person with congenital long QT may be prone to the same hazards and a caution regarding this possibility may be wise.

PVT WITH NORMAL QT PROLONGATION

Brugada Syndrome

Brugada syndrome was initially described by the Brugada brothers as the presence of an injury pattern in leads V_1 and V_2 with ST elevation followed by T-wave inversion (Fig. 13) and a history of syncope and SCD.[45-48] Since then, more has been learned regarding the role of ionic currents, the underlying mechanism and the worldwide prevalence of this potentially malignant syndrome.

The exact preponderance is unknown, but Pokkuri in Japan, Bangungut in the Philippines and Tai Lai in Thailand seem to be the same affliction (Table 1). Mostly seen in young males, death from PVT-VF occurs at night. The ECG abnormalities (Fig. 13) may not always be present. However, Class I agents, such as ajmaline and procainamide, can unmask the abnormality. In many cases, the genes that encode SCN5A can be detected. Quinidine has been identified as a potentially effective agent to prevent SCD in this population. However, ICD remains the most reliable therapy to prevent PVT-VT related deaths in patients with Brugada syndrome.

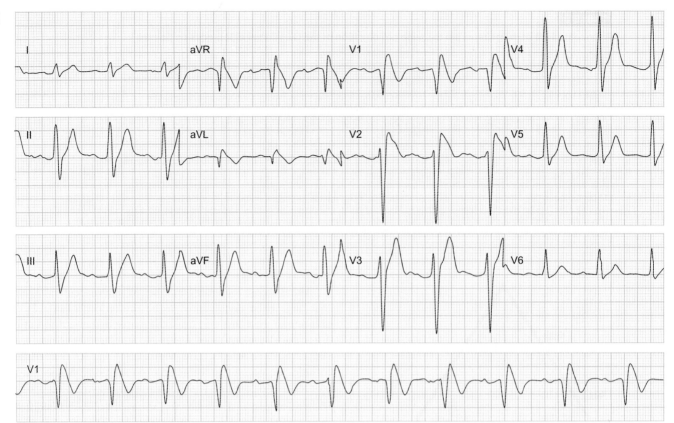

FIGURE 13: Typical 12-lead ECG of Brugada syndrome. The most characteristic features are seen in leads V_1 and V_2. ST elevation and T-wave inversion gives the impression of a right bundle branch block pattern (*Source:* Modified from Dorian P, Bharati S, Myerburg RJ, et al. Ventricular fibrillation. In: Saksena S, Camm AJ (Eds). Electrophysiological Disorders of the Heart. New York: Churchill-Livingston; 2005. pp. 419-53

Active Ischemia

In patients with clinically significant CAD, some degree of ischemia may exist at all times, but a critical degree of ischemia with exercise, spontaneously or with spasm, can induce a PVT-VF. This is a highly malignant arrhythmia and usually fatal unless it stops spontaneously or is terminated. Anti-ischemic therapy and revascularization are the preferred treatment modalities. The tracing in Figure 14 is from a 60-year-old male who underwent coronary artery bypass grafting, was continued on beta-blockers and still had 3–4 episodes of VT per year.[5] He received an ICD, which intervened several times over the years. This occurred primarily due to incomplete revasculari-

zation—partly due to some areas of inoperable disease, not an infrequent clinical scenario.

Acute ischemic-related PVT-VF should be addressed promptly since patients have died while waiting for revascularization. Three decades ago, large infarcts resulting in aneurysms were associated with monomorphic VT. With early intervention and the use of several effective anti-ischemic agents, large infarcts and ventricular aneurysms are less frequently encountered. The PVT seems to be more common. Since it degenerates into VF quickly, the true incidence of PVT is difficult to estimate, but it certainly constitutes a significant cause of the SCD from CAD.

Myocardial Hypertrophy

The VF and consequent SCD remain one of the main causes of cardiovascular death in patients with hypertrophic cardiomyopathy.[49] Apical hypertrophy has a particularly malignant outcome. Syncope, near-syncope and nonsustained VT define a particularly high-risk population. The SCD is seen in both obstructive and nonobstructive forms. High-risk patients should be considered for ICD therapy, both for primary and for secondary prevention of SCD.

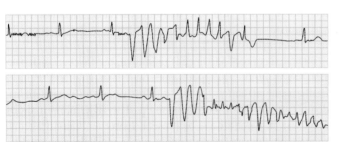

FIGURE 14: Polymorphic ventricular tachycardia (top panel) and onset of VF (bottom panel) in a patient with CAD post-coronary artery bypass surgery. Incomplete revascularization may lead to this and, in patients present with VF, ICD may still be necessary. (*Source:* bottom panel Akhtar M. Clinical spectrum of ventricular tachycardia. Circulation. 1990;82:1561-73, with permission)

LV Noncompaction[50]

Isolated LV noncompaction (LVNC) is a rare myopathy, primarily of autosomal inheritance. The main structural abnormality is intrauterine failure of LV muscle compaction.

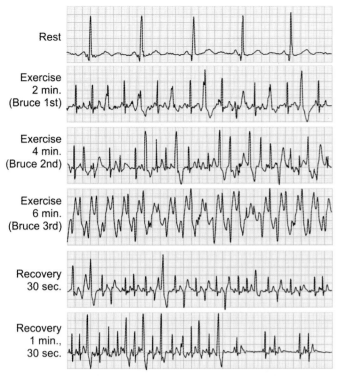

FIGURE 15: Progressive increase in ventricular ectopy as the exercises load increases. The 4th panel shows bidirectional tachycardia, and the last two panels show further polymorphism during recovery phase of exercise (*Source:* Modified from Napolitano C, Priori SG. Catecholaminergic polymorphic ventricular tachycardia and short-coupled Torsades de Pointes. In: Zipes DP, Jalife J (Eds). Cardiac Electrophysiology: From Cell to Bedside, 4th edition. Philadelphia: WB Saunders; 2004. pp. 633-9)

The main clinical manifestations are congestive heart failure and ventricular arrhythmias with around 20% incidence of SCD.

Catecholaminergic PVT[51,52]

Catecholaminergic PVT (CPVT) can be a dominant or recessive inheritance, mostly manifested in childhood or young adults. The heart is structurally normal as is the baseline ECG.

Adrenergic drive brings out characteristic bidirectional [Fig. 15 (4th panel from top)] or PVT. There is a high incidence of SCD (> 30% mortality by age 30). The basis is mutation in the genes, encoding ryanodine receptor 2 (RyR2) or calsequestrin 2 (CASQ2) triggering activity from delayed afterdepolarization due to abnormalities of Ca^{++} handling, which is responsible for arrhythmogenesis. The conversion to PVT is most likely related to transmural dispersion of repolarization between the various myocardial layers. Degeneration to VF is the most likely cause of SCD.

J-Wave Syndromes[12,53,54]

This category includes several entities, where the individuals are prone to arrhythmic death. The primary defect seems to be imbalance of current during Phase 1 of the action potential producing Phase 2 reentry leading to VF. Some examples include Brugada syndrome, early repolarization, short QT syndrome and perhaps many cases of so-called idiopathic VF. Rapid outward current plays a significant role and may be the reason that quinidine, which blocks K^+ current, is effective in preventing recurrence. This subject is covered in greater detail elsewhere in this book.

Idiopathic VF

This fascinating entity is described in greater detail by Belhassan and Viskin, and is associated with identifiable SHD.[55] It is characterized by the occurrence of spontaneous VT with inducible PVT and VF, which respond to oral guideline both in the electrophysiology laboratory (i.e. not inducible after drug) and in the excellent clinical response seen over many years. Nonetheless, as Brugada syndrome and the various J-wave syndrome have been described, it is not clear how many of these cases will continue to be called idiopathic.

PVT IN ASSOCIATION WITH SHORT QT SYNDROME[56,57]

This topic is somewhat new and with very limited experience and follow-up. Figure 16 shows an example of short QT, usually

CHAPTER 35 Clinical Spectrum of Ventricular Tachycardia

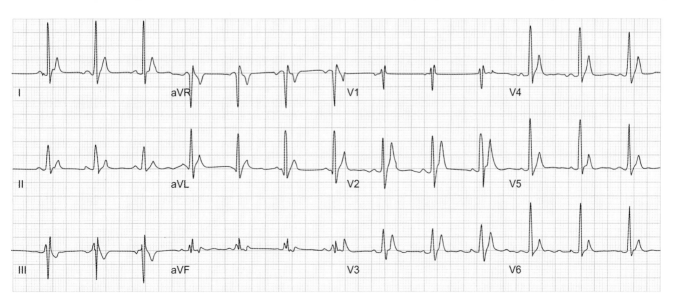

FIGURE 16: Example of a short QT, which can lead to fatal arrhythmia. The coexistence of short QT and Brugada has also been described (*Source:* Bjerregaard P, Gussak I. Short QT syndrome: mechanisms, diagnosis and treatment. Nat Clin Pract Cardiovasc Dis. 2005;2:84-7, with permission)

described as QT less than 300 msec, but some cases with similar genetic mutation had QT of 320 msec. At least five mutations have been described.

The foregoing outline is a summary of VT as the subject is clinically viewed. For a comprehensive review and ACC/AHA/ESC guidelines on work-up and management of VT, the reader is referred to the most recent literature.[17,18]

REFERENCES

1. Wellens HJ, Bar FW, Lie KI. The value of the electrocardiogram in the differential diagnosis of a tachycardia with a widened QRS complex. Am J Med. 1978;64:27-33.
2. Akhtar M, Shenasa M, Jazayeri M, et al. Wide QRS complex tachycardia. Reappraisal of a common clinical problem. Ann Intern Med. 1988;109:905-12.
3. Brugada P, Brugada J, Mont L, et al. A new approach to the differential diagnosis of a regular tachycardia with a wide QRS complex. Circulation. 1991;83:1649-59.
4. Miller JM, Das MK, Arora R, et al. Differential diagnosis of wide QRS complex tachycardia. In: Zipes DP, Jalife J (Eds). Cardiac Electrophysiology: From Cell to Bedside, 4th edition. Philadelphia: W.B. Saunders; 2004. pp. 747-57.
5. Akhtar M. Clinical spectrum of ventricular tachycardia. Circulation. 1990;82:1561-73.
6. Dessertenne F. La tachycardie ventriculaire a deux foyers opposes variables. Arch Mal Coeur Vaiss. 1966;59:263-72.
7. Ruan Y, Wang L. Short-coupled variant of torsade de pointes. J Tongji Med Univ. 2001;21:30-1.
8. Josephson ME, Almendral JM, Buxton AE, et al. Mechanisms of ventricular tachycardia. Circulation. 1987;75:III41-7.
9. Stevenson WG, Soejima K. Catheter ablation of ventricular tachycardia. In: Zipes DP, Jalife J (Eds). Cardiac Electrophysiology: From Cell to Bedside, 4th edition. Philadelphia: W.B. Saunders; 2004. pp. 1087-96.
10. Wellens HJ, Schuilenburg RM, Durrer D. Electrical stimulation of the heart in patients with ventricular tachycardia. Circulation. 1972;46:216-26.
11. Priori SG, Rivolta I, Napolitano C. Genetics of long QT, Brugada and other channelopathies. In: Zipes DP, Jalife J (Eds). Cardiac Electrophysiology: From Cell to Bedside, 4th edition. Philadelphia: W.B. Saunders; 2004. p. 462.
12. Tikkanen JT, Anttonen O, Juntilla MJ, et al. Long-term outcome associated with early repolarization on electrocardiography. New Engl J Med. 2009;361:2529-37.
13. de Bakker JM, van Capelle FJ, Janse MJ, et al. Reentry as a cause of ventricular tachycardia in patients with chronic ischemic heart disease: electrophysiologic and anatomic correlation. Circulation. 1968;77:589-606.
14. Buxton AE, Waxman HL, Marchlinski FE, et al. Role of triple extrastimuli during electrophysiologic study of patients with documented sustained ventricular tachyarrhythmias. Circulation. 1984;69:532-40.
15. Luu M, Stevenson WG, Stevenson LW. Diverse mechanisms of unexpected cardiac arrest in advanced heart failure. Circulation. 1989;80:1675-80.
16. Haberl R, Jilge G, Pulter R, et al. Comparison of frequency and time domain analysis of the signal-averaged electrocardiogram in patients with ventricular tachycardia and coronary artery disease: methodologic validation and clinical relevance. J Am Coll Cardiol. 1988;12:150-8.
17. Zipes DP, Camm AJ, Borggrefe M, et al. ACC/AHA/ESC 2006 Guidelines for management of patients with ventricular arrhythmias and the prevention of sudden cardiac death—executive summary: a report of the American College of Cardiology/American Heart Association Task Force and the European Society of Cardiology Committee of Practice Guidelines (Writing Committee to Develop Guidelines for Management of Patients with Ventricular Arrhythmias and the Prevention of Sudden Cardiac Death) Developed in collaboration with the European Heart Rhythm Association and the Heart Rhythm Society. Eur Heart J. 2006;27:2099-140.
18. Epstein AE, DiMarco JP, Ellenbogen KA, et al. ACC/AHA/HRS 2008 Guidelines for Device-Based Therapy of Cardiac Rhythm Abnormalities: a report of the American College of Cardiology/ American Heart Association Task Force on Practice Guidelines (Writing Committee to Revise the ACC/AHA/NASPE 2002 Guideline Update for Implantation of Cardiac Pacemakers and Antiarrhythmia Devices) developed in Collaboration with the American Association for Thoracic Surgery and Society of Thoracic Surgeons. J Am Coll Cardiol. 2008;51:e1-e62.
19. Tchou PJ, Kadri N, Anderson J, et al. Automatic implantable cardioverter defibrillators and survival of patients with left ventricular dysfunction and malignant ventricular arrhythmias. Ann Intern Med. 1988;109:529-34.
20. Akhtar M, Damato AN, Batsford WP, et al. Demonstration of re-entry within the His-Purkinje system in man. Circulation. 1974;50:1150-62.
21. Caceres J, Jazayeri M, McKinnie J, et al. Sustained bundle branch reentry as a mechanism of clinical tachycardia. Circulation. 1989;79:256-70.
22. Tchou P, Jazayeri M, Denker ST, et al. Transcatheter electrical ablation of right bundle branch: a method of treating macroreentrant ventricular tachycardia attributed to bundle branch reentry. Circulation. 1988;78:246-57.
23. Blanck Z, Dhala A, Deshpande S, et al. Bundle branch reentrant ventricular tachycardia: cumulative experience in 48 patients. J Cardiovasc Electrophysiol. 1993;4:253-62.
24. Narasimhan C, Jazayeri MR, Sra J, et al. Ventricular tachycardia in valvular heart disease: facilitation of sustained bundle-branch reentry by valve surgery. Circulation. 1997;96:4307-13.
25. Merino JL, Carmona JR, Fernández-Lozano I, et al. Mechanisms of sustained ventricular tachycardia in myotonic dystrophy: implications for catheter ablation. Circulation. 1998;98:541-6.
26. Cohen TJ, Chien WW, Lurie KG, et al. Radiofrequency catheter ablation for treatment of bundle branch reentrant tachycardia: results and long-term follow-up. J Am Coll Cardiol. 1991:18:1767-73.
27. Blanck Z, Jazayeri M, Dhala A, et al. Bundle branch reentry: a mechanism of ventricular tachycardia in the absence of myocardial or valvular dysfunction. J Am Coll Cardiol. 1993;22:1718-22.
28. Fontaine G, Fontaliran F, Hébert JL, et al. Arrhythmogenic right ventricular dysplasia. Ann Rev Med. 1999;50:17-35.
29. Nasir K, Bomma C, Tandri H, et al. Electrocardiographic features of arrythmogenic right ventricular dysplasia/cardiomyopathy according to disease severity: a need to broaden diagnostic criteria. Circulation. 2004;110:1527-34.
30. Fontaine G, Fornes P, Hebert JL, et al. Ventricular tachycardia in arrhythmogenic right ventricular cardiomyopathies. In: Zipes D, Jalife J (Eds). Cardiac Electrophysiology: From Cell to Bedside, 4th edition. Philadelphia: W.B. Saunders; 2004. pp. 588-600.
31. Gonska BD, Cao K, Raab J, et al. Radiofrequency catheter ablation of right ventricular tachycardia late after repair of congenital heart defects. Circulation. 1996;94:1902-8.
32. Horton RP, Canby RC, Kessler DJ, et al. Ablation of ventricular tachycardia associated with tetralogy of Fallot: demonstration of bidirectional block. J Cardiovasc Electrophysiol. 1997;8:432-5.
33. Lerman BB, Stein KM, Markowitz SM, et al. Recent advances in right ventricular outflow tract tachycardia. Card Electrophysiol Rev. 1999;3:210-4.
34. Rodriguez LM, Smeets JL, Timmermans C, et al. Predictors for successful ablation of right- and left-sided idiopathic ventricular tachycardia. Am J Cardiol. 1997;79:309-14.

35. Ohe T, Shimomura K, Aihara N, et al. Idiopathic sustained left ventricular tachycardia: clinical and electrophysiologic characteristics. Circulation. 1988:77:560-8.

36. Kottkamp H, Chen X, Hindricks G, et al. Radiofrequency catheter ablation of idiopathic left ventricular tachycardia: further evidenced for microreentry as the underlying mechanism. J Cardiovasc Electrophysiol. 1994;5:268-73.

37. Kanagaratnam L, Tomassoni G, Schweikert R, et al. Ventricular tachycardias arising from the aortic sinus of valsalva: an under-recognized variant of left outflow tract ventricular tachycardia. J Am Coll Cardiol. 2001;37:1408-14.

38. Kamakura S, Shimizu W, Matsuo K, et al. Localization of optimal ablation site of idiopathic ventricular tachycardia from right and left ventricular outflow tract by body surface ECG. Circulation. 1998;98:1525-33.

39. Schwartz PJ, Periti M, Malliani A. The long Q-T syndrome. Am Heart J. 1975;89:378-90.

40. Moss AJ, Zareba W, Benhorin J, et al. ECG T-wave patterns in genetically distinct forms of the hereditary long QT syndrome. Circulation. 1995;92:2929-34.

41. Schwartz PF, Priori SG. Long QT. syndrome: genotype-phenotype correlations. In: Zipes DP, Jalife J (Eds). Cardiac Electrophysiology: From Cell to Bedside, 4th edition. Philadelphia: W.B. Saunders; 2004. pp. 651-9.

42. Shimizu W, Antzelevitch C. Sodium channel block with mexiletine is effective in reducing dispersion of repolarization and preventing torsade de pointes in LQT2 and LQT3 models of the long-QT syndrome. Circulation. 1997;96:2038-47.

43. Kay GN, Plumb VJ, Arciniegas JG, et al. Torsades de pointes: the long-short initiating sequence and other clinical features; observations in 32 patients. J Am Coll Cardiol. 1990;2:806-17.

44. El-Sherif N, Turitto G. Torsade de pointes. In: Zipes DP, Jalife J (Eds). Cardiac Electrophysiology: From Cell to Bedside, 4th edition. Philadelphia: WB Saunders; 2004. pp. 687-99.

45. Brugada P, Brugada J. Right bundle branch block, persistent ST segment elevation and sudden cardiac death: a distinct clinical and electrocardiographic syndrome. A multicenter report. J Am Coll Cardiol. 1992;20:1391-6.

46. Brugada P, Brugada R, Brugada J. The Brugada syndrome. In: Saksena S, Camm AJ (Eds). Electrophysiological Disorders of the Heart. New York: Churchill Livingstone; 2005. pp. 697-703.

47. Antzelevitch C, Brugada P, Borggrefe M, et al. Brugada syndrome: report of the second consensus conference: endorsed by the Heart Rhythm Society and the European Heart Rhythm Association. Circulation. 2005;111:659-70.

48. Dorian P, Bharati S, Meyerburg RJ, et al. Ventricular fibrillation. In: Saksena S, Camm AJ (Eds). Electrophysiological Disorders of the Heart. New York: Churchill Livingstone; 2005. pp. 419-53.

49. Maron BJ, McKenna WJ, Danielson GK, et al. American College of Cardiology/European Society of Cardiology clinical expert consensus document on hypertrophic cardiomyopathy: a report of the American College of Cardiology Foundation Task Force on Clinical Expert Consensus Documents and the European Society of Cardiology Committee for Practice Guidelines. J Am Coll Cardiol. 2003;42:1687-713.

50. Li L, Burke A, Zhang X, et al. Sudden unexpected death due to left ventricular noncompaction of myocardium. Am J Forensic Med Pathol. 2010;31:122-4.

51. Martini B, Buja GF, Canciani B, et al. Bidirectional tachycardia. A sustained form, not related to digitalis intoxication, in an adult without apparent cardiac disease. Jpn Heart J. 1988;29:381-7.

52. Napolitano C, Priori SG. Catecholaminergic polymorphic ventricular tachycardia and short-coupled torsades de pointes. In: Zipes D, Jalife J (Eds). Cardiac Electrophysiology: From Cell to Bedside, 4th edition. Philadelphia: W.B. Saunders; 2004. pp. 633-9.

53. Takagi M, Aihara N, Takahi H, et al. Clinical characteristics of patients with spontaneous or inducible ventricular fibrillation without apparent heart disease presenting with J wave and ST segment elevation in inferior leads. J Cardiovasc Electrophysiol. 2000;11:844-8.

54. Haïssaguerre M, Derval N, Sacher F, et al. Sudden cardiac arrest associated with early repolarization. N Engl J Med. 2008;358:2016-23.

55. Belhassen B, Viskin S. Idiopathic ventricular tachycardia and fibrillation. J Cardiovasc Electrophysiol. 1993;4:356-68.

56. Gussak I, Antzelevitch C. Early repolarization syndrome: clinical characteristics and possible cellular and ionic mechanisms. J Electrocardiol. 2000;33:299-309.

57. Bjerregaard P, Gussak I. Short QT syndrome: mechanisms, diagnosis and treatment. Nat Clin Pract Cardiovasc Med. 2005;2:84-7.

CHAPTER 35

Clinical Spectrum of Ventricular Tachycardia

Chapter 36

Bradycardia and Heart Block

Arthur C Kendig, James B Martins

Chapter Outline

INTRODUCTION

Bradycardia is generally defined as a heart rate less than 50 beats per minute. However, this simple definition is a gross oversimplification of what is a multifaceted and multifactorial issue. Bradycardia is a dichotomy of sorts, in some cases being a marker of excellent cardiovascular fitness, or conversely, a sign of cardiovascular disease, especially when it is symptomatic.

CONDUCTION SYSTEM ANATOMY AND DEVELOPMENT

On the most basic level, the normal specialized electrical tissue is comprised of the sinoatrial (SA) node (dominant pacemaker), atrioventricular (AV) node and His-Purkinje system. Embryologically, the conduction system of the human heart begins very early in development, with an ECG recording at 4–6 weeks gestation being similar to what is seen in an adult.

The SA node, first described by Keith and Flack in 1907, is located in the lateral right atrium in the sulcus terminalis. It is first noted at around 20 days into embryonic development, when a primitive SA node is formed in the slow-conducting inflow region of the heart. The inflow region is initially bilateral, with the developing heart's pacemaker on the left side. By 35 weeks, the SA node becomes a more distinct entity in the posterolateral region of the early four-chambered heart's right atrium, with impulses directed with a posterior to anterior vector, toward the AV node. Even after completion of its development, and into adulthood, the SA node is a heterogeneous structure, and essentially a loose collection of cells. Only a portion of these cells act as initiating pacemakers; the rest conduct the signals sent to them. There is also a hierarchy of pacemakers, with overdrive suppression by those with faster rates, of those with lower rates (the AVN and His-Purkinje).

The AV node itself located along the interatrial septum in the Triangle of Koch—which is composed posteriorly of the tendon of Todaro, and anteriorly by the septal leaflet of the tricuspid valve and inferiorly by the coronary sinus os—is also formed around 5 weeks into embryonic development. Like the SA node, it exhibits its conduction properties in its adult role prior to being noted as a distinct identifiable entity.

The His bundle is located anteriorly to the compact AV node along the interatrial septum and near the AV groove. The Purkinje fibers continue from the His into the ventricles and divide into the right, left anterior and left posterior fascicles. Embryologically, the cells making up the His-Purkinje system are derived from already present cardiac myocytes, differentiating into conduction system cells after exposure to endothelin. Interestingly, in animal models, the conduction system is present and functioning prior to coronary vessel formation.[1–5]

BRADYCARDIA SYNDROMES/DISEASES

IATROGENIC AND NONCARDIAC CAUSES

Before considering intrinsic conduction disease, in light of many patients living with multiple medical comorbidities as well as complex medical regimens being commonplace, it is of utmost importance to consider iatrogenic and noncardiac causes of bradycardia and heart block.

TABLE 1

Common noncardiac and iatrogenic causes of bradycardia and heart block

Cardiac medications	Noncardiac medications	Medical disease
BARBs (including eye drops)	SSRIs	Lyme disease
Calcium channel blockers	Opiates	Renal/Hepatic disease
Digoxin	Succinylcholine Lithium	Hypothyroidism Carotid hypersensitivity
Amiodarone	Cholinesterase inhibitors (e.g. donepezil for Alzheimer's)	Renal/Hepatic disease
Sotalol	Propofol	Endovascular cooling after cardiac arrest
Sodium channel blockers		
Clonidine		

First, in terms of medications, the most common agents related to this issue are those already diagnosed for cardiovascular disease including tachycardias. Examples include beta-adrenergic receptor blockers (BARBs, both ophthalmologic and oral),[6] calcium channel blockers, digoxin[7] and clonidine[8,9] (Table 1).

Noncardiac medications as culprits include lidocaine spray or topical such as is used for endoscopic procedures,[10] selective serotonin reuptake inhibitors (SSRIs) such as escitalopram,[11] cholinesterase inhibitors (via enhancement of vagal tone) commonly used for treatment of Alzheimer's disease[12] and succinylcholine.[13]

Propofol is a commonly used sedation agent which, in rare cases, may lead to the development of propofol infusion syndrome. This includes a sudden-onset of bradycardia and possibly asystole, with other effects such as fatty liver, metabolic acidosis or rhabdomyolysis. Risk factors include prolonged (> 48 hours) use at high doses, patient age less than 19 years and low carbohydrate reserves.[14]

In terms of medical syndromes, potential causes include: hypothyroidism; Lyme disease;[15] endovascular cooling after cardiac arrest;[16] and renal or hepatic disease. The latter two are more related to decreasing medication clearance and metabolism, thus increasing serum drug levels and potentiating a drug's effect. This is especially salient with digoxin and renally cleared BARBs such as atenolol. Again, it is important to note that medication and medical disease-related bradycardia and heart block are potentially reversible, that is why these need to be considered early in the differential diagnosis.

FAMILIAL

Development of the cardiac conduction system does not always occur in a normal fashion. When mutations occur, different syndromes may develop. One example of this (specifically related to sinus bradycardia) is familial sinus bradycardia. In a recent paper, the HCN4 channel (located near the cAMP-binding site) was identified as the mutation causing this syndrome, which acts much like a vagally mediated bradycardia.[17]

Although the cardiac conduction system is primarily derived from myocardial cells and not neural crest cells (which differentiate into neural tissue), there is still a rich two-way interaction with the nervous system communication. In 1867, von Bezold first described cardioinhibitory reflexes initiating from the heart itself. It was found that receptors located primarily in the posterior left ventricle, sensitive to mechanical stretch or certain chemicals, when stimulated, increase parasympathetic and decrease sympathetic tone via the vagus nerve, resulting in—among other reactions—sinus bradycardia.[18]

This mechanism may cause bradycardia commonly in diverse situations, all of which could be called vaso-vagal reactions since they may be triggered by psychiatric stressors like fear or sight of blood as well as volume depletion from many etiologies. The fact that animal models show similar responses with, for example, hemorrhage suggests that this mechanism may be in most or all humans as well. Therefore most physicians will see bradycardia due to this mechanism which is best prevented and treated by increasing vascular volume.

Interestingly, trained athletes, especially elite ones, frequently have asymptomatic bradycardia.[19] Commonly elite athletes may also have orthostatic hypotension. Rarely, vagally mediated bradycardia severe enough to cause presyncope or syncope may also (somewhat paradoxically) be seen in trained athletes, where high vagal tone assists in rapid post-exercise heart rate recovery, but in some cases may go too far in lowering heart rate, causing symptoms.[19] The sinus node as well as the subsidiary pacemakers may be influenced by this vagal tone, at times leading to asystole. Nevertheless, the vagal influence never permanently stops the heart; it only delays its next beat for a matter of seconds. Meantime, in this brief period of time, syncope may occur because of loss of cardiac output as well as peripheral resistance.

CARDIAC TRANSPLANTATION

In post-cardiac transplant patients, bradycardia—specifically sinus bradycardia—occurs in approximately 18% of patients, and ultimately 4–7% require a permanent pacemaker (usually atrial pacing only). One of the primary risk factors for development of sinus bradycardia is ischemic time.[20] Another related risk factor is surgical technique, with biatrial anastomosis (Shumway-Lower) resulting in less ischemic time, but increased risk of physical damage to the SA node, while the bicaval (Wythenshawe) approach keeps the atria intact, but increases ischemic time.[21–24] Other risk factors for post-transplant bradycardia include SA nodal artery lesions and transplant vasculopathy.[25,26]

Due to vagal and sympathetic denervation resulting from the surgical procedure, these patients have relative bradycardia and some degree of chronotropic incompetence, but are somewhat shielded from bradycardia by the standard definition due to high intrinsic heart rate. The transplanted ventricle increases stroke volume to compensate for the lack of sympathetically increased heart rate with exercise; even though cardiac output may be normal at rest the transplant cannot increase HR enough to make up for the lesser heart rate with exercise. Reinnervation can occur, but the extent to which it happens varies from patient to patient.

CLINICAL PRESENTATION

Depending on the patient's heart rate and robustness of so-called "back-up" pacemakers, patients may entirely be asymptomatic, symptomatic with exertion only or at rest. Common symptoms include lightheadedness, dizziness, syncope, palpitations, shortness of breath at rest, dyspnea on exertion, angina, and progressive lower extremity edema.

MEASUREMENT/DIAGNOSIS

The diagnosis of bradycardia, regardless of the mechanism, is primarily made by obtaining an ECG or rhythm strip from surface leads at the time of symptoms. Other times, bradycardia may be found serendipitously by an ECG or telemetry strip performed for other reasons. When a patient's symptoms suggest an arrhythmia of a low rate, occur paroxysmally, and the patient has a normal ECG or rhythm strip at presentation while asymptomatic, monitoring via a Holter (24 or 48 hour) if symptoms occur daily, a 21+ day event recorder if occurring monthly, or if rarely occurring but with significant symptoms at the time of the event, an implantable loop recorder may be appropriate. These methods of measurement are discussed in this textbook in more detail.

Another issue in diagnosing bradycardia is relative bradycardia, also known as chronotropic incompetence. This describes a scenario where at rest, the patient does not demonstrate significant symptoms, but with exertion, is unable to mount an appropriate heart rate to increase cardiac output appropriate for increased needs of exercise. A common definition of this is failure to obtain greater than 85% of age-predicted maximum heart rate with exercise testing. A postulate for an etiology is decreased responsiveness of the heart to increased sympathetic input. Evaluation is primarily via exercise testing. In some cases, direct measurement of cardiac output is performed via right heart catheterization before, during and after temporary pacing at higher rates than baseline; if cardiac output significantly improves with a modest increase in heart rate, then chronotropic incompetence may be assumed.[27]

SINUS NODE DISEASE

SICK SINUS SYNDROME

Sick sinus syndrome (SSS), in its most rudimentary sense, is defined as sinus node dysfunction which results in an inadequate heart rate physiologically, and may include sinus bradycardia, sinus arrest, or sinus node exit block, and may lead to takeover of cardiac pacemaking and atrial contraction by subsidiary intrinsic cardiac pacemaker sites. The mere present of SSS without symptoms is not an indication for any therapy, but cautious use of agents listed in the Table 1.

In a clinicopathological study of six cases of SSS in patients ranging 69–91 years of age, Sugiura et al. found that in patients with SA block and bradycardia-tachycardia syndrome, the SA node and AV node regions showed 70–80% decrease in nodal cells, infiltration of the SA node by connective tissue and left

bundle branch (LBB) fibrosis.[28] SSS has also been reported to be caused by cardiac lipomatosis.[29]

During ageing, the sinus node itself changes. A rat model comparing what was equivalent to a young adult and 69 year old showed that in older animals, the heart rate is lower, the pacemaker action potentials were slower, more widely distributed (enlargement of the SA node), and located more toward the inferior vena cava in the RA. Moreover, histologically, the SA nodal cells demonstrated hypertrophy and extracellular matrix remodeling.[30]

The I(f) "funny" current, although first discovered more than 30 years ago, has recently been found, albeit controversially, to have a significant role in spontaneous cardiac pacemaker activity. Basically, these channels determine the slope of phase 4 (depolarization), thereby playing a role in the frequency of cardiac pacing. A mutation in the HCN4 gene, which encodes this channel, demonstrates sinus bradycardia. Thus an abnormality in this channel may be at least partially at fault for some sinus bradycardias.[31]

Recently, genetic factors related to this disease have been elucidated, specifically SCN5A mutation related functional loss of the sodium channel.[32]

In terms of association with other conduction diseases, a recent retrospective study suggests Brugada-type ECG and Brugada syndrome are associated with SSS; 2.87% had Brugada-type ECGs (0.82% with Type I, and 2.05% with Type II). Generally, in the population at large, in recent studies, the prevalence has ranged from 0.07% (7/10,000) in a Danish population[33] and 0.012% (120/10,000)[34] to 0.14%.[35] Moreover, in the above noted study, during a 7-year follow-up period, 50% of those with Type I and none of those with Type II ECGs experienced VF events. Thus, SSS is associated with an increased prevalence of Brugada-type ECG and Brugada syndrome compared to the general population. This may be associated with the aforementioned SCN5A mutations.

Wu et al. performed EP studies in 38 patients with SSS. The mean sinus pause was 5.6 +/- 2.8 sec. Three predominate groups were discovered. Nine patients had SA block, with sinus node function intrinsically noted during pauses. Seven had unidirectional exit block, and two others bidirectional, all of which had evidence of an atrial impulse to conduct into the SA node and inhibit SA node firing. A second group of 22 patients showed slow 1:1 conduction, second degree SA node exit block, with 17/22 patients showing abnormal sinus node recovery times. A third group had no sinus node electrograms measurable.[36]

Frequently patients will have symptoms shown to be due to sinus bradycardia, but careful clinical evaluation will reveal that symptoms began upon institution of BARBs or other drugs listed in the Table 1. Usually the symptoms will resolve if the offending drug can be discontinued or replaced by one which does not aggravate SSS.

AV NODE DISEASE

PATHOLOGY

The most common cause of permanent AV block is idiopathic bundle branch fibrosis. This may include the main AV bundle and LBB, as a result of aging fibrosis of the cardiac skeleton, referred to as Lev's disease, or in fibrosis of the left and right bundles themselves, referred to as Lenègre's disease, occurring in younger people in certain families. Other etiologies include interruption of the AV node related to aortic or mitral valve calcification, myocardial infarction leading to ischemic damage to the AV node, or cardiomyopathy. Other causes, although rare, include: congenital AV block; infiltration by tumor and surgical or other trauma.[37]

FIRST-DEGREE AV BLOCK

Although a relatively common and seemingly benign finding of a prolonged PR interval (> 200 msec) on ECG, it has recently been postulated that this may precede more advanced AV block, and even itself serve as a marker of increased risk of other arrhythmic and mortality concerns. Cheng described long-term outcomes of patients with first-degree AV block.[38] Within the Framingham Heart Study cohort, and found that when compared to control patients with a prolonged PR interval at baseline had twice the risk of developing atrial fibrillation, three times the risk of requiring a pacemaker and almost one-and-a-half times the risk of all-cause mortality. At this point however, despite these findings, management of these patients with only a prolonged PR interval is unclear.

SECOND-DEGREE AV BLOCK

Second-degree AV block is commonly divided into two varieties, and was first classified in this manner by Woldemar Mobitz in the early 1920s.[39] Type I (Mobitz I, also "Wenckebach" named for Karel Wenckebach who discovered "Wenckebach periodicity" in 1906) second-degree AV block presents as a normal or near-normal PR interval (120–200 msec) which gradually prolongs with successive beats, until only a P wave is seen, and a "dropped" QRS occurs, which is the absence of AV conduction. After a brief reset, the next cycle begins, again with a normal PR interval, progressively lengthening again until a drop occurs. There may be the same number of beats prior to that which is dropped, or at times, variable numbers. Type I basically demonstrates AV nodal decremental conduction.

Type II (Mobitz II) second-degree AV block, similar to Type I, has dropped ventricular beats due to AV block. However, in this scenario, there is no PR lengthening, only dropped beats, which may occur after one, two or any number of normally conducted beats, and may or may not be a consistent number. An easy way to diagnose this mechanism is to evaluate the PR before and after the regular blocked P wave; if the PR after the block is not shorter by more than 20 msec then Type II block must be considered. False Type II may be diagnosed if irregular P-P intervals, owing to sinus arrhythmia or atrial prematures, or frequent junctional prematures (suggesting concealed His extrasystoles) produce block.[40] Patients with Type II block also tend to have concomitant QRS prolongation.

2:1 AV block, due to 2:1 conduction, may be Type I or II, but which one is not able to be ascertained because there is no PR lengthening—or lack thereof—to be seen because block occurs after only one beat. It may be a progression from either. Anatomically, 80% of the time, 2:1 AV block occurs in the His-Purkinje system, and 20% in the AV node itself. Careful

examination of the ECG for more typical 3:2 Type I block will suggest the right mechanism. Interestingly, atropine may increase the degree of AV block.[40–42] The importance of differentiating Type I versus Type II AV block is that even if asymptomatic, the latter requires a permanent pacer, but in the former a permanent pacemaker is not needed unless symptoms are present.

THIRD-DEGREE AV BLOCK

Third-degree AV block is defined as a complete electrical dissociation of the atria and ventricles. The ventricular rhythm in this case, referred to as an escape rhythm, may either be a junctional, which is a normal, narrow-complex rhythm emanating more proximally to the AV node and generally faster (40–60 bpm), or ventricular where the rhythm is abnormal, wide complex and slower (< 30 bpm). Rarely no escape rhythm is present whatsoever.

Treatment entails eliminating or neutralizing reversible causes, such as AV nodal blockers (e.g. BARBs). If a patient has complete heart block and is unstable with symptoms, such as chest pain, shortness of breath, lightheadedness and/or hypotension, then atropine should be given, especially if a junctional escape is present. If not effective, temporary pacing (first transcutaneous, then transvenous) is recommended. If the patient has what appears to be a permanent complete heart block, then permanent pacing is recommended. Of note, some sources state that an escape rhythm of greater than 40 beats per minute is adequate, and is not an indication for permanent pacing. However, as noted in the recent ACC/AHA device therapy guidelines, this arbitrary number is not based on strong data.[43]

PAROXYSMAL AV BLOCK

Paroxysmal AV block has been defined by Lee et al. as "a sudden," "paroxysmal pause-dependent phase 4 AV block occurring in diseased conduction system". It is essentially the change from 1:1 AV conduction, suddenly to complete heart block. There is no official definition for this type of AV block and the prevalence may be underestimated because of this and difficulty in recording this arrhythmia. The most common risk factor is apparently right bundle branch (RBB) block. Since paroxysmal AV block originates in the distal portion of the AV node, it most often is seen in older patients, with the commonest presentation being syncope. As noted above, the mechanism has been postulated to be block due to phase 4 depolarization of the distal AV node, more specifically in the His-Purkinje system itself. Factors differentiating this from vagally mediated complete heart block include rapid or sudden onset, no change in P-R interval, and infranodal versus nodal level of block. Treatment includes pacemaker implantation and removal of culprit AV nodal blocking agents if present.[44]

HEMIBLOCK

Although not necessarily a bradycardia *per se*, or AV block, such as those described above, the hemiblocks (first described by Rosenbaum, et al. in 1968 are nevertheless important findings which may be intricately related to AV block.[45]

First of all, building on the concept of the right and left bundles in the His-Purkinje system, the LBB is generally found to divide into two discrete—yet somewhat interconnected—branches, the anterior and the posterior fascicles. Thus, the ventricular system, including the right bundle, is essentially trifasicular.

The left anterior fascicle, being anteriorly located as the name implies, is the more vulnerable of the two LBBs. For one, there is only a single coronary artery distribution (anterior descending) for blood supply. In addition, this fascicle is smaller and thinner than its posterior counterpart. A left anterior hemiblock (LAH) (also known as a fascicular block) is defined as a leftward axis of less than –45 degrees, an "rS" pattern in II, III, aVF and with a narrow QRS complex. The most common causes include hypertension, cardiomyopathy, VSD closure (spontaneous or iatrogenic), and Lev and Lenegre disease. In the case of the latter two causes, the RBB is commonly affected concurrently, and by the nature of these progressive diseases, patients often eventually develop complete heart block. Generally, without significant coronary artery disease or infarction, the finding of isolated LAH does not appear to portend an increased risk of morbidity or mortality, although LAH is associated with risk of disease in the Framingham study.

The left posterior fascicle is supplied by both the anterior and the posterior descending coronary arteries. This dual blood supply source is beneficial especially in the setting of myocardial infarction, where if one of the supplying coronary arteries is the site of occlusion or stenosis, the fascicle is unlikely to sustain significant ischemic damage, and thus is less prone to infarction and hemiblock. Left posterior hemiblock is defined as a rightward axis of greater than +100 degrees, narrow QRS and an rS in I and aVL. A pure left posterior fascicular block is rare, but tends to be found coexisting with a RBB block. This combination, if occurring in the setting of a myocardial infarction, significantly increases mortality to over 80% within a few weeks after infarction. The risk of progression to complete heart block with this bifascicular block is 42%. Because of the dual-coronary artery supply, however, the cause of the block is more likely due to Lenegre disease, or even Chagas disease in endemic regions.[46]

That said, the concept of trifasicular block is uncommon as opposed to bifasicular block (LAH and RBB block) and concomitant first degree AVB which is usually in the AVN.[40] Patients with LAH and RBB block frequently have no symptoms or VT inducible.[47] Differentiation from trifasicular block is usually easy (lack of symptoms) but exercise testing or EPS may be necessary if a certain diagnosis is necessary.

BUNDLE BRANCH BLOCK

The concept of the existence of the LBB and RBB coming off of the His was first published by Eppinger and Rothberger in 1909.[48]

LEFT BUNDLE BRANCH BLOCK

Left bundle branch (LBB) block is defined grossly as a QRS duration greater than or equal to 120 msec with left axis deviation. As early as 1940, Rasmussen and Moe determined via clinical, ECG, radiography, and necropsy in 100 patients with LBB block, that the most common cause, comprising approximately 72% of cases was left ventricular hypertrophy and/or enlargement (with associated increased weight of the heart), primarily due to hypertension or aortic valve disease.[49] Early data from the Framingham Study had similar findings, including hypertension, "cardiac enlargement" and/or coronary artery disease. It was further noted that the mean age of onset of new LBB block was 62 years of age. The 10-year prognosis was poor, with one-half of these patients expiring due to cardiovascular disease.[50] Other etiologies for LBB block include myocardial infarction, electrolyte abnormalities, and fibrosis (Lev's and Lenegre's disease).[51]

A salient issue with LBB block is in myocardial infarction. It may be the presenting ECG finding for MI. If an old finding, it may hinder interpretation of the ECG in the setting of suspected acute coronary syndrome. The specific method of diagnosing an MI in this setting is discussed in this book.[52]

Moreover, and discussed earlier, LBB block is important in selecting patients with interventricular dyssynchrony who would be candidates for cardiac resynchronization therapy, in that most studies suggest that interventricular dyssynchrony due to LBB block responds better to CRT than those with RBB block.[53,54]

RIGHT BUNDLE BRANCH BLOCK

Right bundle branch (RBB) block is grossly defined as a QRS duration greater than or equal to 120 msec with right axis deviation, and commonly an RSR pattern in lead V_1.

From the same follow-up data from the Framingham Study noted above, patients with new onset RBB block over an 18-year-follow-up period were identified. These patients were more likely to have hypertension prior to the development of RBB block; these patients were 2.5–4 times more likely to have coronary artery disease or congestive heart failure than their age-matched controls. A QRS of greater than or equal to 130 ms with an axis –45° to –90° was associated with increased risk of cardiovascular issues. Common causes of or association with RBB block include pulmonary embolism (acute or chronic), pulmonary hypertension, left sided heart failure causing RV volume or pressure overload, severe MR, pulmonic valve stenosis.

In patients with a new RBB or LBB block associated with high grade AV block during an acute myocardial infarction, permanent pacing is indicated as is infarction with bilateral BB block.

TREATMENT

Treatment of bradycardia and heart block is primarily initiated if there are symptoms such as syncope, lightheadedness, chest pain, shortness of breath and/or evidence of hemodynamic compromise or low cardiac output. Obviously, if offending agents—be it cardiac drugs such as AV nodal blocking agents, digoxin or noncardiac such as opiates—are in use and thought to be the perpetrators, these should be discontinued, if possible. However, if cessation of drug therapy for a reasonable duration of time does not result in improvement, or drug therapy is needed for an indication such as a tachyarrhythmia, then permanent pacing should be considered.

If cessation of an agent does not result in improvement, and a more rapid means of treating bradycardia is needed, the next step would be pharmacologic therapy such as atropine. There are special circumstances, such as BARB toxicity or digoxin toxicity where an antidote of sorts is available, such as glucagon or Digibind, respectively. For more acutely decompensated patients, beta-agonists, such as isoproterenol, may be required until pacing may be initiated.

Beyond pharmacologic measures are the electromechanical therapies. External pacing is considered, but is only of benefit in a very short period of time, due to the unpredictable transcutaneous capture and is poorly tolerated by the patient unless sedated, which itself may perpetuate bradycardia. Temporary pacing is indicated if the above noted therapies are unhelpful and the patient requires more time for conservative measures (holding medications, pharmacologic therapy) to work, or as a bridge to permanent pacing which is commonly not as rapidly available. Permanent pacing is discussed in this book in detail.[43]

REFERENCES

1. Keith A, Flack M. The form and nature of the muscular connections between the primary divisions of the vertebrate heart. J Anat Physiol. 1907;41:172-89.

2. Baruscotti M, Robinson RB. Electrophysiology and pacemaker function of the developing sinoatrial node. Am J Physiol Heart Circ Physiol. 2007;293:H2613-23.

3. Moorman AF, de Jong F, Denyn MM, et al. Development of the cardiac conduction system. Circ Res. 1998;82:629-44.

4. Boullin J, Morgan JM. The development of cardiac rhythm. Heart. 2005;91:874-5.

5. Rossi L. Anatomopathology of the normal and abnormal AV conduction system. Pacing Clin Electrophysiol. 1984;7:1101-7.

6. Calvo-Romero JM, Lima-Rodriguez EM. Bradycardia associated with ophthalmic beta-blockers. J Postgrad Med. 2003;49:186.

7. Mills TA, Kawji MM, Cataldo VD, et al. Profound sinus bradycardia due to diltiazem, verapamil, and/or beta-adrenergic blocking drugs. J La State Med Soc. 2004;156:327-31.

8. Byrd BF 3rd, Collins HW, Primm RK. Risk factors for severe bradycardia during oral clonidine therapy for hypertension. Arch Intern Med. 1988;148:729-33.

9. Golusinski LL Jr, Blount BW. Clonidine-induced bradycardia. J Fam Pract. 1995;41:399-401.

10. Amornyotin S, Srikureja W, Chalayonnavin W, et al. Endoscopy. 2009;41:581-6.

11. van Gorp F, Whyte IM, Isbister GK. Clinical and ECG effects of escitalopram overdose. Ann Emerg Med. 2009;54:404-8.

12. Bordier P, Garrigue S, Barold SS, et al. Significance of syncope in patients with Alzheimer's disease treated with cholinesterase inhibitors. Europace. 2003;5:429-431.

13. Birkenhäger TK, Pluijms EM, Groenland TH, et al. Severe bradycardia after anesthesia before electroconvulsive therapy. J ECT. 2010;26:53-4.

14. Fudickar A, Bein B. Propofol infusion syndrome: update of clinical manifestations and pathophysiology. Minerva Anestesiol. 2009;75:339-44.

15. McAlister HF, Klementowicz PT, Andrews C, et al. Lyme carditis: an important cause of reversible heart block. Ann Intern Med. 1989;110:339-45.

16. Holzer M, Müllner M, Sterz F, et al. Efficacy and safety of endovascular cooling after cardiac arrest: cohort study and Bayesian approach. Stroke. 2006;37:1792-1797.

17. Milanesi R, Baruscotti M, Gnecchi-Ruscone T, et al. Familial sinus bradycardia associated with a mutation in the cardiac pacemaker channel. N Engl J Med. 2006;354:151-7.

18. Mark AL. The Bezold-Jarisch reflex revisited: clinical implications of inhibitory reflexes originating in the heart. J Am Coll Cardiol. 1983;1:90-102.

19. Link MS, Estes NAM. Athletes and arrhythmias. J Cardiovasc Electrophysiol. 2010;21:1-6.

20. Jacquet L, Ziady G, Stein K, et al. J Am Coll Cardiol. 1990;16:832-837.

21. Miyamoto Y, Curtiss El, Kormos RL, et al. Bradyarrhythmias after heart transplantation. Incidence, time, course, and outcome. Circulation. 1990;82:IV313-7.

22. Bernardi L, Valenti C, Wdowczyck-Szuluc J, et al. Influence of type of surgery on the occurrence of parasympathetic reinnervation after cardiac transplantation. Circulation. 1998;97:1368-1374.

23. Deleuze PH, Benvenuti C, Mazzucotelli JP, et al. Orthotopic cardiac transplantation with direct caval anastomosis: is it the optimal procedure? J Thorac Cardiovasc Surg. 1995;109:731-7.

24. el Gamel A, Yonan NA, Grant S, et al. Orthotopic cardiac transplantation: a comparison of standard and bicaval Wythenshawe techniques. J Thorac Cardiovasc Surg. 1995;109:721-730.

25. Rothman SA, Jeevanandam V, Combs WG, et al. Eliminating bradyarrhythmias after orthotopic heart transplantation. Circulation. 1996;94:II278-82.

26. DiBiase A, Tse TM, Schnittger I, et al. Frequency and mechanism of bradycardia in cardiac transplant recipients and need for pacemakers. Am J Cardiol. 1991;67:1385-9.

27. Kawasaki T, Kaimoto S, Sakatani T, et al. Chronotropic incompetence and autonomic dysfunction in patients without structural heart disease. Europace. 2010;12:561-6.

28. Sugiura M, Ohkawa S, Hiraoka K, et al. A clinicopathological study on the sick sinus syndrome. Jpn Heart J. 1976;17:731-41.

29. Kadmon E, Paz R, Kusniec J, et al. Sick sinus syndrome in a patient with extensive cardiac lipomatosis (sinus node dysfunction in lipomatosis). Pacing Clin Electrophysiol 2010;33:513-5.

30. Yanni J, Tellez JO, Sutyagin PV, et al. Structural remodeling of the sinoatrial node in obese old rats. J Mol Cell Cardiol 2010;48:653-62.

31. Verkerk AO, van Ginneken AC, Wilders R. Pacemaker activity of the human sinoatrial node: role of the hyperpolarization-activated current, I(f). Int J Cardiol. 2009;132:318-36.

32. Butters TD, Aslanidi OV, Inada S, et al. Mechanistic links between Na^+ channel (SCN5A) mutations and impaired cardiac pacemaking in sick sinus syndrome. Circ Res. 2010;107:126-37.

33. Pedcini R, Cedergreen P, Theilade S, et al. The prevalence and relevance of the Brugada-type electrocardiogram in the Danish general population: data from the Copenhagen city heart study. Europace. 2010;12:982-6.

34. Patel SS, Anees S, Ferrick KJ. Prevalence of a Brugada pattern electrocardiogram in an urban population in the United States. Pacing Clin Electrophysiol. 2009;32:704-8.

35. Donohoe D, Tehrani F, Jamehdor R, et al. Am Heart Hosp J. 2008;6:48-50.

36. Wu DL, Yeh SJ, Lin FC, et al. Sinus automaticity and sinoatrial conduction in severe symptomatic sick sinus syndrome. J Am Coll Cardiol. 1992;19:355-64.

37. Davies MJ. Pathology of chronic A-V block. Acta Cardiol. 1976;21:19-30.

38. Cheng S, Keyes MJ, Larson MG, et al. Long-term outcomes in individuals with prolonged pr interval or first-degree atrioventricular block. JAMA. 2009;301:2571-7.

39. Silverman ME, Upshaw CB Jr, Lange HW. Woldemar Mobitz and his 1924 classification of second-degree atrioventricular block. Circulation. 2004;110:1162-7.

40. Zipes DP. Second degree atrioventricular block. Circulation. 1979;60:465-72.

41. Barold SS, Hayes DL. Second-degree atrioventricular block: a reappraisal. Mayo Clin Proc. 2001;76:44-57.

42. Barold SS. 2:1 Atrioventricular block: order from chaos. Am J Emerg Med. 2001;19:214-7.

43. Epstein AE, DiMarco JP, Ellenbogen KA, et al. ACC/AHA/HRS 2008 Guidelines for device based therapy of cardiac rhythm abnormalities. Circulation. 2008;117:e350-e408.

44. Lee S, Wellens HJ, Josephson ME. Paroxysmal atrioventricular block. Heart Rhythm. 2009;6:1229-34.

45. Rosenbaum MB, Elizari MV, Lázzari JO. Los Hemibloqueos. Buenos Aires, Argentina: Paidós;1968.

46. Elizari MV, Acunzo RS, Ferreiro M. Hemiblocks revisited. Circulation. 2007;115:1154-63.

47. McAnulty JH, Rahimtoola SH, Murphy E, et al. Natural history of "high-risk" bundle-branch block: final report of a prospective study. NEJM. 1982;307:137-43.

48. Eppinger H, Rothberger CJ. Zur analyse des elektrokardiogramms. Wien Klin Wochenschr. 1909;22;1091-8.

49. Rasmussen H, Moe T. Pathogenesis of left bundle branch block. Br Heart J. 1948;10:141-7.

50. Schneider JF, Thomas Jr HE, Kreger BE, et al. Newly acquired left bundle-branch block: the Framingham study. Annals Int Med. 1979;90:303-10.

51. Haft JI, Herman MV, Gorlin R. Left bundle branch block: etiologic, hemodynamic, and ventriculographic considerations. Circulation. 1971;43:279-87.

52. Sgarbossa EB, Pinski SL, Barbagelata A, et al. Electrocardiographic diagnosis of evolving acute myocardial infarction in the presence of left bundle-branch block. GUSTO-1 (Global utilization of streptokinase and tissue plasminogen activator for occluded coronary arteries) investigators. N Engl J Med. 1996;22:334:481-7.

53. Riccckard J, Kumbhani DJ, Gorodeski EZ, et al. Cardiac resynchronization therapy in non-left bundle branch block morphologies. Pacing Clin Electrophysiol. 2010;33:590-5.

54. Wokhlu A, Rea RF, Asirvatham SJ, et al. Upgrade and de novo cardiac resynchronization therapy: impact of paced or intrinsic QRS morphology on outcomes and survival. Heart Rhythm. 2009;6:1439-47.

Chapter 37

Arrhythmogenic Right Ventricular Dysplasia/Cardiomyopathy

Richard NW Hauer, Frank I Marcus, Moniek GJP Cox

Chapter Outline

INTRODUCTION

Arrhythmogenic right ventricular dysplasia/cardiomyopathy (ARVD/C) is a disease characterized histopathologically by progressive fibrofatty replacement of the myocardium, primarily of the right ventricle (RV).[1-3] Affected individuals typically present between the second and the fourth decade of life with monomorphic ventricular tachycardia (VT) originating from the RV. ARVD/C can be the cause of sudden death in all stages of the disease, but particularly in adolescence.[4] From autopsy studies, it is known that fibrofatty tissue can replace major parts of normal myocardium in teenagers (Fig. 1). Sudden death may occur in the early concealed phase of the disease.

The first series of ARVD/C patients was published in 1982. It was described as a disease in which "the right ventricular musculature is partially or totally absent and is replaced by fatty and fibrous tissue".[1] This disease was initially thought to be a defect in RV development, which is why it was first called "dysplasia". In the past 25 years, increased insight in the development of the disease as well as the discovery of pathogenic mutations involved led to our current understanding that ARVD/C is a genetically determined "cardiomyopathy".[3,5] However, since non-familial sporadic cases occur even after extensive family screening, non-genetic causes cannot be excluded. It is now clear that ARVD/C is a desmosomal disease resulting from defective cell adhesion proteins. Desmosomes maintain mechanical coupling of cardiomyocytes. The first disease-causing gene, encoding the desmosomal protein

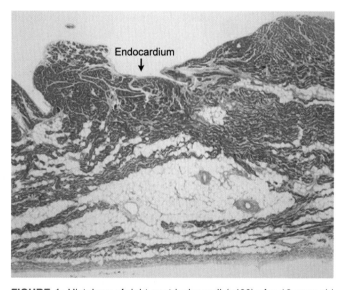

FIGURE 1: Histology of right ventricular wall (x400) of a 13-year-old girl who died suddenly during exercise. AZAN stain with cardiac myocytes (red), collagen (blue) and adipocytes (white). Shown is the typical pattern of ARVD/C with strands of fibrosis reaching all the way to the endocardium (particularly just right of the middle). Bundles of cardiac myocytes are embedded in between the fibrotic strands, particularly in the subendocardial layers. These interconnecting bundles of myocytes give rise to activation delay and re-entrant circuits, the typical electrophysiologic substrate for ventricular arrhythmias in ARVD/C. The large homogeneous subepicardial area of adipose tissue is not arrhythmogenic, although it may be observed in ARVD/C. However, it is a typical feature of the cor adiposum, a non-arrhythmogenic condition

plakoglobin (JUP), was identified in patients with Naxos disease, an autosomal recessive variant of ARVD/C, reported from the Greek island of Naxos.[6] This discovery stimulated research in the direction of other desmosomal genes. Till 2004, only three genes were identified as responsible for the autosomal dominantly inherited ARVD/C.[7-15] Since *RyR2* mutations are typically associated with catecholaminergic polymorphic VT, it is less certain that these *RyR2* mutations are a caused of ARVD/C. The desmoplakin gene (*DSP*) was the first desmosomal protein gene associated with the autosomal dominant form of ARVD/C.[15] It was followed by discovery of mutations in plakophilin-2 (*PKP2*), desmoglein-2 (*DSG2*) and desmocollin-2(*DSC2*), all components of the cardiac desmosome.[16-18] Impaired desmosomal function results in myocardial cell-to-cell uncoupling, followed by cell death and fibrofatty replacement, and thus disruption of the myocardial architecture leading to activation delay and arrhythmias. In a few rare cases, autosomal dominant ARVD/C has been linked to other genes unrelated to the cell adhesion complex, i.e. the genes encoding the cardiac ryanodine receptor (RyR2), the transforming growth factor-β3 gene (*TGFβ3*), and trans-membrane protein 43 (*TMEM43*).[13,14,19] Since *RyR2* mutations are typically associated with catecholaminergic polymorphic VT it is less certain that these *RyR2* mutations are a cause of ARVD/C.

With mutations found in about half of the patients, mainly in desmosomal genes and *PKP2* in particular, ARVD/C is currently considered a genetically determined desmosomal disease.

This chapter provides an overview of ARVD/C, starting from the genetic defects that are responsible for the pathophysiologic mechanisms to clinical diagnosis, treatment and prognosis.

MOLECULAR AND GENETIC BACKGROUND

DESMOSOME STRUCTURE AND FUNCTION

The cellular adhesion junctions in the intercalated disk are vital for the structural and functional integrity of cardiac myocytes. Intercalated disks are located between cardiomyocytes at their longitudinal ends and contain three different kinds of intercellular connections: (1) Desmosomes; (2) Adherens junctions and (3) Gap junctions.

Desmosomes are important for cell-to-cell adhesion and are predominantly found in tissues that experience mechanical stress—the heart and the epidermis. They couple cytoskeletal elements to the plasma membrane. Desmosomes also protect the other components of the intercalated disk from mechanical stress and are involved in structural organization of the intercalated disk. Desmosomes consist of multiple proteins which belong to the following three different families:

1. Transmembranous cadherins (desmogleins and desmo-collins)
2. Linker armadillo repeat proteins (plakoglobin and plako-philin)
3. Plakins (desmoplakin and plectin).

Figure 2 schematically represents the organization of the various proteins in the cardiac desmosome.

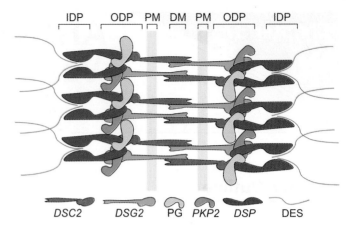

FIGURE 2: Schematic representation of the molecular organization of cardiac desmosomes. The plasma membrane (PM) spanning proteins desmocollin-2 (DSC2) and desmoglein-2 (DSG2) interact in the extracellular space at the dense midline (DM). At the cytoplasmic side, they interact with plakoglobin (PG) and plakophilin-2 (PKP2) at the outer dense plaque (ODP). The PKP2 and PG also interact with desmoplakin (DSP). At the inner dense plaque (IDP), the C-terminus of DSP anchors the intermediate filament desmin (DES) (*Source:* Modified from: Van Tintelen et al. Curr Opin Cardiol. 2007;22:185-92)

Within desmosomes, cadherins are connected to armadillo proteins which interact with plakins. The plakins anchor the desmosomes to intermediate filaments, mainly desmin. They form a three-dimensional scaffold providing mechanical support.

Adherens junctions act as bridges that link the actin filaments within sarcomeres of neighboring cells. These junctions are involved in force transmission and, together with desmosomes, these mechanical junctions act as "spot welds" to create membrane domains that are protected from shear stress caused by contraction of the neighboring cells. Furthermore, they facilitate assembly and maintenance of gap junctions, securing intercellular electrical coupling.

Cardiomyocytes are individually bordered by a lipid bilayer which gives a high degree of electrical insulation. The electrical current that forms the impulse for mechanic contraction travels from one cell to the other via gap junctions. Gap junctions provide electrical coupling by enabling ion transfer between cells. The number, size and distribution of gap junctions all influence impulse propagation in cardiac muscle. Consequently, alterations in function of gap junctions can lead to intercellular propagation disturbances and arrhythmogenesis.[20]

The intercalated disk is an intercellular structure, where desmosomes and adherens junctions not only provide mechanical strength but also protect the interspersed gap junctions, enabling electrical coupling between cells.

DESMOSOMAL DYSFUNCTION AND ARVD/C PATHOPHYSIOLOGY

It is not well known how mutations of desmosomal protein genes are related to the ARVD/C phenotype. Several mechanisms have been proposed.

First, alterations in desmosomal proteins are thought to lead to mechanical uncoupling of myocytes at the intercalated disks, particularly under mechanical stress (e.g. exercise, sports activities, etc.). Mechanical uncoupling will be followed by: (1) Electrical uncoupling due to dysfunction of gap junctions and (2) Cell death with fibrofatty replacement. Both electrical uncoupling and interconnecting bundles of surviving myocardium embedded in the fibrofatty tissue lead to lengthening of conduction pathways and load mismatch. This results in marked activation delay and conduction block, which are pivotal mechanisms for re-entry and thereby VT. Invasive electrophysiologic studies have confirmed that VT in patients with ARVD/C is due to re-entrant circuits in areas of abnormal myocardium.[21] In addition, environmental factors, such as exercise or inflammation from viral infection, could aggravate impaired adhesion and accelerate disease progression. The RV may be more vulnerable to histopathologic alteration than the left ventricle (LV) due to its thinner walls and its normal dilatory response to exercise.

Secondly, recent studies have shown that impairment of cell-to-cell adhesion due to changes in desmosomal components may affect the amount and distribution of other intercalated disk proteins, including connexin 43, the major protein forming gap junctions in the ventricular myocardium.[22-24] This was shown for *DSP* and *JUP* by Western blotting and confocal immuno-fluorescence techniques, but alterations in other desmosomal components, such as *PKP2, DSG2* and *DSC2*, are thought to have similar effects. Changes in number and function of gap junctions will diminish intercellular electrical coupling contributing to intraventricular activation delay.

The third hypothesis involves the canonical Wnt/β-catenin signaling pathway. Plakoglobin can localize both to the plasma membrane and the nucleus. It was demonstrated that disruption of desmoplakin frees plakoglobin from the plasma membrane allowing it to translocate to the nucleus and suppress canonical Wnt/β-catenin signaling. Wnt signaling can inhibit adipogenesis by preventing mesodermal precursors from differentiating into adipocytes.[25] Suppression of Wnt signaling by plakoglobin nuclear localization could, therefore, promote the differentiation to adipose tissue in the cardiac myocardium in patients with ARVD/C.[26]

Finally, since ion channels, like the Na^+ channel, are also located in the intercalated disk, they might be disrupted and contribute to arrhythmogeneity as well.

The pathophysiological mechanisms proposed above are not mutually exclusive and could occur simultaneously.

Two patterns of inheritance have been described in ARVD/C. The most common or classical form of ARVD/C is inherited as an autosomal dominant trait. Naxos disease and Carvajal syndrome are rare, inherited as autosomal recessive. Table 1 summarizes the different genes involved in ARVD/C with the corresponding phenotypes.

AUTOSOMAL RECESSIVE DISEASE

In Naxos disease, affected individuals were found to be homozygous for a 2-base pair deletion in the *JUP* gene.[6] All patients who are homozygous for this mutation have diffuse palmoplantar keratosis and woolly hair in infancy. Children usually have no cardiac symptoms, but may have electro-cardiographic abnormalities and nonsustained ventricular arrhythmias.[27] In one report, an Arab family was found to have an autosomal recessive mutation in the desmoplakin gene that caused ARVD/C with a classical ARVD/C cardiac phenotype, that was also associated with woolly hair, and a pemphigus-

TABLE 1

Mutated genes and concurrent types of autosomal dominant ARVD/C

	Gene	Type of disease
Desmosomal	PKP2	ARVD/C
	DSG2	ARVD/C
	DSC2	ARVD/C
	JUP	Naxos disease*
	DSP	Carvajal syndrome*
		ARVD/C
		LDAC
Non-desmosomal	RyR2	CPVT ARVD/C
	TGF-β	Typical ARVD/C
	TMEM43	ARVD/C

*Autosomal recessive inheritance;
(Abbreviations: CPVT: Catecholaminergic polymorphic VT; LDAC: Left dominant arrhythmogenic cardiomyopathy. See text for other abbreviations. (*Source:* Modified from: Van Tintelen et al. Curr Opin Cardiol. 2007;22:185-92)

like skin disorder.[28] A different autosomal recessive disease, Carvajal syndrome, is associated with a desmoplakin gene mutation. It manifests by woolly hair, epidermolytic palmoplantar keratoderma and cardiomyopathy.[29] The cardiomyopathy of Carvajal syndrome was thought to have a predilection for the LV, but subsequent evaluation of a deceased child revealed typical ARVD/C changes in both ventricles.[24]

AUTOSOMAL DOMINANT DISEASE

Mutations in the gene encoding the intracellular desmosomal component desmoplakin can cause "classic ARVD/C" with a clinical presentation of VT, sudden death as well as LV involvement as the disease progresses.[15,30,31] Desmoplakin gene mutations have also been associated with predominantly left-sided ARVD/C and, as noted above, with autosomal recessive disease.

Various authors identified mutations in the *PKP2* gene as the most frequently observed genetic abnormality. Figure 3 shows the pedigree of a family with a *PKP2* mutation. Incomplete penetrance and clinical variability are well documented. In four studies from different countries, analyzing 56–100 ARVD/C patients each, the following observations were made.[16,32-34] *PKP2* mutations were found in 11–43% of unrelated index patients who fulfilled diagnostic task force criteria for ARVD/C. In a Dutch ARVD/C cohort, 78 of 149 (52%) probands had a pathogenic *PKP2* mutation. This high yield of *PKP2* mutations is partly due to occurrence of founder mutations in the Netherlands. Haplotype analysis previously performed suggested founder mutations were responsible for 4 of the 14 different mutations identified.[34] Among index patients with a positive family history of ARVD/C, 70% had a *PKP2* mutation.[34]

Pilichou et al. screened patients with ARVD/C for mutations in the transmembranous desmosomal component *DSG2*.[17] Among 80 unrelated probands, 26 were found to have *DSP* or *PKP2* mutations. Direct sequencing of *DSG2* in the other 54 patients revealed nine distinct mutations in eight individuals. These individuals demonstrated typical clinical characteristics of ARVD/C. An analogous study of 86 ARVD/C probands

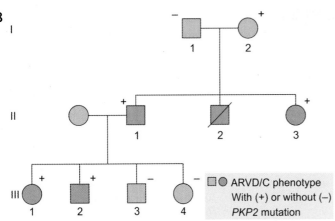

FIGURE 3: Pedigree of family with ARVD/C and *PKP2* mutation. This figure shows incomplete penetrance and variability of clinical expression. Both the 72-year-old grandmother (I:2) and 20-year-old grandson (III:2) are free of any signs of disease, despite carrying the mutation. The proband (II:1) was resuscitated at age 35, his brother (II:2) died suddenly at age 18. Both the proband's sister (II:3) and daughter (III:1) were diagnosed with the disease due to a positive family history, arrhythmias and RV structural abnormalities. The sister (II:3) of the proband has structural and ECG abnormalities, but no symptomatic arrhythmias

identified eight novel *DSG2* mutations in nine probands. Clinical evaluation of family members with *DSG2* mutations revealed a penetrance of 58% using task force criteria from 1994 and 75% using proposed modified criteria.[35] Morphological abnormalities of the RV were present in 66% of gene carriers, LV involvement in 25% and classical right precordial T-wave inversion in only 26%. The authors noted that disease expression of *DSG2* mutations was of variable severity, but that overall penetrance was high and LV involvement prominent.[36]

In *DSC2*, another important transmembranous desmosomal cadherin, two heterozygous mutations (a deletion and an insertion) were identified in 4 of 77 probands with ARVD/C.[18] Finally, a dominant mutation in the plakoglobin (*JUP*) gene has been identified.[37] The identification of so many desmosomal cell adhesion gene abnormalities supports the hypothesis that ARVD/C is predominantly a disease of cell-to-cell coupling.

OTHER NON-DESMOSOMAL GENES

Mutations in the cardiac ryanodine receptor *RyR2*, which is responsible for calcium release from the sarcoplasmic reticulum, have been described in only one Italian ARVD/C family.[13] Affected patients have exercise-induced polymorphic VT.[38] Mutations in *RyR2* have primarily been associated with familial catecholaminergic polymorphic VT without ARVD/C.[19,39] Although the general opinion is that *RyR2* mutations lead to catecholaminergic polymorphic VT without structural abnormalities, the mutations in ARVD/C have been advocated to act differently from those in familial polymorphic VT without ARVD/C.[40-42]

The *TGFβ3* regulates the production of extracellular matrix components and modulates expression of genes encoding desmosomal proteins. The gene has been mapped to chromosome 14. Sequencing studies failed to identify any disease-causing mutations in the exonic regions of *TGFβ3*. This led to screening of the promoter and untranslated regions, where a mutation of the *TGFβ3* gene was found in all clinically affected

members of a large family with ARVD/C.[14] The mutation is predicted to produce an amino acid substitution in a short peptide with an inhibitory role in *TGFβ3* regulation. The implication of these observations is that regulatory mutations resulting in overexpression of *TGFβ3* may contribute to the development of ARVD/C in these families. The *TGFβ* family of cytokines stimulates production of components of the extracellular matrix. It is therefore possible that enhanced *TGFβ* activity can lead to myocardial fibrosis. However, genetic analysis of two other families with ARVD/C failed to identify mutations in any of the regions of the *TGFβ3* gene.

A missense mutation in the *TMEM43* gene was found in 15 unrelated ARVD/C families from a genetically isolated population in New Foundland and caused a fully penetrant, sex-influenced, high risk form of ARVD/C.[19] The *TMEM43* gene contains the response element for PPAR gamma, an adipogenic transcription factor. The *TMEM43* gene mutation is thought to cause dysregulation of an adipogenic pathway regulated by PPAR gamma, which may explain the fibrofatty replacement of myocardium in ARVD/C patients.

EPIDEMIOLOGY

Estimations of the prevalence of ARVD/C in the general population vary from 1:2000 to 1:5000.[43] The real prevalence of ARVD/C, however, is unknown and is presumably higher due to many non-diagnosed and misdiagnosed cases.

The disease appears to be especially common in adolescents and young adults in northern Italy, accounting for approximately 11% of cases of sudden cardiac death overall and 22% in athletes.[44,45] In as many as 20% of sudden deaths occurring in people under 35 years of age, features of ARVD/C were detected at post mortem evaluation.[45] In nearly half of them, no prior symptoms had been reported.

ARVD/C has incomplete penetrance and extremely variable clinical expression. For instance, family screening has identified pathogenic mutation carriers, who had stayed free of any sign of disease up to or over 70 years of age (Fig. 3).

From the genetic aspect, both men and women should be equally affected. However, men are more frequently diagnosed with ARVD/C than women. In a recent large multicenter study, 57% of affected individuals were male.[46] As many women as men show at least some signs of disease, but women more often do not fulfill criteria to meet the diagnosis. Factors explaining this difference in severity of disease expression have not yet been elucidated. It is speculated that (sports) activity or hormonal factors may play a role. Familial disease has been demonstrated in greater than 50% of ARVD/C cases.

CLINICAL PRESENTATION

ARVD/C patients typically present between the second and the fourth decade of life with monomorphic VT originating from RV. However, in a minority of patients, sudden death, frequently at a young age, or RV failure are the first signs. Based on clinicopathologic and patient follow-up studies, four different disease phases have been described for the classical form of ARVD/C, i.e. primarily affecting the RV (Table 2):
1. Early ARVD/C is often described as "concealed" owing to the frequent absence of clinical findings, although minor

TABLE 2

Different phases of disease severity

Phase	Characteristics
1. Concealed	Asymptomatic patients with possibly only minor ventricular arrhythmia and subtle structural changes
2. Overt	Symptoms due to LBBB VT or multiple premature complexes, with more obvious structural RV abnormalities
3. RV failure	With relatively preserved LV function
4. Biventricular	Significant overt LV involvement

ventricular arrhythmias and subtle structural changes may be found. Although patients tend to be asymptomatic, they may nonetheless be at risk of sudden death, mainly during vigourous exercise.

2. The overt phase follows, in which patients suffer from palpitations, syncope and ventricular arrhythmias of left bundle branch block (LBBB) morphology, ranging from isolated ventricular premature complexes to sustained VT and ventricular fibrillation (VF).

3. The third phase is characterized by RV failure due to progressive loss of myocardium with severe dilatation and systolic dysfunction, in the presence of preserved LV function.

4. Biventricular failure occurs due to LV involvement at a later stage. This phase may mimic dilated cardiomyopathy (DCM) and may require cardiac transplantation.

In the initially described classical form of ARVD/C, the RV is primarily affected with possibly (in a later stage) some LV involvement. Two additional patterns of disease have been identified by clinicogenetic characterization of families. These are the left dominant phenotype, with early and predominant LV manifestations, and the biventricular phenotype with equal involvement of both ventricles.

Recent immunohistochemical analysis of human myocardial samples demonstrated that both ventricles are affected by the disease.[47] A marked reduction in immunoreactive signal levels for plakoglobin was observed both in RV and LV, independent of genotype. Thus at a molecular level ARVD/C is a global biventricular disease. However, histologically and functionally overt manifestations of the disease usually start in the RV. The reason for this is still unclear. The most commonly advocated hypothesis is that the thin walled RV is less able to withstand pressure (over)load in the presence of impaired function of mechanical junctions.

CLINICAL DIAGNOSIS

Diagnosis of ARVD/C can be very challenging. Although VF and sudden death may be the first manifestations of ARVD/C, symptomatic patients typically present with sustained VT with LBBB morphology, thus originating from the RV. The occurrence of VT episodes is usually induced by adrenergic stimuli mainly during exercise, especially competitive sports. The ARVD/C is a disease that shows progression over time.

In ARVD/C demonstration of transmural fibrofatty replacement primarily of right ventricular myocardium can be determined at surgery or autopsy (Fig. 1). Predilection sites for these structural abnormalities are the so-called triangle of dysplasia formed by the RV outflow tract, the apex and the subtricuspid region.[1] In clinical practice, diagnosis based on cardiac pathology is not practical. Endomyocardial biopsies have major limitations. Tissue sampling from the affected often thin RV free wall, directed by imaging techniques or voltage mapping, is associated with a slight risk of perforation. Sampling from the interventricular septum is relatively safe. However, the septum is histopathogically rarely affected in ARVD/C. In addition, histology may be classified as normal due to the focal nature of the lesions. Finally, since subendocardial layers are usually not affected in an early stage of the disease, histological diagnosis may be hampered by the nontransmural nature of endomyocardial biopsies.[48]

Clinical diagnosis has been facilitated by a set of clinically applicable criteria for ARVD/C diagnosis defined by a Task Force based on consensus in 1994, and modified in 2010.[49,50] The current Task Force criteria are the essential standard for classification of individuals suspected of ARVD/C. In addition, its universal acceptance contributes importantly to unambiguous interpretation of clinical studies and facilitates comparison of results. The Task Force criteria included six different categories. They are derived into: (1) Global and regional dysfunction and structural alterations; (2) Tissue characterization; (3) Depolarization abnormalities; (4) Repolarization abnormalities; (5) Arrhythmias and (6) Family history, including pathogenic mutations. Within these groups, diagnostic criteria are categorized as major or minor according to their specificity for the disease. In order to fulfill ARVD/C diagnosis it is required to have either two major or one major plus two minor or four minor criteria. From each different group, only one criterion can be counted for diagnosis, even when multiple criteria in one group are present. Table 3 gives an overview of the Task Force criteria which is defined in 2010.

Specific evaluations are recommended in all patients suspected of ARVD/C. Detailed history and family history, physical examination, 12-lead ECG, signal averaged ECG (SAECG), 24-hours Holter monitoring, exercise testing and 2D echocardiography with quantitative wall motion analysis. When appropriate, more detailed analyzes of the RV can be done by cardiac magnetic resonance imaging (MRI). Invasive tests are also useful for diagnostic purposes: RV and LV cineangiography, electrophysiological testing, and endomyocardial biopsies.

GLOBAL AND/OR REGIONAL DYSFUNCTION AND STRUCTURAL ALTERATIONS

Evaluation of RV size and function can be done by various imaging modalities, including echocardiography, cardiac MRI, computed tomography and/or cineangiography. According to the Task Force criteria, major criteria are defined as presence of an akinetic or dyskinetic areas in the RV (Fig. 4) combined with severe dilatation of the RV or RV ejection fraction 40% or lower.[50] With RV cineangiography the finding of only regional akinesia, dyskinesia or aneurysm is considered sufficient for qualification as a major criterion. RV cineangiography has historically been considered the most sensitive method to visualize RV structural abnormalities, with a high specificity of 90%.[51] Compared to cineangiography, the non-invasive

New task force criteria

I. Global and/or regional dysfunction and structural alterations

Major (2D echo)
Regional RV akinesia, dyskinesia or aneurysm
and one of:
- Parasternal long axis view
  RVOT (PLAX) $\geq$ 32 mm
  Corrected for body size
  (PLAX/BSA) $\geq$ 19 mm/m²
- Parasternal short axis view
  RVOT (PSAX) $\geq$ 36 mm
  Corrected for body size
  (PSAX/BSA) $\geq$ 21 mm/m²
- Fractional area change
  (FAC) $\leq$ 33%

Major (MRI)
Regional RV akinesia or dyskinesia or dyssynchronous RV contraction
And one of:
- RV end diastolic volume $\geq$ 110 ml/m² male
  (RVEDV/BSA) $\geq$ 100 ml/m² female
- RV ejection fraction (RVEF) $\leq$ 40%

Major (RV cineangiography)
Regional RV akinesia, dyskinesia or aneurysm

Minor (2D echo)
Regional RV akinesia or dyskinesia
And one of:
- Parasternal long axis view
  RVOT (PLAX) $\geq$ 29–$\leq$ 31 mm
  Corrected for body size
  (PLAX/BSA) $\geq$ 16–$\leq$ 18 mm/m²ⁱ
- Parasternal short axis view
  RVOT (PSAX) $\geq$ 32–$\leq$ 35 mm
  Corrected for body size (PSAX/BSA) $\geq$ 18–$\leq$ 20 mm/m²
- Fractional area change (FAC) $\leq$ 40%

Minor (MRI)
Regional RV akinesia or dyskinesia or dyssynchronous RV contraction
And one of:
- RV end diastolic volume/BSA $\geq$ 100 ml/m² male
                                 $\geq$ 90 ml/m² female
- RV ejection fraction (RVEF) $\leq$ 45%

II. Tissue characterization of wall

Major
Residual myocytes < 60% by morphometric analysis, (or < 50% if estimated), with fibrous replacement of the RV free wall myocardium in at least 1 sample, with or without fatty tissue replacement

Minor
Residual myocytes 60–75% by morphometric analysis, (or 50–65% if estimated), with fibrous replacement of the RV free wall myocardium in at least 1 sample, with or without fatty tissue replacement

III. Repolarization abnormalities

Major
Negative T waves in at least leads V1-3

Minor
Negative T waves only in leads V1 and V2 or in V4-6
In case of complete right bundle branch block: negative T waves in leads V1-4

IV. Depolarization/Conduction abnormalities

Major
Epsilon wave in one of leads V1-3

Minor
Late potentials by signal averaged ECG in at least one of three parameters in the absence of a QRS duration of $\geq$ 110 msec on the standard ECG
- Filtered QRS duration (fQRS) $\geq$ 114 msec
- Duration of terminal QRS
  < 40 µV (LAS) $\geq$ 38 msecs
- RMS voltage of terminal 40 msecs $\leq$ 20 µV
- Terminal activation duration $\geq$ 55 ms

V. Arrhythmias

Major
- (Non-)sustained VT of left bundle branch block morphology with superior axis

Minor
- (Non-)sustained VT of left bundle branch block morphology with inferior axis or unknown axis
- > 500 ventricular extrasystoles/24 hours by Holter

VI. Family history

Major
- ARVD/C confirmed in a first-degree relative who meets current task force criteria
- ARVD/C confirmed pathologically at autopsy or surgery in a first-degree relative
- Identification of a pathogenic mutation associated with ARVD/C

Minor
- History of ARVC/D in a first-degree relative in whom it is not possible or practical to determine if the family member meets current task force criteria
- Premature sudden death (< 35 years) due to suspected ARVD/C in a first-degree relative

(*Source:* Modified from: Marcus FI et al. Circulation. 2010;121:1533-41)·

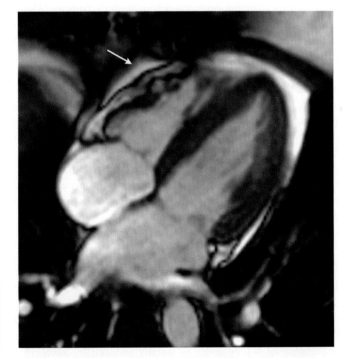

FIGURE 4: An MRI image of ARVD/C patient at end of systole. Dyskinetic areas are visible in the RV free wall (arrow)

technique of echocardiography is widely used and serves as the first-line imaging technique in evaluating patients suspected of ARVD/C and in family screening. Especially with improvement of echocardiographic modalities, such as 3-dimensional echocardiography, strain and tissue Doppler, the sensitivity and specificity of echocardiography have improved in recent years. Cardiac MRI has the unique ability to characterize tissue composition, by differentiating fat from fibrous tissue by using delayed enhancement. However, this technique is expensive, not widely available and requires great expertise to prevent misdiagnosis of ARVD/C.[52] Also; this technique cannot be applied in patients with an implantable cardioverter-defibrillator (ICD). Incorrect interpretation of cardiac MRI is the most common cause of overdiagnosis and physicians should be reluctant to diagnose ARVD/C when structural abnormalities are present only on MRI.[53] Furthermore, it is important to note that the presence of fat in the epimyocardial and midmyocardial layers (without fibrosis) can be a normal finding and should not be considered diagnostic of ARVD/C (Fig. 1).

ENDOMYOCARDIAL BIOPSY

For reasons previously noted, undirected endomyocardial biopsies are infrequently diagnostic. However, it had been included as a major criterion by the Task Force, since the finding of fibrofatty replacement was considered to strongly support any findings derived from other clinical investigations. The rather vague terminology of any "fibrofatty replacement of myocardium" has been quantified. Diagnostic values according to the new Task Force criteria are considered major if histomorphometric analysis of endomyocardial biopsies shows that the number of residual myocytes is below 60% or below 50% by estimation, with fibrous replacement of the RV free wall in at least one sample, with or without fatty tissue replacement.[54] If the number of residual myocytes is higher but still below 75% (morphometric) or below 65% (estimated), only a minor criterion is fulfilled.

ECG CRITERIA

The 12-lead ECG is most important for diagnosis of ARVD/C. Consistent with early electrical uncoupling, ECG changes and arrhythmias may develop before histologic evidence of myocyte loss or clinical evidence of ARVD/C. ECG criteria on depolarization and repolarization have to be obtained during sinus rhythm and while off antiarrhythmic drugs. These drugs may cause misinterpretation of ECG criteria due to their contribution on activation delay and repolarization abnormalities.

DEPOLARIZATION ABNORMALITIES

The RV activation delay is a hallmark of ARVD/C. This delay is reflected by the presence of an epsilon wave, prolonged terminal activation duration (TAD) in the terminal part and after the QRS complex, and also by recording of late potentials on SAECG.

Epsilon waves are defined as low amplitude potentials after and clearly separated from the QRS complex, in at least one of precordial leads, V1-V3 (Fig. 5).[55] This highly specific major criterion is observed in only a small minority of patients.[56,57]

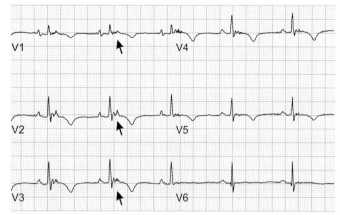

FIGURE 5: Epsilon waves indicated by arrows (also prolonged terminal activation duration; 120 ms) and negative T waves in V1-5

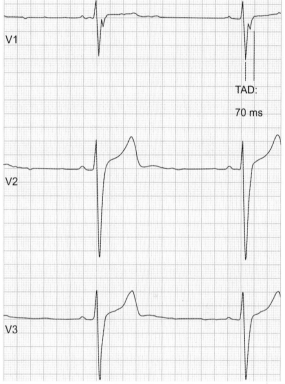

FIGURE 6: Prolonged terminal activation duration (70 ms from nadir of S wave to end of depolarization), *without* epsilon wave. Paper speed 25 mm/s

TAD has been defined as the longest value measured from the nadir of the S wave to the end of all depolarization deflections in V1-V3, thereby including not only the S wave upstroke but also both late and fractionated signals and epsilon waves (Figs 5 and 6).[58] Thus, total activation delay presumably from the RV is conveyed by this new parameter. The TAD is considered prolonged if greater than or equal to 55 ms, and only applicable in the absence of complete right bundle branch block (RBBB). Prolonged TAD, introduced as minor criterion, appears to be equally sensitive as late potential recording and much more sensitive than epsilon waves. Prolonged TAD was recorded in 30 of 42 ARVD/C patients and in only 1 of 27 patients with idiopathic VT.[58] Both epsilon waves and prolonged TAD are measured only in V1-V3, which face the RV outflow

712 tract. Activation delay in other areas of RV is not reflected by these criteria.

The detection of late potentials on SAECG is the surface counterpart of delayed activation or late potentials detected during endocardial mapping in electrophysiologic studies. They are frequently found in patients with documented VT. However, these late potentials can also be observed after myocardial infarction and with other structural heart diseases. Due to this lack of specificity, SAECG abnormalities were considered a minor criterion. For all the depolarization criteria, it is apparent that they will correlate with disease severity. For instance, a positive correlation has been found between late potentials and the extent of RV fibrosis, reduced RV systolic function and significant morphological abnormalities on imaging.[59-61]

REPOLARIZATION ABNORMALITIES

In the new Task Force criteria negative T waves in leads V1, V2 and V3 form a major ECG criterion in the absence of complete RBBB, and only if the patient is older than 14 years of age (Fig. 5). Studies have reported variable prevalences of right precordial T wave inversion, ranging from 19% to 94%.[49,55-57,62] The lower rates are often due to evaluation of family members, while higher rates are seen in series consisting of unrelated index patients. In the recent study by Cox et al. this criterion was identified in 67% of exclusively ARVD/C index patients and in none of the patients with idiopathic VT.[58] T wave inversion can be a normal feature of the ECG in children and in early adolescence. Therefore, this finding is not considered abnormal in persons at the age of 14 years and younger.

In the new Task Force criteria, two minor repolarization criteria were included:
1. Inverted T waves only in leads V1-V2 or in V4-V6 in individuals older than 14 years of age and in the absence of complete RBBB.

2. Inverted T waves in leads V1-V4 in individuals older than 14 years of age in the presence of RBBB. This was included since T wave inversion in RBBB seldom extends to V4 in otherwise healthy individuals.

ARRHYTHMIAS

In ARVD/C, ventricular arrhythmias range from premature ventricular complexes to sustained VT and VF, leading to cardiac arrest.[58,63] Due to their typical origin in the RV, QRS complexes of ventricular arrhythmias show a LBBB morphology. Moreover, the QRS axis indicates the VT origin, i.e. superior axis from the RV inferior wall or apex (major criterion) and inferior axis (minor criterion) from the RV outflow tract (RVOT) (Figs 7 and 8). The VT of LBBB configuration with an unknown axis counts as minor criterion. Patients with extensively affected RV often show multiple VT morphologies.[58,64]

The VF is the mechanism of instantaneous sudden death especially occurring in young people and athletes with ARVD/C, who were often previously asymptomatic. In this subset of patients, VF may occur from deterioration of monomorphic VT, or in a phase of acute disease progression, due to myocyte death and reactive inflammation.[3]

Finally, in the new Task Force criteria the number of premature ventricular complexes on 24-hours Holter recording is reduced to 500 or more for a minor criterion.

FAMILY HISTORY

Before the discovery of pathogenic mutations underlying the disease, it was recognized that ARVD/C often occurs in family members.[1] Having a family member with proven ARVD/C is considered an increased risk for other family members to be affected. Therefore, having a first-degree relative who meets the current Task Force criteria, or having ARVD/C confirmed pathologically at autopsy or during surgery, or identification of a pathogenic mutation in the family, is included as major

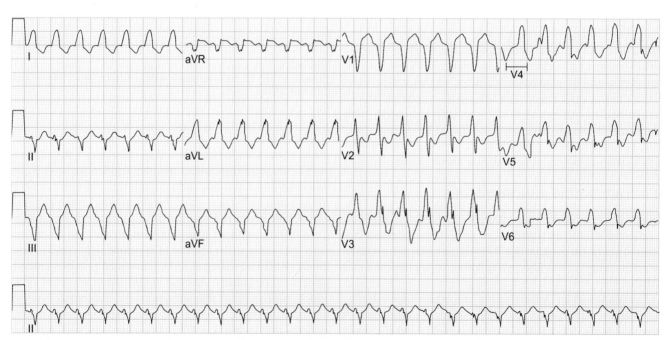

FIGURE 7: An ECG (25 mm/s) from ARVD/C patient with *PKP2* mutation. This VT has an LBBB morphology and superior axis (with positive QRS complex in aVL), thus originating inferiorly from the RV

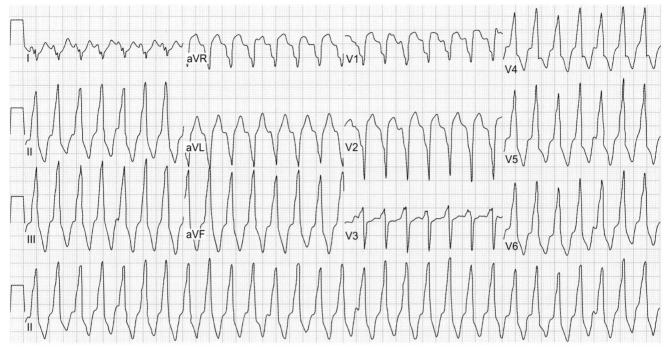

FIGURE 8: An ECG (25 mm/s) from ARVD/C patient without identified mutation. This VT has also LBBB morphology, but with inferior axis, originating from RV outflow tract. Note the typical negative QRS complex in aVL

diagnostic criteria. If a first-degree relative is diagnosed with ARVD/C but does not fulfill the diagnostic criteria, only a minor criterion is counted. Sudden death of a family member under the age of 35 years, presumably but not proven to be due to ARVD/C related arrhythmias, is a minor criterion. Pathologic confirmation of transmural fibrofatty replacement of the RV at autopsy or after surgical resection is considered a major criterion for the diagnosis.[50]

NON-CLASSICAL ARVD/C SUBTYPES

NAXOS DISEASE

All patients who homozygously carry the recessive *JUP* mutation for Naxos disease have diffuse palmoplantar keratosis and woolly hair in infancy. Children usually have no cardiac symptoms, but may have ECG abnormalities and nonsustained ventricular arrhythmias.[6,27] The cardiac disease is 100% penetrant by adolescence, being manifested by symptomatic arrhythmias, ECG abnormalities, right ventricular structural alterations and LV involvement. In one series of 26 patients followed for 10 years, 62% had structural progression of right ventricular abnormalities and 27% developed heart failure due to LV involvement.[27] Almost half of the patients developed symptomatic arrhythmias and the annual cardiac and SCD mortality were 3% and 2.3% respectively, which are slightly higher than seen in autosomal dominant forms of ARVD/C. A minority of heterozygotes has minor ECG and ECG changes, but clinically significant disease is not present.

CARVAJAL SYNDROME

Carvajal syndrome is associated with a *DSP* gene mutation, and is also a recessive disease manifested by woolly hair, epidermo-

lytic palmoplantar keratoderma and cardiomyopathy.[29] All diagnosed patients have been from Ecuador. The cardiomyopathy of Carvajal syndrome was first thought to be mainly left ventricular, with dilated left ventricular cardiomyopathy. A number of the patients with Carvajal syndrome had heart failure in their teenage years, resulting in early morbidity. Further research revealed that the disease is characterized mainly by ventricular hypertrophy, ventricular dilatation and discrete focal ventricular aneurysms. In the RV, focal wall thinning and aneurysmal dilatation were identified in the triangle of dysplasia.

LEFT DOMINANT ARVD/C (LDAC)

As previously mentioned, in classic ARVD/C the histologic process predominantly involves the RV and extends to the LV in more advanced stages.[52,62,65-67] In contrast, patients with left-dominant arrhythmogenic cardiomyopathy (LDAC, also known as left-sided ARVD/C or arrhythmogenic left ventricular cardiomyopathy) have fibrofatty changes that predominantly involve the LV.[68] Clinically, this disease entity is characterized by (infero)lateral T-wave inversion, arrhythmias of LV origin and/or proven LDAC.

Patients may present with arrhythmias or chest pain at ages ranging from adolescence to over 80 years. By cardiac MRI about one-third of patients show a LV ejection fraction less than 50%. Furthermore, MRI with late gadolinium enhancement (LGE) of the LV demonstrated late enhancement in a subepicardial/midwall distribution. Similar to ARVD/C, some patients with LDAC have desmosomal gene mutations (see below).

DIFFERENTIAL DIAGNOSIS

Although the diagnosis in an overt case of ARVD/C is not difficult, early and occasionally late stages of the disease may show similarities with a few other diseases. In particular, differentiation from idiopathic VT originating from the RVOT can be challenging. However, idiopathic RVOT VT is a benign non-familial condition, in which the ECG shows no depolarization or repolarization abnormalities and no RV structural changes can be detected. Furthermore, VT episodes have a single morphology (LBBB morphology with inferior axis) and are usually not reproducibly inducible by premature extrastimuli at programmed stimulation during electrophysiologic studies.[69,70] Idiopathic RVOT VT may be inducible by regular burst pacing and isoproterenol infusion. It is important to differentiate idiopathic RVOT VT from ARVD/C for several reasons. The first is the known genetic etiology in ARVD/C. A genetic abnormality is not present in patients with idiopathic VT originating from the RVOT. Therefore, it has implications with regards to screening of family members. The prognosis of RVOT tachycardia is uniformly excellent with sudden death occurring rarely. Finally, in contrast to ARVD/C, catheter ablation is usually curative in idiopathic RVOT tachycardia.

Another disease mimicking ARVD/C is cardiac sarcoidosis. Sarcoidosis is a disease of unknown etiology, characterized by the presence of noncaseating granulomas in affected tissues, mainly lungs, but heart, skin, eyes, reticuloendothelial system, kidneys and central nervous system can also be affected. The prevalence of this condition varies in different geographical regions, and the disease may also be familial and occurs in specific racial subgroups.[71] Clinical symptoms of cardiac involvement are present in about 5% of all patients with sarcoidosis. The clinical manifestations of cardiac sarcoidosis depend upon the location and extent of granulomatous inflammation and include conduction abnormalities, ventricular arrhythmias, valvular dysfunction and congestive heart failure. Myocardial sarcoid granulomas or areas of myocardial scarring are typically present in the LV and septum of patients with this condition, and the RV can be predominantly affected. The VT associated with right ventricular abnormalities can, therefore, result in diagnostic confusion, especially if there is no systemic evidence of sarcoidosis. Patients can present with clinical features similar to those of ARVD/C including arrhythmias and sudden cardiac death.[72] Cardiac sarcoidosis can be diagnosed definitively by endomyocardial biopsy if granulomas are visualized.[73] To strengthen differentiation from ARVD/C, gadolinium-enhanced MRI may be beneficial by detecting located abnormalities in the septum, which is typical for sarcoidosis but seldom seen in ARVD/C. Active foci of sarcoidosis can be visualized by positron emission tomography (PET) scan. Therapy with corticosteroids is recommended for patients diagnosed with cardiac sarcoidosis. Treatment aims to control inflammation and fibrosis in order to maintain cardiac structure and function.

Myocarditis has to be excluded in patients suspected of ARVD/C. Myocarditis may arise from viral or other pathogens as well as toxic or immunologic insult. In general, endomyocardial biopsy is required to distinguish ARVD/C from myocarditis.

ARVD/C may mimic DCM, especially in the more advanced stages of disease. Patients with DCM usually present with heart failure or thromboembolic disease, including stroke. Since it is uncommon to have sustained VT or sudden death as the initial presenting symptom of DCM, patients with these symptoms should be first suspected of having ARVD/C.

MOLECULAR GENETIC ANALYSIS

It is important to realize that the clinical diagnosis of ARVD/C is based exclusively on fulfillment of the diagnostic Task Force criteria. Mutations underlying the disease show incomplete penetrance and variable clinical expression. Some genetically affected patients may have no signs or symptoms whatsoever, whereas no mutations can be identified in a large minority of clinically diagnosed patients. Therefore, genetic analyzes may not be of any critical diagnostic value for the index patient who meets Task Force criteria, but can be used to identify if family members are predisposed to disease development.

The strategy for genetic testing in ARVD/C is as follows:
Individuals with clinical diagnosis of ARVD/C are the first to be tested. The detection of a pathogenic mutation does not make a clinical diagnosis of ARVD/C. In contrast, if no mutation can be identified in a patient diagnosed with ARVD/C, the clinical diagnosis of ARVD/C is still applicable. If a pathogenic mutation is identified in the proband, parents, siblings and children of this patient can be tested for the mutation via the cascade method. When an (asymptomatic) relative is found to carry a pathogenic mutation, periodic cardiologic screening is required.

Table 1 shows the different genes related to ARVD/C. Currently, DNA analysis for *PKP2, DSG2, DSC2, DSP* and *JUP* is recommended in ARVD/C patients with an appropriate indication for this analysis.

PROGNOSIS AND THERAPY

The prognosis of classical ARVD/C is considerably better than that of patients with sustained VT from left ventricular structural heart disease. However, ARVD/C is a progressive disease and may lead to RV and also LV failure or sudden cardiac death. The death rate for patients with ARVD/C has been estimated at 2.5% per year.[74] Retrospective analysis of clinical and pathologic studies identified several risk factors for sudden death, such as previously aborted sudden death, syncope, young age, malignant family history, severe RV dysfunction and LV involvement.[75,76]

Electrophysiologic induction of VT with LBBB morphology and superior axis is a major diagnostic criterion.[58,64] However, electrophysiologic studies have not proven to be useful in risk stratifying patients with ARVD/C. This was illustrated in a multicenter study of 132 patients with ARVD/C in whom electrophysiologic study was performed prior to ICD implantation.[77] The positive and negative predictive values of VT inducibility for subsequent appropriate device therapy were 49% and 54% respectively.

In addition to symptomatic treatment, prevention of sudden death is the most important therapeutic goal in ARVD/C. Most data on effective treatment strategies refer to retrospective analyzes in single centers with only limited numbers of patients, and results are difficult to compare due to different patient selection and treatment strategies. There is limited data on long-term outcomes and no controlled randomized trials have been performed. International registries have been established, but have not yet reported results on treatment.

Evidence suggests that asymptomatic patients and healthy mutation carriers do not require prophylactic treatment. They should undergo regular cardiac evaluations including 12-lead ECG, 24-hours Holter monitoring, echocardiography and exercise testing for early identification of unfavorable signs. In patients diagnosed with or have signs or symptoms of ARVD/C as well as mutation carriers, specific life style advice is advisable. Sports participation has been shown to increase the risk of sudden death fivefold in ARVD/C patients.[78] Furthermore, excessive mechanical stress, such as during competitive sports activity and training, may aggravate the underlying myocardial abnormalities and accelerate disease progression. Therefore, patients with ARVD/C should be advised against practicing highly competitive and endurance sports, such as running marathons.

Therapeutic options in patients with ARVD/C include antiarrhythmic drugs, catheter ablation and ICD.

Patients with VT have a favorable outcome when they are treated medically and therefore pharmacologic treatment is the first choice. This concerns not only patients who have presented with sustained VT but also patients and family members with nonsustained VT or greater than 500 ventricular extrasystoles on 24-hours Holter monitoring. Since ventricular arrhythmias and cardiac arrest occur frequently during or after physical exercise or may be triggered by catecholamines, antiadrenergic β-blockers are recommended. Sotalol is the drug of first choice. Alternatively, other β-receptor blocking agents, amiodarone and flecainide have all been reported as useful.[79] Efficacy of drug treatment has to be evaluated by serial Holter monitoring and/or exercise testing. This strategy has proven to have better long-term outcome when compared to standard empirical treatment.[79]

Catheter ablation is an alternative in patients who are refractory to drug treatment and have frequent VT episodes with a predominantly single morphology. Marchlinski et al. performed VT ablation in 19 ARVD/C patients by the use of focal and/or linear lesions; in 17 no VT recurred during the subsequent 7±22 months.[80] In a series of 50 consecutive patients studied during 16 years, Fontaine et al. reported a 40% success rate by radiofrequency ablation after multiple ablation sessions, that increased to 81% when fulguration was used additionally.[81] However, these reports are from single centers with highly experienced electrophysiologists, and may not be reproducible in general practice. Catheter ablation is generally considered to be palliative and not curative. Long-term success rates are poor. Due to disease progression, new VTs with different morphologies will usually occur.[82]

Although antiarrhythmic drugs and catheter ablation may reduce VT burden, there is no proof from prospective trials that these therapies will also prevent sudden death. The ICD implantation is indicated in patients who are intolerant of antiarrhythmic drug therapy and who are at serious risk for sudden death. Implantation of an ICD has to be considered in ARVD/C patients with aborted cardiac arrest, intolerable fast VT and those with risk factors as mentioned above.

SUMMARY

Arrhythmogenic right ventricular dysplasia cardiomyopathy is most often a genetically determined disease characterized by fibrofatty replacement of myocardial tissue. Primarily affecting the RV, but extension to the LV occurs, especially in more advanced stages of the disease. At the molecular level, both ventricles are affected, presumably in all stages of the disease. Its prevalence has been estimated to vary from 1:2000 to 1:5000. Patients typically present between the second and the fourth decade of life with exercise induced tachycardia episodes originating from the RV. It is also a major cause of sudden death in the young and athletes.

The causative genes encode proteins of mechanical cell junctions (e.g. plakoglobin, plakophilin-2, desmoglein-2, desmocollin-2, desmoplakin) and account for intercalated disk remodeling. The classical form of ARVD/C is inherited in an autosomal dominant trait, but has variable expression. The rare recessively inherited variants are often associated with palmoplantar keratoderma and woolly hair. The diagnosis is made according to a set of Task Force criteria, based on family history, depolarization and repolarization abnormalities, ventricular arrhythmias with an LBBB morphology, functional and structural alterations of the RV, and fibrofatty replacement in endomyocardial biopsy. Two dimensional echocardiography, cineangiography and magnetic resonance are the imaging tools to visualize structural-functional abnormalities. The main differential diagnoses are idiopathic right ventricular outflow tract tachycardia, myocarditis and sarcoidosis. Palliative therapy consists of antiarrhythmic drugs, catheter ablation and implantable cardioverter defibrillator. Young age, family history of juvenile sudden death, overt left ventricular involvement, VT, syncope and previous cardiac arrest are the major risk factors for adverse prognosis.

REFERENCES

1. Marcus FI, Fontaine GH, Guiraudon G, et al. Right ventricular dysplasia: a report of 24 adult cases. Circulation. 1982;65:384-98.
2. Corrado D, Basso C, Thiene G, et al. Spectrum of clinicopathologic manifestations of arrhythmogenic right ventricular cardiomyopathy/dysplasia: a multicenter study. J Am Coll Cardiol. 1997;30:1512-20.
3. Basso C, Thiene G, Corrado D, et al. Arrhythmogenic right ventricular cardiomyopathy: dysplasia, dystrophy, or myocarditis? Circulation. 1996;94:983-91.
4. Thiene G, Nava A, Corrado D, et al. Right ventricular cardiomyopathy and sudden death in young people. N Engl J Med. 1988;318:129-33.
5. Richardson P, McKenna W, Bristow M, et al. Report of the 1995 World Health Organization/International Society and Federation of Cardiology Task Force on the Definition and Classification of cardiomyopathies. Circulation. 1996;93:841-2.
6. McKoy G, Protonotarios N, Crosby A, et al. Identification of a deletion in plakoglobin in arrhythmogenic right ventricular cardiomyopathy with palmoplantar keratoderma and woolly hair (Naxos disease). Lancet. 2000;355:2119-24.
7. Rampazzo A, Nava A, Miorin M, et al. ARVD4: a new locus for arrhythmogenic right ventricular cardiomyopathy, maps to chromosome 2 long arm. Genomics. 1997;45:259-63.
8. Ahmad F, Li D, Karibe A, et al. Localization of a gene responsible for arrhythmogenic right ventricular dysplasia to chromosome 3p23. Circulation. 1998;98:2791-5.
9. Li D, Ahmad F, Gardner MJ, et al. The locus of a novel gene responsible for arrhythmogenic right-ventricular dysplasia characterized by early onset and high penetrance maps to chromosome 10p12–p14. Am J Hum Genet. 2000;66:148-56.
10. Melberg A, Oldfors A, Blomstrom-Lundqvist C, et al. Autosomal dominant myofibrillar myopathy with arrhythmogenic right

ventricular cardiomyopathy linked to chromosome 10q. Ann Neurol. 1999;46:684-92.

11. Rampazzo A, Nava A, Danieli GA, et al. The gene for arrhythmogenic right ventricular cardiomyopathy maps to chromosome 14q23–q24. Hum Mol Genet. 1994;3:959-62.

12. Severini GM, Krajinovic M, Pinamonti B, et al. A new locus for arrhythmogenic right ventricular dysplasia on the long arm of chromosome 14. Genomics. 1996;31:193-200.

13. Tiso N, Stephan DA, Nava A, et al. Identification of mutations in the cardiac ryanodine receptor gene in families affected with arrhythmogenic right ventricular cardiomyopathy type 2 (ARVD2). Hum Mol Genet. 2001;10:189-94.

14. Beffagna G, Occhi G, Nava A, et al. Regulatory mutations in transforming growth factor-beta3 gene cause arrhythmogenic right ventricular cardiomyopathy type 1. Cardiovasc Res. 2005;65:366-73.

15. Rampazzo A, Nava A, Malacrida S, et al. Mutation in human desmoplakin domain binding to plakoglobin causes a dominant form of arrhythmogenic right ventricular cardiomyopathy. Am J Hum Genet. 2002;71:1200-6.

16. Gerull B, Heuser A, Wichter T, et al. Mutations in the desmosomal protein plakophilin-2 are common in arrhythmogenic right ventricular cardiomyopathy. Nat Genet. 2004;36:1162-4.

17. Pilichou K, Nava A, Basso C, et al. Mutations in desmoglein-2 gene are associated to arrhythmogenic right ventricular cardiomyopathy. Circulation. 2006;113:1171-9.

18. Syrris P, Ward D, Evans A, et al. Arrhythmogenic right ventricular dysplasia/cardiomyopathy associated with mutations in the desmosomal gene desmocollin-2. Am J Hum Genet. 2006;79:978-84.

19. Merner ND, Hodgkinson KA, Haywood AF, et al. Arrhythmogenic right ventricular cardiomyopathy type 5 is a fully penetrant, lethal arrhythmic disorder caused by a missense mutation in the TMEM43 gene. Am J Hum Genet. 2008;82:809-21.

20. Bernstein SA, Morley GE. Gap junctions and propagation of the cardiac action potential. Adv Cardiol. 2006;42:71-85.

21. Ellison KE, Friedman PL, Ganz LI, et al. Entrainment mapping and radiofrequency catheter ablation of ventricular tachycardia in right ventricular dysplasia. J Am Coll Cardiol. 1998;32:724-8.

22. Saffitz JE. Dependence of electrical coupling on mechanical coupling in cardiac myocytes: insights gained from cardiomyopathies caused by defects in cell-cell connections. Ann N Y Acad Sci. 2005;1047:336-44.

23. Kaplan SR, Gard JJ, Protonotarios N, et al. Remodeling of myocyte gap junctions in arrhythmogenic right ventricular cardiomyopathy due to a deletion in plakoglobin (Naxos disease). Heart Rhythm. 2004;1:3-11.

24. Kaplan SR, Gard JJ, Carvajal-Huerta L, et al. Structural and molecular pathology of the heart in Carvajal syndrome. Cardiovasc Pathol. 2004;13:26-32.

25. Ross SE, Hemati N, Longof KA, et al. Inhibition of adipogenesis by Wnt signaling. Science. 2000;289:950-3.

26. Garcia-Gras E, Lombardi R, Giocondo MJ, et al. Suppression of canonical Wnt/beta-catenin signaling by nuclear plakoglobin recapitulates phenotype of arrhythmogenic right ventricular cardiomyopathy. J Clin Invest. 2006;116:2012-21.

27. Protonotarios N, Tsatsopoulou A, Anastasakis A, et al. Genotype-phenotype assessment in autosomal recessive arrhythmogenic right ventricular cardiomyopathy (Naxos disease) caused by a deletion in plakoglobin. J Am Coll Cardiol. 2001;38:1477-84.

28. Alcalai R, Metzger S, Rosenheck S, et al. A recessive mutation in desmoplakin causes arrhythmogenic right ventricular dysplasia, skin disorder, and woolly hair. J Am Coll Cardiol. 2003;42:319-27.

29. Norgett EE, Hatsell SJ, Carvajal-Huerta L, et al. Recessive mutation in desmoplakin disrupts desmoplakin-intermediate filament interactions and causes dilated cardiomyopathy, woolly hair and keratoderma. Hum Mol Genet. 2000;9:2761-6.

30. Bauce B, Basso C, Rampazzo A, et al. Clinical profile of four families with arrhythmogenic right ventricular cardiomyopathy caused by dominant desmoplakin mutations. Eur Heart J. 2005;26:1666-75.

31. Sen-Chowdhry S, Syrris P, McKenna WJ. Desmoplakin disease in arrhythmogenic right ventricular cardiomyopathy: early genotype-phenotype studies. Eur Heart J. 2005;26:1582-4.

32. Syrris P, Ward D, Asimaki A, et al. Clinical expression of plakophilin-2 mutations in familial arrhythmogenic right ventricular cardiomyopathy. Circulation. 2006;113:356-64.

33. Dalal D, Molin LH, Piccini J, et al. Clinical features of arrhythmogenic right ventricular dysplasia/cardiomyopathy associated with mutations in plakophilin-2. Circulation. 2006;113:1641-9.

34. Van Tintelen JP, Entius MM, Bhuiyan ZA, et al. Plakophilin-2 mutations are the major determinant of familial arrhythmogenic right ventricular dysplasia/cardiomyopathy. Circulation. 2006;113:1650-8.

35. Hamid MS, Norman M, Quraishi A, et al. Prospective evaluation of relatives for familial arrhythmogenic right ventricular cardiomyopathy/dysplasia reveals a need to broaden diagnostic criteria. J Am Coll Cardiol. 2002;40:1445-50.

36. Syrris P, Ward D, Asimaki A, et al. Desmoglein-2 mutations in arrhythmogenic right ventricular cardiomyopathy: a genotype-phenotype characterization of familial disease. Eur Heart J. 2007;28:581-8.

37. Asimaki A, Syrris P, Wichter T, et al. A novel dominant mutation in plakoglobin causes arrhythmogenic right ventricular cardiomyopathy. Am J Hum Genet. 2007;81:964-73.

38. Rampazzo A, Beffagna G, Nava A, et al. Arrhythmogenic right ventricular cardiomyopathy type 1 (ARVD1): confirmation of locus assignment and mutation screening of four candidate genes. Eur Hum Genet. 2003;11:69-76.

39. Wehrens XH, Lehnart SE, Huang F, et al. FKBP12.6 deficiency and defective calcium release channel (ryanodine receptor) function linked to exercise-induced sudden cardiac death. Cell. 2003;113:829-40.

40. Bauce B, Nava A, Rampazzo A, et al. Familial effort polymorphic ventricular arrhythmias in arrhythmogenic right ventricular cardiomyopathy map to chromosome 1q42-43. Am J Cardiol. 2000;85:573-9.

41. Priori SG, Napolitano C, Memmi M, et al. Clinical and molecular characterization of patients with catecholaminergic polymorphic ventricular tachycardia. Circulation. 2002;106:69-74.

42. Tiso N, Salamon M, Bagattin A, et al. The binding of the RyR2 calcium channel to its gating protein FKBP12.6 is oppositely affected by ARVD2 and VTSIP mutations. Biochem Biophys Res Commun. 2002;299:594-8.

43. Gemayel C, Pelliccia A, Thompson PD. Arrhythmogenic right ventricular cardiomyopathy. J Am Coll Cardiol. 2001;38:1773-81.

44. Corrado D, Pelliccia A, Bjørnstad HH, et al. Cardiovascular pre-participation screening of young competitive athletes for prevention of sudden death: proposal for a common European protocol. Consensus Statement of the Study Group of Sport Cardiology of the Working Group of Cardiac Rehabilitation and Exercise Physiology and the Working Group of Myocardial and Pericardial Diseases of the European Society of Cardiology. Eur Heart J. 2005;26:516-24.

45. Basso C, Corrado D, Thiene G. Cardiovascular causes of sudden death in young individuals including athletes. Cardiol Rev. 1999;7:127-35.

46. Marcus FI, Zareba W, Calkins HG, et al. Arrhythmogenic right ventricular dysplasia/cardiomyopathy, clinical presentation and diagnostic evaluation: results from the North American multidisciplinary study. Heart Rhythm. 2009;6:984-92.

47. Asimaki A, Tandri H, Huang H, et al. A new diagnostic test for arrhythmogenic right ventricular cardiomyopathy. N Engl J Med. 2009;360:1075-84.

48. Corrado D, Basso C, Thiene G. Arrhythmogenic right ventricular cardiomyopathy: diagnosis, prognosis, and treatment. Heart. 2000;83:588-95.

49. McKenna WJ, Thiene G, Nava A, et al. Diagnosis of arrhythmogenic right ventricular dysplasia/cardiomyopathy. Task Force of the Working Group Myocardial and Pericardial Disease of the European Society of Cardiology and of the Scientific Council on Cardiomyopathies of the International Society and Federation of Cardiology. Br Heart J. 1994;71:215-8.

50. Marcus FI, McKenna WJ, Sherrill D, et al. Diagnosis of arrhythmogenic right ventricular cardiomyopathy/dysplasia: proposed modification of the task force criteria. Circulation. 2010;121:1533-41, Eur Heart J. 2010;31:801-14.

51. White JB, Razmi R, Nath H, et al. Relative utility of magnetic resonance imaging and right ventricular angiography to diagnose arrhythmogenic right ventricular cardiomyopathy. J Interv Card Electrophysiol. 2004;10:19-26.

52. Bluemke DA, Krupinski EA, Ovitt T, et al. MR Imaging of arrhythmogenic right ventricular cardiomyopathy: morphologic findings and interobserver reliability. Cardiology. 2003;99:153-62.

53. Tandri H, Calkins H, Nasir K, et al. Magnetic resonance imaging findings in patients meeting task force criteria for arrhythmogenic right ventricular dysplasia. J Cardiovasc Electrophysiol. 2003;14:476-82.

54. Basso C, Ronco F, Marcus F, et al. Quantitative assessment of endomyocardial biopsy in arrhythmogenic right ventricular cardiomyopathy/dysplasia: an in vitro validation of diagnostic criteria. Eur Heart J. 2008;29:2760-71.

55. Fontaine G, Umemura J, Di Donna P, et al. Duration of QRS complexes in arrhythmogenic right ventricular dysplasia. A new non-invasive diagnostic marker. Ann Cardiol Angeiol (Paris). 1993;42:399-405.

56. Peters S, Trümmel M. Diagnosis of arrhythmogenic right ventricular dysplasia-cardiomyopathy: value of standard ECG revisited. Ann Noninvasive Electrocardiol. 2003;8:238-45.

57. Pinamonti B, Sinagra G, Salvi A, et al. Left ventricular involvement in right ventricular dysplasia. Am Heart J. 1992;123:711-24.

58. Cox MG, Nelen MR, Wilde AA, et al. Activation delay and VT parameters in arrhythmogenic right ventricular dysplasia/cardiomyopathy: toward improvement of diagnostic ECG criteria. J Cardiovasc Electrophysiol. 2008;19:775-81.

59. Nasir K, Rutberg J, Tandri H, et al. Utility of SAECG in arrhythmogenic right ventricle dysplasia. Ann Noninvasive Electrocardiol. 2003;8:112-20.

60. Oselladore L, Nava A, Buja G, et al. Signal-averaged electro-cardiography in familial form of arrhythmogenic right ventricular cardiomyopathy. Am J Cardiol. 1995;75:1038-41.

61. Turrini P, Angelini A, Thiene G, et al. Late potentials and ventricular arrhythmias in arrhythmogenic right ventricular cardiomyopathy. Am J Cardiol. 1999;83:1214-9.

62. Nava A, Bauce B, Basso C, et al. Clinical profile and long-term follow-up of 37 families with arrhythmogenic right ventricular cardiomyopathy. J Am Coll Cardiol. 2000;36:2226-33.

63. Zareba W, Piotrowicz K, Turrini P. Electrocardiographic mani-festations. In: Marcus FI, Nava A, Thiene G (Eds). Arrhythmogenic Right Ventricular Dysplasia/Cardiomyopathy, Recent Advances. Milano: Springer Verlag;2007. pp. 121-8.

64. Cox MG, Van der Smagt JJ, Wilde AA, et al. New ECG criteria in arrhythmogenic right ventricular dysplasia/cardiomyopathy. Circ Arrhythm Electrophysiol. 2009;2:524-30.

65. Tandri H, Saranathan M, Rodriguez ER, et al. Noninvasive detection of myocardial fibrosis in arrhythmogenic right ventricular cardiomyopathy using delayed-enhancement magnetic resonance imaging. J Am Coll Cardiol. 2005;45:98-103.

66. Sen-Chowdhry S, Prasad SK, Syrris P, et al. Cardiovascular magnetic resonance in arrhythmogenic right ventricular cardiomyopathy revisited: comparison with task force criteria and genotype. J Am Coll Cardiol. 2006;48:2132-40.

67. Corrado D, Basso C, Thiene G, et al. Spectrum of clinicopathologic manifestations of arrhythmogenic right ventricular cardiomyopathy/dysplasia: a multicenter study. J Am Coll Cardiol. 1997;30:1512-20.

68. Sen-Chowdhry S, Syrris P, Prasad SK, et al. Left-dominant arrhythmogenic cardiomyopathy: an under-recognized clinical entity. J Am Coll Cardiol. 2008;52:2175-87.

69. Lerman BB, Stein KM, Markowitz SM. Idiopathic right ventricular outflow tract tachycardia: a clinical approach. PACE. 1996;19:2120-37.

70. Markowitz SM, Litvak BL, Ramirez de Arellano EA, et al. Adenosine-sensitive ventricular tachycardia, right ventricular abnormalities delineated by magnetic resonance imaging. Circulation. 1997;96:1192-200.

71. Thomas KW, Hunninghake GW. Sarcoidosis. JAMA. 2003;289:3300-3.

72. Chapelon C, Piette JC, Uzzan B, et al. The advantages of histological samples in sarcoidosis. Retrospective multicenter analysis of 618 biopsies performed on 416 patients. Rev Med Interne. 1987;8:181-5.

73. Ladyjanskaia GA, Basso C, Hobbelink MG, et al. Sarcoid myocarditis with ventricular tachycardia mimicking ARVD/C. J Cardiovasc Electrophysiol. 2010;21:94-8.

74. Fontaine G, Fontaliran F, Hebert J, et al. Arrhythmogenic right ventricular dysplasia. Annu Rev Med. 1999;50:17-35.

75. Hulot JS, Jouven X, Empana JP, et al. Natural history and risk stratification of arrhythmogenic right ventricular dysplasia/cardiomyopathy. Circulation. 2004;110:1879-84.

76. Peters S. Long-term follow-up and risk assessment of arrhythmogenic right ventricular dysplasia/cardiomyopathy: personal experience from different primary and tertiary centres. J Cardiovasc Med. 2007;8:521-6.

77. Corrado D, Leoni L, Link MS, et al. Implantable cardioverter-defibrillator therapy for prevention of sudden death in patients with arrhythmogenic right ventricular cardiomyopathy/dysplasia. Circulation. 2003;108:3084-91.

78. Corrado D, Basso C, Rizzoli G, et al. Does sports activity enhance the risk of sudden death in adolescents and young adults? J Am Coll Cardiol. 2003;42:1959-63.

79. Wichter T, Paul TM, Eckardt L, et al. Arrhythmogenic right ventricular cardiomyopathy. Antiarrhythmic drugs, catheter ablation, or ICD? Herz. 2005;30:91-101.

80. Marchlinski FE, Zado E, Dixit S, et al. Electroanatomic substrate and outcome of catheter ablative therapy for ventricular tachycardia in setting of right ventricular cardiomyopathy. Circulation. 2004;110:2293-8.

81. Fontaine G, Tonet J, Gallais Y, et al. Ventricular tachycardia catheter ablation in arrhythmogenic right ventricular dysplasia: a 16-year experience. Curr Cardiol Rep. 2000;2:498-506.

82. Dalal D, Jain R, Tandri H, et al. Long-term efficacy of catheter ablation of ventricular tachycardia in patients with arrhythmogenic right ventricular dysplasia/cardiomyopathy. J Am Coll Cardiol. 2007;50:432-40.

CHAPTER 37

Arrhythmogenic Right Ventricular Dysplasia/Cardiomyopathy

Long QT, Short QT, and Brugada Syndromes

Seyed Hashemi, Peter J Mohler

Chapter Outline

INTRODUCTION

Over the past two decades, ample information has been accumulated on cellular mechanisms and genetics of arrhythmias in structurally normal heart. The basic pathogenic mechanism for these arrhythmias may involve hereditary disturbances in ionic currents at the cellular level while the heart remains grossly normal. The high rate of sudden death (especially in the young) due to congenital arrhythmias, coupled with the potential availability of preventive measures, mandate the need for higher awareness of the medical community of these potentially lethal arrhythmia syndromes. In this chapter, we will review the current state of understanding of inherited arrhythmias including long QT (LQT) syndrome, short QT (SQT) syndrome and Brugada syndrome. This review focuses on inherited arrhythmias and will not cover acquired LQT syndrome.

LQT SYNDROME

Jervell and Lange-Nielsen, in 1957, firstly described the congenital LQT syndrome in a Norwegian family with four members suffering from prolonged QT, syncope and congenital deafness.[1] Three of the four affected patients died suddenly at the age of 4, 5 and 9 years.[1] Jervell and Lange-Nielsen syndrome, is inherited in an autosomal recessive pattern. Several years later, Romano et al. and Ward et al. independently described a similar syndrome but without deafness and with an autosomal dominant pattern of inheritance.[2,3] The underlying genes for LQT syndrome, however, were not discovered until more recently; in 1995 and 1996, the first

three genes associated with the most common forms of the LQT syndromes (types 1, 2 and 3) were identified.[4–6] Since then, the scientific and medical community has witnessed discovery of hundreds of variants in nearly a dozen genes associated with a wide variety of LQT or related arrhythmia syndromes.

CLINICAL MANIFESTATIONS

The congenital LQT syndrome is a common identifiable cause of sudden death in the presence of structurally normal heart.[7] The natural history of LQT syndrome is highly variable.[8–12] The majority of patients may be entirely asymptomatic with the only abnormality being QT prolongation in the ECG.[8–12] Some gene variant carriers of LQT syndromes may not even display the prolonged QT interval (silent carriers).[13,14] Symptomatic patients typically, present in the first two decades of life including the neonatal period, with recurrent attacks of syncope precipitated by *torsade de pointes* type of ventricular arrhythmias.[8,11] This form of tachycardia is characterized by cyclical changes in the amplitude and, polarity of QRS complexes such that their peak appears to be twisting around an imaginary isoelectric baseline. *Torsade de pointes* may resolve spontaneously, however, it has a great potential to degenerate into ventricular fibrillation and is an important cause of sudden death.[9]

PATHOGENESIS

As the QT interval represents a combination of action potential (AP) depolarization and repolarization, variations in QT

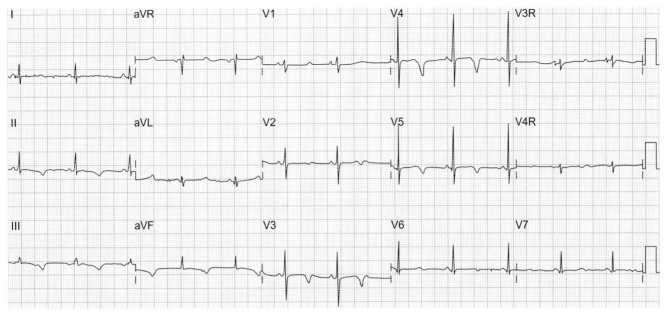

FIGURE 1: LQT1 ECG belongs to a 7-year-old boy with history of cardiac arrest during swimming. Note the prolonged QT with inverted, broad-based and T-wave pattern

interval may arise from the dysfunction of ion channel, responsible for the timely execution of the cardiac AP. A decrease in the outward repolarizing currents (mainly potassium currents) or an increase in the inward depolarizing currents (mainly sodium and calcium) may increase action potential duration (APD) and QT prolongation. The increases in APD result in lengthening of effective refractory period (ERP) that in turn predisposes to the occurrence of early after depolarizations (EADs), due to enhancement of the sodium-calcium exchanger (NCX) current and reactivation of the L-type calcium channels.[15–18] These EADs are known to support ventricular arrhythmias.[16–18]

MOLECULAR GENETICS

Over the last fifteen years, gain- or loss-of-function variants in nearly a dozen genes have been associated with development of LQTS. LQT1 is the most common form of the LQT syndrome and results from loss-of-function variants in *KCNQ1*, which encodes the alpha subunit of I_{Ks}, the cardiac slowly activating delayed-rectifier potassium channel current.[6] The mechanism(s) by which, each variant causes decreased I_{Ks} current varies among the gene variant carriers. Variant sub-units may co-assemble with the wild-type protein and render them defective causing more than 50% loss-of-function (i.e. dominant-negative effect).[19] Alternatively, the variants may result in haploinsufficiency with ~ 50% reduction in protein expression and the resultant current.[19] In addition to the biophysical function (dominant-negative vs haploinsufficiency), the location of variants appears to significantly influence the severity of phenotype. For example, Moss et al. demonstrated significantly higher cardiac event rates in patients with transmembrane variants in *KCNQ1* gene[19] (Fig. 1).

LQT2 results from loss-of-function variants in *KCNH2* (also known as *HERG*), which encodes the alpha-subunit of I_{Kr}, the rapidly activating delayed-rectifier potassium current in the heart.[5] The loss-of-function in the genes responsible for I_{Ks} and

IKr reduces the outward potassium current and prolongs APD, leading to QT prolongation in LQT1 and LQT2, respectively[5,6] (Fig. 2)

LQT3 arises from variants in *SCN5A* that encodes the alpha-subunit of $Na_V1.5$, the primary cardiac voltage-gated sodium-channel.[4] These variants disrupt fast inactivation of $Na_V1.5$ leading to excess late inward sodium current that in turn results in prolonged repolarization and APD.[4] The three most common LQTS, i.e. LQT 1-3, vary significantly in their natural history and clinical presentation, which will be discussed later in this chapter.

Unlike LQT1-3, LQT4 is not caused by an ion channel gene variant. LQT4 arises from variants in *ANK2*, which encodes ankyrin-B in cardiomyocytes.[20] The human *ANK2* gene was the first LQT syndrome gene that was discovered to encode a membrane associated protein (ankyrin-B) rather than an ion channel or channel subunit.[20] Ankyrin-B is an adaptor protein that interacts with several membrane-associated ion channels and transporters in ventricular myocytes including Na^+/K^+ ATPase, Na^+/Ca^{2+} exchanger-1 (NCX1) and IP3 receptors.[20] Dysfunction of Na/K ATPase and NCX1 are associated with a significant increase in $[Ca^{2+}]_i$ transient amplitude, SR calcium load and catecholamine-induced after depolarizations.[20] Abnormal intracellular calcium homeostasis is thought to be the central mechanisms underlying ventricular arrhythmias.[20] Symptomatic patients with specific *ANK2* variants may display significant QT prolongation (mean QTc: 490 ± 30 ms), ventricular tachycardia, syncope and sudden death.[21] However, many variant carriers do not display prolonged QTc, but display other ventricular phenotypes with risk of syncope and death. Additionally, *ANK2* variant carriers may manifest with sinus node dysfunction and/or atrial fibrillation in addition to ventricular arrhythmias and sudden death, hence, the name ankyrin-B syndrome.[20,21] Notably, ventricular phenotypes are often triggered by catecholamines, and thus, ankyrin-B syndrome may ultimately be more appropriately described as a

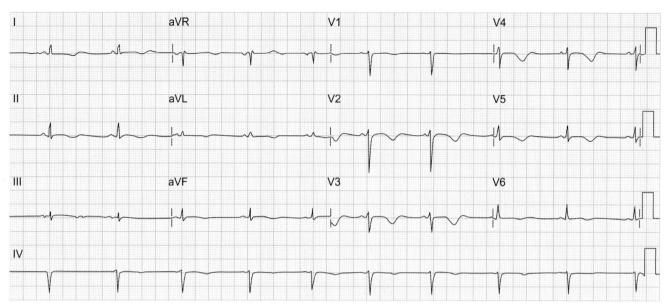

FIGURE 2: LQT2 ECG belongs to a 19-year-old female with history syncope and polymorphic ventricular tachycardia. ECG shows QT prolongation with low-amplitude inverted T-waves

class of catecholaminergic polymorphic ventricular tachycardia (CPVT).

LQT5 and LQT6 arise from loss-of-function variants in *KCNE1* and *KCNE2*, that encode the beta subunit of I_{Ks} and I_{Kr}, respectively (same currents in which the alpha subunit variants cause LQT1 and LQT2).[22–24] Akin to LQT1 and LQT2, these variants reduce outward potassium current leading to subsequent QT prolongation.[22–24]

LQT7 arises from loss-of-function variants in *KCNJ2* that encodes inward rectifying potassium channels (Kir2.1), responsible for I_{K1}.[25] I_{K1} represents the major ion conductance in the later stages of repolarization and during diastole, and reduced I_{K1} is associated with QT prolongation. Linkage studies on patients with LQT7 variants demonstrate a wide range of extra-cardiac findings associated with this form of LQTS.[25,26] These patients suffer from an autosomal dominant multisystem disease, also known as Andersen-Tawil syndrome, characterized by a combination of potassium-sensitive periodic paralysis, cardiac arrhythmia and distinctive facial or skeletal dysmorphic features such as low set ears and micrognathia.[25,26]

LQT8 is related to variants in *CACNA1c* that encodes the alpha-1C subunit of the voltage-gated calcium channel (CaV1.2) responsible for L-type calcium current ($I_{Ca,L}$) in myocytes.[27] These variants are associated with loss of voltage-dependent CaV1.2 inactivation, leading to Ca^{2+} overload and delayed repolarization due to prolonged inward, Ca^{2+} current during the plateau phase of the AP.[27] Similar to LQT7 syndrome, patients with LQT8 variants display a variety of extra-cardiac signs and symptoms (also termed Timothy syndrome) including syndactyly, abnormal teeth, immune deficiency, intermittent hypoglycemia, cognitive abnormalities, autism and baldness at birth[27] consistent with the critical role of $I_{Ca,L}$ in other tissues. Cardiac manifestations include patent foramen ovale (PFO) and septal defects, in addition to ventricular arrhythmias.[28] The condition is severe, with most affected patients dying in early childhood.[27,28]

LQT9 is associated with variants in *CaV3,* that encodes caveolin-3.[29] Caveolins are the principal proteins required for the assembly of caveolae, 50–100 nm membrane invaginations involved in the localization of membrane proteins including $Na_v1.5$ (LQT3 associated channel).[29,30] These variants interfere with the regulatory pathways between caveolin-3 and $Na_v1.5$, disrupting inactivation of $Na_v1.5$, resulting in a gain-of-function effect on late I_{Na}; the same pathological mechanism that underlies LQT3.[29]

LQT10 is linked to variants in *SCN4B*, which encodes $Na_v1.5$ one of four auxiliary subunits of $Na_v1.5$.[31] $Na_v\beta$ dysfunction is associated with a significant increase in late sodium current that affects the terminal repolarization phase of the AP, and prolongs the QT interval by a similar mechanism as LQT3-associated variants in the alpha subunit of $Na_v1.5$.[31]

LQT11 is associated with variants in *AKAP9.* that encodes A-kinase anchoring protein (AKAP), also known as yotiao, involved in the subcellular targeting of protein kinase A (PKA).[32] Yotiao is a PKA targeting protein for multiple cardiac ion channel complexes including the ryanodine receptor, the L-type calcium channel, and the slowly activating delayed rectifier I_{Ks} potassium channel (*KCNQ1*).[32,33] Variants in the *AKAP9* are associated with disruption of the interaction between *KCNQ1* and yotiao, reducing the cAMP-induced phosphorylation of the channel, that in turn eliminates the functional response of the I_{Ks} channel to cAMP, prolongs the APD and QT interval.[32,33] LQT12 is associated with variants in *SNTA1*, which encodes for ?-1syntrophin, a scaffolding protein with multiple molecular interactions including $Na_v1.5$, plasma membrane Ca^{2+}-ATPase (PMCA4b) and neuronal nitric oxide synthase (nNOS).[34] The variants in *SNTA1* are associated with increased direct nitrosylation of $Na_v1.5$ and increased late I_{Na}.[34] Akin to the mechanism in LQT3 syndrome, the increase in late sodium current causes prolonged QT interval.

GENOTYPE-PHENOTYPE CORRELATION STUDIES AND RISK STRATIFICATION STRATEGIES

The pattern of inheritance of LQTS varies depending on the type of the syndrome. Most LQTS are inherited as autosomal dominant Romano-Ward syndrome. LQT syndrome types 1 and 5 (representing variants in alpha and beta subunit of I_{Ks}) are inherited as either autosomal recessive Jervell and Lange-Nielsen or autosomal dominant Romano-Ward syndrome.[35] Additionally, a host of factors may influence disease severity. Recently, the genotype-phenotype correlation studies on the most common forms of LQTS (type 1-3) have allowed for more in-depth understanding of natural history of each variant. For example, Priori et al. prospectively studied a large data base of unselected, consecutively, genotyped patients with LQTS (n = 647) and developed a risk stratification scheme based on gender, genotype and QTc interval after a mean observation period of 28 years.[13] The authors showed that different genotypes may manifest differently in males versus females. For example, the incidence of a first cardiac arrest or sudden death was greater among LQT2 females than LQT2 males and LQT3 males than LQT3 females.[13]

The duration of QT interval may be influenced by the genetic locus, and may also predict the likelihood of future cardiac events (defined as syncope, cardiac arrest or sudden death). In the Priori study, mean QTc was 466 ± 44 msec in LQT1, 490 ± 49 msec in LQT2 and 496 ± 49 msec in LQT3.[13] Event free survival was higher in LQT1 than LQT2 and LQT3.[13] Within each LQTS category, QTc of patients with cardiac events was significantly, longer than asymptomatic patients.[13] Amongst LQT1 patients, mean QTc was 488 ± 47 msec in those with cardiac events versus 459 ± 40 msec in asymptomatic subjects.[13] These data suggest that LQTS may have a normal or near normal QTc and sustain a cardiac event (albeit at a very low rate) and vice versa. However, irrespective of the genotype, the risk of becoming symptomatic was associated with QTc duration; a QTc of 500 msec or more was the most significant predictor of potential cardiac events.[13]

Notably, the percentage of silent variant carriers (those with gene variants but normal QT interval) was higher in the LQT1 (36%) than LQT2 (19%) or LQT3 (10%).[13] Higher percentage of silent carriers in LQT1 may at least partly explain the lower rate of cardiac events in patients with LQT1 compared to LQT2 and LQT3.[14,36-38] The fact that silent variant carriers may have normal QT interval, yet to be at increased risk of cardiac events indicates that LQTS cannot be excluded solely based on ECG findings. Furthermore, the silent carrier state may confer susceptibility of drug-induced QT prolongation and Torsade de pointes arrhythmias.[36,38,39]

Triggers of cardiac events in LQT syndrome have been shown to be largely gene specific. Schwartz et al. studied specific triggers of cardiac events in 670 LQTS patients (types 1, 2 and 3) with known genotype.[40] In LQT1, nearly 80% of cardiac events occurred during physical or emotional stress, whereas LQT3 patients experience 40% of their events at rest or during sleep and only 13% during exercise.[40] In LQT2 patients, the events occurred during emotional stress in 43% of patients. For lethal cardiac events (cardiac arrest and sudden death), the difference among the groups were more dramatic. In LQT1, 68% of lethal events occurred during exercise, whereas this rarely occurred for LQT2 and occurred in only 4% of cases for LQT3.[40] In contrast, 49% and 64% of lethal events occurred during rest/sleep without arousal for LQT2 and LQT3 patients, respectively, whereas this occurred

Criteria	Point
ECG criteria	
QTc	
> 480	3
460–479	2
450–459	1
Torsade de pointes	2
T-wave alternans	1
Notched T-wave in 3 leads	1
Low heart rate for age	0.5
Clinical history	
Syncope with stress	2
Syncope without stress	1
Congenital deafness	1
Family history	
Definite LQT syndrome in family	1
Unexplained SCD < 30 y/o in immediate family	0.5
Scoring	
≤ 1 point = low probability for LQTS	
2–3 points = intermediate probability for LQTS	
≥ 3.5 points = high probability for LQTS	

in only 9% of cases for LQT1 patients.[40] Auditory stimuli particularly clustered among LQT2 patients, whereas swimming as a trigger was more frequent in LQT1 patients.[40] A stunning percentage of patients who experienced their cardiac events during swimming were LQT1.[40]

The T-wave repolarization pattern varies according to genotype. Patients with LQT1 variant positive genotype display a distinct, inverted, broad-based, prolonged T-wave pattern that is different from the low-amplitude and sometimes, notched T-wave observed in LQT2 patients.[41] Both of these repolarization patterns are different from late-appearing T-wave seen in LQT3 patients.[41] Patients with LQT4 genotype display a characteristic notched, biphasic T-wave morphology in ECG.[21]

DIAGNOSIS

The typical case of LQTS, characterized by syncope or cardiac arrest associated with QT prolongation on ECG is fairly straightforward to diagnose. However, borderline cases may be more complex and pose a diagnostic challenge to the practicing clinician. Schwartz and his colleagues devised a diagnostic criteria based on a scoring system first in 1985 and then, updated in 1993.[37,42] Based on this scoring system, a score of one or less indicates low probability for LQTS; 2-3 denotes intermediate probability and higher than 3.5 indicates high probability for LQTS. If a patient receives a score of 2-3, serial ECG and 24-h Holter monitoring may be obtained as the QT interval may vary from time to time.[38] Short-term variability of QT interval has recently been demonstrated to correlate with high risk LQT syndrome.[43]

GENETIC TESTING

The diagnostic criteria based on ECG and clinical history were primarily devised before the human genome project era and therefore, may not always account for many new advances in molecular genetics. As mentioned earlier, individuals may harbor disease-associated variants and yet have normal ECG parameters and QT interval (silent carriers). In select cases, genetic testing and molecular diagnostic methods may complement the ECG and clinical criteria; allowing for screening of proband family members to detect silent variant carriers that may predispose individuals to potential events.[36,39,44,45] For example, HERG inhibition is commonly the mechanism associated with drug-induced QT prolongation, and variants in other ion channel/ion channel modulator genes may also predispose individuals to QT prolongation and ventricular arrhythmias.[36,45,46] Therefore, identifying gene variants that promote arrhythmia susceptibility (either congenital or acquired) may provide important information to a physician in their clinical practice (i.e. avoiding QT prolonging drugs in patients harboring specific channel variants). It is important to note that current genetic testing for arrhythmias may harbor its own drawbacks. For example, false negative results may occur when the patient has a variant in a gene not covered in the testing panel (the relevant gene or gene variant may not have even been discovered!). Moreover, the significance of a positive test result may often be difficult to ascertain. As reviewed by others, it will be critical to continue to define genotype-phenotype relationships to provide additional new data that can be carefully considered when utilizing patient genotype to predict and/or manage clinical phenotypes.

THERAPY

As the risk of cardiac events in LQTS is genotype, age and gender dependent, therapy should be carefully tailored to the individual patients according to their risk factors. According to a recently published study from the International LQTS Registry, beta blocker therapy, significantly, reduces the risk of cardiac events in LQT1 and LQT2 patients.[47] This is not surprising as the most common triggers of cardiac events in LQT1 and LQT2 patients are exercise and emotional stress, respectively.[40] Furthermore, LQT1 patients harbor I_{Ks} dysfunction, which has been shown to activate in higher heart rates and is necessary for QT interval shortening with tachycardia.[6] In contrast, beta blockers may offer limited efficacy among LQT3 patients; as they display further QT prolongation at slower heart rates.[48] Moreover, according to the International LQT Registry data, beta blocker therapy reduces the risk to similar extent in LQT1 and LQT2 patients (67% and 71% risk reduction, respectively).[47] Different beta blockers displayed differential effects in each category of LQTS. Atenolol, but not nadolol, reduced the risk significantly in LQT1 patients, whereas nadolol, but not atenolol was associated with a significant risk reduction in LQT2 patients.[47] Higher risk patients, such as LQT1 males and LQT2 females gained more benefit from beta blocker therapy compared to lower risk subsets. Despite the significant risk reduction with beta blocker therapy, high risk patients experienced considerable residual event rates during beta blocker therapy.[47] History of syncope during beta blocker therapy was associated with higher event rates.[47] LQT2 genotype was associated with significantly higher residual event rates while taking beta blockers compared to LQT1.[47,49]

ICD THERAPY

Insofar, as high risk patients with LQT syndrome continue to have a residual event rate while receiving beta blocker therapy, there may be a need for additional protection against potentially fatal arrhythmias. Current guidelines recommend ICD therapy as a class IIa indication for primary prevention of cardiac events in LQTS patients who experience syncope or ventricular tachycardias during beta blocker therapy.[50] These guidelines provide a class IIb recommendation for ICD therapy in patients with risk factors for SCD, irrespective of medical therapy.[50]

LEFT CARDIAC SYMPATHETIC DENERVATION

Left cardiac sympathetic denervation (LCSD) was introduced in 1971 as the first therapy for LQT syndrome.[51] The contemporary LCSD techniques use extrapleural approach and obviate the need for thoracotomy.[52] A recent study of 147 very high-risk LQTS patients, who underwent LCSD over a span of 35 years (average follow-up period of 8 years) demonstrated that LCSD reduced the number of cardiac events by 91% per patient per year.[52] According to the result from this study, LCSD may be considered in patients with recurrent syncope despite beta-blockade, and in patients, who experience arrhythmia storms with ICD therapy.[52]

GENOTYPE-SPECIFIC THERAPY

As cardiac events may be clustered around exercise or emotional stress in LQT1 patients, these individuals may be advised to avoid competitive sports and/or stressful situations. For example, swimming has previously been particularly discouraged in LQT1 patients. Beta blockers remain the mainstay of therapy in LQT1 syndrome.

In patients with LQT2, maintaining adequate serum potassium level is essential, as I_{Kr} activity may vary with serum potassium levels.[53] Therefore, use of potassium supplements in combination with potassium sparing diuretics may be recommended in LQT2 patients.[53] Since arousal from sleep, especially with a sudden noise may be a triggering a risk factor in LQT2 patients, the use of alarm clock or telephone in the patient's bedroom should also be carefully considered.[40]

Sodium channel blockers have been proposed for gene-specific treatments in LQT3, which is associated with variants in the sodium channel gene (*SCN5A*).[48] Early clinical studies demonstrated efficacy of mexiletine or flecainide in shortening of repolarization period and QT interval.[48] Indeed, ACC/AHA 2006 guidelines for management of patients with ventricular arrhythmias and the prevention of sudden cardiac death recommended sodium channel blockers for treatment of LQT3 patients as a class IIb indication.[54] However, more recently, Ruan et al. in an elegant study, provided *in vitro* cellular evidence that different *SCN5A* variants may display heterogeneous biophysical properties; and the use of sodium channel blockers may be deleterious in selected group of LQT3 patients.[55] The study was prompted by the death of a young child affected by an *SCN5A* variant whose QT interval not only shorten, but also prolonged in response to mexiletine treatment.

SQT SYNDROME

SQT syndrome is a rare channelopathy associated with increased risk of atrial and ventricular arrhythmias. The association of SQT interval with sudden cardiac death was first described near two decades ago by Algra and his colleagues.[56] They reported a two-fold risk of sudden death in patients with a QTc less than 400 milliseconds, as compared with patients with a QTc between 400 and 440 milliseconds.[56] In the year 2000, Gussak et al. reported the first familial cases of idiopathic SQT syndrome associated with paroxysmal atrial fibrillation. A few years later, Gaita et al. described additional cases of SQT syndrome associated with sudden cardiac death.[57] To date, the number of identified patients with SQT syndrome is low.[58,59] However, with increasing awareness of medical community of the relationship of SQT with AF and sudden cardiac death, the prevalence is expected to rise.

CLINICAL MANIFESTATIONS

The clinical manifestations of SQT syndrome include propensity to AF, syncope and sudden death.[57,60,61] In most reported cases, the QTc was less than 320 ms and often less than 340 ms.[62,63] Therefore, it is prudent to suspect SQT syndrome in patients with a QT interval of less than 340 ms and personal and/or family history of lone AF, ventricular fibrillation, syncope or sudden cardiac death. To date, there is no gender predilection for SQT syndrome.[63] Age at onset of symptoms vary widely with reported cases from one year old (sudden infant death syndrome) to age 80 year old.[63] One study reported the mean age at diagnosis of 30 years.[63] Cardiac arrest has been reported to occur both at rest and under stress.[63,64]

MOLECULAR GENETICS

To date, three genes with an association with SQT syndrome have been identified. All three genes encode potassium channel proteins. SQT1 is associated with variants in *KCNH2* (also LQT2 gene), that result in increases in I_{Kr}.[60] SQT2 is associated with variants in *KCNQ1* (also LQT1 gene) that result in increased I_{Ks}.[65] SQT3 is associated with variants in *KCNJ2* (also LQT7 gene) that encodes the inwardly rectifying potassium channel protein, Kir2.1.[66] Gain-of-function variants in *KCNJ2* may result in increased outward I_{K1} current and SQT syndrome type 3.[66]

PATHOGENESIS

Gain-of-function variants in specific cardiac potassium channels may cause acceleration of repolarization and abbreviation of APD leading to shortening of ERP.[60,61,65,66] Shortened refractory period is a well established substrate for re-entrant tachycardias; hence, predisposition to atrial fibrillation and ventricular tachycardias in patients with SQT syndrome.[67] A second proposed mechanism for predisposition to re-entrant arrhythmias in SQT syndrome is the increases in transmural dispersion of repolarization. The ECG of affected individuals has distinctive features including tall, peaked, symmetrical T-waves with prolonged T_{peak}-T_{end}.[68] Prolonged T_{peak}-T_{end} has been proposed to be indicative of augmented transmural dispersion of repolarization.[68] Exaggerated transmural heterogeneity during repolarization forms the substrate for the development of re-entrant arrhythmias.[68] Extramiana and colleagues demonstrated that QT-interval abbreviation in the absence of transmural dispersion of repolarization was not sufficient to induce

ventricular arrhythmias.[68] Therefore, the combination of short refractory periods and increased dispersion of refractoriness may result in patients with SQT syndrome vulnerable to arrhythmias.

DIAGNOSIS

The precise cut-off point for QT interval in SQT syndrome is still somewhat debated. Currently, based on several reports, the upper limit of QT interval suggestive of SQT syndrome is considered 320–340 ms.[62,63] However, the mere presence of SQT interval does not necessarily appear to be sufficient to make the diagnosis. Anttonen et al. screened a population of over 1000 healthy volunteers for SQT interval and followed them up for a mean of 29 years.[69] The prevalence of QTc interval less than 320 ms (very short) and less than 340 ms (short) was 0.10% and 0.4%, respectively.[69] All cause or cardiovascular mortality did not differ between subjects with a very short or SQT interval and those with normal QT intervals (360–450 ms).[69] There were no sudden cardiac deaths, aborted sudden cardiac deaths, or documented ventricular tachyarrhythmias among subjects with SQT interval.[69]

In addition to shortened QT interval, patients with SQT syndrome may display a peculiar ECG morphology.[62,70,71] Affected patients often demonstrate absent ST segment with the T-wave attached to the S-wave.[71,72] A second finding, that is seen in at least about half of the patients, is a tall, peaked, narrow-based T-waves in the right precordial leads.[69,70,72] Another distinctive ECG feature of patients with SQT syndrome is the relatively prolonged T_{peak}-T_{end} interval which may indicate enhanced transmural dispersion of repolarization.[68] Electrophysiological studies have been reported in a limited number of patients with SQT syndrome. Both atrial and ventricular ERP were reported to be shortened.[61,63,73] Furthermore, ventricular tachycardias were inducible in nearly all patients.[61,63,73]

As part of the diagnostic evaluation of SQT syndrome, acquired causes of QT interval shortening are often excluded. Electrolyte/acid-base abnormalities, such as hyperkalemia, hypercalcemia and acidosis, are well known to shorten QT interval. Other causes include hyperthermia and QT shortening medications such as digoxin and mexiletine. Finally, QT measurements are commonly made at heart rates less than 80 beat/min, as the QT interval in SQT syndrome patients may fail to adapt to increase heart rates.

THERAPY

The paucity of SQT syndrome cases may limit the opportunity to systematically study treatment of this recently recognized arrhythmia syndrome. Nonetheless, drugs that block outward potassium current and prolong repolarization seem attractive and have been tested in a limited number of cases. The class Ia anti-arrhythmic agents, quinidine and disopyramide have been demonstrated to prolong QT interval and ventricular ERP and reduce inducibility of ventricular arrhythmias.[63,74–76]

The high incidence of fatal cardiac events associated with SQT suggests the use of ICD therapy, early on, in the management of the symptomatic patients.[62] In asymptomatic patients, however, the indications for ICD may be less clear. Patients with SQT interval and implanted ICD may be at increased risk for inappropriate therapy due to oversensing as a result of the detection of short-coupled and prominent T-waves.[77] Reprogramming of the ICD with adaptation of sensing levels and decay delays without sacrificing correct arrhythmia detection may be helpful in these patients.[77]

BRUGADA SYNDROME

In 1992, Brugada and Brugada described a hereditary arrhythmia syndrome characterized by ST segment elevation in the right precordial leads, right bundle branch block and increased vulnerability to ventricular tachycardias and sudden death in the absence of any structural heart disease.[78] Although the Brugada brothers are the first to formally describe and characterize the syndrome, the history of the syndrome dates back to several decades prior. A similar syndrome manifested as sudden death during sleep frequently after a heavy meal, most often affecting young men, has long been noted in the south Asian culture. The terms sudden unexplained nocturnal deaths (SUND) or sudden unexplained death in sleep (SUDS) are used to explain this folk illness with various local names including *Bangungot* (in Philippines), *Pokkuri* (in Japan) or *Lai Tai* (in Thailand). Although Brugada syndrome seems to be endemic in south-east Asian countries, cohorts of the syndrome have been reported across the world.[79] Currently, Brugada syndrome is considered as a major cause of sudden cardiac death in the young. Timely identification of symptomatic Brugada syndrome patients is important, as implantable cardioverter defibrillators (ICD) may be life-saving in these individuals.

CLINICAL MANIFESTATIONS

Brugada syndrome is characterized by the occurrence of polymorphic ventricular tachycardias in patients with the ECG patterns of a peculiar ST-segment elevation in right precordial leads and **right bundle branch block** (RBBB).[78] An increased propensity to atrial fibrillation and supraventricular arrhythmias has also been reported.[80] Patients with Brugada syndrome have structurally normal hearts; and are typically, otherwise healthy and active.[80] Notwithstanding, recent research suggests that with the use of high resolution magnetic resonance imaging, subclinical structural abnormalities in right ventricle may be identified.[81] Many patients with the syndrome may have the characteristic ECG findings; however, remain asymptomatic until the first arrhythmic episode that may lead to syncope or sudden death. On the other hand, the symptomatic patients with positive ECG findings may transiently display normal ECG which makes the diagnosis more challenging.

GENETICS

Brugada syndrome is a familial arrhythmia syndrome with autosomal dominant pattern of inheritance, incomplete and gender-dependent penetrance. The mean age of clinical manifestations is 40 years with a wide range from infancy to the eighth decade of life.[82,83] Men are affected much more commonly than women with a male to female ratio of 3/1.[82,83] The true prevalence of the disease is unknown. A great deal of work has been published during the last two decades, since the Brugada brothers' authored the initial report.

In 1998, Chen et al. identified the first loss-of-function gene variant related to the Brugada syndrome on *SCN5A,* that encodes cardiac voltage gated sodium channels.[84] Since then, over 100 associated variants have been reported in the literature with 15–30% of them located on *SCN5A* gene.[85,86] Another 11–12% have been attributed to *CACNA1C* and *CACNB2.*[85] Variants in other genes (*GPD1L, SCN1B, KCNE3* and *SCN3B*) likely contribute to the Brugada phenotype, although to a lesser extent.[85] Notably, all the genes discovered to date explain only one-third of Brugada syndrome cases, indicating that there is, still an important amount of work to be done to unravel the genetic basis of this lethal disease.

PATHOGENESIS

In 2001, Antzelevitch et al. proposed the dispersion of repolarization model, which hypothesizes a pathophysiological mechanism of re-entrant arrhythmias in Brugada syndrome.[87] This model is based on the demonstration that the density and kinetics of currents underlying phase-1 of AP (Ito), exhibit transmural dispersal.[88] The Ito current density is more profound in epicardium compared to endocardium.[88] In Brugada syndrome, the impaired sodium influx in epicardial cells is subject to exaggerated Ito defect leading to accentuated AP morphology variability between epicardial cells and endocardial cells. The arrhythmic substrate is, therefore, the result of increased transmural heterogeneity of the currents involved in the phase-I depolarization of the ventricle, enabling local re-excitation via re-entry.[87,89]

DIAGNOSIS

Electrocardiographic signs of Brugada syndrome are classified into three types as follows:[80]
- Type I: Coved ST-segment elevation greater than 2 mm followed by negative T-wave in greater than 1 mm right precordial lead (V1–V3)
- Type 2: Saddleback ST-segment elevation with a high takeoff ST-segment elevation of greater than 2 mm, a trough displaying greater than 1 mm ST-elevation followed by a positive or biphasic T-wave
- Type 3: Saddleback or coved appearance of ST-elevation less than 1 mm, present in greater than 1 mm right precordial lead (V1–V3)

Type 2 ST-segment elevation is less specific and more common in general healthy population.[80] Type 1 (coved type) ST-segment elevation is more specific and more predictive of future arrhythmic events, and is considered the diagnostic ECG abnormality for Brugada syndrome.[80] The coved type ST-elevation is less sensitive owing to its dynamic nature. In up to 50% of patients with coved ST-segment elevation, the ECG may normalize or the ST-segment elevation may convert from the coved type to the saddle type periodically.[80] However, the coved-type ECG pattern, can be unmasked by administration of sodium channel blockers, ajmaline, flecainide or procainamide in the electrophysiology laboratory.[90] Additionally, vagotonic agents and fever are known to bring about the ECG signs when concealed.[91,92]

Brugada syndrome is diagnosed on the basis of a spontaneous or drug-induced type 1 (coved-type), ST-segment elevation in the right precordial leads plus one of the following conditions:[80]

- Documented VF or polymorphic VT
- Unexplained syncope
- Nocturnal agonal respiration
- Inducibility of VT/VF with programmed electrical stimulation
- A family history of SCD at a young age (< 45 years) or a coved-type ECG pattern.

The differential diagnosis of syncope and the ECG abnormalities is broad and the following conditions may be considered and ruled out: atypical right bundle branch block, left ventricular hypertrophy, early repolarization, acute pericarditis, acute myocardial ischemia or infarction, pulmonary embolism, Printzmetal angina, dissecting aortic aneurysm, central or peripheral nervous system abnormalities, Duchenne muscular dystrophy, thiamine deficiency, hyperkalemia, hypercalcemia, arrhythmogenic right ventricular cardiomyopathy, pectus excavatum, hypothermia, or mechanical compression of the right outflow tract (RVOT) as seen with mediastinal tumors or hemopericardium.[80]

PROGNOSIS, RISK STRATIFICATION AND THERAPY

Patients displaying the Brugada syndrome, ECG pattern were initially thought to carry a high risk of cardiac events. The second consensus conference report on Brugada syndrome recommended electrophysiology studies (EPS) as a valuable tool in risk stratifying asymptomatic patients with spontaneous type 1 ECG pattern or with drug induced type 1 ECG pattern plus positive family history of SCD.[80] Subsequent studies, however, have questioned the role of EPS in risk stratification of asymptomatic patients.[93] The role inducibility of ventricular arrhythmias by EPS remains debatable. Recently, the investigators of the FINGER Brugada syndrome registry addressed the long-term prognosis of Brugada syndrome and the role of EPS in risk stratifying asymptomatic patients.[93] In the largest cohort of symptomatic and asymptomatic patients with Brugada syndrome to date, following a 32-month follow-up period of the cohort, they demonstrated the following results:[93]

- The risk of arrhythmic events is low in asymptomatic patients (0.5% event rate per year)
- The presence of symptoms and a spontaneous type 1 ECG are the only independent predictors of arrhythmic events
- Genders, family history of SCD, inducibility of ventricular tachyarrhythmias during EPS and presence of a variant in the *SCN5A* gene, have no predictive value.

In view of these results, the risk stratification strategy proposed in the second consensus report may be revised to reflect the decreased value of EPS as a predictor of future cardiac events. Recommendations to implant ICD at the present time may be limited to symptomatic patients with type 1 ECG pattern. To date, no pharmacologic intervention has been approved for the treatment of Brugada syndrome. However, active research is underway to define potential pharmacologic options to treat this potentially lethal arrhythmia syndrome.[94–96]

ACKNOWLEDGMENTS

The authors thank Drs Ian Law and Nicholas Von Bergen of the University of Iowa Carver College of Medicine for LQT1 and LQT2 ECGs.

REFERENCES

1. Jervell, A, Lange-Nielsen F. Congenital deaf-mutism, functional heart disease with prolongation of the Q-T interval and sudden death. Am Heart J. 1957;54:59-68.
2. Romano C, Gemme G, Pongiglione R. Rare cardiac arrythmias of the pediatric age. II. Syncopal attacks due to paroxysmal ventricular fibrillation (presentation of 1st case in Italian pediatric literature). Clin Pediatr (Bologna). 1963;45:656-83.
3. Ward OC. A new familial cardiac syndrome in children. J Ir Med Assoc. 1964;54:103-6.
4. Wang Q, et al. SCN5A mutations associated with an inherited cardiac arrhythmia, long QT syndrome. Cell. 1995;80:805-11.
5. Curran ME, et al. A molecular basis for cardiac arrhythmia: HERG mutations cause long QT syndrome. Cell. 1995;80:795-803.
6. Wang Q, et al. Positional cloning of a novel potassium channel gene: KVLQT1 mutations cause cardiac arrhythmias. Nat Genet. 1996;12:17-23.
7. Tester DJ, Ackerman MJ. Postmortem long QT syndrome genetic testing for sudden unexplained death in the young. J Am Coll Cardiol. 2007;49:240-6.
8. Schwartz PJ, Periti M, Malliani A. The long Q-T syndrome. Am Heart J. 1975;89:378-90.
9. Moss AJ, Schwartz PJ. Sudden death and the idiopathic long Q-T syndrome. Am J Med. 1979;66:6-7.
10. Moss AJ, Schwartz PJ. Delayed repolarization (QT or QTU prolongation) and malignant ventricular arrhythmias. Mod Concepts Cardiovasc Dis. 1982;51:85-90.
11. Moss AJ, et al. The long QT syndrome: a prospective international study. Circulation. 1985;71:17-21.
12. Moss AJ, et al., The long QT syndrome. Prospective longitudinal study of 328 families. Circulation. 1991;84:1136-44.
13. Priori SG, et al. Risk stratification in the long-QT syndrome. N Engl J Med. 2003;348:1866-74.
14. Mohler PJ, et al. A cardiac arrhythmia syndrome caused by loss of ankyrin-B function. Proc Natl Acad Sci USA. 2004;101:9137-42.
15. Viswanathan PC, Rudy Y. Pause induced early afterdepolarizations in the long QT syndrome: a simulation study. Cardiovasc Res. 1999;42:530-42.
16. Szabo B, et al. Role of Na$^+$:Ca^{2+} exchange current in Cs(+)-induced early afterdepolarizations in Purkinje fibers. J Cardiovasc Electrophysiol. 1994;5:933-44.
17. Keating MT, Sanguinetti MC. Molecular and cellular mechanisms of cardiac arrhythmias. Cell. 2001;104:569-80.
18. Marban E, Robinson SW, Wier WG. Mechanisms of arrhythmogenic delayed and early afterdepolarizations in ferret ventricular muscle. J Clin Invest. 1986;78:1185-92.
19. Moss AJ, et al. Clinical aspects of type-1 long-QT syndrome by location, coding type, and biophysical function of mutations involving the KCNQ1 gene. Circulation. 2007;115:2481-9.
20. Mohler PJ, et al. Ankyrin-B mutation causes type 4 long-QT cardiac arrhythmia and sudden cardiac death. Nature. 2003;421:634-9.
21. Schott JJ, et al. Mapping of a gene for long QT syndrome to chromosome 4q25-27. Am J Hum Genet. 1995;57:1114-22.
22. Schulze-Bahr E, et al. KCNE1 mutations cause jervell and Lange-Nielsen syndrome. Nat Genet. 1997;17:267-8.
23. Splawski I, et al. Mutations in the hminK gene cause long QT syndrome and suppress IKs function. Nat Genet. 1997;17:338-40.

CHAPTER 38

Long QT, Short QT and Brugada Syndromes

24. Abbott GW, et al. MiRP1 forms IKr potassium channels with HERG and is associated with cardiac arrhythmia. Cell. 1999;97:175-87.

25. Tristani-Firouzi M, et al. Functional and clinical characterization of KCNJ2 mutations associated with LQT7 (Andersen syndrome). J Clin Invest. 2002;110:381-8.

26. Lucet V, Lupoglazoff JM, Fontaine B. Andersen syndrome, ventricular arrhythmias and channelopathy (a case report). Arch Pediatr. 2002;9:1256-9.

27. Splawski I, et al. Ca(V)1.2 calcium channel dysfunction causes a multisystem disorder including arrhythmia and autism. Cell. 2004;119:19-31.

28. Splawski I, et al. Severe arrhythmia disorder caused by cardiac L-type calcium channel mutations. Proc Natl Acad Sci USA. 2005;102:8089-96; discussion 8086-8.

29. Vatta M, et al. Mutant caveolin-3 induces persistent late sodium current and is associated with long-QT syndrome. Circulation. 2006;114:2104-12.

30. Palygin OA, Pettus JM, Shibata EF. Regulation of caveolar cardiac sodium current by a single Gsalpha histidine residue. Am J Physiol Heart Circ Physiol. 2008;294:H1693-9.

31. Medeiros-Domingo A, et al. SCN4B-encoded sodium channel beta4 subunit in congenital long-QT syndrome. Circulation. 2007;116:134-42.

32. Chen L, et al. Mutation of an A-kinase-anchoring protein causes long-QT syndrome. Proc Natl Acad Sci USA. 2007;104:20990-5.

33. Summers KM, et al. Mutations at KCNQ1 and an unknown locus cause long QT syndrome in a large Australian family: implications for genetic testing. Am J Med Genet A. 2010152A:613-21.

34. Ueda K, et al. Syntrophin mutation associated with long QT syndrome through activation of the nNOS-SCN5A macromolecular complex. Proc Natl Acad Sci USA. 2008;105:9355-60.

35. Schwartz PJ, et al. The Jervell and Lange-Nielsen syndrome: natural history, molecular basis, and clinical outcome. Circulation. 2006;113:783-90.

36. Mohler PJ, et al. Defining the cellular phenotype of "ankyrin-B syndrome" variants: human ANK2 variants associated with clinical phenotypes display a spectrum of activities in cardiomyocytes. Circulation. 2007;115:432-41.

37. Schwartz PJ. Idiopathic long QT syndrome: progress and questions. Am Heart J. 1985;109:399-411.

38. Schwartz PJ. The congenital long QT syndromes from genotype to phenotype: clinical implications. J Intern Med. 2006;259:39-47.

39. Donger C, et al. KVLQT1 C-terminal missense mutation causes a forme fruste long-QT syndrome. Circulation. 1997;96:2778-81.

40. Schwartz PJ, et al. Genotype-phenotype correlation in the long-QT syndrome: gene-specific triggers for life-threatening arrhythmias. Circulation. 2001;103:89-95.

41. Moss AJ, et al. ECG T-wave patterns in genetically distinct forms of the hereditary long QT syndrome. Circulation. 1995;92:2929-34.

42. Schwartz PJ, et al. Diagnostic criteria for the long QT syndrome. An update. Circulation. 1993;88:782-4.

43. Hinterseer M, et al. Relation of increased short-term variability of QT interval to congenital long-QT syndrome. Am J Cardiol. 2009;103:1244-8.

44. Napolitano C, et al. Evidence for a cardiac ion channel mutation underlying drug-induced QT prolongation and life-threatening arrhythmias. J Cardiovasc Electrophysiol. 2000;11:691-6.

45. Yang P, et al. Allelic variants in long-QT disease genes in patients with drug-associated torsades de pointes. Circulation. 2002;105:1943-8.

46. Sesti F, et al. A common polymorphism associated with antibiotic-induced cardiac arrhythmia. Proc Natl Acad Sci USA. 2000;97:10613-8.

47. Goldenberg I, et al. Beta-blocker efficacy in high-risk patients with the congenital long-QT syndrome types 1 and 2: implications for patient management. J Cardiovasc Electrophysiol, 2010.

48. Schwartz PJ, et al. Long QT syndrome patients with mutations of the SCN5A and HERG genes have differential responses to Na$^+$ channel blockade and to increases in heart rate. Implications for gene-specific therapy. Circulation. 1995;92:3381-6.

49. Priori SG, et al. Association of long QT syndrome loci and cardiac events among patients treated with beta-blockers. JAMA. 2004;292:1341-4.

50. Epstein AE, et al. ACC/AHA/HRS 2008 Guidelines for Device-Based Therapy of Cardiac Rhythm Abnormalities: a report of the American College of Cardiology/American Heart Association Task Force on Practice Guidelines (Writing Committee to Revise the ACC/AHA/NASPE 2002 Guideline Update for Implantation of Cardiac Pacemakers and Antiarrhythmia Devices): developed in collaboration with the American Association for Thoracic Surgery and Society of Thoracic Surgeons. Circulation. 2008;117:e350-408.

51. Moss AJ, McDonald J. Unilateral cervicothoracic sympathetic ganglionectomy for the treatment of long QT interval syndrome. N Engl J Med. 1971;285:903-4.

52. Schwartz PJ, et al. Left cardiac sympathetic denervation in the management of high-risk patients affected by the long-QT syndrome. Circulation. 2004;109:1826-33.

53. Tan HL, et al. Long-term (subacute) potassium treatment in congenital HERG-related long QT syndrome (LQTS2). J Cardiovasc Electrophysiol. 1999;10:229-33.

54. Zipes DP, et al. Guidelines for management of patients with ventricular arrhythmias and the prevention of sudden cardiac death. Executive summary. Rev Esp Cardiol. 2006;59:1328.

55. Ruan Y, et al. Trafficking defects and gating abnormalities of a novel SCN5A mutation question gene-specific therapy in long QT syndrome type 3. Circ Res. 2010;106:1374-83.

56. Algra A, et al. QT interval variables from 24 hour electrocardiography and the two year risk of sudden death. Br Heart J. 1993;70:43-8.

57. Gussak I, et al. Idiopathic short QT interval: a new clinical syndrome? Cardiology. 2000;94:99-102.

58. Patel U, Pavri BB. Short QT syndrome: a review. Cardiol Rev. 2009;17:300-3.

59. Crotti L, et al. Congenital short QT syndrome. Indian Pacing Electrophysiol J. 2010;10:86-95.

60. Brugada R, et al. Sudden death associated with short-QT syndrome linked to mutations in HERG. Circulation. 2004;109:30-5.

61. Hong K, et al. Short QT syndrome and atrial fibrillation caused by mutation in KCNH2. J Cardiovasc Electrophysiol. 2005;16:394-6.

62. Schimpf R, et al. Short QT syndrome. Cardiovasc Res. 2005;67:357-66.

63. Giustetto C, et al. Short QT syndrome: clinical findings and diagnostic-therapeutic implications. Eur Heart J. 2006;27:2440-7.

64. Wolpert C, et al. Clinical characteristics and treatment of short QT syndrome. Expert Rev Cardiovasc Ther. 2005;3:611-7.

65. Bellocq C, et al. Mutation in the KCNQ1 gene leading to the short QT-interval syndrome. Circulation. 2004;109:2394-7.

66. Priori SG, et al. A novel form of short QT syndrome (SQT3) is caused by a mutation in the KCNJ2 gene. Circ Res. 2005;96:800-7.

67. Weiss JN, et al. The dynamics of cardiac fibrillation. Circulation. 2005;112:1232-40.

68. Extramiana F, Antzelevitch C. Amplified transmural dispersion of repolarization as the basis for arrhythmogenesis in a canine ventricular-wedge model of short-QT syndrome. Circulation. 2004;110:3661-6.

69. Anttonen O, et al. Prevalence and prognostic significance of short QT interval in a middle-aged Finnish population. Circulation. 2007;116:714-20.

70. Anttonen O, et al. Differences in twelve-lead electrocardiogram between symptomatic and asymptomatic subjects with short QT interval. Heart Rhythm. 2009;6:267-71.

71. Gussak I, et al. ECG phenomenon of idiopathic and paradoxical short QT intervals. Card Electrophysiol Rev. 2002;6:49-53.

72. Bjerregaard P, Gussak I. Short QT syndrome: mechanisms, diagnosis and treatment. Nat Clin Pract Cardiovasc Med. 2005;2:84-7.

73. Gaita F, et al. Short QT syndrome: a familial cause of sudden death. Circulation. 2003;108:965-70.

74. Gaita F, et al. Short QT syndrome: pharmacological treatment. J Am Coll Cardiol. 2004;43:1494-9.

75. Wolpert C, et al. Further insights into the effect of quinidine in short QT syndrome caused by a mutation in HERG. J Cardiovasc Electrophysiol. 2005;16:54-8.

76. Schimpf R, et al. In vivo effects of mutant HERG K$^+$ channel inhibition by disopyramide in patients with a short QT-1 syndrome: a pilot study. J Cardiovasc Electrophysiol. 2007;18:1157-60.

77. Schimpf R, et al. Congenital short QT syndrome and implantable cardioverter defibrillator treatment: inherent risk for inappropriate shock delivery. J Cardiovasc Electrophysiol. 2003;14:1273-7.

78. Brugada P, Brugada J. Right bundle branch block, persistent ST segment elevation and sudden cardiac death: a distinct clinical and electrocardiographic syndrome. A multicenter report. J Am Coll Cardiol. 1992;20:1391-6.

79. Antzelevitch C, et al. Brugada syndrome: a decade of progress. Circ Res. 2002;91:1114-8.

80. Antzelevitch C, et al. Brugada syndrome: report of the second consensus conference: endorsed by the Heart Rhythm Society and the European Heart Rhythm Association. Circulation. 2005;111:659-70.

81. Catalano O, et al. Magnetic resonance investigations in Brugada syndrome reveal unexpectedly high rate of structural abnormalities. Eur Heart J. 2009;30:2241-8.

82. Brugada J, et al. Long-term follow-up of individuals with the electrocardiographic pattern of right bundle-branch block and ST-segment elevation in precordial leads V1 to V3. Circulation. 2002;105:73-8.

83. Brugada J, Brugada R, Brugada P. Determinants of sudden cardiac death in individuals with the electrocardiographic pattern of Brugada syndrome and no previous cardiac arrest. Circulation. 2003;108:3092-6.

84. Chen Q, et al. Genetic basis and molecular mechanism for idiopathic ventricular fibrillation. Nature. 1998;392:293-6.

85. Campuzano O, Brugada R, Iglesias A. Genetics of Brugada syndrome. Curr Opin Cardiol. 2008;23:176-83.

86. Mohler PJ, et al. Nav1.5 E1053K mutation causing Brugada syndrome blocks binding to ankyrin-G and expression of Nav1.5 on the surface of cardiomyocytes. Proc Natl Acad Sci USA. 2004;101:17533-8.

87. Antzelevitch C. Molecular biology and cellular mechanisms of Brugada and long QT syndromes in infants and young children. J Electrocardiol. 2001;34:177-81.

88. Antzelevitch C. Transmural dispersion of repolarization and the T wave. Cardiovasc Res. 2001;50:426-31.

89. Antzelevitch C, Fish J. Electrical heterogeneity within the ventricular wall. Basic Res Cardiol. 2001;96:517-27.

90. Hong K, et al. Value of electrocardiographic parameters and ajmaline test in the diagnosis of Brugada syndrome caused by SCN5A mutations. Circulation. 2004;110:3023-7.

91. Antzelevitch C, Brugada R. Fever and Brugada syndrome. Pacing Clin Electrophysiol. 2002;25:1537-9.

92. Brugada P, Brugada J, Brugada R. Arrhythmia induction by anti-arrhythmic drugs. Pacing Clin Electrophysiol. 2000;23:291-2.

93. Probst V, et al. Long-term prognosis of patients diagnosed with Brugada syndrome: results from the FINGER Brugada Syndrome Registry. Circulation. 2010;121:635-43.

94. Hermida JS, et al. Hydroquinidine therapy in Brugada syndrome. J Am Coll Cardiol. 2004;43:1853-60.

95. Belhassen B, Glick A, Viskin S. Efficacy of quinidine in high-risk patients with Brugada syndrome. Circulation. 2004;110:1731-7.

96. Viskin S, et al. Empiric quinidine therapy for asymptomatic Brugada syndrome: time for a prospective registry. Heart Rhythm. 2009;6:401-4.

Long QT, Short QT and Brugada Syndromes

Surgical and Catheter Ablation of Cardiac Arrhythmias

Yanfei Yang, David Singh, Nitish Badhwar, Melvin Scheinman

Chapter Outline

SUPRAVENTRICULAR TACHYCARDIA

INTRODUCTION

Supraventricular tachycardias (SVTs) arise from the atrium or atrioventricular (AV) junction and include atrial tachycardia (AT), AV nodal re-entrant tachycardia (AVNRT), AV re-entrant tachycardia (AVRT), atrial flutter (AFL) and atrial fibrillation (AF). Re-entry is the mechanism for the majority of SVTs, while triggered activity and abnormal automaticity are the mechanisms for the others.[1] Paroxysmal SVT (PSVT) denotes a clinical syndrome characterized by SVT associated with sudden onset and termination. The most common causes of PSVT are AVNRT (56%), AVRT (27%) and AT (17%).[2]

Pharmacological management of SVT was used as a first-line approach in the past. However, as knowledge of tachycardia mechanisms and technology advanced, nonpharmacological therapy allows for safe and curative treatment. Current guidelines consider ablation as first-line therapy for most forms of SVT.[3]

HISTORY OF CLINICAL ELECTROPHYSIOLOGIC STUDIES

The modern era of invasive electrophysiologic studies begin with the work of Drs Durrer and Wellens[4,5] who were the first to use programmed electrical stimulation in the heart to define the mechanism(s) of arrhythmias and Dr Scherlag and his colleagues[6] were the first to systematically record the His bundle activity in humans. Drs Durrer and Wellens showed that reciprocating tachycardia could be induced by premature atrial or ventricular stimulation and could be either orthodromic or antidromic; they also defined the relationship of the accessory pathway refractory period to the ventricular response during AF. These workers provided the framework for the use of intracardiac electrophysiological studies to define re-entrant circuit in patients with SVT.[7,8]

CARDIAC-SURGICAL ABLATION

Prior to the era of catheter ablation, patients with SVT that were refractory to medical therapy underwent direct surgical ablation of the AV junction.[9,10] This approach, however, is not appropriate for the management of the patient with AF with rapid conduction over a bypass tract. In 1960s, Durrer and Roos[11] were the first to perform intraoperative mapping and cooling to locate an accessory pathway. Later, using intraoperative mapping, Burchell et al.[12] showed that the accessory pathway conduction could be abolished by injection of procainamide (1967). Sealy and the Duke team were the first to successfully ablate a right free-wall pathway (1968).[13] Dr Iwa of Japan also concurrently demonstrated the effectiveness of cardiac electrosurgery for these patients.[14]

CATHETER ABLATION

The technique of catheter ablation of the AV junction was introduced by Scheinman et al. in 1981.[15] The initial attempts used high energy DC countershocks to destroy cardiac tissue, but expansion of its use to other arrhythmias was limited due to risk of causing diffuse damage from barotrauma. In 1984, Morady and Scheinman introduced a catheter technique for disruption of posteroseptal accessory pathways.[16] This technique was associated with 65% efficacy.[17] Later, successful ablation of nonseptal pathways was reported by Warin et al.[18] The introduction of radiofrequency (RF) energy in the late 1980s[19,20] completely altered catheter ablation procedures. The salient advances in addition to RF energy included much better catheter design, together with better understanding in the mechanism of SVTs.[20-22] A variety of both registry and prospective studies have documented the safety and efficacy of ablative procedures for these patients.[23,24]

Atrioventricular nodal re-entrant tachycardia (AVNRT) is the most common regular, narrow-complex tachycardia. In order to better diagnose this tachycardia and guide the ablation procedure, it is important to understand the anatomy of AVN and the pathophysiology of AVNRT.

ELECTROPHYSIOLOGY OF AVNRT

The seminal findings by Moe and Mendez[25,26] of reciprocal beats in animal models were rapidly applied to humans and introduced just as the field of clinical invasive electrophysiology began to emerge. Early invasive electrophysiologic studies[27,28] attributed AV nodal re-entry as cause of paroxysmal SVT. The work of Dr Ken Rosen and his colleagues[28] demonstrated evidence for dual AV nodal physiology manifest by an abrupt increase in AV nodal conduction time in response to critically timed atrial premature depolarizations. These data served as an excellent supportive compliment to the original observations of Moe and Mendez.[25,26] By the end of the 1970s, the concept of dual AV nodal conduction in humans had been well established.

The working model used to explain the electrophysiological behavior of the AVNRT circuit involves two pathways: one is the so-called "fast pathway" which conducts more rapidly and has a relatively longer refractory period; while the other is the "slow pathway" which conducts slower than the fast pathway but has a relatively shorter refractory period (Fig. 1). The fast pathway constitutes the normal, physiological AV conduction axis.

Traditionally AVNRT has been categorized into typical and atypical forms. Such categorization is based on the retrograde limb of the re-entrant circuit (Fig. 1). Typical AVNRT has antegrade conduction through slow pathway and the retrograde limb is the fast pathway (so-called "slow-fast"); whereas atypical AVNRT shows retrograde conduction via slow pathway, which is less common and includes "fast-slow" and "slow-slow" variants.

In addition, there are several case reports that documented the need to ablate AVNRT from the left annulus or left posteroseptal area.[29,30] One source of LA input is via the left-sided posterior nodal extension.

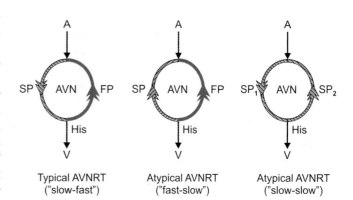

FIGURE 1: A schema of different AVNRT circuits. The broken line indicates the slow pathway (SP) and the solid line represent the fast pathway (FP). (Abbreviations: A: Atrium; V: Ventricle; AVN: Atrioventricular node; His: His bundle)

Ross et al.[31] first introduced nonpharmacologic therapy of AVNRT that involved surgical dissection in Koch's triangle, and their results were confirmed by a number of surgical groups.[32-34] In most patients the retrograde fast pathway (either during tachycardia or ventricular pacing) showed earliest atrial activation over the apex of Koch's triangle while in the minority earliest atrial activation occurred near the CS. This observation nicely compliment the current designation of AVNRT subforms.[35]

CATHETER ABLATION OF AVNRT

In 1989, two groups[36,37] almost simultaneously reported success using high energy discharge in the region of slow pathway. The subsequent use of RF energy completely revolutionized catheter cure of AVNRT. The initial attempts targeted the fast pathway by applying RF energy superior and posterior to the His bundle region (so-called anterior approach) until the prolongation of AV nodal conduction occurred. Initial studies[36-38] showed a success rate of 80–90%, but the risk of AV block was up to 21%. Due to the high-risk of developing AV block, fast pathway ablation is no longer used as the primary approach. Jackman et al.[39] first introduced the technique of ablation of the slow pathway for AVNRT. Ablation of the slow pathway is achieved by applying RF energy at the posterior-inferior septum in the region of the CS_{OS}. This technique can be guided by either discrete potentials[39,40] or via an anatomic approach,[41] both have equal success rate. The safest and most effective approach is to combine anatomic and eletrogram approaches together, in which RF lesions are applied at the posteroseptal sites with slow pathway potentials (Fig. 2). The RF energy is usually applied until junctional ectopics appear and diminish, but at times successful slow pathway ablation may result without eliciting

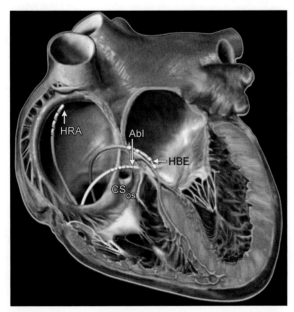

FIGURE 2: Typical slow pathway ablation site. This diagram shows catheter positions for slow pathway ablation in patients with typical AVNRT. The ablation catheter is positioned at the posterior septum just above the CS_{OS}. (Abbreviations: HRA: High right atrium; HBE: His bundle electrogram; Abl: Ablation catheter; CS_{OS}: The ostium of coronary sinus)

the junctional ectopic complexes. The end point for slow pathway ablation involves the proof either that the slow pathway has been eliminated of which there is no more evidence of dual AV nodal physiology (i.e. no AH "jump" with atrial programmed stimulus) or that no more than one AV nodal echo is present.[39]

Among experienced centers the current acute success rate for this procedure is 99% with a recurrence rate of 1.3%, and a 0.4% incidence of AV block requiring a pacemaker.[42] Although the risk of AV block from selective slow pathway ablation in patients with normal baseline PR interval is very low, some reports have suggested that the risk may be higher in patients with pre-existing PR prolongation and/or older age (> 70 years old).[43] In those patients at higher risk, delayed onset of symptomatic AV block can develop and vigilant follow-up may be needed.[43,44] An approach of retrograde fast pathway ablation has been used in patients with baseline PR prolongation and is associated with no delayed development of AV block.[45]

Technologic advances continue to improve the safety of ablation procedures. Besides significantly reducing radiation time to both patient and operator, the development of sophisticated, real-time, 3D mapping systems has allowed for precise localization of the His bundle, reducing the risk of AV block. In addition, cryoablation may be used for slow pathway ablation.[46] The advantage of this technology includes catheter sticking to adjacent endocardium during application of energy, avoiding inadvertent catheter displacement and damage to the node or His bundle. In addition, any AV conduction delay during test ablation is reversible.

WOLFF-PARKINSON-WHITE SYNDROME AND ATRIOVENTRICULAR RE-ENTRANT TACHYCARDIA

HISTORICAL EVOLUTION OF VENTRICULAR PRE-EXCITATION AND AVNRT

The first complete description of WPW syndrome was by Drs Wolff, Parkinson and White in 1930s.[47] They reported 11 patients without structural heart disease who had a short P-R interval, "bundle branch block (BBB)" ECG pattern and episodes of PSVT. At the time, the wide QRS patterns seen in ventricular pre-excitation were thought to be related to a short P-R interval and BBB. Discrete extranodal AV connections accounting for ventricular pre-excitation were initially proposed by Kent[48] and later confirmed by Wood,[49] Öhnell[50] and others.

CARDIAC-SURGICAL CONTRIBUTION

Sealy et al.[13] were the first to successfully ablate a right free-wall pathway. Their subsequent results conclusively showed that a vast majority of patients with the WPW syndrome could be cured by either direct surgical or cryoablation of these accessory pathways. Simultaneously, Iwa et al. also demonstrated the efficacy of cardiac electrosurgery in these patients.[14] He should be credited for being among the first to use an endocardial approach for accessory pathway ablation. The endocardial approach was independently used by the Duke team of Sealy and Cox. Only later was the "closed" epicardial approach reintroduced by Guiraudon.

DEVELOPMENT OF CATHETER ABLATION

The technique of catheter ablation was first introduced by Scheinman and his colleagues in the early 1980s,[15-17] but ablation using DC shocks was limited due to its high-risk of causing diffuse damage from barotrauma. The introduction of RF energy in the late 1980s[19,20] along with better catheter design and the demonstration of accessory pathway (AP) potential for facilitating localization of AP have dramatically improved the safety and efficacy of catheter ablation. The remarkable work of Jackman,[20] Kuck[21] and Calkins[22] ushered in the modern era of ablative therapy for patients with accessory pathways in all locations. A variety of both registry and prospective studies have documented the safety and efficacy of ablative procedures for these patients.[23,24] Nowadays, catheter ablation is the procedure of choice for patients with symptomatic WPW syndrome. In most experienced centers, the success rate is 95–97% with a recurrence rate of approximately 6%.

CLINICAL IMPLICATIONS OF WPW SYNDROME AND AVRT

Patients with WPW syndrome may experience very rapid conduction over the AP during AF. In some patients, ventricular fibrillation (VF) may be the first manifestation of this syndrome.[51] In a symptomatic patient with WPW syndrome, the lifetime incidence of sudden cardiac death (SCD) has been estimated to be approximately 3–4%.[52]

CLASSIFICATION AND LOCALIZATION OF ACCESSORY PATHWAYS

The accessory pathways (APs) are classified into three different types: (1) manifest APs which show a typical WPW pattern on surface ECG; (2) concealed APs are those that lack antegrade conduction but only show retrograde conduction over the APs and (3) a third group known as latent WPW syndrome shows pre-excitation when pacing close to the atrial insertion of the AP.

Precise mapping of APs is critical to the success of ablation procedure. The delta waves and QRS morphologies of the 12-lead ECG in patients with WPW syndrome can help predict the AP location and guide ablation. A successful ablation site can be identified an AP potential (Fig. 3), early onset of local ventricular activation compared to the onset of delta waves on surface ECG during antegrade pre-excitation and fused local atrial and ventricular electrogram.

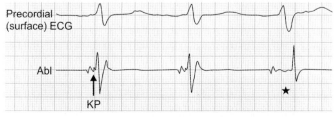

FIGURE 3: Electrogram in sinus rhythm during application of radio-frequency energy. Kent potential (AP potential) on ablation catheter (Abl) disappears (*) and there is abrupt local A-V interval prolongation and a subtle change in the surface QRS, indicating loss of pre-excitation. (Abbreviations: Abl: Ablation catheter; KP: Kent potential)

EFFICACY AND CHALLENGES OF CATHETER ABLATION FOR ACCESSORY PATHWAYS

The majority of the APs are located at the left free wall, 20–30% are located in the posteroseptum, 10–20% along the right free wall and 5–10% at the anteroseptum. The left free-wall APs can be mapped and ablated along the mitral annulus (MA) via either a transseptal or a retrograde transaortic approach. Overall, catheter ablation of left free-wall APs are associated with a high success rate (95%); while ablation of the right free-wall APs is associated with a lower success rate (90%) and a recurrence rate of 14%.[53] The relatively low success rate of right-sided AP ablation is due to the more poorly formed tricuspid annulus (TA) resulting in problems with catheter stability and lack of an accessible right-sided CS-like structure that parallels the TA to facilitate AP localization. Ablation of right-sided APs may be improved by using long deflectable sheaths and a small multipolar mapping catheter placed in the right coronary artery to assist AP mapping.

Ablation of septal APs can be challenging due to the anatomic relationship to the normal conduction system. Therefore, catheter ablation in these areas has the potential risk of producing AV block. The electrogram recorded from the ablation catheter should be carefully assessed and monitored before and during RF delivery. Using 3D electroanatomic mapping (EAM) system to localize the His bundle and track the ablation catheter may prevent or reduce the risk of AV block. Lately cryomapping and cryoablation have improved the safety in difficult cases.[54] Most posteroseptal APs can be ablated from the right side, although up to 20% of the cases require a left-side approach.[55] About 5–17% of the posteroseptal and left posterior APs are located epicardially and require ablation within the CS or middle cardiac vein.[56] Coronary sinus diverticulum may harbor the posteroseptal APs, and CS angiography can confirm such an anomaly. In some patients RF ablation at the neck of the diverticulum may be required to eliminate the APs.[57,58] Applying RF ablation within the CS should be initiated with low energy in order to prevent the risk of perforation and tamponade.

A small percentage of APs are epicardial, suggested by the finding of small or no AP potential during endocardial mapping but with a large AP potential recorded within the CS.[59] Left-side epicardial AP can be successfully ablated within the CS. However, ablation of some epicardial APs may require a percutaneous epicardial approach.[60]

COMPLICATIONS OF CATHETER ABLATION

Overall, catheter ablation of APs is associated with a complication rate of 1–4%, including life-threatening complications (such as perforation, tamponade and embolism) (0.6–0.7%), and procedure-related death (approximately 0.2%).[22,56,61] Complete AV block occurs in about 1% of the patients and is mostly associated with the ablation procedures for septal APs.

FOCAL ATRIAL TACHYCARDIA

Atrial tachycardia (AT) is a group of SVT that is confined to the atrium without involvement of AV node. It is a relatively uncommon arrhythmia, comprising less than 10% of

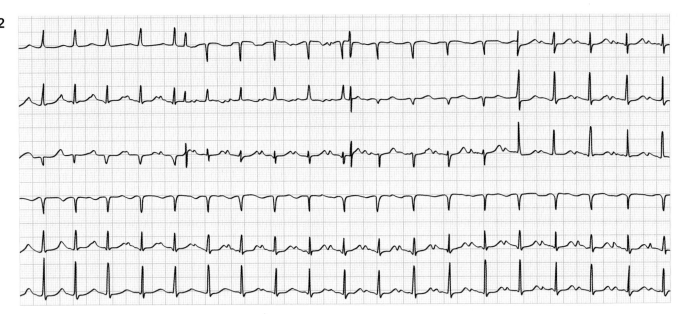

FIGURE 4: Surface ECG in a patient with focal AT arising from the high crista terminalis. Note the P waves in the inferior leads (II, III and aVF) are positive, and negative in V1

symptomatic SVTs encountered in the adult electrophysiological laboratory.[62] However, AT is more common in children (up to 14–23%).[63]

MECHANISMS AND CLASSIFICATIONS OF AT

The AT can be classified into two types: (1) focal AT and (2) macro-re-entry. The mechanism of focal AT can be due to abnormal automaticity or triggered activity. In adults, macro-re-entry is the most common mechanism for AT,[62] while automatic or triggered mechanisms are more common in children.[63]

DIFFERENTIATION OF THE MECHANISMS OF AT

Distinguishing the mechanisms of focal AT may be difficult. In general, a focal AT due to abnormal automaticity tends to have spontaneous initiations or initiation with isoproterenol. It can be suppressed but not terminated by atrial overdrive pacing, and lacks response to adenosine, verapamil or vagal maneuvers.[64,65] The AT with triggered activity can be initiated or terminated by rapid atrial overdrive pacing, and it is sensitive to large-dose of adenosine or vagal maneuvers.[65]

Differentiating focal from macro-re-entrant AT is important to the ablation procedure. Ablation of focal AT is accomplished by targeting the discharging focus (usually it is a single source, except for multifocal AT); whereas ablation of macro-re-entrant AT requires delineation of a critical isthmus that allows for tachycardia perpetuation. Detailed atrial activation mapping, including electrogram and EAM mapping, can distinguish focal from macro-re-entrant AT.

INDICATIONS OF CATHETER ABLATION FOR FOCAL AT

Pharmacologic therapy in patients with focal AT is often ineffective. The proarrhythmia effects of these drugs also limit the long-term efficacy of pharmacologic therapy. Therefore, catheter ablation of focal AT may be considered as a first-line

option, especially in those patients who have incessant tachycardia or baseline ventricular dysfunction.[3]

TECHNIQUES OF CATHETER ABLATION FOR FOCAL AT

Most focal ATs arise from the right atrium (67%), especially from the crista terminalis and TA.[66] Left atrial focal ATs mostly involve the pulmonary veins (PVs) and MA, and less often from the CS, atrial appendages and atrial septum. The surface P wave morphology facilitates the mapping and ablation of AT (Fig. 4). Left-sided ATs require a transseptal approach.

Successful ablation of AT relies on detailed atrial activation mapping during the tachycardia, and use of multipolar catheters and/or 3D EAM systems (Fig. 5).[67,68] A successful ablation site

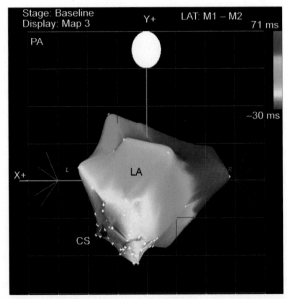

FIGURE 5: A 3D activation map (by CARTO system) of the left atrium (LA) during tachycardia in a patient with a focal AT originating from the CS musculature. The posteroanterior projection (PA) view showed the earliest activation (red area) at the posterior lateral wall

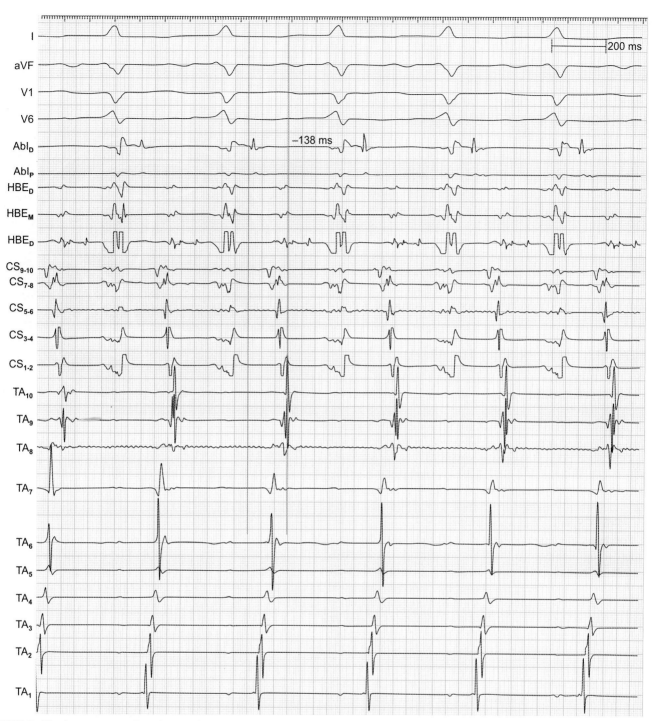

FIGURE 6: Simultaneous recordings from surface leads and catheters placed at ablation site (Abl), His bundle region (HBE), the CS and a 20-pole catheter around the TA with its distal pair of electrodes (TA1) at low lateral TA and proximal at the high septum during tachycardia in a patient with a focal AT originating from inferior TA. Note the earliest atrial activation, which was recorded by the distal ablation catheter, was 138 ms earlier than the onset of surface P waves. The RF delivered at this site abolished the tachycardia without inducibility

can be identified by early local endocardial activation (usually preceding the surface P wave by ≥ 30 ms) and/or low-amplitude, fractionated electrograms (Fig. 6). The RF energy is typically delivered during tachycardia. Acceleration of the tachycardia during ablation is usually a reliable predictor for successful ablation of automatic AT,[69] and noninducibility is the end-point of ablation procedure for focal AT.

Caution should be taken during ablation of focal ATs originating from the areas where important anatomic structures situated such as sinus node and AV node. Lately, cryoablation

has been used for ATs originating from the region of His bundle to reduce the potential risks of AV block.[70]

EFFICACY OF CATHETER ABLATION OF AT

The success rate of ablation for focal AT is about 93% with a recurrence rate of 7%.[71] Left-sided ATs have a lower success rate than the right-sided ATs. Patients with multifocal AT have a higher recurrence rate than those with single tachycardia foci. Also, elder patients and patients with structural heart disease tend to have a higher recurrence rate after initial "successful" ablation.

ATRIAL FLUTTER

CLINICAL IMPLICATIONS OF AFL AND INDICATION FOR CATHETER ABLATION

Atrial flutter is a rapid macro-re-entrant circuit that is confined to either atrium, and bounded by either functional or anatomic barriers. Due to its rapid and regular atrial rate, AFL often produces more rapid ventricular responses. Hence, chronic AFL can result in tachycardia-mediated cardiomyopathy and heart failure. It also predisposes to intracardiac thrombus formation and the risk for stroke. Although antiarrhythmic agents can suppress paroxysmal AFL, the long-term efficacy is poor.[72] Therefore, with technological advances in catheter ablation and better understanding of locating re-entrant circuits, catheter ablation should be considered as first-line treatment for AFL.

HISTORY OF NONPHARMACOLOGIC TREATMENT IN PATIENTS WITH AFL

In the late 1970s, the seminal observations by Waldo and his colleagues, who studied patients with postoperative flutter by means of fixed atrial electrodes, confirmed re-entry as the mechanism of AFL in humans and demonstrated the importance of using entrainment for detection of re-entrant circuits.[73] Klein and Guiraudon mapped two patients with AFL in the operating room found evidence of a large RA re-entrant circuit and the narrowest part of the circuit lay between the TA and the IVC.[74] They successfully treated the flutter by using cryoablation around the CS and surrounding atrium.

Following the report of Klein et al., there appeared several studies using high-energy shocks in an attempt to cure AFL (Saoudi,[75] Chauvin and Brechenmacher[76]). Subsequently both Drs Feld and Cosio almost simultaneously described using RF energy to disrupt cavotricuspid isthmus (CTI) conduction in order to cure patients with AFL. Feld et al. contributed an elegant study using endocardial mapping techniques and entrainment pacing to prove that the area posterior or inferior to the CS was a critical part of the flutter circuit and application of RF energy to this site terminated AFL.[77] Cosio et al. used similar techniques but placed the ablative lesion at the area between the TA and IVC.[78] The latter technique forms the basis for current ablation of CTI dependent flutter.

ABLATION OF CTI DEPENDENT AFLs

In the majority of patients with RA flutter, the CTI is a critical part of the re-entrant circuit. The CTI dependent AFL circuits include those with counterclockwise (CCW) and clockwise (CW) re-entrant circuits around the TA;[79] double-wave re-entry (DWR) which has two wavefronts traveling around the TA simultaneously;[80] lower-loop re-entry (LLR) around the inferior vena cava (IVC)[81-83] and intraisthmus re-entry (IIR).[84,85]

Detailed electrogram mappings as well as entrainment techniques are required to diagnose the flutter circuits. Electrograms recorded from the multielectrode catheter placed around the TA demonstrate the RA activation sequence such as

CCW or CW pattern (Fig. 7A). Entrainment pacing at different atrial sites can help identify the re-entrant circuit and its critical isthmus (Fig. 7B). In addition, using 3D EAM mapping systems can facilitate illustrating the re-entrant circuit and guide catheter ablation over the CTI. A complete linear lesion from TA to IVC

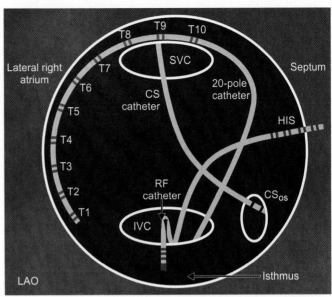

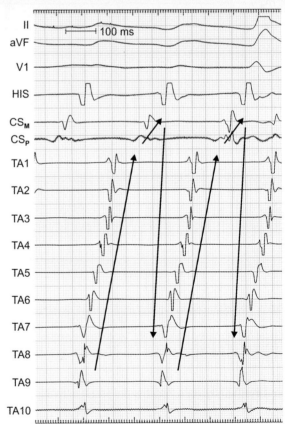

FIGURE 7A: Left panel shows the schema of catheter positions in the left anterior oblique projection (LAO) view during ablation for CTI dependent AFL. A duo-decapolar catheter is positioned along the TA, as well as a quadrupolar catheter at His bundle region and a decapolar catheter inside of the CS. Right panel shows the simultaneous recordings from surface ECG and these catheters. The intracardiac electrogram demonstrates a counterclockwise activation sequence (as shown by the arrows) around the TA

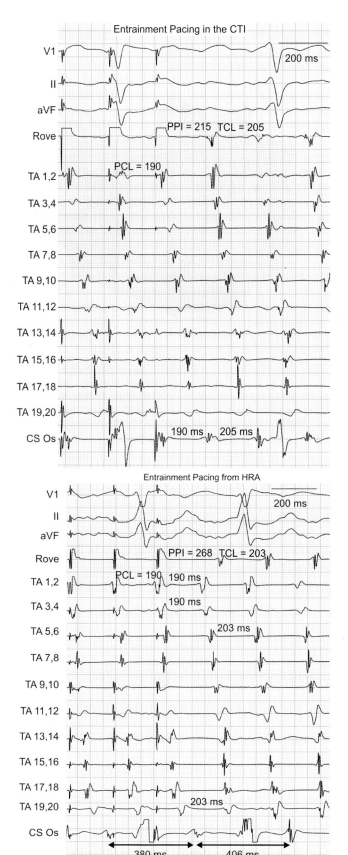

Entrainment Pacing in the CTI

V1

II

aVF

Rove   PPI = 215   TCL = 205

TA 1,2   PCL = 190

TA 3,4

TA 5,6

TA 7,8

TA 9,10

TA 11,12

TA 13,14

TA 15,16

TA 17,18

TA 19,20

CS Os   190 ms   205 ms

200 ms

Entrainment Pacing from HRA

V1

II

aVF

Rove   PPI = 268   TCL = 203

TA 1,2   PCL = 190   190 ms

TA 3,4   190 ms

TA 5,6   203 ms

TA 7,8

TA 9,10

TA 11,12

TA 13,14

TA 15,16

TA 17,18

TA 19,20   203 ms

CS Os

380 ms   406 ms

200 ms

FIGURE 7B: Entrainment pacing from the mapping catheter (Rove) during tachycardia in a patient with clockwise CTI dependent AFL. The left panel shows the difference between PPI and TCL (< 30 ms) when pacing within the CTI, and the atrial activation sequence was same compared to that of the tachycardia, which indicated that the CTI is the critical part of the flutter circuit. The right panel showed the "PPI-TCL" was greater than 30 ms when pacing from the high right atrium (HRA), which suggested that this area is out of the circuit

during AFL results in interrupting the CTI-dependent flutter circuit and terminating the tachycardia.

END-POINT OF CTI ABLATION

Initially it was felt that a good end point for successful CTI ablation was tachycardia termination during RF application. However, many patients suffered recurrences, and eventually it was recognized that it was important to achieve true bidirectional block in the isthmus. Many studies have shown that recurrence rates of AFL are much improved when bidirectional block is achieved.[86] Currently there are many techniques for assessing bidirectional isthmus block.[87-89]

ABLATION OF NON-CTI DEPENDENT AFLs

As shown in Flow chart 1, non-CTI dependent AFL circuit can be classified into two categories: (1) RA and (2) LA flutter circuits. Ablation of non-CTI dependent AFLs can sometimes be challenging, but using 3D EAM system can facilitate the procedure.

RIGHT ATRIAL FLUTTER CIRCUITS

In the RA, non-CTI dependent AFL includes scar-related macro-re-entrant tachycardia and upper loop re-entry (ULR). It has been shown that macro-re-entrant AT can occur in patients with or without atriotomy or congenital heart disease.[82,90,91] In these patients, the 3D electroanatomic voltage maps from the RA often show "scar(s)" or low-voltage area(s) (< 0.2 mV) which act(s) as the central obstacle or channels for the re-entrant circuit. The morphology of surface ECG varies depending on where the scar(s) and low-voltage area(s) are and how the wavefronts exit the circuits. The critical isthmus of the re-entrant circuit can be identified by entrainment pacing, and the electrogram recorded at such a site often shows low-amplitude, fractionated, long duration mid-diastolic potentials. Catheter ablation of scar-related macro-re-entrant tachycardia involves deliver RF energy within the critical channel/isthmus or linear lesion connecting from the scar to an anatomic barrier, such as IVC or super vena cava (SVC).

The ULR is a form of AFL only involving the upper portion of RA with transverse conduction over the CT and wavefront collision occurring at the lower part of RA or within the CTI.[82,92] It was initially felt to involve a re-entrant circuit using the channel between the superior vena cava (SVC), fossa ovalis (FO) and CT.[82] A study by Tai et al. using noncontact mapping technique showed that this form of AFL was a macro-re-entrant tachycardia in the RA free wall with the CT as its functional obstacle.[92] They successfully abolished ULR by linear ablation of the gap in the CT.

LEFT ATRIAL FLUTTER CIRCUITS

Left AFL circuits are often seen in patients post-AF ablation. In recent years, these circuits have been better defined by the use of electroanatomic or noncontact mapping techniques.[93] Cardiac surgery involving the LA or atrial septum can produce various left flutter circuits. But, left AFL circuits also can be found in patients without a history of atriotomy. Electroanatomic maps in these patients often show low voltage or scar areas in

FLOW CHART 1: Nomenclature of atrial flutter (AFL)

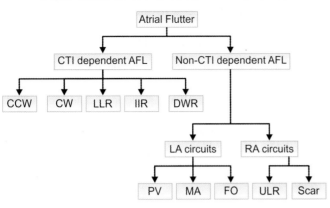

(Abbreviations: CTI: Cavotricuspid Isthmus; CCW: Counterclockwise AFL around the tricuspid annulus (TA); CW: Clockwise AFL around the TA; LLR: Lower Loop Re-entry around inferior vena cava; IIR: Intraisthmus Re-entry; DWR: Double-wave Re-entry around the TA; LA: Left Atrium; RA: Right Atrium; PV: Re-entrant circuit around the Pulmonary Vein (s) with or without scar(s) in the LA; MA: re-entrant circuit around mitral annulus; FO: re-entrant circuit around the fossa ovalis; ULR: Upper Loop Re-entry in the RA)

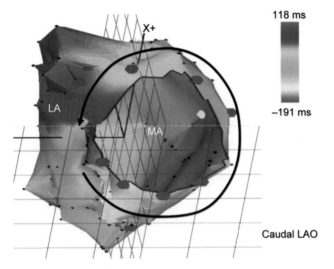

FIGURE 8: A CARTO activation map of the left atrium in a caudal LAO view in a patient with CCW AFL around the mitral annulus (MA). The map shows "early meets late activation" at the spetal MA and the mapped cycle length spanned the TCL. Ablation was completed with a line from the left inferior pulmonary vein (PV) to the MA

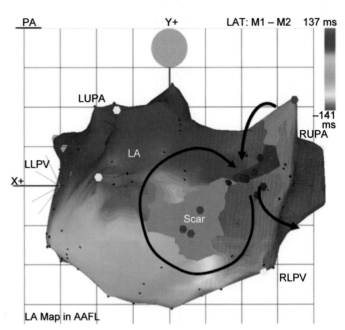

FIGURE 9: A CARTO activation map of the LA in a patient with LA AFL. The map shows a scar over the posterior LA wall. The tachycardia wave front traveled in a "Figure-of-8" pattern around the scar and the right upper pulmonary vein (RUPV) respectively and through the common channel between the scar and the right upper pulmonary vein (RUPV). Successful ablation was achieved with an RF line from the RUPV to the scar. (Abbreviations: LUPV: Left upper pulmonary vein; LLPV: Left lower pulmonary vein; RLPV: Right lower pulmonary vein)

Various left AFL circuits involve the PVs, especially in those patients who underwent AF ablation or those with mitral valve disease. Re-entry can circle around one or more PVs and/or posterior scar or low-voltage area(s).[93,94] In order to cure these complex circuits, 3D EAM is required to reveal the circuit and guide ablation (Fig. 9). Since these circuits are related to low voltage or scar area(s), the surface ECG usually shows low amplitude or flat flutter waves.

In summary, modern mapping techniques allow for identification and successful ablation of complex AFL circuits.

ABLATION OF VENTRICULAR TACHYCARDIA IN PATIENTS WITH STRUCTURAL CARDIAC DISEASE

Ventricular tachycardia (VT) is an important source of morbidity and mortality among patients with ischemic heart disease. Patients with VT and a history of myocardial infarction are at high-risk of recurrent VT, VF and SCD. Internal cardiac defibrillators (ICDs) have become the mainstay of therapy in this patient population and are effective at terminating episodes of VT and VF. Among patients at high-risk for VT and SCD, ICD therapy has been shown to reduce SCD and all-cause mortality.[95-98] Although ICDs are highly effective, they do not prevent VT or VF, and ICD shocks have been associated with decreased quality of life, increased anxiety and depression and increased mortality.[99-105] While antiarrhythmic therapy is frequently used to prevent ICD shocks, its efficacy is limited and frequently associated with untoward side effects.[106,107]

Catheter ablation for scar-based VT has emerged as an important treatment option, particularly among individuals who

the LA, which act as a central obstacle in the circuit. There are several subgroups of left AFLs (Flow chart 1).

Mitral annular AFL involves re-entry around the MA either in a CCW or CW direction (Fig. 8). The surface ECG of MA flutter can mimic CTI-dependent CCW or CW flutter, but with low-amplitude flutter waves in most of the 12 leads.[94] This arrhythmia is more common in patients with structural heart disease. However, it has been described in patients without obvious structural heart disease.[93,94] Electroanatomic voltage map from the LA often shows scar(s) or low-voltage area(s) at the posterior wall as a posterior boundary of this circuit. A linear RF lesion is usually applied at the mitral isthmus, i.e. from the ostium of left lower PV to the lateral MA.[94] Bidirectional mitral isthmus block should be assessed after completing the ablation line.

have received recurrent ICD shocks. Several studies have demonstrated that this approach can reduce the incidence of ICD shocks and/or VT burden.[108-110] In the case of incessant VT or VT storm (three or more episodes within a 24 hour period), catheter ablation can be a lifesaving measure. However, catheter ablation in patients with ischemic heart disease can be technically challenging. Patients with ischemic heart disease and VT are by definition, a vulnerable population, and are often unable to tolerate long procedure-times and VT rates frequently induced during ablation. This section will provide an overview of catheter ablation for patients with scar-related VT. It will review the mechanisms of scar-related VT, indications for ablation and describe the various mapping and ablation techniques commonly employed.

ANATOMIC SUBSTRATE

The vast majority of VT in patients with ischemic heart disease is due to re-entry involving a healed scar. Unidirectional block is a necessary condition for re-entry. Areas of conduction block can be anatomically fixed (present during tachycardia and sinus rhythm) or can be functional (present only during tachycardia).[111] The sites of VT origin are frequently located adjacent to and within scar locations where surviving bundles of muscle fiber can be found. These muscle bundles are isolated from neighboring bundles by strands of fibrous tissue. Endocardial recordings form these sites demonstrate fractionated (low-amplitude and disorganized) potentials which serve as regions of slow conduction and provide the substrate for re-entrant VT (Fig. 10).[112] Although scar based re-entry is the most common arrhythmia associated with ischemic heart disease, other clinical VTs, such as focal tachycardia, bundle branch re-entry and fascicular re-entry, are also observed on occasion.

PATIENT SELECTION

In general, ablation for scar-related VT is reserved for patients with recurrent monomorphic VT and/or frequent ICD shocks.

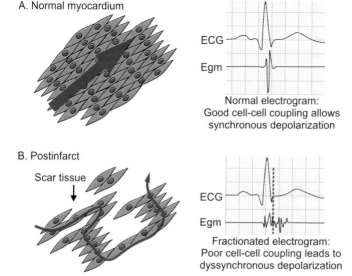

A. Normal myocardium

ECG

Egm

Normal electrogram:
Good cell-cell coupling allows
synchronous depolarization

B. Postinfarct

Scar tissue

ECG

Egm

Fractionated electrogram:
Poor cell-cell coupling leads to
dyssynchronous depolarization

FIGURE 10: Slow conduction through scarred myocardium provides the substrate for re-entry. This is often accompanied by the presence of fractionated electrograms as seen on the right (*Source:* John Miller)

There is, however, a growing interest in performing early or even prophylactic ablation to prevent VT episodes and ICD discharges.[109,110] In general, ablation is not considered for patients with recurrent polymorphic VT. However, it is important to recognize the occasional patient with idiopathic polymorphous VT or VF due to short coupled premature ventricular complexes (PVCs). If the triggering PVC can be identified and ablated in these patients, it may result in cure or significant attenuation of the VT/VF burden.[113]

The most recent American College of Cardiology/American Heart Association Task Force/European Society of Cardiology guidelines for management of patients with ventricular arrhythmias and the prevention of sudden death recommends catheter ablation for VT as adjunctive therapy for patients with an ICD who have had multiple shocks due to sustained VT, not amenable to ICD reprogramming or drug therapy (Class I, level of evidence C).[114] In addition, ablation may be considered as an alternative to long-term drug therapy. A more recent consensus document expands on these guidelines and recommends catheter ablation for patients with structural heart disease in each of the following conditions:

- Symptomatic sustained monomorphic VT (SMVT), including VT terminated by an ICD, that recurs despite antiarrhythmic drug therapy or when antiarrhythmic drugs are not tolerated or not desired.
- Incessant SMVT or VT storm that is not due to a transient reversible cause.
- Patients with frequent PVCs, nonsustained VT (NSVT) or VT that is presumed to cause ventricular dysfunction.
- Bundle branch re-entrant or interfascicular VTs.
- Recurrent sustained polymorphic VT and VF that is refractory to antiarrhythmic therapy when there is a suspected trigger that can be targeted for ablation.[115]

It is generally agreed that the role of catheter ablation for scar-related VT is to reduce a patient's arrhythmic burden. As such, even successful ablations do not obviate the need for an ICD. There have been several studies that have prospectively evaluated the role of catheter ablation for VT.

The multicenter thermocool ventricular tachycardia ablation trial examined the role of catheter ablation for VT in patients with reduced ejection fraction (EF) and recurrent monomorphic VT.[108] Around 231 patients were enrolled and underwent ablation. The median number of VT morphologies per patient was three. All inducible VTs with rates near to or less than the clinical VT were targeted. Ablation abolished all inducible VTs in 49% of patients. At six months, 53% of patients achieved the primary endpoint of freedom from recurrent incessant or sustained VT. In 142 patients with ICDs VT episodes were reduced from a median of 11.5 to 0 (p < 0.0011). The 1-year mortality rate was 18%, with 72.5% of deaths attributed to ventricular arrhythmias or heart failure. The procedure mortality rate was 3%, with no strokes. Although this was a nonrandomized trial, it demonstrated moderate success for VT ablation in carefully selected patients.

Two prospective trials have evaluated the role of VT ablation for the prevention of SMVT. The SMASH-VT trial enrolled 128 subjects with an ICD placed either for secondary prevention (for VF or hemodynamically unstable VT or syncope with inducible VT) or for primary prevention with subsequent delivery of an appropriate ICD therapy.[110] Patients were randomly assigned to defibrillator implantation alone or defibrillator implantation with adjunctive catheter ablation (64 patients in each group). Ablation was performed using a substrate-based approach (see below). The primary end point was survival free from any appropriate ICD therapy. During the mean 23 month follow-up period, appropriate ICD therapy occurred more frequently in the ICD alone group and than in the ablation group (33 vs 12%, P = 0.007). There was a trend toward decreased mortality in the ablation group (9 vs 17%, P = 0.29). Ablation-related complications occurred in three patients (pericardial tamponade, HF requiring prolonged hospitalization and deep venous thrombosis) and there were no procedural deaths.

The VTACH trial, enrolled 110 subjects with stable VT, prior MI and LVEF less than or equal to 50% who were randomly assigned to either catheter ablation plus an ICD or ICD alone.[109] The primary endpoint was the time to first recurrence of VT or VF. After a mean follow-up duration of 22.5 months, time to VF or recurrent VT was longer in the ablation group than in the control group (median 18.6 vs 5.9 months p = 0·045). According to the Kaplan-Meier analysis, 59% of patients in the ablation group and 40% of patients in the control group were free from any VT or VF episode after 12 months. No significant difference in quality of life was found. Ablation-related complications occurred in two patients (transient ST-segment elevation in one patient and a transient cerebral ischemic event in the other) and there were no procedural deaths.

PRIOR TO ABLATION

Since patients with scar-based VT frequently have coronary artery disease (CAD), it is important to understand a patient's coronary anatomy and ischemic burden prior to ablation. Patients with unrevascularized CAD are unlikely to tolerate prolonged periods of VT. It is therefore prudent to obtain a noninvasive or invasive assessment of a patient's coronary anatomy prior to the procedure. Ideally, a patient should be revascularized before catheter ablation. In some instances, revascularization itself may reduce a patient's arrhythmic burden. For some patients, inotropic support, balloon pump or other forms of hemodynamic support (e.g. left ventricular assist-device or extracorporeal membrane oxygenation) may be required to perform the case.[116-118]

Prior to ablation, all patients should undergo a transthoracic echocardiogram to assess for left ventricular thrombus. The presence of thrombus is a contraindication to endocardial VT ablation due to the risk of thrombus dislodgement. In patients without ICDs, preprocedural magnetic resonance imaging (MRI) can be used to guide ablation by identifying areas of scar. Finally patients should be assessed for peripheral arterial disease (PAD) prior to ablation. Frequently, access to the LV is achieved retrogradely across the aortic valve. For patients with extensive PAD a transseptal approach may be more desirable.

12-LEAD LOCALIZATION

Planning for scar-based monomorphic VT ablation first requires analysis of the 12-lead ECG during tachycardia (providing it is available). For re-entrant VT, the QRS morphology represents the exit point of the circuit. In general, VTs arising in the septum (or fascicular system) are more narrow than VTs originating on the free wall. Positive concordance (dominant R wave in all precordial leads) is associated with VTs that exit from the posterior base of the heart. Negative concordance (QS in all precordial leads) is associated with VTs that exit from the anterior left ventricular apex.[119] A left bundle branch block (LBBB) pattern (R < S in lead V1) is observed with VTs from the right ventricle or ventricular septum. Right bundle branch block (RBBB) morphologies (R > S in lead V1) are almost invariably associated with VTs that arise in the left ventricle. In patients with prior infarction, the frontal axis of the VT is also influenced by the location of the VT exit site. The VTs that exit on the inferior wall produce a superiorly directed axis. An inferiorly directed axis usually reflects a VT from the anterior wall. A negative deflection in lead I and AVL indicates a lateral exit.[111] The VTs of epicardial origin typically have a longer QRS duration and slurred QRS upstrokes in the precordial leads.[120]

APPROACH TO ABLATION

The term "mapping" is a broad term that refers to number of electrophysiological techniques that are used to gain insight about the nature and location of an arrhythmia. There are a variety of mapping techniques that are used in scar-based VT ablations. Many of these techniques require the presence of sustained VT. In many instances patients are unable to tolerate sustained VT, and alternative approaches must be taken (see substrate-based ablation below). In order to induce VT, an operator usually performs a pacing stimulation protocol from the right ventricular apex or right ventricular outflow tract (RVOT). Frequently, the resulting VT is not the patient's "clinical VT" (e.g. it may have a different cycle length or morphology). Moreover, many patients will have multiple inducible VTs. Ideally all VTs that are reproducibly inducible and hemodynamically tolerated should be mapped and ablated.

ACTIVATION MAPPING (FOCAL TACHYCARDIAS)

One common form of mapping used in the electrophysiology lab is "activation mapping". This form of mapping is performed while a patient is in VT. To accomplish this, a mapping catheter is maneuvered to different sites in the chamber of interest, focusing on areas suggested by the 12-lead ECG or over scars detected by Echo or MRI. The recording electrode at the catheter tip reflects local myocardial activation. By comparing the timing of the local electrogram to a standard reference (typically the onset of the QRS for VT), a great deal can be learned about the arrhythmia. Activation mapping is of particular use in focal tachycardias where the local electrogram (EGM) typically precedes the onset of the QRS by 20–30 ms at site of the focus. By locating areas with very early EGM-QRS timings the arrhythmia focus can be localized and ablated.

RE-ENTRANT TACHYCARDIA

In contrast to focal VTs, re-entrant VTs demonstrate continuous electrical activity as the wavefront propagates around a circuit. Strictly speaking, there is no "earliest" point in the circuit.[121] Operators frequently use this form of mapping to identify a

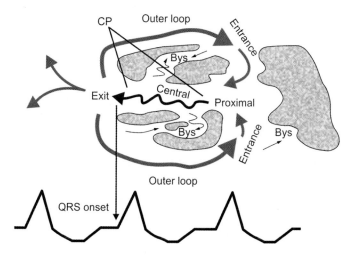

FIGURE 11: Hypothetical VT circuit consisting of a central isthmus with entrance and exit zones. The outer loops course around the scarred areas (border zones) and bystander loops (Bys) are found within the scar. (*Source:* Modified from reference 123)

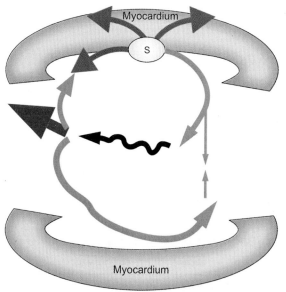

FIGURE 12: Stimulation is performed at an outer loop site (S) in the re-entry circuit that shown in Figure 12. The stimulated orthodromic wavefront propagates through the circuit, resetting the re-entry circuit. After the last stimulus, the pacing site is next depolarized by the orthodromic wavefront that has made one revolution through the circuit. The PPI therefore approximates the TCL. Pacing at this site also directly stimulates surround myocardial tissue. The QRS morphology therefore differs from that of the VT. (*Source:* Modified from reference 123)

critical isthmus (or zone of slow conduction) where the VT is likely to be terminated (Fig. 11). Typically, these sites are characterized by a diastolic electrogram that is low amplitude and fractionated. However, the specificity of isolated diastolic potentials is limited as they can be observed in regions other than a critical isthmus.[122]

ENTRAINMENT MAPPING

During activation mapping it is not uncommon to encounter areas with fractionated diastolic potentials that may or may not be participating in the VT circuit. In order to determine whether such a site is participating in the VT circuit, a technique known as entrainment mapping can be used. Entrainment refers to the continuous resetting of a tachycardia circuit by pacing at a cycle length slightly faster than the tachycardia cycle length (TCL). To demonstrate entrainment, the tachycardia must be accelerated to the pacing cycle length and tachycardia resumption upon cessation of pacing. When pacing from a site remote from the circuit, the pacing impulse travels toward the circuit and penetrates it in two directions. In the antidromic direction, the impulse collides with the previous circulating orthodromic wavefront. In the orthodromic direction, the impulse travels around circuit, resetting the tachycardia. The result of entrainment from a site remote to the VT circuit is QRS fusion where the resulting QRS morphology represents a fusion between the tachycardia circuit and a purely paced beat.

If entrainment is performed from a site within the circuit, the resulting QRS morphology should replicate the VT morphology exactly. This is known as concealed entrainment. If concealed entrainment is observed, several other features can be examined to confirm that the pacing catheter is located within the tachycardia circuit. The stimulus-QRS interval can be compared to the electrogram-QRS interval during VT. These intervals should be similar if pacing is taking place along the circuit (generally within 10 ms).

The post-pacing interval (PPI) refers to the duration between the last pacing stimulus artifact and the return of next local EGM at that pacing site. This represents the time that it takes for the

last orthodromically stimulated wavefront to revolve around the circuit. If pacing is performed from a site within the circuit, the PPI should equal the TCL. A PPI-TCL less than or equal to 30 ms suggests that pacing site is within the VT circuit. Pacing at a site remote from the re-entry circuit can also entrain tachycardia, but in this instance the PPI is equal to the conduction time from the pacing site to the circuit through circuit and back to the pacing site and therefore exceeds the TCL.[123]

The VT model proposed by Stevenson and others have greatly enhanced out understanding about the entrainment of these circuits.[124] The hypothetical VT shown in Figures 11 and 12 depicts a "figure of eight" circuit with a common central isthmus.[123] The common isthmus has an entrance and exit as well as central regions. The QRS complex is inscribed after the wavefront leaves the exit site and begins propagating around the border of the scar around two outer loops. The wavefronts then enter the infarct region through entrances to reach the entrance of the isthmus. Regions that are within scar do not participate in the circuit are labeled as bystanders.

Analysis of the PPI can reveal a great deal about the location of the pacing catheter with respect to this hypothetical circuit. As above, when pacing from within the VT circuit (i.e. from the exit, or critical isthmus) the QRS morphology will be identical to the VT and the PPI-TCL should be less than or equal to 30 ms (Figs 13A to C). Pacing from a bystander site will, however, produce a PPI-TCL that is greater than or equal to 30 ms as it reflects the time for the stimulus to leave the bystander region, propagate around the circuit and return to the site of pacing. In this instance the QRS morphology will resemble the VT so long as the bystander is insulated by scar from surrounding myocardium. Entrainment from the true isthmus

A VT circuit
"Bystander" pathway

VT cycle length

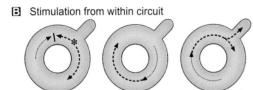

B Stimulation from within circuit

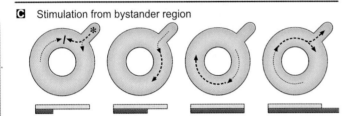

C Stimulation from bystander region

FIGURES 13A TO C: Stimulation during VT is shown: (A) A VT circuit is depicted with an arrow showing the direction of impulse propagation. The impulse also enters a bystander or dead-end pathway to the side. The length of one complete VT cycle is shown as a white bar below; (B) A stimulus (*) is delivered from within the circuit; propagation occurs in the same direction around the circuit path as during VT as well as in the opposite direction, where it collides with the advancing "head" of the prior VT beat (dimmed arrow). A black bar beneath tracks the progress of the stimulated wave front during the figure. At right, the wave front has continued propagating around the circuit until it reaches the site of stimulation. The time required to return to the site of stimulation (the postpacing interval) just equals the VT cycle length (black bar = white bar); (C) A stimulus is given from a bystander pathway. The impulse must travel a short distance to arrive at the circuit, after which it propagates as in (B). However, the PPI (black bar) exceeds the VT cycle length by the time required to exit from and return to the point of stimulation. (*Source:* Modified from reference 138)

will result in stimulus to QRS = mid-diastolic EGM to QRS. Pacing from the innerloop bystander shows that the stimulus to QRS will be greater than EGM to QRS onset. Entrainment from an outerloop site will generally produce a PPI-TCL less than or equal to 30 ms (as it is within the circuit), however, the resulting QRS morphology will represent fusion between the circuit's propagating wavefront and direct depolarization of surrounding myocardium (Figs 13A to C).

Entrainment can also be used to differentiate a diastolic potential that reflects activation of the VT circuit and a "far field potential" which is due to depolarization of tissue remote from the circuit. During entrainment, a potential that is participating the VT circuit will be captured by the entrainment maneuver and will be obscured by the pacing artifact. In contrast, the inability to "entrain" the potential whereby it appears dissociated from the pacing suggests that the potential is a far field electrogram and not part of the VT circuit.

It can be challenging to localize an ideal target for ablation even under the best of circumstances. The size and location of

an isthmus can vary widely depending on a patient's substrate. On most occasions, ablation of a critical portion of a VT circuit requires multiple lesions depending on the volume of the isthmus. While any one of the above mentioned findings (i.e. mid-diastolic potential, concealed entrainment, Stim-QRS ~ EGM-QRS, PPI-TCL < 30 ms) does not itself predict an ideal site for ablation, the presence of multiple findings is likely to increase the rate of success.[125]

ELECTROANATOMIC THREE-DIMENSIONAL MAPPING

The advent of three-dimensional EAM systems, such as CARTO (Biosense Webster, Baldwin Park, CA) or EnSite/NavX (St. Jude Medical, St. Paul, MN), has greatly enhanced the ability to perform complex ablations. Whereas conventional mapping relies on interpretation of intracardiac electrograms and two-dimensional fluoroscopic imaging, EAM provides additional real-time three-dimensional data about a patient's arrhythmogenic substrate. Although there are differences in their underlying technologies, in general, these systems allow operators to determine the spatial orientation of catheters in three-dimensions, delineate anatomic areas of interest, define cardiac chamber geometry and locate areas of scar. In addition, they can be used to create detailed activation maps that help to accurately locate the region and nature of the arrhythmia (e.g. focal versus macro-re-entrant). Given the complexity of the procedure, EAM systems are particularly useful for ablation in patients with scar-based VT.

Both CARTO and EnSite can be used to perform activation mapping during VT. To perform this, a designated catheter is moved to various locations in the chamber of interest. At each point, the mapping software is able to integrate the position of the catheter and the timing of the local electrogram with respect to an arbitrarily designated reference (or fiducial) point. The temporal relationship of the local activation to the reference point is color coded with red generally representing early activation sites, purple representing late activation sites and other colors, such as yellow, green and blue, representing intermediate activation times. This isochronal map is displayed in real-time on a review screen and can be used to distinguish focal from re-entrant arrhythmias. In addition to this, it localizes the source or circuit in the cardiac chamber. Focal arrhythmias generally have a small site of early activation with centrifugal spread away from the source. In contrast, macro-re-entrant rhythms display transitions from early (red) to intermediate (yellow-green-blue) to late (purple) as the wavefront propagates around the circuit with characteristic early-meets-late patterns. By tracing this propagation map around the chamber, the location of the circuit can be visualized.

VOLTAGE MAPPING

Another powerful application of EAM is its ability to delineate areas of scar. Areas of scar typically exhibit low voltage electrograms. A cardiac chamber can be readily mapped by placing a catheter at various locations and recording the signal amplitude. As with endocardial activation, a color-coded voltage scale can be used to display areas of low voltage amplitude, to distinguish between areas of scar, dense scar and relatively

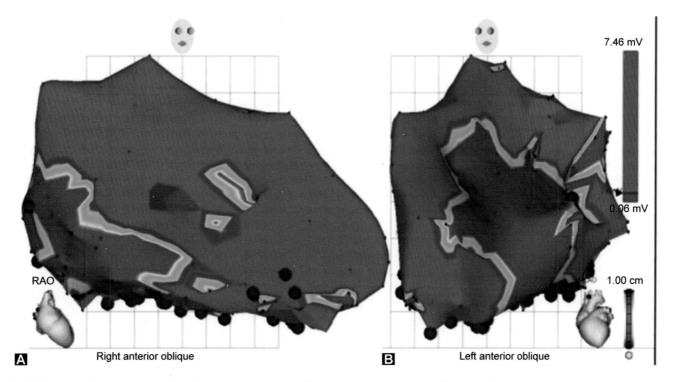

FIGURES 14A AND B: Voltage map of the left ventricle (LV), RAO and LAO view, in an individual with large, healed inferolateral myocardial infarction. Local bipolar electrogram voltage of less than or equal to 0.5 mV has been arbitrarily selected as the threshold for delineating low electrogram amplitude, as seen on the voltage scale on the right. Areas of red coloration represent sites with the lowest electrogram amplitude, with the area of next lowest voltage demarcated by yellow, followed by green, etc. The area colored in magenta indicates normal electrogram voltage. (*Source:* Modified from reference 139)

normal tissue (Figs 14A and B). Voltage mapping is critical for re-entrant VT as the majority of these circuits are intimately related to scar border zones and other anatomic obstacles. Understanding the location and density of scar can be used to perform VT ablations in patients during sinus rhythm (see substrate-based ablation below).

PACE MAPPING

Pace mapping is a useful technique for individuals with hemodynamically unstable VT in whom entrainment or activation mapping is not possible. The 12-lead ECG of the paced site is compared to the 12 lead of the VT. When the paced and comparison QRS morphologies are identical, this is referred to as a 12/12 match. When performing pace mapping, it is essential to confirm that the lead placement for the pace map is identical to the 12 lead used for comparison. Often times, the precordial leads are placed in modified locations during EP studies. If the comparison ECG has been performed outside of the EP lab, alternate lead placement may render an inaccurate pace map.

Pace mapping can be useful for focal VTs where a 12/12 match is presumed to represent the site of origin.[126] However, its utility is somewhat limited in patients with macro-re-entrant VT. In patients with scar-related VT, a perfect or near perfect pace map usually indicates that the catheter is located near the VT exit site. However, ablation at a VT exit site may merely result in shifting the exit to a new location and fail to eliminate the circuit. Ablation at isthmus sites are more likely to be successful, however this can be difficult to perform with pace mapping alone. Regions of functional block that may define

activation pathways during VT may not be present while pacing during sinus rhythm. When pace mapping in a defined isthmus, the stimulated wavefront can propagate in both antidromic and orthodromic directions.[127] The resulting QRS may be a fusion between these two wavefronts and differ from the morphology of the VT circuit under investigation.

Pace mapping can be used to identify areas of slow conduction which are typically found within infarct zones, and may represent positioning in a critical isthmus. When pacing normal myocardium, there is typically little or no delay between the pacing stimulus and the surface ECG complex (S-QRS). Since the isthmus of VT circuit usually represents a zone of slow conduction, pacing from this region can sometimes result in S-QRS delay. Brunckhorst and his colleagues performed pace mapping at 890 sits in 12 patients with postmyocardial infarction VT. Their data demonstrated that areas with S-QRS delay were always localized to an infarct region (as identified by electrogram voltage) and 13 of 14 areas of conduction delay were associated with the isthmus of a re-entrant circuit.[128] In a similar study, this group combined pace mapping data with S-QRS data to localize successful sites of ablation in patients with scar-related VT.[127]

Pace mapping within scar at sites with an isolated diastolic potential during sinus rhythm has also been shown to be an indicator of a critical isthmus (Fig. 15). In one study, application of this strategy resulted in freedom from recurrent VT in 16 of 19 patients (84%) during a mean follow-up period of 10 months.[129] Finally, pace mapping can be useful to define regions within scar that are electrically unexcitable. Soejima and his colleagues demonstrated that in some patients, re-entry circuit isthmuses can be identified by delineation of electrically

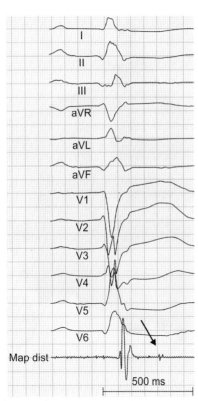

FIGURE 15: Example of an isolated diastolic potential recorded during sinus rhythm within left ventricular scar. (*Source:* Modified from reference 129)

unexcitable scar that defines their borders.[130] The RF ablation in these regions abolished inducible VT in 10 of 14 patients and abolished or markedly reduced spontaneous VT during follow-up.

SUBSTRATE-BASED ABLATION

The term "substrate based ablation" has been used to describe the combination of techniques used to perform VT ablations in patients with hemodynamically unstable VT who cannot tolerate entrainment or activation mapping. The specific protocols for substrate ablation vary from center to center. However, in general, the following steps are taken (Flow chart 2 and Fig. 16):

- A voltage map of the chamber of interest is created such that areas of scar can be defined.
- Areas with diastolic potentials and fractionated electrograms are tagged and noted on the electroanatomic map.
- Pace mapping is performed in multiple areas with particular attention to QRS morphology and S-QRS duration and electrically unexcitable scar.
- Probable VT exit sites as well as isthmuses are identified based on the above information.
- Ablations in regions of potential isthmus sites are undertaken.

Although substrate-based ablation is often performed in patients with poorly tolerated VT, it can also be used in conjunction with other mapping techniques such as entrainment mapping. Substrate mapping may help to operators to identify areas likely to be of particular interest for re-entrant circuits. Following this an operator may induce VT for short periods of time and further localize potential ablation sites.

SAFETY

The VT ablation is complex procedure performed in patients who frequently have advanced illness. These features coupled with long procedure times and extensive ablation in the left-sided circulation creates risk for a myriad of serious complications, including stroke, valvular injury, major bleeding, tamponade, hemodynamic collapse and death. In two prospective trials in which VT ablation was performed for recurrent VT the periprocedural mortality was 2.7–3%.[108,131] The risk of a major complication, such as the ones mentioned above, was 8–10%. The risk of minor complications was 6–7.3%.

The 1998 North American Society of Pacing and Electrophysiology (NASPE) Prospective Catheter Ablation Registry, significant procedural complications were observed in 3.8% of

FLOW CHART 2: Steps of VT ablation

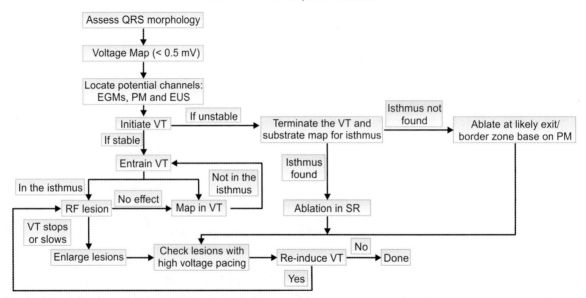

(Abbreviations: EGM: Electrogram; EUS: Electrically unexcitable Scar; PM: Pace-map). (*Source:* Modified from reference 111)

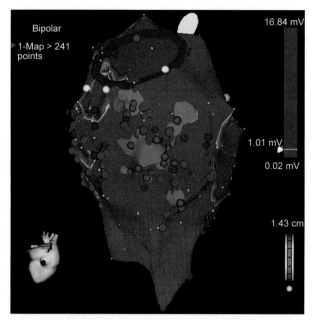

FIGURE 16: Voltage map of the posterior aspect of the left ventricle. Radiofrequency energy was delivered at points marked in red. Sites with an isolated potential during sinus rhythm are marked in blue and sites where there was noncapture are marked in grey[129]

patients undergoing a VT ablation.[132] However, this registry included idiopathic VT patients and the higher complication rates should be expected in sicker patient populations. As with

most complex procedures, complication rates may vary significantly depending on the patient population and operator experience.

EPICARDIAL VT

It is increasingly recognized that VT may arise from the epicardial surface of the heart. Re-entrant epicardial circuits are particularly common among patients with nonischemic cardiomyopathies as well as arrhythmogenic right ventricular dysplasia (ARVD).[133] However, epicardial re-entry has also been documented in 15–23% of patients with postmyocardial infarction VT.[133,134] The presence of an epicardial circuit may be the cause of failure for many endocardially based VT ablations. Various ECG criteria have been proposed to recognize the presence of an epicardial VT circuit.[120,135,136] In general, epicardial circuits manifest a QRS onset that is often slurred, with pseudodelta wave appearance. A pseudodelta wave of more than 34 ms is quite specific for epicardial VT (95%), but less sensitive than an intrinsicoid deflection time of more than 85 ms (defined as the interval measured from the earliest ventricular activation to the peak of the R wave in V2).[120]

Access to the epicardial space can be accomplished by the approach described by Sosa and his colleagues.[134] Using a needle originally designed to enter to epidural space, fluoroscopy is used to approach the epicardium. Contrast injection confirms proper placement of the needle and an introducer sheath is subsequently advanced over a guidewire into the

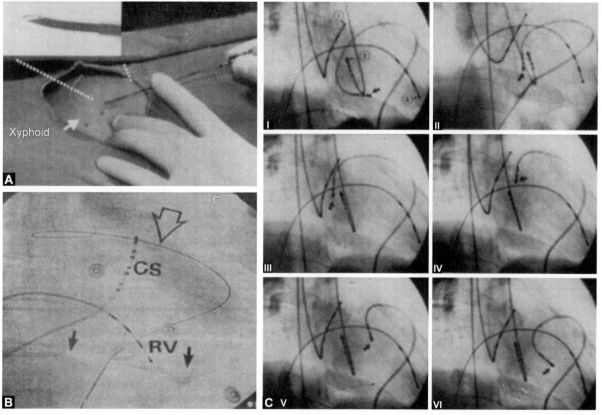

FIGURES 17A TO C: Technique used to insert the mapping and ablation catheter in the pericardial space. (A) A touchy needle is advanced into the pericardial space with the aid of fluoroscopy and contrast injection; (B) A soft guidewire is introduced into the pericardial space (large arrow), where contrast is also present (panel 2). An introducer is then advanced, the guidewire is removed and an ablation catheter is introduced into the pericardial sac to perform epicardial mapping and/or ablation; (C) Demonstrates a right anterior oblique view at 60° obtained by fluoroscopy during epicardial mapping procedure. The epicardial catheter (arrow) is manipulated and placed in different locations of the epicardial space (I to VI), where epicardial electrograms are obtained. (*Source:* Modified from reference 132)

pericardial space (Figs 17A to C). Once access to the pericardial space is achieved, mapping of VT can be performed using methods similar to endocardial ablation. Access to the pericardial space can be challenging in patients with prior cardiac surgery or pericarditis due to the presence of dense adhesions. In these instances, hybrid surgical approaches, such as the use of a subxiphoid window or limited anterior thoracotomy, can be employed to access the epicardium.[137]

The risk of injury to the coronary arteries is a significant concern with epicardial VT ablation and coronary angiography is usually performed to ensure that an ablation site is safe. In addition, the left phrenic nerve courses along the lateral aspect of the left ventricle and pacing should be performed at all ablation sites to confirm the absence of phrenic nerve capture. Sacher and his colleagues recently evaluated the safety of epicardial ablation through retrospective analysis of 156 epicardial VT procedures at three tertiary care centers.[133] Major periprocedural complications occurred in 9% of patients approximately half of which were due to epicardial bleeding. One patient developed asymptomatic right coronary artery stenosis due to cryoablation. There were no periprocedural deaths. It is important to note that these procedures were performed at experienced centers in carefully selected patients. The safety and efficacy of this procedure will likely continue to evolve over the next several years.

IDIOPATHIC VENTRICULAR TACHYCARDIA

Most causes of VT are due to underlying structural heart disease (mainly ischemia or cardiomyopathy). Idiopathic VT (VT in patients without structural heart disease) accounts for 10–20% of VT cases evaluated by electrophysiology centers.[140,141] It is important to recognize these patients as they frequently respond to nonpharmacologic ablative techniques. Idiopathic VT can be broadly classified as polymorphic VT and monomorphic VT (Table 1). In this chapter we will describe the clinical, electrocardiographic (ECG) and electrophysiologic findings for patients with monomorphic idiopathic VT.

OUTFLOW TRACT-VENTRICULAR TACHYCARDIA (OT-VT)

This form of idiopathic VT arises from the outflow tract of the right or the left ventricle. Based on its origin it can be classified

SECTION 4

Electrophysiology

TABLE 1

Idiopathic ventricular tachycardia

Monomorphic ventricular tachycardia	*Polymorphic ventricular tachycardia*
• Outflow tract VT-RVOT-VT, LVOT-VT, aortic cusp VT, Epicardial VT • Fascicular VT-LAF-VT, LPF-VT, Septal VT • Adrenergic monomorphic VT • Annular VT-mitral annular, tricuspid annular	• Long QT syndrome • Brugada syndrome • Short coupled torsades • Short QT syndrome • Catecholaminergic polymorphic VT • Idiopathic VF

(Abbreviations: LAF: Left anterior fascicular; LPF: Left posterior fascicular; LVOT: Left ventricular outflow Tract; RVOT: Right ventricular outflow tract; VF: Ventricular fibrillation; VT: Ventricular tachycardia)

---

as VT that arises from the right ventricular outflow tract (RVOT VT), the left ventricular outflow tract (LVOT VT) and the aortic cusps (Cusp VT) (Table 2).

The RVOT VT is more common in females and is usually seen in third to fifth decade of life while LVOT VT is equally distributed between males and females.[142] Symptoms include palpitations, dizziness, atypical chest pain and syncope. There are three predominant clinical forms of this syndrome: (i) non-sustained repetitive monomorphic VT alternating with periods of sinus rhythm; (ii) paroxysmal exercise-induced sustained VT[143] and (iii) frequent premature ventricular contractions (PVCs) often in a bigeminal fashion. There are also reports of tachycardia-induced cardiomyopathy in patients with a high PVC burden.[144]

RVOT VT

This form of VT is associated with a characteristic ECG morphology of LBBB with inferior axis suggesting origin from the right ventricle outflow tract (Fig. 18). Jadonath et al.[145] evaluated the utility of 12-lead ECG in localizing the site of origin of RVOT VT. A QS pattern in lead avR and monophasic R waves in leads II, III, avF and V6 were noted in each patient at all pacing sites. The anterior sites showed a dominant Q wave or a qR complex in lead I and QS complex in avL. Pacing at

---

TABLE 2

Electrocardiographic findings in outflow tract VT

RVOT VT	*LVOT/aortic cusp VT*

• QS in avR
• Monophasic R wave in II, III, avF, V$_6$
• Septal sites have negative qrs in avL
• Free-wall sites have wider notched qrs in inferior leads and later precordial transition (V$_4$)
• Lead I shows Q wave in anterior sites and dominant R wave in posterior sites
• Phase analysis as measured from the earliest QRS onset to:
  a. Earliest QRS onset is V$_2$
  b. Initial peak/nadir in III $\geq$ 120 ms
  c. Initial peak/nadir in V$_2$ $\geq$ 78 ms
	• Early precordial transition (V$_2$ V$_3$)
	• Taller and broader R wave or RBBB in V$_1$ V$_2$
	• Septal LVOT has dominant Q in V$_1$, qrs II/qrs III > 1
	• Aortomitral LVOT has qR in V$_1$, qrs II/qrs III < 1
	• Cusp VT – notch in V$_5$, lack of S in V$_5$-V$_6$, taller R in inferior leads
	• Lead I – rS in left cusp VT, notched R in noncoronary cusp VT
	• Phase analysis (Cusp VT) as measured from the earliest QRS onset to:
	  d. Earliest QRS onset not in V$_2$
	  e. Initial peak / nadir in III $\leq$ 120 ms
	  f. Initial peak/nadir in V$_2$ $\leq$ 78 ms

(Abbreviations: LVOT: Left ventricular outflow tract; RVOT: Right ventricular outflow tract)

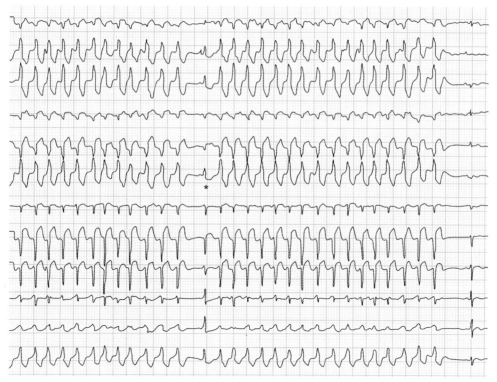

FIGURE 18: Twelve-lead ECG of ventricular tachycardia arising from the right ventricular outflow tract. There is left bundle branch block morphology with late transition (V4) in the precordial leads and an inferior axis in the limb leads. Negative QRS complex in lead avL suggests a septal origin while a q wave in lead I points to anterior focus. Fusion beat is noted in the middle of the tracing (*)

the posterior sites produced a dominant R wave in lead I, QS or R wave in avL and an early precordial transition (R/S ≥ 1 by V3). Coggins et al. showed that septal RVOT VT was associated with negative QRS complex in avL while RVOT VT arising from the lateral wall produced a positive QRS complex in avL.[146] Dixit et al.[147] used pace-mapping techniques to differentiate between RVOT VT arising from the free wall versus the septal wall. They showed that free-wall RVOT VT was associated with wider and notched QRS complexes in the inferior leads and the precordial R wave transition was late (R/S ≥ 1 by V4). Recently OT-VTs arising from near the His-bundle region have been described.[148,149] The characteristic ECG abnormalities for VT arising from this site include a R/RSR' pattern in avL, taller R wave in I, small R waves in inferior leads, taller R waves in V5, V6 and QS pattern in V1 (Fig. 19). Representative example of RVOT VT is shown in Figure 18.

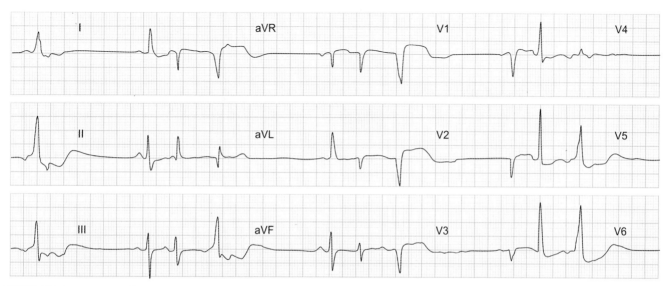

FIGURE 19: Twelve-lead ECG during sinus rhythm showing PVC arising from the para-Hisian region. There is tall R wave in lead I, QS in V1, R in lead II > R in lead III, taller R waves in V5 and V6 and a characteristic rSR in lead avL. Local intracardiac signal at this site preceded the QRS onset by 25 ms

CHAPTER 39

Surgical and Catheter Ablation of Cardiac Arrhythmias

Idiopathic VT may arise just proximal to the outflow tract in the para-Hisian region. This ECG will mimic that of RVOT except for the characteristic rSr1 in avL (Fig. 19).

Idiopathic VT arising from the pulmonary artery (PA) has also been described.[150,151] The origin of VT from the PA is thought to be from remnants of embryonic muscle sleeves that have been noted in amphibian and mammalian outflow tract.[152] This is supported by the presence of a sharp potential at these sites that preceded the onset of ventricular activation during VT.[150] Sekiguchi et al.[151] noted the following ECG characteristics during VT that favor PA VT as compared to RVOT VT: (i) Larger R-wave amplitude in inferior leads; (ii) The ratio of the Q-wave amplitude in avL/avR was larger in the PA group; (iii) Significantly larger R/S amplitude in lead V2 in patients with PA VT than in those with RVOT VT.

LVOT VT

The VT arising from the LVOT shares similar characteristics to the RVOT VT due to a common embryonic origin. This form of VT can be differentiated from the RVOT VT by differences in QRS morphology (Fig. 20). The LVOT VT is suggested by LBBB morphology with inferior axis with small R waves in V1 and early precordial transition (R/S ≥ 1 by V2 or V3) or RBBB morphology with inferior axis[153-156] and presence of S wave in V6.[157,158] The LVOT VT arising from the septal para-Hisian region has an ECG pattern of QS or Qr in V1 with early precordial transition and ratio of QRS in leads II/III greater than 1 while LVOT VT arising from the aortomitral continuity has a characteristic qR pattern in V1 with a ratio of QRS in leads II/III less than or equal to 1.[159]

CUSP VT

Case reports of idiopathic VT with LBBB morphology and inferior axis that failed ablation in the RVOT but were successfully ablated in the left coronary cusp[160,161] were described in 1999. Kanagaratnam et al.[162] reported the ECG characteristics of 12 patients with outflow tract VT that required ablation in the aortic sinus of Valsalva. All patients had LBBB inferior axis morphology with taller monophasic R waves in inferior leads and an early precordial R wave transition by V2 or V3. The VT arising from the left cusp had an rS pattern in lead I, and VT arising from the noncoronary cusp had a notched R wave in lead I. Ouyang et al.[163] evaluated the ECG differences between 8 patients with RVOT VT and 7 patients with VT arising from the aortic sinus cusp (5 from left sinus and 2 from right sinus). They found that a broader R wave duration and a taller R/S wave amplitude in V1 and V2 favored VT arising from the aortic cusp. Yang[164] used phase differences in the 12-lead ECG to differentiate between RVOT VT (32 patients) and aortic cusp VT (15 patients). They showed that RVOT VT was associated with earliest ventricular activation in V2 and a shorter time from onset of ECG to peak/nadir in lead III and V2.

EPICARDIAL VT

Outflow tract VT occasionally arises from the epicardial surface of the heart that requires ablation in the great cardiac vein or via pericardial approach.[148,165-167] Ito et al.[148] showed that the Q wave ratio of avL to avR greater than 1.4 or an S wave amplitude in V1 greater than 1.2 mV was useful in differentiating between epicardial VT from aortic cusp VT. Daniels et al.[167] showed that 9% of the patients with idiopathic VT referred to their institution had an epicardial focus. They found that a

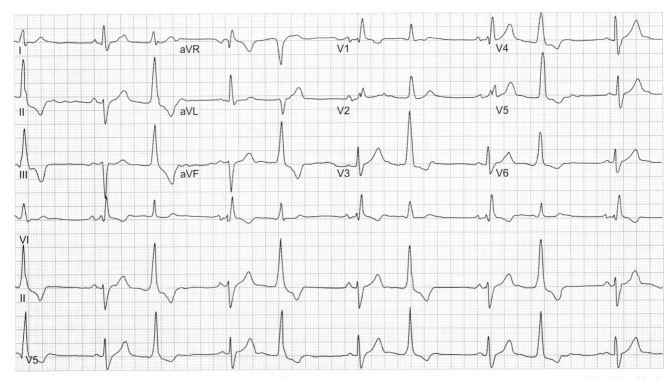

FIGURE 20: Twelve-lead ECG during sinus rhythm showing PVC arising from the left ventricular outflow tract that was successfully ablated in the aortomitral continuity region. There is qR wave in lead V1 that differentiates this from a septal LVOT focus that has a QS or Qr pattern in lead V1

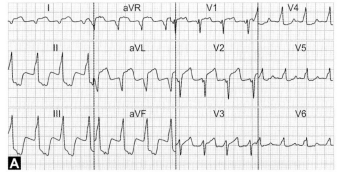

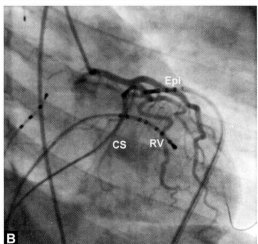

FIGURES 21A AND B: (A) Twelve-lead ECG of VT that was successfully ablated on the epicardial surface of the heart. The precordial maximum deflection index is greater than 55 (calculated by measuring the time from the QRS onset to the earliest maximum deflection (nadir or peak) in precordial leads and dividing it by the total QRS duration). (B) Fluoroscopic view of the catheter position with ablation catheter (Epi) on the epicardial surface of the heart, right ventricular (RV) catheter and coronary sinus catheter (CS). The site of origin of the VT is very close to the left anterior descending (LAD) coronary artery

delayed precordial maximum deflection index greater than or equal to 55 (calculated by measuring the time from the QRS onset to the earliest maximum deflection (nadir or peak) in precordial leads and dividing it by the total QRS duration) differentiates this form of idiopathic epicardial VT from other forms of outflow tract VT (Figs 21A and B). Recently idiopathic VT arising from the crux of the heart has been described that presents as rapid VT usually triggered by exercise and can lead to hemodynamic compromise.[168]

The 12-lead ECG morphology of this VT is similar to that of maximally pre-excited posteroseptal accessory pathways with QRS transition from V1 to V2 and QS complexes in inferior leads (Fig. 22). This can be successfully ablated in the middle cardiac vein or via an epicardial approach.

MANAGEMENT

The majority of the patients with outflow tract VT have a benign course with a very low-risk of sudden death.[169-171] It can be associated with tachycardia-induced cardiomyopathy that improves after successful treatment.[144,172] It is important to differentiate this form of VT from VT associated with arrhythmogenic right ventricular cardiomyopathy (ARVC) that is also associated with LBBB morphology. The ARVC is associated with a worse prognosis and is responsible for sudden death especially in young adults less than 35 years old.[173,174]

Acute termination of RVOT VT can be achieved with adenosine, carotid sinus massage, verapamil and lidocaine. Beta-blockers are especially effective for those with exercise-induced outflow tract VT and a synergistic action is noted with calcium channel blockers. Antiarrhythmic agents like procainamide, flecainide, amiodarone and sotalol are also effective in these patients. There was a trend toward greater efficacy with sotalol in a study of 23 patients with RVOT VT.[175] Nicorandil, a

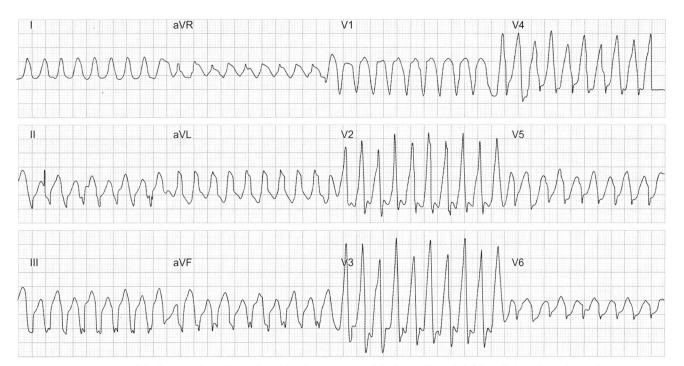

FIGURE 22: Twelve-lead ECG of ventricular tachycardia arising from the crux of the heart. There is left bundle branch block morphology with early transition (V2) in the precordial leads and qs complex in the inferior leads. This matches the 12-lead ECG morphology of maximally pre-excited posteroseptal accessory pathway. This VT was successfully ablated via an epicardial approach

potassium channel opener, has been reported to terminate and suppress adenosine-sensitive VT.[176]

CATHETER ABLATION

Catheter ablation using RF energy to cure patients with outflow tract VT is associated with a high success rate due to the focal origin of this form of VT. The 12-lead ECG is a useful initial guide to localize the site of origin of the tachycardia. Intracardiac mapping to select the optimal site for ablation include activation mapping (earliest local intracardiac electrogram that precedes the onset of surface QRS during VT) and pace mapping (pacing the ventricle from a selected site in sinus rhythm to match the 12-lead morphology of the spontaneous or induced VT). The use of three dimensional (3D) electroanatomical mapping systems reduces fluoroscopic exposure and improves the efficacy of catheter ablation.[177,178] The success rate of catheter ablation for outflow tract VT reported from various series is greater than 90%[132,179] with a recurrence rate of 5% (mainly in the first year). Serious complications include induction of RBBB (2%), cardiac perforation and tamponade (1%); there has been one death reported secondary to complications from RVOT perforation.[146] Ablation for LVOT VT has been associated with occlusion of a coronary artery.[180] Failure of endocardial RF ablation can be due to epicardial location of the VT focus (Fig. 21). Epicardial ablation can be achieved by a subxiphoid technique of pericardial puncture as described by Sosa[181] or by ablating within the great cardiac vein. Coronary angiograms are performed prior to epicardial ablation and ablation in the aortic sinus to avoid ablation close to the coronary arteries that can lead to arterial damage and thrombus formation. Intracardiac echocardiography has also been used to provide real time visualization of the relationship between the ablation site and the coronary arteries during ablation in the aortic sinus.[182]

IDIOPATHIC LEFT VENTRICULAR TACHYCARDIA (ILVT) OR FASCICULAR VT

This form of VT arises from the fascicles in the left ventricle. Based on the QRS morphology and the site of origin it can be classified as left posterior fascicular VT (LPF VT), left anterior fascicular VT (LAF VT) and left upper septal VT (Septal VT).[183]

This form of idiopathic VT was first described by Zipes et al.[184] in 1979 with the following characteristic triad: (i) induction with atrial pacing; (ii) the RBBB morphology with left axis deviation and (iii) occurrence in patients without structural heart disease. In 1981, Belhassen et al.[185] showed that this form of VT could be terminated by verapamil, the fourth identifying feature. In 1988, Ohe et al.[186] described another form of this VT with RBBB and right axis deviation that required ablation in the region of the left anterior fascicle. Shimoike[187] and Nogami[183] described a form of idiopathic VT with narrow QRS that required ablation in the upper LV septum.

The ILVT is typically seen in patients between the ages of 15–40 years with an earlier presentation in females.[142,188-193] Most of the affected patients are males (60–70%). The symptoms include palpitations, fatigue, dyspnea, dizziness and presyncope. Syncope and sudden death are very rare.[188] Most of the episodes occur at rest; however, this form of VT can be triggered by exercise and emotional stress.[193,194] Incessant tachycardia

leading to tachycardia-induced cardiomyopathy has also been described.[191]

ECG RECOGNITION

The baseline 12-lead ECG is normal in most patients or it may show transient T wave inversions related to T wave memory shortly after a tachycardia episode terminates. The 12-lead ECG of left posterior fascicular VT (LPF VT) shows RBBB with left axis deviation suggesting an exit site from the inferoposterior ventricular septum (Fig. 23). Nogami et al.[195] reported 6 patients with left anterior fascicular VT (LAF VT) that showed a RBBB with right axis deviation with the earliest ventricular activation in the anterolateral wall of the LV in all patients. Three patients had a distal type of LAF VT with QS or rS morphology in leads I, V5 and V6 and the other 3 had proximal type of LAF VT with RS or Rs morphology in the same leads. Figure 24 shows PVCs that were successfully ablated at the distal LAF. The QRS duration in fascicular VT varies 140–150 msec and the duration from the beginning of the QRS onset to the nadir of the S-wave (RS interval) in the precordial leads is 60–80 msec unlike VT associated with structural heart disease that is usually associated with longer duration of QRS and RS intervals. This makes it difficult to differentiate fascicular VT from SVT with aberrancy using the criteria based on QRS morphology and RS interval.[196-198]

MANAGEMENT

The long-term prognosis of patients with fascicular VT without structural heart disease is very good. Patients with mild symptoms without medical therapy did not show progression of their arrhythmias in a study of 37 patients with verapamil sensitive VT during an average follow-up of 5.8 years,[190] however those with incessant tachycardia can develop a cardiomyopathy.[191] Acute termination of VT can be achieved with intravenous verapamil (adenosine and Valsalva maneuvers are ineffective). Patients with moderate symptoms can be treated with oral verapamil (120–480 mg/day).

CATHETER ABLATION

The RF catheter ablation is an appropriate management strategy for patients with severe symptoms or those intolerant or resistant to antiarrhythmic therapy. Nakagawa[194] and Wen[199] showed that successful ablation could be performed by targeting the earliest high-frequency Purkinje potential (and not the earliest ventricular activation) during VT and this could be recorded far from the exit site that shows the perfect pace map. Tsuchiya et al.[200] targeted a site recording both a late diastolic potential and a presystolic potential and showed tachycardia termination with catheter pressure at these sites. Nogami et al.[201] used an octapolar catheter to record double potentials during VT from the mid-septal LV and successfully terminated VT during catheter ablation at these sites. Ouyang et al.[202] used a 3D electroanatomical mapping system to record sites with retrograde Purkinje (retro PP) potential during sinus rhythm (sharp low amplitude potentials that followed a Purkinje potential and local ventricular electrogram) in patients with ILVT. They showed that the site recording the earliest retro PP during sinus rhythm correlated with early diastolic potential during VT. They suggest

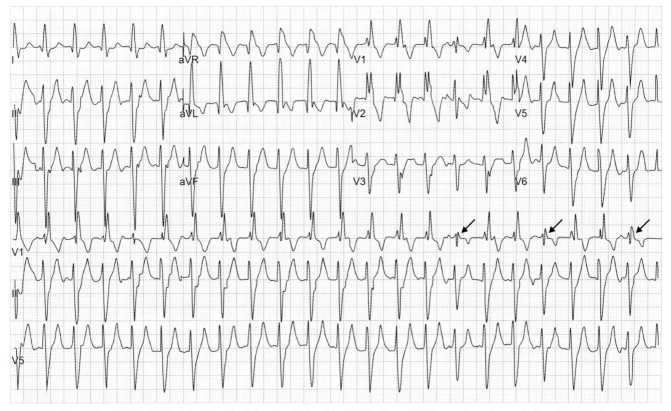

FIGURE 23: Twelve-lead ECG of VT arising from the left posterior fascicle (ILVT) with an RBBB superior axis morphology. The duration of the QRS complex and the RS interval are narrower than that of noted in VT associated with structural heart disease. However, the presence of AV dissociation and fusion beats (arrows) is diagnostic of VT. (*Source:* Modified from Badhwar et al. Idiopathic ventricular tachycardia: diagnosis and management. Curr Probl Cardiol. 2007;32:7-43)

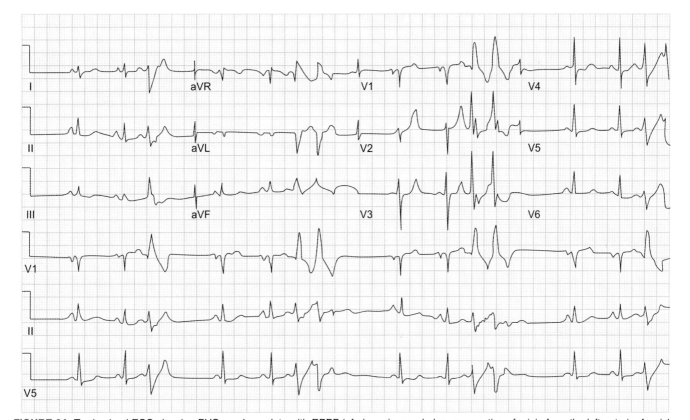

FIGURE 24: Twelve-lead ECG showing PVCs and couplets with RBBB inferior axis morphology suggestive of origin from the left anterior fascicle. The QRS complex in leads I, V5 and V6 show an rS morphology that is consistent with an exit site in the distal part of the left anterior fascicle where this VT was successfully ablated (*Source:* Modified from Badhwar et al. Idiopathic ventricular tachycardia: diagnosis and management. Curr Probl Cardiol. 2007;32:7-43)

that use of the earliest retro PP as a target for ablation when VT cannot be induced in the electrophysiology lab. Chen et al.[203] used a noncontact mapping system to create a successful linear ablation line perpendicular to the wavefront propagation direction of the left posterior fascicle in sinus rhythm in patients with nonsustained or noninducible VT. Ma et al.[204] have used development of a left posterior fascicular block (LPFB) pattern on the surface ECG as an end point for successful ablation in patients with noninducible ILVT. However, most authors have found that successful ablation occurs in majority of the patients without the need for LPFB pattern on the ECG. Long-term success after catheter ablation is more than 92% with rare complications that include mitral regurgitation due to catheter entrapment in the chordae of the mitral valve leaflet and aortic regurgitation due to damage to the aortic valve using a retrograde aortic approach.[146,193,194,199, 205-207]

MITRAL ANNULAR VT

There have been case reports of adenosine sensitive monomorphic VT that was successfully ablated at the anterobasal LV.[208-210] Tada et al.[211] were the first group to describe the prevalence and ECG characteristics of mitral annular VT (MAVT). Their definition was based on the ratio of atrial to ventricular electrograms less than 1 and the amplitude of the atrial and ventricular electrograms greater than 0.08 and 0.5 mV respectively at the successful ablation site.

Tada et al. reported that MAVT was noted in 5% of all the cases of idiopathic VT while Kumagai et al. showed that MAVT accounts for 49% of idiopathic repetitive monomorphic VT arising from the left ventricle (other sites included coronary cusps and inferoseptal region). Patients presented with palpitations and were noted to have repetitive monomorphic VT or frequent monomorphic PVCs. Tachycardia was noted spontaneously or initiated with isoproterenol. Termination was noted with adenosine (10–40 mg) and intravenous verapamil in some patients. The VT entrainment was not observed in any of the sustained episodes.

ECG RECOGNITION

Tada et al.[211] showed that the surface ECG in all patients with MAVT had an RBBB pattern (transition in V1 or V2); S-wave in V6 and monophasic R or Rs in leads V2–V6. They further classified MAVT into three categories depending on the site of origin as being anterolateral (AL) MAVT (58%), posterior (Pos) MAVT (11%) and posteroseptal (PS) MAVT (31%). In AL-MAVT, the polarity of the QRS complex in leads I and avL was negative and positive in the inferior leads; Pos-MAVT and PS-MAVT showed a negative polarity in the inferior leads and positive in leads I and avL. The AL-MAVT and Pos-MAVT showed a longer QRS duration and "notching" in the late phase of the R wave/Q wave in the inferior leads suggesting an origin from the free wall. This feature was not observed in PS-MAVT. Pos-MAVT showed a dominant R in V1 while PS-MAVT had a negative QRS component in V1 (qR, qr, rs, rS or QS). The Q-wave amplitude ratio of lead III to lead II was greater in PS-MAVT than in Pos-MAVT. Figure 25 shows the representative ECG from PVCs arising from the lateral MA. Kumagai et al.[212] illustrated the delta-wave like beginning on the QRS complex during VT and showed a similarity between the MAVT and the maximally pre-excited left-sided accessory pathways in terms of QRS morphology.

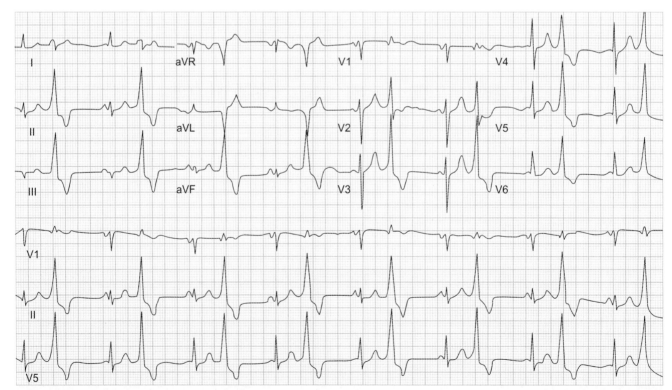

FIGURE 25: Twelve-lead ECG during sinus rhythm showing PVCs arising from the lateral mitral annulus. There is precordial concordance with negative QRS complexes in leads I, avL and inferior axis which is similar to the ECG morphology of a maximally pre-excited accessory pathway located on the lateral mitral annulus

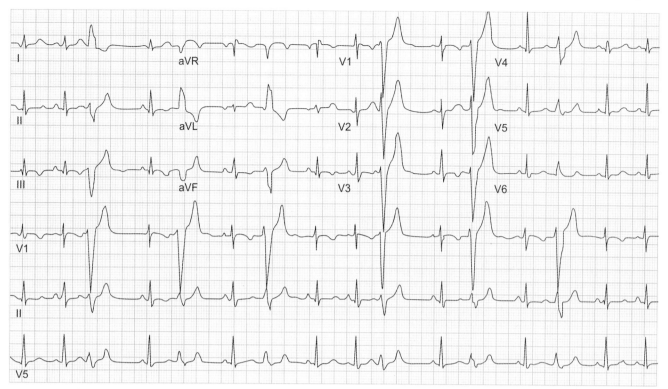

FIGURE 26: Twelve-lead ECG during sinus rhythm showing PVCs arising from the posterolateral tricuspid annulus. There is LBBB in V1 with late transition, left axis and notching in the inferior leads

CATHETER ABLATION

Electrophysiology mapping was performed using activation mapping and pace mapping to localize the site of origin of the VT. All successful sites had an adequate atrial and ventricular electrogram satisfying the criteria for mitral annular origin and a potential was noted before the local ventricular electrogram in most of the patients. Pace mapping was useful in patients with nonsustained tachycardia. Acute success was obtained in all the patients in both the series; however, there was a recurrence rate of 8% in one series.[212]

TRICUSPID ANNULAR VT

Recently VT arising from the TA has been described. This form of VT was noted in 8% of the patients presenting with idiopathic VT.[213] This was preferentially seen to originate from the septal region (74%) than the free wall (26%). Most of the septal VT was seen to arise from the anteroseptal region (72%). The septal VT had an early transition in precordial leads (V3), narrower QRS complexes, Qs in lead V1 with absence of "notching" in the inferior leads while the free-wall VT was associated with late precordial transition (> V3), wider QRS complexes, absence of Q wave in lead V1 and "notching" in the inferior leads (the timing of the second peak of the "notched" QRS complex in the inferior leads corresponded precisely with the left ventricular free-wall activation). Figure 26 shows ECG characteristics of PVCs originating from posterolateral TA. The success rate for catheter ablation of the free-wall VT was 90% as compared to 57% in the septal group due to the presence of junctional rhythm and the likelihood of impairing AV nodal conduction with catheter ablation.

SUMMARY

In summary, VT occurring in patients without structural heart disease accounts for approximately 10–20% of VTs evaluated at large referral centers. It is often difficult to differentiate this form of VT from SVT with aberration based on morphology alone. Depending on tachycardia mechanism the arrhythmia may respond to beta-blockers, Ca^{++} channel blockers or to vagal maneuvers. In addition, these arrhythmias are susceptible to cure by catheter ablation.

REFERENCES

1. Waldo AL, Wit AL. Mechanisms of cardiac arrhythmias. Lancet. 1993;341:1189-93.
2. Porter MJ, Morton JB, Denman R, et al. Influence of age and gender on the mechanism of supraventricular tachycardia. Heart Rhythm. 2004;1:393-6.
3. Blomstrom-Lundqvist C, Scheinman MM, Aliot EM, et al. ACC/AHA/ESC Guidelines for the Management of Patients with Supraventricular Arrhythmias–Executive Summary. A Report of the American College of Cardiology/American Heart Association Task Force on Practice Guidelines and the European Society of Cardiology Committee for Practice Guidelines (Writing Committee to Develop Guidelines for the Management of Patients with Supraventricular Arrhythmias) developed in collaboration with NASPE-Heart Rhythm Society. J Am Coll Cardiol. 2003;42:1493-531.
4. Durrer D, Schoo L, Schuilenburg RM, et al. The role of premature beats in the initiation and the termination of supraventricular tachycardia in the Wolff-Parkinson-White syndrome. Circulation. 1967;36:644-62.
5. Wellens HJ, Schuilenburg RM, Durrer D. Electrical stimulation of the heart in patients with Wolff-Parkinson-White syndrome, type A. Circulation. 1971;43:99-114.

6. Scherlag BJ, Lau SH, Helfant RH, et al. Catheter technique for recording His bundle activity in man. Circulation. 1969;39:13-8.

7. Gallagher JJ, Pritchett ELC, Sealy WC, et al. The preexcitation syndrome. Circulation. 1976;54:571-91.

8. Jackman WM, Friday KJ, Scherlag BJ, et al. Direct endocardial recording from an accessory atrioventricular pathway, localization of the site of block effect of antiarrhythmic drugs and attempt at nonsurgical ablation. Circulation. 1983;68:906-16.

9. Dreifus LS, Nichols H, Morse D, et al. Control of recurrent tachycardia of Wolff-Parkinson-White syndrome by surgical ligature of the A-V bundle. Circulation. 1968;38:1030-6.

10. Edmunds JH, Ellison RG, Crews TL. Surgically induced atrioventricular block as treatment for recurrent atrial tachycardia in Wolff-Parkinson-White syndrome. Circulation. 1969;39:105-11.

11. Durrer D, Roos JP. Epicardial excitation of ventricles in patient with Wolff-Parkinson-White syndrome (type B). Circulation. 1967;35:15-21.

12. Burchell HB, Frye RL, Anderson MW, et al. Atrioventricular and ventriculoatrial excitation in Wolff-Parkinson-White syndrome (type B). Circulation. 1967;36:663-9.

13. Cobb FR, Blumenschein SD, Sealy WC, et al. Successful surgical interruption of the bundle of Kent in a patient with Wolff-Parkinson-White syndrome. Circulation. 1968;38:1018-29.

14. Iwa T, Kazui T, Sugii S, et al. Surgical treatment of Wolff-Parkinson-White syndrom. Kyobu Geka. 1970;23:513-8.

15. Scheinman MM, Morady F, Hess DS, et al. Catheter-induced ablation of the atrioventricular junction to control refractory supraventricular arrhythmias. JAMA. 1982;248:851-5.

16. Morady F, Scheinman MM. Transvenous catheter ablation of a posteroseptal accesory pathway in a patient with the Wolff-Parkinson-White syndrome. N Engl J Med. 1984;310:705-7.

17. Morady F, Scheinman MM, Kou WH, et al. Long-term results of catheter ablation of a posteroseptal accessory atrioventricular connection in 48 patients. Circulation. 1989;79:1160-70.

18. Warin JF, Haissaguerre M, Lemetayer P, et al. Catheter ablation of accessory pathways with a direct approach. Results in 35 patients. Circulation. 1988;78:800-15.

19. Borggrefe M, Budde T, Podczeck A, et al. High frequency alternating current ablation of an accessory pathway in humans. J Am Coll Cardiol. 1987;10:576-82.

20. Jackman WM, Wang XZ, Friday KJ, et al. Catheter ablation of accessory atrioventricular pathways (Wolff-Parkinson-White syndrome) by radiofrequency current. N Engl J Med. 1991;334:1605-11.

21. Kuck KH, Schlüter M, Geiger M, et al. Radiofrequency current catheter ablation of accessory atrioventricular pathways. Lancet. 1991;337:1557-61.

22. Calkins H, Sousa J, El-Atassi R, et al. Diagnosis and cure of the Wolff-Parkinson-White syndrome or paroxysmal supraventricular tachycardias during a single electrophysiologic test. N Engl J Med. 1991;324:1612-8.

23. Scheinman MM. NASPE survey on catheter ablation. Pacing Clin Electrophysiol. 1995;18:1474-8.

24. Hindricks G for the Multicentre European Radiofrequency Survey (MERFS) investigators of the Work Group on Arrhythmias of the European Society of Cardiology. The Multicentre European radiofrequency survey (MERFS): complications of radiofrequency catheter ablation of arrhythmias. Eur Heart J. 1993;14:1644-53.

25. Moe GK, Preston JB, Burlington H. Physiologic evidence for a dual A-V transmission system. Circ Res. 1956;4:357-75.

26. Mendez C, Moe GK. Demonstration of a dual A-V nodal conduction system in the isolated rabbit heart. Circ Res. 1966;19:378-93.

27. Goldreyer BN, Bigger JT. The site of re-entry in paroxysmal supraventricular tachycardia in man. Circulation. 1971;43:15-26.

28. Denes P, Wu D, Dhingra RC, et al. Demonstration of dual A-V nodal pathways in patients with paroxysmal supraventricular tachycardia. Circulation. 1973;48:549-55.

29. Jais P, Haissaguerre M, Shah DC, et al. Successful radiofrequency ablation of a slow atrioventricular nodal pathway on the left posterior atrial septum. Pacing Clin Electrophysiol. 1999;22:525-7.

30. Sousa J, El-Atassi R, Rosenheck S, et al. Radiofrequency catheter ablation of the atrioventricular junction from the left ventricle. Circulation. 1991;84:567-71.

31. Ross D, Johnson D, Denniss A, et al. Curative surgery for atrioventricular junctional ("AV nodal") re-entrant tachycardia. J Am Coll Cardiol. 1985;6:1383-92.

32. Cox J, Holman W, Cain M. Cryosurgical treatment of atrioventricular node re-entrant tachycardia. Circulation. 1987;76:1329-36.

33. Guiraudon GM, Klein GJ, van Hemel N, et al. Anatomically guided surgery to the AV node. AV nodal skeletonization: experience in 26 patients with AV nodal re-entrant tachycardia. Eur J Cardiothorac Surg. 1990;4:464-5.

34. Ruder MA, Mead RH, Smith NA, et al. Comparison of pre- and postoperative conduction patterns in patients surgically cured of atrioventricular node re-entrant tachycardia. J Am Coll Cardiol. 1990;17:397-402.

35. Heidbüchel H, Jackman WM. Characterization of subforms of AV nodal re-entrant tachycardia. Europace. 2004;6:316-29.

36. Haissaguerre M, Warin J, Lemetayer P, et al. Closed-chest ablation of retrograde conduction in patients with atrioventricular nodal re-entrant tachycardia. N Engl J Med. 1989;320:426-33.

37. Epstein LM, Scheinman MM, Langberg JJ, et al. Percutaneous catheter modification of the atrioventricular node: a potential cure for atrioventricular nodal tachycardia. Circulation. 1989;80:757-68.

38. Lee MA, Morady F, Kadish A, et al. Catheter modification of the atrioventricular junction with radiofrequency energy for control of atrioventricular nodal re-entry tachycardia. Circulation. 1991;83:827-35.

39. Jackman WM, Beckman KJ, McClelland JH, et al. Treatment of supraventricular tachycardia due to atrioventricular nodal re-entry by radiofrequency catheter ablation of slow-pathway conduction. N Engl J Med. 1992;327:313-8.

40. Haissaguerre M, Gaita F, Fischer B, et al. Elimination of atrioventricular nodal re-entrant tachycardia using discrete slow potentials to guide application of radiofrequency energy. Circulation. 1992;85:2162-75.

41. Kalbfleisch SJ, Strickberger SA, Williamson B, et al. Randomized comparison of anatomic and electrogram mapping approaches to ablation of the slow pathway of atrioventricular node re-entrant tachycardia. J Am Coll Cardiol. 1994;23:716-23.

42. Morady F. Catheter ablation of supraventricular tachycardia: state of the art. J Cardiovasc Electrophysiol. 2004;15:124-39.

43. Li YG, Gronedfeld G, Bender B, et al. Risk of development of delayed atrioventricular block after slow pathway modification in patients with atrioventricular nodal re-entrant tachycardia and pre-existing prolonged PR interval. Eur Heart J. 2001;22:89-95.

44. Sra JS, Jazayeri MR, Blanck Z, et al. Slow pathway ablation in patients with atrioventricular node re-entrant tachycardia and a prolonged PR interval. J Am Coll Cardiol. 1994;24:1064-8.

45. Lee SH, Chen SA, Tai CT, et al. Atrioventricular node re-entrant tachycardia in patients with a prolonged AH interval during sinus rhythm: clinical features, electrophysiologic characteristics and results of radiofrequency ablation. J Interv Card Electrophysiol. 1997;1:305-10.

46. Skanes AC, Dubuc M, Klein GJ, et al. Cryothermal ablation of the slow pathway for the elimination of atrioventricular nodal re-entrant tachycardia. Circulation. 2000;102:2856-60.

47. Wolff L, Parkinson J, White PD. Bundle-branch block with short P-R interval in healthy young people prone to paroxysmal tachycardia. Am Heart J. 1930;5:685-704.

48. Kent AFS. A conducting path between the right auricle and the external wall of the right ventricle in the heart of the mammal. J Physiol. 1914;48:57.

49. Wood FC, Wolferth CC, Geckeler GD. Histologic demonstration of accessory muscular connections between auricle and ventricle in a case of short P-R interval and prolonged QRS complex. Amer Heart J. 1943;25:454-62.

50. Öhnell RF. Pre-excitation, cardiac abnormality, pathophysiological, pathoanatomical and clinical studies of excitatory spread phenomenon bearing upon the problem of the WPW (Wolff, Parkinson, and White) electrocardiogram and paroxysmal tachycardia. Acta Med Scand. 1944;152:1-167.

51. Timmermans C, Smeets JL, Rodriguez LM, et al. Aborted sudden death in the Wolff-Parkinson-White syndrome. Am J Cardiol. 1995;76:492-4.

52. Munger TM, Parker DL, Hammill SC, et al. A population study of the natural history of Wolff-Parkinson-White syndrome in Olmsted County, Minnesota, 1953-1989. Circulation. 1993;87:866-73.

53. Calkins H, Yong P, Miller JM, et al. Catheter ablation of accessory pathways, atrioventricular nodal re-entrant tachycardia, and the atrioventricular junction: final results of a prospective, multicenter clinical trial. The Atakr Multicenter Investigators Group. Circuilation. 1999;99:262-70.

54. Gaita F, Haissaguerre M, Giustetto C, et al. Safety and efficacy of cryoablation of accessory pathways adjacent to the normal conduction system. J Cardiovasc Electrophysiol. 2003;14:825-9.

55. Calkins H, Langberg J, Sousa J, et al. Radiofrequency catheter ablation of accessory atrioventricular connections in 250 patients. Abbreviated therapeutic approach to Wolff-Parkinson-White syndrome. Circulation. 1992;85:1337-46.

56. Morady F. Catheter ablation of supraventricular arrhythmias: state of the art. Pacing Clin Electrophysiol. 2004;27:125-42.

57. Lesh MD, Van Hare G, Kao AK, et al. Radiofrequency catheter ablation for Wolff-Parkinson-White syndrome associated with a coronary sinus diverticulum. Pacing Clin Electrophysiol. 1991;14:1479-84.

58. Beukema WP, Van Dessel PF, Van Hemel NM, et al. Radiofrequency catheter ablation of accessory pathways associated with a coronary sinus diverticulum. Eur Heart J. 1994;15:1415-8.

59. Langberg JJ, Man KC, Vorperian VR, et al. Recognition and catheter ablation of subepicardial accessory pathways. J Am Coll Cardiol. 1993;22:1100-4.

60. Valderrabano M, Cesario DA, Ji S, et al. Percutaneous epicardial mapping during ablation of difficult accessory pathways as an alternative to cardiac surgery. Heart Rhythm. 2004;1:311-6.

61. Scheinman MM. History of Wolff-Parkinson-White syndrome. Pacing Clin Electrophysiol. 2005;28:152-6.

62. Josephson ME. Clinical cardiac electrophysiology: techniques and interpretations, 3rd edition. Philadelphia, PA: Lippincott Williams and Wilkins; 2002.

63. Garson A Jr, Gillette PC. Electrophysiologic studies of supraventricular tachycardia in children II. Prediction of specific mechanism by noninvasive features. Am Heart J. 1981;102:383-8.

64. Engelstein ED, Lippman N, Stein KM, et al. Mechanism-specific effects of adenosine on atrial tachycardia. Circulation 1994;89:2645-54.

65. Roberts-Thomson KC, Kistler PM, Kalman JM. Atrial tachycardia: mechanisms, diagnosis, and anatomic location. Curr Probl Cardiol. 2005;30:529-73.

66. Kistler PM, Roberts-Thomson KC, Haqqani HM, et al. P-wave morphology in focal atrial tachycardia: development of an algorithm to predict the anatomic site of origin. J Am Coll Cardiol. 2006;48:1010-7.

67. Schmitt C, Zrenner B, Schneider M, et al. Clinical experience with a novel multielectrode basket catheter in right atrial tachycardias. Circulation. 1999;99:2414-22.

68. Natale A, Breeding L, Tomassoni G, et al. Ablation of right and left ectopic atrial tachycardias using a three-dimensional nonfluoroscopic mapping system. Am J Cardiol. 1998;82:989-92.

69. Lesh MD, Kalman JM, Olgin JE. New approaches to treatment of atrial flutter and tachycardia. J Cardiovasc Electrophysiol. 1996;7:368-81.

70. Wong T, Segal OR, Markides V, et al. Cryoablation of focal atrial tachycardia originating close to the atrioventricular node. J Cardiovasc Electrophysiol. 2004;15:838.

71. Tsai CF, Tai CT, Chen SA. Catheter ablation of atrial tachycardia. In: Jalife J, Zipes DP (Eds). Cardiac electrophysiology: from cell to bedside, 4th edition. Philadelphia, PA: Saunders; 2004. pp. 1060-8.

72. Natale A, Newby KH, Pisano E, et al. Prospective randomized comparison of antiarrhythmic therapy versus first-line radiofrequency ablation in patients with atrial flutter. J Am Coll Cardiol. 2000;35:1898-904.

73. Waldo AL, MacLean WAH, Karp RB, et al. Entrainment and interruption of atrial flutter with atrial pacing. Studies in man following open heart surgery. Circulation. 1977;56:737-45.

74. Klein GJ, Guiraudon GM, Sharma AD, et al. Demonstration of macrore-entry and feasibility of operative therapy in the common type of atrial flutter. Am J Cardiol. 1986;57:587-91.

75. Saoudi N, Atallah G, Kirkorian G, et al. Catheter ablation of the atrial myocardium in human type I atrial flutter. Circulation. 1990;81:762-71.

76. Chauvin M, Brechenmacher C. A clinical study of the application of endocardial fulguration in the treatment of recurrent atrial flutter. Pacing and Clin Electrophysiol. 1989;12:219-24.

77. Feld GK, Fleck RP, Chen PS, et al. Radiofrequency catheter ablation for the treatment of human type 1 atrial flutter: identification of a critical zone in the re-entrant circuit by endocardial mapping techniques. Circulation. 1992;86:1233-40.

78. Cosio FG, Lopez-Gil M, Goicolea A, et al. Radiofrequency ablation of the inferior vena cava-tricuspid valve isthmus in common atrial flutter. Am J Cardiol. 1993;71:705-9.

79. Olgin JE, Kalman JM, Fitzpatrick AP, et al. Role of right atrial structures as barriers to conduction during human type I atrial flutter. Activation and entrainment mapping guided by intracardiac echocardiography. Circulation. 1995;92:1839-48.

80. Cheng J, Scheinman MM. Acceleration of typical atrial flutter due to double-wave re-entry induced by programmed electrical stimulation. Circulation. 1998;97:1589-96.

81. Cheng J, Cabeen WR, Scheinman MM. Right atrial flutter due to lower loop re-entry; mechanism and anatomic substrates. Circulation. 1999;99:1700-5.

82. Yang Y, Cheng J, Bochoeyer A, et al. Atypical right atrial flutter patterns. Circulation. 2001;103:3092-8.

83. Zhang S, Younis G, Hariharan R, et al. Lower loop re-entry as a mechanism of clockwise right atrial flutter. Circulation. 2004;109:1630-5.

84. Yang Y, Varma N, Keung EC, et al. Re-entry within the cavotricuspid isthmus: an isthmus dependent circuit. PACE. 2005;28:808-18.

85. Yang Y, Varma N, Badhwar N, et al. Prospective Observations in the Clinical and Electrophysiological Characteristics of Intra-Isthmus Re-entry. J Cardiovasc Electrophysiol. 2010;21:1-8.

86. Poty H, Saoudi N, Nair M, et al. Radiofrequency catheter ablation of atrial flutter. Further insights into the various types of isthmus block: application to ablation during sinus rhythm. Circulation. 1996;94:3204-13.

87. Shah DC, Haissaguerre M, Takahashi A, et al. Differential pacing for distinguishing block from persistent conduction through an ablation line. Circulation. 2000;102:1517-22.

88. Tada H, Oral H, Sticherling C, et al. Double potential along the ablation line as a guide to radiofrequency ablation of typical atrial flutter. J Am Coll Cardiol. 2001;38:750-5.

89. Mangat I, Yang Y, Cheng J, et al. Optimizing the detection of bidirectional block across the flutter isthmus for patients with typical isthmus-dependent atrial flutter. Am J Cardiol. 2003;91:559-64.

90. Kall JG, Rubenstein DS, Kopp DE, et al. Atypical atrial flutter originating in the right atrial free wall. Circulation. 2000;101:270-9.

Surgical and Catheter Ablation of Cardiac Arrhythmias

91. Nakagawa H, Shah N, Matsudaira K, et al. Characterization of re-entrant circuit in macrore-entrant right atrial tachycardia after surgical repair of congenital heart disease: isolated channels between scars allow "focal" ablation. Circulation. 2001;103:699-709.

92. Tai CT, Huang JL, Lin YK, et al. Noncontact three-dimensional mapping and ablation of upper loop re-entry originating in the right atrium. J Am Coll Cardiol. 2002;40:746-53.

93. Jais P, Shah DC, Haissaguerre M, et al. Mapping and ablation of left atrial flutters. Circulation. 2000;101:2928-34.

94. Bochoeyer A, Yang Y, Cheng J, et al. Surface electrocardiographic characteristics of right and left atrial flutter. Circulation. 2003;108:60-6.

95. Moss AJ, Hall WJ, Cannom DS, et al. Improved survival with an implanted defibrillator in patients with coronary disease at high risk for ventricular arrhythmia. Multicenter Automatic Defibrillator Implantation Trial Investigators. N Engl J Med. 1996;335:1933-40.

96. A comparison of antiarrhythmic-drug therapy with implantable defibrillators in patients resuscitated from near-fatal ventricular arrhythmias. The Antiarrhythmics versus Implantable Defibrillators (AVID) Investigators. N Engl J Med. 1997;337:1576-83.

97. Kuck KH, Cappato R, Siebels J, et al. Randomized comparison of antiarrhythmic drug therapy with implantable defibrillators in patients resuscitated from cardiac arrest: the Cardiac Arrest Study Hamburg (CASH). Circulation. 2000;102:748-54.

98. Connolly SJ, Gent M, Roberts RS, et al. Canadian implantable defibrillator study (CIDS): a randomized trial of the implantable cardioverter defibrillator against amiodarone. Circulation. 2000;101:1297-302.

99. Kamphuis HC, de Leeuw JR, Derksen R, et al. Implantable cardioverter defibrillator recipients: quality of life in recipients with and without ICD shock delivery: a prospective study. Europace. 2003;5:381-9.

100. Irvine J, Dorian P, Baker B, et al. Quality of life in the Canadian Implantable Defibrillator Study (CIDS). Am Heart J. 2002;144: 282-9.

101. Schron EB, Exner DV, Yao Q, et al. Quality of life in the antiarrhythmics versus implantable defibrillators trial: impact of therapy and influence of adverse symptoms and defibrillator shocks. Circulation. 2002;105:589-94.

102. Moss AJ, Greenberg H, Case RB, et al. Long-term clinical course of patients after termination of ventricular tachyarrhythmia by an implanted defibrillator. Circulation. 2004;110:3760-5.

103. Poole JE, Johnson GW, Hellkamp AS, et al. Prognostic importance of defibrillator shocks in patients with heart failure. N Engl J Med. 2008;359:1009-17.

104. Aksoz E, Aksoz T, Bilge SS, et al. Antidepressant-like effects of echo-planar magnetic resonance imaging in mice determined using the forced swimming test. Brain Res. 2008;1236:194-9.

105. Daubert JP, Zareba W, Cannom DS, et al. Inappropriate implantable cardioverter-defibrillator shocks in MADIT II: frequency, mechanisms, predictors, and survival impact. J Am Coll Cardiol. 2008;51:1357-65.

106. Connolly SJ, Dorian P, Roberts RS, et al. Comparison of beta-blockers, amiodarone plus beta-blockers, or sotalol for prevention of shocks from implantable cardioverter defibrillators: the OPTIC study: a randomized trial. JAMA. 2006;295:165-71.

107. Pacifico A, Hohnloser SH, Williams JH, et al. Prevention of implantable-defibrillator shocks by treatment with sotalol. d,l-Sotalol Implantable Cardioverter-Defibrillator Study Group. N Engl J Med. 1999;340:1855-62.

108. Stevenson WG, Wilber DJ, Natale A, et al. Irrigated radiofrequency catheter ablation guided by electroanatomic mapping for recurrent ventricular tachycardia after myocardial infarction: the multicenter thermocool ventricular tachycardia ablation trial. Circulation. 2008;118:2773-82.

109. Kuck K-H, Schaumann A, Eckardt L, et al. Catheter ablation of stable ventricular tachycardia before defibrillator implantation in patients with coronary heart disease (VTACH): a multicentre randomised controlled trial. Lancet. 2010;375:31-40.

110. Reddy VY, Reynolds MR, Neuzil P, et al. Prophylactic catheter ablation for the prevention of defibrillator therapy. N Engl J Med. 2007;357:2657-65.

111. Raymond J-M, Sacher F, Winslow R, et al. Catheter ablation for scar-related ventricular tachycardias. Curr Probl Cardiol. 2009;34:225-70.

112. de Bakker JM, van Capelle FJ, Janse MJ, et al. Re-entry as a cause of ventricular tachycardia in patients with chronic ischemic heart disease: electrophysiologic and anatomic correlation. Circulation. 1988;77:589-606.

113. Haïssaguerre M, Shoda M, Jaïs P, et al. Mapping and ablation of idiopathic ventricular fibrillation. Circulation. 2002;106:962-7.

114. Zipes DP, Camm AJ, Borggrefe M, et al. ACC/AHA/ESC 2006 guidelines for management of patients with ventricular arrhythmias and the prevention of sudden cardiac death: a report of the American College of Cardiology/American Heart Association Task Force and the European Society of Cardiology Committee for Practice Guidelines (Writing Committee to Develop Guidelines for Management of Patients with Ventricular Arrhythmias and the Prevention of Sudden Cardiac Death). J Am Coll Cardiol. 2006;48:e247-e346.

115. Aliot EM, Stevenson WG, Almendral-Garrote JM, et al. EHRA/HRS Expert Consensus on Catheter Ablation of Ventricular Arrhythmias: developed in a partnership with the European Heart Rhythm Association (EHRA), a Registered Branch of the European Society of Cardiology (ESC), and the Heart Rhythm Society (HRS); in collaboration with the American College of Cardiology (ACC) and the American Heart Association (AHA). Europace. 2009;11:771-817.

116. Carbucicchio C, Della Bella P, Fassini G, et al. Percutaneous cardiopulmonary support for catheter ablation of unstable ventricular arrhythmias in high-risk patients. Herz. 2009;34:545-52.

117. Dandamudi G, Ghumman WS, Das MK, Miller JM. Endocardial catheter ablation of ventricular tachycardia in patients with ventricular assist devices. Heart Rhythm. 2007;4:1165-9.

118. Friedman PA, Munger TM, Torres N, et al. Percutaneous endocardial and epicardial ablation of hypotensive ventricular tachycardia with percutaneous left ventricular assist in the electrophysiology laboratory. Journal of Cardiovascular Electrophysiology. 2007; 8:106-9.

119. Josephson ME, Callans DJ. Using the twelve-lead electrocardiogram to localize the site of origin of ventricular tachycardia. Heart Rhythm. 2005;2:443-6.

120. Berruezo A, Mont L, Nava S, et al. Electrocardiographic recognition of the epicardial origin of ventricular tachycardias. Circulation. 2004;109:1842-7.

121. Stevenson W, Khan H, Sager P, et al. Identification of re-entry circuit sites during catheter mapping and radiofrequency ablation of ventricular tachycardia late after myocardial infarction. Circulation. 1993;88:1647-70.

122. Kocovic DZ, Harada T, Friedman PL, et al. Characteristics of electrograms recorded at re-entry circuit sites and bystanders during ventricular tachycardia after myocardial infarction. J Am Coll Cardiol. 1999;34:381-8.

123. Stevenson WG, Friedman PL, Sager PT, et al. Exploring postinfarction re-entrant ventricular tachycardia with entrainment mapping. J Am Coll Cardiol. 1997;29:1180-9.

124. Stevenson WG, Khan H, Sager P, et al. Identification of re-entry circuit sites during catheter mapping and radiofrequency ablation of ventricular tachycardia late after myocardial infarction. Circulation. 1993;88:1647-70.

125. El-Shalakany A, Hadjis T, Papageorgiou P, et al. Entrainment/mapping criteria for the prediction of termination of ventricular tachycardia by single radiofrequency lesion in patients with coronary artery disease. Circulation. 1999;99:2283-9.

126. Bogun F, Taj M, Ting M, et al. Spatial resolution of pace mapping of idiopathic ventricular tachycardia/ectopy originating in the right ventricular outflow tract. Heart Rhythm. 2008;5:339-44.

127. Brunckhorst CB, Delacretaz E, Soejima K, et al. Identification of the ventricular tachycardia isthmus after infarction by pace mapping. Circulation. 2004;110:652-9.

128. Brunckhorst CB, Stevenson WG, Soejima K, et al. Relationship of slow conduction detected by pace-mapping to ventricular tachycardia re-entry circuit sites after infarction. J Am Coll Cardiol. 2003;41:802-9.

129. Bogun F, Good E, Reich S, et al. Isolated potentials during sinus rhythm and pace-mapping within scars as guides for ablation of post-infarction ventricular tachycardia. J Am Coll Cardiol. 2006;47:2013-9.

130. Soejima K, Stevenson WG, Maisel WH, et al. Electrically unexcitable scar mapping based on pacing threshold for identification of the re-entry circuit isthmus: feasibility for guiding ventricular tachycardia ablation. Circulation. 2002;106:1678-83.

131. Calkins H, Epstein A, Packer D, et al. Catheter ablation of ventricular tachycardia in patients with structural heart disease using cooled radiofrequency energy: results of a prospective multicenter study. Cooled RF Multi Center Investigators Group. J Am Coll Cardiol. 2000;35:1905-14.

132. Scheinman MM, Huang S. The 1998 NASPE prospective catheter ablation registry. Pacing Clin Electrophysiol. 2000;23:1020-8.

133. Sacher F, Roberts-Thomson K, Maury P, et al. Epicardial ventricular tachycardia ablation a multicenter safety study. J Am Coll Cardiol. 2010;55:2366-72.

134. Sosa E, Scanavacca M, d'Avila A, et al. Nonsurgical transthoracic epicardial catheter ablation to treat recurrent ventricular tachycardia occurring late after myocardial infarction. J Am Coll Cardiol. 2000;35:1442-9.

135. Daniels DV, Lu Y-Y, Morton JB, et al. Idiopathic epicardial left ventricular tachycardia originating remote from the sinus of valsalva: electrophysiological characteristics, catheter ablation, and identification from the 12-lead electrocardiogram. Circulation. 2006;113:1659-66.

136. Vallès E, Bazan V, Marchlinski FE. ECG criteria to identify epicardial ventricular tachycardia in nonischemic cardiomyopathy. Circ Arrhythm Electrophysiol. 2010;3:63-71.

137. Michowitz Y, Mathuria N, Tung R, et al. Hybrid procedures for epicardial catheter ablation of ventricular tachycardia: Value of surgical access. Heart Rhythm. 2010;7:1635-43.

138. Miller JM, Altemose GT, Jayachandran JV. Catheter ablation of ventricular tachycardia in patients with structural heart disease. Cardiol Rev. 2001;9:302-11.

139. Bhakta D, Miller JM. Principles of electroanatomic mapping. Indian Pacing Electrophysiol J. 2008;8:32-50.

140. Brooks R, Burgess JH. Idiopathic ventricular tachycardia. A review. Medicine (Baltimore). 1988;67:271-94.

141. Okumura K, Tsuchiya T. Idiopathic left ventricular tachycardia: clinical features, mechanisms and management. Card Electrophysiol Rev. 2002;6:61-7.

142. Nakagawa M, Takahashi N, Nobe S, et al. Gender differences in various types of idiopathic ventricular tachycardia. J Cardiovasc Electrophysiol. 2002;13:633-8.

143. Altemose GT, Buxton AE. Idiopathic ventricular tachycardia. Annu Rev Med. 1999;50:159-77.

144. Yarlagadda RK, Iwai S, Stein KM, et al. Reversal of cardiomyopathy in patients with repetitive monomorphic ventricular ectopy originating from the right ventricular outflow tract. Circulation. 2005;112:1092-7.

145. Jadonath RL, Schwartzman DS, Preminger MW, et al. Utility of the 12-lead electrocardiogram in localizing the origin of right ventricular outflow tract tachycardia. Am Heart J. 1995;130:1107-13.

146. Coggins DL, Lee RJ, Sweeney J, et al. Radiofrequency catheter ablation as a cure for idiopathic tachycardia of both left and right ventricular origin. J Am Coll Cardiol. 1994;23:1333-41.

147. Dixit S, Gerstenfeld EP, Callans DJ, et al. Electrocardiographic patterns of superior right ventricular outflow tract tachycardias: distinguishing septal and free-wall sites of origin. J Cardiovasc Electrophysiol. 2003;14:1-7.

148. Ito S, Tada H, Naito S, et al. Development and validation of an ECG algorithm for identifying the optimal ablation site for idiopathic ventricular outflow tract tachycardia. J Cardiovasc Electrophysiol. 2003;14:1280-6.

149. Yamauchi Y, Aonuma K, Takahashi A, et al. Electrocardiographic characteristics of repetitive monomorphic right ventricular tachycardia originating near the His-bundle. J Cardiovasc Electrophysiol. 2005;16:1041-8.

150. Timmermans C, Rodriguez LM, Crijns HJ, et al. Idiopathic left bundle-branch block-shaped ventricular tachycardia may originate above the pulmonary valve. Circulation. 2003;108:1960-7.

151. Sekiguchi Y, Aonuma K, Takahashi A, et al. Electrocardiographic and electrophysiologic characteristics of ventricular tachycardia originating within the pulmonary artery. J Am Coll Cardiol. 2005;45:887-95.

152. Moorman AF, Christoffels VM. Cardiac chamber formation: development, genes, and evolution. Physiol Rev. 2003;83:1223-67.

153. Callans DJ, Menz V, Schwartzman D, et al. Repetitive monomorphic tachycardia from the left ventricular outflow tract: electrocardio-graphic patterns consistent with a left ventricular site of origin. J Am Coll Cardiol. 1997;29:1023-7.

154. Kamakura S, Shimizu W, Matsuo K, et al. Localization of optimal ablation site of idiopathic ventricular tachycardia from right and left ventricular outflow tract by body surface ECG. Circulation. 1998;98:1525-33.

155. Krebs ME, Krause PC, Engelstein ED, et al. Ventricular tachycardias mimicking those arising from the right ventricular outflow tract. J Cardiovasc Electrophysiol. 2000;11:45-51.

156. Lamberti F, Calo L, Pandozi C, et al. Radiofrequency catheter ablation of idiopathic left ventricular outflow tract tachycardia: utility of intracardiac echocardiography. J Cardiovasc Electrophysiol. 2001;12:529-35.

157. Hachiya H, Aonuma K, Yamauchi Y, et al. Electrocardiographic characteristics of left ventricular outflow tract tachycardia. Pacing Clin Electrophysiol. 2000;23:1930-4.

158. Tada H, Nogami A, Naito S, et al. Left ventricular epicardial outflow tract tachycardia: a new distinct subgroup of outflow tract tachycardia. Jpn Circ J. 2001;65:723-30.

159. Dixit S, Gerstenfeld EP, Lin D, et al. Identification of distinct electrocardiographic patterns from the basal left ventricle: distinguishing medial and lateral sites of origin in patients with idiopathic ventricular tachycardia. Heart Rhythm. 2005;2:485-91.

160. Shimoike E, Ohnishi Y, Ueda N, et al. Radiofrequency catheter ablation of left ventricular outflow tract tachycardia from the coronary cusp: a new approach to the tachycardia focus. J Cardiovasc Electrophysiol. 1999;10:1005-9.

161. Sadanaga T, Saeki K, Yoshimoto T, et al. Repetitive monomorphic ventricular tachycardia of left coronary cusp origin. Pacing Clin Electrophysiol. 1999;22:1553-6.

162. Kanagaratnam L, Tomassoni G, Schweikert R, et al. Ventricular tachycardias arising from the aortic sinus of valsalva: an under-recognized variant of left outflow tract ventricular tachycardia. J Am Coll Cardiol. 2001;37:1408-14.

163. Ouyang F, Fotuhi P, Ho SY, et al. Repetitive monomorphic ventricular tachycardia originating from the aortic sinus cusp: electrocardiographic characterization for guiding catheter ablation. J Am Coll Cardiol. 2002;39:500-8.

CHAPTER 39

Surgical and Catheter Ablation of Cardiac Arrhythmias

164. Yang Y, Saenz LC, Varosy PD, et al. Analyses of phase differences from surface electrocardiogram recordings to distinguish the origin of outflow tract tachycardia (abstr). Heart Rhythm. 2005;2:S80.

165. Tanner H, Hindricks G, Schirdewahn P, et al. Outflow tract tachycardia with R/S transition in lead V3: six different anatomic approaches for successful ablation. J Am Coll Cardiol. 2005;45:418-23.

166. Meininger GR, Berger RD. Idiopathic ventricular tachycardia originating in the great cardiac vein. Heart Rhythm. 2006;3:464-6.

167. Daniels DV, Lu YY, Morton JB, et al. Idiopathic epicardial left ventricular tachycardia originating remote from the sinus of Valsalva: electrophysiological characteristics, catheter ablation, and identification from the 12-lead electrocardiogram. Circulation. 2006;113:1659-66.

168. Doppalapudi H, Yamada T, Ramaswamy K, et al. Idiopathic focal epicardial ventricular tachycardia originating from the crux of the heart. Heart Rhythm. 2009;6:44-50.

169. Buxton AE, Waxman HL, Marchlinski FE, et al. Right ventricular tachycardia: clinical and electrophysiologic characteristics. Circulation. 1983;68:917-27.

170. Lemery R, Brugada P, Bella PD, et al. Nonischemic ventricular tachycardia. Clinical course and long-term follow-up in patients without clinically overt heart disease. Circulation. 1989;79:990-9.

171. Rowland TW, Schweiger MJ. Repetitive paroxysmal ventricular tachycardia and sudden death in a child. Am J Cardiol. 1984;53:1729.

172. Chugh SS, Shen WK, Luria DM, et al. First evidence of premature ventricular complex-induced cardiomyopathy: a potentially reversible cause of heart failure. J Cardiovasc Electrophysiol. 2000;11:328-9.

173. Thiene G, Nava A, Corrado D, et al. Right ventricular cardiomyopathy and sudden death in young people. N Engl J Med. 1988;318:129-33.

174. Marcus FI, Fontaine GH, Guiraudon G, et al. Right ventricular dysplasia: a report of 24 adult cases. Circulation. 1982;65:384-98.

175. Gill JS, Mehta D, Ward DE, et al. Efficacy of flecainide, sotalol, and verapamil in the treatment of right ventricular tachycardia in patients without overt cardiac abnormality. Br Heart J. 1992;68:392-7.

176. Kobayashi Y, Miyata A, Tanno K, et al. Effects of nicorandil, a potassium channel opener, on idiopathic ventricular tachycardia. J Am Coll Cardiol. 1998;32:1377-83.

177. Gepstein L, Hayam G, Ben-Haim SA. A novel method for nonfluoroscopic catheter-based electroanatomical mapping of the heart. In vitro and in vivo accuracy results. Circulation. 1997;95:1611-22.

178. Fung JW, Chan HC, Chan JY, et al. Ablation of nonsustained or hemodynamically unstable ventricular arrhythmia originating from the right ventricular outflow tract guided by noncontact mapping. Pacing Clin Electrophysiol. 2003;26:1699-705.

179. Joshi S, Wilber DJ. Ablation of idiopathic right ventricular outflow tract tachycardia: current perspectives. J Cardiovasc Electrophysiol. 2005;16:S52-8.

180. Friedman PL, Stevenson WG, Bittl JA, et al. Left main coronary artery occlusion during radiofrequency catheter ablation of idiopathic outflow tract ventricular tachycardia (abstr). Pacing Clin Electrophysiol. 1997;20:1184.

181. Sosa E, Scanavacca M, D'Avila A, et al. Endocardial and epicardial ablation guided by nonsurgical transthoracic epicardial mapping to treat recurrent ventricular tachycardia. J Cardiovasc Electrophysiol. 1998;9:229-39.

182. Cole CR, Marrouche NF, Natale A. Evaluation and management of ventricular outflow tract tachycardias. Card Electrophysiol Rev. 2002;6:442-7.

183. Nogami A. Idiopathic left ventricular tachycardia: assessment and treatment. Card Electrophysiol Rev. 2002;6:448-57.

184. Zipes DP, Foster PR, Troup PJ, et al. Atrial induction of ventricular tachycardia: re-entry versus triggered automaticity. Am J Cardiol. 1979;44:1-8.

185. Belhassen B, Rotmensch HH, Laniado S. Response of recurrent sustained ventricular tachycardia to verapamil. Br Heart J. 1981;46:679-82.

186. Ohe T, Shimomura K, Aihara N, et al. Idiopathic sustained left ventricular tachycardia: clinical and electrophysiologic characteristics. Circulation. 1988;77:560-8.

187. Shimoike E, Ueda N, Maruyama T, et al. Radiofrequency catheter ablation of upper septal idiopathic left ventricular tachycardia exhibiting left bundle branch block morphology. J Cardiovasc Electrophysiol. 2000;11:203-7.

188. German LD, Packer DL, Bardy GH, et al. Ventricular tachycardia induced by atrial stimulation in patients without symptomatic cardiac disease. Am J Cardiol. 1983;52:1202-7.

189. Lin FC, Finley CD, Rahimtoola SH, et al. Idiopathic paroxysmal ventricular tachycardia with a QRS pattern of right bundle branch block and left axis deviation: a unique clinical entity with specific properties. Am J Cardiol. 1983;52:95-100.

190. Klein GJ, Millman PJ, Yee R. Recurrent ventricular tachycardia responsive to verapamil. Pacing Clin Electrophysiol. 1984;7:938-48.

191. Ward DE, Nathan AW, Camm AJ. Fascicular tachycardia sensitive to calcium antagonists. Eur Heart J. 1984;5:896-905.

192. Ohe T, Aihara N, Kamakura S, et al. Long-term outcome of verapamil-sensitive sustained left ventricular tachycardia in patients without structural heart disease. J Am Coll Cardiol. 1995;25:54-8.

193. Kottkamp H, Chen X, Hindricks G, et al. Idiopathic left ventricular tachycardia: new insights into electrophysiological characteristics and radiofrequency catheter ablation. Pacing Clin Electrophysiol. 1995;18:1285-97.

194. Nakagawa H, Beckman KJ, McClelland JH, et al. Radiofrequency catheter ablation of idiopathic left ventricular tachycardia guided by a Purkinje potential. Circulation. 1993;88:2607-17.

195. Nogami A, Naito S, Tada H, et al. Verapamil-sensitive left anterior fascicular ventricular tachycardia: results of radiofrequency ablation in six patients. J Cardiovasc Electrophysiol. 1998;9:1269-78.

196. Akhtar M, Shenasa M, Jazayeri M, et al. Wide QRS complex tachycardia. Reappraisal of a common clinical problem. Ann Intern Med. 1988;109:905-12.

197. Wellens HJ, Bar FW, Lie KI. The value of the electrocardiogram in the differential diagnosis of a tachycardia with a widened QRS complex. Am J Med. 1978;64:27-33.

198. Brugada P, Brugada J, Mont L, et al. A new approach to the differential diagnosis of a regular tachycardia with a wide QRS complex. Circulation. 1991;83:1649-59.

199. Wen MS, Yeh SJ, Wang CC, et al. Successful radiofrequency ablation of idiopathic left ventricular tachycardia at a site away from the tachycardia exit. J Am Coll Cardiol. 1997;30:1024-31.

200. Tsuchiya T, Okumura K, Honda T, et al. Significance of late diastolic potential preceding Purkinje potential in verapamil-sensitive idiopathic left ventricular tachycardia. Circulation. 1999;99:2408-13.

201. Nogami A, Naito S, Tada H, et al. Demonstration of diastolic and presystolic purkinje potentials as critical potentials in a macrore-entry circuit of verapamil-sensitive idiopathic left ventricular tachycardia. J Am Coll Cardiol. 2000;36:811-23.

202. Ouyang F, Cappato R, Ernst S, et al. Electroanatomic substrate of idiopathic left ventricular tachycardia: unidirectional block and macrore-entry within the purkinje network. Circulation. 2002;105:462-9.

203. Chen M, Yang B, Zou J, et al. Non-contact mapping and linear ablation of the left posterior fascicle during sinus rhythm in the treatment of idiopathic left ventricular tachycardia. Europace. 2005;7:138-44.

204. Ma FS, Ma J, Tang K, et al. Left posterior fascicular block: a new endpoint of ablation for verapamil-sensitive idiopathic ventricular tachycardia. Chin Med J (Engl). 2006;119:367-72.

205. Thakur RK, Klein GJ, Sivaram CA, et al. Anatomic substrate for idiopathic left ventricular tachycardia. Circulation. 1996;93:497-501.

206. Lin FC, Wen MS, Wang CC, et al. Left ventricular fibromuscular band is not a specific substrate for idiopathic left ventricular tachycardia. Circulation. 1996;93:525-8.

207. Page RL, Shenasa H, Evans JJ, et al. Radiofrequency catheter ablation of idiopathic recurrent ventricular tachycardia with right bundle branch block, left axis morphology. Pacing Clin Electrophysiol. 1993;16:327-36.

208. Yeh SJ, Wen MS, Wang CC, et al. Adenosine-sensitive ventricular tachycardia from the anterobasal left ventricle. J Am Coll Cardiol. 1997;30:1339-45.

209. Nagasawa H, Fujiki A, Usui M, et al. Successful radiofrequency catheter ablation of incessant ventricular tachycardia with a delta wave-like beginning of the QRS complex. Jpn Heart J. 1999;40:671-5.

210. Kondo K, Watanabe I, Kojima T, et al. Radiofrequency catheter ablation of ventricular tachycardia from the anterobasal left ventricle. Jpn Heart J. 2000;41:215-25.

211. Tada H, Ito S, Naito S, et al. Idiopathic ventricular arrhythmia arising from the mitral annulus: a distinct subgroup of idiopathic ventricular arrhythmias. J Am Coll Cardiol. 2005;45:877-86.

212. Kumagai K, Yamauchi Y, Takahashi A, et al. Idiopathic left ventricular tachycardia originating from the mitral annulus. J Cardiovasc Electrophysiol. 2005;16:1029-36.

213. Tada H, Tadokoro K, Ito S, et al. Idiopathic ventricular arrhythmias originating from the TA: prevalence, electrocardiographic characteristics, and results of radiofrequency catheter ablation. Heart Rhythm. 2007;4:7-16.

CHAPTER 39

Surgical and Catheter Ablation of Cardiac Arrhythmias

Cardiac Resynchronization Therapy

David Singh, Nitish Badhwar

Chapter Outline

INTRODUCTION

Despite major advances in the treatment of systolic heart failure (HF), it continues to enact a large burden on healthcare systems around the world. The estimated direct and indirect cost of HF in the United States alone for 2010 was $39.2 billion. In the United States, 1 out of 5 individuals in the age group of 40 years and above will develop a clinical HF syndrome.[1] Advances in pharmacological therapy, most notably the use of beta-blockers, ace inhibitors, angiotensin receptor blockers and aldosterone antagonists have reduced mortality in this population.[2-7] Despite this, HF patients have a poor prognosis with a 20% annual and nearly 50% five-year mortality rate.[1]

The introduction of device-based therapies including internal cardiac defibrillators (ICD) and cardiac resynchronization therapy (CRT) also known as biventricular (BIV) pacing have transformed the landscape of HF management. Both of these modalities have been independently shown to improve survival among patients with systolic HF.[8-10] Based on estimates between 2001 and 2005, as many as 500,00 CRT devices have been implanted in the United States.[11]

Despite these advances, the prevalence of HF remains high and is estimated to affect 5.8 million individuals in the United States.[12] Paralleling, this has been a rise in HF related hospitalizations.[12] The complexity of acute HF management has increased considerably over the past decades. In addition to an ever-expanding armamentarium of HF medications, device-based therapies have become more sophisticated with each generation. Thus the need for clinicians who are well versed in all the aspects of HF management has never been greater. Proper management of these patients requires an interdisciplinary approach, including intensivists, cardiologists, HF specialists, nurses and electrophysiologists.

CRT: RATIONAL FOR USE

The contractile apparatus of the human heart is influenced by a myriad of factors including the highly coordinated electrical activation of the atria and ventricles. Disruption to this activation pattern [for example, in the case of left bundle branch block (LBBB)] can impede ventricular performance. In advanced HF, it is common to see abnormal electrical conduction which promotes asynchronous activation of the ventricles, reduced cardiac output and, in the long-term, adverse ventricular remodeling.[13] The term mechanical dyssynchrony has been used to describe the loss of synchronized contraction both between and within the right and left ventricles. This phenomenon is usually, but not always, the result of disorganized electrical activation.

Patients with depressed systolic function are more susceptible to the adverse effects of conduction disturbances and mechanical dyssynchrony. Patients with first-degree heart block have suboptimal contribution of atrial systole, less filling time for the LV, and can have diastolic mitral regurgitation (MR)[14,15] Among HF patients, the most common conduction abnormality is LBBB. In LBBB, the electrical activation of the ventricles occurs first through the right bundle to the RV followed by trans-septal conduction that eventually results in activation of the lateral LV myocardium. The delayed contraction of the LV lateral wall occurs during the period of septal relaxation. This results in inefficient LV contraction since the septum and lateral walls fail to move in unison to eject blood. While this may be one of the most common forms of mechanical dyssynchrony, any variation in the timing of regional contraction can impede ventricular performance.

CRT IN PRACTICE

The CRT typically involves placing pacing leads in the right atrium, right ventricle and a branch of the coronary sinus (CS) (Figs 1 and 2). The CRT implantation is performed using a transvenous approach whereby the CS is cannulated and a pacing lead is advanced into a lateral CS branch. The CS lead is also known as the LV lead as it activates LV myocardium. Optimal lead placement is the subject of ongoing research and is dependant on many factors including scar location and the regional mechanics of an individual's ventricle. However, it is generally accepted that optimal placement involves maximal separation of the RV and LV leads ideally in a posterolateral branch of the CS.[16]

The CRT can be utilized to influence several key elements of ventricular performance. The AV interval can be adjusted to optimize ventricular preload. The timing of RV and LV pacing can be adjusted to improve interventricular (VV) dyssynchrony. Intraventricular dyssynchrony (LV) can be improved by coordinating the contraction between the LV septum and the lateral wall. Finally, earlier activation of the lateral wall can help to reduce MR, which is likely related to the improved timing of papillary muscle contraction and augmented dP/dt (Figs 3A and B).[17,18] All of these mechanisms contribute to the improvements in myocardial function associated with CRT.

To date, CRT has demonstrated a number of beneficial effects in patients with advanced systolic HF. Several studies have demonstrated its impact on physiologic endpoints such as improved hemodynamics, reduction in MR, increased ejection fraction, increased blood pressure and reverse remodeling.[10,17-23] In addition, randomized and observational studies have shown that CRT favorably impacts clinical endpoints including, exercise capacity, New York Heart Association (NYHA) functional class, hospitalization rate and quality of life (QOL).[18,21,24-26] More recently, at least one randomized controlled trial (RCT) and a meta-analysis of 14 RCTs have shown that CRT reduces mortality among patients with wide QRS and NYHA class III or IV HF.[26,27] Table 1 illustrates the results of randomized clinical trials of CRT in patients with advanced HF. The following section will detail the results of three landmark trials involving CRT.

MIRACLE STUDY

The multicenter insync randomized clinical evaluation (MIRACLE) trial was the first large scale, prospective, randomized, double-blind trial of CRT.[28] A total of 453 patients with NYHA class III or IV HF, EF less than or equal to 35%, and QRS duration greater than or equal to 130 millisecond were enrolled. Patients were randomized to have the CRT feature turned on or off. At 6 months, patients randomized to CRT on had significant improvement in QOL, 6-minute walking distance (39 meters vs 10 meters, p = 0.005), NYHA functional class (p < 0.001) and exercise treadmill time, EF (+ 4.6 vs – 0.2%, p < 0.001). Furthermore, patients in the CRT on group had significantly fewer hospitalizations (15 vs 7%, p = 0.02) and improved peak oxygen consumption (+ 0.2 vs + 1.1, p = 0009).

COMPANION STUDY

The comparison of medical therapy, pacing and defibrillation in heart failure (COMPANION) study was the first large scale, randomized CRT trial to suggest that in addition to symptomatic improvement, CRT may confer mortality benefit.[25] A total of 1,520 patients with NYHA class III and IV HF due to ischemic or nonischemic causes, and QRS duration greater than or equal to 120 milliseconds were randomized to optimal medical therapy, implantation of CRT device or implantation of a CRT device with defibrillator. The mean follow period was 12 months. As with the MIRACLE trial, COMPANION showed that CRT improved HF symptoms based on exercise tolerance testing and QOL surveys. In addition, there was a significant 20% reduction in the primary composite endpoint of all-cause mortality of hospitalization for any cause among those randomized to the CRT arm as compared to medical therapy. Although patients in the CRT-ICD arm experienced a significant reduction in all-cause mortality (HR 0.64, p = 0.003), the implantation of CRT device alone was associated with a marginally nonsignificant reduction with respect to this endpoint (HR 0.76, p = 0.06).

CARE-HF

The cardiac resynchronization-heart failure (CARE-HF) trial randomly assigned 813 patients with NYHA class III or IV HF (ischemic and nonischemic) with EF less than 35% and QRS prolongation to optimal medical therapy or CRT.[26] Patients with

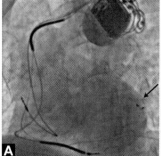 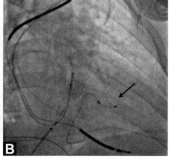

FIGURES 1A AND B: (A) Left anterior oblique; (B) Right anterior oblique fluoroscopic views of a biventricular pacemaker-defibrillator with left ventricular lead positioned in a lateral branch of the coronary sinus (arrows)

TABLE 1

Randomized clinical trials of cardiac resynchronization therapy

Study	Design	No. of patients	Mean follow-up (months)	Results	P value
MUSTIC (NEJM 2001)	Crossover CRT vs no CRT in patients with CHF NYHA III, EF < 35%, QRS > 150 ms, LVEDD > 60 mm, NSR	58	6	Improved 6 MWT QOLHospitalization Peak V_{O2}	< 0.001 < 0.001 < 0.05 < 0.03
MIRACLE (NEJM 2002)	Parallel arms CRT vs no CRT in patients with CHF NYHA III, EF < 35%, QRS > 130 ms, LVEDD > 55 mm, 6 MWT < 450 m, NSR	453	6	Improved 6 MWT NYHA class QOL LVEF Peak V_{O2}	= 0.005 < 0.001 = 0.001 < 0.001 = 0.009
PATH-CHF (JACC 2002)	Crossover CRT (LV or BiV) vs no CRT in patients with CHF NYHA III-IV, EF < 35%, QRS > 120 ms, PR > 150 ms, NSR	41	12	Improved 6 MWT Peak V_{O2} QOL NYHA class LV and BiV had similar improvement	= 0.03 = 0.002 = 0.062 < 0.001
MIRACLE ICD (JAMA 2003)	Parallel arms CRT + ICD vs CRT in patients with CHF NYHA III, EF < 35%, QRS > 130 ms, LVEDD > 55 mm, cardiac arrest due to VT/VF, spontaneous VT or inducible VT/VF, NSR	369	6	Improved NYHA class QOL No change 6 MWT	= 0.007 = 0.02 = 0.36
CONTAK CD (JACC 2003)	Crossover, parallel controlled CRT vs no CRT in patients undergoing ICD implantation with CHF NYHA II-IV, EF < 35%, QRS > 120 ms, NSR, indications for ICD implantation	490	6	Improved 6 MWT Peak V_{O2} LVEF LV volumes No significant change NYHA class QOL HF progression	= 0.043 = 0.030 < 0.001 = 0.02 = 0.10 = 0.40 = 0.35
PATH-CHF II (JACC 2003)	Crossover CRT (LV only) vs no CRT in patients with CHF NYHA II-IV, EF < 30%, QRS > 120 ms, NSR, Peak V_{O2} < 18 ml/min/kg	86	6	Improved 6 MWT QOL Peak V_{O2} No benefit in QRS 120–150 ms	= 0.021 = 0.015 < 0.001
COMPANION (NEJM 2004)	Parallel arms Optimal pharmacological therapy (OPT) vs CRT vs CRT + ICD (CRT-D) in patients with CHF NYHA III-IV, EF ≤ 35%, QRS > 120 ms	1520	16	Death or hospitalization for CHF reduced by 34% in CRT, 40% in CRT-D As compared to OPT	< 0.002 < 0.001
			Stopped early by DSMB	All cause mortality reduced by 36% in CRT-D 24% in CRT	= 0.003 = 0.05
CARE-HF (NEJM 2005)	Open label, randomized Medical therapy vs Medical therapy + CRT in patients with CHF NYHA III-IV, EF ≤ 35%, QRS > 120 ms with dyssynchrony (aortic pre-ejection > 140 ms, interventricular mechanical delay > 40 ms, delayed activation of postlateral LV) QRS > 150 ms (no dyssynchrony evidence needed)	814	29.4	All cause mortality/ hospitalization reduction by 37% in CRT	< 0.001
				All cause mortality reduced by 36% in CRT	< 0.002
				Improvement in QOL LVEF LVESV NYHA class	< 0.01

(Abbreviations: 6 MWT: 6-Minute walking test; AF: Atrial fibrillation; CARE-HF: Cardiac resynchronization-heart failure study group; CHF: Congestive heart failure; CONTAK-CD: CONTAK-Cardiac defibrillator; COMPANION: Comparison of medical therapy, resynchronization, and defibrillation therapies in heart failure study group; CRT: Cardiac resynchronization therapy; DSMB: Data safety monitoring board; EF: Ejection fraction; ICD: Implantable cardioverter-defibrillator; JACC: Journal of American College of Cardiology; JAMA: Journal of American Medical Association; LVEDD: LV end diastolic diameter; LVESV: LV end systolic volume; MIRACLE: Multicenter insync randomized clinical evaluation trial; MUSTIC: Multisite stimulation in cardiomyopathies study group; NEJM: New England Journal of Medicine; NSR: Normal sinus rhythm; NYHA: New York Heart Association; QOL: Quality of life; PACE: Pacing and clinical electrophysiology; PATH-CHF: Pacing therapies in heart failure study group; VT: Ventricular tachycardia; VF: Ventricular fibrillation)

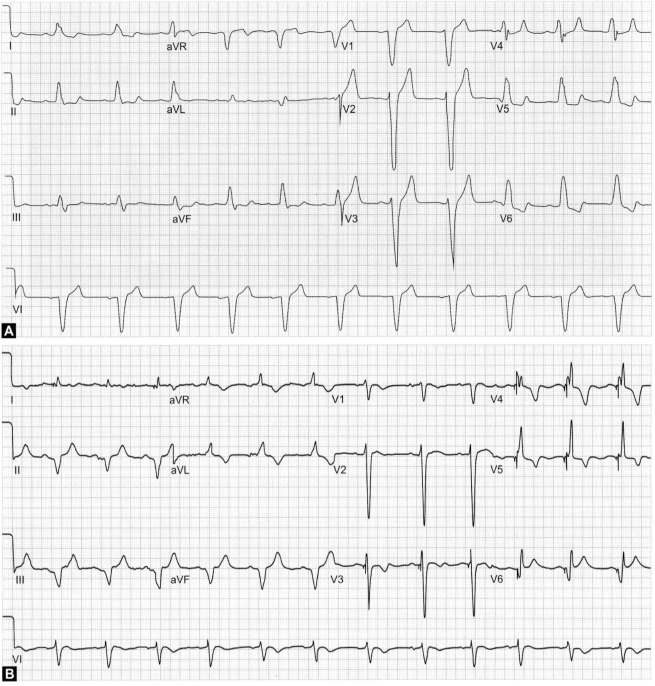

FIGURES 2A AND B: (A) ECG before; (B) ECG after implantation of cardiac resynchronization therapy (CRT) device. Note the considerable QRS narrowing and change in QRS morphology with small Q wave in lead I, positive QRS in aVR that is consistent with biventricular pacing

QRS duration of 120–149 milliseconds were required to have echocardiographic evidence of dyssynchrony for enrollment. There was a 37% reduction in the primary endpoint of death from any cause or unplanned hospitalization for a major cardiac event (p < 0.001). The major secondary endpoint in CARE-HF was all-cause mortality. The CRT was associated with a 36% reduction in this endpoint as compared to medical therapy alone (p < 0.002). As per previous studies, CRT was associated with improvements in a number of parameters including ejection fraction, reverse remodeling, systolic blood pressure, MR and QOL.

SUMMARY OF CRT BENEFIT

These and other trials have provided robust evidence that CRT has a favorable impact on many important physiologic and non-physiologic endpoints in HF. In addition, there is evidence that CRT alone (without back-up defibrillator) reduces mortality. There is some uncertainty about whether CRT coupled to ICD therapy confers additional mortality benefit (in COMPANION, the risk reductions associated with CRT and CRT + ICD were similar). However, due to the wide range of benefits associated with CRT, it is reasonable to combine CRT and ICD therapy in

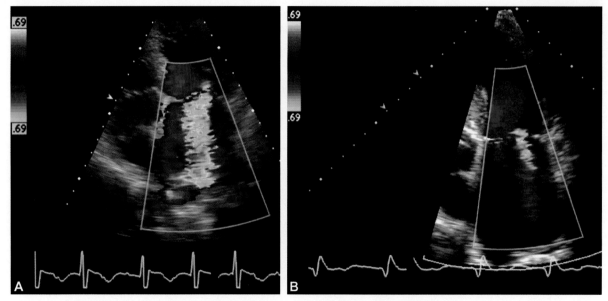

FIGURES 3A AND B: Echocardiographic images (A) and (B) showing significant improvement in mitral regurgitation after cardiac resynchronization therapy (CRT)

patients who meet criteria for both. In accordance with this, the most recent ACC/AHA/HRS guidelines recommend CRT (with or without ICD) in patients who have left ventricular ejection fraction (LVEF) less than 35%, QRS duration more than 120 millisecond, and NHYA III or IV on optimal medical therapy.[29]

PREDICTION OF RESPONSE TO CRT THERAPY

One of the great challenges associated with CRT is how to determine which patients are likely to derive the most benefit. Response to CRT is dependant on the endpoint evaluated. When a clinical endpoint, such as NHYA classification, is used to determine response to CRT, there appears to be a consistent 20–30% nonresponder rate. However, when more objective measures, such as echocardiographic parameters, are employed, nonresponder rates may be closer to 40%.[30-32] It remains unknown whether this discrepancy is related to the placebo effect from device implantation or for some other reason.

The reasons for lack of response include suboptimal HF drug therapy, end stage HF, significant MR and other comorbidities such as obesity. Device-related reasons include ineffective biventricular pacing (BiV), suboptimal atrioventricular (AV) and VV timing, suboptimal LV lead position and absence of mechanical dyssynchrony in selected patients. An illustration of a step-by-step approach to CRT nonresponders is given in Flow chart 1.

IS THERE ADEQUATE BIV CAPTURE?

Optimal delivery of CRT requires continuous ventricular pacing. Although a formal device interrogation may be necessary to assess effective BIV pacing, a great deal can be learned from the surface 12-lead electrocardiogram (ECG). Prior to inspection of the ECG, it is helpful to examine a patient's chest radiograph to determine the position of the RV and LV leads. Several pacing patterns can be observed with: (1) BIV pacing; (2) Complete

BIV capture; (3) Isolated RV capture; (4) Isolated LV capture; (5) Absence of BIV capture (native QRS) and (6) BIV capture with fusion.[33]

Traditional RV pacing (with the RV lead in an apical position) activates the myocardium in an inferior-superior and right-left fashion. The surface ECG therefore usually demonstrates a "superior axis" (negative in the inferior leads) and LBBB. Isolated LV pacing can produce a variety of patterns depending on the location of the LV lead. In general, the activation of the ventricle proceeds from left to right producing a "rightward axis" (negative or initial negative QRS complex in leads I and AVL) and a right bundle branch pattern (RBBB).

The pattern of BIV pacing represents the summed vector of RV and LV lead activation. The ECG pattern of BIV capture can vary widely depending on device programming and the placement of the RV and LV leads. In general BIV capture produces a rightward axis (negative or initial negative in leads I, AVL and positive in aVR) and R greater than S in lead V_1 (Figs 3A and B). The inferior leads (II, III and aVF) can be positive or negative depending on the location of the LV lead. The absence of this pattern should not however be interpreted to mean the loss of BIV capture. Often there is narrowing of the intrinsic QRS complex with BIV pacing. This has been shown to correlate with clinical benefit.[34,35] However, it has also been shown that wide QRS with BIV pacing also correlates with clinical benefit.[36] Hence, the duration of the BIV paced QRS complex cannot be used to assess presence or absence of BIV pacing although a narrower BIV paced QRS (when compared to intrinsic QRS) suggests a good prognosis.

Georger and his colleagues analyzed ECG patterns of patients with CRT and observed a Q wave in lead I in 17 out of 18 patients during BIV pacing.[37] A Q wave in lead I with RV pacing alone was found to extremely uncommon. In this series, the absence of a Q wave in lead I was 100% predictive of loss of LV capture. Although this was a small study, the assessment of lead I may be a simple way to assess the presence of LV capture during BIV pacing.

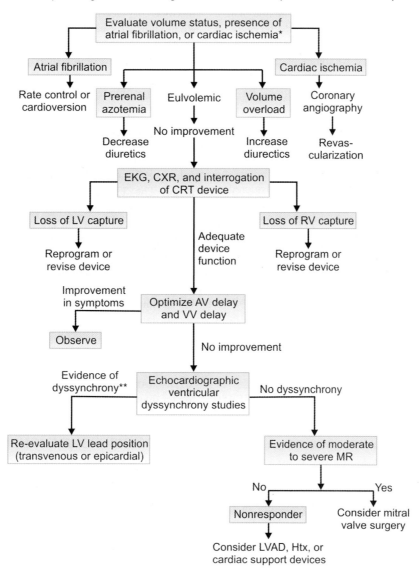

(Abbreviations: AV: Atrioventricular; CXR: Chest X-ray; EKG: Electrocardiogram; Htx: Heart transplant; LV: Left ventricular; LVAD: Left ventricular assist device; MR: Mitral regurgitation; RV: Right ventricular; VV: Interventricular).
*Cardiac ischemia is evaluated in patients with ischemic cardiomyopathy. **Evidence of dyssynchrony includes septal to posterior wall motion delay ≥ 130 ms, intraventricular mechanical delay ≥ 40 ms and tissue Doppler imaging ≥ 65 ms. (*Source:* Modified from Aranda, et al, Management of heart failure after cardiac resynchronization therapy: integrating advanced heart failure treatment with optimal device function. J Am Coll Cardiol. 2005;46:2193-8)

A simple algorithm to assess LV capture among patients with baseline LBBB and RV apical leads was developed by Ammann and his colleagues using leads V_1 and I.[38] An R-S ratio greater than or equal to 1 in lead V_1 reliably detected left ventricular capture. In the absence of this finding, lead I was analyzed. An R-S ratio of less than or equal to 1 suggested the presence of LV capture. The sensitivity of the algorithm to correctly identify loss of left ventricular capture was 94% (95% CI, 88.2–97.7%), and the specificity was 93% (CI, 86.3–95.8%).

Adequate BIV pacing can only occur if the programmed AV delay is shorter than a patient's native PR interval. When BIV output competes with native AV nodal conduction the result is called fusion. In such cases, both the BIV device and native conduction contribute to the ventricular depolarization.

Pseudofusion refers to the phenomena of a pacemaker stimulus that appears to precede ventricular depolarization, but does not contribute to ventricular depolarization. In this case, the QRS complex should be identical to a nonpaced beat. To determine this, it is necessary to compare the ECG in question with a prior ECG that is known to represent nonpaced intrinsic conduction. We recommend performing 12-lead ECG on patients with CRT during their device visit and compare it to previous BIV paced ECG and intrinsic ECG to ensure effective delivery of BIV pacing (Figs 3A and B).

OPTIMIZATION OF CRT DEVICE

Manipulation of AV and VV delays to achieve an optimal hemodynamic response in patients with CRT devices is known as "optimization". Commonly, noninvasive optimization protocols utilize echocardiography to achieve the desired hemodynamic changes. A number of optimization methods have been developed to establish the optimal AV and VV delays using a variety of different echo parameters. Although alterations in AV delay are more established with respect to their hemodynamic benefits, changes in VV delays are more contentious. At least two randomized trials have failed to show benefit associated with optimization of VV delays.[39,40]

Although echo optimization protocols vary widely, they are usually performed by systematically altering the AV and VV delays to achieve a desired hemodynamic response. The AV and VV delay with the best hemodynamic profile is considered to be "optimal". Some of the hemodynamic parameters used for echo optimization include, mitral inflow doppler patterns, time velocity integral of the left ventricular outflow tract (which is proportional to stroke volume), and dP/dt (which can be assessed noninvasively through analysis of continuous wave doppler of an MR jet).[41-43] In addition to echo-guided optimization, a number of other noninvasive optimization techniques have been reported including impedance cardiography, finger plethysmography and radionuclide ventriculography.[44-46] In addition, some CRT devices possess intracardiac electrogram-based (IEGM) algorithms that can determine optimal AV and VV delays.[47]

Although optimization studies have demonstrated improved ejection fraction, NYHA class, QOL, 6-minute walking distance and cardiac hemodynamics, in general, these studies have been small, nonrandomized and frequently lack control groups.[43,48-50] There is therefore no consensus regarding the optimal optimization method or universally accepted protocol for patients with CRT devices. Although some practitioners utilize optimization more frequently, in most institutions, only patients who gain suboptimal benefit from CRT undergo optimization as it can be costly, time-consuming and requires specialized skill and expertise.

ROLE OF DYSSYNCHRONY IMAGING

Cardiac dyssynchrony can occur with respect to atrio-ventricular (A-V) VV delay (RV-LV) or LV. In general, patients with LV dyssynchrony are more likely to response to CRT.[51,52] While QRS duration is a reasonable marker of VV (RV-LV) dyssynchrony; it does not predict LV dyssynchrony (as assessed by echocardiogram) with great accuracy.[53,54]

There have been a number of dyssynchrony criteria that have been shown to predict response to CRT. In general, these trials have been conducted at single centers, with relatively small numbers of patients using a variety of echocardiographic techniques. While a complete review of dyssynchrony parameters is beyond the scope of this paper, a brief review of some of these techniques is provided below.

SEPTAL TO POSTERIOR WALL MOTION DELAY

The LV dyssynchrony was initially assessed with conventional M-Mode echocardiography that measured the delay in contraction between the septum and the posterior wall. This measure is obtained by taking the shortest interval between

the maximal posterior displacement of the septum and the maximal displacement of the left posterior wall using an M-Mode short-axis view of the left ventricle at the level of the papillary muscle. Several observational studies demonstrated that a SPWMD greater than 130 millisecond predicted a favorable response to CRT.[55-57] However, a recent study showed that this technique was not predictive of response to CRT in a larger study cohort.[58]

TISSUE DOPPLER IMAGING

The tissue doppler imaging (TDI) is an echocardiographic technique that uses ultrasound to image the velocity of cardiac tissue. The TDI is used to assess LV dyssynchrony by comparing the time to peak velocity of various myocardial segments. Measurements are obtained for the time to peak systolic velocity (from the onset of QRS complex) in different segments of the LV and the delay between them is used as a marker of LV dyssynchrony (Figs 4A and B). There have been a number of dyssynchrony indices that have been derived using this technique. Initial studies used a four-segment model (septal, lateral, inferior and anterior) and showed that a delay greater than 65 millisecond predicted response to CRT.[59] Yu et al. used a 12-segment model (6 basal and 6 mid segment) and derived an LV dyssynchrony index from the standard deviation of all 12 intervals.[60,61] An LV dyssynchrony index greater than 31 millisecond yielded a sensitivity and specificity of 96 and 78% to predict LV reverse remodeling.[62]

TISSUE SYNCHRONIZATION IMAGING

The tissue synchronization imaging (TSI) builds upon the technique of TDI by transforming the timing of regional peak velocities into color codes (Figs 5A and B). This allows visual identification of regional delay in systole by comparing the color-coding of opposing walls, thus providing rapid identification of dyssynchrony by simple visual evaluation. As with TDI, quantitative assessment of regional delay is possible, and

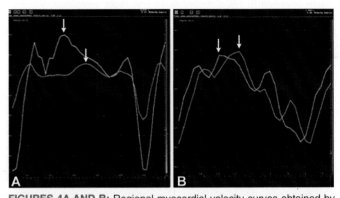

FIGURES 4A AND B: Regional myocardial velocity curves obtained by tissue Doppler imaging (TDI) at the basal septal (yellow) and basal lateral (green) segments. (A) In a patient with left bundle branch block with QRS duration of 180 ms, there was delay in peak systolic contraction (arrows) of 95 ms in the lateral wall compared to the septal wall; (B) After biventricular pacing, there was improvement in synchronicity as reflected by the near overlapping of myocardial velocity curves with a difference of only 20 ms. (*Source:* Modified from Yu et al. Comparison of efficacy of reverse remodeling and clinical improvement for relatively narrow and wide QRS complexes after cardiac resynchronization therapy for heart failure. J Cardiovasc Electrophysiol. 2004;15:1058-65)

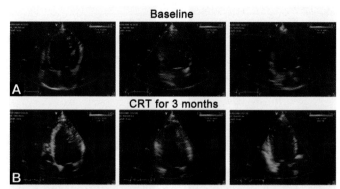

Baseline

CRT for 3 months

FIGURES 5A AND B: Tissue synchronization imaging (TSI) on three apical views showing the presence of extensive regional wall delay in a heart failure patient with prolonged QRS duration. The TSI method was set up to measure the time to peak myocardial systolic velocity (Ts) at ejection phase. The Ts values were then transformed into various color coding depending on the severity of delay, in the sequence of *green, yellow, orange* and *red*. (A) Before cardiac resynchronization therapy (CRT), this patient had severe delay over the basal to mid-lateral wall and the whole septal wall (*red* color in four-chamber view), severe delay over the whole inferior wall (*red* color in two-chamber view) and moderate to severe delay over the whole posterior wall (*orange* to *red* color in long-axis view); (B) Three months after CRT, corresponding views showed dramatic improvement of these delays, with only mild residual delay over the lateral and inferior wall (*green* to *yellow*). (*Source:* Yu C, et al. A novel tool to assess systolic asynchrony and identify responders of cardiac resynchronization therapy by tissue synchronization imaging. J Am Coll Cardiol. 2005;45:677-84)

a number of models have been constructed to define dyssynchrony using variable numbers of myocardial segments. Several studies have demonstrated that TSI (including visual and quantitative parameters) is useful in predicting a response to CRT.[62-64]

STRAIN RATE IMAGING (SRI)

One of the major limitations of TDI is that myocardial velocities may be overestimated or underestimated by translational motion or tethering of the myocardium respectively.[65] Strain imaging overcomes this problem by measuring the actual extent of myocardial deformation in selected regions of the heart. In this manner, it can distinguish between passive motion and active contraction. Myocardial deformation occurs in three dimensions, and strain can therefore be assessed along each axis. Radial strain (RS) represents the myocardial thickening in a short-axis plane; circumferential strain (CS) represents myocardial shortening in a circumferential plane, and longitudinal strain (LS) represents the myocardial shortening in the long-axis plane.[66] Regional differences in strain along any of these axes, can be a marker of LV dyssynchrony. As with other echocardiographic techniques to evaluate dyssynchrony, a number of SRI-derived indices have been shown to predict reverse remodeling and response to CRT.[67-69]

SPECKLED TRACKING

The speckled tracking (ST) is another echocardiographic technique that takes advantage of acoustic markers produced by reflection, scattering and interference of the echo ultrasound beam to assess regional myocardial motion.

Unlike TSI, which relies on tissue Doppler to assess myocardial strain, ST is not limited by angle dependence of the ultrasound transducer. Several studies have validated the used of speckled tracking measured LV dyssynchrony to predict response to CRT.[70-72]

THE PROSPECT TRIAL

One of the major limitations of the studies, such as the ones mentioned above, was that they were for the most part, confined to single centers and contained relatively few numbers of patients. The PROSPECT trial was designed to address these limitations. The PROSPECT was a nonrandomized observational study that sought to identify which of the previously published markers of dyssynchrony could predict response to CRT in a multicenter setting in three major regions (United States, Europe, Hong Kong).[32] A total number of 12 echocardiographic markers of dyssynchrony were evaluated in nearly 500 patients with blinded analysis of dyssynchrony in three core laboratories. Dyssynchrony markers were based on both conventional and tissue Doppler based methods, speckled tracking was not evaluated.

The results of PROSPECT raised several concerns with respect to previously published single-center experiences. The feasibility of image acquisition was a major limitation, particularly for TDI measures. Specifically, the percentage of individual parameters deemed interpretable by the core laboratories was between 37% and 82% for TDI-based tests. Intraoperator and interoperator reproducibility was also a major issue ranging from 3.8 to 24.3% and 6.5 to 72.1% respectively. Most disappointing was that no single parameter appeared to predict response to CRT effectively. Sensitivity for predicting improvement in the clinical composite endpoint ranged from 6 to 74% and specificity ranged from 35 to 92%. For all measured parameters, the area under the ROC curve to predict a positive response was less than or equal to 0.62.

Despite the results of PROSPECT, many investigators and clinicians continue to believe in the utility of dyssynchrony imaging for CRT. In PROSPECT, some investigators have raised concerns about site selection, lack of quality control, lack of adequate training, poor patient selection and poor image acquisition as the factors that might account for the discrepancies between its results and other previously published studies.[73,74] The role of echo-derived dyssynchrony imaging for CRT thus remains uncertain, and future studies will likely be performed to help elucidate this issue.

OTHER DYSSYNCHRONY IMAGING TECHNIQUES

In addition to two-dimensional echocardiography, a myriad of other imaging techniques have been utilized to assess dyssynchrony and/or predict response to CRT.

MAGNETIC RESONANCE IMAGING

The magnetic resonance imaging (MRI) is able to offer an integrated assessment of myocardial viability, function, dyssynchrony, anatomy and scar burden making it an attractive modality for patients in whom CRT is being considered. Advantages of CMR include high spatial resolution and reproducibility, accurate assessment of cardiac chamber size and the ability to assess myocardial deformation in three dimensions. However, it is limited by high-cost, long acquisition times and, for the time being, incompatibility with implanted devices.

Three major CMR techniques have been used to assess LV dyssynchrony. The CMR myocardial tagging is similar to speckled tracking analysis whereby a grid is superimposed onto the myocardial image and myocardial strain is assessed via analysis of grid deformation. The CMR phase-contrast tissue velocity mapping (TVM) allows direct myocardial wall motion measurement similar to TDI (i.e. comparing velocity timing obtained in different regions of the myocardium). Unlike TDI, MR TVM is not limited by the acoustical windows of the chest and can acquire three-directional velocity information of the entire myocardium.[75] Displacement-encoded MRI, or DENSE, is a CMR technique that is similar to TVM. However, instead of coding for velocity, DENSE codes for myocardial displacement which are then used to calculate myocardial strain and dyssynchrony. While these MRI techniques are promising, there is currently little data to support their used in predicting response to CRT.

In addition to the quantification of strain, MRI is particularly useful in the assessment of myocardial scar via a technique known as delayed gadolinium enhancement. A high scar burden has been shown to correlate negatively with response to CRT.[76,77] The location of scar is also an important factor in considering CRT. Bleeker and his colleagues demonstrated that patients with ischemic cardiomyopathy, dyssynchrony and posterolateral scar as assessed by MRI do not respond well to CRT.[78]

NUCLEAR IMAGING

Equilibrium radionuclide angiography (ERNA) and gated SPECT myocardial perfusion imaging (MPI) have also been used to assess VV and LV. The ERNA derived phase image analysis, a functional method based on the first Fourier harmonic fit of the gated blood pool versus radioactivity curve, generates the parameters of amplitude (A) and phase angle (Ø). Amplitude (A) measures the magnitude of regional contraction and phase angle (Ø) represents the timing of regional contraction (Fig. 6). In a healthy heart, all segments of the myocardium should contract during the same phase angle. The mean and standard deviation of LV Ø have been used to characterize LV dyssynchrony[79] and has been used to predict changes in ejection fraction after CRT.[80] More recently, the synchrony (S) [efficiency of contraction in a region of interest (ROI)] and entropy (E) (disorder of contraction in a ROI) parameters have been developed and applied to planar ERNA as a tool for evaluation of LV dyssynchrony.[81] In one study, these parameters were shown to detect mechanical dyssynchrony with low interobserver and intraobserver variability.[82]

The role of ERNA or MPI dyssynchrony imaging represents a promising advance of a well-established myocardial imaging technology. Whether or not it will be useful in predicting response to CRT will need to be assessed in future studies. The role of nuclear imaging for evaluation of scar burden is somewhat better established. As with CMR, MPI has also been

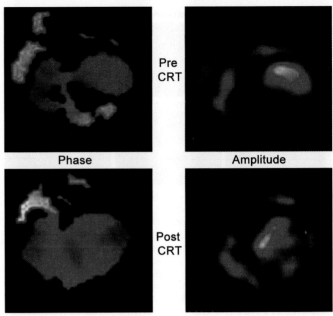

FIGURE 6: Equilibrium radionuclide angiogram (ERNA) images showing phase and amplitude analysis that are used to measure left ventricular dyssynchrony before and after cardiac resynchronization therapy (CRT). Phase analysis shows timing of regional contraction that shows apical dyssynchrony that corrects after CRT. Amplitude analysis reflects magnitude of regional contraction that shows improvement after CRT

used to assess LV scar burden. Similar to MRI studies, scar burden as assessed by SPECT has been shown to correlate negatively with response to CRT.[83-85]

REAL-TIME THREE-DIMENSIONAL ECHOCARDIOGRAPHY

The real-time three-dimensional echocardiography (RT3DE) has emerged as a new technique for assessment of LV dyssynchrony based on evaluation of LV regional volumetric changes.[86] This technique is accomplished by dividing the LV into 17 standard subvolumes and assessing the time for each segment to reach the minimum systolic volume (Tmsv). In a normally contracting heart the Tmsv should occur simultaneously for all myocardial segments. The standard deviation of 16 segments is used to create a dyssynchrony index (DI).[87] Preliminary data from a single center suggests that this technique may be used to predict response to CRT.[87] While RT3DE offers several advantages including accurate assessment of chamber size and volume, angle independence and semi-automated measurement, its application may be limited by translational artifacts and suboptimal image quality which may render the data unreadable.[88]

MULTIDETECTOR COMPUTED TOMOGRAPHY

Preliminary investigations have been performed utilizing computed tomography (CT) to assess LV dyssynchrony. Truong and his colleagues have derived several dyssynchrony indices with 64 slice CT using changes in wall thickness, wall motion and volume overtime.[89] The global LV dyssynchrony metric using changes in LV wall thickness overtime (average of the SD of 6 segments per slice, using all slices) had the best reproducibility with high interobserver and intraobserver reproducibility. Compared to aged-matched controls, patients with systolic HF and wide QRS had a higher DI. This DI was also moderately well correlated with dyssynchrony as measured by 2D speckled tracking and RT3DE. As with MRI, CT assessment can provide additional information about the heart including its chamber size volumetric analysis, and contractile function. One of the unique features of CT is its ability to visualize CS anatomy, which could help operators to determine optimal lead location prior to implantation.

DYSSYNCHRONY SUMMARY

Despite extensive research and the multitude of imaging modalities established to assess myocardial dyssynchrony, its role in CRT remains uncertain. No single dyssynchrony parameter has been shown to conclusively predict response to CRT. While many of the above techniques appear promising, conclusive large-scale trials will need to be performed before dyssynchrony assessment can be incorporated into routine clinical practice. Accordingly, neither the ACC/AHA/HRS guidelines for device-based therapy of cardiac rhythm abnormalities nor the ACC/AHA guidelines for the diagnosis and management of HF recommend the use of dyssynchrony imaging to establish candidacy for CRT.[29,90]

LV LEAD PLACEMENT

The site of placement of the LV lead has also been shown to be an important determinant of the effects of CRT with demonstration of significantly better outcomes with lateral LV pacing as compared to anterior LV pacing.[16] Echocardiogram with TDI has been used to select sites of latest activation in the LV that will be ideal sites for placement of the LV lead.[91] Surgical LV lead placement should be considered when these areas of latest activation do not have a suitable CS branch vein that allows transvenous lead placement.[92-94] We have used multiple gated acquisition scan (MUGA) to identify areas of latest mechanical activation and shown significant improvement in clinical outcomes with imaging guided lead placement as compared to the traditional placement in the lateral LV.[95] Radiographic LV-RV interlead distance has also been shown to predict acute hemodynamic response to CRT as measured by a rise in dP/dt and this can be used to improve the success rate at the time of lead implantation.[96] Placement of the LV lead at areas of LV scarring is unlikely to show response to CRT and can lead to worsening of congestive heart failure (CHF) due to unopposed RV pacing[97] or worsening of ventricular tachycardia.[98] Imaging with PET or contrast enhanced cardiovascular magnetic resonance can identify areas of LV scar preoperatively.

CRT COMPLICATIONS

As with any implantable device there are a myriad of potential complications associated with CRT. In addition to standard device complications, such as infection and bleeding, there are several complications specific to CRT including: CS dissection and perforation, phrenic nerve stimulation and LV lead

dislodgement. In major trials, LV lead dislodgement occurred in 4–6% of the patients.[10,18] The CS sinus dissection or perforation ranged from 0.3 to 4% and 0.8 to 2% respectively.[10,18,25] Management for CS dissection or perforation is usually conservative and, in most instances, CS cannulation can safely be performed several weeks later.

PHRENIC NERVE SIMULATION

The LV lead is frequently positioned in the region of the left phrenic nerve that may in turn lead to diaphragmatic stimulation. Although great care is taken to avoid phrenic nerve stimulation during implantation, subtle changes in lead position as well as postural changes can cause this complication at anytime postimplant. Phrenic nerve stimulation is often easy to recognize by observing the contractions of the abdomen during pacemaker output. Frequently, patients will complain of discomfort that occurs with certain positions or movements. It is sometimes helpful to ask a patient to recreate the setting in which they experience discomfort in order to make the diagnosis. A cardiologist or industry representative should be made immediately aware if the diagnosis of phrenic nerve stimulation is made. Although it is not life threatening, it can be the source of considerable discomfort for a patient. Frequently, a CRT device can be reprogrammed to eliminate phrenic nerve stimulation. At times, however, revision of the LV lead may be necessary.

LOSS OF CRT

As discussed above, it is essential to ensure maximum BiV pacing among patients with CRT devices. There are a number of settings in which maximum BiV pacing can be compromised (Table 2). It is important to recognize the loss of BiV capture in order to maximize the benefits of CRT.

CRT AND VENTRICULAR ARRHYTHMIAS

Several small studies have suggested that CRT may have a role in reducing the incidence of ventricular arrhythmias.[99-101] Although decreasing wall tension and favorable remodeling provide a biological basis for this hypothesis, CRT has not been formally tested in this manner. In many of the large randomized trials of CRT, the impact of CRT on the incidence of VT and

TABLE 2

Causes of loss of biventricular pacing

- Atrial undersensing can be caused by a variety of factors including sinus tachycardia with first-degree AV block, atrial fibrillation and lead dislodgement
- Fusion or pseudofusion (discussed above)
- Ventricular oversensing
- Atrial tachyarrhythmias with rapid ventricular conduction (frequently AF)
- Frequent ventricular ectopy
- Loss of LV capture due to LV pacing threshold increase
- Loss of LV capture due to LV lead dislodgement

VT storm was not systematically studied. However, meta-analysis of five major CRT trials revealed that sudden cardiac death was not significantly reduced by CRT when compared to optimal medical therapy.[102] In all but one of these trials, (CARE-HF) CRT, was not associated with a decreased risk of sudden death.

There is also concern that CRT has been associated with increases in ventricular arrhythmias. There are numerous reported cases of patients developing recurrent ventricular arrhythmias following implantation of a BiV device.[98,103-106] Various mechanisms have been proposed to explain CRT-associated ventricular arrhythmia including LV pacing in close proximity to scar, increases in the transmural dispersion of repolarization (which is proarrhythmic), and alteration of the wavefront of LV activation which is thought to facilitate re-entry.[106,107]

Nayak and his colleagues described a series of 8 out of 191 (4%) patients who developed VT storm (VTS) following BiV implantation.[106] Several observations, such as (1) VTS developed a mean of 16 ± 12.5 days after initiation of BVP, (2) VTS was refractory to intravenous antiarrhythmic medication and was managed by turning off LV pacing and/or radio-frequency catheter ablation and long-term oral antiarrhythmic therapy, (3) of the four patients who refused catheter ablation, three had cessation of VTS after turning off the LV lead; the fourth had the LV lead reprogrammed to a lower output resulting in considerable reduction in the burden of VT and (4) despite elimination of VT, the presence of VTS carried a poor prognosis in that all eight patients subsequently developed refractory CHF, were made in this single-center case-series.

Although reports such as these raise the possibility that CRT may facilitate VT in select patients, this concept has not been firmly established. Nonetheless, clinicians should consider this possibility in patients with BIV devices admitted for incessant VT refractory to antiarrhythmic therapy.

EMERGING CRT INDICATIONS

NARROW QRS

Although the benefits of CRT have been well established in patients with wide QRS duration, its role in patients with normal QRS is less clear. A number of small nonrandomized studies have been conducted which suggest that patients with narrow QRS and dyssynchrony benefit from CRT.[108-111] In addition, Jeevanantham and his colleagues performed a meta-analysis of nonrandomized narrow QRS CRT trials. Pooled data from three studies (totaling 98 patients) found that CRT was associated with improvements in NYHA, LVEF and 6-minute walking distance (6MWD).[112]

The role of CRT in narrow QRS patients was evaluated in a prospective randomized fashion in the RethinQ trial.[113] In this study, 172 patients with LVEF less than 35%, NHYA class III HF, QRS interval of less than 130 millisecond and evidence of mechanical dyssynchrony as measured by echocardiography were randomized to CRT + ICD or ICD-alone groups. No significant difference between these groups was found with respect to the primary endpoint of increase in peak oxygen consumption at 6 months. Additionally, no difference with

respect of echocardiographic evidence of remodeling was observed between the two groups.

Despite these negative results, many clinicians and investigators continue to believe in the value of CRT in narrow QRS HF populations. Some of the criticisms of RethinQ, include, reliance on nonspecific dyssynchrony criteria (TDI-measured opposing wall delay greater than 65 millisecond, short follow-up time and a primary endpoint that was not studied in the major CRT trials. Further clinical trials are currently underway to determine whether alternative study designs may help to elucidate the discrepancies between RethinQ and previous observational studies among patients with HF and narrow QRS durations.[114]

ATRIAL FIBRILLATION

Multiple observational and at least one randomized trial have demonstrated benefit among patients who meet standard criteria for CRT and coexisting atrial fibrillation (AF).[115-118] In these trials, many of the enrolled patients had well-controlled ventricular rates, or else, had undergone prior AV nodal ablation. This underscores the challenges associated with the optimal delivery of BiV pacing in patients with AF. In AF, high ventricular rates may inhibit consistent BiV pacing. In addition, heart rate irregularity may result in fusion or pseudofusion thereby attenuating or eliminating the effects of BiV capture.

To overcome these challenges AV nodal ablation is increasingly utilized in patients with AF who meet criteria for CRT. Although this procedure renders a patient pacemaker-dependant and eliminates AV synchrony, it serves to regularize ventricular performance, and ensures 100% BiV pacing. The net result may be improvement in patient symptoms and beneficial remodeling in patients with HF. In one study, Gasparini and his colleagues prospectively evaluated 673 patients (162 in AF, 511 in sinus rhythm) with LVEF less than or equal to 35%, QRS greater than or equal to 120 millisecond, and NYHA greater than or equal to II.[119] Patients who were deemed to have inadequate BiV capture (arbitrarily determined to be < 85%) underwent AV nodal ablation. Both SR and AF groups showed significant and sustained improvements of all assessed parameters ($p < Û0.001$ for all parameters). However, within the AF group, only patients who underwent ablation showed a significant increase of ejection fraction ($p < 0.001$), reverse remodeling effect ($p < 0.001$) and improved exercise tolerance ($p < 0.001$); no improvements with respect to these parameters were observed in AF patients who did not undergo ablation. Although this strategy has not been evaluated in a randomized prospective fashion, a clinician should consider AV nodal ablation in AF patients with CRT devices, in whom consistent BIV capture cannot consistently be obtained or reliably assessed.

PACEMAKER DEPENDANT PATIENTS

It is well established that RV pacing is associated with hemo-dynamic derangement, the promotion of dyssynchrony and worsening of LV function, particularly among patients with decreased ejection fraction.[120-126] Early evidence that RV pacing may impact clinical endpoints came from analysis of the Mode

Selection Trial (MOST) a 6-year randomized trial of dual chamber rate adaptive pacemaker (DDDR) versus ventricular rate modulated pacing (VVIR) pacing in patients with sinus node dysfunction. Analysis of the trial suggested that the cumulative percent of ventricular paced beats (Cum%VP) was a strong predictor of HF hospitalization in both DDDR and VVIR modes.[125]

Corroborating evidence came from the dual chamber and VVI implantable defibrillator (DAVID) trial in which patients eligible for ICD were randomized to dual chamber universal, rate responsive (DDD/R) pacing at a lower rate of 70 or VVI, at a lower rate of 40 beats/min. The study was terminated prematurely due to an excess of HF and deaths in the DDD/R arm.[123] Subsequent analysis of the DAVID trial suggested that the lowest risk of HF worsening and death was seen in patients randomized to DDD/R with a low Cum%VP.[127]

The findings from these studies provided a therapeutic rational to investigate whether CRT may attenuate the negative impact of chronic long-term RV apical pacing. The Homburg Biventricular Pacing Evaluation (HOBIPACE) was a prospective randomized crossover study of patients with LV dysfunction and need for antibradycardiac pacing.[128] When compared with RV pacing, CRT was found to be superior to RV pacing as it induced reverse LV remodeling with significant reductions in LV end-diastolic and end-systolic volumes and an increase in ejection fraction. In addition, BiV pacing was found to impact favorably on the Minnesota living with HF score, NT-proBNP levels and peak oxygen consumption. The HOBIPACE was a small trial (30 patients) but served to reinforce the notion that RV pacing may particularly be detrimental to patients with pre-existing LV dysfunction.

The role of CRT among patients with normal EF and standard indications for pacing was tested in the pacing to avoid cardiac enlargement (PACE) trial.[129] A total of 177 patients with standard pacing indications in whom a BiV pacemaker was implanted were randomized to BiV pacing or RV apical pacing. The primary endpoints were LVEF and ESV at 12 months. In both groups, devices were programmed to ensure maximum pacing. During a follow-up period of 12 months, no effect on the primary endpoints was observed among those randomized to BiV pacing. However, there was a decline of 6.7 percentage points in LVEF and a 25% increase in left ventricular end-systolic volume in patients who were assigned to right ventricular pacing. The LVEF declined to less than 45% in 9% of the patients in the right-ventricular-pacing group.

While thought provoking, the results of PACE by no means suggest that all patients with pacing indications require a CRT device. First, roughly 40% of patients in each group had sinus node dysfunction. Since the study was designed to force RV pacing in the RV apical pacing group, native AV conduction would have been possible with alternative programming. In many patients, particularly those with sinus node dysfunction, RV pacing can be minimized by the use of extended AV delays, hysteresis and device algorithms that promote native AV conduction.

Second, there is a limited body of evidence that selective site right ventricular pacing (for example, from the RVOT) may be less detrimental than RV apical pacing.[130] It is possible that alternative RV pacing sites may sufficient to prevent adverse remodeling in properly selective patients. This could in theory obviate the need for CRT in patients with normal ejection fraction and AV nodal disease. However, larger clinical trials will need to be conducted to establish this as a viable pacing strategy.

Third, the clinical significance of the volumetric changes observed in the RV pacing group remains unknown. Although these changes are intuitively undesirable, they were not associated with concomitant reductions in 6-minute walking test, QOL or hospitalization for HF. It is possible that with longer follow-up duration, these parameters may have also been adversely affected.

Finally, only 9% of patients in the RV apical pacing group experienced significant reductions in LVEF (< 45%). This suggests that, at one year, the vast majority of patients with normal EF in whom antibradycardic pacing is indicated will not experience steep declines in their cardiac function with RV apical pacing. Accordingly, clinicians might consider initial implantation of an RV lead in these patients with the addition of an LV lead should a patient's EF decline with serial echocardiographic monitoring.

MINIMALLY SYMPTOMATIC HEART FAILURE

The beneficial effect of CRT on ventricular remodeling has prompted investigators to evaluate the role of CRT in patients with depressed ejection fraction and minimal symptoms (NYHA I-II). The resynchronization reverse remodeling in systolic left ventricular dysfunction (REVERSE) trial enrolled 610 patients with NYHA I or II HF, QRS greater than or equal to 120 millisecond and LVEF less than or equal to 40%.[131] All enrollees were implanted with CRT devices +/− ICD. Following implantation, patients were randomized in 2:1 fashion to CRT-on or CRT-off. At 12 months, there was no difference between these groups with respect to the trial's primary endpoint, a clinical composite that assessed worsening of HF through a number of measures including all-cause mortality, heart-failure hospitalizations, crossover due to worsening HF, NYHA class and the patient global assessment. The CRT was however shown to improve left ventricular end-systolic volumes (LVESV), left ventricular end-diastolic volumes (LVEDV) and LVEF.

A prospectively planned two-year follow-up of 262 European participants in REVERSE was also conducted. At two years, comparison of the CRT-on versus CRT-off groups demonstrated that a significantly higher percentage of patients in the latter group had a worsening of HF (34 vs 19% p = 0.01). Improvement in volumetric parameters persisted over this time period. In addition, there was a 12% absolute risk reduction in the time to first hospitalization or death, associated with CRT therapy (p = 0.003).

A similar hypothesis was tested in the MADIT-CRT trial.[132] In this study, 1,820 patients with ischemic or nonischemic cardiomyopathy, EF less than or equal to 30%, QRS greater than or equal to 130 millisecond and NYHA class I or II symptoms were randomly assigned to receive CRT + ICD or ICD alone. The primary end point was death from any cause or nonfatal heart-failure event (whichever came first). After a mean follow-up of 2.5 years, CRT therapy was associated with a significant 34% reduction in the risk of death or nonfatal HF (p = 0.001). The difference between CRT and control groups was driven primarily by a reduced incidence of HF events among those randomized to CRT (23 vs 14% p < 0.001). As with many other CRT trials, CRT was associated with significant improvements in LVESV, LVEDV and EF.

The results of REVERSE and MADIT-CRT suggest that CRT may play a role in delaying HF progression in patients with minimal symptoms. Based on MADIT-CRT, FDA has recently been approved CRT therapy in patients with wide QRS, reduced ejection fraction and NYHA class I and II.

CRT FOR ACUTE DECOMPENSATED HEART FAILURE

Patients with systolic HF who are admitted to the ICU may be candidates for CTR. In these instances, patients who meet current guidelines for CRT implantation should be referred for further evaluation. In general, however, it is preferable to wait until a patient is stabilized, before CRT implantation is undertaken. Rarely, is CRT therapy required in an acute setting for patient stabilization. Although there is little evidence to guide the practice, many clinicians advocate acute implantation of CRT device for patients who meet criteria for implantation and cannot be weaned from inotropic therapies or else are responding poorly to aggressive HF management.[133,134] In this setting, there may be a role for acute CRT implantation as carefully selected patients may acutely respond with dramatic improvement in their clinical status. These cases should be evaluated on an individual basis in concert with consulting cardiologists, electrophysiologists or HF specialists.

SUMMARY

The advent of CRT has been an important development in the management of HF. The results of multiple large-scale clinical trials have consistently demonstrated its favorable impact on symptoms related to HF. In addition, there is mounting evidence that CRT is associated with mortality benefit. Current indications for CRT include patients with wide QRS and ejection fraction less than or equal to 35% with advanced HF despite optimal medical management. Around 30–40% of the patients who are candidates for CRT do not respond. This can be improved by optimizing the device, using imaging to select patients based on dyssynchrony and optimal LV lead placement. In the future, indications for BIV implantation may expand to include select patients with systolic HF and narrow QRS and patients with normal ejection fraction who require chronic RV pacing.

MODIFIED SUMMARY OF GUIDELINES (ACC/AHA/HRS GUIDELINES FOR DEVICE-BASED THERAPY, JACC. 2008;51:E1-62)

Modified by Kanu Chatterjee

Class I: Conditions for which there is evidence and/or general agreement that a given procedure/therapy is useful and effective.

Class II: Conditions for which there is conflicting evidence and/or a divergence of opinion about the usefulness/efficacy of performing the procedure/therapy.

Class IIa: Weight of evidence/opinion is in favor of usefulness/efficacy.

Class IIb: Usefulness/efficacy is less well established by evidence/opinion.

Class III: Conditions for which there is evidence and/or general agreement that a procedure/therapy is not useful/effective and in some cases may be harmful.

Level A (highest): Derived from multiple randomized clinical trials.

Level B (intermediate): Data are on the basis of a limited number of randomized trials, nonrandomized studies or observational registries.

Level C (lowest): Primary basis for the recommendation was expert opinion.

RECOMMENDATIONS FOR PERMANENT PACING IN SINUS NODE DYSFUNCTION (SND)

Class I:
1. Permanent pacemaker implantation is indicated in symptomatic patients with symptomatic bradycardia including frequent symptomatic sinus pauses (Level of Evidence C).
2. Permanent pacemaker implantation is indicated for symptomatic chronotropic incompetence (Level of Evidence C).

Class IIa:
1. Permanent pacemaker implantation is reasonable for SND with heart rate less than 40/bpm, when a clear association between symptoms consistent with bradycardia and actual presence of bradycardia has not been documented (Level of Evidence C).
2. Permanent pacemaker implantation is reasonable in patients with unexplained syncope when SND is documented by electrophysiologic studies (Level of Evidence C).

Class IIb:
1. Permanent pacemaker therapy is reasonable in minimally symptomatic patients with chronic awake heart rate of less than 40/bpm (Level of Evidence C).

RECOMMENDATIONS FOR ACQUIRED ATRIOVENTRICULAR BLOCK IN ADULTS.

Class I:
1. Permanent pacemaker therapy is indicated in patients with third-degree and advanced second-degree AV block even in absence of symptoms (Level of Evidence C).
2. Permanent pacemaker therapy is indicated in patients with third-degree or advanced second-degree AV block in asymptomatic patients with documented period of asystole of 3 seconds or greater (Level of Evidence C).
3. Permanent pacemaker implantation is indicated in patients with third-degree or advanced second-degree AV block developing after AV nodal ablation (Level of Evidence C).
4. Permanent pacemaker therapy is indicated in postcardiac surgery AV block when AV block is unlikely to resolve (Level of Evidence C).
5. Permanent pacemaker treatment is indicated in patients with neuromuscular diseases (e.g. Duchane's and Baker's, limb girdle, peroneal muscular dystrophy) with third-degree or advanced second-degree AV block with or without symptoms (Level of Evidence B).
6. Permanent pacemaker therapy is indicated in symptomatic patients with any type of second degree AV block (Level of Evidence B).
7. Permanent pacemaker therapy is indicated in patients with systolic heart failure with third-degree or infranodal AV block in absence of symptoms related to heart block (Level of Evidence B).
8. Permanent pacemaker implantation is indicated in patients who develop second or third-degree AV block during exercise unrelated to myocardial ischemia (Level of Evidence C).

Class IIa:
1. Permanent pacemaker therapy is reasonable in asymptomatic patients with third-degree, or intra or infra Hisian AV block (Level of Evidence C).
2. Symptom limited exercise test at 3 to 6 weeks after discharge to assess prognosis, activity prescription or evaluation of medical therapy if early exercise test was submaximal.

RECOMMENDATIONS FOR PERMANENT PACING IN CHRONIC BIFASCICULAR BLOCK

Class I:
1. Permanent pacemaker therapy is indicated in patients with bifascicular block with advanced second-degree, intermittent third-degree or alternating bundle-branch block (Level of Evidence B).

Class IIa:
1. Permanent pacemaker implantation is reasonable in patients with bifascicular block with history of syncope when other causes have been excluded (Level of Evidence B).
2. Permanent pacemaker implantation is reasonable in patients with bifascicular block if HV interval is 100 ms or greater documented during electrophysiologic study (Level of Evidence B).

RECOMMENDATIONS FOR PERMANENT PACING AFTER THE ACUTE PHASE OF MYOCARDIAL INFARCTION

Class I:
1. Permanent pacemaker therapy is indicated in post-ST elevation myocardial infarction with intermittent or persistent third-degree, advanced second-degree infranodal AV block or alternating bundle-branch block (Level of Evidence B).
2. Permanent pacemaker therapy is indicated in symptomatic second-degree or third-degree AV block (Level of Evidence C).

RECOMMENDATIONS FOR PERMANENT PACING IN HYPERSENSITIVE CAROTID SINUS SYNDROME AND NEUROCARDIOGENIC SYNCOPE

Class I:
1. Permanent pacemaker implantation is indicated in patients with recurrent syncope due to hypersensitive carotid sinus syndrome with ventricular asystole of 3 seconds or longer (Level of Evidence C).

Class IIa:
1. Permanent pacing is reasonable in patient with hypersensitive carotid sinus syndrome with cardioinhibitory response of 3 seconds or longer without provocative events (Level of Evidence C).

Class IIb:
1. In patients with neurocardiogenic syncope permanent pacemaker therapy may be considered associated cardioinhibitory response occurring spontaneously or during tilt-table test (Level of Evidence B).

RECOMMENDATIONS FOR PACING AFTER CARDIAC TRANSPLANTATION

1. Permanent pacemaker implantation is indicated for inappropriate heart rate response and for Class I indications as in non transplant patients (Level of Evidence C).

Class IIb:
1. Permanent pacemaker therapy can be considered in postcardiac transplant patients with recurrent prolonged bradycardia or inappropriate heart rate response that limits rehabilitation (Level of Evidence C).

RECOMMENDATIONS FOR PACING TO PREVENT TACHYCARDIA

Class I:
1. Permanent pacemaker implantation is indicated for sustained pause-dependent ventricular tachycardia with or without QT prolongation (Level of Evidence C).

Class IIa:
1. Permanent pacemaker implantation is reasonable in high-risk patients with congenital Long QT syndrome (Level of Evidence B).

Class IIb:
1. Permanent pacing may be considered in patients with brady-tachy syndrome with recurrent atrial fibrillation (Level of Evidence B).
2. After discharge for activity counseling and/or exercise training as part of cardiac rehabilitation in patients who have undergone revascularization

Class IIb:
1. In patients with ECG abnormalities of LBBB, pre-excitation syndrome, left ventricular hypertrophy, digoxin therapy, greater than 1 mm resting ST depression. Electronically paced ventricular rhythm.
2. Periodic monitoring in patients who continue to participate in exercise training or cardiac rehabilitation.

Class III:
1. Severe comorbidity likely to limit life expectancy and/or candidacy for revascularization.
2. To evaluate patients with acute myocardial infarction with uncompensated heart failure, cardiac arrythmia or noncardiac conditions that limit the ability to exercise (Level of Evidence C).
3. Predischarge exercise test in patients who had already cardiac catheterization (Level of Evidence C).

ASYMPTOMATIC DIABETIC PATIENTS

Class IIa:
1. Evaluation of asymptomatic patients with diabetes who plan to do vigorous exercise (Level of Evidence C).

Class IIb:
1. Evaluation of patients with multiple risk factors as guide to risk-reduction therapy.
2. Evaluation of asymptomatic men older than 45 years or women older than 55 years who plan to do vigorous exercise or who are involved in an occupation in which exercise impairment may impact public safety or who are at high-risk for CAD.

Class III:
1. Routine screening of asymptomatic men or women.

PATIENTS WITH VALVULAR HEART DISEASE

Class I:
1. In patients with chronic aortic regurgitation for assessment of symptoms and functional capacity in whom it is difficult assess symptoms.

Class IIa:
1. In patients with chronic aortic regurgitation for evaluation of symptoms and functional capacity before participation in athletic activity.
2. In patients with chronic aortic regurgitation for assessment of prognosis before aortic valve replacement in asymptomatic or minimally symptomatic patients with left ventricular dysfunction.

Class IIb:
1. Evaluation of patients with valvular heart disease (see guide lines in valvular heart disease).

Class III:
1. For diagnosis of CAD in patients with moderate to severe valvular heart disease or with LBBB, electronically paced rhythm, pre-excitation syndrome or greater than 1 mm ST depression in the rest ECG.

PATIENTS WITH RHYTHM DISORDERS

Class I:
1. For identification of appropriate settings in patients with rate-adaptive pacemakers.
2. For evaluation of congenital complete heart block in patients considering increased physical activity or participation in competitive sports (Level of Evidence C).

Class IIa:
1. Evaluation of patients with known or suspected exercise-induced arrhythmias.
2. Evaluation medical, surgical or ablation therapy in patients with exercise-induced arrhythmias (including atrial fibrillation).

Class IIb:
1. Investigation of isolated ventricular ectopic beats in middle aged patients without other evidence of CAD.
2. For investigation of prolonged first-degree atrioventricular block or type I second degree Wenckebach, left bundle-branch block, right bundle-branch block or isolated ectopic beats in young persons considering participation in competitive sports (Level of Evidence C).

Class III:
1. Routine investigations of isolated ectopic beats in young patients.

CHAPTER 40 Cardiac Resynchronization Therapy

REFERENCES

1. Lloyd-Jones D, Adams RJ, Brown TM, et al. Heart disease and stroke statistics 2010 update: a report from the American Heart Association. Circulation. 2010;121:e46-215.
2. Rogers WJ, Johnstone DE, Yusuf S, et al. Effect of enalapril on survival in patients with reduced left ventricular ejection fractions and congestive heart failure. N Engl J Med. 1991;325:293-302.
3. CIBIS-II Investigators. The cardiac insufficiency bisoprolol study II: a randomised trial. Lancet. 1999;353:9-13.
4. Packer M, Coats AJ, Fowler MB, et al. Effect of carvedilol on survival in severe chronic heart failure. N Engl J Med. 2001;344:1651-8.
5. Hjalmarson A, Goldstein S, Fagerberg B, et al. Effects of controlled-release metoprolol on total mortality, hospitalizations and well-being in patients with heart failure: the Metoprolol CR/XL Randomized Intervention Trial in congestive heart failure (MERIT-HF). MERIT-HF Study Group. JAMA. 2000;283:1295-302.
6. Pitt B, Remme W, Zannad F, et al. Eplerenone: a selective aldosterone blocker in patients with left ventricular dysfunction after myocardial infarction. N Engl J Med. 2003;348:1309-21.
7. Pitt B, Zannad F, Remme WJ, et al. The effect of spironolactone on morbidity and mortality in patients with severe heart failure. Randomized aldactone evaluation study. N Engl J Med. 1999;341:709-17.
8. Moss AJ, Zareba W, Hall WJ, et al. Prophylactic implantation of a defibrillator in patients with myocardial infarction and reduced ejection fraction. N Engl J Med. 2002;346:877-83.
9. Bardy GH, Lee KL, Mark DB, et al. Amiodarone or an implantable cardioverter-defibrillator for congestive heart failure. N Engl J Med. 2005;352:225-37.
10. Cleland JG, Daubert JC, Erdmann E, et al. The effect of cardiac resynchronization on morbidity and mortality in heart failure. N Engl J Med. 2005;352:1539-49.
11. Reicin G, Miksic M, Yik A, et al. Hospital supplies and medical technology 4Q05. Statistical handbook: growth moderating but outlook remains strong. New York: Morgan Stanley Equity Research; 2005. p. 44.
12. American Heart Association. Heart Disease and Stroke Statistics–2010 Update. Dallas, Texas: American Heart Association; 2010.
13. Auricchio A, Prinzen FW. Update on the pathophysiological basics of cardiac resynchronization therapy. Europace. 2008;10:797-800.
14. Auricchio A, Stellbrink C, Block M, et al. Effect of pacing chamber and atrioventricular delay on acute systolic function of paced patients with congestive heart failure. The pacing therapies for congestive heart failure study group. The guidant congestive heart failure research group. Circulation. 1999;99:2993-3001.
15. Nishimura R, Hayes D, Holmes D, et al. Mechanism of hemodynamic improvement by dual-chamber pacing for severe left ventricular dysfunction: an acute Doppler and catheterization hemodynamic study. J Am Coll Cardiol. 1995;25:281-8.
16. Butter C, Auricchio A, Stellbrink C, et al. Effect of resynchronization therapy stimulation site on the systolic function of heart failure patients. Circulation. 2001;104:3026-9.
17. Breithardt OA, Sinha AM, Schwammenthal E, et al. Acute effects of cardiac resynchronization therapy on functional mitral regurgitation in advanced systolic heart failure. J Am Coll Cardiol. 2003;41:765-70.
18. Abraham WT, Fisher WG, Smith AL, et al. Cardiac resynchronization in chronic heart failure. N Engl J Med. 2002;346:1845-53.
19. Leclercq C, Cazeau S, Le Breton H, et al. Acute hemodynamic effects of biventricular DDD pacing in patients with end-stage heart failure. J Am Coll Cardiol. 1998;32:1825-31.
20. Kass DA, Chen CH, Curry C, et al. Improved left ventricular mechanics from acute VDD pacing in patients with dilated cardiomyopathy and ventricular conduction delay. Circulation. 1999;99:1567-73.
21. St John Sutton MG, Plappert T, Abraham WT, et al. Effect of cardiac resynchronization therapy on left ventricular size and function in chronic heart failure. Circulation. 2003;107:1985-90.
22. Saxon LA, De Marco T, Schafer J, et al. Effects of long-term biventricular stimulation for resynchronization on echocardiographic measures of remodeling. Circulation. 2002;105:1304-10.
23. Yu C, Chau E, Sanderson J, et al. Tissue Doppler echocardiographic evidence of reverse remodeling and improved synchronicity by

simultaneously delaying regional contraction after biventricular pacing therapy in heart failure. Circulation. 2002;105:438-45.

24. Cazeau S, Leclercq C, Lavergne T, et al. Effects of multisite biventricular pacing in patients with heart failure and intraventricular conduction delay. N Engl J Med. 2001;344:873-80.

25. Bristow MR, Saxon LA, Boehmer J, et al. Cardiac-resynchronization therapy with or without an implantable defibrillator in advanced chronic heart failure. N Engl J Med. 2004;350:2140-50.

26. Cleland JG, Daubert JC, Erdmann E, et al. The effect of cardiac resynchronization on morbidity and mortality in heart failure. N Engl J Med. 2005;352:1539-49.

27. McAlister FA, Ezekowitz J, Hooton N, et al. Cardiac resynchronization therapy for patients with left ventricular systolic dysfunction: a systematic review. JAMA. 2007;297:2502-14.

28. Abraham W, Fisher W, Smith A, et al. Cardiac resynchronization in chronic heart failure. N Engl J Med. 2002;346:1845-53.

29. Jessup M, Abraham WT, Casey DE, et al. Focused update: ACCF/AHA guidelines for the diagnosis and management of heart failure in adults. J Am Coll Cardiol. 2009;119:1977-2016.

30. Bleeker GB, Bax JJ, Fung JW, et al. Clinical versus echocardiographic parameters to assess response to cardiac resynchronization therapy. Am J Cardiol. 2006;97:260-3.

31. Birnie DH, Tang AS. The problem of non-response to cardiac resynchronization therapy. Curr Opin Cardiol. 2006;21:20-6.

32. Chung ES, Leon AR, Tavazzi L, et al. Results of the Predictors of Response to CRT (PROSPECT) trial. Circulation. 2008;117:2608-16.

33. Sweeney MO. Programming and follow-up of cardiac resynchronization devices. In: Ellenbogen KA (Ed). Clinical Cardiac Pacing, Defibrillation, and Resynchronization Therapy. Philadelphia: Elsevier; 2007. pp. 1087-140.

34. Molhoek SG, VANE L, Bootsma M, et al. QRS duration and shortening to predict clinical response to cardiac resynchronization therapy in patients with end-stage heart failure. Pacing Clin Electrophysiol. 2004;27:308-13.

35. Lecoq G, Leclercq C, Leray E, et al. Clinical and electrocardiographic predictors of a positive response to cardiac resynchronization therapy in advanced heart failure. Eur Heart J. 2005;26:1094-100.

36. Kashani A, Barold SS. Significance of QRS complex duration in patients with heart failure. J Am Coll Cardiol. 2005;46:2183-92.

37. Georger F SC, Collet B. Specific electrocardiographic patterns may assess left ventricular capture during biventricular pacing. Pacing Clin Electrophysiol. 2002;25:37-41.

38. Ammann P, Sticherling C, Kalusche D, et al. An electrocardiogram-based algorithm to detect loss of left ventricular capture during cardiac resynchronization therapy. Ann Intern Med. 2005;142:968-73.

39. Rao RK, Kumar UN, Schafer J, et al. Reduced ventricular volumes and improved systolic function with cardiac resynchronization therapy: a randomized trial comparing simultaneous biventricular pacing, sequential biventricular pacing, and left ventricular pacing. Circulation. 2007;115:2136-44.

40. Boriani G, Müller CP, Seidl KH, et al. Randomized comparison of simultaneous biventricular stimulation versus optimized interventricular delay in cardiac resynchronization therapy. The resynchronization for the hemodynamic treatment for heart failure management II implantable cardioverter defibrillator (RHYTHM II ICD) study. Am Heart J. 2006;151:1050-8.

41. Jansen AH, Bracke FA, van Dantzig JM, et al. Correlation of echo-Doppler optimization of atrioventricular delay in cardiac resynchronization therapy with invasive hemodynamics in patients with heart failure secondary to ischemic or idiopathic dilated cardiomyopathy. Am J Cardiol. 2006;97:552-7.

42. Barold SS, Ilercil A, Herweg B. Echocardiographic optimization of the atrioventricular and interventricular intervals during cardiac resynchronization. Europace. 2008;10:88-95.

43. Morales MA, Startari U, Panchetti L, et al. Atrioventricular delay optimization by doppler-derived left ventricular dP/dt improves 6-month outcome of resynchronized patients. Pacing Clin Electrophysiol. 2006;29:564-8.

44. Whinnett ZI, Davies JE, Willson K, et al. Haemodynamic effects of changes in atrioventricular and interventricular delay in cardiac resynchronisation therapy show a consistent pattern: analysis of shape, magnitude and relative importance of atrioventricular and interventricular delay. Heart. 2006;92:1628-34.

45. Braun MU, Schnabel A, Rauwolf T, et al. Impedance cardiography as a noninvasive technique for atrioventricular interval optimization in cardiac resynchronization therapy. J Interv Card Electrophysiol. 2005;13:223-9.

46. Burri H, Sunthorn H, Somsen A, et al. Optimizing sequential biventricular pacing using radionuclide ventriculography. Heart Rhythm. 2005;2:960-5.

47. Kamdar R, Frain E, Warburton F, et al. A prospective comparison of echocardiography and device algorithms for atrioventricular and interventricular interval optimization in cardiac resynchronization therapy. Europace. 2010;12:84-91.

48. Hardt SE, Yazdi SH, Bauer A, et al. Immediate and chronic effects of AV-delay optimization in patients with cardiac resynchronization therapy. Int J Cardiol. 2007;115:318-25.

49. Riedlbauchová L, Kautzner J, Frídl P. Influence of different atrioventricular and interventricular delays on cardiac output during cardiac resynchronization therapy. Pacing Clin Electrophysiol. 2005;28:S19-23.

50. Sawhney NS, Waggoner AD, Garhwal S, et al. Randomized prospective trial of atrioventricular delay programming for cardiac resynchronization therapy. Heart Rhythm. 2004;1:562-7.

51. Bax J, Abraham T, Barold S, et al. Cardiac resynchronization therapy: Part 1—issues before device implantation. J Am Coll Cardiol. 2005;46:2153-67.

52. Bax JJ, Bleeker GB, Marwick TH, et al. Left ventricular dyssynchrony predicts response and prognosis after cardiac resynchronization therapy. J Am Coll Cardiol. 2004;44:1834-40.

53. Ghio S, Constantin C, Klersy C, et al. Interventricular and intraventricular dyssynchrony are common in heart failure patients, regardless of QRS duration. Eur Heart J. 2004;25:571-8.

54. Bleeker G, Schalij M, Molhoek S, et al. Relationship between QRS duration and left ventricular dyssynchrony in patients with end-stage heart failure. J Cardiovasc Electrophysiol. 2004;15:544-9.

55. Pitzalis MV, Iacoviello M, Romito R, et al. Ventricular asynchrony predicts a better outcome in patients with chronic heart failure receiving cardiac resynchronization therapy. J Am Coll Cardiol. 2005;45:65-9.

56. Pitzalis MV, Iacoviello M, Romito R, et al. Cardiac resynchronization therapy tailored by echocardiographic evaluation of ventricular asynchrony. J Am Coll Cardiol. 2002;40:1615-22.

57. Sassone B, Capecchi A, Boggian G, et al. Value of baseline left lateral wall postsystolic displacement assessed by M-mode to predict reverse remodeling by cardiac resynchronization therapy. Am J Cardiol. 2007;100:470-5.

58. Marcus GM, Rose E, Viloria EM, et al. Septal to posterior wall motion delay fails to predict reverse remodeling or clinical improvement in patients undergoing cardiac resynchronization therapy. J Am Coll Cardiol. 2005;46:2208-14.

59. Bax J, Bleeker G, Marwick T, et al. Left ventricular dyssynchrony predicts response and prognosis after cardiac resynchronization therapy. J Am Coll Cardiol. 2004;44:1834-40.

60. Yu CM, Chau E, Sanderson JE, et al. Tissue Doppler echocardiographic evidence of reverse remodeling and improved synchronicity by simultaneously delaying regional contraction after biventricular pacing therapy in heart failure. Circulation. 2002;105:438-45.

61. Yu CM, Fung JW, Zhang Q, et al. Tissue Doppler imaging is superior to strain rate imaging and postsystolic shortening on the prediction of reverse remodeling in both ischemic and nonischemic heart failure

after cardiac resynchronization therapy. Circulation. 2004;110:66-73.

62. Yu C, Zhang Q, Fung J, et al. A novel tool to assess systolic asynchrony and identify responders of cardiac resynchronization therapy by tissue synchronization imaging. J Am Coll Cardiol. 2005;45:677-84.

63. Gorcsan J, 3rd, Kanzaki H, Bazaz R, et al. Usefulness of echocardiographic tissue synchronization imaging to predict acute response to cardiac resynchronization therapy. Am J Cardiol. 2004;93:1178-81.

64. Van de Veire NR, Bleeker GB, De Sutter J, et al. Tissue synchronisation imaging accurately measures left ventricular dyssynchrony and predicts response to cardiac resynchronisation therapy. Heart. 2007;93:1034-9.

65. Oh JK, Seward JB, Jamil Tajik A. The Echo Manual, 3rd edition. Philadelphia: Lippincott Williams and Wilkins; 2007.

66. Bogaert J, Rademakers FE. Regional nonuniformity of normal adult human left ventricle. Am J Physiol Heart Circ Physiol. 2001;280: H610-20.

67. Porciani MC, Lilli A, Macioce R, et al. Utility of a new left ventricular asynchrony index as a predictor of reverse remodelling after cardiac resynchronization therapy. Eur Heart J. 2006;27:1818-23.

68. Mele D, Pasanisi G, Capasso F, et al. Left intraventricular myocardial deformation dyssynchrony identifies responders to cardiac resynchronization therapy in patients with heart failure. Eur Heart J. 2006;27:1070-8.

69. Dohi K, Suffoletto MS, Schwartzman D, et al. Utility of echocardiographic radial strain imaging to quantify left ventricular dyssynchrony and predict acute response to cardiac resynchronization therapy. Am J Cardiol. 2005;96:112-6.

70. Delgado V, Ypenburg C, van Bommel RJ, et al. Assessment of left ventricular dyssynchrony by speckle tracking strain imaging comparison between longitudinal, circumferential, and radial strain in cardiac resynchronization therapy. J Am Coll Cardiol. 2008;51:1944-52.

71. Gorcsan J 3rd, Tanabe M, Bleeker GB, et al. Combined longitudinal and radial dyssynchrony predicts ventricular response after resynchronization therapy. J Am Coll Cardiol. 2007;50:1476-83.

72. Suffoletto MS, Dohi K, Cannesson M, et al. Novel speckle-tracking radial strain from routine black-and-white echocardiographic images to quantify dyssynchrony and predict response to cardiac resynchronization therapy. Circulation. 2006;113:960-8.

73. Sanderson JE. Echocardiography for cardiac resynchronization therapy selection. J Am Coll Cardiol. 2009;53:1960-4.

74. Bax JJ, Gorcsan J 3rd. Echocardiography and noninvasive imaging in cardiac resynchronization therapy: results of the PROSPECT (Predictors of Response to Cardiac Resynchronization Therapy) study in perspective. J Am Coll Cardiol. 2009;53:1933-43.

75. Delfino JG, Fornwalt BK, Oshinski JN, et al. Role of MRI in patient selection for CRT. Echocardiography. 2008;25:1176-85.

76. Ypenburg C, Roes SD, Bleeker GB, et al. Effect of total scar burden on contrast-enhanced magnetic resonance imaging on response to cardiac resynchronization therapy. Am J Cardiol. 2007;99:657-60.

77. White JA, Yee R, Yuan X, et al. Delayed enhancement magnetic resonance imaging predicts response to cardiac resynchronization therapy in patients with intraventricular dyssynchrony. J Am Coll Cardiol. 2006;48:1953-60.

78. Bleeker GB, Kaandorp TA, Lamb HJ, et al. Effect of posterolateral scar tissue on clinical and echocardiographic improvement after cardiac resynchronization therapy. Circulation. 2006;113:969-76.

79. Botvinick EH, O'Connell JW, Badhwar N. Imaging synchrony. J Nucl Cardiol. 2009;16:846-8.

80. Kerwin WF, Botvinick EH, O'Connell JW, et al. Ventricular contraction abnormalities in dilated cardiomyopathy: effect of biventricular pacing to correct interventricular dyssynchrony. J Am Coll Cardiol. 2000;35:1221-7.

81. O'Connell JW, Schreck C, Moles M, et al. A unique method by which to quantitate synchrony with equilibrium radionuclide angiography. J Nucl Cardiol. 2005;12:441-50.

82. Wassenaar R, O'Connor D, Dej B, et al. Optimization and validation of radionuclide angiography phase analysis parameters for quantification of mechanical dyssynchrony. J Nucl Cardiol. 2009;16:895-903.

83. Ypenburg C, Schalij MJ, Bleeker GB, et al. Impact of viability and scar tissue on response to cardiac resynchronization therapy in ischaemic heart failure patients. Eur Heart J. 2007;28:33-41.

84. Adelstein EC, Saba S. Scar burden by myocardial perfusion imaging predicts echocardiographic response to cardiac resynchronization therapy in ischemic cardiomyopathy. Am Heart J. 2007;153:105-12.

85. Sciagra R, Giaccardi M, Porciani MC, et al. Myocardial perfusion imaging using gated SPECT in heart failure patients undergoing cardiac resynchronization therapy. J Nucl Med. 2004;45:164-8.

86. Marsan NA, Tops LF, Nihoyannopoulos P, et al. Real-time three dimensional echocardiography: current and future clinical applications. Heart. 2009;95:1881-90.

87. Marsan NA, Bleeker GB, Ypenburg C, et al. Real-time three-dimensional echocardiography as a novel approach to assess left ventricular and left atrium reverse remodeling and to predict response to cardiac resynchronization therapy. Heart Rhythm. 2008;5:1257-64.

88. Hawkins NM, Petrie MC, Burgess MI, et al. Selecting patients for cardiac resynchronization therapy. J Am Coll Cardiol. 2009;53:1944-59.

89. Truong QA, Singh JP, Cannon CP, et al. Quantitative analysis of intraventricular dyssynchrony using wall thickness by multidetector computed tomography. JACC Cardiovasc Imaging. 2008;1:772-81.

90. Epstein AE, Dimarco JP, Ellenbogen KA, et al. ACC/AHA/HRS 2008 guidelines for device-based therapy of cardiac rhythm abnormalities. J Am Coll Cardiol. 2008;51:e1-62.

91. Ansalone G, Giannantoni P, Ricci R, et al. Doppler myocardial imaging to evaluate the effectiveness of pacing sites in patients receiving biventricular pacing. J Am Coll Cardiol. 2002;39:489-99.

92. Dekker AL, Phelps B, Dijkman B, et al. Epicardial left ventricular lead placement for cardiac resynchronization therapy: optimal pace site selection with pressure-volume loops. J Thorac Cardiovasc Surg. 2004;127:1641-7.

93. Koos R, Sinha AM, Markus K, et al. Comparison of left ventricular lead placement via the coronary venous approach versus lateral thoracotomy in patients receiving cardiac resynchronization therapy. Am J Cardiol. 2004;94:59-63.

94. Fernandez AL, Garcia-Bengochea JB, Ledo R, et al. Minimally invasive surgical implantation of left ventricular epicardial leads for ventricular resynchronization using video-assisted thoracoscopy. Rev Esp Cardiol. 2004;57:313-9.

95. Badhwar N, Lee BK, Kumar UN, et al. Utility of equilibrium radionuclide angiograms to guide coronary sinus lead placement in heart failure patients requiring resynchronization therapy (abstract). Western Regional Meeting. Carmel, CA; 2006.

96. Heist EK, Fan D, Mela T, et al. Radiographic left ventricular-right ventricular interlead distance predicts the acute hemodynamic response to cardiac resynchronization therapy. Am J Cardiol. 2005;96:685-90.

97. Kanhai SM, Viergever EP, Bax JJ. Cardiogenic shock shortly after initial success of cardiac resynchronization therapy. Eur J Heart Fail. 2004;6:477-81.

98. Guerra JM, Wu J, Miller JM, et al. Increase in ventricular tachycardia frequency after biventricular implantable cardioverter defibrillator upgrade. J Cardiovasc Electrophysiol. 2003;14:1245-7.

99. Nordbeck P, Seidl B, Fey B, et al. Effect of cardiac resynchronization therapy on the incidence of electrical storm. International Journal of Cardiology. 2010;143:330-6 (Epub. 2009).

100. Walker S, Levy TM, Rex S, et al. Usefulness of suppression of ventricular arrhythmia by biventricular pacing in severe congestive cardiac failure. Am J Cardiol. 2000;86:231-3.

101. Zagrodzky JD, Ramaswamy K, Page RL, et al. Biventricular pacing decreases the inducibility of ventricular tachycardia in patients with ischemic cardiomyopathy. Am J Cardiol. 2001;87:1208-10; A7.

102. Rivero-Ayerza M, Theuns DA, Garcia-Garcia HM, et al. Effects of cardiac resynchronization therapy on overall mortality and mode of death: a meta-analysis of randomized controlled trials. European Heart Journal. 2006;27:2682-8.

103. Combes N, Marijon E, Boveda S, et al. Electrical storm after CRT implantation treated by AV delay optimization. Journal of Cardiovascular Electrophysiology. 2010;21:211-3 (Epub. 2009).

104. Kantharia BK, Patel JA, Nagra BS, et al. Electrical storm of monomorphic ventricular tachycardia after a cardiac-resynchronization-therapy-defibrillator upgrade. Europace. 2006;8:625-8.

105. Bortone A, Macia J-C, Leclercq F, et al. Monomorphic ventricular tachycardia induced by cardiac resynchronization therapy in patient with severe nonischemic dilated cardiomyopathy. Pacing Clin Electrophysiol. 2006;29:327-30.

106. Nayak HM, Verdino RJ, Russo AM, et al. Ventricular tachycardia storm after initiation of biventricular pacing: incidence, clinical characteristics, management, and outcome. Journal of Cardiovascular Electrophysiology. 2008;19:708-15.

107. Fish JM, Brugada J, Antzelevitch C. Potential proarrhythmic effects of biventricular pacing. J Am Coll Cardiol. 2005;46:2340-7.

108. Gasparini M, Regoli F, Galimberti P, et al. Three years of cardiac resynchronization therapy: could superior benefits be obtained in patients with heart failure and narrow QRS? Pacing Clin Electrophysiol. 2007;30:S34-9.

109. Yu C-M, Chan Y-S, Zhang Q, et al. Benefits of cardiac resynchronization therapy for heart failure patients with narrow QRS complexes and coexisting systolic asynchrony by echocardiography. J Am Coll Cardiol. 2006;48:2251-7.

110. Achilli A, Sassara M, Ficili S, et al. Long-term effectiveness of cardiac resynchronization therapy in patients with refractory heart failure and "narrow" QRS. J Am Coll Cardiol. 2003;42:2117-24.

111. Bleeker G, Holman E, Steendijk P, et al. Cardiac resynchronization therapy in patients with a narrow QRS complex. J Am Coll Cardiol. 2006;48:2243-50.

112. Jeevanantham V, Zareba W, Navaneethan S, et al. Meta-analysis on effects of cardiac resynchronization therapy in heart failure patients with narrow QRS complex. Cardiology Journal. 2008;15:230-6.

113. Beshai JF, Grimm RA, Nagueh SF, et al. Cardiac-resynchronization therapy in heart failure with narrow QRS complexes. N Engl J Med. 2007;357:2461-71.

114. [cited; Available from: http://clinicaltrials.gov/ct2/show/NCT00683696]

115. Leon AR, Greenberg JM, Kanuru N, et al. Cardiac resynchronization in patients with congestive heart failure and chronic atrial fibrillation: effect of upgrading to biventricular pacing after chronic right ventricular pacing. J Am Coll Cardiol. 2002;39:1258-63.

116. Linde C, Leclercq C, Rex S, et al. Long-term benefits of biventricular pacing in congestive heart failure: results from the MUltisite STimulation in cardiomyopathy (MUSTIC) study. J Am Coll Cardiol. 2002;40:111-8.

117. Molhoek SG, Bax JJ, Bleeker GB, et al. Comparison of response to cardiac resynchronization therapy in patients with sinus rhythm versus chronic atrial fibrillation. Am J Cardiol. 2004;94:1506-9.

118. Dong K, Shen WK, Powell BD, et al. Atrioventricular nodal ablation predicts survival benefit in patients with atrial fibrillation receiving cardiac resynchronization therapy. Heart Rhythm. 2010;7:1240-5.

119. Gasparini M, Auricchio A, Regoli F, et al. Four-year efficacy of cardiac resynchronization therapy on exercise tolerance and disease progression: the importance of performing atrioventricular junction ablation in patients with atrial fibrillation. J Am Coll Cardiol. 2006;48:734-43.

120. Delgado V, Tops LF, Trines SA, et al. Acute effects of right ventricular apical pacing on left ventricular synchrony and mechanics. Circulation: Arrhythm Electrophysiol. 2009;2:135-45.

121. Lieberman R, Padeletti L, Schreuder J, et al. Ventricular pacing lead location alters systemic hemodynamics and left ventricular function in patients with and without reduced ejection fraction. J Am Coll Cardiol. 2006;48:1634-41.

122. O'Keefe JH, Abuissa H, Jones PG, et al. Effect of chronic right ventricular apical pacing on left ventricular function. Am J Cardiol. 2005;95:771-3.

123. Wilkoff BL, Cook JR, Epstein AE, et al. Dual-chamber pacing or ventricular backup pacing in patients with an implantable defibrillator: the Dual Chamber and VVI Implantable Defibrillator (DAVID) trial. JAMA. 2002;288:3115-23.

124. Sweeney MO, Prinzen FW. A new paradigm for physiologic ventricular pacing. J Am Coll Cardiol. 2006;47:282-8.

125. Sweeney MO, Hellkamp AS, Ellenbogen KA, et al. Adverse effect of ventricular pacing on heart failure and atrial fibrillation among patients with normal baseline QRS duration in a clinical trial of pacemaker therapy for sinus node dysfunction. Circulation. 2003;107:2932-7.

126. Thambo J-B, Bordachar P, Garrigue S, et al. Detrimental ventricular remodeling in patients with congenital complete heart block and chronic right ventricular apical pacing. Circulation. 2004;110:3766-72.

127. Sharma AD, Rizo-Patron C, Hallstrom AP, et al. Percent right ventricular pacing predicts outcomes in the DAVID trial. Heart Rhythm. 2005;2:830-4.

128. Kindermann M, Hennen B, Jung J, et al. Biventricular versus conventional right ventricular stimulation for patients with standard pacing indication and left ventricular dysfunction: the Homburg Biventricular Pacing Evaluation (HOBIPACE). J Am Coll Cardiol. 2006;47:1927-37.

129. Yu C-M, Chan JY-S, Zhang Q, et al. Biventricular pacing in patients with bradycardia and normal ejection fraction. N Engl J Med. 2009;361:2123-34.

130. Albouaini K, Alkarmi A, Mudawi T, et al. Selective site right ventricular pacing. Heart. 2009;95:2030-9.

131. Linde C, Abraham WT, Gold MR, et al. Randomized trial of cardiac resynchronization in mildly symptomatic heart failure patients and in asymptomatic patients with left ventricular dysfunction and previous heart failure symptoms. J Am Coll Cardiol. 2008;52:1834-43.

132. Moss AJ, Hall WJ, Cannom DS, et al. Cardiac-resynchronization therapy for the prevention of heart-failure events. N Engl J Med. 2009;361:1329-38.

133. Herweg B, Ilercil A, Cutro R, et al. Cardiac resynchronization therapy in patients with end-stage inotrope-dependent class IV heart failure. Am J Cardiol. 2007;100:90-3.

134. James KB, Militello M, Barbara G, et al. Biventricular pacing for heart failure patients on inotropic support: a review of 38 consecutive cases. Tex Heart Inst J. 2006;33:19-22.

Ambulatory Electrocardiographic Monitoring

Renee M Sullivan, Brian Olshansky, James B Martins, Alexander Mazur

"...orthodox electrocardiography will always have its uses in the measurement of established heart conditions, but it does not provide an accurate sampling of all-day heart activity any more than the analysis of a single rock provides an accurate sample of a mountain of ore."

Norman J. Holter[1]

Chapter Outline

- Holter Monitoring
- Event Recorders
- Mobile Cardiac Outpatient Telemetry
- Implantable Loop Recorders

- Key Considerations in Selecting a Monitoring Modality
- Guidelines

INTRODUCTION

Ambulatory electrocardiographic (AECG) monitoring, the recording of the electrocardiogram (ECG) over an extended period of time using a portable or implantable recording device, enables the clinician to study dynamic electrocardiographic changes during real-life activities. It is considered to be the cornerstone in the evaluation of patients with suspected cardiac arrhythmias.[2]

The AECG was championed by Norman J Holter in the late 1940s and was introduced into clinical practice in the early 1960s.[1] Early devices consisted of continuous single-lead ECG recordings on a magnetic tape with a storage capacity of only a few hours. The recorded data could be played back at an increased speed for manual review by an operator using a specific analyzer equipped with an oscilloscope. Technological advances in signal recording, processing and transmitting, as well as automatic data analysis, have significantly enhanced the diagnostic capabilities of the ambulatory monitors we use today.

With the advent of digital data acquisition and solid state memory technology, recording devices have been substantially downsized and are now capable of recording and storing high fidelity multichannel continuous electrocardiographic data over several days. Modern computer-based analysis systems use advanced diagnostic software algorithms that provide automatic quantification of a large amount of stored ECG data with calculation of multiple electrocardiographic parameters and generation of arrhythmia counters. In addition, areas of interest in the recordings that require operator review are automatically identified.

With the availability of event recorders that store only a few minutes of ECG when activated manually or automatically, based upon programmed parameters, and the capability of transmitting stored information over the phone, the period of monitoring has been extended to weeks and months. The

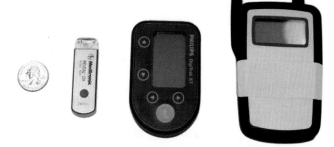

FIGURE 1: Examples of current monitoring devices are pictured next to a quarter, shown as a reference for size. From left to right: an implantable loop recorder; a Holter monitor and an event monitor. This model of the event monitor may also be used as mobile cardiac outpatient telemetry when programmed as such

implantable version of event recorders has further expanded the period of monitoring up to three years. More recently, the development of automatic arrhythmia detection algorithms, as well as wireless communication technology, has enabled continuous ambulatory monitoring with real-time data transfer and analysis. Currently available monitoring modalities include: continuous or Holter monitors, external event (postevent and loop) recorders, implantable loop recorders (ILRs), and mobile cardiac outpatient telemetry (MCOT) (Fig. 1 and Table 1).

This chapter reviews the clinical utility and appropriate cost-effective selection of currently available monitoring modalities based on their advantages, limitations and diagnostic yields in specific populations of patients.

HOLTER MONITORING

Ambulatory Holter monitoring is accomplished with portable battery-operated devices that continuously record multiple

TABLE 1

Characteristics of monitoring modalities

	Recording type	Monitoring period	Event activation	Transmission	Data analysis
Holter monitor	Continuous, full disclosure	Typically 24–48 hours	Manual	Typically none	Delayed
Loop recorder	Intermittent pre-and post-event	Typically up to 30 days	Manual and automatic	Dial-in trans-telephonic	Delayed
Event recorder	Intermittent post-event		Manual	Dial-in trans-telephonic	Delayed
ILR	Intermittent	Up to 3 years	Manual and automatic	Dial-in trans-telephonic or wireless	Delayed
MCOT	Continuous, full disclosure	Individualized, up to 30 days	Manual and automatic	Automatic and dial-in wireless	Immediate

(Abbreviations: ILR: Implantable loop recorder; MCOT: Mobile cardiac outpatient telemetry)

electrocardiographic channels, typically over a 24–48 hours period. Some modern devices can store up to two weeks of continuous ECG data. Holter monitors generally record two to three ECG leads. Although devices that allow for the recording of up to 12 ECG leads are currently available, the clinical advantage of multichannel recordings is not well determined. Manually activated events are marked with timestamps which are linked to patient diaries in an attempt to correlate symptoms with an arrhythmia.

Automatic analysis of the full data set is performed using proprietary software, but a manual over read is generally completed to validate accuracy of the automatic arrhythmia diagnosis. The standard Holter monitor analysis summarizes heart rate trends, along with the presence and frequency of tachyarrhythmias and bradyarrhythmias, atrial and ventricular ectopy, as well as asystolic pauses. With the improved quality of acquired ECG signals in present day recorders, standard ECG measurements including PR and QT intervals, QRS width and variation in ST segments can be assessed accurately. The recorded ECG signals can also be used for more complex analyses including heart rate variability, signal averaged ECG, heart rate turbulence and T wave alternans.

Holter monitoring is generally utilized to detect a cause for symptoms and to diagnose rhythm disturbances that are expected to occur within a 24–48 hour monitoring period (Fig. 2 and Table 2). The major advantage of this modality is the continuous nature of the recording that provides "full disclosure" of the ECG during the monitoring period. This type of information is particularly useful for assessment of ventricular rate response in patients with atrial fibrillation or quantification of arrhythmia burden in patients with frequent ectopy.

Although an effective diagnostic modality in patients with daily symptoms, the diagnostic yield of a Holter monitor is likely to be low, as in the case of infrequent episodes of syncope or palpitations. Depending on patient selection and the length of monitoring, the likelihood of documenting cardiac rhythm during syncope is usually less than 20%; most of the captured events correlate with the absence of significant arrhythmia.[3-5] Patients with palpitations have a diagnosis secured by a Holter monitor more so than patients with syncope but only when the symptoms are frequent and occur during the recording.[6,7] The presence of an asymptomatic arrhythmia in patients with syncope or other symptoms should be interpreted with caution since it may have little clinical meaning. Rarely, an asymptomatic arrhythmia such as Mobitz II or complete atrial-

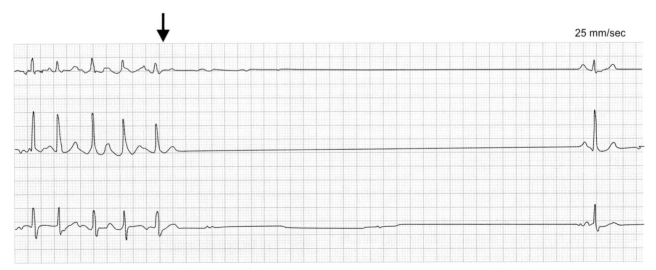

FIGURE 2: A 3-ECG channel Holter monitor recording obtained in a patient with recurrent palpitations and syncope. Note a 6-second sinus pause following termination of atrial fibrillation (arrow)

TABLE 2

Selection of monitoring modalities for common clinical indications

	Holter monitor	Event monitor Looping	Event monitor Non-looping	Implantable loop recorder	Mobile cardiac outpatient telemetry
Syncope					
≥ 1 episode/week	+				+
≥ 1 episode/month		+*			+
< 1 episode/month				+	
Palpitations					
≥ 1 episode/week	+		+		+
≥ 1 episode/month		+	+		+
< 1 episode/month			+	+	
Risk assessment (HCM, CAD, LQTS)	+	+*			
Atrial fibrillation					
Burden	+				+
Rate control	+	+*#			+
AAD monitoring		+*			+

* With auto-trigger capability
\# With an automatic atrial fibrillation algorithm
Abbreviations: AAD: Antiarrhythmic drug; MCOT: Mobile cardiac outpatient telemetry; HCM: Hypertrophic cardiomyopathy; CAD: Coronary artery disease; LQTS: Long QT syndrome

25 mm/sec

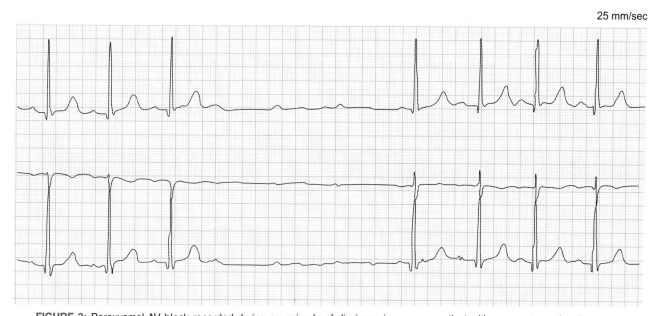

FIGURE 3: Paroxysmal AV block recorded during an episode of dizziness in a young patient with recurrent exertional syncope. The patient has became asymptomatic following placement of a permanent pacemaker

ventricular block, prolonged sinus pauses, or significant QT interval prolongation, among others, may provide a diagnostic clue as to the cause of symptoms (Fig. 3). However, it is always critical to know whether an arrhythmia is temporally linked to a symptom or unnecessary therapy that may fail to provide benefit and cause harm. For instance, although sinus bradycardia may be documented during sleep, sinus bradycardia may not necessarily correlate with symptoms while the patient is awake.

In addition to its diagnostic indications, Holter monitoring may be useful as a screening tool in identifying patients at increased risk for sudden death. The presence of asymptomatic nonsustained ventricular tachycardia may aid in risk stratification in patients with hypertrophic cardiomyopathy or ischemic heart disease and impaired left systolic ventricular function.[8,9] Transient QT interval prolongation and macroscopic T wave alternans are recognized markers of risk for life-threatening ventricular arrhythmias in patients with long QT syndrome.[10] While possible to ascertain from high quality Holter monitor recordings, the clinical utility of heart rate variability, SAECG, heart rate turbulence, microscopic T wave alternans and other complex methods of analyzing continuous ECG recordings remains controversial.

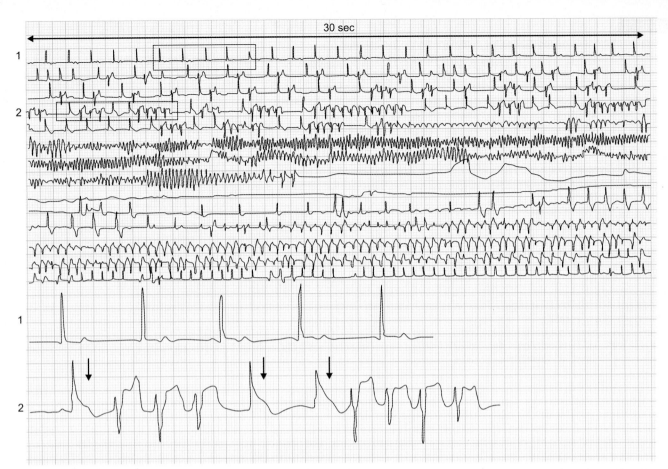

FIGURE 4: Continuous single channel Holter monitor ECG recorded during a prolonged syncopal spell in a 60-year-old patient with recurrent episodes of chest pressure and syncope. The bottom tracings (1 and 2) show selected portions of the ECG (boxes 1 and 2) in an expanded scale. Note transient ST-segment elevation (arrows, bottom tracing 2) followed by a 90-second episode of ventricular fibrillation and a 50-second asystolic pause. Coronary angiography showed mild (40%) narrowing of the right coronary artery

Holter monitoring has a limited role in assessing the efficacy and proarrhythmic response to antiarrhythmic medications due to the relatively short period of recording. Furthermore, conventional Holter recordings require off-line stored ECG processing and, therefore, do not provide immediate notification to the prescribing physician and patient about serious arrhythmic events. In this regard, the MCOT has recently emerged as a promising modality that permits extended periods of monitoring with automatic wireless transmission of arrhythmia events and real-time ECG analysis.[11] Short-term recording periods covered by conventional 24–48 hours Holter monitors are usually insufficient to quantify atrial fibrillation burden following initiation of antiarrhythmic therapy or a catheter ablation procedure.[12]

Detection of myocardial ischemia based upon variations in ST segments is another potential application of Holter monitoring. The ST segment changes on Holter recordings have been associated with adverse outcomes in patients with coronary artery disease in some series[13,14] but not in others.[15] Despite ongoing clinical interest in this area, the role of Holter monitoring in managing patients with coronary artery disease remains ill defined. This is at least in part due to the low specificity of ST segment changes on Holter recordings to predict ischemia as a number of technical and physiological factors may limit interpretation of the ST segment including

body position, nonstandard lead position, medications and changes in autonomic tone. Rarely, Holter monitoring may be useful in the evaluation of patients with suspected variant angina (Fig. 4).

EVENT RECORDERS

Similar to Holter monitors, event recorders are used to correlate symptoms to arrhythmias but over longer periods of time, usually up to one month. Unlike continuous monitors, these devices have limited memory capacity and are capable of storing only short intervals of ECG recordings related to manually or automatically activated events and, therefore, do not provide "full disclosure" data. Data from event recorders are usually transmitted from a patient transtelephonically to a central location for interpretation and dispersal, by either internet transmission or facsimile, to the prescribing physician.

Event recorders are differentiated mainly by the presence or absence of the memory loop recording capability which allows for the storage of ECG recording immediately preceding a triggered event. A loop recorder continuously stores in internal loop memory several minutes of the most recent ECG by overwriting earlier data. Similarly to a Holter monitor, it is connected to the chest with leads and adhesive electrodes. When the patient develops symptoms and activates the device, pre-

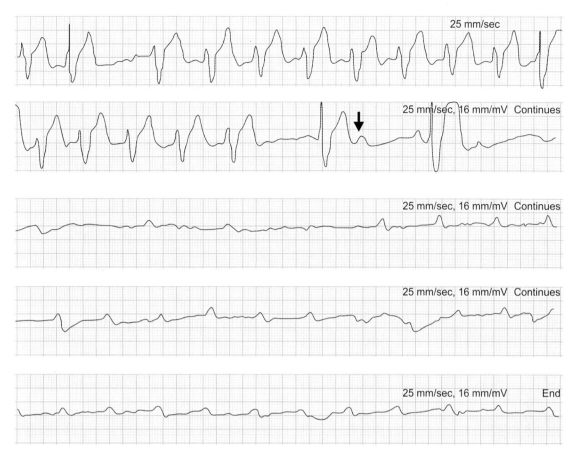

FIGURE 5: A continuous single channel recording automatically captured during an episode of syncope in a patient with recurrent palpitations and syncope. In this case, the patient was not able to activate the loop monitor manually. Note paroxysmal complete AV block with prolonged asystolic pause following termination of atrial fibrillation (arrow)

and postactivation ECG data are stored for several seconds to minutes depending on specific programmable recording time intervals. Some advanced loop monitors also have an auto-trigger capability based on specific algorithms that allow for automatic detection of slow, fast or irregular heart rates, as well as asystolic pauses. This feature is especially useful in the diagnosis of syncopal events when the patient is not able to manually activate the monitor or in the detection of asymptomatic arrhythmia (Fig. 5). It has been shown that the automatic arrhythmia detection capability improves the diagnostic yield of monitoring devices primarily by detecting asymptomatic arrhythmias.[16] A retrospective analysis of a large AECG database showed that clinically significant arrhythmias were detected in 36% of patients using auto-triggered loop recorders as compared to 17% and 6% using manually activated loop recorders and Holter monitors, respectively.[16] The relatively high diagnostic yield of auto-triggered recorders in this study was due to better documentation of asymptomatic atrial fibrillation or transient bradycardia.

"Non-looping" or postevent monitors do not have internal loop memory and record ECG only prospectively following manual activation by the patient. These small handheld or wrist worn monitors that have "built in" electrodes are applied directly to the skin for recording. Since no continuous application of adhesive electrodes is required, long-term compliance is usually better compared to loop recorders. Also, these monitors are ideal for use in patients with sensitivity or allergy to adhesives.

However, given the technical aspects of the device, its clinical application is limited to situations when prompt activation of the device during symptoms is feasible. It is, therefore, not practical for patients with brief symptoms or syncope. Furthermore, lack of internal memory in these devices does not allow for the capturing of the ECG during the onset of arrhythmia, this information may be helpful in understanding the mechanism of some tachyarrhythmias. Finally, "non-looping" monitors do not provide information about asymptomatic arrhythmias. As mentioned earlier, in rare circumstances, detection of asymptomatic arrhythmias may help in guiding appropriate therapy in symptomatic patients. In addition, detection of asymptomatic recurrences plays an important role in assessing the efficacy of medical or interventional rhythm control strategies for atrial fibrillation.

Event recorders are useful in the diagnosis of symptoms (such as palpitations, syncope or pre-syncope) suspected to be directly caused by an arrhythmia that occur at least monthly (Table 2). Extended surveillance with event recorders provides higher diagnostic yield than conventional short-term Holter monitoring and allows symptom-ECG correlation in up to two-thirds of patients with frequent palpitations.[6,7] Similarly, loop recorders have been shown to be superior to Holter monitors in the evaluation of patients with frequent syncope (Fig. 5).[4] However, the relative diagnostic utility of these devices for evaluation of syncope as compared to palpitations is lower because of the unpredictable course of syncopal events.[17] The

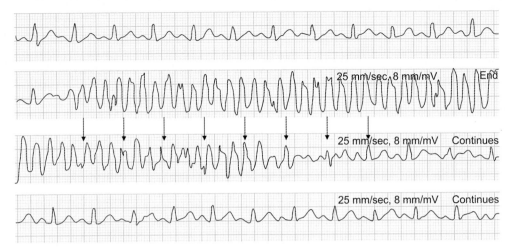

FIGURE 6: An automatically logged asymptomatic event consistent with recording artifact mimicking ventricular tachycardia. Note normal QRS complexes (arrows) "marching through" the artifacts

optimal duration of monitoring remains unclear. Although some studies suggest that 70–90% of arrhythmias are usually diagnosed within the first two weeks of surveillance,[7,18] the extent of the required monitoring period should be individualized depending on the type and frequency of symptoms.

Loop recorders with auto-trigger capability may be useful in the surveillance of patients undergoing medical therapy for arrhythmias or following catheter ablation procedures. In this regard, management of atrial fibrillation is one of the major applications for these devices, since they allow for the detection of asymptomatic recurrences. It is well recognized that atrial fibrillation recurrences are commonly asymptomatic, particularly following catheter ablation procedures.[19,20] Newer devices can detect atrial fibrillation automatically and display daily atrial fibrillation burden, although accuracy of this information needs further validation. However, this modality does not offer live monitoring with real-time data analysis and, therefore, may not be optimal for patients who are at high risk for serious proarrhythmia.

While event recorders have inherent advantages, they have limitations. Recorders without auto-trigger capability rely upon the patient to activate the device at the time of, or directly after, an episode. In one study, using patient activated loop recorders, one quarter of patients were unable to activate the device properly despite previous education and test transmissions.[4] Long-term compliance in wearing loop recorders is usually limited due to the need for application of adhesive electrodes.[5] As noted previously, patients with extremely rare symptoms may not be good candidates for external event recording. Correct interpretation of recording artifacts may be challenging when only a single lead ECG recording is available (Fig. 6).

MOBILE CARDIAC OUTPATIENT TELEMETRY

More recently, MCOT has been introduced into clinical practice. The devices used for MCOT are similar in size to conventional loop recorders and are capable of transmitting ECG data wirelessly, either directly or via a portable data manager (an external cellular telephone-sized device). Some providers use

the same recorder which can be programmed either as a loop or MCOT monitor (Fig. 1). Potential advantages of MCOT over other modalities include continuous live ECG monitoring with automatic arrhythmia recognition and real-time ECG transmission to a central location that operates 24 hours a day and provides immediate notification of the ordering physician and patient about significant events based on prespecified notification criteria, in addition to daily summary reports. Since the ECG is transmitted continuously to a receiver system, there are practically no memory constraints and "full disclosure" data are available for analysis, including quantification of heart rate and arrhythmia burden.

Initial observational experience suggests that MCOT may offer an improved diagnostic yield in patients with symptoms concerning for arrhythmia and may also potentially be useful for outpatient initiation of antiarrhythmic medications, thereby obviating the need for hospitalization.[7,11] A randomized prospective evaluation of patients with symptoms suggestive of arrhythmia showed that symptom-ECG correlation could be obtained in 88% of patients randomized to MCOT, compared to 75% randomized to a patient activated loop recorder.[18] Higher diagnostic yield of MCOT in this study was due to detection of asymptomatic arrhythmia deemed to be clinically significant with atrial fibrillation and nonsustained ventricular tachycardia accounting for the majority of automatically captured events. However, outcome data show that asymptomatic arrhythmia could be used as a surrogate to guide appropriate therapy for symptomatic events are limited.[21]

Although there are potential advantages to this real-time approach to monitoring, more data are needed to define its role in the management of arrhythmia patients. The MCOT is a technologically and operationally demanding modality and, therefore, is substantially more expensive than conventional event recorders. The system requires not only well trained technical personnel but also a physician available 24 hours a day to manage large amounts of ECG data. It remains unclear whether or not this method can provide cost-effective benefit over older technologies, particularly auto-triggered loop recording.

Implantable loop recorders (ILRs) have extended diagnostic capabilities not afforded by external loop recorders and are generally indicated in patients with infrequent symptoms suspicious for cardiac arrhythmia. These small leadless devices are implanted subcutaneously, usually in the left pectoral area, and provide up to three years of continuous monitoring. They record a single bipolar ECG lead from a pair of electrodes embedded into the shell of the device. Despite relatively closely spaced electrodes, P waves and QRS complexes are generally visible. A subcutaneous wire antenna utilized in some new devices may improve quality of recording by providing more flexible electrode configurations and a larger inter-electrode distance.[22] Similar to external loop recorders, ILRs have limited memory capacity (42–48 minutes of compressed ECG signals) and store only short intervals (seconds to minutes) of both patient and automatically activated ECG recordings based on prespecified parameters. Stored data can be retrieved either manually during interrogation with a standard pacemaker programmer or remotely over the phone. Devices with wireless transmission capability (similar to MCOT) have recently become available,[22] although the clinical utility of live monitoring using ILRs has yet to be confirmed because of inherent problems with inappropriate sensing in these devices.

The longer periods of monitoring afforded by ILRs compared to external loop recorders allow for better correlation of events with arrhythmias in patients with rare but serious symptoms. The devices are usually well tolerated and there are no long-term compliance issues. Most data support their use in patients with recurrent unexplained syncope in whom a conventional invasive and noninvasive evaluation has been unrevealing. The reported diagnostic yield in symptom-ECG correlation is 30–88% depending on studied population of patients.[23-26] The diagnostic yield is directly proportional to the frequency of syncope while likelihood of the diagnosis of significant arrhythmia underlying syncopal events is higher in patients with structural heart disease and/or conduction abnormalities.[17] Some data suggest that selected patients with unexplained syncopal events clinically suspicious for arrhythmia may benefit from relatively early utilization of these devices before embarking on the conventional diagnostic, particularly invasive, techniques provided that cardiac conditions associated with high risk of life-threatening arrhythmia are carefully excluded.[27-29]

The ILRs play a relatively limited role in the evaluation of patients with palpitations as compared to syncope. Palpitations usually are a less severe symptom and are more likely to be diagnosed with external recorders or electrophysiologic testing.[17] In one study which randomized 50 patients with infrequent and sustained palpitations to either ILR or a conventional diagnostic approach including external monitoring and electrophysiology testing, the diagnostic yield of ILR was 73% compared to only 21% using the conventional strategy.[30] The ILR guided therapy yielded symptomatic benefit in the majority of patients.

Some observational data suggest that ILRs may be useful in guiding pacemaker therapy in patients with severe and frequent episodes of neurocardiogenic syncope caused by significant bradycardia.[29] However, prospective randomized studies are warranted before this approach can be adopted in routine clinical practice. The ILRs may potentially be helpful in establishing arrhythmic cause of recurrent nonaccidental falls,[31] as well as unexplained episodes of loss of consciousness.[32]

Other emerging areas of application for ILRs are risk stratification of patients with structural or primary arrhythmogenic cardiac conditions who are at high risk for sudden death (hypertrophic and right ventricular cardiomyopathies, myotonic dystrophy, long and short QT syndromes, Brugada syndrome, etc.) as well as long-term management of atrial fibrillation.[17] Automatic algorithms for the diagnosis of atrial fibrillation have been recently introduced, although accuracy of the derived information requires further validation.

With future advent of multiple physiological sensors (such as blood pressure, oxygen saturation, drug concentrations, etc.) implantable monitoring technology may become an invaluable tool in the management of a variety of cardiac and non-cardiac conditions.

Disadvantages of ILRs exist. The major issue remains inappropriate detection of arrhythmia episodes secondary to either undersensing, most commonly due to loss of electrode contact within the device pocket or oversensing due to "noise" (Fig. 7). This may compromise automatic arrhythmia detection either by undersensing of tachyarrhythmia episodes or by saturation of the device memory with inappropriately sensed ECG recordings and thereby precluding storage of true arrhythmia episodes. In a recent study that analyzed a large database of automatically stored ECGs by an ILR, inappropriately detected events were found in 71.9% of all recordings from 88.6% of patients.[33] An ILR is the most expensive of all available monitoring modalities, although some data suggest that it may be more cost effective compared to conventional diagnostic approaches in selected patients with rare, unexplained syncope.[34] The device requires surgical implantation with inherent risk of pocket complications.

KEY CONSIDERATIONS IN SELECTING A MONITORING MODALITY

- Major considerations in the selection of a monitoring modality are type and frequency of symptoms (Table 2). In patients with daily symptoms, a Holter monitor remains a preferred device. External event recorders are useful in patients with less frequent (but at least monthly) symptoms. An ILR is generally reserved for evaluation of rare symptoms, usually unexplained syncope, suggestive of an arrhythmic cause.
- In the case of syncope or brief palpitations, loop memory monitors that allow for capturing of ECG data preceding the activation are required. Recorders with auto-triggered capability or MCOT that do not rely solely on the patient's ability to activate the device during symptoms may help to better secure the diagnosis.
- For detection of asymptomatic arrhythmia recurrences or quantification of arrhythmia burden, as well as in patients who are not able to properly activate the device or transmit recorded ECG data, devices providing continuous, "full

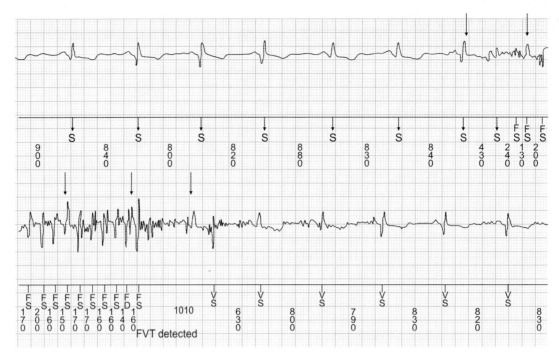

FIGURE 7: An example of inappropriate automatic detection by an implantable loop recorder due to "noise" oversensing. Note normal QRS complexes (arrows) "marching through" nonphysiologic high frequency signals

disclosure", type of information (Holter monitor or MCOT) or event recorders with auto-triggered capability and special arrhythmia algorithms are the most appropriate choice.

- The MCOT offers continuous wireless live ECG monitoring with automatic arrhythmia recognition and immediate notification of the prescribing physician and patient regarding significant arrhythmia events.

(AAA/AHA GUIDELINES FOR AMBULATORY ELECTROCARDIOGRAPHY: EXECUTIVE SUMMARY AND RECOMMENDATIONS, CIRCULATION. 1999;100:886-93) MODIFIED SUMMARY OF GUIDELINES

Modified by Kanu Chatterjee

Class I: Conditions for which there is evidence and/or general agreement that a given procedure/therapy is useful and effective

Class II: Conditions for which there is conflicting evidence and/or a divergence of opinion about the usefulness/efficacy of performing the procedure/therapy

Class IIa: Weight of evidence/opinion is in favor of usefulness/efficacy

Class IIb: Usefulness/efficacy is less well established by evidence/opinion

Class III: Conditions for which there is evidence and/ or general agreement that a procedure/therapy is not useful/effective and in some cases may be harmful

Level A (highest): Derived from multiple randomized clinical trials

Level B (intermediate): Data are on the basis of a limited number of randomized trials, nonrandomized studies or observational registries

Level C (lowest): Primary basis for the recommendation was expert opinion

INDICATIONS FOR AMBULATORY ELECTROCARDIOGRAPHY (AECG) TO ASSESS SYMPTOMS POSSIBLY RELATED TO RHYTHMIC DISTURBANCES

Class I:
1. Patients with unexplained syncope, presyncope or episodic dizziness
2. Patients with unexplained recurrent palpitation

Class IIb:
1. Patients with unexplained episodic shortness of breath, chest pain, or fatigue
2. Patients with neurological events when transient atrial fibrillation or flutter is suspected
3. Patients with persistent symptoms after non-arrhythmogenic cause of syncope, presyncope dizziness or palpitation have been detected and treated

Class III:
1. Patients with symptoms of syncope, presyncope episodic dizziness or palpitation in whom other causes have been established
2. Patients with cerebrovascular accidents without other evidence of arrhythmia

INDICATIONS FOR AECG ARRHYTHMIA DETECTION TO ASSESS RISK FOR FUTURE CARDIAC EVENTS IN PATIENTS WITHOUT SYMPTOMS FROM ARRHYTHMIA

Class I: None

Class IIb:
1. Post-MI patients with LV systolic dysfunction (ejection fraction of 40% or less)
2. Patients with congestive heart failure
3. Patients with idiopathic hypertrophic cardiomyopathy

Class III:
1. Patients who have sustained myocardial contusion
2. Systemic hypertensive patients with LV hypertrophy
3. Post-MI patients with normal LV function
4. Preoperative arrhythmia evaluation of patients for noncardiac surgery
5. Patients with sleep apnea
6. Patients with valvular heart disease

INDICATIONS FOR MEASUREMENT OF HEART RATE VARIABILITY (HRV) TO ASSESS RISK FOR FUTURE CARDIAC EVENTS IN PATIENTS WITHOUT SYMPTOMS FROM ARRHYTHMIA

Class I: None

Class IIb:
1. Post-MI patients with LV dysfunction
2. Patients with congestive heart failure
3. Patients with idiopathic hypertrophic cardiomyopathy

Class III:
1. Post-MI patients with normal LV function
2. Diabetic subjects to evaluate for diabetic neuropathy
3. Patients with rhythmic disturbances that preclude HRV analysis (i.e. atrial fibrillation)

INDICATIONS FOR AECG TO ASSESS ANTIARRHYTHMIC THERAPY

Class I: To assess antiarrhythmic drug response if required

Class IIa: To detect proarrhythmic response in patients at high risk

Class IIb:
1. To assess rate control during atrial fibrillation
2. To document recurrent or asymptomatic nonsustained arrhythmias in outpatients

INDICATIONS FOR AECG TO ASSESS PACEMAKER AND ICD FUNCTION

Class 1:
1. In patients with frequent palpitation, syncope, or presyncope to assess device malfunction
2. To assess the response to adjunctive pharmacotherapy

Class IIb:
1. Evaluation of device function immediately after implantation
2. Evaluation of the rate of supraventricular arrhythmias

Class III:
1. Assessment of device malfunction when it's diagnosis has been already established
2. For routine follow-up in asymptomatic patients

INDICATIONS FOR AECG FOR ISCHEMIA MONITORING

Class IIa: Patients with suspected variant angina

Class IIb:
1. Evaluation of patients with chest pain who cannot exercise
2. Preoperative evaluation for vascular surgery who cannot exercise
3. Patients with known CAD and atypical chest pain syndrome

Class III:
1. Initial evaluation of patients with chest pain who are able to exercise
2. Routine screening of asymptomatic subjects

REFERENCES

1. Holter NJ. New method for heart studies. Science. 1961;134:1214-20.
2. Crawford MH, Bernstein SJ, Deedwania PC, et al. ACC/AHA Guidelines for Ambulatory Electrocardiography. A report of the American College of Cardiology/American Heart Association Task Force on Practice Guidelines (Committee to Revise the Guidelines for Ambulatory Electrocardiography). Developed in collaboration with the North American Society for Pacing and Electrophysiology. J Am Coll Cardiol. 1999;34:912-48.
3. Gibson TC, Heitzman MR. Diagnostic efficacy of 24-hour electrocardiographic monitoring for syncope. Am J Cardiol. 1984;53:1013-7.
4. Sivakumaran S, Krahn AD, Klein GJ, et al. A prospective randomized comparison of loop recorders versus Holter monitors in patients with syncope or presyncope. Am J Med. 2003;115:1-5.
5. Linzer M, Yang EH, Estes NA, et al. Diagnosing syncope. Part 2: Unexplained syncope. Clinical Efficacy Assessment Project of the American College of Physicians. Ann Intern Med. 1997;127:76-86.
6. Kinlay S, Leitch JW, Neil A, et al. Cardiac event recorders yield more diagnoses and are more cost-effective than 48-hour Holter monitoring in patients with palpitations. A controlled clinical trial. Ann Intern Med. 1996;124:16-20.
7. Zimetbaum PJ, Kim KY, Josephson ME, et al. Diagnostic yield and optimal duration of continuous-loop event monitoring for the diagnosis of palpitations. A cost-effectiveness analysis. Ann Intern Med. 1998;128:890-5.
8. Maron BJ, Spirito P. Implantable defibrillators and prevention of sudden death in hypertrophic cardiomyopathy. J Cardiovasc Electrophysiol. 2008;19:1118-26.
9. Moss AJ, Hall WJ, Cannom DS, et al. Improved survival with an implanted defibrillator in patients with coronary disease at high risk for ventricular arrhythmia. Multicenter Automatic Defibrillator Implantation Trial Investigators. N Engl J Med. 1996;335:1933-40.
10. Zareba W, Moss AJ, le Cessie S, et al. T wave alternans in idiopathic long QT syndrome. J Am Coll Cardiol. 1994;23:1541-6.
11. Olson JA, Fouts AM, Padanilam BJ, et al. Utility of mobile cardiac outpatient telemetry for the diagnosis of palpitations, presyncope, syncope and the assessment of therapy efficacy. J Cardiovasc Electrophysiol. 2007;18:473-7.
12. Kottkamp H, Tanner H, Kobza R, et al. Time courses and quantitative analysis of atrial fibrillation episode number and duration after circular plus linear left atrial lesions: trigger elimination or substrate modification: early or delayed cure? J Am Coll Cardiol. 2004;44:869-77.
13. Rocco MB, Nabel EG, Campbell S, et al. Prognostic importance of myocardial ischemia detected by ambulatory monitoring in patients with stable coronary artery disease. Circulation. 1988;78:877-84.
14. Scirica BM, Morrow DA, Budaj A, et al. Ischemia detected on continuous electrocardiography after acute coronary syndrome: observations from the MERLIN-TIMI 36 (Metabolic Efficiency with Ranolazine for Less Ischemia in Non-ST-Elevation Acute Coronary Syndrome-Thrombolysis in Myocardial Infarction 36) trial. J Am Coll Cardiol. 2009;53:1411-21.
15. Nair CK, Khan IA, Esterbrooks DJ, et al. Diagnostic and prognostic value of Holter-detected ST-segment deviation in unselected patients with chest pain referred for coronary angiography: a long-term follow-up analysis. Chest. 2001;120:834-9.
16. Reiffel JA, Schwarzberg R, Murry M. Comparison of auto-triggered memory loop recorders versus standard loop recorders versus 24-hour Holter monitors for arrhythmia detection. Am J Cardiol. 2005;95:1055-9.
17. Brignole M, Vardas P, Hoffman E, et al. Indications for the use of diagnostic implantable and external ECG loop recorders. Europace. 2009;11:671-87.
18. Rothman SA, Laughlin JC, Seltzer J, et al. The diagnosis of cardiac arrhythmias: a prospective multi-center randomized study comparing mobile cardiac outpatient telemetry versus standard loop event monitoring. J Cardiovasc Electrophysiol. 2007;18:241-7.
19. Joshi S, Choi AD, Kamath GS, et al. Prevalence, predictors, and prognosis of atrial fibrillation early after pulmonary vein isolation: findings from 3 months of continuous automatic ECG loop recordings. J Cardiovasc Electrophysiol. 2009;20:1089-94.
20. Pontoppidan J, Nielsen JC, Poulsen SH, et al. Symptomatic and asymptomatic atrial fibrillation after pulmonary vein ablation and the impact on quality of life. Pacing Clin Electrophysiol. 2009;32:717-26.
21. Krahn AD, Klein GJ, Yee R, et al. Detection of asymptomatic arrhythmias in unexplained syncope. Am Heart J. 2004;148:326-32.
22. Jacob S, Kommuri NV, Zalawadiya SK, et al. Sensing performance of a new wireless implantable loop recorder: a 12-month follow up study. Pacing Clin Electrophysiol. 2010;33:834-40.
23. Krahn AD, Klein GJ, Yee R, et al. Use of an extended monitoring strategy in patients with problematic syncope. Reveal investigators. Circulation. 1999;99:406-10.
24. Brignole M, Menozzi C, Moya A, et al. Mechanism of syncope in patients with bundle branch block and negative electrophysiological test. Circulation. 2001;104:2045-50.
25. Menozzi C, Brignole M, Garcia-Civera R, et al. Mechanism of syncope in patients with heart disease and negative electrophysiologic test. Circulation. 2002;105:2741-5.
26. Solano A, Menozzi C, Maggi R, et al. Incidence, diagnostic yield and safety of the implantable loop-recorder to detect the mechanism of syncope in patients with and without structural heart disease. Eur Heart J. 2004;25:1116-9.
27. Krahn AD, Klein GJ, Yee R, et al. Randomized assessment of syncope trial: conventional diagnostic testing versus a prolonged monitoring strategy. Circulation. 2001;104:46-51.

28. Farwell DJ, Freemantle N, Sulke N. The clinical impact of implantable loop recorders in patients with syncope. Eur Heart J. 2006;27:351-6.

29. Brignole M, Sutton R, Menozzi C, et al. Early application of an implantable loop recorder allows effective specific therapy in patients with recurrent suspected neurally mediated syncope. Eur Heart J. 2006;27:1085-92.

30. Giada F, Gulizia M, Francese M, et al. Recurrent unexplained palpitations (RUP) study comparison of implantable loop recorder versus conventional diagnostic strategy. J Am Coll Cardiol. 2007;49:1951-6.

31. Armstrong VL, Lawson J, Kamper AM, et al. The use of an implantable loop recorder in the investigation of unexplained syncope in older people. Age Ageing. 2003;32:185-8.

32. Pezawas T, Stix G, Kastner J, et al. Implantable loop recorder in unexplained syncope: classification, mechanism, transient loss of consciousness and role of major depressive disorder in patients with and without structural heart disease. Heart. 2008;94:e17.

33. Brignole M, Bellardine Black CL, Thomsen PE, et al. Improved arrhythmia detection in implantable loop recorders. J Cardiovasc Electrophysiol. 2008;19:928-34.

34. Krahn AD, Klein GJ, Yee R, et al. Cost implications of testing strategy in patients with syncope: randomized assessment of syncope trial. J Am Coll Cardiol. 2003;42:495-501.

Ambulatory Electrocardiographic Monitoring

Cardiac Arrest and Resuscitation

Christine Miyake, Richard E Kerber

Chapter Outline

OVERVIEW OR BACKGROUND

Cardiopulmonary resuscitation (CPR) guidelines are continuously changing as new evidence and techniques are developed and researched. Despite these advances overall survival from sudden cardiac arrest remains low.[1] The return of spontaneous circulation (ROSC) is directly related to adequate coronary perfusion, while good clinical outcomes are more closely related to adequate vital organ perfusion during and immediately after resuscitation. This chapter covers the most recent understanding of blood flow, current emergency medical services (EMS) out of hospital resuscitation efforts, standard techniques of CPR, basic life support (BLS) and advanced life support (ALS) as well as post-resuscitative care. This chapter does not cover the details of pediatric resuscitation.

EVOLUTION OF CARDIAC RESUSCITATION

Cardiopulmonary resuscitation is a relatively new concept. The idea of artificial blood flow with artificial respirations as a means to restore life, after what appears to be death, was not a concept that came easily. It took many years of trial and error and research to develop the idea that blood can flow without opening the chest and directly massaging the heart. In the 1700s mouth-to-mouth resuscitation was recommended for drowning victims; however, there was no formal training for physicians or any type of EMS.[1] The Society for the Recovery of Drowned Persons became the first organization to deal with sudden and unexpected death; however, it was not until the 1950s that James Elam proved expired air was sufficient to maintain adequate

oxygenation until blood flow was restored or other mechanical means of ventilation could be established.[1] In the late 1800s to early 1900s, external chest compressions were being used sporadically in humans with little scientific research or impact on survival rates. The first documented successful use of external chest compressions was reported by Dr George Crile in 1903.[1] After the landmark paper by Kouwenhoven and Jude in the 1960s, who showed adequate circulation could be achieved with closed chest cardiac massage, CPR guidelines were developed and the American Heart Association (AHA) started a program to train physicians and the general public in the techniques of closed-chest cardiac massage.[2] Prior to this landmark paper, it was believed that the only way to artificially circulate blood was to open the chest and perform direct cardiac massage. Since then the AHA has established the standards of care for CPR. The AHA re-evaluates its recommendations and updates the guidelines as new information and research become available.

The mechanism of forward blood flow during CPR has been the subject of much debate and research. There have been two proposed mechanisms most widely recognized: (1) the "thoracic pump model" and (2) the "cardiac pump model". The thoracic pump model postulates that blood flows during closed chest cardiac massage, or CPR, due to an increase in intrathoracic vascular pressure that exceeds extrathoracic vascular pressures. This theory was postulated by Weale and Rothwell-Jackson in 1962. They showed almost equivalent increases in arterial and venous pressures in animals during closed chest CPR.[3] Blood flow is in the proper direction due to venous valves that prevent retrograde flow. The heart is essentially passive with the valves

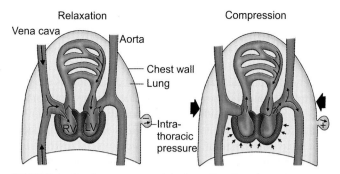

FIGURE 1: Cardiac pump model of cardiopulmonary resuscitaton. (*Source:* Modified from Luce JM, Cary JM, Ross BK, et al. New developments in cardiopulmonary resuscitation. JAMA. 1980;244:1366-70)

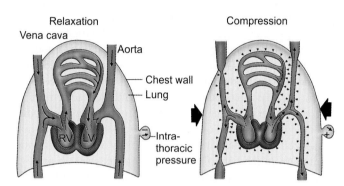

FIGURE 2: Thoracic pump model of cardiopulmonary resuscitation. (*Source:* Modified from Luce JM, Cary JM, Ross BK, et al. New developments in cardiopulmonary resuscitation. JAMA. 1980;244:1366-70)

remaining open due to equal pressure from all sides during compression (Fig. 1). The cardiac pump model, proposed by Kouwenhoven et al., states that flow occurs due to compression of the heart between the sternum and the spine.[2] Flow is maintained in the proper direction due to the mitral valve staying closed during systole or the compression phase. With release of the chest compression the heart expands, the mitral and tricuspid valves open and the heart fills with blood (Fig. 2). In 1993, Redberg et al. performed transesophageal echocardiography on 20 patients during resuscitation in an attempt to determine if cardiac size changed and if the mitral valve opened during diasystole or the release phase of CPR. They found a reduction of ventricular cavity size with compression and mitral valve opening during cardiac release, supporting the cardiac pump theory.[4] Multiple other studies have used ultrasound in an attempt to determine the mechanism of blood flow with mixed results. Studies done on animal models are difficult to extrapolate to humans and many of the human studies show conflicting results without much correlation with survival rates. Both mechanisms may occur, especially during prolonged resuscitation, when the myocardium becomes edematous and stiffer, which might make the heart less compressible favoring the thoracic pump mechanism. While it is still uncertain exactly which mechanism is correct or if it is a combination of both, it is known that the quality and rate of chest compression is extremely important for increasing rates of survival from sudden cardiac arrest.

Using electricity for cardioversion and defibrillation in order to terminate dysrhythmias has been used worldwide for many years. Its origins began in 1775 when Abildgaard demonstrated that stunned chickens can be revived by electrical shocks to the head and heart.[5] In 1899, Prevost and Batelli showed that dogs in ventricular fibrillation (VF) could be restored to a normal rhythm by electric shocks.[6] Then in the 1900s the Consolidated Edison Company of New York began funding research on the mechanisms and treatments of electrical accidents.[6] This allowed extensive research into the electrical mechanisms of heart function and, as a consequence, ways in which electricity can be used to restore proper function in the setting of electrical dysfunction. Human defibrillation began in an operating room in 1947 when Beck administered electrical shocks to the exposed heart (open chest defibrillation) to terminate VF.[7] The first closed chest defibrillation was not achieved until 1965 by Zoll et al.; prior to this a few successful attempts with direct cardiac defibrillation were reported.[8] After Kouwenhoven et al. developed closed-chest cardiac massage, the AHA started a program to train physicians with the techniques of advanced CPR that included CPR as well as electrical defibrillation.[2,6] Types of defibrillators and mechanism of defibrillation are discussed later in this chapter.

CARDIOPULMONARY ARREST

Sudden cardiac arrest is still a major public health problem and a leading cause of death in the United States. It is important when discussing resuscitation strategies from sudden cardiac arrest to define what is meant by "sudden", "cardiac arrest" and "death". The epidemiologic definition of "sudden" is usually defined by less than 1 hour from onset of symptoms to terminal clinical event which could include: death, loss of detectable pulse or cessation of breathing. This definition does not take into account unwitnessed events. The World Health organization has included in its definition of "sudden" unwitnessed deaths that occur less than 24 hours prior to discovery of the victim. "Death" is defined as an absolute irreversible event; this is a biologic, legal and literal definition. "Cardiac arrest" can be reversible and is defined as the cessation of pump function. If the patient is unable to be resuscitated or resuscitation is not performed then the event becomes irreversible and is considered sudden cardiac death. Cardiovascular collapse is defined as loss of effective blood flow either due to cardiac dysfunction or loss of vascular function.

Approximately 10% of all emergency department visits are cardiac related.[6] Cardiac causes are by far the most common cause of sudden cardiac arrest. Ventricular tachycardia (VT) and VF account for the vast majority of sudden death cases. Other causes of sudden death include intracranial hemorrhage, pulmonary embolism, drug overdose, lung disease, aortic dissection or rupture, trauma and drowning. Atherosclerotic disease is the leading cause of death in the United States and in addition it carries significant morbidity, disability and loss of productivity. Atherosclerotic disease is present to some extent in all adult patients, but genetic background and lifestyle risk factors, such as cigarette smoking, sedentary lifestyles and high fat diets, put patients at higher risk for developing significant atherosclerotic disease complications or death. The initiating event is usually injury to the vascular endothelium leading to accumulation of macrophages and lipids at the site of injury. Plaque formation then occurs which can subsequently rupture leading to clot formation compromising blood flow through the arterial lumen. Decreased blood flow or complete occlusion leads to myocardial ischemia, hypoxia, acidosis and infarction. The consequences of arterial occlusion depend upon the availability of collateral blood flow and the size of the area of myocardium supplied by the occluded vessel. Risk factors for increasing plaque formation include: genetic predisposition, hypercholesterolemia, diabetes, hypertension, smoking, male gender and postmenopausal status in women.

The AHA estimates that there are 300,000 out of hospital cardiac arrests each year.[1] Unfortunately survival rates are extremely low. Of those that do survive, more than half have poor neurologic outcomes.[9] According to the AHA, an average of 31.4% of out of hospital cardiac arrest patients receive bystander CPR, of which 60% are treated by EMS.[1] Immediate CPR can substantially improve a victim's chance of survival. Increasing survival rates involves many factors including measuring outcomes and improving "weak links" in the chain of survival. The AHA uses four "links" in the "chain of survival" for victims of sudden cardiac arrest: (1) early recognition of the emergency and activation of emergency medical services; (2) early bystander CPR; (3) early defibrillation if indicated and (4) early ALS and post-resuscitative care. Quality rescuer education and frequency of retraining are also critical factors.

The cardiopulmonary resuscitation is highly accessible and requires little medical training and no equipment but out of hospital cardiac arrest survival rates remain low. Many studies have documented that only 15–30% of victims receive bystander CPR. The EMS often takes 6–7 minutes or longer to arrive at the scene; each minute that passes without blood flow to vital organs decreases the victims' chance of survival. Many theories have been proposed to explain the hesitation to perform CPR by bystanders even when they are trained. One explanation is the concern bystanders have performing mouth-to-mouth resuscitation. The complexity of the guidelines and instructional materials may prevent bystanders from performing CPR. The fear of poor performance or failure may also prevent many from even attempting. Legal liability is also a concern of many individuals because they may not be aware of "good Samaritan" laws that provide some protection for rescuers.

Every 5 years the AHA revises its guidelines for resuscitation care. The 2005 revision placed greater emphasis on compressions and de-emphasized ventilations. This change was studied after its initiation and found an increase in survival rates suggesting less interruption of chest compressions improves outcomes.[10,11] The bigger problem and concern was the need to increase bystander performed CPR. Given the concerns bystanders have of performing mouth-to-mouth resuscitation several studies were conducted to evaluate the outcome differences between compression only CPR and standard CPR with ventilations. Svensson et al. conducted a randomized prospective study comparing the two groups.[12] They found no significant difference in survival rates of compression only CPR and standard CPR for witnessed out of hospital cardiac arrest victims. This along with other studies prompted the AHA to change its recommendations for the 2010 guidelines to compression only CPR for witnessed out of hospital cardiac

arrest victims. Two main conclusions can be currently drawn from these studies: (1) first and foremost CPR needs to be performed as quickly as possible and (2) quality compressions with minimal interruption need to occur. The 2010 AHA guidelines for pulseless arrest are discussed later in this chapter.

Implementation of new guidelines does improve outcomes; however, expediting guideline implementation is challenging. It can take several years for new guidelines to be implemented; barriers to implementation include: delays in instruction, technology upgrades, and difficulties with coordination of medical direction, government agencies and participation in research.

EMERGENCY MEDICAL SERVICES

The credit for developing the first EMS system seems to go to Napoleon's Surgeon-in-Chief, Barron Jean Larrey. He noted that wounded soldiers were left unattended until the fighting ceased, after which rescue teams would enter the battlefield and care for the wounded. He was convinced that if the wounded were attended to sooner, mortality rates would improve. He positioned medical transport teams closer to the battlefield to remove the injured soldiers. During the American Civil War the medical director of the Army of the Potomac, Jonathan Letterman, organized horse-drawn trains to rapidly remove wounded soldiers from the battlefield to field hospitals set-up nearby.[13]

During the first half of the 20th century most civilian transports were performed by morticians. There were no government regulations or financial support. The poor state of emergency medical response and treatment along with recommendations for improvement were first published by the National Safety Council's Traffic Conference after surveying several cities across the United States on how injuries from traffic accidents were handled.[14] In 1966, a second national survey by the National Academy of Sciences-National Research Council was used to complete the "White Paper" entitled Accidental Death and Disability: the Neglected Disease of Modern Society.[15] The issues brought forth in this paper along with public concern pushed congress to draft legislation that enabled the US Department of Transportation and the National Highway Traffic Safety Administration (NHTSA) to develop a national program to improve emergency medical care.[16] In 1973, the US Senate passed the EMS Systems Act which gave federal funding to improve regional EMS systems.[17] Currently all states have an administrative department that governs EMS activities and assists in the planning, licensing and development of standards of practice.

Each state is responsible to ensure that their citizens receive prompt emergency medical care. The National Highway Safety Administration has made recommendations and guidelines for the implementation of an EMS system and course curriculum training for care providers. At a minimum EMS, programs should have these ten components: (1) Regulation and Policy— this should include comprehensive legislation, regulations and operational policies and procedures to provide emergency medical and trauma care services; (2) Resource Management— the state should establish a central lead agency that identifies, categorizes and coordinates resources necessary for the overall system implementation and operation; (3) Human Resources and Training—the EMS system must have trained persons to perform the required tasks, including first responders, emergency medical technicians (EMTs), communications, physicians, nurses, hospital administrators and planners; (4) Transportation—reliable and safe ambulance transportation is critical for an effective EMS system; (5) Facilities—proper facilities that are accessible are required to ensure high-quality care and these must be available in a timely manner. Hospital resources and capabilities need to be designated and known in advance and agreements need to be established between facilities to ensure patients receive treatment at the closest, most appropriate facility; (6) Communications—an effective communication system is needed to provide a means for persons to access resources, mobilize units, manage and coordinate those resources to provide care in a timely fashion; (7) Trauma Systems—a designated trauma system needs to be established to provide high quality, effective patient care; (8) Public Information and Education—public awareness and education of the EMS system is essential for proper access to occur; (9) Medical Direction—physician involvement is critical for a system to provide high quality and proper care. Physicians must delegate responsibilities to non-physician providers; protocols need to be developed, implemented and have continuous oversight with audits and evaluations. Immediate medical direction by a physician should be available at all times to ensure quality patient care and (10) Evaluation—evaluation is required to provide improvement in the system as new medical knowledge is obtained.[18] Table 1 summarizes all these ten components.

Not all EMS systems operate in similar fashion. System designs need to accommodate the needs of the local community or jurisdiction. The system may be served by a private or public agency, it may provide BLS services only or both BLS and ALS. Responses to 911 calls may be in the form of single-tiered, multi-tiered or first responder only. Currently not all systems incorporate record keeping, data collection or auditing programs. This puts these systems at a disadvantage due to their inability to improve patient care through changes in protocol, tracking

those changes to ensure proper implementation and demonstrating a true impact on patient care.

Public agencies are the responsibility of local governments; many of these systems use fire departments to provide EMS services. Providers are then cross trained as firefighter or paramedics. Some public EMS systems are separate entities referred to as municipal third-service systems. Some communities may combine public agencies such as EMS, fire and police services with one director or administrator. Funding public EMS systems may be tax based or a combination of use fees plus government funding. Medical oversight is usually provided by an appointed physician or medical control board.

Private agencies that provide EMS services may be locally owed, hospital based or operated by large corporations. Most private agencies are funded by user fees; some government subsidies may be provided; however, depending on the local needs and percent of uninsured population. Some systems have multiple agencies, public or private, providing services to the same area. These systems may have varying ways of allocating calls, such as rotational coverage or zone coverage.

Single-tier systems provide the same level of personnel and equipment irrelevant of call types, for example all BLS or all ALS. A multi-tiered system dispatches different levels, BLS or ALS depending on the nature of the call. Cost differences are debated and may depend on the community being served. It may prove to be cost effective to have a single ALS system providing consistent advanced care avoiding the potential to under-triage a call and send a lower BLS unit when an ALS unit is actually required. This can be difficult to fund as paramedics are more costly to staff than EMTs. First responders are usually part of any system and consist of police or firefighter who may arrive at the scene prior to the ambulance.

Individual states are responsible for drafting recognized provider levels, testing and recertification requirements. The NHTSA provides recommendations for a national standard curriculum. Basic provider levels include: First responder, emergency medical technician-basic (EMT-B), emergency medical technician-intermediate (EMT-I) and paramedic. The BLS and ALS refer to type of emergency care provided. The BLS or BLS services involve life-saving skills such as bag-valve-mask ventilation, oral and nasal airway use, CPR training, bleeding control techniques, basic fracture care or splinting and childbirth assistance. The use of an automated external defibrillator (AED) is also often included in BLS training. The ALS includes BLS training but also incorporates more advanced airways such as intubation, laryngeal mask airway (LMA) use and the use of rapid sequence intubation (RSI) medications. They also include cardiac medications for the resuscitation of cardiac arrest victims. Details about BLS and ALS are to be discussed later in this chapter.

First responder training is typically done for all personnel, such as firefighters and police officers, who might be the first to respond to an emergency. Many bystanders may also be first responder trained. First responders can provide limited life-saving procedures such as CPR, Heimlich maneuver, spinal immobilization and basic bleeding control measures. Most first responders receive 40 hours of didactic instruction and 16–36 hours required for refresher training as recommended by the NHTSA.[19]

TABLE 1

Components needed for EMS system operation

Regulation and policy	Legislation, regulations and operational policies and procedures
Resource management	Lead agency identifies categorizes and coordinates resources
Human resources and training	Trained persons to perform required tasks
Transportation	Reliable and safe ambulances
Facilities	Proper and accessible with known hospital capabilities
Communication	Communication system for resource allocation
Trauma system	Predetermined for timely access
Public information and education	Public awareness/education for proper utilization of resources
Medical direction	Physician directed protocols and oversight
Evaluation	Provide improvement and implementation of new medical knowledge

TABLE 2

Summary of EMS provider levels

Training level	Personnel	Skills	Education
First responder	Personnel first on scene: Police/Firefighters/Bystanders	Limited life-saving procedures: CPR, Heimlich	40 hours didactic training
EMT-B	Minimum level of training to staff ambulance	First responder + immobilization techniques and use of oxygen, auto injection medications, albuterol	100–125 hours training including laboratory
EMT-I	EMT-B plus some advanced resuscitation techniques	EMT-B + LMA, IV line with fluid resuscitation, defibrillator use	300–400 hours training with clinical/field rotations
Paramedic	Most advanced prehospital training	EMT-I + ACLS, RSI, ECG interpretation, limited medication administration, IO	1100–1200 hours training: didactic + laboratory 250–300 hours clinical 250–300 hours field

The EMT-B is the minimal level of training required to staff an ambulance. It incorporates the skill of a first responder as well as some training in patient assessment, immobilization procedures and the use of oxygen administration. Depending on the state, some incorporate the use of life saving cardiac medications such as epinephrine given subcutaneously with auto injection, albuterol via nebulizer and intravenous (IV) fluids. The NHTSA recommends 100–125 hours of training that includes laboratory training.[20] The EMT-B usually also includes training in the use of AED.

Emergency Medical Technician-Intermediate (EMT-I) is trained in the skills of first responder and EMT-B plus more advanced techniques of care such as laryngeal mask airway, endotracheal intubation, IV line with fluid resuscitation and are trained in the use of a defibrillator. The EMT-I approaches the level of training of a paramedic but with less education and in most cases less cost. The NHTSA recommends 300–400 hours of initial education that combines classroom education as well as clinical training through hospital and field rotations.[21] Some states are removing the EMT-I level of training to simplify the training process.

Paramedics have the highest level of prehospital training. Their training includes all BLS training plus advanced cardiac life support (ACLS) training that includes the use of RSI medications, use of 12 lead ECG and its basic interpretation, defibrillator use, many medications including cardiac medications, pain medications and antiseizure medications. Paramedics are also trained in the use of alternative access lines such as the use of intraosseous access. Training also includes more advanced emergent delivery techniques such as neonatal resuscitation for emergency deliveries. The NHTSA recommends 1100–1200 hours of training that include 500–600 hours of classroom and laboratory time, 250–300 clinical hours in the hospital and 250–300 hours of field training.[22] All levels of training require some level of continuing medical education and refresher training. Table 2 summarizes prehospital personnel training levels.

BASIC LIFE SUPPORT

Basic life support is the first step and the foundation for saving lives from sudden cardiac arrest. It involves immediate recognition, activation of emergency response system, performing high-quality CPR and rapid defibrillation when appropriate.[23] The BLS also involves basic trauma and other medical techniques that have not been covered in this chapter. The more people who are trained in BLS the better survival rates can be since witnessed arrest victims would receive CPR sooner. It is not the intention of this chapter to provide complete instruction on the performance of CPR; interested individuals should seek a certified AHA BLS or ACLS classes for complete training and instruction.

ROLE OF BYSTANDERS

The role of bystanders in sudden cardiac arrest is extremely important in the "chain of survival". Bystanders can perform 3 of the 4 links in the chain of survival and greatly impact a victim's chance of survival with good neurologic outcome. Bystanders are important for recognition and EMS activation, perform immediate CPR and apply and use an AED for defibrillation. Kitamura et al.[24] conducted a prospective, observational study in Japan which evaluated the effects of nationwide dissemination of public-access AEDs on the rate of survival of out of hospital cardiac arrest victims. Nationwide access to AEDs resulted in earlier administration of shocks by laypersons and an increase in survival at one month with minimal neurologic impairment. The new 2010 AHA guidelines for BLS emphasize immediate chest compressions without delay for rescue breathing and application of an AED as soon as it is available.

EMERGENCY MEDICAL SERVICES ACTIVATION

Immediate activation of EMS is extremely important for the survival of sudden cardiac arrest victims. In many communities the time interval for EMS arrival is 7–8 minutes. This means that for the first several minutes the chances of survival for the victim is in the hands of bystanders. The sooner EMS can arrive at the scene the sooner victims can receive ACLS and post-resuscitative care. The BLS algorithm has been simplified: immediate activation of the emergency response system and initiate chest compressions for any unresponsive adult victim who is not breathing normally.[23] The previous recommendation of "Look, Listen and Feel" step was too time consuming and inconsistent between rescuers. Lay rescuers should not attempt to check for a pulse as even trained healthcare providers often incorrectly assess the presence or absence of a pulse especially if blood pressure is extremely low.[23] Chest compression performed on a patient with a heart beat is rarely associated with significant injury.[25] Many arrest victims will have gasping respirations or appear to be having a seizure. Lay rescuers should be instructed to start CPR immediately on any unresponsive victim who appears to be struggling to breathe given the unusual presentations of sudden cardiac arrest.

DISPATCHER ASSISTED CARDIOPULMONARY RESUSCITATION

When dispatchers receive a 911 call of a witnessed sudden cardiac arrest they are encouraged to instruct the lay rescuer to perform "hands-only" (compression only) CPR. Compression only CPR is much easier to perform and prevents delays in providing chest compressions. Positioning the head, attaining a seal for mouth-to-mouth or assembling a bag mask can take time and as such this delay has been found to decrease overall survival rates. In 2005, the AHA published new guidelines for cardiac arrest victims in which chest compressions were emphasized before first defibrillation. Placing electrode pads and analyzing rhythm all take time during which the victim is not receiving CPR. It was believed that the lack of immediate chest compressions and the delay in CPR during the "3 stacked shocks" that were previously advised for cardiac arrest due to VF or unstable or pulseless VT was decreasing vital organ blood flow and contributing to poor outcomes. After implementation of the 2005 AHA guidelines multiple studies found significant improvement in survival rates.[10,26,27]

COMPRESSION ONLY CARDIOPULMONARY RESUSCITATION

Changing chest compression ratios, emphasizing more compressions and less ventilation was a controversial topic at the 2005 International Consensus Conference on Resuscitation and a major change to the AHA 2005 guidelines for CPR. Recent studies have demonstrated an increase in survival from out of hospital cardiac arrest resulting from improved quality of CPR, with adequate rate and depth and minimizing interruptions by avoiding excessive ventilations and "stacking shocks".[26-30] During the time between 2005 and 2010 the AHA has been studying ways to simplify CPR and increase its use by laypersons due to the fact that survival rates of out of hospital cardiac arrest remain low.[1] Compression only CPR for most adults for out of hospital cardiac arrest has been shown to achieve similar outcomes to those who receive standard CPR with rescue breathing.[12,31-34] Thus, bystanders are encouraged and directed by dispatch to perform compression only CPR until the arrival of EMS. Starting the procedure with compressions only eliminates the step that most laypersons have difficulty with: opening the airway and giving rescue breaths. However, children rarely arrest from a primary cardiac cause and thus for the pediatric cardiac arrest victim, rescue breathing may be much more important. Pediatric cardiac resuscitation has not been covered in this chapter.

The newest change to the AHA guidelines for CPR will be changing from "A-B-C" (airway, breathing, circulation) to "C-A-B" (chest compressions, airway, breathing).[23] The change will not be an easy one to make. Everyone who has ever learned CPR will have to be re-educated. The vast majority of sudden cardiac arrest patients arrest from VF or pulseless VT, and these patients have improved survival from immediate high quality CPR with early defibrillation.[23] When a collapse is witnessed by a lone rescuer the AHA now advises to confirm unresponsiveness, activate the emergency response system and then begin chest compressions with a rate of 100 per minute for adults with a depth of at least 2 inches, allowing complete recoil of the chest after each compression. Proper hand position is two fingerbreadths above the xiphoid-sternal notch. For the lay person it is easier to understand "center of the chest between the nipples". The first compression cycle should be 30 compressions in length. Early application of an AED or defibrillator should be done as soon as another rescuer is available. Ventilations should be given with 2 breaths after 30 compressions with minimal interruption of compressions. Bystander or dispatcher assisted CPR should be performed with compressions only if a barrier device is not available and there is concern about exposure. Once a "shockable" rhythm is identified and a defibrillator or AED has been applied a shock should be delivered. After the shock is delivered CPR should be started immediately without checking for a pulse or rhythm. After 2 minutes of CPR there should be a pause for a rhythm and pulse check. Healthcare providers should tailor the sequence of actions to the most likely cause of the arrest. In a known drowning, for example, conventional CPR with rescue breathing would be more important. Children and newborn infants are more likely to suffer a respiratory cause of arrest and would also benefit from the conventional A-B-C sequence of resuscitation. Children and infant CPR is performed slightly differently and is not covered in this chapter.

Rescue breathing should be performed with a head tilt chin lift maneuver or jaw thrust if trauma is suspected. A bag valve mask or other barrier should be used if available. More advanced airway techniques have been discussed below. Rescue breaths should be given quickly, minimizing interruption of chest compressions.

MECHANICAL DEVICES FOR CARDIOPULMONARY RESUSCITATION

Mechanical devices for adult CPR have been developed for several reasons. It is possible that mechanical devices may perform CPR better than standard CPR. Mechanical devices are also useful for long transports to prevent rescuer fatigue. The longer a rescuer performs CPR, the more the quality decreases as the rescuer becomes tired. Several studies have shown improved coronary perfusion pressures with mechanical devices. However no studies have shown improved survival with any mechanical device compared to standard CPR.[35-41] Decreased quality of chest compressions with time is however well recognized.[42] It is recommended that rescuers performing CPR change often during the resuscitation and if a long transport is to occur a mechanical device should be considered to be used to prevent rescuer fatigue as well as free up the rescuer to perform other duties. More study is needed to effectively evaluate the use of mechanical CPR devices.

USE OF AUTOMATIC EXTERNAL DEFIBRILLATORS

Automatic external defibrillators are small, portable, battery operated devices that allow providers to defibrillate cardiac arrest victims without interpretation of an electrocardiographic waveform. Laypersons can use the device with minimal or no training, as audible and visual prompts are incorporated into the machine. It is well known that the earlier a victim is defibrillated the better chance of survival. Studies of placement of the devices where it was easily accessible have shown improvement in the survival rate of out of hospital cardiac arrest victims.[24] Most in-hospital defibrillators are now equipped with AED technology to help improve the time to first shock by allowing those untrained or uncertain to use the device.

When a victim is recognized and the emergency medical system is activated CPR should be started. Once the AED is available, the device should be placed by the patient's head for easy access and operation. The AED's power should be turned on which initiates a self check by the machine. The machine then instructs the user in its use. It will begin by advising to attach the electrode pads to the patient. There are pictures on the electrode pads for proper placement on the chest wall. The electrode pads should be placed on the right upper chest just below the clavicle and the left lower lateral chest below the nipple. The chest wall should be dry when the electrode pads are applied. The AED will then analyze the rhythm; some devices require a button to be pushed to analyze the rhythm. The CPR should continue uninterrupted as much as possible during set-up and application of the electrode pads. During analysis of the rhythm the patient should not be touched. The AED will then advise if a shock is indicated or if CPR should be continued. If shock is advised then the machine will indicate to "charge" then will wait for the user to push the "shock" button. Before the shock is initiated everyone must be clear of the patient. After the shock is initiated CPR should be started immediately and not be delayed to analyze the rhythm and check for a pulse. This is a deviation from past AHA guidelines and if the AED is old it may not be programmed appropriately, but CPR should be initiated after the shock in any case. If return of circulation occurs then airway or breathing assistance should be maintained until more definitive care arrives. The cycle of shock, 2 minutes of CPR then rhythm or pulse check should continue until advanced interventions are available.

PACEMAKER OR AUTOMATIC IMPLANTABLE CARDIOVERTER DEFIBRILLATOR PATIENT IN CARDIAC ARREST

If a patient has an implantable device such as a defibrillator or pacemaker, care should be taken to avoid placing electrode paddles or pads on the device; placement should be at least 1 inch away to avoid any potential artifact interference during rhythm analysis and potential damage to the device from defibrillation. There is little danger to a rescuer performing CPR from an implantable automatic internal defibrillator. If the defibrillator fires during CPR the rescuer may feel a slight electrical shock; however, it is not harmful. Pacemaker problems can occur from defibrillation or cardioverson, although this is rare, including damage to the circuitry resulting in complete dysfunction or inappropriate pacing or defibrillation. It is not necessary to turn off the devices during CPR; however, if it is indicated or to alleviate fears of the resuscitation team a circular magnet is needed. For an automatic implantable cardioverter defibrillator (AICD), the magnet is placed over the upper right-hand corner, if left in place for 30 seconds the AICD is turned off. The magnet is then removed. Placing the magnet back for 30 seconds will turn the AICD back on. If a magnet is placed on a pacemaker, it changes the pacemaker to a set predetermined rate in an asynchronous mode. It will pace at the predetermined rate without trying to sense an intrinsic rhythm or coordinate its pacing. All patients who present with a cardiac dysrhythmia and have a pacemaker or AICD in place should receive an interrogation of the device by a cardiologist, trained nurse or technician following the resuscitation. This can be helpful in determining the cause of the arrest as well as ensuring proper pacemaker or AICD function and reprogramming.

COMPLICATIONS OF CARDIOPULMONARY RESUSCITATION

Cardiopulmonary resuscitation is performed to save the life of the victim; however, it is not without complications. Resuscitation teams need to be aware of the potential complications in order to provide better care to a patient whose resuscitation is not going well or for those who deteriorate post-resuscitation. Many studies have been conducted in an attempt to determine the rate of complication from CPR. The most common complication found was sternal and rib fractures with a rate of 25–30%. Other complications include: anterior mediastinal hemorrhage, upper airway complications, abdominal organ injuries and lung injuries.[43-48]

Rib and sternal fractures are the most common complications of even well performed CPR.[45] The sternum may become separated from the ribs during the first several compression cycles and the anterior ribs during this time can be fractured. Most commonly this does not cause permanent problems for the patient but will be painful during recovery. Sometimes the fractured ribs can puncture or injure the lung leading to a tension pneumothorax. If a patient during resuscitation becomes difficult to bag it is important to consider pneumothorax as the cause. If a pneumothorax occurs this can quickly lead to tension for patients who are receiving positive pressure ventilation. Tension pneumothorax interferes with cardiac filling during diastole or the release phase of CPR and can lead to pulseless electrical activity (PEA). Providers need to decompress the chest quickly. To decompress the chest a chest tube needs to be placed, but this can take time during which the patient may continue to deteriorate. While obtaining the supplies and placing a chest tube a needle thoracotomy should be performed. This is performed by placing a large gauge (14-G is preferred) angio-catheter in the second intercostal space on the anterior chest in the midclavicular line. A rush of air should be heard releasing the pressure on the heart allowing for proper filling. The needle can then be removed leaving the plastic catheter in place until a chest tube is in place. If a patient is very large with a thick chest wall a spinal needle may be used instead. While sternal and rib fractures are common complications of CPR they rarely cause any problems for the resuscitation. However, better CPR technique leads to a lower rate of complication.

During a resuscitation attempt many patients will develop gastric distention from either mouth-to-mouth or other rescue breathing prior to intubation. Patients may vomit from this gastric distention or from the resuscitation itself, which can lead to aspiration, especially before a definitive airway can be achieved. An endotracheal tube does not completely occlude the airway and fluid may still pass the endotracheal tube balloon; however, intubation does prevent large amounts of fluid and food particles from being aspirated. If aspiration occurs the patient is at risk for pneumonitis from the acidic contents.

Abdominal organ injury from CPR is not a common complication, but can occur. The most common organ injured is the liver; liver lacerations can occur due to fractured ribs and from CPR performed with the hands too low on the anterior chest. Splenic lacerations have also been known to occur. If a post-resuscitation patient becomes acutely hypotensive, one must consider liver or splenic lacerations as a potential source of hemorrhage. Bowel injury or perforation can also occur.

Fatal bleeding following CPR and the initiation of thrombolytic therapies is not a common complication. Even despite multiple rib fractures most patients do not suffer fatal hemorrhage.[49] Concern over the possible bleeding risks of thrombolytic agents should not preclude providers from thrombolysis following post-cardiac arrest if it is medically indicated for the treatment of acute coronary syndrome (ACS).

ADVANCED CARDIAC LIFE SUPPORT

OVERVIEW-STATISTICS OF SUCCESS

Advanced cardiac life support includes high quality BLS and interventions that can prevent cardiac arrest in the setting of ACSs, treat cardiac arrest and improve outcomes after the cardiac arrest patient is resuscitated. During any resuscitation the healthcare provider must recognize and treat reversible causes of cardiac arrest. The "4 Hs and 4 Ts" are known causes and possible complications of cardiac arrest. These are listed in Table 3. The new AHA 2010 guidelines for the "Chain of Survival" includes "Part 9: Post-Cardiac Arrest Care" emphasizing comprehensive multidisciplinary care beginning with the recognition of cardiac arrest and concludes with hospital discharge, but may carry beyond to prevent future cardiac complications.[23]

ADVANCED AIRWAY MANAGEMENT

The new 2010 AHA guidelines for ACLS have new recommendations for airway management that include: the use of quantitative waveform capnography for confirmation and continuous monitoring of endotracheal tube placement for adults, the use of supraglottic advanced airways as alternative to endotracheal intubation and they no longer recommend the routine use of cricoid pressure during airway management.[23]

TABLE 3

Reversible causes of cardiac arrest

Five Hs	Five Ts
Hypoxia	Toxins
Hypovolemia	Tamponade
Hydrogen ion (acidosis)	Tension pneumothorax
Hypokalemia/hyperkalemia	Thrombosis, pulmonary
Hypothermia	Thrombosis, coronary

(*Source*: Neumar RE, Ottto CS, Link MS, et al. Guidelines for cardiopulmonary resuscitation and emergency cardiovascular care. Part 8: Adult advanced cardiovascular life support. Circulation. 2010;122(Suppl. 3):S729-67)

Endotracheal intubation is the recommended airway of choice for all patients needing invasive ventilation management or airway protection due to alteration in mentation, airway swelling or any other injuring that may compromise the upper airways. The possibility of spinal injury is a relative contra-indication of direct laryngoscopy orotracheal intubation; however, if a patient requires endotracheal intubation for life-saving reasons then one must perform the procedure with as much spinal immobilization as possible without interfering with the intubation procedure. Interested individuals should seek a certified ACLS course for instruction on endotracheal intubation.

The difficult airway where intubation fails can be due to prominent upper incisors, inability to extend the neck, extremely large tongue, swelling, blood or secretions in the airway, small lower jaw, inability to completely open the mouth, tumors or any other unusual anatomy. Some patients despite normal-appearing anatomy without complicated history may pose an unexpected challenge to intubate. For those experienced and skilled in the practice of endotracheal intubation it is still the best airway; however, intubation is also a motor skill that requires practice and for those providers in the EMS system who may not be very experienced airway adjuncts are extremely important. Good bag-valve-mask (BVM) ventilation is the first technique and probably the most important to know. BVM, however, can cause gastric distention and does not protect the airway from aspiration. The most common adjunct supraglottic airways include the LMA, Combitube and King LT. An ideal airway should be rapidly and reliably inserted with minimal training, control ventilation, protect against aspiration and be able to be inserted with ongoing chest compressions. No one device provides all of these things but the LMA, Combitube and King LT are easy to use and found to be useful as adjunct airways for the inexperienced.[50] Multiple mannequin studies have found that most out of hospital providers prefer the King LT as easier and faster to insert.[51-54]

PHARMACEUTICAL INTERVENTIONS

Pharmaceutical interventions for cardiac arrest victims are a controversial subject. There is no evidence that any medications given during cardiac arrest that have lead to any improvement in survival to hospital discharge.[55,56] The most important factors in survival are high quality CPR and early defibrillation. When pharmaceutical therapies are to be used it is important to continue high quality CPR with minimal interruptions in compressions for line placement and intubation. The medications used during CPR should assist in potentiating the return of circulation, enhance cardiac function, support blood pressure and shunt blood toward vital organs.[57] Drug therapy regimens should ultimately increase survival to discharge and not just increase initial resuscitation rates which may only result in unsalvageable patients with transient cardiac activity.[55,56] The AHA includes several medications in their Advanced Cardiovascular Life Support Pulseless Algorithm.

Epinephrine

Epinephrine is a mixed alpha and beta adrenergic receptor agonist. Alpha agonists are potent vasopressors and increase systemic vascular resistance which results in elevated aortic diastolic pressure which then increases coronary and carotid blood flow. However, epinephrine may increase myocardial workload and decrease endocardial perfusion, compromising cardiac tissue. The recommendation of the AHA is 1 mg of epinephrine on every 3–5 minutes for pulseless VT or VF and asystole. High-dose epinephrine does not enhance long-term outcome, can be detrimental and should not be used.[58]

Vasopressin

Vasopressin is a naturally occurring polypeptide produced from cells within the hypothalamus. When administered in pharmacologic dosages it acts as a peripheral vasoconstrictor. Vasopressin has also a longer half-life than epinephrine, about 10–20 minutes. Studies on the use of vasopressin in sudden cardiac arrest have not shown any greater benefit than epinephrine on long-term survival in sudden cardiac arrest.[59-63] If vasopressin is used, the AHA recommendation is 40 units IV in lieu of epinephrine for the first or second dose.

Lidocaine

Lidocaine increases uniformity of the action-potential duration and refractory period and can terminate reentrant rhythms. Lidocaine is given as a bolus of 1 mg/kg. The AHA recommends its administration after epinephrine, vasopressin and amiodarone have been tried. A second loading dose of 1 mg/kg can be given 10–15 minutes after the first one.

Amiodarone

Amiodarone is an antiarrhythmic agent that lengthens the cardiac action potential, prolongates refractoriness of the myocytes and decreases cardiac oxygen consumption. Amiodarone also improves cardiac pump performance, dilates coronary arteries, causes peripheral arterial vasodilatation and increases coronary blood supply. It does have the side effect of decreasing systemic vascular resistance and causing hypotension. The ALIVE trial showed significant improvement in terminating VF and increasing survival to hospital admission in the prehospital setting over the use of lidocaine; however, it is unclear if there is any long-term benefit from its use.[64,65] The AHA does have amiodarone in its guidelines for the use of refractory VF or VT in their pulseless arrest algorithm. The recommended dosing is 300 mg IV bolus with a second dose of 150 mg IV if needed.

Procainamide

Procainamide is a sodium channel-blocking antiarrhythmic medication that prolongs the refractory period and slows conduction through the myocardial conduction system. There are very few studies addressing the use of procainamide during pulseless cardiac arrest. Procainamide must be infused slowly; therefore, its practical use during cardiac arrest is limited. Procainamide must be avoided in patients with torsades de pointes. More study is needed to determine if procainamide has any long-term benefits for pulseless cardiac arrest. The AHA recommends procainamide for stable wide-QRS tachycardia but not for pulseless cardiac arrest.

Atropine

Atropine is a competitive antagonist of acetylcholine at muscarinic receptors. For cardiac arrest patients or those with symptomatic bradycardia, parasympathetic tone is increased due to vagal stimulation. Atropine blocks the depressant effect of the vagus nerve at the sinus and AV nodes. The AHA, however, has removed atropine from its 2010 guidelines for PEA or asystole ACLS Cardiac Arrest Algorithm due to a lack of any evidence showing therapeutic benefit.[66,67]

Magnesium Sulfate

If reversible causes of cardiac arrest are identified and treated patient outcomes improve. Magnesium deficiency can precipitate refractory VF. No prospective clinical trials have been published that show any change in long-term outcome from the routine use of magnesium in cardiac arrest patients except those with hypomagnesemia and patients in trosades de pointes. The recommended dose in cardiac arrest is 1–2 g diluted in 10 ml D5W given IV.

Calcium Chloride

Calcium chloride is not recommended for routine use in pulseless cardiac arrest unless there is an identifiable reason such as known hypocalcemia, hyperkalemia or calcium channel blocker toxicity. Increases in intracellular calcium potentiate myocardial ischemic injury. Canine myocardial cells were investigated and found to have increased uptake of calcium after myocardial ischemia followed by reperfusion, the mechanism of this uptake has not been established but could be a concern for ischemic cellular injury.[68] For hyperkalemia and calcium channel blocker overdose the recommended dosing is 500–1,000 mg IV.

Morphine and Oxygen

The new 2010 ACLS guidelines from the AHA do not recommend the routine administration of oxygen for all ACS patients. The recommendation is to use oxygen to keep saturations greater than 94%. For cardiac arrest patients, 100% oxygen should be used during resuscitation but weaned down in the post-resuscitation period. Morphine is indicated for ST elevation myocardial infarction and when a patient's chest pain is unresponsive to nitrates. Caution should be used when administering to unstable angina or non-ST elevation myocardial infarction patients.

DEFIBRILLATION OR CARDIOVERSION

Defibrillation is a procedure where controlled electrical energy is applied to the myocardium either through the chest wall or through directly on the heart and is designed to terminate an unstable or pulseless rhythm. Defibrillators are divided into two main types: (1) Manual and (2) Automatic. The AEDs were discussed earlier. Manual defibrillators require the provider to obtain and interpret an electrocardiogram and determine if: (1) defibrillation is necessary; (2) select an energy level and (3) decide if synchronization should be used. The goal of defibrillation is to uniformly depolarize a majority of the myocardium and terminate the abnormal dysrhythmia. Once electrical activity is reset and the myocardium regains its excitability, the SA node will presumptively reinitiate normal pacing and the myocardium can begin coordinated rhythmic contractions.

There are currently three basic theories of defibrillation. (1) The "critical mass" theory hypothesizes that the electrical current depolarizes a "critical mass" of myocardium and that the remaining myocardium that is not depolarized is inadequate to sustain the dysrhythmia. Zipes et al.[69] studied VF in dogs and found that successful defibrillation occurred most often when the electrodes were placed in the right ventricular apex and the posterior base of the left ventricle and least often when delivered between the two right ventricular electrodes;[69] (2) The theory of "upper limit of vulnerability" hypothesizes that the most important factor in defibrillation is achieving a critical current density throughout the ventricular myocardium that not only stops the fibrillation fronts but also does not reinitiate fibrillation by the same mechanism by which a shock during the vulnerable period of sinus or paced rhythm initiates fibrillation;[70] (3) It was found that the strength of shocks that stopped inducing VF were similar to the strength of shocks at the defibrillation threshold.[70] The theory of "extension of refractoriness" hypothesizes the shock prolongs the refractoriness in most of the myocardium so the fibrillation wavefronts cannot propagate.[71] Post-shock response durations, from shock to repolarization, were significantly longer in successful defibrillations than for unsuccessful defibrillation.[71] The "critical mass" theory may be important in both the "extension of refractoriness" and "upper limit of vulnerability" hypothesizes.

Defibrillators are classified by the type of waveforms they produce. Monophasic defibrillators send an electrical wave from one electrode to the other in only one direction. With biphasic defibrillators the electrode potential is reversed in midshock so the current reverses direction (Fig. 3). The waveform can also be classified by the way the current flows and terminates during the "discharge" period with respect to time on an x-y Cartesian plot—rapid or gradual at onset and termination. If the wave has a rapid rise to a peak and then a gradual decline to baseline it is considered a damped sinusoidal waveform. If the waveform has a rapid rise and then a rapid descent, it is considered a truncated waveform (Fig. 3). In 1962, Lown introduced the monophasic damped sinusoidal waveform for defibrillation and it remained the standard waveform for defibrillation for 30 years.[72] More recently studies have shown improved rates of terminating VF using biphasic truncated exponential (BTE) waveforms compared to monophasic damped sinusoidal waveforms. The BTE waveform also causes fewer post-shock

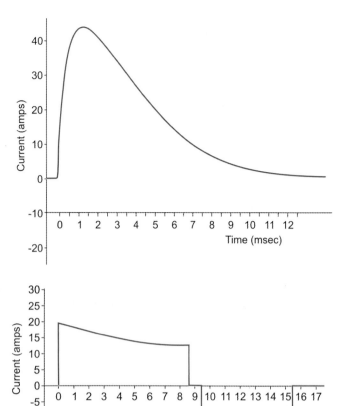

FIGURE 3: Monophasic vs Biphasic waveforms. The monophasic waveform is damped and the biphasic waveform is truncated. (*Source:* Modified from Deakin CD, Nolan JP, Sunde KJ, et al. European resuscitation council guidelines for resuscitation 2010 Section 3. Electrical therapies: automated external defibrillation, cardioversion and pacing. Resuscitation. 2010;81:1293-304)

arrhythmias with less myocardial damage.[73-78] The second phase of the biphasic shock also removes excess charge left on the myocardial cells after the first shock, a process called "charge burping".[79]

Biphasic defibrillators require lower energy levels to terminate VF or VT; the lower energy levels result in a decreased chance of myocardial damage and also allow smaller machines to be built. This technology has allowed portable battery operated AEDs to be developed and placed in public areas for use by lay rescuers. Public access to AEDs has increased survival rates for out of hospital cardiac arrest by decreasing time to first shock as discussed earlier in the chapter.[24,80]

Minimizing transthoracic impedance increases success rates of defibrillation. Paddle force, paddle orientation, a couplant, such as conductive gel use, shaving the chest and lung volumes, can all affect the transthoracic impedance. It is important that gel is applied when using hand-held paddles; without conductive gel the transthoracic impedance is extremely high resulting in poor current flow and decreased defibrillation success. Care must be taken not to smear the gel across the chest between the paddles as this could cause the current to flow through the low impedance path of the gel away from the heart.[81] Breast tissue can also increase impedance; therefore, the paddles or pads should be placed adjacent to or under the breast. Commercially

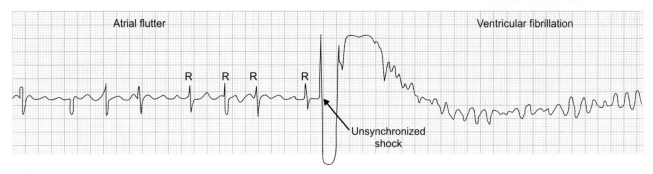

FIGURE 4: Induction of ventricular fibrillation by unsynchronized shock occurring on the vulnerable T-wave. (*Source:* Modified with permission from Kerber RE. Transchest cardioversion: Optimal technique. In Tacker WA (Ed). Defibrillation of the Heart. St Louis, USA: Mosby-Year Book; 1994. pp. 46-81)

available biphasic defibrillators are able to automatically adjust voltages and pulse duration to compensate for high or low transthoracic impedance. Monophasic defibrillators do not have this capability and result in considerable variability in delivered waveform depending on transthoracic impedance. "Smart" biphasic defibrillators can alter the waveform duration and/or voltage of the two pulses individually and instantaneously to optimize performance.

While defibrillation is a life-saving procedure it is not without risk. There are three basic risks: (1) risk to the patient; (2) risk to the user and (3) risk to equipment or environment. Care must be taken to minimize these risks.

Risk to the Patient

Defibrillators are equipped with "synchronization" mode which allows the user to avoid unintended delivery of a shock to the "T" wave of the ECG [which can induce VF, (Fig. 4)]. The user must be sure, when using a manual defibrillator, to appropriately use the synchronization for cardioversion of stable dysrhythmias but must avoid its use in unstable or pulseless rhythms, such as VF or polymorphic VT, where there will not be a discrete "R" wave to synchronize on and the device will not fire, thereby causing a delay until the synchronizer is disabled.

The energy level applied to the myocardium from defibrillation can cause damage manifest as myocardial necrosis and functional damage evident as atrioventricular conduction disturbances.[82] Chest wall impedance also posses challenges to delivery of safe defibrillation; high impedance results in a wide waveform with lower current, low impedance results in a narrow waveform with high current. Excessive current runs the risk of myocardial damage and low current may be inadequate to achieve defibrillation. As discussed earlier electrode orientation, electrode placement, chest hair and lung volumes can all affect impedance.

Incorrectly displayed asystole can occur when paddles or gel pads are used to display the ECG tracing due to electrical voltage "offset". This "false" asystole display can last long enough to mislead rescuers. If asystole is displayed it must be confirmed immediately by attaching the standard ECG electrodes; therefore, whenever possible gel pads or paddles should not be used for ECG display or monitoring.[83]

After transthoracic shocks first-degree skin burns are common.[84] Current flows preferentially to the edges of the electrodes increasing the thermal temperature causing skin burns mostly around the edges. New electrode pads are designed to decrease thermal temperatures at the contact site and therefore decrease skin burns.[85]

Risk to the Environment or Equipment

An increasing number of patients requiring CPR and defibrillation or cardioversion have implantable pacemakers or defibrillators. It is recommended that placement of paddles or pads are at least 12–15 cm from the device to help prevent damage to the implantable device. Although this risk is very low, it is possible that the electrical energy can be transferred down the lead wires damaging the wires and preventing proper defibrillation.[86-88]

Risks to the Rescuer

Risks to the rescuer during cardioversion or defibrillation are difficult to quantify. It is estimated that injury to paramedics was 1 per 1,700 without significant morbidity or mortality.[89] Recent clinical studies have measured current flow through rescuers who have deliberately placed themselves in the current pathway during cardioversion of atrial fibrillation; measured current flow through the rescuers was trivial and no injury occurred.[90] It has been suggested that the traditional admonition to "clear" the patient before delivering a defibrillating shock is therefore unnecessary, providing gloves are worn and self-adhesive paddles are used.[91] However the AHA recommends that all personnel stand clear during shock delivery. There is also no significant evidence documenting that performing CPR on a patient with an implantable cardiac defibrillator is harmful to the rescuer; therefore, CPR should be performed as usual but the device may be turned off as described earlier in the chapter when a magnet becomes available. The most common rescuer injuries are musculoskeletal related.

VF or VT-stable vs unstable: Ventricular fibrillation is always pulseless and, therefore, an unstable rhythm; CPR should be started immediately and defibrillation should be performed as soon as possible. The 2010 AHA guidelines recommend immediate CPR then defibrillation followed by more immediate CPR, minimizing pauses and "hands off" time. The monophasic energy recommendation is 360 J. Biphasic waveform defibrillator configurations differ among manufacturers and none have been directly compared to humans, therefore, the AHA recommends using the manufacturer's recommendations for energy dose on biphasic machines. Since no optimal biphasic energy level has been determined the AHA does not make any definitive recommendation for the selected energy for subsequent biphasic defibrillation attempts. If subsequent shocks are required then the energy levels should be equivalent or higher than the first shock.

Ventricular tachycardia can be either unstable or stable. If the rhythm does not produce a blood pressure sufficient to maintain mentation then CPR should be started with defibrillation as soon as possible. If the patient with VT has a pulse with tolerable blood pressures then elective cardioversion is recommended, as soon as possible to prevent deterioration to a pulseless rhythm. Cardioversion is always performed using synchronized shocks, which avoids shock delivery during the relative refractory period of the cardiac cycle when the shock is most likely to induce VF. Monomorphic VT has been found to convert with lower energy and current during cardioversion than polymorphic VT which behaves more like VF.[92] Amiodarone administration for persistent VF or VT has been found to be relatively safe but ineffective for the acute termination of sustained VT.[93] Amiodarone is administered at a dose of 300 mg IV bolus.

Atrial fibrillation or supraventricular tachycardia: Atrial dysrhythmias and other tachycardias may require urgent cardioversion due to hypotension or pulmonary edema. Treatment of the cause of the arrhythmia may restore sinus rhythm or prevent recurrence. Causes include hyperthyroidism, pulmonary embolism, congestive heart failure and valve disorders. Table 4 lists some of the causes of wide and narrow tachycardia. Factors that may influence immediate and long-term success of cardioversion include the type of tachycardia, underlying cause of the dysrhythmia, and duration of the dysrhythmia. The AHA recommends initial biphasic energy doses of 120–200 J for atrial fibrillation; the monophasic energy dose should be 200 J. Atrial flutter and other supraventricular rhythms require less energy and a starting dose of 50–100 J of monophasic or biphasic with increasing step wise dosing is often sufficient. Synchronization is required for cardioversion. Table 4 summarizes classification of tachycardia.

Defibrillation or cardioversion in pacemaker or AICD patients: As described earlier in the chapter, defibrillation with pacemakers and AICDs in place pose little risk to the patient and the rescuer; however, some precautions are indicated. Placement of the pads or paddles should be in an anterior-posterior or anterior-lateral locations avoiding overlap with the device if at all possible. Delay in defibrillation should not occur due to an implantable device. Pacemaker spikes with unipolar pacing may confuse AED software and prevent VF from being recognized.[67] As soon as more advanced equipment and personnel are available the rhythm should be analyzed.

CESSATION OF RESUSCITATION

Termination of resuscitation is difficult for all providers of cardiac arrest patients but it can become especially difficult for emergency medical personnel in the prehospital setting. There are ethical, legal and cultural factors that need to be taken into consideration when deciding the need for termination of resuscitation. Initiation of resuscitation may conflict with a patient's desires or may not be in the best interest of the patient and in some instances resuscitation may not be the best use of limited resources. The public in general overestimates the probability of survival from cardiac arrest and even most physicians cannot accurately predict mortality rates of sudden cardiac arrest.

The 2010 AHA guidelines give some guidance for termination of resuscitation efforts in adults with out of hospital cardiac arrest. The AHA has developed the "BLS termination of resuscitation rule"; if all the following criteria are met then there is no indication for ambulance transport: (1) arrest was not witnessed by and EMS provider or first responder; (2) no ROSC after three complete rounds of CPR and AED analysis and (3) no AED shocks delivered. The "ALS termination of resuscitation rule" states if all the following criteria are met then termination of resuscitation before transport is indicated: (1) arrest not witnessed by anyone; (2) no bystander CPR provided; (3) no ROSC after complete ALS care in the field and (4) no shocks delivered. Implementation of these rules usually includes contacting the EMS medical control. EMS providers should be trained in sensitive communication with family members about outcomes. Collaboration with hospital EDs, medical coroner's office, online medical directors and the police are necessary. These rules have been validated for adult out of hospital cardiac arrest victims in multiple EMS settings across the United States, Canada and Europe.[67,94-96] Implementation of these rules reduces the rate of unnecessary hospital transports which can place providers and the public at risk from road traffic hazards, decrease unnecessary exposures from potential biohazards and decrease costs.

The decision to terminate resuscitative efforts is never an easy one. While guidelines are available, all providers including first responders, EMS personnel and physicians need to take into consideration many factors when deciding to terminate efforts. It is clear that resuscitation should not be started for

TABLE 4

Classification of tachycardias

- Narrow–QRS-complex (SVT) tachycardias (QRS < 0.12 second), listed in order of frequency
  — Sinus tachycardia
  — Atrial fibrillation
  — Atrial flutter
  — AV nodal re-entry
  — Accessory pathway–mediated tachycardia
  — Atrial tachycardia
  — Multifocal atrial tachycardia (MAT)
  — Junctional tachycardia
- Wide–QRS-complex tachycardias (QRS ≥ 0.12 second)
  — Ventricular tachycardia (VT) and ventricular fibrillation (VF)
  — SVT with aberrant conduction
  — Pre-excitation tachycardias [Wolff-Parkinson-White (WPW) syndrome]
  — Ventricular paced rhythms

(*Source*: Neumar RW, Otto CS, Link MS, et al. American Heart Association guidelines for cardiopulmonary resuscitation and emergency cardiovascular care. Part 8: Adult advanced cardiovascular life support. Circulation. 2010;122(Suppl. 3):S729-67)

victims who have a valid do not resuscitate (DNR), newborn premature infants less than 23 weeks gestation and victims who present with obvious signs of death such as: rigor mortis, decapitation or dependent lavidity.

POST-RESUSCITATION CARE

Post-resuscitative care is a new section in the 2010 AHA guidelines for CPR. The goal is to emphasize an organized multidisciplinary program that focuses on optimizing neurologic, hemodynamic and metabolic function that may provide an increase in survival to hospital discharge.[67] Patients should be cared for in a multidisciplinary environment with angiography and interventional capabilities and a team capable of caring for patients with multiorgan dysfunction.

CARDIOPULMONARY SUPPORT

Once circulation is restored oxygen should be weaned down to lowest required to maintain oxygen greater than 94%, to avoid hyperoxia. The 2010 international consensus on CPR and ECC science with treatment recommendations found harmful effects of hyperoxia after ROSC.[67,97] An oxyhemoglobin of 100% can correspond to a PaO_2 anywhere between 80 and 500. With return of circulation a "post-arrest syndrome" often presents that requires proper inotropic support and monitoring. Standard vasopressor treatment is indicated to improve patient hemodynamics. Many patients will develop multisystem organ dysfunction and this must be anticipated and treated in a timely fashion.

CARDIAC INTERVENTIONS

The goal of interventions is to prevent further myocardial necrosis and left ventricular dysfunction leading to heart failure. Percutaneous coronary intervention (PCI) will provide patients with ST elevation myocardial infarction the most favorable outcomes, even in out of hospital cardiac arrest where overall survival remains low.[98-101] For those patients without obvious ST elevations an ischemic cardiac etiology may still be a reasonable assumption given the insensitivity or possible misleading electrocardiogram following cardiac arrest; more study is needed to determine if this subgroup of patients would benefit from intervention.[100] Patients should be transferred or taken from the scene to a facility that is capable of providing a comprehensive post-cardiac arrest treatment system of care that includes advanced cardiac interventions even if they have received thrombolytic therapy at a less capable institution. Early PCI following thrombolysis is associated with reduced recurrence of ischemia and reinfarction without increased risk of major hemorrhage.[102,103]

THERAPEUTIC HYPOTHERMIA

Predicting neurologic outcomes post-cardiac arrest is challenging. Therapeutically induced mild hypothermia after successful initial resuscitation has been studied and found to improve neurologic outcome in comatose cardiac arrest survivors and to decrease overall mortality.[104-107] Methods of inducing hypothermia to 33°C for 24 hours include: external ice, blankets through which cold water continuously circulates,

cold IV saline and endovascular coils.[108,109] Interventions to rapidly reduce body temperature during CPR have been shown to improve defibrillation success and ROSC in animal models; however, limited clinical experience has been favorable.[110-113] Improving patients' final functional outcome also involves early recognition and treatment of treatable neurologic disorders such as seizures. Seizures may be difficult to diagnose in the hypothermia induced patient due to neuromuscular blockade use that is designed to prevent shivering. It is therefore important to have electroencephalographic monitoring during this coma induced state. To date there have not been any diagnostic evaluations or tools found that consistently predict neurologic outcome in post-cardiac arrest patients. There is limited evidence to guide clinical decisions and, therefore, best clinical judgment with family discussion should be used to make decisions regarding withdraw of life support.

SUMMARY

Cardiopulmonary resuscitation from sudden cardiac arrest is challenging. Since 1960, our impact on patient survival from out of hospital cardiac arrest has changed very little. What we do know is that high quality, minimally interrupted CPR that is started immediately upon recognition is extremely important for improving patient survival. Rate and depth of compressions is the key to high quality CPR. Providers who do not perform CPR often should have frequent retraining. The AHA guidelines for 2010 have been simplified to help improve compliance and to emphasize compressions over other interventions in the field to help improve the number of patients who receives bystander CPR; this includes compression only CPR for those who may be unwilling or unable to perform conventional CPR. Many fears that potential rescuers have may be alleviated with education and debriefing which may improve first responder or bystander initiation of resuscitation. Continuous evaluations and re-education should be implemented in all levels from the prehospital setting to hospital resuscitation teams, to improve resuscitation performance with an emphasis on CPR quality and team work. Continued research is required in all areas of resuscitation from prehospital to hospital discharge to improve survival and neurologic outcomes.

REFERENCES

1. CPR and Sudden Cardiac Arrest Fact Sheet. American Heart Association. Available from www.heart.org [Accessed October, 2010].
2. Kouwenhoven WB, Jude JR, Knickerbocker CG. Closed chest cardiac massage. JAMA. 1960;173:1064-7.
3. Weale FE, Rothwell-Jackson RL. Cardiac massage. Lancet. 1962; 7237:990-2.
4. Redberg RF, Tucker KJ, Cohen TJ, et al. Physiology of blood flow during cardiopulmonary resuscitation. A transesophageal echocardiographic study. Circulation. 1993;88:534-42.
5. Driscoll TE, Ratnoff OD, Nygard OF. The remarkable Dr. Abildgaard and countershock. Ann Internal Med. 1975;83:878-82.
6. American Heart Association. History of CPR. Available from www.heart.org [Accessed October, 2010].
7. Beck CS, Pritchard WH, Feil HS. Ventricular fibrillation of long duration abolished by electric shock. J Am Med Assoc. 1947;135:985-6.

8. Zoll P, Linenthal A, Gibson W, et al. Termination of ventricular fibrillation in man by externally applied electrical countershock. NEJM. 1956;254:727-32.

9. Young BG. Neurologic prognosis after cardiac arrest. NEJM. 2009;361:605-11.

10. Sayre MR, Cantrell SA, White LJ, et al. Impact of the 2005 American Heart Association cardiopulmonary resuscitation and emergency cardiovascular care guidelines on out-of-hospital cardiac arrest survival. Prehosp Emerg Care. 2009;13:469-77.

11. Hinchey PR, Myers JB, Lewis R, et al. Improved out-of-hospital cardiac arrest survival after the sequential implementation of 2005 AHA guidelines for compressions, ventilations and induced hypothermia: the Wake County experience. Ann Emerg Med. 2010;56:358-61.

12. Svensson L, Bohm K, Castren M, et al. Compression-only CPR or standard CPR in out of hospital cardiac arrest. NEJM. 2010;363:434-42.

13. Boyd DR. The conceptual development of EMS systems in the United States. Emerg Med Serv. 1982;11:19-23.

14. Hampton OP. Transportation of the injured: a report. Bull Am Coll Surg. 1960;45:55-9.

15. Division of Medical Sciences, National Academy of Sciences-National Research Council: accidental death and disability: the neglected disease of modern society. Washington DC: US Government Printing Office; 1966.

16. National Highway Safety Act of 1966, Public Law 89-564, Washington DC: 89th US Congress; 1966.

17. Emergency Medical Services Systems Act of 1973, Public law 93-154, Washington DC: 93rd US Congress; 1973.

18. US Department of Transportation-National Highway Traffic Safety Administration: Highway Safety Program Guideline No 11 Emergency Medical Services, 2009 [www.nhtsa.gov].

19. US Department of Transportation-National Highway Traffic Safety Administration: First responder: National standard curriculum, 1997 [www.nhtsa.gov].

20. US Department of Transportation-National Highway Traffic Safety Administration: Emergency Medical Technician-Basic: National standard curriculum, 1997 [www.nhtsa.gov].

21. US Department of Transportation-National Highway Traffic Safety administration: Emergency Medical Technician-Intermediate: National Standard Curriculum, 1999 [www.nhtsa.gov].

22. US Department of Transportation-National Highway Traffic Safety Administration: Emergency Medical Technician-Paramedic: National Standard Curriculum, 2004 [www.nhtsa.gov].

23. Executive Summary: 2010 American Heart Association Guidelines for Cardiopulmonary resuscitation. Circulation. 2010. Available from www.circ.ahajournals.org [Accessed October, 2010]

24. Kitamura T, Iwami T, Kawamura T, et al. Nationwide public-access defibrillation in Japan. NEJM. 2010;362:994-1004.

25. White L, Roger J, Bloomingdale M, et al. Dispatcher-assisted cardiopulmonary resuscitation: risks for the patients not in cardiac arrest. Circulation. 2010;121:91-7.

26. Iwami T, Nichol G, Hiraide A, et al. Continuous improvements in "chain of survival" increased survival after out-of-hospital cardiac arrests: a large-scale population-based study. Circulation. 2009;119:728-34.

27. Rea TD, Helbock M, Perry S, et al. Increasing use of cardio-pulmonary resuscitation during out-of-hospital ventricular fibrillation arrest: survival implications of guideline changes. Circulation. 2006;114:2760-5.

28. Hollenberg J, Herlitz J, Lindqvist J, et al. Improved survival after out-of-hospital cardiac arrest is associated with an increase in proportion of emergency crew-witnessed cases and bystander cardiopulmonary resuscitation. Circulation. 2008;118:389-96.

29. Lund-Kordahl I, Olasveengen TM, Lorem T, et al. Improving outcome after out-of-hospital cardiac arrest by strengthening weak links of the Chain of Survival: quality of advanced life support and post-resuscitation care. Resuscitation. 2010;81:422-6.

30. Bobrow BJ, Clark LL, Ewy GA, et al. Minimally interrupted cardiac resuscitation by emergency medical services for out-of-hospital cardiac arrest. JAMA. 2008;299:1158-65.

31. Iwami T, Kawamura T, Hiraide A, et al. Effectiveness of bystander-initiated cardiac-only resuscitation for patients with out-of-hospital cardiac arrest. Circulation. 2007;116:2900-7.

32. Ong ME, Ng FS, Anushia P, et al. Comparison of chest compression only and standard cardiopulmonary resuscitation for out-of-hospital cardiac arrest in Singapore. Resuscitation. 2008;78:119-26.

33. Bohm K, Rosenqvist M, Herlitz J, et al. Survival is similar after standard treatment and chest compression only in out-of-hospital bystander cardiopulmonary resuscitation. Circulation. 2007;116:2908-12.

34. Rea TD, Fahrenbruch C, Culley L, et al. CPR with chest compression alone or with rescue breathing. NEJM. 2010;363:423-33.

35. Dickinson ET, Verdile VP, Schneider RM, et al. Effectiveness of mechanical versus manual chest compressions in out-of-hospital cardiac arrest resuscitation: a pilot study. Am J Emerg Med. 1998;16:289-92.

36. Ward KR, Menegazzi JJ, Zelenak RR, et al. A comparison of chest compressions between mechanical and manual CPR by monitoring end-tidal PCO_2 during human cardiac arrest. Ann Emerge Med. 1993;22:669-74.

37. Larsen AI, Hjornevik AS, Ellingsen CL, et al. Cardiac arrest with continuous mechanical chest compression during percutaneous coronary intervention. A report on the use of the LUCAS device. Resuscitation. 2007;75:454-9.

38. Wik L, Bircher NG, Safar P. A comparison of prolonged manual and mechanical external chest compression after cardiac arrest in dogs. Resuscitation. 1996;32:241-50.

39. Niemann JT, Rosborough JP, Kassabian L, et al. A new device producing manual sternal compression with thoracic constraint for cardiopulmonary resuscitation. Resuscitation. 2006;69:295-301.

40. Timerman S. Cardoso LF, Ramires JA, et al. Improved hemodynamic performance with a novel chest compression device during treatment of in-hospital cardiac arrest. Resuscitation. 2004;61:273-80.

41. Axelsson C, Nestin J, Svensson L, et al. Clinical consequences of the introduction of mechanical chest compression in the EMS system for the treatment of out-of-hospital cardiac arrest—a pilot study. Resuscitation. 2006;71:47-55.

42. Hightower D, Thomas SH, Stone CK, et al. Decay in quality of closed-chest compressions over time. Ann Emerg Med. 1995;26:300-3.

43. Fitchet A, Neal R, Bannister P. Splenic trauma complicating cardiopulmonary resuscitation. BMJ. 2001;322:480-1.

44. Bedell SE, Fulton EJ. Unexpected findings and complications at autopsy after cardiopulmonary resuscitation (CPR). Arch Intern Med. 1986;146:1725-8.

45. Lederer W, Mair D, Rabi W, et al. Frequency of rib and sternum fractures associated with out-of-hospital cardiopulmonary resuscitation is underestimated by conventional chest X-ray. Resuscitation. 2004;60:157-62.

46. Hoke RS, Chamberlain D. Skeletal chest injuries secondary to cardiopulmonary resuscitation. Resuscitation. 2004;63:327-38.

47. Boz B, Erdur B, Acar K, et al. Frequency of skeletal chest injuries associated with cardiopulmonary resuscitation: forensic autopsy. Ulus Trauma Acil Cerrahi Derg. 2008;14:216-20.

48. Krisher JP, Fine EG, Davis JH, et al. Complications of cardiac resuscitation. Chest. 1987;92:287-91.

49. Scholz KH, Tebbe U, Hermann C, et al. Frequency of complications of cardiopulmonary resuscitation after thrombolysis during acute myocardial infarction. Am J Cardiol. 1992;69:724-8.

50. Cook TM, Hommers C. New airways for resuscitation? Resuscitation. 2006;69:371-87.

51. Russi CS, Hartley MJ, Buresh CT. A pilot study of the King LT supralaryngeal airway use in a rural Iowa EMS system. Int J Emerg Med. 2008;1:135-8.

52. Burns JB, Branson R, Barnes SL, et al. Emergency airway placement by EMS providers: comparison between the King LT supralaryngeal airway and endotracheal intubation. Prehosp Disaster Med. 2010;25:92-5.

53. Tumpach EA, Lutes M, Ford D, et al. The King LT versus the combitube: flight crew performance and preference. Prehosp Emerg Care. 2009;13:324-8.

54. Murray MJ, Vermeulen MJ, Morrison LJ, et al. Evaluation of prehospital insertion of the laryngeal mask airway by primary care paramedics with only classroom mannequin training. CJEM. 2002;4:338-43.

55. Herlitz J, Ekstrom L, Wennerblom B, et al. Adrenaline in out-of-hospital ventricular fibrillation: does it make any difference? Resuscitation. 1995;29:195-201.

56. Olasveengen TM, Sunde K, Brunbarg C, et al. Intravenous drug administration during out-of-hospital cardiac arrest: a randomized trial. JAMA. 2009;302:2222-9.

57. White SJ, Himes D, Rouhani M, et al. Selected controversies in cardiopulmonary resuscitation. Semin Respir Crit Care Med. 2001;22:35-50.

58. Brown CG, Martin DR, Pepe PE, et al. A comparison of standard-dose and high-dose epinephrine in cardiac arrest outside the hospital the multicenter high-dose epinephrine study group. NEJM. 1992;327:1051-5.

59. Guevniaud PY, David JS, Chamzy E, et al. Vasopressin and epinephrine vs epinephrine alone in cardiopulmonary resuscitation. NEJM. 2008;359:21-30.

60. Mentzelopoulos SD, Zakynthinos SG, Tzoufi M, et al. Vasopressin, epinephrine and corticosteroids for in-hospital cardiac arrest. Arch Intern Med. 2009;169:15-24.

61. Morris DC, Dereczyk BE, Grzybowski M, et al. Vasopressin can increase coronary perfusion pressure during human cardiopulmonary resuscitation. Acad Emerge Med. 1997;4:878-83.

62. Lindner KH, Prengel AW, Brinkmann A, et al. Vasopressin administration in refractory cardiac arrest. Ann Intern Med. 1996;124:1061-4.

63. Stiell IG, Hebert PC, Wells GA, et al. Vasopressin versus epinephrine for in-hospital cardiac arrest: a randomized controlled trial. Lancet. 2001;358:105-9.

64. Gonzalez ER, Kannewurf BS, Ornato JP. Intravenous amiodarone for ventricular arrhythmias: overview and clinical use. Resuscitation. 1998;39:33-42.

65. Kudenchuk PJ, Cobb LA, Copass MK, et al. Amiodarone for resuscitation after out-of-hospital cardiac arrest due to ventricular fibrillation. NEJM. 1999;341:871-8.

66. Coon GA, Clinton JE, Ruiz E. Use of atropine for brady-asystolic prehospital cardiac arrest. Ann Emerg Med. 1981;10:462-7.

67. Highlights of the 2010 American Heart Association Guidelines for CPR and ECC. Available from www.static.org/eccguidelines [Accessed December 2010].

68. Shen AC, Jennings RB. Kinetics of calcium accumulation in acute myocardial ischemic injury. Am J Pathol. 1972;67:441-52.

69. Zipes DP, Fischer J, King RM, et al. Termination of ventricular fibrillation in dogs by depolarizing a critical amount of myocardium. Am J Cardiol. 1975;36:37-44.

70. Malkin RA, Souza JJ, Ideker RE. The ventricular defibrillation and upper limit of vulnerability dose-response curves. J Cardiovasc Electrophysiol. 1997;8:895-903.

71. Tovar OH, Jones JL. Relationship between "extension of refractoriness" and probability of successful defibrillation. Am J Physiol. 1997;272:H1011-9.

72. Lown B, Neuman J, Amarasinghem R. Comparison of alternating current with direct current electroshock across closed chest. Am J Cardiol. 1962;10:223-7.

73. Behr JC, Hartley LL, York DK, et al. Truncated exponential versus damped sinusoidal waveform shocks for transthoracic defibrillation. Am J Cardiology. 1996;78:1242-5.

74. Bardy GH, Marchlinski F, Sharma A, et al. Multicenter comparison of truncated biphasic shocks and standard damped sine wave monophasic shocks for transthoracic ventricular fibrillation. Circulation. 1996;94:2507-14.

75. Schneider JT, Martens PR, Paschen H, et al. Multicenter, randomized controlled trial of 150-J biphasic shocks compared with 200 to 360-J monophasic shocks in the resuscitation of out-of-hospital cardiac arrest victims. Circulation. 2000;102:1780-7.

76. Van Alem AP, Chapman FW, Lank P, et al. A prospective, randomized and blinded comparison of first shock success of monophasic and biphasic waveforms in out-of-hospital cardiac arrest. Resuscitation. 2003;58:17-24.

77. Tang W, Weil MH, Sun S, et al. The effects of biphasic and conventional monophasic defibrillation on postresuscitation myocardial function. J Am Coll Cardiol. 1999;34:815-22.

78. Martens PR, Russel JK, Wolcke B, et al. Optimal response to cardiac arrest study: defibrillation waveform effects. Resuscitation. 2001;49:233-43.

79. White RD, Kerber RE. Ventricular fibrillation and defibrillation: experimental and clinical experience with waveforms and energy. Textbook of Emergency Cardiovascular Care CPR. Philadelphia Lippincott, Williams and Wilkins; 2009. pp. 222-31.

80. The Public Access Defibrillation Trial Investigators. Public access defibrillation and survival after out-of-hospital cardiac arrest. NEJM. 2004;351:637-46.

81. Caterine MR, Yoerger DM, Spencer KT, et al. Effect of electrode position and gel-application technique on predicted transcardiac current during transthoracic defibrillation. Ann Emerg Med. 1997;29:588-95.

82. Kerber RE. Transthoracic cardioversion and defibrillation. Cardiac Electrophysiology Zipes and Jalife, 4th edition. Philadelphia: Saunders; 2004. pp. 966-9.

83. Chamberlain D. Gel pads should not be used for monitoring ECG after defibrillation. Resuscitation. 2000;43:159-60.

84. Pagan-Carlo LA, Stone MS, Kerber RE. Nature and determinants of skin burns after transthoracic cardioversion. AM J Cardiol. 1997;79:689-91.

85. Meyer PF, Gadsby PD, Van Sickle D, et al. Impedance-gradient electrode reduces skin irritation induced by transthoracic defibrillation. Med Biol Eng Comput. 2005;43:225-9.

86. Waller C, Callies F, Langenfeld H. Adverse effects of direct current cardioversion on cardiac pacemakers and electrodes. Is external cardioversion contraindicated in patients with permanent pacing systems? Europace. 2004;6:165-8.

87. Aylward P, Blood R, Tonkin A. Complications of defibrillation with permanent pacemaker in situ. Pacing Clin Elctrophysiol. 1979;2:462-4.

88. Manegold JC, Israel CW, Ehrlich JR. et al. External cardioversion of atrial fibrillation in patients with implanted pacemaker or cardioverter-defibrillator systems: a randomized comparison of monophasic and biphasic shock energy application. Eur Heart J. 2007;28:1668-9.

89. Gibbs W, Eisenberg M, Damon SK. Dangers of defibrillation: injuries to emergency personnel during patient resuscitation. Am J Emerg Med. 1990;8:101-4.

90. Lloyd MS, Heeke BS, Walter PF, et al. Hands-on defibrillation. An analysis of electrical current flow through rescuers in direct contact with patients during biphasic external defibrillation. Circulation. 2008;117:2510-4.

91. Kerber RE. "I'm clear, you're clear, everybody's clear" A tradition no longer necessary for defibrillation? Circulation. 2008;117:2435-6.

92. Kerber RE, Olshansky B, Waldo AL, et al. Ventricular tachycardia rate and morphology determine energy and current requirements for transthoracic cardioversion. Circulation. 1992;85:158-63.

93. Marill KA, DeSouza IS, Nishijima DK, et al. Amiodarone is poorly effective for the acute termination of ventricular tachycardia. Ann Emerg Med. 2006;47:217-24.

94. Ong ME, Jaffey J, Stiell I, et al. Comparison of termination-of-resuscitation guidelines for basic life support: defibrillator providers in out-of-hospital cardiac arrest. Ann Emerg Med. 2006;47:337-43.

95. Morrison LJ, Verbeek PR, Vermeulen MJ, et al. Derivation and evaluation of a termination of resuscitation clinical prediction rule for advanced life support providers. Resuscitation. 2007;74:266-75.

96. Sherbino J, Keim SM, Davis DP. Clinical decision rules for termination of resuscitation in out-of-hospital cardiac arrest. J Emerg Med. 2010;38:80-6.

97. Kilgannon JH, Jones AE, Shapiro NI, et al. Association between arterial hyperoxia following resuscitation from cardiac arrest and in-hospital mortality. JAMA. 2010;303:2165-71.

98. Reynolds JC, Callaway CW, Khoudary SR, et al. Coronary angiography predicts improved outcome following cardiac arrest: propensity-adjusted analysis. J Intensive Care Med. 2009;24:179-86.

99. Lettieri C, Savonitto S, De Servi S, et al. Emergency percutaneous coronary intervention in patients with ST-elevation myocardial infarction complicated by out-of-hospital cardiac arrest: early and medium-term outcome. Am Heart J. 2009;157:569-75.

100. Garot P, Lefevre T, Eltchaninoff H, et al. Six-month outcome of emergency percutaneous coronary intervention in resuscitated patients after cardiac arrest complicating ST-elevation myocardial infarction. Circulation. 2007;115:1354-62.

101. Kern KB, Rahman O. Emergent percutaneous coronary intervention for resuscitated victims of out-of-hospital cardiac arrest. Catheter Cardiovasc Interv. 2010;75:616-24.

102. D'Souza SP, Marnas MA, Fraser DG, et al. Routine early coronary angioplasty versus ischemia-guided angioplasty after thrombolysis in acute ST-elevation myocardial infarction: a meta-analysis. Eur Heart J. 2010; online publication October 28, 2010.

103. Sanchez P, Fernandez-Aviles F. Routine early coronary angioplasty after thrombolysis in acute ST-elevation myocardial infarction: lysis is not the final step. Eur Heart J. 2010; online publication December 22, 2010.

104. The Hypothermia Cardiac Arrest Study Group. Mild therapeutic hypothermia to improve the neurologic outcome after cardiac arrest. NEJM. 2002;346:549-56.

105. Bernard SA, Gray TW, Buist MD, et al. Treatment of comatose survivors of out of hospital cardiac arrest with induced hypothermia. NEJM. 2002;346:557-63.

106. Arrich J, Holzer M, Herkner H, et al. Hypothermia for neuro-protection in adults after cardiopulmonary resuscitation. Conchrane Database Syst Rev. 2009;4:CD004128.

107. Lee R, Asare K. Therapeutic hypothermia for out-of-hospital cardiac arrest. Am J Health Syst Pharm. 2010;67:1229-37.

108. Cheung KW, Green RS, Magee KD. Systematic review of randomized controlled trials of therapeutic hypothermia as a neuro-protectant in post cardiac arrest patients. CJEM. 2006;8:329-37.

109. Boddicker KA, Zhang Y, Zimmerman B, et al. Hypothermia improves defibrillation success and resuscitation outcomes from ventricular fibrillation. Circulation. 2005;111:3195-201.

110. Staffey KS, Dendi R, Kerber RE, et al. Liquid ventilation with perfluorocarbons facilitates resumption of spontaneous circulation in a swine cardiac arrest model. Resuscitation. 2008;78:77-84.

111. Riter HG, Brooks LA, Kerber RE, et al. Intra-arrest hypothermia: Both cold liquid ventilation with perfluorocarbons and cold intravenous saline rapidly achieve hypothermia, but only cold liquid ventilation improves resumption of spontaneous circulation. Resuscitation. 2009;80:561-6.

112. Boller M, Lampe JW, Katz JM, et al. Feasibility of intra-arrest hypothermia induction: a novel nasopharyngeal approach achieves preferential brain cooling. Resuscitation. 2010;81:1025-30.

113. Busch HJ, Eichwede F, Fodisch M, et al. Safety and feasibility of nasopharyngeal evaporative cooling in the emergency department setting in survivors of cardiac arrest. Resuscitation. 2010;81:943-9.

Chapter 43

Risk Stratification for Sudden Cardiac Death

Dwayne N Campbell, James B Martins

Chapter Outline

- Healthy Athletes
- Brugada Syndrome
- Long QT Interval Syndrome
- Early Repolarization
- Short QT Syndrome
- Catecholamine Polymorphic Ventricular Tachycardia
- Wolff-Parkinson-White Syndrome

- Arrhythmogenic Right Ventricular Cardiomyopathy
- Hypertrophic Cardiomyopathy
- Marfan Syndrome
- Noncompaction
- Congenital Heart Disease
- Non-ischemic Cardiomyopathy
- Coronary Artery Disease

INTRODUCTION

Sudden death is overwhelmingly a cardiac etiology [sudden cardiac death (SCD)] defined as unexpected death occurring within one hour of symptoms.[1] The heart rhythm causing SCD is most frequently ventricular tachycardia (VT) or ventricular fibrillation (VF). Assessing risk is not trying to predict the future, but to plan for the possibility of this disaster with cost effective strategies; the most comprehensive discussion of individual assessment was published almost a decade ago and yet is still largely valid.[1] As Myerberg and Castellanos[2] have so aptly depicted this problem, the groups of patients where we think we know what to do to prevent SCD account for a small fraction of the total number; hence our need to continue looking to improve risk assessment. Our approach is to aid the clinician with the most recent scientifically based risk assessment to guide clinical judgment. The most frustrating aspects of this effort are that the first symptom of many entities may be SCD and that after a decade of reports little better risk assessment is available.

Many noninvasive as well as invasive procedures are available to help the clinician to evaluate the risk of SCD. A partial list includes signal averaged electrocardiogram (ECG), heart rate variability and turbulance, and T-wave alternans.[3] Unfortunately while these assessments have excellent basic background in theory, they do not pan out in studies of even the most common ischemic heart disease with congestive heart failure. However, we find studies revealing important simple clinical ways to help patients in specific categories. In general most SCDs involve patients with previous cardiac arrest or syncope or a family history of SCD.

HEALTHY ATHLETES

We start with those most healthy athletes which would apriori be the least likely to succumb to SCD. Surprisingly there was a 2.5-fold increase in SCD in an Italian athletic population, compared to non-athletes.[4] Some high profile deaths in professional sports have lead international groups to make recommendations which disagree.[5] The Bethesda conference recommends careful physical and history to include family occurrence of syncope and SCD. Symptoms of palpitations, syncope or seizure, especially during exercise, require further work up to identify the cause. Parenthetically, simple orthostatic dizziness due to vasodilatation is very common in elite athletes and needs to be separated from other symptoms. However, the European Society of Cardiology Consensus recommends routine ECGs, based on a reduction in SCD in athletes in Italy, but which is now reduced to the frequency observed in most other countries including the US.[6,7] However, this reduction was an uncontrolled observation.[8] Clearly standard evaluations based on good scientific criteria must be developed to protect athletes, without being overly invasive. Here we hope to give evidence based data that can inform all parties in this endeavor including the patient (athlete) and family.

Athletes may by virtue of their training actually develop a unique set of cardiac findings, different from untrained persons of the same age, which need to be appreciated as normal for sport. These include asymptomatic slower heart rates and second degree AV block at rest, but normal rate and rhythm with exercise.[9] Although we are only beginning to understand that ECG and echocardiographgic (ECHO) criteria may have to be altered in athletes such criteria change may depend on race.[10] A recent controlled study involving ECG screening in 510 athletes using ECHO as the standard increased specificity of screening from 5 to 10 of 11 documented ECHO abnormalities, but at the expense of increasing false positives from 5.5% to 16.9%. This study used standard ECG criteria published by European society of cardiology.[11] As expected such screening will significantly add to the cost of case finding.[12] One of six athletes would be expected to have an abnormal screening ECG, but only about 1% of all would have a cardiac abnormality capable of causing SCD. Annual cost estimates for ECG screening and follow-up exceeded $126 million. False-positive ECGs accounted for 98.8% of follow-up costs. Similar evaluation schemes have been used for soccer with similar outcomes.[13] While 4.8% soccer players had potentially abnormal ECGs, only 1% had clearly abnormal evaluations preventing participation in the 2006 world cup.

Recently an international group recommended an entity specific ECG screening approach that may deal with the risk-cost ratio.[14] They made recommended limits on the ECG changes attributable to training in athletes, including incomplete right bundle branch block (RBBB), differentiating it from Brugada and early repolarization (pre-SCD findings, see below), eliminating incomplete RBBB as a risk factor. On the contrary ST sement depression, right atrial disease, ventricular hypertrophy, bundle branch block, QRS greater than 110 millisecond, QTc greater than 500 and lesser than 380 millisecond should prompt a further work up since these findings are not physiological in athletes. Thus the ECG will identify inherited electrical as well as structural heart diseases, which will apply to screening anyone with a family history of SCD including athletes.

BRUGADA SYNDROME

Electrocardiogram (ECG) screening has the potential for identification of electrical disorders which could lead to SCD, although there is not much evidence that athletes would be affected by these entities. Brugada syndrome is one such disorder;[15] it is an autosomal dominantly inherited disease producing a high-risk-associated ECG with a coved appearance of ST segment elevation (2 mm) in the right precordial leads; this pattern has (4.7-fold increase risk) predictive accuracy for SCD in meta analysis of 947 patients (Veltmann 09). However, in a patient with this ECG finding, syncope may predict SCD with a hazard ratio (HR) = 2.5–6.4 for SCD.[16] Males are 3.5 times at more risk than females and there is clustering of patients with the syndrome from South-east Asia. No other factors are reproducibly predictive including positive family history or abnormal EPS.[17]

LONG QT INTERVAL SYNDROME

Long QT interval syndrome has been well reviewed in general population[18] as well as in athletes. New data collectively suggest that the magnitude of the QT prolongation is highly predictive.[16] The younger age, the shorter the QT of risk, so in the first decade risk occurs at QTc > 500: HR = 2.12, the second decade QTc > 530: HR = 2.3. In adults the diagnosis is made with a QTc > 480, but the risk in adults is incrementally greater the larger the QTc: QTc 500–549: HR = 3.3 while QTc > 550: HR = 6.4. In children males are at higher risk, while after puberty females are at higher risk.[16] Genotyping, to confirm ECG types, may be abnormal in 70% of cases; some subtypes of LQT1, LQT2 and LQT3 may have more risk than others.[16] LQT1 should not compete particularly in swimming. Similar to Brugada, the addition of syncope to the QT increases risk of SCD to 2.7–18 times those without syncope. A recent report suggests that a simple standing QT measurement will confirm a diagnosis of

long QT especially in LQT2 patients.[19] Therapy with ICD is indicated if symptoms cannot be controlled with beta blocker therapy and or cervicothoracic sympathectomy. ICD may be appropriate if there is a strong family history of SCD or inability to take beta blockers.[20]

EARLY REPOLARIZATION

Early repolarization on the ECG has been implicated in the etiology of SCD although the mechanism is unclear.[21] However, the occurrence of this finding in normal athletes with an apparently good prognosis make it a rather difficult risk assessment tool except perhaps when it is localized in the inferior leads in middle aged subjects.[22] Recently it is suggested that early repolarization localized to the lateral ECG leads is benign associated with athletic training, while localization to inferior leads is intermediate and localization to inferior, lateral and right precordial ECG is more high-risk for SCD.[23]

SHORT QT SYNDROME

Short QT syndrome[16] known only since 2000 has little patient data from which to guide assessment. Certainly a patient with QTc less than 350 and resuscitated SCD should have a defibrillator, but even syncope is not predictive of SCD unless in the presence of a markedly positive family history.

CATECHOLAMINE POLYMORPHIC VENTRICULAR TACHYCARDIA

Catecholamine polymorphic VT[16] is a well studied and strikingly reproducible syndrome of exercise facilitated VT with multiple morphologies associated with mutations in ryanodine (autosomal dominant) or calsequestrin (autosomal recessive). Exercise induced bidirectional ventricular ectopy and bidirectional VT makes the diagnosis and therapy with beta adrenergic blockers is indicated with ICD implantation if VT cannot be suppressed. Left upper thoracic chain sympathectomy may prevent ICD shocks. Genetic testing showing mutations in a family member are at risk of syncope and SCD, which may be prevented by beta blockers, has been shown to significantly reduce them. Flecainide may also be protective of VT. Family history of the syndrome does not predict SCD.

WOLFF-PARKINSON-WHITE SYNDROME

Pre-excitation of the ventricle by non-atrioventricular nodal structures when producing symptoms is called Wolff-Parkinson-White (WPW) syndrome. WPW is a well known entity found in 1% of individuals recently reviewed. It is clear that patients with rapid tachycardia symptoms need therapeutic ablation. However, the recommendation for ablation in order for asymptomatic persons with pre-excitation alone to participate in competitive athletics seems inappropriately invasive when the risk of pre-excitation alone is unclear. Prospective studies have not identified the presence of asymptomatic pre-excitation as a risk [24,25], although in children multiple pathways and rapidly conducting pathways (causing deterioration of supraventricular tachycardia to VT and VF) may suggest danger on follow-up.[26] Even electrophysiological study (EPS) identifying the functional characteristics of rapidly conducting pathways do not predict the occurrence of SCD due to rarity of SCD (0.1%) in asymptomatic pre-excitation. Therefore, asymptomatic pre-excitation does not warrant EPS and ablation. Expert opinions on certain sports, such as sky-diving or occupations such as airline piloting suggest EPS and ablation for rapidly conducting pathways.

Electrical syndromes, however, do not account for most of sudden deaths in young people. In Italy, the top three causes of SCD in athletes were arrhythmogenic right ventricular cardiomyopathy (ARVC) (22%), coronary atherosclerosis (18%) and anomalous origin of a coronary artery (12%). In the US predominant structural cardiac abnormalities identified in the military population were coronary artery abnormalities (61%), myocarditis (20%) and hypertrophic cardiomyopathy (HCM) (13%). An anomalous coronary artery accounted for one-third (21 of 64 recruits) of the cases in this cohort, and, in each, the left coronary artery arose from the right sinus of Valsalva, coursing between the pulmonary artery and the aorta. So the populations are different. Recommendations include attention to young persons who complain of angina.

ARRHYTHMOGENIC RIGHT VENTRICULAR CARDIOMYOPATHY

Arrhythmogenic right ventricular cardiomyopathy (ARVC) is an autosomal dominantly inherited disease involving molecular regulation of basic cell to cell adhesion, and production of fat, fibrous tissue and apoptosis, which results in VT and VF.[27] A specific list including major and minor criteria has been published including fibrofatty replacement of the RV, ECG depolarization (epsilon wave)/repolarization changes (with T-wave inversions in the right precordium), VT with a LBBBM and atrial fibrillation, and family history.[28,29] Of interest is the fact that the disease can be quiescent for years in youth but progresses to symptomatic disease with time. The highest risk occurs in patients having been resuscitated from SCD, with syncope at a young age or extreme involvement of the RV and LV. The primary prevention management of patients and their families is complex because of variable penetrance.[30] It was hoped that genetic testing would be an effective way to stratify risk.[31] Although eight causative genes have been identified, up to 50% of cases do not have genetic markers. Thus good clinical judgment is necessary since risk factors may be hidden, but progressive.[32,33] Since competitive sports may provoke VT/VF, exercise must be curtailed and beta blockers and sotalol may effectively prevent VT.

HYPERTROPHIC CARDIOMYOPATHY

Hypertrophic cardiomyopathy (HCM) is the most common cause of SCD in people in the US below the age of 25 years, particularly in athletes, with incidence of about 1%.[34] Clearly interdiction of competitive sports for such a patient would make the best sense. However, even though the arrhythmogenic substrate of myocardial disarray is clear, our ability to predict SCD is flawed due to apparent dormancy despite the presence of substrate. After years of attempts to prevent SCD with drugs although improving symptoms, it is concluded that this approach has never proved effective. Clearly a survivor

of SCD can be treated with an ICD, but indications for primary prevention are not clear, particularly since 60% of ICD treated patient do not have VT/VF in 5 years after resuscitation from SCD.[29,35] Risk factors commonly cited have not been well proven until recently, particularly because the evidence was taken from "appropriate" ICD shocks, which are not the same as SCD (a VT which is shocked is only seconds long and may (had no ICD intervention taken place) have only been non-sustained and not cause syncope or SCD.[36] Syncope has clearly been shown on follow-up of untreated patients to predict SCD.[37] Combinations of studies taken together have recently suggested that the aforementioned risk stratification data may be true[38] including VT nonsustained: HR = 2.2–3.6 (95% confidence); syncope: HR = 0.97–4.4; extreme LVH (wall thickness > 3 cm): HR = 1.8–4.4; hypotension on exercise HR = 0.6–2.0 and family history of SCD = 1.2–1.4. Also combinations of risk factors produced a higher HR than individual ones. Aggravating factors including atrial fibrillation, ischemia, genotype and exercise do not show risk, but LVOT gradient may increase risk.

MARFAN SYNDROME

Marfan syndrome is a connective tissue disorder caused by mutations in genes encoding supporting scaffold for elastin. Its prevalence is between 1 in 5,000 or 10,000. It causes SCD, produced by aortic dissection, rupture and pericardial tamponade.[39] Risk stratification for this outcome is based on ECHO measurement of aortic root greater than 50–55 mm.[40] SCD without dissection are reported and ventricular arrhythmias are thought to be the cause;[41] mitral valve prolapse is a common component of Marfan's syndrome but LV dilatation is the associated finding suggesting risk in Marfan's patients with ventricular ectopy and VT. Unfortunately LV dilatation is not commonly found in sporadic cases of SCD with only MVP studied at autopsy.[42] However, SD can occur without cardiac cause due to the elongated odontoid causing pressure on the cerebellum and medulla owing to alantoaxial hypermobility.[43]

NONCOMPACTION

Noncompaction of the left ventricle is a potentially arrhythmogenic condition diagnosable with ECHO which is presently not well understood. It is a cause of SCD which may be appropriately treated with ICD but follow-up shocks occur as frequently in primary as secondary prevention cases,[44] EPS does not predict ICD therapy for VT/VF. It is not clear which patients in absence of resuscitated VT/VF would benefit from ICD implantation.[20] There is simply no information to risk stratify this group at this time, since many patients with the disorder have a benign course.[45]

CONGENITAL HEART DISEASE

Congenital heart disease (CHD) afflicts approximately 75 of 1,000 live births. Significant advances in the treatment of CHD over past 50 years have allowed the majority of afflicted children to reach adulthood. The number of adults with CHD now exceeds that of children and is expected to increase with further advances.[46] SCD is the most common cause of death in these patients, occurring usually by the third or forth decade of life. The incidence, estimated at 0.09% per year, represents up to a 100-fold increased risk compared to age matched controls.[47] SCD is especially likely in patients with repaired cyanotic and left heart obstructive lesions. In a recent report of over 8,000 patients with CHD, the majority of SCD occurred out of hospital (62%), at rest (only 7% SCD occurred during exercise), and demonstrated seasonal variation with the nadir occurring in summer (22%) and peak in the fall (33%).[48] Predictors of mortality in patients with CHD include New York Heart Association (NYHA) functional class greater than one, cyanosis, age (postsurgical repair) and complexity of malformations.[49,50] There are virtually no prospective or randomized clinical trials of risk stratification. Patients with CHD presenting with cardiac arrest, sustained symptomatic VT or syncope and have significant systemic ventricular dysfunction are stratified as high-risk and ICD therapy is generally recommended.[20] Three special groups are associated with the highest risk of SCD including patients treated with Mustard/Senning procedures, Fontan procedures and repaired tetralogy of Fallot (TOF).[51] In the latter incidence of SCD is approximately 0.15% per year, risk factors include QRS greater than 180 millisecond , older age at repair, transannular right ventricular outflow tract patch, left ventricular dysfunction, frequent ectopy and inducible sustained VT, with poor specificity. Although reduced left ventricular (EF < 35%) function is the strongest risk factor for SCD in ischemic heart disease (see below), there is debate as to whether such findings should be extended to patients with CHD.[52,53] Systemic ventricular dysfunction (such as in corrected transposition) has been demonstrated in numerous observational studies and registries to identify CHD patients at risk for SCD. Studies evaluating the efficacy of ICD therapy in CHD patients have usually been observational and retrospective.[54,55] Beyond secondary prevention scenarios risk stratification in the CHD population must be done on an individual basis combining available diagnostic data with sound clinical judgment and weighing the risk and benefits of a particular intervention.[56]

NON-ISCHEMIC CARDIOMYOPATHY

Non-ischemic cardiomyopathy (NICM) is the primary etiology in 10–15% of SCDs and accounts for the second largest number of SCDs from cardiac causes behind coronary artery disease (CAD).[57] NICM is characterized by biventricular dilatation and impaired ventricular contractility without CAD. Mortality rates in this patient population range from 12–13% at three years to 20% at five years.[29,58,59] Like ischemic heart disease, numerous diagnostic techniques exist to risk stratify without careful data to identify high-risk patients would benefit from existing interventions (ICDs); in fact the majority of the major primary prevention trials enrolling patients with NICM failed to demonstrate definitive benefit to ICD therapy.[59] The primary risk stratifying approach utilized was a combination of quantitative left ventricular function assessment and functional status based on NYHA functional class. Cardiomyopathy Trial (CAT), Amiodarone versus Implantable Cardioverter-defibrillator Study (AMIOVERT), Defibrillators in Non-Ischemic Cardiomyopathy Treatment Evaluation (DEFINITE)

Trial and SCD in Heart Failure Trials (SCD-HEFT) failed to demonstrate significant mortality benefit of ICDs in patients with NICM.[59] The Comparison of Medical, Therapy, Pacing and Defibrillation in Heart Failure (COMPANION) did demonstrate benefit (significantly lower risk of death from any cause compared to medical therapy HR=0.5 P=0.015 but no significant benefit in the primary end point of the study which was a composite of death from any cause or hospitalization for any cause) of ICDs in patients with NICM treated with biventricular pacing.[60] However, the Cardiac resynchronization-Heart Failure (Care-HF) trial which enrolled 813 patients, a majority with NICM, EF < 35%, NYHA class III to IV, QRS > 149 or QRS 120–149 with evidence of dyssynchrony did demonstrate a significant benefit of CRT alone in decreasing mortality (36% p < 0.003) to the same extent as in the CRT-D arm of the COMPANION trial (36% p < 0.003).[61] Interestingly in Care-HF the presence of NICM predicted a better outcome. However, 36% of the deaths in the pacing only arm of the COMPANION trial were attributed to SCD similar to the 35% in the CRT arm CARE-HF trial; these deaths might have been prevented with an ICD.[62] A meta-analysis of the pooled data from the ICD trials (1854 patients) demonstrated 31% reduction in all cause mortality with ICD therapy compared to medical therapy.[63] Thus current guidelines recommend placement of ICDs in patients with NICM, EF less than 35% and NYHA Class II–III symptoms.[20] A number of noninvasive diagnostic methods for risk stratifying patients with NICM have recently been reviewed[64,65] with the exception of syncope, EF and NYHA functional class, no significant data exists for other methods of identifying patients that would benefit from available therapies.[65,66]

CORONARY ARTERY DISEASE

Coronary artery disease (CAD) accounts for (or is the underlying condition in) 65–80% of patients presenting with SCD. Depending on age group 13–50% of CAD deaths are SCD with coronary occlusion the most common.[57] In general the incidence of SCD in a population depends on the incidence of CAD.[57] In recent years, the steady decrease in mortality due to CAD has correlated with the decrease in SCD, although the prevalence of CAD has increased.[67] Medical therapy directed at treating CAD, in particular beta blockers and renin angiotensin system modifiers (ACE inhibitors ARBs, Aldosterone antagonist) have been demonstrated to decrease the incidence of SCD.[68] Traditional risk factors of CAD (HTN, DM, smoking, hypercholesterolemia) identify patients at risk for ischemic heart disease and hence SCD (with obesity, DM and smoking showing an increased proportion of deaths that are sudden).[29] However, these factors do not discriminate among CAD patients, those at high-risk.[69]

Risk stratification in patients immediately postmyocardial infarction is particularly difficult, especially in patients with impaired ventricular function.[29] These patients may have a particularly high-risk of SCD despite optimal medical therapy. To date no risk stratification strategy exists that utilizes invasive or noninvasive diagnostic testing that can identify patients that would benefit from advanced therapies (ICDs) within the first 40 days of infarction.[70] Both the Defibrillator in Acute

Myocardial Infarction Trial (DINAMIT) and the Immediate Risk-Stratification Improves Survival (IRIS) Trial failed to demonstrated any overall mortality benefit with ICD use.[70] Similarly in a substudy of the MADIT 2 Trial, no survival benefit was found in this population if the time interval from index infarct was within 18 months.[71] In the home use of external automated defibrillators for SCD trial (HAT) no mortality benefit was noted over conventional resuscitation methods in high-risk post-MI patients.[72] Current ICD guidelines reflect these results.[20]

The previously mentioned factors stratifying patients at high risk with NICM also identify CAD patients. So, NYHA functional class higher than 2, EF less than 35 and syncope identify patients who benefit from ICDs.[20] Unlike NICM, there may be utility of invasive electrophysiologic testing in patients with CAD. In the MUSTT and MADIT clinical trials sustained VT/VF during EPS, in addition to LV dysfunction (EF $\leq$ 40%) and presence of NSVT on ambulatory testing, identified patients that benefited from prophylactic ICD therapy.[20] In addition, invasive EP testing is recommended in patients with remote history of myocardial infarction and symptoms suggestive of VT, including palpitations syncope and presyncope.[29] If sustained VT/VF is induced then ICD therapy is usually recommended.[20] Although a positive EPS identifies patients with CAD at high-risk of SCD who benefit from advanced therapies a negative study in patients with severe LV dysfunction less than 30% does not necessarily indicate a good prognosis.[29,73]

Although LV function can identify patients at high-risk of sudden death it does not discriminate well between those at high-risk and those at low-risk of sudden death.[64] The risk of sudden death or cardiac arrest increased by 21% for every 5% decrease in left ventricular function. However, this is a U shaped relationship, in that as EF decreases deaths due to pump failure increase as arrhythmic deaths decrease.[64,74] Recently risk stratification test studied in the Cardiac Arrhythmias and Risk Stratification after Acute Myocardial Infarction (CARISMA) study and the Alternans Before Cardioverter Defibrillator (ABCD) trial were compared to a "coin toss" high-risk (heads) and low-risk (tails).[75] Compared to LVEF (NPV 94% PPV 9% HR 1.3) in CARISMA study population the coin toss performed only mildly worst (NPV 92% PPV 8%).[75,76] It was noted that the coin toss (HR 1 in both populations) has no role in risk stratification as net correct reclassification would always be zero. This comparison demonstrates the limitation of individual risk stratification test for SCD to adequately stratify patients. An alternative approach is a multi-tiered risk stratification strategy similar to that utilized by the SHAPE task force for athero-sclerosis.[77,78] To date there have been no prospective studies utilizing such an approach.

SUMMARY

We have reviewed the available data on risk stratification in major entities encountered by clinicians. Generally good clinical judgment can be enhanced by the published knowledge; in addition to a history of SCD, symptoms of syncope or arrhythmogenic dizziness predict likely risk of SCD in most disorders. A family history of SCD may also inform such an evaluation. An ECG abnormality coupled with the above may focus additional evaluation such as exercise testing in appropriate patients. Documentation of structural heart disease by ECHO confirms risk in various population groups. Normal ECG and ECHO may exclude risk in many groups. Further research is needed to clarify the specific risk in more rare diseases. Unfortunately based on our experience with CAD, it is not likely we will find easy risk stratifiers in many disease states.

REFERENCES

1. Priori SG, Aliot E, Blomstrom-Lundqvist C, et al. Task force on sudden cardiac death of the european society of cardiology. Eur Heart J. 2001;22:1374-450.
2. Myerberg RJ, Castellanos A. Sudden cardiac death In: Zipes DP, Jalife J (Eds). Cardiac Electrophysiology from Cell to Bedside, 5th edition. Philadelphia: Saunders, Elsevier; 2009.
3. Zipes DP, Jalife J (Editors). Cardiac Electrophysiology from Cell to Bbedside, 5th edition. Philadelphia: Saunders, Elsevier; 2009.
4. Corrado D, Basso C, Rizzoli G, et al. Does sports activity enhance the risk of sudden death in adolescents and young adults? J Am Coll Cardiol. 2003;42:1959-63.
5. Pelliccia A, Zipes DP, Maron BJ. Bethesda conference #36 and the european society of cardiology consensus recommendations revisited a comparison of U.S. and european criteria for eligibility and disqualification of competitive athletes with cardiovascular abnormalities. J Am Coll Cardiol. 2008;52:1990-6.
6. Maron BJ, Doerer JJ, Haas TS, et al. Sudden deaths in young competitive athletes: analysis of 1866 deaths in the United States, 1980-2006. Circulation. 2009;119:1085-92.
7. Perez M, Fonda H, Le VV, et al. Adding an electrocardiogram to the pre-participation examination in competitive athletes: a systematic review. Curr Probl Cardiol. 2009;34:586-662.
8. Maron BJ, Haas TS, Doerer JJ, et al. Comparison of US and Italian experiences with sudden cardiac deaths in young competitive athletes and implications for preparticipation screening strategies. Am J Cardiol. 2009;104:276-80.
9. Link MS, Mark Estes NA. Athletes and arrhythmias. J Cardiovasc Electrophysiol; 2010.
10. Rawlins J, Carre F, Kervio G, et al. Ethnic differences in physiological cardiac adaptation to intense physical exercise in highly trained female athletes. Circulation. 2010;121:1078-85.
11. Baggish AL, Hutter AM Jr, Wang F, et al. Cardiovascular screening in college athletes with and without electrocardiography: a cross-sectional study. Ann Intern Med. 2010;152:269-75.
12. O'Connor DP, Knoblauch MA. Electrocardiogram testing during athletic preparticipation physical examinations. J Athl Train. 2010;45:265-72.
13. Thunenkotter T, Schmied C, Dvorak J, et al. Benefits and limitations of cardiovascular pre-competition screening in international football. Clin Res Cardiol. 2010;99:29-35.
14. Corrado D, Pelliccia A, Heidbuchel H, et al. Section of Sports Cardiology, European Association of Cardiovascular Prevention and Rehabilitation, Working Group of Myocardial and Pericardial Disease, European Society of Cardiology. Recommendations for interpretation of 12-lead electrocardiogram in the athlete. Eur Heart J. 2010;31:243-59.
15. Brussey T, Brugada R, Brugada J, et al. The brugada syndrome. In: DP Zipes, J Jalife (Eds). Cardiac Electrophysiology from Cell to Bedside, 5th edition. Philadelphia: Saunders; 2009.
16. Veltmann C, Schimpf R, Borggrefe M, et al. Risk stratification in electrical cardiomyopathies. Herz. 2009;34:518-27.
17. Probst V, Veltmann C, Eckardt L, et al. Long-term prognosis of patients diagnosed with brugada syndrome: results from the FINGER brugada syndrome registry. Circulation. 2010;121:635-43.

18. Schwartz P, Crotti L. Long QT and short QT syndromes. In: DP Zipes, J Jalife (Eds). Cardiac Electrophysiology from Cell to Bedside, 5th edition. Philadelphia: Saunders, Elsevier; 2009.

19. Viskin S, Postema PG, Bhuiyan ZA, et al. The response of the QT interval to the brief tachycardia provoked by standing: a bedside test for diagnosing long QT syndrome. J Am Coll Cardiol. 2010;55:1955-61.

20. Epstein AE, DiMarco JP, Ellenbogen KA, et al. ACC/AHA/HRS 2008 guidelines for device-based therapy of cardiac rhythm abnormalities: a report of the American College of Cardiology/ American Heart Association Task Force on Practice Guidelines (writing committee to revise the ACC/AHA/NASPE 2002 guideline update for implantation of cardiac pacemakers and antiarrhythmia devices) developed in collaboration with the american association for thoracic surgery and society of thoracic surgeons. J Am Coll Cardiol. 2008;51:e1-e62.

21. Haissaguerre M, Derval N, Sacher F, et al. Sudden cardiac arrest associated with early repolarization. N Engl J Med. 2008;358:2016-23.

22. Tikkanen JT, Anttonen O, Junttila MJ, et al. Long-term outcome associated with early repolarization on electrocardiography. N Engl J Med. 2009;361:2529-37.

23. Antzelevitch C, Yan GX. J wave syndromes. Heart Rhythm. 2010;7:549-58.

24. Tischenko A, Fox DJ, Yee R, et al. When should we recommend catheter ablation for patients with the wolff-parkinson-white syndrome? Curr Opin Cardiol. 2008;23:32-7.

25. Santinelli V, Radinovic A, Manguso F, et al. Asymptomatic ventricular preexcitation: a long-term prospective follow-up study of 293 adult patients. Circ Arrhythm Electrophysiol. 2009;2:102-7.

26. Santinelli V, Radinovic A, Manguso F, et al. The natural history of asymptomatic ventricular pre-excitation a long-term prospective follow-up study of 184 asymptomatic children. J Am Coll Cardiol. 2009;53:275-80.

27. Fontaine G, Charron P. Arrhythmogenic right ventricular cardio-myopathies. In: DP Zipes, J Jalife (Eds). Cardiac Electrophysiology from Cell to Bedside, 5th edition. Philadelphia: Saunders, Elsevier; 2009.

28. Muthappan P, Calkins H. Arrhythmogenic right ventricular dysplasia. Prog Cardiovasc Dis. 2008;51:31-43.

29. European Heart Rhythm Association, Heart Rhythm Society, Zipes DP, et al. ACC/AHA/ESC 2006 guidelines for management of patients with ventricular arrhythmias and the prevention of sudden cardiac death: a report of the American College of Cardiology/ American Heart Association Task Force and the European Society of Cardiology Committee for Practice Guidelines (writing committee to develop guidelines for management of patients with ventricular arrhythmias and the prevention of sudden cardiac death). J Am Coll Cardiol. 2006;48:e247-e346.

30. Sen-Chowdhry S, Morgan RD, Chambers JC, et al. Arrhythmogenic cardiomyopathy: etiology, diagnosis, and treatment. Annu Rev Med. 2010;61:233-53.

31. Hershberger RE, Cowan J, Morales A, et al. Progress with genetic cardiomyopathies: screening, counseling, and testing in dilated, hypertrophic, and arrhythmogenic right ventricular dysplasia/ cardiomyopathy. Circ Heart Fail. 2009;2:253-61.

32. Boldt LH, Haverkamp W. Arrhythmogenic right ventricular cardio-myopathy: diagnosis and risk stratification. Herz. 2009;34:290-7.

33. Basso C, Corrado D, Marcus FI, et al. Arrhythmogenic right ventricular cardiomyopathy. Lancet. 2009;373:1289-300.

34. Maron BJ. Contemporary insights and strategies for risk stratification and prevention of sudden death in hypertrophic cardiomyopathy. Circulation. 2010;121:445-56.

35. Maron BJ, Spirito P, Shen WK, et al. Implantable cardioverter-defibrillators and prevention of sudden cardiac death in hypertrophic cardiomyopathy. JAMA. 2007;298:405-12.

36. Ellenbogen KA, Levine JH, Berger RD, et al. Are implantable cardioverter defibrillator shocks a surrogate for sudden cardiac death in patients with nonischemic cardiomyopathy? Circulation. 2006;113:776-82.

37. Spirito P, Autore C, Rapezzi C, et al. Syncope and risk of sudden death in hypertrophic cardiomyopathy. Circulation. 2009;119: 1703-10.

38. Christiaans I, van Engelen K, van Langen IM, et al. Risk stratification for sudden cardiac death in hypertrophic cardiomyopathy: systematic review of clinical risk markers. Europace. 2010;12:313-21.

39. Pearson GD, Devereux R, Loeys B, et al. Report of the national heart, lung, and blood institute and national marfan foundation working group on research in marfan syndrome and related disorders. Circulation. 2008;118:785-91.

40. Stout M. The marfan syndrome: implications for athletes and their echocardiographic assessment. Echocardiography. 2009;26:1075-81.

41. Yetman AT, Bornemeier RA, McCrindle BW. Long-term outcome in patients with marfan syndrome: is aortic dissection the only cause of sudden death? J Am Coll Cardiol. 2003;41:329-32.

42. Anders S, Said S, Schulz F, et al. Mitral valve prolapse syndrome as cause of sudden death in young adults. Forensic Sci Int. 2007;171:127-30.

43. MacKenzie JM, Rankin R. Sudden death due to atlantoaxial subluxation in marfan syndrome. Am J Forensic Med Pathol. 2003;24:369-70.

44. Kobza R, Steffel J, Erne P, et al. Implantable cardioverter-defibrillator and cardiac resynchronization therapy in patients with left ventricular noncompaction. Heart Rhythm. 2010.

45. Lofiego C, Biagini E, Pasquale F, et al. Wide spectrum of presentation and variable outcomes of isolated left ventricular non-compaction. Heart. 2007;93:65-71.

46. Khairy P. EP challenges in adult congenital heart disease. Heart Rhythm. 2008;5:1464-72.

47. Yap SC, Harris L. Sudden cardiac death in adults with congenital heart disease. Expert Rev Cardiovasc Ther. 2009;7:1605-20.

48. Zomer AC, Uiterwaal CSPM, Velde ETvd, et al. Circumstances of death in adult congenital heart disease. J Am Coll Cardiol. 2010;55:A41.E393.

49. Trojnarska O, Grajek S, Katarzynski S, et al. Predictors of mortality in adult patients with congenital heart disease. Cardiol J. 2009; 16:341-7.

50. Oechslin EN, Harrison DA, Connelly MS, et al. Mode of death in adults with congenital heart disease. Am J Cardiol. 2000;86:1111-6.

51. Triedman JK. Arrhythmias in adults with congenital heart disease. Heart. 2002;87:383-9.

52. Silka MJ, Bar-Cohen Y. Should patients with congenital heart disease and a systemic ventricular ejection fraction less than 30% undergo prophylactic implantation of an ICD? Patients with congenital heart disease and a systemic ventricular ejection fraction less than 30% should undergo prophylactic implantation of an implantable cardioverter defibrillator. Circ Arrhythm Electrophysiol. 2008;1:298-306.

53. Triedman JK. Should patients with congenital heart disease and a systemic ventricular ejection fraction less than 30% undergo prophylactic implantation of an ICD? Implantable cardioverter defibrillator implantation guidelines based solely on left ventricular ejection fraction do not apply to adults with congenital heart disease. Circ Arrhythm Electrophysiol. 2008;1:307-16; discussion 316.

54. Khairy P, Harris L, Landzberg MJ, et al. Implantable cardioverter-defibrillators in tetralogy of fallot. Circulation. 2008;117:363-70.

55. Khairy P, Harris L, Landzberg MJ, et al. Sudden death and defibril-lators in transposition of the great arteries with intra-atrial baffles: a multicenter study. Circ Arrhythm Electrophysiol. 2008;1:250-7.

56. Walsh EP. Practical aspects of implantable defibrillator therapy in patients with congenital heart disease. Pacing Clin Electrophysiol. 2008;31:S38-40.

57. Lee KK, Al-Ahmad A, Wang PJ, et al. Epidemiology and etiologies of sudden cardiac death. In: PJ Wang, A Al-Ahmad, HH Hsia, PC Zei (Eds). Ventricular arrhythmias and sudden cardiac death. Oxford, UK: Blackwell Futura; 2009.

58. Dec GW, Fuster V. Idiopathic dilated cardiomyopathy. N Engl J Med. 1994;331:1564-75.

59. Cevik C, Nugent K, Perez-Verdia A, et al. Prophylactic implantation of cardioverter defibrillators in idiopathic nonischemic cardio-myopathy for the primary prevention of death: a narrative review. Clin Cardiol. 2010;33:254-60.

60. Bristow MR, Saxon LA, Boehmer J, et al. Cardiac-resynchronization therapy with or without an implantable defibrillator in advanced chronic heart failure. N Engl J Med. 2004;350:2140-50.

61. Cleland JG, Daubert JC, Erdmann E, et al. The effect of cardiac resynchronization on morbidity and mortality in heart failure. N Engl J Med. 2005;352:1539-49.

62. Ellenbogen KA, Wood MA, Klein HU. Why should we care about CARE-HF? J Am Coll Cardiol. 2005;46:2199-203.

63. Desai AS, Fang JC, Maisel WH, et al. Implantable defibrillators for the prevention of mortality in patients with nonischemic cardiomyopathy: a meta-analysis of randomized controlled trials. JAMA. 2004;292:2874-9.

64. Goldberger JJ, Cain ME, Hohnloser SH, et al. American Heart Association/American College of Cardiology Foundation/Heart Rhythm Society scientific statement on noninvasive risk stratification techniques for identifying patients at risk for sudden cardiac death: a scientific statement from the american heart association council on clinical cardiology committee on electrocardiography and arrhythmias and council on epidemiology and prevention. Circulation. 2008;118:1497-518.

65. Okutucu S, Oto A. Risk stratification in nonischemic dilated cardiomyopathy: current perspectives. Cardiol J. 2010;17:219-29.

66. Grimm W, Christ M, Sharkova J, et al. Arrhythmia risk prediction in idiopathic dilated cardiomyopathy based on heart rate variability and baroreflex sensitivity. Pacing Clin Electrophysiol. 2005;28:S202-6.

67. Chugh SS, Reinier K, Teodorescu C, et al. Epidemiology of sudden cardiac death: clinical and research implications. Prog Cardiovasc Dis. 2008;51:213-28.

68. Das MK, Zipes DP. Antiarrhythmic and nonantiarrhythmic drugs for sudden cardiac death prevention. J Cardiovasc Pharmacol. 2010;55:438-49.

69. El-Sherif N, Khan A, Savarese J, et al. Pathophysiology, risk stratification, and management of sudden cardiac death in coronary artery disease. Cardiol J. 2010;17:4-10.

70. Estes NA, 3rd. The challenge of predicting and preventing sudden cardiac death immediately after myocardial infarction. Circulation. 2009;120:185-7.

71. Wilber DJ, Zareba W, Hall WJ, et al. Time dependence of mortality risk and defibrillator benefit after myocardial infarction. Circulation. 2004;109:1082-4.

72. Bardy GH, Lee KL, Mark DB, et al. Home use of automated external defibrillators for sudden cardiac arrest. N Engl J Med. 2008;358:1793-804.

73. Lopera G, Curtis AB. Risk stratification for sudden cardiac death: current approaches and predictive value. Curr Cardiol Rev. 2009;5:56-64.

74. Solomon SD, Zelenkofske S, McMurray JJ, et al. Sudden death in patients with myocardial infarction and left ventricular dysfunction, heart failure, or both. N Engl J Med. 2005;352:2581-8.

75. Goldberger JJ. The coin toss: implications for risk stratification for sudden cardiac death. Am Heart J. 2010;160:3-7.

76. Huikuri HV, Raatikainen MJ, Moerch-Joergensen R, et al. Prediction of fatal or near-fatal cardiac arrhythmia events in patients with depressed left ventricular function after an acute myocardial infarction. Eur Heart J. 2009;30:689-98.

77. Naghavi M, Falk E, Hecht HS, et al. From vulnerable plaque to vulnerable patient—part III: executive summary of the screening for heart attack prevention and education (SHAPE) task force report. Am J Cardiol. 2006;98:2H-15H.

78. Bailey JJ, Berson AS, Handelsman H, et al. Utility of current risk stratification tests for predicting major arrhythmic events after myocardial infarction. J Am Coll Cardiol. 2001;38:1902-11.

Chapter 44

Cardiocerebral Resuscitation for Primary Cardiac Arrest

Jooby John, Gordon A Ewy

Chapter Outline

INTRODUCTION

Out-of hospital cardiac arrest (OHCA) claims hundreds of thousands of lives each year.[1,2] Despite this enormous public health problem, and the promulgation of standards and guidelines, with also numerous updates of guidelines (Fig. 1), the aggregate survival rate of OHCA of 7.6% has not significantly changed in almost three decades.[3] Likewise there is little data to indicate that guidelines have improved in-hospital survival. A large medicare database of over 400,000 elderly patients revealed that even in-hospital survival after cardiopulmonary resuscitation (CPR) has been unchanged for the period from 1992 to 2005.[4]

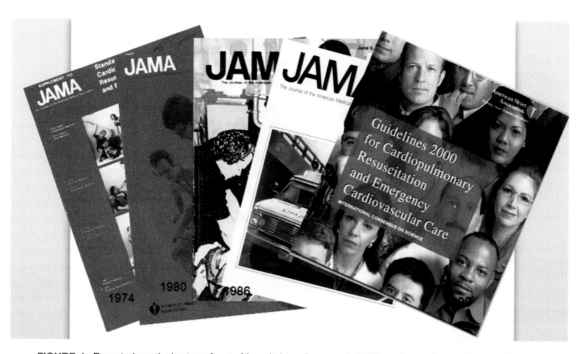

FIGURE 1: Reported survival rates of out-of-hospital cardiac arrests 7.6% unchanged over the past 30 years

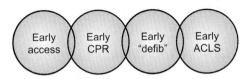

FIGURE 2: Cardiopulmonary resuscitation "chain of survival" (*Source:* Modified from Cummings, et al. Circulation. 1991;83:1832)

The major limitation of the chain of survival (Fig. 2) was the necessity for "early" initiation of each link.[5] However, in retrospect its failure to recognize that gasping was common during the first few minutes of primary cardiac arrest often prevented "early" recognition, its insistence on mouth-to-mouth ventilation as the initial intervention precluded most bystanders from providing "early" CPR, and many factors, including traffic congestion in larger cities, precluded "early" defibrillation. In addition, the prescription of endotracheal intubation as the initial step in advanced cardiac lift support (ACLS), and the use of automated external defibrillators for the proscribed "stacked" shocks further delayed or interrupted essential chest compressions; all contributed to poor survival rates.[6]

Survival was especially poor in large metropolitan cities. A 2005 report revealed a rate of neurologically intact survival from OHCA of 1.4% in Los Angeles, similar to survival rates previously reported from Chicago, New York City and Detroit.[7,8] Survival is better in areas where the incidence of bystander CPR is high and the emergency medical system (EMS) response times are short.[9] Unfortunately these "links" are rare, so new approaches were needed.

In this chapter we have discussed recent insights into the physiology of cardiac arrest and resuscitation and present a new approach to the management of cardiac arrest developed by our University of Arizona Sarver Heart Center Resuscitation Research Group, called Cardiocerebral Resuscitation (CCR) (Fig. 3). The CCR has been shown to markedly improve survival of patients with OHCA with survival rates of 38% or better in the subset of patients who have greatest chance of survival; those with witnessed arrest and a shockable rhythm (Fig. 4).[10-12]

ETIOLOGY AND PATHOPHYSIOLOGY OF CARDIAC ARREST

Cardiac arrest is either primary or secondary. The emphasis of this chapter is on primary cardiac arrest. The CCR is not recommended for arrests secondary to hypoxia from drowning or respiratory failure. However, it much be emphasized that not all cardiac arrest in individuals under the age of 18 years are respiratory.

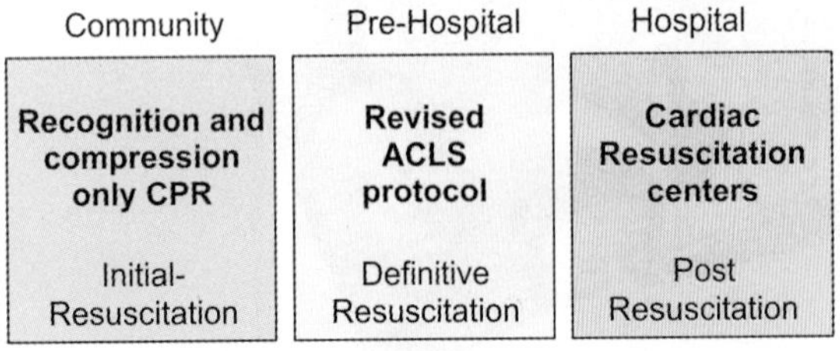

Community   Pre-Hospital   Hospital

Recognition and compression only CPR	Revised ACLS protocol	Cardiac Resuscitation centers
Initial-Resuscitation	Definitive Resuscitation	Post Resuscitation

FIGURE 3: Cardiocerebral resuscitation "The New CPR" for primary cardiac arrest

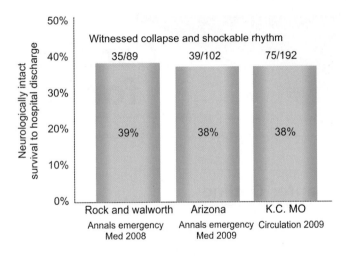

FIGURE 4: Cardiocerebral resuscitation for OHCA. Witnessed collapse and shockable rhythm

PRIMARY CARDIAC ARREST IN CHILDREN AND ADOLESCENTS

Respiratory arrests are the reason for the majority of cardiac arrests in children, and should be treated according to guidelines.[13] However, primary cardiac arrest also occurs in children and adolescents in the presence of diverse pathologies such as the prolonged QT syndrome, the cardiomyopathy of arrhythmogenic right ventricular dysplasia (ARVD), Brugada syndrome, anomalous coronary arteries or commotio cordis [where a blow to the precordium at the peak of the electrocardiographic T wave can result in ventricular fibrillation (VF)]. Accordingly, chest compression only (CCO) CPR is the best approach to bystander CPR in children and adolescence when the cardiac arrest is primary.

Primary cardiac arrest is recognized by an unexpected, witnessed (seen or heard) collapse in an individual who is not responsive. As emphasized in this chapter, many individuals with primary cardiac arrest continue to have spontaneous ventilation, and checking for the presence or absence of an arterial pulse by bystanders is no longer recommended.[13]

PATHOPHYSIOLOGY OF PRIMARY CARDIAC ARREST

One minute into persistent VF or pulseless VT, coronary blood flow comes to a standstill, and minutes later carotid blood flow (and therefore cerebral perfusion) becomes nil.[14] The ensuing equalization of systemic pressures in the arterial and venous beds takes place, resulting in the so-called "mean circulatory filling pressure" described by Guyton.[15] This shift in blood volume from higher pressure arterial system to the low pressure venous system results in "acute distension of the right ventricle" originally described by Professor Stig Steen in open chest swine.[16] This phenomenon is perhaps best illustrated by closed chest imaging techniques (Fig. 5).[17,18] The resultant pericardial restraint produces a constrictive pericardial condition, and even with defibrillation poor contractility occurs due to the lack of stretch of the myocardial fibers.[19] This sequence helps to explain why chest compressions (to decompress the heart to relieve pericardial

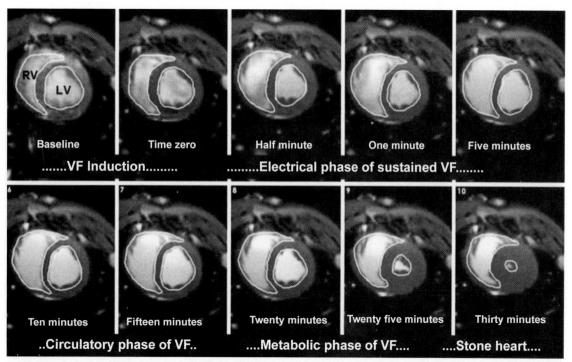

FIGURE 5: Development of the "Stone Heart" after prolonged VF (*Source:* Sorrell VL, Altbach MI, Kern KB, et al. Images in cardiovascular medicine. Continuous cardiac magnetic resonance imaging during untreated ventricular fibrillation. Circulation. 2005;111:e294)

restraint) are often necessary for successful generations of an arterial pressure following defibrillation.

Untreated VF results in a progressive decrease in left ventricular volumes until a state of extreme myocardial contraction develops (referred to as stone heart). This sequence has also been demonstrated by magnetic resonance imaging (MRI) in closed chest animal models of VF[17] (Fig. 5).

CORONARY PERFUSION PRESSURES DURING RESUSCITATION EFFORTS

Several observations lead the University of Arizona Sarver Heart Center Resuscitation Research Group almost two decades ago to advocate of CCO CPR. One of the most important was the observation during our early (1980s) experimental studies that survival from prolonged VF arrest was related to the coronary perfusion pressure (CPP) generated by chest compressions (Fig. 6).[20] The CPP is defined as the difference between the

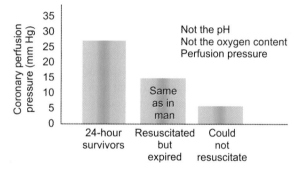

FIGURE 6: Survival from prolonged VF arrest in experimental studies was related to pressure generated by chest compressions. (*Source:* Kern, Ewy, Voorhees, Babbs, Tacker. Resuscitation. 1988;16:241-50; Paradis, et al. JAMA .1990;263:1106)

aortic and the right atrial pressures during the release phase "diastole" of closed chest cardiac compression (Fig. 7).[21] The CPP is the pressure gradient that is responsible for antegrade coronary flow. Similar to normal sinus rhythm where most blood flow through the coronary arteries occurs in diastole, during chest compressions for cardiac arrest, most coronary blood flow occurs during "compression diastole" or the release phase of chest compressions. During life the pressures in the myocardium, the ventricle and the aorta are similar during ventricular systole and therefore there is very little coronary blood flow. But during diastole, the aortic valve closes, the pressure is higher in the aorta than in the myocardium, and thus most of the coronary blood flow to the myocardium occurs during diastole. During chest compression for cardiac arrest, the pressure in the heart and aorta are similar. But during the release phase the aortic valve closes[22] and the pressure in the aorta is higher than the right atrium, so antegrade coronary blood flow occurs during the release phase of chest compressions. During cardiac arrest and resuscitation efforts, the amount of coronary flow is predominantly related to the amount of arterial pressure generated by chest compressions. We found that one had to generate a minimal CPP of 15 mm Hg for return of spontaneous circulation (ROSC) in our experimental studies.[20] Of interest is the fact that this was the same value found by Norman Paradis in his measurements during resuscitation efforts in man (Fig. 6).[21] Of note in their report there were no survivors![21]

The CPP is built up slowly with the initiation of chest compressions during resuscitation efforts for cardiac arrest, such that the first few compressions often do not generate a significant CPP (Fig. 8). The CPP is a surrogate for myocardial cellular perfusion and has been shown to be a determinant of survival in prolonged VF.[20,23-25] Obviously to generate an adequate

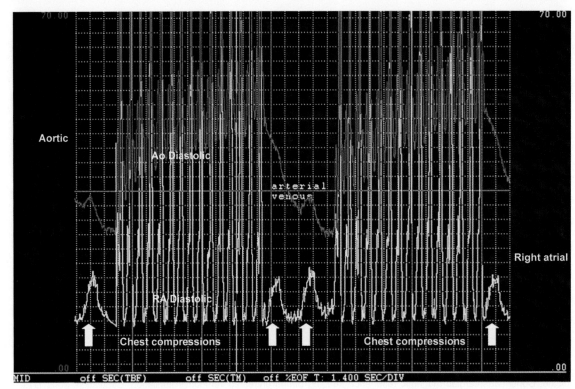

FIGURE 7: The difference between the aortic and the right atrial pressures during the released phase "diastole" of closed chest cardiac compression is termed as coronary perfusion pressure

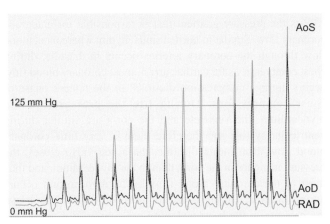

FIGURE 8: Simultaneous recording of aortic and right atrial pressures during first 15 external chest compressions in swine in cardiac arrest due to ventricular fibrillation. Note how initial compressions do not generate much of a pressure (*Source:* Modified from Ewy GA. Circulation. 2005;111:2134-42)

coronary perfusion pressure, one is usually generating an adequate cerebral perfusion pressure as the CPP produced during resuscitation efforts for cardiac arrest relates to neurologically intact survival as well. However, all who survive for 24 hours are not neurologically intact.[26]

When chest compressions are interrupted for even 4 seconds, the CPP decays and with it myocardial perfusion. The coronary perfusion gradient has to be re-established once again when compressions are restarted (Fig. 7). This is a key element in understanding why continuous chest compression (CCC) or CCO CPR results better survival. The CPP gradient, once

established, is not interrupted and therefore cellular perfusion is maintained.[23,24,27]

ASSISTED VENTILATION IN PRIMARY CARDIAC ARREST

The technique of closed chest "cardiac massage" for cardiac arrest was first published in 1960 and, since the survival rate in this initial report was 70% (14/20), it quickly became the preferred technique for both in-hospital and prehospital treatment of cardiac arrest.[28] In their early teachings, the authors, Kouwenhoven, Knickerbocker and Jude said that, "assisted ventilation was not necessary as the victim gasped" during closed chest compression.[29] Seven of their initial 20 reported patients received chest-compression only without assisted ventilation.[28]

Nevertheless, influential individuals advocated bystander mouth-to-mouth assisted ventilations for cardiac as well as for respiratory arrests.[30,31] The possible justifications for this view were: (1) the emphasis of therapy for out-of-hospital arrests was historically based on the resuscitation of drowning victims; (2) it was thought that lay individuals could not reliably differentiate between respiratory and cardiac arrest; (3) gasping was not appreciated as a common event in primary cardiac arrest and (4) studies by Safer and his associates in volunteers given drugs to produce temporary paralysis showed that without assisted ventilation, their blood gases rapidly deteriorated.[31] Unfortunately it was not recognized that the explanation was that these subjects were not in cardiac arrest, and had normal cardiac outputs; therefore, their arterial blood quickly became unsaturated without assisted ventilation. In contrast, with sudden onset VF in primary cardiac arrest, the arterial blood is fully

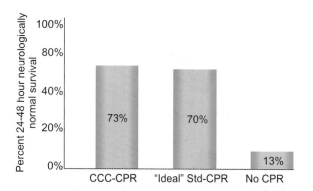

FIGURE 9: "CPR" for VF arrest, 6 different publications, in 169 non-paralyzed swine, between 1993 and 2002 (*Source:* University of Arizona Sarver Heart Center Resuscitation Research Group)

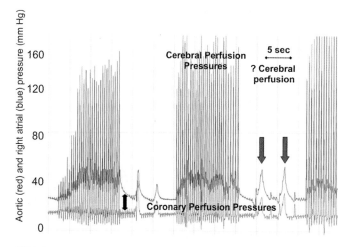

FIGURE 10: Hemodynamics of simulated single rescuer performing 30:2 compression: ventilations in experimental animal with realistic 16 sec. interruption of chest compressions for mouth-to-mouth ventilations

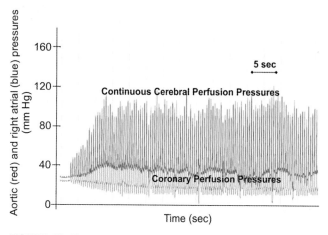

FIGURE 11: Hemodynamics of simulated single rescuer performing continuous chest compressions in experimental animal

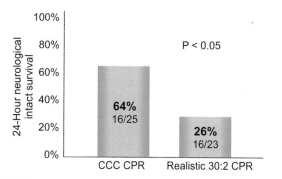

FIGURE 12: Survival following simulated single lay rescuer scenario of primary cardiac arrest (4–6 minutes untreated VF followed by bystander CPR; at 12 min, all received ACLS) (*Source:* Ewy GA, Zuercher M, Hilwig RW, et al. Circulation. 2007;116:2525)

oxygenated and remains so for several minutes, because it is not circulating. Nevertheless closed chest cardiac massage was merged with mouth-to-mouth to form what became known as cardiopulmonary resuscitation or CPR.[32]

By 1966, standardized methods of training and performance criteria for the administration of CPR had been advocated and published. A few years later the American Heart Association (AHA) adopted CPR as one of its main focus areas, developed standards for CPR and emergency cardiac care (ECC) and spearheaded a campaign to disseminate the techniques of CPR to the public and both CPR and ECC to professionals. Until the 2008 scientific advisory, all previous guidelines recommended mouth-to-mouth or so-called "rescue breathing" as the initial step for bystander initiated CPR.[33]

Years of defibrillation and resuscitation research led the senior author and his associates to advocate CCO CPR decades ago.[27,34-37] In our experimental laboratory, survival was better with CCO CPR than not doing anything until the simulated arrival of the paramedics and definite treatment. As our studies progressed, we were somewhat surprised to find that survival with CCO CPR was equivalent to "ideal" guidelines advocated CPR where each series of chest compressions were interrupted by 4 seconds to deliver the "two quick breaths" of "rescue breathing" (Fig. 9).[27,36]

In 2000, it was documented that recently certified lay individuals interrupted chest compressions for 16 seconds to deliver the two recommended "rescue breaths."[38] Subsequent experimental studies from our laboratories showed that survival was better with CCO CPR than with guidelines recommend CPR when each set of 15 compressions were interrupted a realistic 16 seconds to simulate the interruptions necessary for mouth-to-mouth ventilations.[24] Subsequently the AHA and International Liaison Committee on Resuscitation (ILCOR) changed the recommended compression to ventilation ratio to 30:2.[13] This recommendation was based on "consensus" as there was no data to support this recommendation. Accordingly, in our experimental laboratory, we then compared survival from simulated OHCA with CCO CPR and guidelines (30:2) CPR, and found that survival to be better with continuous chest compression CPR (Figs 10 to 12).[39] If lay individuals interrupted chest compressions an average of 16 seconds to provide the two recommended rescue breaths, could medical students who were younger provide these breaths quicker? How about the

professionals, the paramedics? As shown in (Fig. 13) no one can provide mouth-to-mouth rescue breaths rapidly.[40,41]

NOT FOLLOWING GUIDELINES FOR PRIMARY CARDIAC ARREST

Years of defibrillation and resuscitation research and continuing analysis of the resuscitation literature and our failure to be able

CHAPTER 44 Cardiocerebral Resuscitation for Primary Cardiac Arrest

Lay public:
16 ± 1 seconds
Assar, et al. Resuscitation
2000;45:7-15

Medical students:
14 ± 1 seconds
Heidenreich, et al. Resuscitation
2004;62:283-9

Paramedics:
10 ± 1 seconds
Higdon et al. Resuscitation
2006;71:34-9

FIGURE 13: Interruptions of chest compressions by single rescuer CPR for guidelines recommended 2 quick mouth-to-mouth ventilations

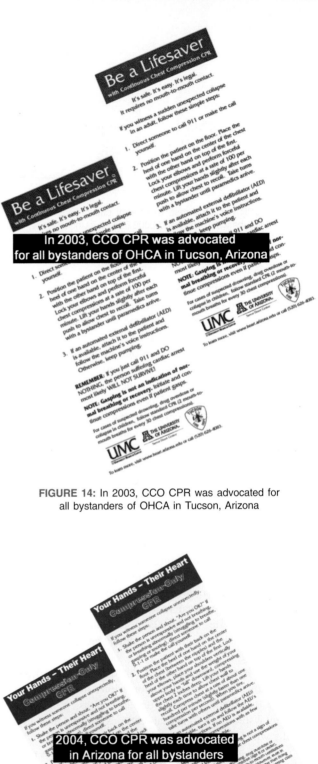

FIGURE 14: In 2003, CCO CPR was advocated for all bystanders of OHCA in Tucson, Arizona

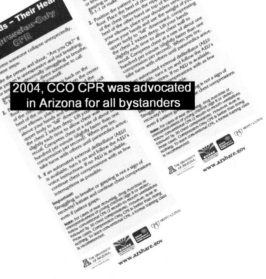

FIGURE 15: 2004, CCO CPR was advocated in Arizona for all bystanders

to influence guidelines led the senior author to conclude in 2003 that we could no longer in good conscience follow the AHA and ILCOR guidelines of 2000.[36,37] We announced our intensions[37] and explained our approach[36,42] Our new approach was called CCR, due to its focus on the maintaining blood flow to the heart (cardio) and the brain (cerebral) during primary cardiac arrest by near continuous chest compressions prior to defibrillation, a necessary components of neurologically intact survival.[36] The CCR deemphasizes the early ventilation or "pulmonary" component of traditional CPR and attempts to minimize other possible detrimental aspects of positive pressure ventilation.[36]

The community (Fig. 3) component of CCR included CCO CPR. In 2003, CCO CPR was advocated in Tucson, AZ, with free training, local radio spots and newspaper interviews, and inserts into utility bills (Fig. 14). In 2004, with Dr Benjamin Bobrow and his statewide SHARE program a statewide effort was initiated in Arizona to encourage CCO CPR.[43] This was a multiple facet approach to training and information was dissemination in multiple venues that included websites (www.azshare.gov) and (www.heart.arizona.edu), celebrity endorsement, online video training, free in-person training in many setting and locations throughout the state, training kits sent to all 6–12th grade schools in Arizona, inserts mailed in utility bills (Fig. 15), tables set up at health and safety fairs by various departments (e.g. Fire, etc.), newspaper articles, editorials, local radio spots and interviews. To determine the effect of this effort, a statewide reporting system was developed.[44] In October 2008, the AHA published a science advisory, recommending CCO (Hands-Only CPR) for lay individuals untrained in CPR.[33]

Between 1 January 2005 and 31 December 2009 we analyzed the results of this five years effort, published as "chest compression-Only CPR by Lay Rescuers and Survival from Out-of-hospital cardiac arrest" in the Journal of the American Medical Association in 2010.[45] After excluding bystander CPR provided by health care professionals or arrests that occurred in a medical facility, 4,415 patients with OHCA were analyzed.[45] Survival to hospital discharge was 5.2% for no bystander CPR group, 7.8% for conventional CPR and 13.3% for CCO CPR (Fig. 16).[45] Survival to hospital discharge of those most likely to survive, those with witnessed arrest and a shockable rhythm on arrival of the Emergency medical services (EMS) personnel, was 17.6% in the no CPR group, 17.7% for conventional CPR

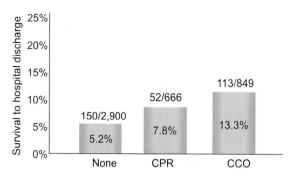

FIGURE 16: Effect of bystander CPR for OHCA on survival in Arizona (2005–2010) (*Source:* Modified from Bobrow, et al. JAMA. 2010)

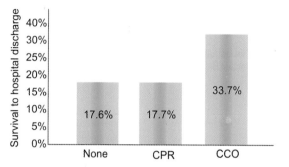

FIGURE 17: Bystander CPR for OHCA in Arizona (2005–2010) Witnessed/Shockable OHCA (*Source:* Modified from Bobrow, et al. JAMA. 2010)

and 33.7% for CCO CPR (Fig. 17).[45] There was no adverse effect of CCO CPR in the subgroup less likely to survive, witnessed arrest but without a shockable rhythm.[45]

This is the first prospective observational study to show that CCO CPR resulted in improved survival of patients with OHCA.[45] However, the first observational study to find that survival was better with lay individuals performing CCO CPR was the SOS-KANTO study which found that the survival of those individuals most likely to survive, witnessed arrest and a shockable rhythm was 11% for those receiving chest compressions plus mouth-to-mouth ventilations versus 19% for those receiving CCO (Fig. 18).[46] This study is of interest, for several reasons, including the fact that a bystander technique that had not been advocated nor taught was more effective than one that has been guidelines advocated for decades, and in which

untold thousands of man-hours had been spent teaching and untold thousands of dollars spent advocating over the past several decades.

To date (2010), there are three reported randomized trials of dispatcher instructed CPR where one group was instructed in guidelines CPR of chest compressions plus mouth-to-mouth ventilations, and the other in CCO CPR. The first was by Hallstrom and his associates who reported in 2000 that the survival was 14.6% in those receiving chest compressions only CPR and 10.4% in those receiving instructions in chest compression and ventilations.[47] Since there were only 520 patients in the study, the difference were not significant and therefore the guidelines were not changed. However, this finding, published in 2000, encouraged the University of Arizona Sarver Heart Center Resuscitation Research Group in our decision in 2003 not to follow the AHA and ILCOR 2000 guidelines.

The other two recently reported studies of patients with OHCA, one from Sweden and the other from Seattle and London, both found no statistically difference in survival.[48,49] In the study from Sweden in which 620 patients received dispatch directed compression-only CPR and 656 received standard CPR, the survival was 8.7% compression-only and 7.0% for standard CPR. These authors concluded that overall "this study lends further support to the hypothesis that compression-only CPR, which is easier to learn and to perform, should be considered the preferred method for CPR for patients with cardiac arrest."[48]

Rea and his associates from Seattle also reported on dispatch directed chest compression alone (981 patients) versus chest compression plus rescue breathing (960 patients) and found that survival to hospital discharge with favorable neurological outcome was 14.4% with chest compression alone and 11.5% in the CC plus rescue breathing group (p = 0.13).[49] However, their prespecified subgroup analysis showed a trend toward a higher proportion of patients survived to hospital discharge with chest compressions alone compared to chest compressions plus rescue breathing (15.5% vs 12.3%) and for those with a shockable rhythm 31.0% versus 25.7%.[49]

THE PUBLIC HAS MADE UP ITS MIND

In our statewide Arizona study, it was of interest to find that from 2005 to 2010, lay rescuer CPR only increased from 28.2% to 39.9% (Fig.19).[45] This was rather disappointing.

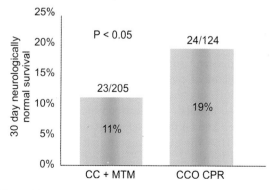

FIGURE 18: SOS-KANTO: Subset of patients with witnessed arrest and shockable rhythm (*Source:* Modified from Nagao et al. for the SOS-KANTO. The Lancet. 2007:369;920)

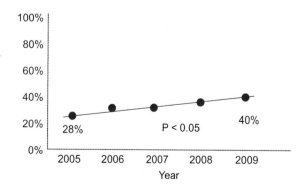

FIGURE 19: Incidence of bystander CPR for OHCA in Arizona (2005–2010) (*Source:* Modified from Bobrow, et al. JAMA. 2010)

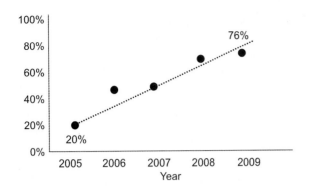

FIGURE 20: Bystander CPR for OHCA in Arizona (2005–2010): Percent of lay CPR providers who performed CCO-CPR (*Source:* Modified from Bobrow, et al. JAMA. 2010)

However, of those performing bystander CPR, the proportion of CPR that was CCO CPR increased from 19.6% to 75.9% (Fig. 20).[45] This indicates to us that the public has made up its mind. When encouraged they are much more likely to perform CCO CPR.

INCREASING THE PREVALENCE OF BYSTANDER RESUSCITATION EFFORTS

However, the fear or concern about mouth-to-mouth breathing is not the only reason a bystander may not initiate resuscitation efforts. We must address all of their concerns (Fig. 21) if we are to increase the prevalence of bystander resuscitation.[50]

INCREASING THE ABILITY TO PROMPTLY IDENTIFY PRIMARY CARDIAC ARREST

The prompt recognition of primary cardiac arrest is essential to any program to improve survival of patients with out-of-hospital cardiac arrest. The recommendation used by cardiocerebral resuscitation is the unexpected, witnessed (seen or heard) collapse in an individual who is not responsive. Note that this recommendation does not say anything about spontaneous ventilations. The reason for this is that one of the major impediments to the prompt recognition of primary cardiac arrest is the fact that subjects with cardiac arrest, rats, swine and humans have a high frequency of gasping after cardiac arrest (Fig. 22). Failure to recognize this fact delays the recognition of primary cardiac arrest (Fig. 23) lists the description of breathing abnormalities that have been described by witnesses of patients with cardiac arrest. Continued normal breathing for the first minute following cardiac arrest (Fig. 22) has only recently been observed in swine by the University of Arizona

• Fear/concern: mouth-to-mouth contact	~20%
• Fear/concern: harming person	~20%
• Fear/concern: legal consequences	~20%
• Fear/concern: not performing properly	~20%
• Physically unable to perform CPR	~20%

FIGURE 21: Is fear or concern about MTM contact the only deterrent to bystander CPR? (*Source:* Coons SJ, Guy MC. Resuscitation. 2009;80: 334-40) This study was designed and funded by the Sarver Heart Center University of Arizona College of Medicine and SHARE

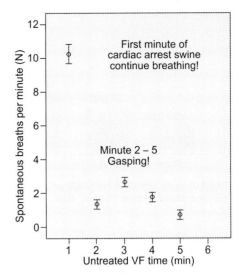

FIGURE 22: Recent unexpected finding (*Source:* Modified from Zuercher Ewy, Hillwig, et al. BioMedCentral Cardiovascular Disorders. 2010)

• Gasping	• Agonal breathing
• Snoring	• Barely breathing
• Gurgling	• Labored breathing
• Moaning	• Noisy breathing
• "Normal" breathing	• Heavy breathing
	• Abnormal breathing

FIGURE 23: Spontaneous ventilatory activity in patients with primary cardiac arrest

Sarver Heart Center Resuscitation Research Group.[51] However, gasping is well know and has been described in animals to begin during the second minute of VF arrest, and has a classical crescendo-decrescendo frequency pattern, of about 1,3,2,1 gasps per minutes (Fig. 22) and is no longer present six or more minutes after the onset of VF arrest, unless chest compressions provides enough blood flow to the brainstem to continue gasping.[52] Physician scientists refer to this phenomenon as gasping or agonal breathing, but lay people may refer to this phenomenon with other terms (Fig. 23).[53]

One of the reasons that assisted ventilation is often not necessary even during prolonged CCO CPR is that effective chest compression provides enough flood flow to the brainstem to maintain this primitive respiratory response.

THE THREE PHASES OF VENTRICULAR FIBRILLATION (VF)

To better understand some of the rationale for the second or pre-hospital phase of cardiocerebral resuscitation, one needs to appreciate not only the pathophysiology of cardiac arrest outlined above but also the electrophysiology of VF.

It has been known for decades that survival rates decrease by about 7–10% for every minute that a patient spends in untreated VF.[6] In the absence of chest compressions, after roughly 12 minutes, defibrillation for VF is rarely effective.[54] Our understanding of the therapy for VF was helped by the three-phase time sensitive concept of untreated VF, articulated by Weisfeldt and Becker in 2002 (Fig. 24).[54] This concept

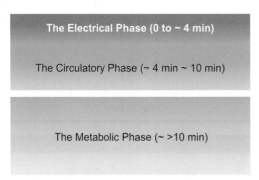

FIGURE 24: 3-Phase time-sensitive model of cardiac arrest due to ventricular fibrillation (*Source:* Modified from Weisfeldt ML, Becker LB. JAMA. 2002;288:3035-8)

• Not witnessed	16%
• Witnessed but no bystander CPR	36%
• Witnessed and bystander CPR	52%

FIGURE 25: Prevalence of VF on arrival of EMS in out-of-hospital cardiac arrest in Arizona (*Source:* Data from 1,296 cardiac arrest in Arizona Voluntary reporting SHARE Program: Data collected October 2004 to April 2006 Bobrow, Clark, Ewy, Kern, Sanders)

divides VF into an electrical phase (around 0–4 minutes), circulatory phase (roughly 4–10 minutes) and a metabolic phase (> 10 minutes). This model helps us to understand why specific therapies need to be tailored to timelines.

Electrical Phase (0–4 minutes)

In this initial phase of VF, there is enough myocardial adenosine triphosphate (ATP) and other energy stores that defibrillation alone is adequate to restore a perfusing rhythm.[55] Patients defibrillated within seconds by an ICD or minutes by an AED often return to a perfusing stable rhythm since they are in the electrical phase of VF arrest. Chest compressions can prolong this so-called electrical phase of VF. As a prototype, the city of Seattle, WA, USA, has an average EMS response time of about 5 minutes, with a bystander CPR rate of over 60%. This translates into patients being defibrillated in the electrical phase and consequently having some of the best survival rates from OHCA anywhere in the United States.[9]

Circulatory Phase (4–10 minutes)

Conversely, once the markedly underperfused fibrillating ventricle uses up a significant portion of its energy stores, defibrillation, even if successful results in pulseless electrical activity (PEA) or asystole.[56] Prolonged untreated VF is manifested electrocardiographically by decreasing amplitude of the VF wave form with a transition to "fine" fibrillation waves on the electrocardiogram (ECG). Defibrillation in the absence of chest compressions is rarely successful in this phase of VF. However, if the CPP is re-established by chest compressions, the resultant perfusion of the myocardium allows the formation of new myocardial energy which makes the myocardium more responsive to defibrillation (Fig. 24) and less likely to deteriorate to PEA or asystole (Fig. 25). Thus chest compressions can prolong the electrical phase of VF.

Most OHCA patients are found in the circulatory phase of VF upon arrival of EMS personnel. For instance, the average time to response in the city of Tucson, Arizona, was 6 minutes 34 seconds[42], placing the patient precisely in the circulatory phase. A defibrillation first strategy in these patients is likely to result in a nonperfusing rhythm like PEA or asystole.[56] In this situation, preshock chest compressions have been demonstrated to increase the likelihood of successful defibrillation in a swine model.[57] A study from Seattle in humans showed increased survival when chest compressions were uniformly performed for 90 seconds prior to defibrillation.[58] In a similar study, Wik and his associates found survival to be improved with 3 minutes of chest compressions prior to defibrillation.[59] Based on these studies, for individuals encountered in the circulatory phase of untreated VF arrest, we prescribed, as part of cardiocerebral resuscitation, a period of 2 minutes of chest compressions prior to the first defibrillation attempt.[36] This was done first due to a compromise between the duration of chest compressions studied by Cobb et al. and by Wik et al. and because the senior author as well as we did not want the paramedics to use their watches to determine the duration of chest compressions prior to delivering the first shock. Two hundred chest compressions at 100 per minutes would be two minutes.[36] A recent report from the resuscitation outcomes consortium also confirmed improved survival in humans with preshock chest compressions, and interestingly they found that survival was greatest in the subgroup who received 2 minutes of chest compressions prior to the first attempted defibrillation.[60]

Metabolic Phase (> 10 minutes from Onset of Untreated Cardiac Arrest)

This third and terminal phase of untreated VF is universally associated with diminishing odds of successful defibrillation and neurologically intact survival. End organ damage has already set in with irreversible cellular impairment. Ischemic and reperfusion injuries are believed to predominate at this stage. Strategies that may delay the onset of irremediable damage during this phase of untreated VF include hypothermia.

CARDIOCEREBRAL RESUSCITATION; PREHOSPITAL COMPONENT

The initial approach to the prehospital component of CCR was implemented in Tucson, AZ, in late 2003 (Figs 26 to 28).[36,37,42] We announced our intensions and gave our rational for no longer following the National and International CPR and EMS guidelines (Fig. 29).[36,37] The CCR was predominantly based

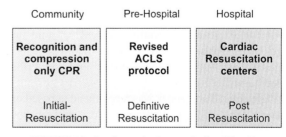

FIGURE 26: Cardiocerebral resuscitation "The New CPR" for primary cardiac arrest

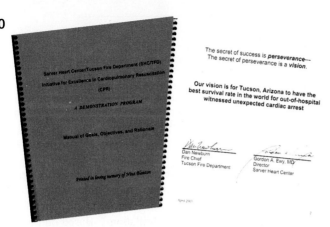

FIGURE 27: Manual of Goals, Objective, and Rationale

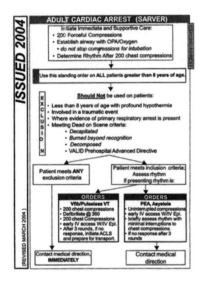

FIGURE 28: Tucson Fire Department

ELSEVIER

Resuscitation. 2003;58:271

RESUSCITATION

w.elsevier.com/locate/resuscitation

A new approach for out-of-hospital CPR: a bold step forward
gordon A. Ewy [1]*

Special Report

Cardiocerebral resuscitation
The new cardiopulmonary resuscitation

Gordon A. Ewy, MD

"Why is that every time I press n his chest he opens his eyes, every time I stop to breathe for him he goes back to sleep?"

Circulation. 2005;111:2134-42

FIGURE 29: Sources of National and International CPR and EMS guidelines

- Interruptions in CPR for paramedic endotracheal intubations in 100 OHCA
- Median duration of 1st endotracheal Intubation was 47 seconds
- Almost one-third exceeded 1 minute
- One-fourth exceeded 3 minutes

FIGURE 30: Interruptions of chest compressions for endotracheal intubation (*Source:* Modified from Wang, et al. Annals of Emergency Medicine. 2009;54:645)

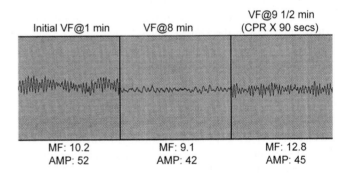

Initial VF@1 min — MF: 10.2 AMP: 52

VF@8 min — MF: 9.1 AMP: 42

VF@9 1/2 min (CPR X 90 secs) — MF: 12.8 AMP: 45

FIGURE 31: Untreated, the VF waveform decreased in amplitude with time. Following 90 seconds of chest compressions, the frequency and amplitude of the VF waveform increases

on our findings of the importance of uninterrupted chest compressions during cardiac arrest, and on ours or others findings that following the 2000 AHA and ILCOR guidelines, EMS paramedics/firefighters were performing chest compressions only half of the time while they were on the scene.[61,62]

We initially did not allow endotracheal intubation based our clinical observations that chest compressions were often interrupted for prolonged periods of time, even by well trained individuals attempting endotracheal intubation. This assumption proved to be correct as documented in a recent study by Wang and his associates (Fig. 30).[63]

We advocated chest compressions prior to defibrillation based on our experimental finding (Fig. 31),[64] and on the observations by Cobb et al. and Wik et al. that in patients with prolonged VF arrest, chest compressions prior to defibrillation improved survival.[58,59,65]

A single defibrillator shock was recommended based on the long interruptions of chest compressions for "stacked shocks". This approach also proved to be correct. Rae and his associates found increased survival in humans with single rather than stacked shocks, and subsequently this recommendation was made in the guidelines.[66]

In our experimental laboratory we found that chest compressions immediately after defibrillation shocks improved survival, and this approach was also subsequently advocated in 2005 guidelines.[13]

In 2004, the adverse affects of hyperventilation were reported by Aufderheide and his colleagues (Fig. 32). We had previously reported that during in-hospital cardiac arrests, physicians, in their excitement, were ventilating at an average rate of 37 per minute.[67] Aufderheide and his associates documented that paramedics were ventilating at this same rapid rate.[68] Accordingly we eliminated bag-mouth-ventilation and substituted "passive ventilation" as part of cardiocerebral resuscitation.[69,70] In 2004, after visiting us, Dr Mike Kellum and his associates instituted CCR (Fig. 33) in Rock and

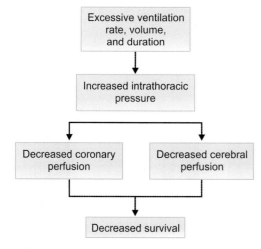

FIGURE 32: Consequence of excessive ventilation

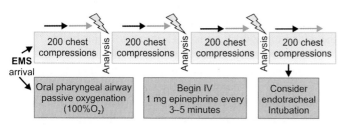

FIGURE 33: Cardiocerebral resuscitation. Goal: minimally interrupted chest compressions, avoiding hyperventilation, and early administration of epinephrine

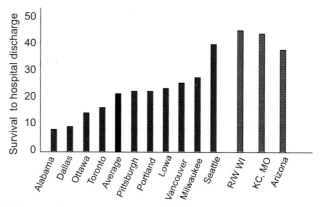

FIGURE 34: Survival to hospital discharge (%) of patients with VF arrest ROC 2005 Guidelines (all VF) vs cardiocerebral resuscitation (Witnessed VF)

Walworth Counties of Wisconsin.[10,36,71,72] The CCR (Figs 26 and 33), although advocating CCO CPR for bystanders, in the reports from Kellum et al. the intervention was essentially the "prehospital (Fig. 26) portion". Its initial component consisted of two hundred chest compressions. While this was being preformed, endotracheal intubation was not allowed, but rather an oral-pharyngeal airway, a non-rebreather mask, and high flow oxygen was administered.[72] A single shock was followed immediately by another 200 continuous chest compressions. After the single shock the EMS personnel were instructed not to feel for a pulse, nor evaluate the rhythm by looking at an ECG. These analyses were allowed, only after the first 400 chest compressions (4 minutes into ACLS). Equally important was the fact that only a single defibrillator shock, at maximal defibrillator output, was allowed.[10,36,72] Intravenous (IV) epinephrine was administered as soon as possible.[36,72]

In 2005, the rational for CCR was presented by the senior author to EMS medical directors in Arizona, and some chose to institute CCR in their cities. In part due to the enthusiasm of EMS personnel and in part in response to the statewide Save Hearts in Arizona Research and Education Program (SHARE) spearheaded by Dr Benjamin Bobrow, Director of the Arizona Department of Health Emergency Care and Trauma Service, CCR was expanded to a statewide effort.[11] In 2006, the senior author was invited to Kansas city, MO, to advocate cardio-cerebral resuscitation.[12,73]

As shown in Figure 4, survival of the subset of patients more likely to survive, those with witnessed arrest and a shockable

rhythm on arrival of EMS personnel, averaged 38% with CCR in all three of these areas. Then compared to arguably some of the better EMS systems in the United States and Canada, the resuscitation outcomes consortiums (ROC), survival with CCR was better than that advocated by the 2005 national and international guidelines for CPR and EMS care (Fig. 34).[1] There is a caveat with this comparison in that the results of CCR are for witnessed arrest and a shockable rhythm, whereas the results reported by ROC was for VF arrest.[1]

DRUG THERAPY IN CARDIAC RESUSCITATION

Epinephrine is a first line agent for a cardiac arrest and is used in all forms of cardiac arrest. Epinephrine causes immediate peripheral vasoconstriction by its α-adrenergic effect, and thereby during chest compressions for cardiac arrest, increases coronary and cerebral perfusion.[74-76] An IV epinephrine dose of 1 mg is administered ever 3–5 minutes till ROSC has been recommended. Since the time from onset of cardiac arrest to IV administration of epinephrine in the field is prolonged, there is a trend to the increasing use of intraosseous (IO) injections.

Vasopressin, which causes peripheral vasoconstriction through V1a receptors on vascular smooth muscle, is a more controversial drug. A large randomized trial of epinephrine or vasopressin showed no difference in survival between the two groups.[77] A 2005 meta analysis also failed to show any benefit of vasopressin over epinephrine.[78] Since the half-life of vasopressin is 10–20 minutes, it is administered as on one time 40U IV dose. Some have recommended epinephrine as the first vasopressor, followed by vasopressin as the second vasopressors in an effort to decrease the number of epinephrine doses.[10] Since it is the alpha adrenergic effect of epinephrine that is beneficial during resuscitation efforts, this approach could decrease the theoretical adverse effects of excessive beta adrenergic effects of frequent epinephrine doses. Others have recommended epinephrine alone, in efforts to simplify the regimen of EMS personnel. Experimental studies have suggested that vasopressin contributes to postresuscitation myocardial dysfunction, but not survival.[79]

Amiodarone and to a lesser extent lidocaine are anti-arrhythmic drugs of choice for pulseless VT/VF, especially of presumed ischemic etiology. Amiodarone was superior to lidocaine in the ALIVE trial, and had been the recommended

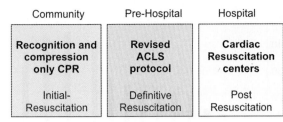

FIGURE 35: Cardiocerebral resuscitation "The New CPR" for primary cardiac arrest

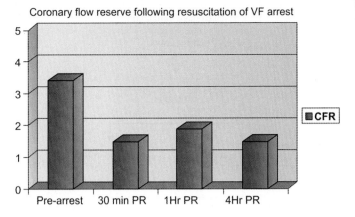

FIGURE 36: Coronary flow reserve (CFR) remained significantly below normal (ratio of 2:4) throughout the 4-hr postresuscitation period (*Source:* Modified from Kem KB, et al. Univ. AZ College Medicine)

first line antiarrhythmic agent for VF/VT arrest.[80,81] Amiodarone is administered as a single 300 mg IV push, followed by, if necessary, another 150 mg IV push.

The largest controlled trial (TROICA) of thrombolytics in cardiac arrest, involving 1,050 patients, was prematurely terminated due to a lack of benefit.[82]

For postresuscitation hypotension, dopamine should be considered. Intra-aortic balloon pumping was not found to be helpful in our experimental laboratory.[83]

CARDIAC RESUSCITATION CENTERS

A more recently advocated third component of CCR is Cardiac Resuscitation Centers (Fig. 35). Cardiac Resuscitations Centers are proposed to improve therapy of resuscitated but comatose patients following cardiac arrest. Although neurologic function after prolonged cardiac arrest is of major concern, there is almost always other organ dysfunction as well. In its 2008 consensus statement, ILCOR termed this as the "post cardiac arrest syndrome".[84]

The clinical manifestation of the post cardiac arrest syndrome can include hypoxic encephalopathy, myocardial dysfunction, aspiration pneumonia, ischemic gut injury, ischemic hepatopathy, renal dysfunction as well as peripheral limb ischemia. Generalized activation of immunological and coagulation cascades occur. Relative adrenal insufficiency,[85] glycemia,[86] and ventilator associated pneumonia are common. Seizures/myoclonus, consequent to hypoxic brain injury, is seen in up to 40% of resuscitated patient and should be treated promptly with anticonvulsants. Coronary flow reserve remains below normal for at least 4 hours in animal models (Fig. 36).

In Arizona, hospitals were encouraged to become designated as Cardiac Resuscitation Centers.[87] To be designated, a hospital has 24/7 capability for therapeutic hypothermia, early cardiac catheterization and indicated percutaneous intervention, glucose management protocols, provide hemodynamic optimization, prophylaxis therapy for stress ulcers, infection and venous thrombosis prophylaxis, and assessment for relative adrenal insufficiency, and be willing to submit their outcomes (which are subsequently not identified in statewide outcome reporting). In an effort to further improve survival from cardiac arrest, requirements for evidence based termination of resuscitation including at least a 72–hour moratorium for termination of care following therapeutic hypothermia, a protocol to address organ donation, and these hospitals are encouraged to have a community out-reach program to promote bystander CCO CPR for primary cardiac arrest.

In Arizona, the SHARE program has studied the impact of prehospital transport intervals on survival from OHCA and found that bypassing a hospital to bring resuscitated but comatose patient to a Cardiac Resuscitation Center (provided the added transport time is < 15 minutes) is justifiable.[88]

Neurologically intact survival is the ultimate goal of resuscitation treatment strategies and is reflected in the inclusion of "cerebral" in "cardiocerebral resuscitation". Resuscitated patients require close monitoring in an intensive care unit setting as they are prone to repeat hemodynamic instability as well as recurrent cardiac arrhythmias.

THERAPEUTIC MILD HYPOTHERMIA

One of the most encouraging approaches to resuscitated cardiac arrest patients with coma is therapeutic controlled mild hypothermia [89.6–93.2°F (32–34°C)]. Two decisive randomized trials have established hypothermia as an integral part of postresuscitation care.[89,90] The hypothermia after cardiac arrest (HACA) study group performed the largest randomized clinical trial of hypothermia to date. Barnard et al. also studied adult patients with out-of-hospital cardiac arrest from VF. Hypothermia has been shown to be safe in patient with cardiogenic shock,[91] where the benefit appears to be even more robust. In 2007, a Norwegian report emphasized aggressive early hypothermia and early coronary angiography in patients who were comatose after OHCA, and demonstrated an increase in survival increased from 26% to 56% with the implementation of this protocol.[92] Based on randomized trial data, approximately 6 patients need to be treated with therapeutic hypothermia to gain one neurologically intact survivor.

The mechanism of action of hypothermia is unknown, but is thought to be related to its inhibitory effect on adverse enzymatic and chemical reactions that are initiated by the global ischemia. Continuous temperature monitoring is an essential part of therapeutic hypothermia as undershooting or overshooting can lead to malignant arrhythmias.[93] Transesophageal temperature monitoring is reported to be more reliable that urinary bladder monitoring.

Early institution of hypothermia in the field is recommended.[94] If available, the rapid administration of 2,000 ml of cold (4°C) normal saline is recommended.[95,96] If available, especially in hot environments, the application of ice packs to the groin, axilla and neck are considered.

The ILCOR, taking into account the increasing evidence, issued an advisory statement in 2003 recommending that unconscious adult patients with spontaneous circulation after out-of-hospital cardiac arrest should be cooled to 89.6–93.2°F (32–34°C) for 12–24 hours when the initial rhythm was VF. Similar recommendations were echoed in more recent guidelines.[13]

Electrolyte abnormalities, coagulation disturbances and alteration of drug metabolism have all been described as complications of therapeutic hypothermia. There is no data supporting one method of cooling over the other.

There are, at present, no reliable predictive tools that can be used in comatose patients to distinguish who will or will not wake up. The best prognostic sign postresuscitation recovery is the return of consciousness. Recent unpublished observation suggests that one should wait at least 72 hours after therapeutic hypothermia before making the decision to discontinue therapy.

MYOCARDIAL ISCHEMIA CAUSING CARDIAC ARREST

The recommendation for early catheterization and possible early percutaneous coronary intervention is based on the fact that about 50% of adult patients with VF arrest may have an acute myocardial infarction as the underlying etiology.[97] Unfortunately, in the postresuscitation state, neither clinical nor electrocardiographic findings are predictors of an acute coronary occlusion. In one study, 48% of patients who had no obvious noncardiac cause and had undergone coronary angiography after resuscitation from out-of-hospital cardiac arrest were found to have had an acute coronary occlusion.[98]

This has led to the concept of bundled postresuscitation care, with standardized protocol for patients with OHCA, including hypothermia and emergent coronary angiography.[87]

ENDING RESUSCITATIVE EFFORTS

For services delivering advanced cardiac life support in England, the Recognition of Life Extinct (ROLE) guidelines state that "resuscitation attempts should be terminated when the patient remains in asystole despite full advanced life support procedures for more than 20 minutes". The AHA guidelines state that "resuscitation efforts should be continued" until "reliable criteria indicating irreversible death are present".[99] Morrison et al. found that only 0.5% of arrest victims survived if: (1) there was no ROSC; (2) no shocks were administered; (3) the arrest was not witnessed by EMS personnel; (4) when response time greater than 8 minutes was retrospectively added to the prediction rule, the survival rate was 0.3% and (5) when not bystander witnessed no one survived.[100] However, practice patterns vary widely and no single consensus has been established as the gold standard for ending resuscitation efforts.

SUMMARY

The classic "chain of survival" identifies five fundamental links in resuscitation: early warning, early cardiopulmonary resuscitation by witnesses, early defibrillation, early advanced life support and care of the post-arrest patient. Despite all the

advances, until recently there has only been a weak trend toward improved survival to hospital discharge.[3] The CCR is a new approach that has been shown to improve survival. It consists of a community approach, which emphasizes early recognition, including the frequency of gasping post witnessed cardiac arrest and early CCO CPR.[36] A Prehospital approach for primary cardiac arrest prohibits early endotracheal intubation, requires prompt initiation of minimally interrupted chest compressions before rhythm analysis or after an indicated single shock and the prompt administration of epinephrine.

The CCR now has human survival outcome data and will likely succeed traditional CPR as the preferred management of primary cardiac arrest.[10-12]

REFERENCES

1. Nichol G, Thomas E, Callaway CW, et al. Regional variation in out-of-hospital cardiac arrest incidence and outcome. JAMA. 2008; 300:1423-31.
2. Atwood C, Eisenberg MS, Herlitz J, et al. Incidence of EMS-treated out-of-hospital cardiac arrest in Europe. Resuscitation. 2005;67:75-80.
3. Sasson C, Rogers MA, Dahl J, et al. Predictors of survival from out-of-hospital cardiac arrest: a systematic review and meta-analysis. Circ Cardiovasc Qual Outcomes. 2010;3:63-81.
4. Ehlenbach WJ, Barnato AE, Curtis JR, et al. Epidemiologic study of in-hospital cardiopulmonary resuscitation in the elderly. N Engl J Med. 2009;361:22-31.
5. Cummins RO, Ornato JP, Thies WH, et al. Improving survival from sudden cardiac arrest: the "chain of survival" concept. A statement for health professionals from the Advanced Cardiac Life Support Subcommittee and the Emergency Cardiac Care Committee, American Heart Association. Circulation. 1991;83:1832-47.
6. American Heart Association Guidelines 2000 for cardiopulmonary resuscitation and emergency cardiovascular care: international consensus on science. Circulation. 2000;102:I1-I348.
7. Eckstein M, Stratton SJ, Chan LS. Cardiac arrest resuscitation evaluation in Los Angeles: CARE-LA. Ann Emerg Med. 2005;45:504-9.
8. Dunne RB, Compton S, Zalenski RJ, et al. Outcomes from out-of-hospital cardiac arrest in Detroit. Resuscitation. 2007;72:59-65.
9. Becker L, Gold LS, Eisenberg M, et al. Ventricular fibrillation in King County, Washington: A 30-year perspective. Resuscitation. 2008;79:22-7.
10. Kellum MJ, Kennedy KW, Barney R, et al. Cardiocerebral resuscitation improves neurologically intact survival of patients with out-of-hospital cardiac arrest. Ann Emerg Med. 2008;52:244-52.
11. Bobrow BJ, Ewy GA, Clark L, et al. Passive oxygen insufflation is superior to bag-valve-mask ventilation for witnessed ventricular fibrillation out-of-hospital cardiac arrest. Ann Emerg Med. 2009;54:656-62.
12. Garza AG, Gratton MC, Salomone JA, et al. Improved patient survival using a modified resuscitation protocol for out-of-hospital cardiac arrest. Circulation. 2009;119:2597-605.
13. International consensus on cardiopulmonary resuscitation and emergency cardiovascular care science with treatment recommendations. Resuscitation. 2005;67:181-341.
14. Andreka P, Frenneaux MP. Haemodynamics of cardiac arrest and resuscitation. Curr Opin Crit Care. 2006;12:198-203.
15. Guyton AC, Polizio D, Armstrong GG. Mean circulatory filling pressure measured immediately after cessation of heart pumping. Am J Physiol. 1954;179:261-7.
16. Steen S, Liao Q, Pierre L, et al. The critical importance of minimal delay between chest compressions and subsequent defibrillation: a haemodynamic explanation. Resuscitation. 2003;58:249-58.

17. Sorrell VL, Altbach MI, Kern KB, et al. Images in cardiovascular medicine. Continuous cardiac magnetic resonance imaging during untreated ventricular fibrillation. Circulation. 2005;111:e294.

18. Sorrell VL, Bhatt RD, Berg RA, et al. Cardiac magnetic resonance imaging investigation of sustained ventricular fibrillation in a swine model with a focus on the electrical phase. Resuscitation. 2007;73: 279-86.

19. Frenneaux M. Cardiopulmonary resuscitation-some physiological considerations. Resuscitation. 2003;58:259-65.

20. Kern KB, Ewy GA, Voorhees WD, et al. Myocardial perfusion pressure: a predictor of 24-hour survival during prolonged cardiac arrest in dogs. Resuscitation. 1988;16:241-50.

21. Paradis NA, Martin GB, Rivers EP, et al. Coronary perfusion pressure and the return of spontaneous circulation in human cardiopulmonary resuscitation. JAMA. 1990;263:1106-13.

22. Higano ST, Oh JK, Ewy GA, et al. The mechanism of blood flow during closed chest cardiac massage in humans: transesophageal echocardiographic observations. Mayo Clin Proc. 1990;65:1432-40.

23. Kern KB, Hilwig RW, Berg RA, et al. Efficacy of chest compression-only BLS CPR in the presence of an occluded airway. Resuscitation. 1998;39:179-88.

24. Kern KB, Hilwig RW, Berg RA, et al. Importance of continuous chest compressions during cardiopulmonary resuscitation: improved outcome during a simulated single lay-rescuer scenario. Circulation. 2002;105:645-9.

25. Berg RA, Sanders AB, Kern KB, et al. Adverse hemodynamic effects of interrupting chest compressions for rescue breathing during cardiopulmonary resuscitation for ventricular fibrillation cardiac arrest. Circulation. 2001;104:2465-70.

26. Kern KB, Ewy GA, Sanders AB, et al. Neurologic outcome following successful cardiopulmonary resuscitation in dogs. Resuscitation. 1986;14:149-55.

27. Berg RA, Kern KB, Hilwig RW, et al. Assisted ventilation does not improve outcome in a porcine model of single-rescuer bystander cardiopulmonary resuscitation. Circulation. 1997;95:1635-41.

28. Kouwenhoven WB, Jude JR, Knickerbocker GG. Closed-chest cardiac massage. JAMA. 1960;173:1064-7.

29. Kouwenhoven WB, Jude JR, Knickerbocker GB. Demonstration of the technique of CPR for New York Society of Anesthesiologist 1960s (Copy of demonstration provided on CD by JR Jude).

30. Safar P. Ventilatory efficacy of mouth-to-mouth artificial respiration; airway obstruction during manual and mouth-to-mouth artificial respiration. J Am Med Assoc. 1958;167:335-41.

31. Safar P, Brown TC, Holtey WJ, et al. Ventilation and circulation with closed-chest cardiac massage in man. JAMA. 1961;176:574-6.

32. Standards for cardiopulmonary resuscitation (CPR) and emergency cardiac care (ECC). II: Basic life support. JAMA. 1974;227:833-68.

33. Sayre MR, Berg RA, Cave DM, et al. Hands-only (compression-only) cardiopulmonary resuscitation: a call to action for bystander response to adults who experience out-of-hospital sudden cardiac arrest: a science advisory for the public from the American Heart Association Emergency Cardiovascular Care Committee. Circulation. 2008;117:2162-7.

34. Ewy GA. Cardiopulmonary resuscitation-strengthening the links in the chain of survival. N Engl J Med. 2000;342:1599-601.

35. Kern K, Hilwig R, Berg R, et al. Assisted ventilation during "bystander" CPR in a swine acute myocardial infarction model does not improve outcome. Circulation. 1997;96:4364-71.

36. Ewy GA. Cardiocerebral resuscitation: the new cardiopulmonary resuscitation. Circulation. 2005;111:2134-42.

37. Ewy GA. A new approach for out-of-hospital CPR: a bold step forward. Resuscitation. 2003;58:271-2.

38. Assar D, Chamberlain D, Colquhoun M, et al. Randomized controlled trials of staged teaching for basic life support. 1. Skill acquisition at bronze stage. Resuscitation. 2000;45:7-15.

39. Ewy GA, Zuercher M, Hilwig RW, et al. Improved neurological outcome with continuous chest compressions compared with 30:2 compressions-to-ventilations cardiopulmonary resuscitation in a realistic swine model of out-of-hospital cardiac arrest. Circulation. 2007;116:2525-30.

40. Heidenreich JW, Higdon TA, Kern KB, et al. Single-rescuer cardiopulmonary resuscitation: 'two quick breaths'-an oxymoron. Resuscitation. 2004;62:283-9.

41. Higdon TA, Heidenreich JW, Kern KB, et al. Single rescuer cardiopulmonary resuscitation: can anyone perform to the guidelines 2000 recommendations? Resuscitation. 2006;71:34-9.

42. Kern KB, Valenzuela TD, Clark LL, et al. An alternative approach to advancing resuscitation science. Resuscitation. 2005;64:261-8.

43. Bobrow BJ, Spaite DW, Mullins T, et al. The impact of state and national efforts to improve bystander CPR rates in Arizona. Circulation. 2009;120:S1443.

44. Bobrow BJ, Vadeboncoeur TF, Clark L, et al. Establishing Arizona's statewide cardiac arrest reporting and educational network. Prehosp Emerg Care. 2008;12:381-7.

45. Bobrow B, Spaite D, Berg R, et al. Chest compression-only CPR by lay rescuers and survival from out-of-hospital cardiac arrest. JAMA. 2010 (In press).

46. SOS-KANTO. Cardiopulmonary resuscitation by bystanders with chest compression only (SOS-KANTO): an observational study. The Lancet. 2007;369:920-6.

47. Hallstrom A, Cobb L, Johnson E, et al. Cardiopulmonary resuscitation by chest compression alone or with mouth-to-mouth ventilation. N Engl J Med. 2000;342:1546-53.

48. Svensson L, Bohm K, Castren M, et al. Compression-only CPR or standard CPR in out-of-hospital cardiac arrest. N Engl J Med. 2010;363:434-42.

49. Rea TD, Fahrenbruch C, Culley L, et al. CPR with chest compression alone or with rescue breathing. N Engl J Med. 2010;363:423-33.

50. Coons SJ, Guy MC. Performing bystander CPR for sudden cardiac arrest: behavioral intentions among the general adult population in Arizona. Resuscitation. 2009;80:334-40.

51. Zuercher M, Ewy GA, Hilwig RW, et al. Continued breathing followed by gasping or apnea in a swine model of ventricular fibrillation cardiac arrest. BMC Cardiovasc Disord. 2010;10:36.

52. Zuercher M, Ewy GA. Gasping during cardiac arrest. Curr Opin Crit Care. 2009;15:185-8.

53. Bobrow BJ, Zuercher M, Ewy GA, et al. Gasping during cardiac arrest in humans is frequent and associated with improved survival. Circulation. 2008;118:2550-4.

54. Weisfeldt ML, Becker LB. Resuscitation after cardiac arrest: a 3-phase time-sensitive model. JAMA. 2002;288:3035-8.

55. Kern KB, Garewal HS, Sanders AB, et al. Depletion of myocardial adenosine triphosphate during prolonged untreated ventricular fibrillation: effect on defibrillation success. Resuscitation. 1990;20: 221-9.

56. Ewy GA. Defining electromechanical dissociation. Ann Emerg Med. 1984;13:830-2.

57. Berg RA, Hilwig RW, Ewy GA, et al. Precountershock cardiopulmonary resuscitation improves initial response to defibrillation from prolonged ventricular fibrillation: a randomized, controlled swine study. Crit Care Med. 2004;32:1352-7.

58. Cobb LA, Fahrenbruch CE, Walsh TR, et al. Influence of cardiopulmonary resuscitation prior to defibrillation in patients with out-of-hospital ventricular fibrillation. JAMA. 1999;281:1182-8.

59. Wik L, Hansen TB, Fylling F, et al. Delaying defibrillation to give basic cardiopulmonary resuscitation to patients with out-of-hospital ventricular fibrillation: a randomized trial. JAMA. 2003;289:1389-95.

60. Bradley SM, Gabriel EE, Aufderheide TP, et al. Survival increases with CPR by emergency medical services before defibrillation of out-of-hospital ventricular fibrillation or ventricular tachycardia: observations from the Resuscitation Outcomes Consortium. Resuscitation. 2010;81:155-62.

61. Valenzuela TD, Kern KB, Clark LL, et al. Interruptions of chest compressions during emergency medical systems resuscitation. Circulation. 2005;112:1259-65.

62. Wik L, Kramer-Johansen J, Myklebust H, et al. Quality of cardiopulmonary resuscitation during out-of-hospital cardiac arrest. JAMA. 2005;293:299-304.

63. Wang HE, Simeone SJ, Weaver MD, et al. Interruptions in cardiopulmonary resuscitation from paramedic endotracheal intubation. Ann Emerg Med. 2009;54:645-52.

64. Berg RA, Hilwig RW, Kern KB, et al. Precountershock cardio-pulmonary resuscitation improves ventricular fibrillation median frequency and myocardial readiness for successful defibrillation from prolonged ventricular fibrillation: a randomized, controlled swine study. Ann Emerg Med. 2002;40:563-70.

65. Valenzuela TD. Priming the pump—can delaying defibrillation improve survival after sudden cardiac death? JAMA. 2003;289:1434-6.

66. Rea TD, Helbock M, Perry S, et al. Increasing use of cardio-pulmonary resuscitation during out-of-hospital ventricular fibrillation arrest: survival implications of guideline changes. Circulation. 2006;114:2760-5.

67. Milander MM, Hiscok PS, Sanders AB, et al. Chest compression and ventilation rates during cardiopulmonary resuscitation: the effects of audible tone guidance. Acad Emerg Med. 1995;2:708-13.

68. Aufderheide TP, Lurie KG. Death by hyperventilation: a common and life-threatening problem during cardiopulmonary resuscitation. Crit Care Med. 2004;32:S345-51.

69. Hayes MM, Ewy GA, Anavy ND, et al. Continuous passive oxygen insufflation results in a similar outcome to positive pressure ventilation in a swine model of out-of-hospital ventricular fibrillation. Resuscitation. 2007;74:357-65.

70. Steen S, Liao Q, Pierre L, et al. Continuous intratracheal insufflation of oxygen improves the efficacy of mechanical chest compression-active decompression CPR. Resuscitation. 2004;62:219-27.

71. Ewy GA, Kern KB, Sanders AB, et al. Cardiocerebral resuscitation for cardiac arrest. Am J Med. 2006;119:6-9.

72. Kellum MJ, Kennedy KW, Ewy GA. Cardiocerebral resuscitation improves survival of patients with out-of-hospital cardiac arrest. Am J Med. 2006;119:335-40.

73. Ewy GA. Do modifications of the American Heart Association guidelines improve survival of patients with out-of-hospital cardiac arrest? Circulation. 2009;119:2542-4.

74. Redding JS, Pearson JW. Evaluation of drugs for cardiac resusci-tation. Anesthesiology. 1963;24:203-7.

75. Otto CW, Yakaitis RW, Ewy GA. Effect of epinephrine on defibrilla-tion in ischemic ventricular fibrillation. Am J Emerg Med. 1985;3:285-91.

76. Attaran RR, Ewy GA. Epinephrine in resuscitation: curse or cure? Future Cardiology. 2010;6:473-82.

77. Wenzel V, Krismer A, Arntz H, et al. A comparison of vasopressin and epinephrine for out-of-hospital cardiopulmonary resuscitation. N Engl J Med. 2004;350:105-13.

78. Aung K, Htay T. Vasopressin for cardiac arrest: a systematic review and meta-analysis. Arch Intern Med. 2005;165:17-24.

79. Kern KB, Heidenreich JH, Higdon TA, et al. Effect of vasopressin on postresuscitation ventricular function: unknown consequences of the recent guidelines 2000 for cardiopulmonary resuscitation and emergency cardiovascular care. Crit Care Med. 2004;32:S393-7.

80. Dorian P, Cass D, Schwartz B, et al. Amiodarone as compared with lidocaine for shock-resistant ventricular fibrillation. N Engl J Med. 2002;346:884-90.

81. Kudenchuk PJ, Cobb LA, Copass MK, et al. Amiodarone for resuscitation after out-of-hospital cardiac arrest due to ventricular fibrillation. N Engl J Med. 1999;341:871-8.

82. Bottiger BW, Arntz HR, Chamberlain DA, et al. Thrombolysis during resuscitation for out-of-hospital cardiac arrest. N Engl J Med. 2008;359:2651-62.

83. Kern KB. Postresuscitation myocardial dysfunction. Cardiol Clin. 2002;20:89-101.

84. Neumar RW, Nolan JP, Adrie C, et al. Post-cardiac arrest syndrome: epidemiology, pathophysiology, treatment, and prognostication. A consensus statement from the International Liaison Committee on Resuscitation (American Heart Association, Australian and New Zealand Council on Resuscitation, European Resuscitation Council, Heart and Stroke Foundation of Canada, InterAmerican Heart Foundation, Resuscitation Council of Asia, and the Resuscitation Council of Southern Africa); the American Heart Association Emergency Cardiovascular Care Committee; the Council on Cardiovascular Surgery and Anesthesia; the Council on Cardiopulmonary, Perioperative, and Critical Care; the Council on Clinical Cardiology; and the Stroke Council. Circulation. 2008;118:2452-83.

85. Hekimian G, Baugnon T, Thuong M, et al. Cortisol levels and adrenal reserve after successful cardiac arrest resuscitation. Shock. 2004;22:116-9.

86. Calle PA, Buylaert WA, Vanhaute OA. Glycemia in the post-resuscitation period. The Cerebral Resuscitation Study Group. Resuscitation.1989;17:S181-8; discussion S199-206.

87. Bobrow BJ, Kern KB. Regionalization of postcardiac arrest care. Curr Opin Crit Care. 2009;15:221-7.

88. Spaite DW, Bobrow BJ, Vadeboncoeur TF, et al. The impact of prehospital transport interval on survival in out-of-hospital cardiac arrest: implications for regionalization of post-resuscitation care. Resuscitation. 2008;79:61-6.

89. Bernard SA, Gray TW, Buist MD, et al. Treatment of comatose survivors of out-of-hospital cardiac arrest with induced hypothermia. N Engl J Med. 2002;346:557-63.

90. HACA Study Group. Mild hypothermia to improve the neurologic outcome after cardiac arrest. N Engl J Med. 2002;346:549-56.

91. Skulec R, Kovarnik T, Dostalova G, et al. Induction of mild hypothermia in cardiac arrest survivors presenting with cardiogenic shock syndrome. Acta Anaesthesiol Scand. 2008;52:188-94.

92. Sunde K, Pytte M, Jacobsen D, et al. Implementation of a standardised treatment protocol for post resuscitation care after out-of-hospital cardiac arrest. Resuscitation. 2007;73:29-39.

93. Merchant RM, Abella BS, Peberdy MA, et al. Therapeutic hypothermia after cardiac arrest: unintentional overcooling is common using ice packs and conventional cooling blankets. Crit Care Med. 2006;34:S490-4.

94. Bernard S, Buist M, Monteiro O, et al. Induced hypothermia using large volume, ice-cold intravenous fluid in comatose survivors of out-of-hospital cardiac arrest: a preliminary report. Resuscitation. 2003;56:9-13.

95. Kim F, Olsufka M, Carlbom D, et al. Pilot study of rapid infusion of 2 L of 4°C normal saline for induction of mild hypothermia in hospitalized, comatose survivors of out-of-hospital cardiac arrest. Circulation. 2005;112:715-9.

96. Kim F, Olsufka M, Longstreth WT, et al. Pilot randomized clinical trial of prehospital induction of mild hypothermia in out-of-hospital cardiac arrest patients with a rapid infusion of 4 degrees C normal saline. Circulation. 2007;115:3064-70.

97. Engdahl J, Abrahamsson P, Bang A, et al. Is hospital care of major importance for outcome after out-of-hospital cardiac arrest? Experience acquired from patients with out-of-hospital cardiac arrest resuscitated by the same emergency medical service and admitted to one of two hospitals over a 16-year period in the municipality of Goteborg. Resuscitation. 2000;43:201-11.

98. Spaulding SM, Joly L-M, Rosenberg A, et al. Immediate coronary angiography in survivors of out-of-hospital cardiac arrest. N Engl J Med. 1997;336:1629-33.

99. ROLE. http://www.asancep.org.uk/JRCALC/publications/doc/ROLE_Most_Final_March2003.pdf

100. Morrison LJ, Visentin LM, Kiss A, et al. Validation of a rule for termination of resuscitation in out-of-hospital cardiac arrest. N Engl J Med. 2006;355:478-87.

CORONARY HEART DISEASES

Coronary Heart Disease: Risk Factors

Bilal Aijaz, Vera Bittner

Chapter Outline

INTRODUCTION

Cardiovascular disease (CVD) remains the leading cause of death in the United States and many other parts of the world and results in substantial disability and loss of productivity. Coronary heart disease (CHD) and stroke are the leading contributors to this heavy CVD burden. The exact mechanisms underlying development of CVD still remain to be fully described. However, through population-based studies starting in the 1940s and 1950s and intervention trials later, multiple risk factors for the development of CVD have been identified. The term 'risk factor' was in fact first used in the context of CHD.[1] A risk factor is any personal, environmental, psychosocial or genetic characteristic that gives an individual a higher likelihood of developing a particular disease. Even though the risk factor is a mere statistical association to an outcome, the current use of the term 'risk factor' often implies causalty. On the other hand, a 'risk marker' has association with a disease but a cause and effect relationship either does not exist or remains to be proven. These terms have evolved over the years and are non-uniformly used in the literature.

Cardiovascular disease risk factors are generally categorized into traditional/conventional and novel/emerging risk factors (Table 1). Risk factors can be inherited or acquired, some are modifiable and others are not. Risk factors may be defined dichotomously by their presence or absence or measured as a continuous variable.

The treatment of CVD risk factors has contributed to the fall in CVD mortality in the past 30 years, at least in developed countries.[2] At the same time, the prevalence of CVD and heart failure has increased due to higher survival rates and an aging population. More recent data suggest that we have reached a plateau in CVD mortality, which correlated with the obesity and physical inactivity epidemics. This highlights the challenge of CVD management: both identification and effective treatment of risk factors are required. Despite identification of patients at risk for CHD, significant gaps remain in implementing treatment. For instance, up to 15–20% of high risk patients discharged from the hospital, such as those with acute coronary syndrome, are not initiated on recommended combination therapy of aspirin, beta-blocker, statin and angiotensin

TABLE 1

Risk factors for cardiovascular disease

Traditional risk factors	
Modifiable	*Non-modifiable*
• Hypertension • Diabetes • Hyperlipidemia • Obesity • Tobacco use • Physical inactivity	• Age (male ≥ 45 years, female ≥ 55 years) • Gender • Family history of premature coronary artery disease*
Selected emerging risk factors	
• C-reactive protein • Small LDL particles • Lipoprotein(a) • Homocysteine • Lipoprotein-associated phospholipase A2 • Coagulation and hemostatic factors • Apolipoproteins A and B • White blood cell count	
(*Definite myocardial infarction or sudden death before 55 years of age in father or other male first-degree relative or before 65 years of age in mother or other female first-degree relative)	

TABLE 2

WHO principles for screening*

1. Condition screened should be an important health problem
2. There should be a suitable test for diagnosis
3. There should be an accepted treatment
4. Facilities for diagnosis and treatment should be available
5. The screening should be cost-effective
6. There should be a recognizable latent stage
7. The natural history should be adequately understood
8. Case finding should be a continuous process

(*Source:* Wilson JMG, Junger G. Principles and practice of screening for disease. Public Health Pap. Geneva: World Health Organization; 1968)

converting enzyme inhibitors. Fewer are referred to comprehensive risk reduction programs like cardiac rehabilitation suggesting that lifestyle risk factors are even less likely to be addressed.[3] As our quest for finding new risk factors and development of new therapeutic strategies is ongoing, we also have to devise ways to uniformly implement effective risk factor treatment.

CHD SCREENING AND PREVENTION

The high lifetime risk of CHD warrants population wide screening for prevention and treatment. The long lag time between the onset of atherosclerosis and its related morbidity and mortality allows for detection and early intervention. Screening involves routine evaluation of asymptomatic people. The widely accepted World Health Organization (WHO) criteria for screening of disease are summarized in Table 2. Screening should be cost-effective with the goal of detecting, not excluding, disease. Using established risk factors, a significant percentage of 'at risk' individuals can be screened as a target for preventive strategies.[4]

Three to five levels of prevention are described in the context of CVD (Table 3), often with dissimilar definition. The Centers for Disease Control and Prevention describe a simple classification with three levels of prevention.[5] Primordial prevention or health promotion targets the population without risk factors and aims to prevent the development of risk factors. The goal of primary prevention is to prevent the development of CVD in individuals with one or more risk factors. Secondary prevention involves patients with established clinical disease with the goal to prevent recurrent CVD events and their complications. A fourth level referred to as tertiary prevention targets late stages of the disease with the goal of restoration and rehabilitation.

TABLE 3

Levels of prevention in cardiovascular disease

1.	Primordial prevention	Prevention of the risk factors for disease
2.	Primary prevention	Reduction in incidence of disease
3.	Secondary prevention	Reduction in the prevalence or consequence of disease
4.	Tertiary prevention	Reductions in complications or disability, rehabilitation or restoration of function

CLUSTERING AND MULTIPLICATIVE EFFECTS OF RISK FACTORS

Initially, risk factors for CHD, such as diabetes, hypertension and hyperlipidemia, were targeted and treated individually. However, risk factors often occur in clusters and show a multiplicative effect rather than a simple additive effect. This has important implications for treatment. Most persons in a population have moderate elevation in multiple risk factors rather than an extremely high level of any single risk factor. Similarly, most cardiovascular events occur in individuals with mild to moderate abnormality in multiple risk factors. Targeting only high levels of individual risk factors will target only a small fraction of the population. Various expert groups stress the concept of 'comprehensive risk factor management'.

CHD RISK ESTIMATION

Despite our knowledge and understanding of many CHD risk factors, a clinical challenge is to effectively predict risk of CHD in individuals to allow appropriate and cost-effective treatment. Risk estimates are also used to raise awareness about CHD, determine population attributable risk to target specific public health measures, and to communicate risk to patients.

Coronary heart disease risk estimation measures the likelihood of a person developing a serious cardiovascular event over a specific follow-up time. Several multivariable models exist to predict the risk for future CHD and CVD (Table 4), many derived from the Framingham cohorts. Risk estimation results are critically dependent on the time frame of prediction. Earlier risk scores predicted short-term and medium-term risk of ≤ 10 years. More recently, long-term and lifetime risk estimation algorithms have been developed.[6,7] Risk estimation also depends on the endpoint chosen, for instance, CHD versus overall cardiovascular risk[8] and within CHD, 'hard events' such as myocardial infarction and CHD death or 'hard and soft endpoints' which also include angina pectoris and revascularization.

Refining and improving risk prediction is a major area of research in cardiovascular medicine. Key issues related to CVD risk estimation include the optimal time frame for risk assessment (short term, long term or lifetime), development of age-specific absolute risk models, defining cut offs for different risk categories, determining eligibility for pharmacological treatment, integration of imaging modalities to detect atherosclerosis and determining whether using a particular risk score will eventually result in better patient outcomes.

FRAMINGHAM RISK SCORE (FRS)

FRS and National Cholesterol Education Program's Third Adult Treatment Panel update (NCEP ATP III) are the most widely used risk scores (Table 4). FRS predicts the 10-year risk of CHD using a multivariable mathematical model of risk.[9] The calculator is available at: (http://www.framinghamheartstudy.org/risk/hrdcoronary.html). The NCEP ATP III risk assessment tool predicts the 10-year risk of hard CHD (myocardial infarction and coronary death).[10] The calculator is available at: (http://hp2010.nhlbihin.net/atpIII/calculator.asp?usertype=prof). Intensity of risk factor treatment is guided by the magnitude of absolute risk. Absolute risk is divided into three risk categories:

TABLE 4

Risk prediction scores for cardiovascular disease

Risk score (year)	Study summary	Variables	End point
Framingham Risk Score (1998)	5,209 men and women, ages 30–62 yrs Follow-up 10 yrs 10-year risk	Age, diabetes, smoking, hypertension, total cholesterol and LDL-C	All CHD
Framingham Risk Score for General Cardiovascular Disease (2008)	Men and women, ages 30–74 yrs without CVD at baseline Follow-up 12 yrs 10-year risk	Age, diabetes, smoking, treated and untreated systolic blood pressure, total cholesterol, HDL-C BMI replacing lipids in a simpler model	CVD (coronary death, myocardial infarction, coronary insufficiency, angina, ischemic stroke, hemorrhagic stroke, transient ischemic attack, peripheral artery disease, heart failure)
Reynolds Risk Score (2007)	24,558 women, age ≥ 45 yrs without CVD Median follow-up 10.2 yrs 10-year risk	Age, hemoglobin A_{1C}, smoking, systolic blood pressure, HDL-C, hs-CRP, total cholesterol, parental history of myocardial infarction at < 60 years	Global CVD (Composite end-point of cardiovascular death, myocardial infarction, ischemic stroke and coronary revascularization)
Reynolds Risk Score, men (2008)	10,724 men, ages 50–80 yrs 10-year risk	Age, hemoglobin A_{1C}, smoking, systolic blood pressure, HDL-C, hs-CRP, total cholesterol, parental history of myocardial infarction at < 60 years	Global CVD (Composite end-point of cardiovascular death, myocardial infarction, ischemic stroke and coronary revascularization)
Third Report of NCEP Adult Treatment Panel (2002, Update 2004)	Uses Framingham Risk Score 10-year risk	Variables same as Framingham risk score. Diabetes is considered a CVD equivalent	Hard CHD (CHD death and non-fatal myocardial infarction)
SCORE (2003)	205, 178 persons, ages 45–64 yrs 10-year risk	Age, cholesterol, smoking, systolic blood pressure Individuals with > 5% 10-year risk are defined as high risk	CVD death
QRISK (2007)	Derivation cohort 1.28 million patients, age 35–74 yrs. Median follow-up 6.5 years 10-year risk	Age, body mass index, ratio of total cholesterol to HDL-cholesterol, family history of premature cardiovascular disease, smoking, systolic blood pressure, deprivation score	CVD (myocardial infarction, ischemic stroke, transient ischemic attack and coronary heart disease)
Prospective cardiovascular Münster (PROCAM) (2002)	5,389 men, age 35–65 yrs 10-year follow-up	Age, LDL-C, smoking, HDL-C, systolic blood pressure, family history of premature myocardial infarction, diabetes mellitus, triglycerides Score 0 to > 60 with score > 53 defined as high risk (> 20% 10-year risk of cardiac event)	Hard CHD (sudden cardiac death or a definite fatal or nonfatal myocardial infarction)
Rasmussen Score (2003)	396 individuals	Blood pressure, N terminal proBNP, electrocardiogram, carotid intima-media thickness, microalbuminuria, treadmill exercise blood pressure, left ventricular ultrasound left ventricular mass index, small and large artery elasticity, optic fundoscopy for retinal vasculature	

(Abbreviations: CVD: Cardiovascular disease; CHD: Coronary heart disease; LDL-C: Low density cholesterol; HDL-C: High density cholesterol; hs-CRP: High-sensitivity C-reactive protein; NCEP: National cholesterol education program)

CHAPTER 45

Coronary Heart Disease: Risk Factors

high, intermediate and low risk (Table 5). High risk individuals include those with established CHD, diabetes, stroke, peripheral vascular disease or with multiple risk factors without established CHD, but a 10-year risk of CHD events greater than or equal to 20%. Certain individuals are considered 'very high-risk' and, according to the NCEP ATP III update,[11] they should be the target of more intensive lipid lowering therapy. This group includes individuals with established CVD in the presence of multiple major risk factors, especially if uncontrolled, or patients with acute coronary syndromes.

The FRS predicts major CHD events well in different populations.[12] Limitations of FRS are that it was developed exclusively in Caucasians. FRS does not include family history, obesity and psychosocial factors, which are important risk factors for CVD. FRS calculates only CHD risk and not the complete risk of other CVD processes including stroke, heart failure and peripheral vascular disease. The data used in the original Framingham Heart Study precede the obesity and physical inactivity epidemic. FRS is heavily influenced by age[13] and gender. For instance, most non-smoking men less than

TABLE 5

Risk categories for 10-year risk of coronary heart disease

Risk category definition	
High risk	CHD or CHD risk equivalent* or ≥ 2 risk factors[†] and 10-year predicted risk of ≥ 20%
Moderately high risk	≥ 2 Risk factors and 10-year predicted risk of 10–20%
Moderate risk	≥ 2 Risk factors and 10-year predicted risk of ≥ 10%
Low risk	0–1 Risk factor

*Peripheral arterial disease, diabetes mellitus; [†]Risk factors include cigarette smoking, hypertension (blood pressure ≥ 140/90 mm Hg or on antihypertensive medication), low high-density lipoprotein cholesterol (< 40 mg/dL), family history of premature CHD (CHD in male first-degree relative < 55 years of age; CHD in female first-degree relative < 65 years of age) and age (men ≥ 45 years; women ≥ 55 years)

45 years and almost all women less than 65 years of age have a 10-year risk of less than 10%. Despite some limitations, FRS is the most widely used and validated risk assessment tool and is able to provide remarkably good discrimination for the majority of individuals.[14]

EUROPEAN RISK SCORES

Since FRS is based on a North American sample, in Europe different risk scores were established including the Systematic Coronary Risk Evaluation (SCORE) project and the QRESEARCH cardiovascular RISK algorithm (QRISK). The SCORE[15] has been adopted by the Joint European Societies' guidelines on CVD prevention. The SCORE risk prediction system uses only fatal CVD as the outcome measure. The risk chart provides more detail for middle-aged persons in whom the risk changes with age. Separate charts are available for higher and lower risk areas in Europe. Individuals with a 10-year risk of CVD death of 5% or more are considered at an *increased risk* and qualify for intensive risk factor management.[16] A newer, computer-based tool for total risk estimation, which operates using the SCORE data, is called the HEARTSCORE (http://www.heartscore.org/eu/high/Pages/Welcome.aspx). The QRISK[17] algorithm was developed using the QRESEARCH database. The QRISK score includes family history of premature CHD, body mass index (BMI) and social deprivation that are not part of the FRS. A 2008 update (QRISK 2 score) contains additional variables including renal disease, atrial fibrillation and rheumatoid arthritis.[18]

NEWER RISK SCORES

Newer risk scores were developed in an attempt to overcome limitations of FRS and to incorporate emerging risk factors for CVD. A risk score's ability to reclassify patients at intermediate risk for CHD into higher risk for more aggressive management or lower risk categories for reassurance may clinically be useful. Some risk factor algorithms have eliminated laboratory based testing to reduce cost and increase availability, in particular to the primary care physicians, who are generally the first contact for the majority of the low-to-intermediate risk population.

The Reynolds risk score[19] for women was developed in 24,558 women from the Women's Health Study. In addition to traditional subject-reported risk factors, it incorporates family history of myocardial infarction, high-sensitivity C-reactive protein (hs-CRP) and hemoglobin A_{1C}. In the original study, Reynolds risk score was able to reclassify 40–50% of intermediate risk women into higher or lower risk categories. Later, a Reynolds risk score for men was developed in a cohort of 10,724 men from the Physicians Health Study II. This risk score reclassified 18% of men into a higher or lower risk category.[20] The risk calculator is available at http://www.reynoldsriskscore.org.

A general CVD risk prediction model was developed by D'Agostino et al.[8] using the original and offspring cohorts of the Framingham study. The risk estimation is for all CVD events compared to only CHD events in FRS. The investigators formulated two separate risk scoring models: one based on standard risk factors including laboratory variables and another using only non-laboratory based clinical variables. This risk assessment tool also presents the concept of 'vascular age' of an individual. Vascular age is the chronological age with optimal risk factors that gives the same predicted risk as that of the individual whose risk is being estimated. Currently, there are no established cut-offs for what is considered high risk when using global risk score. Published studies have used a 10-year risk of a CVD event of greater than 20% as the cut-off. To overcome the limitation of short-term risk prediction, recently, long-term and lifetime risk estimation algorithms have been developed.[7] Lifetime risk estimation may be useful for younger patients who have low short-term risk but high lifetime risk. In fact, data from the National Health and Nutrition Examination Survey 2003 to 2006 suggest that over 50% of US adults with a low 10-year risk have a high lifetime risk of CVD.[21] Initiating earlier treatment may result in substantial benefit over the life of these individuals but also potentially exposes them to long-term pharmacological therapy, of which the safety and cost-effectiveness is not fully established.

In contrast to the traditional approach of identifying risk factors for CVD, others have proposed direct assessment of the presence and severity of atherosclerosis/vascular disease. Cohn et al. developed the Rasmussen score[22] based on ten parameters including imaging modalities such as echocardiogram and carotid ultrasound. Similarly, the Screening for Heart Attack Prevention and Education (SHAPE) Task Force issued a consensus statement recommending that all asymptomatic men (45–75 years) and women (55–75 years) with a 10-year risk of CHD greater than 5% should undergo noninvasive imaging to detect subclinical CHD.[23] The SHAPE task force II is currently working to update to these guidelines.

MEASURES TO EVALUATE RISK PREDICTION MODELS

Several metrics exist to help clinicians evaluate the performance and utility of risk prediction scores including discrimination, calibration and reclassification.[24] Discrimination is the ability of a model to separate those with or without disease. The C statistic or area under the receiver operating characteristic (ROC) curve is widely used to report the discrimination ability of a risk score. It indicates the probability of a randomly selected case having a higher score than a noncase. For instance, a C statistic of 0.80 predicts that a patient with disease will have a higher score compared to a healthy patient 80% of the time. 1.0 is perfect discrimination and 0.5 is random chance. A C statistic greater than 0.70 is considered an acceptable level of discrimination. The C statistic does not quantitate the difference of risk between the case and the noncase. Large odds ratios or relative risks are required to achieve an acceptable C statistic score.

Calibration of a test determines its ability to accurately predict the absolute level of risk by comparing the predicted to the observed event rate. A good model will have an observed event rate close to the predicted rate. A test may have good discrimination but poor calibration. Generally, a model cannot have a perfect discrimination and be perfectly calibrated at the same time.

Other measures include likelihood ratio tests and Bayes information criterion which are sensitive assessments, used as initial measures to ascertain the global fit of the model.[25] These assess the ability of a score to predict disease incidence better than by chance alone. A penalty is paid for the number of variables included. A risk score's ability to reclassify individuals from one risk category to another is also used to evaluate the utility of the model. Both the net reclassification improvement (NRI) (difference between appropriate reclassification and inappropriate reclassification) and how much the individual moved in order to be reclassified (termed the integrative discrimination index or IDI) are important when using reclassification.

TRADITIONAL CHD RISK FACTORS

NON-MODIFIABLE RISK FACTORS FOR CHD

Certain risk factors for CHD are non-modifiable including age, male gender and family history of CHD. Although these risk factors are non-modifiable, they are an essential part of the risk prediction algorithms and identification of patients at higher risk for CHD events. Based on the Framingham Heart Study and NCEP ATP III recommendations, a positive family history of premature CHD is defined as a coronary event in parents before age 55 years in men and 65 years in women. Parental CHD, on an average, doubles the risk of CHD in an adult offspring. CVD in siblings also increases the risk of incident CVD even after adjustment for traditional risk factors and parental history of CVD. Compared to parental CVD, sibling CVD is reported to be a stronger predictor of CVD.[26] The reported variability in risk with family history of CVD is possibly due to recall bias, difference in family size and referral bias.[26]

MODIFIABLE RISK FACTORS FOR CHD

Lifestyle Risk Factors

Lifestyle risk factors including physical inactivity, diet and psychosocial factors are established risk factors for CHD and carry considerable public health importance as targets for intervention. In the INTERHEART study,[27] healthy lifestyle behavior including eating fruits and vegetables, exercising regularly and avoiding smoking led to 80% lower relative risk for myocardial infarction.

Smoking: Cigarette smoking is an important risk factor not only for CVD but also due to its impact on non-cardiovascular morbidity and mortality. It is the single most important preventable cause of disease and early death.[28] Smoking is a major public health threat in low-to-middle income countries where CVD is already on the rise.

Cigarette smoking has several detrimental effects on the cardiovascular system including increase in heart rate and blood pressure, increased thrombogenesis, endothelial dysfunction, increased plaque instability and less favorable effects on lipids. These processes lead to a proinflammatory state and atherosclerosis. Cigarette smoking also decreases high density lipoprotein cholesterol (HDL-C) levels. These effects are directly proportional to the amount of tobacco smoked. There is no evidence that using filters or other barriers reduces the risk. Smoking cigars and pipe raises the risk of CHD, as does passive smoking. It is unclear if decreasing, but not quitting, tobacco use provides any benefit or not.[29] Quitting smoking both for asymptomatic persons and those with established CVD is an extremely effective preventive measure for decreasing CVD mortality. Past smokers continue to reduce their risk over 10 years and eventually reach that of a non-smoker. For secondary prevention, patients who quit smoking decrease their risk of recurrent myocardial infarction by 50%.[30] Patients who quit smoking after coronary artery bypass have better survival and lower rates of angina and hospital admissions compared to patients who continue to smoke.[31]

In the clinical setting, it is important that every patient undergoes a full assessment of smoking status. This includes amount, type and duration of cigarette smoking, any other tobacco products used, social and family environment and reason for smoking. Physicians should assess the patient's knowledge about specific harmful effects of smoking on the cardiovascular system. Practitioners can use the clinical practice guidelines issued by the US Department of Health and Human Services to effectively intervene on tobacco users. The five steps recommended for intervention, referred to as the 5As, are summarized in Table 6. It is important to continue to address

TABLE 6

The 5As for intervention for tobacco dependence*

1.	Ask about tobacco use	Identify and document tobacco use status for every patient at every visit
2.	Advise to quit	In a clear, strong and personalized manner urge every tobacco user to quit
3.	Assess willingness to make a quit attempt	Is the tobacco user willing to make a quit attempt at this time?
4.	Assist in quit attempt	For the patient willing to make a quit attempt, use counseling and pharmacotherapy to help him or her quit
5.	Arrange follow-up	Schedule follow-up contact, preferably within the first week after the quit date

(*Fiore et al. Treating Tobacco Use and Dependence: Clinical Practice Guideline. Rockville, MD: US Dept of Health and Human Services; 2000)

smoking cessation at every visit. Physicians can also use the opportunity at the time of an acute myocardial infarction to provide smoking cessation counseling, as patients are more likely to be motivated to quit. Multiple options exist to help with smoking cessation including providing self-help materials to patients,[32] behavioral counseling[33] and group therapy. Support from spouse and family may also be important. Data regarding acupuncture and hypnotherapy for smoking cessation is inconsistent and these are not currently recommended. Physicians should be aware of different pharmacological therapy options available including several nicotine preparations, the anti-depressant drug bupropion and the more recently introduced medication vareniciline. In most patients, smoking cessation is associated with only mild weight gain. Any deleterious effects of even modest-to-major weight gain are likely minor compared to the harmful effects of continued smoking.[34] At a public health and policy level, restricting smoking in public places and at work, limiting tobacco advertising and promotion, and preventing tobacco sales to minors are some of the ways by which tobacco use can be decreased.

Physical inactivity: Physical activity is any bodily movement that expends energy. It is generally measured by self-reporting or occasionally by activity monitors. Cardiorespiratory fitness is a physiological characteristic of a person measured by exercise testing. Regular physical activity improves cardiorespiratory fitness. Any planned physical activity with the intent of improving one's health or fitness is considered exercise. It is important to note that not all physical activity is exercise.

Physical inactivity is an important and increasingly common lifestyle factor contributing to the global burden of CVD. Data from several lines of investigation link physical inactivity to CHD morbidity and mortality. Physical inactivity and excess caloric intake have greatly contributed to the global obesity epidemic. Physical activity exerts multiple cardiovascular benefits including decreased risk of developing hypertension, insulin resistance, and dyslipidemia and beneficial effects on endothelial function and thrombogenesis. The minimum recommended level of physical activity includes moderate intensity exercise for 30 minutes on at least 5 days of the week. The daily 30 minutes can be accumulated in as little as 10-minute sessions and may include walking, cycling, gardening, elliptical, swimming, recreational sports, etc. There are no recommendations for the maximum amount of physical activity and the 'optimal' level likely varies among different individuals and the endpoint desired (metabolic change vs peak fitness). Nearly half of the population fails to meet even the recommended minimum physical activity.[35] The small amount of excess risk reported with vigorous physical activity is negligible compared to the beneficial effects of regular physical activity. In patients with established CHD, physical activity and cardiac rehabilitation decrease risk of future coronary events and mortality.[36]

Guidelines to help physicians evaluate physical activity level and counsel appropriately have been published.[37] Physicians should assess the level of physical activity (both leisure time and at work) for all patients. Physical activity can be measured by recall questionnaire, diary or using a pedometer. Exercise prescriptions can provide more specific instructions to help with compliance. Referral to exercise programs or rehabilitation centers should be made as appropriate.

Nutrition: Diet is an important risk factor for CVD and also directly influences multiple CVD risk factors. Several dietary factors including the intake of fruits, vegetables, fatty acids, fiber, alcohol, excess salt and the ratio of carbohydrates, fat and lipids have been studied in relation to CHD risk (Table 7). Both epidemiological studies and intervention trials have demonstrated the importance of a balanced diet for CHD prevention.

Dietary lipids have an important role in the formation of atheromatous plaque. Diets, high in saturated and trans-fatty acids, are linked to higher rates of CHD.[38] Saturated fatty acids increase low density lipoprotein cholesterol (LDL-C) concentration. The principal source of saturated fatty acids is animal products and some commercially prepared meals. Consumption of polyunsaturated fatty acids decreases LDL-C. Primary food sources of polyunsaturated fatty acids include vegetable oil, soya bean and rapeseed. Eicosapentaenoic acids (EPA) and docosahexaenoic acids (DHA) are members of the n-3 fatty acid group derived from fish oil. Intake of EPA and DHA reduces plasma triglycerides, increases HDL-C and has beneficial effects on the cardiovascular system. Multiple proposed mechanisms for the benefit of fish consumption and omega-3 fatty acids include anti-inflammatory, antiarrhythmic and antithrombotic effects.[39] Guidelines recommend less than 30% of total calories from dietary fat and less than 7% from saturated fats.[40,41] Dietary primary prevention trials show benefit of reduced saturated fatty acid intake and increase in polyunsaturated fat intake on clinical cardiovascular endpoints.[42] Such dietary data should not be extrapolated to include intake of corresponding supplements.

High sodium intake is linked to hypertension, CHD and death. Current recommendations for the general population are to consume less than 5–6 gm of salt daily (equivalent of roughly 2,000–2,400 mg of sodium).[41,43] A diet rich in fiber and natural products, fruits and vegetables decreases risk of CHD.[38] The idea of combining foods or different diets, a portfolio, to achieve cholesterol control was suggested in the 1990s. The dietary portfolio contains four main elements including soy, nuts, viscous fibers and plant sterols and has been shown to reduce cholesterol.[44]

Nutrition is often neglected when counseling about CVD prevention and treatment. Health care providers quote lack of time and knowledge as barriers to successful nutrition counseling. Misleading information from the media is compounded by the lack of clinical trials. Despite patient counseling, the results are often disappointing in bringing substantial change in nutrition habits. In general, a cardioprotective or healthy diet is well balanced and includes different food sources. It should include the recommended amounts of fatty acids and sodium. The diet should be rich in fruits, vegetables, whole grains and high fiber foods. Fish should be consumed at least twice weekly.[40] A balanced diet also helps to maintain a healthy body weight. Consultation with a dietitian should be sought whenever available.

Obesity: Obesity is an independent risk factor for CVD and increases mortality. Obesity is also associated with multiple other

TABLE 7

Select studies involving dietary interventions and cardiovascular outcomes

Reference, Year, Study design, Duration (N)	Study population	Intervention	Outcome	Results
Dasinger ML, et al. Comparison of Atkins, Ornish, Weight Watchers and Zone diets for weight loss and heart disease risk reduction, 2005, RCT, 12 months (N = 160)	160 adults aged 22–72 yrs	Assigned to Atkins, Zone, Weight Watchers or Ornish diets	1 year changes in baseline weight and cardiac risk factors, and self-selected dietary adherence rates per self-report	Modest weight loss and reduction in total/HDL-C, C reactive protein, insulin without any significant difference among different diets
Howard BV, et al. Low fat dietary pattern and risk of cardiovascular disease, 2006, RCT, 8.1 yrs (N = 48,835)	48,835 post-menopausal women aged 50–79 yrs	Assigned to reduced fat, high fruits, vegetables and grains group or a comparison group	Fatal and nonfatal CHD, fatal and nonfatal stroke, and CVD (composite of CHD and stroke)	No difference in CVD, CHD or stroke
Hooper L, et al. Dietary fat intake and prevention cardiovascular disease: Systematic review, 2001, Meta-analysis, at least 6 months of follow-up	27 studies (30,902 persons years of observation) included	Advice about reducing or modifying dietary fat intake	Total and cardiovascular mortality and cardiovascular morbidity	Small reduction in total mortality 0.98; 95% confidence of interval 0.86–1.12) and cardiovascular mortality (0.91; 0.77–1.07). Cardiovascular events reduced by 16% (0.84; 0.72–0.99)
Hooper L, et al. Omega 3 fatty acids for prevention and treatment of cardiovascular disease, 2004, meta-analysis of RCTs and cohort studies, follow-up for at least 6 months, (N = 36,913)	36,913 participants from 48 RCTs and 41 cohort studies	Dietary or supplemental omega 3 fatty acids	Total mortality, cardiovascular events or cancers	No reduction in end point in persons taking additional omega 3 fats
de Lorgeril M, et al. Mediterranean diet, traditional risk factors, and the rate of cardiovascular complications after myocardial infarction: Final report of the Lyon Diet Heart Study, 1999, RCT, 5 yrs (N = 423)	423 patients with CHD	Mediterranean diet versus western prudent	Composite endpoints of cardiac death and nonfatal myocardial infarction. Additional endpoints also included (unstable angina, stroke, heart failure, pulmonary or peripheral embolism	Significant reduction in composite end point (risk ratio 0.28, 0.015–0.53)
Sacks FM, et al. Effects on blood pressure of reduced dietary sodium and the dietary approaches to stop hypertension (DASH) Diet, 2001, RCT, 5 yrs (N = 412)	412 participants	Comparing DASH diet (rich in vegetables, fruits and low-fat dairy products) to typical western diet	Reduction in blood pressure	DASH diet with a low sodium level led to a mean systolic blood pressure reduction of 7.1 mm Hg in participants without hypertension, and 11.5 mm Hg in participants with hypertension
Liu S, et al. Fruit and vegetable intake and risk of cardiovascular disease: The Women's Health Study, 2000, Prospective observational, 5 yrs (N = 39,876)	39,876 female health professionals without CVD or cancer	Assessing fruit and vegetable intake	Nonfatal myocardial infarction, stroke, percutaneous transluminal coronary angioplasty, coronary artery bypass graft or death due to CVD	Significant inverse association between fruit and vegetable intake and CVD risk. Compared to median serving of 2.6/day the relative risk in those consuming 10.2 servings/day was 0.68 (0.51, 0.92; P = 0.01).
Tuttle KR, et al. Comparison of low-fat versus Mediterranean-style dietary intervention after first myocardial infarction (from The Heart Institute of Spokane Diet Intervention and Evaluation Trial), 2008, RCT, 46 months (N = 202)	202 patients with CHD	Comparison of Mediterranean diet, low fat diet and controls	Reduction in cardiovascular event and morality after first myocardial infarction	Primary outcome did not differ between Mediterranean and low fat diets but was significantly lower in either diet compared to the usual diet with adjusted odd ratio of 0.28 (0.13–0.63, p = 0.002)
Swain JF, et al. Characteristics of the diet patterns tested in the optimal macronutrient intake trial to prevent heart disease (OmniHeart): options for a heart-healthy diet, 2008, RCT, 19 weeks (N = 164)	164 participants with prehypertension and hypertension	Comparison of carbohydrate rich, high protein and high fat diet	Estimated cardio-vascular risk	All three diets reduced blood pressure, total and low-density lipoprotein cholesterol levels, and estimated CHD risk

(Abbreviations: RCT: Randomized controlled trial; CHD: Coronary heart disease; CVD: Cardiovascular disease; HDL-C: High density lipoprotein cholesterol)

TABLE 8

Effects of obesity on different organ systems and diseases

- Increase heart rate, blood volume and cardiac output
- Left ventricular hypertrophy
- Diastolic dysfunction
- Obesity cardiomyopathy and congestive heart failure
- Arrhythmias
- Venous stasis and insufficiency
- Pulmonary thromboembolism
- Endothelial dysfunction
- Hypertension
- Dyslipidemia
- Insulin resistance
- Proinflammatory state
- Sleep apnea
- Pulmonary hypertension
- Stroke
- Coronary heart disease

TABLE 10

Ethnic specific values for abnormal waist circumference

Ethnic group/region	Waist circumference	
North America	Male	$\geq$ 102 cm
	Female	$\geq$ 88 cm
Europe	Male	$\geq$ 94 cm
	Female	$\geq$ 80 cm
South Asians	Male	$\geq$ 90 cm
	Female	$\geq$ 80 cm
Chinese	Male	$\geq$ 90 cm
	Female	$\geq$ 80 cm
Japanese	Male	$\geq$ 90 cm
	Female	$\geq$ 90 cm
South and Central America	Use South Asian recommendations	
Middle East (Arab) and Eastern Mediterranean	Use European recommendations	

CVD risk factors (Table 8), which in turn adversely affects the heart.[45] Obesity has reached epidemic proportions in many industrialized countries and its prevalence continues to increase, posing a major global health problem. Prevalence of childhood and adolescent obesity is also on the rise. Sedentary lifestyle, ease of access to food, increase in portion size and caloric intake are important reasons for the current obesity epidemic. Genetic factors and certain other environmental factors also predispose some individuals to excess weight.

Mechanisms by which obesity is associated with CVD are not completely understood. Adipocytes act as an endocrine organ and may play a central role in the pathogenesis through the release of adipocytokines. The role of different fat depots is also under active research. Several measures exist to define obesity, the commonest being BMI. The BMI is calculated as weight (kg)/height (m²). Obesity is defined as BMI of greater than or equal to 30 (Table 9). Other indexes of obesity include waist circumference and waist-hip ratio, increases in which are also linked to adverse cardiovascular outcomes. Different cut-offs for abnormal waist circumferences according to ethnicity are summarized in Table 10. Both BMI and waist circumference should be recorded for overall risk assessment and tracked over time as a vital sign.

Weight loss can prevent and improve obesity related risk factors and CVD. Interventions for weight management include dietary changes, increased physical activity, pharmacological therapy and surgical treatment. A weight reducing diet combined

TABLE 9

Classification of obesity by body mass index

Body mass index (kg/m²)	
• Underweight	< 18.5
• Normal	18.5–24.9
• Overweight	25.0–29.9
• Obesity Class	
— I	30.0–34.9
— II	35.0–39.9
— III	$\geq$ 40

with exercise can result in significant weight loss.[46] Reduction in calorie intake, regardless of the proportion of macronutrients (fats, proteins or carbohydrates), results in clinically meaningful weight loss.[47]

Despite great interest in pharmacotherapy for obesity, its clinical use is limited by modest weight loss, high relapse rate and side effects of the medications. Fenfluramine and dexfenfluramine were withdrawn due to their adverse effects on heart valves. Orlistat, a gastrointestinal lipase inhibitor, induces weight loss by decreasing fat absorption.[48] It is FDA approved and is available also for over the counter use for weight loss. Common side effects include oily stools, diarrhea and gas. Rimonabant, a selective cannabinoid-1 receptor blocker, improved weight and cardiovascular risk factors,[49] but was not approved in the United States over concerns about psychiatric side effects and did not reduce cardiovascular events in one large clinical trial.[50]

Surgical treatment for obesity includes various malabsorptive or restrictive procedures. In patients who have failed an adequate diet and exercise program, with severe obesity (BMI $\geq$ 40) or medically complicated obesity with a BMI greater than or equal to 35, bariatric surgery may be considered.[51,52] Long-term follow-up of patients after bariatric surgery continues to show weight loss, improvement in CVD risk factors and lower mortality.[53]

Psychosocial factors: Several psychosocial factors are associated with increased risk of CVD including depression, stress, anxiety, social isolation, lack of social support and stress at work.[54] In a meta-analysis, depression was shown to increase the risk of CHD by 64%.[55] In the MRFIT study greater depressive symptoms were associated with increased 18-year mortality.[56] Depression especially after coronary events is not only common but also increases the incidence of recurrent coronary event by threefold.[57] Lower socioeconomic class and adverse events in life are also associated with CVD. Poor socio-economic status is linked to increased risk of CHD through multiple mechanisms including unhealthy diet, lack of access to health care, excessive stress and tobacco use.

Type A behavior with associated hostility and anger raises the risk of CHD.[58] Social isolation and lack of social support may increase the risk of CHD by 2–3 fold in men and 3–5 fold in women.[59] Marital discord worsens prognosis in acute coronary syndrome. Psychosocial risk factors tend to cluster in the same individuals and groups; for instance, job stress is linked to depression, hostility, anger and social isolation. This compounds the risk of CVD.

Psychosocial factors raise the risk of CVD through several mechanisms including greater likelihood of unhealthy behaviors such as smoking, alcohol and drug use and increased calorie intake and direct physiologic effects such as increased platelet activation and increase in inflammatory cytokines[60] and neuroendocrine reactivity[61] to stress.

Management of psychosocial risk factors is challenging in part due to the difficulty in defining an individual's level of risk and in part due to complex treatment. Moreover, the influence of these factors in any individual may change over time. Few trials show benefits of behavioral intervention on CVD risk or outcomes. Meditation decreases blood pressure and carotid artery intimal thickness in men. Extended cardiac rehabilitation (stress management combined with physical training and cooking sessions) improved depression, anxiety and quality of life at one year in patients with CHD.[62] In the Recurrent Coronary Prevention Project, behavioral counseling resulted in reduced type A behavior and decrease in cardiac risk.[63] Behavioral treatment in The Enhancing Recovery in Coronary Heart Disease (ENRICHD) trial reduced depression and social isolation in post-MI patients, but did not improve survival.[64] To reduce psychosocial risk factors, emphasis needs to be placed on modifying stress, improving quality of life and recognizing and treating depression and other mood disorders.

Hypertension

Hypertension defined as a blood pressure of greater than or equal to 140/90 mm Hg is a major risk factor for CVD. In fact, there is a strong, graded relationship between blood pressure and fatal coronary events: risk doubles for every 20 mm Hg increase in systolic blood pressure or 10 mm Hg increase in diastolic blood pressure. Various mechanisms by which hypertension leads to coronary events include hemodynamic stress on blood vessels and heart, increased myocardial oxygen demand, diminished coronary blood flow and impaired endothelial function. Several trials have shown reduction in cardiovascular morbidity and mortality by reduction in blood pressure.[65]

The seventh report of the Joint National Committee (JNC) on prevention, detection, evaluation, and treatment of high blood pressure recommends a treatment goal of less than 140/90 mm Hg for all individuals, however, in patients with CHD, renal insufficiency, congestive heart failure, peripheral vascular disease and diabetes a stricter goal of less than 130/80 mm Hg is recommended.[66] Treatment of pre-hypertension (blood pressure 120–139/80–89 mm Hg) with Candesartan reduced the risk of incident hypertension in the TROPHY trial.[67] Whether lowering of blood pressure to 'normal' (< 120/80 mm Hg) is beneficial is not clear. The next JNC guidelines are expected to be released in 2012.

Nonpharmacological interventions such as dietary modification,[68] moderation of alcohol consumption, smoking cessation, increasing physical activity and weight loss improve blood pressure and are recommended for any level of hypertension. Multiple drug classes exist to treat hypertension including beta blockers, calcium channel blockers, diuretics, angiotensin converting enzyme inhibitors, angiotensin receptor blockers, renin inhibitors, vasodilators and centrally acting agents. First-line therapy is usually tailored to drug availability, cost, comorbid medical conditions and side effect profile of medications. Blood pressure lowering is more important than the choice of drug class. In a meta-analysis of 29 randomized controlled trials,[69] Turnbull et al. found that there were no significant differences in the primary endpoint of major cardiovascular events between regimens based on angiotensin converting enzyme inhibitors, calcium antagonists, diuretics or beta-blockers.

Hyperlipidemia

There is a strong positive association between total cholesterol and LDL-C and CVD risk. Elevated triglycerides and low HDL-C are also independent risk factors for CVD. Individuals with severely elevated levels of LDL-C due to genetic abnormalities show premature atherosclerosis. Conversely, individuals with certain loss of function variants of the PCSK9 gene, who have moderate life-long reduction in LDL-C, have up to 88% reduction in risk of CHD.[70] Different mechanisms by which LDL-C increases CHD include delivery of cholesterol to blood vessels, proinflammatory properties, role in plaque formation and plaque instability. High levels of HDL-C convey reduced risk of CHD. HDL-C exerts its protective effects on the cardiovascular system through numerous mechanisms including reverse cholesterol transport, antioxidant properties, inhibition of apoptosis and dysfunction of endothelial cells and inhibition of LDL oxidation.[71] Low HDL-C and elevated triglycerides frequently occur with the presence of small dense LDL particles. This pattern of dyslipidemia is referred to as diabetic or atherogenic dyslipidemia.

Elevated LDL-C is the primary target for therapy and reduction in LDL-C substantially reduces CHD risk. In patients with elevated triglycerides (≥ 200 mg/dL), non-HDL-C (total cholesterol minus HDL-C) is a secondary target for therapy due to a strong association with CHD risk.[72] Non-HDL-C highly correlates with levels of apolipoprotein B which is the major apolipoprotein of all major atherogenic lipoproteins. The non-HDL-C treatment goal is 30 mg/dL higher than LDL-C.

Lifestyle changes are important for management of hyperlipidemia including reduction in intake of saturated fats and cholesterol, increasing fiber intake, increasing physical activity and weight reduction. Pharmacological therapy is required to treat hyperlipidemia in many patients. The availability of HMG-CoA reductase inhibitors (statins) has revolutionized treatment for both primary and secondary prevention of CVD. Multiple large randomized controlled clinical trials have shown benefits of using statins for treatment of hyperlipidemia with an estimated 20–40% reduction in major cardiovascular events and mortality.[73] The reduction in risk for an individual depends both on their initial overall risk for CVD as well as the degree of elevation in cholesterol, in particular

LDL-C. Statins are usually first-line agents but combination therapy is sometimes required when LDL-C elevation is pronounced or multiple lipid abnormalities are present. Available agents include bile acid sequestrants, nicotinic acid, fibrates, ezetimibe or high doses of EPA/DHA. For low HDL-C, after controlling LDL-C and instituting lifestyle changes, niacin or fibrates can be used. Caution should be used when combining fibrate therapy with statins as it increases the risk of myopathy. Markedly elevated triglyceride levels (> 500 mg/dl) should be treated to prevent pancreatitis. The next NCEP guidelines are expected to be released in 2012.

Diabetes Mellitus

Diabetes is a strong and independent risk factor for CVD. Whether diabetes confers a risk of events similar to that of established CHD is controversial,[74,75] but current guidelines consider diabetes a CHD equivalent. Mechanisms by which diabetes causes CHD include increase in platelet aggregability, increase in inflammatory mediators, impaired endothelial function, dyslipidemia, increase in highly small, dense highly atherogenic LDL-C, among others.

Intensive glycemic control (hemoglobin A_{1C} ~7%) prevents microvascular complications but the impact on macrovascular complications including cardiovascular events is less well established. Recent large trials including the ACCORD[76] and ADVANCE[77] failed to show benefit of tighter control of diabetes (Hemoglobin A_{1C} < 6–6.5%) compared to usual glycemic control (Hemoglobin A_{1C} 7–7.9%) on major cardiovascular events. The American Diabetes Association and other major societies recommend a target Hemoglobin A_{1C} goal of less than 7%.[78]

Lifestyle interventions for prevention and treatment of diabetes are well established and are the recommended initial strategy.[79,80] Several different classes of drugs exist for treatment of diabetes the details of which are beyond the scope of this chapter.

Alcohol

Numerous prospective studies have suggested an inverse relation between moderate alcohol consumption (1–2 drinks per day) and CHD.[81] Mechanisms by which alcohol may exert beneficial effects on CHD include antioxidant effects, increase in HDL-C and antithrombotic action.[82] It is unclear if any particular type of alcoholic beverage is more protective. At the same time, alcohol use is associated with several health problems including cardiomyopathy, sudden cardiac death, cardiac arrhythmias, hypertension and stroke. Alcohol is an addictive substance and abuse of it remains a major public health problem.

Due to limitations of observational data, lack of clinical trials and the health hazards associated with its use, alcohol intake is not recommended as a cardioprotective strategy.[83] For patients with current or past abuse, systemic diseases including hepatic or cardiac problems, it is best to advise against alcohol use. On a case-by-case basis, for individuals who drink, 1–2 drinks per day for men and 1 drink for women is acceptable to advise.

EMERGING RISK FACTORS

More than a hundred non-traditional or emerging risk factors have been reported.[84] Whether they independently predict risk of CHD or add incremental information to existing risk factors continues to generate controversy and poses an obstacle to their incorporation into risk assessment and routine clinical practice. For a risk factor to be accurate and effective in predicting risk, it must meet certain criteria: It must have a strong, consistent association with the disease in a dose-response manner that is biologically plausible. It should be measured easily with acceptable reference values. It should be an independent predictor of major CHD events. It should reclassify a substantial number of individuals who were previously stratified by traditional risk factors and the results should be generalizable to different population groups.[14] Before a novel risk factor or marker is incorporated into guidelines, its predictive value must be tested in multiple ways in different populations.

A recent US Preventive Services Task Force Recommendation Statement concludes that the current evidence is insufficient to assess the balance of benefits and harms of using non-traditional risk factors for screening asymptomatic men and women.[14,85] Similarly, NCEP ATP III guidelines do not recommend routine use of emerging risk factors for risk assessment.

The emerging risk factors include both laboratory-based tests for biomarkers of atherosclerosis and noninvasive imaging modalities for detecting atherosclerosis. Some of the more commonly used emergent risk factors will briefly be reviewed.

HIGH-SENSITIVITY C-REACTIVE PROTEIN (hs-CRP)

hs-CRP has been extensively studied to help in risk stratification for CHD events. CRP is an acute phase reactant that is made by the liver. Inflammatory conditions result in a rise in CRP levels. Several CVD risk factors are also associated with higher levels of CRP. For cardiovascular risk prediction, an hs-CRP assay exists with levels less than 1.0 mg/L considered low risk, between 1.0–3.0 as intermediate risk and greater than 3.0 as high risk. hs-CRP independently predicts coronary events,[86] however, the risk is modest with about 1.5 times elevated risk of coronary events in patients with CRP greater than 2.0, after adjustment for traditional CHD risk factors.[87] The American Heart Association and Centers for Disease Control and Prevention endorse using hs-CRP as an optional test to help with further classification in particular of those patients who are at intermediate risk by FRS (Class IIa).[88]

Weight loss, physical activity, smoking cessation, cholesterol therapy with statins and niacin all decrease hs-CRP levels. In a subgroup of the Air Force/Texas Coronary Atherosclerosis Prevention Study (AFCAPS/Tex-CAPS) study Ridker et al.[89] showed that participants with LDL-C below and hs-CRP above the median benefited from lovastatin therapy [relative risk, 0.58 (0.34, 0.98)] in contrast to those participants with both LDL-C and hs-CRP below the median whose coronary events were not reduced [relative risk, 1.08 (0.56–2.08)]. Results from the randomized controlled JUPITER trial[90] suggest that hs-CRP could be used to select patients (women $\geq$ 60 years, men $\geq$ 50 years) for primary prevention with statins. For secondary prevention, a sub-analysis from the PROVE IT study showed that lowering hs-CRP in patients with acute coronary syndrome with statins resulted in lower risk of future coronary events.[91]

LIPOPROTEIN (A) [LP(A)]

Lp(a) consists of an LDL particle linked to an apo A polypeptide chain. Levels of Lp(a) are genetically determined. There are no observed gender differences but racial differences exist. Whether Lp(a) is causally linked to CHD remains controversial.[92] A recent study using genetic data suggested causal relation of elevated Lp(a) to myocardial infarction.[93]

The European Atherosclerosis Society recommends screening for Lp(a) in patients at intermediate or high risk for CHD.[94] Levels of Lp(a) less than 50 mg/dL were recommended as the treatment goal using niacin, while acknowledging that randomized controlled trials are lacking. A North American panel endorsed testing for Lp(a) in patients who are moderate to high risk according to FRS, and decreasing the LDL-C treatment goal by 30 mg/dL in patients with high levels of Lp(a) (> 200 ng/mL).[95]

HYPERHOMOCYSTEINEMIA

Homocysteine is an intermediary product of methionine metabolism. Homocysteine can cause endothelial dysfunction and result in a procoagulant state. Many cross-sectional and prospective observational studies report a positive association between homocysteine levels and CVD. Untreated patients who are homozygous for homocystinuria have serum homocysteine concentrations five times above normal and increased risk of vascular events.

Dietary intake of folate, vitamin B6 and B12 affect homocysteine levels. Despite observational data linking homocysteine to CVD, multiple randomized controlled trials using supplementation with vitamin B12 and folic acid showed no reduction in the risk of major cardiovascular events in patients with or without preexisting vascular disease.[96,97] The 2007 American Heart Association guidelines for prevention of CVD in women recommend against using folic acid supplementation, with or without B6 and B12 for CVD prevention.[98]

LIPOPROTEIN-ASSOCIATED PHOSPHOLIPASE A2 (LP-PLA2)

Lp-PLA2 is an enzyme expressed by inflammatory cells in atherosclerotic plaques. In observational and epidemiological studies, Lp-PLA2 was modestly associated with an increased risk of CHD.[99] There is an approximately 10% increase in coronary events per one standard deviation higher Lp-PLA2 activity and mass. In one study[100] Lp-PLA2 increased the ROC curve minimally suggesting some clinical improvement in risk discrimination. Even though the FDA has approved a test for Lp-PLA2 for CHD, there is no trial evidence to date that Lp-PLA2 modification changes risk. A randomized controlled trial (STABILITY) involving the Lp-PLA2 inhibitor darapladib is expected to be reported in late 2012.

TABLE 11

Hemostatic factors associated with cardiovascular disease

- Fibrinogen
- Fibrin D-dimer
- Factor VII
- Factor VIII
- Plasminogen activator inhibitor
- Tissue plasminogen activator
- von Willebrand factor antigen
- Activated partial thromboplastin time
- Thrombin-antithrombin
- Activated protein C ratio

APOLIPOPROTEIN B

Apoliporotein B (Apo B) is a structural component of several lipoprotein particles which are atherogenic. Standardized assays for measurement of Apo B are available. Apo B is associated with increased risk of CHD.[101] Whether Apo B measurement predicts CHD risk beyond commonly assessed risk factors in the FRS is uncertain.[102]

Plasma Apo B levels may be useful as a treatment target. A target value of less than 85 mg/dL for patients at high risk for CHD is proposed by the Canadian Cardiovascular Society.[103] American Association of Clinical Chemistry recommends a treatment goal of less than 80 mg/dL in patients whose target LDL-C by NCEP ATPIII guidelines is less than 100 mg/dL.[104]

FIBRINOGEN AND OTHER HEMOSTATIC FACTORS

Several hemostatic factors involved in coagulation and fibrinolysis are associated with increased risk of CHD[105] (Table 11). Fibrinogen levels in the upper third of the control distribution are associated with a 2.0–2.5 times excess risk of future CVD.[106] The current assays are not standardized and whether fibrinogen and other hemostatic factors add to traditional risk factors is unclear. Physical activity can decrease levels of fibrinogen but there is no evidence from randomized trials that fibrinogen modification by lifestyle or pharmacological therapy decreases CHD events.

SUB-CLINICAL ATHEROSCLEROSIS

Detecting sub-clinical atherosclerosis with noninvasive imaging modalities has generated great interest. This is distinct from the general 'risk factor' concept. Whether early detection of atherosclerosis should lead to modification in therapy and whether such modification in therapy offers clinical benefit is not clear.

The presence of calcium in coronary arteries correlates with atherosclerosis and is measured using cardiac tomographic imaging. Coronary artery calcium (CAC) score, which quantifies the extent of coronary calcium, is reported as percentiles of calcification according to age and sex. A 'negative' test has a CAC score of 0 and is associated with a low risk of subsequent coronary events. Numerous studies show that CAC testing is an independent predictor of coronary events in both men and women, from multiple racial and ethnic groups.[107,108] CAC score has high sensitivity and negative predictive value for angiographically obstructive CAD but its positive predictive value is low.[24] To date, it is unclear whether CAC testing should lead to change in therapy if that results in a favorable impact on clinical outcomes. Cost and radiation exposure also limit widespread CAC screening. CAC score may be used in select intermediate risk patients for further risk stratification.

Vascular intimal thickening is one of the earliest changes of atherosclerosis. Carotid arteries can easily be visualized because of their location and using ultrasound techniques the intima-media thickness can be determined noninvasively, without exposure to radiation. Increased carotid intima-media thickness is an independent predictor of cardiovascular risk.[109] Carotid intima-media thickness also correlates with multiple CVD risk factors.[110] Statin treatment decreases Carotid intima-media thickness. There is lack of consensus on examination techniques and reference standards for quantifying intima-media thickness.[85] Recently, the American Society of Echocardiography published a consensus statement proposing standardization of imaging and measurement protocols.[111] Correct patient selection, assessment of clinical benefit of treatment and lack of outcome data limits widespread use at present.

Ankle brachial index is a noninvasive test to diagnose and assess the severity of peripheral vascular disease. It is the ratio of systolic blood pressure in the ankle, measured at the level of the posterior tibial or dorsalis pedis artery, to that of the brachial artery. A lower value of ankle brachial index is not only an indicator for the severity of peripheral vascular disease but also correlates independently with major coronary events and stroke.[112,113] When used in conjunction with FRS, a low ankle brachial index (≤ 0.90) approximately doubled the risk of cardiovascular events and death.[114]

At a population level, the best approach currently is probably to use the traditional risk factors for CHD screening. It is generally agreed that the established risk factors for CHD have very good ability to discriminate those at risk for CHD and account for over 90% of population attributable risk.[27] We need to ensure that the traditional risk factors and risk prediction tools are applied routinely in clinical practice. At the same time, clinicians should be aware of the emerging risk factors and may use their clinical judgment to use additional screening modalities to better gauge an individual patient's risk.

TRANSLATING RISK FACTOR SCREENING INTO EVENT REDUCTION

It is our responsibility to fully implement strategies to ensure that any risk factors identified are fully treated. Barriers to such implementation exist at the physician, patient, system and societal level.[115] Physicians can, through better communication and education, ensure better adherence to risk factor reduction strategies. Specific verbal and written instructions and prompt follow-up can help increase adherence. Monitoring progress goals and providing feedback can help patients stay on track, particularly with lifestyle modifications. There should be open communication between the specialists and primary care physicians. Enabling easy access to electronic medical records from index hospitalization as well as specialist visits should help primary care physicians to deliver risk factor reduction treatment on a long-term basis.

REFERENCES

1. Kannel WB, Dawber TR, Kagan A, et al. Factors of risk in the development of coronary heart disease—Six-year follow-up experience. The Framingham Study. Ann Intern Med. 1961;55:33-50.
2. Hunink MG, Goldman L, Tosteson AN, et al. The recent decline in mortality from coronary heart disease, 1980-1990. The effect of secular trends in risk factors and treatment. JAMA. 1997;277:535-42.
3. Brown TM, Hernandez AF, Bittner V, et al. Predictors of cardiac rehabilitation referral in coronary artery disease patients: findings from the American Heart Association's Get With The Guidelines Program. J Am Coll Cardiol. 2009;54:515-21.
4. Stamler J, Stamler R, Neaton JD, et al. Low risk-factor profile and long-term cardiovascular and noncardiovascular mortality and life expectancy: findings for 5 large cohorts of young adult and middle-aged men and women. JAMA. 1999;282:2012-8.
5. Mensah GA, Dietz WH, Harris VB, et al. Prevention and control of coronary heart disease and stroke—Nomenclature for prevention approaches in public health: a statement for public health practice from the Centers for Disease Control and Prevention. Am J Prev Med. 2005;29:152-7.
6. Lloyd-Jones DM, Leip EP, Larson MG, et al. Prediction of lifetime risk for cardiovascular disease by risk factor burden at 50 years of age. Circulation. 2006;113:791-8.
7. Pencina MJ, D'Agostino RB, Sr, Larson MG, et al. Predicting the 30-year risk of cardiovascular disease: the Framingham heart study. Circulation. 2009;119:3078-84.
8. D'Agostino RB, Sr, Vasan RS, Pencina MJ, et al. General cardiovascular risk profile for use in primary care: the Framingham Heart Study. Circulation. 2008;117:743-53.
9. Wilson PW, D'Agostino RB, Levy D, et al. Prediction of coronary heart disease using risk factor categories. Circulation. 1998;97:1837-47.
10. Expert Panel on Detection, Evaluation and Treatment of High Blood Cholesterol in Adults. Executive Summary of the Third Report of the National Cholesterol Education Program (NCEP) Expert Panel on Detection, Evaluation, and Treatment of High Blood Cholesterol in Adults (Adult Treatment Panel III). JAMA. 2001;285:2486-97.
11. Grundy SM, Cleeman JI, Merz CN, et al. Implications of recent clinical trials for the National Cholesterol Education Program Adult Treatment Panel III Guidelines. J Am Coll Cardiol. 2004;44:720-32.
12. D'Agostino RB, Sr, Grundy S, Sullivan LM, et al. Validation of the Framingham coronary heart disease prediction scores: results of a multiple ethnic groups investigation. JAMA. 2001;286:180-7.
13. Ridker PM, Cook N. Should age and time be eliminated from cardiovascular risk prediction models? Rationale for the creation of a new national risk detection program. Circulation. 2005;111:657-8.
14. US Preventive Services Task Force. Using nontraditional risk factors in coronary heart disease risk assessment: US Preventive Services Task Force Recommendation Statement. Ann Intern Med. 2009;151:1-38.
15. Conroy RM, Pyörälä K, Fitzgerald AP, et al. Estimation of ten-year risk of fatal cardiovascular disease in Europe: the SCORE project. Eur Heart J. 2003;24:987-1003.
16. Graham I, Atar D, Borch-Johnsen K, et al. European guidelines on cardiovascular disease prevention in clinical practice: executive summary. Eur Heart J. 2007;28:2375-414.
17. Hippisley-Cox J, Coupland C, Vinogradova Y, et al. Derivation and validation of QRISK: a new cardiovascular disease risk score for the United Kingdom: prospective open cohort study. BMJ. 2007;335:136.

18. Hippisley-Cox J, Coupland C, Vinogradova Y, et al. Predicting cardiovascular risk in England and Wales: prospective derivation and validation of QRISK2. BMJ. 2008;336:a332.

19. Ridker PM, Buring JE, Rifai N, et al. Development and validation of improved algorithms for the assessment of global cardiovascular risk in women: the Reynolds Risk Score. JAMA. 2007;297:611-9.

20. Ridker PM, Paynter NP, Rifai N, et al. C-reactive protein and parental history improve global cardiovascular risk prediction: the Reynolds Risk Score for men. Circulation. 2008;118:2243-51, 2244p following 2251.

21. Marma AK, Berry JD, Ning H, et al. Distribution of 10-year and lifetime predicted risks for cardiovascular disease in US adults: findings from the National Health and Nutrition Examination Survey 2003 to 2006. Circ Cardiovasc Qual Outcomes. 2010;3:8-14.

22. Cohn JN, Hoke L, Whitwam W, et al. Screening for early detection of cardiovascular disease in asymptomatic individuals. Am Heart J. 2003;146:679-85.

23. Naghavi M, Falk E, Hecht HS, et al. From vulnerable plaque to vulnerable patient—Part III: executive summary of the Screening for Heart Attack Prevention and Education (SHAPE) Task Force report. Am J Cardiol. 2006;98:2H-15H.

24. Greenland P, Lloyd-Jones D. Defining a rational approach to screening for cardiovascular risk in asymptomatic patients. J Am Coll Cardiol. 2008;52:330-2.

25. Cook NR. Use and misuse of the receiver operating characteristic curve in risk prediction. Circulation. 2007;115:928-35.

26. Murabito JM, Nam BH, D'Agostino RB, Sr, et al. Accuracy of offspring reports of parental cardiovascular disease history: the Framingham Offspring Study. Ann Intern Med. 2004;140:434-40.

27. Yusuf S, Hawken S, Ounpuu S, et al. Effect of potentially modifiable risk factors associated with myocardial infarction in 52 countries (the INTERHEART study): case-control study. Lancet. 2004;364:937-52.

28. Mackay J, Mensah G. WHO Atlas of Heart Disease and Stroke. Geneva: Nonserial WHO Publication; 2004.

29. Stead LF, Lancaster T. Interventions to reduce harm from continued tobacco use. Cochrane Database Syst Rev. 2007;CD005231.

30. Hermanson B, Omenn GS, Kronmal RA, et al. Beneficial six-year outcome of smoking cessation in older men and women with coronary artery disease. Results from the CASS registry. N Engl J Med. 1988;319:1365-9.

31. Cavender JB, Rogers WJ, Fisher LD, et al. Effects of smoking on survival and morbidity in patients randomized to medical or surgical therapy in the Coronary Artery Surgery Study (CASS): 10-year follow-up. CASS Investigators. J Am Coll Cardiol. 1992;20:287-94.

32. Lancaster T, Stead LF. Self-help interventions for smoking cessation. Cochrane Database Syst Rev. 2005;CD001118.

33. Lancaster T, Stead LF. Individual behavioural counselling for smoking cessation. Cochrane Database Syst Rev. 2005;CD001292.

34. Williamson DF, Madans J, Anda RF, et al. Smoking cessation and severity of weight gain in a national cohort. N Engl J Med. 1991;324:739-45.

35. National Center for Chronic Disease Prevention and Health Promotion Behavioral Risk Factor Surveillance System. Adults with 30+ minutes of moderate physical activity five or more days per week, or vigorous physical activity for 20+ minutes three or more days per week. Prevalence and Trends Data for Physical Activiy. 2009.

36. Witt BJ, Jacobsen SJ, Weston SA, et al. Cardiac rehabilitation after myocardial infarction in the community. J Am Coll Cardiol. 2004;44:988-96.

37. US Department of Health and Human Services. Physical Activity Guidelines for Americans; 2008.

38. Hu FB, Willett WC. Optimal diets for prevention of coronary heart disease. JAMA. 2002;288:2569-78.

39. Hu FB, Bronner L, Willett WC, et al. Fish and omega-3 fatty acid intake and risk of coronary heart disease in women. JAMA. 2002;287:1815-21.

40. Lichtenstein AH, Appel LJ, Brands M, et al. Diet and lifestyle recommendations revision 2006: a scientific statement from the American Heart Association Nutrition Committee. Circulation. 2006;114:82-96.

41. Prevention of cardiovascular disease: guideline for assessment and management of cardiovascular risk. World Health Organization; 2007.

42. Turpeinen O, Karvonen MJ, Pekkarinen M, et al. Dietary prevention of coronary heart disease: the Finnish Mental Hospital Study. Int J Epidemiol. 1979;8:99-118.

43. Krauss RM, Eckel RH, Howard B, et al. AHA Dietary Guidelines: revision 2000: a statement for healthcare professionals from the Nutrition Committee of the American Heart Association. Circulation. 2000;102:2284-99.

44. Jenkins DJ, Josse AR, Wong JM, et al. The portfolio diet for cardiovascular risk reduction. Curr Atheroscler Rep. 2007;9:501-7.

45. Poirier P, Giles TD, Bray GA, et al. Obesity and cardiovascular disease: pathophysiology, evaluation, and effect of weight loss: an update of the 1997 American Heart Association Scientific Statement on Obesity and Heart Disease from the Obesity Committee of the Council on Nutrition, Physical Activity, and Metabolism. Circulation. 2006;113:898-918.

46. Avenell A, Brown TJ, McGee MA, et al. What interventions should we add to weight reducing diets in adults with obesity? A systematic review of randomized controlled trials of adding drug therapy, exercise, behaviour therapy or combinations of these interventions. J Hum Nutr Diet. 2004;17:293-316.

47. Sacks FM, Bray GA, Carey VJ, et al. Comparison of weight-loss diets with different compositions of fat, protein, and carbohydrates. N Engl J Med. 2009;360:859-73.

48. Sjöström L, Rissanen A, Andersen T, et al. Randomised placebo-controlled trial of orlistat for weight loss and prevention of weight regain in obese patients. European Multicentre Orlistat Study Group. Lancet. 1998;352:167-72.

49. Pi-Sunyer FX, Aronne LJ, Heshmati HM, et al. Effect of rimonabant, a cannabinoid-1 receptor blocker, on weight and cardiometabolic risk factors in overweight or obese patients: RIO-North America: a randomized controlled trial. JAMA. 2006;295:761-75.

50. Topol EJ, Bousser MG, Fox KA, et al. Rimonabant for prevention of cardiovascular events (CRESCENDO): a randomised, multicentre, placebo-controlled trial. Lancet. 2010;376:517-23.

51. Snow V, Barry P, Fitterman N, et al. Pharmacologic and surgical management of obesity in primary care: a clinical practice guideline from the American College of Physicians. Ann Intern Med. 2005;142:525-31.

52. North American Association for the Study of Obesity (NAASO) and the National Heart, Lung aBIN. Practical Guide to the Identification, Evaluation, and Treatment of Overweight and Obesity in Adults; 2000.

53. Sjöström L, Narbro K, Sjöström CD, et al. Effects of bariatric surgery on mortality in Swedish obese subjects. N Engl J Med. 2007;357:741-52.

54. Rosengren A, Hawken S, Ounpuu S, et al. Association of psychosocial risk factors with risk of acute myocardial infarction in 11119 cases and 13648 controls from 52 countries (the INTERHEART study): case-control study. Lancet. 2004;364:953-62.

55. Rugulies R. Depression as a predictor for coronary heart disease. A review and meta-analysis. Am J Prev Med. 2002;23:51-61.

56. Gump BB, Matthews KA, Eberly LE, et al. Depressive symptoms and mortality in men: results from the multiple risk factor intervention trial. Stroke. 2005;36:98-102.

57. Welin C, Lappas G, Wilhelmsen L. Independent importance of psychosocial factors for prognosis after myocardial infarction. J Intern Med. 2000;247:629-39.

58. Williams JE, Paton CC, Siegler IC, et al. Anger proneness predicts coronary heart disease risk: prospective analysis from the atherosclerosis risk in communities (ARIC) study. Circulation. 2000;101:2034-9.

59. Bunker SJ, Colquhoun DM, Esler MD, et al. Stress and coronary heart disease: psychosocial risk factors. Med J Aust. 2003;178:272-6.

60. Rothermundt M, Arolt V, Peters M, et al. Inflammatory markers in major depression and melancholia. J Affect Disord. 2001;63:93-102.

61. Suarez EC, Kuhn CM, Schanberg SM, et al. Neuroendocrine, cardiovascular, and emotional responses of hostile men: the role of interpersonal challenge. Psychosom Med. 1998;60:78-88.

62. Karlsson MR, Edström-Plüss C, Held C, et al. Effects of expanded cardiac rehabilitation on psychosocial status in coronary artery disease with focus on type D characteristics. J Behav Med. 2007;30:253-61.

63. Friedman M, Thoresen CE, Gill JJ, et al. Alteration of type A behavior and its effect on cardiac recurrences in post myocardial infarction patients: summary results of the recurrent coronary prevention project. Am Heart J. 1986;112:653-65.

64. Berkman LF, Blumenthal J, Burg M, et al. Effects of treating depression and low perceived social support on clinical events after myocardial infarction: the Enhancing Recovery in Coronary Heart Disease Patients (ENRICHD) Randomized Trial. JAMA. 2003;289:3106-16.

65. Neal B, MacMahon S, Chapman N, et al. Effects of ACE inhibitors, calcium antagonists, and other blood-pressure-lowering drugs: results of prospectively designed overviews of randomised trials. Blood pressure lowering treatment trialists' collaboration. Lancet. 2000;356:1955-64.

66. Chobanian AV, Bakris GL, Black HR, et al. The Seventh Report of the Joint National Committee on Prevention, Detection, Evaluation, and Treatment of High Blood Pressure: the JNC 7 report. JAMA. 2003;289:2560-72.

67. Julius S, Nesbitt SD, Egan BM, et al. Feasibility of treating prehypertension with an angiotensin-receptor blocker. N Engl J Med. 2006;354:1685-97.

68. Svetkey LP, Simons-Morton DG, Proschan MA, et al. Effect of the dietary approaches to stop hypertension diet and reduced sodium intake on blood pressure control. J Clin Hypertens (Greenwich). 2004;6:373-81.

69. Turnbull F, Collaboration BPLTT. Effects of different blood-pressure-lowering regimens on major cardiovascular events: results of prospectively-designed overviews of randomised trials. Lancet. 2003;362:1527-35.

70. Cohen JC, Boerwinkle E, Mosley TH, Jr, et al. Sequence variations in PCSK9, low LDL, and protection against coronary heart disease. N Engl J Med. 2006;354:1264-72.

71. Natarajan P, Ray KK, Cannon CP. High-density lipoprotein and coronary heart disease: current and future therapies. J Am Coll Cardiol. 2010;55:1283-99.

72. Cui Y, Blumenthal RS, Flaws JA, et al. Non-high-density lipoprotein cholesterol level as a predictor of cardiovascular disease mortality. Arch Intern Med. 2001;161:1413-9.

73. Baigent C, Keech A, Kearney PM, et al. Efficacy and safety of cholesterol-lowering treatment: prospective meta-analysis of data from 90,056 participants in 14 randomised trials of statins. Lancet. 2005;366:1267-78.

74. Haffner SM, Lehto S, Rönnemaa T, et al. Mortality from coronary heart disease in subjects with type 2 diabetes and in nondiabetic subjects with and without prior myocardial infarction. N Engl J Med. 1998;339:229-34.

75. Bulugahapitiya U, Siyambalapitiya S, Sithole J, et al. Is diabetes a coronary risk equivalent? Systematic review and meta-analysis. Diabet Med. 2009;26:142-8.

76. Gerstein HC, Miller ME, Byington RP, et al. Effects of intensive glucose lowering in type 2 diabetes. N Engl J Med. 2008;358:2545-59.

77. Patel A, MacMahon S, Chalmers J, et al. Intensive blood glucose control and vascular outcomes in patients with type 2 diabetes. N Engl J Med. 2008;358:2560-72.

78. Executive Summary. Standards of medical care in diabetes—2010. Diabetes Care. 2010;33(Suppl. 1):S4-S10.

79. Pi-Sunyer X, Blackburn G, Brancati FL, et al. Reduction in weight and cardiovascular disease risk factors in individuals with type 2 diabetes: one-year results of the look AHEAD trial. Diabetes Care. 2007;30:1374-83.

80. Knowler WC, Barrett-Connor E, Fowler SE, et al. Reduction in the incidence of type 2 diabetes with lifestyle intervention or metformin. N Engl J Med. 2002;346:393-403.

81. Hvidtfeldt UA, Tolstrup JS, Jakobsen MU, et al. Alcohol intake and risk of coronary heart disease in younger, middle-aged, and older adults. Circulation. 2010;121:1589-97.

82. Tolstrup J, Jensen MK, Tjønneland A, et al. Prospective study of alcohol drinking patterns and coronary heart disease in women and men. BMJ. 2006;332:1244-8.

83. Goldberg IJ, Mosca L, Piano MR, et al. Nutrition Committee, Council on Epidemiology and Prevention and Council on Cardiovascular Nursing of the American Heart Association. AHA Science Advisory: wine and your heart: a science advisory for healthcare professionals from the Nutrition Committee, Council on Epidemiology and Prevention, and Council on Cardiovascular Nursing of the American Heart Association. Circulation. 2001;103:472-5.

84. Brotman DJ, Walker E, Lauer MS, et al. In search of fewer independent risk factors. Arch Intern Med. 2005;165:138-145.

85. Helfand M, Buckley DI, Freeman M, et al. Emerging risk factors for coronary heart disease: a summary of systematic reviews conducted for the US Preventive Services Task Force. Ann Intern Med. 2009;151:496-507.

86. Tsimikas S, Willerson JT, Ridker PM. C-reactive protein and other emerging blood biomarkers to optimize risk stratification of vulnerable patients. J Am Coll Cardiol. 2006;47:C19-C31.

87. Danesh J, Wheeler JG, Hirschfield GM, et al. C-reactive protein and other circulating markers of inflammation in the prediction of coronary heart disease. N Engl J Med. 2004;350:1387-97.

88. Pearson TA, Mensah GA, Alexander RW, et al. Markers of inflammation and cardiovascular disease: application to clinical and public health practice: a statement for healthcare professionals from the Centers for Disease Control and Prevention and the American Heart Association. Circulation. 2003;107:499-511.

89. Ridker PM, Rifai N, Clearfield M, et al. Measurement of C-reactive protein for the targeting of statin therapy in the primary prevention of acute coronary events. N Engl J Med. 2001;344:1959-65.

90. Ridker PM, Danielson E, Fonseca FA, et al. Rosuvastatin to prevent vascular events in men and women with elevated C-reactive protein. N Engl J Med. 2008;359:2195-207.

91. Ridker PM, Cannon CP, Morrow D, et al. C-reactive protein levels and outcomes after statin therapy. N Engl J Med. 2005;352:20-8.

92. Danesh J, Collins R, Peto R. Lipoprotein(a) and coronary heart disease. Meta-analysis of prospective studies. Circulation. 2000;102:1082-5.

93. Kamstrup PR, Tybjaerg-Hansen A, Steffensen R, et al. Genetically elevated lipoprotein(a) and increased risk of myocardial infarction. JAMA. 2009;301:2331-9.

94. EAS Consensus Panel Lp(a). Cardiovascular risk reduction in atherogenic dyslipidemia: beyond LDL-C and statins. EAS Press release; 2010.

95. Davidson MH, Corson MA, Alberts MJ, et al. Consensus panel recommendation for incorporating lipoprotein-associated phospholipase A2 testing into cardiovascular disease risk assessment guidelines. Am J Cardiol. 2008;101:51F-7F.

96. Lonn E, Yusuf S, Arnold MJ, et al. Homocysteine lowering with folic acid and B vitamins in vascular disease. N Engl J Med. 2006;354:1567-77.

97. Albert CM, Cook NR, Gaziano JM, et al. Effect of folic acid and B vitamins on risk of cardiovascular events and total mortality among women at high risk for cardiovascular disease: a randomized trial. JAMA. 2008;299:2027-36.

98. Mosca L, Banka CL, Benjamin EJ, et al. Evidence-based guidelines for cardiovascular disease prevention in women: 2007 update. J Am Coll Cardiol. 2007;49:1230-50.

99. Thompson A, Gao P, Orfei L, et al. Lipoprotein-associated phospholipase A(2) and risk of coronary disease, stroke, and mortality: collaborative analysis of 32 prospective studies. Lancet. 2010;375:1536-44.

100. Folsom AR, Chambless LE, Ballantyne CM, et al. An assessment of incremental coronary risk prediction using C-reactive protein and other novel risk markers: the atherosclerosis risk in communities study. Arch Intern Med. 2006;166:1368-73.

101. Thompson A, Danesh J. Associations between apolipoprotein B, apolipoprotein AI, the apolipoprotein B/AI ratio and coronary heart disease: a literature-based meta-analysis of prospective studies. J Intern Med. 2006;259:481-92.

102. Ingelsson E, Schaefer EJ, Contois JH, et al. Clinical utility of different lipid measures for prediction of coronary heart disease in men and women. JAMA. 2007;298:776-85.

103. McPherson R, Frohlich J, Fodor G, et al. Canadian Cardiovascular Society position statement—Recommendations for the diagnosis and treatment of dyslipidemia and prevention of cardiovascular disease. Can J Cardiol. 2006;22:913-27.

104. Contois JH, McConnell JP, Sethi AA, et al. Apolipoprotein B and cardiovascular disease risk: position statement from the AACC Lipoproteins and Vascular Diseases Division Working Group on Best Practices. Clin Chem. 2009;55:407-19.

105. Smith A, Patterson C, Yarnell J, et al. Which hemostatic markers add to the predictive value of conventional risk factors for coronary heart disease and ischemic stroke? The caerphilly study. Circulation. 2005;112:3080-7.

106. Ernst E, Resch KL. Fibrinogen as a cardiovascular risk factor: a meta-analysis and review of the literature. Ann Intern Med. 1993;118:956-63.

107. Lakoski SG, Greenland P, Wong ND, et al. Coronary artery calcium scores and risk for cardiovascular events in women classified as 'low risk' based on Framingham risk score: the multi-ethnic study of atherosclerosis (MESA). Arch Intern Med. 2007;167:2437-42.

108. Detrano R, Guerci AD, Carr JJ, et al. Coronary Calcium as a Predictor of Coronary Events in Four Racial or Ethnic Groups. 2008;358:1336-45.

109. Folsom AR, Kronmal RA, Detrano RC, et al. Coronary artery calcification compared with carotid intima-media thickness in the prediction of cardiovascular disease incidence: the Multi-Ethnic Study of Atherosclerosis (MESA). Arch Intern Med. 2008;168:1333-9.

110. O'Leary DH, Bots ML. Imaging of atherosclerosis: carotid intima-media thickness. Eur Heart J. 2010;31:1682-9.

111. James HS, Claudia EK, Hurst RT, et al. Use of Carotid Ultrasound to Identify Subclinical Vascular Disease and Evaluate Cardiovascular Disease Risk: a Consensus Statement from the American Society of Echocardiography Carotid Intima-Media Thickness Task Force Endorsed by the Society for Vascular Medicine. Journal of the American Society of Echocardiography: official publication of the American Society of Echocardiography. 2008;21:93-111.

112. Newman AB, Shemanski L, Manolio TA, et al. Ankle-arm index as a predictor of cardiovascular disease and mortality in the Cardiovascular Health Study. The Cardiovascular Health Study Group. Arterioscler Thromb Vasc Biol. 1999;19:538-45.

113. Resnick HE, Lindsay RS, McDermott MM, et al. Relationship of high and low ankle brachial index to all-cause and cardiovascular disease mortality: the strong heart study. Circulation. 2004;109:733-9.

114. Fowkes FG, Murray GD, Butcher I, et al. Ankle brachial index combined with Framingham Risk Score to predict cardiovascular events and mortality: a meta-analysis. JAMA. 2008;300:197-208.

115. Pearson TA, Blair SN, Daniels SR, et al. AHA Guidelines for Primary Prevention of Cardiovascular Disease and Stroke: 2002 Update: consensus Panel Guide to Comprehensive Risk Reduction for Adult Patients Without Coronary or Other Atherosclerotic Vascular Diseases. American Heart Association Science Advisory and Coordinating Committee. Circulation. 2002;106:388-91.

Chapter 46

Changing Focus in Global Burden of Cardiovascular Diseases

Rajeev Gupta, Prakash C Deedwania

Chapter Outline

- CVD in High Income Countries
- Low and Middle Income Countries
- Risk Factors
- Global Response for Combating CVD

INTRODUCTION

Cardiovascular diseases (CVD), such as coronary heart disease (CHD) and stroke, are the most important causes of mortality and morbidity worldwide. Globally the burden of these diseases has shifted from high to middle and presently to low income countries. These diseases peaked in high income countries of Western Europe and North America in the middle of last century and have been declining there ever since. A decline is also observed, albeit at a lower pace, in many middle income countries in Eastern Europe and South America. However, in almost all low income countries of Asia, Central and South America and Africa, these diseases are increasing. In terms of absolute numbers the patients with these diseases are many times more in low income countries, such as China, India, Pakistan and Bangladesh, as compared to all other regions of the globe. This article summarizes burden of CVD, especially CHD, in high income countries and increasing burden of these diseases in middle and low income countries. We also enumerate the reasons for decline in mortality and morbidity from CVD in high income countries. Also suggested are policy actions and clinical measures for preventing and controlling these diseases in low income countries, the new focus in global CVD epidemiology.

CVD IN HIGH INCOME COUNTRIES

Globally, there is an uneven distribution of CVD mortality (Fig. 1). The lowest age-adjusted mortality rates are in the industrialized high income countries whereas the highest rates today are found in Eastern Europe and a number of low and middle income countries. For example, age-standardized mortality rates for CVD are in excess of 500 per 100,000 in Russia and Egypt; between 400 and 450 for South Africa, India, Pakistan and Saudi Arabia; and around 300 for Brazil and China. This is in contrast to rates between 100 and 200 per 100,000 for Australia, Japan, France and the United States. About 15% of world population lives in high income countries that include the United States, Canada, Australia, New Zealand, Western European countries in the European Union and Japan. The

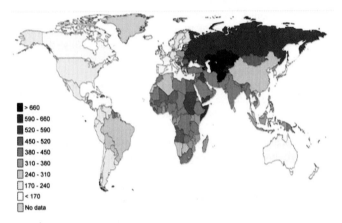

> 660
590 - 660
520 - 590
450 - 520
380 - 450
310 - 380
240 - 310
170 - 240
< 170
No data

FIGURE 1: Cardiovascular mortality patterns in different countries. There is substantial variation in age-adjusted mortality rates. (*Source:* US Institute of Medicine Report, 2010)

epidemic of CVD has reached mature levels in these countries. Majority of CVD events occur in men and women greater than 70 years of age, there is low premature mortality and low morbidity. In the United States there has been a gradual decline in mortality from all forms of CVD, CHD and strokes, beginning 1970s (Fig. 2).

Examination of CHD mortality trends across countries reveals considerable variability in the shape and magnitude of CHD epidemics since the 1950s. Trends are not consistent even among countries or within the same geographic region. In general, the disease and mortality incidence increased, peaked and then fell significantly in many countries (Fig. 2). There are rising patterns, where rates have steadily increased indicating an ongoing epidemic; and a flat pattern, where CHD mortality rates have remained relatively low and stable. The rise-and-fall pattern is most notable in high income Anglo-Celtic, Nordic and Western European countries as well as in the United States and Australia. In these countries, CHD mortality rates peaked in the 1960s or early 1970s and have since fallen precipitously by an average of about 50%. The rising pattern of CHD is most notable in Eastern European and former Soviet countries, where

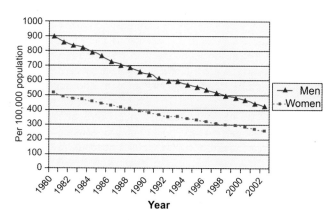

FIGURE 2: Declining mortality from coronary heart disease in USA. Trends in age-adjusted mortality rates for adults less than 35 years (*Source:* Modified from Ford, Capewell. J Am Coll Cardiol. 2007;50:2128-32)

mortality rates have continued to increase at an alarming pace and where the highest mortality rates ever recorded are currently being observed. Although data on CVD mortality trends in low income countries are scarce, an increasing trend, which is similar to the rising pattern in Eastern European nations, is observed in many of these countries such as China and India. By contrast, CHD mortality rates in Japan and several European Mediterranean countries have remained relatively low, following the flat pattern. Epidemiological transition, which is change in disease profile with societal changes, is responsible for changing disease patterns. Initially defined as changing disease profiles with aging and modernization, this is now considered a dynamic process with five distinct phases. These phases of epidemiological transition are shown in Table 1.

The theory of epidemiological transition was initially described by Omran. He described a progressive state of transition in evolution of communicable diseases in populations and hypothesized that the non-communicable disease epidemic also follows a similar trend. He postulated that in the initial phase, characterized by poverty, the diseases are related mainly to undernutrition and infection and death occurs at younger ages

(Fig. 3A). With socioeconomic progress the diseases patterns change and infections are replaced with degenerative diseases. Gillum in early 1990s modified this schema after study of hypertension and stroke among the blacks in USA. He postulated that in a population initial lifestyle changes associated with affluence lead to increase in salt and fat intake leading to epidemic of hypertension, hypercholesterolemia and later to CVD. More socioeconomic evolution leads to positive changes in lifestyle with control of smoking, high blood pressure and cholesterol levels. This is associated with decline in CVD (Fig. 3B). The present phase in developed countries is characterized by massive increases in obesity and the metabolic syndrome that is poised to lead to a second wave of CVD epidemic (Fig. 3C). Recent studies have shown that despite increasing obesity, the metabolic syndrome and diabetes in developed countries the cardiovascular mortality has continued to decline due to greater decline in smoking and better control of hypertension and hypercholesterolemia (Fig. 3D).

The decline in CVD mortality in high income European and North American countries has followed two phases. The first phase of decline from 1970 to 1990s was due to population based measures for risk factor control initiated by changes in policies on smoking, substitution of vegetable oils for animal fats and physical activity promotion. The second phase of decline from 1990s to date is ascribed to better management of risk factors and acute CVD syndromes and short-term as well as long-term use of evidence based pharmacotherapies and coronary interventions or coronary bypass surgeries. Public healthcare financing and strengthening of primary, secondary and tertiary care are important in this regard. Influence of policy changes on CVD mortality in different countries is summarized in Table 2. It is observed that in countries where population based tobacco control policies, salt and fat control strategies and focused control of multiple CVD risk factors (mainly hypertension and hypercholesterolemia) by physicians have been actively pursued there has been a significant decline in CVD incidence varying from 50% to 90% over a 25–30 year period. In middle income countries of Eastern Europe where such initiatives were delayed there has been a lesser decline (20–40%).

LOW AND MIDDLE INCOME COUNTRIES

Researchers project that by 2030 non-communicable diseases will account for more than two-thirds of deaths worldwide; CVD alone will be responsible for more deaths in low income countries than infectious diseases (including HIV/AIDS, tuberculosis and malaria), maternal and perinatal conditions and nutritional disorders combined. Thus, CVD is today the largest single contributor to global mortality and will continue to dominate mortality trends in the future. Global deaths from non-communicable and CVD will continue to rise over the next 10 years, with sub-Saharan Africa expected to see the highest relative increase.

World Health Organization (WHO) estimates that chronic diseases—mainly cardiovascular disease, cancer, chronic respiratory diseases and diabetes—cause more than 60% of all deaths. In absolute terms it has been estimated that, in 2005, the total number of CVD deaths (mainly CHD, stroke and

TABLE 1

Epidemiological transition in disease patterns with societal progress and aging

Stage of transition	Societal development	Disease patterns
Stage I	Stage of pestilence and famine, < 10% urban	Infection and undernutrition related diseases
Stage II	Stage of early development, 10–30% urban	Receding infective pandemics and emerging lifestyle habits
Stage III	Increasing urbanization and migration, 30–50% urban	Degenerative and lifestyle diseases
Stage IV	Stabilized population, > 50–60% urban	Age of delayed degenerative diseases
Stage V	Stage of social and economic upheavals in a stabilized population, > 60% urban	Increasing stress and lifestyle related diseases

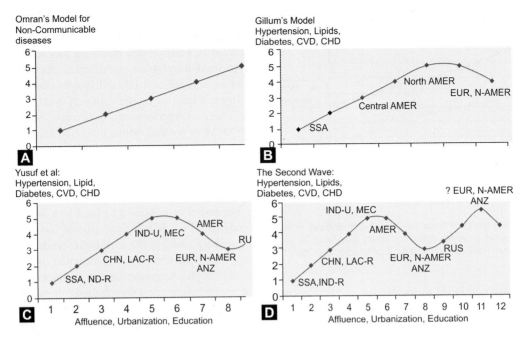

Omran's Model for Non-Communicable diseases

A

Gillum's Model Hypertension, Lipids, Diabetes, CVD, CHD

North AMER

EUR, N-AMER

Central AMER

SSA

B

Yusuf et al: Hypertension, Lipid, Diabetes, CVD, CHD

IND-U, MEC

AMER

CHN, LAC-R

RU

EUR, N-AMER ANZ

SSA, ND-R

C

The Second Wave: Hypertension, Lipids, Diabetes, CVD, CHD

? EUR, N-AMER ANZ

IND-U, MEC

AMER

CHN, LAC-R

RUS

EUR, N-AMER ANZ

SSA, IND-R

D

Affluence, Urbanization, Education

FIGURES 3A TO D: Models of epidemiological transition and CVD mortality in different countries. (A) In the initial phase the chronic non-communicable diseases are considered a continuum and it is projected to progressively increase with increasing civilization. With socioeconomic progress the diseases patterns change and infections are replaced with degenerative diseases; (B) Gillum postulated that in a population initial lifestyle changes associated with affluence lead to increase in salt and fat intake leading to epidemic of hypertension, hypercholesterolemia and later to cardiovascular diseases. More socioeconomic evolution leads to positive changes in lifestyle with control of smoking, high blood pressure and cholesterol levels. This is associated with decline in cardiovascular diseases. The present phase in high income countries is characterized by massive increases in obesity and the metabolic syndrome that is poised to lead to a second wave of CVD epidemic; (C and D) Recent studies have shown that despite increasing obesity, the metabolic syndrome and diabetes in developed countries the cardiovascular mortality has continued to decline due to greater decline in smoking and better control of hypertension and hypercholesterolemia. (Abbreviations: SSA: Sub-Saharan Africa; AMER: Americas; EUR: Europe; CHN: China; IND: India; RUS: Russia; ANZ: Australia-New Zealand; U: Urban; R: Rural)

rheumatic heart disease) had increased globally to 17.5 million from 14.4 million in 1990. Of these, 7.6 million were attributed to CHD and 5.7 million to stroke. More than 80% of the deaths occurred in low and middle income countries. It was also estimated that there will be about 20 million CVD deaths in 2015, accounting for 31% of all deaths worldwide. This increase in CVD is due to a number of causes which include the following: (i) conquest of deaths in childhood and infancy from nutritional deficiencies and infection; (ii) urbanization with increasing levels of obesity; (iii) increasing longevity of the population so that a higher proportion of individuals reaches the age when they are subject to chronic diseases and (iv) increasing use of tobacco worldwide. In most countries in the world other than those in the West, the burden of disease is still due to a combination of infections and nutritional disorders as well as those due to chronic diseases. This double burden of disease poses a challenge that is not only medical and epidemiological, but also social and political.

Disease burden in a given country can be estimated using a variety of processes including national vital registration systems using physician certified cause-of-death data, sample registration surveys using trained enumerators and verbal autopsy instruments, epidemiological assessment using prevalence and incidence data and estimates derived from empirical modeling. Presently in most of the low and middle income countries global trends in CVD are based on models that use country-specific data from a diverse range of developed and developing countries including those of the European Union,

Saudi Arabia, Pakistan, South Africa, China, Indonesia, Mexico, India and the United States. Over the past decade, the quality and availability of country-specific data on CVD risks, incidence and mortality has increased. What emerges are nationally derived data on risks and CVD outcomes. Therefore, in many developing countries, the lack of country-specific data on risks and CVD outcomes is less of an impediment to policy development and action. Nonetheless, before beginning a discussion of CVD trends and risk factor incidence around the world and in specific countries and regions, it is important to note several persistent limitations with the available data. Although, many countries have established health surveillance systems with death registration data, the quality of the data collected varies substantially across countries.

Mortality rates generally appear to be most closely linked to a country's stage of epidemiological transition. Epidemiological transition, a concept first proposed by Omran in the 1970s, refers to the changes in the predominant forms of disease and mortality burdening a population that occurs as its economy and health system develops as described above (Table 1, Figs 3A to D). In underdeveloped countries at the early stages of epidemiological transition, infectious diseases predominate, but as the economy, development status and health systems of these countries improve, the population moves to a later stage of epidemiological transition and chronic non-communicable diseases become the predominant causes of death and disease.

Although this general pattern connecting trends in causes of mortality and stage of development can be observed, it is

TABLE 2

Changes in policy and practice in European, North American and other countries that led to decline in CVD mortality

Country	Political agenda		Risk factor prevention			Better risk factor and disease management				Decline in CVD mortality	
	Strengthening of healthcare systems for acute and chronic CVD care	Public healthcare financing and insurance	Tobacco control policies	Food-modification initiatives	Physical activity promotion	Chronic diseases/CVD focused physician education	Aggressive population based pharmacological risk factor control	CVD focused primary care	CVD focused secondary/tertiary care	Period evaluated	Percent change
Western Europe	++++	++++	+++	++	++	++++	++	+++	+++	1970-2000	(-) 40-45%
Finland	++++	++++	+++	++	+++	++++	++	+++	+++	1972-2007	(-) 75-80%
Germany	++++	++++	+++	++	+++	++++	++	+++	+++	1980-2000	(-) 39-50%
Spain	++++	++++	+++	+++	+++	++++	++	+++	+++	1970-2000	(-) 48-50%
England	++++	++++	+++	++	++	++++	+++	++++	+++	1984-2004	(-) 48-52%
Australia	++++	++++	+++	++	++	++++	+++	++++	+++	1968-2000	(-) 83%
USA	+++	++	++	++	++	++++	++++	+++	++++	1970-2000	(-) 60%
Russia	++	+++	++	+	+	+++	++	++	+++	1970-2000	(-) 10%
Eastern Europe	++	++	++	++	++	+++	++	++	++	1985-2000	(-) 16%
China	+	+++	+	++	++	++	+	+	++	1985-2004	(+) 27-50%
India	+	+	++	0	0	+	0	0	+++	No data	—

Scale of 0 to 4+.

CHAPTER 46   Changing Focus in Global Burden of Cardiovascular Diseases

difficult to make generalized observations about CHD mortality trends for most low and middle income regions. This is due to limited trending data from many low and middle income countries as well as considerable country-to-country variability within regions. The data are strongest from Latin America, where several countries, such as Argentina, Brazil, Chile and Cuba, have experienced decline in CHD mortality rates in the past several decades. However, with the exception of Argentina, where rates declined by more than 60% between 1970 and 2000, the declines have generally occurred more recently (in the 1980s and 1990s) and have been less dramatic (between 20% and 45%) than those in high income countries. By contrast, the epidemic in Mexico appears to be worsening, with CHD mortality rates increasing by more than 90% between 1970 and 2000. Mortality rates in Peru have remained relatively low, following the flat pattern. In Asia, some high income countries, such as Singapore, have followed the rise-and-fall pattern, while CHD deaths in other countries (such as the Philippines, urban China and India) appear to be rising. Although trending data for most of Africa is not available, it has been reported that mortality rates for CVD and diabetes are rising in South Africa.

Because there can be so much variability in the nature of CVD epidemics within regions it is concluded that the most prudent strategy when grouping countries in similar epidemiological situations is to group according to CVD mortality pattern rather than by geographic region (Fig. 4). In India and China, the two major countries of the world, there is variable nature of epidemiological transition in different geographic regions. In rural areas of these countries infectious diseases are still predominant causes of deaths while in urban regions chronic non-communicable diseases predominate. The epidemic of CVD and CHD may have evolved in some highly developed social and ethnic groups in these countries which is similar to the countries of North America and West Europe.

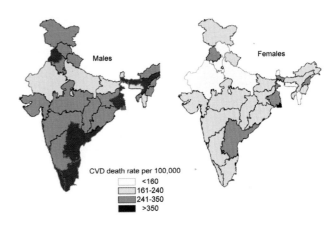

FIGURE 5: Geographic variation in cardiovascular mortality in different states of India in men and women according to Million Death Study in India (2009)

The geographic heterogeneity of CVD mortality rates in India and China are shown in Figures 5 and 6. In India, reliable mortality data using vital registration systems do not exist and there is paucity of data from other national sources. Mortality data from Registrar General of India prior to 1998 were poorly compiled and obtained from predominantly rural populations where vital registration varied from 5% to 15%. The first phase of the Million Death Study has reported mortality statistics from all Indian states using National Sample Registration System units. Causes of deaths in more than 113,000 subjects from about 1.1 million homes were analyzed using a validated verbal autopsy instrument. CVD were the single largest cause of deaths in men (20.3%) as well as women (16.9%) and led to 1.7–2.0 million deaths annually. The prospective phase of this study shall provide more information about trends in mortality from various causes. More robust vital registration systems need to be developed in India. Similar trends in CVD mortality are predicted from other countries of South Asia.

In China it has been observed that CVD are major causes of mortality (stroke and CHD in that order). Using Markov model and InterASIA study data the future risk factor trends in China were projected based on prior trends. CVD (CHD and stroke) in adults ages 35–84 years was projected from 2010 to 2030 and with risk factor levels held constant, projected annual

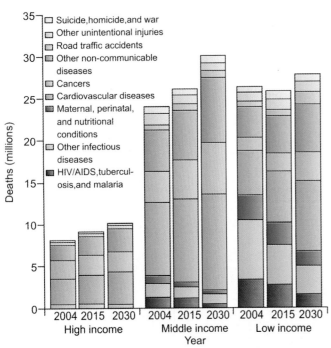

FIGURE 4: Trends in mortality from cardiovascular and other diseases in high, middle and low income countries. (*Source:* Modified from World Health Report, WHO, 2008)

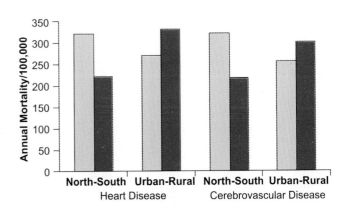

FIGURE 6: Variation in cardiovascular mortality in northern vs southern and urban vs rural regions of China. (*Source:* Modified from He et al. N Engl J Med. 2005;353:1124-34)

cardiovascular events increased by greater than 50% between 2010 and 2030 based on population aging and growth alone. Projected trends in blood pressure, total cholesterol, diabetes (increases) and active smoking (decline) would increase annual CVD events by an additional 23%, an increase of approximately 21.3 million cardiovascular events and 7.7 million cardiovascular deaths over 2010 to 2030. Aggressively reducing active smoking in Chinese men to 20% prevalence in 2020 and 10% prevalence in 2030 or reducing mean systolic blood pressure by 3.8 mm Hg in men and women would counteract adverse trends in other risk factors by preventing cardiovascular events and 2.9–5.7 million total deaths over two decades. It has been concluded that aging and population growth will increase cardiovascular disease by more than a half over the coming 20 years and projected unfavorable trends in blood pressure, total cholesterol, diabetes and body mass index may accelerate the epidemic.

The evolving epidemic of CVD in low and middle income countries and increasing burden of these diseases threatens to overwhelm their strapped health systems and cripple their fragile economies. CVD accounts for large burden from chronic diseases in low and middle income countries. This is especially true in urban centers of countries, such as China and India, where CVD is now the leading cause of disability. Increasing disability adjusted life years (DALYs) lost from CVD has been projected by WHO (Table 3). Hospital-based statistics have revealed an increasing burden of CVD patients (acute CHD and stroke) in low and middle income countries. WHO has predicted that DALYs lost from CVD as well as CHD shall double in both men and women in India. Another method to assess the burden of disease is analysis of CHD and stroke prevalence studies. In India, it has been reported that CHD diagnosed using history and ECG changes trebled in both urban and rural adults from mid-1960s to 2000s to 10% and 5% respectively. Similar trends are observed for stroke prevalence. There are no long-term prospective CHD incidence data. Stroke incidence registries using population-based surveillance have reported that annual incidence of strokes is increasing in these countries especially China (Fig. 7). Cross sectional studies provide only limited information of burden of diseases but can provide empirical assessment regarding increasing trends but have multiple limitations. There is need for properly designed prospective studies in different countries to correctly identify trends in incidence of CVD.

RISK FACTORS

Risk factors for CVD have been extensively studied in developed countries. Multiple prospective studies have reported that smoking, high LDL cholesterol, low HDL cholesterol, hypertension and type 2 diabetes are major proximate risk factors. All these are caused by abnormal lifestyles characterized by sedentary habits, over-nutrition and stress. Scientific articles from the 1970s and 1980s suggest hypertension, cholesterol, poor nutrition, obesity, smoking, physical inactivity and psychosocial stress as the leading factors contributing to CVD and CHD. Tobacco use has been the most reliably documented and historical trends in CVD mortality and tobacco use in the United States from 1900 to 1990 closely mirror each other, with both rates increasing through the 1950s, followed by a precipitous fall beginning in the 1960s. There is a strong epidemiological, experimental, clinical and randomized trial evidence of support for some other risk factors such as high LDL cholesterol, low HDL cholesterol and hypertension, and control of them. In the United Kingdom, a 38 year follow-up of men showed that baseline differences in tobacco use, high blood pressure and cholesterol were associated with a 10- to 15-year shorter life expectancy from age 50. This study has significance for developing countries since many of the baseline levels of risk common in the late 1960s in the United Kingdom are the norm in many developing countries today.

The increase in CHD and stroke in low and middle income countries is largely an urban phenomenon and only now a rapid rise in rural population has been reported. There are no prospective studies from these countries that have identified risk factors of importance in either urban or rural populations. The case-control INTERHEART study conducted in 52 countries worldwide, with a large representation from low income countries, reported that standard risk factors, such as smoking,

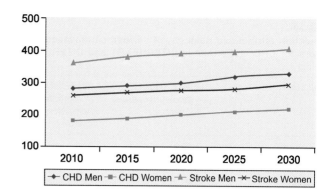

FIGURE 7: Projections for crude event rates (per 100,000) of CHD and hemorrhagic stroke in Chinese men and women ages 35–84 years projected from 2010 to 2030. (*Source:* Modified from Moran et al. Circ Cardiovasc Qual Outcomes. 2010;3:243-52)

TABLE 3

DALYs lost due to cardiovascular disease in low and middle income countries (in millions)

	1990	2002	2005	2015	2020	2030
China	22.9	25.4	25.4	25.5	26.1	27.1
India	23.4	30.7	32.2	35.2	37.4	41.6
Sub-Saharan Africa	11.6	11.7	12.7	16.1	17.97	22.8
Latin America/Caribbean	7.8	8.6	9.1	10.3	10.91	12.1

TABLE 4

Population attributable risks (%) of various cardiovascular risk factors for CHD and stroke in INTERHEART and INTERSTROKE studies

Risk factor	INTERHEART (acute myocardial infarction)	INTERSTROKE (thrombotic or hemorrhagic strokes)
Apolipoprotein A/B ratio	49.2	24.9
Hypertension	17.9	34.6
Smoking	35.7	18.9
Diabetes	9.9	5.0
High waist-hip ratio	20.1	26.5
Psychosocial stress	32.5	9.8
Regular physical activity	12.2	28.5
Diet	13.7	18.8
Alcohol intake	6.7	3.8
Cardiac causes	—	6.7

abnormal lipids, hypertension, diabetes, high waist-hip ratio, sedentary lifestyle, psychosocial stress and lack of consumption of fruits and vegetables, explained more than 90% of acute CHD events. Preliminary data from the INTERSTROKE study reported that these risk factors explained more than 90% of thrombotic and hemorrhagic strokes. However, population attributable risks are different for CHD and stroke (Table 4). There are only a few prospective studies that provide more direct insight into the causes of recent increase in CVD incidence and mortality in low and middle income countries. For example, in a study on the rise of CHD mortality in Beijing from 1984 to 1990, it was reported that blood lipid increase were the largest contributor—responsible for 77% of increased CHD mortality. Another likely contributor is a rise in smoking. There has been a steady rise in global cigarette consumption since the 1970s, which is expected to continue over the next decade if current trends continue.

An emerging body of evidence suggests that rapid dietary changes associated with nutritional transition, along with a decrease in levels of physical activity in many rapidly urbanizing societies, also may play a particularly important role in the rise of CVD observed in developing countries. The nutritional transition currently occurring in many low and middle income countries has created a new phenomenon in which it is not uncommon to see both undernutrition and obesity coexist in the same population. Epidemiological evidence suggests that dietary changes associated with the nutritional transition, specifically the increasing consumption of energy-dense diets high in unhealthy fats, oils, sodium and sugars, have contributed to an increase in CVD incidence in low and middle income countries. It is now clear that both smoking as well as obesity reduce life span by 10 years and cause equal CVD risk (Fig. 7).

Traditionally, monitoring of dietary consumption trends in low and middle income countries has been difficult due to poor availability of quality data. The Food and Agricultural Organization (FAO) of the United Nations examines trends in the amounts of various foods that are produced, which can serve as a rough proxy for consumption. This measure usually overestimates consumption, but trends remain valid indicators of the broad changes underway. FAO data indicate that the total kilocalorie intake per capita per day in many low and middle income countries as well as the consumption of animal products and some tropical oils (e.g. palm oil)—major sources of saturated fat—have been increasing.

Multiple epidemiological studies to identify prevalence of CHD and stroke risk factors have been performed in different low and middle income countries. Although many studies suffer from multiple biases inherent to population based prevalence studies, large regional studies, have provided important information. Tobacco production as well as consumption has been increasing rapidly in China and India. Prevalence of hypertension defined using earlier and more recent criteria has increased in both urban and rural populations and presently in urban adult subjects, it is prevalent in 25–40%. Lipids levels are increasing and serial studies from a north India city reported increasing mean levels of total, LDL and non-HDL cholesterol and triglycerides and decreasing HDL cholesterol. Although there are large regional variations in prevalence of diabetes, it has more than quadrupled in the last 20 years in urban as well as rural areas. Studies have reported increasing obesity as well as truncal obesity, increasing sedentary lifestyle and psychosocial stress. Trends in major CVD risk factors (smoking, obesity, hypertension, dyslipidemia and diabetes) in India are shown in Figures 8 and 9.

Social determinants of CVD have been inadequately studied in low income countries. There are multiple determinants that include the social gradient, stress, early life events, social exclusion, work conditions, unemployment, lack of social support, addiction including alcohol, tobacco use and smoking, food quality, lack of urban transport and illiteracy and low educational status. All these determinants have been extensively studied in high income countries where a direct correlation of CVD and risk factors with increasing levels of these determinants has been found. Low income countries suffer from social inequality and one of the highest income differentials within the countries are found in India and China. The inequality index (Gini coefficient of economists) is low in high income countries, such as Sweden, Norway and countries of West Europe, and is very high in Central and South American, East and South Asian and African countries (Fig. 10). The inequality is also increasing in these countries. All these countries also have a huge burden of cardiovascular risk factors and CVD.

GLOBAL RESPONSE FOR COMBATING CVD

Tackling the global epidemic of CVD needs policies that combine sound knowledge of prevention and good clinical care and also deal with the allocation of resources for both individual level and community level preventive strategies. The former involves dealing with high-risk individuals through appropriate medical and therapeutic interventions. The latter involves societal level changes including laws that curb the use of tobacco and strategies that promote physical activities and appropriate nutrition. Prevention and control from all types of CVD including CHD is a three pronged process:

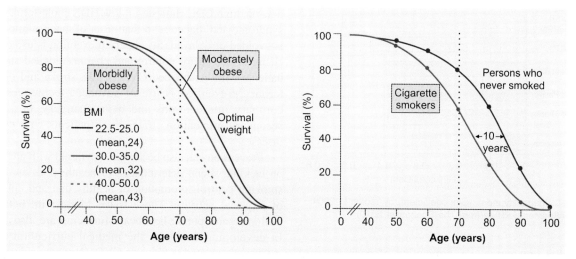

FIGURE 8: Influence of obesity and smoking on survival. (*Source:* Modified from Peto and Jha. N Engl J Med. 2010;362:855-7)

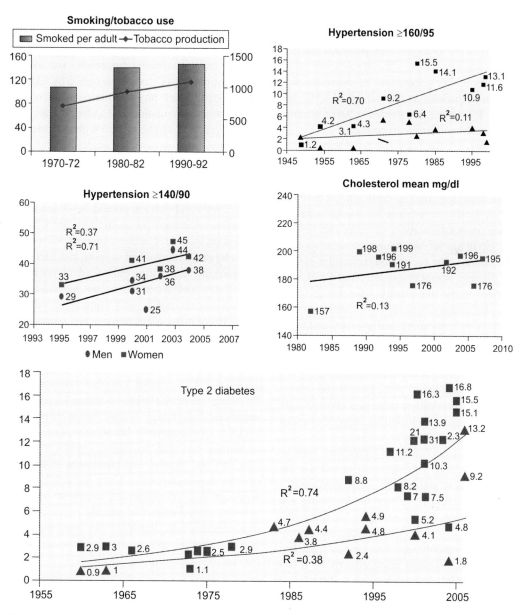

FIGURE 9: Secular trends in prevalence of major coronary risk factors in India. All the four major risk factors: smoking, hypertension, hypercholesterolemia and diabetes show a significant increase, both in urban (square marker) and rural (triangular marker) populations

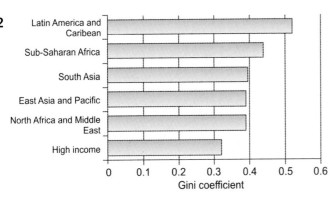

FIGURE 10: Inequality index (Gini coefficient) by region in 2004 (*Source:* Modified from The Economist 2010)

- Primordial prevention, i.e. prevention of occurrence of proximate CVD risk factors by lifestyle changes that involve control of three major risk factor determinants (smoking and tobacco use, physical inactivity and poor quality diet).
- Primary prevention, which is focused on control of proximate risk factors, dyslipidemia, hypertension and diabetes, using lifestyle changes and pharmacological measures.
- Secondary prevention, i.e. prevention of occurrence of second CVD event in patients with established CHD and stroke using lifestyle changes and evidence based pharmacotherapies and cardiovascular interventions.

Progression of CVD is a continuum and prevention extends across all stages of the diseases. Propensity to development of risk factors is either genetic or begins in early antenatal and postnatal period, risk behaviors start in early adolescence and young adulthood, risk factors commence in young to middle ages and depending on accumulation of risks the disease manifests in middle age in low income countries and at an older age in high income countries. The prevention continuum extends across all phases of disease. Social determinants of CVD, such as social organization, early life events, life course social gradient and hierarchy, unemployment, work environment, transport, social support and cohesion, food, poverty and social exclusion and low literacy, influence individual health behaviors and influence primordial, primary as well as secondary prevention. Primary prevention is focused on control of risk factors using both population-based and clinic-based control strategies while secondary prevention strategies involve acute and long-term disease management including lifestyle changes, revascularization and pharmacotherapy.

The decline in mortality from CVD in high income countries is almost all due to population wide decrease in risk factors, better risk factor management and better disease management strategies. Primordial prevention is focused on decreasing risk factor load in the population using strategies for increasing awareness and access through education regarding smoking and tobacco cessation, dietary modulation (low fat and high fruit and vegetables intake) and increased physical activity. It also involves addressing the social determinants of health through improvement in daily living conditions, fair distribution of power, money and resources and continuous upgradation of knowledge, monitoring and skills. Primary prevention is directed towards control of CVD risk factors, such as smoking, hyper-

tension, high LDL cholesterol, low HDL cholesterol, metabolic syndrome and diabetes, so that onset of manifestation of CVD is avoided or delayed. Secondary prevention is use of lifestyle changes, risk factor control and pharmacological strategies in patients with established CVD (CHD, stroke and others) and tertiary prevention is use of advanced techniques, such as coronary interventions and bypass surgery, in addition to secondary prevention strategies in patients with established disease.

Prevention can also be seen as a pyramid with greatest focus on tackling social determinants of health, policies directed to smoking control, promotion of healthy diet and enhancement of physical activity. These issues along with better health insurance and public healthcare financing are also important. In developing countries the medical curriculum has to be extensively revised to focus on CVD. Conventional primary and secondary prevention which involve control of risk factors and better disease management also contribute to CVD mortality decline.

Approaches must be comprehensive and integrated which means investing in and combining measures that reduce the risks associated with poverty and implementing strategies that take a holistic and preventative approach. The evidence shows that the majority of CVD can be prevented by addressing risk factors like unhealthy diet, physical inactivity, alcoholism and tobacco use at policy, population and individual levels. Those that are non-preventable can be treated with essential medicines. While medicines, such as aspirin, penicillin and insulin, to control diseases and morphine to relieve pain have been on the WHO essential medicines list for years, the reality is that they remain beyond the reach of many. Funding models for HIV/AIDS, tuberculosis and malaria should be expanded to allow for the provision of essential medicines for CVD. Strategies for prevention include effective national CVD control program with financial and management support, risk factor control programs on smoking cessation, enhanced physical activity, dietary modulation and better risk factor and disease management.

A 10-point policy and clinical initiative that combines strategies of primordial, primary and secondary prevention and can be implemented in low and middle income countries is hereby suggested. The policies should focus on (i) improvement in socioeconomic status and literacy; (ii) implementation of national CVD control program; (iii) adequate healthcare financing and public health insurance for preventive and curative treatment; (iv) change in educational curriculum with focus on CVD; (v) smoking and tobacco control program; (vi) promotion of healthy diet with legislative control of saturated fats, trans fats, salt and alcohol and promotion of fruits and vegetables; (vii) increased physical activity through better urban planning, worksite and school-based interventions; (viii) aggressive primary prevention for control of smoking, hypertension, dyslipidemia and diabetes; (ix) implementation of evidence based acute care and (x) effective long-term care for secondary prevention.

CONCLUSION

Cardiovascular diseases are major pubic health problems worldwide. The diseases peaked in mid 1970s in high income countries and age-adjusted mortality is declining in these countries since then. On the other hand the epidemic is increasing in low income countries and is established in middle income countries. Standard cardiovascular risk factors that are rampant worldwide are important in genesis of the disease. The risk factors include societal factors, primordial lifestyle factors (smoking, poor diet and physical inactivity) and primary proximate risk factors (smoking, hypertension, lipid abnormalities and diabetes). The reasons for rise and fall in CVD in high income countries have been well documented and include prevention and control of risk factors, better medical management of acute CVD events, better long term care and judicious use of advanced interventional techniques. On the other hand in low income countries rapid increase in urbanization and affluence is fuelling the increase in risk factors and increase in CVD mortality and morbidity. Tackling the epidemic of CVD in low and middle income countries is a global priority and needs policy response from governments and clinical response from medical institutions and physicians.

BIBLIOGRAPHY

1. Abegunde DO, Mathers CD, Adam T, et al. The burden and costs of chronic diseases in low-income and middle-income countries. Lancet. 2007;370:1929-38.
2. Burke GL, Bell RA. Global trends in cardiovascular disease. In: Wong ND, Black HR, Gardin JM. (Eds). Preventive Cardiology, 2nd edition. New York: McGraw Hill; 2005. pp. 22-43.
3. Deedwania PC, Gupta R. East Asians and South Asians, and Asian and Pacific-Islander Americans. In: Wong ND, Black HR, Gardin JM. (Eds). Preventive Cardiology, 2nd edition. New York: McGraw Hill; 2005. pp. 456-72.
4. Ford ES, Ajani UA, Croft JB, et al. Explaining the decrease in US deaths from coronary disease 1980-2000. N Engl J Med. 2007;356:2388-98.
5. Fuster V, Kelly BB, Board for Global Health. Promoting cardiovascular health in developing world: a critical challenge to achieve global health. Washington: Institute of Medicine; 2010.
6. Gaziano T. Cardiovascular disease in the developing world and its cost-effective management. Circulation. 2005;112:3547-53.
7. Gersh B, Mayosi B, Sliwa K, et al. The epidemic of cardiovascular diseases in the developing world: global implications. Eur Heart J. 2010;31:642-8.
8. Gupta R, Joshi PP, Mohan V, et al. Epidemiology and causation of coronary heart disease and stroke in India. Heart. 2008;94:16-26.
9. Gupta R, Gupta KD. Coronary heart disease in low socioeconomic status subjects in India: an evolving epidemic. Indian Heart J. 2009;61:358-67.
10. Kesteloot H, Sans S, Kromhout D. Dynamics of cardiovascular and all-cause mortality in Western and Eastern Europe between 1970 and 2000. Eur Heart J. 2006;27:107-13.
11. Marmot MG, Friel S, Bell R, et al. Closing the gap in a generation: health equity through action on the social determinants of health. Lancet. 2008;372:1661-9.
12. Smith SC, Jackson R, Pearson TA, et al. Principles for national and regional guidelines on cardiovascular disease prevention: a scientific statement from the World Heart and Stroke Forum. Circulation. 2004;109:3112-21.
13. World Health Organization. Prevention of cardiovascular disease. Guidelines for risk assessment and management of cardiovascular risk. Geneva: World Health Organization; 2007.

Changing Focus in Global Burden of Cardiovascular Diseases

Chapter 47

Evaluation of Chest Pain

Kirsten E Fleischmann, Raveen Pal

Chapter Outline

SCOPE

Chest pain is a common presenting symptom for patients visiting family physicians, general internists, cardiologists and emergency physicians. In 2009, there were 8 million visits to the emergency room alone due to chest pain.[1] Although chest pain is most often benign,[2] it may represent the symptoms of a life threatening process, such as myocardial infarction (MI) or aortic dissection, so a low threshold for prompt investigation is prudent. Indeed, heart disease is the leading cause of death in the United States. In 2009, an estimated 785,000 had a new heart attack, while approximately 470,000 had a recurrent heart attack.[3] This high incidence has resulted in the development of programs directed to both the general public and the general medical practitioners to promote awareness of the signs and symptoms of heart disease and the indications for further investigation of chest pain. Fortunately, through increased awareness and improved therapies, mortality from heart disease has decreased steadily in the last few decades.[4]

This chapter reviews the history and differential diagnosis of chest pain, the physical findings associated with cardiac ischemic pain and the role of various investigations in the further investigation and management of chest pain.

HISTORY

Chest pain has an extensive differential diagnosis, so the clinical history is critical in establishing the pre-test probability of any given diagnosis and to guide subsequent test decisions. Testing then refines this risk further into a post-test risk. Finally, the history is an important part of the physician patient interaction that helps patients to establish trust and provides the physician with important social information about the patient that may impact their management.

DIFFERENTIAL DIAGNOSIS

Chest pain has an extensive differential diagnosis. It may be useful to think of the differential diagnosis of chest pain by system (Table 1).

The first step in the management of chest pain is to rule out an immediate life threatening cause. Once stable vitals have been established and if the patient is not in extremis, it is reasonable to proceed with a more detailed history and physical examination, helping to differentiate among the various etiologies. The history includes the description of the pain itself and the patient's medical history and risk factors.

TABLE 1

Differential diagnosis of chest pain by system

- Cardiac
  — Angina
  — MI
  — Pericarditis/Myocarditis
  — Aortic dissection
- Musculoskeletal
- Gastrointestinal
  — Esophageal spasm
  — Reflux
  — Cholecystitis
  — Pancreatitis
- Pulmonary
  — Pulmonary embolus
  — Pneumothorax
  — Pneumonia
  — Pulmonary hypertension
- Neuropathic
  — Shingles
  — Costochondritis
  — Cervical spine
- Psychiatric

PATIENT'S DESCRIPTION

Description of patient's presenting symptoms should include details of location, radiation, quality, intensity, onset, duration, and exacerbating and alleviating factors.

LOCATION

Location of pain (retrosternal, epigastric, shoulder) can be useful to determine the source. A discrete location of pain, especially if reproducible with palpation, makes a musculoskeletal origin more likely. Epigastric pain more commonly has a gastrointestinal (GI) etiology, although ischemia, particularly in the inferior distribution, can sometimes mimic GI symptoms. Pain that follows a nerve distribution may be attributable to shingles. In general, location of pain is a poor discriminator.[5]

RADIATION

Radiation of pain to the jaw, neck, shoulders, arms or back can be useful in assessing the likely cause of chest pain. Pain radiating to the jaws or neck or arms is classically associated with cardiac ischemia. Radiation to the back is classically associated with aortic dissection. This feature can be used to rule in cardiac ischemia with a greater likelihood.[6]

QUALITY

Description of chest pain by the patient can be helpful. Angina may be described in many ways. However, most often it is described as a dull ache, squeezing or heaviness. Pain that is sharp or stabbing in nature is less likely to be ischemic in origin. Pain that is referred to as burning is more suggestive of a GI etiology. Classically, the pain of aortic dissection has been described as a tearing sensation. These various descriptors can help raise or lower suspicion for various causes of pain.

INTENSITY

Pain severity is typically graded on a scale of 1 to 10. However, recent data suggest that pain due to myocardial ischemia has a wide range of intensities and that severity is not useful to discriminate source of chest discomfort.[7] Thus, pain severity is most useful to grade relief from pain or change from previous episodes.

ASSOCIATED SYMPTOMS

Shortness of breath, diaphoresis, nausea and dizziness are symptoms that often accompany cardiac ischemia.

ONSET OF PAIN

Sudden onset versus gradual onset is a useful differentiating feature. Aortic dissection and pulmonary embolism tend to have sudden onsets. More gradual and escalating pain is more typical of cardiac ischemia. Cardiac ischemic pain tends to occur with activity. Also, cardiac pain has been reported to occur more frequently in the morning when sympathetic tone is highest.

DURATION

The length of symptoms is a useful piece of information. Pain that is brief and sharp, and conversely pain that is prolonged and unremitting for days, are both less likely to be ischemic in origin.

ALLEVIATING AND AGGRAVATING FACTORS

Pain with a pleuritic component that worsens with position or with respiration suggests a pericardial or respiratory etiology. Pain that worsens following meals, or at night after lying down, and is relieved with oral antacid preparations, suggests a GI etiology. Pain that is exacerbated by exertion or strong emotion is more typical of cardiac ischemia. While it is classically taught that pain relieved with nitroglycerin is suggestive of cardiac ischemia, it can also be esophageal in origin, limiting its usefulness as a distinguishing feature.[8]

It is important to recognize that, while pain descriptors make various etiologies of pain more or less likely, there is no perfect discriminator. Various studies have shown a wide range of likelihood ratios for different symptoms and signs.[9,10] Furthermore, elderly,[11] female[12,13] and diabetic[14] patients have been found to have more atypical symptoms. Thus, while the medical history can help to narrow the differential diagnosis and determine the next most appropriate steps in management, no one symptom is definitive.

ANGINA

Angina is a medical term derived from the classical Greek word "ankhon" meaning to strangle or choke. Angina pectoris is chest pain due to lack of blood flow to the heart, or cardiac ischemia. The first ischemic chest pain was described by Heberden in 1798; a painful sensation in the chest accompanied by a strangling sensation. This description remains largely unchanged today. Angina is still classically described as a dull, heavy, pressure-like sensation in the retrosternal area. Since angina is caused by inadequate blood flow to the myocardium, which is innervated by the vagus nerve, there is a visceral nature to the pain that does not allow clear localization. It is broadly localized to the central chest area. Occasionally, patients will make a fist on top of their retrosternal area; this has been given the moniker the Levine sign, and may be associated with ischemia. Pain can radiate to the jaw, neck or shoulders. The intensity varies quite significantly and lasts for a few minutes to half an hour. (Please see the section "History").

Angina is due to a fixed coronary artery stenosis, less commonly dynamic coronary artery stenosis and spasm or small vessel disease, that does not allow adequate blood flow, and thus oxygen delivery, to the myocardium. Therefore, it is usually brought on by exercise, emotional exertion, or even after large meals; states that result in increased heart rate (HR) and/or blood pressure (BP) and, therefore, have increased myocardial oxygen demands. Coronary blood flow is increased during exercise, but oxygen extraction is not, since it is already at maximal levels. Therefore, oxygen delivery to the myocardium is directly proportional to vessel size. If there is a fixed coronary artery stenosis that limits blood flow, it, in effect, limits oxygen delivery to the myocardium. Thus, in states requiring increased myocardial oxygen, there is an imbalance between oxygen delivery and demand.

Double product (HR times BP) is an indirect marker of myocardial oxygen consumption in patients with fixed coronary stenosis, because it incorporates two variables that affect oxygen consumption. First, the systolic pressure developed by the ventricular wall (Laplace's law tension = pressure x radius/wall thickness) and second, the HR which determines diastolic filling time, during which the majority of coronary blood flow occurs. Since the degree of stenosis determines the amount of blood flow, the amount of physical activity that elicits angina appears to be related to the severity of stenosis rather than the number of stenoses.

Diurnal variation in angina has been reported. It can sometimes be reported consistently with sleep. It is speculated that this is due to the increased venous return to the heart in the supine position, which results in increased LV size, and therefore LV wall tension (Laplace's law), resulting in increased oxygen demand. Angina can also classically be reported as a morning phenomenon. It is thought that this is related to increased sympathetic activity following waking which results in increased HR and BP. These variables together result in increased oxygen demand with less delivery, resulting in angina. Angina is classically relieved with rest or the use of sublingual nitroglycerin. Nitroglycerin relaxes the vascular tone resulting in dilation of coronary vasculature, resulting in increased flow to the myocardium. This, at least temporarily, alleviates the oxygen delivery imbalance and relieves pain. It also decreases myocardial oxygen demand resulting from decreased left ventricular (LV) end-diastolic volume.

Diamond and Forrester [15] developed a simple classification scheme to determine the pre-test likelihood that a patient's pain was cardiac ischemic in origin. Patient's age and sex was recorded and their symptoms were divided into typical, atypical, non-cardiac and asymptomatic. Typical angina (definite) was described as: (1) substernal chest discomfort with a characteristic quality and duration; (2) provoked by exertion or emotional stress and (3) relieved by rest or NTG. Atypical angina

(probable) met two of the above characteristics, and so-called noncardiac chest pain met one or none of the typical anginal characteristics. Based on age, gender and symptom description, the pre-test likelihood of angina was determined. This system continues to provide a rapid and reasonably reliable estimate of the likelihood that a patient's symptoms are reflective of coronary artery disease (CAD).

PAST MEDICAL HISTORY

Once the chest pain description has been clearly classified, risk factors for the development of CAD should be determined. Large population studies, like Framingham, followed participants prospectively and determined their risk of developing CAD depending on their medical conditions. From this cohort study, currently established cardiac risk factors include age, cigarette smoking, hyperlipidemia, diabetes and hypertension.[16,17] These clinical features are incorporated into a risk score (Fig. 1) that determines if a patient is at low (< 10%), intermediate (10% to < 20%) or high (≥ 20%) risk for the development of atherosclerosis over the next 10 years.[18] In addition, pre-established histories of kidney disease and coronary vascular, cerebrovascular or peripheral vascular disease are high-risk indicators. An alternate, revised risk score is the Reynolds risk score. This score incorporates all of the Framingham risk factors, but adds family history of CAD and requires a high sensitivity CRP determination.[19]

While risk factors increase the risk of underlying CAD, they have not been shown to predict whether an individual presentation of chest pain is or is not cardiac ischemic in origin.[20-22] A classic history, ECG finding and/or biomarker findings supersede clinical risk factor prediction.

PHYSICAL EXAMINATION

Following a history, the next step is to incorporate the patient's physical examination findings into a clinical decision making process. The physical examination starts with a general assessment of appearance. It is important to observe if the patient is in distress, diaphoretic, working hard to breath, pale or cyanotic. Concurrently vital signs, such as HR, BP and rhythm, should be recorded. Normal sinus rhythm is regular and between 60 and 100 beats per minute. The BP should be performed in both arms to detect discrepancies that may heighten suspicion for dissection or peripheral vascular disease. Respiratory rate and oxygen saturation should all be done routinely. An anatomical approach with review of the patient's head and neck area may reveal signs of hypercholesterolemia—specifically arcus senilis in patients under 50, xanthelasma and xanthomas in the feet. A fundoscopic exam may reveal signs of longstanding hypertension (pruning of arterioles distally, arteriovenous nicking, flame-shaped hemorrhages, optic head edema) or diabetes (hard exudates, microaneurysms, retinopathy).

A complete cardiovascular examination including inspection, palpation and auscultation should be completed. The carotid pulsation is palpated for volume and contour. Then all of the peripheral pulses (brachial, radial, renal, femoral, popliteal and dorsalis pedis) are palpated and areas overlying the carotid and femoral pulses auscultated for bruits. The jugular venous pressure (JVP) is examined for height and contour.

FIGURE 1: Framingham risk score calculation. (*Source:* Wilson, et al. Circulation. 1998;97:1837-47)

Step 1

Age		
Years	LDL pts	Chol pts
30–34	–1	[–1]
35–39	0	[0]
40–44	1	[1]
45–49	2	[2]
50–54	3	[3]
55–59	4	[4]
60–64	5	[5]
65–69	6	[6]
70–74	7	[7]

Step 2

LDL-C		
(mg/dl)	(mmol/L)	LDL pts
< 100	< 2.59	-3
100-129	2.60-3.36	0
130-159	3.37-4.14	0
160-190	4.15-4.92	1
≥ 190	≥ 4.92	2

Cholesterol		
(mg/dl)	(mmol/L)	Chol pts
< 160	< 4.14	[-3]
160-199	4.15-5.17	[0]
200-239	5.18-6.21	[1]
240-279	6.22-7.24	[2]
≥ 280	≥ 7.25	[3]

Step 3

HDL-C			
(mg/dl)	(mmol/L)	LDL pts	Chol pts
< 35	< 0.90	2	[2]
35-44	0.91-1.16	1	[1]
45-49	1.17-1.29	0	[0]
50-59	1.30-1.55	0	[0]
≥ 60	≥ 1.56	-1	[-2]

Step 4

Blood pressure					
Systolic (mm Hg)	Diastolic (mm Hg)				
	< 80	80-84	85-89	90-99	≥ 100
< 120	0 [0] pts				
120-129		0 [0] pts			
130-139			1 [1] pts		
140-159				2 [2] pts	
≥ 160					3 [3] pts

Note: When systolic and diastolic pressures provide different estimates for point scores, use the higher number

Step 5

Diabetes		
	LDL pts	Chol pts
No	0	[0]
Yes	2	[2]

Step 6

Smoker		
	LDL pts	Chol pts
No	0	[0]
Yes	2	[2]

Step 7

(Sum from steps 1-6)

Adding up the points

Age _____

LDL-C or Chol _____

HDL-C _____

Blood pressure _____

Diabetes _____

Smoker _____

Point total _____

Step 8

(Determine CHD risk from point total)

CHD Risk			
LDL Pts total	10 Yr CHD Risk	Chol Pts Total	10 Yr CHD Risk
< -3	1%		
-2	2%		
-1	2%	[< -1]	[2%]
0	3%	[0]	[3%]
1	4%	[1]	[3%]
2	4%	[2]	[4%]
3	6%	[3]	[5%]
4	7%	[4]	[7%]
5	9%	[5]	[8%]
6	11%	[6]	[10%]
7	14%	[7]	[13%]
8	18%	[8]	[16%]
9	22%	[9]	[20%]
10	27%	[10]	[25%]
11	33%	[11]	[31%]
12	40%	[12]	[37%]
13	47%	[13]	[45%]
≥ 14	≥ 56%	[≥ 14]	[≥ 53%]

Step 9

(compare to average person your age)

Comparative Risk			
Age (years)	Average 10 Yr CHD Risk	Average 10 Yr Hard* CHD Risk	Low** 10 Yr CHD Risk
30-34	3%	1%	2%
35-39	5%	4%	3%
40-44	7%	4%	4%
45-49	11%	8%	4%
50-54	14%	10%	6%
55-59	16%	13%	7%
60-64	21%	20%	9%
65-69	25%	22%	11%
70-74	30%	25%	14%

Key	
Color	Relative risk
Green	Very low
White	Low
Yellow	Moderate
Rose	High
Red	Very high

* Hard CHD events exclude angina pectoris

** Low risk was calculated for a person the same age, optimal blood pressure, LDL-C 100-129 mg/dl or cholesterol 160-199 mg/dl, HDL-C 45 mg/dl for men or 55 mg/dl for women, non-smoker, no diabetes

Risk estimates were derived from the experience of the Framingham Heart Study, a predominantly Caucasian population in Massachusetts, USA

Auscultation of the patient with chest pain usually reveals normal sounding first and second heart sounds. The S2 may demonstrate paradoxical splitting during active myocardial ischemia for the same reason as a left bundle branch block (LBBB); the delayed LV ejection time due to dysfunctional myocardium results in a later aortic component resulting in lack of splitting or paradoxical splitting of S2. The S3 can be heard, if there is associated heart failure, due to rapid and high volume LV filling. Actively ischemic myocardium also has decreased ventricular compliance, resulting in an audible S4.

Auscultation for systolic and diastolic murmurs is important in the aortic, tricuspid, pulmonic and mitral areas. The most common murmur heard in patients with CAD is one of mild mitral regurgitation due to ischemia and papillary muscle dysfunction. In particular, the murmurs secondary to acute complications of MIs, including acute mitral regurgitation, ventricular septal defect and free wall rupture, are important to seek. Also, the murmur of aortic regurgitation, which may suggest an aortic dissection, is important to rule out and may be accentuated by auscultation at end expiration with the patient sitting forward. Finally, the discovery of a pericardial rub may lend support to an alternate diagnosis of chest pain namely pericarditis.

The respiratory exam is an important part of a chest pain examination. There may be crepitations or crackles heard in the lower lung fields or throughout the lung fields depending on the degree of edema present. Crepitations localized to one focal area with evidence of consolidation may be more representative of an infectious process such as pneumonia. Active wheeze may represent bronchoconstriction, although pulmonary edema can present with wheezing as well. Finally an examination of the abdomen, searching for liver capsule tenderness, abdominal aorta size and epigastric pain on palpation should be completed (please see the section "Physical Examination").

Most commonly, the physical exam of a patient with stable CAD is quite benign. In the routine investigation of chest pain, the physical exam is most important in ruling out an imminent life threatening cause requiring immediate investigation or intervention.

INVESTIGATIONS

CHEST X-RAY

The chest radiograph is a routine diagnostic test in the assessment of patients with chest pain. The cardiac silhouette may be enlarged due to LV chamber enlargement, resulting in a high cardiac:thoracic (C:T) ratio. Longstanding hypertension or LV dysfunction can lead to left atrial enlargement, suggested by flattening of the left heart border, splaying of the left and right bronchus, or by a double right heart border. The right ventricle (RV) may also be enlarged due to infarction, volume overload or pulmonary hypertension and is marked by loss of the retrosternal airspace in the lateral projection. Right atrial enlargement is seen by a prominent right heart border.[23] Aortic arch, aortic valve and mitral valve calcification can be viewed on plain radiographs and are associated with increased risk of atherosclerosis.[24] Coronary artery calcification is difficult to visualize on plain radiographs, but if present is also a high risk indicator of coronary atherosclerosis. There may be signs of congestive heart failure; plethoric pulmonary arteries, peribronchiolar cuffing, interstitial edema, Kerley B lines and blunting of the costophrenic angles with pleural effusions. There may be signs of pulmonary hypertension, prominent pulmonary arteries with rapid pruning, with right atrial and/ or RV enlargement.

Chest radiograph is most commonly normal in a patient with anginal chest pain, but may be helpful in identifying a non-cardiac diagnosis or to diagnose complications of acute cardiac ischemia. In patients with aortic dissection, there may be a wide mediastinum, pericardial effusion or displacement of calcium from the soft tissue border of the aorta. In pulmonary embolus, there may be RV and pulmonary artery enlargement, a Westermark sign (a zone of avascular tissue), or Hampton's hump (wedge-shaped density along the periphery consistent with infarction).[25] Clear signs of an infiltrative process, a pneumothorax or a mediastinal mass may also help to direct the diagnosis.

ECG

The resting electrocardiogram (ECG) is normal in up to half of individuals who present with undifferentiated chest pain. A normal ECG is very useful in reducing the probability of acute coronary syndromes (ACS).[26,27] However, a retrospective series of patients presenting to an outpatient cardiology clinic for evaluation of recent chest pain showed that up to 30% of patients ultimately diagnosed with unstable angina (UA) had a normal ECG.[28]

An abnormal ECG may reveal the presence of Q waves suggesting a previous MI. However, it is important to note that prior MI may not result in the presence of a Q wave and that the presence of Q waves is not pathognomic of infarction, particularly if seen in leads III, V1 and V2.

Changes in the ST segment are important to pursue. Elevation of more than 1 mm in two or more consecutive leads is highly concerning for acute transmural infarction and requires immediate evalution for possible intervention. ST flattening and ST depression are also commonly witnessed and are also highly suggestive of ischemia. The only changes seen on an ECG may be T wave flattening or inversion. Deep symmetric T wave inversion in the anterior precordial leads is referred to as Wellen's sign, a marker of LAD territory ischemia. The presence of ST elevation, Q waves, ST depression, T wave inversion or new conduction defects all significantly increase the risk of chest pain being cardiac ischemic in origin.[27,29]

Comparison with a prior ECG and serial ECGs are very helpful in the interpretation of ECG changes. Patients may have longstanding non-specific ST segment flattening. The presence of the same findings during an episode of chest pain in a patient with a previously normal ECG is far more concerning. Subtle ECG changes which are transient during an episode of chest discomfort are highly suspicious for cardiac ischemic changes. Finally alternate causes of ST and T waves changes, such as pericarditis, metabolic states, digitalis effect or hypertrophic cardiomyopathy, should always be considered.

LABORATORY INVESTIGATIONS

Laboratory biomarkers can be useful for determining diagnosis as well as prognosis in cardiac disease. In addition to this, biomarkers help to identify the subset of patients most likely to benefit from more aggressive therapeutic interventions. As myocardium becomes ischemic and necrotic, the myocardial cell membrane integrity is compromised resulting in leakage of intracellular enzymes. While there are multiple enzymes (myoglobin, creatine kinase, troponins) that are specific to muscle cell compromise, there are only a few enzymes, such as troponins T and I, that are specific to cardiac muscle cells. The presence of these enzymes in the blood stream implies loss of specifically cardiac muscle.

Creatine kinase (CK) has multiple isoforms such as MM, BB and MB. The MB form is most concentrated in cardiac muscle. In the past, unfractionated CK or CK-MB were the primary cardiac markers used in the evaluation of ACS. The CK-MB is limited by its specificity since it can also be released by strain or damage to skeletal muscles and it is occasionally present in normal healthy individuals.[30] Troponin detection is the current key tool in the diagnosis of MI. The troponin complex is composed of Troponin T, I and C. The Troponin I (TnI) and Troponin T (TnT) of cardiac myofibrils are distinct from those of skeletal muscles. Therefore, if cardiac myofibrils undergo damage, cardiac-specific TnI or TnT is released into the bloodstream.[31] Troponins have both greater specificity and greater sensitivity for small amounts of cardiac damage than CK-MB.[32] Troponin elevation without CK-MB elevation has been found to be associated with evidence of focal myocardial necrosis. One study estimated that 30% of patients who presented with rest pain, and without ECG changes, would have been diagnosed as having UA rather than non ST elevation myocardial infarction (NSTEMI), based on CK-MB alone versus TnI or TnT. It is important to distinguish between detection of myocardial damage and the cause of myocardial damage. While myocardial strain or damage can be inferred by the release of TnI or TnT into the bloodstream, myocardial strain can be secondary to many causes other than ACS and underlying

CAD. Congestive heart failure, chronic kidney disease, LV hypertrophy and extreme exercise are all common alternate explanations for an elevated troponin. Elevated levels of TnI or TnT also provide useful prognostic information. Patients with elevated levels of TnI or TnT are at increased risk of death, irrespective of whether the troponin elevation is identified as having a cardiac cause or not.[33,34] When elevated troponin is due to CAD, the amount of troponin released is related to the amount of damaged myocardium. Larger amounts of troponin release are associated with increased risk of death.[35,36] Troponin elevation can also help to identify the subset of patients presenting with ACS who will benefit from GpIIb/IIIa inhibitor treatment[37] and LMWH treatment.[38] Only patients who were biomarker positive showed a lower risk of death or MI when treated with these more aggressive medications. Cardiac biomarkers have varying kinetics with respect to their release into the bloodstream and, thus, their availability to detection. Therefore, it is critical to correlate the presence or absence of a particular biomarker in the blood stream with the onset of the patient's symptoms. While myoglobin is the earliest detectable biomarker, its lack of specificity limits its utility. CK is present in the bloodstream as quickly as 2–4 hours after the onset of damage. As compared with troponins, CK levels peak more quickly (24 hours) and clear much more quickly. Troponins are typically not present until 6 hours after the onset of damage, they take 5–7 days to peak and can persist for 10–14 days. These timelines are important in determining presence of damage and whether or not recurrence of pain is associated with recurrence of damage. Thus, if troponin is negative immediately after, or within the first 6 hours after, an episode of pain, it must be repeated, so that it is being measured at least 8–10 hours after pain in order to ensure that it is in fact negative. Furthermore, it is important to understand that troponin levels may be persistently elevated after an episode of cardiac damage. Thus, if a patient has an MI on day one and then experiences more pain on day 5, a single elevated troponin may simply represent residual biomarker from the incident MI, not a recurrent MI. If serial troponin levels are increasing, however, this would be consistent with a recurrent ischemic event.

ESTIMATION OF RISK

As aforementioned, the Framingham and Reynolds risk scores are population based risk scores that predict an individual's risk of having a heart disease event in the longer term.

However, other scores have been developed that address the more acute risk of adverse events in patients with ACS. Risk of death or other adverse outcome based on initial presentation has been assessed in multiple large trials. The thrombolysis in myocardial infarction (TIMI) risk score is one score that assesses 7 aspects of the history and physical examination to predict the risk of adverse outcome. Age more than 64 years, greater than 3 CAD risk factors (family history, hypertension, increased cholesterol, diabetes, smoking), known CAD (stenosis > 50%), aspirin use in the last 7 days, recent (< 24 hours) severe angina, increased cardiac markers and ST deviation on ECG greater than or equal to 0.5 mm are each assigned a single point. The risk of death, MI or urgent revascularization by 14 days based on this score ranges from 5% to 41%.[39]

Another score, the Grace risk score, derived from a population with undifferentiated chest pain, incorporates age, HR, systolic BP, Killip class (degree of pulmonary edema/shock), presence of ST deviation on ECG, cardiac arrest, creatinine and elevated cardiac biomarkers to predict in-hospital mortality. It has been shown to be predictive of both shorter (30 days) and longer term (1 year) mortality.[40]

One limitation of these scores is that they have been derived from trial populations that tend to exclude very high and very low risk patients. So, their application to all patients is unclear. Also, known high-risk indicators, such as kidney dysfunction, are not included since these patients tend to be excluded from the clinical trials from which these scores are derived. Finally, regression models used to derive these prediction scores can result in statistical significance, but not necessarily clinical meaning.

Thus, while these scores can be used to determine, how aggressively a patient should be treated with medications and interventions, clinical judgment must always be factored in.

DIAGNOSTIC TESTING

Several testing modalities are available to help determine whether an individual patient's chest pain is due to CAD or ischemia. The main distinction among testing modalities is functional versus anatomic testing. Functional tests investigate the effect of stress on the myocardium, while anatomic tests image the coronary arteries that provide blood flow to the myocardium. Functional tests generally employ stress in the form of exercise (treadmill or bicycle) or pharmaceutical agents (dipyridamole, dobutamine and adenosine). There are many combinations of these stress and imaging modalities. The most commonly applied stress test is the treadmill electrocardiogram test (ETT), which involves stress in the form of ambulation and electrocardiography as the main assessment tool. It is important to understand that each test has its own sensitivity and specificity for the detection of CAD. Thus, depending on the pre-test likelihood of a patient's having CAD, a test will further increase or decrease that probability.

The choice of stress test often relates to patient factors that make either a test inappropriate or uninterpretable. For example, treadmill stress testing is generally inappropriate in a person unable to exercise, or with ACS, unstable arrhythmia, symptomatic heart failure, acute aortic dissection, acute pericarditis/myocarditis, or acute pulmonary embolism. Additional relative contraindications include known left main disease, uncontrolled systolic hypertension at rest, severe aortic stenosis or dynamic LV outflow obstruction, high-grade atrioventricular block, and severe peripheral vascular disease. Testing would be uninterpretable in someone with resting ECG abnormalities (ST-T shift, LBBB, digitalis effect, accessory pathways, paced rhythm) that interfere with assessment for ischemia, and limited exercise capacity or beta-blocker use may blunt the ability to elevate HR to diagnostic level and therefore reduce sensitivity.

If a patient is unable to exercise, a pharmaceutical agent can be used to simulate exercise. The most common agents used are dipyridamole, adenosine and dobutamine. These agents are mostly used in conjunction with nuclear perfusion imaging, although echocardiography has also been performed.

Dobutamine is a positive inotrope that increases both the HR and the strength of contraction, resulting in ischemia if a stenosis is present. It is most commonly paired with echocardiography. The choice of a pharmaceutical agent is also affected by the patient's clinical factors. Dipyridamole can worsen bronchospasm and heart block, while dobutamine can cause or exacerbate paroxysmal arrhythmia. LBBB and paced rhythms can cause significant artifact in nuclear perfusion images and abnormal septal motion in dobutamine stress echocardiograms, but are still considered preferable to exercise electrocardiogram alone. Differences in cost, local availability and local expertise may also drive testing decisions.[41]

TREADMILL EXERCISE STRESS TESTING

An ETT involves ambulation on a treadmill according to a specified protocol. The most common is the Bruce protocol that involves an increase in speed and inclines every 3 minutes.[42,43] The test is continued until the patient fatigues, the target HR (85% of peak HR) is achieved, or concerning symptomatic, electrocardiographic or hemodynamic changes are noted.

It is imperative to consider the pre-test probability of CAD in the patient prior to the application of a stress test. In a classic study of patients with a wide range of pre-test likelihoods of CAD (7–87%) based on chest pain description, a positive ETT only increased the pre-test risk by 6–20% and a negative ETT decreased the post-test risk by only 2–28%.[44] This is in part due to limitations in the diagnostic performance of ETT. A large meta-analysis of ETT, in comparison to angiography as the gold standard, showed a wide variation in the sensitivity and specificity of ETT. These researchers found that the mean sensitivity was 68% ± 16%; range, 23–100% and mean specificity, 77% ± 17%; range, 17–100%. When the analysis was restricted to those patients who agreed to both tests prior to either examination, the sensitivity was 50% and the specificity was 90%.[45] In a more recent study of ETT, the sensitivity of treadmill exercise testing alone was 45%, with a specificity of 85%.[46] However, in populations with a low pre-test likelihood of CAD, the specificity of ST-segment depression for detecting CAD decreased to the range of only 60%. Specificity can be increased by increasing the amount of ST segment depression required for a positive study from 1 mm to 2 mm. However this comes at the risk of decreased sensitivity.

The ETT can also be used to provide prognostic information with the calculation of a Duke treadmill score. This score incorporates total exercise time, degree of ST segment deviation and presence/absence of anginal symptoms to predict risk of future cardiac events and death. This score can also be used to diagnostically predict the likelihood of CV disease. Patients with high-risk scores (< -11) were associated with a 74% chance of 3 vessel or left main disease. However use of the score does not improve the sensitivity of the test.[47]

These studies all highlight the limitations of ETT and the need for judicious application of the test to the appropriate population and the need for clinical correlation. If the history of chest discomfort is non-anginal in nature, but an ETT is ordered, there is an approximately 40% chance that it will be falsely positive resulting in further unnecessary testing. Alternatively, if the history is very suggestive of anginal discomfort, but the ETT is negative, further testing may still be warranted.

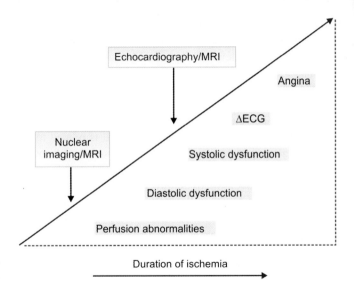

FIGURE 2: Diagrammatic representation of the ischemic cascade with increasing time from onset of ischemia (as with increasing heart rate and BP with exercise stress). Regional hypoperfusion (that can be detected by nuclear imaging) occurs early, followed by diastolic and systolic functional abnormalities (that can be detected by echocardiography), culminating with ECG changes of ischemia and angina. (*Source:* Schuijf JD, Shaw LJ, Wijns W, et al. Cardiac imaging in coronary artery disease: differing modalities. Heart. 2005;91:1110-7)

STRESS TESTING WITH MYOCARDIAL IMAGING

The addition of myocardial imaging increases the sensitivity and specificity to ETT alone. This increased accuracy is due to the changes seen in the ischemic cascade. As exercise progresses, a supply demand mismatch develops. The myocardium requires increased oxygen supply, but myocardial blood flow (supply) is limited, presumably due to a coronary artery stenosis. This decrease in myocardial perfusion is followed by diastolic and then systolic changes. Finally, electrocardiographic changes and symptoms occur (Fig. 2). The earliest change in decreased myocardial perfusion can be detected by the nuclear perfusion imaging.

In addition to adding an imaging modality, exercise can be simulated by pharmaceutical means. Pharmaceutical stress tests are always conducted with myocardial imaging as well as ECG monitoring due to the poor diagnostic performance of pharmacologic stress ECG alone.

STRESS MYOCARDIAL PERFUSION IMAGING

Single photon emission computed tomography (SPECT) utilizes a nuclear tracer, delivered intravenously, to image perfusion of the myocardium. Images are taken of the myocardium at rest and following stress (exercise or vasodilator). Rest and stress images are compared to each other to detect areas of reversible defects, indicating areas of ischemia.

In a pooled analysis of 44 studies, exercise SPECT had a sensitivity of 87% (95% CI, 86–88%) but a specificity of only 64% (95% CI, 60–68%) (i.e. more false positives).[48] The incremental improvement in test performance over exercise ECG was 1.49. In another study of 33 pooled results, the sensitivity for detecting CAD (≥ 50% stenosis) averaged 87% and specificity, derived from patients referred for cardiac catheterization who had normal angiograms, averaged 73%. In addition, the normalcy rate, or the percentage of patients with normal results who had less than 5% chance of disease, was 91%. This means 91% of patients with a low pre-test probability of disease (< 5%) had normal SPECTs. Normalcy rate reduces the referral bias inherent in specificity determinations that use a negative coronary angiogram as gold standard. The diagnostic performance of pharmacologic vasodilator (dipyridamole or adenosine) stress imaging tests were comparable to those of exercise stress imaging with a sensitivity of 89% and specificity of 75%.[49] The sensitivity (85%) and specificity (72%) of dobutamine stress myocardial perfusion imaging (MPI) for diagnosis of CAD in a study of 13 pooled results was also similar. The reported sensitivity and specificity for CAD detection by exercise, dipyridamole and dobutamine myocardial perfusion imaging are comparable.

Stress myocardial imaging has several advantages; it does not necessarily require myocardium to become ischemic since it detects differential perfusion to produce an abnormal result. Stress data can be obtained at peak stress rather than immediately post exercise, if a pharmacological stress is used. It also allows determination of the location and the extent of CAD. The disadvantages are that only LV volumes and ejection fraction can be obtained and no other cardiac structures are assessed. The imaging protocols are longer and take multiple sessions for rest and peak imaging. Radioactive tracers are employed with the inherent risks of radiation exposure. There can be false positives due to attenuation from diaphragmatic or breast tissue in addition to artifactual defects due to LBBB, and false positives due to overlap with liver or gut uptake of tracer and spatial resolution is low. Finally, defects are seen in comparison to normally perfused myocardium; therefore, balanced ischemia or diffusely reduced blood flow can result in relatively normal appearing scans which can "miss" significant underlying CAD.

POSITRON EMISSION TOMOGRAPHIC PERFUSION IMAGING

Positron emission tomographic (PET) perfusion imaging is an alternative to SPECT imaging. PET perfusion imaging involves the administration of Rubidium (Rb-82) and of a glucose analog, fluorine-18-deoxyglucose (FDG). The Rb-82 distributes in perfused vascular spaces while FDG is metabolized by viable tissue. Rb-82 has a very short half-life (78 seconds) and must be generated just prior to administration. The stress must be in the form of a vasodilator. In a pooled analysis comparing PET to SPECT, the sensitivity and specificity of Rb-82 PET for detection of CAD are 91% and 90% respectively compared to 83% and 72%.[50] The diagnostic accuracy of PET was 89% versus 79% with SPECT.[51]

There are a number of advantages of PET relative to SPECT. Some of these include:

- Attenuation correction is more easily performed.
- PET has higher spatial and contrast resolution, which potentially yields better specificity and improved multi-vessel disease identification, with determination of perfusion and viability simultaneously.
- PET can quantify myocardial blood flow in ml/min/g, so that coronary flow reserve can be assessed. This permits better identification of diffuse CAD since tracer uptake can be homogeneous, reflective of balanced ischemia.

There are important limitations to PET as well. Given the short half-life, only vasodilator stress can be used. In addition, a generator is required as well as a PET scanner making it an expensive and less commonly available test.

STRESS TESTING WITH ECHOCARDIOGRAM IMAGING

Echocardiography is a versatile tool that can be used with treadmill, bicycle or arm ergonometer and dipyridamole, adenosine or dobutamine stress modalities. The addition of echocardiography to an exercise stress protocol increases both sensitivity and specificity.[48] If pharmaceutical stress is used in conjunction with echocardiography, dobutamine has the best combination of sensitivity and specificity compared with dipyridamole and adenosine echocardiography or SPECT (Table 2).[52]

There are many advantages to stress echocardiography. It is non-invasive, inexpensive, portable, and does not involve the use of radioactive tracers. It can also be used to define structural heart disease that may provide alternative explanations for symptoms. Stress echocardiography's limitations are that the endocardium can be difficult to visualize, peak images are

TABLE 2

Weighted mean sensitivities and specificities of stress studies

Pharmacologic test	Studies	Subjects	Mean age (y)	CAD (%)	MI (%)	Men (%)	Sensitivity (% [95% CI])	Specificity (% [95% CI])
Adenosine echocardiography	6	516	65	73	31	71	72 (62–79)	91 (88–93)
Adenosine SPECT	9	1,207	63	80	17	59	90 (89–92)	75 (70–79)
Dipyridamole echocardiography	20	1,835	56	67	15	72	70 (66–74)	93 (90–95)
Dipyridamole SPECT	21	1,464	60	71	31	77	89 (84–93)	65 (54–74)
Dobutamine echocardiography*	40	4,097	59	70	26	66	80 (77–83)	84 (80–86)
Dobutamine SPECT	14	1,066	58	66	9	63	82 (77–87)	75 (70–79)
Total	120[†]	10,817						

*One dobutamine echocardiographic study not included here because only multivessel disease was examined.
[†]Total number of tests exceeds the number of studies reviewed because some studies examined more than one pharmacologic test.
(*Source:* Kim C, et al. Pharmacologic stress testing for coronary disease diagnosis: a meta-analysis. Am Heart J. 2001;142:934-44)

difficult to acquire due to rapid breathing and cardiac motion, a truly ischemic response resulting in abnormal wall motion is required for detection of ischemia, quality of imaging is operator dependent, and finally there is significant inter-observer variability in interpretation depending on reader experience.[53] Some of the current limitations of stress echocardiography are being addressed with the use of contrast and the advent of three-dimensional imaging. Intravenous (IV) contrast administration has been shown to improve endocardial border recognition, making previously non-diagnostic images interpretable.[54,55] In addition, three-dimensional echocardiography has made image acquisition less angle dependent and made assessment more reproducible and accurate.[56,57]

COMPARISON OF MPI TO STRESS ECHO

Most studies compare two or, at most, three tests to each other. No study has compared all possible diagnostic tests in the same population. One cost-effectiveness study compared ETT, SPECT, planar thallium imaging, dobutamine stress echocardiography (DSE) and PET. This study showed that while SPECT had higher sensitivity, DSE had higher specificity. In this analysis, due to its higher specificity, stress echo was the most cost effective test. The non-invasive test with the highest sensitivity and specificity was PET and it was cost-effective (Table 3).[58]

Another pooled analysis, comparing stress myocardial perfusion imaging to stress echocardiography had similar findings; that myocardial perfusion imaging offered higher sensitivity (84% vs 80%), but specificity was lower (77% vs 86%) than stress echocardiography. However, using normalcy rate as a substitute for specificity, resulted in a false-positive rate of only 10%.[59] The largest meta-analysis of 44 studies compared these modalities and found that comparing exercise echocardiogram performance to exercise SPECT, the exercise echocardiogram was associated with better discriminatory power (1.18; 95% CI, 0.71–1.65), when adjusted for age, publication

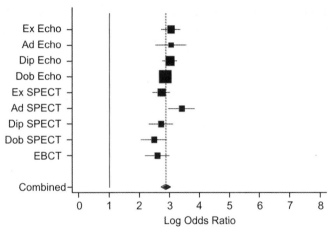

FIGURE 3: Log odds of various stress test modalities. (*Source:* Heijenbrok-kal MH, Fleischmann KE, Hunink MG. Stress echocardiography, stress single-photon-emission computed tomography and electron beam computed tomography for the assessment of coronary artery disease: a meta-analysis of diagnostic performance. Am Heart J. 2007;154:415-23)

year, and a setting including known CAD. The incremental improvement in performance over exercise stress was greater for echo (3.43; 95% CI, 2.74–4.11) than for SPECT (1.49; 95% CI 0.91-2.08).[48]

Clearly, the addition of an imaging component, either nuclear perfusion or echocardiography, to ETT confers greater sensitivity and specificity to ETT alone (Fig. 3). The application of nuclear perfusion imaging versus stress echo, however, depends on pre-test probability, patient factors, local availability, expertise and cost.

All these various studies demonstrate similar themes. The addition of an imaging component to any form of stress increases the sensitivity and specificity of that test. Overall, stress echocardiography tends toward increased specificity, while stress nuclear imaging may tend toward increased sensitivity.

TABLE 3

Pooled sensitivities and specifities of noninvasive tests

Diagnostic test	Sensitivity (Range)*	Specificity (Range)*	Studies (n)	Patients (n)`	Patients with Coronary Disease (%)	Sensitivity for Left Main or Three-Vessel Disease	Studies (n)	Patients (n)
Planar thallium imaging	0.79 (0.70–0.94)	0.73 (0.43–0.97)	6	510	66	0.93	2	72
Single-photon emission computed tomography	0.88 (0.73–0.98)	0.77 (0.53–0.96)	8	628	70	0.98	3	92
Echocardiography†	0.76 (0.40–1.00)	0.88 (0.80–0.95)	10	1174	64	0.94	4	115
Positron emission tomography	0.91 (0.69–1.00)	0.82 (0.73–0.88)	3	206	68	Not available		
Exercise electrocardiography‡	0.68	0.77	132	24074	66	0.86	48	

*Range of sensitivity and specificity reported in individual studies
†Test characteristics for echocardiography are based on pooled studies of dobutamine, dipyridamole, and exercise as stressors. Pooling only studies that used dobutamine as a stressor gave similar results, with a sensitivity of 0.76 and a specificity of 0.87 for all coronary disease
‡Sensitivity of exercise electrocardiography for detection of all coronary artery disease is based on a meta-analysis that included 144 studies for estimates of sensitivity and 132 studies for specificity. Exercise electrocardiography results for sensitivity in left main and three-vessel disease were based on another meta-analysis. No studies of positron emission tomography reported sensitivity for left main and three-vessel disease.
(*Source:* Garber AM, Solomon NA. Cost-effectiveness of alternative test strategies for the diagnosis of coronary artery disease. Ann Intern Med. 1999;130:719-28)

However, various forms of stress imaging tests have generally similar diagnostic log odds ratios and overall diagnostic performance.[60] While PET has improved sensitivity and specificity over both stress echocardiography and stress nuclear, the cost and lack of availability limits its use.

NONINVASIVE COMPUTED TOMOGRAPHIC ANGIOGRAPHY

Computed tomographic angiography (CTA) is a promising technology that allows direct visualization of coronary arteries without an invasive procedure. Intravenous contrast is delivered through a peripheral IV and images are rapidly acquired within a 10 second breath-hold.

The original CTA scanners were electron beam CTs (EBCT), which still have the advantage of superior temporal resolution, but have quite limited spatial resolution. Currently CTA is performed by multi-detector CT (MDCT) scanners which are capable of a high degree of both spatial and temporal resolution. A 64 detector array is the current standard allowing a 0.5 mm discrimination.

There have been three recent trials assessing the accuracy and precision of 64-MDCT in relation to invasive angiography. Core-64 studied 291 patients undergoing both CTA and invasive coronary angiography. In comparison to invasive coronary angiography, CTA had a sensitivity of 85% and specificity of 90%, resulting in a PPV = 91% and NPV = 83%.[61] Another study found that in 230 patients having both procedures there was a sensitivity of 95%, and a specificity of 83%. The positive and negative predictive values were 64% and 99% respectively.[62] The third large trial comparing the diagnostic accuracy of CTA to invasive coronary angiography found a similar sensitivity of 99%, but a much lower specificity of only 64%, resulting in an NPV of 97% and a PPV of 86%.[63] These studies all demonstrate that the main utility of CTA is its negative predictive value in ruling out obstructive CAD in symptomatic low- to intermediate-risk patients.

In addition to its diagnostic use, CTA also has incremental prognostic value, beyond standard risk factors, in assessing future risk of coronary events or death.[64-66] However, whether CTA should be used to narrow risk stratification and whether any additional testing is cost-effective in routine use are currently unclear.

The advantage that CTA provides is an anatomical picture without requiring an invasive procedure with its small but definite risks of vascular access complication, stroke, arrhythmia, ischemia or death. It is useful for detecting coronary anomalies, assessing patency of coronary artery bypass grafts, and ruling out CAD in symptomatic patients with low to intermediate risk of CAD and equivocal stress test results.[67]

Computed tomographic angiography has shown promising results in the triage of patients with chest pain in the emergency department,[68,69] as a first test in the investigation of chest pain,[70,71] and as compared to invasive catheterization in patients with low pre-test probability of CAD.[72] CTA has also been compared to MPI as a first test in the detection of coronary disease. It has been shown to be more diagnostic and more economical in small, single-center, non-randomized studies.[68,71] However, the positive predictive value of CTA is low resulting in potentially unnecessary invasive angiograms in low-risk populations. Therefore, the appropriate use of CTA in the diagnosis of CAD is not yet established and is undergoing evaluation.[73,74]

INVASIVE CORONARY ANGIOGRAPHY

The current gold standard for the detection of CAD is invasive coronary angiography. In the event that the clinical history is highly suspicious for ischemic pain, and non-invasive tests are negative or equivocal, the definitive test is a coronary angiogram. It is also the test of first choice in situations where pre-test likelihood is high and in most cases of ACS.[41]

The limitations of invasive coronary angiography are that it is invasive and therefore carries various risks, although small, of vascular access complications, heart attack, arrhythmia, stroke and death. It requires a dedicated facility and is costly. It requires the use of intra-arterial contrast and radiation with their respective side effects. Finally, it does not provide information with respect to the functional significance of visual coronary stenosis, which is especially important for lesions of borderline severity, although the addition of fractional flow reserve assessment can be helpful in this regard. The advantages are that it provides a definitive diagnosis[75] and it allows for a therapeutic intervention to be carried out within the diagnostic procedure.[76] It should be recognized that definitive diagnosis of CAD with invasive angiography is limited to epicardial vessel disease. There are a minority of patients with clearly ischemic symptoms and no epicardial vessel disease, who may have small vessel disease.[77] Thus, even with the gold standard in the diagnosis of CAD, clinical context must be considered.

SUMMARY

In summary, the evaluation and management of patients with chest pain is not always straightforward. Initial evaluation includes a thorough medical history incorporated with physical exam findings. Biomarker evaluation helps to risk stratify patients into low, intermediate or high-risk categories. This risk stratification process determines the most appropriate further testing to be conducted and results should be interpreted in the context of the individual patient's risk.

MODIFIED SUMMARIES OF GUIDELINES
(Testing of Low-risk Patients Presenting to the Emergency Department with Chest Pain. A Scientific Statement from the American Heart Association. Circulation 2010;122:756-76)

Kanu Chatterjee

THE MAGNITUDE OF THE PROBLEM

There are more than 8 million visits to emergency department (ED) annually for chest pain or other symptoms suggesting myocardial ischemia. This is the second most frequent cause of ED visits in adults.

Less than 5% of patients presenting with chest pain have ST-segment elevation myocardial infarction (STEMI). Approximately 25% of patients have non-ST-segment elevation acute coronary syndrome (NSTEMI/UA).

HIGH LIKELIHOOD OF ACS

- History—Accelerating tempo of ischemic symptoms in preceding 48 hours
- Character of pain—Prolonged ongoing (> 20 min) rest pain
- Clinical findings—Hemodynamic pulmonary edema, new or worsening mitral regurgitation, S3 or new/worsening rales, hypotension, bradycardia, tachycardia, age greater than 75 years
- ECG—ST-segment changes greater than 0.05 mV, new or presumed new bundle-branch block, sustained ventricular tachycardia
- Cardiac markers—Elevated troponin.

INTERMEDIATE LIKELIHOOD OF ACS

- History—Prior MI or cerebrovascular disease, or CABG; prior aspirin use
- Character of pain—Prolonged (> 20 min) rest angina now resolved with moderate or high likelihood of CAD, rest angina (< 20 min or relieved with rest or nitroglycerin)
- Clinical findings—Greater than 70 years
- ECG—T-wave inversions greater than 0.2 mV, pathologic Q waves
- Cardiac markers—Normal troponin.

LOW LIKELIHOOD OF ACS

- Character of pain—New-onset or progressive Canadian Cardiovascular System III or IV angina during the past 2 weeks without prolonged (> 20 min) rest pain but with moderate or high likelihood of CAD
- ECG—Normal or unchanged ECG during an episode of chest pain
- Cardiac markers—Normal troponin.

CARDIAC CAUSES OF ACUTE CHEST PAIN

Cardiovascular Causes of Chest Pain

Angina

- Location: Usually substernal, can be epigastric, intercapular, shoulders, frequently difficult to localize (localize—finger sign)
- Quality: Pressure, heaviness, squeezing, indigestion
- Radiation: One or both the arms, upper back, neck, epigastrium, shoulder, lower jaw (not upper jaw or head, lower back, lower abdomen or lower extremity)
- Duration: 1-10 minutes (not a few seconds or hours)
- Aggravating or relieving factors: Exercise, cold weather, emotional stress heavy meals; heavy meals, relieved by rest or nitroglycerin (not diagnostic)
- Associated symptoms or signs: Dyspnea, S4, MR murmur

Pericarditis

Physical examination:
- Pericardial rub

Diagnostic tests:
- ECG
- TTE if necessary

Acute Aortic Dissection

Physical examination:
- Auscultation for AR
- Findings for tamponade

Diagnostic tests:
- ECG
- Chest X-ray
- CT, MRI, TEE

Pulmonary Embolism

Physical examination:
- Findings for right heart failure
- Pulmonary hypertension
- Pleural rub

Diagnostic tests:
- ECG
- Chest X-ray
- Dimers
- CT
- V/Q scan

NONCARDIAC CAUSES OF ACUTE CHEST PAIN

- Gastrointestinal—Esophageal reflux, peptic ulcer biliary disease, pancreatitis
- Musculoskeletal—Costochondritis, cervical disk disease
- Psychological—Anxiety, depression

CONFIRMATORY TEST SELECTION IN ACCELERATED DIAGNOSTIC PROTOCOLS

- Exercise Treadmill Testing
- Myocardial imaging—Pharmacologic stress nuclear perfusion imaging, positron emission tomography, stress echocardiography
- Computed tomography coronary angiography.
- Magnetic resonance imaging.

FOLLOW-UP OF PATIENTS WITH NEGATIVE CHEST PAIN UNIT EVALUATIONS

All patients should be followed in the cardiology clinic for appropriate investigations and treatments.

MODIFIED SUMMARY OF GUIDELINES
ACC/AHA 2007 Guidelines on Perioperative Cardiovascular Evaluation and Care for Non Cardiac Surgery Circulation 2007;1971-96)

Kanu Chatterjee

Class I: Conditions for which there is evidence and/or general agreement that a given procedure or treatment is useful and effective.

Class II: Conditions for which there is conflicting evidence and/or divergence of opinion about the usefulness/efficacy of a procedure or treatment.

Class IIa: Weight of evidence/opinion is in favor of usefulness/efficacy.

Class IIb: Usefulness/efficacy is well established by evidence/opinion.

Class III: Conditions for which there is evidence and/or general agreement that the procedure/treatment is not useful/effective and in some cases may be harmful.

Level of evidence A: The presence of multiple randomized clinical trials.

Level of evidence B: The presence of a single randomized trial or nonrandomized studies.

Level of evidence C: Expert consensus.

High-risk procedure (e.g. Aortic aneurysm surgery).

Intermediate-risk procedure (e.g. Carotid surgery).

Low-risk procedure (e.g. Cataract surgery).

PREOPERATIVE NONINVASIVE EVALUATION OF LEFT VENTRICULAR FUNCTION

Class IIa:
- Patients with dyspnea (level of evidence: C)
- Patients with current or prior heart failure (level of evidence: C)

Class IIb:
- Reassessment of left ventricular function in clinically stable patients in whom the diagnosis is not well established (level of evidence: C)

Class III:
- Routine perioperative evaluation of left ventricular function (level of evidence: B)

PREOPERATIVE RESTING 12-LEAD ECG

Class I:
- Patients with at least one clinical risk factor (level of evidence: B)
- Patients with known coronary artery disease, peripheral arterial disease
- Cerebrovascular disease who are undergoing intermediate-risk surgical procedures (level of evidence: C)

Class IIa:
- Patients with no clinical risk factors undergoing vascular surgical procedures (level of evidence: B)

Class IIb:
- In patients with at least one clinical risk factor who are undergoing intermediate-risk operative procedures (level of evidence: B)

Class III:
- Asymptomatic patients undergoing low-risk surgical procedures (level of evidence: B)

RECOMMENDATIONS FOR NONINVASIVE STRESS TESTING BEFORE NONCARDIAC SURGERY

Class I:
- Patients with active cardiac conditions (level of evidence: B)

Class IIa:
- Recommended in patients with 3 or more clinical risk factors and poor functional capacity who require vascular surgery (level of evidence: B)

Class IIb:
- In patients with at least 1 or 2 clinical risk factors and poor functional capacity who require intermediate-risk noncardiac surgery (level of evidence: B)
- In patients with at least 1 or 2 clinical risk factors and good functional capacity who are undergoing vascular surgery (level of evidence: B)

Class III:
- In patients with no clinical risk factors undergoing intermediate-risk noncardiac surgery (level of evidence: C)
- In patients undergoing low-risk noncardiac surgery (level of evidence: C)

RECOMMENDATIONS FOR PREOPERATIVE CORONARY REVASCULARIZATION WITH CORONARY ARTERY BYPASS GRAFTING OR PERCUTANEOUS CORONARY INTERVENTION

Class I:
- In patients with stable angina who have significant left coronary artery stenosis (level of evidence: A)
- In patients with stable angina who have 3-vessel disease (level of evidence: A)
- In patients with stable angina who have 2-vessel disease (level of evidence: A)
- In patients with high-risk unstable angina or non-ST-segment elevation myocardial infarction (level of evidence: A)
- In patients with acute ST-elevation MI (level of evidence: A)

Class IIa:
- Patients in whom percutaneous intervention (PCI) is appropriate for relief of cardiac symptoms and who need elective noncardiac surgery (level of evidence: B)
- It is reasonable to continue aspirin if it is at all possible in patients who had drug-eluting coronary artery stents who require urgent surgical procedures

Class IIb:
- In patients the usefulness of coronary revascularization is not well established (level of evidence: C)
- In patients the usefulness of coronary revascularization is not well established for low-risk ischemic patients with an abnormal dobutamine stress echocardiogram (level of evidence: B)

Class III:
- Routine prophylactic coronary revascularization in patients with stable coronary artery disease (level of evidence: B)
- Elective noncardiac surgery is not recommended within 4"6 weeks in patients receiving bare-metal stents or within 12 months in patients receiving drug-eluting stents in whom aspirin or clopidogrel will need to be discontinued (level of evidence: B)
- Elective noncardiac surgery is not recommended within 4 weeks of coronary revascularization with balloon angioplasty (level of evidence: B)

RECOMMENDATIONS FOR BETA-BLOCKER MEDICAL THERAPY

Class I:
- Beta blockers should be continued if the patients had been on beta blocker therapy (level of evidence: C)
- Beta blockers should be given in the high-risk patients (level of evidence: B)

Class IIa:
- Beta blockers are recommended in patients with suspected or established coronary artery disease (level of evidence: B)
- Beta blockers are probably recommended for patients in whom preoperative assessment for vascular surgery identifies high cardiac risk, as defined by more than one clinical risk factor(level of evidence: B)
- Beta blockers are probably recommended in whom preoperative assessment identifies coronary heart disease or high cardiac risk as identified by the presence of more than one clinical risk factor (level of evidence: B)

Class IIb:
- The usefulness of beta blockers is uncertain for patients who are undergoing either intermediate-risk procedures or vascular surgery in whom preoperative assessment identifies a single clinical risk factor (level of evidence: C)
- The usefulness of beta blockers is uncertain in patients undergoing vascular surgery with no clinical risk factors who are not currently taking beta blockers (level of evidence: B)

Class III:
- Beta blockers should not be given in patients undergoing surgery who have absolute contraindications to beta blockers (level of evidence: C)

RECOMMENDATIONS FOR STATIN THERAPY

Class I:
- For patients currently taking statins and scheduled for noncardiac surgery statins should be continued (level of evidence: B)

Class IIa:
- For patients undergoing vascular surgery with or without clinical risk factors, statin use is reasonable (level of evidence: C)

Class IIb:
- For patients with at least one clinical risk factor who are undergoing intermediate-risk procedures (level of evidence: C)

RECOMMENDATIONS FOR ALPHA-2 AGONISTS

Class IIb:
- Alpha-2 agonists for perioperative control of hypertension may be considered for patients with known CAD or at least one clinical risk factor who are undergoing surgery (level of evidence: B)

Class III:
- Alpha-2 agonists should not be given to patients undergoing surgery who have contraindications for alpha-2 agonists

RECOMMENDATIONS FOR PREOPERATIVE INTENSIVE CARE MONITORING

Class IIb:
- Should be restricted to a very few patients who are unstable and who have multiple comorbid conditions (level of evidence: B)

RECOMMENDATIONS FOR USE OF VOLATILE ANESTHETIC AGENTS

Class IIa:
- May be useful in stable patients at risk of myocardial ischemia (level of evidence: B)

RECOMMENDATIONS FOR PROPHYLACTIC INTRAOPERATIVE NITROGLYCERIN

Class IIb:
- The usefulness of intraoperative nitroglycerin to prevent myocardial ischemia has not been established. It should be used with caution as vasodilatation and hypotension may occur (level of evidence: C)

RECOMMENDATIONS FOR USE OF TRANSESOPHAGEAL ECHOCARDIOGRAPHY (TEE)

Class IIa:
- The emergency use of TEE is reasonable to determine the cause of persistent hemodynamic abnormality (level of evidence: C)

RECOMMENDATIONS FOR MAINTENANCE OF BODY TEMPERATURE

Class I:
- Maintenance of normothermia is indicated during most procedures except in patients with mild hypothermia is indicated (e.g. during high aortic cross-clamping) (level of evidence: B)

RECOMMENDATIONS FOR PERIOPERATIVE CONTROL OF BLOOD GLUCOSE CONCENTRATION

Class IIa:
- It is reasonable to control blood sugar in diabetics or in patients with acute hyperglycemia during high-risk surgical procedures

Class IIb:
- The usefulness of strict control of blood glucose remains in uncertain in patients who are not planned to be in intensive care units (level of evidence: C)

RECOMMENDATIONS FOR PERIOPERATIVE USE OF PULMONARY ARTERY CATHETERS

Class IIb:
- May be reasonable in patients at risk for major hemodynamic disturbances during high-risk noncardiac surgical procedures (e.g. liver transplantation) provided proper interpretations of hemodynamics can be made by persons with the knowledge of hemodynamics (level of evidence: B)

Class III:
- Routine use of pulmonary artery catheters for noncardiac surgical procedures (level of evidence: A)

RECOMMENDATIONS FOR INTRAOPERATIVE AND POSTOPERATIVE USE OF ST-SEGMENT MONITORING

Class IIa:
- To monitor for myocardial ischemia in patients with known CAD or those undergoing vascular surgery (level of evidence: B)

Class IIb:
- In patients with single or multiple risk factors for CAD (level of evidence: B)

RECOMMENDATIONS FOR SURVEILLANCE FOR PERIOPERATIVE MI

Class I:
- Postoperative troponin measurement is recommended in patients with ECG changes or chest pain typical of acute coronary syndrome (level of evidence: C)

Class IIb:
- Routine measurement of postoperative troponin is not well established in clinically stable patients who had vascular and intermediate-risk surgery (level of evidence: C)

Class III:
- Postoperative measurement of troponin is not recommended in asymptomatic stable patients who had high-risk surgery (level of evidence: C)

REFERENCES

1. Pitts SR, Niska RW, Xu J, et al. National Hospital Ambulatory Medical Care Survey: 2006 emergency department summary. Natl Health Stat Report. 2008;7:1-38.

2. Klinkman MS, Stevens D, Gorenflo DW. Episodes of care for chest pain: a preliminary report from MIRNET. Michigan Research Network. J Fam Pract. 1994;38:345-52.

3. NCHS, Health Data Interactive. 2010.

4. Yeh RW, et al. Population trends in the incidence and outcomes of acute myocardial infarction. N Engl J Med. 2010;362:2155-65.

5. Everts B, et al. Localization of pain in suspected acute myocardial infarction in relation to final diagnosis, age and sex, and site and type of infarction. Heart Lung. 1996;25:430-7.

6. Goodacre S, et al. How useful are clinical features in the diagnosis of acute, undifferentiated chest pain? Acad Emerg Med. 2002;9: 203-8.

7. Eriksson B, Vuorisalo D, Sylven C. Diagnostic potential of chest pain characteristics in coronary care. J Intern Med. 1994;235:473-8.

8. Diercks DB, et al. Changes in the numeric descriptive scale for pain after sublingual nitroglycerin do not predict cardiac etiology of chest pain. Ann Emerg Med. 2005;45:581-5.

9. Swap CJ, Nagurney JT. Value and limitations of chest pain history in the evaluation of patients with suspected acute coronary syndromes. JAMA. 2005;294:2623-9.

10. Rollag A, Jonsbu J, Aase O, et al. Standardized use of simple criteria from case history improves selection of patients for cardiac-care unit (CCU) admission. J Intern Med. 1992;232:299-304.

11. Bayer AJ, Chadha JS, Farag RR, et al. Changing presentation of myocardial infarction with increasing old age. J Am Geriatr Soc. 1986;34:263-6.

12. Milner KA, Frunk M, Richards S, et al. Gender differences in symptom presentation associated with coronary heart disease. Am J Cardiol. 1999;84:396-9.

13. Cunningham MA, Lee TH, Cook EF, et al. The effect of gender on the probability of myocardial infarction among emergency department patients with acute chest pain: a report from the Multicenter Chest Pain Study Group. J Gen Intern Med. 1989;4:392-8.

14. Caracciolo EA, Chaitman BR, et al. Diabetics with coronary disease have a prevalence of asymptomatic ischemia during exercise treadmill testing and ambulatory ischemia monitoring similar to that of nondiabetic patients. An ACIP database study. ACIP Investigators. Asymptomatic Cardiac Ischemia Pilot Investigators. Circulation. 1996;93:2097-105.

15. Diamond GA, Forrester JS, Hirsh H, et al. Application of conditional probability analysis to the clinical diagnosis of coronary artery disease. J Clin Invest. 1980;65:1210-21.

16. Kannel WB, Dawber TR, Kagan A, et al. Factors of risk in the development of coronary heart disease-six year follow-up experience. The Framingham Study. Ann Intern Med. 1961;55:33-50.

17. Dawber TR, Kannel WB. The Framingham study. An epidemiological approach to coronary heart disease. Circulation. 1966;34:553-5.

18. Wilson PW, D'Agostino RB, Levy D, et al. Prediction of coronary heart disease using risk factor categories. Circulation. 1998;97:1837-47.

19. Ridker PM, Buring JE, Rifai N, et al. Development and validation of improved algorithms for the assessment of global cardiovascular risk in women: the Reynolds Risk Score. JAMA. 2007;297:611-9.

20. Jayes RL Jr, Beshansky JR, D'Agostino RB, et al. Do patients' coronary risk factor reports predict acute cardiac ischemia in the emergency department? A multicenter study. J Clin Epidemiol. 1992;45:621-6.

21. Goldman L, Weinstein MC, Goldman PA, et al. 27th Bethesda Conference: matching the intensity of risk factor management with the hazard for coronary disease events. Task Force 6. Cost effectiveness of assessment and management of risk factors. J Am Coll Cardiol. 1996;27:1020-30.

22. Lee TH. Chest pain in the emergency department: uncertainty and the test of time. Mayo Clin Proc. 1991;66:963-5.

23. Webb WR, Charles BH. Thoracic Imaging: Pulmonary and Cardiovascular Radiology; 2005.

24. Iribarren C, Sidney S, Sternfeld B, et al. Calcification of the aortic arch: risk factors and association with coronary heart disease, stroke and peripheral vascular disease. JAMA. 2000;283:2810-5.

25. Worsley DF, Alavi A, Aronchick JM, et al. Chest radiographic findings in patients with acute pulmonary embolism: observations from the PIOPED Study. Radiology. 1993;189:133-6.

26. Lee TH, Cook EF, Weisberg M, et al, Acute chest pain in the emergency room. Identification and examination of low-risk patients. Arch Intern Med. 1985;145:65-9.

27. Panju AA, Hennelgarn BR, Guyatt GH, et al. The rational clinical examination. Is this patient having a myocardial infarction? JAMA. 1998;280:1256-63.

28. Norell M, Lythall D, Coghlan G, et al. Limited value of the resting electrocardiogram in assessing patients with recent onset chest pain: lessons from a chest pain clinic. Br Heart J. 1992;67:53-6.

29. Rude RE, Pook WK, Muller JE, et al. Electrocardiographic and clinical criteria for recognition of acute myocardial infarction based on analysis of 3,697 patients. Am J Cardiol. 1983;52:936-42.

30. Adams JE, Abendschein DR, Jaffe AS. Biochemical markers of myocardial injury. Is MB creatine kinase the choice for the 1990s? Circulation. 1993;88:750-63.

31. Adams JE 3rd, Border G, Davila-Roman V, et al, Cardiac troponin I. A marker with high specificity for cardiac injury. Circulation. 1993;88:101-6.

32. Saenger AK, Jaffe AS. Requiem for a heavyweight: the demise of creatine kinase-MB. Circulation. 2008;118:2200-6.

33. Babuin L, Vasile VC, Rio Perez JA, et al. Elevated cardiac troponin is an independent risk factor for short- and long-term mortality in medical intensive care unit patients. Crit Care Med. 2008;36:759-65.

34. Heidenreich PA, Alloggiamento T, Melsop K, et al. The prognostic value of troponin in patients with non-ST elevation acute coronary syndromes: a meta-analysis. J Am Coll Cardiol. 2001;38:478-85.

35. Ohman EM, Armstrong PW, Chirstenson PW, et al. Cardiac troponin T levels for risk stratification in acute myocardial ischemia. GUSTO IIA Investigators. N Engl J Med. 1996;335:1333-41.

36. Antman EM, Tanasijevic MJ, Thompson B, et al. Cardiac-specific troponin I levels to predict the risk of mortality in patients with acute coronary syndromes. N Engl J Med. 1996;335:1342-9.

37. Inhibition of the platelet glycoprotein IIb/IIIa receptor with tirofiban in unstable angina and non-Q-wave myocardial infarction. Platelet Receptor Inhibition in Ischemic Syndrome Management in Patients Limited by Unstable Signs and Symptoms (PRISM-PLUS) Study Investigators. N Engl J Med. 1998;338:1488-97.

38. Antman Elliot M. Low-molecular-weight heparin during instability in coronary artery disease, Fragmin during instability in coronary artery disease (FRISC) study group. Lancet. 1996;347:561-8.

39. Antman EM, Cohen M, Bernink PJ, et al. The TIMI risk score for unstable angina/non-ST elevation MI: A method for prognostication and therapeutic decision making. JAMA. 2000;284:835-42.

40. Granger CB, Goldberg RJ, Dabbous O, et al. Predictors of hospital mortality in the global registry of acute coronary events. Arch Intern Med. 2003;163:2345-53.

41. Gibbons RJ, Chatterjee K, Daley J, et al. ACC/AHA/ACP-ASIM guidelines for the management of patients with chronic stable angina: a report of the American College of Cardiology/American Heart Association Task Force on Practice Guidelines (Committee on Management of Patients with Chronic Stable Angina). J Am Coll Cardiol. 1999;33:2092-197.

42. Bruce RA, Lovejoy FW Jr, et al. Normal respiratory and circulatory pathways of adaptation in exercise. J Clin Invest. 1949;28:1423-30.

43. Bruce RA, Pearson R, et al. Variability of respiratory and circulatory performance during standardized exercise. J Clin Invest. 1949;28: 1431-8.

44. Weiner DA, Ryan TJ, McCabe CH, et al. Exercise stress testing. Correlations among history of angina, ST-segment response and prevalence of coronary-artery disease in the coronary artery surgery study (CASS). N Engl J Med. 1979;301:230-5.

45. Gianrossi R, Detrano R, Mulvihill D, et al. Exercise-induced ST depression in the diagnosis of coronary artery disease. A meta-analysis. Circulation. 1989;80:87-98.

46. Froelicher VF, Lehmann KG, Thomas R, et al. The electrocardiographic exercise test in a population with reduced workup bias: diagnostic performance, computerized interpretation, and multi-variable prediction. Veterans Affairs Cooperative Study in Health Services #016 (QUEXTA) Study Group. Quantitative Exercise Testing and Angiography. Ann Intern Med. 1998;128:965-74.

47. Shaw LJ, Peterson ED, Shaw LK, et al. Use of a prognostic treadmill score in identifying diagnostic coronary disease subgroups. Circulation. 1998;98:1622-30.

48. Fleischmann KE, Hunink MG, Kuntz KM, et al. Exercise echocardiography or exercise SPECT imaging? A meta-analysis of diagnostic test performance. JAMA. 1998;280:913-20.

49. Klocke FJ, Baird MG, Lorell BH, et al. ACC/AHA/ASNC guidelines for the clinical use of cardiac radionuclide imaging-executive summary: a report of the American College of Cardiology/American Heart Association Task Force on Practice Guidelines (ACC/AHA/ASNC Committee to Revise the 1995 Guidelines for the Clinical Use of Cardiac Radionuclide Imaging). Circulation. 2003;108:1404-18.

50. Beanlands RS, Chow BJ, Dick A, et al. CCS/CAR/CANM/CNCS/CanSCMR joint position statement on advanced noninvasive cardiac imaging using positron emission tomography, magnetic resonance imaging and multidetector computed tomographic angiography in the diagnosis and evaluation of ischemic heart disease—executive summary. Can J Cardiol. 2007;23:107-19.

51. Bateman TM, Heller GV, McGhie AL, et al. Diagnostic accuracy of rest/stress ECG-gated Rb-82 myocardial perfusion PET: comparison with ECG-gated Tc-99m sestamibi SPECT. J Nucl Cardiol. 2006;13:24-33.

52. Kim C, Kwok YS, Heagerty P, et al. Pharmacologic stress testing for coronary disease diagnosis: a meta-analysis. Am Heart J. 2001;142:934-44.

53. Picano E, Lattanzi F, Orlandini A, et al. Stress echocardiography and the human factor: the importance of being expert. J Am Coll Cardiol. 1991;17:666-9.

54. Dolan MS, Riad K, El-Shafei A, et al. Effect of intravenous contrast for left ventricular opacification and border definition on sensitivity and specificity of dobutamine stress echocardiography compared with coronary angiography in technically difficult patients. Am Heart J. 2001;142:908-15.

55. Plana JC, Mikati A, Dokainish H, et al. A randomized cross-over study for evaluation of the effect of image optimization with contrast on the diagnostic accuracy of dobutamine echocardiography in coronary artery disease: the OPTIMIZE Trial. JACC Cardiovasc Imaging. 2008;1:145-52.

56. Ahmad M. Real-time three-dimensional dobutamine stress echocardiography: a valuable adjunct or a superior alternative to two-dimensional stress echocardiography? J Am Soc Echocardiogr. 2009;22:443-4.

57. Yoshitani H, Takeuchi M, Mor-AviV, et al. Comparative diagnostic accuracy of multiplane and multislice three-dimensional dobutamine stress echocardiography in the diagnosis of coronary artery disease. J Am Soc Echocardiogr. 2009;22:437-42.

58. Garber AM, Solomon NA. Cost-effectiveness of alternative test strategies for the diagnosis of coronary artery disease. Ann Intern Med. 1999;130:719-28.

59. Schinkel AF, Bax JJ, Geleijnse ML, et al, Noninvasive evaluation of ischaemic heart disease: myocardial perfusion imaging or stress echocardiography? Eur Heart J. 2003;24:789-800.

60. Heijenbrok-Kal MH, Fleischmann KE, Hunink MG. Stress echocardiography, stress single-photon-emission computed tomography and electron beam computed tomography for the assessment of coronary artery disease: a meta-analysis of diagnostic performance. Am Heart J. 2007;154:415-23.

61. Miller JM, Rochitte CE, Dewey M, et al. Diagnostic performance of coronary angiography by 64-row CT. N Engl J Med. 2008;359:2324-36.

62. Budoff MJ, Dowe D, Jollis JG, et al. Diagnostic performance of 64-multidetector row coronary computed tomographic angiography for evaluation of coronary artery stenosis in individuals without known coronary artery disease: results from the prospective multicenter ACCURACY (Assessment by Coronary Computed Tomographic Angiography of Individuals Undergoing Invasive Coronary Angiography) trial. J Am Coll Cardiol. 2008;52:1724-32.

63. Meijboom WB, Meijs MS, Schuiif JD, et al, Diagnostic accuracy of 64-slice computed tomography coronary angiography: a prospective, multicenter, multivendor study. J Am Coll Cardiol. 2008;52:2135-44.

64. Chow BJ, Wells GA, Chen L, et al. Prognostic value of 64-slice cardiac computed tomography severity of coronary artery disease, coronary atherosclerosis, and left ventricular ejection fraction. J Am Coll Cardiol. 2010;55:1017-28.

65. Min JK, Shaw LJ, Devereux RB, et al. Prognostic value of multi-detector coronary computed tomographic angiography for prediction of all-cause mortality. J Am Coll Cardiol. 2007;50:1161-70.

66. Ostrom MP, Gopal A, Ahmadi N, et al. Mortality incidence and the severity of coronary atherosclerosis assessed by computed tomography angiography. J Am Coll Cardiol. 2008;52:1335-43.

67. Hendel RC, Patel MR, Kramer CM, et al. ACCF/ACR/SCCT/SCMR/ASNC/NASCI/SCAI/SIR 2006 appropriateness criteria for cardiac computed tomography and cardiac magnetic resonance imaging: a report of the American College of Cardiology Foundation Quality Strategic Directions Committee Appropriateness Criteria Working Group, American College of Radiology, Society of Cardiovascular Computed Tomography, Society for Cardiovascular Magnetic Resonance, American Society of Nuclear Cardiology, North American Society for Cardiac Imaging, Society for Cardiovascular Angiography and Interventions, and Society of Interventional Radiology. J Am Coll Cardiol. 2006;48:1475-97.

68. Ladapo JA, Hoffmann U, Bamberg F, et al. Cost-effectiveness of coronary MDCT in the triage of patients with acute chest pain. AJR Am J Roentgenol. 2008;191:455-63.

69. Hoffmann U, Bamberg F, Chae CU, et al. Coronary computed tomography angiography for early triage of patients with acute chest pain: the ROMICAT (Rule Out Myocardial Infarction using Computer Assisted Tomography) trial. J Am Coll Cardiol. 2009;53:1642-50.

70. Ladapo JA, Jaffer FA, Hoffmann U, et al. Clinical outcomes and cost-effectiveness of coronary computed tomography angiography in the evaluation of patients with chest pain. J Am Coll Cardiol. 2009;54:2409-22.

71. Min JK, Kang N, Shaw LJ, et al. Costs and clinical outcomes after coronary multidetector CT angiography in patients without known coronary artery disease: comparison to myocardial perfusion SPECT. Radiology. 2008;249:62-70.

72. Halpern EJ, Savage MP, Fischman DL, et al. Cost-effectiveness of coronary CT angiography in evaluation of patients without symptoms who have positive stress test results. AJR Am J Roentgenol. 2010;194:1257-62.

73. Douglas PS. Prospective Imaging Study for Evaluation of Chest Pain; 2010.

74. Hachamovitch R, et al. The study of myocardial perfusion and coronary anatomy imaging roles in CAD (SPARC): design, rationale, and baseline patient characteristics of a prospective, multicenter observational registry comparing PET, SPECT, and CTA for resource utilization and clinical outcomes. J Nucl Cardiol. 2009;16:935-48.

75. Levin DC. Invasive evaluation (coronary arteriography) of the coronary artery disease patient: clinical, economic and social issues. Circulation. 1982;66:III 71-9.

76. Smith SC Jr, Dove JT, Jacobs AK, et al. ACC/AHA guidelines for percutaneous coronary intervention (revision of the 1993 PTCA guidelines)-executive summary: a report of the American College of Cardiology/American Heart Association task force on practice guidelines (Committee to revise the 1993 guidelines for percutaneous trans-luminal coronary angioplasty) endorsed by the Society for Cardiac Angiography and Interventions. Circulation. 2001;103: 3019-41.

77. Mosseri M, Yarom R, Gotman MS, et al. Histologic evidence for small-vessel coronary artery disease in patients with angina pectoris and patent large coronary arteries. Circulation. 1986;74:964-72.

Chapter 48

Acute Coronary Syndrome I
(Unstable Angina and Non-ST-Segment Elevation Myocardial Infarction): Diagnosis and Early Treatment

Saket Girotra, Theresa M Brennan

Chapter Outline

INTRODUCTION

Each year, more than 1.3 million patients are admitted to hospitals throughout the United States with an acute coronary syndrome (ACS); unstable angina (UA) and non-ST-elevation myocardial infarction (NSTEMI) account for 60–70% of all those admissions.[1] Recognizing that everyone with an ACS is not admitted to a hospital, one can appreciate the magnitude of this problem.

The UA/NSTEMI constitutes a subset of the clinical syndrome of ACS that is usually, but not always, caused by atherosclerotic coronary artery disease (CAD). In the spectrum of ACS, UA/NSTEMI is defined by an accelerated or unstable clinical syndrome consistent with angina, with electro-cardiographic changes consistent with ischemia and/or positive biomarkers of necrosis (e.g. troponin), in the absence of ST-segment elevation.

PATHOPHYSIOLOGY

ETIOLOGY

The physiology of myocardial ischemia is simply an imbalance between coronary supply and myocardial demand. Any factor leading to decreased flow or increased demand may offset this delicate balance of supply and demand, and result in myocardial ischemia.

Although chronic stable angina is most commonly secondary to an obstructive coronary stenosis that has developed over years, ACS on the other hand occurs due to an acute event that is most commonly associated with a morphologic change in a previously nonobstructive plaque. This event is usually a result of the abrupt development of plaque rupture or erosion at an unstable plaque with resultant thrombus formation. This occurs through a series of events related to innate plaque characteristics and/or external factors. Consequently, plaque composition rather than degree of luminal stenosis is the major predisposing factor.

Less commonly, acute ischemic events (i.e. ACS) may be precipitated in patients with chronic stable angina by an increase in myocardial workload (increased demand). These may include but are not limited to hemodynamic stress imposed by surgery, hypoxia, anemia, significant hypertension, tachycardia, hyperthyroidism, etc. In this case, the treatment must focus on what is driving the increased in myocardial work. The ACS can also occur in the setting of coronary vasospasm. Coronary vasospasm may occur in the large epicardial vessels, in which case there is generally nonobstructive CAD at the site of the spasm, or in the microcirculation (with angiographically normal epicardial vessels). The spasm may be precipitated by the presence of superimposing environmental triggers such as medications (e.g. vasoconstrictors, triptans, etc.), illicit drugs (e.g. cocaine, methamphetamines, etc.), or may occur in a patient who has an underlying vasoactive disorder (Raynaud's phenomenon or migraine headaches) or endothelial dysfunction. These episodes may have a circadian pattern, occurring commonly in the early morning hours, are more likely in smokers and, although seen commonly at rest, may be precipitated by exercise (although not reproducibly so, as is the case in chronic stable CAD), or even hyperventilation. Finally, progressive atherosclerosis may lead to acceleration in coronary ischemic symptoms, although this is less common, and may be most commonly seen with coronary stent restenosis.

VULNERABLE PLAQUE

Despite a common pathophysiologic pathway, atherosclerotic lesions are heterogeneous in their risk for rupture. The lesions that are at highest risk for rupture are referred to as unstable or vulnerable plaques. These typically consist of a large lipid laden core (> 40% of the total plaque volume),[2] a thin fibrous cap, with a dense infiltration of monocytes and macrophages, with abundant production of matrix metalloproteinases, a loss of smooth muscle cells and a decrease in stabilizing collagen. These characteristics make them more prone to rupture when compared to the fibrous, collagen-rich plaques. Since these plaques are generally not flow limiting, they may escape identification by stress testing and even angiography as at times the vessel will remodel in a positive way and maintain the lumen size. Once plaque disruption occurs, the highly thrombogenic, lipid-rich core is exposed and thrombogenic tissue factors and vasoconstrictors are released into the local circulation. This is followed by activation and aggregations of platelets with formation of a thrombus at the site of rupture. This may lead to various degrees of acute narrowing of the vessel lumen. In patients with UA/NSTEMI, this process falls short of complete vessel occlusion but results in ischemia to the distal territory that is manifested by new (or a change in) symptoms, ischemic electrocardiographic changes and/or biomarker elevation. It has been estimated that up to 75% of vulnerable lesions resulting in ACS and sudden cardiac death are secondary to plaque rupture; the remaining lesions have plaque erosion as the precipitating event.[2]

Multiple lines of evidence suggest that the "culprit" lesion responsible for ACS is frequently nonobstructive prior to the rupture. Data from the Coronary Artery Surgery Study (CASS) evaluated progression of disease among non-bypassed arteries. They found that lesions with greatest severity of stenosis had a higher likelihood of progression to occlusion compared to nonobstructive lesions. However, given that there were many more nonobstructive lesions within an individual's coronary artery tree, the majority of coronary occlusions at follow-up were accounted for by lesions that were nonobstructive at baseline.[3,4] Furthermore, studies have also shown that many patients with ACS do not have an acute collateral filling of the infarct related artery suggesting that the acute event occurred in a lesion that was not previously hemodynamically significant.[5]

SYSTEMIC FACTORS (VULNERABLE PATIENT)

The predisposition to plaque rupture and, thus, the development of ACS and sudden cardiac death may not solely be a manifestation of the plaque itself; other "systemic" factors play an important role. The systemic inflammatory response, changes in local shear stress (sudden and abrupt changes in blood velocity), or chronic and recurrent changes in shear stress may result in fatigue of the fibrous cap leading to rupture.[6] Prothrombotic states (e.g. transient hypercoagulability from smoking, dehydration, infection, cocaine, malignancy, etc.) could facilitate progression of thrombosis once the plaque has eroded/ruptured.[7] One study showed that the levels of neutrophil myeloperoxidase (a marker of inflammation) were significantly increased in both right and left coronary arteries and the femoral artery in patients with ACS compared to stable angina, or variant angina.[8] In addition, this elevation was independent of site of the culprit lesion. Finally, it is now a well-recognized phenomenon that patients presenting with ACS may have more than one "culprit lesion".[9] In these patients and others seen in routine practice, there is a lesion that appears to be causing the clinical syndrome of ACS, based on degree of obstruction or electrocardiogram (ECG) changes (the "culprit lesion"). In addition, the patient will have one or more lesions that appear irregular, ulcerated, hazy and/or thrombotic suggesting an active, acute process. Multiple active lesions in a single individual suggest a systemic impact. Thus, systemic factors are important, perhaps equally so, in determining the individual's predisposition to acute changes in plaques that herald the onset of ACS.

Finally, histologic evaluation supports that the progression of atherosclerosis, perhaps at an accelerated rate, may be subsequent to healing of previously ruptured plaques. The acute event of rupture of the plaque may have had no clinically apparent impact, but the healing of these may result in more rapid luminal narrowing.[10] This suggests that the rupture of the atherosclerotic plaque, in and of itself, may be insufficient to lead to ACS.

Atherosclerosis with positive remodeling maintains lumen patency despite, at times, significant plaque burden. Coronary angiography is, therefore, inherently limited in its ability to estimate atherosclerotic burden in the setting of positive remodeling which preserves a normal lumen diameter. Extensive plaque may be visualized by intravascular ultrasound, CT angiography, or postmortem examination in these patients, that is not apparent, or underestimated by coronary angiography. Newer technologies including intravascular ultrasound with virtual histology, optical coherence tomography (OCT), angioscopy, thermography, positron emission tomography (PET) and magnetic resonance imaging (MRI) are being studied to help us identify the "vulnerable plaque" in the potentially vulnerable patient. Until then, our ability to prevent ACS altogether remains limited.

ROLE OF PLATELETS AND COAGULATION SYSTEM

Platelets play a central role in vascular hemostasis and thrombosis, and our understanding of the mechanisms involved in platelet activation (Fig. 1A), aggregation and its integration with the coagulation cascade (Fig. 1B) has paved the way for the development of several new and investigational drugs that target some key pathways. While an extensive review of the different mechanisms involved in platelet response to vascular injury is outside the scope of this chapter, a brief overview is warranted.

Plaque disruption exposes subendothelial collagen, and platelets adhere to the exposed collagen via surface glycoprotein receptors. This interaction is mediated by von Willebrand factor

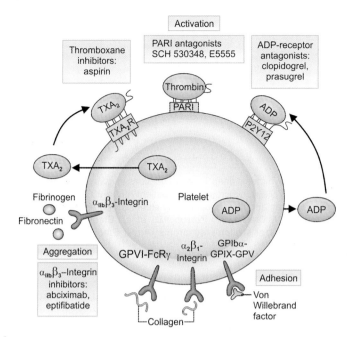

FIGURE 1A: Platelet surface receptors and targets of antiplatelet therapy. (*Source:* Modified from Mackman N. Triggers, targets and treatments for thrombosis. Nature. 2008;451:914-8[9])

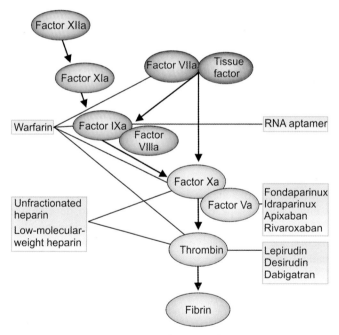

FIGURE 1B: The coagulation pathway and targets of anticoagulation medications. (*Source:* Modified from Mackman N. Triggers, targets and treatments for thrombosis. Nature. 2008;451:914-8[9])

(vWF) and results in adhesion to the subendothelium. Simultaneously, release of tissue factor activates the coagulation cascade with production of thrombin. Thrombin is a very potent activator of human platelets and initiates platelet activation via interaction of proteinase activator receptor 1 (PAR 1) and proteinase activator receptor 4 (PAR 4). A number of intracellular events are triggered that result in platelet activation and degranulation. Platelet granules release among other substances ADP, which is an agonist on two important receptors; the P2Y1 and P2Y12 receptors. This amplifies the platelet

activation response by a positive feedback mechanism. The latter receptor is the target of clopidogrel, prasugrel and ticagrelor. In addition, activation of platelets leads to influx of calcium in the cytosol which activates phospholipase A_2; this enzyme releases phospholipids, which leads to the formation of thromboxane A_2 (TXA_2) via the cyclooxygenase (COX) pathway. Aspirin inhibits this activation pathway. The downstream action of platelet activation is a marked increased surface expression of glycoprotein IIb/IIIa which through the binding with fibrinogen, resulting in platelet aggregation and the development of a platelet rich hemostatic plug. The different glycoprotein IIb/IIIa inhibitors exert their antiplatelet action by inhibiting this binding. Thereby, the rupture of an unstable plaque may lead to abrupt change in coronary luminal area by the aggressive development of a platelet-rich thrombus. Within this pathway, there are multiple sites of potential inhibition that are targets of the medications considered to be standard of care in the treatment of patients with ACS.

CLINICAL FEATURES

Anginal chest pain is the cardinal symptom of ischemic coronary disease. The pain is typically described as deep or poorly localized pain that is reproducibly associated with physical exertion or emotional stress, and is promptly relieved with rest or nitroglycerin. It may radiate to the jaw, neck, back or arm(s) and may be associated with shortness of breath, nausea, lightheadedness or diaphoresis. In patients with UA/NSTEMI, episodes of angina may be severe or prolonged, may be provoked by minimal exertion or may even occur at rest. Many patients do not describe angina as "chest pain" but may describe it as a discomfort; this distinction may be important while interviewing patients as they may deny having pain, but will admit to having discomfort. This pain/discomfort is typically not localized, but rather, is diffuse and in most cases not severe. Others may have no chest discomfort at all and may only experience pain in jaw, neck, arm, shoulder, back or epigastrium. Occasionally, patients may present without any discomfort, instead they may experience unexplained shortness of breath, diaphoresis, nausea, lightheadedness or even syncope as their presenting symptom.[11-13] Such atypical presentations may account for about one-third of all patients who present to the hospital with an ACS.[14] Atypical symptoms are particularly common among the elderly, women, diabetics and patients with heart failure. It is important to recognize that the term "atypical" refers only to the reality that the symptoms are not classical/typical, but does not exclude the diagnosis of ischemia as the etiology of these symptoms. Finally, the angina symptoms may not be relieved with, only partially relieved with, or relieved with rapid recurrence, with rest or nitroglycerin.

In comparison, features that are generally not characteristic of acute myocardial ischemia include: (1) Pleuritic chest pain; (2) Pain localized at the tip of the finger particularly over the left ventricular (LV) apex or costochondral junction; (3) Pain reproduced with movement or palpation and (4) Pain lasting for a few seconds. Although these four types of chest discomfort are not generally ischemic in origin, there is no single characteristic that clearly defines, or excludes the diagnosis of ACS.

The relief of chest pain with nitroglycerin does not always predict CAD as the cause. In a study, up to 41% of patients without CAD had relief of chest pain with nitroglycerin.[15] Due to its effect on smooth muscle relaxation, nitroglycerin may relieve chest pain that may be on account of esophageal spasm, etc. At the same time, relief of chest pain with a "GI cocktail" does not preclude the diagnosis of CAD either.

Finally, knowledge of a patient's risk factors is very important in determining the pretest probability of ACS. Information regarding presence of known CAD, peripheral arterial disease (PAD), hypertension, diabetes, hyperlipidemia, tobacco use, obesity, physical inactivity and/or a family history of premature cardiovascular disease as well as other non-traditional risk factors (e.g. connective tissue diseases, renal failure, etc.) must be sought.[16-18] At least one traditional risk factor is present in as many as 90% of patients with a coronary event.

PHYSICAL EXAMINATION

A normal physical examination is common in patients with ACS and does not exclude this diagnosis. More importantly, findings on the physical examination can help to assess the hemodynamic impact of the ischemic insult. The signs and symptoms, such as cool, clammy skin, diaphoresis, sinus tachycardia, significant bradycardia, S3 or S4, mitral regurgitation murmur and bibasilar rales, may herald the onset of cardiogenic shock even before the development of frank hypotension. Such patients are at a high risk and may require urgent coronary angiography and admission to a coronary intensive care unit (CICU). The physical examination may also be useful in identifying the precipitating causes such as anemia, thyrotoxicosis, uncontrolled blood pressure, and may also helpful in identifying important comorbid conditions (e.g. lung disease, malignancy, etc.) that influence medical decision-making. Occasionally, physical findings might suggest an alternative diagnosis, such as aortic dissection, pericarditis, cholecystitis, etc. and therefore the importance of physical examination cannot be overemphasized.

ELECTROCARDIOGRAM

A 12-lead electrocardiogram (ECG) is an integral part of the initial evaluation of a patient with ACS. In addition to identifying candidates for reperfusion (e.g. STEMI patients), it also provides prognostic information.[19] It is, therefore, a powerful tool in the evaluation and the treatment of patients with possible ACS and should be obtained in all patients with chest pain or angina equivalent, within 10 minutes of arrival to the hospital.

Typical ECG findings that are consistent with ischemia in patients with UA/NSTEMI include the presence of ST-segment depression (at least 0.5 mm in at least two contiguous leads), transient ST changes or presence of T wave inversions. However, up to 20% of patients with an NSTEMI, confirmed by cardiac enzymes, have no diagnostic ischemic ECG changes. While isolated T wave inversion is nonspecific, the finding of symmetric deep T wave inversion (> 2 mm) in multiple precordial leads is usually associated with severe critical stenosis of the proximal left anterior descending artery (Wellen's syndrome) (Fig. 2).[20] Such patients should be

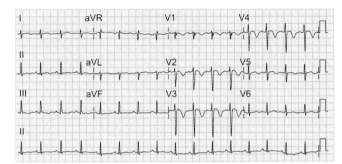

FIGURE 2: Symmetric deep T wave inversions involving multiple precordial leads (Wellen's syndrome). This patient had a 90% stenosis in his proximal left anterior descending artery stenosis. (*Source:* Modified from Rhinehardt J, Brady WJ, Perron AD, et al. Electrocardiographic manifestations of Wellen's syndrome. Am J Emerg Med. 2002;20: 638-43)

promptly referred for cardiac consultation, and early coronary angiography. An ECG finding with ST depression less than 0.5 mm is less specific for the diagnosis of ACS. A normal ECG decreases but does not eliminate the possibility of ACS. Approximately up to 4% of patients with chest pain and a normal ECG are later diagnosed with UA/NSTEMI.[21] It is well known that infarcts in the distribution of the left circumflex coronary artery can be electrocardiographically silent on the standard 12-lead ECG. In these situations, posterior leads (V7–V9) may help to uncover ischemia involving the posterior wall. In some patients, the ECG changes may be dynamic. Therefore the finding of a normal initial ECG in a patient where the clinical suspicion is high should always prompt serial ECG evaluation (along with cardiac biomarker testing), especially if the ECG was obtained after the symptoms have resolved.

It is always helpful to compare a current ECG with a previous one, if available, to note subtle changes, or pseudo-normalization (the change from a previously inverted T wave to now a normal appearing upright T wave). Also, development of ischemic changes, while a patient is experiencing chest discomfort, which resolve if the patient becomes asymptomatic, is highly suggestive of cardiac ischemia and increases the likelihood of underlying significant CAD.

BIOMARKERS

Creatinine Kinase

Creatinine kinase (CK) has been the most commonly used biochemical markers among patients with ACS worldwide. The MB isoenzyme has greater specificity for myocardial tissue compared to total CK (which may be elevated in neurological or skeletal muscle disorders as well). The CK-MB levels peak at 10–18 hours after injury and usually remain elevated up to 72 hours after which they return to baseline (Fig. 3). Due to its shorter half-life, CK and CK-MB elevation is particularly useful in detecting episodes of reinfarction. It should be remembered that CK is cleared by the kidneys and thus may be chronically elevated in renal failure in patients and may not be indicative of an acute myocardial infarction (AMI).

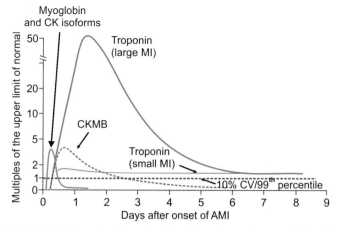

FIGURE 3: Timing of release of various biomarkers after acute ischemic myocardial infarction. (*Source:* Modified from Kumar, et al. Acute coronary syndromes: diagnosis and management, Part 1. Mayo Clin Proc. 2009;84(10):917-38)

Troponin

Cardiac troponins have gained widespread acceptance, and have largely replaced CK-MB as the biomarkers of choice for detecting myocardial injury. This is due to their high sensitivity and specificity to the heart muscle as well as the commercial availability of a rapid, inexpensive and reproducible test. Troponin is a multimer that is composed of three subunits: (1) Troponin (Tn) T, (2) Tn I and (3) Tn C. Only Tn T and Tn I are commercially available as diagnostic tests. Since normal individuals should not have any detectable levels, levels higher than 99th percentile of a normal population of subjects are used as a cutoff for troponin elevation.

Troponin levels do not increase until at least 6 hours after the onset of the infarct; therefore, a negative test during this period should be repeated after a period of 4–6 hours (Fig. 3). Also, the longer half-life of troponin (5–14 days) limits its usefulness in detecting reinfarction. In these situations, CKD and CK-MB are more reliable.

Among patients with symptoms consistent with UA, the presence of troponin elevation identifies patients with NSTEMI. It is estimated that up to 25% of patients with UA who have normal CK-MB levels would be classified as having NSTEMI based on troponin assay.[22] It must be emphasized, however, that the availability of an easy to order test should not replace clinical judgment. Troponins are specific markers of myocardial injury, but they do not automatically imply ischemia as the cause of injury (e.g. myocarditis, heart failure, cardiac contusion, etc.).[23] Therefore one must interpret the results of biomarker elevation in the context of the clinical syndrome.

RISK STRATIFICATION—PUTTING IT ALL TOGETHER TO DETERMINE THE OPTIMAL TREATMENT STRATEGY

Patients presenting with chest pain or angina equivalent, consistent with possible UA/NSTEMI are heterogeneous in terms of their risk of mortality. Therefore, appropriate risk stratification is of paramount importance.

Early risk assessment must be twofold. Firstly, one must determine the likelihood that the clinical syndrome is related to coronary ischemia and evaluate whether the course of symptoms are accelerated. This is performed by a focused history assessing whether the clinical presentation is consistent with angina. In order to do so, one must understand the clinical characteristics that are typical of angina (described previously) and be aware of the potential for atypical presentations of angina. In addition, one must consider the overall risk factors that the individual patient will have CAD by assessing patient's risk factors (known CAD, PAD, hypertension, diabetes, hyperlipidemia, smoking, family history of premature CAD, obesity, physical inactivity, chronic renal failure and the presence of a connective tissue disease or rheumatoid arthritis).[16-18,24] Next, one must consider findings on the ECG and available laboratory testing. Finally, one must consider the likelihood of alternative diagnoses.

Based upon this, a patient may be classified into one of the following groups:
- Definite ACS (clinical symptoms consistent with angina, and electrocardiogram (ECG) changes consistent with ischemia and/or positive troponin, or patients with known stable angina with acceleration in the pattern of the angina).
- Possible ACS (clinical symptoms consistent with angina, but lack of ECG changes or positive troponin).
- Stable angina (clinical symptoms consistent with angina, without a pattern of acceleration or instability).
- Noncardiac chest pain (clinical symptoms that are not consistent with angina and lack of ECG changes or positive troponins, especially with a documented noncardiac cause).

Patients with definite ACS require hospitalization and further evaluation and treatment as described here. Patients with possible ACS require further evaluation in a monitored setting such as a chest pain observation unit or a monitored telemetry unit. In the chest pain observation unit, ECG and cardiac markers are repeated after 3–8 hours (pending institutional protocol and the time elapsed from the onset of discomfort) and if negative the patient will undergo a provocative (stress) or anatomic (CT) test to assess coronary ischemia as the etiology of the syndrome. If the evaluation is negative, the patient may be discharged with recommendations for risk factor modification as appropriate and follow-up as necessary. Patients with a presumed diagnosis of noncardiac chest must have an evaluation to determine other life-threatening noncoronary diagnoses (e.g. pulmonary embolism, aortic dissection, pneumonia, etc.). Of course, the identification of a noncardiac cause should prompt appropriate treatment. If any of the tests suggests the diagnosis of ACS, the patient will be admitted for further evaluation and therapy. Patients with stable angina may be discharged home with increased medical therapy to follow-up as an outpatient.

Second, one must perform early risk stratification in those patients with possible/definite ACS to tailor treatment intensity according to patient's risk for early morbidity and mortality. The estimation of risk in ACS involves incorporating information from several prognostic variables which include history, physical findings, ECG changes and troponin, and is further discussed below.

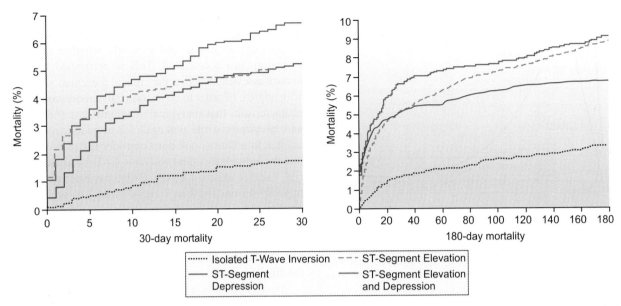

FIGURE 4: Risk of 30-day and 180-day mortality according to ECG changes at presentation in patients with NSTEMI. (*Source:* Modified from Savonitto S et al. Admission ECG changes and the impact on 30- and 180-day mortality. JAMA. 1999;281:707-13)

HISTORY

The risk for short-term and long-term mortality increases with advancing age among patients with UA/NSTEMI.[25] Prior history of CAD increases the likelihood of obstructive and multivessel CAD. While traditional risk factors are important in assessing the likelihood of ACS as discussed above, they are less important in predicting short-term mortality except history of diabetes[26] and/or extra cardiac PAD,[27] both of which increase the short-term risk. Similarly, patients who present with hemodynamic compromise (advanced Killip Class) have a significantly higher risk of death and should be treated with aggressive use of antithrombotics and early use of invasive angiography.[28]

ELECTROCARDIOGRAM

Multiple studies have shown that the electrocardiogram (ECG) provides valuable prognostic information among patients with ACS. The patient with ACS and an ECG showing dynamic ST segment changes or left bundle branch block (LBBB) have the highest risk of death while patients with isolated T wave inversions or normal ECG have a lower risk of death. This association is independent of the remaining clinical findings and the patient risk factors (Fig. 4).[29,30] The association of Wellen's T waves with critical proximal left anterior descending artery stenosis has been previously discussed. These patients if left untreated are at a high risk for developing extensive anterior wall myocardial infarction, significant morbidity and death. Once recognized, urgent coronary angiography should be pursued in these patients.[20]

CARDIAC BIOMARKERS

Elevation in troponin is a strong predictor of short-term mortality with a gradient of risk according to the level of troponin

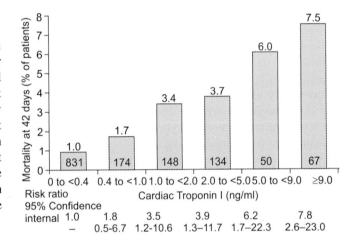

FIGURE 5: Mortality rates at 42 days according to the level of cardiac troponin I. (*Source:* Modified from Antman EM, Tanasijevic MJ, Thompson B, et al. Cardiac-specific troponin I levels to predict the risk of mortality in patients with acute coronary syndromes. N Engl J Med. 1996;335:1342-9)

elevation (Fig. 5),[22] and it is incorporated into all of the risk prediction tools that are currently available. Therefore, the utility of the test is not just limited to diagnosis; an elevated troponin level implies a worse prognosis regardless of etiology, even among those patients later identified to have no epicardial CAD.[31,32] Thus, troponin elevation is considered as an important marker of risk and identifies patients who may be candidates for more aggressive treatment (see risk stratification below).

During the past decade, inflammation has been recognized to play an important role in the pathogenesis of ACS. Consequently, attention has been focused on biomarkers of inflammation, of which C-reactive protein (CRP) is the most widely studied. Elevated CRP detected by a high sensitivity assay (hs-CRP) has been strongly associated with increased risk

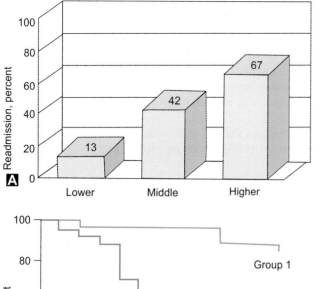

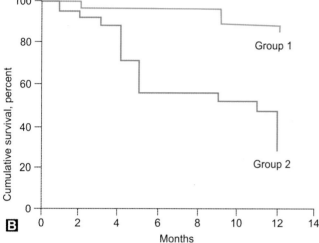

TABLE 1

TIMI risk score

- Age > 65 years
- Chest pain in previous 24 hours
- Three major risk factors (diabetes, hypertension, hyperlipidemia, family history of ischemic heart disease and current smoking)
- Aspirin use in last 7 days
- Known coronary stenosis > 50%
- ST segment deviation > 0.5 mm or new left bundle branch block on initial ECG
- Elevated troponin level

(Score: One point is awarded for each parameter)

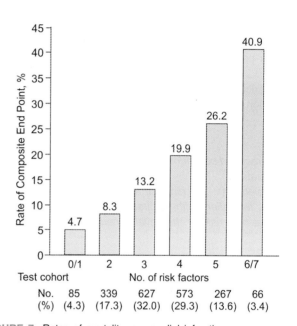

Test cohort	0/1	2	3	4	5	6/7
No.	85	339	627	573	267	66
(%)	(4.3)	(17.3)	(32.0)	(29.3)	(13.6)	(3.4)

FIGURES 6A AND B: The incidence of readmission for unstable angina or myocardial infarction during follow-up correlates with the serum concentration of CRP measured at discharge in patients with unstable angina. (A) Patients in upper tertile of serum CRP (≥ 0.87 mg/dL) had significantly more events during follow-up than patients in the middle (0.26–0.86 mg/dL) or lower (≤ 0.25 mg/dL) tertiles. (B) The 1-year survival free of readmission for myocardial infarction or unstable angina was lower in patients with increased serum CRP at discharge compared to those with normal levels. (*Source:* Modified from Biasucci LM, Liuzzo G, Grillo RL, et al. Elevated levels of C-reactive protein at discharge in patients with unstable angina predict recurrent instability. Circulation. 1999;99:855-60)

FIGURE 7: Rates of mortality, myocardial infarction, severe recurrent myocardial ischemia that prompted urgent revascularization according to TIMI risk score. (*Source:* Modified from Antman EM, Cohen M, Bernink PJ, et al. The TIMI risk score for unstable angina/non-ST elevation MI: a method for prognostication and therapeutic decision-making. JAMA. 2000;284:835-42)

of short-term mortality, and identifies patients with normal troponin levels who are at an increased risk of death and recurrent ischemic events (e.g. recurrent ischemia/hospitalization, reinfarction and death) (Figs 6A and B).[33,34] Similarly, elevated levels of B-type natriuretic peptide (BNP) have also been shown to provide powerful prognostic information across the entire spectrum of ACS for both short-term and long-term mortality in a number of studies.[35,36]

Since multiple variables are predictive of risk in UA/NSTEMI patients, several groups have developed comprehensive multivariable risk models that incorporate information from several predictor variables into a score for the purpose of determining intensity of initial treatment and prognosis. The most commonly used risk score in the United States is the thrombolysis in myocardial infarction (TIMI) risk score, which incorporates information from seven variables (Table 1).[37] The TIMI risk score enables identification of high-risk patients that

are at increased risk of death, and recurrent myocardial infarction (MI) and thus would benefit from aggressive therapies and early invasive treatment (Fig. 7). Other risk scores, such as the GRACE and PURSUIT are also available, and may be better at predicting mortality, but are more complex.[38,39]

EARLY MEDICAL THERAPY

The following section discusses early medical therapy in patients with ACS with special emphasis on UA/NSTEMI. At the end of each section, recommendations from the American College of Cardiology (ACC) and the American Heart Association (AHA) 2007 guidelines, and the more recent 2011 focused updates on the management of patients with UA/NSTEMI are included wherever appropriate.[40,41] Indications for use are divided into Class I (should be performed/administered), Class II (reasonable to or may consider performing/administering) and

Class III (should NOT perform/administer due to the lack of benefit and/or potential for harm). The reader is directed to the guidelines for a detailed discussion and the reasoning for these recommendations.

GENERAL MEASURES

Based on the risk of future events, patients with a presumed diagnosis of UA/NSTEMI may be admitted to a coronary care unit (high risk), a telemetry unit (intermediate or low risk) or may be managed in a chest pain observation unit (low risk). Continuous telemetry monitoring should be available to detect dysrhythmias.

Even though not rigorously studied, oxygen supplementation is frequently used to provide adequate supply of oxygen, especially to the patients with oxygen saturations of 90% or below. The patients should be on bed rest during the early evaluation process.

> The American College of Cardiology (ACC)/American Heart Association (AHA) guidelines recommend:
>
> **Class I**
>
> - *Bed rest and continuous ECG monitoring during the initial evaluation.*
> - *Supplemental oxygen if arterial saturation is less than 90%, for patient with respiratory distress or patient who are at high risk for the development of hypoxemia.*

NITRATES

These agents are donors of nitric oxide (NO), which causes activation of cyclic guanylyl cyclase pathway resulting in an increase in intracellular cyclic guanosine monophosphate (cGMP). This leads to vasodilation, primarily in the venous bed with decrease in venous return and cardiac preload. Additional mechanisms include coronary vasodilation and improvement in blood flow to ischemic areas. Finally, a reduction in platelet aggregation has also been proposed as a potentially beneficial mechanism.[42]

Patients with ACS should receive a sublingual nitroglycerin (0.4 mg) or a buccal spray which may be repeated every 5 minutes for a total of 3 doses. If pain persists, then intravenous nitroglycerin should be initiated at a dose of 10 microgram/minute and rapidly titrated up (every 3–5 minutes) to achieve pain relief or until relative hypotension develops. There is no absolute maximum dose of nitroglycerin, although doses above 200 microgram/minute have not generally been shown to provide additional benefit. Nitrates should not be used in patients who have recently ingested type 5 phosphodiesterase inhibitors (e.g. sildenafil, tadalafil, etc.) as it may result in dangerous and reportedly fatal hypotension. Men and patients with known pulmonary hypertension should be questioned regarding recent use of these agents. Once the acute pain episode has resolved oral or, less commonly, topical nitrates may be used to prevent recurrences of symptomatic ischemic episodes. It must be remembered that patients should ultimately have a nitrate free period of at least 8–10 hours to prevent the development of tachyphylaxis, but generally in the first 24 hours after presentation, nitroglycerin may be continued for pain relief and prevention.

Evidence for the effect of nitrates in reducing long-term mortality is generally lacking.[43,44] Therefore, the primary role of chronic nitrates in ACS patients is relief of pain acutely in patients who have angina that is refractory to other effective medications (e.g. aspirin, clopidogrel, β-blockers, etc.).

> The American College of Cardiology (ACC)/American Heart Association (AHA) guidelines recommend:
>
> **Class I**
>
> - *Sublingual nitroglycerin every 5 minutes for 3 doses to relieve symptoms.*
> - *Intravenous nitroglycerin for up to 48 hours in patients with refractory symptoms of ischemia, or heart failure or continued hypertension despite medical therapy, provided use of nitroglycerin does not preclude the use of other mortality-reducing agents (β-blockers or ACE inhibitors).*
>
> **Class III**
>
> Use of nitrates should be avoided in:
> - *Systolic pressure less than 90 mm Hg or a 30 mm Hg drop from baseline.*
> - *Significant bradycardia or tachycardia in absence of heart failure.*
> - *Suspected right ventricular infarction.*
> - *Patient has taken a phosphodiesterase inhibitor for erectile dysfunction in previous 24 hours for sildenafil or 48 hours for tadalafil.*

MORPHINE

Morphine sulfate used in a dose of 1–4 mg intravenously is a useful adjunctive therapy for pain relief among patients with ACS. In addition to its potent analgesic effect, morphine results in venodilation and reduction in cardiac preload—this effect is particularly beneficial in patients with pulmonary edema. In addition, due to its anxiolytic effect, it helps to relieve agitation and has a calming effect in such patients; therefore, decreasing their myocardial oxygen demand. Some patients may develop hypotension which generally responds to supine positioning and/or volume challenge. Rarely, respiratory depression may develop that responds to reversal with naloxone.

> The American College of Cardiology (ACC)/American Heart Association (AHA) guidelines recommend:
>
> **Class IIA**
>
> - *Morphine sulfate may be used for symptom control in addition to other medical therapy for ischemia.*

BETA BLOCKERS

These drugs act by blocking the effect of catecholamines on β1-receptors of the heart which results in slowing of the heart rate, and reduction of contractility thereby reducing myocardial oxygen consumption. Slowing of the heart rate is beneficial as it helps in prolonging diastole thereby improving coronary perfusion.

In the absence of contraindications, patients with ACS should be treated with β-blockers at initial presentation. Oral dosing is appropriate although it is reasonable to use intravenous dosing in patients who are persistently hypertensive. Contraindications to the use of β-blockers include: (1) Signs of heart failure; (2) Evidence of low-output state; (3) Increased risk for cardiogenic shock and (4) Other relative contraindications (first degree AV block with PR interval > 0.24 seconds, any 2nd or 3rd degree AV block, reactive airway disease or active asthma). A history of chronic obstructive pulmonary disease (COPD) should not preclude use of β-blockers; however, one should select a short-acting agent that is cardioselective (e.g. metoprolol).

While the use of β-blockers acutely in ACS is widespread, the data supporting this practice are based on older trials.[45,46] In the modern era, role of β-blockers in ACS was studied in the clopidogrel and metoprolol in myocardial infarction trial/second chinese cardiac study (COMMIT/CCS-2) trial. This large trial (45,852 patients with AMI with a majority of patients with STEMI) found no difference in the risk of a composite outcome of death, reinfarction, shock or cardiac arrest among patients treated with early metoprolol (intravenous up to 15 mg followed by 200 mg daily) compared to placebo for a period of 30 days. While risk of reinfarction and ventricular fibrillation was significantly lower with β-blockers; this was counterbalanced with a significantly increased risk of cardiogenic shock.[47] Based on this trial, caution must be exercised in the use of intravenous β-blockers acutely in the setting of an AMI particularly in patients with decompensated heart failure or who are at high risk of developing cardiogenic shock.

The American College of Cardiology (ACC)/American Heart Association (AHA) guidelines recommend:

Class I

- *Oral β-blockers be given in the first 24 hours after presentation if no contraindication are present.*
- *Intravenous β-blockers be considered only in patients without heart failure, evidence of low cardiac output state, relative contraindications (asthma and heart block) or multiple risk factors for development of cardiogenic shock (age > 70 years, systolic blood pressure of < 120 mm Hg, sinus rhythm with heart rates > 110 or < 60, and prolonged time from onset of ischemia to presentation).*

CALCIUM CHANNEL BLOCKERS

These drugs inhibit the inward flux of calcium via L-type calcium channels and thus inhibit both myocardial and vascular smooth muscle contraction. Agents in this class have diverse effects—the dihydropyridines (nifedipine and amlodipine) predominantly cause vasodilation by relaxation of vascular smooth muscle; the non-dihydropyridines (verapamil and diltiazem) have additional predominant negative inotropic and chronotropic actions. Calcium channel blockers that slow the heart rate may be used for the relief of angina in patients with angina refractory to nitrates and β-blockers, in patients with contraindications to β-blockers, in those with vasospastic angina,

or in those with hypertension. The side effects include bradycardia, worsening of heart block, hypotension and heart failure respectively.

Both diltiazem[48] and verapamil[49] have been studied in the setting of AMI and have been shown to reduce recurrent MI and death. Importantly though, both agents were associated with an increase in the risk of death among patients with AMI and LV systolic dysfunction or congestive heart failure (CHF) and, therefore, should not be used in these patients.[50] Nifedipine, which is a predominant vasodilator and does not lower the heart rate (but may cause a reflex tachycardia), is also associated with increased mortality in the absence of β-blockade and should not be used in patients with ACS.[51] The newer agents (amlodipine and felodipine) have not been directly studied in UA/NSTEMI patients, but have otherwise been found to be safe in patients with CAD and LV dysfunction.[52,53] Amlodipine and felodipine may be used as additional agents for blood pressure control in the subacute and chronic stages of the treatment.

Overall, the role of calcium channel blockers is primarily for symptomatic relief when β-blockers cannot be used or for the treatment of hypertension or persistent symptoms despite maximal therapy with β-blockers and nitrates. One must use caution when combining high doses of β-blockers with calcium channel blockers due to the risk of sinus node and AV block, and depression of LV function.

The American College of Cardiology (ACC)/American Heart Association (AHA) guidelines recommend:

Class I

- *Non-dihydropyridine agents may be considered if persistent ischemia and no contraindications (heart failure) despite maximal dosing of nitrates and β-blocker.*

Class III

- *Avoid immediate release dihydropyridine calcium channel blockers in absence of a β-blocker.*

ANTIPLATELET AGENTS

Potent antiplatelet therapy is the cornerstone of management of UA/NSTEMI given what has been previously described regarding the central role of platelets/thrombus in the pathophysiology of ACS.

Aspirin

For more than 50 years, aspirin has been the cornerstone of antiplatelet therapy and occupies a prominent role even today. It irreversibly acetylates the platelet enzyme COX-1 and thus prevents the generation of TXA2 from arachidonic acid thereby blocking the activation of platelets (Fig. 1). Aspirin is rapidly absorbed in the buccal mucosa (when chewed) and the stomach and the small intestine, achieving platelet inhibition within 15–60 minutes.[54] Even though aspirin chemically has a short plasma half-life, the antiplatelet action lasts for the lifetime of the platelet (7–10 days), due to irreversible inhibition of COX-1 enzyme.

To date, there have been four large-scale randomized trials that have demonstrated greater than 50% reduction in the risk of recurrent MI or death in patients with UA/NSTEMI.[55-58] The benefit begins as early as the first day of treatment. An initial dose of 162–325 mg daily followed by 75–162 mg daily for secondary prevention is recommended. However, considerable controversy surrounds the optimal dose of aspirin for long-term use in patients for secondary prevention. This controversy is mainly engendered by observational studies that have suggested no difference in efficacy in death or MI prevention, but a higher risk of bleeding with higher doses (> 200 mg) of aspirin.[59,60] To address this, a large randomized trial to examine clinical outcomes in more than 25,000 ACS patients referred for an invasive strategy who were randomized to aspirin at a dose of 300–325 mg versus 75–100 mg was recently completed. The trial did not show any difference in clinical efficacy endpoint or the risk of major bleeding between the two aspirin groups.[61] Thus, all UA/NSTEMI patients should receive aspirin as soon as possible after hospital presentation and this should be continued indefinitely.

The concept of "aspirin resistance" has emerged in the past decade. Based on small studies, 2–8% of patients have a limited antiplatelet effect (as assessed by in vitro platelet function studies) despite being on aspirin therapy. Two recently published meta-analyses showed a strong association with laboratory defined aspirin resistance and a higher risk of recurrent cardiovascular events in these patients.[62,63] Limitations of these meta-analyses include varied prevalence of aspirin resistance, small sample size of included studies, inability to account for noncompliance and possibly publication bias. Increasing the dose of aspirin from 81 mg to 325 mg may result in more complete antiplatelet response in these patients.[64] Routine monitoring of platelet function and adjustment of aspirin dose based on test results maybe an effective strategy that has not been evaluated in larger trials. Consideration of aspirin resistance should be given to any patient presenting with stent thrombosis.

The American College of Cardiology (ACC)/American Heart Association (AHA) guidelines recommend:

Class I

- *Aspirin (dose of 162–325 mg) should be given as soon as possible to all patients without a contraindication (allergy or active bleeding), and continued indefinitely.*

Adenosine Dinucleotide Phosphate Receptor Antagonists

The adenosine dinucleotide phosphate (ADP) is an important platelet agonist which exerts its action by binding to the P2Y12 receptors on the surface of the platelets (Fig. 1). The result of ADP signaling through the P2Y12 receptor pathway is the amplification of degranulation and ultimately platelet aggregation.[65] This is achieved by enhanced surface expression and affinity of platelet glycoprotein IIb/IIIa protein which interacts with fibrinogen and vWF to result in platelet aggregation. Consequently, several drugs have been developed that target the inhibition of this pathway.

Clopidogrel

It is a thienopyridine that causes irreversible inhibition of the P2Y12 receptor and thus prevents ADP binding to its molecular target on the platelet surface. Clopidogrel is a prodrug and requires metabolic activation by cytochrome P450s to its active metabolite. Clopidogrel has largely replaced ticlopidine (the first agent in this class, now rarely used) as the latter was associated with an increased risk of hematologic complications such as neutropenia and thrombotic thrombocytopenic purpura.[66]

The landmark clopidogrel in unstable angina to prevent recurrent events (CURE) trial showed that clopidogrel in addition to aspirin, heparin and other standard therapy was beneficial in preventing death, MI or stroke in UA/NSTEMI patients.[67] The benefit occurred as early as 24 hours and continued for up to 1 year in the study. Although clopidogrel is indicated in patients who are treated with stents,[68] the vast majority of patients in the CURE trial were not treated with stents, suggesting that clopidogrel results in a significant reduction in ischemic endpoints among patients with UA/NSTEMI regardless of treatment strategy (i.e. invasive vs conservative).[69,70] More recently, a higher loading dose of clopidogrel (600 mg) followed by a maintenance dose of 150 mg daily for 6 days and then 75 mg daily was compared to standard dose (loading dose 300 mg followed by 75 mg daily) in a large multinational trial involving high-risk ACS patients. While the overall trial results did not show a significant reduction in the combined endpoint of cardiovascular death, MI or stroke at 30 days, the subgroup of patients who underwent percutaneous coronary intervention (PCI) and received higher dose clopidogrel had lower rates of the primary outcome and stent thrombosis; this benefit was largely offset by increased risk of bleeding.[61]

Bleeding risk: Not surprisingly, antiplatelet inhibition with clopidogrel is associated with an increased risk of major bleeding. This is of particular concern among patients who are identified as candidates for bypass surgery. In the CURE trial, the increased coronary artery bypass grafting (CABG) related bleeding risk was only confined to those patients who did not discontinue clopidogrel for at least 5 days; bleeding was not increased among those who discontinued clopidogrel for greater than 5 days. Therefore, it is recommended that clopidogrel be discontinued at least 5 days before planned/elective surgery, if possible. After bypass surgery, clopidogrel should be resumed whenever feasible and continued for a period of up to 1 year. To avoid delaying surgery in a patient who may have multivessel or left main disease, some physicians withhold clopidogrel treatment acutely in an ACS patient until coronary anatomy is defined.[71] While this delayed approach avoids the increased bleeding risk in approximately 10% of patients with UA/NSTEMI who undergo CABG, it deprives all patients of the significant benefit from ischemic events or death that early initiation of clopidogrel affords.[69,70] It has been suggested that for every 1,000 UA/NSTEMI patients who are treated with early clopidogrel, 10–12 deaths, MIs or stroke would be prevented compared to delayed use, at the cost of 1 excess major bleeding (CABG-related) assuming that all clopidogrel treated patients

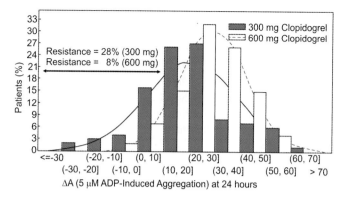

FIGURE 8: Distribution of ADP-induced platelet aggregation at 24 hours according to 300 mg and 600 mg of clopidogrel loading dose. (*Source:* Modified from Gurbel PA, Bliden KP, Hayes KM, et al. The relation of dosing to clopidogrel responsiveness and the incidence of high post-treatment platelet aggregation in patients undergoing coronary stenting. J Am Coll Cardiol. 2005;45:1392-6)

continued the drug until surgery.[72] Thus the risk-benefit ratio favors early use of clopidogrel in most patients.

Clopidogrel Resistance

The antiplatelet response of clopidogrel shows considerable interindividual variability (Fig. 8).[73] This may be overcome by higher loading doses.[74] The variability in response is clinically relevant—patients who achieve lower platelet inhibition on clopidogrel (hyporesponders) have been shown to have an increased risk for adverse cardiac events including death in multiple studies.[75,76] This is of particular concern among patients treated with stents where clopidogrel hyporesponsiveness may be associated with increased risk of developing stent thrombosis. It is well established that stent thrombosis leads to significant morbidity (e.g. recurrent MI, rehospitalization, etc.) and mortality (at least 30–40% risk of death), and thus all measures should be taken to avoid it.[77,78]

Clopidogrel is a prodrug that undergoes enzymatic conversion to its metabolically active form by the cytochrome P450 family of enzymes. As a result, polymorphism of the cytochrome P450 enzymes explain much of the observed variability in clopidogrel response in populations.[79-82] Most of the evidence points toward CYP2C19*2 allele, a loss of function allele, that results in reduced activity of the enzyme and lower antiplatelet effect of clopidogrel. Polymorphisms in the CYP2C19 gene are quite common and are reported in approximately 30% of whites, 40% of blacks and over 55% of east Asians.[83] Likewise inhibitors of cytochrome P450 enzymes (e.g. omeprazole)[84] have been suggested to cause reduced antiplatelet activity among clopidogrel treated patients; however, the impact of this finding on clinical outcomes remains uncertain.[85]

At this time, genetic testing is being evaluated as a strategy to identify patients with clopidogrel resistance as is the use of platelet function assays in guiding treatment strategy (higher dose of clopidogrel vs prasugrel). There is no definitive data at this time to suggest population-wide screening of the genetic polymorphism, or evaluation of platelet reactivity. As well, the effect of the combination of clopidogrel and proton pump inhibitors on clopidogrel effect is under investigation.

The American College of Cardiology (ACC)/American Heart Association (AHA) guidelines recommend:

Class I

Clopidogrel loading dose (at least 300 mg) with continued daily dosing (75 mg daily) should be administered:

- *As alternative antiplatelet therapy for patients intolerant/allergic to aspirin.*
- *As 2nd antiplatelet therapy in patients on aspirin with planned initial conservative approach for at least 1 month, and preferably 1 year.*
- *As 2nd antiplatelet agent in patients on aspirin in medium to high-risk patients with planned early invasive approach for at least 1 month, and preferably 1 year.*

Class IIb

- *Patients with definite UA/NSTEMI and undergoing PCI, a loading dose of clopidogrel 600 mg followed by a higher maintenance dose of 150 mg daily for 6 days, and then 75 mg daily may be reasonable in patients who are not at a high risk of bleeding.*
- *Clopidogrel may be considered beyond 15 months in patients receiving drug-eluting stents.*

PLATELET FUNCTION AND GENETIC TESTING

Class IIb

- Platelet function testing to determine platelet inhibitory response in patients with UA/NSTEMI (or, after ACS and PCI) on thienopyridine therapy may be considered if results of testing may alter management.
- Genotyping for a CYP2C19 loss of function variant in patients with UA/NSTEMI (or, after ACS and with PCI) on clopidogrel therapy might be considered if results of testing may alter management.

Newer Antiplatelet Agents

Prasugrel: Variability in the dose response of standard dose clopidogrel has led to an interest in the development of newer agents. Prasugrel is an oral thienopyridine drug and is less dependent on the cytochrome P450 enzymes for metabolic activation. After a loading dose of 60 mg, prasugrel reaches peak action within 30 minutes. Compared to clopidogrel (75 mg), prasugrel (10 mg) achieves more rapid and complete platelet inhibition with significantly less interindividual variability in its response; this is partly due to lesser dependence on the cytochrome P450 enzymes for metabolic activation.[86]

The clinical efficacy of prasugrel was studied in the TRITON-TIMI trial.[87] In this study, treatment with prasugrel (60 mg loading dose followed by 10 mg maintenance dose) was compared to clopidogrel (300 mg loading dose followed by 75 mg maintenance dose) in 13,608 high-risk ACS patients

(10,074 patients with UA/NSTEMI). Prasugrel treatment was associated with a significant reduction in the primary endpoint of death from cardiovascular causes, nonfatal MI or nonfatal stroke when compared to standard dose clopidogrel (9.9% vs 12.1%, p < 0.001). However, this was at the cost of a significantly increased risk of major bleeding (2.4% vs 1.8%, P value = 0.03) and life threatening bleeding (1.4% vs 0.9%, P value = 0.01) among prasugrel treated patients. As a result, overall mortality was not different in between the two groups at 15 months. Post-hoc analysis revealed that patients with prior stroke or transient ischemic attack (TIA) had net harm on prasugrel, while those 75 years or older and also those with body weight less than 60 kg did not have a net benefit on prasugrel.

Given the greater potency and lesser interindividual variability on inhibition of platelet function, prasugrel is a reasonable alternative in patients with recurrent events on clopidogrel therapy (clopidogrel hyporesponders). There are currently no systematic data on resistance to prasugrel or its clinical impact. While a case report of a patient who had persistently high on-treatment platelet reactivity to prasugrel is described, the clinical significance of this finding was not conclusively demonstrated.[88]

Prasugrel was recently approved by the FDA with a warning against its use in patient's age greater than 75 years, body weight less than 60 kg and prior history of TIA or stroke.

The American College of Cardiology (ACC)/American Heart Association (AHA) guidelines recommend:

Class I

Prasugrel loading dose (60 mg) followed by a maintenance dose (10 mg) should be given:

- *As 2nd antiplatelet agent in patients on aspirin in medium to high-risk patients with planned early invasive approach for at least 1 month and preferably 1 year.*
- *Prasugrel 60 mg loading dose promptly upon presentation in patients with UA/NSTEMI for whom PCI is planned, before definition of coronary anatomy if both the risk for bleeding is low and the need for CABG is considered unlikely.*

Class IIb

- *Prasugrel may be considered beyond 15 months in patients receiving drug-eluting stents.*

Class III

Prasugrel should be avoided in patients with:
- *Prior history of TIA or stroke, for whom PCI is planned.*

Ticagrelor: Ticagrelor is a non-thienopyridine, directly acting oral ADP receptor antagonist that reversibly binds to the P2Y12 receptor, with a stronger and more rapid antiplatelet effect than clopidogrel.[89] Unlike prasugrel and clopidogrel, it does not require metabolic activation, and its effect is reversed within 12–24 hours of drug discontinuation.

In the recently published study of platelet inhibition and patient outcomes (PLATO) trial, treatment with ticagrelor (180 mg loading dose, followed by 90 mg twice daily maintenance dose) was associated with a 16% relative reduction in the risk of cardiovascular events when compared to standard dose clopidogrel in high-risk ACS patients without a significantly increased risk of major bleeding. Even though the trial was not powered for mortality, patients randomized to ticagrelor also had a lower risk of all cause mortality (4.5% vs 5.9%, p < 0.001). An increased risk of dyspnea and bradycardia was noted among ticagrelor treated patients, which has been attributed to its modulation of adenosine receptors.[90]

At the time of writing of this chapter, the FDA has not approved ticagrelor for use in ACS.

Glycoprotein IIb/IIIa inhibitors: These medications block the final common pathway of platelet activation and aggregation and thereby prevent platelet aggregation initiated from a variety of stimuli (Fig. 1). Drugs which are currently available include: (1) Abciximab: a recombinant murine monoclonal antibody against the human GP IIb/IIIa receptor. Abciximab binds to this receptor tightly and inhibits platelet aggregation for days after the drug infusion is discontinued. (2) Eptifibatide: a cyclic peptide inhibitor with a rapid onset and short half-life (1–2.5 hours). Therefore it requires a continuous infusion for sustained response. (3) Tirofiban: a non-peptide Gp IIb/IIIa antagonist with a half-life of 4 hours.

The role of Gp IIb/IIIa inhibitors in the contemporary management of UA/NSTEMI continues to evolve. Numerous studies have shown that glycoprotein IIb/IIIa inhibitors reduce the risk of periprocedural MI, recurrent ischemia and death when used in patients with ACS.[91-95] This benefit reached statistical significance due predominantly to reduction in recurrent ischemic events. This has been confirmed in a large meta-analysis of all contemporary studies.[96] This benefit is particularly seen in higher risk patients, e.g. troponin positive patients,[97,98] those with dynamic ST changes or recurrent angina,[91] diabetic patients[99] or those with TIMI risk-score greater than 4.[37] In addition, in high-risk patients, the benefit seems to be present even in a subset of those patients who have been pretreated with clopidogrel and are given the medication as an adjunct during PCI.[92] In contrast, low-risk patients or those who are treated with an initial conservative strategy derive a very modest benefit with these drugs which may be counterbalanced by a significantly increased risk of major and life threatening bleeding.[96] Consequently, careful patient selection is important in identifying those who have the greatest likelihood for benefit.

Optimal timing of Gp IIb/IIIa inhibition continues to remain uncertain. Traditionally, two treatment strategies have been advocated: (1) Use as adjunctive therapy in the catheterization lab at the time of PCI or (2) As upstream therapy early in the course of ACS. While earlier studies have suggested a benefit of upstream therapy before PCI in these patients, these studies were performed in the era when clopidogrel was not widely used and rates of early angiography and revascularization were low. More recent data from two large randomized studies (ACUITY and EARLY-ACS) have not shown any benefit of routine upstream use of eptifibatide compared to delayed provisional use at the time of angiography in these patients, thus arguing that for most patients adjunctive use at the time of PCI may be most appropriate.[100,101]

Currently, all three agents have been approved for use as adjunctive PCI therapy; however, only eptifibatide and tirofiban have been approved for use as upstream therapy. This is because in a large trial of upstream therapy, abciximab was associated with no benefit and a trend toward harm.[93] Concomitant use of aspirin and heparin is recommended with glycoprotein IIb/IIIa inhibitors. Since bleeding risk may be substantial with combination therapies and is frequently due to excess dosing,[102] careful attention should be paid when using these drugs especially in patients who are at a heightened risk of bleeding (e.g. elderly, patients with renal disease, patients with small BMI, etc.). Thrombocytopenia occurs in about 0.5% of patients treated with glycoprotein IIb/IIIa inhibitors necessitating the need for platelet monitoring. This routinely resolves after cessation of therapy.

The American College of Cardiology (ACC)/American Heart Association (AHA) guidelines recommend:

Use of a Gp IIb/IIIa receptor inhibitor (in addition to aspirin) in patients with UA/NSTEMI when:

Class I

- *Medium- to high-risk patients in whom an initial invasive strategy is planned either upstream or at the time of PCI (alternative to thienopyridines, preferred agents: eptifibatide or tirofiban).*
- *An initial conservative strategy is planned, but patient develops recurrent ischemia, heart failure or significant arrhythmias prior to the patient having urgent diagnostic angiography (alternative to clopidogrel).*

Class IIa

- *Patients in whom an initial conservative strategy is planned and who have recurrent discomfort with aspirin, clopidogrel and anticoagulants.*
- *Patient in whom PCI is planned, glycoprotein IIb/IIIa inhibitors may be started particularly in high-risk patients (e.g. troponin positive).*
- *Patients in whom PCI is planned, it is reasonable to omit glycoprotein IIb/IIIa drugs when bivalirudin is selected and at least 300 mg of clopidogrel has been administered at least 6 hours prior.*

Class IIb

- *Upstream therapy in high-risk patients already receiving aspirin and clopidogrel in whom an initial invasive strategy is planned (troponin positive, diabetes or significant ST segment depression) and who do not have a high risk of bleeding.*

Class III

Avoidance of the upstream use of Gp IIb/IIIa inhibitors:
- *Upstream use of abciximab in patients in whom coronary intervention in not planned.*
- *Low-risk patients (TIMI risk score < 2) or those at high risk of bleeding already receiving aspirin and clopidogrel.*

In addition to the medications that inhibit platelet activation and aggregation, medications that inhibit the coagulation cascade remain an important part of the treatment armamentarium.

Heparin

Unfractionated heparin (UFH) is the most commonly used medication in the setting of ACS. It is a glycosaminoglycan with polysaccharide side chains of varying lengths. It binds to antithrombin which results in a conformational change in the latter, thereby inactivating factor IIa (thrombin) and Xa. In clinical practice, only one-third of a given dose of heparin binds to antithrombin. Heparin also binds to several other plasma proteins which results in variability of dose response. Therefore, the anticoagulant effect of heparin should be closely monitored by measurement of activated partial thromboplastin time (APTT). The variability in action, need for close monitoring and the potential for heparin-induced thrombocytopenia makes heparin a suboptimal antithrombotic medication.

In a meta-analysis of patients with UA/NSTEMI, treatment with heparin was associated with a non-significant 33% relative reduction in the composite outcome of death or MI.[103]

Low-Molecular Weight Heparin

Low-molecular weight heparins (LMWH) are derived from heparin by chemical modification of the polysaccharide side chains. Enoxaparin is the most widely used LMWH in the United States. Compared to UFH, it is a more potent anti-Xa agent which inhibits generation of thrombin more effectively. Also, its greater bioavailability and lower plasma protein binding allows for a convenient subcutaneous dosing and predictable dose response and therefore does not require routine monitoring of anticoagulant effect. Anticoagulant activity of LMWH drugs cannot be reliably monitored using the APTT. Rather, it requires the measurement of anti-Xa activity and these assays are not as widely available. The standard dose of 1 mg/kg subcutaneous twice daily provides effective anticoagulant effect. The incidence of heparin induced thrombocytopenia is significantly lower compared to the UFH. Since LMWH are cleared by the kidney, the dose should be adjusted or altogether avoided in patients with renal dysfunction depending on their glomerular filtration rate. Also, dose response may be unpredictable in morbidly obese patients and therefore enoxaparin should generally be avoided in these patients.

Two early studies[104,105] compared enoxaparin to UFH in UA/NSTEMI patients and both found that enoxaparin was superior with a lower risk of death, MI or recurrent angina. The overall benefit was slightly offset with a slightly higher risk of bleeding with enoxaparin. In more recent studies,[106,107] which enrolled a higher risk group of patients showed that enoxaparin was noninferior but not superior to UFH. These divergent findings are likely due to more widespread use of additional antiplatelet drugs (clopidogrel, and/or Gp IIb/IIIa) and greater use of early invasive approach in the more recent studies. In fact, studies suggest that UA/NSTEMI patients undergoing initially conservative management derived much greater benefit with enoxaparin when compared to the UFH. In contrast, in patients who underwent an early invasive approach, the results were very similar between the UFH and the enoxaparin group.[108] The greater bleeding associated with enoxaparin has been suggested as a possible explanation. This finding along with the complexity of monitoring the level of anticoagulant activity in the catheterization lab has prevented the widespread adoption of enoxaparin for adjunctive therapy at the time of PCI.

Fondaparinux

Fondaparinux is a synthetic pentasaccharide. It is an anti-Xa agent and does not have any direct effect on thrombin. This drug has predictable metabolism and can be conveniently dosed once a day by subcutaneous injection without any need for monitoring.

A large study comparing fondaparinux 2.5 mg/day to enoxaparin 1 mg/kg twice a day found the two medications to be similar with respect to the primary efficacy endpoint (death, MI, refractory ischemia—5.9% with fondaparinux vs 5.8% with enoxaparin at day 9) with a nearly 50% lower risk of bleeding in the fondaparinux group.[109] This translated into an overall lower 30-day mortality rate in the fondaparinux treated patients in this trial (2.9% vs 3.5%, p = 0.02). However, inclusion of patients with elevated creatinine and use of supplemental UFH may have resulted in greater bleeding in enoxaparin treated group, and biased the results in favor of fondaparinux. Also, fondaparinux was associated with a significantly higher risk of acute thrombosis in those undergoing PCI. Due to these concerns, the use of fondaparinux among ACS patients is not widespread.

Direct Thrombin Inhibitors

Bivalirudin: Bivaliridin is a synthetic analog derived from hirudin. It has direct action on thrombin, and therefore differs from heparin in that it does not require a cofactor (antithrombin) for its action. It directly inactivates thrombin including clot-bound thrombin. It also does not bind any plasma proteins and therefore has predictable pharmacokinetics. It does not result in complications such as thrombocytopenia.

The REPLACE-2 trial studied bivalirudin monotherapy in patients undergoing elective PCI compared to UFH and eptifibatide and found similar rates of ischemic events and death with significantly lower rates of bleeding in the bivalirudin treated patients.[110] Although this was a PCI trial, between 40% and 45% of patients had UA or MI as indication for the PCI. Subsequently, the ACUITY trial evaluated bivalirudin therapy in moderate- to high-risk UA/NSTEMI patients undergoing early invasive treatment. The trial had a complex design, but the principal findings of this trial were that bivalirudin monotherapy was not inferior to combination therapy with glycoprotein IIb/IIIa inhibitor with UFH, enoxaparin or bivalirudin for the prevention of major adverse cardiovascular events. At the same time, bivalirudin mono-therapy was associated with a nearly 50% lower risk of bleeding.[100] Cost-effectiveness studies have found that despite higher medication costs, bivalirudin alone is cost-saving when compared to heparin and eptifibatide in moderate to high-risk NSTEMI patients.[111]

The American College of Cardiology (ACC)/American Heart Association (AHA) guidelines recommend:

Class I

Anticoagulation therapy in addition to antiplatelet therapy in patients with UA/NSTEMI as soon as possible with:
- *Enoxaparin or unfractionated heparin, or consider bivalirudin or fondaparinux in patients with a planned invasive strategy.*
- *Enoxaparin or fondaparinux in patients with a planned conservative strategy with fondaparinux being the preferred agent in patients with an increased risk of bleeding.*
- *Discontinue anticoagulant after PCI with uncomplicated procedures.*

Warfarin

Several studies have examined the role of warfarin in combination with aspirin in patients with ACS.[112,113] More recent studies have suggested a benefit of carefully monitored oral warfarin at a goal INR of 2.0–2.5 along with aspirin in reducing the combined endpoint of death, MI or stroke.[113] However, the contemporary role of warfarin is limited given the established role of clopidogrel in these patients particularly in those who receive PCI with a coronary stent. In the patient without a coronary stent, who may have another indication for warfarin, the combination of aspirin and warfarin may be preferable. The "triple" antithrombotic therapy (e.g. aspirin, clopidogrel and warfarin) has not been prospectively studied, and is likely to be associated with a greater risk of bleeding. This is not an infrequent consideration in a patient who receives a coronary stent, and also has another strong indication to be on warfarin (e.g. atrial fibrillation with a high CHADS2 score, or mechanical valve). Guidelines recommend using low dose of aspirin (75–162 mg aspirin), close monitoring of INR to a goal of 2.0–2.5, and use of clopidogrel for the shortest recommended duration based on type of stent (Class IIb).

The American College of Cardiology (ACC)/American Heart Association (AHA) guidelines recommend:

Class IIb

- *When triple-combination therapy is necessary based on clear clinical indications, consider using low dose of aspirin (75–162 mg aspirin), close monitoring and careful regulation of INR to a goal of 2.0–3.0, and use of clopidogrel for the shortest recommended duration based on type of stent.*

EARLY INVASIVE OR INITIAL CONSERVATIVE STRATEGY

An early invasive strategy involves performing coronary angiography within the first 24–48 hours of admission with the intent of performing revascularization with PCI or CABG, as appropriate. An initial conservative strategy involves initial medical management as outlined below with coronary angiography reserved for patients who have recurrent ischemia or a high-risk stress test despite medical therapy.

A number of randomized trials have compared early invasive strategy to an initial conservative strategy and the results have been mixed.[114-120] In a meta-analysis of contemporary trials, an early invasive strategy was associated with a 25% lower risk of death compared to initial conservative strategy.[121,122] A consistent finding in studies is that an early invasive strategy affords greatest benefit in high-risk patients especially those with elevated troponin, ST-segment deviation or higher TIMI risk score (> 3). While a study examining gender differences in treatment benefit suggested that low-risk women with UA/NSTEMI (negative biomarkers cardiac necrosis) may be potentially harmed with an early invasive strategy.[123] A heterogeneous study population with different standard medical regimens and a varied proportion of patient's actually undergoing revascularization in each group are important limitations of this study. It is clear that additional investigations to further clarify the gender differences in outcomes with different treatment strategies are warranted.

The specific issues regarding PCI in patients with ACS, particularly those with NSTEMI are: (1) The use of bare metal versus drug eluting stent at the time of PCI, and (2) The timing of angiography and intervention. The data on safety and efficacy of drug eluting stents versus bare metal stents for this population (UA/NSTEMI) are somewhat sparse, are mostly based on registry data (not randomized trials) and are conflicting. Presently there is no clear contraindication for either, but further randomized trials are recommended.[124,125]

Recent studies have addressed the issue of optimal timing of PCI in UA/NSTEMI patients, specifically the role of early intervention. The timing of intervention in acute coronary syndrome (TIMACS) study showed that early intervention within 24 hours (median time, 14 hours) did not result in a reduction in risk of death, recurrent MI or stroke in the first 6 months) when compared to delayed intervention more than 36 hours (median time, 50 hours). The subgroup analyses suggested a benefit of early intervention among high-risk patients (GRACE risk score > 140).[126] A second study compared very early intervention (within 6 hours) versus prolonged medical treatment or "cooling off" for 3–5 days with aspirin, heparin, clopidogrel and tirofiban among patients with chest discomfort and ischemic ECG changes and/or positive biomarkers. The study found no difference in events between these groups.[118] Lastly, a French study examined a strategy of planned immediate intervention (median time from randomization to sheath insertion was 70 minutes) versus a planned delayed intervention strategy (median time, 21 hours) and found no difference in the primary endpoint of peak troponin elevation, or in the secondary endpoint of death, MI or urgent revascularization within 30 days.[127] Thus, existing data do not support a strategy for immediate intervention for patients with UA/NSTEMI (unlike that for STEMI). At the same time, there is no inherent benefit in delaying revascularization with PCI after a "cooling off" period. The data suggest that the patient should be taken, in a timely manner, to the cardiac catheterization lab for angiography and planned intervention as deemed medically appropriate.

The American College of Cardiology (ACC)/American Heart Association (AHA) guidelines recommend:

Class I

- *An early invasive strategy in patients with refractory angina, or hemodynamic or electrically instability.*
- *An early invasive strategy in patients who have been stabilized with medical therapy, who are without comorbidities or contraindications to angiography or coronary intervention, and who have an increased risk of future events.*

Class IIa

- *Early invasive strategy (within 12–24 hours of admission) over a delayed invasive strategy for initially stabilized high-risk patients with UA/NSTEMI. For patients not at high risk, a delayed invasive approach is reasonable.*

Class IIb

- *An initial conservative strategy in patients at increased risk of future events (high risk) stabilized with medical therapy, who are without comorbidities or contraindications to angiography or coronary intervention, based on physician and patient preference.*
- *An early invasive strategy in patients with chronic renal failure, specifically with Stage II or Stage III CKD—there is not enough data for recommendations for more advanced stages of CKD.*

Class III

Avoidance of an early invasive strategy in patients with:
- *Extensive comorbidities in whom the risk of revascularization outweigh the benefits.*
- *Acute chest discomfort and a low likelihood of ACS.*
- *No plan to consent for revascularization regardless of the findings on angiography.*

REVASCULARIZATION

Revascularization in patients with UA/NSTEMI may improve symptoms, quality of life, reduce ischemic complications or improve survival depending on the clinical circumstance. The need for revascularization depends on several factors which include patient age and more importantly functional status, serious comorbidities, expected survival, coronary anatomy, LV function and V, viability and severity of symptoms. Available alternatives for revascularization include PCI and CABG. The choice of revascularization strategy for patients with coronary disease has been a moving target with ongoing advances in technology, and the indications may continue to evolve.

In general, the indications for revascularization (and for CABG vs PCI) for patients with UA/NSTEMI are similar to those in patients with stable angina, with the exception of patients who may be candidates for CABG, based on anatomy, but has urgent/emergent need for infarct-related artery (IRA) revascularization for poor TIMI flow or threatened closure of

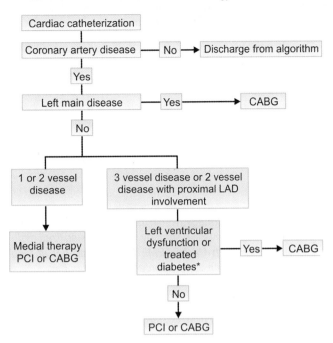

*There is conflicting information about these patients. Most consider CABG to be preferable to PCI

(*Source:* Modified from Anderson JL, Adams CD, Antman EM, et al. ACC/AHA 2007 guidelines for the management of patients with unstable angina/non ST-elevation myocardial infarction: a report of the American College of Cardiology/American Heart Association Task Force on Practice Guidelines. Circulation. 2007;116:e148-304)

the vessel. In this instance, PCI of the IRA to stabilize the patient, with subsequent consideration of further need for revascularization, should be performed. The high-risk patients with left main (> 50%) or three vessel disease, two-vessel disease with proximal LAD stenosis, diabetics with multivessel disease, and multivessel disease with LV dysfunction are better suited for CABG provided surgery can be performed with an acceptable risk (Flow chart 1).[128,129] An important issue that frequently influences timing of bypass surgery in these patients is the use of thienopyridines which increase the risk of CABG-related bleeding. Therefore, these drugs should be discontinued to allow for dissipation of the antiplatelet effect (clopidogrel 5 days, prasugrel 7 days) in an elective setting. However, clinical judgment should be exercised in making this decision in more emergent case (e.g. severe left main disease or recurrent ischemia) where the need for urgent revascularization may outweigh the risks of bleeding. Finally, while some studies have suggested an increased risk in CABG-related mortality in the first 3–5 days after an MI, recent data from the National Cardiovascular Data Registry found no difference in mortality in UA/NSTEMI patients undergoing early (within 48 hours) versus late CABG (after 48 hours). Thus, delaying surgery might increase resource use without improving outcomes.[130]

For other high-risk patients with less severe CAD, PCI may be an appropriate alternative to surgical revascularization particularly if the lesions are amenable to PCI. The angiographic success rate of PCI is generally more than 95%; further reduction in acute ischemic complications may be achieved with

adjunctive use of glycoprotein IIb/IIIa inhibitors, clopidogrel and/or other antithrombotic drugs. Among low-risk patients, survival benefit with revascularization is less apparent from the available data and medical therapy alone may be appropriate. In such patients, revascularization may be considered for the treatment of symptoms that are refractory to optimal medical therapy, and for improvement in quality of life. It must be remembered that the modest benefit with revascularization in these patients must be counterbalanced with procedural risk.

The American College of Cardiology (ACC)/American Heart Association (AHA) guidelines recommend:

Class I

- *Early invasive strategy with angiography and PCI within 12–24 hours of admission.*
- *Early invasive PCI strategy in high-risk patients without serious comorbidity and who have amenable lesions for PCI.*
- *The PCI or CABG in patients with 1 or 2 vessel CAD with or without proximal LAD but with a large viable at-risk territory.*
- *The PCI or CABG in patients with multivessel CAD and suitable anatomy with normal LV function and no diabetes.*

Class II

PCI in patients with:
- *Vein graft lesions who are poor candidates for reoperation.*
- *Left main stenosis (> 50%) in patients who are not CABG candidates or who require emergent intervention for hemodynamic instability.*
- *No high-risk features who have single vessel CAD, or patients with multivessel CAD who have at least one lesion to be dilated with decreased likelihood of success.*
- *Considered in patients with two or three vessel disease amenable to percutaneous intervention with proximal LAD disease who have neither treated diabetes nor decreased LV systolic function.*

PCI or CABG in patients with:
- *One or two vessel CAD with or without proximal LAD stenosis but with moderate-sized viable at-risk territory.*
- *One vessel CAD with significant proximal LAD stenosis.*

Class III

PCI in patients with:
- *One or two vessel CAD without proximal LAD stenosis, with no ischemic symptoms or evidence of ischemia on stress testing.*

PCI in patients without high-risk features, in absence of a trial of medical therapy, and with:
- *Small sized at-risk territory.*
- *Lesions with low likelihood of success in treatment.*
- *High procedural risk of morbidity or mortality.*
- *Lesions that are not hemodynamically significant (< 50%).*
- *Significant left main CAD and are candidates for CABG.*
- *Stable patient with persistent occlusion of infarct-related artery.*

The American College of Cardiology (ACC)/American Heart Association (AHA) guidelines recommend:

Class I

CABG in patients with:
- *Significant left main CAD (> 50%).*
- *Three vessel CAD, especially patients with LVEF less than 50%.*
- *Two vessel CAD with significant proximal LAD stenosis and either LVEF less than 50% or ischemia on stress testing.*
- *Poor or no options for PCI who have ongoing ischemia refractory to medical therapy.*
- *UA/NSTEMI patients on thienopyridines, in whom CABG is planned and can be delayed, thienopyridines should be discontinued to allow dissipation of the antiplatelet effect (clopidogrel 5 days, prasugrel 7 days) unless the need for revascularization and the net effect of thienopyridines outweighs the risk of bleeding.*

Class II

CABG in patients with:
- *Multivessel disease who have diabetes and who will have an internal mammary graft during CABG.*
- *Single or two-vessel CAD, without proximal LAD stenosis, but with a modest sized at-risk territory and PCI option is poor and not possible.*
- *Need for repeat CABG when there are multiple vein graft stenosis and the graft to the LAD has a significant stenosis.*

Class III

CABG in patients with:
- *Single or two-vessel CAD without proximal LAD stenosis, with no ischemic symptoms or evidence of ischemia on stress testing.*

SUMMARY AND CONCLUSIONS

Over the past few years, there has been a tremendous growth in our understanding of the biology of atherosclerosis and the mechanisms that lead to ACS, one of the most dreaded consequences of coronary atherosclerosis. At the same time, important breakthroughs have emerged with development of new medications and treatment protocols that have improved patient outcomes. Diagnosis of ACS hinges on a careful assessment which includes a detailed history, physical examination, ECG and levels of cardiac biomarkers. The initial management of ACS includes initial medical stabilization with relief of pain, dual antiplatelet and antithrombotic therapy with consideration for early invasive treatment and revascularization. Early risk stratification is a very important tool that allows identification of patients who are at a high risk for short-term mortality; these patients benefit the most from aggressive management including thienopyridines, glycoprotein IIb/IIIa inhibitors and early invasive treatment. Revascularization should be considered in high-risk patients, and the choice of revascularization strategy and its timing depends on a patient's

clinical condition, coronary anatomy and associated comorbidities.

REFERENCES

1. Lloyd-Jones D, Adams RJ, Brown TM, et al. Heart disease and stroke statistics—2010 update: a report from the American Heart Association. Circulation. 2010;121:e46-215.
2. Davies MJ. The composition of coronary-artery plaques. N Engl J Med. 1997;336:1312-4.
3. Giroud D, Li JM, Urban P, et al. Relation of the site of acute myocardial infarction to the most severe coronary arterial stenosis at prior angiography. Am J Cardiol. 1992;69:729-32.
4. Alderman EL, Corley SD, Fisher LD, et al. Five-year angiographic follow-up of factors associated with progression of coronary artery disease in the Coronary Artery Surgery Study (CASS). CASS Participating Investigators and Staff. J Am Coll Cardiol. 1993;22:1141-54.
5. Hackett D, Davies G, Maseri A. Preexisting coronary stenoses in patients with first myocardial infarction are not necessarily severe. Eur Heart J. 1988;9:1317-23.
6. Falk E, Shah PK, Fuster V. Coronary plaque disruption. Circulation. 1995;92:657-71.
7. Naghavi M, Libby P, Falk E, et al. From vulnerable plaque to vulnerable patient: a call for new definitions and risk assessment strategies: Part II. Circulation. 2003;108:1772-8.
8. Buffon A, Biasucci LM, Liuzzo G, et al. Widespread coronary inflammation in unstable angina. N Engl J Med. 2002;347:5-12.
9. Goldstein JA, Demetriou D, Grines CL, et al. Multiple complex coronary plaques in patients with acute myocardial infarction. N Engl J Med. 2000;343:915-22.
10. Burke AP, Kolodgie FD, Farb A, et al. Healed plaque ruptures and sudden coronary death: evidence that subclinical rupture has a role in plaque progression. Circulation. 2001;103:934-40.
11. Abidov A, Rozanski A, Hachamovitch R, et al. Prognostic significance of dyspnea in patients referred for cardiac stress testing. N Engl J Med. 2005;353:1889-98.
12. Goff DC, Sellers DE, McGovern PG, et al. Knowledge of heart attack symptoms in a population survey in the United States: The REACT Trial. Rapid Early Action for Coronary Treatment. Arch Intern Med. 1998;158:2329-38.
13. Hayden M, Pignone M, Phillips C, et al. Aspirin for the primary prevention of cardiovascular events: a summary of the evidence for the U.S. Preventive Services Task Force. Ann Intern Med. 2002;136:161-72.
14. Canto JG, Shlipak MG, Rogers WJ, et al. Prevalence, clinical characteristics, and mortality among patients with myocardial infarction presenting without chest pain. JAMA. 2000;283:3223-9.
15. Henrikson CA, Howell EE, Bush DE, et al. Chest pain relief by nitroglycerin does not predict active coronary artery disease. Ann Intern Med. 2003;139:979-86.
16. Greenland P, Knoll MD, Stamler J, et al. Major risk factors as antecedents of fatal and nonfatal coronary heart disease events. JAMA. 2003;290:891-7.
17. Vasan RS, Sullivan LM, Wilson PW, et al. Relative importance of borderline and elevated levels of coronary heart disease risk factors. Ann Intern Med. 2005;142:393-402.
18. Maradit-Kremers H, Crowson CS, Nicola PJ, et al. Increased unrecognized coronary heart disease and sudden deaths in rheumatoid arthritis: a population-based cohort study. Arthritis Rheum. 2005;52:402-11.
19. Savonitto S, Ardissino D, Granger CB, et al. Prognostic value of the admission electrocardiogram in acute coronary syndromes. JAMA. 1999;281:707-13.
20. de Zwaan C, Bar FW, Janssen JH, et al. Angiographic and clinical characteristics of patients with unstable angina showing an ECG

pattern indicating critical narrowing of the proximal LAD coronary artery. Am Heart J. 1989;117:657-65.

21. Slater DK, Hlatky MA, Mark DB, et al. Outcome in suspected acute myocardial infarction with normal or minimally abnormal admission electrocardiographic findings. Am J Cardiol. 1987;60:766-70.

22. Antman EM, Tanasijevic MJ, Thompson B, et al. Cardiac-specific troponin I levels to predict the risk of mortality in patients with acute coronary syndromes. N Engl J Med. 1996;335:1342-9.

23. Jaffe AS, Babuin L, Apple FS. Biomarkers in acute cardiac disease: the present and the future. J Am Coll Cardiol. 2006;48:1-11.

24. Doria A, Iaccarino L, Sarzi-Puttini P, et al. Cardiac involvement in systemic lupus erythematosus. Lupus. 2005;14:683-6.

25. Bach RG, Cannon CP, Weintraub WS, et al. The effect of routine, early invasive management on outcome for elderly patients with non-ST-segment elevation acute coronary syndromes. Ann Intern Med. 2004;141:186-95.

26. Roffi M, Chew DP, Mukherjee D, et al. Platelet glycoprotein IIb/IIIa inhibitors reduce mortality in diabetic patients with non-ST-segment-elevation acute coronary syndromes. Circulation. 2001;104:2767-71.

27. Cotter G, Cannon CP, McCabe CH, et al. Prior peripheral arterial disease and cerebrovascular disease are independent predictors of adverse outcome in patients with acute coronary syndromes: are we doing enough? Results from the Orbofiban in Patients with Unstable Coronary Syndromes-Thrombolysis In Myocardial Infarction (OPUS-TIMI) 16 study. Am Heart J. 2003;145:622-7.

28. Khot UN, Jia G, Moliterno DJ, et al. Prognostic importance of physical examination for heart failure in non-ST-elevation acute coronary syndromes: the enduring value of Killip classification. JAMA. 2003;290:2174-81.

29. Petrina M, Goodman SG, Eagle KA. The 12-lead electrocardiogram as a predictive tool of mortality after acute myocardial infarction: current status in an era of revascularization and reperfusion. Am Heart J. 2006;152:11-8.

30. Westerhout CM, Fu Y, Lauer MS, et al. Short- and long-term risk stratification in acute coronary syndromes: the added value of quantitative ST-segment depression and multiple biomarkers. J Am Coll Cardiol. 2006;48:939-47.

31. Ohman EM, Armstrong PW, Christenson RH, et al. Cardiac troponin T levels for risk stratification in acute myocardial ischemia. GUSTO IIA Investigators. N Engl J Med. 1996;335:1333-41.

32. Dokainish H, Pillai M, Murphy SA, et al. Prognostic implications of elevated troponin in patients with suspected acute coronary syndrome but no critical epicardial coronary disease: a TACTICS-TIMI-18 substudy. J Am Coll Cardiol. 2005;45:19-24.

33. Morrow DA, Rifai N, Antman EM, et al. C-reactive protein is a potent predictor of mortality independently of and in combination with troponin T in acute coronary syndromes: a TIMI 11A substudy. Thrombolysis in myocardial infarction. J Am Coll Cardiol. 1998;31:1460-5.

34. Biasucci LM, Liuzzo G, Grillo RL, et al. Elevated levels of C-reactive protein at discharge in patients with unstable angina predict recurrent instability. Circulation. 1999;99:855-60.

35. de Lemos JA, Morrow DA, Bentley JH, et al. The prognostic value of B-type natriuretic peptide in patients with acute coronary syndromes. N Engl J Med. 2001;345:1014-21.

36. James SK, Lindahl B, Siegbahn A, et al. N-terminal pro-brain natriuretic peptide and other risk markers for the separate prediction of mortality and subsequent myocardial infarction in patients with unstable coronary artery disease: a Global Utilization of Strategies To Open occluded arteries (GUSTO)-IV substudy. Circulation. 2003;108:275-81.

37. Antman EM, Cohen M, Bernink PJ, et al. The TIMI risk score for unstable angina/non-ST elevation MI: a method for prognostication and therapeutic decision making. JAMA. 2000;284:835-42.

38. Eagle KA, Lim MJ, Dabbous OH, et al. A validated prediction model for all forms of acute coronary syndrome: estimating the risk of 6-month postdischarge death in an international registry. JAMA. 2004;291:2727-33.

39. Granger CB, Goldberg RJ, Dabbous O, et al. Predictors of hospital mortality in the global registry of acute coronary events. Arch Intern Med. 2003;163:2345-53.

40. Anderson JL, Adams CD, Antman EM, et al. ACC/AHA 2007 guidelines for the management of patients with unstable angina/non ST-elevation myocardial infarction: a report of the American College of Cardiology/American Heart Association Task Force on Practice Guidelines (Writing Committee to Revise the 2002 Guidelines for the Management of Patients With Unstable Angina/Non ST-Elevation Myocardial Infarction): developed in collaboration with the American College of Emergency Physicians, the Society for Cardiovascular Angiography and Interventions, and the Society of Thoracic Surgeons: endorsed by the American Association of Cardiovascular and Pulmonary Rehabilitation and the Society for Academic Emergency Medicine. Circulation. 2007;116:e148-304.

41. Wright RS, Anderson JL, Adams CD, et al. 2011 ACCF/AHA Focused Update of the Guidelines for the Management of Patients With Unstable Angina/Non-ST-Elevation Myocardial Infarction (Updating the 2007 Guideline): a report of the American College of Cardiology Foundation/American Heart Association Task Force on Practice Guidelines. Circulation. 2011 [Epub ahead of print].

42. Radomski MW, Palmer RM, Moncada S. Endogenous nitric oxide inhibits human platelet adhesion to vascular endothelium. Lancet. 1987;2:1057-8.

43. GISSI-3: effects of lisinopril and transdermal glyceryl trinitrate singly and together on 6-week mortality and ventricular function after acute myocardial infarction. Gruppo Italiano per lo Studio della Sopravvivenza nell'infarto Miocardico. Lancet. 1994;343:1115-22.

44. ISIS-4: a randomised factorial trial assessing early oral captopril, oral mononitrate, and intravenous magnesium sulphate in 58,050 patients with suspected acute myocardial infarction. ISIS-4 (Fourth International Study of Infarct Survival) Collaborative Group. Lancet. 1995;345:669-85.

45. Gottlieb SO, Weisfeldt ML, Ouyang P, et al. Effect of the addition of propranolol to therapy with nifedipine for unstable angina pectoris: a randomized, double-blind, placebo-controlled trial. Circulation. 1986;73:331-7.

46. Yusuf S, Peto R, Lewis J, et al. Beta blockade during and after myocardial infarction: an overview of the randomized trials. Prog Cardiovasc Dis. 1985;27:335-71.

47. Chen ZM, Pan HC, Chen YP, et al. Early intravenous then oral metoprolol in 45,852 patients with acute myocardial infarction: randomised placebo-controlled trial. Lancet. 2005;366:1622-32.

48. Gibson RS, Boden WE, Theroux P, et al. Diltiazem and reinfarction in patients with non-Q-wave myocardial infarction. Results of a double-blind, randomized, multicenter trial. N Engl J Med. 1986;315:423-9.

49. Effect of verapamil on mortality and major events after acute myocardial infarction (the Danish Verapamil Infarction Trial II—DAVIT II). Am J Cardiol. 1990;66:779-85.

50. The effect of diltiazem on mortality and reinfarction after myocardial infarction. The Multicenter Diltiazem Postinfarction Trial Research Group. N Engl J Med. 1988;319:385-92.

51. Furberg CD, Psaty BM, Meyer JV. Nifedipine. Dose-related increase in mortality in patients with coronary heart disease. Circulation. 1995;92:1326-31.

52. Packer M, O'Connor CM, Ghali JK, et al. Effect of amlodipine on morbidity and mortality in severe chronic heart failure. Prospective Randomized Amlodipine Survival Evaluation Study Group. N Engl J Med. 1996;335:1107-14.

53. Cohn JN, Ziesche S, Smith R, et al. Effect of the calcium antagonist felodipine as supplementary vasodilator therapy in patients with chronic heart failure treated with enalapril: V-HeFT III. Vasodilator-Heart Failure Trial (V-HeFT) Study Group. Circulation. 1997;96:856-63.

54. Patrono C, Baigent C, Hirsh J, et al. Antiplatelet drugs: American College of Chest Physicians Evidence-Based Clinical Practice Guidelines (8th Edition). Chest. 2008;133:199S-233S.

55. Risk of myocardial infarction and death during treatment with low dose aspirin and intravenous heparin in men with unstable coronary artery disease. The RISC Group. Lancet. 1990;336:827-30.

56. Cairns JA, Gent M, Singer J, et al. Aspirin, sulfinpyrazone, or both in unstable angina. Results of a Canadian multicenter trial. N Engl J Med. 1985;313:1369-75.

57. Lewis HD, Davis JW, Archibald DG, et al. Protective effects of aspirin against acute myocardial infarction and death in men with unstable angina. Results of a Veterans Administration Cooperative Study. N Engl J Med. 1983;309:396-403.

58. Theroux P, Ouimet H, McCans J, et al. Aspirin, heparin, or both to treat acute unstable angina. N Engl J Med. 1988;319:1105-11.

59. Peters RJ, Mehta SR, Fox KA, et al. Effects of aspirin dose when used alone or in combination with clopidogrel in patients with acute coronary syndromes: observations from the Clopidogrel in Unstable angina to prevent Recurrent Events (CURE) study. Circulation. 2003;108:1682-7.

60. Topol EJ, Easton D, Harrington RA, et al. Randomized, double-blind, placebo-controlled, international trial of the oral IIb/IIIa antagonist lotrafiban in coronary and cerebrovascular disease. Circulation. 2003;108:399-406.

61. Mehta SR, Bassand JP, Chrolavicius S, et al. Dose comparisons of clopidogrel and aspirin in acute coronary syndromes. N Engl J Med. 2010;363:930-42.

62. Krasopoulos G, Brister SJ, Beattie WS, et al. Aspirin "resistance" and risk of cardiovascular morbidity: systematic review and meta-analysis. BMJ. 2008;336:195-8.

63. Snoep JD, Hovens MM, Eikenboom JC, et al. Association of laboratory-defined aspirin resistance with a higher risk of recurrent cardiovascular events: a systematic review and meta-analysis. Arch Intern Med. 2007;167:1593-9.

64. Mirkhel A, Peyster E, Sundeen J, et al. Frequency of aspirin resistance in a community hospital. Am J Cardiol. 2006;98:577-9.

65. Michelson AD. Antiplatelet therapies for the treatment of cardiovascular disease. Nat Rev Drug Discov. 2010;9:154-69.

66. Bertrand ME, Rupprecht HJ, Urban P, et al. Double-blind study of the safety of clopidogrel with and without a loading dose in combination with aspirin compared with ticlopidine in combination with aspirin after coronary stenting: the clopidogrel aspirin stent international cooperative study (CLASSICS). Circulation. 2000;102:624-9.

67. Yusuf S, Zhao F, Mehta SR, et al. The clopidogrel in unstable angina to prevent recurrent events trial I. Effects of clopidogrel in addition to aspirin in patients with acute coronary syndromes without ST-segment elevation. N Engl J Med. 2001;345:494-502.

68. Steinhubl SR, Berger PB, Mann Iii JT, et al. Early and sustained dual oral antiplatelet therapy following percutaneous coronary intervention: a randomized controlled trial. JAMA. 2002;288:2411-20.

69. Mehta SR, Yusuf S, Peters RJ, et al. Effects of pretreatment with clopidogrel and aspirin followed by long-term therapy in patients undergoing percutaneous coronary intervention: the PCI-CURE study. Lancet. 2001;358:527-33.

70. Yusuf S, Mehta SR, Zhao F, et al. Early and late effects of clopidogrel in patients with acute coronary syndromes. Circulation. 2003;107:966-72.

71. Cannon CP. What is the optimal timing of clopidogrel in acute coronary syndromes? Crit Pathw Cardiol. 2005;4:46-50.

72. Fox KAA, Mehta SR, Peters R, et al. Benefits and risks of the combination of clopidogrel and aspirin in patients undergoing surgical revascularization for Non-ST-Elevation Acute Coronary Syndrome: The clopidogrel in unstable angina to prevent Recurrent ischemic Events (CURE) Trial. Circulation. 2004;110:1202-8.

73. Serebruany VL, Steinhubl SR, Berger PB, et al. Variability in platelet responsiveness to clopidogrel among 544 individuals. J Am Coll Cardiol. 2005;45:246-51.

74. Gurbel PA, Bliden KP, Hayes KM, et al. The relation of dosing to clopidogrel responsiveness and the incidence of high post-treatment platelet aggregation in patients undergoing coronary stenting. J Am Coll Cardiol. 2005;45:1392-6.

75. Matetzky S, Shenkman B, Guetta V, et al. Clopidogrel resistance is associated with increased risk of recurrent atherothrombotic events in patients with acute myocardial infarction. Circulation. 2004;109:3171-5.

76. Sibbing D, Braun S, Morath T, et al. Platelet reactivity after clopidogrel treatment assessed with point-of-care analysis and early drug-eluting stent thrombosis. J Am Coll Cardiol. 2009;53:849-56.

77. Buonamici P, Marcucci R, Migliorini A, et al. Impact of platelet reactivity after clopidogrel administration on drug-eluting stent thrombosis. J Am Coll Cardiol. 2007;49:2312-7.

78. Mauri L, Hsieh WH, Massaro JM, et al. Stent thrombosis in randomized clinical trials of drug-eluting stents. N Engl J Med. 2007;356:1020-9.

79. Collet JP, Hulot JS, Pena A, et al. Cytochrome P450 2C19 polymorphism in young patients treated with clopidogrel after myocardial infarction: a cohort study. Lancet. 2009;373:309-17.

80. Mega JL, Close SL, Wiviott SD, et al. Cytochrome P450 genetic polymorphisms and the response to prasugrel: relationship to pharmacokinetic, pharmacodynamic, and clinical outcomes. Circulation. 2009;119:2553-60.

81. Simon T, Verstuyft C, Mary-Krause M, et al. Genetic determinants of response to clopidogrel and cardiovascular events. N Engl J Med. 2009;360:363-75.

82. Shuldiner AR, O'Connell JR, Bliden KP, et al. Association of Cytochrome P450 2C19 Genotype With the Antiplatelet Effect and Clinical Efficacy of Clopidogrel Therapy. JAMA. 2009;302:849-57.

83. Desta Z, Zhao X, Shin JG, et al. Clinical significance of the cytochrome P450 2C19 genetic polymorphism. Clin Pharmacokinet. 2002;41:913-58.

84. Gilard M, Arnaud B, Cornily JC, et al. Influence of omeprazole on the antiplatelet action of clopidogrel associated with aspirin: the randomized, double-blind OCLA (Omeprazole CLopidogrel Aspirin) study. J Am Coll Cardiol. 2008;51:256-60.

85. Writing Committee M, Abraham NS, Hlatky MA, et al. ACCF/ACG/AHA 2010 Expert Consensus Document on the Concomitant Use of Proton Pump Inhibitors and Thienopyridines: a focused update of the ACCF/ACG/AHA 2008 Expert Consensus Document on Reducing the Gastrointestinal Risks of Antiplatelet Therapy and NSAID Use: a report of the American College of Cardiology Foundation Task Force on Expert Consensus Documents. Circulation. 2010;122:2619-33.

86. Wiviott SD, Trenk D, Frelinger AL, et al. Prasugrel compared with high loading- and maintenance-dose clopidogrel in patients with planned percutaneous coronary intervention: the Prasugrel in Comparison to Clopidogrel for Inhibition of Platelet Activation and Aggregation-Thrombolysis in Myocardial Infarction 44 trial. Circulation. 2007;116:2923-32.

87. Wiviott SD, Braunwald E, McCabe CH, et al. Prasugrel versus clopidogrel in patients with acute coronary syndromes. N Engl J Med. 2007;357:2001-15.

88. Silvano M, Zambon CF, De Rosa G, et al. A case of resistance to clopidogrel and prasugrel after percutaneous coronary angioplasty. J Thromb Thrombolysis. 2011;31:233-4.

89. Cannon CP, Husted S, Harrington RA, et al. Safety, tolerability, and initial efficacy of AZD6140, the first reversible oral adenosine diphosphate receptor antagonist, compared with clopidogrel, in patients with non-ST-segment elevation acute coronary syndrome: primary results of the DISPERSE-2 trial. J Am Coll Cardiol. 2007;50:1844-51.

90. Serebruany VL, Atar D. The PLATO trial: do you believe in magic? Eur Heart J. 2010;31:764-7.

91. Inhibition of the platelet glycoprotein IIb/IIIa receptor with tirofiban in unstable angina and non-Q-wave myocardial infarction. Platelet Receptor Inhibition in Ischemic Syndrome Management in Patients Limited by Unstable Signs and Symptoms (PRISM-PLUS) Study Investigators. N Engl J Med. 1998;338:1488-97.

92. Kastrati A, Mehilli J, Neumann FJ, et al. Abciximab in patients with acute coronary syndromes undergoing percutaneous coronary intervention after clopidogrel pretreatment: the ISAR-REACT 2 randomized trial. JAMA. 2006;295:1531-8.

93. Simoons ML. Effect of glycoprotein IIb/IIIa receptor blocker abciximab on outcome in patients with acute coronary syndromes without early coronary revascularisation: the GUSTO IV-ACS randomised trial. Lancet. 2001;357:1915-24.

94. Inhibition of platelet glycoprotein IIb/IIIa with eptifibatide in patients with acute coronary syndromes. The PURSUIT Trial Investigators. Platelet Glycoprotein IIb/IIIa in Unstable Angina: Receptor Suppression Using Integrilin Therapy. N Engl J Med. 1998;339:436-43.

95. Randomised placebo-controlled trial of abciximab before and during coronary intervention in refractory unstable angina: the CAPTURE Study. Lancet. 1997;349:1429-35.

96. Boersma E, Harrington RA, Moliterno DJ, et al. Platelet glycoprotein IIb/IIIa inhibitors in acute coronary syndromes: a meta-analysis of all major randomised clinical trials. Lancet. 2002;359:189-98.

97. Hamm CW, Heeschen C, Goldmann B, et al. Benefit of abciximab in patients with refractory unstable angina in relation to serum troponin T levels. c7E3 Fab Antiplatelet Therapy in Unstable Refractory Angina (CAPTURE) Study Investigators. N Engl J Med. 1999;340:1623-9.

98. Heeschen C, Hamm CW, Goldmann B, et al. Troponin concentrations for stratification of patients with acute coronary syndromes in relation to therapeutic efficacy of tirofiban. PRISM Study Investigators. Platelet Receptor Inhibition in Ischemic Syndrome Management. Lancet. 1999;354:1757-62.

99. Theroux P, Alexander J, Pharand C, et al. Glycoprotein IIb/IIIa receptor blockade improves outcomes in diabetic patients presenting with unstable angina/non-ST-elevation myocardial infarction: results from the Platelet Receptor Inhibition in Ischemic Syndrome Management in Patients Limited by Unstable Signs and Symptoms (PRISM-PLUS) study. Circulation. 2000;102:2466-72.

100. Stone GW, McLaurin BT, Cox DA, et al. Bivalirudin for patients with acute coronary syndromes. N Engl J Med. 2006;355:2203-16.

101. Giugliano RP, White JA, Bode C, et al. Early versus delayed, provisional eptifibatide in acute coronary syndromes. N Engl J Med. 2009;360:2176-90.

102. Alexander KP, Chen AY, Roe MT, et al. Excess dosing of antiplatelet and antithrombin agents in the treatment of non-ST-segment elevation acute coronary syndromes. JAMA. 2005;294:3108-16.

103. Oler A, Whooley MA, Oler J, et al. Adding heparin to aspirin reduces the incidence of myocardial infarction and death in patients with unstable angina. A meta-analysis. JAMA. 1996;276:811-5.

104. Cohen M, Blaber R, Demers C, et al. The Essence Trial: Efficacy and Safety of Subcutaneous Enoxaparin in Unstable Angina and Non-Q-Wave MI: A Double-Blind, Randomized, Parallel-Group, Multicenter Study Comparing Enoxaparin and Intravenous Unfractionated Heparin: Methods and Design. J Thromb Thrombolysis. 1997;4:271-4.

105. Antman EM, McCabe CH, Gurfinkel EP, et al. Enoxaparin prevents death and cardiac ischemic events in unstable angina/non-Q-wave myocardial infarction. Results of the thrombolysis in myocardial infarction (TIMI) 11B trial. Circulation. 1999;100:1593-601.

106. Blazing MA, de Lemos JA, White HD, et al. Safety and efficacy of enoxaparin vs unfractionated heparin in patients with non-ST-segment elevation acute coronary syndromes who receive tirofiban and aspirin: a randomized controlled trial. JAMA. 2004;292:55-64.

107. Ferguson JJ, Califf RM, Antman EM, et al. Enoxaparin vs unfractionated heparin in high-risk patients with non-ST-segment elevation acute coronary syndromes managed with an intended early invasive strategy: primary results of the SYNERGY randomized trial. JAMA. 2004;292:45-54.

108. de Lemos JA, Blazing MA, Wiviott SD, et al. Enoxaparin versus unfractionated heparin in patients treated with tirofiban, aspirin and an early conservative initial management strategy: results from the A phase of the A-to-Z trial. Eur Heart J. 2004;25:1688-94.

109. Yusuf S, Mehta SR, Chrolavicius S, et al. Comparison of fondaparinux and enoxaparin in acute coronary syndromes. N Engl J Med. 2006;354:1464-76.

110. Lincoff AM, Bittl JA, Harrington RA, et al. Bivalirudin and provisional glycoprotein IIb/IIIa blockade compared with heparin and planned glycoprotein IIb/IIIa blockade during percutaneous coronary intervention: REPLACE-2 randomized trial. JAMA. 2003;289:853-63.

111. Pinto DS, Stone GW, Shi C, et al. Economic evaluation of bivalirudin with or without glycoprotein IIb/IIIa inhibition versus heparin with routine glycoprotein IIb/IIIa inhibition for early invasive management of acute coronary syndromes. J Am Coll Cardiol. 2008;52:1758-68.

112. Hurlen M, Smith P, Arnesen H. Effects of warfarin, aspirin and the two combined, on mortality and thromboembolic morbidity after myocardial infarction. The WARIS-II (Warfarin-Aspirin Reinfarction Study) design. Scand Cardiovasc J. 2000;34:168-71.

113. van Es RF, Jonker JJ, Verheugt FW, Deckers JW, Grobbee DE. Aspirin and coumadin after acute coronary syndromes (the ASPECT-2 study): a randomised controlled trial. Lancet. 2002;360:109-13.

114. Invasive compared with non-invasive treatment in unstable coronary-artery disease: FRISC II prospective randomised multicentre study. FRagmin and Fast Revascularisation during InStability in Coronary artery disease Investigators. Lancet. 1999;354:708-15.

115. Cannon CP, Weintraub WS, Demopoulos LA, et al. Comparison of early invasive and conservative strategies in patients with unstable coronary syndromes treated with the glycoprotein IIb/IIIa inhibitor tirofiban. N Engl J Med. 2001;344:1879-87.

116. Fox KA, Poole-Wilson PA, Henderson RA, et al. Interventional versus conservative treatment for patients with unstable angina or non-ST-elevation myocardial infarction: the British Heart Foundation RITA 3 randomised trial. Randomized Intervention Trial of unstable Angina. Lancet. 2002;360:743-51.

117. Lagerqvist B, Husted S, Kontny F, et al. A long-term perspective on the protective effects of an early invasive strategy in unstable coronary artery disease: two-year follow-up of the FRISC-II invasive study. J Am Coll Cardiol. 2002;40:1902-14.

118. Neumann FJ, Kastrati A, Pogatsa-Murray G, et al. Evaluation of prolonged antithrombotic pretreatment ("cooling-off" strategy) before intervention in patients with unstable coronary syndromes: a randomized controlled trial. JAMA. 2003;290:1593-9.

119. Spacek R, Widimsky P, Straka Z, et al. Value of first day angiography/angioplasty in evolving non-ST segment elevation myocardial infarction: an open multicenter randomized trial. The VINO study. Eur Heart J. 2002;23:230-8.

120. Wallentin L, Lagerqvist B, Husted S, et al. Outcome at 1 year after an invasive compared with a non-invasive strategy in unstable coronary-artery disease: the FRISC II invasive randomised trial. FRISC II Investigators. Fast revascularisation during instability in coronary artery disease. Lancet. 2000;356:9-16.

121. Mehta SR, Cannon CP, Fox KA, et al. Routine vs selective invasive strategies in patients with acute coronary syndromes: a collaborative meta-analysis of randomized trials. JAMA. 2005;293:2908-17.

122. Hoenig MR, Aroney CN, Scott IA. Early invasive versus conservative strategies for unstable angina and non-ST elevation myocardial infarction in the stent era. Cochrane Database Syst Rev. 2010;3: CD004815.

123. O'Donoghue M, Boden WE, Braunwald E, et al. Early invasive vs conservative treatment strategies in women and men with unstable angina and non-ST-segment elevation myocardial infarction: a meta-analysis. JAMA. 2008;300:71-80.

124. Mahmoudi M, Delhaye C, Waksman R. Safety and efficacy of drug-eluting stents and bare-metal stents in acute coronary syndrome. Cardiovasc Revasc Med. 2011 [Epub ahead of print].

125. Suh HS, Song HJ, Choi JE, et al. Drug-eluting stents versus bare-metal stents in acute myocardial infarction: a systematic review and meta-analysis. Int J Technol Assess Health Care. 2011;27:11-22.

126. Mehta SR, Granger CB, Boden WE, et al. Early versus delayed invasive intervention in acute coronary syndromes. N Engl J Med. 2009;360:2165-75.

127. Montalescot G, Cayla G, Collet JP, et al. Immediate vs delayed intervention for acute coronary syndromes: a randomized clinical trial. JAMA. 2009;302:947-54.

128. Kushner FG, Hand M, Smith SC, et al. 2009 Focused Updates: ACC/AHA Guidelines for the Management of Patients With ST-Elevation Myocardial Infarction (Updating the 2004 Guideline and 2007 Focused Update) and ACC/AHA/SCAI Guidelines on Percutaneous Coronary Intervention (Updating the 2005 Guideline and 2007 Focused Update): a report of the American College of Cardiology Foundation/American Heart Association Task Force on Practice Guidelines. J Am Coll Cardiol. 2009;54:2205-41.

129. Smith SC, Feldman TE, Hirshfeld JW, et al. ACC/AHA/SCAI 2005 Guideline Update for Percutaneous Coronary Intervention: a report of the American College of Cardiology/American Heart Association Task Force on Practice Guidelines (ACC/AHA/SCAI Writing Committee to Update the 2001 Guidelines for Percutaneous Coronary Intervention). J Am Coll Cardiol. 2006;47:e1-121.

130. Parikh SV, de Lemos JA, Jessen ME, et al. Timing of in-hospital coronary artery bypass graft surgery for non-ST-segment elevation myocardial infarction patients results from the National Cardiovascular Data Registry ACTION Registry-GWTG (Acute Coronary Treatment and Intervention Outcomes Network Registry-Get With The Guidelines). JACC Cardiovasc Interv. 2010;3:419-27.

Chapter 49

Acute Coronary Syndrome II
(ST-Elevation Myocardial Infarction and Post Myocardial Infarction): Complications and Care

Theresa M Brennan, Patricia Lounsbury, Saket Girotra

Chapter Outline

INTRODUCTION

Nearly 400,000 patients suffer from an ST-elevation myocardial Infarction (STEMI) every year in the United States.[1] It is a life-threatening event and a true medical emergency.[1] The risk of morbidity and mortality associated with STEMI increases with greater amount of myocardium at risk, delay in reperfusion, lack of collaterals to the infarct related artery (IRA), previous cardiovascular disease co-morbidities (e.g. diabetes, renal failure, etc.) and abnormal thrombolysis in myocardial infarction (TIMI) flow postreperfusion. It is estimated that at least 15% of patients, with a confirmed myocardial infarction (MI), die acutely and that 70% of these deaths occur prior to arrival at a hospital.[1] Based on 2006 data, 181,000 people in the United States died of STEMI. Among survivors, it is estimated that the average MI results in 15 years of life lost.[1]

The time from onset of symptoms to reperfusion is an extremely important factor on overall mortality (Fig. 1).[2,3] The success of restoration of normal flow in the IRA after primary percutaneous intervention was directly related to the ischemic time (i.e. symptom onset to initial balloon).[2] The relative risk of death increased by 1.075 for every 30-minute increase in symptom onset to balloon time.[2] Therefore, we must not only treat STEMI patients rapidly and appropriately when they arrive at our facilities, but we must also educate all patients on the signs and symptoms of an MI and the urgency of seeking medical treatment. In addition, patients must be educated to utilize the emergency medical transport system, instead of utilizing private transportation to the emergency facility. This allows for the prehospital treatment protocols that have been developed and utilized within communities to be effective in facilitating rapid reperfusion.

The reader should compare and contrast the evaluation and management of STEMI patients with UA/NSTEMI patients described in the Chapter 48. At the end of each section, recommendations from the American College of Cardiology (ACC) and the American Heart Association (AHA) 2004 guidelines[4] for the management of patients with STEMI, and

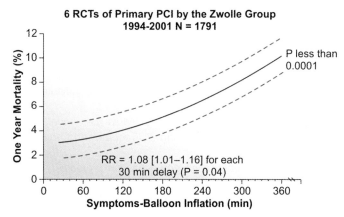

FIGURE 1: Symptom onset to balloon time and mortality in primary PCI for ST-elevation myocardial infarction. The relationship between time-to-treatment and 1 year mortality, as continuous functions, was assessed using a quadratic regression model. The dotted lines represent 95% confidence intervals of the predicted mortality. (Abbreviations: RCT: Randomized controlled trial; PCI: Percutaneous coronary intervention) (*Source:* Modified from DuLuca G, Suryapranate H, Ottervanger JP, et al. Time delay to treatments and mortality in primary angioplasty for acute myocardial infarction: every minute of delay counts. Circulation. 2004;109:1223-5)

the focused updates in 2007 and 2009[5,6] are included wherever appropriate. In addition, reference is also made to respective 2007 guidelines[7] for UA/NSTEMI and the 2011 focused update[8] wherever appropriate. Indications for use are divided into Class I (should be performed or administered), Class II (reasonable or may consider performing or administering) and Class III (should not perform or administer due to the lack of benefit and/or potential for harm). The reader is directed to the guidelines for a detailed discussion and the reasoning for these recommendations.

PATHOPHYSIOLOGY

The pathophysiology of STEMI is most commonly associated with acute rupture of a vulnerable plaque. This has been discussed in detail in Chapter 48 "Acute Coronary Syndrome I: Unstable Angina and Non-ST Segment Elevation Myocardial Infarction". Patients who present with UA/NSTEMI do not, in general, have sustained thrombotic vessel occlusion secondary to this plaque rupture. When this sustained occlusion occurs, STEMI results and the treatment strategy is focused on restoring flow as rapidly as possible as discussed later.

STENT THROMBOSIS

With the advent of stenting, particularly drug-eluting stent use, a second major etiology of STEMI, is stent thrombosis. The pathophysiology of early (within 24 hours of the procedure) stent thrombosis is related to mechanical complications, such as edge dissection or malapposition or under sizing of the stent, decreased flow in the target vessel at procedure end, or physical aspects of the vessel including visible thrombus during the procedure, intermediate lesions (50–70%) distal to the treated lesion, and stents placed at a bifurcation. After any coronary intervention, one must also be aware of potential for acute coronary syndrome (ACS), secondary to procedural complications due to mechanical trauma at the site of treatment

as well as remote to the treated site (e.g, guide catheter or wire trauma). For early postcoronary intervention patients who develop STEMI, the interventional center must have a protocol for rapid assessment and immediate return to the catheterization laboratory for rapid restoration of flow.

The risk, of stent thrombosis continues after the initial periprocedural time period. Registry data with follow-up mean of 30 months demonstrated that 2.1% of patients presented with confirmed stent thrombosis. The risk of stent thrombosis decreases over time with 32% occurring within 24 hours, 41.2% occurring after 24 hours, but within 30 days, 13.3% at 31days to 1 year, 13.5% were beyond 1 year. This registry suggested no difference in numbers of stent thrombosis in bare metal stents compared to drug eluting stents.[9] With bare metal stenting, the risk of stent thrombosis is elevated above the long-term baseline for up to 1 month, but for drug eluting stents, this time of increased risk may be to 1 year and perhaps beyond.

The majority of subacute stent thromboses occur in patients who discontinue the necessary dual antiplatelet therapy early. Therefore, patients with stenting in the previous year, who present with STEMI in the territory of the previously treated vessel, must be questioned about compliance with their antiplatelet regimen. This questioning has direct impact on procedural strategies (if repeat stenting is necessary), and post interventional antiplatelet therapy.

In addition, characteristics of the patient (including prothrombotic states, the presence of malignancy, etc.) may significantly increase the risk.[9] Finally, aspirin and/or clopidogrel resistance may increase the risk of stent thrombosis.[10-13] Again, differentiation between noncompliance and resistance is very important in the management of patients. Data regarding resistance to antiplatelet therapy, particularly clopidogrel, including recent identification of genetic mutations in the cytochrome P450 pathway (CYP2C19 loss of function alleles), have been implicated in the increased risk of cardiovascular events and stent thrombosis in compliant patients.[14] This has been thoroughly discussed in Chapter 48 "Acute Coronary Syndrome I: Unstable Angina and Non-ST Segment Elevation Myocardial Infarction".

COCAINE OR METHAMPHETAMINE

Cocaine or methamphetamine-associated STEMI must be considered in all patients. Although, it may be more common to see illicit-drug associated cardiovascular events in younger patients, one must have a suspicion in all patients and take a careful history regarding cocaine or methamphetamine use. Urine toxicology testing must be considered especially patients with few or no risk factors for coronary artery disease (CAD). Most events occur early, but the illicit-drug may be a factor up to a few days after use. The ST-elevation may be a result of coronary vasoconstriction, commonly diffuse, without obstructive CAD, obstructive CAD related to repeated use and/or risk factors for CAD with or without plaque rupture, or related to myopericarditis related to the illicit-drug use. Patients using illicit-drugs may have other associated cardiovascular effects including dysrhythmia, aortic dissection, or stroke.

Other etiologies of STEMI include vasospasm, thrombo-emboli (originating from a mechanical valve, the left atrium in a patient with atrial fibrillation, left ventricular (LV) thrombus, etc.) and stent restenosis with or without associated thrombus.

CLINICAL PRESENTATION

Patients with diagnosis of STEMI will present with symptoms consistent with ACS (see Chapter 48 "Acute Coronary Syndrome I: Unstable Angina and Non-ST Segment Elevation Myocardial Infarction"). Those with STEMI, though, have a higher likelihood of early complications including hemodynamic instability and shock, atrial and ventricular dysrhythmias and sudden cardiac death. Therefore, early evaluation including prehospital evaluation and timely determination of optimal reperfusion is essential.

PREHOSPITAL ASSESSMENT

The development of community or regional based STEMI protocols between emergency medical services (EMS), emergency rooms and the interventional cardiology catheterization labs is critical for optimal treatment of STEMI. The advent of systems that allow for high quality digital transmission of a 12-lead electrocardiogram (ECG) from the field facilitates early recognition of STEMI and infield treatment including thrombolysis. When a STEMI patient is to be transported to a facility with capability to perform primary angioplasty [percutaneous coronary intervention (PCI) center], activation of the cardiac catheterization laboratory team while the patient is in the field, decreases time to reperfusion and improves likelihood of TIMI III flow in the IRA.[15,16] This decrease in time leads to equalization of door to balloon (D2B) times between normal working hours and after hours or weekends when the interventional team may not be onsite. Thus, early in field activation of the interventional laboratory team allows for an overall decrease in D2B times and an improvement in patient outcomes.[15,16]

Alternatively, if the patient is not near a PCI center, a determination of need for full-dose thrombolysis can be performed by qualified physicians at the accepting facility after the checklist of contraindications is reviewed by EMS paramedics. When this thrombolytic therapy is given in the field, the time to therapy can be decreased by up to 40% depending on the location of the patient and time to the accepting facility.[17] Thrombolysis in the field, though, requires advanced training, clear protocols and ongoing quality assessment which limit the ability for this to be widespread.

It is also important to recognize that if primary angioplasty or stenting is to be performed, transport of the patient directly to a PCI center is optimal, even if it results in bypassing a non-PCI center.[18] Recent statewide protocols have been changed, including in the predominantly rural state of Iowa, to bypass small critical access hospitals and take the patient directly to a PCI center. This decreases overall transport time to the PCI center by eliminating time spent transporting the patient to and having the patient evaluated at a hospital that is not able to perform primary PCI and in many instances does not have a STEMI protocol to optimize D2B times. This direct transport to a PCI center improves time to reperfusion and thus improves outcomes.

The American College of Cardiology (ACC)/American Heart Association (AHA) guidelines recommend:

Class I

Community based programs be developed and instituted to include:
- *Quality focused multidisciplinary teams (personnel from EMS and hospitals including PCI centers and non-PCI centers)*
- *Prehospital identification and activation protocols*
- *PCI center protocols for STEMI*
- *Non-PCI center protocols for transfer of STEMI patients.*

Class II

Prehospital thrombolysis protocols be established and utilized if:
- *Either physician or full-time paramedics with ECG interpretation training are present in ambulance, and who work with dedicated hospital based STEMI program with ongoing continual quality improvement.*

EMERGENCY ROOM EVALUATION

It is expected that when a patient presents to a facility with chest pain, or other symptoms consistent with MI, that an ECG be performed and read by a qualified physician as soon as possible, but always within 10 minutes of arriving at that facility. If the electrocardiogram (ECG) is not diagnostic but the clinical scenario is consistent, the ECG must be repeated in no more than 10 minutes to assess for changes or evolution. If EKG is consistent with a STEMI (Figs 2 to 14) then, reperfusion must be the primary focus. A brief and rapid clinical evaluation for contraindications to reperfusion therapies and identification of other medical disorders, (particularly aortic dissection with compromise of a coronary artery resulting in STEMI) must be performed. In addition, it is prudent to evaluate the patient for emergency PCI, by rapidly assessing anticoagulation status, any history of contrast allergy and potential vascular access. This evaluation should not delay the reperfusion course. If the patient is not in a PCI Center, arrangements for transfer and/or consideration of thrombolysis should begin immediately.

The American College of Cardiology (ACC)/American Heart Association (AHA) guidelines recommend:

Class I

- *Hospitals should establish multidisciplinary teams with protocols for rapid triage and delivery of therapy including determination and delivery of reperfusion strategy*
- *The ECG within 10 minutes of arrival, with repeat in 5–10 minutes if ongoing symptoms and initial ECG is not diagnostic of STEMI*
- *Emergency room provider must rapidly obtain a focused history and physical examination to evaluate likelihood of STEMI and contraindications to reperfusion strategies.*

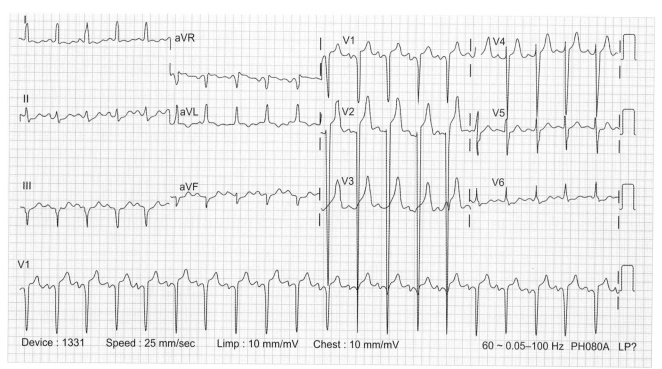

FIGURE 2: A 65-year-old patient who was in hospital undergoing evaluation for chest discomfort, developed recurrent chest pain and ECG was done within minutes. Patient has baseline j-point elevation in the anterior precordium likely due to LVH, but T waves are markedly different from previous and are tall and peaked consistent with hyper acute T waves. Note also the beginnings of subtle ST abnormalities in the inferior and lateral leads (V6 and aVF). Patient was taken to cardiac catheterization lab and had a thrombotic occlusion of the proximal left anterior descending (LAD) coronary artery

Electrocardiogram

The ECG is the essential tool in the assessment and risk stratification of patients presenting with chest pain.[19] The presence of ST-elevation on ECG denotes STEMI in greater than 80% of patients and can assist in the localization of the MI into anterior, inferior (with or without posterior and/or right ventricular (RV) involvement) and lateral.[20] The remaining 20% of patients with apparent ST-elevation may have: vasospasm, myopericarditis, takotsubo cardiomyopathy, LV hypertrophy and/or hypertrophic cardiomyopathy, ventricular preexcitation (Wolff-Parkinson-White syndrome) hyperkalemia, or a normal variant. It must be recognized that the clinical picture is very important in determining etiology of the ST-elevation, particularly when the ECG is not classic for STEMI (shape of ST segments, lack of reciprocal changes, etc.).

The first change in the ECG that occurs during vessel occlusion is upright, peaked and symmetric T waves (commonly referred to as hyper acute).[21] The duration of this change, in the presence of persistent occlusion, is short (in minutes) and, therefore, is rarely seen clinically.[22] If present, subtle reciprocal abnormalities may be seen increasing the suspicion for acute myocardial infarction (AMI) (Fig. 2). The subsequent evolution is to the development of ST-elevation. The shape of the ST-segment (coving or straightening of the segment compared to a normal concave upward segment), and the presence of reciprocal changes (ST-depressions) in the leads opposite the ST-elevation are strongly supportive of STEMI as the etiology of the ST-elevation.

The presence of ST-elevation in V1–V3 signifies anteroseptal STEMI or if involving V4, V5 and V6, anterolateral STEMI resulting from occlusion of the LAD coronary artery. Presence of ST-elevation in aVL suggests involvement of a high diagonal and thus a proximal LAD occlusion. In either case, the diagnosis of STEMI is supported by ST-depressions in II, III and aVF (reciprocal changes). In a patient with a large LAD that "wraps" around the apex of the heart and supplies a significant portion of the inferior wall, or with occlusion of the left main coronary artery, one may see ST-elevation in II, III and aVF as well (Figs 3 and 4).

The presence of ST-elevation in V5, V6 and I and aVL suggests a high lateral MI and may signify occlusion of a large ramus intermedius, very proximal obtuse marginal from the left circumflex or early diagonal coronary artery from the left anterior descending coronary artery (Fig. 5).

The ST-elevation in II, III and aVF signifies inferior MI (Fig. 6). In inferior STEMI, reciprocal changes (ST-depressions) can be seen in I, aVL and V1–V3. The presence of ST-elevation in III greater than in II suggests right coronary artery (RCA) occlusion versus occlusion of a dominant left circumflex coronary artery (LCX). The determination of RCA versus LCX involvement is important to the cardiac interventionalist in preparing the procedural protocol in the catheterization lab, but is also very important to the treating physician in that only with RCA occlusion can one potentially have coexistence of RVMI (Fig. 7). In addition, the presence of ST-elevation of at least 1 mm in V1 suggests that this occlusion is in the proximal RCA and thus, involves the right ventricle.[23] A more complex

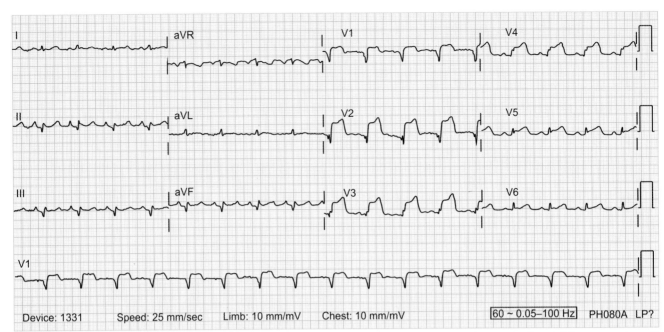

FIGURE 3: A 56-year-old patient with drug eluting stent to mid left anterior descending coronary artery that wrapped around the apex and supplied the inferior wall, one week prior who presented now after cardiac arrest. Note the shape and extent of the ST-elevation in all the precordial leads, but not in I, or aVL; this consistent with mid LAD occlusion. In addition, there are no reciprocal changes, but the shape of the ST segments is quite consistent with injury, and the clinical scenario consistent with STEMI. Coronary angiography showed stent thrombosis and patient was noted to have been noncompliant with dual antiplatelet therapy prior to this event

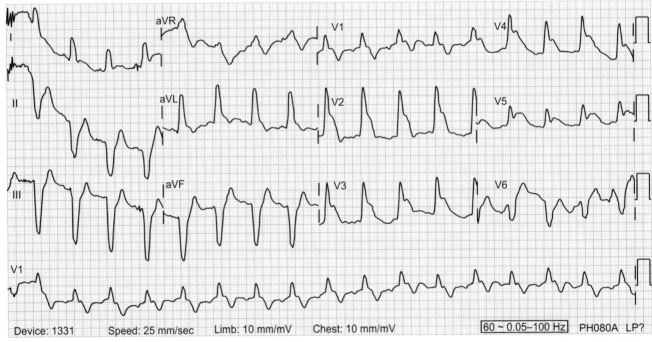

FIGURE 4: A 46-year-old patient presented with chest pain, became hemodynamically unstable and progressed to cardiac arrest. The ECG was obtained just prior to arrest; note the diffuse ST-elevation in the presence of an RBBB. Note the lack of expected ST-segments (discordant to the QRS), in the precordial leads with the RBBB. Coronary angiography showed left main coronary artery occlusion

algorithm exists to assist in differentiating the culprit artery in inferior MI.[24] Finally, the presence of RV infarction can be identified with high accuracy by obtaining right sided ECG leads in which the precordial leads V3–V6 are placed in the same interspace positions, but to the right of the sternum, mirroring their normal position. The presence of at least 1 mm of ST-elevation in lead V4R signifies RVMI.[25] The identification of RVMI is imperative as the medical treatment as well as the prognostic significance of RVMI differs from the general population of STEMI patients, as has been discussed later.

True posterior wall MI (without inferior involvement) is challenging to diagnose on ECG as these patients may present

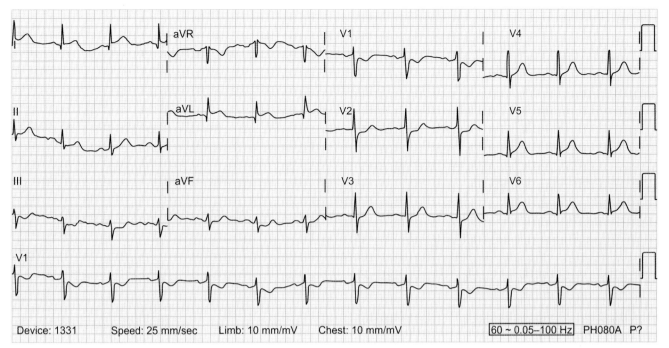

FIGURE 5: A 71-year-old patient presented with chest and jaw pain. Note ST-elevation in V5, V6, I and aVL with reciprocal changes is most prominent in V1 and V2. Coronary angiography showed 99% thrombotic lesion in large ramus intermedius

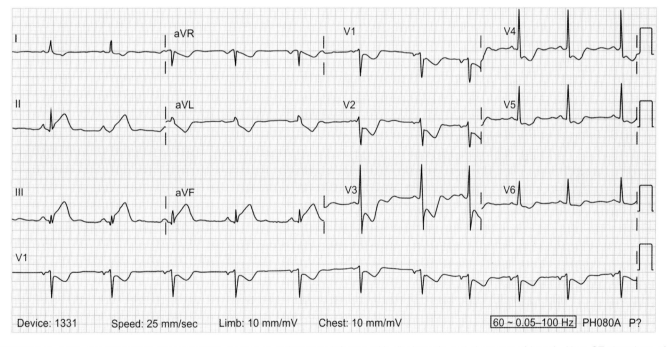

FIGURE 6: A 76-year-old patient presents with chest pain radiating to left arm with diaphoresis and shortness of breath. Note ST-elevations of similar magnitude in II and III, and significant ST-depressions throughout the precordial leads that are likely reciprocal, but may be manifestation of posterior STEMI or remote ischemia given the patients left main coronary artery lesion. Coronary angiogram showed occlusion on distal RCA with 65% left main coronary artery lesion

with ST-depressions in leads V1–V3 that are mirror images of the ST-elevations posteriorly (Fig. 8) or may present with no ECG changes (Fig. 9). There may be occlusion of the mid to distal LCX, or of a large posterolateral branch of the circumflex or the RCA that is electrocardiographically silent on the standard 12-lead ECG. Therefore, true posterior wall infarction should be considered in all patients who present with ongoing chest discomfort and persistent ST-depressions in these V1–V3, or no ECG changes at all. One should consider posterior infarction in any patient with typical angina, a normal ECG and persistent chest discomfort despite optimal medical therapy. To better assess, one can obtain posterior ECG leads by placing leads V7, V8 and V9 in the 5th interspace posteriorly around the chest. The presence of ST-elevations in these leads assists in the

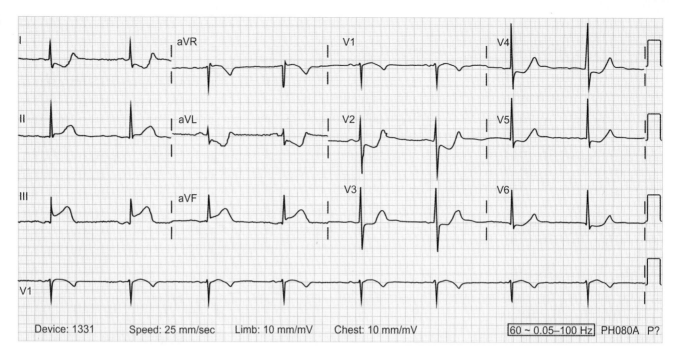

Device: 1331   Speed: 25 mm/sec   Limb: 10 mm/mV   Chest: 10 mm/mV   60 ~ 0.05–100 Hz PH080A P?

FIGURE 7: A 52-year-old patient presented with chest pain and shortness of breath. He developed hypotension and bradycardia after nitroglycerin was administered; this required IV fluid bolus and initiation of dopamine. Note sinus bradycardia with ST-elevation in III of greater magnitude than in II, lack of ST-depression in V1 and reciprocal changes in I and aVL. Clinical scenario, angiogram and EKG are consistent with and inferoposterior STEMI with RV infarction. Coronary angiography showed thrombotic occlusion of the proximal right coronary artery. Patient developed significant RV dysfunction post MI

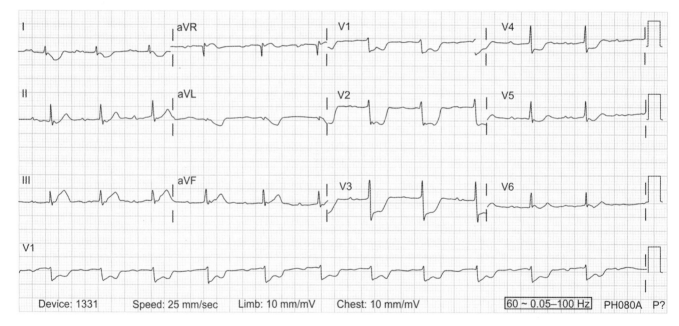

Device: 1331   Speed: 25 mm/sec   Limb: 10 mm/mV   Chest: 10 mm/mV   60 ~ 0.05–100 Hz PH080A P?

FIGURE 8: A 43-year-old patient presented with chest tightness and left neck pain. Shortly after presentation became unstable with hypotension and respiratory failure. Note significant ST-depressions in the anterior leads that, in this case, signify a true posterior infarct. In light of the patient's instability, the diagnosis was readily made (versus consideration of anterior ischemia) and posterior leads were not obtained. Coronary angiogram showed thrombotic occlusion at the origin of the left circumflex coronary artery with thrombus extending into, but not obstructing the left main coronary artery

diagnosis of posterior STEMI and allows for the physician to initiate a reperfusion strategy. As well, assessment with a transthoracic echocardiogram looking for a new wall motion abnormality may assist in determining need for immediate reperfusion.

In the presence of a right bundle branch block (RBBB) ST-elevation is identifiable (Fig. 4). In the presence of a left bundle branch block (LBBB) (Fig. 10), STEMI diagnosis is more complex. First, the presence of a new or presumed LBBB in the clinical scenario of ongoing symptoms of ACS should

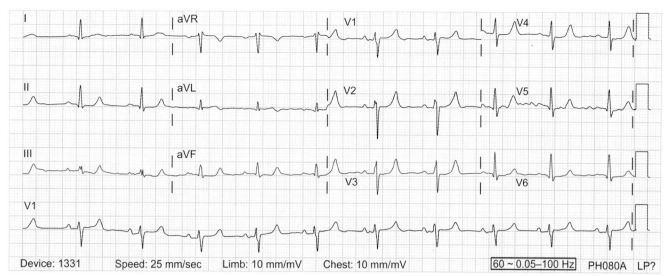

FIGURE 9: A 43-year-old patient post-remote coronary artery bypass graft (CABG) presented with ongoing chest discomfort that was not responsive to nitroglycerin at high doses, in addition to standard medical therapy. Note ECG without significant ST abnormality, in this case, consistent with the potentially electrically silent posterolateral wall MI. Coronary angiogram showed previously known right posterior descending coronary artery occlusion, with new mid RCA occlusion, supplying only the right posterolateral coronary artery myocardial territory

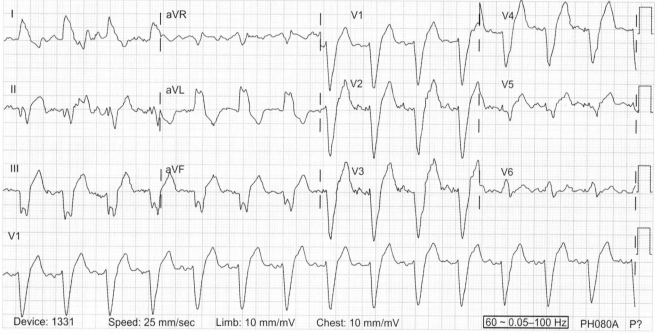

FIGURE 10: A 51-year-old patient presents with chest pain and new LBBB (compared to ECG 4 months prior). Note LBBB, new, with no other criteria for STEMI. Coronary angiography showed no culprit vessel for STEMI. The troponins were negative on serial examination. Despite the fact that this patient did not have STEMI, the emergent coronary angiogram was the correct diagnostic evaluation in the given clinical scenario

prompt strong and rapid consideration of vessel occlusion or MI (STEMI-equivalent). This patient should be considered for reperfusion therapy. In a patient with a known LBBB, there are diagnostic criteria for acute STEMI: greater than or equal to 1 mm of ST-elevation that is concordant (in the same direction as the QRS), greater than or equal to 1 mm ST-depression in lead V1, V2 or V3, and greater than or equal to 5 mm ST-elevation that is discordant (opposite direction of the QRS). The presence of any degree of ST-elevation that is concordant is not found with an LBBB; therefore, this criterion is highly specific for the diagnosis of acute MI in the presence of an LBBB, but it is

not necessary. The presence of ST-depressions in the precordial leads should as well be considered a specific marker of MI in the patient with an LBBB. The presence of discordant ST-elevation should significantly raise the physician's suspicion, but one may consider confirmatory evaluation (i.e. transthoracic echocardiogram, etc.)[26]

One should not be "distracted by the obvious and remarkable abnormality" of ST-elevation when reading the ECG. The rapid recognition of STEMI is laudable and necessary, but the entire ECG must be interpreted in order that the patient should be cared for optimally. Learners should develop an organized

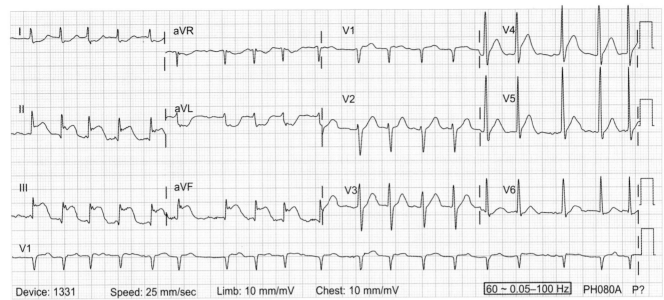

Device: 1331   Speed: 25 mm/sec   Limb: 10 mm/mV   Chest: 10 mm/mV   60 ~ 0.05–100 Hz   PH080A   P?

FIGURE 11: A 48-year-old patient presented with chest pain. An ECG shows atrial fibrillation with rapid ventricular response, with inferior ST-elevations and is consistent with RV involvement given the ST-elevations greater in III than II, and the lack of ST depression in V1. Coronary angiography was attempted with failure to engage the coronary arteries due to aortic dissection with involvement of the right coronary ostium resulting in inferior STEMI. After dissection was repaired, and coronary artery bypass graft (CABG) performed to the distal RCA, patient had significant RV dysfunction resulting in cardiogenic shock, requiring right ventricular assist device placement

system for reading the ECG beginning with the rhythm and continuing through the assessment of the QT interval. If one does not, the potential for this "distraction" exists, and will prompt the reader to miss other important aspects of the ECG, particularly the rhythm (Fig. 11). In the setting of AMI, sinus bradycardia, advance heart block and atrial and ventricular dysrhythmias may exist that require identification and at times specific treatment. In addition, the presence of accelerated idioventricular rhythm may signal reperfusion.

Finally, the reader must understand the evolution of the ECG in the hours and days after MI. Acutely after reperfusion, the ST-segments will return to or toward normal, and the T waves may initially appear normalized. In the following hours, the T waves will invert and may appear biphasic (Figs 12 to 14). These QRS and T wave changes are a part of the typical evolutionary process of the ECG after MI and should not be interpreted as a clinical change, in the absence of symptoms. If symptoms are present, these, usually marked abnormalities, will inhibit electrocardiographic evaluation to varying degrees.

Persistent ST elevation and the development of Q waves in the infarcted territory signals significant myocardial necrosis. ST-elevations that persist for days to weeks may signal the

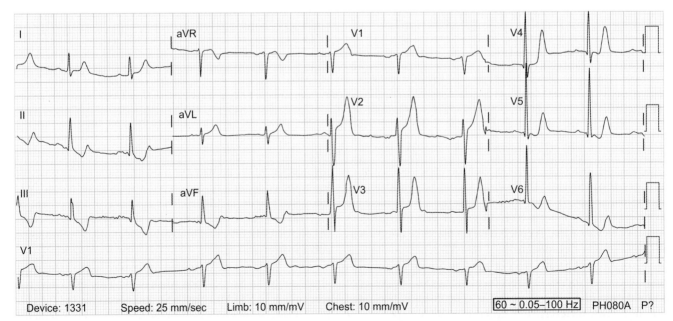

Device: 1331   Speed: 25 mm/sec   Limb: 10 mm/mV   Chest: 10 mm/mV   60 ~ 0.05–100 Hz   PH080A   P?

FIGURE 12: The figure demonstrates tall peaked T waves with associated ST-elevation in the anterior leads, and reciprocal depressions in the inferior leads. Coronary angiography done rapidly after onset of symptoms, showed 99% proximal left anterior descending coronary artery

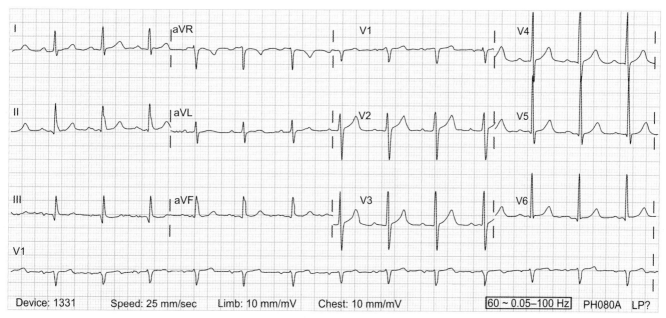

I   aVR   V1   V4

II   aVL   V2   V5

III   aVF   V3   V6

V1

Device: 1331   Speed: 25 mm/sec   Limb: 10 mm/mV   Chest: 10 mm/mV   60 ~ 0.05–100 Hz   PH080A   LP?

FIGURE 13: This figure is immediately after successful stenting of the lesion. Note normalization of the ST-segments and T waves

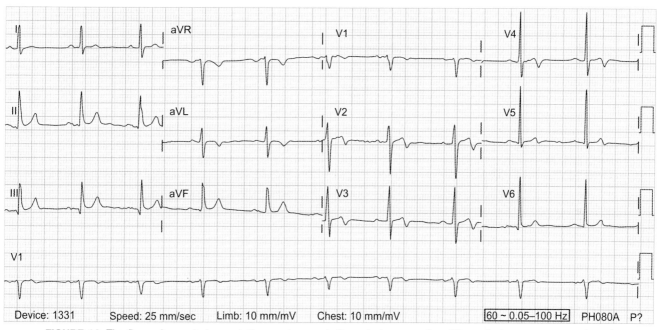

I   aVR   V1   V4

II   aVL   V2   V5

III   aVF   V3   V6

V1

Device: 1331   Speed: 25 mm/sec   Limb: 10 mm/mV   Chest: 10 mm/mV   60 ~ 0.05–100 Hz   PH080A   P?

FIGURE 14: The figure demonstrates evolutionary changes in the anterior precordium. The patient was asymptomatic and these changes were not related to recurrent ischemia but were normal evolution after anterior MI

development of a ventricular aneurysm, defining nonviable myocardium. The lack of Q waves is in general a testament to early reperfusion and myocardial salvage.

Other Early Diagnostic Evaluation

Further evaluation with laboratory studies, portable chest X-ray, echocardiography, etc. should be done, if they do not delay reperfusion and if there is a clear clinical indication (evaluation for aortic dissection, etc.). Laboratory studies sent on arrival to the emergency room are helpful in assessing electrolytes (particularly potassium), renal function, hemoglobin, platelets and coagulation status. Urine toxicology screen should

be considered on all patients, particularly those with few or no risk factors for CAD; this can be done after reperfusion. Biomarkers should be sent, but the reader must remember that elevation in the biomarker takes time (see the chapter "Acute Coronary Syndrome I: Unstable Angina and Non-ST Segment Elevation Myocardial Infarction") and a normal initial troponin in a patient with is quite common. The lack of elevation in troponin at presentation should not alter the physicians plan for reperfusion therapy in the early presenters. Portable chest X-ray (CXR) should be used to evaluate other etiologies of chest discomfort, such as aortic dissection, or when the diagnosis of STEMI is unclear. It is unnecessary to obtain a CXR to diagnose pulmonary edema, as this will be evident on examination.

A bedside echocardiogram is helpful in patients in which the diagnosis is unclear or there is concern that anterior ST-depressions are a marker of posterior wall infarction.

The American College of Cardiology (ACC)/American Heart Association (AHA) guidelines recommend:

Class I

- *Laboratory examinations should be performed but should not delay delivery of reperfusion therapy*
- *Troponin should be used as the optimal biomarker:*
  - *Abnormal cardiac biomarkers should not be necessary to proceed with reperfusion therapy*
  - *Portable chest X-ray should be performed as possible, but should not delay reperfusion therapy unless the physician suspects a clinical condition (i.e. aortic dissection) that would be a contraindication for reperfusion*
  - *Imaging of the aorta via transthoracic or transesophageal echocardiography, chest CT or MRI should be performed if there is significant concern for aortic dissection as etiology of syndrome.*

REPERFUSION

Reperfusion is the primary treatment of patients who present with STEMI. Medical therapy should be instituted as a reperfusion strategy is being put in place. The decision to perform primary PCI or administer a thrombolytic agent must be made and carried out rapidly in order to salvage as much myocardium as possible, and therefore prevent morbidity and mortality. Institutional protocols should be in place to allow for this decision to be made rapidly by the treating physician. These protocols must take into consideration the availability of each strategy and the estimated time to delivery of the appropriate care. The standard of care is D2B (patient arrival to first balloon inflation in the catheterization laboratory) of less than 90 minutes and door to needle (patient arrival to administration of thrombolytic agent) of less than 30 minutes. Again, although these times are standards of care, the physician must aim for these times to be as low as is possible. Presently the time begins with the patient's entry to the emergency room. Ideally this "door" time should begin with first medical contact (i.e. paramedic, etc.). Protocols should be continually reviewed and include discussion between local paramedics, emergency room physicians and the interventional cardiologists regarding potential to eliminate delays in delivery of each patient's appropriate reperfusion strategy and thus to optimize time to reperfusion.

The following is a discussion of the data to support each strategy, thrombolysis versus primary PCI. Although there are situations in which emergency coronary artery bypass graft (CABG) is the optimal reperfusion strategy in certain individual patients, these are rare. The time necessary to mobilize the operating room and reperfuse the patient is always excessive. Emergency CABG should be considered only in patients with critical left main CAD who have reperfused at the time of angiography (done with intent to perform PCI) and continue to demonstrate hemodynamic stability, or in patients with a large at-risk territory in whom PCI was attempted and is unsuccessful. Again, these scenarios are rare.

From this discussion, the physician should recognize the indications and contraindications to each strategy and be able to determine the most appropriate therapy for each individual patient based on the time from onset of symptoms, specific patient clinical status and contraindications, and the time to availability of primary PCI (within a PCI center vs need for transport and the time this will require).

THROMBOLYSIS

Available thrombolytics approved for use in STEMI have included: Streptokinase, Alteplase, Reteplase and Tenecteplase (TNK).

1. Streptokinase is a naturally occurring polypeptide obtained from the culture of group C beta hemolytic *Streptococcus*. It binds to plasminogen creating an active complex and thereby facilitates the transformation of plasminogen to plasmin resulting in fibrinolysis and proteolysis. It is therefore not specific to fibrin cleavage. It is antigenic and although significant allergic reactions are rare, repeat administration, even years after initial administration, increases the risk of serious allergic reaction. Approximately up to 10% may develop a rash and patients may develop hypotension during infusion. The half-life is 80 minutes.[27]

2. Alteplase is a reproduction of a naturally occurring tissue plasminogen activator (tPA) that is manufactured by recombinant technology. It is fibrin specific (does not have proteolytic effects) and the bound alteplase or fibrin compound has a high affinity for plasminogen. It does not have the side effect of hypotension, and allergic reactions are rare. The half-life is short (3–4 minutes). The use of IV heparin with alteplase during STEMI results in increased patency and less reocclusion.[27]

3. Reteplase is a recombinant plasminogen activator (rPA) that has less affinity for fibrin and a longer half-life than alteplase.[27]

4. Tenecteplase (TNK-tPA) is a genetically engineered plasminogen activator. The half-life is longer allowing for single bolus dosing which is advantageous in STEMI. In addition, it has less clinical intracranial bleeding than alteplase, though has been shown to have equal efficacy with respect to major adverse cardiac endpoints.[27,28] Therefore, TNK is preferred based on its equal efficacy, and decreased risk of intracranial hemorrhage. In the United States, TNK is the most widely used lytic agent for STEMI today. Comparison and contrast of these four agents are provided in Table 1.[4]

FACILITATED PERCUTANEOUS CORONARY INTERVENTION

Facilitated percutaneous coronary intervention (PCI) (upstream administration of partial dose GpIIb/IIIa inhibitor or full or partial dose thrombolytic or a combination thereof with plan for emergent PCI), in ambulance or at a non-PCI center prior to transfer for planned immediate PCI, has not been shown to improve mortality and in many instances led to increased

TABLE 1

Comparison of approved thrombolytic agents

	Streptokinase	Alteplase	Reteplase	Tenecteplase
Dose	1.5 MU over 30–60 minutes	Up to 100 mg in 90 minutes (weight based)	10 U × 2 each 30–50 mg over 2 minutes	Weight based
Bolus administration	No	No	Yes	Yes
Antigenic	Yes	No	No	No
Allergic reactions	Yes (hypotension)	No	No	No
Systemic fibrinogen depletion	Marked	Mild	Moderate	Minimal
~ 90 minutes patency rate	50%	75%	75%	75%
%TIMI 3 flow at 90 minutes	32	54	60	63
Approximate cost per dose (2004)	$613	$2974	$2750	$2833 for 50 mg (US$)

(*Source:* ACC/AHA guidelines for the management of patients with ST-elevation myocardial infarction. Circulation. 2004;110:588-636)

morbidity (increased need for revascularization, increased reinfarction rates and increased major bleeding complications).[29,30] Although the strategy would seem helpful in improving vessel patency, and some studies have shown this to be true (infarct-related artery patency is improved with some protocols), this has not been translated to a decrease in major adverse cardiovascular events (MACE).[31-34] Facilitated PCI for STEMI cannot be recommended.

> The American College of Cardiology (ACC)/American Heart Association (AHA) guidelines 2009 update removed the recommendation regarding facilitated PCI given the lack of convincing benefit.

Full Dose Thrombolytic Agent

Full dose thrombolytic as primary reperfusion therapy has been shown to improve mortality in patients with STEMI, compared to standard medical therapy. Both Second International Study of Infarct Survival (ISIS-2) (comparing the addition of streptokinase to aspirin vs placebo)[35] and Gruppo Italiano per lo Studio della Streptochinasi nell'Infarto Miocardico (GISSI)[36] showed that streptokinase was effective in reducing the incidence of death. In addition, ISIS-2 showed benefit in the addition of aspirin to streptokinase in the reduction in reinfarction, stroke and death.[35] Further studies have shown that accelerated dose alteplase (t-PA) had a greater benefit than streptokinase.[37] This study also showed that the administration of IV heparin was superior to subcutaneous heparin with alteplase. Notably the reduction of events with t-PA over streptokinase (death or disabling stroke), although significant, was just 1%. Given the cost difference between streptokinase and t-PA and this apparent small benefit, this study launched significant discussion regarding the cost or benefit of the use of accelerated t-PA over streptokinase, the financial impact this would have on hospitals, particularly smaller hospitals.

Secondly, data from this study[37] showed the greatest benefit in patients who are less than 75 years of age and also with an anterior infarction. A meta-analysis of large thrombolytic trials[38] further characterized that there was an overall 18% reduction in 35 days mortality with thrombolysis (with the benefit being

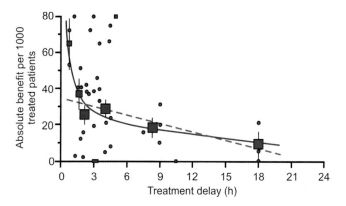

FIGURE 15: Absolute 35 days mortality reduction versus treatment delay: small closed dots—information from trials included in FTT analysis; open dots—information from additional trials; small squares—data beyond scale of x/y cross. The linear (34·7–1·6x) and non-linear (19·4–0·6x+29·3x−1) regression lines are fitted within these data, weighed by inverse of the variance of the absolute benefit in each datapoint. The four black squares: average effects in six time-to-treatment groups (areas of squares are inversely proportional to variance of absolute benefit described). (*Source:* Modified from Boersma E, Maas ACP, Deckers JW, et al. Early thrombolytic treatment in acute myocardial infarction: reappraisal of the golden hour. Lancet. 1996;348:771-5)

seen between 2–35 days, due to an excess number of deaths in the treatment arm in days 0 and 1). This benefit was seen in patients with STEMI and LBBB but not MI with EKG showing ST depressions. In patients with anterior STEMI versus inferior STEMI, the relative risk reduction was not different, but given the higher overall risk of the anterior STEMI patients, the absolute benefit was greater in patients presenting with anterior ST-elevation. Patients had a gradual decrease in benefit of thrombolysis with time from onset of symptoms, with the greatest benefit from delivery of drug within the first hour and a non-statistically significant benefit of only 1% overall when medication was administered greater than 12 hours from time of onset of symptoms.[38] This absolute mortality reduction over time has been confirmed (Figs 15 to 17).[39] Therefore, in patients who present to a non-PCI center with STEMI in the first hour after onset of symptoms (commonly referred to as the "golden hour"), strong consideration should be given to the

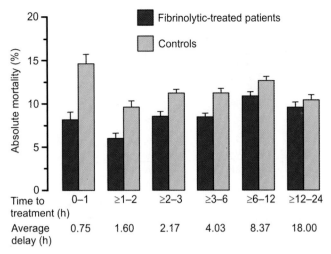

FIGURE 16: Mortality at 35 days among fibrinolytic-treated and control patients, according to treatment delay. (*Source:* Modified from Boersma E, Maas ACP, Deckers JW, et al. Early thrombolytic treatment in acute myocardial infarction: reappraisal of the golden hour. Lancet. 1996;348: 771-5)

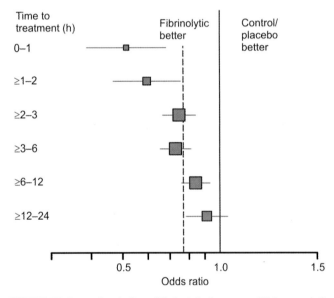

FIGURE 17: Proportional effect of fibrinolytic therapy on 35 days mortality according to treatment delay. (*Source:* Modified from Boersma E, Maas ACP, Deckers JW, et al. Early thrombolytic treatment in acute myocardial infarction: reappraisal of the golden hour. Lancet. 1996;348:771-5)

administration of thrombolytic for maximal myocardial salvage. The older patients had a higher overall mortality with STEMI and also had greatest risk of therapy. Therefore, although there was a trend to greater mortality reduction in the young, the absolute mortality reductions were similar for young and old. For multiple populations, men and women, diabetics and non-diabetics, young and old, anterior versus inferior STEMI, there was an absolute risk reduction with lysis compared to standard medical therapy.[38]

Established contraindications are noted in Table 2.[4] All patients, being considered for the use of thrombolysis for reperfusion in STEMI, should be evaluated for the presence of contraindications and thus the risk or benefit of this therapy should be determined.

TABLE 2

Contraindications and cautions for fibrinolysis in ST-elevation myocardial infarction

Absolute contraindications
- Any prior ICH
- Known structural cerebral vascular lesion (e.g. arteriovenous malformation)
- Known malignant intracranial neoplasm (primary or metastatic)
- Ischemic stroke within 3 months
- Suspected aortic dissection
- Active bleeding or bleeding diathesis (excluding menses)
- Significant closed-head or facial trauma within 3 months

Relative contraindications
- History of chronic, severe, poorly controlled hypertension
- Severe uncontrolled hypertension on presentation (SBP >180 mm Hg or DBP > 110 mm Hg)[†]
- History of prior ischemic stroke greater than 3 months
- History of dementia, or known intracranial pathology not covered in contraindications
- Traumatic or prolonged (> 10 minutes) CPR or major surgery (< 3 weeks)
- Recent (within 2–4 weeks) internal bleeding
- Noncompressible vascular punctures
- For streptokinase: prior exposure (> 5 days ago) or prior allergic reaction to these agents
- Pregnancy
- Active peptic ulcer
- Current use of anticoagulants: the higher the INR, the higher the risk of bleeding

(Abbriviations: ICH: Intracranial Hemorrhage; SBP: Systolic Blood Pressure; DBP: Diastolic Blood Pressure; CPR: Cardiopulmonary Resuscitation; INR: International Normalized Ratio; MI: Myocardial Infarction)
[†]Could be an absolute contraindication in low-risk patients with MI
(*Source:* Modified from ACC/AHA guidelines for the management of patients with ST-elevation myocardial infarction. Circulation. 2004;110: 588-636)

The American College of Cardiology (ACC)/American Heart Association (AHA) guidelines recommend:

Class I

Thrombolysis should be considered in patients with STEMI (or LBBB) without contraindications, who:
- *Present within 12 hours of onset of symptoms and*
- *Are at a non-PCI center when transfer to a PCI center will result in greater than 90 minutes from first medical contact, or have a greater than 60 minutes probable difference between initiation of thrombolytic and angioplasty at a PCI center*

Class II

Thrombolysis (with stipulations as above) when:
- *True posterior infarct is likely*
- *Patient presents in 12–24 hours after onset of symptoms, but with persistent symptoms and ECG consistent with STEMI*

Class III

Avoid thrombolytics:

- *When patient presents in greater than 24 hours after STEMI and has no ischemic symptoms*
- *Patient has only ST depressions on ECG, and no evidence of true posterior infarct.*

Clinically, reperfusion after administration of thrombolytic is demonstrated when the patient has some or all of the following characteristics: resolution of ischemic symptoms, improvement in ST elevation by at least 50% and the presence of a notable reperfusion rhythm (accelerated idioventricular rhythm). Angiographically, reperfusion is noted with reestablishment of TIMI 3 (normal) flow in the IRA. Angiographically, failure of thrombolysis occurs in nearly 40% of patients treated with thrombolytics (i.e. ~ 60% of patients have TIMI 3 flow in the infarct-related artery at 90 minutes).[40] In addition, it is clear that reperfusion (defined as improvement in ST-elevation), leads to improved mortality in the first 30 days.[41] Therefore, if reperfusion does not occur, it is essential that this be recognized by the physician and that continued efforts to attain normal flow in the IRA be instituted.

Rescue PCI is superior to both conservative medical therapy and repeat thrombolysis in patients who fail thrombolysis (with failure defined as reduction of < 50% of the ST elevation at 90 minutes).[42] In contrast to previous trials, stents were used more commonly as part of rescue PCI strategy. Furthermore, decision to perform PCI was not based solely on lack of TIMI3 flow; degree of residual stenosis was also considered consistent with modern clinical practice.[42] Given this data, it is recommended that high-risk patients who present to a non-PCI center, and receive thrombolytic therapy, be considered for transport as soon as possible to the nearest PCI center in order that, if necessary, they may receive rescue PCI with stenting of the IRA, in a timely manner. The high-risk patients are defined as: extensive ST elevation, anterior STEMI, new LBBB, previous MI, Killip class greater than 2, previous EF less than or equal to 35%,[43] or inferior STEMI with systolic blood pressure less than 100 mm Hg, heart rate more than 100 bpm, or greater than 2 mm ST depression, or at least 1 mm ST elevation in right sided lead V4 (indicative of RV involvement).[44]

The American College of Cardiology (ACC)/American Heart Association (AHA) guidelines recommend:

Class I

- *Transfer of high-risk patients, extensive ST elevation, anterior STEMI, new LBBB, previous MI, Killip class greater than 2, previous EF less than or equal to 35%, or inferior STEMI with systolic blood pressure less than 100 mm Hg, heart rate more than 100 bpm, or greater than 2 mm ST depression, or at least 1 mm ST elevation in right sided lead V4 indication RV involvement. From a non-PCI center to the nearest PCI center immediately after thrombolysis*
- *Consideration of transfer, as soon as possible, in patients who have received thrombolysis and are not at high risk to the nearest PCI center after thrombolysis for PCI as needed*

- *Coronary angiography with intent to perform revascularization be performed in patients after treatment with thrombolysis who have:*
  - *Cardiogenic shock and who are reasonable candidates for revascularization (Class I if age ≤ 75, and Class II if age > 75)*
  - *Severe congestive heart failure (CHF) or pulmonary edema*
  - *Hemodynamically significant dysrhythmias*
  - *Hemodynamic or electrical instability*
  - *Persistent ischemic type symptoms*
  - *Failure of lysis and large myocardium at risk, anterior STEMI, or*
  - *Inferior STEMI with evidence of RV involvement*

Class III

- *Avoid planned (in absence of the above clinical parameters) immediate PCI in patients having received full dose thrombolytics*

Elective Angiography and PCI after Successful Thrombolysis

In patients with apparent reperfusion after thrombolysis for STEMI, the consideration of invasive angiography and revascularization is based on the clinical features of the patient. Patients who develop recurrent ischemic symptoms or threatened reocclusion of the vessel have an increased mortality both at 30 days and at 2 years. During hospitalization PCI has been shown to decrease recurrent MI and 2 year mortality.[45] Patients who develop shock, severe CHF, including pulmonary edema, or hemodynamically significant ventricular dysrhythmias during hospitalization should be considered for invasive angiography, and revascularization by PCI or coronary artery bypass grafting as appropriate.

Elective angiography and PCI in patients receiving thrombolysis have been studied with variable results. The TRANSFER AMI trial[44] studied high-risk patients with STEMI, receiving TNK within 2 hours of symptom onset, with transfer to a PCI center for planned elective PCI within 6 hours. Mean time to angiography was 3 hours in the invasive group and 33 hours in the medical therapy group. The primary endpoint of death, reinfarction, CHF, severe recurrent ischemia and shock was significantly less in the invasive group with no significant difference in bleeding. The majority of this benefit was in recurrent ischemia and infarct. The GRACIA-1 trial[46] studied patients who presented with STEMI, received thrombolysis, and were not at high risk, in contrast to the previous trial. They showed that in the invasive group (with angiography at 6–24 hours after lysis) patients had less need for revascularization and hospitalization, but primary endpoints at 30 days were similar. At 1 year the combined event rate of death and nonfatal reinfarction was statistically significant in favor of the invasive approach, but the majority of this was due to reinfarction. In addition, they found no increase in bleeding events and showed a significantly decreased length of stay (LOS) at the time of the initial event. Therefore, elective PCI, after apparent successful thrombolysis, is reasonable in that there is no increase in cardiac events or in bleeding, and it may decrease the index hospitalization LOS and prevent recurrent hospitalizations due to recurrent ischemia or reinfarction.

The issue of late (24 hours to 30 days) elective PCI of a persistently occluded IRA has been addressed.[47] There is no data to suggest a benefit of this approach, in absence of symptoms.

The American College of Cardiology (ACC)/American Heart Association (AHA) guidelines recommend:

Class IIb

- *Elective coronary angiography with the intent to perform PCI in STEMI patients (who have received successful thrombolysis) in the absence of high-risk features noted above*
- *The PCI of a lesion, that is hemodynamically significant, but not 100% occluded, within 24 hours after STEMI*

Class III

- *There is no indication for PCI of an occluded IRA for 24 hours or more after STEMI in a patient without symptoms, hemodynamic or electrical instability, or evidence of severe ischemia.*

PRIMARY CORONARY INTERVENTION

Reperfusion (vessel patency) can be accomplished at higher rates with primary coronary intervention than with thrombolysis in patients presenting with STEMI. Studies have shown that the majority of patients are candidates for this reperfusion strategy, and it is superior to full dose thrombolysis with statistically significant decrease in rates of death, nonfatal MI and stroke.[48,49] In addition to improved rates of reperfusion, this strategy also offers the ability to risk stratify patients by evaluation of the remainder of the coronary anatomy, thus allowing for optimal treatment post MI and allows for evaluation of hemodynamics and cardiac filling pressures as needed. Finally patients who have cardiogenic shock have the greatest benefit from primary coronary intervention versus thrombolysis.[50]

Today coronary intervention is done with the great majority of patients receiving coronary stents, not just angioplasty alone. Available data shows that primary coronary stenting is superior to primary coronary angioplasty in patients with STEMI with decreased major adverse cardiac events at 30 and 180 days.[51,52] The greatest benefit was in recurrent ischemia and need for revascularization. The previously discussed meta-analysis showing benefit from PCI compared to thrombolysis also demonstrated that the benefit of PCI with stents versus thrombolysis (compared to primary coronary angioplasty) was maintained (Fig. 18).[49]

It should be noted that this data is valid only in centers with experienced interventionalists and laboratories with protocols maintaining D2B times as short as possible (and always less than 90 minutes). Patients who present to a PCI center with STEMI, in absence of contraindications should undergo emergency angiography with intent to perform PCI, unless there are extenuating circumstances that will not allow for the patient to have a D2B time of less than 90 minutes. In patients who present to a non-PCI center, the choice of thrombolysis versus transfer of patients for PCI becomes more complex. Studies have been performed to assess the impact of transfer on outcomes.

These studies suggest that transfer of patients for PCI with arrival at the PCI center within 90–120 minutes of arrival at the transferring center has statistical benefit in the primary endpoint of death, reinfarction and stroke.[53-55] The greatest benefit of timely transfer for primary PCI over thrombolytics was in achieving lower rates of reinfarction.[53] At the same time, ensuring timely reperfusion in patients undergoing transfer to a PCI center requires substantial investment in developing sophisticated systems of care and treatment protocols which may not be feasible for all hospitals and communities.[53]

The American College of Cardiology (ACC)/American Heart Association (AHA) guidelines recommend:

Class I

- *The STEMI patients undergo PCI (when presenting to a capable PCI-center) within 90 minutes from first medical contact*
- *The STEMI patients presenting to a PCI center without the capability for expert, prompt intervention with primary PCI within 90 minutes of first medical contact should receive thrombolytic therapy unless contraindicated*
- *The STEMI patients presenting to a center without PCI capability and who cannot be transferred to a PCI center and undergo PCI within 90 minutes of first medical contact should receive thrombolytic therapy within 30 minutes of hospital presentation unless contraindicated.*

EARLY MEDICAL THERAPY

GENERAL MEASURES

As reperfusion therapy is being arranged, medical therapy must be initiated; this medical therapy mirrors that has been discussed for UA/NSTEMI in the chapter "Acute Coronary Syndrome I: Unstable Angina and Non-ST Segment Elevation Myocardial Infarction". Oxygen should be administered. Patients should be placed on continuous telemetry and all transport must be monitored with a defibrillator and emergency medications immediately available. As soon as STEMI is diagnosed, in a PCI center, preparation must be made for emergency transport into the cardiac catheterization laboratory.

The American College of Cardiology (ACC)/American Heart Association (AHA) guidelines recommend:

Class I

- *Supplemental oxygen should be given to patients with desaturation below 90%*

Class II

- *It is reasonable to consider supplemental oxygen to all STEMI patients for first 6 hours.*

NITRATES

In order to decrease the vasoconstriction which is associated with STEMI, nitroglycerin (SL and IV as necessary) should be given. Care should be taken in the STEMI patient as abrupt changes in hemodynamics may occur. In addition, the reader

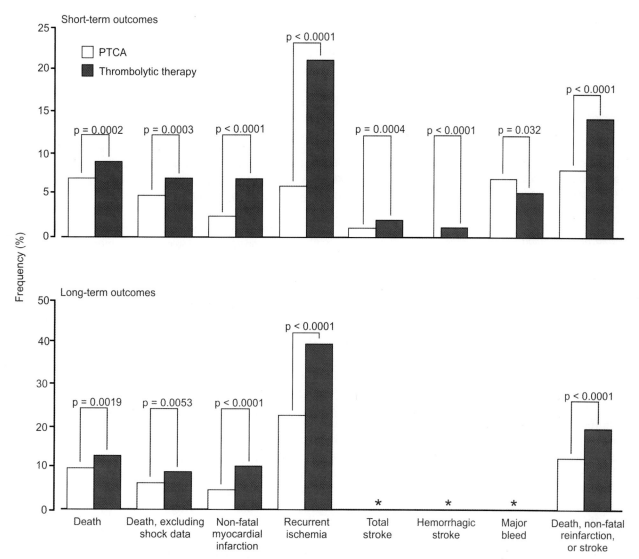

FIGURE 18: Percutaneous coronary intervention (PCI) versus fibrinolysis for ST-elevation myocardial infarction (STEMI). The short-term (4–6 weeks) and long-term outcomes for the various endpoints shown are plotted for patients with STEMI randomized to PCI or fibrinolysis for reperfusion in 23 trials (N = 7739) (*Source:* Modified from Keeley EC, Boura JA, Grines CL. Primary angioplasty versus intravenous thrombolytic therapy for acute myocardial infarction: a quantitative review of 23 randomized trials. Lancet. 2003;361:13-20)

should be well aware of the potential hypotension and hemodynamic collapse that may occur in a patient with a RV infarction who receives nitroglycerin and avoid the use of nitrates in these patients.

The American College of Cardiology (ACC)/American Heart Association (AHA) guidelines recommend:

Class I

- *Nitroglycerin 0.4 mg sl every 5 minutes for 3 doses and then consider IV nitroglycerin for ongoing ischemic symptoms, hypertension or for management of pulmonary congestion*

Class III

- *Nitrates should be avoided in patients with:*
  - *Systolic blood pressure less than 90 mm Hg or more than 30 mm Hg below baseline*

- *Severe bradycardia (< 50 bpm)*
- *Tachycardia (> 100 bpm)*
- *Suspected RV infarction*
- *Use of type 5 phosphodiesterase inhibitors in last 24–48 hours*

Note: The guideline notes that these are used in men for erectile dysfunction, but the reader should be aware of the increasing use of sildenafil for patients with pulmonary hypertension.

MORPHINE

Morphine can serve as analgesia and thereby decreases the generalized anxiety and apprehension that is common in STEMI patients. One must be aware of the potential for hypotension associated with morphine dosing, and be aware of potential treatment of this with placing the patient supine and potentially raising the lower extremities to improve venous return and administering a fluid bolus (neither to be performed in the patient with pulmonary edema). Morphine will also have a positive effect on patients presenting with STEMI and pulmonary edema to decrease venous return and improve respiratory status.

The uses of nonsteroidal anti-inflammatory agents for analgesia are to be avoided.

> The American College of Cardiology (ACC)/American Heart Association (AHA) guidelines recommend:
>
> **Class I**
> - *Administration of morphine sulfate 2–4 mg IV with repeated dosing of 2–8 mg every 5–15 minutes as needed*
> - *Discontinue all nonaspirin NSAID agents*
>
> **Class III**
> - *Avoid all nonaspirin NSAID agents.*

ANTIPLATELET AGENTS

If not already given, the patient must receive aspirin therapy at a dose of 162–325 mg, chewed. The importance of aspirin cannot be underestimated, and therefore, if the physician is not certain that aspirin has been taken by the patient at home, or was given in the ambulance, it should be given without delay.

Thienopyridines are effective in decreasing MACE in patients presenting with STEMI as is seen in patients with UA/NSTEMI. The COMMIT-CCS trial showed that a combination of aspirin 162 mg daily and clopidogrel 75 mg daily was superior to aspirin alone in prevention of death, re-infarction and stroke in patients with acute MI (majority of the treated patients had STEMI). This benefit was seen regardless of reperfusion strategy (thrombolysis or primary PCI). Notably the risks of major bleeding and cerebral bleeding were not statistically different between the two groups.[56] The CLARITY-TIMI 28 trial randomized patients with STEMI who underwent reperfusion with thrombolytics to clopidogrel (loading dose 300 mg followed by 75 mg daily) or placebo. All patients received aspirin. The trial showed a significant reduction in the primary endpoint of death, recurrent MI and occluded artery on angiogram, without a significant increase in bleeding. Additionally, there was a reduction in the need for urgent revascularization.[57] Based on these studies, it is recommended to administer clopidogrel at arrival to all STEMI patients who are 75 years old or younger.

A discussion of clopidogrel resistance can be found in the Chapter 48 "Acute Coronary Syndrome I: Unstable Angina and Non-ST Segment Elevation Myocardial Infarction". Also included in that chapter was a discussion of reluctance of some physicians to administer clopidogrel to MI patients until coronary anatomy is defined. Although clopidogrel does increase the risk of bleeding should a patient need to undergo CABG emergently, that scenario is becoming increasingly rare given the advances in modern interventional techniques and the rapidity with which reperfusion can be achieved with PCI compared to CABG. Therefore, we recommend pre-treatment of all STEMI patients with clopidogrel if no contraindications exist.

The TRITON-TIMI 38 trial[58] studied patients with ACS randomized to prasugrel (60 mg load, then 10 mg daily) or clopidogrel (300 mg load, then 75 mg daily). All patients received standard medical therapy. Reperfusion strategies in the subgroup of STEMI patients included primary PCI or thrombolysis followed by later secondary elective PCI 12 hours to 14 days later). In the STEMI subgroup who received prasugrel, there was a significant reduction in the primary event of cardiovascular death, nonfatal MI and nonfatal stroke, and in the secondary endpoint of cardiovascular death, MI and need for urgent target vessel revascularization at 30 days with persistence to 15 months. The rate of stent thrombosis was decreased with prasugrel. Prasugrel is therefore quite attractive for use in STEMI patients as it has faster onset of action, and in the STEMI subgroup there was no increase in bleeding compared to clopidogrel.

> The American College of Cardiology (ACC)/American Heart Association (AHA) guidelines recommend:
>
> **Class I**
> - *Clopidogrel loading dose of 300–600 mg as early as possible, before or at PCI*
> - *Prasugrel 60 mg as soon as possible for primary PCI*
> - *Discontinuation of clopidogrel for 5 days and prasugrel for 7 days prior to elective CABG*
>
> **Class III**
> - *Avoidance of prasugrel in STEMI patients undergoing primary PCI who have a history of a stroke or transient ischemic attack (TIA).*

Unlike in the UA/NSTEMI patient, the benefit of upstream glycoprotein IIb/IIIA inhibitors has not definitively been demonstrated. These may be useful as adjunctive therapy during primary PCI for STEMI, although the most recent studies in which patients received dual oral antiplatelet therapy are small and fail to show a significant benefit. One study, HORIZONS AMI suggested a potentially increased incidence of net clinical events (particularly a higher risk of bleeding) when glycoprotein IIb/IIIa receptor blockers with heparin or bivalirudin was compared to bivalirudin alone.[59]

> The American College of Cardiology (ACC)/American Heart Association (AHA) guidelines recommend:
>
> **Class II**
> - *Administration of glycoprotein IIb/IIIa receptor blockers (abciximab or eptifibatide) at the time of primary PCI in selected patients with STEMI*
> - *Administration of glycoprotein IIb/IIIa receptor blockers as a part of preparatory medication regimen in STEMI patients being taken to the cardiac cath lab is of uncertain benefit.*

ANTICOAGULATION

Anticoagulation therapy should be administered in all STEMI patients who are without absolute contraindication. The choice of anticoagulant may be, in part, based on the reperfusion strategy, but in all cases full systemic anticoagulation with either unfractionated heparin or low molecular weight heparin or bivalirudin is beneficial.[59] Anticoagulation should continue for

48 hours in patients treated with thrombolysis. In patients who undergo primary PCI, anticoagulation may be discontinued after the procedure, unless there is another indication (i.e. intra-aortic balloon pump, LV thrombus, mechanical valve, etc.). Data for bivalirudin suggests that it be used predominantly in the catheterization laboratory during PCI.

The American College of Cardiology (ACC)/American Heart Association (AHA) guidelines recommend:

Class I

- All STEMI patients receive, in addition to aspirin and a thienopyridine:
  — Unfractionated heparin upstream and during primary PCI or
  — Bivalirudin during primary PCI either alone, or after the use of heparin prior to arriving in the catheterization lab

Class II

- Bivalirudin for patients undergoing primary PCI for STEMI who have a high risk of bleeding.

BETA BLOCKERS

Beta blockers should be given orally, with reservation of IV beta blockade for hypertensive or tachycardic patients with ongoing chest pain. Based on the COMMIT study, IV beta blockade should be avoided in patients at high risk for cardiogenic shock, those with systolic blood pressures below 105 mm Hg, and those who are more than 75 years old, due to a higher risk of hypotension and increased mortality.[5,60] In the case of a patient with suspected cocaine- or methamphetamine-associated STEMI, one should not use beta blockers as there is a physiologic concern about unopposed alpha constriction and worsening of the clinical scenario.

The American College of Cardiology (ACC)/American Heart Association (AHA) guidelines recommend:

Class I

- Oral beta blockers be administered within the first 24 hours after STEMI in patients without:
  — Congestive heart failure
  — Evidence of poor cardiac index
  — Increased risk for cardiogenic shock, defined as an increased number of these risk factors: age more than 70 years old, systolic pressure less than 120 mm Hg, heart rate more than 100 or less than 60 bpm or prolonged ischemic time.
  — Heart block (PR > 240 ms or second or third degree AV block)
  — Active asthma or known significant reactive airway disease
  — If not given in the first 24 hours, that oral beta blockers be considered for secondary prevention
  — Patients with moderate or severe LV dysfunction receive beta blockers as secondary prevention

---

Class II

- Intravenous (IV) beta blockers in hypertensive patients with no contraindications above

Class III

- Avoid IV beta blockers in patients with:
- Acute congestive heart failure
- Evidence of poor cardiac index
- Increased risk for cardiogenic shock, age more than 70 years old, systolic pressure less than 120 mm Hg, heart rate more than 100 or less than 60 bpm or prolonged ischemic time
- Heart block (PR > 240 ms or second or third degree AV block)
- Active asthma or known significant reactive airway disease.

POST MYOCARDIAL INFARCTION CARE

ASSESSMENT OF LEFT VENTRICULAR EJECTION FRACTION

All patients following an MI must have assessment of LV ejection fraction (LVEF). This not only guides medical therapy but also provides prognostic information. It has long been known that decreased LVEF post MI and increased end systolic volume are markers for increased risk of development of CHF and death.[61-63] Abnormal LVEF (< 40%) portends an overall poor prognosis in the post MI patient (Fig. 19).[62] In addition, when comparing multiple variables and prognosis, decreased EF is the single most significant predictor of mortality. The presence of multivessel disease and the development of clinical heart failure, as well, did increase the likelihood of mortality, although to a lesser degree (Fig. 20).[63]

The choice of imaging modalities available today to assess EF, include: left ventriculography, transthoracic echocardiography, radionuclide imaging, CT and magnetic resonance imaging (MRI). Each modality offers additional information that may be helpful to the clinician and each is limited by patient-specific factors. Left ventriculography done at the time of coronary angiography offers the additional measurement of LV end diastolic pressure, assessment of mitral regurgitation and assessment for ventricular septal defect, location and relative size. It is limited by the need for radiation, iodinated contrast (important considerations in the presence of decompensated heart failure and/or with renal insufficiency) and inability to visualize wall motion in all territories (unless biplane capabilities are available or a second contrast injection is performed).

Echocardiography offers the ability to not only assess the LVEF but also to assess for wall motion abnormalities in all territories, detects LV thrombus, ventricular septal defect, noninvasive estimate of pulmonary artery pressures, RV systolic function, pericardial effusion and importantly to assess for preexisting or post MI valvular abnormalities. Echocardiographic imaging is limited at times by the patient's body habitus (obesity, large breasts, etc.), and in patients with significant obstructive lung disease. In addition, the assessment of EF is to some extent subjective.

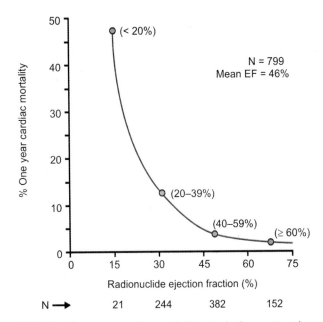

FIGURE 19: One year cardiac mortality rate in four categories of radionuclide ejection fraction (EF) determined before discharge. (*Source:* Modified from The Multicenter Postinfarction Research Group. Risk stratification and survival after myocardial infarction. N Engl J Med. 1983;309(6):331-6)

Radionuclide ventriculography offers a more objective LVEF and right ventricular ejection fraction (RVEF) assessment and can assess wall motion in all territories. It does not provide additional data, and is limited by the radiation exposure to the patient.

Cardiac MRI, done in facilities with expertise, offers the ability to assess wall motion, LVEF and RVEF (and is now the gold standard for EF assessment). Precise evaluation of VSD and other structural abnormalities (including assessment of aortic disease, pericardial disease, LV mass and LV thrombus) can be performed with cardiac MRI. Of great value, is the potential to assess the infarct zone (versus peri-infarct), the amount of scar (versus viability) and presence of inflammation and infiltration. However, MRI is the optimal

test for these assessments. The MRI test is limited in patients with metal implants, patients who have significant claustrophobia (in whom sedation is a poor option or in patients who will require high levels of sedation to overcome the claustrophobic symptoms, thus inhibiting the necessary breath hold for the test) and in patients who have renal insufficiency who require IV gadolinium for assessment of LV structure (viability, infiltration, inflammation, etc.). Therefore, the physician must choose the optimal study for each patient with the goal to first assess EF and then to assess other clinical parameters as deemed most necessary.

The American College of Cardiology (ACC)/American Heart Association (AHA) guidelines recommend:

Class I

- *The LVEF assessment in all STEMI/NSTEMI patients*
- *A noninvasive assessment of EF in patients who are not scheduled to undergo left ventriculography*

STRESS TESTING PRIOR TO DISCHARGE

Stress testing should be considered to assess areas of at-risk myocardium in the patient who has received successful thrombolysis, who presented late with presumed completed infarct and did not receive reperfusion therapy, who presented with ACS non-STEMI who has been chosen for a conservative medical therapy approach and in the patient who has an indeterminate lesion noted on coronary angiography during the index hospitalization. The choice of stress testing includes exercise treadmill testing with or without imaging (echocardiography or nuclear perfusion) or chemical stress testing with dobutamine or dipyridamole/adenosine/regadenosine (depending on the institutional practice) with echocardiography or nuclear perfusion. In depth descriptions of these tests can be found in the chapter on Stress Testing and will not be reviewed here. It should be noted, although, that if a patient has an interpretable ECG and are able to undergo exercise testing, this

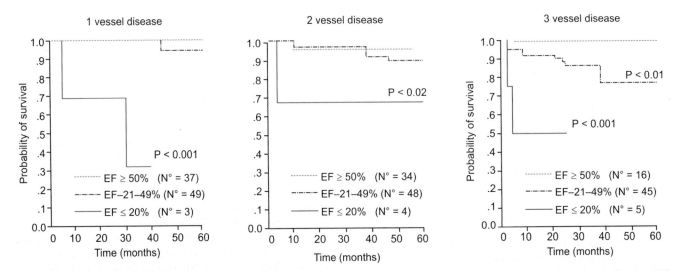

FIGURE 20: Kaplan-Meier survival curves of patients with 1-vessel, 2-vessel and 3-vessel disease, stratified according to ejection fraction (EF). Caution should be taken with interpretation of the class of patients with EF less than 20% due to the very small numbers in these groups. (*Source:* Modified from Sanz G, Castañer A, Betriu A, et al. Determinants of prognosis in survivors of myocardial infarction: a prospective clinical angiographic study. N Engl J Med. 1982;306(18):1065-70)

should be preferred to chemical stress as it provides information regarding heart rate and blood pressure response, and peak exercise workload that is important for the treating physician.

The American College of Cardiology (ACC)/American Heart Association (AHA) guidelines recommend:

Class I

- *Exercise testing in:*
  - *Low-risk patients with ACS (this does not include patients with ECG changes or positive biomarkers)*
  - *Intermediate risk patients with ACS (this may include patients with an abnormal resting ECG or a slight increase in troponins) who have been without ischemia (at rest or with low-level activity) or heart failure within the preceding 12–24 hours*
  - *The STEMI patients in hospital or early post discharge who have not during the index hospitalization and have no plan to proceed directly to coronary angiography and intervention, and are without high-risk features*

Class III

- *Avoid stress testing in STEMI patients who have not undergone reperfusion within 2–3 days of STEMI*
- *Post MI patients who have unstable post-infarction angina, decompensated heart failure, ventricular dysrhythmias, or other absolute contraindications to stress testing*
- *Patients who have planned coronary angiography pending*

CORONARY ANGIOGRAPHY AND REVASCULARIZATION

In patients who present with ACS, the decision for emergent and early angiography and intervention has been discussed in this chapter as well as in Chapter 48 "Acute Coronary Syndrome I: Unstable Angina and Non-ST Segment Elevation Myocardial Infarction". In patients who have not undergone early angiography, the need for angiography and possible intervention prior to discharge must be addressed. The potential contraindications should be evaluated and considered, including the patient's willingness to consent to both coronary angiography and potential revascularization. If no absolute or limiting relative contraindications exist, the following patients should be considered appropriate. In patients who present without STEMI, if any high-risk feature is identified on presentation, including accelerated or rest anginal symptoms, evidence of heart failure or hemodynamic instability, dynamic ECG changes or positive biomarkers for MI, one should strongly consider coronary angiography. In patients who have recurrent ischemic symptoms in hospital, particularly those who have angina at rest or are refractory to medical therapy, or those with post-infarction angina, coronary angiography is indicated. Patients with a decrease in EF or those with evidence of heart failure during hospitalization should undergo angiography. In addition, in patients who have undergone stress testing, a positive test with a significant amount of at-risk myocardium should prompt angiography. In addition, the previously reviewed indications for STEMI patients post lysis.

The American College of Cardiology (ACC)/American Heart Association (AHA) guidelines recommend:

Class I

- *Prompt angiography in patients with ACS (NSTEMI) who have failed intensive medical treatment*
- *Coronary angiography in STEMI patients with:*
  - *Recurrent myocardial ischemia*
  - *Intermediate or high-risk features on stress testing*
  - *Before surgical treatment of a mechanical complication of MI (acute MR, VSD or LV aneurysm repair) in a hemodynamically stable patient*
  - *Hemodynamic instability*
  - *Heart failure during hospitalization, but with normal EF*
- *PCI in patients with any high-risk features (recurrent angina, elevated cardiac biomarkers for infarction, new ST depressions, symptoms of heart failure, high-risk findings on stress testing, hemodynamic instability, ventricular dysrhythmias, PCI within preceding 6 months, prior CABG, high-risk score on presentation, or decreased LVEF) if lesion amenable and no contraindication*
- *PCI (or CABG) as indicated based on lesion morphology and patient characteristics as per the guidelines for PCI or CABG*

Class II

- *Early angiography (within 12–24 hours from admission) in initially stabilized high-risk patient with UA/NSTEMI*
- *Coronary angiography in STEMI patients with:*
  - *Patients who have STEMI suspected to not be secondary to CAD (i.e. emboli, spasm, etc.)*
  - *Diabetes, decreased EF (or ≤ 40%, heart failure, history of PCI or CABG, or ventricular dysrhythmia)*
  - *As a routine strategy post-successful thrombolysis*
- *PCI of left main stenosis greater than 50% in patients who are not eligible for CABG (or who require PCI emergently due to hemodynamic compromise)*
- *PCI in a patient with a hemodynamically significant lesion greater than 24 hours after STEMI as a part of an invasive approach (in a patient who has had successful lysis)*
  - *Chapter 48 stent or drug*

Class III

- *Coronary angiography in patients who are not candidates for revascularization*
- *Non-LAD lesion PCI or CABG in patients with no current symptoms (or symptoms that are unlikely to be secondary to ischemia) and no inducible ischemia on stress testing*
- *PCI in patients with no high-risk features, no trial of medical therapy and:*
  - *A small at-risk territory on stress testing*
  - *Likelihood of successful PCI is low in the lesion to be treated*
  - *Procedural morbidity or mortality is excessively high*
  - *No lesions greater than 50% stenosed (with exception on LM stenosis who are not eligible for CABG)*
  - *Stable post-NSTEMI patients with a persistently occluded infarct related vessel*

CHAPTER 49 · Acute Coronary Syndrome II

Patients who require revascularization, should undergo this without avoidable delay (although there is a lack of data to suggest urgent coronary angiography in stable ACS, non-STEMI patients).[64] The exception to this is in the patient who requires nonurgent CABG who has been given clopidogrel or prasugrel (see section on thienopyridines), who has acutely reversible renal failure,[65] and who has had STEMI in which consideration of 3–7 days delay to CABG is recommended.[66] There is an increase in hospital mortality early after MI in patients undergoing CABG with mortality rates of 11.8% if within 6 hours, 9.5% between 6 hours and 1 day and 2.8% after 1 day. Patients with a transmural MI had a higher mortality up to 7 days post MI. Therefore, nonurgent CABG should be delayed for 5–7 days after clopidogrel or prasugrel respectively, until renal function improves and for up to 7 days in STEMI patients.

The physician should recognize that although the bleeding risk in patients on clopidogrel and prasugrel is increased, there is no data to suggest that aspirin should be held at the time of CABG. As a matter of fact administration of aspirin in the patient's undergoing CABG is a Class I indication. Therefore, aspirin should be continued without interruption in all patients undergoing CABG.

The American College of Cardiology (ACC)/American Heart Association (AHA) guidelines recommend:

Class I

- *Aspirin should not be withheld prior to CABG*
- *Elective CABG should be delayed for 5 days in patients on clopidogrel and 7 days in patients on prasugrel*
- *In STEMI patients, CABG mortality is increased in the first 3–7 days after infarct*
- *The Risk/Benefit ratio must be assessed (presence or lack of symptoms, hemodynamic stability, presences of dysrhythmias and extent of MI and likelihood of recovery in short-term with medical therapy):*
  - *Stable patients with normal EF may undergo CABG within several days of infarct*
  - *If critical anatomy does not exist consideration of CABG may be done after the index hospitalization*

COMPLICATIONS

RIGHT VENTRICULAR INFARCTION

The involvement of the right ventricle in patients presenting with inferior wall STEMI portends a poor prognosis.[25] Data suggests that in hospital mortality is increased from 5% (without RV infarct) to 31% (with RV infarct). In addition, the major complications of cardiogenic shock, high-grade AV block (both transient and requiring permanent pacemaker placement) and ventricular dysrhythmias, increased from 28% to 64% respectively.[25] The identification of RV infarction is critical in the care of the patient with an inferior wall MI and therefore the presenting ECG should be scrutinized for the criteria noted previously. In addition, the use of a right-sided ECG is strongly encouraged. These patients are not only at higher risk but also are much more sensitive to optimal cardiac preload. Therefore, optimizing volume status and consideration of IV fluid challenge should be performed. One should avoid the use of nitroglycerin

in patients with suspected or diagnosed RV infarction. These patients not uncommonly will require inotropic support (dobutamine or epinephrine infusion preferred) and therefore one should be very cautious with beta blockers in these patients as administration may precipitate hemodynamic collapse.

The American College of Cardiology (ACC)/American Heart Association (AHA) guidelines recommend:

Class I

- *Right sided ECG in patients presenting with inferior STEMI and hemodynamic compromise*
- *Patient with STEMI and RV infarction/ischemia have therapy with:*
  - *Early reperfusion*
  - *Correction of bradycardia and AV block*
  - *Optimal RV preloading conditions, consider IV fluid challenge*
  - *Optimal RV afterload (i.e. treatment of LV dysfunction)*
  - *Inotropic support as necessary*

Class II

- *Up to 4 weeks delay to CABG in patient with RV dysfunction*

HEART FAILURE OR CARDIOGENIC SHOCK AND MECHANICAL COMPLICATIONS AFTER A MYOCARDIAL INFARCTION

The incidence of heart failure and frank shock is increased in patients presenting with STEMI, but is certainly a complication of NSTEMI as well. Patients with MI complicated by heart failure have a high mortality, approaching 50% in some studies. Patients with heart failure should have aggressive treatment of ischemia or infarct. As already described, patients with cardiogenic shock achieve greater benefit with primary PCI compared to thrombolysis.[50] As noted in the previous section, RV infarct or failure can be the etiology of heart failure and shock, and should be considered in all patients with shock and inferior wall MI. Assessment of LVEF early in treatment is necessary to determine if the clinical heart failure is secondary to systolic or diastolic dysfunction and to guide both medical and revascularization therapy.

In addition to severe LV or RV dysfunction as etiology of heart failure or shock, the physician should be aware of the mechanical complications of MI and the expected timing of these. Although these are thoroughly covered elsewhere in this text and the reader is encouraged to read this chapter; briefly the three major complications resulting in hemodynamic compromise and collapse include acute papillary muscle rupture resulting in acute mitral regurgitation, acute ventricular septal rupture and LV free wall rupture. These complications require emergent evaluation and treatment, with surgery being the mainstay of treatment in all patients. In preparation for surgical intervention, patients with acute mitral regurgitation or ventricular septal defect may benefit from intra-aortic balloon pump (IABP) support. The patient with ventricular free wall rupture has an extremely high mortality, but may benefit from emergent pericardiocentesis to decrease the hemodynamic impact of the elevated pericardial pressures, as the operating team or room is being mobilized.

Supplemental oxygen, morphine, nitrates and diuresis may improve symptomatic pulmonary edema. Beta blockers should be avoided early in acute heart failure complicating MI. The use of a pulmonary artery catheter may help to guide medical therapy. An IABP may be necessary in patients with refractory heart failure or shock. More aggressive support may be required with LV assist devices, including Impella, TandemHeart and implantable left ventricular assist device (LVAD). Ultimately the patient who has refractory heart failure may need consideration of heart transplantation.

The American College of Cardiology (ACC)/American Heart Association (AHA) guidelines recommend:

Class I

- *For post MI heart failure:*
  - *Oxygen supplementation if oxygen saturation is less than 90%*
  - *Morphine sulfate for patients with pulmonary congestion*
  - *Nitrates for patients with pulmonary congestion unless systolic blood pressure is 30 mm Hg below baseline or less than 100 mm Hg*
  - *Diuretic for patients with pulmonary congestion and volume overload*
  - *Beta blockers should be considered at low dose with gradual titration upwards prior to discharge*
  - *Aldosterone blockers should be considered in patients without contraindication*
  - *Transthoracic echocardiogram should be performed urgently to assess LV and RV systolic function and exclude mechanical complications of MI*
- *Intra-aortic balloon counterpulsation if:*
  - *Cardiogenic shock is not readily reversed with medical therapy or revascularization*
  - *Patient has low cardiac output state*
  - *Recurrent ischemia refractory to medical therapy and hemodynamic instability, poor LVEF, or a large at-risk territory of myocardium. Consideration should be given to urgent revascularization in these patients*
- *Early revascularization for STEMI patients in the age of less than 75 years old who:*
  - *Develop shock within 36 hours of STEMI*
  - *Are suitable for revascularization that can be accomplished within 18 hours and*
  - *Do not have contraindication or reason not to pursue revascularization (i.e. Patient wishes, futility, etc.)*

Class II

- *Pulmonary artery catheter placement:*
  - *To guide therapy of STEMI patients with cardiogenic shock*
  - *In STEMI patients with hypotension unresponsive to IV fluid challenge*
  - *When mechanical complication of MI are suspected*
- *Early revascularization for STEMI patients in the age of 75 years old or more who:*
  - *Develop shock within 36 hours of STEMI*

- *Are suitable for revascularization that can be accomplished within 18 hours and*
- *Do not have contraindication or reason not to pursue revascularization (i.e. Patient wishes, futility, etc.)*

DYSRHYTHMIAS

In the early phase of STEMI (first 24–48 hours), ventricular dysrhythmias can occur related to the ischemic event. The patient should be supported during this time with the main goal being reperfusion, normalization of electrolytes and treatment of any heart failure. Cardioversion should be performed if the patient has ventricular fibrillation (VF), sustained and hemodynamically significant ventricular tachycardia (VT), or VT associated with angina or pulmonary edema. Recurrence may require antiarrhythmic therapy with IV amiodarone or IABP placement. The reader should recognize the benefit of IABP for the treatment of refractory ventricular dysrhythmias. Treatment of premature ventricular complexes or nonsustained ventricular tachycardia (NSVT) is not recommended unless there is impact on hemodynamics. In the absence of significant heart failure, up titration of beta blockers may improve ventricular ectopy.

Sustained ventricular dysrhythmias that occur after 48 hours (without recurrent ischemia/infarct, decompensated CHF or other precipitant), in general, require long-term therapy including but not necessarily limited to internal cardioverter/defibrillator placement (ICD). These patients may require antiarrhythmic medication to prevent repetitive ICD discharges.

The American College of Cardiology (ACC)/American Heart Association (AHA) guidelines recommend:

Class I

- *Cardioversion for VF, polymorphic VT or monomorphic VT without pulse, or associated with angina, pulmonary edema or hypotension and*
- *Amiodarone 150 mg bolus over 10 minutes with repeat as needed and consideration of full loading dose of 1 mg/minute over 6 hours and then 0.5 mg/minute over 18 hours, not to exceed 2.2 g in 24 hours for patients with monomorphic VT associated with angina, pulmonary edema or hypotension*
- *ICD may be considered in patients with VF or hemodynamically significant VT greater than 48 hours after STEMI provided that this is not felt to be secondary to recurrent ischemia or reinfarction*

Class II

- *Amiodarone 300 mg IV bolus over 10 minutes be considered when VF or pulseless VT is refractory to cardioversion, in preparation for repeat cardioversion*
- *Correction of electrolyte abnormalities (goal potassium > 4.0 mEq/L and magnesium > 2.0 mg/dL) to prevent further VT/VF*
- *ICD placement in patient with LVEF of 30% or less and with STEMI greater than 1 month prior and last revascularization greater than 90 days prior*

Class III

- *Avoidance of routine prophylactic antiarrhythmic medications for:*
  - *— All STEMI patients undergoing thrombolysis*
  - *— Suppression of ectopy or NSVT*
  - *— Accelerated idioventricular rhythms*
- *Avoid of ICD in patients with early VT/VF (< 48 hours), or who have an LVEF greater than 40% at 1 month post MI.*

As previously mentioned, particularly with patients with inferior MI (with or without RV infarction), bradycardia and heart block may complicate the MI and require permanent pacemaker placement. Transient bradycardia or heart block should be treated supportively, and may require short-term temporary transvenous pacemaker placement if hemodynamically significant.

The American College of Cardiology (ACC)/American Heart Association (AHA) guidelines recommend:

Class I

- *Temporary pacemaker placement for medically refractory symptomatic sinus bradycardia, sinus bradycardia with heart rate less than 40 bpm associated with hypotension or sinus pause of greater than 3 seconds*
- *Consideration of permanent pacemaker placement for sinus node dysfunction should follow ACC/AHA guidelines for pacemaker placement*
- *Permanent pacemaker placement for:*
  - *— Second degree AV block (below the His-Purkinje system) with bilateral bundle branch block*
  - *— Third degree block within or below the His-Purkinje system*
- *All patients requiring permanent pacemaker placement post MI should be assessed for indications for ICD implantation*

Class II

- *Permanent pacemaker placement for persistent second or third degree AV block at the level of the AV node*

Class III

- *Avoid permanent pacemaker placement for:*
  - *— First degree AV block in the presence of bundle branch block*
  - *— Transient AV block*
  - *— New left anterior fascicular block.*

Other dysrhythmias may occur during the index hospitalization for STEMI, including atrial fibrillation, atrial flutter or SVT. These should be treated appropriately with consideration of cardioversion early given the more tenuous status of these patients. In patients with heart failure and atrial fibrillation or flutter, consideration should be given to the use of digoxin for ventricular rate control.

RECURRENT CHEST DISCOMFORT

The reader should be aware of potential etiologies of recurrent chest discomfort post MI. Recurrent ischemia or infarction must always be a consideration. The ECG evaluation during symptoms and monitoring of cardiac biomarkers of necrosis should be used for diagnosis of recurrent ischemia or reinfarction. Unfortunately each of these presents a difficulty. Not uncommonly patients have a persistently abnormal ECG, or an ECG consistent with evolution of infarct, limiting the ability to confidently assess for acute or dynamic changes. In addition, the longer half-life of troponin prevents accurate determination of reinfarction in the first 10–14 days after MI; therefore, creatine kinase (CK and CK MB) which rises and falls more rapidly may be needed. Stress testing may be appropriate, if not previously performed and repetition of coronary angiography may be necessary to assess patency of stented vessels.

Post MI pericarditis may occur early after MI (within the first 4 days) or late, generally after discharge (Dressler's syndrome). It is diagnosed by characteristic pain, a pericardial rub on auscultation, ECG changes (which may be obscured in the early post MI period), presence of a small effusion on echocardiography and improvement with anti-inflammatory agents. Early pericarditis is associated with late index presentation, longer ischemic times prior to reperfusion, larger infarct and failed PCI.[67] Despite the fact that this association exists, the presence of early pericarditis alone does not seem to have any implications on short- or long-term prognosis.[67] Late pericarditis or Dressler's syndrome is very uncommon today given the improved success with reperfusion therapies.

Pericarditis may be treated with higher dose of aspirin or indomethacin. Colchicine is another option, as is the use of steroids, although steroids are not preferred in the early post MI period due to potential inhibition of the normal scarring that occurs in the infarcted zone. This decrease in appropriate scar formation at the site of the infarct can potentially increase the risk of myocardial rupture.

As patients are hospitalized for ACS, and thus are immobile, they are at increased risk for deep venous thrombosis (DVT) and pulmonary embolism. Patients with a prolonged hospital course (particularly those with CHF), patients with heparin-induced thrombocytopenia and thrombosis, or other hypercoagulable states should be anticoagulated to prevent DVT. Pulmonary embolism should be considered in all patients with pleuritic-type chest discomfort, shortness of breath that is unexplained, or sudden hemodynamic change not associated with a cardiovascular change. Treatment should proceed with full anticoagulation if not contraindicated.

SPECIAL CONSIDERATIONS

DIABETES

The diabetic population is unique with respect to ACS and have been shown to have worse short-term and long-term outcomes after an MI compared to non-diabetics. It is also known that they require more aggressive efforts at primary and secondary prevention. In addition, hyperglycemia during hospitalization has been associated with worse outcomes. Although the 2004 guidelines recommended aggressive glucose control with IV insulin to normalize blood glucose as a Class I indication, that recommendation has been downgraded to a Class II indication based on a recent study showing higher mortality in aggressively treated patients.[5,6]

> The American College of Cardiology (ACC)/American Heart Association (AHA) guidelines recommend:
>
> ### Class II
>
> - *Use of an insulin-based regimen to achieve and maintain glucose levels less than 180 mg/dL, while avoiding hypoglycemia.*

WOMEN

In general, women present with ACS at an older age than men and have the potential to have a more atypical presentation. They should be treated in similar manner to their male counterparts in the setting of ACS. Many of the early trials for ACS did not include a significant percentage of women. There is no clear data, that MI therapy should be significantly different for women than for men, except for the discontinuation of hormone replacement therapy. Due to the smaller body size of women, there may be increased risk of bleeding with standard dosing of antiplatelet medications and anticoagulants. This should be considered when treating the female patient.

> The American College of Cardiology (ACC)/American Heart Association (AHA) guidelines recommend:
>
> ### Class I
>
> - *Women with ACS:*
>   - *Should be managed similarly as men*
>   - *May need dose adjustment for antiplatelet and anti-coagulation therapy based on smaller body surface area*
>   - *Have similar indications for noninvasive testing (and similar prognostic value if imaging is used) compared to men*
>   - *Are recommended for early invasive strategy if at high risk*
>   - *Are recommended for conservative medical strategy if at low risk*
>   - *Should not have initiation of, and should have discontinuation of previously prescribed, hormone replacement therapy after an MI.*

ELDERLY

Patients should not have care withheld or altered based on age alone. The recommendations made in this chapter and in the guidelines, in certain areas, are based on data from studies that suggested either a decreased benefit or an increased risk in patients who are elderly. The premorbid functional class of the patient, as well as their associated comorbidities should guide therapy to a greater degree than age alone.

ACUTE CORONARY SYNDROME WITH COCAINE (AND METHAMPHETAMINE) USE

Cocaine as an etiology of ACS has been discussed earlier in this chapter. As the pathophysiology of cocaine induced ischemia or infarct may not be related to obstructive CAD, its management is somewhat different. Coronary vasodilators are the mainstay of therapy. However, the potential unopposed alpha constriction that may occur when beta blockers are given is a concern. Finally, although patients with cocaine use may have risk factors for CAD and develop a ruptured plaque to cause ACS, a significant portion do not have ACS secondary to platelet aggregation or thrombus formation. Therefore, the previous discussions regarding invasive approach to UA/NSTEMI and the use of antiplatelet medications, anticoagulants and thrombolytics may be less applicable in this population. Finally, methamphetamine use is on the rise and, although is not addressed directly in the guidelines, one may consider applying a similar approach in these patients as well.

> The American College of Cardiology (ACC)/American Heart Association (AHA) guidelines recommend:
>
> ### Class I
>
> - *Use of nitroglycerin and calcium channel blockers for the patients with ischemic-type chest discomfort and ST-depressions after cocaine use*
> - *Immediate coronary angiography with intent to perform primary PCI as necessary, should be performed if ST-elevation persists after coronary vasodilators*
> - *Thrombolytics should be considered in the above patient if coronary angiography is not possible*
>
> ### Class II
>
> - *Nitroglycerin or calcium channel blockers in patients after cocaine use, with ischemic-type chest discomfort with no or minimal ECG changes*
> - *Coronary angiography in patients after cocaine use if persistent ischemic-type chest discomfort and ST-depressions or isolated T wave inversions and lack of response to nitroglycerin or calcium channel blockers*
> - *Management of ACS patients after the use of methamphetamines be similar to patients after cocaine use*
> - *Use of combined alpha and beta blocking agents (labetalol) for patients with hypertension or sinus tachycardia, after the administration of nitroglycerin and/or calcium channel blockers*
>
> ### Class III
>
> - *Coronary angiography in patients after using cocaine who presented with chest discomfort and have no ST-segment or T-wave changes on ECG, negative biomarkers for necrosis and a negative stress test*

POST MYOCARDIAL INFARCTION DEPRESSION

Patients with depression after MI have a significantly worse prognosis compare to those who do not. Specifically, there is an increased risk of mortality at 6 months. This impact on prognosis is equivalent to the impact of high Killip class or previous MI.[68] In addition, mortality at 4 months was elevated even in patients with mild depression and the increase in mortality correlated with the degree of depression.[69,70]

Interestingly, the impact of depression seems to be solely related to mortality, not to the frequency of recurrent events. In addition, there does not appear to be a definitive study showing that medical treatment of the depression has a favorable impact.[71] Therefore, the physician should recognize the potential increase in incidence of depression in the patient post MI, and the increase in mortality associated with this diagnosis. Routine assessment of patients for the symptoms of depression should be a part of post MI care, both before and after discharge. Given that there is presently no data that treatment is either beneficial or harmful, medical therapy and counseling should be recommended as with any other patient with depression.

SURVIVORS OF OUT OF HOSPITAL CARDIAC ARREST

Out of hospital cardiac arrest is a complication of acute MI and, unlike in-hospital arrest, the prognosis is very poor with less than 10% rates of survival to discharge with any meaningul neurologic function.[72] Neurologic prognosis is worse if arrest is unwitnessed, occurs at home (versus in a public place), results in increased time to resuscitation, as well as in patients with advanced age and the initial rhythm of asystole or PEA compared to VF or VT. The cause of death is less commonly due to cardiogenic shock or recurrent dysrhythmias and more commonly related to complications of the anoxic brain injury (anoxic encephalopathy, sepsis, ventilator associated pneumonia, multiorgan failure, etc.). Thus prevention of brain injury has to be a focus of care for post MI patients who arrest prior to arrival at the hospital. The mainstay of this care today is induced therapeutic hypothermia. Patients are intentionally cooled to 32–34°C for 12–24 hours. In order to accomplish this, the patients must be paralyzed and sedated. Commercially available systems are available, and cold saline infusion is delivered to accomplish cooling. Two large randomized trials studied the use of therapeutic hypothermia in patients who were successfully resuscitated with out of hospital cardiac arrest due to VF and were comatose on arrival to the hospital. Both studies showed a significant improvement in survival and favorable neurologic outcome at the time of discharge.[73,74] Notably, in practice, patients who undergo cooling have a higher likelihood of hemodynamic and electric instability. These must be treated supportively with some tolerance of mild perturbations and then the addition of medications and occasionally IABP. There is an increased risk of coagulopathy. This should be considered in the patient who is at higher risk of bleeding due to thrombocytopenia, elevated INR or active bleeding. The American Heart Association Guidelines for Cardiopulmonary Resuscitation and Emergency Cardiovascular Care Science, published within the last few months, clearly recommends consideration of therapeutic hypothermia in comatose patients presenting after cardiac arrest. This recommendation is made with recognition that although there is apparent benefit, the specifics of timing, duration and optimal patient selection require further study.[75]

CONTINUED MEDICAL THERAPY FOR PATIENTS WITH A MYOCARDIAL INFARCTION

INHIBITION OF THE RENIN-ANGIOTENSIN-ALDOSTERONE AXIS

Angiotensin converting enzyme (ACE) inhibitors have been thoroughly studied in patients with heart failure.[76-79] The data show that they are indicated and beneficial in patients post MI who have a decreased LV systolic function (defined as LVEF ≥ 40%), or who have chronic kidney disease, diabetes or hypertension. The guidelines recommend against the routine use of IV ACE inhibitors, except in refractory hypertension.

Angiotensin receptor blockers should be considered in patients who are intolerant to ACE inhibitors (i.e. cough, angioedema, etc.) and have either a decrease in LVEF or who have hypertension requiring treatment, or as a primary option (versus ACE inhibitors) in these patients.[79-81]

Blood pressure reduction with the medications (beta blockers, nitrates, ACE inhibitors or angiotensin receptor blockers as first line, calcium channel blockers and thiazides as second line, etc.) and lifestyle changes to include diet (including reduction in sodium intake), exercise and weight reduction in attempt to attain ideal body weight should be a part of the patients discharge planning. The goal of blood pressure is less than 140/90 (with more stringent goal of < 130/80 blood pressure in patients with diabetes mellitus or chronic kidney disease).

The use of an aldosterone antagonist has been well established in heart failure[82] and has been shown to improve mortality and morbidity in patients who have had an AMI complicated by LV systolic dysfunction and heart failure.[83] Therefore, patients with decreased LVEF (≥ 40%) and who do not have significant decrease in renal function or elevation in potassium, who are post MI should be considered for initiation of eplerenone 25 mg daily in the beginning on 3–14 days and titrated up to 50 mg as tolerated.

The American College of Cardiology (ACC)/American Heart Association (AHA) guidelines recommend:

Class I

- ACE inhibitors should be administered to post MI patients with:
  — An EF less than or equal to 40%
  — Diabetes
  — Hypertension (Goal of <140/90 blood pressure in general and < 130/80 blood pressure in patients with chronic kidney disease or diabetes mellitus)
  — Chronic kidney disease
  — Increased risk for the recurrence of cardiovascular events (i.e. continued elevated risk due to poorly controlled risk factors)[84]
  — Normal EF with risk factors under control, at the discretion of the physician and patient (reasonable to administer)
- Angiotensin receptor blocker should be administered to post MI patients with:

- — The LVEF less than or equal to 40% who are intolerant to ACE inhibitor
- — Hypertension who are ACEI in tolerant
- — Systolic dysfunction who are already on ACE inhibitor
- Aldosterone receptor blocker should be administered to post MI patients with:
  - — The LVEF less than or equal to 40% and either diabetes or heart failure, but without significant renal dysfunction (Creatinine < 2.5 mg/dL in men and 2.0 mg/dL in women)

Class III

- The IV ACE inhibitor use in patient with MI due to the risk of hypotension (may be considered to control refractory hypertension)

LIPID MANAGEMENT

Although there is a clear benefit from several medications we prescribe for patients with cardiovascular disease, as providers, we must remember that the "prescription" of a heart healthy diet combined with a regular exercise program is highly beneficial to and essential for our patients. The diet has been shown, by itself and with exercise to lower low density lipoprotein (LDL) cholesterol, decrease progression of CAD (and potentially lead to regression) and reduce cardiovascular events.[85-88] However, the majority of CAD patients, are not able to either follow these stringent diets or intense physical exercise regimens and are unable to attain their lipid goal with these lifestyle changes alone. Patients with recent ACS have the lowest target LDL, at less than 70 mg/dL, which is extremely difficult to achieve for most of the patients, without medications.[89,90]

It is clear from multiple studies that lipid lowering with 3-hydroxy-3-methyl-glutaryl-coenzyme A (HMG CoA) reductase inhibitors (statins) prevents cardiovascular events both primarily (prior to first event) and secondarily (after diagnosis of atherosclerotic cardiovascular disease).[91-93] Early and aggressive use of statins (atorvastatin 80 mg daily) decreases risk in the early (as early as 16 weeks post ACS)[94-96] and late period post MI (after 4 months with simvastatin 40 mg up titrated to 80 mg/dL at 1 month).[97] These benefits remain long term.[98]

Reduction in LDL is important for reducing progression of atherosclerosis over long term. However, the relatively early benefit with statins as noted in major trials suggests that additional mechanisms besides LDL lowering may be involved. In fact, multiple "pleiotropic" effects of statins have been studied. These effects include: stabilization of the vulnerable plaque, improvement in endothelial function, decrease in inflammation both in the plaque itself (less macrophages and decreased metalloproteinase production by macrophages and decreased cell death within the plaque) and systemically (by decreasing expression of chemokines and inflammatory cytokines, lowering of clinical markers of inflammation—highly sensitive C-reactive protein) and decreased thrombogenesis.[99]

Full fasting lipid panel should be measured as soon as possible after admission. It must be recognized by the physician that LDL cholesterol decreases, significantly, after MI and to a lesser extent with unstable angina. This decreased level will underestimate true baseline level and the needed reduction based on diet, exercise and medication. The absolute decrease in any given patient is variable, but the decrease itself is generally significant and can approach 50%.[100]

It is recommended that a statin medication be initiated in patients who have no contraindication, early after the diagnosis of ACS (as early as day 1), and no later than at the time of discharge. In addition to the early effects of statins, the initiation of this medication at the time of the ACS event, improves long-term compliance.[101]

Niacin has been shown to decrease the risk of recurrent nonfatal MI in patients with a previous history of MI,[102] and is a consideration in the statin intolerant patient. The AIM-HIGH trial, which is presently ongoing, will look at patients with optimal LDL levels on a statin, plus placebo versus extended release niacin.[103]

Omega 3 fatty acids are beneficial in lowering triglycerides and thus raising HDL, both as an increase in dietary intake and as a supplement. The supplemental use of omega 3 fatty acids has been shown to prevent sudden cardiac death in patients with previous MI.[104] The addition of omega 3 fatty acids should be considered in patients post MI with elevated triglycerides.

The American College of Cardiology (ACC)/American Heart Association (AHA) guidelines recommend:

Class I

- Assessment of lipids within 24 hours of presentation and initiation of medications prior to discharge
- Dietary changes (education) to reduce intake of saturated fats (< 7% of calories), trans fats and cholesterol (< 200 mg/dL)
- Promote daily physical activity and weight management
- The HMG CoA reductase inhibitors, in absence of contraindications:
  - — In UA/NSTEMI, regardless of baseline
  - — In UA/NSTEMI/STEMI patients with LDL greater than 100 mg/dL (it is reasonable to use medications to achieve LDL < 70 mg/dL—Class II)
- Treatment of triglycerides, if between 200 and 499 mg/dL, and non-HDL (total cholesterol minus HDL) if greater than 130 mg/dL is reasonable
- Treatment of triglycerides if greater than 500 mg/dL with fibrates or niacin should be a first priority

Class II

- Increase dietary intake of omega 3 fatty acids or supplement (up to 1 g/dL if triglycerides are normal, 4 g/dL if triglycerides are elevated)
- Addition of niacin or fibrates (beware of increased incidence of side effects with combination therapy) to treat low HDL (< 40 mg/dL) or elevated triglycerides (> 200 mg/dL) after LDL lowering therapy is instituted.

GLUCOSE MANAGEMENT

It is well established that diabetics have an increased risk of cardiovascular events. Unfortunately, to date, there have not been any definitive randomized trials to show that intensive glucose control in established diabetics has a benefit on reduction in major adverse cardiovascular events. On the contrary, the ACCORD study was stopped prematurely due to an excess mortality in the intensive treatment group.[105]

The United Kingdom Prospective Diabetes study, in contrast, looked at new diabetics and assigned them to conventional therapy, (diet alone) versus an intensive glucose control arm with sulfonylurea or insulin. Findings from this study showed that intensive treatment of type 2 diabetes with a sulfonylurea or insulin resulted in a lower incidence of microvascular complications (e.g., neuropathy, retinopathy, and nephropathy) without a significant reduction in macrovascular events (e.g., myocardial infarction). Aggressive control of blood pressure on the other hand was shown to have a beneficial impact on the risk of macrovascular complications. In the subgroup of patients treated with metformin however, notable reduction in the risk of microvascular and macrovascular complications was noted.[106]

Based on this data, one should consider aggressive glucose control in new diabetics, but recognize that intensive control in long-term diabetics may have a negative impact on cardiovascular events and mortality. More data is clearly necessary to determine optimal level of glycemic control and the type of therapy to be used in patients with long-term diabetes.

Finally, it is clear that aggressive risk modification should occur in patients with diabetes particularly with blood pressure and lipid management.[107,108]

The American College of Cardiology (ACC)/American Heart Association (AHA) guidelines recommend:

Class I

- *Initiate lifestyle modification and pharmacotherapy with goal of near normal HbA1c*
- *Aggressive modification of other risk factors (weight loss, exercise, blood pressure control, lipid management, etc.)*
- *Care coordination for management of diabetes with primary care physician or endocrinologist*

SMOKING CESSATION

Continued tobacco smoking in patients with CAD significantly increases the risk of reinfarcton and death.[109] Compliance with smoking cessation increases when initiated at the time of an event (MI or CABG).[110] Smoking cessation decreased the relative risk of mortality by 36% and significantly decreased the risk of nonfatal cardiac events, in a meta-analysis of studies performed in patients with previous cardiovascular events.[111] The relative risk of death is decreased by half in women smokers who quit compared to those who continued to smoke, and these curves begin to separate within the first year. The incidence of reinfarction trended toward a decrease, but this was not statistically significant in this study.[112]

Secondhand or passive smoke increases the risk of developing CAD, cardiovascular events and cardiovascular mortality, and should be avoided.[113] Patients and their family members (particularly the spouse and other smokers residing in the same residence) should be counseled on the deleterious effects of secondhand smoke and on the inability of the patient to discontinue smoking in the presence of ongoing smokers. Given the multiple bans on smoking in the community, the likelihood of the patient encountering with unavoidable smoking in the workplace has decreased.

Smoking cessation is a difficult task for most of the patients. It is a duty of the caregiver (physician, nurse and cardiac rehabilitation specialist) to discuss with the patient about the negative impacts of smoking on his or her cardiovascular and overall health. The patient must first recognize these impacts and understand the necessity of smoking cessation. Counseling is a mainstay of smoking cessation. This should occur at multiple levels, including prior to and also after discharge. Successful discontinuation of tobacco use is dependent on the patient making a determination that cessation is necessary. The direct discussion between patient and physician is a first step in the patient making a determination of need to quit and this counseling increases the likelihood of cessation.[114] Ongoing counseling will occur in cardiac rehabilitation and is also available via telephone and internet through the "QUITNOW" program. The patients should be encouraged to utilize these resources.

The addition of pharmacotherapy to counseling is beneficial. Adding nicotine replacement therapy has been shown to increase the likelihood of cessation.[114] Nicotine replacement therapy is clearly safe in patients with stable angina and considered safe in patients after ACS (safer than continued smoking), particularly if revascularized.[115] Patients should be counseled on the avoidance of combining nicotine replacement therapy with continued active smoking.

Bupropion is at least as effective as nicotine replacement therapy in smoking cessation.[116,117] Consideration may be given to combined therapy, in some patients, although there was not a statistically significant difference when compared to bupropion alone. The smoker should be encouraged to choose a "quit date" and then to begin the bupropion 1 week prior at a dose of 150 mg/dL for 3 days, then 150 mg twice per day for at least 12 weeks and up to 6 months. There is efficacy data for the single daily 150 mg dose in some studies and therefore it can be considered as an option. Bupropion can decrease seizure threshold and thus should not be given in patients with a seizure disorder.[118]

Varenicline is a partial agonist of the nicotinic acetylcholine receptor and thus decreases the withdrawal symptoms.[27] Varenicline has been compared to bupropion in randomized controlled trials and it is superior to use both for short-term and long-term smoking cessation.[119,120] There have been reported cases of suicidal ideation and/or new aggressive or erratic behaviors in patients taking varenicline. The FDA therefore has issued a warning that varenicline may increase the risk of serious neuropsychiatric symptoms in patients. Physicians should assess the risk or benefit of this therapy, use caution in prescribing and educate patients and their families regarding symptoms that should prompt discontinuation of the medication and when to seek medical evaluation (including changes in behavior, aggression, decreased mood or increased anxiety or agitation, or suicidal ideation).

Small studies have suggested the increased efficacy and safety of combined varenicline and bupropion, as well as varenicline with nicotine replacement.[121,122] One should consider reserving this therapy for patients with low risk of side effects and continued interest in cessation despite lack of success with either medication alone.

Class I

- *Smoking cessation and avoidance of environmental smoke at home and work with a stepwise strategy:*
  - *Ask the patient about exposure (smoking and exposure to secondhand smoke)*
  - *Advise counsel regarding cessation of smoking and avoidance of secondhand smoke*
  - *Assess willingness to quit, and barriers (including smokers in environment) and continually asses success rate at follow-up visits*
  - *Assist with pharmacologic agents as necessary*
  - *Arrange follow-up and cardiac rehabilitation*

DISCHARGE

Optimal length of stay for a patient with an MI is dependent on the patient's clinical status, the need for monitoring and completion of the evaluation. Although length of stay has progressively decreased over time, ultimately there will be a point at which it cannot decrease further or patient safety will be impacted. Low-risk patients (defined as patients age < 70 years old who were without heart failure, major dysrhythmias, three-vessel CAD, or need for IABP and with EF > 45%, a successful PCI and CK/MB-fraction values < two times the upper limit of the reference value at the discharge) were discharged in 48–72 hours after admission without significant morbidity or mortality at 6 weeks (0% mortality and 0.6% morbidity), or 6 months (0.5% mortality and 2% morbidity).[123] Notably, at least in this study, the risk stratification is not impacted by the patients original presentation, particularly whether the patient presents with NSTEMI or STEMI. Patients with a complicated course will require longer stay. Predischarge planning should occur early in the hospital stay in order for the patient to be ready for discharge as early as their medical condition allows. The average length of stay for a patient with MI is 3–5 days.

NITRATES

Although there is no data to show a mortality benefit in patients treated with nitrates chronically, it is important that all patients with CAD have rescue nitroglycerin available to them. This can be delivered in tablet (sublingual) or spray form. Patients should be given a prescription at discharge and be educated on its use. The standard instructions are to use nitroglycerin at the onset of angina, and repeat in every 5 minutes as needed. The patient should be instructed to call 911 if requiring a third dose. It is important that patients understand the indications for use, and be educated on "their angina" as many patients will have either atypical angina, or have difficulty in differentiating angina from other chest or epigastric symptoms. In addition, it is appropriate to educate the patient on the side effects, including hypotension (instructing patients to sit or lie down when taking nitroglycerin, if possible) and the potential for headache and to let them know about the serious interaction with type 5 phosphodiesterase inhibitors.

Class I

- *The use of nitrates to limit ischemic symptoms.*

CARDIAC REHABILITATION AND SECONDARY PREVENTION OF CORONARY HEART DISEASE FOR PATIENTS WITH MYOCARDIAL INFARCTION

Over the past two decades, there has been tremendous progress in pharmacological therapies, sophisticated technology-based diagnostic and therapeutic procedures for the treatment of cardiovascular diseases. As survival from acute events has improved, a greater number of men and women with prevalent cardiovascular disease are at increased risk for future events and thus, may suffer significant physical and psychological disability. Secondary prevention strategies focused on lifestyle modification, diet, exercise and medical therapy are an integral part of disease management and have been discussed. Cardiac rehabilitation is a very important (and underutilized) multi-disciplinary intervention that provides comprehensive services focused on exercise training and important life style modifications for a patient with cardiovascular disease. It helps to limit the functional and psychological impact of the illness and to prevent future events.

Cardiac rehabilitation can begin as soon as an eligible inpatient stabilizes after AMI, PCI, CABG surgery, valve surgery, heart transplant or acute coronary syndrome. Inpatient rehabilitation, known as Phase I, is intended to prevent deconditioning from hospitalization, ready the patient for referral to an outpatient cardiac rehabilitation program, assess for activity tolerance, prescribe activity for the period immediately following hospital discharge, and begin patient teaching for secondary prevention.

Outpatient cardiac rehabilitation, also known as Phase II, is a standard of care following MI, PCI, CABG surgery, valve surgery, heart transplant, and for those with stable angina. It is designed to limit the physiological and psychological effects of MI, reduce the risk of sudden cardiac death and reinfarction, control cardiac symptoms, stabilize or reverse the atherosclerotic process, and enhance patients' psychosocial and vocational status.[124,125] Secondary prevention, essential in contemporary care of patients with heart disease, is a key element of cardiac rehabilitation.[126]

Phase II cardiac rehabilitation begins with referral into a program as soon as possible post MI, followed by baseline patient assessment, including exercise, nutritional and psychosocial assessments. Patients are then provided appropriate individualized nutritional counseling, aggressive risk factor management, psychosocial intervention as needed, and monitored exercise training by a qualified multidisciplinary team, typically composed of experienced registered nurses, exercise physiologists, physical therapists, a registered dietitian and psychologist or social worker. Patients are strongly encouraged to attend several sessions (up to 36 and sometimes more), the number of which is determined by complications, risk category and progress in meeting goals. Medicare, medicaid and most private insurance companies reimburse for Phase II cardiac rehabilitation. Some insurance plans have recently implemented co-payments that have made CR prohibitively expensive. However, many Medicare patients carry supplemental insurance that assist with co-payments that have recently risen substantially since 2010.

The benefits of Phase II cardiac rehabilitation are impressive, multifaceted and interrelated, and are attained by implementing the following components:

- *Exercise training*: Supervised monitored exercise is carried out in a group setting (typically no more than 4 patients per staff member) after individual exercise assessment. The exercise prescription, recommended by the staff and approved by the physician, includes aerobic and strength training with various modes of exercise equipment based on the patient's goals and abilities. The initial exercise assessment is comprised of an exercise test not to exceed 70% of age-predicted maximum heart rate for the post MI patient, 85% for the non-MI patient, or a rating of perceived exertion (RPE) of 14 (Borg 6–20 scale), absence of angina or ECG signs of ischemia and arrhythmias. From that initial assessment, the exercise prescription is written considering heart rate parameters, avoidance of angina and/or ECG signs of ischemia and RPE. On the first evaluation, patients achieve a peak level of anywhere between 1.6 and 13.5 METs[*] (METs are estimated metabolic equivalent units where 1 MET = oxygen consumption of 3.5 ml/kg/minute), depending on age, physical conditioning prior to the event and severity of cardiac diagnosis. Patients then progress by gradually increasing the aerobic exercise duration (up to 60 minutes) as well as the workload. Typically patients are able to begin aerobic training at 50% or more of their peak MET level on admission. The typical patient is training at the level at which they tested on admission at least by mid-point in the program. Aerobic training includes exercise on treadmills, bicycles, elliptical trainers, arm ergometers and other modes. Strength training begins as soon as possible in Phase II based on the patient's diagnosis, surgical status (and clearance from surgeon) and blood pressure response to exercise.

  The exercise training increases a patient's peak oxygen uptake by 11–36%, with the greatest improvement in the most deconditioned individuals.[124,126,127] At the University of Iowa CHAMPS (cardiac rehabilitation program) the final exercise evaluation showed a mean improvement in estimated METs of 53%[†] (range 2.2–21.5 METs).

  In addition, exercise increases high density lipoprotein, lowers triglycerides, and helps with weight loss and blood pressure control. Specifically designed exercise programs enable patients to safely return to occupational demands as well as attain recreational goals.

- *Nutritional counseling*: For most patients, lipid management, blood pressure lowering and weight control are important goals. Baseline data are collected concerning usual caloric intake, saturated and trans fat consumption, eating habits,

fruits and vegetables consumption, carbohydrate and alcohol consumption. Patient-specific goals are delineated.

- *Weight management*: Not only is obesity an independent risk factor for cardiovascular disease, it adversely impacts other risk factors.[128] Calculation of the body mass index, measurement of the waist circumference, frequent body weights and patient history help the dietitian establish short-term and long-term goals appropriate for the patient and specific risk factors.

- *Blood pressure (BP) management*: Resting, orthostatic and exercise BPs are routinely and regularly obtained in cardiac rehabilitation programs. Weight management, sodium restriction when indicated, other dietary interventions, and exercise all work to lower the BP. Optimal blood pressure is accomplished through these lifestyle changes, in conjunction with interaction with the physician for optimal medical therapy.

- *Lipid management*: Dietary counseling aimed at specific lipid and/or blood glucose abnormalities are provided, followed and coordinated with the patient's physician. This allows the patient to reach lipid goals with lifestyle alteration and medical management.

- *Diabetes management*: Diabetes mellitus is an independent risk factor for cardiovascular disease. Management of the diabetic patient in terms of exercise and diet are imperative for secondary prevention. Self-monitoring skills are taught as well as practiced and take on special significance for the insulin-dependent patient on a diet and exercise regimen. For example, patients are taught how to recognize hypoglycemia and ways to avoid this during exercise. In addition, they are taught ideal blood sugar control based on individual pathology, exercise intensity, body weight loss and medications.

- *Tobacco cessation*: Current smoking, smokeless tobacco and secondhand smoke are addressed with appropriate cessation interventions. Relapse prevention is taught and patient follow-up is implemented.

- *Psychosocial intervention*: Depression and hostility, common in patients with MI, have been shown to increase the risk of coronary heart disease as well as impede recovery. Participation in Phase II cardiac rehabilitation has been shown to markedly improve these profiles[129] through counseling and exercise. Compared with older (mean ± SD age 75 ± 3 years) patients, young (mean ± SD age, 48 ± 6 years) patients have been shown to have higher scores for anxiety and hostility and slightly more depression symptoms. Following phase II cardiac rehabilitation, younger patients have shown markedly improved scores for depression, anxiety and hostility.[130] At the University of Iowa CHAMPS, the 9-Symptom Checklist is used to assess depression on admission and discharge. From July 2000 through November 2010, 1,170 patients took the admission 9-Symptom Checklist for a mean score of 6.53. The 701 patients took the test at the time of discharge with a mean score of 3.48. Patients with scores of 6 or more, which may indicate other

---

[*]Based on data compiled at the University of Iowa CHAMPS Phase II cardiac rehabilitation from 2000 to 2010, n = 1,123)
[†]Matched pairs analysis of 704 consecutive patients who finished Phase II cardiac rehabilitation from 2000 to 2010 showed a mean difference of 2.84 METs from first test (mean 5.28 METs) to final test (mean 8.12 METs)

depressive syndrome, who took the admission and discharge assessment (n = 283) demonstrated significant improvement with a mean admission score of 10.71 to a mean discharge score of 5.75. It is important to note that this occurred without the use of antidepressant medications.

After completion of Phase II cardiac rehabilitation, patients are urged to enter maintenance programs, also known as Phases III and IV, for long-term risk factor modification. These programs are typically not covered by insurance and have less staff supervision. The ECG monitoring is not done routinely, and the staff to patient ratio is higher than in Phase II.

Advantages of Cardic Rehabilitation

Meta-analyses of randomized controlled trials of exercise-based rehabilitation for patients with coronary heart disease have confirmed numerous benefits. Compared with usual care, cardiac rehabilitation was associated with a reduction of all-cause mortality [odds ratio (OR) = 0.80; 95% confidence interval (CI): 0.68–0.93] as well as cardiac mortality [OR = 0.74; 95% CI: 0.61–0.96]. In addition, lipids and smoking cessation were positively impacted with greater reductions in total cholesterol, triglycerides and reduction of systolic blood pressure (weighted mean difference, -3.2 mm Hg; 95% CI: -5.4 to -0.9 mm Hg).[131]

Patients age of 65 years and/or older benefit from a strong dose-response relationship between the number of sessions and positive long-term outcomes at 4 years. Those who completed 36 sessions had lower death and MI rates than those who completed fewer sessions.[132] Specifically, patients who attended 36 sessions had a 14%, 22%, and 47% lower risk of death compated to those who attended 24 sessions, 12 sessions and only 1 session, respectively.[132] The beneficial impact of cardiac rehabilitation on the incidence of new MI was also similar.[132] In addition, studies have demonstrated a clear cost-effectiveness ratio for cardiac rehabilitation programs for the post MI patient.[133-135]

Utilization of Cardiac Rehabilitation in the United States

With such impressive outcomes, the expectation is that participation in cardiac rehabilitation would be high. However, this is not the case. The use of cardiac rehabilitation is relatively low among Medicare beneficiaries. An analysis of 267,427 beneficiaries 65 years of age or older revealed that overall, cardiac rehabilitation was utilized by only 13.9% of patients hospitalized for AMI and 31% of patients who underwent coronary artery bypass graft surgery. The use of cardiac rehabilitation varied from 6.6% in Idaho to the highest rates of 53.5%, 48.9% and 46.5% in Nebraska, South Dakota, and Iowa respectively with the highest rates clustered in the northern central states of the United States.[136]

At University of Iowa, cardiac rehabilitation is a standing order following MI, PCI, CABG, and valve surgery. Since its inception in 1990, the program has enjoyed among the highest referral and participation rates in the United States. The development of a culture of cardiac rehabilitation as an integral part of the cardiac patient's care, fosters these high referral and participation rates. It is clear that hospitals and physician

practices should embrace the "culture of cardiac rehab" to best serve their cardiac patients.

With decreases in mortality, morbidity and cardiac risk factors enjoyed by patients who complete cardiac rehabilitation, analyses suggest that greater utilization of cardiac rehabilitation in the United States would be highly cost-effective.[137,138] It has been proposed that referral to and completion of cardiac rehabilitation be included as a quality indicator for organizations such as the ACC, the AHA, the Agency for Health Care Research and Quality, the National Committee for Quality Assurance and the Joint Commission on Accreditation of Health Care Organizations as a way to increase the use of cardiac rehabilitation.[136]

Predischarge Education

Education must occur before discharge regarding importance of recurrence of symptoms, diet, exercise, smoking cessation, medication compliance and continuing cardiac rehabilitation as an outpatient. The patient must have a follow-up appointment scheduled prior to discharge. The timing of this appointment depends on the medical stability of the patient and can vary 1–6 weeks after discharge. The patient should clearly understand how to contact someone in the healthcare team (who will continue long-term follow-up with the patient) if there are questions, concerns or symptoms after discharge.

The physician should understand that the patient will have many questions regarding resumption of normal daily activity after ACS. In the patient with an uncomplicated course, activities of daily living (showering, dressing, normal walking, etc.) should be resumed immediately dictated by symptoms. Driving can be resumed within 1 week, with this limitation being predominantly related to concern for complications from femoral access for PCI.

Returning to normal sexual activity is anxiety provoking for the patient and should be discussed prior to discharge. This is, of course, a topic that the patient may not be comfortable bringing to the attention of the physician. Therefore, it should be normal practice for the physician, nurse and/or rehab specialist to discuss prior to discharge. Sexual activity may resume within 1–2 weeks after discharge in a symptoms limited approach, or be addressed during the early course of phase II CR in the patient with concerns or with decreased functional capacity.

Return to work is a decision to be made by the treating physician (in consultation with the patient's cardiac rehabilitation specialist) and should be based on the overall clinical status of the patient (lack symptoms of ischemia, heart failure or dysrhythmia), the patient's premorbid functional status and the physical nature of the patient's job. It is reasonable to consider return to work within 2 weeks in the low-risk post MI patient (age < 70 years old, normal EF and optimal revascularization),[139] specifically those who are able to exercise to more than 7 METs on a symptom limited exercise treadmill test.[140] This study also suggested that patients with an EF less than 40% who were able to exercise to 7 METs without symptoms or ECG changes, and did not have any evidence of electrical instability could return to normal activities, including work at 2 weeks.[140]

This time frame also allows for the patients to begin cardiac rehabilitation in order to assess their overall function status and anginal symptoms with activity. In the patients who are at low risk and have a sedentary and low stress job, it may be reasonable to return to work after the first rehabilitation session. In a patient with a high physical workload, or high stress job, one should consider longer convalescence, focused education regarding stress reduction, and a "back to work evaluation" that is tailored to the patient's myocardial work demands (lifting, etc.). Data suggests that older age, manual labor jobs, unmarried status (poor social network) and the presence of anxiety and depression, but not necessarily the severity of the event, may increase the likelihood of a patient not returning to work after MI.[141,142]

SUMMARY

In summary, STEMI is a life-threatening event and a true medical emergency. It is important that physicians and patients alike recognize that time is muscle. Patients should be educated regarding symptoms, and the necessity to utilize the emergency medical transport system (911), if they have accelerated or rest symptoms that are consistent with an MI. At the time of arrival, the team must be prepared to rapidly evaluate the patient and make quick decisions regarding reperfusion. Protocols should be in place, and routinely reviewed, as this is an area of medicine where we as clinicians can make a great difference in the outcome of these patients. One must remain vigilant to recognize and manage complications especially with an acute change in patient's clinical status. Risk factors for recurrence of future cardiovascular events must be recognized during hospitalization and every effort should be made towards ameliorating that risk. Recommendations should include lifestyle modification (diet, physical activity, smoking cessation), and medications to treat hypertension, hyperlipidemia, diabetes as well as the sequelae of the current insult (heart failure). Finally, we must prepare our patients to adapt to this changing event. Cardiac rehabilitation program is an important multi-disciplinary intervention focused on exercise training, and lifestyle modification that can have a significant impact in returning patients back to a normal life and positively impact their outcomes.

REFERENCES

1. Lloyd-Jones D, Adams RJ, Brown TM, et al. Heart disease and stroke statistics-2010 update: a report from the American Heart Association. Circulation. 2010;121:e46-215.
2. De Luca G, Suryapranata H, Ottervanger JP, et al. Time delay to treatments and mortality in primary angioplasty for acute myocardial infarction. Circulation. 2004;109:1223-5.
3. Indications for fibrinolytic therapy in suspected acute myocardial infarction: collaborative overview of early mortality and major morbidity results from all randomised trials of more than 1000 patients. Fibrinolytic Therapy Trialists' (FTT) Collaborative Group. Lancet. 1994;343:311-22.
4. ACC/AHA guidelines for the management of patients with ST-elevation myocardial infarction—executive summary: a report of the American College of Cardiology/American Heart Association Task Force on Practice Guidelines (Writing Committee to Revise the 1999 Guidelines for the Management of Patients with Acute Myocardial Infarction). Circulation. 2004;110:588-636.
5. Antman EM, Hand M, Armstrong PW, et al. 2007 Focused Update of the ACC/AHA 2004 Guidelines for the Management of Patients with ST-Elevation Myocardial Infarction. American College of Cardiology/American Heart Association Task Force on Practice Guidelines. Circulation. 2008;117:296-329.
6. Kushner FG, Hand M, Smith SC, et al. 2009 Focused Updates: ACC/AHA Guidelines for the Management of Patients with ST-Elevation Myocardial Infarction (Updating the 2004 Guideline and 2007 Focused Update) and ACC/AHA/SCAI Guidelines on Percutaneous Coronary Intervention (Updating the 2005 Guideline and 2007 Focused Update): a report of the American College of Cardiology Foundation/American Heart Association Task Force on Practice Guidelines. Circulation. 2009;120:2271-306.
7. Anderson JL, Adams CD, Antman EM, et al. ACC/AHA 2007 Guidelines of the Management of Patients with Unstable Angina/Non-ST-Elevation Myocardial Infarction. A report of the American College of Cardiology/American Heart Association Task Force on Practice Guidelines (Writing Committee to Revise the 2002 Guidelines for the Management of Patients with Unstable Angina/Non-ST-Elevation Myocardial Infarction). Circulation. 2007;116:e148-304.
8. Wright RS, Anderson JL, Adams CD, et al. 2011 ACCF/AHA Focused Update of the Guidelines for the Management of Patients with Unstable Angina/Non-ST-Elevation Myocardial Infarction (Updating the 2007 Guideline). J Am Coll Cardiol. 2011;57:1920-59 [Epub 2011].
9. Van Werkum JW, Heestermans AA, Zomer AC, et al. Predictors of coronary stent thrombosis. The Dutch Stent Thrombosis Registry. J Am Coll Cardiol. 2009;52(16)1399-409.
10. Ivandic BT, Sausemuth M, Ibrahim H, et al. Dual antiplatelet drug resistance is a risk factor for cardiovascular events after percutaneous coronary intervention. Clin Chem. 2009;55:1171-6.
11. Jung H, Sir JJ. Recurrent myocardial infarction due to one subacute and two very late thrombotic events of the drug-eluting stent associated with clopidogrel resistance. J Invasive Cardiol. 2011;23: e15-8.
12. Sweeny JM, Gorog DA, Fuster V. Antiplatelet drug 'resistance'. Part 1: mechanisms and clinical measurements. Nat Rev Cardiol. 2009;6:273-82.
13. Gorog DA, Sweeny JM, Fuster V. Antiplatelet drug 'resistance'. Part 2: laboratory resistance to antiplatelet drugs—fact or artifact? Nat Rev Cardiol. 2009;6:365-73.
14. Collet JP, Hulot JS, Pena A, et al. Cytochrome P450 2C19 polymorphism in young patients treated with clopidogrel after myocardial infarction: a cohort study. Lancet. 2009;373:309-17.
15. Grosgurin O, Plojoux J, Keller PF, et al. Prehospital emergency physician activation of interventional cardiology team reduces door-to-balloon time in ST-elevation myocardial infarction. Swiss Med Wkly. 2010;140:228-32.
16. Rao A, Kardouh Y, Darda S, et al. Impact of the prehospital ECG on door-to balloon time in ST elevation myocardial infarction. Catheter Cardiovasc Interv. 2010;75:174-8.
17. McLean S, Wild S, Connor P, et al. Treating ST elevation myocardial infarction by primary percutaneous coronary intervention, in-hospital thrombolysis and prehospital thrombolysis. An observational study of timelines and outcomes in 625 patients. Emerg Med J. 2011;28:230-6.
18. Terkelsen CJ, Christiansen EH, Sorensen JT, et al. Primary PCI as the preferred reperfusion in STEMI: it is a matter of time. Heart. 2009;95:362-9.
19. Nikus K, Pahlm O, Wagner G, et al. Electrocardiographic classification of acute coronary syndromes: a review by a committee of the International Society for Holter and Non-Invasive Electrocardiology. J Electrocard. 2010;43:91-103.
20. Zimetbaum PJ, Josephson ME. Use of the electrocardiogram in acute myocardial infarction. N Eng J Med. 2003;348:933-40.
21. Dressler W, Roesler H. High T waves in the earliest stage of myocardial infarction. Am Heart J. 1947;34:627-45.
22. Madias JE. The earliest electrocardiographic sign of acute transmural myocardial infarction. J Electrocardiol. 1977;10:193-6.

23. Herz I, Assali AR, Adler Y, et al. New electrocardiographic criteria for predicting either the right or left circumflex artery as the culprit coronary artery in inferior wall acute myocardial infarction. Am J Cardiol. 1997;80:1343-5.

24. Fiol M, Cygankiewicz I, Carrillo A, et al. Value of electrocardiographic algorithm based on the "ups and downs" of ST in assessment of a culprit artery in evolving inferior wall acute myocardial infarction. Am J Cardiol. 2004;94:709-14.

25. Zehender M, Kasper W, Kauder E, et al. Right ventricular infarction as an independent predictor of prognosis after acute inferior myocardial infarction. N Eng J Med. 1993;328:981-8.

26. Sgarbossa EB, Pinski SL, Barbagelata A, et al. Electrocardiographic diagnosis of evolving acute myocardial infarction in the presence of left bundle-branch block. GUSTO-1 (Global Utilization of Streptokinase and the Tissue Plasminogen Activator for Occluded Coronary Arteries) Investigators. N Eng J Med. 1996;334:481-7.

27. Micromedex 2.0. Copyright Thompson Reuters; 2011.

28. Van De Werf F, Adgey J, Ardissino D, et al. On behalf of the ASSENT-2 Investigators. Single-bolus tenecteplase compared with front-loaded alteplase in acute myocardial infarction: the ASSENT-2 double-blind randomised trial. Lancet. 1999;354:716-22.

29. Assessment of the Safety and Efficacy of a New Treatment Strategy with Percutaneous Coronary Intervention ASSENT-4 PCI Investigators. Primary versus tenecteplase-facilitated percutaneous coronary intervention in patients with ST-segment elevation acute myocardial infarction (ASSENT-4 PCI): randomised trial. Lancet. 2006;267:569-78.

30. Keeley EC, Boura JA, Grines CL. Comparison of primary and facilitated percutaneous interventions for ST-elevation myocardial infarction: quantitative review of randomised trials. Lancet. 2006;367:579-88.

31. Eitel I, Franke A, Schuler G, et al. ST-segment resolution and prognosis after facilitated versus primary percutaneous coronary intervention in acute myocardial infarction: a meta-analysis. Clin Res Cardiol. 2010;99:1-11.

32. Kiernan TJ, Ting HH, Gersh BJ. Facilitated percutaneous coronary intervention: current concepts, promises and pitfalls. Eur Heart J. 2007;28:1545-53.

33. Ellis SG, Tendera M, de Belder MA, et al. on behalf of the FINESSE Investigators. Facilitated PCI in patients with ST-elevation myocardial infarction. N Engl J Med. 2008;358:2205-17.

34. Van't Hof AW, Ten Berg J, Heestermans T, et al. on behalf of the ongoing tirofiban in myocardial infarction evaluation (On-TIME) 2 study group. Prehospital initiation of tirofiban in patients with ST-elevation myocardial infarction undergoing primary angioplasty (On-TIME 2): a multicenter, double-blind, randomized controlled trial. Lancet. 2008;372:537-46.

35. Randomised trial of intravenous streptokinase, oral aspirin, both, or neither among 17,187 cases of suspected acute myocardial infarction: ISIS-2. ISIS-2 (Second International Study of Infarct Survival) Collaborative Group. Lancet. 1988;2:349-60.

36. Effectiveness of intravenous thrombolytic treatment in acute myocardial infarction. Gruppo Italiano per lo Studio della Streptochinasi nell'Infarto Miocardico (GISSI). Lancet. 1986;1:397-402.

37. An international randomized trial comparing four thrombolytic strategies for acute myocardial infarction. The Gusto investigators. N Engl J Med. 1993;329:673-82.

38. Indications for fibrinolytic therapy in suspected acute myocardial infarction: collaborative overview of early mortality and major morbidity results from all randomised trials of more than 1000 patients. Fibrinolytic Therapy Trialists' (FTT) Collaborative Group. Lancet. 1994;343:311-22.

39. Boersma E, Maas AC, Deckers JW, et al. Early thrombolytic treatment in acute myocardial infarction: reappraisal of the golden hour. Lancet. 1996;348:771-5.

40. Cannon CP, Gibson CM, McCabe CH, et al. TNK-tissue plasminogen activator compared with front-loaded alteplase in acute myocardial infarction: results of the TIMI 10B trial. Circulation. 1998;98:2805-14.

41. de Lemos JA, Braunwald E. ST segment resolution as a tool for assessing the efficacy of reperfusion therapy. J Am Coll Cardiol. 2001;38:1283-94.

42. Gershlick AH, Stephens-Lloyd A, Hughes S, et al. for the REACT Trial Investigators. Rescue angioplasty after failed thrombolytic therapy for acute myocardial infarction. N Engl J Med. 2005;353:2758-68.

43. Di Mario C, Dudek D, Piscione F, et al. on behalf of the CARESS-in-AMI Investigators. Immediate angioplasty versus standard therapy with rescue angioplasty after thrombolysis in the Combined Abciximab Reteplase Stent Study in Acute Myocardial Infarction (CARESS-in-AMI): an open, prospective, randomised, multicentre trial. Lancet. 2008;371:559-68.

44. Cantor WJ, Fitchett D, Borgundvaag B, et al. on behalf of the TRANSFER-AMI Trial Investigators. Routine early angioplasty after fibrinolysis for acute myocardial infarction. N Engl J Med. 2009;360:2705-18.

45. Gibson CM, Karha J, Murphy SA, et al. on behalf of the TIMI Study Group. Early and long-term clinical outcomes associated with reinfarction following fibrinolytic administration in the thrombolysis in myocardial infarction trials. J Am Coll Cardiol. 2003;42:7-16.

46. Fernandez-Aviles F, Alonso JJ, Castro-Beiras A, et al. on behalf of the Gracia (Grupo de Analisis de la Cardiopatia Isquemica Aguda) Group. Routine invasive strategy within 24 hours of thrombolysis versus ischaemia-guided conservative approach for acute myocardial infarction with ST-segment elevation (GRACIA-1): a randomized controlled trial. Lancet. 2004; 364:1045-53.

47. Hochman JS, Lamas GA, Buller CE, et al. On behalf of the Occluded Artery Trial Investigators. Coronary intervention for persistent occlusion after myocardial infarction. N Engl J Med. 2006;355:2395-407.

48. Weaver WD, Simes RJ, Betriu A, et al. Comparison of primary coronary angioplasty and intravenous thrombolytic therapy for acute myocardial infarction: a quantitative review. JAMA. 1997;278: 2093-8.

49. Keeley EC, Boura JA, Grines CL. Primary angioplasty versus intravenous thrombolytic therapy for acute myocardial infarction: a quantitative review of 23 randomised trials. Lancet. 2003;361:13-20.

50. Hochman JS, Sleeper LA, Webb JG, et al. on behalf of the SHOCK Investigators. Early revascularization in acute myocardial infarction complicated by cardiogenic shock. N Engl J Med. 1999;341:625-34.

51. Antoniucci D, Santoro GM, Bolognese L, et al. A clinical trial comparing primary stenting of the infarct-related artery with optimal primary angioplasty for acute myocardial infarction: results from the Florence Randomised Elective Stenting in Acute Coronary Occlusion (FRESCO) trial. J Am Coll Cardiol. 1998;31:1234-9.

52. Grines CL, Cox DA, Stone GW, et al. on behalf of the Stent Primary Angioplasty in Myocardial Infarction Study Group. Coronary angioplasty with or without stent implantation for acute myocardial infarction. Stent Primary Angioplasty in Myocardial Infarction Study Group. N Engl J Med. 1999;341:1949-56.

53. Andersen HR, Nielsen TT, Rasmussen K, et al. on behalf of the DANAMI-2 Investigators. A comparison of coronary angioplasty with fibrinolytic therapy in acute myocardial infarction. N Engl J Med. 2003;349:733-42.

54. Pinto DS, Kirtane AJ, Nallamothu BK, et al. Hospital delays in reperfusion for ST-elevation myocardial infarction: implications when selecting a reperfusion strategy. Circulation. 2006;114:2019-25.

55. Nallamothu BK, Bates ER. Percutaneous coronary intervention versus fibrinolytic therapy in acute myocardial infarction: is timing (almost) everything? Am J Cardiol. 2003;92:824-6.

56. Chen ZM, Jiang LX, Chen YP, et al. on behalf of the COMMIT (ClOpidogrel and Metoprolol in Myocardial Infarction Trial) collaborative group. Addition of clopidogrel to aspirin in 45,852 patients with acute myocardial infarction: randomized placebo controlled trial. Lancet. 2005;366:1607-21.

57. Sabatine MS, Cannon CP, Gibson CM, et al. On behalf of the CLARITY-TIMI 28 Investigators. Addition of clopidogrel to aspirin and fibrinolytic therapy for myocardial infarction with ST-segment elevation. N Engl J Med. 2005;352:1179-89.

58. Montalescot G, Wiviott SD, Braunwald E, et al. On behalf of the TRITON-TIMI 38 investigators. Prasugrel compared with clopidogrel in patients undergoing percutaneous coronary intervention for ST-elevation myocardial infarction (TRITON-TIME 38): double-blind, randomised controlled trial. Lancet. 2009;373:723-31.

59. Stone GW, Witzenbichler B, Guagliumi G, et al. On behalf of the HORIZONS-AMI Trial Investigators. Bivalirudin during primary PCI in acute myocardial infarction. N Engl J Med. 2008;358:2218-30.

60. Chen ZM, Pan HC, Chen YP, et al. On behalf of the COMMIT (Clopidogrel and Metoprolol in Myocardial Infarction Trial) collaborative group. Early intravenous then oral metoprolol in 45,852 patients with acute myocardial infarction: randomized placebo-controlled trial. Lancet. 2005;366:1622-32.

61. White HD, Norris RN, Brown MA, et al. Left ventricular end-systolic volume as the major determinant of survival after recovery from myocardial infarction. Circulation. 1987;76:44-51.

62. The Multicenter Post Infarction Research Group. Risk stratification and survival after myocardial infarction. N Engl J Med. 1983;309:331-6.

63. Sanz G, Castañer A, Betriu A, et al. Determinants of prognosis in survivors of myocardial infarction: a prospective clinical angiographic study. N Engl J Med. 1982;306:1065-70.

64. Montalescot G, Cayla G, Collet JP, et al. for the ABOARD investigators. Immediate vs delayed intervention for acute coronary syndromes. JAMA. 2009;302:947-54.

65. Cooper WA, O'Brien SM, Thourani VH, et al. Impact of renal dysfunction on outcomes of coronary artery bypass surgery: results from the Society of Thoracic Surgeons National Adult Cardiac Database. Circulation. 2006;113:1063-70.

66. Lee DC, Oz MC, Weinberg AD, et al. Optimal timing of revascularization: transmural versus nontransmural acute myocardial infarction. Ann Thorac Surg. 2001;71:1197-202.

67. Imazio M, Negro A, Belli R, et al. Frequency and prognostic significance of pericarditis following acute myocardial infarction treated by primary percutaneous coronary intervention. Am J Cardiol. 2009;103:1525-9.

68. Frasure-Smith N, Lesperance F, Talajic M. Depression following myocardial infarction. Impact on 6-month survival. JAMA. 1993;270:1819-25.

69. Bush DE, Ziegelstein RC, Tayback M, et al. Even minimal symptoms of depression increase mortality risk after acute myocardial infarction. Am J Cardiol. 2001;88:337-41.

70. Carney R, Blumenthal JA, Catellier D, et al. Depression as a risk factor for mortality after acute myocardial infarction. Am J Cardiol. 2003;92:1277-81.

71. Taylor CB, Youngblood ME, Catellier D, et al. Effects of antidepressant medication of morbidity and mortality in depressed patients after myocardial infarction. Arch Gen Psych. 2005;62:792-8.

72. de Vreede-Swagemakers JJ, Gorgels AP, Dubois-Arbouw WI, et al. Out-of-hospital cardiac arrest in the 1990s: a population-based study in the Maastricht area on incidence, characteristics and survival. J Am Coll Cardiol. 1997;30:1500-5.

73. Hypothermia after Cardiac Arrest Study Group. Mild therapeutic hypothermia to improve the neurologic outcome after cardiac arrest. N Engl J Med. 2002;346:549-56.

74. Bernard SA, Gray TW, Buist MD, et al. Treatment of comatose survivors of out-of-hospital cardiac arrest with induced hypothermia. N Engl J Med. 2002;346:557-63.

75. Field JM, Hazinski MF, Sayre MR, et al. 2010 American Heart Association Guidelines for Cardiopulmonary Resuscitation and Emergency Cardiovascular Care Science. Circulation. 2010;122: S639-933.

76. ISIS-4: a randomised factorial trial assessing early oral captopril, oral mononitrate, and intravenous magnesium sulphate in 58,050 patients with suspected acute myocardial infarction. ISIS 4 (Fourth International Study of Infarct Survival) Collaborative Group. Lancet. 1995;345:669-85.

77. GISSI-3: effects of lisinopril and transdermal glyceryl trinitrate singly and together on 6-week mortality and ventricular function after acute myocardial infarction. Gruppo Italiano per lo Studio della Sopra-vvivenza nell'infarto Miocardico. Lancet. 1994;343:1115-22.

78. Pfeffer MA, Braunwald E, Moye LA, et al. On behalf of the SAVE Investigators. Effect of captopril on mortality and morbidity in patients with left ventricular dysfunction after myocardial infarction. Results of the survival and ventricular enlargement trial. N Engl J Med. 1992;327:669-77.

79. Hess G, Preblick R, Hill J, et al. Effects of angiotensin-converting enzyme inhibitor or angiotensin receptor blocker therapy after hospital discharge on subsequent rehospitalization for acute myocardial infarction and heart failure. Congest Heart Fail. 2009;15:170-5.

80. Dickstein K, Kjekshus J. On behalf of the OPTIMAAL Steering Committee of the OPTIMAAL Study Group. Effects of losartan and captopril on mortality and morbidity in high-risk patients after acute myocardial infarction: the OPTIMAAL randomised trial. Optimal Trial in Myocardial Infarction with Angiotensin II Antagonist Losartan. Lancet. 2002;360:752-60.

81. Pfeffer MA, McMurray JJ, Velazquez EJ, et al. On behalf of the Valsartan in Acute Myocardial Infarction Trial Investigators. Valsartan, captopril, or both in myocardial infarction complicated by heart failure, left ventricular dysfunction, or both. N Engl J Med. 2003;349:1893-906.

82. Pitt B, Zannad F, Remme WJ, et al. On behalf of the Randomized Aldactone Evaluation Study Investigators. The effect of spironolactone on morbidity and mortality in patients with severe heart failure. Randomized Aldactone Evaluation Study Investigators. N Engl J Med. 1999;341:709-17.

83. Pitt B, Remme W, Zannad F, et al. On behalf of the Eplerenone Post-Acute Myocardial Infarction Heart Failure Efficacy and Survival Study Investigators. Eplerenone, a selective aldosterone blocker, in patients with left ventricular dysfunction after myocardial infarction. N Engl J Med. 2003;348:1309-21.

84. Yusuf S, Sleight P, Pogue J, et al. Effects of an angiotensin-converting-enzyme inhibitor, ramipril, on cardiovascular events in high risk patients. The Heart Outcomes Preventive Evaluation Study Investigators. N Engl J Med. 2000;342:145-53.

85. Watts GF, Lewis B, Brunt JN, et al. Effects on coronary artery disease of lipid-lowering diet, or diet plus cholestyramine, in the St Thomas' Atherosclerosis Regression Study (STARS). Lancet. 1992;339:563-9.

86. de Lorgeril M, Renaud S, Mamelle N, et al. Mediterranean alpha-linolenic acid-rich diet in secondary prevention of coronary heart disease. Lancet. 1994;343:1454-9.

87. Ornish D, Brown SE, Scherwitz LW, et al. Can lifestyle changes reverse coronary heart disease? The Lifestyle Heart Trial. Lancet. 1990;336:129-33.

88. Schuler G, Hambrecht R, Schlierf G, et al. Regular physical exercise and low-fat diet. Effects on progression of coronary artery disease. Circulation. 1992;86:1-11.

89. Expert panel on detection, evaluation, and treatment of high blood cholesterol in adults. Executive Summary of the Third Report of the National Cholesterol Education Program (NCEP) Expert Panel on Detection, Evaluation, and Treatment of High Blood Cholesterol in

Adults (Adult Treatment Panel III). J Am Med Assoc. 2001;285:2486-97.

90. Grundy SM, Cleeman JI, Merz CN, et al. Implications of recent clinical trials for the National Cholesterol Education Program Adult Treatment Panel III guidelines. Circulation. 2004;110:227-39.

91. The Scandinavian Simvastatin Survival Study Group. Randomised trial of cholesterol lowering in 4444 patients with coronary heart disease: the Scandinavian Simvastatin Survival Study (4S). Lancet. 1994;344:1383-9.

92. Sacks FM, Pfeffer MA, Moye LA, et al. on behalf of the Cholesterol and Recurrent Events Trial investigators. The effect of pravastatin on coronary events after myocardial infarction in patients with average cholesterol levels. N Engl J Med. 1996;335:1001-9.

93. Heart Protection Study Collaborative Group. MRC/BHF Heart Protection Study of cholesterol lowering with simvastatin in 20,536 high-risk individuals: a randomised placebo-controlled trial. Lancet. 2002;360:7-22.

94. Cannon CP, Braunwald E, McCabe CH, et al. on behalf of the Pravastatin or Atorvastatin, Evaluation and Infection Therapy—Thrombolysis in Myocardial Infarction 22 Investigators. Intensive versus moderate lipid lowering with statins after acute coronary syndromes. N Engl J Med. 2004;350:1495-504.

95. Stenestrand U, Wallentin L. On behalf of the Swedish Register of Cardiac Intensive Care (RIKS-HIA). Early statin treatment following acute myocardial infarction and 1 year survival. J Am Med Assoc. 2001;285:430-6.

96. Schwartz GG, Olsson AG, Ezekowitz MD, et al. on behalf of the Myocardial Ischemia Reduction with Aggressive Cholesterol Lowering (MIRACL) Study Investigators. Effects of atorvastatin on early recurrent ischemic events in acute coronary syndromes: the MIRACL study: a randomized controlled trial. JAMA. 2001;285:1711-8.

97. de Lemos JA, Blazing MA, Wiviott SD, et al. on behalf of the A to Z Investigators. Early intensive vs a delayed conservative simvastatin strategy in patients with acute coronary syndromes: phase Z of the A to Z trial. JAMA. 2004;292:1307-16.

98. Pedersen TR, Cater NB, Faergeman O, et al. Comparison of atorvastatin 80 mg/day versus simvastatin 20 to 40 mg/day on frequency of cardiovascular events late (five years) after acute myocardial infarction [from the Incremental Decrease in Endpoints through Aggressive Lipid Lowering (IDEAL) trial]. Am J Cardiol. 2010;106:354-9.

99. Rosenson RS. Pluripotential mechanisms of cardioprotection with HMG-CoA reductase inhibitor therapy. Am J Cardiovasc Drugs. 2001;1:411-20.

100. Rauoof MA, Iqbal K, Mir MM, et al. Measurement of plasma lipids in patients admitted with acute myocardial infarction or unstable angina pectoris. Am J Cardiol. 2001;88:165-7.

101. Smith CS, Cannon CP, McCabe CH, et al. Early initiation of lipid-lowering therapy for acute coronary syndromes improves compliance with guideline recommendations: observations from the Orbofiban in Patients with Unstable Coronary Syndromes (OPUS-TIMI 16) trial. Am Heart J. 2005;149:444-50.

102. Canner PL, Berge KG, Wenger N, et al. Fifteen years mortality in Coronary Drug Project patients: long-term benefit with niacin. J Am Coll Cardiol. 1986;8:1245-55.

103. The AIM-HIGH Investigators. The role of niacin in raising high-density lipoprotein cholesterol to reduce cardiovascular events in patients with atherosclerotic cardiovascular disease and optimally treated low-density lipoprotein cholesterol: baseline characteristics of study participants. The Atherothrombosis Intervention in Metabolic syndrome with low HDL/high triglycerides: Impact on Global Health outcomes (AIM-HIGH) trial. Am Heart J. 2011;161:538-43.

104. Marchioli R, Barzi F, Bomba E, et al. on behalf of the GISSI Prevenzione Investigators. Early protection against sudden death by polyunsaturated fatty acids after myocardial infarction; a time-course analysis of the results of the Gruppo Italiano per lo Studio della Sopravvivenza nell'infarto Miocardico (GISSI)-Prevenzione. Circulation. 2002;105:1897-903.

105. Gerstein HC, Miller ME, Byington RP, et al. The Action to Control Cardiovascular Risk in Diabetes study Group. Effects of Intensive Glucose lowering in Type 2 Diabetes. N Engl J Med. 2008;358:2545-59.

106. Intensive blood-glucose control with sulphonylureas or insulin compared with conventional treatment and risk of complications in patients with type 2 diabetes (UKPDS 33). UK Prospective Diabetes Study (UKPDS) Group. Lancet.1998;352:837-53.

107. Gaede P, Vedel P, Larsen N, et al. Multifactorial intervention and cardiovascular disease in patients with type 2 diabetes. N Engl J Med. 2003;348:383-93.

108. National Heart lung and Blood Institute. (2003).The Seventh Report of the Joint National Committee on Prevention, Detection, Evaluation, and Treatment of High Blood Pressure (JNC 7). [online] NHLBI website. Available from http://www.nhlbi.nih.gov/guidelines/hypertension/. [Accessed December, 2003].

109. Goldenberg I, Jonas M, Tenenbaum A, et al. on behalf of the Bezafibrate Infarction Prevention Study Group. Current smoking, smoking cessation, and the risk of sudden cardiac death in patients with coronary artery disease. Arch Intern Med. 2003;163:2301-5.

110. Smith PM, Burgess E. Smoking cessation initiated during hospital stay for patients with coronary artery disease: a randomized controlled trial. CMAJ. 2009;180:1297-303.

111. Critchley J, Capewell S. Smoking cessation for the secondary prevention of coronary heart disease. Cochrane Database Syst Rev. 2004;CD003041.

112. Johansson S, Bergstrand R, Pennert K, et al. Cessation of smoking after myocardial infarction in women: effects on mortality and reinfarctions. Am J Epidemiol. 1985;121:823-31.

113. The Health Consequences of Involuntary Exposure to Tobacco Smoker. A Report of the Surgeon General. 2006. [online] Available from http://www.surgeongeneral.gov/library/secondhandsmoke/report/fullreport.pdf. [Accessed 2006].

114. Lancaster T, Stead L. Physician advice for smoking cessation. Cochrane Database Syst Rev. 2004.

115. Rigotti NA, Thorndike AN, Regan S, et al. Bupropion for smokers hospitalized with acute cardiovascular disease. Am J Med. 2006;119:1080-7.

116. Lancaster T, Stead L, Silagy C, et al. Effectiveness of interventions to help people stop smoking: findings from the Cochrane Library. BMJ. 2000;321:355-8.

117. Jorenby DE, Leischow SJ, Nides MA, et al. A controlled trial of sustained-release bupropion, a nicotine patch, or both for smoking cessation. N Engl J Med. 1999;340:685-91.

118. Hurt RD, Sachs DP, Glover ED, et al. A comparison of sustained-release bupropion and placebo for smoking cessation. N Engl J Med. 1997;337:1195-202.

119. Gonzales D, Rennard SI, Nides M, et al. On behalf of the Varenicline Phase 3 Study Group. Varenicline, an alpha 4 beta 2 nicotinic acetylcholine receptor partial agonist, vs sustained-release bupropion and placebo for smoking cessation: a randomized controlled trial. JAMA. 2006;296:47-55.

120. Jorenby DE, Hays JT, Rigotti NA, et al. On behalf of the Varenicline Phase 3 Study Group. Efficacy of varenicline, an alpha4beta2 nicotinic acetylcholine receptor partial agonist, vs placebo or sustained-release bupropion for smoking cessation: a randomized controlled trial. JAMA. 2006;296:56-63.

121. Ebbert JO, Croghan IT, Sood A, et al. Varenicline and bupropion sustained-release combination therapy for smoking cessation. Nicotine Tob Res. 2009;11:234-9.

122. Ebbert JO, Burke MV, Hays JT, et al. Combination treatment with varenicline and nicotine replacement therapy. Nicotine Tob Res. 2009;11:572-6.

123. Branca G, Capodanno D, Capranzano P, et al. Early discharge in acute myocardial infarction after clinical and angiographic risk assessment. J Cardiovasc Med. 2008;9:858-61.

124. Wenger NK, Froelicher ES, Smith LK, et al. AHCPR Supported Guidelines. Clinical Practice Guideline Number 17: Cardiac Rehabilitation. US Dept of Health and Human Services. Public Health Service. Agency for Health Care Policy and Research. National Heart, Lung, and Blood Institute, October 1995. AHCPR publication No. 96-0672.

125. Balady GJ, Ades PA, Comoss P, et al. Core components of cardiac rehabilitation/secondary prevention programs: a statement for healthcare professionals from the American Heart Association and the American Association of Cardiovascular and Pulmonary Rehabilitation Writing Group. Circulation. 2000;102:1069-73.

126. Leon AS, Franklin BA, Costa F, et al. Cardiac rehabilitation and secondary prevention of coronary heart disease: an American Heart Association Scientific Statement from the Council on Clinical Cardiology (Subcommittee on Exercise, Cardiac Rehabilitation, and Prevention) and the Council on Nutrition, Physical Activity, and Metabolism (Subcommittee on Physical Activity), in collaboration with the American Association of Cardiovascular and Pulmonary Rehabilitation. Circulation. 2005;111:369-76.

127. Ades PA. Cardiac rehabilitation and secondary prevention of coronary heart disease. N Engl J Med. 2001;345:892-902.

128. Wenger NK. Current status of cardiac rehabilitation. J Am Coll Cardiol. 2008;51:1619-31.

129. Artham SM, Lavie CJ, Milani RV. Cardiac rehabilitation programs markedly improve high-risk profiles in coronary patients with high psychological distress. Southern Med J. 2008;101:262-7.

130. Lavie CJ, Milani RV. Adverse psychological and coronary risk profiles in young patients with coronary artery disease and benefits of formal cardiac rehabilitation. Arch Intern Med. 2006;166:1878-83.

131. Taylor RS, Brown A, Ebrahim S, et al. Exercise-based rehabilitation for patients with coronary heart disease: systematic review and meta-analysis of randomized controlled trials. Am J Med. 2004;116:682-92.

132. Hamill BG, Curtis LH, Schulman KA, et al. Relationship between cardiac rehabilitation and long-term risks of death and myocardial infarction among elderly Medicare beneficiaries. Circulation. 2010;121:63-70.

133. Briffa TG, Eckermann SD, Griffiths AD, et al. Cost-effectiveness of rehabilitation after an acute coronary event: a randomized controlled trial. Med J Aust. 2005;183:450-5.

134. Papadakis S, Reid RD, Coyle D, et al. Cost-effectiveness of cardiac rehabilitation program delivery models in patients at varying cardiac risk, reason for referral, and sex. Eur J Cardiovasc Prev Rehabil. 2008;15:347-53.

135. Oldridge N, Furlong W, Feeny D, et al. Economic evaluation of cardiac rehabilitation soon after acute myocardial infarction. Am J Cardiol. 1993;72:154-61.

136. Suaya JA, Shepard DS, Normand ST, et al. Use of cardiac rehabilitation by Medicare beneficiaries after myocardial infarction or coronary bypass surgery. Circulation. 2007;116:1653-62.

137. Ades P, Pashkow F, Nestor J. Cost-effectiveness of cardiac rehabilitation after myocardial infarction. J Cardiopulm Rehabil. 1997;17:222-31.

138. Lee A, Strickler G, Shepard DS. The economics of cardiac rehabilitation: a review of the literature. J Cardiopulm Rehabil. 2007;27:135-42.

139. Grines CL, Maarsalese D, Brodie B, et al. On behalf of the PAMI investigators. Safety and cost-effectiveness of early discharge after primary angioplasty in low risk patients with acute myocardial infarction. J Am Coll Cardiol. 1998;31:967-72.

140. Kovoor P, Lee AK, Carrozzi F, et al. Return to full normal activities including work at two weeks after acute myocardial infarction. Am J Cardiol. 2006;97:952-8.

141. Isaaz K, Coudrot M, Sabry MH, et al. Return to work after acute ST-elevation myocardial infarction in the modern era of reperfusion by direct percutaneous coronary intervention. Arch Cardiovasc Dis. 2010;103:310-6.

142. Waszkowska M, Szymczak W. Return to work after myocardial infarction: a retrospective study. Int J Occup Med Environ Health. 2009;22:373-81.

Management of Patients with Chronic Coronary Artery Disease and Stable Angina

Prakash C Deedwania, Enrique V Carbajal

Chapter Outline

INTRODUCTION

Ischemic heart disease (IHD), usually due to underling coronary artery disease (CAD), remains the leading cause of mortality in the United States and in developed countries.[1,2] In many patients with IHD, stable angina seems to be the initial clinical manifestation. Additionally, many patients who survive a nonfatal acute coronary syndrome (ACS), such as unstable angina or an acute myocardial infarction (MI), go onto experience anginal symptoms after such an acute event.[3] It can be estimated that there are 30 cases of stable angina for every patient with MI who is hospitalized.[1] This estimate, however, does not include patients who do not seek medical attention for their chest pain or whose chest pain has a noncardiac cause. Overall, it is estimated that more than 10 million Americans suffer from stable angina. Stable angina is important not only because of its high prevalence, but also because of its associated morbidity and mortality.

In many patients, anginal symptoms could be disabling and frightening, and present a challenge for the clinician on a frequent basis. Effective treatment for symptom control in patients with chronic stable angina is an essential therapeutic goal to improve quality of life and clinical outcomes. Angina occurs, whenever there is myocardial ischemia due to an imbalance between myocardial perfusion and myocardial oxygen demand. In most patients myocardial ischemia occurs due to a flow limiting coronary stenotic lesion secondary to atherosclerotic process. However, it is important to recognize that although the high grade stenotic lesions are responsible for the impaired coronary blood flow, it is the less stenotic (< 50% stenosis), so-called, "vulnerable" plaques that seem to be responsible for most cases of ACS. Therefore, the treatment of patients with chronic stable angina should not only aim at relief of symptoms by correcting the imbalance between myocardial oxygen demand and supply, but it should also be directed towards stabilization of the vulnerable plaque to reduce the risk of future coronary events.

There two major goals of therapy in patients with chronic stable angina: relief of symptoms and reduction in cardiac morbidity and mortality. There are multiple medical and revascularization modalities available for treatment of anginal symptoms, however, recent data suggest that current therapies are not universally effective in controlling symptoms and most do not reduce cardiovascular events. For example, studies have shown that despite optimal revascularization many patients continue to experience anginal symptoms and as many as two-thirds of the patients might require one or more antianginal drugs.[1,3] It is also known that persistence of symptoms in patients with stable angina is associated with impaired quality of life.[4] Additionally, despite a strong push for routine revascularization in most patients with stable angina, there is little evidence that such strategy improves survival in patients with stable CAD.

CURRENT THERAPEUTIC APPROACHES FOR STABLE ANGINA

There are multiple therapeutic modalities currently available for treatment of anginal symptoms in patients with stable CAD. These include antianginal drugs and myocardial revascularization procedures. Until recently, the antianginal drug therapy primarily consisted of nitrates, beta-blockers and calcium channel blockers (CCB). Although antianginal drug therapy is effective in most patients, it is not infrequent that many patients are subjected to percutaneous or surgical revascularization. In the following section, we will discuss currently available treatment modalities for stable angina, and examine their effectiveness in controlling symptoms as well as their impact on cardiovascular outcomes.

ANTIANGINAL DRUG THERAPY

Several antianginal agents primarily nitrates, beta-blockers and CCB (Table 1) have been used in the management of symptoms in patients with chronic CAD and stable angina pectoris.[1,2,5-7] Although these drugs have been found to be effective antianginal agents, there is lack of data on the effect of such therapies on clinical outcomes including MI and death in patients with chronic CAD and stable angina.[1,5,6] Despite the popularity of nitrates and beta-blockers in patient with angina, these drugs have not been evaluated in prospective randomized clinical trials regarding their impact on hard clinical end points such as myocardial infarction and cardiac death.

NITRATES

Nitrates exert their beneficial effects primarily by venodilatation resulting in venous pooling of blood, which reduces ventricular volume and cardiac work and chamber size (Table 1). Nitrates are also systemic as well as coronary arterial vasodilators; however, to what extent these effects account for their antianginal efficacy is not well established (except in patients with coronary artery spasm). It is well established that sublingual nitroglycerine is the most effective therapy for relief of anginal symptoms and all patients with anginal symptoms should be given sublingual nitroglycerin. The long acting nitrates are often prescribed as prophylactic antianginal drugs and are particularly effective in patients who are nitrate responders. However, because of the problem of nitrate tolerance during long term therapy, it is essential to use eccentric dosing scheme which provides a minimum of 10–12 hours nitrate free interval.[1,5,6] Although effective in symptom control, nitrate therapy has not been evaluated regarding impact on cardiovascular outcomes. Some of the important side effects/limitations of nitrates and other antianginal drugs in the treatment of stable angina are shown in Table 2.

BETA-BLOCKERS

Beta-blockers have been found to be effective antianginal therapy by increasing exercise tolerance and decreasing the frequency and severity of anginal episodes.[1,2,5,6,8] Beta-blockers exert their effects through a reduction in myocardial oxygen demand which includes a decrease in ventricular inotropy, decreased heart rate and a decrease in the maximal velocity of myocardial fiber shortening. Therapy with beta-blockers has been associated with a reduced risk of death (sudden and non-sudden) and reduced risk of MI in patients who survived an acute MI. However, it is not known whether similar benefit would occur in stable angina patients without prior MI.

TABLE 1

Pharmacologic actions of antianginal drugs

Class	Heart rate	Arterial pressure	Venous return	Myocardial contractility	Coronary flow
β-blockers	↓	↓	↔	↓	↔
DHP CCB	↑*	↓	↔	↓	↑
Non-DHP CCB	↓	↓	↔	↓	↑
Long acting nitrates	↑/↔	↓	↓	↔	↑
Ranolazine†	↔	↔	↔	↔	↔

*Except amlodipine
†Late Na + channel blocker
(Abbreviations: ↓: Decrease, ↔: No effect; ↑: Increase

TABLE 2

Side effects, precautions and contraindications of antianginal drugs

	Beta-blockers	Nitrates	Calcium channel blockers	Ranolazine
Side effects	• Hypotension • Syncope • Sexual dysfunction • Fatigue • Depression	• Hypotension • Syncope • Headache • Tolerance	• Hypotension • Flushing • Dizziness • Edema • Fatigue	• Dizziness • Headache • Constipation • Nausea
Precautions/ contraindications	• Bradycardia • AV conduction problems • Sick sinus syndrome • Peripheral vascular disease • COPD	• Left ventricular outflow tract obstruction • Erectile dysfunction (concomitant use of PDE5 inhibitors)	• Bradycardia • AV conduction problems • Sick sinus syndrome • Heart failure • LV dysfunction	• Use with QT prolonging drugs • Significant liver disease • Contraindicated with strong CYP3A4 inhibitors (ketoconazole, clarithromycin, or nelfinavir) and CYP3A inducers (rifampin, phenobarb)

Although no prospective, randomized controlled trial (RCT) has evaluated the effect of therapy with beta-blocker(s) on clinical outcomes in patients with chronic CAD and stable angina, there is limited data available regarding the impact of beta-blocker therapy on clinical outcomes in asymptomatic, or minimally symptomatic patients with CAD. The atenolol silent ischemia study (ASIST)[9] evaluated the effects of atenolol on clinical outcomes and ischemia during daily life in patients with documented CAD who were asymptomatic, or minimally symptomatic [Canadian cardiac society classification (CCS) class I or II]. Compared to placebo, treatment with atenolol was associated with a significantly lower risk (11.1% vs 25.3%, respectively) of the primary combined end point that included death, resuscitation from ventricular tachycardia/fibrillation (VT/VF), nonfatal MI, hospitalization for unstable angina, aggravation of angina requiring known antianginal therapy, or need for myocardial revascularization during the follow-up period of 12 months. There was no difference between the treatment groups on the incidence of individual hard end points such as death and nonfatal MI most likely due to a lack of power to identify significant differences. Table 2 illustrates some of the limitations/side effects of beta-blocker therapy in the treatment of stable angina.

CALCIUM CHANNEL BLOCKERS

Calcium channel blockers (CCB) are potent coronary and systemic arterial vasodilators, and these agents reduce blood pressure as well as cardiac contractility. CCBs have been shown to increase coronary blood flow and are highly effective antianginal agents in patients with coronary artery spasm. CCBs have become popular in treatment of patients with angina primarily because of the relatively lower incidence of side effects. However, like other antianginal drugs, their impact on cardiovascular outcomes in patients with stable CAD and angina has not been systematically evaluated in RCT. There is limited information available from the "a coronary disease trial investigating outcome with nifedipine gastrointestinal therapeutic system" (ACTION) study,[10] which evaluated the effects of the long acting CCB nifedipine (nifedipine GITS) on the combined end point defined as death, acute MI, refractory angina, congestive heart failure, nonfatal stroke, or need for peripheral arterial revascularization in patients with stable symptomatic CAD. Compared to placebo, therapy with nifedipine GITS was associated with similar rates of the combined primary end point, as well as the individual end points of death, MI and stroke. Therapy with nifedipine GITS was associated with a small, but statistically significant, reduction in the "softer" end points of need for coronary angiography and need for coronary artery bypass graft surgery (CABGS). The important side effects and limitation of CCB are shown in Table 2.

NEWER ANTIANGINAL DRUGS

Although there has been lack of development of newer antianginal drugs during the past 25 years, recently several new drugs with unique mechanism of action have been introduced for treatment of patients with stable angina. In the following section, we will discuss two of these agents that have recently become available or about to become available to the clinician for the treatment of patients with stable angina.

RANOLAZINE

Ranolazine is the newest drug recently approved by the Food and Drug Administration (FDA) for use in the initial or supplementary treatment of patient with chronic angina.[11,12] Although the precise mechanism of ranolazine is not established, it is thought to be related to selective late sodium channel blockade. The findings from clinical trials that have evaluated ranolazine suggest that its antianginal effect is different than that of currently available conventional antianginal medications, as it is neither a coronary vasodilator, nor it is associated with reduction in hemodynamic parameters (e.g. heart rate, blood pressure, preload and inotropy) (Table 1).[13-15]

Several clinical trials have evaluated the antianginal efficacy of ranolazine in patients with confirmed diagnosis of CAD and inducible ischemia on treadmill exercise test. These trials have demonstrated that ranolazine used either as monotherapy, or as an add-on therapy to traditional antianginal drugs, including beta-blocker, CCB or nitrates, improves not only anginal symptoms, but also associated with improved performance during exercise testing. Based on the results of these trials ranolazine was initially approved for clinical use only in patients who had persistent anginal symptoms despite use of traditional antianginal drugs. This limited indication was primarily due to the concern about its safety related to the prolongation of the QT interval. However, this limited indication has now been expanded to unrestricted use of ranolazine in all patients with stable angina. This was possible primarily because of the safety of ranolazine demonstrated in a large cohort of high risk patients with ACS enrolled in the metabolic efficiency with ranolazine for less ischemia in non-ST-elevation acute coronary syndromes (MERLIN)-TIMI 36 study.[11,12]

The MERLIN trial also provided additional data regarding the antianginal efficacy of ranolazine. In the analysis of the pre-specified group of patients with history of chronic angina before an ACS,[12] in the MERLIN-TIMI 36 study, the long term effects of ranolazine on modification of antianginal therapy as well as improvement in the exercise duration during a stress test performed at the 8 months follow-up period was evaluated. Compared to patients on placebo, treatment with ranolazine was associated with: a significant improvement in anginal symptoms, need for additional antianginal drugs and longer exercise duration. Additionally, in this cohort of patients with prior history of angina, ranolazine was associated with a significantly lower risk of the primary combined end point at the 1 month follow-up (23.3% vs 19.8%, respectively P = 0.039) and at 12 months (29.4% vs 25.2%, respectively P = 0.017). This risk reduction was primarily due to a reduction in the rate of recurrent ischemia at 1 month (17.2% vs 13.7%, respectively P = 0.015) and at 12 months (21.1% vs 16.5%, respectively P = 0.002). However, at 12 months treatment with ranolazine did not significantly reduce the risk of CV death or MI (12.5% vs 11.9%, respectively).[11,12]

The findings from the available studies indicate that ranolazine is a safe and well tolerated antianginal medication. Ranolazine is effective in patients who continue to experience angina despite optimized treatment with other conventional antianginal agents. Ranolazine can also be safely used in patients with compromised hemodynamic parameters (e.g. baseline bradycardia and/or risk of developing significant hypotension). Furthermore, ranolazine can be used safely in patients with diabetes, COPD, LV dysfunction/heart failure and in those patients requiring Phosphodiesterase-5 inhibitor such as Sildenafil. Compared to other antianginal drugs, ranolazine has fewer side effects (Table 2).

IVABRADINE

Ivabradine is a newer drug that has been evaluated in patients with chronic CAD and stable angina (BEAUTIFUL. Lancet. 2008;372(9641):807-16). Ivabradine is a specific inhibitor of the I-f channels in the sinoatrial node. As a result, it is considered a pure heart rate lowering agent in patients with sinus rhythm. Ivabradine does not seem to have an effect on blood pressure, myocardial inotropy, intracardiac conduction, or ventricular repolarization (BEAUTIFUL. Lancet. 2008;372(9641):807-16). Ivabradine is an agent that seems effective in reducing myocardial ischemia, and in controlling symptoms in patients with chronic stable angina pectoris who are in sinus rhythm primarily by reducing heart rate. There have been several clinical trials that have evaluated the role of ivabradine as monotherapy, as well as an add-on therapy, and have shown its effectiveness in controlling anginal symptoms as well as increasing the exercise performance. In addition, the data from a large randomized clinical trial in patients with stable CAD and LV systolic dysfunction showed that treatment with ivabradine was associated with reduced incidence of CAD related outcomes in the subgroup of patients with resting heart rate 70 bpm or greater.[16]

COMBINATION THERAPY

Combination therapy is often necessary for adequate symptom control in many patients with stable angina. It is important to realize that the best combination therapy is the one that provides maximum symptoms relief with relatively few adverse effects. In general, combination therapy should utilize a beta-blocker with nitrate, or CCB based on patient's underlying comorbid conditions. Such combination may allow the clinician to use lower doses of each agent to achieve symptom control with minimal side effects. Additionally, several studies have shown effectiveness of ranolazine when added to standard therapy with beta-blockers, CCB and nitrates. Ranolazine has been particularly found to be quite useful in patients who remain symptomatic despite optimal doses of older established antianginal drugs. However, there has not been a systematic evaluation of combination therapy on hard clinical end points in patients with stable angina.

OTHER DRUGS IN PATIENTS WITH STABLE ANGINA AND CHRONIC CAD

ANGIOTENSIN CONVERTING ENZYME INHIBITORS

Because of the well demonstrated vasculoprotective effects of angiotensin converting enzyme inhibitors (ACEI), two recent studies evaluated their effects in patients with stable CAD or diabetes, and at least one other cardiovascular factor.[17,18] The heart outcomes prevention evaluation (HOPE) trial[17] evaluated the effect of ramipril 10 mg daily in a high risk population characterized by patients with history of CAD, stroke, peripheral vascular disease, or diabetes, and at least one other cardio-

vascular risk factor (hypertension, elevated total cholesterol levels, low high-density lipoprotein cholesterol levels, cigarette smoking or documented microalbuminuria). These patients had no prior history of heart failure and had no evidence of depressed LV systolic function. Compared to placebo, treatment with the ACEI was associated with a significantly lower absolute risk (17.8% vs 14%, respectively) of experiencing the composite end point (MI, stroke or CV death) as well as a significantly lower risk of each individual end point.[17] Secondary end points were death from any cause, admission to hospital for congestive heart failure, or unstable angina, complications related to diabetes and cardiovascular revascularization.[17] Compared to placebo, the ramipril arm underwent significantly fewer cardiovascular revascularizations (18.3% vs 16%, P = 0.002) and experienced fewer complications related to diabetes (7.6% vs 6.4%, P = 0.03). The incidence of other secondary end points was similar between the groups.

The European trial on reduction of cardiac events with perindopril in stable coronary artery disease (EUROPA) study[18] evaluated the effect of another ACEI, perindopril, on clinical outcomes in patients with stable CAD and angina. In this study, compared to placebo, the therapy with perindopril resulted in a relatively small but significantly lower risk (9.9% vs 8%, respectively) of the composite end point (NFMI, CV death, or resuscitated arrest). Of the individual end points only the risk of NFMI was significantly lower during therapy with perindopril.

A meta-analysis of six studies,[19] including the HOPE and the EUROPA, evaluated the effect of ACEI therapy in patients with CAD, and preserved LV systolic function. The findings from this meta-analysis revealed that, compared to placebo, therapy with an ACEI was associated with a modest, statistically significant favorable effect resulting in reduced rates of CV death, all cause mortality and nonfatal MI.

Based on the findings of these two trials and the findings of the recent meta-analysis, an ACEI should be considered in stable patients who are considered to be at high risk of cardiovascular events, and in patients with stable CAD and angina pectoris.

LIPID LOWERING THERAPY

A number of studies during the last two decades have shown that lipid lowering therapy with statins not only reduces the risk of major acute coronary events (MACE) but it also reduces the need for revascularization as well as decreases the signs and symptoms of myocardial ischemia in patients with angina pectoris.[20-24]

The atorvastatin versus revascularization treatment (AVERT)[22] trial was a randomized study that evaluated the impact of lipid lowering therapy on outcomes in patients, with stable CAD and angina, who received atorvastatin and compared them to patients who underwent percutaneous myocardial revascularization with or without stent implantation. Treatment with atorvastatin 80 mg daily was associated with a lower risk of the primary composite end point defined as at least one of the following: death from cardiac causes, resuscitation after cardiac arrest, nonfatal MI, cerebrovascular accident, CABGS, angioplasty, and worsening angina with objective evidence resulting in hospitalization. There was no difference between the treatment groups in rates of cardiac death, nonfatal MI, or need for CABGS. It is important to note that, as expected, treatment with percutaneous coronary angioplasty (PTCA) was associated with significantly greater improvement in the severity of anginal symptoms as assessed by CCS. The quality of the AVERT study was not as robust compared to the previous trials, since it was conducted in an unmasked manner and was unclear if randomization was concealed.

Recently, several clinical trials have specifically evaluated the role of lipid lowering therapy with a statin as anti-ischemic therapy in patients with stable CAD. The Scandinavian simvastatin survival study (4S)[25] is one of the earlier studies that revealed the potential antianginal property of statin therapy. In this trial, 4444 patients with dyslipidemia and coronary heart disease (CHD) were randomized to receive treatment with placebo, or simvastatin during a period of 5.4 years. In a post hoc analysis, treatment with simvastatin, compared to placebo, was associated with a 26% reduction in new angina, or worsening angina, and a 37% reduction in the need to undergo revascularization. Furthermore, the simvastatin group treated with simvastatin, experienced a significant reduction in the risk of new or worsening intermittent claudication.

There is evidence from clinical assessment which suggests that the anti-ischemic efficacy of statins is comparable to that of the more established pharmacological antianginal medications. The double-blind atorvastatin amlodipine (DUAAL) trial [26] compared the anti-ischemic effects of atorvastatin with that of the CCB amlodipine. After treatment for 24 weeks, both treatments resulted in a similar significant reduction in myocardial ischemia detected during ambulatory electrocardiography (AECG) and exercise testing. The marked decrease in the frequency of angina and the use of nitroglycerin was seen during treatment with amlodipine, which was equivalent to the effect seen during the treatment with atorvastatin. These findings lead to the conclusion that atorvastatin was a similar antianginal agent as amlodipine.[26]

In addition, there is evidence in the medical literature showing a favorable influence of statins on myocardial ischemia in patients with CHD. The vascular basis for the treatment of myocardial ischemia study[23] of patients with dyslipidemia, stable CHD and documented ischemia on stress testing or on AECG showed that 12 months of treatment with a statin using either intensive or moderate dosing strategies led to a significant reduction in the duration of ischemia and on the frequency of anginal episodes. Statin therapy also resulted in a significant improvement in exercise duration prior to onset of ischemia on the ECG.

Another major clinical trial, the study assessing goals in the elderly (SAGE)[27] compared intensive (atorvastatin 80 mg daily) to moderate (pravastatin 40 mg daily) statin therapy in nearly 900 patients with CHF and at least one documented episode of myocardial ischemia on AECG. After 1 year of follow-up, the trial demonstrated that statin therapy, using either intensive or moderate dosing strategies, was associated with a significant 37% reduction in the total duration of myocardial ischemia on AECG, a benefit that was evident as early as 3 months into the study. Similar to the findings in the Vascular Basis Study, there was no significant difference between treatment groups in the total duration of ischemia despite a greater cholesterol reduction in those who received intensive statin therapy[27]. However, a trend towards fewer occurrences of major adverse cardiac events

was also seen in the intensive lipid-lowering arm. Remarkably, high-dose atorvastatin was associated with a significant 77% reduction in total mortality. These findings suggest that the magnitude of LDL lowering that seems effective in the stabilization of vulnerable plaque and in the reduction of adverse clinical events may show a continuous relationship. When taken in context of the clinical outcomes utilizing revascularization and aggressive drug evaluation (COURAGE) trial[28] the results of these studies suggest that treatment with a statin in patients with chronic stable angina not only reduces the risk of future coronary events, but such therapy also has the potential of reducing myocardial ischemia and the associated symptoms. Therefore, it is recommended that all patients with chronic, stable angina should be treated with a statin to a goal of reducing LDL-C less than 70 mg/dl.

ROLE OF MYOCARDIAL REVASCULARIZATION

Myocardial revascularization (revascularization) has been evaluated and compared to medical treatments in patients with chronic stable angina. Revascularization includes CABGS and PTCA with or without stent deployment [percutaneous revascularization (PCI)]. Although revascularization provides relief of anginal symptoms, it seems to abolish anginal episodes in a minority of patients. A significant proportion of patients will continue to experience anginal symptoms after revascularization. Furthermore, revascularization procedures are often performed in asymptomatic patients with the intent of reducing the incidence of coronary events and cardiac death in patients with stable CAD. However, little data exists to support such benefit.

COMPARISON OF REVASCULARIZATION WITH PHARMACOLOGICAL ANTIANGINAL THERAPY

During the past four decades several studies[28-52] have compared the impact of pharmacological antianginal therapy versus revascularization in patients with chronic CAD and stable angina. In general, the results of these studies have shown that revascularization is usually more effective in symptom control compared to the conventional antianginal drug therapy. However, it is important to note that since the earlier time when many of the previous trials were conducted, the medical therapy of patients with stable angina has improved considerably with the routine use of beta-blockers, antiplatelet agents, ACEI and lipid lowering therapy particularly with statins, and as such the result of those earlier trials might not be applicable and pertinent today. A number of recent trials using these drugs have shown that medical therapy may be as effective as revascularization in controlling symptoms and, when aggressive risk factor modification is implemented, such strategy is also effective in reducing the risk of future coronary events in patients with chronic CAD and stable angina.[29,51,52] In the following section we will first review the results of the earlier randomized clinical trials with myocardial revascularization and then discuss the recently completed trials that compared the contemporary medical therapy (including comprehensive and aggressive risk factor modification) with the state-of-the-art revascularization procedure in stable CAD patients.

Three of the earlier major randomized CABGS studies: the VA cooperative study of surgery for coronary arterial occlusive disease (VACSS),[29-35] the European coronary surgery study (ECSS),[36-41] and the National Heart, Lung, and Blood Institute coronary artery surgery study (CASS)[42-46] were conducted on patients with angina and stable CAD. The CASS trial also included a group of post MI asymptomatic patients.

In these initial CABGS trials, all randomized patients continued to receive medical measures as needed to assist with control of anginal symptoms. In the VACSS, ECSS, and CASS studies, structured antianginal therapies were not provided, dosages were not controlled, and medical treatment was provided according to individual clinical practice patterns, thereby making the comparisons between pharmacological therapy and revascularization less meaningful. The VACSS and CASS trials included short and long acting nitrates as well as propranolol as antianginal agents. In the ECSS antianginal therapy was left to the clinical judgment of the care provider. Also, in all three trials, management of coronary risk factors was suggested but not enforced.

Applying an intention-to-treat (ITT) analysis approach, the VACSS, ECSS and CASS trials revealed similar mortality rates between the patients randomized to undergo CABGS, and the patients randomized to receive pharmacological antianginal therapy.[32,37,44-46] Only the ECSS showed that during long term follow-up there was a small, but statistically significant improvement in mortality rate with CABGS compared to medical therapy at some points in time.[37] The rates of MI in these trials were similar between the patients who underwent CABGS, compared to patient who did not undergo CABGS.[35,41,43] Surprisingly, the VACSS study reported a small, but statistically significant, increase in the incidence of nonfatal MI among patients who underwent CABGS compared to patients randomized to receive medical therapy.[35]

Each of these trials identified, on post hoc analyses, high risk subgroups that include patients with left main coronary (LMC) artery involvement,[30,31] patients with three-vessel CAD[36] and impaired LV function,[30,31] patients with p-LAD greater than 75% stenosis as a part of two-vessel or three-vessel CAD,[36] and patients with three-vessel CAD and LVEF less than 50%.[42,43]

The first official report by the VACSS described outcomes on the relatively small (n = 113) subgroup of patients with involvement of the LMC.[30] Although compared to medical therapy, CABGS was associated with a significant lower mortality risk (29.3% vs 7.1%, respectively) by 36 months of follow-up the mortality difference between the two groups was not statistically significant. The loss of significance is likely related to the initial small size of the subgroup and to progressive reduction in the size of the subgroup due to mortality during follow-up. In a subsequent report,[33] patients were further sub-grouped into those with a LMC showing a 50–75% stenosis (n = 47) and those with a LMC stenosis greater than 75% (n = 44). The subgroup with a LMC showing a 50–75% stenosis revealed no difference in mortality between the CABGS and no CABGS arms. However, the sub-analysis of the 44 patients with a LMC showing greater than 75% stenosis revealed a statistically significant reduction (17% vs 52%, respectively) in mortality among CABGS patients compared to patients randomized to medical therapy. Based on the findings from these

small subgroups,[30,33] a recommendation to offer CABGS was issued for patients receiving medical therapy. Subsequently, it became standard clinical practice to perform CABGS in patients with LMC showing greater than 50% stenosis. Since these results were published, no further attempts have been made to confirm, in a prospective randomized trial, the results of the VACSS in the subgroup of patients with involvement of the LMC. Interestingly, in the ECSS trial the post hoc analysis of the subgroup with LMC involvement revealed no difference in mortality between the CABGS and the no CABGS arms.[37]

In a different report, the VACSS evaluated another subgroup, this time without LMC involvement. This was the subgroup with three-vessel CAD plus impaired LV function.[35] In this angiographic high risk subgroup, compared to the medical therapy arm, CABGS improved survival up to 132 months of follow-up, after which this difference disappeared.

The ECSS evaluated the subgroups with two-vessel and three-vessel CAD.[36,38-40] In the subgroup with two-vessel CAD, there was no difference in mortality between the CABGS and medical therapy groups.[36,38-40] However, in the subgroup with three-vessel CAD, there was a statistically significant difference in survival favoring the CABGS group.[37] Further sub-analyses of the two-vessel CAD subgroup was carried out to separate the patients into those with either greater than or equal to 50% stenosis of the proximal LAD (p-LAD) and those without p-LAD involvement (< 50% stenosis) of the p-LAD.[39] This analysis revealed that in patients with two-vessel CAD plus p-LAD involvement CABGS, compared to medical therapy, was associated with a relatively small, but statistically significant, reduced mortality rate. When the sub-analysis was carried out with the p-LAD showing either greater than or equal to 75% stenosis, therapy with CABGS, compared to medical therapy, was associated with an even smaller, but statistically significant, improved survival.[41] Following these sub-analyses, the subgroup with p-LAD involvement (≥ 50% stenosis) and presence of two-vessel or three-vessel CAD was evaluated.[37] This sub-analysis revealed that CABGS, compared to medical therapy, was associated with a significantly lower mortality rate. Based of this sub-analysis,[37] patients with p-LAD involvement were identified as a high risk subgroup that appeared to derive benefit from therapy with CABGS.

In contrast, in the CASS trial, analysis of the subgroup with LAD involvement (≥ 70% stenosis in its proximal, mid, or distal sections) revealed no difference in mortality rates between patients randomized to undergo CABGS, and those randomized to medical therapy.[45] Additionally, in the CASS study CABGS compared to medical therapy was associated with improved survival in the subgroup with LVEF less than 50% as well as in the subgroup with LVEF less than 50% plus three-vessel involvement. In these two subgroups, the improved survival with CABGS became statistically significant at 84 months follow-up.[44,45] However, the analysis at 120 months in the subgroup with LVEF less than 50% plus three-vessel involvement, the survival benefit of CABGS was not significant anymore. Except for these findings, there was no difference in mortality between the treatment arms in patients sub-grouped by 1v, 2v or 3v involvement.[44,46] Based on these findings patients with LVEF less than 50% plus three-vessel involvement were identified as a high risk subgroup that appeared to benefit from therapy with CABGS.

Based on the angiographic profiles considered to confer higher risk to the various subgroups in the VACSS, ECSS and CASS studies, recommendations for treatment with CABGS were put into practice guidelines for patients with chronic CAD and stable angina who met a similar high risk angiographic criteria. Of the several subgroups identified by angiography as being at high risk, only the subgroup with p-LAD involvement was subsequently evaluated in a prospective manner in the medicine, angioplasty or surgery study (MASS-1).[47,48]

MEDICAL THERAPY VERSUS PERCUTANEOUS REVASCULARIZATION OR STRATEGIES COMPARING INVASIVE VERSUS OPTIMAL MEDICAL THERAPY

Several studies have evaluated the role of CABGS, PTCA/PCI, or medical treatment in patients with stable CAD. These include the asymptomatic cardiac ischemia pilot (ACIP),[31,32] the MASS trials,[47,48,51] the COURAGE trial[28] and the bypass angioplasty revascularization investigation 2 diabetes (BARI 2D) trial.[52]

The ACIP study[49,50] evaluated the effects of medical or revascularization (PTCA or CABGS) treatment strategies in patients with stable angiographic CAD ($\geq$ 50% stenosis) with or without angina, myocardial ischemia on AECG, and evidence of ischemia on an exercise treadmill test or pharmaceutical stress perfusion study. In this complex, partly blinded study, the three treatment strategies were angina-guided medical therapy; angina-guided plus AECG ischemia-guided medical therapy; and myocardial revascularization of major coronary arteries. Use of one or more unblinded antianginal medication(s) for control of symptoms was necessary in 77%, 70% and 39% of the treatment arms respectively. The primary end point was complete suppression of ischemia on 48 hours AECG. Secondary clinical outcomes at 12 months included death, MI, cardiac arrest, unstable angina, sustained ventricular tachycardia and congestive heart failure. Compared to the medical therapy arms, myocardial revascularization was associated with a significantly greater proportion of patients free of ischemia on AECG. However, compared to the medical therapy arms, revascularization therapy was associated with a similar risk of MI or stroke. Compared to angina-guided medical therapy only, revascularization was associated with a significantly lower mortality rate (4.4% vs 0.0%, respectively). Although, mortality rates were similar between the two medical treatment arms and between the revascularization and angina-guided plus AECG-guided medical therapy (1.6%).[49,50]

The MASS trial compared the effect of these therapies in patients with proximal-LAD (MASS-1)[47,48] and in patients with multi-vessel CAD (MASS-2).[51] In the MASS trials, all patients were placed on an optimal medical regimen that included: nitrates, aspirin, beta-blockers, CCB, ACEI, or a combination of these drugs. In addition, a statin along with a low-fat diet was provided on an individual basis.[47,48,51]

In the prospective MASS-1 trial[47,48] in patients with p-LAD involvement ($\geq$ 80% stenosis) compared to PTCA and medical therapy, CABGS was associated with a modest benefit on the combined outcome that consisted of cardiac death, MI, or angina requiring revascularization (the benefit was predominantly related to a reduced frequent need for subsequent revascularization).[47,48] It is important to note that compared to CABGS,

medical therapy was associated with a similar reduction in the risk of hard events (mortality or MI). Treatment with PTCA appeared to be an inferior option compared to the other treatment strategies.

In the MASS-2 trial[51] of patients with stable multi-vessel CAD, there was no difference in mortality between the medical therapy, medical therapy plus PTCA, and medical therapy plus CABGS groups. The group treated with medical therapy plus CABGS had the best outcome for the primary end point that consisted of cardiac death, Q-wave MI, or anginal symptoms requiring revascularization. The group with medical therapy plus PTCA appeared to have the worse outcome due to increased risk of MI as well as higher mortality.

Only a few trials have carefully examined the strategy of initial angiography/revascularization versus medical therapy in patients with stable CAD and angina pectoris.[53-58] The trial of invasive versus medical therapy in elderly patients (TIME)[55,56] with chronic symptomatic coronary-artery disease was a prospective, randomized, multi-center study in patients aged 75 years or more with angina CCS class II or more despite treatment with either two or more antianginal drugs. This study compared the invasive strategy of left-heart catheterization followed by either PCI or CABGS, with a strategy of optimized medical therapy with aimed at increase in the number of antianginal drugs and their doses to reduce anginal pain as much as possible. Additionally, antiplatelet agents and lipid-lowering drugs were advised. Compared to optimum medical therapy, the invasive strategy was associated with a lower risk of admission for ACS that required revascularization. However, compared to optimum medical therapy, the invasive strategy was associated with a similar risk of the hard end point of death or MI.

The second randomized intervention treatment of angina (RITA-2) trial[57,58] was designed to compare the effects of initial strategies of coronary angioplasty or conservative (medical) care over a follow-up of 5 years or more. Compared to medical treatment for symptom relief, treatment with PTCA was associated with similar risk of the primary combined end point (death or definite MI) or secondary hard end point (death). The pattern of unstable angina was similar in both groups. Although both groups remained symptomatic, an early intervention with PTCA was associated with greater, albeit temporary, symptomatic improvement in angina.

The COURAGE trial compared the clinical efficacy of PCI plus optimal medical therapy (OMT) versus OMT alone in patients with stable CAD.[28] OMT consisted of therapy with a beta-blocker and, when needed, diltiazem and aggressive management of risk factors for CAD. During the median follow-up of 55 months the OMT and the OMT plus PCI groups had similar rates of the primary combined (death and nonfatal MI) outcome (18.5% vs 19.0%, respectively) (Fig. 1). As expected a significantly greater proportion of patients in the PCI group were angina-free at 12 months (57% vs 50%, respectively, P = 0.005), however, this benefit was lost at 3 years (59% vs 56%, respectively) (Fig. 2).[59]

The BARI 2D trial[52] in patients with diabetes, CAD, and classic angina compared the effects of prompt revascularization by discretionary CABGS or PCI to medical therapy alone on clinical outcomes. During the 5-year follow-up there was no difference between the medical therapy and revascularization

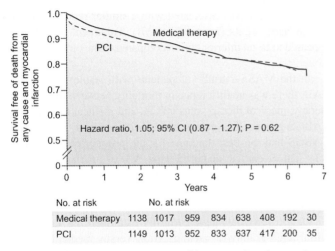

FIGURE 1: The estimated 4.6 year rate of the composite primary outcome of death from any cause and nonfatal myocardial infarction was 19.0% in the PCI group and 18.5% in the medical therapy group. (*Source:* Modified from reference 28, with permission)

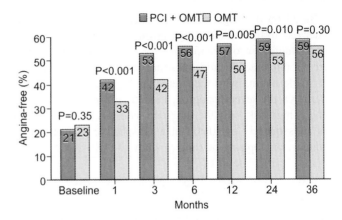

FIGURE 2: Freedom from angina over time as assessed with the angina-frequency scale of the Seattle angina questionnaire, according to treatment group. (Abbreviations: OMT: Optimal medical therapy; PCI: Percutaneous coronary intervention). (*Source:* Modified from reference 59, with perission)

groups on the risk (13.5% vs 13.2%, respectively) of the primary outcome (all cause-death), or the risk of MI (11.6% vs 10.0%, respectively), or the risk of stroke (2.8% vs 2.6%, respectively) (Figs 3A to D).

The above discussion of the early revascularization trials as well as the recent revascularization trials in patients with stable CAD have provided data that confirm the impression that, compared to medical treatment, revascularization has resulted

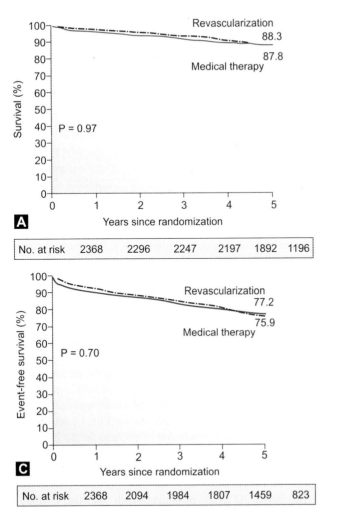

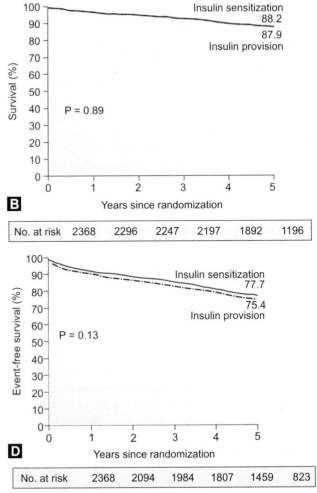

FIGURES 3A TO D: Rates of survival and freedom from major cardiovascular events. (A) There was no significant difference in rates of survival between the revascularization group and the medical therapy group and (B) between the insulin sensitization group and the insulin-provision group. (C) The rates of major cardiovascular events (death, myocardial infarction, or stroke) also did not differ significantly between the revascularization group and the medical therapy group or (D) between the insulin sensitization group and the insulin provision group. (*Source:* Modified from reference 52, with permission)

in similar rates of hard clinical outcomes in the main groups. The consistent benefit of revascularization, compared to medical treatment, appears to be a more striking, albeit temporary, improvement in anginal discomfort.

CONCLUSION

There are many therapeutic options available for the treatment of anginal symptoms in patients with stable CAD. These options include nitrates, beta-blockers, CCB, and ranolazine. Although combination therapy is often necessary for symptomatic relief, there has been no evaluation of the effects of combination antianginal therapy on hard clinical end points in such patients. Recent trials have shown that medical therapy is as effective as revascularization in controlling symptoms and, along with aggressive risk factor modification, is highly effective in reducing the risk of future coronary events. There is need for more definitive outcomes studies which examine the role of existing therapies (including aggressive and comprehensive risk factor modification), and newer antianginal agents with the state-of-the-art revascularization procedure in high risk patients with stable CAD and chronic angina.

GUIDELINES
ACC/AHA/ACP-ASIM GUIDELINES FOR THE MANAGEMENT OF PATIENTS WITH CHRONIC STABLE ANGINA: EXECUTIVE SUMMARY AND RECOMMENDATIONS CIRCULATION 1999; 99:2829-48

Kanu Chatterjee

Class I: Conditions for which there is evidence and /or general agreement that a given procedure or treatment is useful and effective.

Class II: Conditions for which there is conflicting evidence and/or a divergence of opinion about the usefulness/efficacy of a procedure or treatment.

Class IIa: Weight of evidence/opinion is in favor of usefulness/efficacy.

Class IIb: Usefulness/efficacy is less well established by evidence/opinion.

Class III: Conditions for which there is evidence and/or general agreement that the procedure/treatment is not useful/effective and in some cases may be harmful.

Level of Evidence A: The presence of multiple randomized clinical trials.

Level of Evidence B: The presence of a single randomized trial or nonrandomized studies.

Level of Evidence C: Expert consensus.

RECOMMENDATIONS FOR PHARMACOTHERAPY TO PREVENT MI AND REDUCE SYMPTOMS

Class I
1. Aspirin in the absence of contraindications (Level of Evidence A).
2. Beta-blockers as initial therapy in absence of contraindications in patients with prior MI (Level of Evidence A).
3. Beta-blockers as initial therapy in absence of contraindications in patients without prior MI (Level of Evidence B).
4. Heart rate regulating calcium channel antagonists and/or long-acting nitrates as initial therapy when beta-blockers are contraindicated (Level of Evidence B).
5. Heart rate regulating calcium channel antagonists and/or long-acting nitrates in combination with beta-blockers when initial treatment with beta-blockers is not successful (Level of Evidence B).
6. Heart rate regulating calcium antagonists and/or long-acting nitrates as a substitute for beta-blockers if initial treatment with beta-blockers leads to unacceptable side effects (Level of Evidence C).
7. Sublingual nitroglycerin or nitroglycerin spray for the immediate relief of angina (Level of Evidence C).
8. Lipid-lowering therapy in patients with documented or suspected CAD and LDL cholesterol > 130 mg/dl with a target LDL of < 100 mg/dl (Level of Evidence A).

Class IIa
1. Clopidogrel when aspirin is absolutely contraindicated (Level of Evidence B).
2. Long-acting heart rate regulating calcium channel blocking agents instead of beta-blockers as initial therapy (Level of Evidence B).
3. Lipid-lowering therapy in patients with documented or suspected CAD and LDL cholesterol between 100 and 129 mg /dl, with a target of 100 mg/dl (Level of Evidence B).

Class IIb
1. Low-intensity anticoagulation with warfarin in addition to aspirin (Level of Evidence B).

Class III
1. Dipyridamole (Level of Evidence B).
2. Chelation therapy (Level of Evidence B).

1. Gibbons R, Abrams J, Chatterjee K, et al.(2002). ACC/AHA 2002 guideline update for the management of patients with chronic stable angina: a report of the American College of Cardiology/American Heart Association Task Force on Practice Guidelines (Committee to update the 1999 guidelines for the management of patients with chronic stable angina). [online] Available from www.acc.org/clinical/guidelines/stable/stable.pdf.

2. Fox K, Garcia MA, Ardissino D, et al. Guidelines on the management of stable angina pectoris: executive summary: the task force on the management of stable angina pectoris of the european society of cardiology. Eur Heart J. 2006;27:1341-81.

3. Holubkov R, Laskey WK, Haviland A, et al. Angina 1 year after percutaneous coronary intervention: a report from the NHLBI dynamic registry. Am Heart J. 2002;144:826-33.

4. Rumsfeld JS, Magid DJ, Plomondon ME, et al. History of depression, angina and quality of life after acute coronary syndromes. Am Heart J. 2003;145:493-9.

5. Abrams J. Clinical practice. Chronic stable angina. N Engl J Med. 2005;352:2524-33.

6. Abrams J, Thadani U. Therapy of stable angina pectoris: the uncomplicated patient. Circulation. 2005;112:e255-9.

7. Opie LH, Commerford PJ, Gersh BJ. Controversies in stable coronary artery disease. Lancet. 2006;367:69-78.

8. Reiter MJ. Cardiovascular drug class specificity: beta-blockers. Prog Cardiovasc Dis. 2004;47:11-33.

9. Pepine C, Cohn P, Deedwania P, et al. Effects of treatment on outcome in mildly symptomatic patients with ischemia during daily life. The Atenolol Silent Ischemia Study (ASIST). Circulation. 1994;90:762-8.

10. Poole-Wilson PA, Lubsen J, Kirwan BA, et al. A coronary disease trial Investigating outcome with nifedipine gastrointestinal therapeutic system investigators. Effect of long-acting nifedipine on mortality and cardiovascular morbidity in patients with stable angina requiring treatment (ACTION trial): randomised controlled trial. Lancet. 2004;364:849-57.

11. Morrow D, Scirica BM, Karwatowska-Prokopczuk E, et al. Effects of ranolazine on recurrent cardiovascular events in patients with non-ST-elevation acute coronary syndromes: the MERLIN-TIMI 36 randomized trial. JAMA. 2007;297:1775-83.

12. Wilson SR, Scirica BM, Braunwald E, et al. Efficacy of ranolazine in patients with chronic angina observations from the randomized, double-blind, placebo-controlled MERLIN-TIMI (Metabolic Efficiency With Ranolazine for Less Ischemia in Non-ST-Segment Elevation Acute Coronary Syndromes) 36 trial. J Am Coll Cardiol. 2009;53:1510-6.

13. Dobesh PP, Trujillo TC. Ranolazine: a new option in the management of chronic stable angina. Pharmacotherapy. 2007;27:1659-76.

14. Stone PH. Ranolazine: new paradigm for management of myocardial ischemia, myocardial dysfunction, and arrhythmias. Cardiol Clin. 2008;26:603-14.

15. Keating GM. Ranolazine: a review of its use in chronic stable angina pectoris. Drugs. 2008;68:2483-503.

16. Fox K, Ford I, Steg PG, et al. Ivabradine for patients with stable coronary artery disease and left-ventricular systolic dysfunction. (BEAUTIFUL): a randomised, double-blind, placebo-controlled trial. Lancet. 2008;372:807-16.

17. Yusuf S, Sleight P, Pogue J, et al. Effects of an angiotension-converting-enzyme inhibitor, Ramipril on cardiovascular events in high-risk patients. The heart outcomes prevention evaluation study investigators. N Engl J Med. 2000;342:145-53.

18. Fox KM. Efficacy of perindopril in reduction of cardiovascular events among patients with stable coronary artery disease: randomised, double-blind, placebo-controlled, multicentre trial (the EUROPA study). Lancet. 2003;362:782-8.

19. Al-Mallah MH, Tleyjeh IM, Abdel-Latif AA, et al. Angiotensin-converting enzyme inhibitors in coronary artery disease and preserved left ventricular systolic function: a systematic review and meta-analysis of randomized controlled trials. J Am Coll Cardiol. 2006;47:1576-83.

20. Randomised trial of cholesterol lowering in 4444 patients with coronary heart disease: the Scandinavian Simvastatin Survival Study (4S). Lancet. 1994;344:1383-9.

21. Schwartz GG, Olsson AG, Ezekowitz MD, et al. Effects of atorvastatin on early recurrent ischemic events in acute coronary syndromes: the MIRACL study: a randomized controlled trial. JAMA. 2001;285:1711-8.

22. Pitt B, Waters D, Brown WV, et al. Aggressive lipid-lowering therapy compared with angioplasty in stable coronary artery disease. Atorvastatin versus Revascularization Treatment Investigators. N Engl J Med. 1999;341:70-6.

23. Stone PH, Lloyd-Jones DM, Kinlay S, et al. Vascular Basis Study Group. Effect of intensive lipid lowering with or without antioxidant vitamins, compared with moderate lipid lowering on myocardial ischemia in patients with stable coronary artery disease: the vascular basis for the treatment of myocardial ischemia study. Circulation. 2005;111:1747-55.

24. Deedwania PC. Effect of aggressive versus moderate lipid-lowering therapy on myocardial ischemia: the rationale, design, and baseline characteristics of the Study Assessing Goals in the Elderly (SAGE). Am Heart J. 2004;148:1053-9.

25. Pedersen T, Kjekshus J, Pyorala K, et al. Effect of simvastatin on ischemic signs and symptoms in the Scandinavian simvastatin survival study (4S). Am J Cardiol. 1998;81:333-5.

26. Deanfield JE, Sellier P, Thaulow E, et al. Potent anti-ischaemic effects of statins in chronic stable angina: incremental benefit beyond lipid lowering? Eur Heart J. 2010;31:2650-9.

27. Deedwania P, Stone PH, Bairey Merz CN, et al. Effects of intensive versus moderate lipid-lowering therapy on myocardial ischemia in older patients with coronary heart disease: results of the study assessing goals in the elderly (SAGE). Circulation. 2007;115:700-7.

28. Boden WE, O'Rourke RA, Teo KK, et al. Optimal medical therapy with or without PCI for stable coronary disease. N Engl J Med. 2007;356:1503-16.

29. Takaro T, Hultgren HN, Detre KM, et al. Effects of intensive versus moderate lipid-lowering therapy on myocardial ischemia in older patients with coronary heart disease results of the study assessing goals in the elderly (SAGE). Circulation. 1975;52:143.

30. Takaro T, Hultgren HN, Lipton MJ, et al. The VA cooperative randomized study of surgery for coronary arterial occlusive disease II. Subgroup with significant left main lesions. Circulation. 1976;54:III 107-17.

31. Detre K. Eleven-year survival in the veterans administration randomized trial of coronary bypass surgery for stable angina. The veterans administration coronary artery bypass surgery cooperative study group. N Engl J Med. 1984;311:1333-9.

32. Peduzzi P, Kamina A, Detre K. Twenty-two-year follow-up in the VA cooperative study of coronary artery bypass surgery for stable angina. Am J Cardiol. 1998;81:1393-9.

33. Takaro T, Peduzzi P, Detre KM, et al. Survival in subgroups of patients with left main coronary artery disease. Veterans Administration Cooperative Study of Surgery for Coronary Arterial Occlusive Disease. Circulation. 1982;66:14-22.

34. Murphy ML, Hultgren HN, Detre K, et al. Treatment of chronic stable angina. A preliminary report of survival data of the randomized Veterans Administration cooperative study. N Engl J Med. 1977;297;621-7.

35. Eighteen-year follow-up in the Veterans Affairs cooperative study of coronary bypass surgery for stable angina. The VA coronary artery bypass surgery cooperative study group. Circulation. 1992;86:121-30.

36. Coronary artery bypass surgery in stable angina pectoris: survival at two years. European Coronary Surgery Study Group. Lancet. 1979;1:889-93.

37. Varnauskas E. Twelve-year follow-up of survival in the randomized European coronary surgery study. N Engl J Med. 1988;319:332-7.

38. Prospective randomised study of coronary artery bypass surgery in stable angina pectoris. Second interim report by the European Coronary Surgery Study Group. Lancet. 1980;2:491-5.

39. Prospective randomized study of coronary artery bypass surgery in stable angina pectoris: a progress report on survival. Circulation. 1982;65:67-71.

40. Long-term results of prospective randomised study of coronary artery bypass surgery in stable angina pectoris. European Coronary Surgery Study Group. Lancet. 1982;2:1173-80.

41. Varnauskas E. Survival, myocardial infarction, and employment status in a prospective randomized study of coronary bypass surgery. Circulation. 1985;72:V90-101.

42. The principal investigators of CASS and their associates. The national heart, lung and blood institute coronary artery surgery study (CASS). Circulation. 1981;63:I 1-81.

43. Myocardial infarction and mortality in the coronary artery surgery study (CASS) randomized trial. N Engl J Med. 1984;310:750-8.

44. Killip T, Passamani E, Davis K. Coronary artery surgery study (CASS): a randomized trial of coronary bypass surgery. Eight years follow-up and survival in patients with reduced ejection fraction. Circulation. 1985;72:V102-9.

45. Alderman EL, Bourassa MG, Cohen LS, et al. Ten-year follow-up of survival and myocardial infarction in the randomized coronary artery surgery study. Circulation. 1990;82:1629-46.

46. Coronary artery surgery study (CASS): a randomized trial of coronary artery bypass surgery. Survival data. Circulation. 1983;68:939-50.

47. Hueb WA, Bellotti G, deOliveira SA, et al. The Medicine, Angioplasty or Surgery Study (MASS): a prospective, randomized trial of medical therapy, balloon angioplasty or bypass surgery for single proximal left anterior descending artery stenoses. J Am Coll Cardiol. 1995;26:1600-5.

48. Hueb W, Soares P, Almeida DeOliveira S, et al. Five-year follow-op of the medicine, angioplasty or surgery study (MASS): a prospective, randomized trial of medical therapy, balloon angioplasty or bypass surgery for single proximal left anterior descending coronary artery stenosis. Circulation. 1999;100:II 107-13.

49. The ACIP investigators. Asymptomatic cardiac ischemia pilot study (ACIP). Am J Cardiol. 1992;70:744-7.

50. Rogers WJ, Bourassa MG, Andrews TC, et al. Asymptomatic Cardiac Ischemia Pilot (ACIP) study: outcome at 1 year for patients with asymptomatic cardiac ischemia randomized to medical therapy or revascularization. The ACIP Investigators. J Am Coll Cardiol. 1995;26:594-605.

51. Hueb W, Soares PR, Gersh BJ, et al. The medicine, angioplasty or surgery study (MASS-II): a randomized, controlled clinical trial of three therapeutic strategies for multivessel coronary artery disease: one-year results. J Am Coll Cardiol. 2004;43:1743-51.

52. BARI 2D Study Group, Frye RL, August P, et al. A randomized trial of therapies for type 2 diabetes and coronary artery disease. N Engl J Med. 2009;360:2503-15.

53. Spargias KS, Cokkinos DV. Medical versus interventional management of stable angina. Coron Artery Dis. 2004;15:S5-10.

54. Parisi AF, Folland ED, Hartigan PA. A comparison of angioplasty with medical therapy in the treatment of single-vessel coronary artery disease. Veterans Affairs ACME Investigators. N Engl J Med. 1992;326:10-6.

55. The TIME Investigators. Trial of invasive versus medical therapy in elderly patients with chronic symptomatic coronary-artery disease (TIME): a randomised trial. Lancet. 2001;358:951-7

56. Pfisterer M, Buser P, Osswald S, et al. Outcome of elderly patients with chronic symptomatic coronary artery disease with an invasive vs optimized medical treatment strategy. One-year results of the randomized TIME trial. JAMA. 2003;289:1117-23.

57. Coronary angioplasty versus medical therapy for angina: the second Randomised Intervention Treatment of Angina (RITA-2) trial. RITA-2 trial participants. Lancet. 1997;350:461-8.

58. Henderson RA, Pocock SJ, Clayton TC, et al. Seven-year outcome in the RITA-2 trial: coronary angioplasty versus medical therapy. J Am Coll Cardiol. 2003;42:1161-70.

59. Weintraub WS, Spertus JA, Kolm P, et al. Effect of PCI on quality of life in patients with stable coronary disease. N Engl J Med. 2008;359:677-87.

Management of Patients with Chronic Coronary Artery Disease and Stable Angina

Variant Angina

Reza Ardehali, John Speer Schroeder

Chapter Outline

INTRODUCTION

The term "variant angina" was coined by Prinzmetal in 1959 when he and his co-workers published a description of three patients that varied from traditional exertional or Heberden's angina.[1,2] The prime "variant" features were typical of angina pectoris except that it occurred at rest or during sleep rather than during exertion and an electrocardiogram (ECG) during an episode of chest pain showed ST segment elevation suggestive of an acute myocardial infarction (MI) rather than ST segment depression. However, resolution of the pain by sublingual nitroglycerine spontaneously resulted in resolution of the abnormal ST segment elevation. The authors proposed that this syndrome was most likely due to temporary occlusion of a large diseased coronary artery, due to local spasm or an intermittent "increased tonus".

Previous observers have also commented on the possibility of spasm of coronary artery causing or contributing to the angina pectoris syndrome. Osler observed that angina pectoris was associated with changes in the arterial wall that were organic or functional.[3] Then, in 1941, Wilson and Johnston reported a patient with ST segment elevation in ECG leads II, III and AVF during spontaneous episodes of chest pain and observed that the attendant myocardial ischemia is due to a change in caliber of coronary arteries affected, rather than an increase in work of the heart.[4]

Variant angina pectoris was considered a relatively rare problem until the advent of coronary arteriography in the early 1970s, when it was observed that as many as 10% of patients with rest or unstable angina have a normal or relatively normal coronary arteriogram.[5] The initial work of Prinzmetal was supported by MacAlpin and his colleagues who reported angiographic findings in 20 patients of variant angina.[6] Subsequently, the introduction of a provocative test for Prinzmetal's angina allowed more precise definition, characterization and understanding of the syndrome.[7] Many of Prinzmetal's theories about the pathophysiology of variant angina have turned out to be remarkably perceptive.

This chapter focuses on variant angina rather than discuss the multiple angina syndrome in which coronary artery spasm may play a role, such as cardiac syndrome X, coronary microvascular disease, inherited thrombophilia or cocaine use.

INCIDENCE AND PREDISPOSING RISK FACTORS

Between 10% and 30% of patients who undergo coronary angiogram are found to have arteriographically normal coronary arteries.[8,9] Despite a normal angiogram, the presence of angina and ischemic ECG findings suggests a cardiac origin for chest pain. It is difficult to identify the precise incidence of variant angina, as different authorities have used different diagnostic tests and criteria to define it. There may also be racial variations in incidence. Large studies from France and North America have found an incidence of 12.3% and 4% positive ergonovine testing,[10,11] whereas a smaller Japanese group reported an incidence of 32.3% using intracoronary acetylcholine.[12] The variability in these reports highlights the differences between patient populations. Although no definitive risk factors have yet been identified, several studies have suggested a number of genetic and environmental risk factors that predispose people to coronary spasm and variant angina (Table 1).[13]

TABLE 1

Predisposing factors

- Racial predisposition
- Age and sex
- Cigarette smoking
- Insulin resistance
- Hormonal variation
- Classic coronary artery disease risk factors

PATHOPHYSIOLOGY

The original hypothesis by Prinzmetal and his colleagues that stated angina is induced by a transient increase in coronary vasomotor tone has been convincingly confirmed by angiographic studies. In contrast to exertion-induced angina pectoris in which the pain and myocardial ischemia reflect an inadequate increase in coronary blood flow through the diseased coronary vessel as myocardial work and oxygen demand increase, variant angina occurs due to a transient reduction in coronary flow. This reduction in flow due to a decrement in vessel diameter can be abrupt and transient causing myocardial ischemia angina symptoms. Although this etiology has been proposed for many years, and repeatedly demonstrated experimentally, the first patient with documented spontaneous coronary spasm during coronary arteriography was reported by Oliva and his co-workers in 1973.[14] Since that time, numerous investigators have observed and reported focal coronary artery spasm occurring either spontaneously or after provocation during coronary arteriography.[15,16] There is little doubt that this focal spasm is responsible for the reduction in coronary flow and causes transient transmural myocardial ischemia, resulting the chest pain or variant angina. The coronary spasm tends to be focal and frequently occurs at an area of atherosclerosis plaque or abnormality in the vessel. MacAlpin and his associates have reported that the focal spasm tends to occur in the same area on repeated occasions and in an area of atherosclerotic plaque during both spontaneous and provoked spasm.[17] The spasm can occur in any of the coronary arteries, although the right coronary artery and, to a lesser degree, the left anterior descending coronary artery are the ones most commonly involved. Patients with very severe coronary artery spasm have been observed to have spasm in more than one vessel or for the spasm to involve a greater length of the vessel. Incomplete occlusion of the vessel has been observed repeatedly. This may cause nontransmural myocardial ischemia in the area supplied by the vessel, resulting ST segment depression or even silent ischemia in these patients. It is believed, however, that this nontransmural ischemia is simply part of the spectrum of coronary artery spasm and that causes for occasionally incomplete spasm are the same as those for complete occlusion of a vessel.

Stress cardiomyopathy or takotsubo cardiomyopathy is a disorder associated with transient left ventricular dysfunction that occurs usually after a stressful event in patients who may or may not have atherosclerotic disease. Several studies have suggested that coronary vasospasm can lead to left ventricular wall-motion abnormalities resembling those in stress-cardiomyopathy.[18,19] It has been shown that substantially elevated plasma catecholamine levels is seen in stress cardiomyopathy.[20,21] This observation could be particularly relevant in inducing coronary vasospasm. However, whether there is a direct cause-effect relationship between coronary vasospasm and stress-cardiomyopathy remains unknown. Furthermore, global coronary vasospasm cannot explain the common variant of stress-cardiomyopathy, which mainly involves apical ballooning with basal sparing.

There are three questions regarding the pathophysiology of coronary artery spasm:

1. Why does the spasm tend to occur in a localized area of the vessel?
2. What initiates or precipitates the spasm?
3. What are the underlying molecular mechanisms?

First, the fact that spasm tends to occur in areas of abnormality or atherosclerotic plaques suggests a local hyperreactivity in the wall of the coronary artery. It has been observed that patients with variant angina tend to have recurrent episodes in the same location, suggesting that this is a local abnormality or hyperreactivity to some vasoconstrictive influence rather than to a generalized hyperreactivity or abnormality in the innervation or level of sympathetic tone of coronary vessels. Ginsburg and his co-workers have reported that in human coronary arteries, areas containing atherosclerotic plaques tend to be more reactive to some vasoconstrictive influences such as histamine in comparison to areas that are not involved with the atherosclerotic process.[22] These studies have been confirmed by other investigators and suggest that a local abnormality may be responsible for the spasm. In addition, it has been recognized that varying provocative agents can precipitate coronary artery spasm in an individual patient. This would suggest that it is not the agent but an abnormality in vasoreactivity in the area where the spasm occurs which is responsible for the spasm and the clinical symptoms.

Second, what are the precipitating causes of this focal spasm in an area of local increased vasoreactivity? Many hypotheses have been proposed including increased vagal tone during sleep. This hypothesis has been supported by the use of methacholine inducing coronary spasm in some reports.[23,24] However, the mechanism for the actual vasoconstrictor triggering of the focal spasm during this period is not understood. Other authors have proposed that the focal spasm occurs at times of increased vagal tone when there is unopposed withdrawal of sympathetic tone such as during sleep or after exercise. Other hypotheses have centered around the general or local release of vasoconstrictive substances such as thromboxane A_2 or sympathomimetic amines; however, these theories would not explain the focality of the spasm.

It is most likely that two circumstances are required to have typical variant angina. One is a local hyperreactivity of a segment of coronary artery, and the other is abnormal release or triggering of the vasoconstrictive influence.

CLINICAL PRESENTATION

The typical patient with variant angina reports recurrent episodes of angina pectoris that are typical in their character, distribution and responsiveness to nitroglycerine. They tend to be younger compared to those with classic stable or unstable angina secondary to atherosclerotic disease. The pain is substernal, with a tight, constricting pressure sensation in the chest that may radiate into the neck, jaw, teeth or inner aspect of the left and/or right arm. Occasionally, patients report the pain occurring predominantly in the jaw or arm with minimal or no chest pain. The pain typically awakens the patients at night or in the early morning hours and can be very severe. Other episodes may occur after arising in the early morning or at other times of the day during rest. In addition to the unprovoked episodes, approximately 50% of patients also report at least some angina related to physical exertion or excitement, but these episodes may occur after cessation of the activity rather than at its peak. Although the circadian nature of the attacks usually remains similar for a given patient, the frequency and severity of the episodes tend to be highly variable and cyclical. Many patients report general worsening of their symptoms during periods of emotional stress in their lives.

The angina usually resolves spontaneously after a few minutes but may last much longer. Response to sublingual nitroglycerine tends to be excellent; in fact, the diagnosis should be questioned if there is not a rapid response to either oral or sublingual nitrates. Patients may complain of anxiety or shortness of breath during the angina if the pain is prolonged and causes transient left ventricular dysfunction and pulmonary venous congestion. In fact, transient left ventricular apical ballooning (LVAB) cardiomyopathy, which leads to severe myocardial dysfunction may occur in the presence of normal coronary arteries on angiography. A recent report demonstrated reproduction of LVAB and coronary spasm in the catheterization laboratory during acetylcholine testing.[25]

In addition to a careful history and characterization of the pain, one should look for other features of the variant angina syndrome and for manifestation of other vasospastic phenomena. Most patients present between ages of 35–50 years. There is a female predominance and a frequent smoking history, and most patients acknowledge stress or tension either in their personal life or job. There is frequently a history of migraine headache in the patient or his/her family. Complaints of Raynaud's phenomenon are common, and some patients simply complain that their hands and feet have been cold all of their lives.

A high index of suspicion for variant angina is important since these patients may themselves attribute their chest pains to nerves and unless the diagnosis of variant angina is being considered many of these patients are diagnosed as having psychogenic chest pain. The report that the chest pain awakens them from sleep is one of the most important clues that this is a medical problem rather than a psychological one.

DIAGNOSIS

HISTORY AND PHYSICAL EXAMINATION

The hallmark of a patient with variant angina is the history of spontaneous or unprovoked episodes of typical angina pectoris. At times when the patient is not having variant angina, examination is usually normal or unrelated to variant angina syndrome. During an episode of pain, the patient may manifest symptoms of pain, sweating, tachycardia or increased blood pressure in response to the pain. Ventricular arrhythmias are common. The patient with right coronary spasm may have varying degrees of atrioventricular (AV) block. More severe or prolonged episodes of myocardial ischemia may result in manifestations of left ventricular dysfunction, such as an S_3 or S_4 gallop rhythm, bibasilar rales or pulmonary congestion or a transient murmur of mitral insufficiency due to ischemic papillary muscle dysfunction. The diagnosis, however, although suspected on the basis of history and physical examination must be confirmed on the ECG and preferably during coronary arteriography.

Laboratory Findings

It is not easy to distinguish variant angina from coronary artery disease due to atherosclerosis based on laboratory data. Since coronary spasms may cause transient occlusion of the vessel, prolonged episodes of myocardial ischemia may lead to release of cardiac biomarkers. Recent studies have demonstrated elevated levels of circulating inflammatory cells, including white blood cells (WBC) and monocytes, as well as high levels of plasma *C-reactive protein* (CRP) and *interleukin-6 (*IL-6) among patients with variant angina.[26,27]

NONINVASIVE STUDIES

ECG Studies

To establish the diagnosis of typical variant angina, it is essential to observe transient ST segment elevation on an ECG during an episode of spontaneous angina pectoris. The ECG abnormalities occur in the areas supplied by the artery that is undergoing coronary spasm and is transiently occluded. The ST segment elevation can be either minimal or at times very dramatic, nearly obscuring the QRS complex and appearing to be the initial ECG manifestation of an acute transmural MI (Figs 1A and B). However, the ST segment elevation resolves with the administration of sublingual nitroglycerin. It is not unusual to see ventricular arrhythmias or even ventricular tachycardia or complete heart block during an episode of severe coronary artery spasm. Since the episodes of pain tend to occur at night and spontaneously, it may be difficult to record an ECG during a severe episode of pain. There are several alternative approaches to this in order to establish a diagnosis.

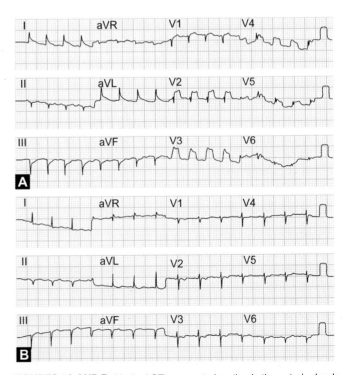

FIGURES 1A AND B: Marked ST segment elevation in the anterior leads of a 12-lead ECG during angina caused by spasm of the left anterior descending artery induced by 0.1 mg ergonovine maleate (A) and after nitroglycerin (B). (*Source:* Modified from Schroeder JS (Ed). Invasive Cardiology. Philadelphia, FA Daving, 1984. pp. 83-96)

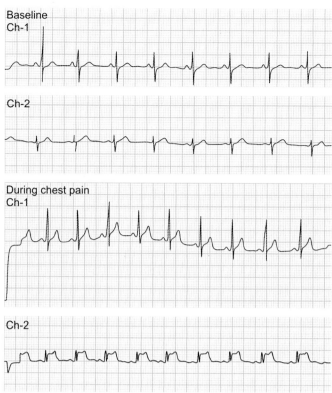

FIGURE 2: Two-channel ambulatory ECG recordings during pain-free period (upper panel) and during angina (lower panel). (*Source:* Modified from Schroeder JS (Ed). Invasive Cardiology. Philadelphia, FA Daving, 1984. pp. 83-96)

Ambulatory ECG Monitoring

If the patient is having frequent or daily episodes of chest pain, ambulatory ECG recordings may be effective in establishing the diagnosis. A two-channel recorder with sufficiently low frequency response to detect 0.1 mV changes is essential. By recording two channels, that is, one inferior and one anterior lead, ST segment elevation reflecting spasm of either the right or left anterior descending coronary artery may be observed (Fig. 2). In addition, patients who complain of syncope or palpitation may have arrhythmias or heart block documented during chest pain as well (Fig. 3).

At other times, patients may have minimal or no chest pain during the episode reflecting silent ischemia as detected on the ECG. In these patients there may be episodes of transient ST segment depression or even occasionally ST segment elevation that are brief and so do not come to clinical attention or result in complaints of angina. In order to establish a diagnosis of variant angina, it is preferable to have at least one episode of ST segment elevation in association with a complaint of or observed chest pain.

Self-Initiated Transtelephonic ECG Monitoring

Since many patients with angina have infrequent or unpredictable chest pain that is not suitable for diagnosis by ambulatory ECG monitoring, several studies have reported the use of transtelephonic transmission of an ECG during symptomatic chest pain.[28-30] Here, a transtelephonic device, such as cardiobeeper (Survival Technology) or cardiophone (Nihon Kohden), can be used to transmit one or two leads of an ECG during chest pain.[29,30] The episode can either be stored on certain units for subsequent transmission or be transmitted by telephone directly during chest pain and recorded for subsequent analysis. It is essential that a baseline transmission be taken for comparison owing to the highly variable nature of ST segment shifts. This system is quite helpful when it is positive, particularly if ST segment elevation is observed (Fig. 4). However, due to the single lead nature of the transmission system and the difficulty in ascertaining how severe the symptomatic episode of chest pain was, a negative test does not rule out a diagnosis of variant angina.

In-Hospital ECG Recording

Despite multiple attempts some patients elude establishment of a diagnosis of variant angina as outpatient because of the difficulty in obtaining a suitable ECG during chest pain. In these patients, it may be feasible to establish the diagnosis by hospitalizing the patient and attaching a 12-lead ECG to monitor the patient overnight. The patient can be instructed to push the record button if chest pain occurs in order to record a 12-lead ECG before nitroglycerine is administered or before the pain resolves spontaneously. This approach does not require support

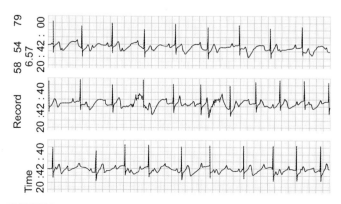

FIGURE 3: Computer printout of Holter ECG recording showing transient second-degree heart block. (*Source:* Modified from Ginsburg R, Schroeder JS, Harrison DC. Coronary artery spasm: pathophysiology, clinical presentations diagnostic approaches and rational treatment. West J Med 1982;136:398)

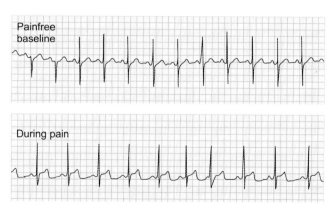

FIGURE 4: ST segment elevation compared with baseline, documented by transtelephonic ECG transmission during chest pain. (*Source:* Modified from Schroeder JS (Ed). Invasive Cardiology. Philadelphia, FA Daving, 1984. pp. 83-96)

CHAPTER 51

Variant Angina

from other medical personnel or the availability of a telephone, and it can be useful in the difficult-to-diagnose patient.

Treadmill Exercise Testing

Although the typical patient with variant angina who has relatively normal coronary arteries will have a negative treadmill exercise test and no exertional evidence of chest pain, there are several subgroups of patients who may have abnormalities during exercise testing. One group of patients may have coronary artery spasm that occurs shortly after cessation of exercise. The typical patient does very well during the treadmill test and has relatively normal exercise tolerance in the absence of any ST segment abnormalities. Once exercise has stopped, the onset of variant angina is noted within the first 5 minutes and at this time ST segment elevation is present. For this reason the ECG leads should be left on patient for at least 10 minutes post exercise. Another group of patients may have coronary artery spasm superimposed on a severely occlusive atherosclerotic lesion. These patients typically complain of effort-induced angina as well and can be identified by detecting either ST segment depression during low level exercise testing or poor exercise tolerance or even exercise-induced hypotension. It is essential that these patients who have ST segment depression plus a history of unprovoked and spontaneous angina undergo coronary arteriography to rule out severe proximal occlusive coronary artery disease.

Radionucleotide Scintigraphy

Several studies have demonstrated the utility of perfusion scintigraphy in detecting variant angina. Single-photon computed tomography (SPECT) and ^{123}I-β-methyl-p-iodophenyl pentadecanoic acid (BMIPP) and ^{123}I-metaiodobenzylguanidine (MIBG) scintigraphy have been used as non-invasive techniques to determine the presence and location of coronary spasm.[31,32] Furthermore, ^{13}N-ammonia positron emission tomography (PET) is an accurate method for myocardial blood flow quantification and presence of microvasculature defect.[33] Clinical utility of these tests need to be confirmed by larger studies.

CORONARY ARTERIOGRAPHY

Since unprovoked angina may be the first manifestation of unstable angina reflecting an extremely severe proximal coronary artery occlusion or early thrombotic occlusion, it is generally recommended that all patients with rest or unprovoked angina undergo coronary arteriography. This study allows definition of the severity of the coronary artery disease and assists in separating the severe occlusive coronary patient who may require angioplasty or surgery from the patient with variant angina who has normal coronary arteries and will respond to medical therapy.

Unless the patient gives a history suggestive of severe occlusive coronary disease, that is, either progressively severe effort angina or risk factors of coronary disease suggesting that this may not be variant angina, it is important to stop all anti-anginal medications for at least 24 hours prior to coronary arteriography. Nitroglycerine can be used for treatment of spontaneous episodes of pain until 1 hour prior to the procedure.

It is particularly important that all long-acting nitrates and transcutaneously applied nitrates, such as nitrate patches and calcium antagonists, be stopped. If the patient is having frequent episodes of pain, this should be done in the hospital under close medical observation.

Routine coronary arteriography is first accomplished to determine whether the patient has severe coronary artery disease and unstable angina or he has mild disease or completely normal vessels and, therefore, falls into the suspect variant angina group. Occasionally a patient will have a spontaneous episode of angina during the arteriogram and documentation of complete or incomplete focal spasm associated with the patient's typical chest pain will help establish the diagnosis. It is helpful to apply radiolucent electrode pads on the chest wall for a complete 12-lead ECG prior to start of arteriogram if variant angina is suspected. A three-channel 12-lead ECG machine can then be attached, and if the patient has angina or has complaints that suggest angina during the arteriogram, ST segment changes can be documented on the ECG. In most cases the patient will not have a spontaneous episode of chest pain, and after documentation of non-occlusive coronary disease or normal coronary arteries, it may be necessary to proceed with provocative testing (Fig. 1).

PROVOCATIVE TESTINGS

Intravenous administration of ergonovine was commonly used to provoke coronary arterial spasm in cardiac catheterization laboratory. However, due to several reports of irreversible coronary spasm and arrhythmias induced by ergonovine, many centers use methacholine as their standard provocative testing. The mechanism by which methacholine may precipitate coronary spasm is not clearly understood. One theory is that spasm results from direct stimulation of cholinergic muscarinic receptors on peripheral vascular smooth muscle, which then results in an abrupt fall in blood pressure with reflex-mediated increase in sympathetic tone. Compared to ergonovine, which acts through serotogenic receptors, the duration of acetylcholine effects is significantly shorter which makes it more attractive agent to use.

A common protocol used by many centers is summarized below.[34] It is essential to anticipate the need for acetylcholine testing so that informed consent, cessation of anti-anginal medication, and proper preparation of the patient can be accomplished prior to documentation of normal coronary vessel or insufficient coronary disease to explain the patient's rest angina. The sequential protocol includes injection of acetylcholine chloride in incremental doses of 20, 50 and 80 mg in 10 ml normal saline into the right coronary artery and 20, 50 and 100 mg into the left coronary artery over 20 seconds with at least a 3-minute interval between each injection. Patients are asked to report any chest pain graded on a scale of 1–10. A standard 12-lead ECG must record every 30 seconds. One minute after each injection, or when chest pain or significant ischemic ST changes appear, coronary arteriogram are obtained.

DIFFERENTIAL DIAGNOSIS

The most important group of patients to consider in the differential diagnosis at the time that a patient presents with

TABLE 2

Clinical characteristics of angina subtypes

	Stable	Unstable	Variant
Chest pain			
Character	Typical	Typical	Typical
Onset	Exertion	Rest/Exertion	Rest
ECG during	ST depression	ST depression	ST elevation
Pain		Occasional ST	Occasional ST
Elevation depression arteriography	Coronary CAD	Severe CAD	Normal or mild CAD
(Abbreviation: CAD: Coronary artery disease)			

rest or nocturnal chest pain is those with unstable or crescendo angina due to severe underlying coronary artery disease (Table 2). Although most of these patients will have a history of known coronary artery disease or effort angina in the past, a few patients will present de novo with this syndrome. Factors that will be helpful in evaluating this patient are the presence of coronary artery disease risk factors, presence of an old MI on ECG, and persistent ECG evidence of ischemia, which would suggest a persistent occlusion or partial occlusion rather than a transient occlusion due to coronary spasm. In patients who have not had previous coronary arteriography, it is essential to proceed with this evaluation to rule out tight occlusion or preinfarction angina.

Most troublesome is the patient who develops typical chest pain in response to acetylcholine testing but does not have demonstrable significant focal spasm on coronary arteriography or major ST-segment changes on ECG. The pathophysiology of chest pain in many of these patients is poorly understood. Esophageal spasm has been proposed as a cause, although results of studies with acetylcholine provocation during esophageal manometry have been difficult to interpret. These patients may have spasm of intramural vessels or have small vessel coronary disease due to endothelial dysfunction that is poorly understood at this time.

Finally, it is important to remember that the coronary spasm generally responds extremely well to either sublingual or intravenous nitroglycerine. In the patient with persistent ST-segment elevation, the early phase of acute MI must be considered and ruled out.

MANAGEMENT

MEDICAL THERAPY

Acute treatment of the chest pain episode is generally sublingual nitroglycerine. This is highly effective treatment, which almost always reverses the spasm. In fact, the diagnosis of transient coronary spasm should be questioned if there is not an excellent response to the nitroglycerine. Other sublingual nitrate preparations may be useful as well in terminating the acute attack.

Long-acting oral nitrates have long been used for prophylaxis in patients with variant angina.[35] Oral agents, such as isosorbide dinitrate, extended release form and nitroglycerine paste, have all been reported to be effective. The primary limiting

factor with use of prophylactic nitrate therapy is the suspected development of tolerance in these patients, although it has been poorly documented in long-term clinical trials. Another limiting factor is the fact that many patients require high doses of nitrates for prophylaxis, which may lead to a significant frequency of adverse side effects, particularly headache and hypotension at a dose level that will prevent the spontaneous episodes of chest pain and angina. Controlled trials of nitrate efficacy for prophylaxis have been limited. Hirai and his colleagues demonstrated that simultaneous administration of an angiotensin II and type 1 receptor blockers suppressed the development of nitrate tolerance during transdermal nitroglycerine therapy.[36] They suggested that increased oxidative stress induced by activation of angiotensin II may be important in the development of nitrate tolerance. Hill and his co-workers reported on a double-blind randomized crossover comparison of nifedipine versus isosorbide dinitrate in 19 patients with variant angina.[37] There was a 72% decrease in angina frequency during nifedipine therapy and a 63% decrease during isosorbide dinitrate therapy compared with placebo. The authors concluded that the two agents were approximately equally effective in this particular trial. Intravenous administration of isosorbide dinitrate at a dose of 1.25–5.0 mg/hr has been reported to be effective in patients in whom oral agents did not control recurrent episodes of angina. In addition, sodium nitroprusside has been reported to be effective, but the adverse side effects of hypotension must be monitored carefully in this patient group.

Alpha-adrenergic blockers, such as phenoxybenzamine or phentolamine, have also been reported to be effective in preventing repeated episode of coronary artery spasm in variant angina patients.[35] The mechanism proposed is simply blockade of coronary artery α-receptors, resulting in prevention of focal spasm. Although these agents have been reported to be effective, it was common to have to achieve doses that cause significant orthostatic hypotension before they were effective in preventing episodes of coronary spasm. For this reason, these treatments have generally been abandoned with the advent of demonstrated excellent efficacy of the calcium blockers.

Treatment of Arrhythmias

Patients may either develop heart block due to spasm of the right coronary artery or ventricular arrhythmias, including sustained ventricular tachycardia, due to spasm of the right, circumflex or left anterior descending coronary arteries. These arrhythmias generally occur in the setting of either myocardial ischemia or reperfusion when the spasm is broken or resolves spontaneously. For this reason antiarrhythmic drugs are not very effective and treatment should be directed at the treatment or prevention of the focal coronary spasm. Patients who have episodes of second- or third-degree heart block and syncope who have not responded to prophylactic therapy with calcium blockers will benefit from a demand pacemaker. Additionally, patients with ischemia associated ventricular fibrillation, who continue to have ischemia despite treatment, should receive an implantable cardioverter-defibrillator.[38]

Calcium Antagonists

Calcium channel blockers have dramatically improved the success of therapy and most likely improved the long-term prognosis for patients with variant angina. The calcium antagonists block the influx of ionized calcium via slow channels during the plateau phase of action potential. This blocking action is more potent at the calcium channel of the vascular smooth muscle cells than of the myocardial cells. This differential effect allows relaxation of vascular smooth muscle at therapeutic concentrations of the drug, which results in minimal negative inotropic activity. The calcium antagonists, therefore, cause a decrease in coronary vascular tone and reactivity, which results in increase in coronary flow. These agents also appear to block the abnormal hyperreactivity or spasm of coronary vessels, which is the cause of variant angina. Clinical trials with calcium antagonists have conclusively shown marked reduction in angina frequency during therapy with calcium antagonists.

Diltiazam, nifedipine and verapamil are all effective for prophylaxis in variant angina. These agents have been proven efficacious in double-blind randomized clinical trials with 50–70% reduction in angina frequency and nitroglycerine consumption compared with a placebo control. Endo and his colleagues first reported, in 1975, that diltiazam was effective for prophylaxis of variant angina.[39] After initial experience with this agent in Japan, subsequent studies in the United States have confirmed that diltiazam is not only efficacious but also safe for short- and long-term efficacy in variant angina. Rosenthal and his co-workers reported on a total of 13 patients with documented coronary spasm and variant angina who completed a prospective randomized dose-finding crossover study of diltiazam, 120 mg/day and 240 mg/day, versus placebo, each given for a 2-week period.[40] The 240 mg/day dose of diltiazam resulted in a decrease in pain of 79% to 50% (P = 0.03) and a significant decrease in angina frequency from 1.6 to 0.4 episodes per day, with similar reductions in nitroglycerine consumption. There was no evidence for a rebound phenomenon when the diltiazam was abruptly changed to placebo, and there were no significant adverse side effects. These findings were confirmed by other investigators, including Pepine and his colleagues, who studied a similar group of patients in whom 64% had either complete or partial resolution of their angina during therapy with diltiazam.[41] Diltiazam has also been shown to be effective for long-term treatment of these patients without evidence of either tolerance or rebound. Rosenthal and his co-workers reported later reported on the long-term efficacy of diltiazam

in 16 patients with clinical variant angina.[42] This 44 weeks study involved eleven 28-day cycles with one random placebo period during the first five cycles and one during the last six cycles. There was a 73% decrease in angina frequency in phase I and a 55% decrease compared with placebo in phase II. In addition, marked disease attenuation was noted. Thus, diltiazam is effective as long-term therapy without evidence of drug tolerance developing.

Open-label experience with the patients who have been on diltiazam shows similar results. We first reported on 36 patients who were followed in the Stanford coronary artery spasm clinic for 6 months or more.[43] During a mean of 7.5 months of diltiazam therapy, angina frequency was reduced from 21.5 to 1.3 attacks per week on either 240 mg or 360 mg of diltiazam daily (Fig. 5). Pain break-through occurred a mean of 1.7 times during the 17.5-month follow-up and tended to be a short duration and related to episodes of stress in patient's life. Six patients had trace to 1+ pedal edema, but no other adverse side effects were reported. Thus, diltiazam appears to be effective for short- and long-term prophylaxis for variant angina.

Nifedipine for prophylaxis of Printzmetal's variant angina was first reported by Hosoda and his associates in 1975.[44] These uncontrolled studies reported a dramatic reduction in angina frequency. Testing of this agent in the United States was first reported by Antman and his colleagues in 1980.[45] In an open-label study of 127 patients with documented coronary spasm and variant angina, doses of 40–160 mg/day resulted in a 63% of patients being completely relieved by of their angina. Furthermore, a total of 87% of patients had 50% or more reduction in the frequency of angina. The authors reported that approximately 5% of patients had to terminate therapy due to adverse side effects. Although few controlled studies of this agent have been reported, it is clear that this is a highly effective

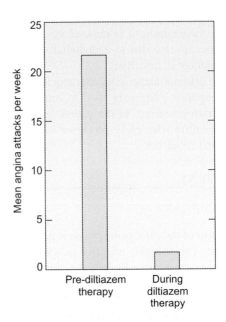

FIGURE 5: Response of 36 patients with angina due to documented coronary arterial spasm during medical therapy with long-acting nitrates (pre-diltiazem) and after therapy with 240 to 360 mg/day of diltiazem. (*Source:* Modified from Schroeder JS, Lamb IH, Ginsberg R et al, Diltiazem for long-term therapy of coronary arterial spasm. Am J Cardiol. 1982;49:533).

drug for prophylaxis of variant angina. It has also been demonstrated in the cardiac catheterization laboratory to block spasm during provocation with ergonovine maleate. With regard to long-term responses, Hill and his co-workers reported on 26 patients who had angina due to coronary spasm who completed a crossover study comparing nifedipine with isosorbide dinitrate.[46] Of the 18 patients who had a short-term beneficial response to nifedipine, 14 were followed for an average of 9.4 months on long-term nifedipine therapy. Overall, 80% of patients had a 50% or more decrease in angina frequency. Three patients did have a marked increase in angina at 9, 14 and 3 months after initiation of therapy, requiring hospitalization. In addition, nifedipine was discontinued in two patients and the dose was decreased in three additional patients due to significant adverse side effects. The authors reported that adverse effects were common, but reduction of dosing usually diminished the unwanted effects of the drug.

Verapamil has also been reported to be effective in carefully controlled randomized trials. Johnson and his colleagues reported on the prophylactic use of verapamil in 16 patients with variant angina over a 9-month period.[47] During the treatment period with verapamil, the angina frequency decreased from 12.6 to 1.7 pain episodes per week with similar decreases in nitroglycerine consumption. Holter monitoring showed marked reduction in episodes of ST-segment deviation from 33.1 to 7.1 deviations per week while on active therapy.[48] The authors concluded that verapamil was an effective drug for therapy of variant angina, but it should be noted that 14 of the 16 patients were also receiving oral isosorbide dinitrate, mean dose 105 mg/day, with a range of 120–200 mg given in four to six divided doses.

There have been very few comparative studies of the efficacy of calcium blockers for treatment of variant angina. The only study that has attempted to compare these agents was a survey of 11 cardiology institutes in Japan where investigators were asked to comment on their impression of the efficacy of nifedipine, diltiazam and verapamil.[49] Efficacy rates were assessed at 94% for nifedipine, 90.8% for diltiazam and 85.7% for verapamil. These agents also tended to be more effective in patients with normal or near normal coronary arteries rather than in patients with coronary disease. It is interesting, however, that verapamil was reported as markedly effective in only 10.7% of patients compared with 80.5% for diltiazam and 77.2% nifedipine. The authors also reported that in 15 patients on a combination of nifedipine and diltiazam that 73.3% had a markedly effective response.

Other studies have attempted to compare calcium antagonists with long-acting nitrates. Ginsburg and his co-workers reported on 12 patients who were entered into a randomized double-blind study comparing nifedipine, mean dose 82 mg/day, with isosorbide dinitrate, mean dose 66 mg/day. Treatment of the 12 patients resulted in a total of 161 patients-days that were available for analysis.[50] During baseline there was an average 1.1 angina attacks per day on placebo, which fell to 0.28 per day during nifedipine treatment and to 0.39 per day during isosorbide dinitrate treatment (Fig. 6). There is no statistical difference between these two responses. A number of adverse side effects occurred with headache being the most prominent during isosorbide dinitrate treatment in 81%

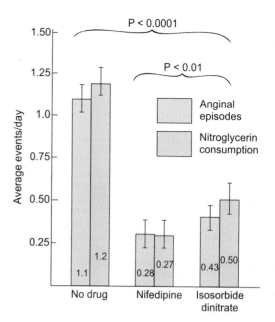

FIGURE 6: Comparison of nifedipine versus isosorbide dinitrate drug efficacy in variant angina therapy in terms of reduction of anginal episodes and sublingual nitroglycerin consumption. (*Source:* Modified from Ginsburg R, Lamb IH, Schroeder JS, et al. Randomized double-blind comparison of nifedipine and isosorbide dinitrate therapy in variant angina pectoris due to coronary arrtery spasm. Am J Heart J. 1982;103:44.)

of patients and dependent edema occurring in 33% patients during nifedipine treatment. Significant adverse side effects requiring cessation of therapy occurred in two patients on nifedipine and in three patients on isosorbide dinitrate. The authors concluded that both these agents were effective but that nifedipine was preferred by majority of patients. Ascherman and his colleagues reported on a randomized double-blind comparison of nifedipine and isosorbide in patients with variant angina.[51] Seventeen patients with documented variant angina were randomized to 20 mg/day of nifedipine versus 120 mg/day of isosorbide dinitrate. The design included a placebo-run-in period and two 6-weeks crossover period of treatment. They demonstrated that mean frequency of angina decreased from 43 attacks per week during placebo period to 4 per week with isosorbide dinitrate and 8 with nifedipine. They also concluded both nifedipine and isosorbide dinitrate in their slow release formulation are effective in the treatment of variant angina.

Patients who are refractory to treatment with oral calcium channel blockers will respond to intravenous isosorbide dinitrate or intravenous nitroglycerine. However, in the medically refractory patient, consideration should be given to combining diltiazam and nifedipine, gradually increasing the combined dose to limit adverse effects.

Beta-blockers have been reported to occasionally be detrimental or to aggravate variant angina. Robertson and his colleagues reported that both 160 mg and 640 mg propranolol per day were associated with significantly prolonged angina episodes compared with findings in control groups.[52] Tilmant studied 11 patients on placebo, diltiazam, propranolol or a combination.[53] Propranolol resulted in increased frequency and duration of angina attacks, but when diltiazam was added, this adverse effect disappeared. Therefore, β-blockers are generally not recommended for the patients with variant angina, although

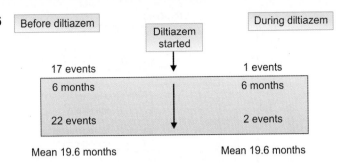

FIGURE 7: Total cardiovascular events (myocardial infarction, sudden death, or hospitalization to rule out myocardial infarction) in 43 patients with documented coronary artery spasm. Events are noted for the 6 months immediately before and after initiation of diltiazem therapy, as well as during the mean 19.6 months before and after initiation of diltiazem therapy. (*Source:* Modified from Schroeder JS, Lamb IH, Bristow MR, et al. Prevention of cardiovascular events in variant angina by long-term diltiazem therapy. J Am Coll Cardiol, 1983;1:1507)

they can be used for demand-related angina in the setting of occlusive coronary artery disease if calcium antagonists are given concurrently.

Is there any evidence that long-term use of calcium antagonists may affect the long-term prognosis of these patients? We previously reported on 43 patients with variant angina and compared their cardiovascular event rate after beginning diltiazam therapy with that at an equal time prior to therapy.[54] Cardiovascular events defined as MI, sudden death and hospitalization for prolonged angina were decreased significantly during both the 6 and mean 19.6 months of therapy compared with a similar period prior to the initiation of therapy. When the data were analyzed by the binomial principle, 22 events occurred during the 19.6 months before therapy and 2 events on therapy (Fig. 7). No patient died during the follow-up period, and there were reports of a dramatic decrease in angina frequency of approximately 94%. Although this was a retrospective study, the marked reduction in events during drug therapy suggested a protective effect and these patients benefit from long-term therapy from this drug. Due to the marked improvement in angina symptoms, it is sometimes difficult to assess how long the patients should be treated with calcium antagonists. Most authors recommend that the patients be treated at least 1 year with gradual reduction in calcium antagonist therapy after that if the patient remains pain free. We have found that flares in angina frequency occur at times of emotional stress and the patients may need increases in their dosing.

SURGICAL AND PERCUTANEOUS INTERVENTION

Although the calcium antagonists are highly effective for prophylaxis in this patient group, an occasional patient has severe unrelenting spasm despite maximal medical therapy. Some authors have reported coronary bypass grafting in such patients with the hypothesis that the graft can bypass the area of focal spasm and result in sufficient perfusion even when spasm occurs.[55] However, those patients who have severe coronary spasm may have a more diffuse process. Subsequent reports indicate that the spasm may involve or propagate distal to the area of the insertion of the bypass graft, and this approach

is generally no longer applied in this patient group. Nordstrom and his co-workers reported on persistence of chest pain despite coronary bypass grafts and a relatively high occlusion rate or postoperative infarction rate.[56] Due to the possibility of sympathetic nervous system-induced spasm, plexectomy at the time of aortocoronary bypass grafting has been reported in an effort to more completely denervate the vessel.[57] Although many of these patients seem to improve, it has been difficult to assess short- and long-term efficacy of these procedures. Prior to the introduction of calcium antagonists, Clark and his colleagues reported on four patients who underwent cardiac denervation because of unrelenting coronary spasm with myocardial ischemia and/or ventricular arrhythmias.[58] Two of their four patients die, but the two survivors did have good short-term relief of the coronary spasm.

Percutaneous transluminal coronary angioplasty (PTCA) has also been proposed as effective therapy for variant angina.[59] However, the success rate for PTCA in variant angina has been variable. As Gruntzig stated "coronary spasm and balloons do not mix".[60] The reason is obvious; if an artery is spastic in one location, manipulation of that artery may lead to more intense spasms. The advent of stents offered a more ideal approach. Corcos and his co-workers reported on 21 patients with variant angina of whom 17 also had effort-induced angina.[61] All patients had single-vessel disease with 60–95% stenotic lesions present. Angioplasty was successful in 19 patients, but only 8 remained free of angina. The restenosis rate appeared to be higher in those patients who had calcium antagonists discontinued after the procedure (80%) compared with those who continued the drug (21%). During a mean follow-up of 33 months, 20 patients were free of angina with 75% of all anti-anginal medications. Therefore, where there is a fixed stenotic coronary lesion related to focal coronary spasm, angioplasty and calcium antagonists may be effective therapies. Martí and his co-workers reported on 22 patients with documented variant angina, 5 who were refractory to pharmacologic treatment and underwent PTCA.[62] Of the 5 patients, the investigators observed coronary spasm recurrence proximal or distal to the stent in 4 patients (2 during the stent implantation procedure and the other 2 in the coronary care unit within 48 hours post procedure). Three patients required additional stenting and the fourth patient improved with pharmacologic treatment. The authors concluded that although PTCA may be an alternative therapy for patients with recurrent variant angina refractory to medical treatment, spasm recurrence in other segments of the treated vessel is common and immediate and continued surveillance is important.

NATURAL HISTORY AND PROGNOSIS

The long-term outlook for patients with variant angina has been reported as quite variable, most likely because of differences in the degree of underlying coronary disease and the advent of calcium channel blockers as the cornerstone of medical therapy. Severi reported on 138 patients with variant angina who were followed for up to 8 years.[63] Only 9 of 107 patients had normal coronary arteries, and the majority had greater than 50% stenosis of at least one major vessel. Coronary vasospasm was demonstrated in only 37 of the patients at the time of coronary arteriography. They reported that 28 patients had an acute MI and 5 patients died within 1 month of hospital admission. The authors then followed the 133 remaining patients, of whom 120 were treated medically and 13 surgically. In the medically treated group, 7 patients died during the follow-up period and symptoms generally became less frequent and severe. Over 50% of patients remained asymptomatic for at least 12 months by the end of year 4. The author noted a general correlation between the severity of the underlying coronary disease and the poor prognosis.

The prognosis of patients with variant angina in the absence of significant coronary artery disease appears to be relatively good.[64] Bory and his colleagues studied 277 successive patients with coronary spasm and normal or near normal coronary arteries for a median follow-up of 7.5 years.[65] While they reported that recurrent angina was common (39%), cardiac death and MI were relatively infrequent and occurred in only 3.6% and 6.5% respectively.

The prognosis of variant angina in patients with multivessel spasm is believed to be poor. Onaka and his colleagues evaluated the clinical manifestation of ischemic episodes in patients with variant angina and normal coronary arteries.[66] They concluded that anginal attacks due to sequential and simultaneous multivessel spasm were more dangerous than those involving single-vessel spasms. The observed pattern of spasm in patients with multivessel involvement included:

- Migratory spasm, which is spasm at a different site on different occasions,
- Spasm that sequentially affected two different sites, and
- Simultaneous spasm at more than one site.

In conclusion, variant angina is characterized by considerable variability of symptoms and response to treatment. Spontaneous remission is frequent outcome in many patients, but numerous studies have convincingly demonstrated that patients with variant angina and no or mild coronary disease do extremely well if they have long-term therapy with a calcium channel blocker. For this reason, we recommend that patients continue medication for at least 1–2 years and then that it be tapered slowly and that medication be added at any time that there is a recurrence of symptoms.

REFERENCES

1. Prinzmetal M, Kennamer R, Merliss R, et al. A variant form of angina pectoris; preliminary report. Am J Med. 1959;27:375-88.
2. Prinzmetal M, Ekmekci A, Kennamer R, et al. Variant form of angina pectoris, previously undelineated syndrome. JAMA. 1960;174:1794-800.
3. Osler W. Lumleian lectures on angina pectoris. Lancet. 1910;1:697-701.
4. Wilson FN, Johnston FD. The occurrence in angina pectoris of electrocardiographic changes similar in magnitude and in kind to those produced by myocardial inlarelion. Am Heart J. 1941;22:64.
5. Scanlon PJ, Niemichas R, Moran JF, et al. Accelerated angina pectoris: clinical, hemodynamic, arteriographic and therapeutic experience in 85 patients. Circulation. 1973;47:19-26.
6. MacAlpin RN, Kattus AA, Alvaro AB. Angina pectoris at rest with preservation of exercise capacity: Prinzmetal's variant angina. Circulation. 1973;47:946-58.
7. Schroeder JS, Bolen JL, Quint RA, et al. Provocation of coronary spasm with ergonovine maleate: new test with results in 57 patients undergoing coronary arteriography. Am J Cardiol. 1977;40:487-91.
8. Proudfit WL, Shirey EK, Sones FM. Selective cine coronary arteriography. Correlation with clinical findings in 1,000 patients. Circulation. 1966;33:901-10.
9. Phibbs B, Fleming T, Ewy GA, et al. Frequency of normal coronary arteriograms in three academic medical centers and one community hospital. Am J Cardiol. 1988;62:472-4.
10. Bertrand ME, LaBlanche JM, Tilmant PY, et al. Frequency of provoked coronary arterial spasm in 1,089 consecutive patients undergoing coronary arteriography. Circulation. 1982;65:1299-306.
11. Harding MB, Leithe ME, Mark DB, et al. Ergonovine maleate testing during cardiac catheterization: a 10-year perspective in 3,447 patients without significant coronary artery disease or Prinzmetal's variant angina. J Am Coll Cardiol. 1992;20:107-11.
12. Sueda S, Ochi N, Kawada H, et al. Frequency of provoked coronary vasospasm in patients undergoing coronary arteriography with spasm provocation test of acetylcholine. Am J Cardiol. 1999;83:1186-90.
13. Mishra PK. Variations in presentation and various options in management of variant angina. Eur J Cardiothorac Surg. 2006;29:748-59.
14. Oliva PB, Potts DE, Pluss RG. Coronary arterial spasm causing Prinzmetal's variant angina. N Engl J Med. 1973;288:745-51.
15. Schroeder JS, Silverman JF, Harrison DC. Right coronary artery spasm causing Prinzmetal's variant angina. Chest. 1974;65:573-7.
16. Maseri A, Pesola A, Marzilli M, et al. Coronary vasospasm in angina pectoris. Lancet. 1977;1:713-7.
17. MacAlpin RN. Relation of coronary arterial spasm to sites 01 organic stenosis. Am J Cardiol. 1980;46:143-53.
18. Angelini P. Transient left ventricular apical ballooning: a unifying pathophysiologic theory at the edge of Prinzmetal angina. Catheter Cardiovasc Interv. 2008;71:342-52.
19. Haghi D, Suselbeck T, Wolpert C. Severe multivessel coronary vasospasm and left ventricular ballooning syndrome. Circ Cardiovasc Interv. 2009;2:268-9.
20. Nef HM, Möllmann H, Elsässer A. Takotsubo cardiomyopathy (apical ballooning). Heart. 2007;93:1309-15.
21. Wittstein IS, Thiemann DR, Lima JA, et al. Neurohumoral features of myocardial stunning due to sudden emotional stress. N Engl J Med. 2005;352:539-48.
22. Ginsburg R, Bristow MR, Schroeder JS, et al. Effects of pharmacologic agents on isolated human coronary arteries. In: Santamore WP, Bove AA (Eds). Coronary Artery Disease. Baltimore: Urban and Schwarzenberg; 1982. pp. 103-15.
23. Endo M, Hiroswaka K, Kancko N, et al. Prinzmetal's variant angina: coronary arteriogram and left ventriculögram during angina attack induced by methacholine. N Engl J Med. 1976;294:252-5.
24. Stang JM, Kolibash AJ, Schorling JB, et al. Methacholine provocation 01 Prinzmetal's variant angina pectoris: a revised perspective. Clin Cardiol. 1982;5:393-402.
25. Angelini P. Transient left ventricular apical ballooning: a unifying pathophysiologic theory at the edge of Prinzmetal angina. Catheter Cardiovasc Interv. 2008;71:342-52.
26. Li JJ, Zhang YP, Yang P, et al. Increased peripheral circulating inflammatory cells and plasma inflammatory markers in patients with variant angina. Coron Artery Dis. 2008;19:293-7.
27. Koh KK, Moon TH, Song JH, et al. Comparison of clinical and laboratory findings between patients with diffuse three-vessel coronary artery spasm and other types of coronary artery spasm. Cath Cardiovasc Diag. 1996;37:132-9.
28. Ginsburg R, Lamb IH, Schroeder JS, et al. Long-term transtelephonic monitoring in variant angina. Am Heart J. 1981;102:196-201.
29. Maas R, Brockhoff C, Patten M, et al. Prinzmetal angina documented by transtelephonic electrocardiographic monitoring. Circulation. 2001;103:2766.
30. Shimada M, Akaishi M, Asakura K, et al. Usefulness of the newly developed transtelephonic electrocardiogram and computer-supported response system. J Cardiol. 1996;27:211-7.

31. Watanabe K, Takahashi T, Miyajima S, et al. Myocardial sympathetic denervation, fatty acid metabolism, and left ventricular wall motion in vasospastic angina. J Nucl Med. 2002;43:1476-81.

32. Ha JW, Lee JD, Jang Y, et al. 123I-MIBG myocardial scintigraphy as a non-invasive screen for the diagnosis of coronary artery spasm. J Nucl Cardiol. 1998;5:591-7.

33. Graf S, Khorsand A, Gwechenberger M, et al. Typical chest pain and normal coronary angiogram: cardiac risk factor analysis versus PET for detection of microvascular disease. J Nucl Med. 2007;48:175-81.

34. Sueda S, Kohno H, Fukuda H, et al. Limitations of medical therapy in patients with pure coronary spastic angina. Chest. 2003;123:380-6.

35. Schroeder JS, Rosenthal S, Ginsburg R, et al. Medical therapy of Prinzmetal's variant angina. Chest. 1980;78:231-3.

36. Hirai N, Kawano H, Yasue H, et al. Attenuation of nitrate tolerance and oxidative stress by an angiotensin II receptor blocker in patients with coronary spastic angina. Circulation. 2003;108:1446-50.

37. Hill JA, Feldman RL, Pepine CJ, et al. Randomized double-blind comparison of nifedipine and isosorbide dinitrate in patients with coronary arterial spasm. Am J Cardiol. 1982;49:431-8.

38. Meisel SR, Mazur A, Chetboun I, et al. Usefulness of implantable cardioverter-defibrillators in refractory variant angina pectoris complicated by ventricular fibrillation in patients with angiographically normal coronary arteries. Am J Cardiol. 2002;89:1114-6.

39. Endo M, Kanda I, Hosoda S, et al. Prinzmetal's variant form of angina pectoris. Circulation. 1975;52:33-7.

40. Rosenthal SJ, Ginsburg R, Lamb IH, et al. The efficacy of diltiazem for control of symptoms of coronary arterial spasm. Am J Cardiol. 1980;46:1027-32.

41. Pepine CJ, Feldman RL, Whittle J, et al. Effects of diltiazem in patients with variant angina: a randomized double-blind trial. Am Heart J. 1981;101:719-25.

42. Rosenthal SJ, Lamb IH, Schroeder JS, et al. Long-term efficacy of diltiazem for control of symptoms of coronary artery spasm. Circ Res. 1983;52:153-7.

43. Schroeder JS, Lamb IH, Ginsburg R. Diltiazem for long-term therapy of coronary arterial spasm. Am J Cardiol. 1982;49:533-7.

44. Hosoda S, Kasanuki H, Mityata K, et al. Results of clinical investigation of nifedipine in angina pectoris with special reference to its therapeutic efficacy in attacks at rest. In: Hishimoto K, Kimura E, Kobayshi T (Eds). Proceedings of International Nifedipine "Adalat" Symposium: New Drug Therapy of Ischemic Heart Disease. Tokyo: University of Tokyo Press; 1975. pp. 185-9.

45. Antman E, Muller J, Goldberg S, et al. Nifedipine therapy for coronary spasm: experience in 127 patients. N Engl J Med. 1980;302(23):1269-73.

46. Hill JA, Feldman RL, Pepine CJ, et al. Randomized double-blind comparison of nifedipine and isosorbide dinitrate in patients with coronary arterial spasm. Am J Cardiol. 1982;49:431-8.

47. Johnson SM, Mauritson DR, Hillis LD, et al. Verapamil in the treatment of Prinzmetal's variant angina: a long-term, double-blind, randomized trial (abstr). Am J Cardiol. 1981;47:399.

48. Johnson SM, Mauritson DR, Willerson JT, et al. Verapamil administration in variant angina pectoris. JAMA. 1981;245:1849-51.

49. Kimura E, Kishida H. Treatment of variant angina with drugs: a survey of 11 cardiology institutes in Japan. Circulation. 1981;63:844-8.

50. Ginsburg R, Lamb IH, Schroeder JS, et al. Randomized double-blind comparison of nifedipine and isosorbide dinitrate therapy in variant angina pectoris due to coronary artery spasm. Am Heart J. 1981;103:44-9.

51. Aschermann M, Bultas J, Karetová D, et al. Randomized double-blind comparison of isosorbide dinitrate and nifedipine in variant angina pectoris. Am J Cardiol. 1990;65:46J-49J.

52. Robertson RM, Wood AJ, Vaughn WK, et al. Exacerbation of vasotonic angina pectoris by propranolol. Circulation. 1982;65:281-5.

53. Tilmant PY, La Blanche JM, Thieuleux FA, et al. Detrimental effect of propranolol in patients with coronary arterial spasm countered by combination with diltiazem. Am J Cardiol. 1983;52:230-3.

54. Schroeder JS, Lamb IH, Bristow MR, et al. Prevention of cardiovascular events in variant angina by long-term diltiazem therapy. J Am Coll Cardiol. 1983;1:1507-11.

55. Shubrooks SJ, Bete JM, Hutter AM, et al. Variant angina pectoris: clinical and anatomic spectrum and results of coronary bypass surgery. Am J Cardiol. 1975;36:142-7.

56. Nordstrom LA, Lillehei JP, Adicoff A, et al. Coronary artery surgery for recurrent ventricular arrhythmias in patients with variant angina. Am Heart J. 1975;89:236-41.

57. Bertrand ME, LaBlanche JM, Tilmant PY. Treatment of Prinzmetal's variant angina. Role of medical treatment with nifedipine and surgical coronary revascularization combined with plexectomy. Am J Cardiol. 1981;47:174-8.

58. Clark DA, Quint RA, Mitchell RL, et al. Coronary artery spasm. J Thorac Cardiovasc Surg. 1977;73:332-9.

59. Leisch F, Herbinger W, Brucke P. Role of percutaneous transluminal coronary angioplasty in patients with variant angina and coexistent coronary stenosis refractory to maximal medical therapy. Clin Cardiol. 1984;7:654-9.

60. Clark DA. The fight against coronary spasm—one more weapon. Cathet Cardiovasc Diagn. 1997;42:444.

61. Corcos T, David PR, Bourassa MG, et al. Percutaneous transluminal coronary angioplasty for the treatment of variant angina. J Am Coli Cardiol. 1985;5:1046-54.

62. Martí V, Ligero C, García J, et al. Stent implantation in variant angina refractory to medical treatment. Clin Cardiol. 2006;29:530-3.

63. Severi S, Davies G, Maseri A, et al. Long-term prognosis of "variant" angina with medical treatment. Am J Cardiol. 1980;46:226-32.

64. Lanza GA, Sestito A, Sgueglia GA, et al. Current clinical features, diagnostic assessment and prognostic determinants of patients with variant angina. Int J Cardiol. 2007;118:41-7.

65. Bory M, Pierron F, Panagides D, et al. Coronary artery spasm in patients with normal or near normal coronary arteries. Long-term follow-up of 277 patients. Eur Heart J. 1996;17:1015-21.

66. Onaka H, Hirota Y, Shimada S, et al. Clinical observation of spontaneous anginal attacks and multivessel spasm in variant angina pectoris with normal coronary arteries: evaluation by 24-hour 12-lead electrocardiography with computer analysis. J Am Coll Cardiol. 1996;27:38-44.

Chapter 52

Cardiogenic Shock in Acute Coronary Syndromes

Sanjay K Shah, Eugen Ivan, Andrew D Michaels

Chapter Outline

INTRODUCTION

Cardiogenic shock, a syndrome of organ hypoperfusion secondary to cardiac failure, complicates ST-segment elevation myocardial infarction (STEMI) in 5–8% of cases.[1] Although less common, cardiogenic shock complicates 2.9% cases of non-ST elevation myocardial infarction and 2.1% of those with unstable angina.[2] Hemodynamic features of this syndrome include hypotension, reduced cardiac output and elevated right- or left-sided filling pressures (Table 1). Pre-shock or shock with end-organ hypoperfusion may be manifest as decreased urine output (oliguria), mental obtundation and/or cool extremities. Although shock is usually caused by left ventricular (LV) pump dysfunction secondary to a large area of LV ischemia or infarction, there is increasing data that neurohormonal or systemic inflammatory response syndrome (SIRS) may be a causative mechanism of shock in acute coronary syndromes (ACS). Other clinical entities must be considered when evaluating shock in the setting of ACS. Mechanical complications of myocardial infarction that can cause shock include right ventricular (RV) infarction, cardiac tamponade secondary to free wall rupture, papillary muscle ischemia or infarction and ventricular septal defect. Additionally, entities that may mimic ACS and present with shock should be considered. Takotsubo cardiomyopathy, acute myopericarditis, hypertrophic cardiomyopathy and acute aortic dissection can present with ST-segment elevation in the absence of significant coronary artery disease.[1]

INCIDENCE

Historically, cardiogenic shock was reported to occur in 7.5% of patients who presented with acute myocardial infarction.[3]

More recent observational studies from the 1990s indicate that the incidence of cardiogenic shock in acute myocardial infarction is roughly 6%.[4] Patients who develop cardiogenic shock are more likely be older and have had a history of myocardial infarction, ischemic heart disease, prior coronary artery bypass graft (CABG) surgery, stroke, diabetes, heart failure, anterior infarction location and bundle branch block.[5,6] Indeed, 48% had significant left anterior descending disease in the Should We Emergently Revascularize Occluded Coronaries for Cardiogenic Shock (SHOCK) trial.[7] Patients who develop cardiogenic shock have a higher prevalence of underlying three-vessel disease or left main disease.[8]

MORTALITY

Prior to the routine use of thrombolytics and percutaneous coronary intervention (PCI) in the setting of STEMI, the in-hospital mortality rate for myocardial infarction complicated by

TABLE 1

Clinical and hemodynamic features of cardiogenic shock

Clinical
- Hypotension: Systolic blood pressure ≤ 90 mm Hg
- Impaired organ perfusion: Oliguria, cold clammy skin, mental obtundation

Hemodynamics
- Systolic blood pressure ≤ 90 mm Hg
- Cardiac index ≤ 2.2 l/min/m^2
- Primary LV failure: Pulmonary capillary wedge pressure ≥ 18 mm Hg with right atrial pressure lower than pulmonary capillary wedge pressure
- Primary RV failure: Right atrial pressure ≥ 15 mm Hg with pulmonary capillary wedge pressure less than right atrial pressure

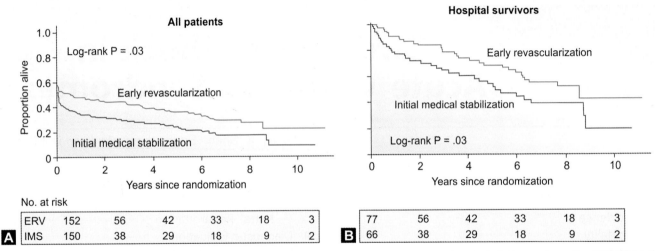

FIGURES 1A AND B: Kaplan-Meier long-term survival of all patients and those surviving to hospital discharge from the SHOCK trial[12] (*Source*: Hochman JS, Sleeper LA, Webb JG, et al. Early revascularization and long-term survival in cardiogenic shock complicating acute myocardial infarction. JAMA. 2006;295:2511-5)

cardiogenic shock was 70–80%.[3] A more recent analysis of the National Registry of Myocardial Infarction database showed a progressive decline in in-hospital mortality (from 60.3% to 47.9% during 1994–2004) in association with increased use of primary PCI for patients with STEMI complicated by cardiogenic shock.[9] Similar improvements in in-hospital mortality were noted in a Swiss observational study.[10] Similar trends in decreased mortality were noted in analysis of the long-term outcomes of the SHOCK trial, a trial that compared initial medical stabilization to early revascularization. At 1 year, survival was lower for those treated with intensive medical therapy (46.7%) compared to those treated with early revascularization (33.3%).[11] Similarly, a follow-up analysis at 6 years of the SHOCK trial showed advantages in survival in the total cohort (32.8% vs 19.6%) and among those who were alive at hospital discharge (62.4% vs 44.4%) for those randomized to the early revascularization group compared with those randomized to the intensive medical therapy group (Figs 1A and B).[12]

PREDICTORS OF CARDIOGENIC SHOCK

Predictors of short-term mortality from cardiogenic shock include advanced age, male gender, Killip class, low systolic blood pressure, anterior location of infarction, increased heart rate, pre-existing cardiac risk factors, prior infarction or angina and previous CABG.[13] In the GUSTO-1 study, age was the greatest predictor of 30-day mortality. For every 10-year increase in age, there was a 47% greater risk of developing shock.[13,14] In an analysis of the TRIUMPH data, creatinine clearance, systolic blood pressure and number of vasopressors were significant predictors of mortality at 30 days in those who underwent successful PCI.[15] In addition, several studies have shown that PCI and glycoprotein IIb/IIIa inhibitor use were associated with decreased mortality.[16,17] In a substudy of the SHOCK trial, three-vessel disease was associated with worse outcome, as was the presence of the left main or saphenous vein graft as the infarct related artery.[18] If the infarct related artery was the left circumflex or the left anterior descending, this was associated with an intermediate mortality, and the right coronary artery was

associated with the best outcome.[8] In a 6-year follow-up of the SHOCK trial, an initial medical stabilization strategy, reduced LV ejection fraction, advanced age and increased serum creatinine were associated with long-term mortality.[12]

PATHOPHYSIOLOGY

The primary cause of cardiogenic shock in ACS is LV dysfunction secondary to infarction and ischemia. Patients with predominantly diastolic dysfunction from ischemia may present with cardiogenic shock. When ischemia or infarction affects a large portion of the LV myocardium, stroke volume and consequently cardiac output decrease. With impairment in the pumping function of the left ventricle, tachycardia ensues to try to maintain cardiac output. However, due to inability to maintain cardiac output, hypotension ensues. In addition, LV filling pressures increase due to pump failure (Figs 2A to C). These compensatory mechanisms beget further ischemia as tachycardia decreases the diastolic filling of the coronary arteries, while hypotension and increased LV filling pressures decrease coronary perfusion pressure, which causes further ischemia leading to a downward spiral. Previous studies suggested that cardiogenic shock ensued when 40–50% of the LV myocardium was infarcted.[19] However, the average ejection fraction in the SHOCK trial was roughly 30%.[20] Although this was measured during the patient's acute presentation when the patients were often on inotropes or had intra-aortic balloon pump (IABP) support, this did not differ significantly from the ejection fraction measured 2 weeks following the incident event. In addition, in the SHOCK trial there was improved ejection fraction in survivors, suggesting that at least part of the myocardium was ischemic and not infarcted.[21]

In addition to the hemodynamic effects of shock, decreased cardiac output stimulates increased sympathetic discharge. In addition, hypotension stimulates the release of renin and angiotensin. Catecholamine stimulation leads to tachycardia and increased systemic vascular resistance. While preserving cardiac output by inotropy, and increasing coronary blood flow by increased systemic vascular resistance, this comes at the cost of increased afterload. Similarly, the renin angiotension system

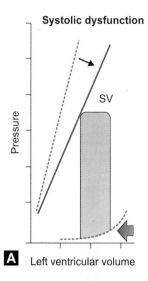
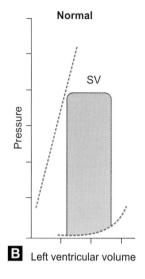
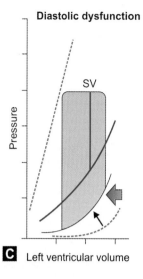

Systolic dysfunction — A — Left ventricular volume (Pressure)

Normal — B — Left ventricular volume (Pressure)

Diastolic dysfunction — C — Left ventricular volume (Pressure)

FIGURES 2A TO C: Schematic pressure-volume loops illustrate the mechanisms for increased LV diastolic pressure and lower cardiac output in systolic and diastolic dysfunction: (A) in cardiogenic shock patients with systolic dysfunction; (B) contractility is reduced compared to normals and (C) cardiogenic shock patients with diastolic dysfunction, the major mechanism of increased diastolic filling pressure is increased ventricular stiffness resulting in an upward and leftward shift in the end-diastolic pressure-volume relationship (*Source*: Chatterjee K, McGlothlin D, Michaels A. Analytic reviews: Cardiogenic shock with preserved systolic function: A reminder. J Intensive Care Med. 2008;23:355-66)

causes deleterious affects by increasing systemic vascular resistance and by fluid retention, further compromising coronary blood flow and increasing filling pressures. These compensatory mechanisms exacerbate the physiology by increasing fluid retention and biventricular filling pressures, causing increased heart rate and systemic vascular resistance, further leading to worsening of the clinical picture.[1]

Through these mechanisms, it would be expected that cardiogenic shock would be invariably associated with a high systemic vascular resistance. This, however, is not the case; there is growing data that the cause of cardiogenic shock complicating acute myocardial infarction is multifactorial, including a syndrome of SIRS with accompanied leukocytosis, fever and reduced systemic vascular resistance (Fig. 3). In the SHOCK trial, 18% manifested signs of SIRS. This group had a median SVR that was within the normal range. Of this group, 74% were culture positive.[22] It has been postulated that passive venous congestion of the gut causes bacterial translocation, which leads to SIRS. One study revealed that a majority of patients with cardiogenic shock had elevated levels of procalcitonin, a marker of an infective process.[23] In addition, TNF-α and IL-6 have been shown to be elevated in patients with acute myocardial infarction who develop shock while in the hospital. These markers, which have cardiodepressant properties, have been shown to be predictive of death and shock.[24] Additionally, nitric oxide (NO) and inducible nitric oxide synthase (iNOS) may be related to SIRS. iNOS and NO are increased in myocardial infarction.[25] NO may lead to excessive vasodilation and contribute to SIRS and consequently to shock. Although trials of the iNOS inhibitor L-MMMA showed no mortality benefit in the setting of cardiogenic shock, there was a significant increase in blood pressure shortly after infusion compared with placebo, suggesting a possible role of iNOS in the development of cardiogenic shock.[26,27]

PATHOLOGY

Pathologic cardiac examinations of patients who died of cardiogenic shock reveal areas of infarct expansion and extension. Infarct expansion occurs to areas of the noninfarcted ventricle after a large infarct, often after extensive anterior infarction. This may occur due to mechanical effects or due to shock with further coronary ischemia in remote areas. Often the most susceptible areas are "watershed" areas adjacent to area of necrosis. One landmark autopsy study revealed that infarct extension occurred in 18 of 22 autopsies analyzed.[19] In addition, there is infarct extension due to reocclusion of patent arteries, propagation of intracoronary thrombi, or from ischemia secondary to cardiogenic shock itself.[28,29]

OTHER CARDIAC CAUSES OF CARDIOGENIC SHOCK

The evaluation of cardiogenic shock in ACS involves exclusion of other cardiac causes of shock in the setting of ACS, including RV infarction, ventricular septal rupture (VSR), ischemic mitral regurgitation and cardiac rupture.

RIGHT VENTRICULAR INFARCTION

Right ventricular infarction may cause cardiogenic shock. Most commonly associated with inferior myocardial infarction, isolated RV infarction occurs in roughly 5% of cases of cardiogenic shock. Mortality in the SHOCK registry was only slightly lower in those with cardiogenic shock from RV versus LV failure.[30] There is typically RV volume overload with decreased LV preload. LV volume is not only decreased due to decreased RV function, but due to a shift of the interventricular septum to the LV from RV volume overload and increased end diastolic pressure.[31]

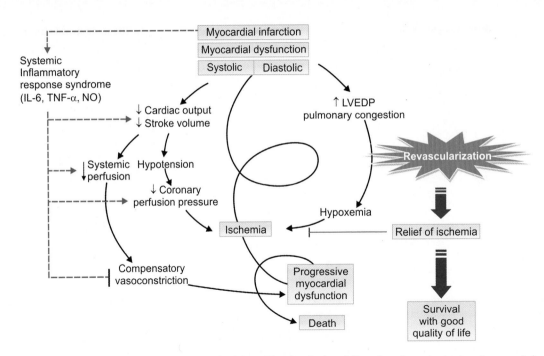

FIGURE 3: The current concept of cardiogenic shock pathophysiology. The classic description of cardiogenic shock pathogenesis is shown in black. Myocardial injury causes systolic and diastolic dysfunction. A decrease in cardiac output leads to a decrease in systemic and coronary perfusion. This exacerbates ischemia causes cell death in the infarct border zone and the remote zone of myocardium. Inadequate systemic perfusion triggers reflex vasoconstriction, which is usually insufficient. Systemic inflammation may play a role in limiting the peripheral vascular compensatory response and may contribute to myocardial dysfunction. Whether inflammation plays a causal role or is only an epiphenomenon remains unclear. Revascularization leads to relief of ischemia. It has not been possible to demonstrate an increase in cardiac output or ejection fraction as the mechanism of benefit of revascularization; however, revascularization does significantly increase the likelihood of survival with good quality of life (Abbreviations: IL-6-Interleukin-6; TNF-α: Tumor necrosis factor-α; LVEDP: LV end-diastolic pressure)[1] (*Source*: Reynolds HR, Hochman JS. Cardiogenic shock: Current concepts and improving outcomes. Circulation. 2008;117:686-97)

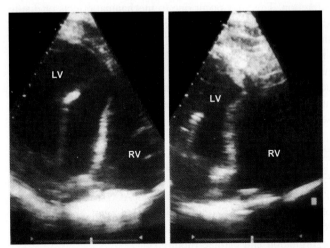

FIGURE 4: Transthoracic two-dimensional echocardiograms from a dog model of RV infarction. Before infarction, both LV and RV volumes were normal (left panel). After infarction, the right ventricle is dilated, while the LV end-diastolic volume is decreased. Leftward diastolic shift of the interventricular septum is evident (Abbreviations: RV: Right ventricle; LV: Left ventricle)[33] (*Source*: Modified from Chatterjee K, McGlothlin D, Michaels A. Analytic reviews: Cardiogenic shock with preserved systolic function: A reminder. J Intensive Care Med. 2008;23:355-66)

Historically, treatment has been volume resuscitation; however, this may impair LV filling. Ideally, RV diastolic pressures should be maintained between 10 mm Hg and 14 mm Hg to maintain RV stroke index.[32] The clinical presentation shows features of cardiogenic shock, evidence of right heart failure and the absence of pulmonary congestion. Elevated jugular venous pressure with a positive Kussmaul's sign, clear lungs,

an RV S3 gallop and lack of increased intensity of P2, suggest RV infarct as the diagnosis. There is usually inferior ST elevation and elevation in V1 and V3R–V4R. Echocardiography usually reveals RV hypokinesis with dilatation, with relatively preserved LV ejection fraction (Fig 4). Treatment involves opening the infarct related artery and supportive medical measures.[33]

VENTRICULAR SEPTAL RUPTURE

Ventricular septal rupture is a rare complication of acute myocardial infarction, occurring in 0.2% of patients in the GUSTO-1 cohort.[34] Risk factors for development of a post-MI VSD include older age, female sex, absence of previous angina or infarction, late time to revascularization and systemic hypertension. VSDs occur with either anterior or inferior myocardial infarctions. VSDs associated with anterior infarction are usually apical in location, whereas those associated with inferior infarction are in the basal septum (Fig. 5). Rupture can occur within the first 24 hours in large infarctions associated with intramural hematomas, or 3–5 days later due to coagulation necrosis.[35] Usually patients present with cardiogenic shock and biventricular failure with a loud holosystolic murmur that is heard best at the lower left sternal border often associated with a thrill. The defect can be diagnosed with echocardiography, ventriculography or catheterization to document a left-to-right shunt in the right ventricle (Fig. 6).[36]

Previously, this defect was surgically closed via patch closure. However recent series have used a technique of surgical exclusion with improved outcomes.[37] Percutaneous closure has been attempted with mixed results.[38]

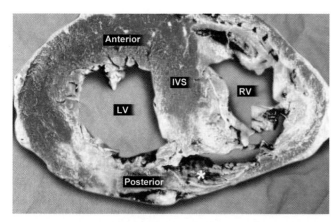

FIGURE 5: Gross findings from a patient with a posterior ventricular septal defect. There is an infarction involving the basal inferior septum, the basal posteroinferior wall, and the right ventricle. The ventricular septal rupture (star) is complex, with an irregular tract at the junction of the inferior wall and the interventricular septum[35] (Abbreviations: RV: Right ventricle; IVS: Interventricular septum) (*Source*: Modified from Birnbaum Y, Fishbein MC, Blanche C, et al. Ventricular septal rupture after acute myocardial infarction. N Engl J Med. 2002;347:1426-32)

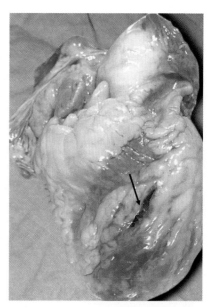

FIGURE 7: Cardiac rupture syndromes complicating ST-elevation myocardial infarction STEMI. Anterior myocardial rupture in an acute infarct (arrow), resulting in death from tamponade (*Source*: Modified from Schoen FJ. The heart. In: Kumar V, Abbas AK, Fausto N (Eds). Robbins and Cotran Pathologic Basis of Disease, 7th edn. Philadelphia: Saunders; 2005)

Rupture usually leads to hemopericardium and death from cardiac tamponade. However there is spectrum of presentations depending on whether or not the rupture is contained. Patients can present with "pericardial" pain, nausea, hypotension and nonspecific symptoms.[43] This is usually followed by pulseless electrical activity and death. Rupture can be diagnosed by transthoracic echocardiography.[44] Survival depends on recognition of tamponade, prompt pericardiocentesis and immediate surgical repair. Medical stabilization includes intravenous resuscitation, vasopressor or inotropic support and IABP support prior to surgical repair.[41,43,45]

MITRAL REGURGITATION

Acute severe mitral regurgitation from severe papillary dysfunction or papillary muscle rupture is a rare, life-threatening complication of acute myocardial infarction (Figs 8 and 9). This complication usually affects the posteromedial papillary muscle, which has its sole blood supply from the posterior descending artery. The anterolateral papillary muscle usually has dual blood supply from the left circumflex and left anterior descending.[36] Usually occurring 2–7 days postinfarction, most patients have relatively modest sized areas of infarction with poor collaterals.[46] Sudden onset of severe mitral regurgitation is associated with decreased forward output and stroke volume, increased pulmonary venous congestion, pulmonary edema and signs of hypoperfusion. On examination, patients have a new holosystolic murmur, often with an associated palpable and audible S3 and S4. The murmur may not extend to the second heart sound due to reduction of regurgitation in late systole because of rapid equalization of LV and left atrial pressures. Echocardiography usually confirms the diagnosis. Pulmonary artery catheterization reveals a large V wave in the pulmonary capillary wedge tracing. Definitive surgical treatment with mitral repair or replacement should be performed. Prior to surgical treatment, vasodilators

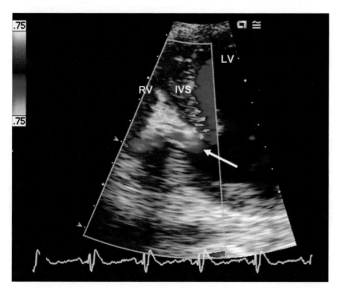

FIGURE 6: Doppler echocardiography demonstrating a post-MI ventricular septal defect with left-to-right flow (arrow) (Abbreviations: LV: Left ventricle; IVS: Interventricular septum; RV: Right ventricle)

CARDIAC RUPTURE

Cardiac rupture occurs in less than 1% of patients who present with acute myocardial infarction (Fig. 7). Cardiac rupture usually involves the anterior or lateral walls. Risk factors for cardiac rupture include female sex, advanced age and systemic hypertension.[39] Cardiac rupture usually occurs in patients without previous myocardial infarction who suffer a transmural infarct. Often, the time to reperfusion therapy is very long. It rarely occurs in patients who have well collateralized or thickened ventricles.[40] Cardiac rupture usually occurs in the first 5 days after myocardial infarction but can occur up to 3 weeks after infarction.[41] It is preceded by infarct expansion, with thinning of the necrotic area.[42] Rupture can occur from a tear in the wall, or it can occur from a dissecting hematoma.[41]

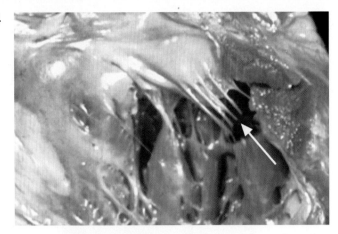

FIGURE 8: Complete rupture of a necrotic papillary muscle (arrow) in a post-infarction patient

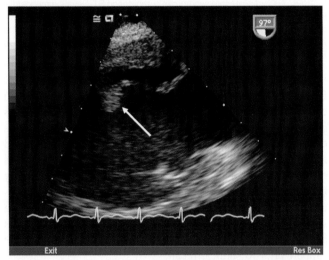

FIGURE 9: Two-dimensional echocardiography illustrates rupture of the posteromedial papillary muscle (arrow) in a patient presenting in cardiogenic shock from acute severe mitral regurgitation

can be used to stabilize the patient. Intravenous sodium nitroprusside can produce dramatic hemodynamic improvement.[33] Vasopressors should be avoided as they increase the regurgitant volume and further impair forward cardiac output. In severe hemodynamic compromise, IABP is indicated to improve cardiac output, decrease regurgitant volume and preserve coronary perfusion.[45]

DIAGNOSTIC EVALUATION

Cardiogenic shock can often be suspected by the presence of signs of shock in the setting of acute myocardial infarction (Table 1). Further testing should be performed to confirm the diagnosis of cardiogenic shock given that there is considerable overlap with other causes of shock. Echocardiography is an invaluable tool for evaluating biventricular dysfunction and excluding mechanical complications of myocardial infarction as a cause of cardiogenic shock. However image quality can be suboptimal due to mechanical ventilation, body habitus, chest deformities or positioning. Pulmonary artery catheterization is

often useful, especially in patients who do not have prompt recovery from a shock state with reperfusion to guide further therapy. Invasive arterial monitoring is essential to guide further therapy.[45]

In addition to a diagnostic tool, echocardiography can be used as a tool to prognosticate patients. In a substudy of the SHOCK trial, echocardiography was performed on 169 subjects. The only echocardiographic variables predictive of mortality were ejection fraction and mitral regurgitation.[21] Those that were alive at 1 year had a mean ejection fraction of 34% versus 28% in those that died. For those with an ejection fraction less than 28%, mortality at 1 year was 24% compared to 56% with an ejection fraction greater than or equal to 28%. Similarly, those with no or mild mitral regurgitation had improved survival compared to those with more significant regurgitation.[21]

MEDICAL MANAGEMENT

The mainstay of medical management for cardiogenic shock includes inotropic and vasopressor agents.[45,46] Although dopamine and dobutamine improve the hemodynamics acutely in cardiogenic shock, there is no data to suggest that they improve survival. These agents increase myocardial oxygen demand, which may worsen supply-demand mismatch in an already failing heart. Although norepinephrine is often a second-line agent given its potent alpha effects, it is useful in patients who have a normal systemic vascular resistance in cardiogenic shock. Recent data suggest that the role of dopamine may need to be reconsidered as there is evidence that treatment with dopamine increases short-term mortality in comparison with those treated with norepinephrine.[47] Pure alpha agents are contraindicated in cardiogenic shock as they increase afterload and further depress cardiac output. Vasodilators may be useful in preshock states; however, they are not recommended as lone agents once shock has ensued as they can lead to further hypotension, thus decreasing coronary blood flow.[48] Vasodilators may be useful when used together with IABP or inotropes; however, there are no trials that have evaluated this strategy. Loop diuretics should be used when there is pulmonary congestion.

MECHANICAL SUPPORT

Considering the profound hemodynamic alterations that are germane to cardiogenic shock, adjunctive mechanical circulatory support is often needed.[1] Several devices are available for mechanical circulatory support in cardiogenic shock. They include IABP, TandemHeart (CardiacAssist, Inc., Pittsburgh, PA), Impella (Abiomed, Inc., Danvers, MA) and surgically implanted left ventricular assist devices (LVAD). While there are significant differences between the mode of action, hemodynamic support and available literature concerning each device, the common objective is maintenance of adequate blood pressure, tissue perfusion and oxygenation. Although not intended to be an exhaustive review of all modalities historically used for mechanical circulatory support, this section will highlight current devices that are most frequently employed in this clinical situation, their indications, limitations and future trends. Devices have been discussed in chronological order of their development.

The IABP was developed by a team led by Dr Adrian Kantrowitz. The first clinical implant was performed at Maimonides Hospital, Brooklyn, New York in October 1967 for a 48-year-old woman who was in cardiogenic shock unresponsive to traditional therapy.[49] An IABP was inserted by a cut-down of the left femoral artery. Pumping was performed for approximately 6 hours. Shock reversed and the patient was subsequently discharged home.

The size of the original balloon catheter was 15 French, but eventually 7–9 French balloons were developed. The balloon was initially inserted through a surgical cut-down of the femoral artery, requiring a second operation for removal of the balloon catheter. Since 1979, percutaneous placement of the balloon has been adopted using the Seldinger technique. Sequential design improvements have led to a decrease in device diameter (and therefore smaller sheaths are required for insertion, reducing vascular complications), more precise algorithms for triggering, requiring less user input and adjustments and fiber-optic sensors, which allow more precise waveform detection.

Intra-aortic balloon pump (IABP) has become the most common method of mechanical cardiac assistance in ACS today. It is commonly inserted via a transfemoral approach, with the tip placed in the descending aorta, just distal to the left subclavian artery, using fluoroscopic landmarks and with the distal end of the balloon superior to the ostia of the renal arteries. This is most commonly accomplished in the cardiac catheterization laboratory, but successful insertion of the pump may be performed at the bedside (generally in the intensive care unit) and in the operating room. Inflation and deflation are synchronized to the patient's cardiac cycle. Inflation occurs at the onset of diastole, resulting in proximal and distal displacement of blood volume in the aorta. Deflation occurs just prior to the onset of systole, resulting in reduced LV afterload. Advantages of the IABP include widespread availability and ease of use, as well as familiarity with its mode of action in most catheterization labs and intensive care units.

Use of an IABP improves coronary and peripheral perfusion during diastolic balloon inflation, and augments LV performance during systolic balloon deflation with an acute decrease in afterload. Accurate timing of inflation and deflation provides optimal support.

Contraindications for IABP insertion include severe aortic insufficiency, aortic dissection and severe peripheral vascular disease. Complications associated with IABP have decreased in the modern era, likely due to miniaturization of the device. In the largest series, the overall and major complication rates were 7.2% and 2.8% respectively.[50] Risk factors for complications include female sex, small body size and peripheral vascular disease.

Despite over four decades of use, high-quality scientific evidence supporting clinical use of intra-aortic balloon counterpulsation from randomized clinical trials still lags behind its widespread clinical adoption. To date, there are no randomized clinical trials of IABP performed specifically for STEMI complicated by cardiogenic shock, and only a few (relatively small) randomized clinical trials have studied IABP therapy in STEMI. The American College of Cardiology and

TABLE 2

ACC/AHA recommendations for cardiogenic shock*

Class 1A: Primary percutaneous coronary intervention (PCI) is recommended for patients < 75 years, with ST elevation or LBBB or who develop shock within 36 hours of MI and are suitable for revascularization that can be performed within 18 hours of shock.
Class 1.1a: Primary PCI is reasonable for selected patients 75 years or older with ST elevation or LBBB or who develop shock within 36 hours of MI and are suitable for revascularization that can be performed within 18 hours of shock.
Class 1A: Intra-aortic ballon pulsation when cardiogenic shock is not quickly reversed with pharmacologic therapy.

*ACC/AHA Revision of Guidelines for the management of STEMI. Circulation. 2004;110.

American Heart Association STEMI guidelines list IABP therapy in cardiogenic shock as a class IB recommendation.[51] The European Society of Cardiology STEMI guidelines also strongly recommend supportive treatment with an IABP in cardiogenic shock patients (Table 2).[52]

Although widely adopted by the clinical community and endorsed by official guidelines, the efficacy of IABP use in cardiogenic shock has come under significant scrutiny lately. A recent systematic review and meta-analysis from 2009 challenged established guidelines, and found that there is insufficient evidence endorsing the current guideline recommendation for the use of IABP therapy in the setting of STEMI complicated by cardiogenic shock.[53] Two separate meta-analyses were performed, the first including seven randomized trials comprising 1,009 patients with STEMI, and the second including nine cohort studies of STEMI patients with cardiogenic shock (n = 10,529). IABP showed neither a 30-day survival benefit nor improved LV ejection fraction, while being associated with significantly higher stroke and bleeding rates. In patients treated with thrombolysis, IABP was associated with an 18% [95% confidence interval (CI), 16–20%; p = 0.0001] decrease in 30-day mortality, but the effect was confounded due to significantly higher revascularization rates in IABP patients compared to patients without support. However, in patients treated with primary PCI, IABP was associated with a 6% (95% CI, 3–10%; p = 0.0008) increase in 30-day mortality. The authors concluded that the pooled randomized data do not support IABP use in patients with high-risk STEMI. The meta-analysis of cohort studies in the setting of STEMI complicated by cardiogenic shock supported IABP therapy adjunctive to thrombolysis. In contrast, the observational data did not support IABP therapy adjunctive to primary PCI. All available observational data concerning IABP therapy in the setting of cardiogenic shock is importantly hampered by bias and confounding.

LEFT VENTRICULAR ASSIST DEVICE

Surgically implanted left ventricular assist devices (LVADs) are another option for mechanical support in cardiogenic shock patients. Manufactured by a variety of companies, these devices remove blood through a cannula placed at the LV apex and return blood to the ascending aorta. These devices have extensively been used for other indications, such as bridge-to-transplant, post-cardiac surgery recovery and as destination therapy in patients with severe heart failure who are not candidates for transplantation. LVADs provide significant augmentation of cardiac output with preload reduction. In cardiogenic shock patients, surgically implanted LVADs have generally been used as a bridge to cardiac transplantation. In the largest reported LVAD series to date, 74% of 49 patients survived to transplantation, and 87% of transplanted patients survived to hospital discharge after receiving a variety of surgical LVADs.[54]

However they are not widely used in cardiogenic shock due to their lack of availability at many institutions (even those providing primary PCI) as well as the logistical challenges involved in assembling an operating team and room in a short time frame.

TANDEMHEART

TandemHeart (CardiacAssist, Inc., Pittsburgh, PA) received United States FDA clearance in 2003, as a percutaneous circulatory assist system. The system consists of a 21 French inflow cannula, an extracorporeal centrifugal pump rotating at up to 7,500 rpm, a femoral outflow cannula (15F–17F), and a microprocessor-based pump controller, which can provide an output of up to 4 l/min (Fig. 10). Its inflow cannula draws blood from the left atrium (via femoral vein access and transseptal puncture), and its outflow cannula returns blood to the femoral artery in a retrograde fashion.

Limitations of the device include the need for a large (21 French) cannula size, leading to frequent peripheral vascular compromise, potential for a residual left-to-right shunt due to the transseptal approach, need for atrial cannulation, which has a higher risk of wall suction disruptions (compared to a direct ventricular approach), and limited forward flow through the pump circuit.

In one small, randomized, multicenter trial comparing the IABP to the TandemHeart for cardiogenic shock in a patient population comprised mostly of acute MI patients (of which the majority were failing treatment with an IABP at enrollment), Burkhoff et al. showed significant increases in cardiac index (CI) and mean arterial blood pressure and a significant decrease in pulmonary capillary wedge pressure in those randomized to TandemHeart compared with those randomized to IABP.[55] Overall, 30-day survival and severe adverse events were not significantly different between the two groups, although the study was underpowered to detect a mortality difference. However, the incidence of bleeding and distal leg ischemia was higher in the TandemHeart arm. A single-center study of comparable size reached similar conclusions.[56]

In clinical practice, the complexity of the cannulation, the transseptal technique, and the need for full anticoagulation has limited its use to the most experienced institutions.

IMPELLA

The Impella 2.5 (Abiomed, Inc., Danvers, MA) is a catheter-mounted axial flow miniature pump, capable of delivering up to 2.5 l/min of blood from the left ventricle, across the aortic valve, and into the aortic root. It has only one cannula (functioning as both inflow and outflow) positioned across the aortic valve, and contiguous to the integrated motor that comprises the largest-diameter section of the catheter (12 French) (Fig. 11). Control and power supply to the device are delivered via the Impella console.

An infusion pump controls a purge system designed to keep blood from entering the motor compartment.

Unlike the IABP, the Impella device does not require synchronization with ventricular activity. Since the pump delivers nonpulsatile flow, there is no need for timing of the

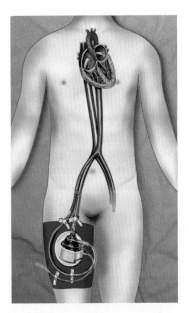

FIGURE 10: The TandemHeart system uses a 21 French intake cannula placed in the left atrium using a transseptal approach, and a 15F–17F femoral arterial return cannula (*Source*: Modified from Kar B, Forrester M, Gemmato C, et al. Use of the TandemHeart percutaneous ventricular assist device to support patients undergoing high-risk percutaneous coronary intervention. J Invasive Cardiol. 2006;18:93-6)

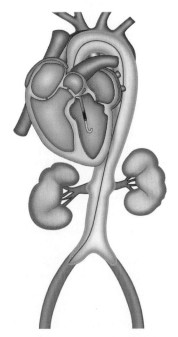

FIGURE 11: The Impella 2.5 device is positioned in the left ventricle in a retrograde fashion across the aortic valve. Blood is removed from the left ventricle and pumped into the ascending aorta (*Source*: http://abiomedtraining.com/QSV/Video1/index.html)

device with the cardiac cycle. Impella 2.5 was approved for use in the United States in June 2008, while the Impella 5 l/min device (Impella 5.0 and Left Direct) was approved for use in the United States in April 2009.

The device is inserted using a modified monorail technique under direct fluoroscopic control. After arterial access is achieved, the 13 French peel-away sheath is positioned. A coronary diagnostic catheter (typically JR4, Multipurpose, or AL1) and, subsequently, a 0.018-inch guidewire are placed across the aortic valve into the left ventricle. Once the guidewire is across the aortic valve, the coronary catheter is removed, and the Impella catheter is advanced to the left ventricle.

Verification of positioning is accomplished by using both a pressure lumen adjacent to the motor as well as motor current monitoring. The device is placed using fluoroscopic guidance to avoid kinking the catheter and compromising the purge lumen. With the device positioned in the left ventricle, the wire is removed, and the device is started at the lowest performance level. Subsequently, once stable positioning and performance have been confirmed, performance characteristics can be adjusted to the desired level.

Implantation time for the Impella device has been reported in a study by Seyfarth et al., and compared to the IABP in a cardiogenic shock patient population.[57] IABP implantation times ranged 6–22 minutes (mean = 14 minutes), while Impella implantation time was 14–31 minutes (mean = 22 minutes; p = 0.40). This ISAR-SHOCK study examined the hemodynamic changes produced by an Impella device compared to an IABP.[57] CI after 30 minutes of support was significantly increased in patients with the Impella 2.5, compared with patients with IABP (Impella: change in CI 0.49 ± 0.46 l/min/m^2; IABP: change in CI 0.11 ± 0.31 l/min/m^2; p = 0.02). Overall 30-day mortality was 46% in both groups, but the study was underpowered for clinical outcomes.

Questions that await clarification from larger randomized trials pertain to the higher incidence of hemolysis (as assessed by measurements of free hemoglobin, which was significantly higher in Impella patients in the first 24 hours), and the higher need for transfusion of packed red blood cells and fresh-frozen plasma in the Impella group (red blood cells: Impella 2.6 ± 2.7 U vs IABP 1.2 ± 1.9 U, p = 0.18; and fresh-frozen plasma: Impella 1.8 ± 2.5 U vs IABP: 1.0 ± 1.7 U, p = 0.39).[58] A major limitation of the trial is the lack of data on major bleeding, which would be expected to be higher in the Impella arm. This could be inferred both from the higher use of blood products (above), as well as the need to use a 13 French sheath for the Impella device (as opposed to 8 French for IABP).

An industry-sponsored clinical trial in the acute MI patient population, RECOVER II, is testing the ability of the device to restore stable hemodynamics, reduce infarct size to improve residual cardiac function, and reduce overall mortality from cardiogenic shock relative to existing treatment modes (IABP).[59] Currently, the trial is still in the recruitment phase (ClinicalTrials.gov identifier: NCT00562016).

REVASCULARIZATION

The question as to whether cardiogenic shock patients would benefit from emergent mechanical coronary revascularization by PCI or CABG (as opposed to aggressive medical therapy) was first answered by the landmark SHOCK trial.[20] In this study, 302 patients were randomly assigned to either initial medical stabilization (150 patients) or emergent revascularization (152 patients). The use of IABP was high (86% in both groups), and a large proportion of patients in the medical stabilization arm received thormbolytics (63%). Although 30-day mortality was not significantly different between the groups, 6-month mortality was lower in the revascularization group than in the medical-therapy group (50.3% vs 63.1%, p = 0.027).

At 1 year, there was a 13% absolute increase in survival for patients assigned to early revascularization, and this benefit was sustained up to 3 years (67% relative improvement in mortality).[12] Although incomplete, another randomized study[60] demonstrated a similar benefit. Numerous registries, including the SHOCK Registry,[30] have strengthened the assertion that early mechanical revascularization is beneficial in cardiogenic shock patients.

Which particular method of mechanical coronary revascularization should be chosen for cardiogenic shock patients: PCI or CABG? PCI has the advantage of wider availability in the community and generally shorter reperfusion times. If successful, timely PCI confers a survival advantage, an important consideration since the SHOCK trial demonstrated a trend toward reduced clinical benefit if reperfusion was delayed. Nonetheless, a reduction in mortality was seen if revascularization was performed even after 48 hours from myocardial infarction and 18 hours after the onset of shock.[61] In this subanalysis of the SHOCK trial, mortality was 38% if TIMI III flow was achieved, but rose to 55% with TIMI II flow, and TIMI I or 0 was always fatal. A retrospective review of 10-year trends in Swiss hospitals showed that more frequent use of PCI in ACS patients without initial cardiogenic shock was associated with a decrease in incidence of cardiogenic shock.[62] Unsuccessful PCI has consistently been shown to be associated with significantly worse outcomes.[63] Adjunctive pharmacological treatment to PCI (GPIIb/IIIa inhibitors) have independently been associated with improved outcomes in patients undergoing PCI in the large ACC-National Cardiovascular Data Registry,[64] and in a small subset of cardiogenic shock patients in a randomized trial using abciximab.[65]

A history of previous myocardial infarction or failed thrombolysis is generally viewed as conferring a worse prognosis. Although some studies cite the presence of multi-vessel disease as being an adverse predictor, others do not.[62] Nonetheless the prevalence of multivessel disease is very high in cardiogenic shock patients (87% in the SHOCK trial). Therefore the question of performing complete versus culprit vessel revascularization is quite important, yet not entirely clarified. Despite having a high prevalence of multivessel disease, most patients in the SHOCK trial (87%) underwent single-vessel PCI, although the proportion of those undergoing multivessel PCI rose steadily as the study was progressing. One-year survival was only 20% after a single-stage multivessel procedure, compared to 55% after single-vessel PCI. It is not clear if these observations might be due to the low utilization rate of stents (34%), since stenting has been correlated with improved outcomes in multiple registries.[64]

CABG has historically been able to achieve complete revascularization in a larger proportion of patients and was used in 37.5% of patients in the SHOCK trial. Patients having left main and multivessel disease were more likely to undergo CABG. Despite the possibility of selection bias, overall outcomes with PCI and CABG were equivalent for both survival and quality of life. Outside of randomized studies, emergent CABG is much less likely to be used as an initial revascularization method (under 10%).[66]

REFERENCES

1. Reynolds HR, Hochman JS. Cardiogenic shock: current concepts and improving outcomes. Circulation. 2008;117:686-97.

2. Hasdai D, Harrington RA, Hochman JS, et al. Platelet glycoprotein IIb/IIIa blockade and outcome of cardiogenic shock complicating acute coronary syndromes without persistent ST-segment elevation. J Am Coll Cardiol. 2000;36:685-92.

3. Goldberg RJ, Gore JM, Alpert JS, et al. Cardiogenic shock after acute myocardial infarction. Incidence and mortality from a community-wide perspective, 1975 to 1988. N Engl J Med. 1991;325:1117-22.

4. Goldberg RJ, Gore JM, Thompson CA, et al. Recent magnitude of and temporal trends (1994-1997) in the incidence and hospital death rates of cardiogenic shock complicating acute myocardial infarction: the second national registry of myocardial infarction. Am Heart J. 2001;141:65-72.

5. Lindholm MG, Kober L, Boesgaard S, et al. Cardiogenic shock complicating acute myocardial infarction; prognostic impact of early and late shock development. Eur Heart J. 2003;24:258-65.

6. Berger PB, Tuttle RH, Holmes DR Jr, et al. One-year survival among patients with acute myocardial infarction complicated by cardiogenic shock, and its relation to early revascularization: results from the GUSTO-I trial. Circulation. 1999;99:873-8.

7. French JK, Harkness S, Sleeper L, et al. Cardiogenic shock without flow-limiting angiographic coronary artery disease: (from the Should We Emergently Revascularize Occluded Coronary Arteries for Cardiogenic Shock Trial and Registry). Am J Cardiol. 2009;104:24-8.

8. Sanborn TA, Sleeper LA, Webb JG, et al. Correlates of one-year survival inpatients with cardiogenic shock complicating acute myocardial infarction: angiographic findings from the SHOCK trial. J Am Coll Cardiol. 2003;42:1373-9.

9. Babaev A, Frederick PD, Pasta DJ, et al. Trends in management and outcomes of patients with acute myocardial infarction complicated by cardiogenic shock. JAMA. 2005;294:448-54.

10. Jeger RV, Radovanovic D, Hunziker PR, et al. Ten-year trends in the incidence and treatment of cardiogenic shock. Ann Intern Med. 2008;149:618-26.

11. Hochman JS, Sleeper LA, White HD, et al. One-year survival following early revascularization for cardiogenic shock. JAMA. 2001;285:190-2.

12. Hochman JS, Sleeper LA, Webb JG, et al. Early revascularization and long-term survival in cardiogenic shock complicating acute myocardial infarction. JAMA. 2006;295:2511-5.

13. Hasdai D, Califf RM, Thompson TD, et al. Predictors of cardiogenic shock after thrombolytic therapy for acute myocardial infarction. J Am Coll Cardiol. 2000;35:136-43.

14. Hasdai D, Holmes DR Jr, Califf RM, et al. Cardiogenic shock complicating acute myocardial infarction: predictors of death. GUSTO Investigators. Global Utilization of Streptokinase and Tissue-Plasminogen Activator for Occluded Coronary Arteries. Am Heart J. 1999;138:21-31.

15. Katz JN, Stebbins AL, Alexander JH, et al. Predictors of 30-day mortality in patients with refractory cardiogenic shock following acute myocardial infarction despite a patent infarct artery. Am Heart J. 2009;158:680-7.

16. Klein LW, Shaw RE, Krone RJ, et al. Mortality after emergent percutaneous coronary intervention in cardiogenic shock secondary to acute myocardial infarction and usefulness of a mortality prediction model. Am J Cardiol. 2005;96:35-41.

17. Chan AW, Chew DP, Bhatt DL, et al. Long-term mortality benefit with the combination of stents and abciximab for cardiogenic shock complicating acute myocardial infarction. Am J Cardiol. 2002;89:132-6.

18. Wong SC, Sanborn T, Sleeper LA. Angiographic findings and clinical correlates in patients with cardiogenic shock complicating acute myocardial infarction: a report from the SHOCK trial registry. Should we emergently revascularize occluded coronaries for cardiogenic shock? J Am Coll Cardiol. 2000;36:1077-83.

19. Alonso DR, Scheidt S, Post M, et al. Pathophysiology of cardiogenic shock. Quantification of myocardial necrosis, clinical, pathologic and electrocardiographic correlations. Circulation. 1973;48:588-96.

20. Hochman JS, Sleeper LA, Webb JG, et al. Early revascularization in acute myocardial infarction complicated by cardiogenic shock. SHOCK investigators. Should we emergently revascularize occluded coronaries for cardiogenic shock. N Engl J Med. 1999;341:625-34.

21. Picard MH, Davidoff R, Sleeper LA, et al. Echocardiographic predictors of survival and response to early revascularization in cardiogenic shock. Circulation. 2003;107:279-84.

22. Kohsaka S, Menon V, Lowe AM, et al. Systemic inflammatory response syndrome after acute myocardial infarction complicated by cardiogenic shock. Arch Intern Med. 2005;165:1643-50.

23. Zhang C, Xu X, Potter BJ, et al. TNF-alpha contributes to endothelial dysfunction in ischemia/reperfusion injury. Arterioscler Thromb Vasc Biol. 2006;26:475-80.

24. Theroux P, Armstrong PW, Mahaffey KW, et al. Prognostic significance of blood markers of inflammation in patients with ST-segment elevation myocardial infarction undergoing primary angioplasty and effects of pexelizumab, a C5 inhibitor: a substudy of the COMMA trial. Eur Heart J. 2005;26:1964-70.

25. Wildhirt SM, Dudek RR, Suzuki H, et al. Involvement of inducible nitric oxide synthase in the inflammatory process of myocardial infarction. Int J Cardiol. 1995;50:253-61.

26. Alexander JH, Reynolds HR, Stebbins AL, et al. Effect of tilarginine acetate in patients with acute myocardial infarction and cardiogenic shock: the TRIUMPH randomized controlled trial. JAMA. 2007;297:1657-66.

27. Dzavik V, Cotter G, Reynolds HR, et al. Effect of nitric oxide synthase inhibition on haemodynamics and outcome of patients with persistent cardiogenic shock complicating acute myocardial infarction: a phase II dose-ranging study. Eur Heart J. 2007;28:1109-16.

28. Hands ME, Rutherford JD, Muller JE, et al. The in-hospital development of cardiogenic shock after myocardial infarction: incidence, predictors of occurrence, outcome and prognostic factors. The MILIS study group. J Am Coll Cardiol. 1989;14:40-6.

29. Leor J, Goldbourt U, Reicher-Reiss H, et al. Cardiogenic shock complicating acute myocardial infarction in patients without heart failure on admission: incidence, risk factors, and outcome. SPRINT study group. Am J Med. 1993;94:265-73.

30. Jacobs AK, Leopold JA, Bates E, et al. Cardiogenic shock caused by right ventricular infarction: a report from the SHOCK registry. J Am Coll Cardiol. 2003;41:1273-9.

31. Brookes C, Ravn H, White P, et al. Acute right ventricular dilatation in response to ischemia significantly impairs left ventricular systolic performance. Circulation. 1999;100:761-7.

32. Berisha S, Kastrati A, Goda A, et al. Optimal value of filling pressure in the right side of the heart in acute right ventricular infarction. Br Heart J. 1990;63:98-102.

33. Chatterjee K, McGlothlin D, Michaels A. Analytic reviews: cardiogenic shock with preserved systolic function: a reminder. J Intensive Care Med. 2008;23:355-66.

34. Crenshaw BS, Granger CB, Birnbaum Y, et al. Risk factors, angiographic patterns, and outcomes in patients with ventricular septal defect complicating acute myocardial infarction. GUSTO-I (Global Utilization of Streptokinase and TPA for Occluded Coronary Arteries) trial investigators. Circulation. 2000;101:27-32.

35. Birnbaum Y, Fishbein MC, Blanche C, et al. Ventricular septal rupture after acute myocardial infarction. N Engl J Med. 2002;347:1426-32.

36. Reeder G. Identification and treatment of complications of myocardial infarction. Mayo Clinic Proceedings. 1995;70:880-4.

37. David TE, Dale L, Sun Z. Postinfarction ventricular septal rupture: repair by endocardial patch with infarct exclusion. J Thorac Cardiovasc Surg. 1995;110:1315-22.

38. Thiele H, Kaulfersch C, Daehnert I, et al. Immediate primary transcatheter closure of postinfarction ventricular septal defects. Eur Heart J. 2009;30:81-8.

39. Patel MR, Meine TJ, Lindblad L, et al. Cardiac tamponade in the fibrinolytic era: analysis of > 100,000 patients with ST-segment elevation myocardial infarction. Am Heart J. 2006;151:316-22.

40. Mann JM, Roberts WC. Rupture of the left ventricular free wall during acute myocardial infarction: analysis of 138 necropsy patients and comparison with 50 necropsy patients with acute myocardial infarction without rupture. Am J Cardiol. 1988;62:847-59.

41. Antman E. ST-elevation myocardial infarction: management. In: Libby P, Bonnow RO, Mann DL, Zipes DP. (Eds). Braunwald's Heart Disease: A Textbook of Cardiovascular Medicine, 8th edn. Philadelphia: Saunders; 2008. pp. 1233-99.

42. Lesser JR, Johnson K, Lindberg JL, et al. Images in cardiovascular medicine. Myocardial rupture, microvascular obstruction, and infarct expansion: elucidation by cardiac magnetic resonance. Circulation. 2003;108:116-7.

43. Oliva PB, Hammill SC, Edwards WD. Cardiac rupture: a clinically predictable complication of acute myocardial infarction: report of 70 cases with clinicopathologic correlations. J Am Coll Cardiol. 1993;22:720-6.

44. McMullan MH, Maples MD, Kilgore TL Jr, et al. Surgical experience with left ventricular free wall rupture. Ann Thorac Surg. 2001;71:1894-8.

45. Antman EM, Anbe DT, Armstrong PW, et al. ACC/AHA guidelines for the management of patients with ST-elevation myocardial infarction-executive summary: a report of the American College of Cardiology/American Heart Association Task Force on Practice Guidelines. Circulation. 2004;110:588-636.

46. Lavie CJ, Gersh BJ. Mechanical and electrical complications of acute myocardial infarction. Mayo Clin Proc. 1990;65:709-30.

47. De Backer D, Biston P, Devriendt J, et al. Comparison of dopamine and norepinephrine in the treatment of shock. N Engl J Med. 2010;362:779-89.

48. Nieminen MS, Bohm M, Cowie MR, et al. Executive summary of the guidelines on the diagnosis and treatment of acute heart failure: the task force on acute heart failure of the European Society of Cardiology. Eur Heart J. 2005;26:384-416.

49. Kantrowitz A, Tjønneland S, Freed PS, et al. Initial clinical experience with intra-aortic balloon pumping in cardiogenic shock. JAMA. 1968;203:113-18.

50. Urban PM, Freedman RJ, Ohman EM. In-hospital mortality associated with the use of intra-aortic balloon counterpulsation. Am J Cardiol. 2004;94:181-85.

51. Kushner FG, Hand M, Smith SC Jr, et al. 2009 focused updates: ACC/AHA guidelines for the management of patients with ST-elevation myocardial infarction (updating the 2004 guideline and 2007 focused update) and ACC/AHA/SCAI guidelines on percutaneous coronary intervention (updating the 2005 guideline and 2007

52. Van de Werf F, Bax J, Betriu A, et al. Management of acute myocardial infarction in patients presenting with persistent ST-segment elevation: the task force on the management of ST-segment elevation acute myocardial infarction of the European Society of Cardiology. Eur Heart J. 2008;29:2909-45.

focused update): a report of the American College of Cardiology Foundation/American Heart Association Task Force on Practice Guidelines. Circulation. 2009;120:2271-306.

53. Sjauw KD, Engström AE, Vis MM, et al. A systematic review and meta-analysis of intra-aortic balloon pump therapy in ST-elevation myocardial infarction: should we change the guidelines? Eur Heart J. 2009;30:459-68.

54. Leshnower BG, Gleason TG, O'Hara ML, et al. Safety and efficacy of left ventricular assist device support in postmyocardial infarction cardiogenic shock. Ann Thorac Surg. 2006;81:1365-70.

55. Burkhoff D, Cohen H, Brunckhorst C, et al. A randomized multicenter clinical study to evaluate the safety and efficacy of the TandemHeart percutaneous ventricular assist device versus conventional therapy with intra-aortic balloon pumping for treatment of cardiogenic shock. Am Heart J. 2006;152:459 (e461-8).

56. Thiele H, Sick P, Boudriot E, et al. Randomized comparison of intra-aortic balloon support with a percutaneous left ventricular device in patients with revascularized acute myocardial infarction complicated by cardiogenic shock. Eur Heart J. 2005;26:1276-83.

57. Seyfarth M, Sibbing D, Bauer I, et al. A randomized clinical trial to evaluate the safety and efficacy of a percutaneous left ventricular assist device versus intra-aortic balloon pumping for treatment of cardiogenic shock caused by myocardial infarction. J Am Coll Cardiol. 2008;52:1584-8.

58. Henriques JP, Remmelink M, Baan J Jr, et al. Safety and feasibility of elective high-risk percutaneous coronary intervention procedures with left ventricular support of the Impella Recover LP 2.5. Am J Cardiol. 2006;97:990-2.

59. Dixon SR, Henriques JP, Mauri L, et al. A prospective feasibility trial investigating the use of the Impella 2.5 system in patients undergoing high-risk percutaneous coronary intervention (The PROTECT I Trial): initial US experience. J Am Coll Cardiol Interv. 2009;2:91-6.

60. Urban P, Stauffer JC, Bleed D, et al. A randomized evaluation of early revascularization to treat shock complicating acute myocardial infarction: the (Swiss) Multicenter Trial of Angioplasty for Shock: (S)MASH. Eur Heart J. 1999;20:1030-8.

61. Webb JG, Lowe AM, Sanborn TA, et al. Percutaneous coronary intervention for cardiogenic shock in the SHOCK trial. J Am Coll Cardiol. 2003;42:1380-6.

62. Jeger RV, Radovanovic D, Hunziker PR, et al. Ten-year trends in the incidence and treatment of cardiogenic shock. Ann Intern Med. 2008;149:618-26.

63. Sutton AGC, Finn P, Hall JA, et al. Predictors of outcome after percutaneous treatment for cardiogenic shock. Heart. 2005;91:339-44.

64. Klein LW, Shaw RE, Krone RJ, et al. Mortality after emergent percutaneous coronary intervention in cardiogenic shock secondary to acute myocardial infarction and usefulness of a mortality prediction model. Am J Cardiol. 2005;96:35-41.

65. Montalescot G, Barragan P, Wittenberg O, et al. Platelet glycoprotein IIb/IIIa inhibition with coronary stenting for acute myocardial infarction. N Engl J Med. 2001;344:1895-903.

66. Babaev A, Frederick PD, Pasta DJ, et al. Trends in management and outcomes of patients with acute myocardial infarction complicated by cardiogenic shock. JAMA. 2005;294:448-54.

Chapter 53

Acute Right Ventricular Infarction

James A Goldstein

Chapter Outline

INTRODUCTION

Based on early experiments of right ventricular (RV) performance, it was felt for many years that RV contraction was unimportant in the circulation and that, despite loss of RV contraction, pulmonary flow could be generated by a passive gradient from a distended venous system and active right atrial contraction.[1] However, recognition of the profound hemodynamic effects of RV systolic dysfunction became evident during the 1970s with the description of severe RV infarction (RVI), resulting in severe right heart failure, clear lungs and hypotension low output despite intact global left ventricular (LV) systolic function.[2-4] Nearly 50% of patients with acute ST elevation inferior myocardial infarction (IMI) suffer concomitant RVI, which is associated with higher in-hospital morbidity and mortality related to hemodynamic and electrophysiologic complications.[5-7] Although the magnitude of hemodynamic derangements is related to the extent of RVFW contraction abnormalities,[7] some patients tolerate severe RV systolic dysfunction without hemodynamic compromise whereas others develop life-threatening low output, emphasizing that additional factors modulate the clinical expression of RVI. Importantly, the term RV "infarction" is to an extent a misnomer. For in most cases acute RV ischemic dysfunction appears to represent viable myocardium which recovers over time, especially following successful reperfusion and even after prolonged occlusion.[8-10]

This chapter will review the pathophysiology, hemodynamics, natural history and management of patients with IMI complicated by RVI. Importantly, we will highlight five key areas in which advances may impact catheterization and laboratory management of these acutely ill patients, including:

- The relationship between the site of right coronary artery (RCA) occlusion and the presence and magnitude of right heart ischemia and its complications.
- The pathophysiologic mechanisms leading to hemodynamic compromise and their relevance to pharmacologic and mechanical interventions.
- Bradyarrhythmias and tachyarrhythmias complicating management during acute occlusion and reperfusion.
- The concept that RV "infarction" is actually a misnomer, for even severe acute ischemic RV dysfunction is nearly always reversible.
- The compensatory mechanisms maintaining hemodynamic performance under conditions of profound RV pump function.
- The benefits of mechanical reperfusion therapy on hemodynamics and clinical outcome, even after prolonged occlusion and in patients with severe shock.

PATTERNS OF CORONARY COMPROMISE RESULTING IN RVI

Significant RVI nearly always occurs in association with acute transmural inferior-posterior LV myocardial infarction (MI) and the RCA is always the culprit vessel,[11] typically a proximal occlusion compromising flow to one or more of the major RV branches (Figs 1 and 2). In contrast, distal RCA occlusions or circumflex culprits that spare RV branch perfusion rarely

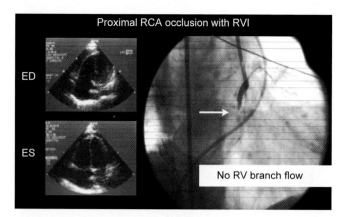

FIGURE 1: Patient with a proximal right coronary artery (right panel, arrow) compromising the right ventricular branches and resulting in severe RVI, indicated on echo as severe RV free wall dysfunction and depressed global RV performance at end systole (ES) and marked RV dilation at end diastole (ED)

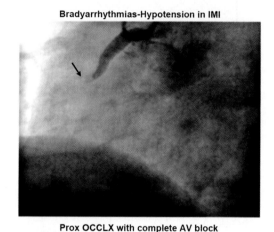

FIGURE 2: Patient with proximal right coronary artery occlusion (arrow) complicated by third-degree AV block. (*Source*: Goldstein JA, et al. Coronary Artery Disease. 2005;16:267, with permission)

compromise RV performance.[9] Occasionally, isolated RVI may develop from occlusion of a nondominant RCA or selective compromise of RV branches during percutaneous interventions.

At necropsy, RVI inscribes a "tripartite" signature consisting of LV inferior-posterior wall, septal and posterior RV free wall (FW) necrosis contiguous with the septum.[12] However, it is important to emphasize that these autopsy patterns do not reflect the vast majority of patients who survive acute RVI, for even in the absence of reperfusion of the infarct-related artery, most patients with severe ischemic RV dysfunction manifest spontaneous early hemodynamic improvement and later recovery of RV function.[7-10] In fact, chronic right heart failure attributable to RVI is rare. Thus, the term RV "infarction" is to an extent a misnomer, as in most cases acute RV ischemic dysfunction appears to represent predominantly viable

myocardium. These responses are in marked contrast to the effects of ischemia on the LV.[13-15]

RIGHT VENTRICULAR MECHANICS AND OXYGEN SUPPLY-DEMAND

The right and left ventricles differ markedly in their anatomy, mechanics, loading conditions and metabolism, therefore it should not be surprising that they have strikingly different oxygen supply and demand characteristics,[16-18] and thus manifest disparate responses to ischemic insults. The LV is a thick-walled pressure pump. In contrast, the pyramidal-shaped RV with its thin crescentic free wall is designed as a volume pump, ejecting into the lower resistance pulmonary circulation. RV systolic pressure and flow are generated by RVFW shortening and contraction toward the septum from apex to outflow tract.[7,18] The septum is an integral architectural and mechanical component of the RV chamber and, even under physiologic conditions, LV septal contraction contributes to RV performance. The RV has a more favorable oxygen supply-demand profile than the LV. RV oxygen demand is lower owing to lesser myocardial mass, preload and afterload.[16,17] RV perfusion also is more favorable, due to the dual anatomic supply system from left coronary branches. Also, the RVFW is thinner, develops lower systolic intramyocardial pressure and faces less diastolic intracavitary pressure, and lower coronary resistance favors acute collateral development to the RCA.[19]

EFFECTS OF ISCHEMIA ON RV SYSTOLIC AND DIASTOLIC FUNCTION

Proximal RCA occlusion compromises RVFW perfusion, resulting in RVFW dyskinesis and depressed global RV performance reflected in the RV waveform by a sluggish, depressed and systolic waveform (Figs 3 and 4).[8,11,20-22] RV systolic dysfunction diminishes transpulmonary delivery of LV preload, leading to decreased cardiac output despite intact LV contractility. Biventricular diastolic dysfunction contributes to hemodynamic compromise.[20-24] The ischemic RV is stiff and dilated early in diastole, which impedes inflow leading to rapid diastolic pressure elevation. Acute RV dilatation and elevated diastolic pressure shift the interventricular septum toward the volume-deprived LV, further impairing LV compliance and filling. Abrupt RV dilatation within the noncompliant pericardium elevates intrapericardial pressure, the resultant constraint further impairing RV and LV compliance and filling. These effects contribute to the pattern of equalized diastolic pressures and RV "dip-and-plateau" characteristic of RVI.[20-24]

DETERMINANTS OF RV PERFORMANCE IN SEVERE RVI

IMPORTANCE OF SYSTOLIC VENTRICULAR INTERACTIONS

Despite the absence of RVFW motion, an active albeit depressed RV systolic waveform is generated by systolic interactions mediated by primary septal contraction and through mechanical displacement of the septum into the RV cavity associated with paradoxical septal motion (Fig. 1).[8,22-24] In the LV, acute ischemia results in regional dyskinesis; such dyssynergic segments are stretched in early isovolumic systole by neighboring contracting segments through regional intraventricular interactions that dissipate the functional work of these neighboring regions.[25] The ischemic dyskinetic RVFW behaves similarly and must be stretched to the maximal extent of its systolic lengthening through interventricular interactions before providing a stable buttress upon which actively contracting segments can generate effective stroke work, thereby impose a mechanical disadvantage that reduce contributions to cardiac performance.[17,22-24] The compensatory contributions of LV septal contraction are emphasized by the deleterious effects of LV septal dysfunction, which exacerbates hemodynamic compromise associated with RVI.[24] In contrast, inotropic stimulation enhances LV septal contraction and thereby augments RV performance through augmented compensatory systolic interactions.

COMPENSATORY ROLE OF AUGMENTED RIGHT ATRIAL CONTRACTION

The hemodynamic benefits of augmented atrial contraction to performance of the ischemic LV are well documented.[26] Similarly, augmented RA booster pump transport is an important compensatory mechanism that optimizes RV performance and cardiac output.[21-23] When RVI develops from occlusions compromising RV but sparing RA branches, RV diastolic dysfunction imposes increased preload and afterload on the right atrium, resulting in enhanced RA contractility that augments RV filling and performance. This is reflected in the RA waveform as a "W" pattern characterized by a rapid upstroke and increased peak A wave amplitude, sharp X descent reflecting enhanced atrial relaxation and blunted Y descent owing to pandiastolic RV dysfunction (Figs 3A to C).

DELETERIOUS IMPACT OF RIGHT ATRIAL ISCHEMIA

Conversely, more proximal RCA occlusions compromising atrial, as well as RV branches result in ischemic depression of atrial function, which compromises RV performance and cardiac output.[21-23] RA ischemia manifests hemodynamically as more severely elevated mean RA pressure and inscribes an "M" pattern in the RA waveform characterized by a depressed A wave and X descent, as well as blunted Y descent (Figs 4A and B). Ischemic atrial involvement is not rare, with autopsy studies documenting atrial infarction in up to 20% of cases of ventricular infarction, with RA involvement five times commoner than left.[27,28] Under conditions of acute RV dysfunction, loss of augmented RA transport due to ischemic depression of atrial contractility or AV dyssynchrony precipitates more severe hemodynamic compromise.[21-23] RA dysfunction decreases RV filling, which impairs global RV systolic performance, thereby resulting in further decrements in LV preload and cardiac output. Impaired RA contraction diminishes atrial relaxation; thus RA ischemia impedes venous return and right heart filling owing to loss of atrial suction associated with atrial relaxation during the X descent.

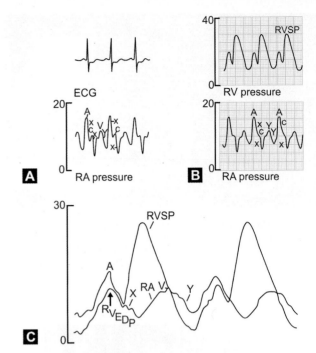

FIGURES 3A TO C: Hemodynamic recordings from a patient with right atrial (RA) pressure W pattern, timed to ECG (A) and RV pressures (B and C). Peaks of W are formed by prominent A waves with an associated sharp "X" systolic descent, followed by a comparatively blunted "Y" descent. Peak RV systolic pressure (RVSP) is depressed, RV relaxation is prolonged, and there is a dip and rapid rise in RV diastolic pressure. (*Source*: Goldstein et al. Circulation. 1990;82:259, with permission)

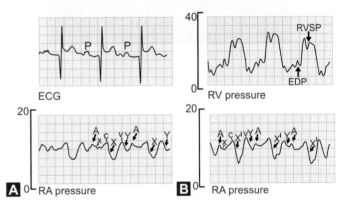

FIGURES 4A AND B: RA pressure M pattern timed to electrocardiogram (A) and RV pressure (B). M pattern comprises a depressed A wave, X descent before a small C wave, a prominent "X" descent, a small V wave and a blunted Y descent. Peak RVSP is depressed and bifid (arrows) with delayed relaxation and an elevated end-diastolic pressure (EDP) (all pressures are measured in mm Hg). (*Source*: Goldstein et al. Circulation. 1990;82:259)

NATURAL HISTORY OF ISCHEMIC RV DYSFUNCTION

Although RVI may result in profound acute hemodynamic effects, arrhythmias and higher in-hospital mortality, many patients spontaneously improve within 3–10 days regardless of the patency status of the infarct-related artery.[9,10] Furthermore, global RV performance typically recovers with normalization within 3–12 months. Moreover, chronic unilateral right heart failure secondary to RVI is rare. This favorable natural history of RV performance is in marked contrast to the effects of coronary occlusion on segmental and global LV function.[13-15] Observations from experimental animal studies confirm spontaneous recovery of RV function despite chronic RCA occlusion attributable to the more favorable oxygen supply-demand characteristics of the RV in general and the beneficial effects of collaterals in particular.[29] Similarly, in patients with chronic proximal RCA occlusion, RV function is typically maintained at rest and augments appropriately during stress.[10] The relative resistance of the RVFW to infarction is undoubtedly attributable to more favorable oxygen supply-demand characteristics. Preinfarction angina appears to reduce the risk of developing RVI, possibly due to preconditioning.[19]

EFFECTS OF REPERFUSION ON ISCHEMIC RV DYSFUNCTION

Although RV function may recover despite persistent RCA occlusion, acute RV ischemia contributes to early morbidity and mortality.[5-7] Furthermore, spontaneous recovery of RV contractile function and hemodynamics may be slow. The beneficial effects of successful reperfusion in patients with predominant LV infarction are well documented.[43,44] Observations in experimental animals[30] and in humans[8,31-33] now demonstrate the beneficial effects of reperfusion on recovery of RV performance. In patients, successful mechanical reperfusion of the RCA including the major RV branches leads to immediate improvement in and later complete recovery of RVFW function and global RV performance (Figs 5 and 6). Reperfusion-mediated recovery of RV performance is associated with excellent clinical outcome (Fig. 7). In contrast, failure to restore flow to the major RV branches is associated with lack of recovery of RV performance and refractory hemodynamic compromise leading to high in-hospital mortality, even if flow was restored in the main RCA. Findings now also demonstrate that successful mechanical reperfusion leads to superior late survival of patients with shock due to predominant RVI versus those with LV shock.[33]

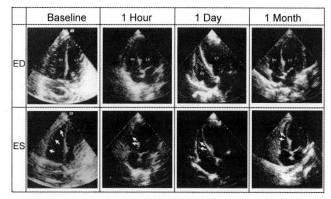

Right heart ischemia

FIGURE 6: Echocardiographic images from a patient with acute IMI and RV ischemia undergoing successful angioplasty. End-diastolic and end-systolic images obtained at baseline show severe RV dilatation with reduced LV diastolic size. At ES, there was RVFW dyskinesis (arrows), intact LV function and compensatory paradoxical septal motion. One hour after angioplasty, there was striking recovery of RVFW contraction (arrows), resulting in marked improvement in global RV performance and markedly increased RV size and LV preload. At one day, there was further improvement in RV function (arrows), which at one month was normal. RV denotes right ventricle while LV denotes left ventricle. (*Source:* Bowers et al. N Eng J Med. 1998;338:933, with permission)

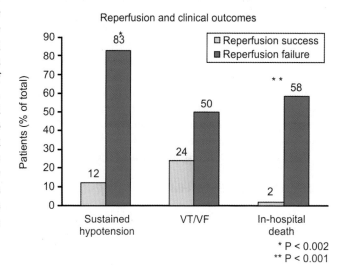

Reperfusion and clinical outcomes

FIGURE 7: Bar graphs demonstrating benefits of successful reperfusion versus reperfusion failure with respect to reduced arrhythmias, sustained hypotension and in-hospital survival. (*Source:* Bowers et al. N Eng J Med. 1998;338:933, with permission)

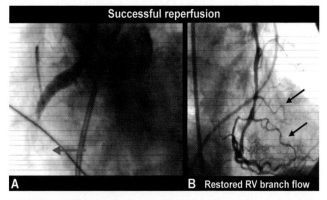

FIGURES 5A AND B: Angiogram showing successful reperfusion in patient with right ventricular infarction who underwent primary angioplasty. (A) Total occlusion of the right coronary artery proximal to RV branches (arrow) in a patient before angiography, and (B) after angioplasty shows complete reperfusion in the right main coronary artery including the major RV branches (arrows). (*Source:* Bowers et al. N Eng J Med. 1998;338: 933, with permission)

Although evidence suggests that patients with IMI benefit from timely thrombolytic reperfusion, the specific short-term and long-term responses of those with RVI have not been adequately evaluated. Some thrombolytic studies suggested that RV function improves only in patients in whom RCA patency is achieved,[34-36] whereas others report little benefit.[37,38] More recent prospective reports demonstrate that successful thrombolysis imparts survival benefit in those with RV involvement and that failure to restore infarct-related artery patency is associated with persistent RV dysfunction and increased mortality.[38] Unfortunately, patients with RVI appear to be particularly resistant to fibrinolytic recanalization, owing to proximal RCA occlusion with extensive clot burden which, together with impaired coronary delivery of fibrinolytic agents is attributable to hypotension.[38] There also appear to be a higher incidence of reocclusion following thrombolysis of the RCA. It is important to consider RVI separately in the elderly. Early reports suggested that elderly patients with RVI suffer 50% in-hospital mortality and that hemodynamic compromise in such cases is irreversible. However, recent studies now document the majority of elderly RVI patients undergoing successful mechanical reperfusion survive, including those with hemodynamic compromise.[32]

RHYTHM DISORDERS AND REFLEXES ASSOCIATED WITH RVI

BRADYARRHYTHMIAS AND HYPOTENSION

High-grade atrioventricular (AV) block and bradycardia-hypotension without AV block commonly complicate IMI and have been attributed predominantly to the effects of AV nodal ischemia and cardioinhibitory (Bezold-Jarisch) reflexes arising from stimulation of vagal afferents in the ischemic LV inferoposterior wall.[39-42] Patients with acute RVI are at increased risk for both high-grade AV block and bradycardia-hypotension without AV block.[5,42] Recent findings now document that during acute coronary occlusion, bradycardia-hypotension and AV block are far more common in patients with proximal RCA lesions (Fig. 2) inducing RV and LV inferior-posterior ischemia, compared to more distal occlusions compromising LV perfusion, but sparing the RV branches.[43] These observations suggest that the ischemic right heart may elicit cardioinhibitory-vasodilator reflexes. In patients with IMI, whose rhythm and blood pressure were stable during occlusion, similar bradycardic-hypotensive reflexes may be elicited during reperfusion[43,44] and also appear to be more common with proximal lesions (Fig. 8).

VENTRICULAR ARRHYTHMIAS

Patients with RVI are prone to ventricular tachyarrhythmias,[5,45] which should not be unexpected given that the ischemic RV is often massively dilated.[45] Autonomic denervation in the peri-infarct area may also play a role.[46] In patients with RVI, VT/VF may develop in a trimodal pattern, either during acute occlusion, abruptly with reperfusion or later.[45] However, successful mechanical reperfusion dramatically reduces the incidence of malignant ventricular arrhythmias,[8,45] presumably through improvement in RV function, which lessens late VT/VF. Occasionally, RVI may be complicated by recurrent malignant arrhythmias and in some cases intractable "electrical storm" (Fig. 9), possibly due to sustained severe RV dilatation.[45]

MECHANICAL COMPLICATIONS ASSOCIATED WITH RVI

Patients with acute RVI may suffer additional mechanical complications of acute infarction that may compound hemo-dynamic compromise and confound the clinical hemodynamic picture. Ventricular septal rupture is a particularly disastrous complication, adding substantial overload stress to the ischemically dysfunctional RV, precipitating pulmonary edema,

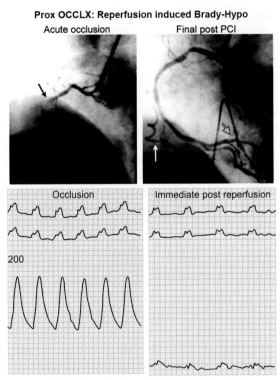

FIGURE 8: Patient with a proximal right coronary artery (left panel, arrow) compromising the RV branches (right panel, solid arrow) as well as the LV and atrioventricular nodal branches (right panel, open arrow), who developed profound repefrusion-induced bradycardia-hypotension. During occlusion there was sinus rhythm with normal blood pressure. Reperfusion by primary percutaneous transluminal coronary angioplasty resulted in abrupt but transient sinus bradycardia with profound hypotension. PCI denotes percutaneous coronary intervention. (*Source*: Goldstein JA et al. Coronary Artery Disease. 2005;16:269, with permission)

elevating pulmonary pressures and resistance and exacerbating low output.[47] Surgical repair is imperative, but may be technically difficult owing to extensive necrosis involving the LV inferior-posterior free wall, septum and apex. Catheter closure of such defects may be possible. Severe right heart dilatation and diastolic pressure elevation associated with RVI may stretch open a patent foramen ovale, precipitating acute right-to-left shunting manifest as systemic hypoxemia or paradoxical emboli.[48] Most PFO complications abate following successful mechanical reperfusions, as right heart pressures diminish with recovery of RV performance; rarely, some may require percutaneous closure.[49] Severe tricuspid regurgitation may also complicate RVI, developing as a result of primary papillary muscle ischemic dysfunction or rupture, as well as secondary functional regurgitation attributable to severe RV and tricuspid valve annular dilatation.[50]

CLINICAL PRESENTATIONS AND EVALUATION

Right ventricular infarction is often silent as only 25% of patients develop clinically evident hemodynamic manifestations.[7] Patients with severe RVI but preserved global LV function may be hemodynamically compensated, manifest by elevated JVP but clear lungs, normal systemic arterial pressure and intact perfusion. When RVI leads to more severe hemodynamic compromise, systemic hypotension and hypoperfusion result. Patients with IMI may initially present without evidence of

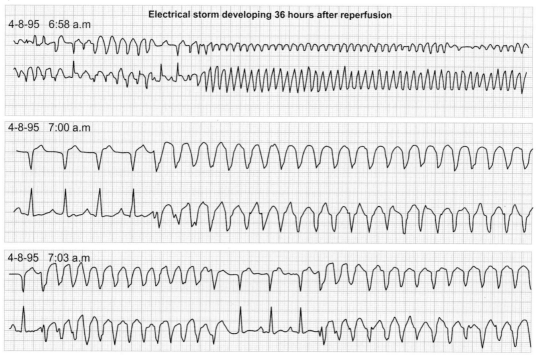

FIGURE 9: Patient with acute RVI who developed intractable ventricular arrhythmias 36 hours following otherwise successful mechanical reperfusion. The patient had sustained marked RV dilatation and dysfunction

hemodynamic compromise, but subsequently develop hypotension precipitated by preload reduction attributable to nitroglycerin[51] or associated with bradyarrhythmias.[43] When RVI develops in the setting of global LV dysfunction, the picture may be dominated by low output and pulmonary congestion, with right heart failure.

NONINVASIVE AND HEMODYNAMIC EVALUATION

Although ST segment elevation and loss of R wave in the right-sided ECG leads (V_{3R} and V_{4R}) are sensitive indicators of the presence of RVI,[52,53] they are not predictive of the magnitude of RV dysfunction nor its hemodynamic impact. Echocardiography is the most effective tool for delineation of the presence and severity of RV dilatation and depression of global RV performance. Echo also delineates the extent of reversed septal curvature that confirms the presence of significant adverse diastolic interactions, the degree of paradoxical septal motion indicative of compensatory systolic interactions, and the presence of severe RA enlargement which may indicate concomitant ischemic RA dysfunction and/or tricuspid regurgitation.

Invasive hemodynamic assessment of the extent and severity of right heart ischemic involvement has been extensively discussed.

DIFFERENTIAL DIAGNOSIS OF RVI

Important clinical entities to consider in patients who present with acute low output hypotension, clear lungs and disproportionate right heart failure include cardiac tamponade, acute pulmonary embolism, severe pulmonary hypertension, right heart mass obstruction and acute severe tricuspid regurgitation; entities including constrictive pericarditis or restrictive cardiomyopathy present a similar picture but are not

TABLE 1

Differential diagnosis of hypotension with disproportionate right heart failure

- RVI
- Cardiac tamponade
- Acute pulmonary embolus
- Acute tricuspid regurgitation
- Pulmonary hypertension with RV failure
- Acute MI with LV failure
- Right heart mass obstruction
- Constriction/Restriction

acute processes (Table 1). The general clinical presentation of chest pain with acute IMI, together with echocardiographic documentation of RV dilatation and dysfunction, effectively excludes tamponade, constriction and restriction. Acute massive pulmonary embolism may also mimic severe RVI and, since the unprepared RV cannot acutely generate elevated RV systolic pressures (> 50–55 mm Hg), severe pulmonary hypertension may be absent. In such cases, absence of inferior LV myocardial infarction by ECG and echo point to embolism, easily confirmed by CT or invasive angiography. Severe pulmonary hypertension with RV decompensation may mimic severe RVI, but delineation of markedly elevated PA systolic pressures by Doppler or invasive hemodynamic monitoring excludes RVI, in which RV pressure generation is depressed. Acute primary tricuspid regurgitation should be evident by echocardiography, typically due to infective endocarditis with obvious vegetations.

THERAPY

Therapeutic options for the management of right heart ischemia (Table 2) follow directly from the pathophysiology discussed. Treatment modalities include: (1) restoration of physiologic

TABLE 2

RVI: Therapeutic algorithm

- Optimize oxygen supply-demand
- Establish physiological rhythm
- Optimize preload
- Inotropic stimulation for persistent low output
- Mechanical support devices:
  — IABP for refractory hypotension
  — RVAD
  — Reperfusion by primary PCI

rhythm; (2) optimization of ventricular preload; (3) optimization of oxygen supply and demand; (4) parenteral inotropic support for persistent hemodynamic compromise; (5) reperfusion and (6) mechanical support with intra-aortic balloon counterpulsation and RV assist devices.

PHYSIOLOGIC RHYTHM

Patients with RVI are particularly prone to the adverse effects of bradyarrhythmias. The depressed ischemic RV has a relatively fixed stroke volume, as does the preload-deprived LV. Therefore, biventricular output is exquisitely heart rate dependent, and bradycardia even in the absence of AV dyssynchrony may be deleterious to patients with RVI. For similar reasons, chronotropic competence is critical in patients with RVI. However, not only are such patients notoriously prone to reflex-mediated frank bradycardia, they often manifest a relative inability to increase the sinus rate in response to low output, owing to excess vagal tone, ischemia or pharmacologic agents. Given that the ischemic RV is dependent on atrial transport, the loss of RA contraction due to AV dyssynchrony further exacerbates difficulties with RV filling and contributes to hemodynamic compromise.[7,21,22] Although atropine may restore physiologic rhythm in some patients, temporary pacing is often required. Although ventricular pacing alone may suffice, especially if the bradyarrhythmias are intermittent, some patients require AV sequential pacing.[53] However, transvenous pacing can be difficult due to issues with ventricular sensing, presumably related to diminished generation of endomyocardial potentials in the ischemic RV. Manipulating catheters within the dilated ischemic RV may also induce ventricular arrhythmias.[54] Intravenous aminophylline may restore sinus rhythm in some patients with atropine-resistant AV block, a response likely reflecting reversal of ischemia-induced adenosine elaboration.[55,56]

OPTIMIZATION OF PRELOAD

In patients with RVI, the dilated, noncompliant RV is exquisitely preload dependent, as is the LV, which is stiff but preload deprived. Therefore, any factor that reduces ventricular preload tends to be detrimental. Accordingly, vasodilators and diuretics are contraindicated. Although experimental animal studies of RVI demonstrate hemodynamic benefit from volume loading,[57] clinical studies have reported variable responses to volume challenge.[58-60] These conflicting results may reflect a spectrum of initial volume status in patients with acute RVI, with those patients who are relatively volume-depleted benefiting, and those who are more replete manifesting a flat response to fluid resuscitation. Nevertheless, an initial volume challenge is appropriate for patients manifesting low output without pulmonary congestion, particularly if the estimated central venous pressure is less than 15 mm Hg. For those unresponsive to an initial trail of fluids, determination of filling pressures and subsequent hemodynamically monitored volume challenge may be appropriate. Caution should be exercised to avoid excessive volume administration above and beyond that documented to augment output, since the right heart chambers may operate on a "descending limb" of the Starling curve, resulting in further depression of RV pump performance as well as inducing severe systemic venous congestion. Abnormalities of volume retention and impaired diuresis may be related in part to impaired responses of the atrial natriuretic factor.[61]

ANTI-ISCHEMIC THERAPIES

Treatment of RVI should focus on optimizing oxygen supply and demand to optimize recovery of both LV and RV function and LV function. However, most anti-ischemic agents exert hemodynamic effects, which may be deleterious in patients with RVI. Specially, beta-blockers and some calcium channel blockers may reduce heart rate and depress conduction, thereby increasing the risk of bradyarrhythmias and heart block in these chronotropically dependent patients. The vasodilator properties of nitrates and calcium channel blockers may precipitate hypotension. In general, these drugs should be avoided in patients with RVI.

REPERFUSION THERAPY

The beneficial effects of successful reperfusion on RV function and clinical outcome, as well as the demonstrated efficacy and advantages of primary angioplasty versus thrombolysis in patients with acute right heart ischemic dysfunction have been discussed.

INOTROPIC STIMULATION

Parenteral inotropic support is usually effective in stabilizing hemodynamically compromised patients not fully responsive to volume resuscitation and restoration of physiologic rhythm.[7,23,58] The mechanisms by which inotropic stimulation improve low output and hypotension in patients with acute RVI have not been well studied. However, experimental animal investigations suggest that inotropic stimulation enhances RV performance by increasing LV septal contraction, which thereby augments septal-mediated systolic ventricular interactions.[23] Although an inotropic agent, such as Dobutamine, that has the least deleterious effects on afterload, oxygen consumption and arrhythmias is the preferred initial drug of choice, patients with severe hypotension may require agents with pressor effects (such as Dopamine) for prompt restoration of adequate coronary perfusion pressure. The "inodilator" agents, such as milrinone, have not been studied in patients with RVI, but their vasodilator properties could exacerbate hypotension.

MECHANICAL ASSIST DEVICES

Intra-aortic balloon pumping may be beneficial in patients with RVI and refractory low output and hypotension. Although there is little research to shed light on the mechanisms by which it exerts salutary effects, balloon assist likely does not directly improve RV performance, but stabilizes blood pressure and thereby improves perfusion pressure throughout the coronary tree in severely hypotensive patients. Since RV myocardial blood flow is dependent on perfusion pressure, balloon pumping may therefore also improve RV perfusion and thereby benefit RV function, particularly if the RCA has been recanalized or if there is collateral supply to an occluded vessel. Intra-aortic balloon pumping may also potentially improve LV performance in those patients with hypotension and depressed LV function. Since performance of the dysfunctional RV is largely dependent on LV septal contraction, RV performance may also benefit. Recent reports suggest that percutaneous RV assist devices can improve hemodynamics in patients with refractory life-threatening low output, thereby providing the reperfused RV a bridge to recovery.[62]

SUMMARY

Acute RCA occlusion proximal to the RV branches results in RVFW dysfunction. The ischemic, dyskinetic RVFW exerts mechanically disadvantageous effects on biventricular performance. Depressed RV systolic function leads to a diminished transpulmonary delivery of LV preload, resulting in reduced cardiac output. The ischemic RV is stiff, dilated and volume dependent, resulting in pandiastolic RV dysfunction and septally mediated alterations in LV compliance, exacerbated by elevated intrapericardial pressure. Under these conditions, RV pressure generation and output are dependent on LV septal contraction and paradoxical septal motion. Culprit lesions distal to the RA branches augment RA contractility and enhance RV filling and performance. Bradyarrhythmias limit the output generated by the rate-dependent ventricles. Ventricular arrhythmias are common, but do not impact short-term outcomes if mechanical reperfusion is prompt. Patients with RVI and hemodynamic instability often respond to volume resuscitation and restoration of physiologic rhythm. Vasodilators and diuretics should generally be avoided. In some patients, parenteral inotropes are required. The RV is relatively resistant to infarction and usually recovers even after prolonged occlusion. However, prompt reperfusion enhances recovery of RV performance and improves the clinical course and survival of patients with ischemic RV dysfunction.

REFERENCES

1. Starr I, Jeffers WA, Meade RH. The absence of conspicuous increments of venous pressure after severe damage to the right ventricle of the dog, with a discussion of the relation between clinical congestive failure and heart disease. Am Heart J. 1943;26:291-301.
2. Cohn JN, Guiha NH, Broder MI, et al. Right ventricular infarction. Clinical and hemodynamic features. Am J Cardiol. 1974;33:209-14.
3. Lorell B, Leinbach RC, Pohost GM, et al. Right ventricular infarction: clinical diagnosis and differentiation from cardiac tamponade and pericardial constriction. Am J Cardiol. 1979;43:465-71.
4. Zehender M, Kasper W, Kauder E, et al. Right ventricular infarction as an independent predictor of prognosis after acute inferior myocardial infarction. N Engl J Med. 1993;328:981-8.
5. Jacobs AK, Leopold JA, Bates E, et al. Cardiogenic shock caused by right ventricular infarction: a report from the SHOCK registry. J Am Coll Cardiol. 2003;41:1273-9.
6. Goldstein JA. State of the art review: pathophysiology and management of right heart ischemia. J Am Coll Cardiol. 2002;40:841-53.
7. Bowers TR, O'Neill WW, Grines C, et al. Effect of reperfusion on biventricular function and survival after right ventricular infarction. N Engl J Med. 1998;338:933-40.
8. Dell'Italia LJ, Lembo NJ, Starling MR, et al. Hemodynamically important right ventricular infarction: follow-up evaluation of right ventricular systolic function at rest and during exercise with radionuclide ventriculography and respiratory gas exchange. Circulation. 1987;75:996-1003.
9. Lim ST, Marcovitz P, Pica M, et al. Right ventricular performance at rest and during stress with chronic proximal occlusion of the right coronary artery. Am J Cardiol. 2003;92:1203-6.
10. Bowers TR, O'Neill WW, Pica M, et al. Patterns of coronary compromise resulting in acute right ventricular ischemic dysfunction. Circulation. 2002;106:1104-9.
11. Andersen HR, Falk E, Nielsen D. Right ventricular infarction: frequency, size and topography in coronary heart disease: a prospective study compromising 107 consecutive autopsies from a coronary care unit. J Am Coll Cardiol. 1987;10:1223-32.
12. Bush LR, Buja LM, Samowitz W, et al. Recovery of left ventricular segmental function after long-term reperfusion following temporary coronary occlusion in conscious dogs. Circ Res. 1983;3:248-63.
13. O'Neill WW, Timmis GC, Bourdillon PD, et al. A prospective randomized clinical trial of intracoronary streptokinase versus coronary angioplasty for acute myocardial infarction. N Engl J Med. 1986;314:812-8.
14. Bates ER, Califf RM, Stack RS, et al. Thrombolysis and angioplasty in myocardial infarction (TAMI-1) trial: influence of infarct location on arterial patency, left ventricular function and mortality. J Am Coll Cardiol. 1989;1:12-8.
15. Kusachi S, Nishiyama O, Yasuhara K, et al. Right and left ventricular oxygen metabolism in open-chest dogs. Am J Physiol. 1982;243:H761-6.
16. Ohzono K, Koyanagi S, Urabe Y, et al. Transmural distribution of myocardial infarction: difference between the right and left ventricles in a canine model. Cir Res. 1986;59:63-73.
17. Santamore WP, Lynch PR, Heckman JL, et al. Left ventricular effects on right ventricular developed pressure. J Appl Physiol. 1976;41:925-30.
18. Shiraki H, Yoshikawa U, Anzai T, et al. Association between preinfarction angina and a lower risk of right ventricular infarction. N Engl J Med. 1998;338:941-7.
19. Goldstein JA, Vlahakes GJ, Verrier ED, et al. The role of right ventricular systolic dysfunction and elevated intrapericardial pressure in the genesis of low output in experimental right ventricular infarction. Circulation. 1982;65:513-22.
20. Goldstein JA, Barzilai B, Rosamond TL, et al. Determinants of hemodynamic compromise with severe right ventricular infarction. Circulation. 1990;82:359-68.
21. Goldstein JA, Harada A, Yagi Y, et al. Hemodynamic importance of systolic ventricular interaction augmented right atrial contractility and atrioventricular synchrony in acute right ventricular dysfunction. J Am Coll Cardiol. 1990;16:181-9.
22. Goldstein JA, Tweddell JS, Barzilai B, et al. Right atrial ischemia exacerbates hemodynamic compromise associated with experimental right ventricular dysfunction. J Am Coll Cardiol. 1991;18:1564-72.
23. Goldstein JA, Tweddell JS, Barzilai B, et al. Importance of left ventricular function and systolic interaction to right ventricular performance during acute right heart ischemia. J Am Coll Cardiol. 1992;19:704-11.
24. Akaishi M, Weintraum WS, Schneider RM, et al. Analysis of systolic bulging: mechanical characteristics of acutely ischemic myocardium in the conscious dog. Circ Res. 1986;8:209-17.
25. Rahimtoola SH, Ehsani A, Sinno MZ, et al. Left atrial transport function in myocardial infarction. Am J Med. 1975;9:686-94.
26. Cushing EH, Feil HS, Stanton EJ, et al. Infarction of the cardiac auricles (atria): clinical, pathological, and experimental studies. Br Heart. 1942;4:17-34.

27. Lasar EJ, Goldberger JH, Peled H, et al. Atrial infarction: diagnosis and management. Am Heart J. 1988;6:1058-63.

28. Laster SB, Shelton TJ, Barzilai B, et al. Determinants of the recovery of right ventricular performance following experimental chronic right coronary artery occlusion. Circulation. 1993;88:696-708.

29. Laster SB, Ohnishi Y, Saffitz JE, et al. Effects of reperfusion on ischemic right ventricular dysfunction: disparate mechanisms of benefit related to duration of ischemia. Circulation. 1994;90:1398-409.

30. Kinn JW, Ajluni SC, Samyn JG, et al. Rapid hemodynamic improvement after reperfusion during right ventricular infarction. J Am Coll Cardiol. 1995;26:1230-4.

31. Hanzel G, Merhi WM, O'Neill WW, et al. Impact of mechanical reperfusion on clinical outcome in elderly patients with right ventricular infarction. Coronary Artery Disease. 2006;17:517-21.

32. Brodie BR, Stuckey TD, Hansen C, et al. Comparison of late survival in patients with cardiogenic shock due to right ventricular infarction versus left ventricular pump failure following primary percutaneous coronary intervention for ST-elevation acute myocardial infarction. Am J Cardiol. 2007;99:431-5.

33. Schuler G, Hofmann M, Schwarz F, et al. Effect of successful thrombolytic therapy on right ventricular function in acute inferior wall myocardial infarction. Am J Cardiol. 1984;54:951-7.

34. Braat SH, Ramentol M, Halders S, et al. Reperfusion with streptokinase of an occluded right coronary artery: effects on early and late right ventricular ejection fraction. Am Heart J. 1987;113:257-60.

35. Roth A, Miller HI, Kaluski E, et al. Early thrombolytic therapy does not enhance the recovery of the right ventricle in patients with acute inferior myocardial infarction and predominant right ventricular involvement. Cardiology. 1990;77:40-9.

36. Giannitsis E, Potratz J, Wiegand U, et al. Impact of early accelerated dose tissue plasminogen activator on in-hospital patency of the infarcted vessel in patients with acute right ventricular infarction. Heart. 1997;77:512-6.

37. Zeymer U, Neuhaus KL, Wegscheider K, et al. Effects of thrombolytic therapy in acute inferior myocardial infarction with or without right ventricular involvement. J Am Coll Cardiol. 1998;32:876-81.

38. Adgey AAJ, Geddes JS, Mulholland C, et al. Incidence, significance, and management of early bradyarrhythmia complicating acute myocardial infarction. Lancet. 1968;2:1097-101.

39. Tans A, Lie K, Durrer D. Clinical setting and prognostic significance of high degree atrioventricular block in acute inferior myocardial infarction: a study of 144 patients. Am Heart J. 1980;99:4-8.

40. Wei JY, Markis JE, Malagold M, et al. Cardiovascular reflexes stimulated by reperfusion of ischemic myocardium in acute myocardial infarction. Circulation. 1983;67:796-801.

41. Mavric Z, Zaputovic L, Matana A, et al. Prognostic significance of complete atrioventricular block in patients with acute inferior myocardial infarction with and without right ventricular involvement. Am Heart J. 1990;19:823-8.

42. Goldstein JA, Lee DT, Pica MC, et al. Patterns of coronary compromise leading to bradyarrhythmias and hypotension in inferior myocardial infarction. Coronary Artery Disease. 2005;16:265-74.

43. Gacioch GM, Topol EJ. Sudden paradoxic clinical deterioration during angioplasty of the occluded right coronary artery in acute myocardial infarction. J Am Coll Cardiol. 1989;14:1202-9.

44. Ricci JM, Dukkipati SR, Pica MC, et al. Malignant ventricular arrhythmias in patients with acute right ventricular infarction undergoing mechanical reperfusion. Am J Cardiol. 2009;104:1678-83.

45. Elvan A, Zipes D. Right ventricular infarction causes heterogeneous autonomic denervation of the viable peri-infarct area. Circulation. 1998;97:484-92.

46. Moore CA, Nygaard TW, Kaiser DL, et al. Postinfarction ventricular septal rupture: the importance of location of infarction and right ventricular function in determining survival. Circulation. 1986;74:45-55.

47. Laham RJ, Ho KK, Douglas PS, et al. Right ventricular infarction complicated by acute right-to-left shunting. Am J Cardiol. 1994;74:824-6.

48. Gudipati CV, Nagelhout DA, Serota H, et al. Transesophageal echocardiographic guidance for balloon catheter occlusion of patent foramen ovale complicating right ventricular infarction. Am Heart J. 1991;121:919-22.

49. Korr KS, Levinson H, Bough E, et al. Tricuspid valve replacement for cardiogenic shock after acute right ventricular infarction. JAMA. 1980;244:1958-60.

50. Ferguson JJ, Diver DJ, Boldt M, et al. Significance of nitroglycerin-induced hypotension with inferior wall acute myocardial infarction. Am J Cardiol. 1989;64:311-4.

51. Braat SH, Brugada P, deZwaan C, et al. Value of electrocardiogram in diagnosing right ventricular involvement in patients with acute inferior wall myocardial infarction. Br Heart J. 1983;49:368-72.

52. Klein HO, Tordjman T, Ninio R, et al. The early recognition of right ventricular infarction: diagnostic accuracy of the electrocardiographic V₄R lead. Circulation. 1983;67:558-65.

53. Topol EJ, Goldschlager N, Ports TA, et al. Hemodynamic benefit of atrial pacing in right ventricular myocardial infarction. Ann Intern Med. 1982;6:594-7.

54. Wesley RC, Lerman BB, DiMarco JP, et al. Mechanism of atropine-resistant atrioventricular block during inferior myocardial infarction: possible role of adenosine. J Am Coll Cardiol. 1986;8:1232-4.

55. Goodfellow J, Walker PR. Reversal of atropine-resistant atrioventricular block with intravenous aminophylline in the early phase of inferior wall acute myocardial infarction following treatment with streptokinase. Eur Heart J. 1995;16:862-5.

56. Goldstein JA, Vlahakes GJ, Verrier ED, et al. Volume loading improves low cardiac output in experimental right ventricular infarction. J Am Coll Cardiol. 1983;2:270-8.

57. Dell'Italia LJ, Starling MR, Blumhardt R, et al. Comparative effects of volume loading, dobutamine, and nitroprusside in patients with predominant right ventricular infarction. Circulation. 1985;72:1327-35.

58. Siniorakis EE, Nikolaou NI, Sarantopoulos CD, et al. Volume loading in predominant right ventricular infarction: bedside hemodynamics using rapid response thermistors. Eur Heart J. 1994;15:1340-7.

59. Ferrario M, Poli A, Previtali M, et al. Hemodynamics of volume loading compared with Dobutamine in severe right ventricular infarction. Am J Cardiol. 1994;74:329-33.

60. Robalino BD, Petrella RW, Jubran FY, et al. Atrial Natriuretic factor in patients with right ventricular infarction. J Am Coll Cardiol. 1990;15:546-53.

61. Giesler GM, Gomez JS, Letsou G, et al. Initial report of percutaneous right ventricular assist for right ventricular shock secondary to right ventricular infarction. Catheter Cardiovasc Interv. 2006;68:263-6.

62. Atiemo AD, Conte JV, Heldman AW. Resuscitation and recovery from acute right ventricular failure using a percutaneous right ventricular assist device. Catheter Cardiovasc Interv. 2006;66:78-82.

Chapter 54

Surgical Therapy in Chronic Coronary Artery Disease

Joss Fernandez, Samad Hashimi, Karam Karam, Jose Torres, Robert Saeid Farivar

Chapter Outline

TECHNIQUE OF SURGICAL THERAPY FOR CHRONIC CORONARY ARTERY DISEASE

Surgical management of coronary artery disease (CAD) has evolved over the last few decades from patients undergoing revascularization through full sternotomy and cardiopulmonary bypass (CPB) to off-pump revascularization and introduction of robotics for revascularization. The modern performance of aorto-coronary bypass by Favolaro at the Cleveland Clinic and the subsequent payment for coronary artery bypass grafting (CABG) by Medicare led to the impetus for the development of modern hospitals, with intensive care units, cardiac catheterization labs for diagnosis and treatment, and the evolution of heart failure specialization. Surgical revascularization has had far reaching applications and allowed the field of cardiothoracic surgery to evolve from its infancy.

While no two surgeons will perform any CABG in the exact same way, it has largely become routine. The standard coronary revascularization is approached through a median sternotomy. This approach has the advantage of allowing global access to the heart and allows harvesting the internal thoracic artery (left internal mammary artery—LIMA), which is used as a conduit. The standard CPB circuit consists of a venous drainage [either through a right atrial cannula, bicaval (SVC and IVC) cannulation, or femoral venous cannulation depending on the operation] and an arterial inflow cannula after full heparinization. Typically a two stage venous cannula is used in the right atrium for CABG, whereas entry into the cardiac chambers uses bicaval cannulation. Venous blood is collected in a reservoir and

circulated through a heat exchanger/oxygenator and returned, circulated though an arterial filter and returned to the patient via an arterial cannula.

Myocardial protection has evolved over the past four decades. Over the years, numerous ways have evolved to allow better myocardial protection. The goal is to allow a bloodless field, minimize myocardial energy demand and decrease the extent of ischemia/reperfusion. The basic mode of cardioplegia requires rapid arrest of the heart with a high potassium substrate, mild hypothermia (32C), appropriate buffering solutions and avoiding depletion of intracellular substrate. Induction of immediate cardiac arrest after aorta has been cross-clamped minimizes depletion of high-energy phosphates by mechanical work. Potassium is the most common agent used and produces rapid arrest. Hypothermia protects ischemic myocardium by decreasing heart rate, slows the rate of high-energy phosphate degradation and decreases oxygen consumption. Buckberg's seminal experiments documented that the warm beating heart uses approximately 20 cc O_2/g myocardial tissue. The warm fibrillating heart consumed 16–20 cc, the cold fibrillating heart approximately 8 cc and the still potassium arrested heart approximately 4 cc. Thus, various strategies have evolved to induce a diastolic arrested cold heart for the perfomance of CABG.

Buffering of cardioplegia is necessary to prevent intracellular acidosis associated with surgically induced myocardial ischemia. Maintaining tissue pH of 6.8 or greater is associated with adequate protection. Hence, frequent infusion of cardioplegia every 10–20 min are necessary to prevent intracellular acidosis. Bicarbonate, phosphate, aminosulfonic acid, trishydroxymethylaminomethane (THAM) and histidine buffers have all been utilized as cardioplegia additives to modulate the pH. To avoid intracellular edema, cardioplegia solution is isotonic in the range of 290–330 mOsm/L or slightly hyperosmolar. Over the years numerous cardioplegia solutions have been utilized ranging from crystalloid to blood to a mixture of the two.

Cardioplegia is infused either antegrade through the aortic root and in normal fashion through the coronary arteries or alternatively in a retrograde fashion through a cannula placed in the coronary sinus. Cardioplegia then flows retrograde through the coronary veins and into the coronary arteries. In a heart with significant CAD, most surgeons will employ a combination of the two techniques. Retrograde cardioplegia has the advantage of being distal to proximal stenoses, but is relatively poor for protection of the right heart. An advantage of retrograde is that it minimizes the interruption of the procedure, since there is no need for a competent aortic valve to administer cardioplegia.

At the University of Iowa, the conduct of a CABG is as follows:
- Median sternotomy.
- Harvesting internal thoracic artery(ies) and saphenous vein.
- After heparinization, cannulating aorta and right atrium.
- Ascending aorta is cross clamped, cardioplegia is infused down the aortic root to induce diastolic arrest. After 5 cc/kg is administered antegrade, an additional 5 cc/kg is administered retrograde. The pericardial well is cooled with iced saline.
- The right coronary vessel is bypassed first, followed by the obtuse marginals and diagonals. Distals are performed first.
- Each bypassed vessel is infused with cardioplegia.
- Cardioplegia is also given antegrade/retrograde every 10–20 min.
- Proximal anastomosis on the aorta is performed followed by the internal thoracic artery to LAD (if LAD needs to be bypassed).
- Potassium is discontinued. Air is evacuated from both the aorta and the ventricles as the heart starts to contract and the clamp is removed from the aorta.
- Hemostasis is confirmed and the patient is weaned from CPB.
- Temporary pacing wires are placed.
- Hemostasis is assured. Drainage tubes are placed and the sternum is closed followed by skin and subcutaneous layers.

INDICATIONS FOR SURGICAL CORONARY REVASCULARIZATION ADVANTAGES OF CABG OVER MEDICAL TREATMENT

The techniques of coronary artery bypass used today were first described in the 1960s. It was not until the 1970s that three major trials were conducted, establishing CABG superiority over medical management in only a select subset of patients. The CASS, VA-CABSCSG and European CSS trials randomized patients with stable angina to either contemporary medical management or CABG. Recent improvements in cardioprotection during CPB and a significant increase in the number of arterial grafts used have lead to an improvement in outcomes.

On the other hand, statin therapy, aspirin and beta-blocker use was not standard of care at the time. Despite significant improvements in both medical and surgical management with reductions in mortality the major findings generated by these landmark studies remain in place.

The Coronary Artery Surgery Study (CASS) was designed to assess the effect of coronary artery bypass surgery on mortality and selected nonfatal end points.[1] Around 780 patients with stable ischemic heart disease were randomly assigned to receive surgical or nonsurgical treatment. At 5 years, a significant difference could not be established between the two management strategies. Annual mortality rates in patients with single-, double- and triple-vessel disease who were in the surgical group were 0.7%, 1.0% and 1.5%; the corresponding rates in patients in the medical group were 1.4%, 1.2% and 2.1%. However, the subset of patients with left ventricular ejection fraction (LVEF) less than 50% treated surgically had a statistically significant difference in survival (61% vs 79%) at 10 years. The excellent survival rates observed both in CASS patients assigned to receive medical and those assigned to receive surgical therapy and the similarity of survival rates in the two groups of patients in this randomized trial lead to the conclusion that patients similar to those enrolled in this trial can safely defer bypass surgery until symptoms worsen to the point that surgical palliation is required if they have preserved (ejection fraction > 50%) left ventricular function.[1]

The Veterans Affairs Coronary Artery Bypass Surgery Cooperative Study Group (VA-CABSCSG) randomly assigned 686 patients with stable angina to medical or surgical treatment at 13 hospitals and followed for an average of 11.2 years. Similar to the CASS trial, the VA trial was not able to demonstrate a significant survival advantage in low-risk patients. However, a group of high-risk patients was defined which clearly had a survival advantage when treated surgically. A statistically significant difference in survival suggesting a benefit from surgical treatment was found in patients who were subdivided into high-risk subgroups defined by either angiographic criteria, clinical criteria or by a combination. The angiographically defined high-risk group consisted of patients with three-vessel disease and impaired left ventricular function. At 7 years, this group demonstrated survival of 52% in the medically treated patients versus 76% in surgically treated patients; at 11 years, 38% and 50%, respectively. The clinically defined high-risk group consisted of patients with at least two of the following: resting ST depression, history of myocardial infarction (MI), or history of hypertension. At 7 years, this group demonstrated survival of 52% in the medical group versus 72% in the surgical group; at 11 years, 36% versus 49%, respectively. The third group consisted of patients with combined angiographic and clinical risk factors. This group had a survival rate at 7 years of 36% in the medical group versus 76% in the surgical group; at 11 years, 24% versus 54%, respectively (VA-CABSCSG).

The European Coronary Surgery Study randomized 767 men with good left ventricular function to either early coronary bypass surgery or medical therapy. At the projected 5-year follow-up there was a higher survival rate in the group assigned to surgical treatment than in the group assigned to medical treatment (92.4% vs 83.1%). The survival advantage diminished during the subsequent 7 years but still favored the surgical treatment group (70.6% vs 66.7%).

In the 1970s and 1980s, studies tested whether CABG would improve the survival in patients with CAD who had acute myocardial infarction (AMI). These trials showed no better and possibly lower survival rates with CABG than with conservative treatment. Operative revascularization is unlikely to occur within 6 hours of the infarct. As a result, emergency CABG for AMI has been replaced by percutaneous revascularization. Randomized studies have been done with patients admitted to the hospital with unstable angina to see if they may live longer with CABG. The VA Study of Unstable Angina found no overall benefit from surgery. However, they discovered a statistically significant difference favoring CABG at 8 years in the high-risk subgroup and a statistically significant advantage favoring medical treatment in the low-risk subgroup.

COMPARING CABG TO PTCA

The modern era of coronary revascularization is marked by the hotly debated role of percutaneous versus surgical revascularization. Comparisons have been difficult due to evolving technologies. Nevertheless, several principals have emerged that currently define the patient which would benefit the most from surgical revascularization. In the 1990s several randomized trials compared angioplasty techniques with CABG. It became clear that although the survival rates were similar revascularization and anginal rates were much higher in the percutaneous groups.

The ERACI,[2] RITA,[3] BARI,[4] GABI,[5] EAST[6] and CABRI[7] trials failed to demonstrate a significant advantage of CABG or PTCA in mortality or in the frequency of MI. However, patients who had bypass surgery were more frequently free of angina and required fewer additional reinterventions than patients who had coronary angioplasty. These finding were held up to 10 years after revascularization in the BARI trial. The BARI trial, although, was able to demonstrate a survival advantage in patients with diabetes undergoing surgical revascularization.

In a similar vein, trials comparing percutaneous bare metal stenting with CABG have not demonstrated a mortality difference despite increased revascularization rates with percutaneous techniques. In the ARTS I trial[8] there was no difference in mortality (8.0% vs 7.6%) or the rate of the combined endpoint of death, MI, or stroke (18.2% vs 14.9%) at five years. However, event-free survival was lower with stenting due to a significant increase in the need for repeat revascularization (21% vs 4% at one year, 27% vs 7% at three years, and 30% vs 9% at five years). Among stented patients in the ARTS I trial, two groups had worse outcomes: those with incomplete revascularization and patients with diabetes. The Stent or Surgery (SoS) trial[9] is unique in establishing a mortality advantage to surgical revascularization in nondiabetic patients. At six years, mortality was significantly higher in the PCI group (10.9% vs 6.8%). It is not clear if this difference was at least in part by chance since there was a larger number of cancer deaths in the stenting group. The ERACI II trial randomized 450 patients to undergo either or CABG.[10] At 5-years follow-up, patients initially treated with PCI had similar survival and freedom from nonfatal AMI than those initially treated with CABG (92.8% vs 88.4% and 97.3% vs 94%, respectively). Freedom from repeat revascularization procedures (PCI/CABG)

was significantly lower with PCI compared with CABG (71.5% vs 92.4%). Freedom from major adverse cardiac event was also significantly lower with PCI compared with CABG (65.3% vs 76.4%; p = 0.013). The study concluded that there were no survival benefits from any revascularization procedure; however, patients initially treated with CABG had better freedom from repeat revascularization procedures and from major adverse coronary event.[10]

The effort to reduce the revascularization rate of percutaneous techniques has resulted in the production of drug-eluting stents (DES). Recent trials have compared DES to CABG. The SYNTAX is currently the only head to head comparison of DES to CABG. The SYNTAX trial[11] randomly assigned 1,800 patients with three-vessel or left main CAD to either CABG or PCI with DES. All patients were eligible for either procedure and were treated with the intention of complete revascularization. After 12 months follow-up the composite primary endpoint (death from any cause, stroke, MI or repeat revascularization) was significantly higher in the PCI group (17.8% vs 12.4%). This was the result mostly of more frequent revascularizations with PCI (13.5% vs 5.9%). The secondary endpoint of the rate of death, stroke or MI were similar (7.6% for PCI vs 7.7% for CABG). More complete revascularization was achieved with CABG (63% vs 57%).

Coronary artery bypass surgery is superior to percutaneous techniques in reducing angina and revascularization rates. This has not translated into a survival advantage except in a select subset of patients. Specifically, the BARI[4] and ARTs I trial[8] demonstrated a survival advantage in diabetics. There has also been established a survival advantage in patients with greater than 95% stenosis of left anterior descending artery and at least 2 vessel disease[11,12] [CABG vs PTCA, Heart 95:1061–6, J Am Coll Cardiol. 53:2389–403, Circulation 119:1013–20, Circulation—11-SEP-2007; 116(Suppl. 11):I200–6].

THE CHANGING CABG POPULATION

Analysis of the patient population undergoing CABG over the last decade has revealed a threefold increase in octogenarians. There also has been a concommitant increase in comorbidities including obesity, hypertension reduced ejection fraction. Despite these worsening comorbidities mortality outcomes were unchanged (Table 1). (PMID 20399675)

WHEN CABG MAY BE INDICATED

The goal of coronary revascularization is to delay or prevent the complications of coronary disease and in turn prolong life

TABLE 1

Progression of worsening comorbidities by decade based on Society of Thoracic Surgery Database CABG mortality

Risk factor	1980	1990	2000
LVEF	62%	51%	45%
Female	17%	27%	33%
Reoperative	2%	9%	14%
Urgent/Emergent	4%	27%	38%
Abbreviation: LVEF: Left Ventricular Ejection Fraction			

and alleviate symptoms. Patients who have symptoms despite maximal medical management or who have coronary anatomy for which revascularization has been proven to have a survival benefit should be considered for revascularization in the absence of any contraindications such as a nonresectable cancer or severe dementia. The choice of revascularization strategy is based on the patient comorbidities and extent of disease.

Early trials comparing CABG to percutaneous techniques demonstrated lower rates of freedom from restenosis with angioplasty or stenting. Despite the need for subsequent repeat revascularization or CABG after PTCA survival rates were similar. The SYNTAX trial and observations from the ARTS II, ERACI III, the New York State registry and the Beijing registry all demonstrated higher rates of revascularization following PTCA despite the use of a DES.

The findings of these and other trials have lead to the following ACC/AHA guidelines for CABG. Bypass surgery is recommended in the following patients:

- Significant left main coronary artery (LMCA) stenosis (> 50%)
- Greater than 70% stenosis of the proximal left anterior descending and circumflex arteries (left main equivalent)
- Three-vessel disease, especially if EF less than 50%
- Two-vessel disease with significant proximal LAD stenosis, EF less than 50% (proximal to the first septal perforators of the left anterior descending artery)

CABG should be considered in the patients with proximal LAD stenosis with one vessel disease with an extensive area of ischemia despite an EF greater than 50% and in those with one- or two-vessel disease even without proximal LAD disease if there is a moderate to large area of at risk myocardium. Patients with diabetes mellitus, as shown in the BARI and ARTS I trials, likely benefit from CABG over PTCA due to the higher rate of repeat revascularization.

Based on the subgroup analysis of the SYNTAX trial and the smaller Le Mans registry it may be reasonable to offer a patient who is poor surgical candidate with left main disease and well preserved left venticular function either CABG or PCI depending upon anatomic factors.[13]

Other indications for surgical revascularization include ischemia on physiological studies or significant coronary stenosis prior to other major cardiac surgery, congenital anomalies, such as aberrant left coronary artery, that are associated with sudden death. No guidelines may substitute for the collaboration between the patient, cardiologist and cardiac surgeons at each individual institution to ensure informed consent and meet the needs of each individual patient.

The indications for surgical revascularization after MI are similar to that of patients with stable angina. Prolonging the interval between acute MI and CABG reduces the risks of perioperative complications. Patients who have an LVEF of greater than 30% may proceed with CABG at any point after the MI is complete but in general at least a minimum of 48 hours. Patients with an EF less than 30% should be stablized for a period of one week prior to revascularization. The generalized edema surrounding infarcted tissue can technically aggravate an operation, and thus a certain amount of judgment is required in timing an intervention after MI. Data now exists that postponing revascularization 5 days after the contrast load from angiography to lessen kidney injury.

WHEN CABG IS NOT INDICATED

Given the success of rapid percutaneous revascularization emergency CABG does not play a role for AMI. In the 1970s and 1980s, studies tested whether CABG would improve the survival in patients with CAD who had AMIs within a few hours to days. These trials showed no better and possibly lower survival rates with CABG than with conservative treatment, so emergency CABG for AMI was abandoned.

Single vessel disease that is not left main or proximal LAD (proximal defined as proximal to first septal perforator) is often best managed by medical therapy or PTCA in the symptomatic patient. The CASS[1] and VA-CABSCSG trials[14] failed to demonstrate an advantage over medical mangement in patients with single vessel disease. Futhermore, the New York State registry demonstrates a survival disadvantage for single vessel disease when compared to PTCA. On the other hand patients with proximal LAD and an EF less than 50% have a significant survival advantage especially if revascularization is performed using the internal mammary artery. Similarly, two-vessel CAD should not undergo CABG without a diminished EF or proximal LAD disease. Lastly, patient with three-vessel disease who have a good left ventricular function and have mild reversible ischemia can safely be managed medically.

RISK FACTORS FOR IN-HOSPITAL MORTALITY FOLLOWING CABG

The perioperative and in-hospital mortality rate after CABG continues to improve with advancements in perioperative care and prevention. The risks associated with CABG are highly dependent upon patient comorbidities (Table 2), hospital procedure volumes and whether or not concomitant procedures are performed with CABG. Models to predict perioperative risks have been developed. One of the most widely used algorithms was developed by the Society of Thoracic Surgeons (STS).[15] This proprietary algorithm incorporates 26 variables including age, sex and comorbidities as well as the severity and acuity of presentation. Another proposed algorithm, the EuroSCORE, has widely been used in Europe. One analysis compared the performance of the STS Database with the EuroSCORE in predicting the survival of 4,497 patients undergoing isolated CABG between 1996 and 2001.[16] Overall 30 days mortality was 1.9%, and was accurately predicted by both risk scores, although, the EuroSCORE had significantly greater discriminatory power. The STS continues to gather new data to permit progressive algorithm revision. There is general consensus that the Euroscore tends to over estimate risk.[16] Other models include the Cleveland Clinic Model, the New York Model, ACEF (Age, Creatinine, Ejection Fraction). The Mayo Clinic Risk Score (MCRS)[17] is unique in that it may be used to provide a risk prediction for either PCI or CABG. First developed using patients undergoing PCI, the MCRS was shown to correlate with the STS Database for observed in-hospital mortality.[17] However, when compared to the 26 variable STS algorithm, its performance was inferior.

TABLE 2

Logistic regression analysis of early postoperative CABG mortality risk factors

	Patient risk factor	Logistic	Regression
Coefficient p value OR Age	0.0511	< 0.0001	1.052
Female Gender	0.3548	0.0005	1.426
Hemodynamic instability	1.2128	< 0.0001	3.363
Shock	2.0533	< 0.0001	7.794
Athero – carotid dz	0.04685	< 0.0001	1.598
Aortoiliac dz	0.7428	< 0.0001	2.102
Calcified asc ao	0.4816	0.0008	1.619
Previous MI < 6h	0.6174	0.0174	1.854
Malignant ventricular arrythmia	0.8056	< 0.0001	2.238
CHF same admission	0.9587	< 0.0001	2.608
CHF previously	0.8088	< 0.0001	2.245
Renal Failure (Cr>2)	1.0615	< 0.0001	2.891
Previous open heart	1.2167	< 0.0001	3.376

MODIFIABLE RISK FACTORS

The American College of Cardiology/American Heart Association (ACC/AHA) guidelines on bypass surgery address general recommendations for preventive measures to minimize the risk of both morbidity and mortality after CABG. These include the use of perioperative aspirin, beta-blockers and statin therapy. Further recommendation on reducing surgical site infection included the appropriate use of prophylactic antimicrobials and strict glycemic control. Health care reform in the United States of America and changes in payment strategy have incorporated some of these measure as part of the Surgical Care Improvement Project (SCIP).

Aspirin 325 mg should be administered to all patients without a contraindication perioperatively to reduce in-hospital mortality and to enhance graft patency after CABG. Concerns of excess bleeding in patients undergoing CABG while under aspirin therapy were raised by two randomized trials in the early 1990s.[18,19] Since, there has been an accumulation of overwhelming data supporting the use of perioperative aspirin. The same 1991 Veterans Administration Cooperative Study that found increased bleeding with aspirin showed that although there was no difference in saphenous vein graft occlusion between the two groups at an average of eight days after surgery (7.4% vs 7.8%), there was a trend toward a lower rate of occlusion of internal mammary artery grafts (0% vs 2.4%, p = 0.08) for the group receiving aspirin preoperatively.[18] A systematic review from the Antiplatelet Trialists' Collaboration concluded that antiplatelet therapy, particularly if given early, was associated with improved graft patency at an average of one year after surgery.[20] A large case patient-control patient study of 8,641 consecutive undergoing isolated CABG procedures performed between July 1987 and May 1991 demonstrated that preoperative aspirin use appeared to be associated with a decreased risk of mortality in CABG patients without significant increase in hemorrhage, blood product requirements, or related morbidities.[21] In a retrospective study published in 2005 of 1,636 consecutive patients undergoing CABG surgery; 80% of patients had taken aspirin within the five days before surgery, all patients received postoperative aspirin six hours after surgery and all patients received an internal mammary artery graft. Preoperative aspirin was associated with a significant reduction in postoperative in-hospital mortality 1.7% versus 4.4% without an increased in bleeding rate. Furthermore, a prospective study of 5,065 patients undergoing coronary bypass surgery, of whom 5,022 survived the first 48 hours after surgery demonstrated a reduced risk of death and ischemic complications involving the heart, brain, kidneys and gastrointestinal tract. Among patients who received aspirin (up to 650 mg) within 48 hours after revascularization, subsequent mortality was 1.3%, as compared with 4.0% among those who did not receive aspirin during this period (P < 0.001). Aspirin therapy was associated with a 48% reduction in the incidence of MI (2.8% vs 5.4%, P < 0.001), a 50% reduction in the incidence of stroke (1.3% vs 2.6%, P = 0.01), a 74% reduction in the incidence of renal failure (0.9% vs 3.4%, P < 0.001), and a 62% reduction in the incidence of bowel infarction (0.3% vs 0.8%, P = 0.01).

The perioperative use of statin has been associated with a reduction in mortality following CABG. The Multicenter Study of Perioperative Ischemia (McSPI) Epidemiology II Study[22] was a prospective, longitudinal study of 5,436 patients undergoing coronary artery bypass graft surgery between November 1996 and June 2000 at 70 centers in 17 countries. Following multivariate analysis, this study concluded that preoperative statin therapy was independently associated with a significant reduction in the risk of early cardiac death after primary, elective coronary bypass surgery (0.3% vs 1.4%; P < 0.03).[22] Discontinuation of statin therapy after surgery was independently associated with a significant increase in late all-cause mortality (2.64% vs 0.60%; P < 0.01). Others have associated statin therapy with a reduction in need for RRT following CABG.[23] Investigators at the Texas Heart Institute performed a retrospective cohort study of patients undergoing primary CABG surgery with CPB (n = 1,663) between January 1, 2000 and December 31, 2001. They did not find a risk reduction in in-hospital morbidities including postoperative MI, cardiac arrhythmias, stroke or renal dysfunction. Nevertheless, they found that preoperative statin therapy was independently associated with a significant reduction in the composite endpoint of 30-day all-cause mortality and stroke (7.1% vs 4.6%; P < 0.05).[24]

Perioperative uses of beta-blockers have been associated with a reduction in atrial arrhythmias and reduced short-term mortality. A review of 629,877 patients undergoing isolated CABG between 1996 and 1999 at 497 US and Canadian sites revealed that patients who received beta-blockers had lower 30-day mortality than those who did not 2.8% versus 3.4%. Patients with LVEF of less than 30%, however, had a trend toward higher mortality rate.[25]

Regardless of diabetic status, glycemic control plays a large role in postoperative morbidity and mortality. Postoperative glycemic control is an established standard to reduce sternal wound infection rates and in-hospital mortality. The largest randomized trial of surgical ICU patient randomized to intensive insulin therapy included patients undergoing CABG. Patients undergoing intensive insulin therapy had a reduction in in-hospital mortality (7% vs 11%).[26] Postoperative CABG patients should be treated with continuous insulin to maintain a glucose between 100 mg/dL and 140 mg/dL.

Intraoperative glycemic control has also been studied. A direct benefit from intraoperative glycemic control has not been elucidated in nondiabetics receiving continuous insulin therapy. In a study of 400 patients randomly assigned to receive continuous insulin infusion to maintain intraoperative glucose levels between 4.4 mmol/l (80 mg/dL) and 5.6 mmol/l (100 mg/dL) or conventional treatment. The intensive therapy group experienced nonstatisically significant increase in deaths and strokes. On the other hand, patients with diabetes who receive a continuous solution of glucose, insulin and potassium (GIK) appear to benefit. Patients were randomly assigned to a GIK or No-GIK group. The GIK group received an infusion through a central line consisting of 500 ml D5W with 80 U of regular insulin and 40 mEq of KCl infused at 30 ml/h. Patients receiving intraoperative GIK had a significantly lower incidence of atrial fibrillation, a shorter length of stay, and at two years less recurrent ischemia (5% vs 19%), fewer wound infections (1% vs 10%), and lower mortality (2% vs 10%).[27] Further research regarding the goals of intraoperative glycemic control is needed.

Carotid duplex ultrasound to identify severe carotid artery stenosis may be warranted in patients at risk for cerbrovascular disease including those with prior history of stroke, transient ischemic attack, carotid bruit or age greater than 65. The management of concomitant carotid stenosis during coronary artery revascularization surgery continues to be controversial. Nevertheless, patients with symptomatic carotid disease should undergo carotid revascularization prior to or during CABG. Patients with asymptomatic carotid stenosis greater than 80% may also benefit from revascularization prior to or concomitantly with CABG.

The in-hospital mortality after CABG has been shown by some groups to be related to the volume of CABG procedures performed at the hospital. In an analysis of over 900,000 CABG procedures in the Medicare database between 1994 and 1999, the adjusted in-hospital or 30-day mortality was inversely related to hospital volume ranging from 6.1% for hospitals performing less than 230 procedures per year to 4.8% when the volume was greater than 849 procedures per year.[28] In a report on over 200,000 procedures from the Society of Thoracic Surgeons (STS) National Cardiac Database between January 2000 and December 2001, the overall operative mortality was 2.7%. The mortality rate ranged from 3.5% for hospitals performing less than or equal to 150 procedures per year to 2.4% for hospitals performing greater than 450 procedures per year.[29]

The use of the LIMA is associated with a higher graft patency rate and a lower perioperative mortality. In 21,873 consecutive, isolated, first-time coronary artery bypass graft procedures from 1992 through 1999, the crude odds ratio for death (LIMA vs no LIMA) was 0.26 (95% confidence intervals, 0.22, 0.31; P: < 0.001). LIMA grafts were protective across all major patient and disease subgroups, and in any age group.[30] In the STS database, non-use of the LIMA in any subgroup is tracked. The data for a free LIMA are almost as compelling as an *in situ* LIMA graft.

In general, patients undergoing elective CABG should continue a beta-blocker, statin and antiplatelet therapy perioperatively. Perioperative morbidity is further reduced by appropriate antiobiotic selection which may require MRSA screening. Glycemic control with postoperative insulin drips may further reduce surgical site infections. The use of the internal mammary as a conduit reduces postoperative mortality. Patients at risk for stroke should undergo preoperative carotid ultrasonography. Hospital volume may affect patient outcomes.

NONMODIFIABLE RISK FACTORS

Age is a predictor of operative mortality. Moreover, CABG is more frequently being performed on the elderly. Fortunately, the operative mortality in the elderly continues to decline. In one study 3,330 consecutive patients age 70 years and older were evaluated. The operative mortality reduced from 7.2% in 1982–1986 to 4.4% in 1987–1991. The prevalence of elderly patients rose from 16.2% to 19.5% during the same time periods.[31] Octogenarians also fare worse than younger patients. Around 725 out of 15,070 patients greater than or equal to 80 years of age underwent CABG between 1996 and 2001 in four Canadian centers were reviewed. Death was higher among the octogenarians (9.2% vs 3.8%; p < 0.001), as was the rate of stroke (4.7% vs 1.6%, p < 0.001).[32] The difference amongst patients undergoing elective surgery was not statistically significant.

Gender is an independent risk factor for complications after both CABG and PCI. Women experience greater complications and early mortality after revascularization. When adjusted for comorbidities this difference declines but still persists. It is unclear if gender along or concommitent risk factors including decreased coronary size and latter presentation which are responsible for these differences.[33]

After adjustment for comorbidities, redo CABG remains a predictor of operative mortality. 13,436 patients undergoing isolated CABG procedures between June 1, 2001 and May 31, 2008 were analyzed. Operative mortality was 4.8% for redo CABG and 1.8% for first-time CABG (p < 0.001). After adjustment, redo status remained a predictor for operative mortality, MI and prolonged ventilation.[34] Patients that undergo urgent or emergent CABG fair worse than there elective counterparts. A meta-analysis of studies stratifying patients undergoing elective versus urgent or emergency CABG demonstrated that the mortality rate was significantly lower in the elective CABG (1.5% vs 1.8%, p < 0.05).[35] Left ventricular dysfunction and heart failure is one of the most important independent predictors of operative mortality and other major adverse events after CABG. Outcome data were collected prospectively on 20,614 patients undergoing isolated coronary operations during 1982–1997. The operative mortality varied from less than 2% with an LVEF greater than 40% to 3.5–4% with an LVEF between 20% and 40% to approximately 8% with an LVEF less than 20%. Traditionally LMCA stenosis has been viewed as a risk factor for mortality after CABG. Swedish investigators noted that this was no longer the case after 1995. During 1970–1984, early mortality was 5.8% in patients with LMCA stenosis compared with 1.5% in patients without LMCA stenosis. The corresponding rates during 1995–1999 were 2% versus 2.2%, respectively.[36] The authors attribute this change to perioperative care.

Mortality following CABG rises sharply in proportion to renal dysfunction. Even minor renal impairment (Cr > 1.5) is associated with a higher mortality. A prospective study of 4,403 consecutive patients undergoing first-time isolated CABG were divided based on preoperative renal function. There were 458 patients with a serum creatinine 130–199 μ/mol/l or 1.47–2.25 mg/dL (mild renal dysfunction group) and 3,945 patients with a serum creatinine less than 130 μ/mol/l (< 1.47 mg/dL). Operative mortality was higher in the mild renal dysfunction group (2.1% vs 6.1%; P < 0.001) Overall there is a 2–3 fold increase in mortality with renal insufficiency. Part of the risk comes from arrhythmias that are difficult to manage from electrolyte imbalances rather than strict fluid management. In fact, patients with known renal failure on dialysis tend to do better than those with worsening renal insufficiency after CABG.

In general, older female patients with left ventricular dysfunction and renal dysfunction undergoing reoperative emergent CABG carry the highest perioperative risk.

OUTCOMES OF SURGERY

GRAFT PATENCY

Short-term graft patency is dependent on technical issues such as graft type, handling of the graft, the quality of the anastomosis, runoff, competitive flow and the size of the target vessel. Long-term patency may be influenced by technical factors but is predominately determined by neointimial hyperplasia and progression of athersclerotic disease. A short arterial bypass to a large target with good runoff provides for the best patency. A review of CABGs performed on 930 patients revealed that the best conduits were the bilaterally internal mammary arteries. One-year patency rate of the left internal thoracic artery, right internal thoracic artery, radial artery, gastroepiploic artery and saphenous vein graft was 96.1%, 92.0%, 69.5%, 81.4% and 82.6%, respectively.[37] One-year patency rates of in situ and free right internal artery graft were not significantly different. One-year patency rate of the radial artery was significantly worse than that of the free right internal thoracic artery graft and saphenous vein graft. The patency rate of saphenous vein grafts may be expect to be 50% at 10 years. Australilian investigators randomized patients younger that 70 years to either radial artery or free right internal thoracic artery and patients older than 70 years to radial artery or saphenous vein grafts. At 5.5 years the patencies were similar in the two groups.[38] Thus in older patients the saphenous vein graft may be a suitable alternative. The benefit of radial arterial grafts may not be seen until after 10 years when half of saphenous grafts have failed. As conduit for coronary artery bypass the LIMA bypass to the left anterior descending artery has supplanted all others as the gold standard (Fig. 1).

LIMA bypassing to the left anterior descending artery the most durable form of revascularization. Several studies have demonstrated that 90% of Internal mammary artery conduits are patent after 20 years. The internal thoracic artery has been shown to be equally resistant to atherosclerosis and maintains its patency as a pedicled conduit and as an in situ graft from the aorta to the left anterior descending coronary artery. Additionally, multiple studies have demonstrated multiple benefits in addition to prolonged graft patency including decreased incidence of reoperation, increased median interval of reoperation from eight to twelve years, and event-free

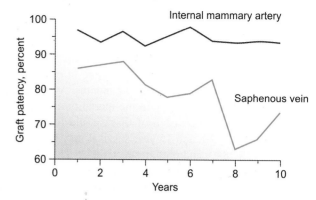

FIGURE 1: Ten-year graft patency for internal mammary artery and saphenous vein grafts[39]

survival. Loop et al. found that patients who had only vein grafts had a 1.61 times greater risk of death throughout the 10 years, as compared with those who received an internal-mammary-artery graft. In addition, patients who received only vein grafts had 1.41 times the risk of late MI, 1.25 times the risk of hospitalization for cardiac events, 2.00 times the risk of cardiac reoperation and 1.27 times the risk of all late cardiac events, as compared with patients who received internal-mammary-artery grafts. They also showed in 2,509 consecutive patients who underwent reoperation for myocardial revascularization at the Cleveland Clinic during a 20-year period (1967–1987).[40] Several factors associated with improved 10-year actuarial survival including age younger than 65 years, mild angina, no major comorbidity, no left main CAD, good left ventricular performance and the use of the internal thoracic artery graft.

As a result of the success of the LIMA as a excellent conduit there has been enusthiasm to use bilateral internal mammary arteries.[41] Unfortunately anatomical constraints limit the usefulness of the right internal thoracic artery as in situ graft. Instead it is often used as a free graft. Furthermore, use of bilateral internal mammary arteries may be of no survival benefit, 67% versus 64% at 15 years (Fig. 2). This comes at the cost of slightly increase sternal wound infection presumably due to revascularization especially in diabetics, 4.8% versus 1.2% with only one mammary used.[41]

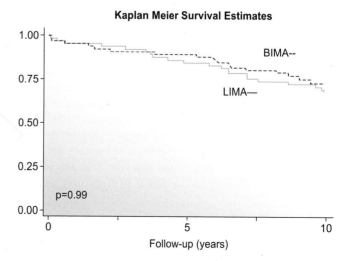

FIGURE 2: Survival of propensity-matched CABG patients who received LIMA or BIMA grafts

The long-term survival of patients undergoing isolated CABG, may be divided into three hazard phases. Following the initial perioperative period there is a rapidly decline in risk of death that plateaus between 6 months and 12 months. After the first year there is a slow gradual rise in the mortality rate which is likely the result of progression of disease and lose of graft patency. The 1-, 5-, 10- and 15-year survival may be expected to be 97%, 92%, 81% and 66%, respectively.[42] The use of the internal thoracic artery to left anterior descending coronary bypass has protective affect increasing 10-year survival up 90%.[39] This is likely the result of increase patency rates. The benefit of CABG is most accentuated in patients with diminished left ventricular function, multivessel disease and diabetes. Nevertheless, these comorbidites continue to affect the survival rate of patients despite CABG. Patients requiring reoperation for CAD do not fair as well with 10-year survival of 65%.

LEFT VENTRICULAR FUNCTION

Increased regional perfusion after CABG results in improved systolic function. It is not unusual to see improvement in wall motion abnormalities of hypokinetic, akinetic and even dyskinetic segment. With improved systolic function, maximal exercise capacity is improved along with functional capacity. Improvement in global function is dependent on complete revascularization. A lack of increase in excercise capacity usually translates into a missed vessel to be bypassed. Late loss of regional wall motions may be the result of graft occlusion or restenosis. Despite improved perfusion and function CABG does not decrease frequency or severity of exercise induced or resting ventricular arrythmias. These are likely due to scar which is uneffected by revascularization. Patients with EF less than 50% and/or large areas of regional malperfusion benefit the most from complete revascularization with CABG. Patient with very low EF less than 30% need to be carefully evaluated with cardiac MRI, PET scan or other imaging modality to determine if there is viable myocardium to revascularize, since risk may outweigh benefit as the EF approaches 20%.

RELIEF OF ANGINAL SYMPTOMS

The Medicine, Angioplasty or Surgery Study-II (MASS-II),[43] compared medical therapy, PCI and CABG. In addition to demonstrating reduction in revascularization in patients undergoing CABG, it demonstrated a 25% incidence of recurrent angina as compared with a 6% in patients undergoing CABG. These effects are reduced by the use of DES as demonstrated by the ARTS II trial. Freedom from recurrent angina is dependent on graft patency and progression of disease. Revascularization using the internal mammary artery is associated with an increase in the symptom-free period from 50% at 10 years w/vein grafts to 70% at 10 years using a LIMA.

QUALITY OF LIFE

Operative procedures have generally been judged based on their effectiveness and safety. Patients nowadays are much better informed and evaluate cardiovascular procedures not only on safety, efficacy and durability but also on the length of hospitalization, pain, postoperative recovery of function and improvement in their quality of life (QOL).[44] Several methods have been used to assess a patient's QOL both before and after operative intervention yet there is no universal agreement as to what QOL means or how it can be measured. Health related QOL is a reflection of the way a patient perceives and reacts to their health status and to nonmedical aspects of their lives (i.e. jobs, family, friends).[45] Major aspects of most QOL surveys include assessment of physical functioning, emotional status, cognitive performance, social functioning, general perception of health and well-being, and disease specific symptoms. One of the main goals of revascularization is to relieve symptoms of angina and improve physical activity. This in turn can affect work, leisure, social and sexual activities, and mood. Most studies have demonstrated improved functional status within 6 months of surgery. Improvements in general health status, 1 year postoperatively, seem to compare favorable with age-matched controls.[45] CABG has been shown to have a better 1-year physical functioning status compared to patients who receive PCI.[46] However, not everyone benefits to same degree from revascularization. Elderly patients and women have limited functional capacity and suffer more comorbidities. Although they benefit from a symptomatic standpoint as much as younger patients, they have less benefit from a QOL standpoint.[47] Women also seem to be at increased risk of subjective cognitive difficulties, increased anxiety and decreased ability to perform tasks of daily living. Patients with multivessel disease have also been shown to have a better QOL 12 months after surgery versus medical management perhaps related to less episodes of angina or heart failure symptoms. There is no significant difference between the conventional CABG and OPCAB in relation to QOL.

MAJOR CLINICAL TRIALS IN CHRONIC CORONARY ARTERY DISEASE

CABG VERSUS MEDICAL MANAGEMENT

CASS (1983)

CASS[1] is a randomized controlled clinical trial with an associated registry. It was designed to assess the effect of coronary artery bypass surgery on mortality and selected nonfatal endpoints. Around 780 patients with stable ischemic heart disease were randomly assigned to receive surgical (n = 390) or nonsurgical treatment (n = 390). At 5 years, the average annual mortality rate in patients assigned to surgical treatment was 1.1%. The annual mortality rate in those receiving medical therapy was 1.6%. Annual mortality rates in patients with single-, double- and triple-vessel disease who were in the surgical group were 0.7%, 1.0% and 1.5%; the corresponding rates in patients in the medical group were 1.4%, 1.2% and 2.1%. The differences were not statistically significant. Of the nearly 75% with an ejection fraction of at least 50%, the annual mortality rates in patients in the surgical group with single-, double- and triple-vessel disease were 0.8%, 0.8% and 1.2% and corresponding rates in the medical group were 1.1%, 0.6% and 1.2%. The annual rate of bypass surgery in patients who were initially assigned to receive medical treatment was 4.7%. The excellent survival rates observed both in CASS patients assigned to receive medical and those assigned to receive surgical therapy, and the similarity of survival rates in the two groups of patients in this randomized trial leads to the conclusion that patients similar to those enrolled in this trial can safely defer bypass surgery until symptoms worsen to the point that surgical palliation is required if they have preserved left ventricular function.

VA-CABSCSG (1984)

The Veterans Affairs Coronary Artery Bypass Surgery Cooperative Study Group[14] randomly assigned 686 patients with stable angina to medical or surgical treatment at 13 hospitals and followed for an average of 11.2 years. For all patients and for the 595 without left main coronary-artery disease, cumulative survival did not differ significantly at 11 years according to treatment. The 7-year survival rates for all patients were 70% with medical treatment and 77% with surgery (P = 0.043), and the 11-year rates were 57% and 58%, respectively. A statistically significant difference in survival suggesting a benefit from surgical treatment was found in patients without left main coronary-artery disease who were subdivided into high-risk subgroups defined angiographically, clinically or by a combination of angiographic and clinical factors: (1) high angiographic risk (three-vessel disease and impaired left ventricular function)—at 7 years, 52% in medically treated patients versus 76% in surgically treated patients (P = 0.002); at 11 years, 38% and 50%, respectively (P = 0.026); (2) clinically defined high risk (at least two of the following: resting ST depression, history of MI, or history of hypertension)—at 7 years, 52% in the medical group versus 72% in the surgical group (P = 0.003); at 11 years, 36% versus 49%, respectively (P = 0.015) and (3) combined angiographic and clinical high risk—at 7 years, 36% in the medical group versus 76% in the surgical group (P = 0.002); at 11 years, 24% versus 54%, respectively (P = 0.005).[14]

European CSS (1988)

The European Coronary Surgery Study randomized 767 men with good left ventricular function to either early coronary bypass surgery or medical therapy.[48] At the projected 5-year follow-up there was a higher survival rate in the group assigned to surgical treatment than in the group assigned to medical treatment (92.4% vs 83.1%). The survival advantage diminished during the subsequent 7 years but still favored the surgical treatment group (70.6% vs 66.7%).

PCI VERSUS MEDICAL MANAGEMENT

ACME (1992)

A comparison of angioplasty with medical therapy is a prospective randomized control veterans administration study,[49] 212 patients with documented ischemia and a single coronary artery stenosis ranging from 70% to 99% in one epicardial coronary artery and with exercise-induced myocardial ischemia were randomly assigned either to undergo PTCA or to receive

medical therapy and were evaluated monthly. After 6 months, they found that there was no mortality difference in either treatment group, but percutaneous intervention provided more complete angina relief with fewer medications and better QOL scores, as well as longer exercise duration on stress testing, than medical therapy. But among the 100 angioplasty patients, 19 underwent repeat PCI, and 7 underwent CABG during the first 6 months, compared with 11 angioplasty procedures and no CABG in the patients randomized to medical therapy. Additionally, it was demonstrated that nearly half of all patients assigned to initial medical therapy were asymptomatic at 6 months. Because this modest symptomatic benefit was achieved at such a large procedural and financial cost, patients who are either asymptomatic or have mild symptoms should have objective evidence of ischemia prior to PCI.

RITA-2

In the Randomized Intervention Treatment of Angina-2 (RITA-2) trial,[50] of 1,018 patients from the United Kingdom and Ireland with stable angina, 514 were randomized to medicine, receiving antianginal medications and optimal medical therapy and 504 to PTCA. One-third of the 1,018 patients had two-vessel disease and 7% had three-vessel disease. At a median follow-up of 2.7 years, the primary endpoints of death or MI had occurred twice as often in the PTCA group (6.3% vs 3.3%, p < 0.02, CI of 0.4–5.7%). Surgical revascularization was required during the follow-up interval in 7.9% of the PTCA group, and repeat angioplasty was required in 11%. In the medical group, 23% of patients required revascularization mostly due to worsening symptoms. Angina improved in both groups, but more in the PTCA group. There was a 16.5% absolute excess of grade 2 or worse angina in the medical group 3 months after randomization (p < 0.001), which attenuated to 7.6% after 2 years. Angina relief and exercise tolerance were improved to a greater degree in the patients undergoing angioplasty but this difference disappeared by three years.

TIMI-IIIB

The Thrombolysis in Myocardial Ischemia (TIMI)-IIIB clinical trial[51] enrolled 1,473 patients who received conventional anti-ischemic medical therapies. It compared the efficacy of t-PA with early invasive versus early conservative strategies in patients with unstable angina and non-Q-wave MI. In this large study of patients with unstable angina and non-Q-wave MI, the incidence of death and nonfatal infarction or reinfarction was low but not trivial after 1 year (4.3% mortality, 8.8% nonfatal infarction). The incidence of death or nonfatal infarction for the t-PA- and placebo-treated groups was similar after 1 year (12.4% vs 10.6%, p = 0.24). The incidence of death or nonfatal infarction was also similar after 1 year for the early invasive and early conservative strategies (10.8% vs 12.2%, p = 0.42). This study found that an early invasive management strategy was associated with slightly more coronary angioplasty procedures but equivalent numbers of bypass surgery procedures than was a more conservative early strategy of catheterization, in which revascularization was performed only when there were signs of recurrent ischemia. No difference was seen in death or nonfatal infarction, or both, after 1 year, according to strategy assignment, but fewer patients in the early invasive strategy group underwent later repeat hospital admission (26% vs 33%, p = 0.001). According to these results, either strategy appears to be acceptable for treatment of patients with unstable angina and non-Q-wave MI; in this regard, physicians have latitude in individualizing care for such patients. In the patients with unstable angina and non-Q-wave MI, thrombolytic therapy did not reduce mortality or morbidity.[51]

CABG VERSUS MULTIVESSEL PTCA (TRIALS COMPARING)

BARI (1997)

The Bypass Angioplasty Revascularization Investigation (BARI)[4] compared the effectiveness of CABG versus PTCA in 1829 highly symptomatic patients with two or three-vessel coronary disease and an anatomy that was deemed equally suitable for revascularization with either technique. Outcomes have been published at 5-, 7- and 10-year follow-up. There was no significant difference in cumulative survival between CABG and PTCA (89% vs 86%, 84% vs 81% and 73% vs 71%, respectively) or cardiac survival between the two groups. Survival rates in the two treatment arms were similar in most patient subgroups, with the exception of diabetes. Revascularization occurred significantly less often in the CABG group (8% vs 54%, 13% vs 60% and 23% vs 77%, respectively). Angina occurred less frequently in the CABG group in the first year but was equivalent at ten years.

RITA (1993)

The Randomized Intervention Treatment of Angina (RITA) trial[52] randomly assigned 1,011 patients, 45% of whom had single vessel disease, to either PTCA or CABG. After a median follow-up of 6.5 years, the rates of death or nonfatal infarction for PTCA or CABG were the same (17% vs 16%). Angina was consistently higher in the PTCA group, 26% of whom required CABG, and 19% of whom required another PTCA.

ERACI (1993)

The ERACI trial[2] (Argentine Randomized Trial of Percutaneous Transluminal Coronary Angioplasty versus Coronary Artery Bypass Surgery in Multivessel Disease) randomized 127 patients who had multivessel CAD and clinical indications for myocardial revascularization to undergo coronary angioplasty (n = 63) or bypass surgery (n = 64). At 3-year follow-up freedom from combined cardiac events (death, Q-wave MI, angina and repeat revascularization procedures) was significantly greater for the bypass surgery group than the coronary angioplasty group (77% vs 47%; p < 0.001). There were no differences in overall (4.7% vs 9.5%; p = 0.5) and cardiac (4.7% vs 4.7%; p = 1) mortality or in the frequency of MI (7.8% vs 7.8%; p = 0.8) between the two groups. However, patients who had bypass surgery were more frequently free of angina (79% vs 57%; p < 0.001) and required fewer additional reinterventions (6.3% vs 37%; p < 0.001) than patients who had coronary angioplasty. Of note the cumulative cost at 3-year follow-up was greater for the bypass surgery group than for the coronary angioplasty group.

GABI (1994)

The German Angioplasty Bypass Surgery Investigation (GABI)[5] was a multicenter study of patients in whom complete revascularization of at least two major vessels supplying different myocardial regions was deemed clinically necessary and technically feasible. Patients with totally occluded arteries supplying viable myocardium were excluded. At 12 months, no significant differences existed between the two groups with respect to Q-wave MI, severe angina, or freedom from angina. However, the total reintervention rate was lower with surgery (6% vs 44%).

EAST (1994)

In the Emory Angioplasty versus Surgery Trial (EAST)[6,53] nearly 400 patients with multivessel disease (most patients had normal left ventricular function) were randomly assigned to either PTCA or CABG. At 3-year follow-up no significant differences were found with respect to the combined endpoint of mortality, Q-wave MI, or large thallium perfusion defect. However, patients treated with CABG had fewer additional procedures at three years (2% vs 23%). After 8-year follow-up, the combined endpoint was the same in the two groups (79% vs 83% for CABG).[53]

CABRI (1995)

The Europe-based multicenter Coronary Angioplasty versus Bypass Revascularization Investigation (CABRI)[7] compared CABG to PTCA in 1,054 patients. There was a similar mortality rate (2.7% vs 3.9%) in the two groups at one year. However, patients assigned to PTCA required more repeat procedures (34% vs 7%) and had a higher incidence of clinically significant angina (relative risk 1.54). Restenosis after PTCA only partially accounted for this difference; of greater importance was the higher likelihood of residual disease after PTCA compared with CABG.

TRIALS COMPARING CORONARY ARTERY BYPASS GRAFTING VERSUS PERCUTANEOUS CORONARY TRANSLUMINAL ANGIOPLASTY USING BARE METAL STENT

ARTS I (2001)

In the ARTS I trial,[8] 1,205 patients (17% diabetics) with multivessel disease were randomly assigned to undergo BMS implantation or bypass surgery, usually with an arterial graft, when a cardiac surgeon and an interventional cardiologist agreed that the same extent of revascularization could be achieved with either procedure. Complete revascularization was significantly more likely to be achieved with CABG (84% vs 71%). There was no difference in mortality (8.0% vs 7.6%) or the rate of the combined endpoint of death, MI or stroke (18.2% vs 14.9%) at five years. However, event-free survival was lower with stenting due to a significant increase in the need for repeat revascularization (21% vs 4% at one year, 27% vs 7% at three years, and 30% vs 9% at five years). Among stented patients in the ARTS I trial, two groups had worse outcomes: those with incomplete revascularization and patients with diabetes.

SoS (2002)

The SoS trial[9] randomly assigned 988 patients with multivessel coronary disease to CABG or PCI with bare metal stent. At a median follow-up of two years, PCI was associated with a significantly higher rate of repeat revascularization (21% vs 6%) with CABG. At six years, mortality was significantly higher in the PCI group (10.9 vs 6.8; hazard ratio 1.66, 95% CI 1.08–2.55). It is not clear if this difference was at least in part by chance since there was a larger number of cancer deaths in the stenting group.

ERACI II (2001)

The ERACI II trial randomized 450 patients to undergo either PCI (n = 225); or CABG (n = 225). Clinical follow-up during five years was obtained in 92% of the total population after hospital discharge.[10] At 5-year follow-up, patients initially treated with PCI had similar survival and freedom from nonfatal AMI than those initially treated with CABG (92.8% vs 88.4% and 97.3% vs 94%, respectively, p = 0.16). Freedom from repeat revascularization procedures (PCI/CABG) was significantly lower with PCI compared with CABG (71.5% vs 92.4%, p = 0.0002). Freedom from major adverse cardiac event was also significantly lower with PCI compared with CABG (65.3% vs 76.4%; p = 0.013). The study concluded that there were no survival benefits from any revascularization procedure; however, patients initially treated with CABG had better freedom from repeat revascularization procedures and from major adverse coronary event.

TRIALS COMPARING CORONARY ARTERY BYPASS GRAFTING VERSUS PERCUTANEOUS CORONARY TRANSLUMINAL ANGIOPLASTY USING DES

SYNTAX (2009)

The SYNTAX trial[11] randomly assigned 1,800 patients with three-vessel or left main CAD to either CABG or PCI with DES. All patients were eligible for either procedure and were treated with the intention of complete revascularization. After 12 months follow-up the composite primary endpoint (death from any cause, stroke, MI or repeat revascularization) was significantly higher in the PCI group (17.8% vs 12.4%). This was the result mostly of more frequent revascularizations with PCI (13.5% vs 5.9%). The secondary endpoint of the rate of death, stroke or MI were similar (7.6 for PCI vs 7.7 for CABG). More complete revascularization was achieved with CABG (63% vs 57%).

ERACI III Registry (2006)

The ERACI III[54] registry consisted of 225 patients who would have met the ERACI II trial inclusion criteria and underwent drug-eluting stenting. The primary endpoint was 3-year major cardiac or cerebrovascular events. ERACI III-DES patients (n = 225) were compared with the BMS (n = 225) and CABG (n = 225) arms of ERACI II. Patients treated with DES were older, more often smokers, more often high risk by EuroSCORE and less frequently had unstable angina. They also received more stents than the BMS-treated cohort. Major adverse event rates

at 3 years were similar in DES and CABG-treated patients (22.7%, P = 1.0). Death or nonfatal MI at 3 years trended higher in the DES (10.2%) than BMS cohort (6.2%, P = 0.08) and lower than in CABG patients (15.1%, P = 0.07).

ARTS II Registry (2008)

The ARTS II registry[55] compared differences in outcomes between sirolimus-eluting stents (SES) in 607 patients with the 1,205 patients from the ARTS I trial. The primary outcome was a composite of all-cause mortality, any MI or cerebrovascular event, or any reintervention. After 3 years freedom from revascularization was 85.5% in patient receiving SES compared to 93.4% with CABG in ARTS I. Conclusions must be tempered since this was not a head-to-head comparison, as the CABG patients were historical controls from the original ARTS I trial.

The New York State Registry (2008)

This registry included 17,400 patients in New York State[12] who underwent CABG or drug-eluting stenting between October 1, 2003 and December 31, 2004. In comparison with treatment with a drug-eluting stent, CABG was associated with lower 18-month rates of death and of death or MI both for patients with three-vessel disease and for patients with two-vessel disease (92.7% vs 94.0% and 94.6% vs 96.0%, respectively). Unfortunately, the design for this registry allows for significant selection bias with the inclusion of unstable patients in the stenting arm.[12]

The Beijing Registry (2009)

A report from Beijing evaluated 3,720 consecutive patients with multivessel disease who underwent isolated CABG surgery or received DES between April 1, 2004 and December 31, 2005. Patients who underwent CABG (n = 1,886) were older and had more comorbidities than patients who received DES (n = 1,834). Patients receiving DES had considerably higher 3-year rates of target-vessel revascularization. DES were also associated with higher rates of death (adjusted hazard ratio, 1.62; 95% confidence interval, 1.07–2.47) and MI (adjusted hazard ratio, 1.65; 95% confidence interval, 1.15–2.44).

SUMMARY

The goal of medical therapy or revascularization is to prevent the complications of CAD, by decreasing the mortality and morbidity associated with cardiac disease and alleviating symptoms. Both CABG and PCI may diminish anginal symtoms, and reduce major adverse cardiac events. In general, patients managed with CABG and PCI have similar combined outcomes of death, MI and stroke. Revascularization rates, although, are higher with PCI. Major clinical trials comparing PCI to CABG have helped stratify patients. The decision to proceed with a specific revascularization strategy is dependent on the coronary anatomy, myocardial function, patient risk factors, patient preference and local expertise. Most patients with single- or two-vessel disease and normal ejection fraction are best managed with PCI unless the proximal left anterior descending artery is involved with a high-grade stenosis. Patients with multivessel disease or left main disease associated with impaired left venticular systolic function benefit most from CABG. Patients with diabetes mellitus, as shown in the BARI and ARTS I trials, benefit from CABG over stenting, especially if they have left ventricular dysfunction. Patient with unprotected left main CAD who are reasonable surgical candidates should be treated with CABG. The use of DES in three-vessel or left main CAD is associated with similar 1 year death, stroke or MI rates at the cost of less complete and more frequent revascularization. Modern day management of chronic CAD requires a frank and integrated discussion between the patient, cardiologist and cardiac surgeon.

REFERENCES

1. Coronary Artery Surgery Study (CASS). A randomized trial of coronary artery bypass surgery. Survival data. Circulation. 1983;68: 939-50.

2. Rodriguez A, et al. Argentine randomized trial of percutaneous transluminal coronary angioplasty versus coronary artery bypass surgery in multivessel disease (ERACI): in-hospital results and 1-year follow-up. ERACI Group. J Am Coll Cardiol. 1993;22:1060-7.

3. Coronary angioplasty versus coronary artery bypass surgery: the Randomized Intervention Treatment of Angina (RITA) trial. Lancet. 1993;341:573-80.

4. Chaitman BR, et al. Myocardial infarction and cardiac mortality in the Bypass Angioplasty Revascularization Investigation (BARI) randomized trial. Circulation. 1997;96:2162-70.

5. Hamm CW, et al. A randomized study of coronary angioplasty compared with bypass surgery in patients with symptomatic multivessel coronary disease. German Angioplasty Bypass Surgery Investigation (GABI). N Engl J Med. 1994;331:1037-43.

6. King SB, 3rd, et al. A randomized trial comparing coronary angioplasty with coronary bypass surgery. Emory Angioplasty versus Surgery Trial (EAST). N Engl J Med. 1994;331:1044-50.

7. First-year results of CABRI (Coronary Angioplasty versus Bypass Revascularisation Investigation). CABRI Trial Participants. Lancet. 1995;346:1179-84.

8. Serruys PW, et al. Five-year outcomes after coronary stenting versus bypass surgery for the treatment of multivessel disease: the final analysis of the Arterial Revascularization Therapies Study (ARTS) randomized trial. J Am Coll Cardiol. 2005;46:575-81.

9. Booth J, et al. Randomized, controlled trial of coronary artery bypass surgery versus percutaneous coronary intervention in patients with multivessel coronary artery disease: six-year follow-up from the Stent or Surgery Trial (SoS). Circulation. 2008;118:381-8.

10. Rodriguez A, et al. Argentine Randomized Study: coronary Angioplasty with Stenting versus Coronary Bypass Surgery in patients with Multiple-Vessel Disease (ERACI II): 30-day and one-year follow-up results. ERACI II Investigators. J Am Coll Cardiol. 2001;37:51-8.

11. Serruys PW, et al. Percutaneous coronary intervention versus coronary-artery bypass grafting for severe coronary artery disease. N Engl J Med. 2009;360:961-72.

12. Hannan EL, et al. Drug-eluting stents vs coronary-artery bypass grafting in multivessel coronary disease. N Engl J Med. 2008;358:331-41.

13. Buszman PE, et al. Early and long-term results of unprotected left main coronary artery stenting: the LE MANS (Left Main Coronary Artery Stenting) registry. J Am Coll Cardiol. 2009;54:1500-11.

14. Eleven-year survival in the Veterans Administration randomized trial of coronary bypass surgery for stable angina. The Veterans Administration Coronary Artery Bypass Surgery Cooperative Study Group. N Engl J Med. 1984;311:1333-9.

15. Edwards FH, Clark RE, Schwartz M. Coronary artery bypass grafting: the Society of Thoracic Surgeons National Database experience. Ann Thorac Surg. 1994;57:12-9.

16. Nilsson J, et al. Early mortality in coronary bypass surgery: the EuroSCORE versus The Society of Thoracic Surgeons risk algorithm. Ann Thorac Surg. 2004;77:1235-9.

17. Singh M, et al. Mayo Clinic Risk Score for percutaneous coronary intervention predicts in-hospital mortality in patients undergoing coronary artery bypass graft surgery. Circulation. 2008;117:356-62.

18. Goldman S, et al. Starting aspirin therapy after operation. Effects on early graft patency. Department of Veterans Affairs Cooperative Study Group. Circulation. 1991;84:520-6.

19. Sethi GK, et al. Implications of preoperative administration of aspirin in patients undergoing coronary artery bypass grafting. Department of Veterans Affairs Cooperative Study on Antiplatelet Therapy. J Am Coll Cardiol. 1990;15:15-20.

20. Collaborative overview of randomised trials of antiplatelet therapy—II: Maintenance of vascular graft or arterial patency by antiplatelet therapy. Antiplatelet Trialists' Collaboration. BMJ. 1994;308: 159-68.

21. Dacey LJ, et al. Effect of preoperative aspirin use on mortality in coronary artery bypass grafting patients. Ann Thorac Surg. 2000;70:1986-90.

22. Collard CD, et al. Preoperative statin therapy is associated with reduced cardiac mortality after coronary artery bypass graft surgery. J Thorac Cardiovasc Surg. 2006;132:392-400.

23. Huffmyer JL, et al. Preoperative statin administration is associated with lower mortality and decreased need for postoperative hemodialysis in patients undergoing coronary artery bypass graft surgery. J Cardiothorac Vasc Anesth. 2009;23:468-73.

24. Pan W, et al. Statins are associated with a reduced incidence of perioperative mortality after coronary artery bypass graft surgery. Circulation. 2004;110:II45-9.

25. Ferguson TB, Jr, Coombs LP, Peterson ED. Preoperative beta-blocker use and mortality and morbidity following CABG surgery in North America. JAMA. 2002;287:2221-7.

26. van den Berghe G, et al. Intensive insulin therapy in the critically ill patients. N Engl J Med. 2001;345:1359-67.

27. Lazar HL, et al. Tight glycemic control in diabetic coronary artery bypass graft patients improves perioperative outcomes and decreases recurrent ischemic events. Circulation. 2004;109:1497-502.

28. Birkmeyer JD, et al. Hospital volume and surgical mortality in the United States. N Engl J Med. 2002;346:1128-37.

29. Peterson ED, et al. Procedural volume as a marker of quality for CABG surgery. JAMA. 2004;291:195-201.

30. Leavitt BJ, et al. Use of the internal mammary artery graft and in-hospital mortality and other adverse outcomes associated with coronary artery bypass surgery. Circulation. 2001;103:507-12.

31. Ivanov J, et al. Fifteen-year trends in risk severity and operative mortality in elderly patients undergoing coronary artery bypass graft surgery. Circulation. 1998;97:673-80.

32. Baskett R, et al. Outcomes in octogenarians undergoing coronary artery bypass grafting. CMAJ. 2005;172:1183-6.

33. Kim C, et al. A systematic review of gender differences in mortality after coronary artery bypass graft surgery and percutaneous coronary interventions. Clin Cardiol. 2007;30:491-5.

34. Yap CH, et al. Contemporary results show repeat coronary artery bypass grafting remains a risk factor for operative mortality. Ann Thorac Surg. 2009;87:1386-91.

35. Nalysnyk L, et al. Adverse events in coronary artery bypass graft (CABG) trials: a systematic review and analysis. Heart. 2003;89: 767-72.

36. Jonsson A, et al. Left main coronary artery stenosis no longer a risk factor for early and late death after coronary artery bypass surgery—An experience covering three decades. Eur J Cardiothorac Surg. 2006;30:311-7.

37. Fukui T, et al. Graft selection and one-year patency rates in patients undergoing coronary artery bypass grafting. Ann Thorac Surg. 2010;89:1901-5.

38. Hayward PA, et al. Comparable patencies of the radial artery and right internal thoracic artery or saphenous vein beyond 5 years: results

from the Radial Artery Patency and Clinical Outcomes trial. J Thorac Cardiovasc Surg. 2010;139:60-5.

39. Loop FD, et al. Influence of the internal-mammary-artery graft on 10-year survival and other cardiac events. N Engl J Med. 1986;314: 1-6.

40. Loop FD, et al. Reoperation for coronary atherosclerosis. Changing practice in 2509 consecutive patients. Ann Surg. 1990;212:378-85.

41. Lytle BW, et al. Two internal thoracic artery grafts are better than one. J Thorac Cardiovasc Surg. 1999;117:855-72.

42. Sergeant P, Blackstone E, Meyns B. Validation and interdependence with patient-variables of the influence of procedural variables on early and late survival after CABG. K.U. Leuven Coronary Surgery Program. Eur J Cardiothorac Surg. 1997;12:1-19.

43. Hueb W, et al. The medicine, angioplasty, or surgery study (MASS-II): a randomized, controlled clinical trial of three therapeutic strategies for multivessel coronary artery disease: one-year results. J Am Coll Cardiol. 2004;43:1743-51.

44. Kapetanakis EI, et al. Comparison of the quality of life after conventional versus off-pump coronary artery bypass surgery. J Card Surg. 2008;23:120-5.

45. Duits AA, et al. Prediction of quality of life after coronary artery bypass graft surgery: a review and evaluation of multiple, recent studies. Psychosom Med. 1997;59:257-68.

46. Szygula-Jurkiewicz B, et al. Health related quality of life after percutaneous coronary intervention versus coronary artery bypass graft surgery in patients with acute coronary syndromes without ST-segment elevation. 12-month follow-up. Eur J Cardiothorac Surg. 2005;27:882-6.

47. Markou AL, et al. Changes in quality of life, physical activity, and symptomatic status one year after myocardial revascularization for stable angina. Eur J Cardiothorac Surg. 2008;34:1009-15.

48. Varnauskas E. Twelve-year follow-up of survival in the randomized European Coronary Surgery Study. N Engl J Med. 1988;319:332-7.

49. Parisi AF, Folland ED, Hartigan P. A comparison of angioplasty with medical therapy in the treatment of single-vessel coronary artery disease. Veterans Affairs ACME Investigators. N Engl J Med. 1992;326:10-6.

50. Henderson RA, et al. Seven-year outcome in the RITA-2 trial: coronary angioplasty versus medical therapy. J Am Coll Cardiol. 2003;42:1161-70.

51. Anderson HV, et al. One-year results of the Thrombolysis in Myocardial Infarction (TIMI) IIIB clinical trial. A randomized comparison of tissue-type plasminogen activator versus placebo and early invasive versus early conservative strategies in unstable angina and non-Q wave myocardial infarction. J Am Coll Cardiol. 1995;26: 1643-50.

52. Henderson RA, et al. Long-term results of RITA-1 trial: clinical and cost comparisons of coronary angioplasty and coronary-artery bypass grafting. Randomised Intervention Treatment of Angina. Lancet. 1998;352:1419-25.

53. King SB, 3rd, et al. Eight-year mortality in the Emory Angioplasty versus Surgery Trial (EAST). J Am Coll Cardiol. 2000;35:1116-21.

54. Rodriguez AE, et al. Revascularization strategies of coronary multiple vessel disease in the Drug Eluting Stent Era: osne year follow-up results of the ERACI III Trial. EuroIntervention. 2006;2:53-60.

55. Serruys PW, et al. Three-year follow-up of the ARTS-II—Sirolimus-eluting stents for the treatment of patients with multivessel coronary artery disease. EuroIntervention. 2008;3:450-9.

Index

Entries from figures/flow charts and tables are represented by locators with *italics* suffix "*f*" and "*t*", respectively.